DIAGNOSTIC IMAGING
ORTHOPAEDICS

RZW

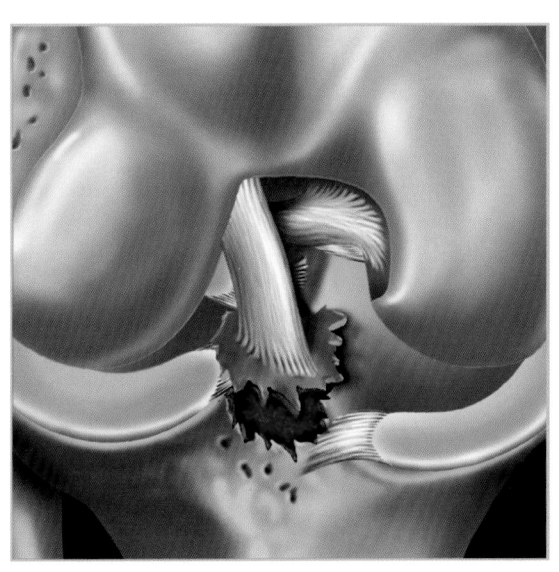

i

DIAGNOSTIC IMAGING
ORTHOPAEDICS

David W. Stoller, MD, FACR

Director, California Advanced Imaging and MRI
California Pacific Medical Center

Director, National Orthopaedic Imaging Associates
San Francisco, California

Director, Musculoskeletal MRI
California Pacific Medical Center

Phillip F. J. Tirman, MD

Director, California Advanced Imaging
California Pacific Medical Center

Director, National Orthopaedic Imaging Associates
San Francisco, California

Director, Musculoskeletal MRI
California Pacific Medical Center

Miriam A. Bredella, MD

Department of Radiology
University of California San Francisco
San Francisco, California

Salvador Beltran, MD

Medical Illustrator

Robert M. Branstetter III, MD

Diversified Radiology of Colorado
Denver, Colorado

Simon C. P. Blease, MD, FRCR

Honorary Senior Clinical Lecturer
University of Bristol
United Kingdom

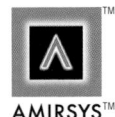

AMIRSYS™
A medical reference publishing company

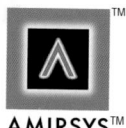

AMIRSYS™

A medical reference publishing company

First Edition

Text - Copyright David W Stoller MD 2004

Drawings - Copyright Amirsys Inc 2004

Compilation - Copyright Amirsys Inc 2004

Composition by Amirsys Inc, Salt Lake City, Utah

Printed by Friesens, Altona, Manitoba, Canada

ISBN: 0-7216-2920-2

Notice and Disclaimer

Library of Congress Cataloging-in-Publication Data

Stoller, David W.
  Diagnostic imaging, orthopaedics / David W. Stoller, Phillip F.J.
Tirman, Miriam A. Bredella ; Salvador Beltran, medical illustrator.—
1st ed.
      p. ; cm.
Includes bibliographical references and index.
  ISBN 0-7216-2920-2
1. Musculoskeletal system—Radiography—Atlases. 2. Diagnostic
imaging—Atlases.
  [DNLM: 1. Musculoskeletal System—radiography—Atlases. 2.
Diagnostic Imaging—methods—Atlases. 3. Orthopedic
Procedures—methods—Atlases. WE 17 S875d 2004] I. Title:
Orthopaedics. II. Tirman, Phillip F. J. III. Bredella, Miriam A. IV.
Title.

RC925.7.S767 2004
616.7'07572—dc22

                    2003062915

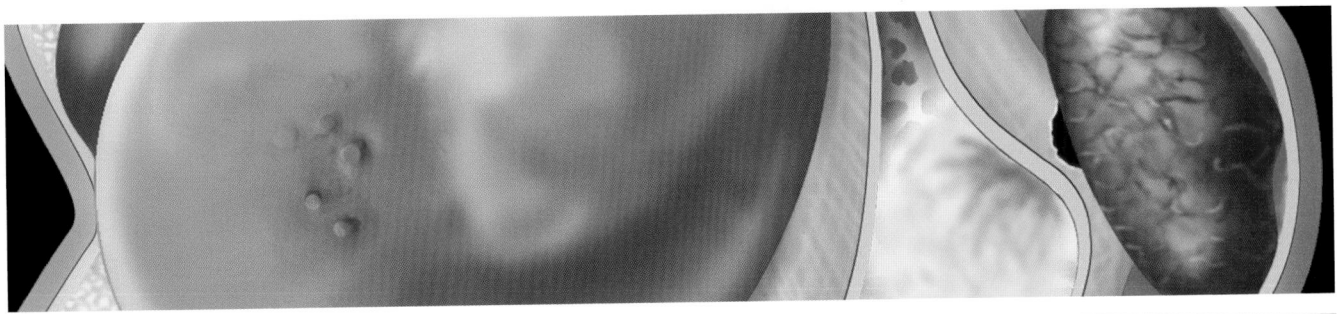

CONTRIBUTORS

David W. Stoller, MD, FACR
Director, California Advanced Imaging and MRI
California Pacific Medical Center

Director, National Orthopaedic Imaging Associates
San Francisco, California

Director, Musculoskeletal MRI
California Pacific Medical Center

Phillip F. J. Tirman, MD
Director, California Advanced Imaging
California Pacific Medical Center

Director, National Orthopaedic Imaging Associates
San Francisco, California

Director, Musculoskeletal MRI
California Pacific Medical Center

Miriam A. Bredella, MD
Department of Radiology
University of California San Francisco
San Francisco, California

Salvador Beltran, MD
Medical Illustrator

Robert M. Branstetter III, MD
Diversified Radiology of Colorado
Denver, Colorado

Simon C. P. Blease, MD, FRCR
Consultant Musculoskeletal Radiologist
Med-Tel International Corporation
McLean, Virginia
Honorary Senior Clinical Lecturer
University of Bristol
United Kingdom

Jana M. Crain, MD
Medical Director
National Orthopaedic Imaging Associates

Niku P. Wasudev, MD
Musculoskeletal MRI
National Orthopaedic Imaging Associates

James O. Johnston, MD
Professor Orthopaedic Oncology
University of California, San Francisco
Director Orthopaedic Oncology
Kaiser South San Francisco

DIAGNOSTIC IMAGING: ORTHOPAEDICS

The imaging, orthopedics and sports medicine communities have been waiting a long time for a new "**Stoller**". We at Amirsys and Elsevier are proud to present a precedent-setting, image- and graphics-packed series that debuts with a brand-new work by David Stoller and colleagues. This splendid work represents the textbook of the twenty-first century: Not your old-fashioned, dense prose exposition with comparatively few images. The unique bulleted format of the *Diagnostic Imaging* books allow our authors to present approximately twice the information and four times the images per diagnosis, compared to the old-fashioned traditional prose textbook.

These richly illustrated books will cover all major body areas and follow a similar format. The same information is in the same place: Every time! A welcome innovation is the new visual differential diagnosis "thumbnail" that provides at-a-glance looks at entities that can mimic the diagnosis in question. "Key Facts" boxes provide a succinct summary for quick, easy review. In short, this is a product designed with you, the reader, in mind. Today's typical practice settings demand efficiency in both image interpretation and learning. We think you'll find the *Diagnostic Imaging* format a highly efficient and wonderfully rich resource. Enjoy!

Anne G. Osborn, MD
Executive Vice-President and Editor-in-Chief, Amirsys

H. Ric Harnsberger, MD
Chairman and CEO, Amirsys Inc

David W. Stoller, MD, FACR
Editor Diagnostic Imaging Orthopaedics

x

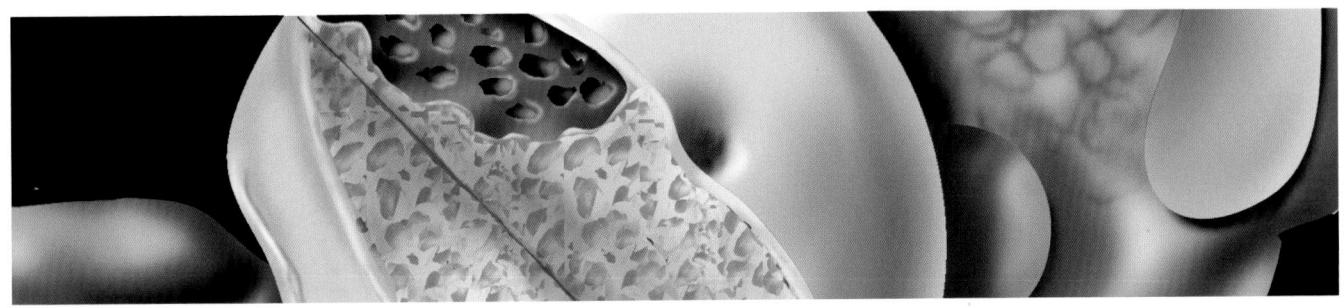

FOREWORD

Over the last 20 years, MR imaging has become a significant diagnostic test performed in orthopaedic and sports medicine. Surgeons have come to depend on this modality to provide crucial information, which assists not only in understanding the underlying pathology, but also in making the critical decision regarding surgical intervention. With the rapid growth and sophistication of MR technology, MR imaging is an indispensable step in the workup of patients with joint disorders and sports injuries. It has especially become important in the evaluation and treatment of professional athletes who often depend on quick and accurate diagnosis in order that they can resume their activities.

Diagnostic Imaging in Orthopaedics is an invaluable text to orthopedists and radiologists alike. This thousand-page text contains over 550 color illustration plates and over 1000 radiographic images. Each radiographic diagnosis is discussed in outline format with thumbnail images of other differential considerations. While the unique correlative color illustrations for each diagnosis allow the reader to better understand anatomy and mechanism of disease, the concise yet complete format of the textbook allows for quick reference in the clinical setting.

Dr. Stoller has successfully expanded the collaboration between orthopedic surgeons and radiologists with *Diagnostic Imaging in Orthopaedics* as exemplified by the representative images and correlative discussions of topics including pathophysiology, anatomy, and patient management. Not only does this text focus on orthopaedic diagnosis involving the appendicular skeleton, but he also covers bone, soft tissue, and marrow tumors. Many of the techniques and applications described in this text were either originated or improved by Dr. Stoller and his co-authors. This comprehensive text is the first of its kind in encompassing an understanding of orthopaedics with correlative color illustrations and therefore will become an invaluable reference and establish a higher standard of imaging for orthopaedists and radiologists.

W. Dilworth Cannon Jr., MD
Professor of Clinical Orthopaedic Surgery
UCSF Sports Medicine Center
University of California
San Francisco, California

PREFACE

Joint efforts from the fields of radiology and orthopaedics have continued to define the growing indications and current issues for the use of MR in orthopaedics and sports medicine. Since the mid-1980's, skeletal radiology has undergone an accelerated transformation with the infusion of MR technology and applications. Credit is acknowledged to my early contemporaries including Jerrold H. Mink, M.D. and John V. Crues III, M.D. Our collaborative research in 1984-5 helped contribute to the initial MR applications for the meniscus; and thus, hastened the integration of MR in routine musculoskeletal imaging.

Diagnostic Imaging Orthopaedics represents the culmination of a collaborative vision I share with Anne Osborn, M.D. and Ric Harnsberger, M.D. to further and improve the landscape of education of residents, fellows, academic institutions, and private practice centers of excellence. This text reflects the manner in which the authors presently utilize MR in clinical imaging and explains the reliance of MR applications over CT and US in the appendicular joints. Each diagnosis consists of a classic color illustration and MR image. Differential diagnosis thumbnails are provided as a reference guide to help address related topics without competing or distracting the reader from the image galleries for each diagnosis. The outline style of writing not only provides more information than a comparable prose format, but also allows the reader to rapidly scan information in selected subsections or within the key facts box.

Our team has performed an excellent job in organizing the orthopaedic topics into nine categories: six chapters concerning the appendicular joints and three chapters addressing marrow, bone and soft tissue tumors. Salvador Beltran, M.D. has provided one of the largest correlative collections of superbly illustrated orthopaedic pathology in color found in a single text.

Diagnostic Imaging Orthopaedics is a comprehensive and current reference that addresses the growing need of radiologists, orthopedists, and sports medicine physicians to understand and incorporate new clinical applications of bone and joint imaging into their practices.

David W Stoller, MD
Director, California Advanced Imaging and MRI
California Pacific Medical Center

Director, National Orthopaedic Imaging Associates
San Francisco, California

Director, Musculoskeletal MRI
California Pacific Medical Center

ACKNOWLEDGMENTS

Illustrations
Salvador Beltran, MD

Art Direction and Design
Richard Coombs, MS
Lane R. Bennion, MS
James A. Cooper, MD

Image/Text Editing
Mingqian Huang, MD
Melissa Morris
Cassie Dearth
Kaerli Main

Medical Text Editing
Mingqian Huang, MD
Richard H. Wiggins III, MD
Karen L. Salzman, MD
Bernard Chow, MD
Janaki N. Ramanathan, MD

Research Contributors
Lesley J. Anderson, MD
Frank M. Crnkovich, MD
David M. Lichtman, MD
Richard D. Ferkel, MD
Wesley M. Nottage, MD

Technological Assistance
Christopher Govea, MD
Philip Tran, MD
Margie Garbarino, CRT, ARRT, (R,MR)
Peter R. Osuna

Manuscript Preparation
Mingqian Huang, MD
Susan Bybee, CRT, ARRT, (R,MR)

Image Contribution
Mel Senac, MD
Rob Campbell, MD
Andrew Grainger, MD
John Feller, MD
Oliver Cuitanic, MD
Britta Gooding, MD

Production Director
Pattie R. Dawson

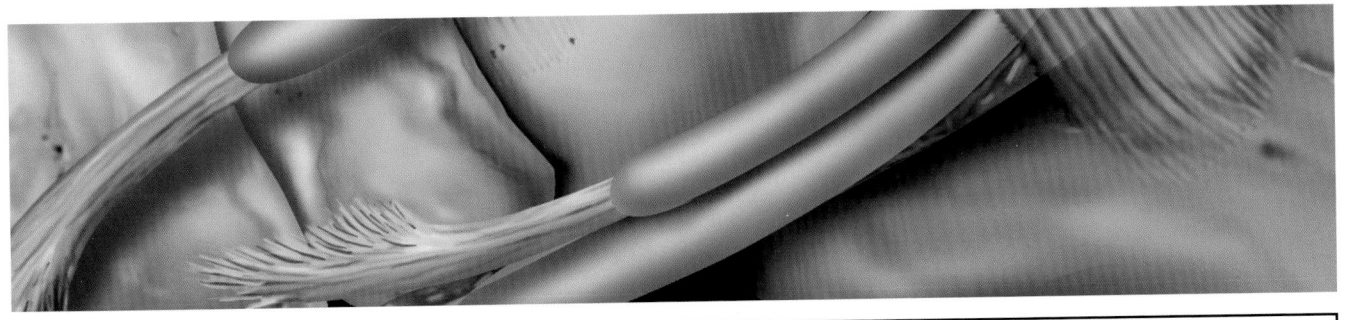

SECTIONS

Weissbuch

RRW

1

2

3

4

5

6

7

8

9

i

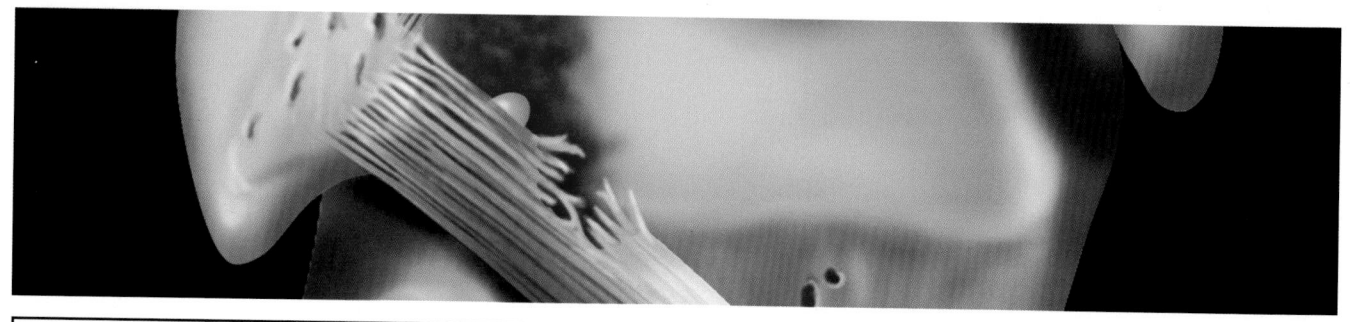

TABLE OF CONTENTS

SECTION 9: Soft Tissue Tumors

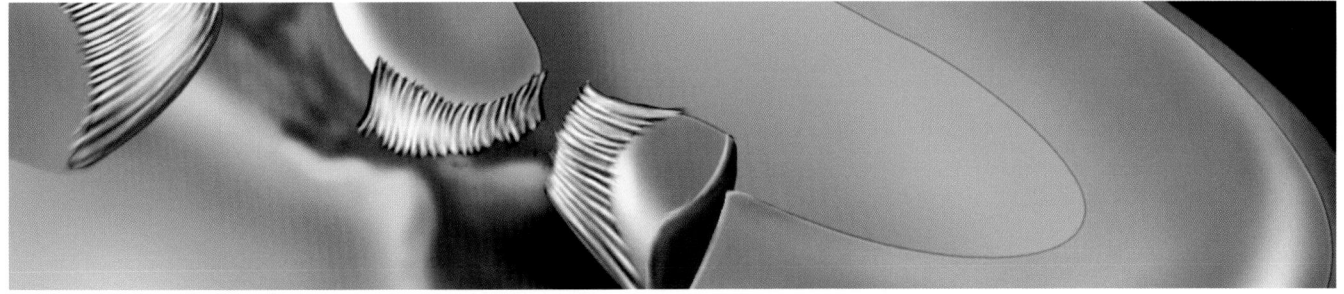

DEFINITION OF TERMS

T1WI

- T1 Weighted Image
- Includes spin echo (SE), fast spin echo (FSE) and gradient echo (GRE)
- Used to show hypointense signal in sclerosis and subchondral edema
- Marrow fat signal is hyperintense on T1 weighted images

T2WI

- T2 Weighted Image
- Includes SE and FSE sequences
- T2 FSE used to evaluate the rotator cuff (complementing FS PD FSE images) by differentiating tendinosis and tears
- T2 FSE application limited because of hyperintense fat signal, (FS PD FSE used more commonly for this reason)
- FS T2 FSE produces an image with poor SNR (signal-to-noise) with TE values of greater than 60 msec

PDWI

- Proton Density Weighted or Intermediate Weighted Image
- Long TR and short TE images
- High SNR
- Useful for articular cartilage evaluation as an alternative to FS PD FSE
- May obscure sclerosis or marrow edema due to poor marrow fat contrast compared to T1WI or FS PD FSE

FS PD FSE

- Fat Suppressed Proton Density Weighted Fast Spin Echo
- Evaluates marrow edema, articular cartilage, ligaments, tendons, synovium, and meniscal morphology
- Commonly used sequence for all appendicular joint imaging
- Often referred to as FS T2 FSE although TE values are typically less than 60 msec
- TR values greater than or equal to 3000 msec
- TE values of 40-50 msec to optimize image quality

GRE

- Gradient Echo
- Reverse gradient polarity to rephrase protons and form echoes
- Usually used to create images with T2* contrast
- T2* contrast used to evaluate TFC (triangular fibrocartilage), patellar tendon, intrameniscal signal, subscapularis tendon and chondrocalcinosis

- Also used when fat suppression fails with FSE sequences
- Sensitive to magnetic field inhomogeneties, paramagnetics and ferromagnetic micrometallic artifacts compared to SE and FSE (secondary to gradient rephrasing)

ZIP

- Zero-fill Interpolation Processing
- Reconstruction technique to enhance apparent image resolution without actually creating resolution

STIR (SHORT TI INVERSION RECOVERY)

- Inversion Recovery Fat Suppressed Spin Echo Pulse Sequence
- Initial 180 degree inversion pulse prior to 90 degree pulse
- STIR has more uniform fat suppression because IR is less sensitive to magnetic field inhomegeneties and off center field-of-view (FOV) effects
- Used when FS PD FSE not available or when fat suppression inadequate in FSE images
- T1 & T2 contrast additive in STIR however SNR is low secondary to reduced transverse magnetization
- Limited by prolonged scan times

T1 C+

- Intravenous contrast administration in conjunction with fat suppression to increase the conspicuity of synovium vascularity, inflammation and tumors
- Also used to improve visualization of intraarticular structures by delayed enhancement of joint fluid without the benefit of capsular distension

ABER

- Abduction External Rotation position of the shoulder to optimize visualization of the inferior glenohumeral ligament labral complex (IGLLC), biceps labral complex (BLC) and articular surface of the rotator cuff

MR ARTHRO

- MR arthrography
- Dilute intraarticular MR contrast agent and saline or non-ionic contrast
- Distend joint capsule to improve visualization of intraarticular and capsular structures
- Used in selective applications for the shoulder, wrist, hip, elbow and knee
- Used in conjunction with T1 fat suppression and FS PD FSE sequences

DIAGNOSTIC IMAGING
ORTHOPAEDICS

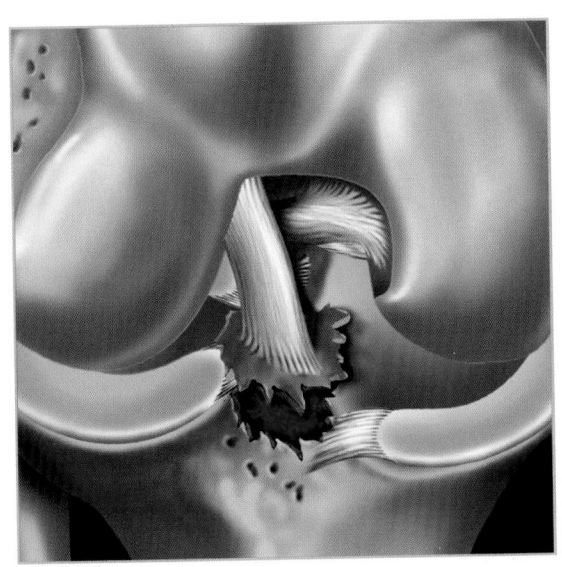

SECTION 1: Shoulder

ROTATOR CUFF TENDINOPATHY

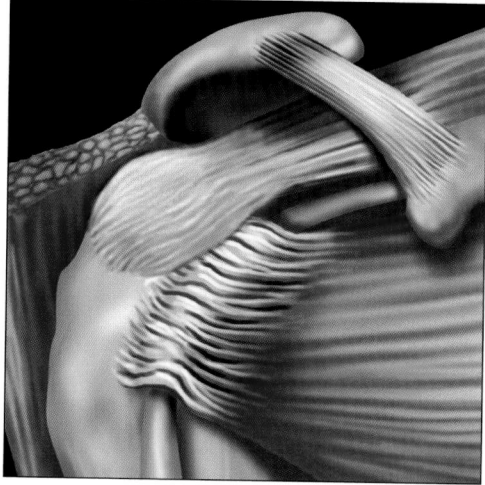

Coronal graphic shows thickening and degeneration of the distal aspect of the supraspinatus tendon, consistent with tendinopathy.

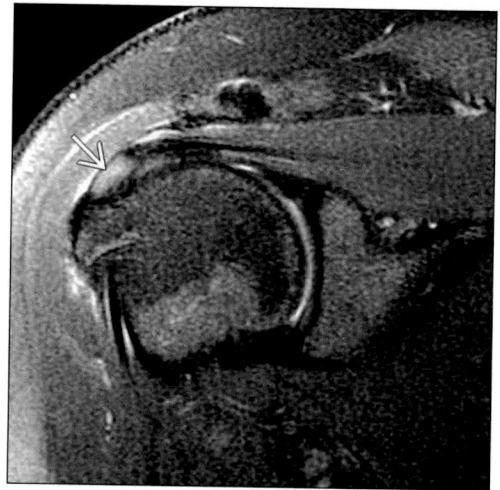

Coronal FS PD FSE MR shows thickening and increased signal intensity (arrow) of the distal supraspinatus tendon, representing tendinopathy (tendinosis).

TERMINOLOGY

Abbreviations and Synonyms
- Rotator cuff (RTC) impingement, subacromial impingement, supraspinatus impingement
- Rotator cuff tendinitis (tendinosis), supraspinatus tendinitis, shoulder periarthritis, painful shoulder syndrome

Definitions
- Collagenous degeneration of the rotator cuff tendons most commonly involving the supraspinatus tendon

IMAGING FINDINGS

General Features
- Best diagnostic clue: Thickened inhomogeneous rotator cuff tendon with increased signal intensity on all pulse sequences
- Location: Anterior leading edge of supraspinatus
- Size: Tendon thickened but may be thinned by attrition
- Morphology
  - Thickened, inhomogeneous tendon with visible surface fraying
  - Tendon torn or partially torn in advanced cases with fluid entering defect

Radiographic Findings
- Radiography
  - Acromial remodeling/sclerosis + acromioclavicular (AC) joint hypertrophy
  - Acromial spurs (impingement)
  - Humeral head subchondral sclerosis/cysts

MR Findings
- T1WI
  - Thickened tendon with intermediate signal intensity
    - Heterogeneous tendon(s) signal
  - Intermediate signal intensity in the long head of biceps tendon with associated tendinosis
  - Hypointense to intermediate signal intensity in thickened or fluid containing subacromial - subdeltoid bursa
- T2WI
  - Increased signal intensity of tendon on PD FSE, FS PD FSE, STIR & T2* GRE
    - Heterogeneous tendon(s) signal
  - Hyperintense tendon degeneration on FS PD FSE
    - FS PD FSE visualizes tendon degeneration as hyperintense while T2 FSE shows degeneration as low to intermediate in signal
  - +/- Hyperintense effusion (glenohumeral joint)
  - Hyperintense (fluid signal intensity) bursitis
    - Subacromial/subdeltoid
    - Subcoracoid - esp. with anterior pathology

DDx: Rotator Cuff Tendinopathy

Normal tendon	Partial Tear	Bursal Part Tear	Full Tear	Cuff Strain
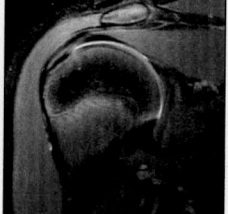	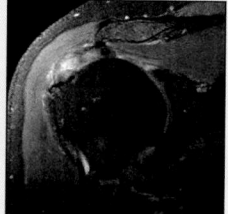	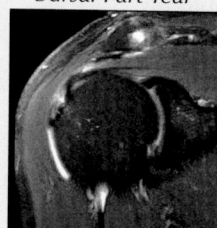	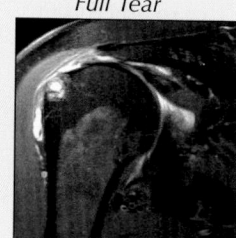	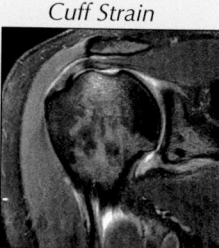
Cor FS PD FSE	Cor FS PD FSE	Cor FS PD FSE	Cor FS PD FSE	Cor FS PD FSE

ROTATOR CUFF TENDINOPATHY

Key Facts

Terminology
- Collagenous degeneration of the rotator cuff tendons most commonly involving the supraspinatus tendon

Imaging Findings
- Best diagnostic clue: Thickened inhomogeneous rotator cuff tendon with increased signal intensity on all pulse sequences
- Increased signal intensity of tendon on PD FSE, FS PD FSE, STIR & T2* GRE

Top Differential Diagnoses
- Calcific Tendinitis
- Intratendinous Cyst
- Magic Angle Artifact
- Normal Variations
- Partial Thickness Tears
- Full Thickness Tears
- Posterosuperior Glenoid Impingement
- Microinstability

Pathology
- Overuse, degeneration and tearing of the rotator cuff - intrinsic theory
- Secondary to impingement syndrome - extrinsic theory

Clinical Issues
- Painful even without tendon tear
- Most common reason for MRI referral of the shoulder

Diagnostic Checklist
- FS PD FSE may overestimate cuff pathology (tendinosis mistaken for a cuff tear)

- o +/- AC arthritis + acromial spurs
  - ▪ Chondromalacia (surface defects, hyperintense hyaline articular cartilage & marrow edema)
- o Prominence of greater tuberosity + subcortical cystic change
- o Post dislocation findings in case of tendinopathy due to supraspinatus strain
  - ▪ Hyperintense bone marrow edema with +/- hypointense fractures
  - ▪ Bankart, Hill-Sachs fracture
- Type III (hooked) acromion
- MR arthrography
  - o No cuff defect identified

Ultrasonographic Findings
- Thickened decreased echogenicity/hypoechoic
- Tears directly visible
- Less sensitive for partial thickness tears
- Advantage - allows dynamic evaluation with pain correlation

Imaging Recommendations
- Best imaging tool: MRI
- Protocol advice
  - o Coronal, sagittal FS PD FSE and T2 FSE are both required
    - ▪ Tears best seen on coronal and sagittal images

DIFFERENTIAL DIAGNOSIS

Calcific Tendinitis
- Form of tendinopathy
- Tendon thickened and with decreased signal intensity on all pulse sequences
  - o Calcium hydroxyapatite within hypointense cuff tendon(s)
  - o Hypointense calcium deposit
- +/- Hyperintense surrounding edema on T2WI
- +/- Adjacent bursitis

Intratendinous Cyst
- Thickened tendon, cyst visible on T2WI
  - o Hyperintense on T2WI

- Associated with partial tear of rotator cuff
- Elongated

Magic Angle Artifact
- Leads to artifactual increased signal at curved portion of tendon without thickening on short TE sequences
- 55 degrees to external magnetic field
- Affects biceps tendon, supraspinatus tendon and labrum

Normal Variations
- Muscle/tendon overlap
  - o In internal rotation
  - o Muscle fibers, esp. posteriorly may extend to the tendon insertion

Partial Thickness Tears
- Fluid within but not transversing tendon
- Hyperintense partial defect on T2WI
  - o Bursal (Bursal Part Tear)
  - o Interstitial
  - o Articular

Full Thickness Tears
- +/- Impingement
- Hyperintense defect on T2WI
- Anterior aspect often involved as in tendinopathy
  - o Tendinopathy often precursor to tear

Posterosuperior Glenoid Impingement
- Internal impingement
- Posterosuperior cuff, labrum, humeral head
  - o Triad of findings
- Overuse
- Throwing athletes
- +/- Occupational risk

Microinstability
- Superior labrum, MGL (middle glenohumeral ligament), anterior cuff abnormalities
- Usually partial supraspinatus tear
- Abnormal movement of shoulder joint results

ROTATOR CUFF TENDINOPATHY

PATHOLOGY

General Features
- General path comments: Common degenerative, pain producing disorder
- Etiology
  - Overuse, degeneration and tearing of the rotator cuff - intrinsic theory
  - Secondary to impingement syndrome - extrinsic theory
    - Subacromial spur formation
    - AC joint osteoarthritis
    - Type 3 (hooked) acromion
    - Lateral/anterior downsloping acromion
    - Os acromiale
  - Acute but usually in the setting of preexisting tendinosis
  - Eccentric tensile overload of the rotator cuff tendons
  - Begins where load is greatest on tendon - on articular side of anterior insertion of the supraspinatus tendon
  - Combination of extrinsic, intrinsic, and biomechanical factors
  - Collagen vascular diseases along with tendinosis of other tendons
- Epidemiology
  - Shoulder pain is 3rd most common cause of musculoskeletal pain syndrome
    - After low back pain (LBP) and cervical pain
  - 7-25% in Western general population

Gross Pathologic & Surgical Features
- Thickened, indurated tendon
- Loss of integrity of tendon in partially torn (bursal, articular or interstitial) and through-and-through torn tendons
- Partial tear may be on the bursal surface, articular surface or interstitial

Microscopic Features
- Collagen degeneration without influx of inflammatory cells: "Tendinosis" is preferred term over tendinitis
- Increase in collagen type III
  - Protein involved in healing and repair
- Increase in glycosaminoglycan and proteoglycan
- Tendon cell apoptosis (cell death) within supraspinatus
- Mucoid/eosinophilic/fibrillary degeneration and scarring
- Angiofibroblastic hyperplasia

Staging, Grading or Classification Criteria
- Impingement
  - Stage I: Reversible edema & hemorrhage typically in active patient ≤ 25 years
  - Stage II: Fibrosis and tendinitis
  - Stage III: Degeneration & rupture often associated with osseous changes in patients > 40 years
- Burkhart's cable/crescent theory of cuff tears
  - Cable = thickened supraspinatus tissue connecting anterior & posterior tendon edges medially
    - Well-perfused
    - Identified histologically
    - Separates musculotendinous junction from crescent
  - Crescent = lateral portion of supraspinatus tendon at risk for most cuff tears
    - Cuff tears in this lateral location may respond to debridement

CLINICAL ISSUES

Presentation
- Most common signs/symptoms
  - Progressive onset of shoulder pain
    - Pain, weakness, and loss of shoulder motion common
    - Pain over anterolateral part of the shoulder worsened by overhead activities in impingement
    - Night pain
- Clinical profile
  - Pain in athletics (internal impingement)
    - Younger patient population
- Painful even without tendon tear
- Most common reason for MRI referral of the shoulder
- Posttraumatic continued pain

Demographics
- Age: Peak: > 40 years for impingement, most common 55 years
- Gender: M:F = 1:1 or slight female predominance

Natural History & Prognosis
- Insidious onset of pain in adult patient with impingement syndrome
- +/- Progression to tear

Treatment
- Physical therapy
- Corticosteroids via injection to decrease inflammation
- Subacromial decompression for impingement

DIAGNOSTIC CHECKLIST

Image Interpretation Pearls
- FS PD FSE may overestimate cuff pathology (tendinosis mistaken for a cuff tear)
- T2 FSE (without fat suppression) is used to show the diminished signal in tendinosis as compared to the hyperintensity of a true cuff tear

SELECTED REFERENCES

1. Teefey SA et al: Ultrasonography of the rotator cuff. A comparison of ultrasonographic and arthroscopic findings in one hundred consecutive cases. J Bone Joint Surg Am 82(4):498-504, 2000
2. Gartsman GM: Arthroscopic management of rotator cuff disease. J Am Acad Orthop Surg 6(4):259-66, 1998
3. Cohen RB et al: Impingement syndrome and rotator cuff disease as repetitive motion disorders. Clin Orthop (351):95-101,1998
4. Fritz RC et al: MR imaging of the rotator cuff. Magn Reson Imaging Clin N Am 5(4):735-54, 1997
5. Neer CD et al: Cuff-tear arthropathy. J Bone Joint Surg 65(9):1232-44, 1983

ROTATOR CUFF TENDINOPATHY

IMAGE GALLERY

Typical

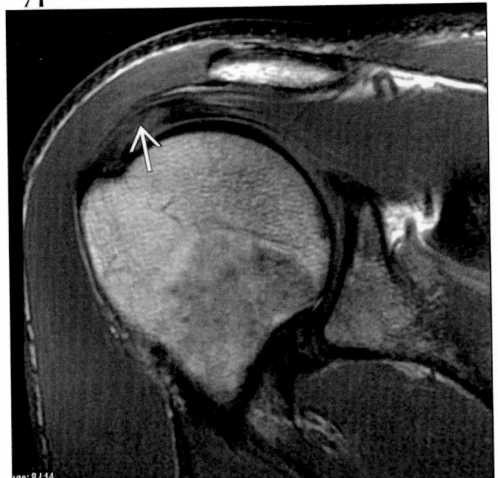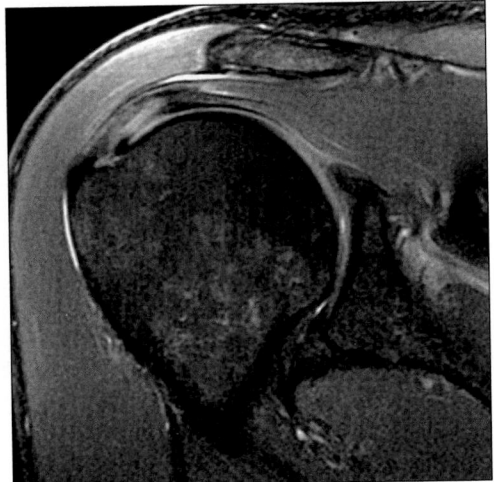

(Left) Coronal PD FSE MR shows increased signal intensity within the supraspinatus critical zone (arrow), consistent with tendinopathy. *(Right)* Coronal FS PD FSE MR shows increased signal of the critical zone, consistent with tendinopathy & articular surface fraying. This sequence visualizes tendinosis as hyperintense.

Typical

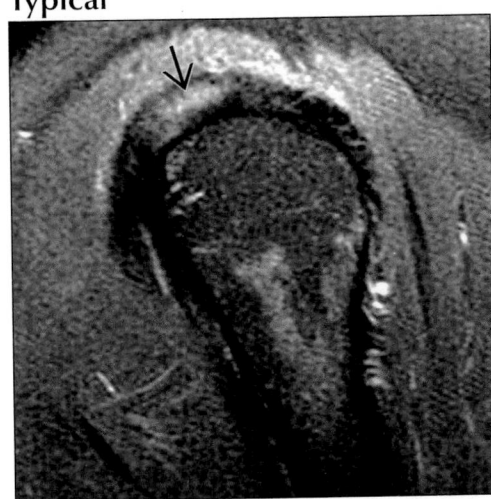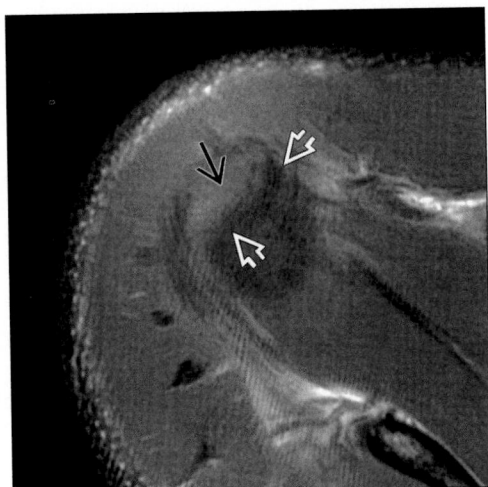

(Left) Sagittal FS PD FSE MR shows thickening and increased signal intensity (arrow) within the supraspinatus, consistent with tendinopathy. *(Right)* Axial PD FSE MR shows increased signal intensity (arrow) within the lateral supraspinatus tendon (crescent area where cuff tears occur). Note the rotator cable (open arrows).

Typical

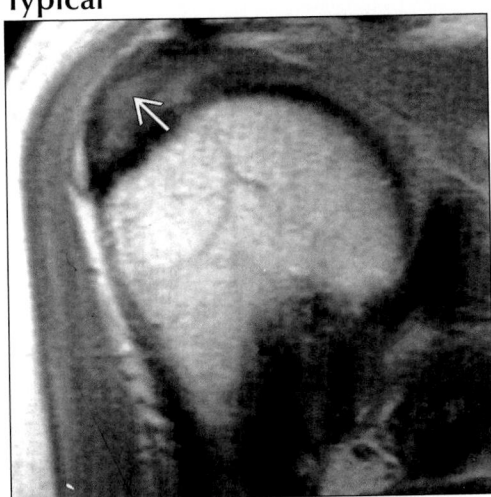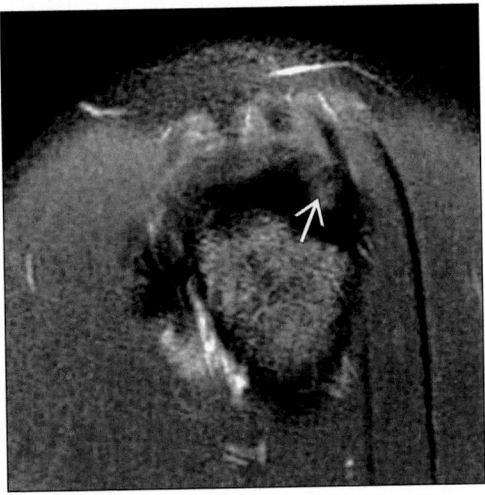

(Left) Coronal PD FSE MR shows marked thickening (arrow) of the posterior aspect of the supraspinatus tendon, consistent with tendinopathy. The patient has PSGI (posterior superior glenoid impingement). *(Right)* Sagittal FS PD FSE MR shows tendinopathy (arrow) predominantly affecting the posterior cuff tendon.

ROTATOR CUFF PARTIAL THICKNESS TEAR

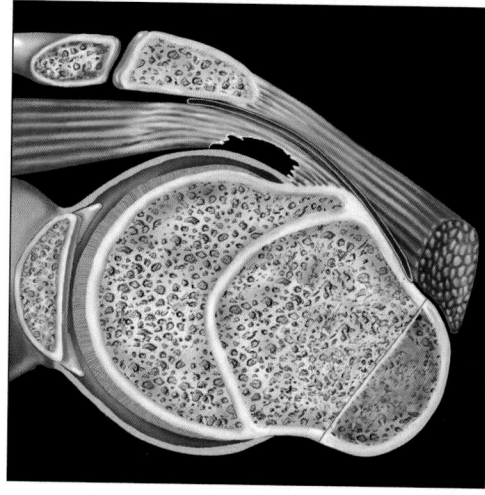

Coronal graphic shows a partial undersurface tear of the supraspinatus tendon involving the critical zone.

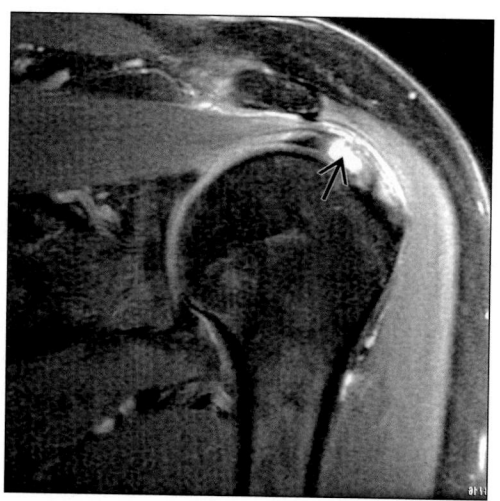

Coronal FS PD FSE MR shows an articular surface partial tear (arrow) of the supraspinatus involving the critical zone.

TERMINOLOGY

Abbreviations and Synonyms
- Partial rotator cuff tear (PRTC Tear)

Definitions
- Incomplete (partial) tear of tendon of rotator cuff
  - Supraspinatus tendon most common
  - Three types
    - Bursal surface
    - Interstitial (within substance - noncommunicating)
    - Articular surface

IMAGING FINDINGS

General Features
- Best diagnostic clue
  - Incomplete tear or gap in the RTC tendon filled with joint bursal fluid, +/- granulation tissue
  - FS PD FSE or T2WI
- Location: Supraspinatus (SST) bursal or articular surfaces or within tendon
- Size: Varies from fraying to large dissecting partial tear
- Morphology
  - Irregularity (fraying) to flap morphology

  - +/- Anatomically sealed (closed) in the adducted shoulder imaging position

Radiographic Findings
- Radiography
  - Findings associated with impingement
    - Acromial spurs
    - Type III (hooked) acromion
    - Humeral head (HH) arthritic changes of greater tuberosity
    - Acromioclavicular (AC) degenerative changes

MR Findings
- T1WI
  - Thickening of RTC tendons, of intermediate signal intensity
  - Calcifications in the supraspinatus, infraspinatus or teres minor = calcific tendinitis
  - Hypointense bone impaction (Hill-Sachs) - anterior dislocation
    - Rotator cuff strain associated
  - Marrow containing acromial spur (marrow fat)
- T2WI
  - Fluid signal intensity filling an incomplete gap in the tendon
    - FS PD FSE
    - Gap - articular surface or bursal surface
    - Interstitial, noncommunicating gap
  - +/- Fluid within the subacromial bursa

DDx: Rotator Cuff Partial Thickness Tear

Ca++ Tendinitis	RTC Tear	Tendinopathy

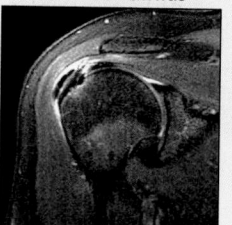 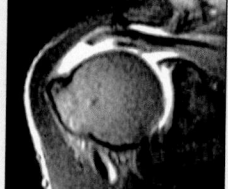 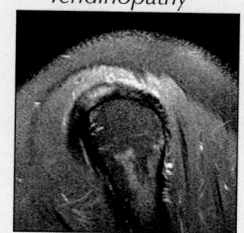

Cor FS PD FSE	Cor T1 Arthro.	Sag FS PD FSE

ROTATOR CUFF PARTIAL THICKNESS TEAR

Key Facts

Terminology
- Incomplete (partial) tear of tendon of rotator cuff
- Bursal surface
- Interstitial (within substance - noncommunicating)
- Articular surface

Imaging Findings
- Incomplete tear or gap in the RTC tendon filled with joint bursal fluid, +/- granulation tissue
- Findings associated with impingement

Top Differential Diagnoses
- Intratendinous Cyst
- Full Thickness Tear without Visible Communication
- Calcific Tendinitis (Ca++ Tendinitis)
- Rotator Cuff Tendinopathy
- Adhesive Capsulitis

Pathology
- Acute strain
- Chronic microtrauma/persistent strain

Clinical Issues
- Pain with abduction flexion maneuvers/impingement tests
- Shoulder pain with use of RTC after trauma
- Partial tears are more painful than full thickness tears

Diagnostic Checklist
- Partial tear in setting of intramuscular cyst
- Interstitial partial tear with fluid in the tendon not communicating with joint or bursa
- Identify fluid on FS PD FSE, and use the T2 FSE sequence to differentiate tendinosis from partial tear

---

- Increased signal intensity on FS PD FSE
  - +/- Fluid within the subcoracoid
    - Anterior supraspinatus tear, rotator interval tear
    - Subcoracoid impingement
  - Intermediate signal intensity in long head of biceps tendon, + associated tendinosis
  - Hyperintense effusion
  - FS PD FSE
    - Sensitive for evaluating partial tears
  - +/- Retraction and degeneration of the tendon edges
    - Articular or bursal surface partial
  - Hypointense bone impaction (Hill-Sachs) - post anterior dislocation
    - Rotator cuff strain commonly associated
  - Fluid within the substance of the tendon between layers in interstitial tear
    - No communication with surface
    - Not seen at arthroscopy
- T1 C+: Enhancement of granulation tissue indicating partial tear (imbibition)
- MR arthrography
  - Arthrography: Contrast may fill tear if articular surface communicates with joint

Ultrasonographic Findings
- Decreased echogenicity and thinning of partially torn region
- Lost of convexity of tendon/bursa interface in bursal surface partial tears
- Calcium = hyperechoic foci + shadowing

Imaging Recommendations
- Best imaging tool
  - MRI
    - FS PD FSE (hyperintense for tendinosis & partial tears)
    - T2 FSE (hyperintense for partial tears and not tendinosis)
- Protocol advice
  - FS PD FSE and T2 FSE coronal and sagittal images
  - +/- MR arthrography

DIFFERENTIAL DIAGNOSIS

Intratendinous Cyst
- Associated with partial tears
- Thickened tendon
- Cyst visible on T2WI
  - Hyperintense smoothly marginated/elongated mass
- Cyst usually flattened

Full Thickness Tear without Visible Communication
- +/- Closed by granulation
- +/- Closed by fibrosis/adhesions
- Uncommon
- Technique
  - Non fat saturation sequences may be less sensitive

Calcific Tendinitis (Ca++ Tendinitis)
- Calcium hydroxyapatite
  - Hypointense on all pulse sequences
- Deposit not visible in following conditions
  - Hypointense deposit within hypointense tendon
  - Quiescent lesions (silent phase)
- +/- Surrounding hyperintense edema on T2WI

Rotator Cuff Tendinopathy
- Thickened hyperintense (T2WI) tendons
- +/- Impingement
- No tear
- +/- Chronic repetitive microtrauma/impingement

Adhesive Capsulitis
- Thickened hyperintense capsule
  - Axillary pouch inferior glenohumeral ligament (IGHL)
  - Rotator interval
- Frozen shoulder
- +/- Cuff tear

ROTATOR CUFF PARTIAL THICKNESS TEAR

PATHOLOGY

General Features
- General path comments
  - Three types partial tears of RTC
    - Articular surface partial tear - most common, associated with classical impingement
    - Interstitial - not seen at arthroscopy
    - Bursal surface
  - Partial thickness tears cause muscle contraction pain similar to other partial tendon injuries (Achilles tendon, extensor carpi radialis brevis)
  - Pain with reflex inhibition of muscle action and loss of strength
  - Partial tear fiber detachment makes muscle less effective for proprioception function
  - Altered cuff function - HH ascends under deltoid contraction
  - Impinging cuff between HH & coracoacromial arch causative
  - Abrasion of cuff occurs with altered humeroscapular motion = cuff degeneration
- Etiology
  - Acute strain
  - Chronic microtrauma/persistent strain
  - Impingement syndromes
  - Collagen vascular diseases along with tears of other tendons
  - Altered concavity compression leading to microtrauma
- Epidemiology: Incidence of partial thickness tears 32-37% after 40 years
- Associated abnormalities
  - Intratendinous cyst
  - Posterosuperior labral fraying/tears internal impingement
  - Posterosuperior humeral head chronic impaction internal impingement
  - Bankart and Hill-Sachs anterior dislocation
  - SLAP tears associated with articular surface partial tears both anterior (SLAC lesion) and posterior (posterior peelback lesion) subclassification of type II SLAP lesions

Gross Pathologic & Surgical Features
- Thickened, indurated tendon edges
- Loss of integrity of tendon collagen fibers
- Hemorrhage in interstitial tears

Microscopic Features
- Collagen degeneration without influx of inflammatory cells
- Inflammatory cells in adjacent bursa = bursitis
- Increased levels of smooth muscle actin (SMA)
  - SMA-positive cells + glycosaminoglycan and proteoglycan promote retraction of torn fibers

Staging, Grading or Classification Criteria
- Type I - superficial capsular fraying, small local area, < 1 cm
- Type II - mild fraying, some failure of tendon fibers, < 2 cm
- Type III - moderate fragmentation and fraying, often involves entire SST surface, usually < 3 cm
  - Partial articular supraspinatus tendon avulsion (PASTA) lesion
- Type IV - severe tear with fraying, fragmentation and flap
  - Often involves more than one tendon

CLINICAL ISSUES

Presentation
- Most common signs/symptoms
  - Pain with abduction flexion maneuvers/impingement tests
  - Shoulder pain with use of RTC after trauma
  - Partial tears are more painful than full thickness tears
- Clinical profile: Athlete, patient after 40 years of age with impingement

Demographics
- Age
  - Younger athlete in case of internal impingement
  - Older than 40 years in subacromial impingement
- Gender: M = F, M > F in throwing athletes and heavy laborers

Natural History & Prognosis
- Insidious onset of pain in adult patient with impingement syndrome
- Sudden onset of pain in acute traumatic event
- Most partial tears progress to full thickness tears within 2 years
- May heal with cessation of impingement activities/physical therapy (PT)

Treatment
- PT for minor partial tears
- Arthroscopic debridement for more extensive tears
  - Subacromial decompression for bursal surface tears and acromial degenerative change

DIAGNOSTIC CHECKLIST

Consider
- Partial tear in setting of intramuscular cyst
- Interstitial partial tear with fluid in the tendon not communicating with joint or bursa

Image Interpretation Pearls
- Identify fluid on FS PD FSE, and use the T2 FSE sequence to differentiate tendinosis from partial tear

SELECTED REFERENCES
1. Kibler WB et al: Clinics in sports medicine. current concepts in tendinopathy. vol 22. W.B. Saunders, Philadelphia PA, 791-812, 2003
2. Read JW et al: Shoulder ultrasound: Diagnostic accuracy for impingement syndrome, rotator cuff tear, and biceps tendon pathology. J Shoulder Elbow Surg 7(3):264-71, 1998
3. Tirman PF et al: Posterosuperior glenoid impingement of the shoulder: Findings at MR imaging and MR arthrography with arthroscopic correlation. Radiology 193(2):431-6, 1994

ROTATOR CUFF PARTIAL THICKNESS TEAR

IMAGE GALLERY

Typical

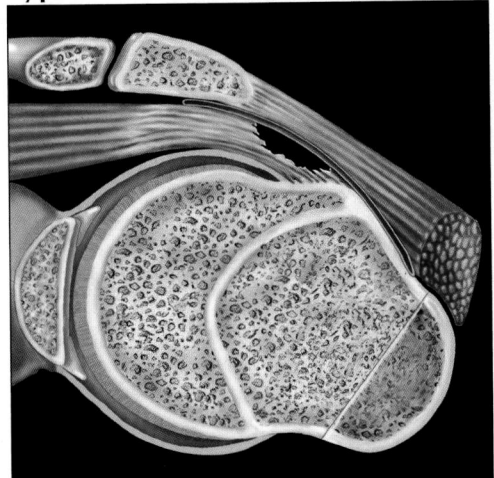 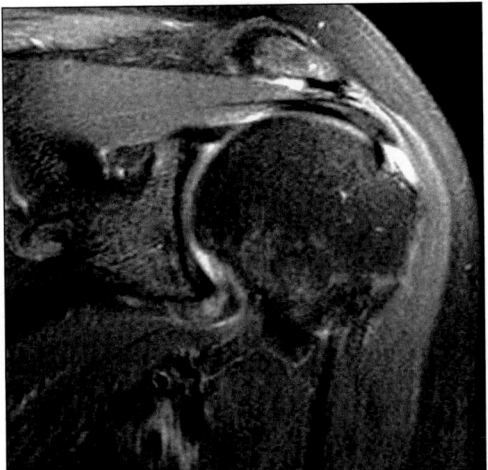

(Left) Coronal graphic shows a bursal surface partial tear with reactive bursal changes. (Right) Coronal FS PD FSE MR shows a bursal surface partial tear of the supraspinatus tendon distal insertion.

Typical

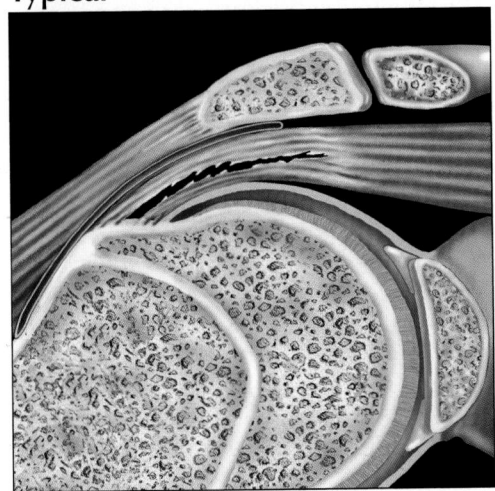 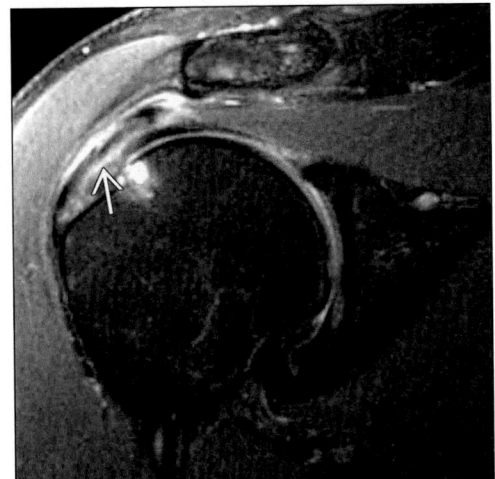

(Left) Coronal graphic shows an interstitial delamination partial tear. (Right) Coronal FS PD FSE MR shows interstitial delamination partial tear (arrow). There are associated degenerative changes of the humeral head.

Typical

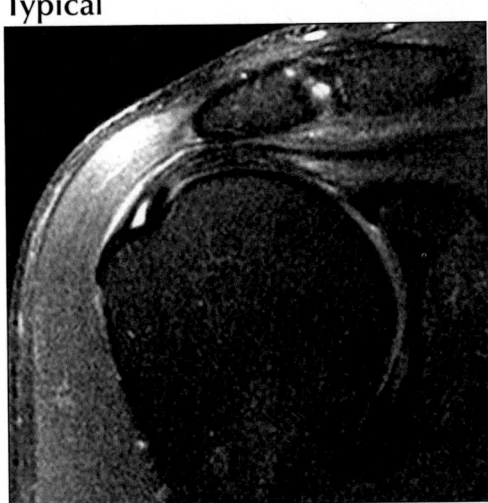 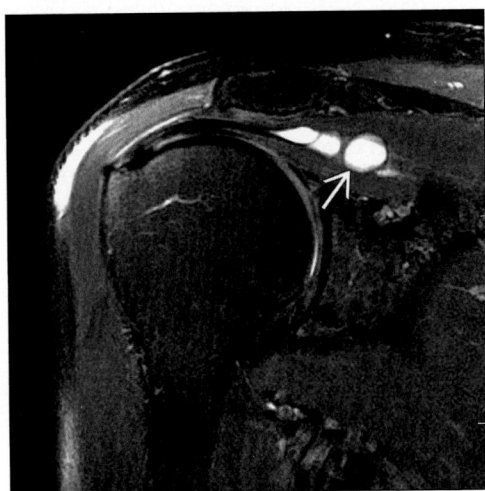

(Left) Coronal FS PD FSE MR shows an interstitial delamination partial tear with fluid signal intensity within the substance of the distal tendon. (Right) Coronal FS PD FSE MR shows multiloculated intramuscular hyperintense cyst (arrow) dissecting from myotendinous junction. There is associated partial cuff tearing. Intramuscular cysts are associated with RTC tears (particularly partial).

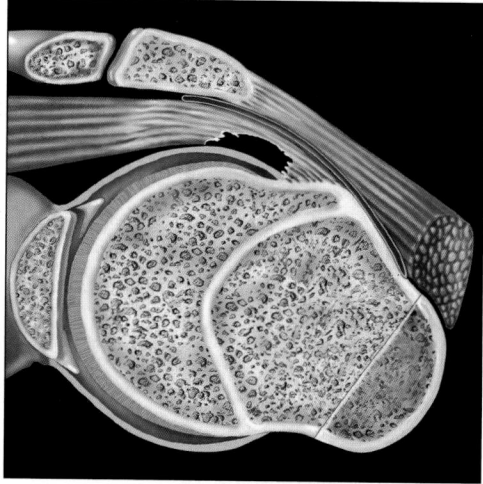

Coronal graphic shows an undersurface partial cuff lesion and a posterosuperior glenoid labral tear.

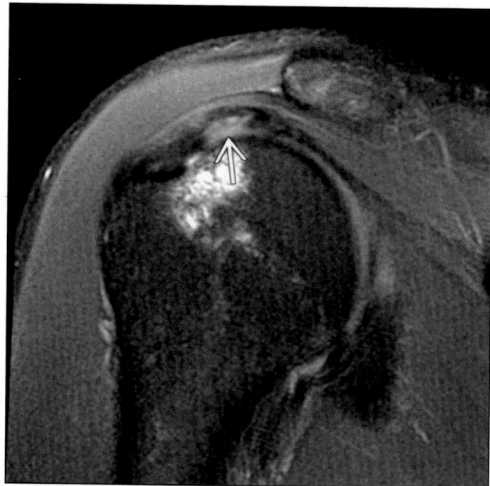

Coronal FS PD FSE MR shows an undersurface posterior supraspinatus tendon tear (arrow) + posterior superior labral fraying and cystic degenerative changes of posterosuperior humeral head.

TERMINOLOGY

Abbreviations and Synonyms
- Posterosuperior glenoid impingement (PSGI), internal impingement

Definitions
- Impingement of undersurface, posterior supraspinatus and anterior undersurface infraspinatus by posterosuperior labrum and humeral head (HH)
- Overhead throwing athletes and occupations which require overhead work (ABER - abduction external rotation)
- Posterior peelback - posterosuperior labral tear
  - Subclassification of type II SLAP lesion
  - Also referred to as internal impingement and includes associated undersurface tear of cuff at junction of supraspinatus and infraspinatus

IMAGING FINDINGS

General Features
- Best diagnostic clue: Triad of undersurface rotator cuff (RTC), posterosuperior labrum and HH damage
- Location: Posterosuperior aspect of glenoid and rotator cuff

- Size: Minimal fraying to full thickness tears of RTC, posterosuperior labrum and osteochondral impaction of posterosuperior HH
- Morphology: Thickened irregular tendon, frayed labrum, degenerative change - HH

Radiographic Findings
- Radiography
  - May be normal
  - +/- Subcortical cystic changes, posterosuperior humeral head
    - Mimics Hill-Sachs deformity

CT Findings
- NECT
  - +/- Cystic changes, posterosuperior humeral head
  - Posteroinferior calcification in throwing athlete
    - Bennett lesion
- CT arthrography
  - Posterosuperior labral fraying, +/- tear
  - Undersurface posterior supraspinatus/anterior infraspinatus partial tear
    - Contrast extends into tear
    - Coronal/sagittal reconstructions helpful

MR Findings
- T1WI
  - Thickened increased signal posterior supraspinatus and anterior infraspinatus = tendinosis

DDx: Internal Impingement, Shoulder

Teres Minor Tear	Partial Tear	Anterior Instab	RTC Tear	Ca++ Tendinitis

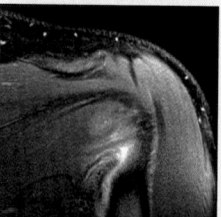 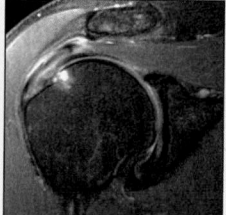 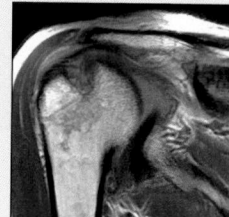 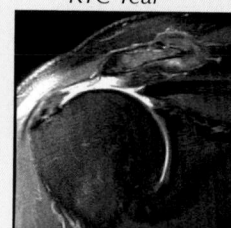 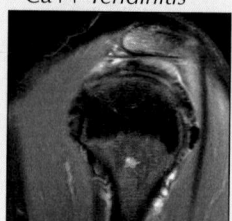

Cor STIR MR	Cor FS PD FSE	Cor PD FSE MR	Cor FS PD FSE	Sag FS PD FSE

INTERNAL IMPINGEMENT, SHOULDER

Key Facts

Imaging Findings
- ABER (abduction and external rotation) imaging demonstrates undersurface tears

Top Differential Diagnoses
- Subacromial Impingement
- SLAP Lesions - without RTC Pathology
- Microinstability - Affects Anterior Leading Edge RTC
- Anterior Instability/Subluxation
- Hidden Lesion
- Calcific Tendinitis
- Supraspinatus Tear

Pathology
- General path comments: Dynamic compression of the posterior superior aspect of RTC between posterosuperior labrum and HH

- Degeneration and tearing of the supraspinatus and infraspinatus tendon due to sheer forces secondary to friction between the posterosuperior RTC, labrum and HH during overhead throwing activities
- Epidemiology: Young athletes and adults performing overhead motion

Clinical Issues
- Most common signs/symptoms: Pain with abduction and external rotation
- Athletes participating in overhead throwing sports
- Non athletes who frequently abduct and externally rotate the arm (occupational)

Diagnostic Checklist
- Primary impingement, and SLAP lesion

  - o Junction of articular surface of supraspinatus and infraspinatus
  - o Posterosuperior labral surface irregularity, hyperintensity = fraying
  - o +/- Tear of posterosuperior labrum
    - Increased signal intensity or avulsion
  - o Posterosuperior humeral head irregularity with
    - +/- Hypointense sclerosis
    - +/- Hypointense subchondral cysts
- T2WI
  - o Undersurface tear of posterior supraspinatus and anterior infraspinatus: Hyperintense
  - o +/- Visible partial to complete tear - disrupted fibers
    - Partial articular surface or interstitial tear
    - +/- Surrounding hyperintense edema
  - o Full thickness tear in more advanced cases
  - o Posterosuperior humeral head chondromalacia
    - Hyperintense (FS PD FSE)
    - +/- Surface defect
  - o Normal "bare area" of posterosuperior humeral head devoid of cartilage may be located adjacent to point of contract between humeral head and glenoid
  - o Subchondral cystic changes
    - +/- Hyperintense
    - Similar location as Hill-Sachs lesion
  - o Fraying +/- tearing of the posterosuperior glenoid labrum
    - Surface irregularity, hyperintensity
    - T2 not as sensitive as short TE sequences (T1, T2* GRE, PD)
  - o Inferior glenohumeral ligament and anterior inferior labral injuries associated as IGL is under tension during abduction and external rotation
- STIR
  - o Less spatial resolution compared to FS PD FSE
  - o Necessary at low field strength as fat saturation important for detecting subtle edema
- MR arthrography
  - o Posterosuperior labral fraying, +/- tear demonstrated by contrast outline
  - o ABER (abduction and external rotation) imaging demonstrates undersurface tears

- Uncovering posterosuperior labrum with improved visualization
- "Touching" of cuff to labrum on ABER view not correlated with PSGI (seen in asymptomatic shoulders)
- Demonstrates any nondisplaced/healed/partial healed anterior inferior labral tear
- ABER places traction on IGHLC (inferior glenohumeral ligament complex)
  - o Chondromalacia outlined by contrast
    - Surface irregularity
    - +/- Defect of cartilage

Imaging Recommendations
- Best imaging tool: MRI
- Protocol advice: ABER imaging helps define associated articular sided cuff lesion

DIFFERENTIAL DIAGNOSIS

Subacromial Impingement
- History is usually suggestive of internal impingement
  - o Athlete involved in overhead throwing activities
  - o Instability may be present
  - o Subluxation while throwing

SLAP Lesions - without RTC Pathology
- Superior labral tear
- Propagate outside superior labrum
- + Speed's test (bicipital resistance), O'Briens test (anterosuperior pain in labral tear)
- +/- Flap component
- Hyperintense signal abnormality on short TE sequences within biceps anchor
- Hyperintensity within substance of biceps anchor specific finding on T2WI

Microinstability - Affects Anterior Leading Edge RTC
- Anterior supraspinatus tear
  - o Undersurface
- +/- Superior labrum tear

- Hyperintense tear of cuff on T2WI
- +/- Middle glenohumeral (MGHL) tear

Anterior Instability/Subluxation

- +/- Anterior inferior labral tear
  - Bankart lesion
  - Bankart variation
  - +/- Small nondisplaced tear in case of subluxation
- +/- Bankart fracture, Hill-Sachs lesion

Hidden Lesion

- Rotator interval
- Biceps instability
- Superior glenohumeral ligament (SGHL)/coracohumeral ligament (CHL) abnormality
- +/- Subscapularis tear

Calcific Tendinitis

- Hypointense calcium deposit (calcium hydroxyapatite) on all pulse sequences
  - Obscured within hypointense cuff tendon(s)
- +/- Hyperintense surrounding edema on T2WI
- +/- Adjacent bursitis

Supraspinatus Tear

- +/- Impingement
- Hyperintense defect on T2WI
- Anterior aspect often involved as opposed to PSGI
  - PSGI extends to involve anterior cuff in advanced cases

PATHOLOGY

General Features

- General path comments: Dynamic compression of the posterior superior aspect of RTC between posterosuperior labrum and HH
- Etiology
  - Degeneration and tearing of the supraspinatus and infraspinatus tendon due to sheer forces secondary to friction between the posterosuperior RTC, labrum and HH during overhead throwing activities
  - Glenoid rim comes in contact with the deep surface of the tendon in 120° abduction, retropulsion, and extreme external rotation
    - Late cocking phase in throwers
    - External rotation of biceps causes posterior peelback lesion
- Epidemiology: Young athletes and adults performing overhead motion
- Associated abnormalities: +/- Anterior instability

Gross Pathologic & Surgical Features

- Tendinosis and tearing of supraspinatus, infraspinatus, labrum
  - Humeral head impaction
- Cuff tendon is indurated, inflamed, frayed or torn
- Degenerative fraying and/or tearing of the posterosuperior labrum = posterior peelback lesion

Microscopic Features

- Degeneration and varying degrees of inflammation associated with rotator cuff tendons and posterosuperior labrum

- Chondral degeneration and thinning, subchondral sclerosis, and geode formation of the posterosuperior humeral head

CLINICAL ISSUES

Presentation

- Most common signs/symptoms: Pain with abduction and external rotation
- Clinical profile
  - Athletes participating in overhead throwing sports
  - Non athletes who frequently abduct and externally rotate the arm (occupational)
  - Varying degrees of RTC disease both and shoulder instability (positive physical examination signs)

Demographics

- Age: Adolescent (athlete), adult (occupational)
- Gender: M > F

Natural History & Prognosis

- Typically improves with rest, RTC strengthening

Treatment

- Physical therapy
- Arthroscopic debridement of rotator cuff and labral fraying
- Repair of rotator cuff tear
- Humeral derotational osteotomy
  - Absence of instability is required

DIAGNOSTIC CHECKLIST

Consider

- Primary impingement, and SLAP lesion

Image Interpretation Pearls

- Posterior articular sided RTC pathology in throwing athlete

SELECTED REFERENCES

1. Matsen FA III: Rotator cuff. The Shoulder. 3rd ed. WB Saunders, Philadelphia PA, 1998
2. Resnick D: Shoulder. Internal derangements of joints: Emphasis on MR imaging. WB Saunders, Philadelphia PA, 163-333, 1997
3. Hawkins RH et al: Nonoperative treatment of rotator cuff tears. Clin Orthop (321):178-88, 1995
4. Tirman PF et al: Posterosuperior glenoid impingement of the shoulder: Findings at MR imaging and MR arthrography with arthroscopic correlation. Radiology 193(2):431-6, 1994

INTERNAL IMPINGEMENT, SHOULDER

IMAGE GALLERY

Typical

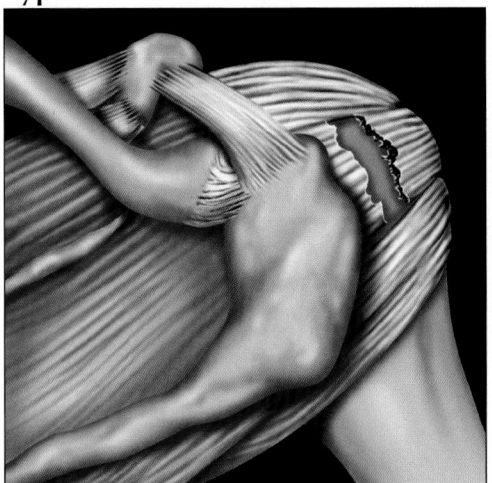
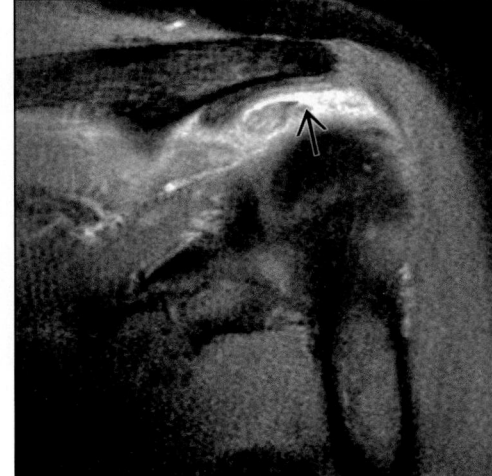

(Left) Coronal graphic demonstrates tearing of the infraspinatus tendon which can be seen with posterosuperior impingement. This undersurface cuff tear usually involves the anterior articular surface of the infraspinatus. *(Right)* Coronal STIR MR demonstrates a tear (arrow) of the infraspinatus/posterior supraspinatus in a patient with posterosuperior glenoid impingement.

Typical

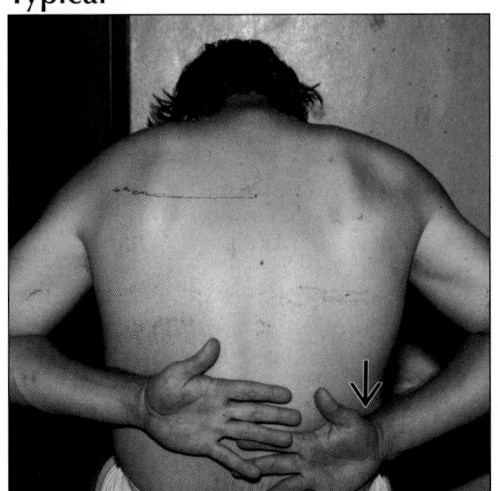
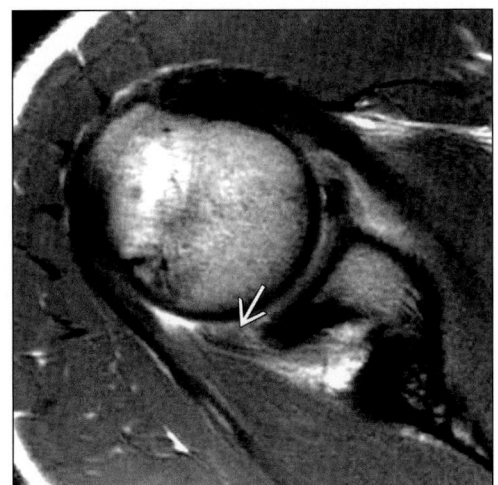

(Left) Clinical photograph of a baseball pitcher demonstrates posterior contracture and inability to raise throwing hand - R hand (arrow) symmetrically with the left hand. Note the shoulder asymmetry. *(Right)* Axial PD FSE MR demonstrates synovitis (arrow) within the posterosuperior aspect of the joint. There is associated labral fraying, sclerosis of the posterosuperior glenoid and cystic changes in the posterolateral humeral head.

Typical

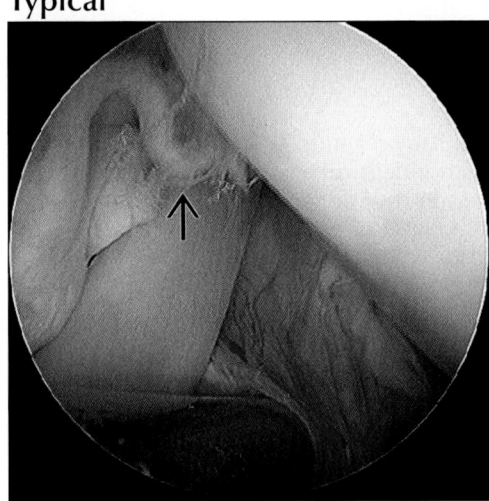
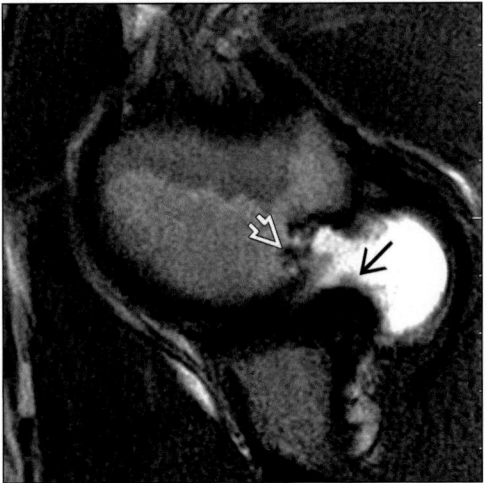

(Left) Sagittal oblique arthroscopic view demonstrates an undersurface rotator cuff tear (arrow) adjacent to the humeral head (right side). *(Right)* T2 FSE ABER shows internal impingement in professional throwing athlete, including posterior peelback subtype SLAP II lesion (arrow), undersurface supraspinatus fraying & humeral head impaction (open arrow).

ROTATOR CUFF FULL THICKNESS TEAR

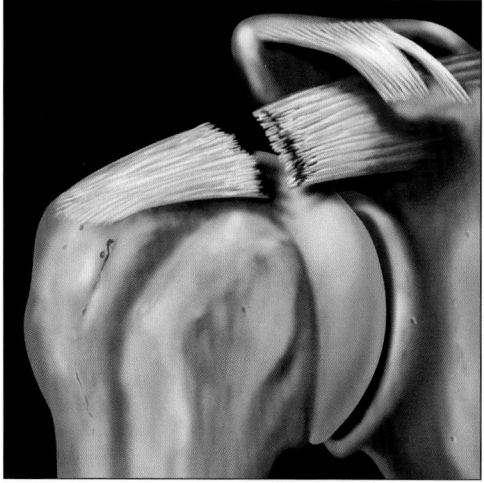

Coronal graphic shows a full thickness tear through the mid substance of the supraspinatus tendon.

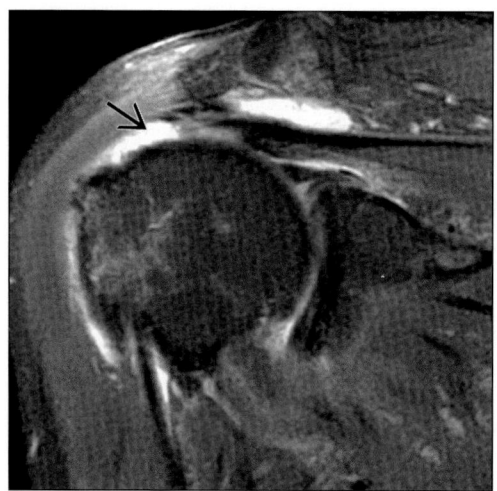

Coronal FS PD FSE MR shows full thickness tear (arrow) of the distal aspect of supraspinatus tendon with retraction & reactive subacromial bursitis. There is secondary adhesive capsulitis.

TERMINOLOGY

Abbreviations and Synonyms
- Rotator cuff (RTC) tear, supraspinatus (SST) tear

Definitions
- Tear of one of the tendons of rotator cuff
  - Supraspinatus tendon most common
- Tendon defect extends to both articular & bursal surfaces

IMAGING FINDINGS

General Features
- Best diagnostic clue: Tear or gap in RTC tendon, +/- joint bursal fluid, fibrosis and/or granulation tissue
- Location
  - Insertional tear within rotator crescent
    - Rotator crescent: Lateral more avascular portion of cuff; at risk for tear
  - Extensive tear involving crescent and cable
    - Rotator cable: More vascularized tissue medial to the crescent which joins anterior & posterior margins of RTC
    - Biomechanically less stable
- Size
  - Millimeter to several centimeters
  - Anterior-posterior, medial-lateral
- Morphology
  - Gap in thickened irregular hyperintense tendon
    - +/- Thinning
  - Repairable tears
    - Crescent within the distal tendon at insertion
    - U-shaped extensive tear
    - L-shaped tear indicates a longitudinal component
  - Massive tear: > 5 cm not repaired
    - Debridement if associated with fatty atrophy of the muscle
    - Surgical repair uncommon

Radiographic Findings
- Radiography
  - Acromial spurs
  - Type III (hooked) acromion
  - Acromioclavicular (AC) arthritis
  - Humeral head (HH) flattening or hypertrophy
  - HH greater tuberosity cysts
  - Superior HH migration

MR Findings
- T1WI
  - Thickened indistinct tendon
    - Tear edges not delineated on T1WI
  - Calcifications in the supraspinatus, infraspinatus or teres minor in cases of calcific tendinitis
    - Hypointense calcium deposits

DDx: Rotator Cuff Full Thickness Tear

Adhesive Capsul	AC Joint Dz	Partial Tear	RA	Tendinopathy
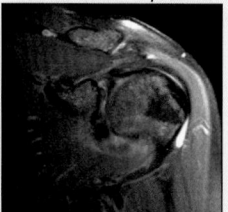	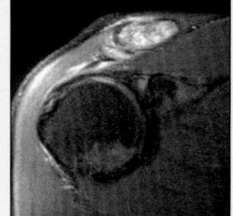	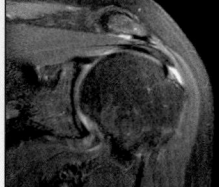	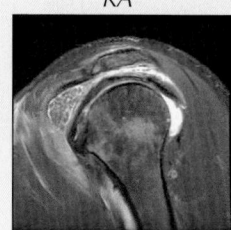	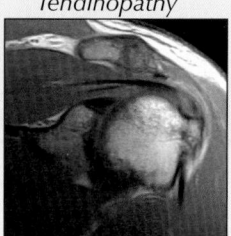
Cor FS PD FSE	Cor FS PD FSE	Cor FS PD FSE	Sag FS PD FSE	Cor PD FSE MR

ROTATOR CUFF FULL THICKNESS TEAR

Key Facts

Imaging Findings
- Insertional tear within rotator crescent
- Retraction and degeneration of tendon edges
- Full thickness tear associated with fatty atrophy of muscles chronic cases (fat signal on T1WI)

Top Differential Diagnoses
- Intratendinous Cyst
- Partial Tear of Rotator Cuff
- Adhesive Capsulitis
- Acromioclavicular Arthritis
- Rheumatoid Arthritis (RA)
- Rotator Cuff Tendinopathy

Pathology
- General path comments: Tear occurring in otherwise degenerated tendon due to chronic overuse

- Overuse, degeneration and complete tearing of RTC
- +/- Secondary to impingement (hooked acromion, overuse) or acute trauma
- Shoulder pain 7-25% of general population

Clinical Issues
- Pain with impingement test
- Insidious onset of pain, continuously increases with time - impingement

Diagnostic Checklist
- Assess tendons involved, status of tendon edges, status of biceps tendon and muscle atrophy
- Identify fluid signal intensity especially on FS PD FSE and PD and STIR sequences

- T2WI
  - Hyperintense fluid signal intensity filling a gap in the tendon
    - T2 FSE & FS PD FSE
  - Bald spot sign
    - Hyperintense fluid "bald spot" within hypointense tendon "head of hair"
    - Sagittal, axial T2WI
  - Fluid in subacromial bursa
    - Increased signal intensity on T2 FSE & FS PD FSE
    - Fluid may also be visualized in bursa without a cuff tear
  - Hyperintense (fluid signal intensity) bursitis
    - Subacromial/subdeltoid fluid or bursal thickening
    - Subcoracoid - esp. anterior tears and rotator interval tears
  - Hyperintense effusion
- Retraction and degeneration of tendon edges
- Full thickness tear associated with fatty atrophy of muscles chronic cases (fat signal on T1WI)
- Intermediate signal intensity in long head of biceps tendon - in tendinosis
- AC arthritis
  - AC joint hypertrophy
  - Chondromalacia (surface defects, hyperintense hyaline articular cartilage defects)
- Type III acromion - impingement

Ultrasonographic Findings
- Focal tendon interruption
- Fluid-filled gap (hypoechoic)
- Loss of convexity of tendon/bursa interface
- Hypoechoic tendon
- Tendon retraction
- Uncovered cartilage sign
- Calcium = hyperechoic foci + shadowing

Imaging Recommendations
- Best imaging tool: MRI
- Protocol advice
  - FS PD FSE & T2 FSE
    - FS PD FSE more sensitive for tendinosis
    - T2 FSE more specific for tears

  - Coronal, sagittal and axial images

DIFFERENTIAL DIAGNOSIS

Intratendinous Cyst
- Thickened tendon
- Cyst (hyperintense mass) visible on T2WI
  - Cyst usually flattened
- Associated with partial tear of the cuff

Partial Tear of Rotator Cuff
- Incomplete tendon defect
- Fluid within not traversing tendon
- Hyperintense partial defect on T2WI
  - Bursal, interstitial, articular
- Low grade (superficial), intermediate grade (< 50% of cuff thickness), and high grade (> 50% of cuff thickness)

Adhesive Capsulitis
- Thickened hyperintense capsule
  - Axially pouch inferior glenohumeral ligament (IGHL) involved
  - Rotator interval (synovitis)
- Frozen shoulder
- +/- Cuff tear

Acromioclavicular Arthritis
- Anterosuperior pain
- Lidocaine injection challenge - diagnostic
- Hyperintense edema on T2WI
- Chondromalacia (hyperintense T2 +/- defects)
- +/- Hyperintense T2 subchondral cysts

Rheumatoid Arthritis (RA)
- Inflammatory arthritides
- Hyperintense (PD/T2) synovitis
  - Thickened synovium
- +/- Rice bodies
  - Bursae
- +/- Rheumatoid factor

ROTATOR CUFF FULL THICKNESS TEAR

Rotator Cuff Tendinopathy
- Thickened (T2WI) cuff tendons
  - Hyperintense on FS PD FSE
  - Intermediate on T2 FSE
- +/- Impingement
- No tear
- +/- Chronic repetitive microtrauma/impingement

PATHOLOGY

General Features
- General path comments: Tear occurring in otherwise degenerated tendon due to chronic overuse
- Etiology
  - Overuse, degeneration and complete tearing of RTC
  - +/- Secondary to impingement (hooked acromion, overuse) or acute trauma
  - Collagen vascular diseases with tears of other tendons
  - Acutely in the setting of preexisting tendinosis, acute trauma
- Epidemiology
  - Shoulder pain 7-25% of general population
    - Full thickness tears - lower percentage
  - Shoulder pain in 10/1000 population
    - Peaks at 25/1000 population (42-46 years)
  - > 60 years - 28% demonstrate full thickness tears
  - Cadaver studies: Incidence of full thickness tears 18-26%
  - MRI studies: Tears in 34% of asymptomatic individuals of all ages
- Associated abnormalities
  - Hill-Sachs deformity - anterior dislocation
  - Patients > 40 years supraspinatus tear after anterior dislocation
  - Biceps tendinosis/tears/SLAP lesions with microinstability

Gross Pathologic & Surgical Features
- Involved tendons
  - Supraspinatus, infraspinatus, subscapularis
- Thickened, indurated tendon edges
- Defect in tendon
- Tendon retraction & atrophy with large/chronic tears

Microscopic Features
- Preexisting collagen degeneration without influx of inflammatory cells
  - "Tendinosis" is preferred term over tendinitis
- Associated tendinosis
  - Muscoid, eosinophilic and fibrillary degeneration
- Fatty infiltration of muscle tissue in chronically torn tendons

Staging, Grading or Classification Criteria
- Classification by size
  - Measure retraction
    - Small < 1 cm
    - Medium or moderate < 3 cm
    - Large 3 to 5 cm
    - Massive > 5 cm
  - Tear measured on coronal (medial to lateral) and sagittal (anterior to posterior) images

CLINICAL ISSUES

Presentation
- Most common signs/symptoms
  - Pain with impingement test
    - Hand on unaffected shoulder and gradual forward flexion of the affected shoulder
- Clinical profile
  - Insidious onset of pain, continuously increases with time - impingement
  - Pain in athletics - internal impingement - younger patient, athlete, occupation
  - Continued pain post trauma

Demographics
- Age: Peak age > 40 years
- Gender: M ≥ F

Natural History & Prognosis
- Insidious onset of pain in adult patient with impingement syndrome
- May heal with cessation of impingement activities/physical therapy
- Large tear: Cuff arthropathy

Treatment
- Level of activity, cause of tear
- Impingement
  - Subacromial decompression (acromioplasty)
  - Tendon repair unless massive cuff tear or tear associated with atrophy
- Massive cuff tears and associated with atrophy - debridement occasionally repair
- Repaired arthroscopically small tear crescent
- Mini-open repair partial tears > 50% thickness of the cuff
  - + Small to moderate sized tears

DIAGNOSTIC CHECKLIST

Consider
- Tear after trauma especially status post anterior dislocation in patient > 40 years
- Assess tendons involved, status of tendon edges, status of biceps tendon and muscle atrophy

Image Interpretation Pearls
- Identify fluid signal intensity especially on FS PD FSE and PD and STIR sequences
- A non fat suppressed sequence (T2 FSE) is required to distinguish between tendinosis and tear

SELECTED REFERENCES
1. Severud EL et al: All-arthroscopic versus mini-open rotator cuff repair: A long-term retrospective outcome comparison. Arthroscopy 19(3):234-8, 2003
2. Ruotolo C et al: Surgical and nonsurgical management of rotator cuff tears. Arthroscopy 18(5):527-31, 2002
3. Handelberg FW: Treatment options in full thickness rotator cuff tears. Acta Orthop Belg 67(2):110-5, 2001
4. Murrell GA et al: Diagnosis of rotator cuff tears. Lancet 357(9258):769-70, 2001

ROTATOR CUFF FULL THICKNESS TEAR

IMAGE GALLERY

Typical

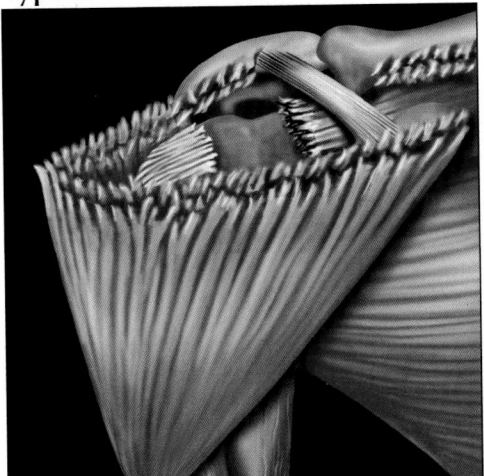 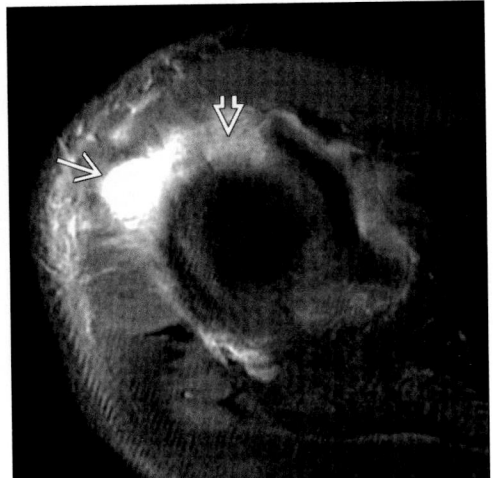

(Left) Coronal graphic shows rupture of the deltoid muscle (most often seen in post-operative patients) and underlying rupture of the supraspinatus tendon. *(Right)* Axial FS PD FSE MR shows tear of the lateral deltoid (arrow) and tearing of the supraspinatus tendon (open arrow).

Typical

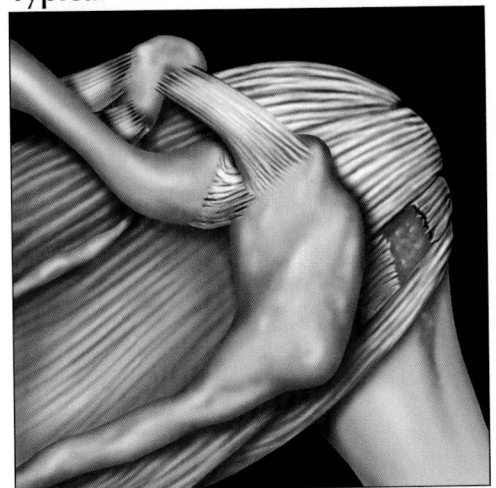 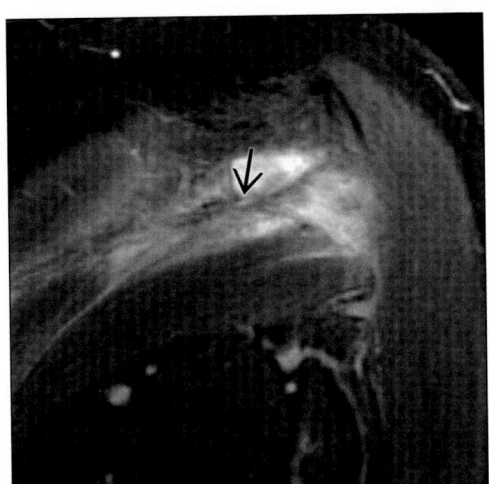

(Left) Coronal graphic shows a tear of the infraspinatus component of the rotator cuff. This is often seen in posterosuperior (internal) glenoid impingement (PSGI). *(Right)* Coronal FS PD FSE MR shows a tear of the infraspinatus tendon (arrow).

Typical

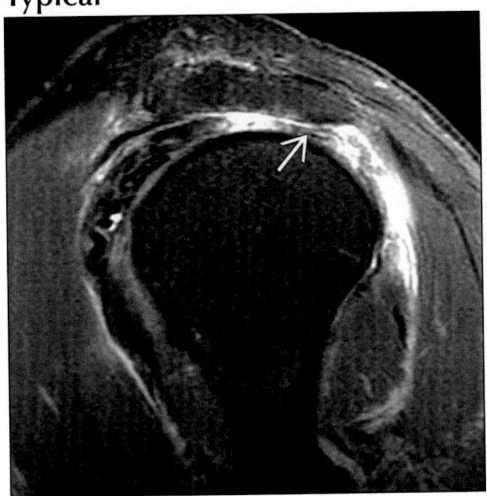 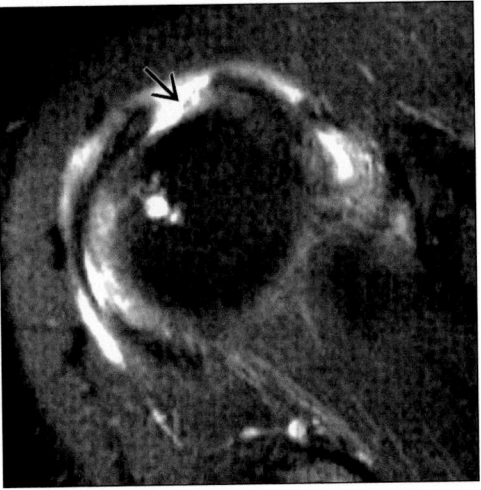

(Left) Sagittal FS PD FSE MR shows tearing of the posterior supraspinatus and infraspinatus (arrow) in a patient with posterosuperior (internal) glenoid impingement (PSGI). *(Right)* Axial FS PD FSE MR shows a full thickness tear (arrow) of the supraspinatus tendon.

ROTATOR INTERVAL TEARS

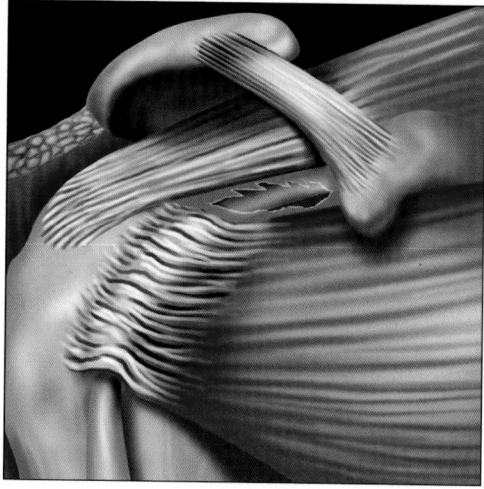

Coronal graphic shows a tear of the bursal aspect of the rotator interval (coracohumeral ligament component). The biceps tendon is visualized through the tear.

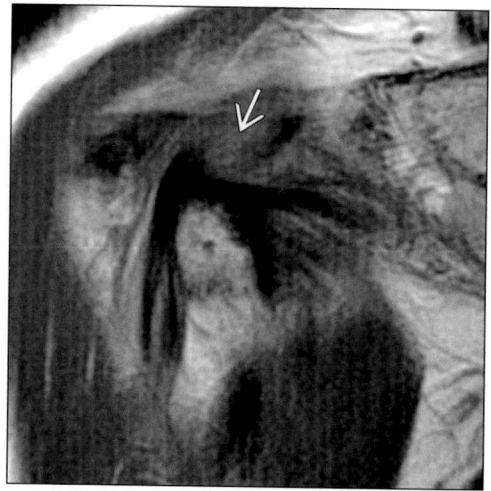

Coronal PD FSE MR shows a tear of the rotator interval with tendinosis of the biceps tendon (arrow). Magic angle contributes to the hyperintensity of the biceps tendon.

TERMINOLOGY

Abbreviations and Synonyms
- Rotator interval (RI)

Definitions
- Subtype of rotator cuff tear
- Tear or lax enlarged capsule between the supraspinatus and subscapularis tendons
- RI lesions: Spectrum of injuries from biceps anchor to rotator interval capsule to the bicipital groove
  - Range: Lax RI capsule, small holes, lesions in which most of the RI capsule is torn
- RI limits flexion and external rotation
- Disruptions of the superior glenohumeral/coracohumeral ligament complex = hidden RI lesion
- RI = tunnel through which long head of biceps travels from its origin on supraglenoid tubercle

IMAGING FINDINGS

General Features
- Best diagnostic clue
  - Tear of RI between supraspinatus tendon (SST) and subscapularis with hemorrhage/edema

- Arthrography shows leak of contrast through RI with intact SST and subscapularis
- Location
  - Interval between the SST and subscapularis tendon
  - Triangular space with apex centered at transverse humeral ligament over the biceps sulcus
    - Greatest width located at base of coracoid process
  - Posterior margin SST, anterior margin subscapularis
  - Roof of interval: Fibers from SST and subscapularis
  - Floor of interval: SST, subscapularis and portion of the superior glenohumeral ligament (SGHL/SGL), joint capsule, coracohumeral ligament (CHL)
- Size
  - Tear may be small (slit like) or large split in integrity of cuff
    - Collagenous fibers of the SST and subscapularis are contiguous through the RI
- Morphology: Tear represents irregular disruption of RI (usually roof)

Radiographic Findings
- Radiography
  - Subcortical cysts of lesser tuberosity with subcoracoid impingement
  - Normal radiographic findings

MR Findings
- T1WI

DDx: Rotator Interval Tears

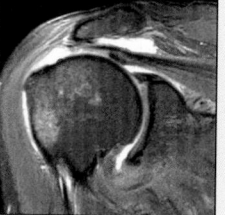

RTC Tear

Cor FS PD FSE

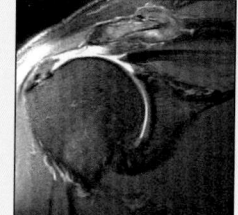

RTC Tear

Cor FS PD FSE

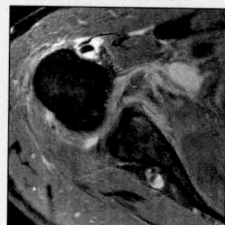

Anterior Instabil

Ax FS PD FSE

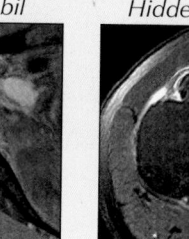

Hidden Lesion

Ax FS PD FSE

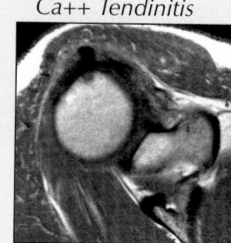

Ca++ Tendinitis

Ax PD FSE MR

ROTATOR INTERVAL TEARS

Key Facts

Terminology
- RI lesions: Spectrum of injuries from biceps anchor to rotator interval capsule to the bicipital groove

Imaging Findings
- Tear of RI between supraspinatus tendon (SST) and subscapularis with hemorrhage/edema

Top Differential Diagnoses
- Rotator Cuff Tear (RTC Tear)
- Adhesive Capsulitis
- Anterior Instability (Anterior Instab)/Multidirectional Instability (MDI)
- Hidden Lesion
- Calcific Tendinitis (Ca++ Tendinitis)

Pathology
- Associated with posterior and inferior instability and posttraumatic anterior instability
- Limitation of external rotation if fibrosis present

Clinical Issues
- Limited external rotation - type I interval lesion
- Inferior instability, posterior or MDI - type II interval lesion
- MDI - lax RI with capacious capsule

Diagnostic Checklist
- Consider RI "hidden lesion" if biceps tendinosis + subluxation present
- FS PD FSE sagittal images are sensitive to synovitis and abnormal fluid extension across the rotator interval

- o Thickened roof of RI + variable degrees of intermediate signal intensity = adjacent synovitis
- o Intermediate signal tendinosis +/- subluxation of long head of biceps (LHB) with "hidden lesion"
- T2WI
  - o +/- Irregular high signal tear of SGHL/CHL complex - "hidden lesion" of the RI
  - o Hyperintense fluid in subacromial and often subcoracoid bursa = reactive bursitis
  - o Visible tear of RI (roof)
    - Disruption of fibers
    - Hyperintense edema
  - o Thickened roof of RI with surrounding edema
  - o +/- Associated tear of adjacent supraspinatus tendon
    - Hyperintense discontinuous fibers
    - RI tear in this case represents anterior extension of a SST tear
  - o Hyperintense subchondral cysts of lesser tuberosity with subcoracoid impingement
- MR arthrography
  - o Leakage of contrast through the tear of the RI
    - Intact SST and subscapularis

Imaging Recommendations
- Best imaging tool: MRI and MR arthrography
- Protocol advice: MR arthrography for small isolated RI tears, FS PD FSE or PD images

DIFFERENTIAL DIAGNOSIS

Rotator Cuff Tear (RTC Tear)
- Superior subscapularis tendon tears without RI involvement
- Anterior SST tears without involvement of RI
  - o Difficult to differentiate
- +/- Supraspinatus labral instability pattern (SLIP) lesion
- +/- Superior labrum anterior-posterior (SLAP) lesion
- Partial or full thickness RTC tear
  - o PASTA (partial articular supraspinatus tendon avulsion) lesion

Adhesive Capsulitis
- Type I interval lesion
- Axillary pouch - inferior glenohumeral ligament (IGHL), RI thickened synovium
- Frozen shoulder

Anterior Instability (Anterior Instab)/Multidirectional Instability (MDI)
- Type II interval lesion
- +/- Bankart, Hill-Sachs lesion
- Fall on outstretched hand (FOOSH)

Hidden Lesion
- SGHL/CHL dysfunction
- Represents type II of RI lesion
- Biceps instability

Calcific Tendinitis (Ca++ Tendinitis)
- Calcium hydroxyapatite
  - o Hypointense on all pulse sequences
- Deposit not visible in following conditions
  - o Hypointense deposit within hypointense tendon
  - o Especially quiescent lesions (silent phase)
- +/- Surrounding hyperintense edema on T2WI

PATHOLOGY

General Features
- General path comments
  - o Lesion isolated from supraspinatus tear
  - o Associated with posterior and inferior instability and posttraumatic anterior instability
  - o Limitation of external rotation if fibrosis present
    - Contracture/fibrosis of RI +/- = chronic adhesive capsulitis
    - +/- Tear of capsule
- Etiology
  - o Subacromial or subcoracoid impingement may lead to RI tear/dysfunction
    - Isolated RI lesion - subcoracoid > subacromial impingement
  - o Acute traumatic injury (esp. anterior dislocation)

ROTATOR INTERVAL TEARS

- Forced internal rotation on externally rotated arm - acute traumatic etiology
- Congenital laxity of the RI capsule or absence of the CHL and SGHL
  - Predispose increased humeral head translation anteriorly and posterior-inferiorly
  - Enlargement of RI and instability
- Epidemiology
  - Rare lesion in isolation
  - Distal subscapularis tendon disruptions with rotator cuff pathology = 35%
- Associated abnormalities
  - Multidirectional instability
    - Treatment = plication of RI
  - Posterior/inferior instability
    - RI important for posterior stability
    - Contracture - limited external rotation (tear - to fibrosis)
  - RI hidden lesion
  - RI lesions (tears) associated with anterior dislocations
  - Microinstability
  - Superior labrum anterior cuff (SLAC) lesions

Gross Pathologic & Surgical Features
- Disruption of collagen fibers
- Fibrotic contracture
- Hypertrophic synovitis

Microscopic Features
- Inflammatory changes in superficial bursal area, fibrosis
- Influx of PMNs with inflammation

Staging, Grading or Classification Criteria
- Type I interval lesion - inflammatory changes in superficial bursal area
  - Contracted state
  - Subcoracoid impingement and anterior pain without instability
- Type II interval lesion - extensive inflammation of deeper tissues in the RI
  - Unstable condition after anterior dislocation
  - Enlargement or tear of RI

CLINICAL ISSUES

Presentation
- Most common signs/symptoms
  - Limited external rotation - type I interval lesion
  - Inferior instability, posterior or MDI - type II interval lesion
- Clinical profile
  - Athlete after acute sprain - traumatic RI tear
  - Chronic impingement + LHB abnormalities
    - Anterior RTC tear in impingement patient
    - +/- "Hidden lesion"
  - MDI - lax RI with capacious capsule

Demographics
- Age
  - Younger patient - acute traumatic event
  - > 40 years - impingement
- Gender

- Multidirectional instability: F > M
- Acute traumatic abnormality: M > F

Natural History & Prognosis
- +/- Progression of tear requires repair - active patient
- Type II treated initially with strengthening physical therapy or arthroscopy
  - Failure of conservative treatment

Treatment
- Conservative: Physical therapy
- Release of fibrotic tissue - type I RI lesion
- Arthroscopic repair or plication if type II RI lesion

DIAGNOSTIC CHECKLIST

Consider
- Anterior cuff tear
- RI lesion rare in isolation
- Consider RI "hidden lesion" if biceps tendinosis + subluxation present

Image Interpretation Pearls
- Arthrography may show contrast leakage in case of intact SST in isolated tear of RI
- FS PD FSE sagittal images are sensitive to synovitis and abnormal fluid extension across the rotator interval

SELECTED REFERENCES

1. Burkhart SS et al: Traumatic glenohumeral bone defects and their relationship to failure of arthroscopic Bankart repairs: Significance of the inverted-pear glenoid and the humeral engaging Hill-Sachs lesion. Arthroscopy 7:677-94, 2000
2. Dumontier C et al: Rotator interval lesions and their relation to coracoid impingement syndrome. J Shoulder Elbow Surg 8:130-5, 1999
3. Treacy SH et al: Rotator interval closure: An arthroscopic technique. Arthroscopy 13:103-6, 1997
4. Le Huec JC et al: Traumatic tear of the rotator interval. J Shoulder Elbow Surg 5:41-6, 1996
5. Field LLD et al: Isolated closure of rotator interval defects for shoulder instability. Am J Sports Med 23:556-63, 1995
6. Walch G et al: Tears of the supraspinatus tendon associated with "hidden" lesions of the rotator interval. J Shoulder Elbow Surg 3:353-60, 1994
7. Harryman DT et al: The role of the rotator interval capsule in passive motion and stability of the shoulder. J Bone Joint Surg Am 74:53-66, 1992
8. Grauer JD et al: Biceps tendon and superior labral injuries. Arthroscopy 8:488-97, 1992
9. Nobuhara-K et al: The rotator interval lesion. Clin-Orthop (223):44-50, 1987

ROTATOR INTERVAL TEARS

IMAGE GALLERY

Typical

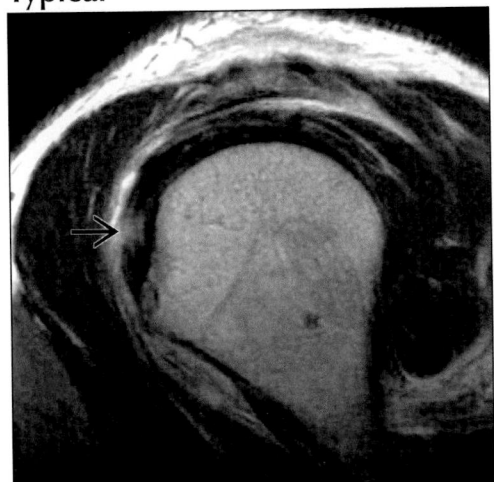 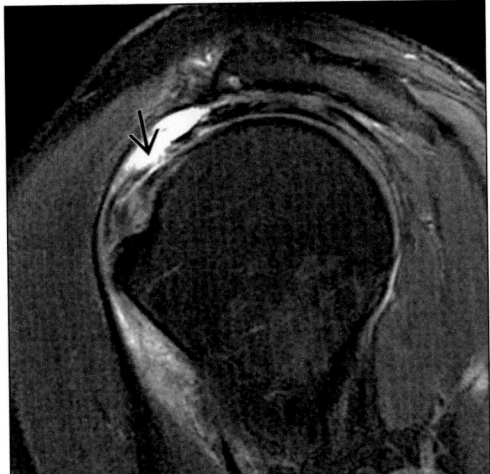

(Left) Sagittal T2 FSE MR shows a hyperintense tear (arrow) of the rotator interval anteriorly. *(Right)* Sagittal FS PD FSE MR shows a tear (arrow) of the anterior aspect of the supraspinatus tendon extending to involve the rotator interval.

Typical

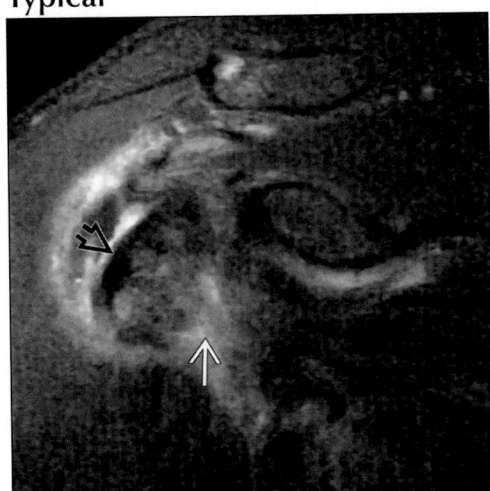 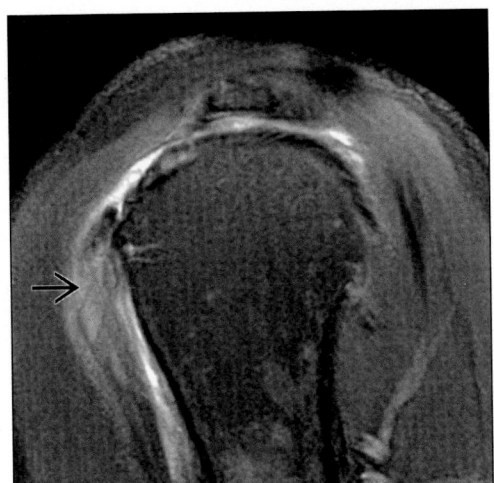

(Left) Coronal FS PD FSE MR shows a tear of the rotator interval with exposure of the biceps tendon (open arrow). There is surrounding bursitis and a tear of the subscapularis tendon (arrow). *(Right)* Sagittal FS PD FSE MR shows marked tendinosis and degenerative fraying/tearing of the biceps tendon (arrow) in association with a rotator interval tear.

Typical

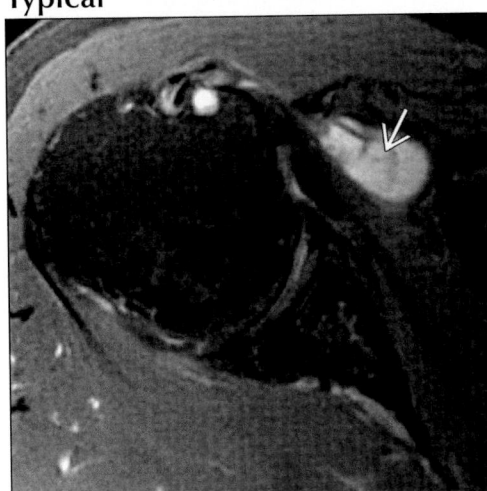 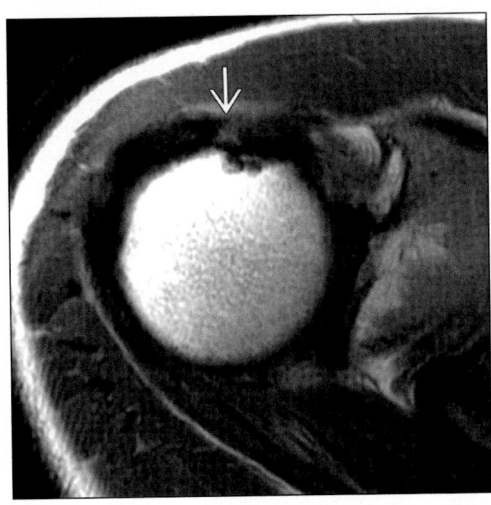

(Left) Axial FS PD FSE MR shows fluid (arrow) within the subcoracoid bursa indicating subcoracoid bursitis. Subcoracoid bursitis is found with rotator interval tears and anterior rotator cuff tears. *(Right)* Axial PD FSE MR shows a tear of the rotator interval (arrow) at the level of the superior aspect of the bicipital groove.

MICROINSTABILITY, SHOULDER

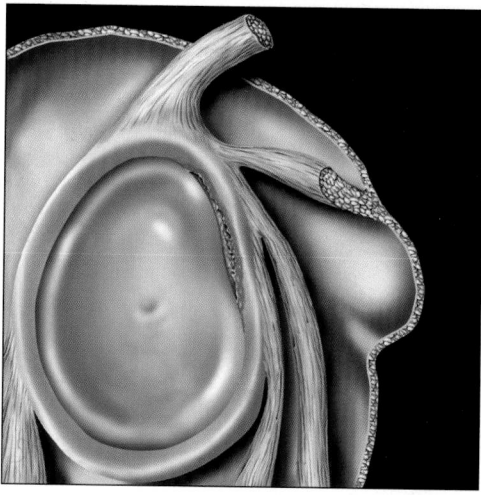

Sagittal graphic shows a tear of the anterior superior labrum.

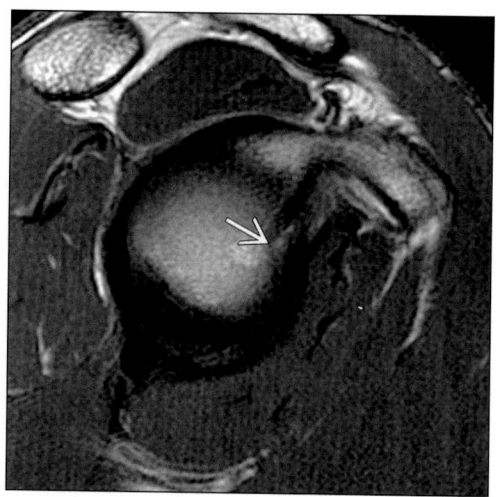

Sagittal PD FSE MR shows a tear of the anterosuperior labrum (arrow) associated with adjacent glenoid chondromalacia.

TERMINOLOGY

Abbreviations and Synonyms
- Microinstability (MI)

Definitions
- Lesions within anterior superior half of shoulder, primarily centered around rotator interval (RI)
  - Microinstability refers: Coracoid limits anterior translation and acromion & rotator cuff (RTC) limits superior translation
  - Spectrum of lesions include
    - Superior glenohumeral ligament (SGHL) avulsion or laxity
    - Middle glenohumeral ligament (MGHL/MGL) avulsion
    - Superior labrum anterior cuff (SLAC) lesion
    - Classic superior labrum anterior to posterior tear (SLAP)
    - Posterior peelback SLAP II variation
    - RI lesions

IMAGING FINDINGS

General Features
- Best diagnostic clue: Anterior RTC fraying/tearing and biceps anchor tear

- Location: Lesions that involve the RI, biceps anchor, superior labrum, MGHL insertion, RTC
- Size: Varies from fraying to frank tearing involving an area of a few centimeters
- Morphology: Varies from discrete tears to fraying, thickening, edematous structures

Radiographic Findings
- Radiography
  - Small subchondral cysts of the superior glenoid with SLAP lesions
  - Cystic (degenerative) change at superior aspect of lesser tuberosity especially with subcoracoid impingement

CT Findings
- NECT: Cystic change due to abnormal concavity compression of the humerus/instability leading to abnormal contact
- CT arthrography: +/- Torn labrum and cuff

MR Findings
- T1WI: Thickened irregular anterior cuff, mild increase in signal
- T2WI
  - Hyperintense fluid signal intensity within or involving attachment of the superior labrum at the biceps anchor - SLAP lesion
  - +/- Irregular, torn MGHL

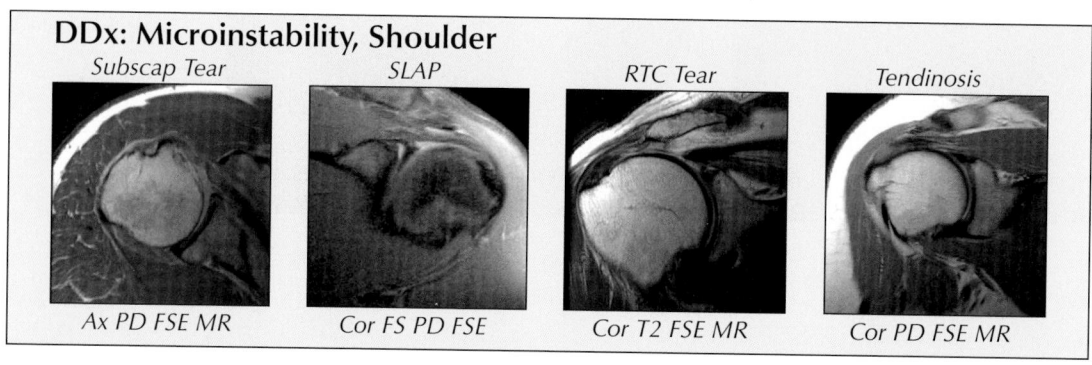

DDx: Microinstability, Shoulder

Subscap Tear	SLAP	RTC Tear	Tendinosis
Ax PD FSE MR	Cor FS PD FSE	Cor T2 FSE MR	Cor PD FSE MR

MICROINSTABILITY, SHOULDER

Key Facts

Terminology
- Spectrum of lesions include
- Superior glenohumeral ligament (SGHL) avulsion or laxity
- Middle glenohumeral ligament (MGHL/MGL) avulsion
- Superior labrum anterior cuff (SLAC) lesion
- Classic superior labrum anterior to posterior tear (SLAP)
- Posterior peelback SLAP II variation
- RI lesions

Imaging Findings
- Best diagnostic clue: Anterior RTC fraying/tearing and biceps anchor tear

Top Differential Diagnoses
- Anterior Instability
- Classic Impingement
- Subcoracoid Impingement
- Hidden Lesion
- SLAP Lesion
- Subscapularis Tear
- Supraspinatus Tear (RTC Tear)
- Supraspinatus Tendinopathy

Clinical Issues
- RTC (cuff tendinitis) or parascapular pain

Diagnostic Checklist
- Consider microinstability when clinical diagnosis is impingement with MRI findings of superior labral/MGHL/SGHL pathology

---

- Hyperintense, thickened, +/- discontinuous fibers
  - Increased signal, tear of LHBT (long head biceps tendon)
  - Fluid signal intensity filling a gap in the supraspinatus tendon (SST)
    - Partial tear/gap common
- STIR
  - Less spatial resolution than FS PD FSE
  - More homogeneous in presence of metal (post-op)
- MR arthrography
  - Sensitive to articular surface RTC tear and labral tearing

Imaging Recommendations
- Best imaging tool: MRI/MR arthrography
- Protocol advice
  - FS PD FSE & PD FSE
  - T2* GRE for intralabral signal on axial images

DIFFERENTIAL DIAGNOSIS

Anterior Instability
- Associated with RI tears
- +/- Bankart or Bankart variation lesions
- +/- Hill-Sachs lesion

Classic Impingement
- Hooked acromion
- +/- Supraspinatus tear
- Anterior supraspinatus involved

Subcoracoid Impingement
- Coracoid on subscapularis tendon/lesser tuberosity
- +/- Subscapularis tear
- +/- Lesser tuberosity cysts

Hidden Lesion
- Biceps instability
- SGHL/CHL (coracohumeral ligament) abnormality
- +/- Subscapularis tear

SLAP Lesion
- Superior labrum tear

- +/- Biceps anchor instability
- +/- Microinstability
- Tear may propagate

Subscapularis Tear
- +/- Anterior dislocation
- +/- Posterior dislocation
- +/- Lesser tuberosity fracture or avulsion
- May result from classical impingement

Supraspinatus Tear (RTC Tear)
- +/- Impingement
- +/- Anterior dislocation
  - > 40 years old
- Thickened increased signal intensity tendon with fluid signal intensity gap - T2WI

Supraspinatus Tendinopathy
- +/- Impingement
- Overuse syndrome
- Thickened increased signal intensity tendon without fluid signal intensity gap - T2WI

PATHOLOGY

General Features
- General path comments
  - Classic SLAP + multiple pathologic lesions in superior shoulder
  - Superior labral anterior cuff (SLAC)
    - SGHL/interval failure
    - Rotator cuff articular lesion secondary to abnormal translation and chafing on glenoid rim
    - Requires both an anterior cuff lesion (fraying/partial tear) and ligamentous laxity (detachment or stretching)
  - Posterior peelback
    - Acquired tight posterior capsule
    - Peelback SLAP lesion
    - Tight posterior band lifts humeral head up and posteriorly
  - Lax anterior capsule secondary to posterior shift of humeral head

MICROINSTABILITY, SHOULDER

- Etiology
  - Traction forces in overhead position - SLAP, SLAC
  - Roll around seat belt during accident - SLAC
  - Fall on abducted arm - SLAP variations
  - "Throwing out" of arm - MGHL injury
  - Professional overhand athletes (posterior peelback SLAP with posterior superior instability)
- Epidemiology: Approximately 6% of shoulder patients seen by orthopedists

Gross Pathologic & Surgical Features
- Biceps anchor failure (classic SLAP)
- Posterior biceps peelback SLAP
- Anterior superior labral detachments (anterior component of a SLAP II in SLAC)
- Superior glenohumeral ligament laxity/tear
- Middle glenohumeral ligament detachment (straight anterior instability)
- Articular partial thickness cuff lesions
- Arthroscopic findings in microinstability
  - Superior labral detachment/labral extensions (synovial reaction, chondral erosion)
  - Capsular (SGHL, MGHL) tears/laxity
  - Laxity of rotator interval
  - Articular sided rotator cuff partial thickness lesions (non-crescentic location in avascular lateral portion of cuff)
- Arthroscopic findings in posterior peelback
  - Displaceable vertex of biceps
  - Associated rotator cuff tear (posterior undersurface at junction of supraspinatus and infraspinatus)
  - Posterior component of a SLAP II lesion

Microscopic Features
- Fibrocartilaginous degeneration and/or tear of the superior labrum/biceps anchor - SLAP/SLAC
- Collagen degeneration without influx of inflammatory cells
  - "Tendinosis" is preferred term over tendinitis; RTC degeneration/tear
  - Cuff tendinopathy associated with an increase of type II collagen, glycosaminoglycan, proteoglycan and smooth muscle actin (SMA)
    - Activation of intracellular protein kinases results in tendon cell apoptosis (cell death), a weaker collagenous matrix and tendon tear

Staging, Grading or Classification Criteria
- Microinstability SLAP II subtypes
  - Classic SLAP (superior labral anterior-to-posterior)
  - SLAC lesion with anterior component of SLAP II + articular sided anterior supraspinatus tear
  - Posterior peelback with posterior component of SLAP II + posterior partial thickness articular sided cuff tear (also described as posterior superior microinstability)
  - Rotator interval defects
    - SGHL (superior glenohumeral ligament)
    - CHL (coracohumeral ligament)

CLINICAL ISSUES

Presentation
- Most common signs/symptoms
  - RTC (cuff tendinitis) or parascapular pain
  - Subjective feeling of slipping when not in abduction external rotation (ABER) position
  - Extension and superior movement of humeral head with the arm abducted is predictive pre-op test
  - Impingement like pain
- Clinical profile
  - Athletes or workers participating in overhead activities
  - Patient after acute trauma

Demographics
- Age: Young adults/adults
- Gender: M > F

Natural History & Prognosis
- Often improves with cessation of repetitive motions leading to disorder
- Post trauma
  - Respond to conservative therapy
  - Arthroscopic treatment

Treatment
- Conservative
  - Reduce pain and inflammation (NSAIDs), restoring range of motion, strengthening (physical therapy)
- Surgical
  - Tighten (imbricate) RI if lax
  - Repair attachment of SGHL and/or MGHL if detached/displaced
  - Repair SLAP/biceps anchor if detached

DIAGNOSTIC CHECKLIST

Consider
- Consider microinstability when clinical diagnosis is impingement with MRI findings of superior labral/MGHL/SGHL pathology
- Not all articular sided cuff lesions represent microinstability

Image Interpretation Pearls
- FS PD FSE and PD FSE images to demonstrate the spectrum of changes
- Consider MR arthrography for subtle changes

SELECTED REFERENCES

1. Miller M et al: Clinics in sports medicine. Cell death and tendinopathy. vol 22. 4th ed. Philadelphia PA, W. B. Saunders, 693-702, 791-812, 2003
2. Ruotolo C et al: Surgical and nonsurgical management of rotator cuff tears. Arthroscopy 18(5):527-31, 2002
3. Murrell GA et al: Diagnosis of rotator cuff tears. Lancet 357(9258):769-70, 2001
4. Stoller DW et al: Magnetic resonance imaging in orthopaedics and sports medicine. vol 1. 2nd ed. Philadelphia PA, J.B. Lippincott, 597-742, 1997

MICROINSTABILITY, SHOULDER

IMAGE GALLERY

Typical

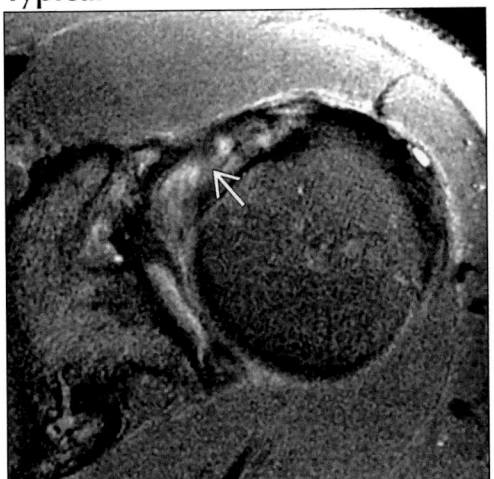 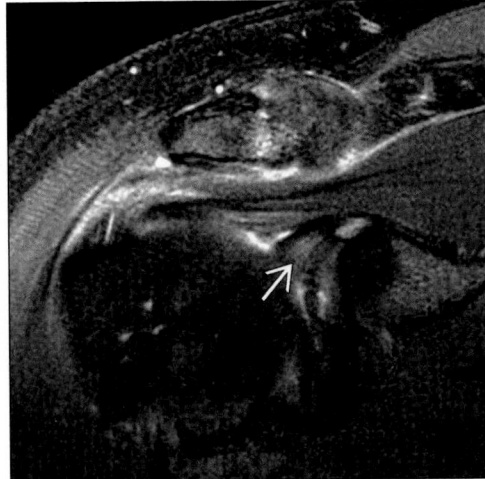

(Left) Axial FS PD FSE MR shows biceps tendinosis (arrow) and degenerative fraying as well as tearing of the superior labrum. There was undersurface rotator cuff tearing in this patient with microinstability. *(Right)* Coronal FS PD FSE MR shows tearing of superior labrum (arrow), moderate tendinosis and interstitial partial tearing + articular surface fraying of supraspinatus tendon. There was fraying of the middle glenohumeral attachment (not shown).

Typical

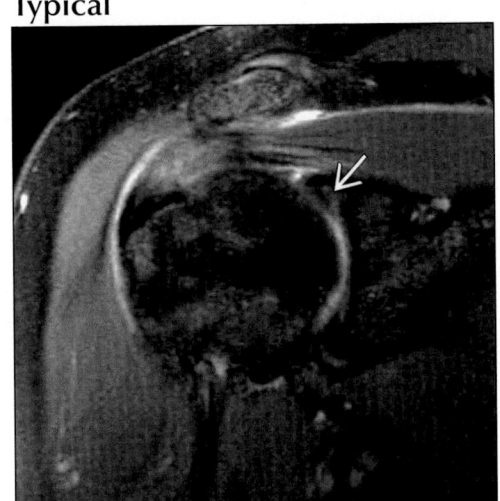 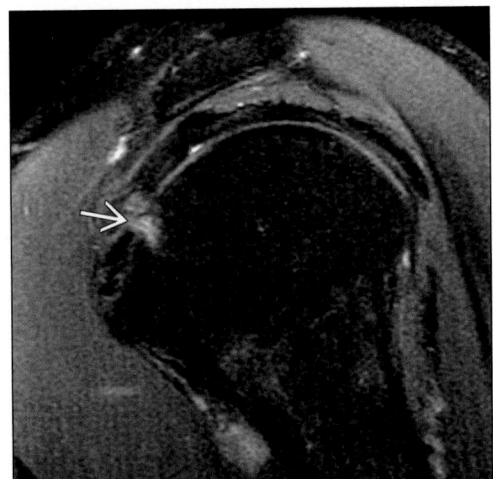

(Left) Coronal FS PD FSE MR shows marked thickening/tendinosis and partial tearing of the supraspinatus tendon (arrow) in association with a SLAP lesion in a patient with microinstability. *(Right)* Sagittal FS PD FSE MR shows thickening and edema (arrow) of the superior glenohumeral ligament attachment adjacent to the biceps in a patient with microinstability. This could represent a hidden lesion.

Typical

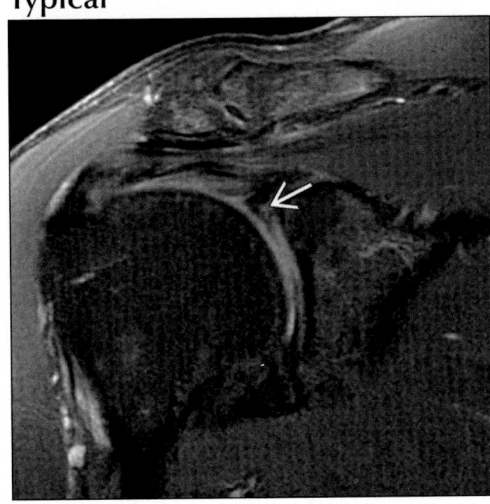 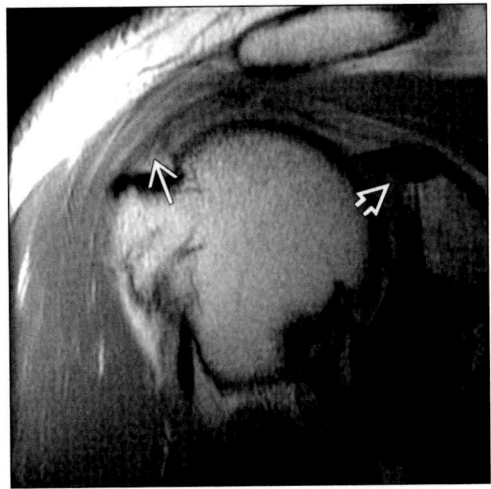

(Left) Coronal FS PD FSE MR shows partial undersurface tearing of the distal anterior supraspinatus tendon in association with an anterior SLAP II lesion (arrow), or SLAC lesion (superior labrum anterior cuff). *(Right)* Coronal PD FSE MR shows a SLAC lesion with articular sided supraspinatus fraying/partial tear (arrow) and anterior component of a SLAP II lesion (open arrow).

ROTATOR CUFF POST-OPERATIVE REPAIR

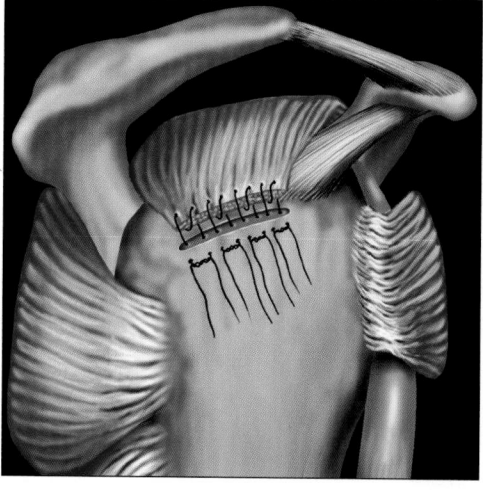

Coronal graphic shows sutures within a repaired supraspinatus tendon.

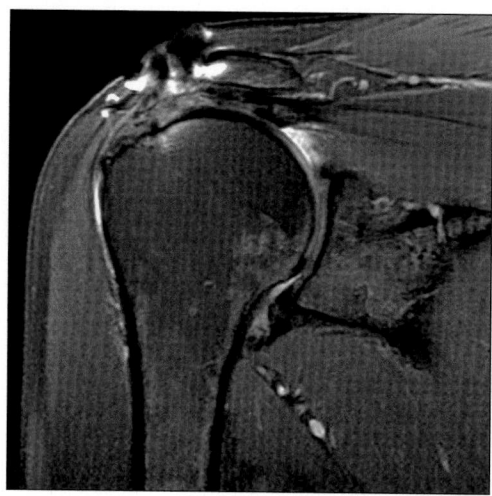

Coronal FS PD FSE shows an intact supraspinatus tendon repair. Note diffuse increased signal intensity & irregularity of intact tendon - common findings of recently post-op rotator cuff.

TERMINOLOGY

Abbreviations and Synonyms
- Rotator cuff repair, rotator cuff operative treatment

Definitions
- Operative (open or arthroscopic) repair or debridement of the RTC tendons

IMAGING FINDINGS

General Features
- Best diagnostic clue
  - Micrometallic artifact within decreased signal intensity rotator cuff tendon on all pulse sequences
    - Indicates surgery has been performed
    - "Trough" at level of the greater tuberosity where repaired tendon is attached
  - Disruption of repair results in discontinuous fibers
    - + Hemorrhage and generalized increased signal intensity on T2WI
    - +/- Retraction
- Location: Rotator cuff (RTC) tendons
- Size: Tears small partial to large complete disruptions
- Morphology
  - Normal tendon appears as linear decreased signal intensity structure attaching to greater tuberosity

  - Similar to normal RTC +/- micrometallic artifact

Radiographic Findings
- Radiography
  - +/- Post acromioplasty changes
    - Acromioplasty: Transforms type II (curved) and type III (anterior inferior hook) acromions into a type I (flat) acromion
  - +/- Trough of lateral aspect of greater tuberosity
  - +/- Sclerosis and/or cysts of greater tuberosity indicative of chronic impingement syndrome

CT Findings
- CT arthrography
  - Contrast extending through defect of retear into the subacromial bursa

MR Findings
- T1WI
  - Thickened tendon with moderate increased signal in cases of degeneration without tear
  - Torn tendon may be difficult to visualize on T1WI
- T2WI
  - Tendon-to-tendon or tendon-to-bone repair
    - Intermediate signal intensity of repaired tendon
    - Associated granulation tissue
  - Fluid signal intensity filling a gap in tendon retear
  - Micrometallic artifact

DDx: Rotator Cuff Post-Operative Repair

Biceps Tenodesis	Loose Hardware	Loose Hardware	Perthes Lesion	P Op Os Acromiale
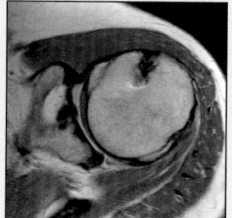	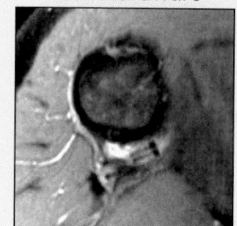	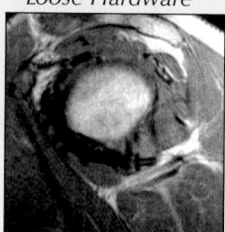	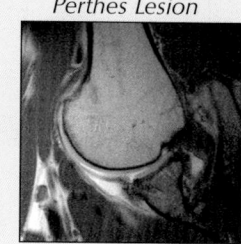	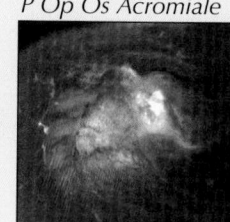
Ax PD FSE MR	*Ax STIR MR*	*Sag PD FSE MR*	*PD FSE MR ABER*	*Ax FS PD FSE*

ROTATOR CUFF POST-OPERATIVE REPAIR

Key Facts

Imaging Findings
- Micrometallic artifact within decreased signal intensity rotator cuff tendon on all pulse sequences
- Fluid signal intensity filling a gap in tendon retear
- Variable retraction and degeneration of tendon edges in retear

Top Differential Diagnoses
- Intact but not Water Tight Tendon After Repair
- Post Op Change not Including Rotator Cuff
- Loose Hardware
- Instability
- Os Acromiale

Pathology
- Rotator cuff tears are repaired utilizing arthroscopic technique, miniopen procedure or open procedure

- Retear occurring in otherwise repaired but also degenerated tendon
- Retear +/- trauma
- Preexisting collagen degeneration without influx of inflammatory cells: "Tendinosis" is preferred term over tendinitis

Clinical Issues
- Recurrent pain especially with impingement test
- Consider repair if patient with persistent pain is unresponsive to conservative measures and muscle dysfunction interferes with daily activities

Diagnostic Checklist
- Retear after trauma
- MR arthrography is helpful in the post operative setting to demonstrate the morphology of the tendon

- Variable retraction and degeneration of tendon edges in retear
- In chronic, low signal intensity retears (granulation tissue) need to evaluate tendon morphology
- Full thickness tear, +/- fatty atrophy of muscles in chronic cases
  - Decreased cuff size, associated with fatty atrophy and retraction
  - Secondary superior ascent of humeral head in direct contact with acromion
- +/- Fluid within the subcoracoid bursa
  - Anterior supraspinatus tears and rotator interval tears
  - Normal communication of fluid across rotator interval post arthroscopy
- Hyperintense effusion + subacromial fluid in bursa
  - Common in immediate post-op period
- Intermediate signal intensity in the long head of biceps tendon + associated tendinosis
- Calcifications in supraspinatus, infraspinatus or teres minor = calcific tendinitis
  - Hypointense deposits
- Flattened undersurface of anterior acromion after acromioplasty
- Tear obscured if micrometallic (ferromagnetic) artifact present
- Deltoid detachment as a complication of cuff repair
- STIR
  - Decreased spatial resolution
  - Artifact decreased
- T2* GRE: Susceptibility artifact from metal exaggerated
- T1 C+: Granulation and bursae will enhance even in the absence of tear
- MR arthrography
  - Contrast extending through defect of retear into subacromial bursa

Imaging Recommendations
- Best imaging tool: MRI/MR arthrography
- Protocol advice: T2 FSE, FS PD FSE +/- STIR for characterization of RTC

DIFFERENTIAL DIAGNOSIS

Intact but not Water Tight Tendon After Repair
- Arthrography shows contrast extending into subacromial bursa
- Common finding after repair
- Perforation site difficult to visualize

Post Op Change not Including Rotator Cuff
- Biceps tenodesis
- Mumford procedure - distal clavicle resection
  - Often accompanies acromioplasty
- Labral repair
- Superior labrum anterior-posterior (SLAP) repair
- Metallic or micrometallic artifact in location other than RTC

Loose Hardware
- Loose hardware in joint
- Arthrography helpful
- Some anchors prone to migration
  - SLAP repair
- Evaluate dependent recesses
- Sometimes erode out of joint into adjacent structures

Instability
- Anterior instability
  - Bankart lesion
  - Bankart variants
    - Anterior labral ligamentous periosteal sleeve avulsion (ALPSA)
    - Perthes
- Humeral avulsion of glenohumeral ligament (HAGL), inferior glenohumeral ligament (IGL) tears
- Relevant history
- Fall on outstretched hand (FOOSH) injury

Os Acromiale
- Failure of fusion of ossification center
- Predisposes to rotator cuff tear
- Diagnosis and treatment important

ROTATOR CUFF POST-OPERATIVE REPAIR

- ○ Acromioplasty of os acromiale inadequate (P Op Os Acromiale)
- ○ Resection or fixation required

Deltoid Dehiscence

- Status post open/mini open procedure
- May become redetached
- Discontinuous fibers at acromion attachment site
  - ○ + Hyperintensity on T2WI
- Weakness with abduction

PATHOLOGY

General Features

- General path comments
  - ○ Rotator cuff tears are repaired utilizing arthroscopic technique, miniopen procedure or open procedure
  - ○ Retear occurring in otherwise repaired but also degenerated tendon
  - ○ Retear +/- trauma
- Etiology
  - ○ Tendon repair - tear in association with a healthy muscle belly (non fatty atrophy)
  - ○ Tears in previously repaired tendons occur in variety of circumstances
    - Acute trauma
    - Recurrent impingement/chronic microtrauma
    - Hardware failure (especially if trough repair)
- Epidemiology
  - ○ Shoulder pain 7-25% in western population
    - Full thickness tears less common
  - ○ > 60 years - 28% demonstrate full thickness tears
- Associated abnormalities
  - ○ Greater tuberosity fractures with trauma
  - ○ Degenerative arthritis
  - ○ Labral tears

Gross Pathologic & Surgical Features

- Thickened, indurated tendon edges
- Loss of tendon integrity with post repair tear

Microscopic Features

- Preexisting collagen degeneration without influx of inflammatory cells: "Tendinosis" is preferred term over tendinitis
- Fibrosis/granulation after repair
- Fatty infiltration of muscle tissue in chronically torn tendons
  - ○ Indication for debridement rather than repair especially for large tendons

CLINICAL ISSUES

Presentation

- Most common signs/symptoms
  - ○ Recurrent pain especially with impingement test
  - ○ Consider repair if patient with persistent pain is unresponsive to conservative measures and muscle dysfunction interferes with daily activities
  - ○ Recurrent night pain associated with retear
  - ○ Recurrent weakness seen with retear

- ○ Hand on the unaffected shoulder and gradual forward flexion the of shoulder producing pain = positive impingement test
- Clinical profile
  - ○ Post operative rotator cuff repair patient
    - +/- Pain with retear
    - +/- Impingement symptoms

Demographics

- Age: Peak age: > 40 years (especially for impingement)
- Gender: M ≥ F

Natural History & Prognosis

- Recurrent partial tear may heal with cessation of impingement activities/physical therapy (PT)
- Recurrent tear often requires second repair
- Repairs of small to moderate size tears = excellent prognosis

Treatment

- Physical therapy
- Revision surgery

DIAGNOSTIC CHECKLIST

Consider

- Retear after trauma
- The presence of contrast material in the subacromial bursa is a normal finding if the repair was not "water tight"

Image Interpretation Pearls

- MR arthrography is helpful in the post operative setting to demonstrate the morphology of the tendon

SELECTED REFERENCES

1. Ruotolo C et al: Surgical and nonsurgical management of rotator cuff tears. Arthroscopy 18(5):527-31, 2002
2. Weber SC et al: Complications associated with arthroscopic shoulder surgery. Arthroscopy 18(2 Suppl 1):88-95, 2002
3. Handelberg FW: Treatment options in full thickness rotator cuff tears. Acta Orthop Belg 67(2):110-5, 2001
4. Goutallier D et al: Impact of fatty degeneration of the supraspinatus and infraspinatus muscles on the prognosis of surgical repair of the rotator cuff. Rev Chir Orthop Reparatrice Appar Mot 85(7):668-76, 1999
5. Neviaser RJ: Evaluation and management of failed rotator cuff repairs. Orthop Clin North Am 28(2):215-24, 1997
6. Tirman PF et al: A practical approach to imaging of the shoulder with emphasis on MR imaging. Orthop Clin North Am 28(4):483-515, 1997
7. Bigliani LU et al: Operative treatment of failed repairs of the rotator cuff. J Bone Joint Surg Am 74(10):1505-15, 1992

ROTATOR CUFF POST-OPERATIVE REPAIR

IMAGE GALLERY

Typical

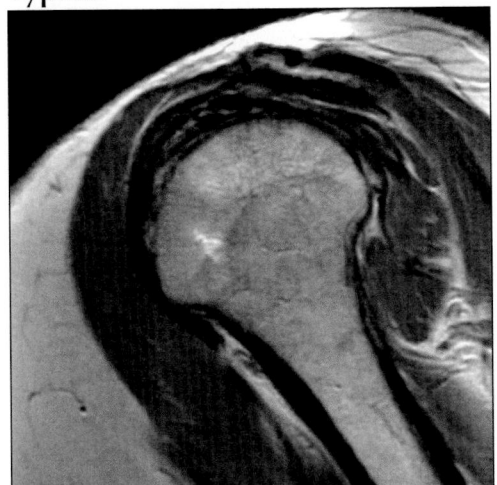 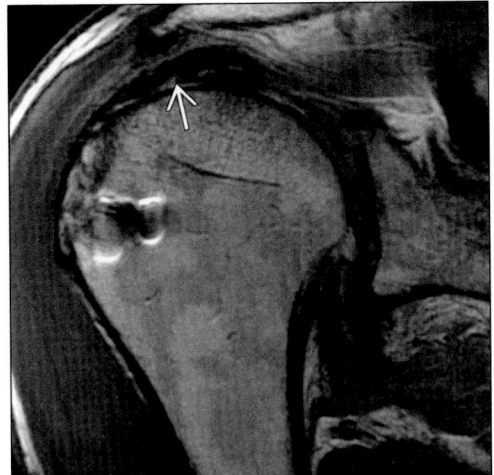

(Left) Sagittal PD FSE MR shows post-operative changes of an acromioplasty with resulting type I acromion. *(Right)* Coronal PD FSE MR shows a repaired rotator cuff tendon with partial tearing of the undersurface and retraction of the partially torn undersurface (arrow). The superior surface was intact.

Variant

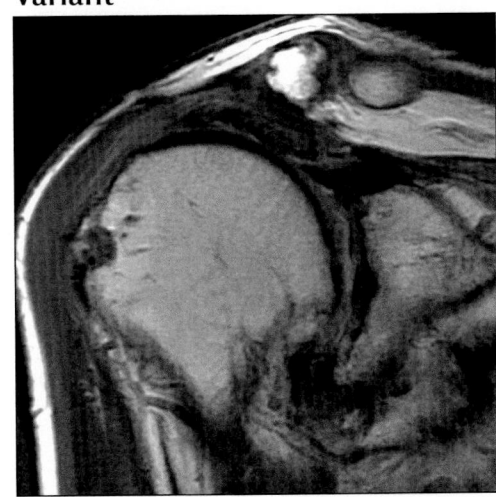 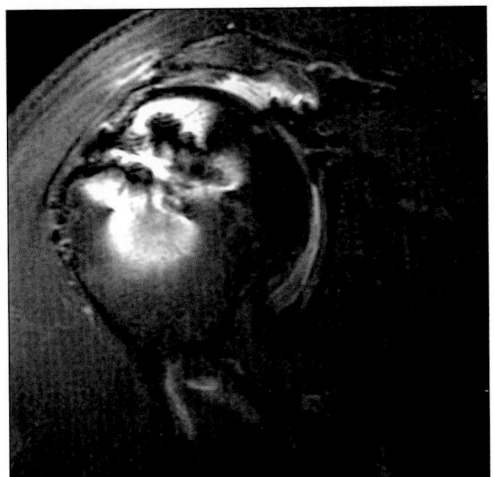

(Left) Coronal PD FSE MR shows a retorn rotator cuff with retraction. Note the developing degenerative changes of the joint. *(Right)* Coronal FS PD FSE MR shows a retear of the supraspinatus. Note the exaggerated metallic artifact due to the use of frequency selective fat saturation.

Variant

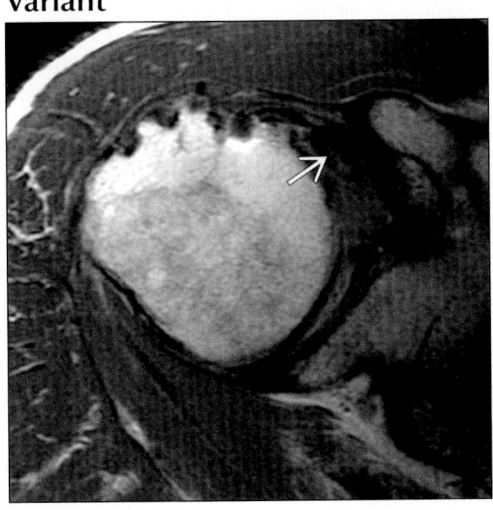 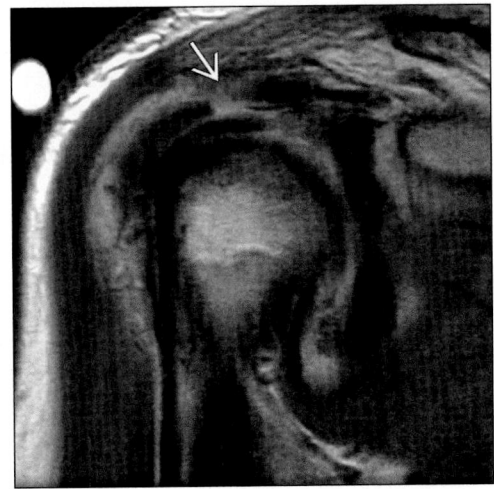

(Left) Axial PD FSE MR shows a dislocation of the long head of the biceps tendon (arrow) in a post-operative patient. Note the post-operative changes of the greater tuberosity. The patient also had a retear of the supraspinatus. *(Right)* Coronal PD FSE MR shows a tear of the anterior supraspinatus tendon and rotator interval (arrow). The biceps tendon anchor is degenerated and frayed.

ROTATOR CUFF CALCIFIC TENDINITIS

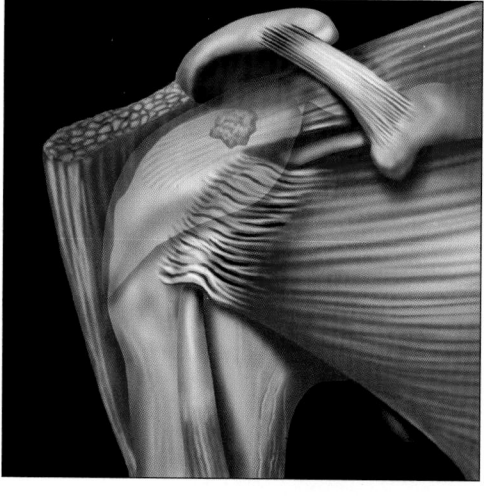

Coronal graphic shows focus of calcific tendinitis within supraspinatus tendon. Note subacromial bursitis & surrounding edema (common) as in silent phase with elevation of subacromial bursa.

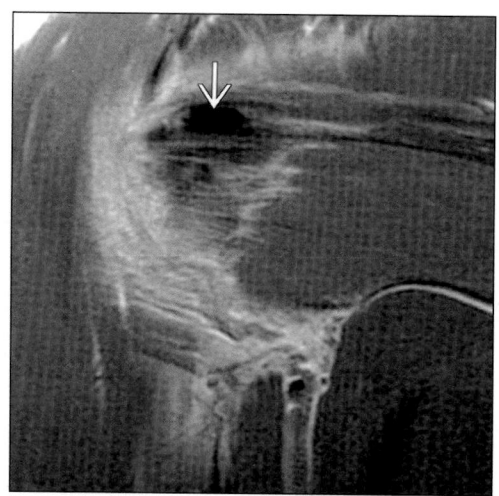

Coronal PD FSE MR of mechanical phase of calcific tendonitis shows at least 3 foci of hypointense (arrow) hydroxyapatite within infraspinatus tendon with surrounding edema.

TERMINOLOGY

Abbreviations and Synonyms
- Calcium hydroxyapatite deposition disease (HADD), peritendinitis, calcifying bursitis, periarthropathy

Definitions
- Deposits of calcium hydroxyapatite - in rotator cuff tendons

IMAGING FINDINGS

General Features
- Best diagnostic clue
  - Globular decreased signal intensity mass (all pulse sequences) of rotator cuff (RTC) tendons, often surrounded by edema or partial tear
    - Calcific deposit may be occult at MRI
- Location
  - Supraspinatus (SST) most commonly affected > infraspinatus (IST) > teres minor (TM) > subscapularis (SSC)
  - Periarticular soft tissues in addition to tendons
    - Ligaments
    - Capsule
    - Bursae

- Size: Varies from small (mm) deposition to several cm in size
- Morphology
  - Globular
    - Hood-like configuration
    - Linear
    - Angular
    - Round shapes

Radiographic Findings
- Radiography
  - Calcific deposits: Increased density on radiography, CT
  - Appearance of calcification depends on location and radiographic view obtained
    - In internal rotation posterior calcifications are seen (infraspinatus, teres minor deposits)
  - Routine views including
    - Anteroposterior views with shoulder in internal/external rotation
    - Axillary view
    - Supraspinatus outlet view (lateral view of scapula)
  - Focal well-defined deposit to diffuse, homogeneous, amorphous, fluffy deposit with poor margins

CT Findings
- NECT
  - Focal well-defined calcific deposits: Increased density

DDx: Rotator Cuff Calcific Tendinitis

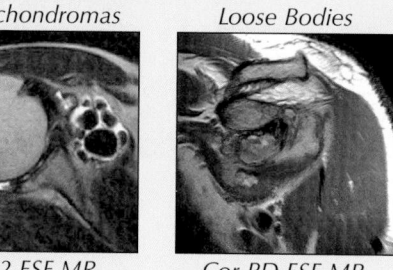

Osteochondromas	Osteochondromas	Loose Bodies
Ax T1WI MR	Ax T2 FSE MR	Cor PD FSE MR

ROTATOR CUFF CALCIFIC TENDINITIS

Key Facts

Imaging Findings

- Globular decreased signal intensity mass (all pulse sequences) of rotator cuff (RTC) tendons, often surrounded by edema or partial tear
- Calcific deposits: Increased density on radiography, CT
- Hyperintense edema may present around hypointense calcium deposits
- Associated tears not common compared to pericalcific edema

Top Differential Diagnoses

- Degenerative Calcification in Torn Tendon
- Loose Bodies
- Osteochondromatosis

Pathology

- Mechanical block if calcific deposit large enough

Clinical Issues

- Chronic mild pain especially in formative and resting phases
- Mechanical symptoms may be present
- Clinical profile: Discovered during imaging examination of shoulder in asymptomatic patients
- Resolve and heal spontaneously
- Needling, aspiration, and lavage if symptomatic
- Surgical treatment helpful in recalcitrant cases

Diagnostic Checklist

- Hydroxyapatite deposits have the same signal as normal cuff tendons

---

- o Dense, granular, well-demarcated calcifications
  - ▪ Indistinct calcification indictor of acute symptoms

MR Findings

- T1WI
  - o Hypointense homogeneous signal
  - o +/- Adjacent thickened tendon
- T2WI
  - o Hyperintense edema may present around hypointense calcium deposits
    - ▪ Associated tears not common compared to pericalcific edema
  - o Hyperintense subacromial-subdeltoid fluid
- T2* GRE
  - o Calcifications may bloom due to susceptibility
  - o Sensitive sequence for identification of hydroxyapatite
- T1 C+: Perilesional edema may enhance due to inflammation
- Globular decreased signal intensity of the calcifications deposit on all pulse sequences
- No involvement of articular cartilage
- MR arthrography
  - o +/- Partial rotator cuff tear

Ultrasonographic Findings

- Increased echogenicity mass with shadowing
- More sensitive and accurate than radiographs and MRI

Nuclear Medicine Findings

- Bone Scan: Calcific deposit may take up tracer

Imaging Recommendations

- Best imaging tool
  - o Ultrasound
  - o MRI: Accuracy 95%
- Protocol advice
  - o Experienced ultrasonographic technologist
  - o PD, T2* GRE or FS PD, T2 FSE

DIFFERENTIAL DIAGNOSIS

Degenerative Calcification in Torn Tendon

- Degenerative calcification generally smaller than calcific tendinitis
- Chemical composition is different
- Age group slightly older than HADD

Loose Bodies

- +/- Chondral defect nidus
- +/- Osteoarthritis
- Hypointense structure within joint on all pulse sequences
- +/- Marrow fat signal intensity center (T1WI, PDWI) - vs. sclerosis
  - o Hypointense on FS PD FSE
- Osteochondral lesions

Osteochondromatosis

- Synovial metaplasia
- Cartilage bodies, +/- osseous bodies
- Multiple bodies in joint

PATHOLOGY

General Features

- General path comments
  - o Mechanical block if calcific deposit large enough
  - o Housewives and clerical workers affected
  - o Crystalline hydroxyapatite: Not typical Ca++ of degenerative disease of tendons
  - o HADD often asymptomatic
- Etiology
  - o Avascular change
  - o Trauma
  - o Abnormal mineral metabolism
- Epidemiology
  - o 3-20% of painless shoulders and 7% of painful shoulders
  - o 13-47% bilateral

ROTATOR CUFF CALCIFIC TENDINITIS

Gross Pathologic & Surgical Features
- Macroscopic clumps of calcification often surrounded by indurated inflamed tendon
  - Intraosseous loculation
    - Unusual intraosseous extension of calcific deposit into the greater tuberosity of the humerus
    - Cystic lesions of humerus
  - Dumbbell loculation
    - Dumbbell appearance of the subbursal deposit beneath the coracoacromial (CA) ligament

Microscopic Features
- Crystalline hydroxyapatite in tendon
- Tendon often edematous with influx of inflammatory cells (esp. in resorptive phase)
- Macrophages and multinuclear giant cells present during resorptive phase
- Fibroblasts present in postcalcic phase

Staging, Grading or Classification Criteria
- Calcific tendinitis
  - Formative phase: Fibrocartilaginous transformation with deposit of calcium
    - Deposit chalk-like
  - Resting phase: No enlargement, +/- pain, may cause mechanical symptoms if large
  - Resorptive phase: Inflammation with cells resorbing calcium
    - Leak into bursa (subbursal and intrabursal rupture)
    - May be very symptomatic
    - Described as toothpaste like
    - Usually self limited
  - Postcalcic phase: Tendon integrity reconstituted
- Moseley classification
  - Silent phase
    - Calcium salts deposited in the tendons in the arterial anastomosis of the critical zone
    - Often asymptomatic
  - Mechanical phase
    - Calcifications increase in volume causing increased intratendinous stress and causing pain
    - +/- Bursitis
    - Intrabursal rupture: Intrabursal rupture of the tendinous or subbursal collection; associated with severe pain
    - Subbursal rupture: Partial extrusion of the calcific deposit beneath the bursa; +/- complete expulsion of the deposit from the tendon
  - Adhesive periarthritis phase
    - Tendinous calcification + adhesive bursitis

CLINICAL ISSUES

Presentation
- Most common signs/symptoms
  - Chronic mild pain especially in formative and resting phases
  - Mechanical symptoms may be present
  - Painful in resorptive phase
- Clinical profile: Discovered during imaging examination of shoulder in asymptomatic patients

Demographics
- Age: Incidence 30-50 years
- Gender: F > M

Natural History & Prognosis
- Resolve and heal spontaneously
- Progress, causing symptoms and requiring treatment
- Milwaukee shoulder
  - Destructive arthrography with hydroxyapatite deposits and rotator cuff tears

Treatment
- Needling, aspiration, and lavage if symptomatic
- Extracorporeal shock wave therapy (ECSW) may be helpful
- Surgical treatment helpful in recalcitrant cases

DIAGNOSTIC CHECKLIST

Consider
- Globular hypointense signal (T1 & T2WI) in tendon, bursa or capsular tissue

Image Interpretation Pearls
- Hydroxyapatite deposits have the same signal as normal cuff tendons
- T2* GRE will increase conspicuity of hypointense calcifications relative to soft tissues including tendons

SELECTED REFERENCES

1. Rupp S et al: Preoperative ultrasonographic mapping of calcium deposits facilitates localization during arthroscopic surgery for calcifying tendinitis of the rotator cuff. Arthroscopy 14(5):540-2, 1998
2. Uhthoff HK et al: Calcific tendinopathy of the rotator cuff: Pathogenesis, diagnosis, and management. J Am Acad Orthop Surg 5(4):183-191, 1997
3. Farin PU et al: Consistency of rotator-cuff calcifications. Observations on plain radiography, Sonography, computed tomography, and at needle treatment. Invest Radiol 31(5):300-4, 1996
4. Loew M et al: Relationship between calcifying tendinitis and subacromial impingement: A prospective radiography and magnetic resonance imaging study. J Shoulder Elbow Surg 5(4):314-9, 1996
5. Riley GP et al: Prevalence and possible pathological significance of calcium phosphate salt accumulation in tendon matrix degeneration. Ann Rheum Dis 55(2):109-15, 1996
6. Jim YF et al: Coexistence of calcific tendinitis and rotator cuff tear: an arthrographic study. Skeletal Radiol 22(3):183-5, 1993
7. Re LP Jr Karzel RP: Management of rotator cuff calcifications. Orthop Clin North Am 24(1):125-32, 1993
8. Moseley HF: Shoulder lesions. Edinburgh London, E&S Livingstone, 99, 1969

ROTATOR CUFF CALCIFIC TENDINITIS

IMAGE GALLERY

Typical

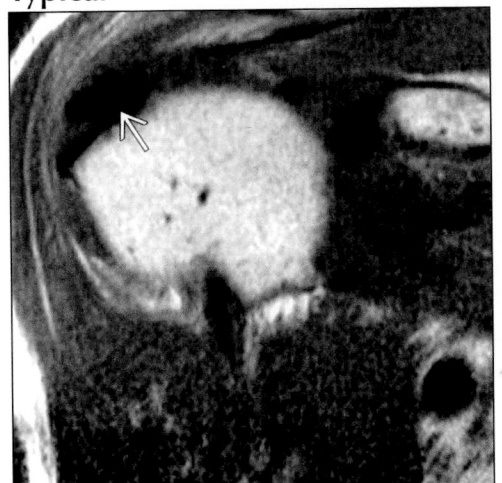 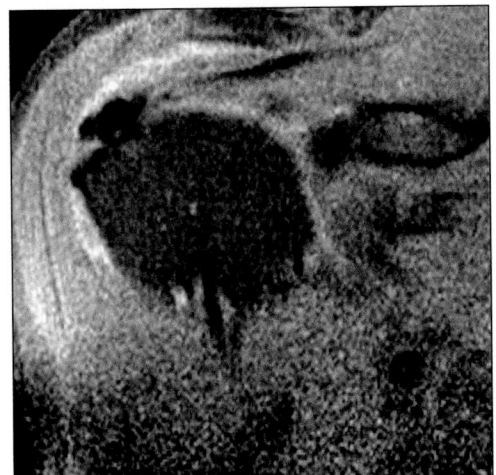

(Left) Coronal PD FSE MR shows clump-like calcification (arrow) within the supraspinatus tendon, consistent with the silent phase of calcific tendinitis. *(Right)* Coronal FS PD FSE MR shows hypointense clumped calcification with subacromial bursal hyperintensity.

Typical

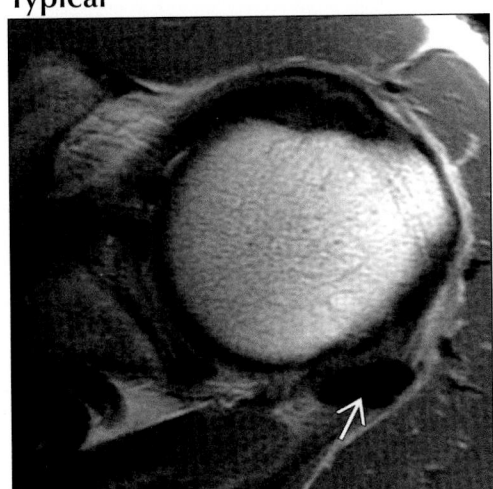 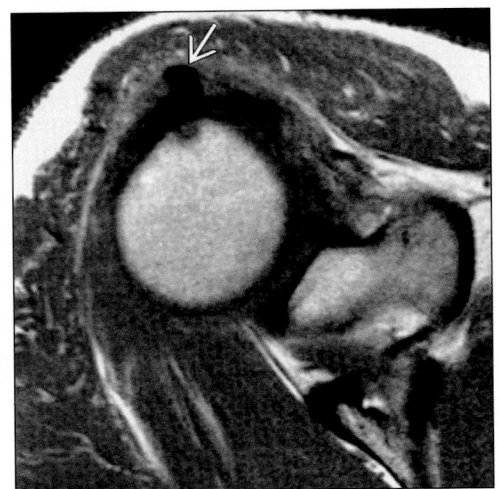

(Left) Axial PD FSE MR shows a large clump of calcification (arrow) within the infraspinatus tendon, consistent with calcific tendinitis. There is extension into the bursa. *(Right)* Axial PD FSE MR shows calcific tendinitis (arrow) within the supraspinatus tendon with extension of the calcium into the bursa. In the mechanical phase, there may be associated bursal elevation.

Typical

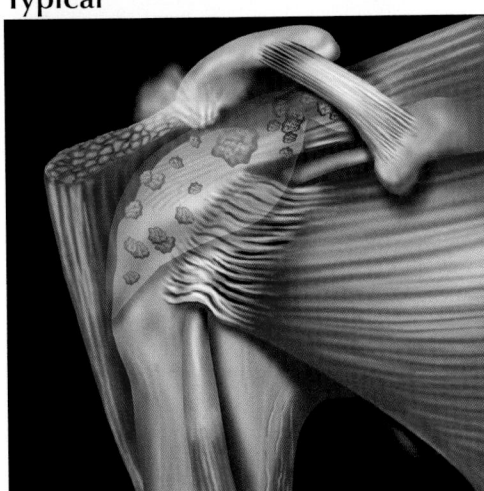 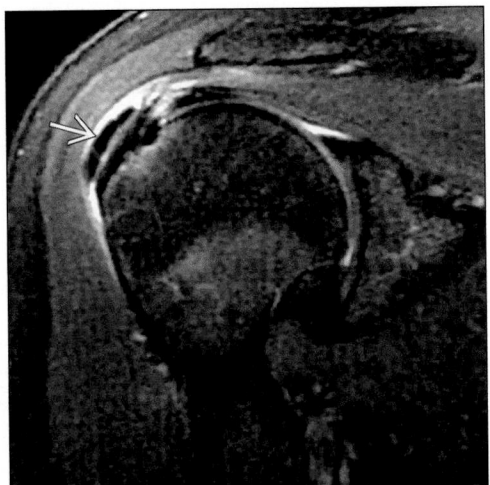

(Left) Coronal graphic shows the mechanical phase of calcific tendinitis with bursal rupture of calcium and reactive bursitis. Calcific deposits are present within the subacromial/subdeltoid bursa. *(Right)* Coronal FS PD FSE MR shows mechanical phase of calcific tendinitis with extension of calcification (arrow) into the hyperintense bursa.

PARSONAGE-TURNER SYNDROME

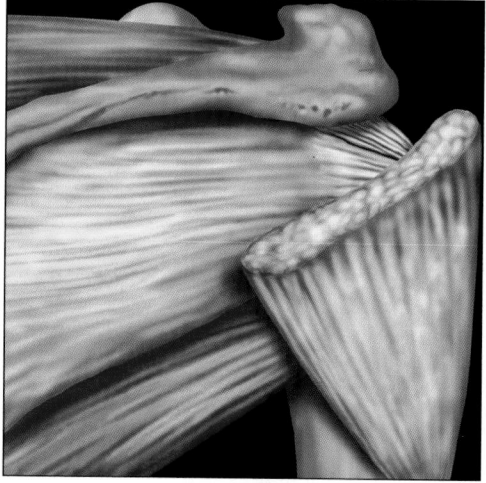

Coronal graphic shows denervation changes within the deltoid and teres minor muscles.

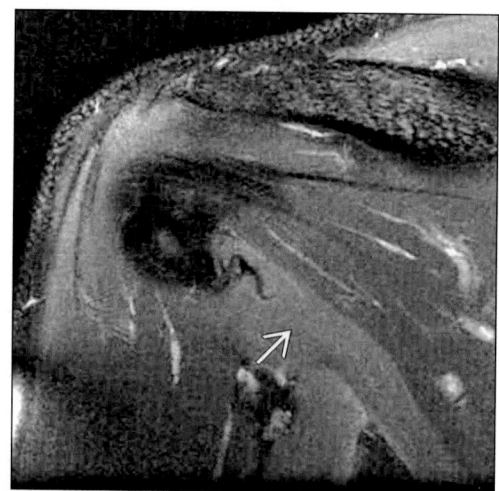

Coronal FS PD FSE MR shows denervation changes within the teres minor (arrow), deltoid and the triceps tendon in a patient with idiopathic brachial neuritis/Parsonage-Turner syndrome.

TERMINOLOGY

Abbreviations and Synonyms
- PTS, neuralgic amyotrophy, acute brachial neuritis, acute brachial radiculitis, nontraumatic neuropathy, shoulder girdle syndrome

Definitions
- Idiopathic denervation syndrome of the shoulder musculature
- More than one nerve distribution may be involved
- Denervation affects mainly the lower motor neurons of the brachial plexus and/or individual nerves or nerve branches

IMAGING FINDINGS

General Features
- Best diagnostic clue
  - Increased signal within muscle bellies on FS PD FSE/PD WI in patient with muscle weakness
    - = Acute to subacute changes
  - Fatty atrophy - chronic cases
- Location
  - Muscles of the shoulder girdle
    - Rare distal form involving the forearm/wrist muscles described

- Size
  - Muscles may be swollen and slightly enlarged in acute and subacute phase
  - Muscles - atrophic in chronic phase
- Morphology
  - Slightly enlarged muscle bellies maintaining shape without focal alteration
    - Acute, subacute
  - Atrophic muscle bellies
    - Chronic, fatty atrophy

CT Findings
- NECT
  - Fatty infiltration in chronic cases
    - Decreased attenuation - fat
    - Often streaky

MR Findings
- T1WI
  - Streaky regions of fat signal in association with small size of muscles in chronic cases (fatty atrophy)
  - Decreased in signal - early phases = edema
- T2WI
  - Increased signal intensity (T2) in muscles of acute and subacute denervation
  - +/- Nerve distribution pattern
  - +/- Muscle enlargement: Acute, subacute
  - +/- Muscle atrophy, slight increase in signal: Chronic, fatty atrophy

DDx: Parsonage-Turner Syndrome

RTC Partial Tear	RTC Tear	PSGI	SSN Denervation	Non Comm Cyst
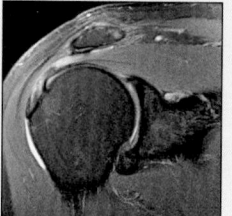	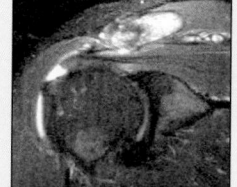	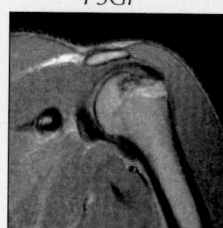	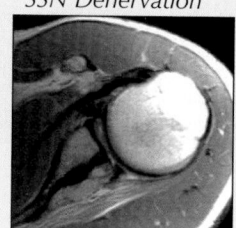	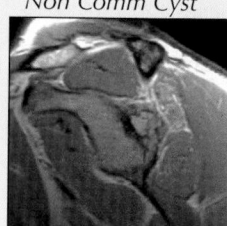
Cor FS PD FSE	Cor FS PD FSE	Cor PD/Intermed	Ax PD FSE	Sag PD FSE MR

PARSONAGE-TURNER SYNDROME

Key Facts

Imaging Findings
- Increased signal within muscle bellies on FS PD FSE/PD WI in patient with muscle weakness
- +/- Muscle enlargement: Acute, subacute
- +/- Muscle atrophy, slight increase in signal: Chronic, fatty atrophy

Top Differential Diagnoses
- Traumatic Neurapraxia
- Nerve Severing
- Cervical Spine Disease (Neuropathy)
- Diabetic Neuropathy
- Nonspecific Myositis
- Trauma to Muscle Belly
- Carcinomatous or Granulomatous Brachial Plexus Infiltration

- Nerve Compression
- Rotator Cuff Tear

Pathology
- Neuritis of mainly lower motor neurons of the brachial plexus

Clinical Issues
- Abrupt onset of pain, may follow recent illness, surgery, immunization, or trauma

Diagnostic Checklist
- Other causes of denervation such as posttraumatic neurapraxia
- FS PD FSE and STIR sequences are sensitive for hyperintensity in early and subacute cases

---

- o FS PD FSE
  - Increased signal intensity (increased cellular water) within muscle
- PD/Intermediate: Increased signal intensity in muscles in acute and subacute cases = swelling
- STIR
  - o Similar contrast as FS PD FSE
  - o Less spatial resolution
- T1 C+: Muscle bellies enhance in acute and subacute phase
- MRI abnormalities appear after approximately 2 weeks

Imaging Recommendations
- Best imaging tool
  - o FS PD FSE or STIR in acute or subacute phase
  - o PD, T1 in chronic atrophic phase
- Protocol advice: T1 and FS PD FSE in axial, coronal and sagittal planes

DIFFERENTIAL DIAGNOSIS

Traumatic Neurapraxia
- Posttraumatic
- Transient in most cases
- Leads to denervation changes of affected muscles
- Traction with resulting hemorrhage/edema

Nerve Severing
- Disrupts function
- Possibility of resumed function
  - o Depends on proximity of severed ends
  - o Axon (recovers) vs. cell body (cell death)
- History of laceration
  - o Regeneration does not occur with disruption of the axon, its myelin sheath and connective tissue elements

Cervical Spine Disease (Neuropathy)
- Radiculitis/radiculopathy
- Radiating pain from neck
- +/- Weakness of muscles supplied by compressed nerves
- +/- Muscle signal changes

Diabetic Neuropathy
- Ischemic neuropathy
- +/- Single nerve involvement
- +/- Osseous changes

Nonspecific Myositis
- Muscle signal increased on FS PD images, muscle dysfunction
- Usually not within a single nerve distribution pattern
- +/- Infection/fasciitis
- +/- Strain injury

Trauma to Muscle Belly
- Muscle signal increased on FS PD images = edema
- No single nerve distribution pattern
- History is critical

Carcinomatous or Granulomatous Brachial Plexus Infiltration
- Metastatic disease
- Usually with known primary disease
- Pancoast's tumor
- +/- Brachial plexitis

Nerve Compression
- Extrinsic compression
- Mass
  - o Benign: Cyst, lipoma
  - o Malignant
- Thickened fibrotic transverse scapular ligament
- Single nerve distribution

Rotator Cuff Tear
- Shoulder weakness secondary to tendon tear
- Generalized shoulder pain vs. anterior shoulder pain (impingement)
- +/- Proprioceptive loss
- +/- Impingement
  - o Classical subacromial
  - o Posterosuperior glenoid impingement (PSGI)
- Visible tear - fluid signal on T2WI

PARSONAGE-TURNER SYNDROME

PATHOLOGY

General Features
- General path comments
  - Neuritis of mainly lower motor neurons of the brachial plexus
  - +/- Individual nerves or nerve branches
- Etiology
  - Immune-mediated inflammatory reaction against nerve fibers
  - Possible causes include: Infection, surgery, trauma, childbirth, vaccinations, systemic illness
- Epidemiology: > 1% of general population
- Associated abnormalities: Rare distal form affecting arm, forearm, wrist and hand

Gross Pathologic & Surgical Features
- Denervation changes within the affected muscles
- Swollen muscle belly - early and subacute
- Fatty atrophy - chronic

Microscopic Features
- Enlarged extracellular fluid space = early and subacute
- Fatty infiltration = chronic
- Myofibers atrophy - small and angular with early denervation

Staging, Grading or Classification Criteria
- Early, subacute: ~ 3-6 months
- Chronic - corresponds to fatty atrophy

CLINICAL ISSUES

Presentation
- Most common signs/symptoms
  - Abrupt onset of pain, may follow recent illness, surgery, immunization, or trauma
  - Followed by weakness, and possible numbness
- Clinical profile
  - Up to 50% report viral illness or vaccination that occurred days or weeks prior to the onset of symptoms
  - Pain: Sharp, throbbing and intense at onset
    - Pain duration: Few hours to several weeks

Demographics
- Age: 3 months - 74 years
- Gender: M:F = 2-4:1
- Ethnicity: Seen in Native American population with increased frequency

Natural History & Prognosis
- Majority resolves
  - Up to over a year
- Residual denervation in 10-20% after 2 years

Treatment
- Conservative treatment - physical therapy
- Nerve grafting/tendon transfers for patients without adequate recovery by 2 years
  - Surgery to improve shoulder abduction

DIAGNOSTIC CHECKLIST

Consider
- Other causes of denervation such as posttraumatic neurapraxia

Image Interpretation Pearls
- FS PD FSE and STIR sequences are sensitive for hyperintensity in early and subacute cases

SELECTED REFERENCES

1. Helms CA: The impact of MR imaging in sports medicine. Radiology 224(3):631-5, 2002
2. Simon JP et al: Parsonage-Turner syndrome after total-hip arthroplasty. J Arthroplasty 16(4):518-20, 2001
3. Petit E et al: Bilateral phrenic involvement disclosing Parsonage Turner syndrome. Rev Neurol (Paris) 156(4):403-4, 2000
4. Auge WK et al: Parsonage-Turner syndrome in the Native American Indian. J Shoulder Elbow Surg 9(2):99-103, 2000
5. Saleem F et al: Neuralgic amyotrophy (Parsonage-Turner syndrome): An often misdiagnosed diagnosis. J Pak Med Assoc 49(4):101-3, 1999
6. Helms CA et al: Acute brachial neuritis (Parsonage-Turner syndrome): MR imaging appearance-report of three cases. Radiology 207(1):255-9, 1998
7. Sallomi D et al: Muscle denervation patterns in upper limb nerve injuries: MR imaging findings and anatomic basis. AJR 171(3):779-84, 1998

PARSONAGE-TURNER SYNDROME

IMAGE GALLERY

Typical

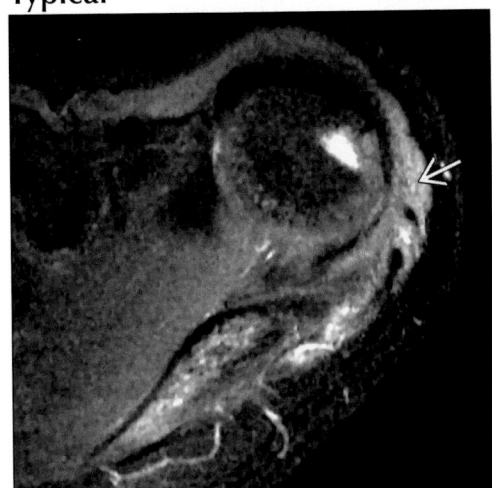
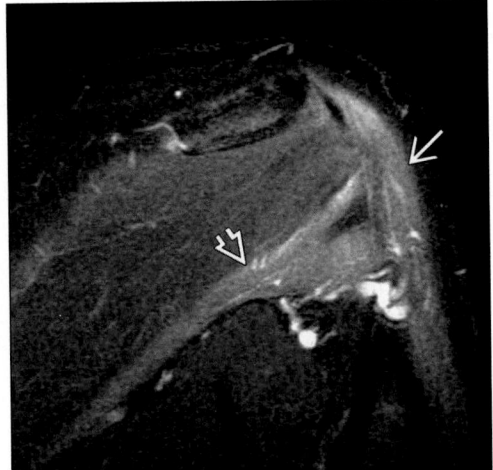

(Left) Axial STIR MR shows increased signal intensity within the deltoid (arrow), consistent with denervation change. *(Right)* Coronal STIR MR in the same patient shows the denervation changes within the deltoid (arrow) and within the teres minor (open arrow) — axillary nerve distribution.

Typical

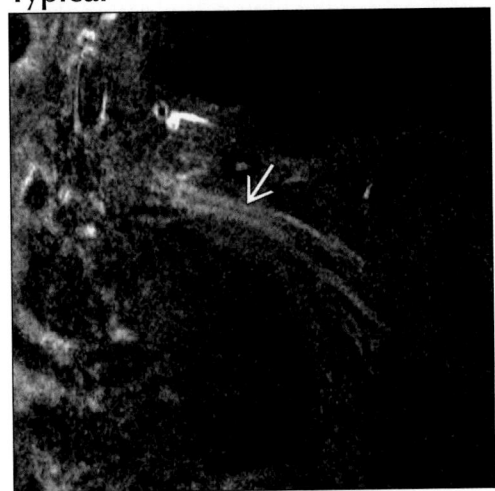
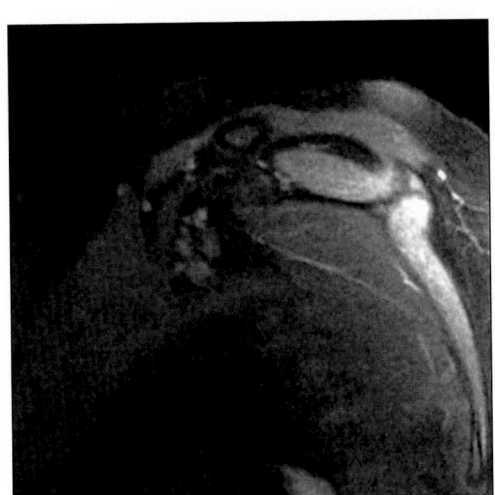

(Left) Coronal STIR MR of chest shows increased signal intensity within brachial plexus (arrow) indicating neuritis in a patient with Parsonage-Turner syndrome. *(Right)* Sagittal STIR MR in the same patient shows denervation changes in the supraspinatus and infraspinatus.

Typical

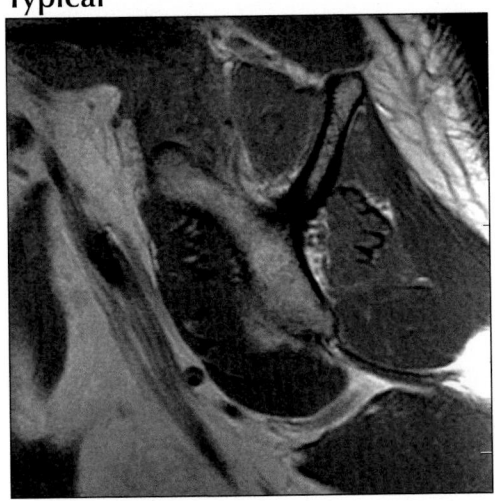
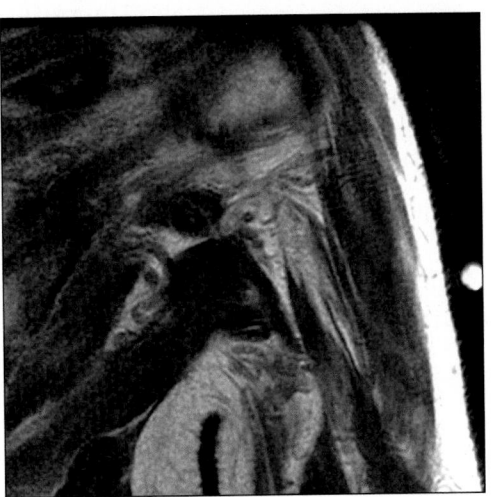

(Left) Sagittal PD FSE MR demonstrates denervation changes in the shoulder girdle muscles. *(Right)* Coronal PD FSE in a patient with Parsonage-Turner syndrome and deltoid weakness shows the changes of denervation.

SUBSCAPULARIS RUPTURE

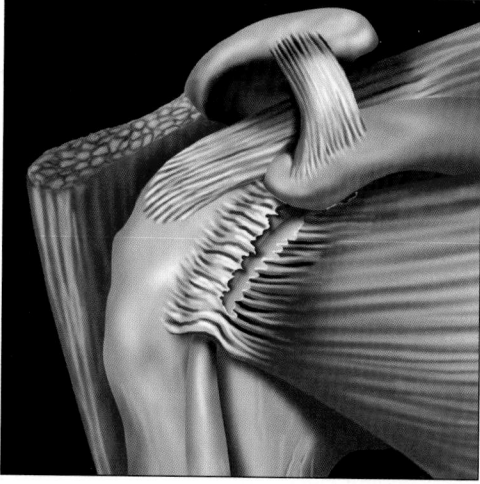

Coronal graphic shows an extensive tear of the insertion site of the subscapularis tendon adjacent to the rotator interval.

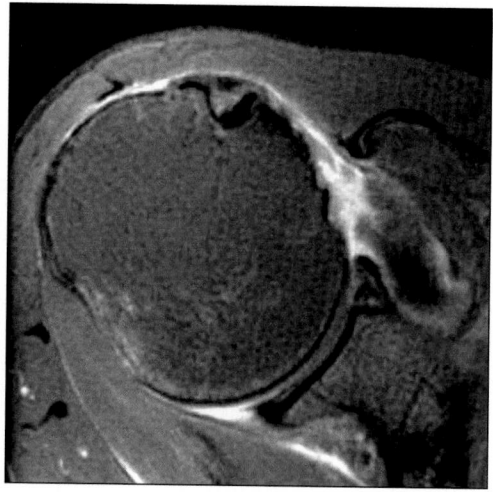

Axial FS PD FSE MR shows a full thickness tear of the subscapularis tendon with retraction. There is synovitis within the tendon gap.

TERMINOLOGY

Definitions
- Subscapularis rupture secondary to anterior shoulder dislocation (> 40 years old)
- Subscapularis rupture secondary to posterior dislocation
- In association with tearing of the other components of the rotator cuff
- Subcoracoid impingement

IMAGING FINDINGS

General Features
- Best diagnostic clue: Tear or gap in subscapularis tendon, filled with fluid/hemorrhage or granulation tissue
- Location
  - Interruption of the normal course of the hypointense tendon
  - Distal tear
- Size: Range from millimeters to centimeters
- Morphology
  - Gap in thickened irregular tendon
    - Tendon may be thinned
  - Thickened tendon with intrasubstance (interstitial) partial tear

- Partial tear of distal tendon with delamination and retraction of deep fibers

Radiographic Findings
- Radiography
  - Lesser tuberosity fracture when associated with posterior dislocation
    - Lesser tuberosity avulsion fracture can occur with intact subscapularis tendon after posterior dislocation
  - Lesser tuberosity cystic degenerative changes when associated with subcoracoid impingement

CT Findings
- NECT
  - Cyst in lesser tuberosity
  - Prominent coracoid in subcoracoid impingement

MR Findings
- T1WI
  - Thick inhomogeneous tendon, intermediate signal
  - Hypointense edema in lesser tuberosity, Bankart, reverse Bankart, Hill-Sachs, reverse Hill-Sachs fractures
    - Bankart fracture: Fracture of anteroinferior glenoid (bony Bankart lesion)
    - Reverse Bankart fracture: Posterior glenoid rim fracture
    - Hill-Sachs: Posterolateral humeral head fracture

DDx: Subscapularis Rupture

HAGL	Ad Capsulitis	HAGL	Chondromatosis	Hidden Lesion
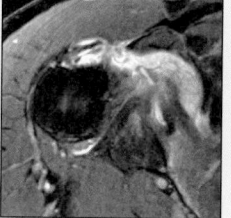	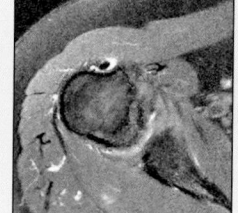	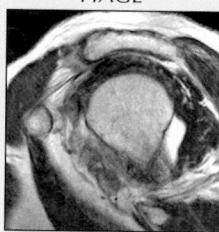	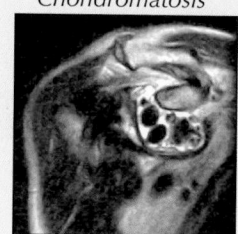	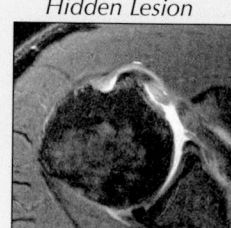
Ax FS PD FSE	Ax FS PD FSE	Sag T2 FSE MR	Cor T2 FSE MR	Ax FS PD FSE

SUBSCAPULARIS RUPTURE

Key Facts

Terminology
- Subscapularis rupture secondary to anterior shoulder dislocation (> 40 years old)

Imaging Findings
- Hyperintense fluid signal intensity filling a gap in the tendon; visualized with FS PD FSE

Top Differential Diagnoses
- Tendinosis without Rupture
- Hidden Lesion
- HAGL Lesion
- Debris in Subscapularis Recess
- Rotator Interval Lesion
- Axillary Neurapraxia
- Adhesive Capsulitis

Pathology
- Isolated tear after anterior dislocation especially in patients > 40 years
- With or without avulsion of lesser tuberosity in patient after posterior dislocation
- Preexisting degeneration as seen with subacromial impingement
- Subcoracoid impingement

Clinical Issues
- Patients > 40 years of age presenting with 1st time anterior dislocation
- Secondary to posterior dislocation at any age

Diagnostic Checklist
- After trauma, especially in older patient

- Reverse Hill-Sachs: Anteromedial humeral head fracture
- T2WI
  - Hyperintense fluid signal intensity filling a gap in the tendon; visualized with FS PD FSE
  - Tendon edges frayed and increased in signal
  - Underlying capsular tear
  - +/- Rotator interval hidden lesion
    - Hyperintense superior glenohumeral/coracohumeral ligament (SGHL/CHL), +/- tear
    - +/- Biceps subluxation/dislocation medially
  - +/- Hyperintense cysts of lesser tuberosity
  - +/- Hyperintense edema of lesser tuberosity with fracture
    - +/- Hypointense fracture line
    - Avulsion or impaction
  - +/- Hill-Sachs fracture in case of anterior/posterior dislocation
  - +/- Reverse Hill-Sachs fracture if posterior dislocation
  - +/- Humeral avulsion of glenohumeral ligament (HAGL) lesion
- T2* GRE: Greatest sensitivity of tendon degeneration compared to other pulse sequences
- Partial tear: Fluid entering a segment of tendon
  - Intrasubstance
  - Deep fibers
- Through-and-through (full thickness) tear
  - Fluid extending through gap in tendon with variable retraction
  - Demonstrated on axial images

Imaging Recommendations
- Best imaging tool: MRI
- Protocol advice
  - FS PD FSE axial images
  - T2* GRE sensitive to subscapularis tendon degeneration and tear
    - As used in the axial plane
    - Not utilized in coronal plane to avoid false positive findings of supraspinatus/infraspinatus tears

DIFFERENTIAL DIAGNOSIS

Tendinosis without Rupture
- No evidence of gap
- Acute traumatic history
- Thickened increased signal intensity tendon on T2* GRE
  - Short TE sequences

Hidden Lesion
- Partial subscapularis tear, superior aspect
- Biceps instability
- +/- Biceps tendinosis
- "Hidden" at arthroscopy (difficult to visualize)
- SGHL/CHL dysfunction/tear

HAGL Lesion
- Humeral avulsion of inferior glenohumeral ligamentous complex (IGHLC)
- Associated with anterior dislocation
- "J" sign of avulsion of humeral attachment of inferior glenohumeral ligament (IGL) on coronal images
  - IGL hyperintensity on T2WI
- Subscapularis tear/partial tear often present

Debris in Subscapularis Recess
- Loose bodies
- Osteochondromatosis (chondromatosis)
- +/- Glenoid, humeral head chondral defects
- +/- Trauma
- Fluid in recess adjacent to subscapularis may mimic tear/partial tear (esp. on coronals)

Rotator Interval Lesion
- +/- Involvement of superior subscapularis
- CHL/SGHL involved
- +/- Anterior supraspinatus tear
- +/- Subcoracoid impingement

Axillary Neurapraxia
- Clinical diagnosis after anterior dislocation
- Subscapularis tear often misdiagnosed as axillary neurapraxia
  - After anterior dislocation

SUBSCAPULARIS RUPTURE

- Hyperintensity in teres minor and deltoid on FS PD FSE/STIR MR
- + Electromyograph (EMG) findings

Adhesive Capsulitis
- Thickened edematous capsule
- Hyperintense on T2WI
- Frozen shoulder
- +/- Secondary (known disorders)

PATHOLOGY

General Features
- General path comments
  - Important stabilizer of anterior joint
  - "Weak link" in older patients rupturing after dislocation
  - Rupture after dislocation
  - Susceptible to chronic overuse
  - Anterior fibers of subscapularis merge with the CHL and traverse bicipital groove
    - Majority of subscapularis fibers may tear but maintain position
  - Subscapularis + superior glenohumeral ligament and coracohumeral ligament stabilize biceps tendon
    - Tears = hidden lesion
- Etiology
  - Isolated tear after anterior dislocation especially in patients > 40 years
  - With or without avulsion of lesser tuberosity in patient after posterior dislocation
  - Preexisting degeneration as seen with subacromial impingement
  - Subcoracoid impingement
- Epidemiology
  - ~ 30% of older patients after first time anterior dislocation
  - Uncommon with posterior dislocation
    - Posterior dislocation accounts for ~ 5% of all shoulder dislocations
  - 2% of rotator cuff tears involve subscapularis
  - Extension of rotator cuff tear
    - Supraspinous (79%)
    - Infraspinous (56%)
  - Bicipital dislocations
    - 49% of subscapularis tears

Gross Pathologic & Surgical Features
- Disruption in integrity (loss of collagen fiber bundles) of tendon in partial and complete tendon tears

Microscopic Features
- Disruption of tendon fiber bundles in partially torn & through-and-through tendon tears
  - Decrease tensile strength in degeneration
    - Decrease in total collagen content
- Fatty infiltration of muscle tissue in chronically torn tendons

CLINICAL ISSUES

Presentation
- Most common signs/symptoms

- Shoulder pain after dislocation
- Insidious onset of pain when associated with impingement/chronic overuse
- Clinical profile: Clinical positive lift-off test (inability to lift hand against resistance from small of back)
- Secondary to posterior dislocation especially in the case of tonic-clonic seizures
- May be misdiagnosed clinically as axillary neurapraxia

Demographics
- Age
  - Patients > 40 years of age presenting with 1st time anterior dislocation
  - Secondary to posterior dislocation at any age
- Gender: M > F

Natural History & Prognosis
- Sudden trauma leads to complete rupture
- ± Surgical repair

Treatment
- Open surgical repair

DIAGNOSTIC CHECKLIST

Consider
- After trauma, especially in older patient

Image Interpretation Pearls
- FS PD FSE and T2* GRE in axial plane to appreciate retraction, tendinosis and associated biceps pathology

SELECTED REFERENCES

1. Beall DP et al: Association of biceps tendon tears with rotator cuff abnormalities: Degree of correlation with tears of the anterior and superior portions of the rotator cuff. AJR 180(3):633-9, 2003
2. Burkhart SS et al: Arthroscopic subscapularis tendon repair: Technique and preliminary results. Arthroscopy 18(5):454-63, 2002
3. Tung GA et al: Subscapularis tendon tear: Primary and associated signs on MRI. J Comput Assist Tomogr 25(3):417-24, 2001
4. Travis RD et al: Technique for repair of the subscapularis tendon. Orthop Clin North Am 32(3):495-500, 2001
5. Stoller DW et al: Magnetic resonance imaging in orthopaedics and sports medicine. vol 1. 2nd ed. Philadelphia PA, J.B. Lippincott, 597-742, 1997
6. Tirman PF et al: A practical approach to imaging of the shoulder with emphasis on MR imaging. Orthop Clin North Am 28(4):483-515, 1997
7. Tirman et al: Humeral avulsion of the anterior shoulder stabilizing structures after anterior shoulder dislocation: Demonstration by MRI and MR arthrography. Skeletal Radiol 25(8):743-8, 1996
8. Neviaser RJ et al: Recurrent instability of the shoulder after age 40. J Shoulder Elbow Surg 4(6):416-8, 1995
9. Patten RM: Tears of the anterior portion of the rotator cuff (the subscapularis tendon): MR imaging findings. AJR 162(2):351-4, 1994

SUBSCAPULARIS RUPTURE

IMAGE GALLERY

Typical

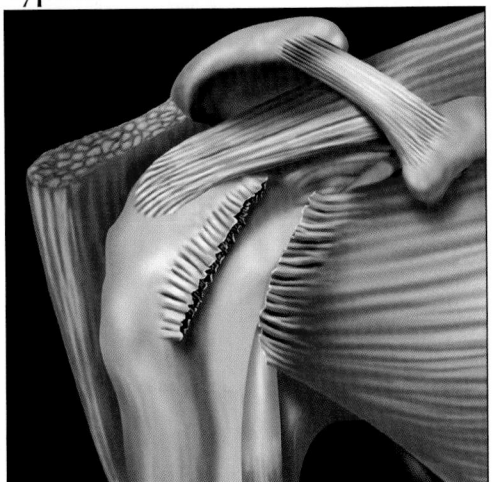
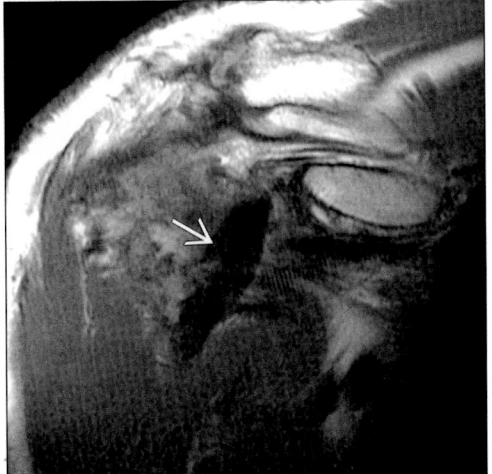

(Left) Coronal graphic shows a full thickness tear of the subscapularis tendon with dislocation of the biceps tendon due to biceps instability. *(Right)* Coronal PD FSE MR shows a tear of the subscapularis tendon with dislocation of the biceps *(arrow)* from the bicipital groove.

Typical

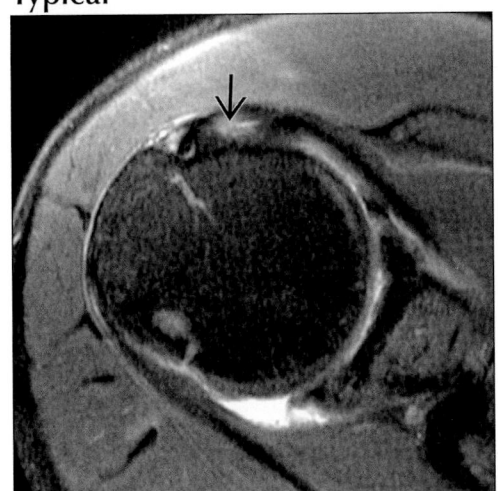
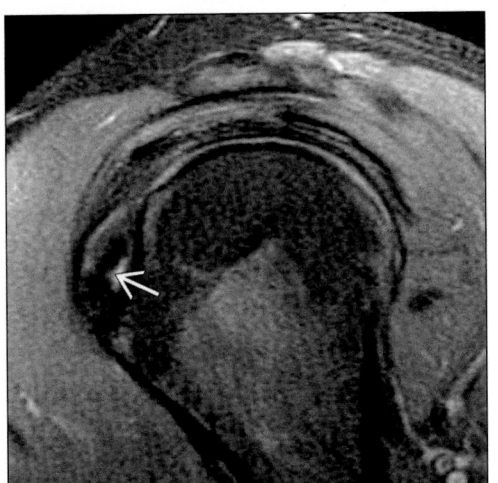

(Left) Axial FS PD FSE MR shows a partial tear *(arrow)* of the distal aspect of the subscapularis tendon. *(Right)* Sagittal FS PD FSE MR shows a partial tear of the distal aspect of the subscapularis tendon *(arrow)* in this patient with pain on internal rotation — a clinical test for subscapularis dysfunction.

Typical

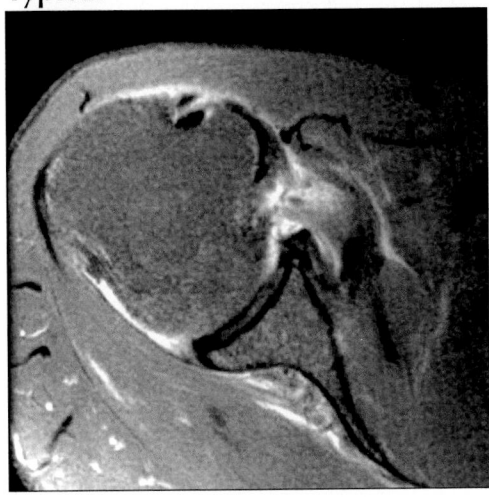
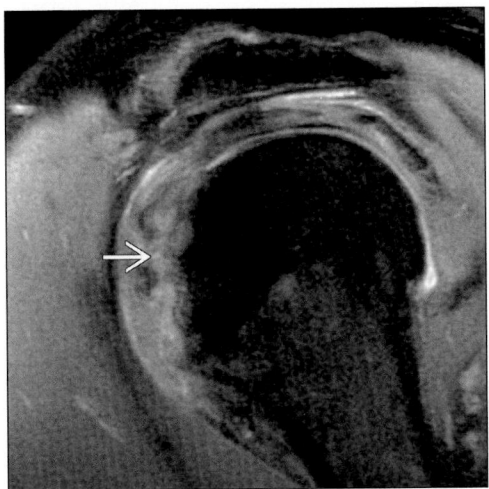

(Left) Axial FS PD FSE MR shows a full thickness tear of the subscapularis tendon with retraction and debris in the gap. *(Right)* Sagittal FS PD FSE MR shows a full thickness tear *(arrow)* of the subscapularis tendon from the lesser tuberosity.

PECTORALIS MAJOR TEAR

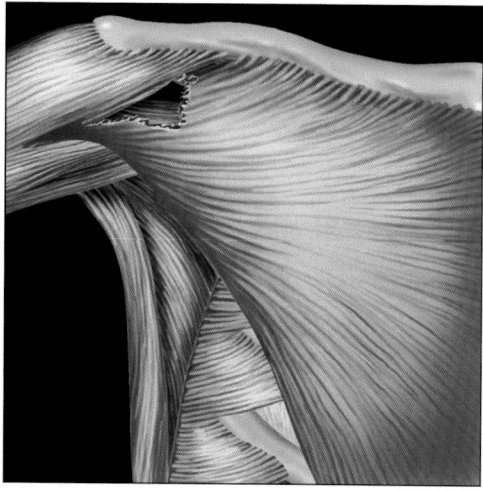

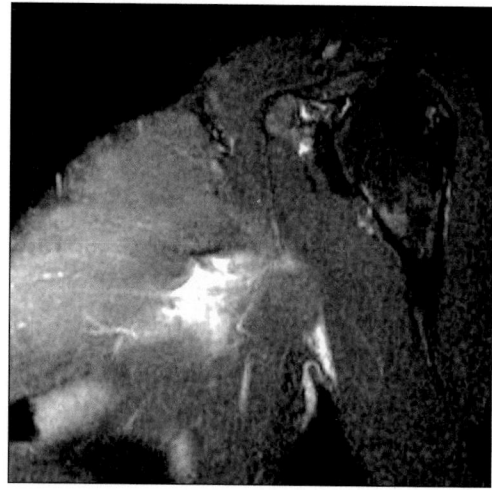

Coronal graphic shows a tear of the pectoralis major tendon with retraction from the humerus.

Coronal STIR MR shows a tear of pectoralis tendon with retraction. There is a surrounding hematoma which is of increased signal intensity.

TERMINOLOGY

Abbreviations and Synonyms
- Muscle strain
- Muscle pull

Definitions
- Disruption of pectoralis myotendinous unit at the humeral insertion site
- 2 major portions of the tendon
  - Sternal (sternocostal) head: Originates from sternum
  - Clavicular head: Originates from undersurface of the clavicle

IMAGING FINDINGS

General Features
- Best diagnostic clue: High signal on FS PD FSE or STIR at pectoralis major tendon tear site
- Location: Anterior chest wall and upper arm
- Size: Variable from physically undetectable myofibrillar tears to full thickness defect of muscle belly
- Morphology
  - Variable tendinous defect
    - +/- Hematoma
  - Avulsion of musculotendinous junction

- Uncommon
  - Avulsion of enthesis
  - Several anatomical variants which may be unusual cause of injury (e.g., accessory insertions adjacent to median nerve)
- Myotendinous junction partial and full thickness tears of the long head of the biceps tendon may mimic pectoralis major tendon tears clinically
  - Pain localized to the same anatomic area

Radiographic Findings
- Radiography: Flake avulsion from lateral lip of bicipital groove if enthesis fails (rare)

CT Findings
- NECT
  - Soft tissue swelling of anterior chest wall
  - Late finding: Calcified hematoma and soft tissue defects, indicating focal muscle atrophy and scarring

MR Findings
- T1WI
  - Decreased marrow signal in clavicle, sternum or ribs indicating response to strain
  - Muscle enlargement, +/- low signal zones indicating subacute hematoma
  - Low signal in myofascial region indicating perifascial edema
- T2WI

DDx: Pectoralis Major Tear

Surg Neck Fx	HAGL Lesion	Scapular Fracture	Sur Neck Fx Impac
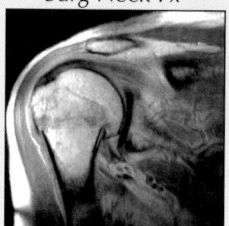	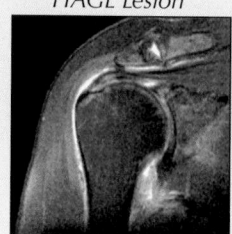	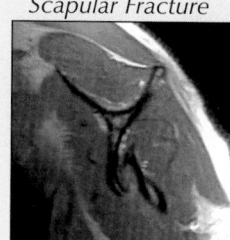	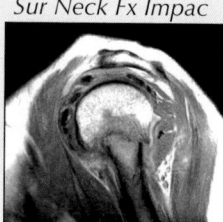
Cor PD FSE MR	*Cor STIR MR*	*Sag PD FSE MR*	*Sag PD FSE MR*

PECTORALIS MAJOR TEAR

Key Facts

Terminology
- Disruption of pectoralis myotendinous unit at the humeral insertion site

Imaging Findings
- Best diagnostic clue: High signal on FS PD FSE or STIR at pectoralis major tendon tear site
- Location: Anterior chest wall and upper arm
- Several anatomical variants which may be unusual cause of injury (e.g., accessory insertions adjacent to median nerve)

Top Differential Diagnoses
- Pectoralis Minor, Latissimus Dorsi or Subscapularis Inferior Glenohumeral Ligament Injuries
- Fracture
- Manubrium-Sternum Dislocation

Pathology
- Resisted forced abduction and external rotation
- Heavy lifting (bench press weightlifting)
- Most injuries involve musculotendinous junction or distal tendon insertion
- Partial tears most common

Clinical Issues
- Pain (severe onset in acute rupture)
- Weakness (weak internal rotation)
- Deformity, especially on attempted contraction

Diagnostic Checklist
- Anomalous anatomy may cause unexpected collateral injury (e.g., to median nerve)

   - o Increased marrow signal in clavicle, sternum or ribs indicating edema
      - Visualization improved by using FS sequence
   - o High signal at humeral insertion indicating tendon tears
      - Insertion to lateral lip of bicipital groove
   - o High signal within muscle indicating site of tear, +/- moderate internal signal indicating fresh hematoma
   - o High signal in perifascial zone and subcutaneous fat
- STIR
   - o Sensitive for bony injury
   - o High signal areas in marrow space
   - o Sensitive to edema within muscle
   - o Useful for homogeneous fat saturation at large fields of view
   - o Useful at low field strength
- Normal myotendinous unit hypointense on T1 & T2WI

Ultrasonographic Findings
- Acute injuries with edema may show only subtle high echogenicity zones
- Larger injuries show low echogenicity zones representing physical defect within muscle + acute hemorrhage
- Muscle activation may show increased size of defect
- Organizing hematoma becomes hyperechoic
- Chronic hematomata become very hypoechoic
- Hyperechoic scar tissue and hyperechoic calcification (late stage)
- Hypoechoic edema plus visualized separation at humeral enthesis

Imaging Recommendations
- Best imaging tool: MRI
- Protocol advice
   - o FS PD FSE or STIR sensitive for edema associated with tear
   - o Axial and coronal FS PD FSE or STIR

DIFFERENTIAL DIAGNOSIS

Pectoralis Minor, Latissimus Dorsi or Subscapularis Inferior Glenohumeral Ligament Injuries
- Deep upper outer chest pain
- MRI diagnostic
- Rare injuries
- Usually sports related

Fracture
- Rib
- Scapula
- Sternum
- Humerus
   - o Anatomic neck
   - o Surgical neck
   - o Hill-Sachs
   - o Bankart
   - o +/- Comminution
- Fractures in proximity of muscle may mimic pectoralis major pain, disability

Manubrium-Sternum Dislocation
- Pathology located center of chest rather than lateral chest or proximal humerus
- +/- Radiating pain from sternum
- CT/MR diagnostic
- Direct trauma
- Myotendinous long head of biceps strain
   - o Associated with pectoralis tear
   - o Mimics pectoralis injury if biceps strain is isolated

PATHOLOGY

General Features
- General path comments
   - o Relevant anatomy of pectoralis major tendon
      - Broad bilaminar tendon
      - Insertion - lateral lip of bicipital groove
      - Two heads - sternocostal and clavicular

PECTORALIS MAJOR TEAR

- Upper clavicular head forms anterior tendon insertion
- Sternocostal head forms posterior tendon insertion
- Sternocostal head - produces anterior axillary fold prominence with spiral layering of muscle fibers
- Sternocostal head more susceptible to avulsion than clavicular head
- Pectoralis - innervated by medial and lateral pectoral nerves (from medial and lateral cords)
- Pectoralis - functions in adduction and medial rotation of the humerus
- Etiology
  - Resisted forced abduction and external rotation
  - Forceful contraction with arm adducted, flexed and internally rotated
  - Rupture in bench press weightlifting
    - Overload of short inferior fibers in eccentric phase of lifting (sternal head failure)
    - Direct blow (sternoclavicular head)
- Epidemiology
  - Heavy lifting (bench press weightlifting)
  - Recreational weight lifting
- Distribution
  - Most injuries involve musculotendinous junction or distal tendon insertion
  - Partial tears most common
  - Combined sternal and clavicular head injuries more common than individual head injuries
  - Silent injuries in the elderly

Gross Pathologic & Surgical Features
- Tearing of muscle fibers
- Bleeding and hematoma formation
- Deformity from retraction of muscle bellies or tendon avulsion
- Partial or incomplete rupture
- Strains of muscle belly or musculotendinous junction
- Avulsion - type
  - At or adjacent to humeral insertion

Microscopic Features
- Disruption of myofibrillar structure
- Vascular rupture with hemorrhage
- Myotendinous separation
- Inflammatory cell infiltration
- Gradual replacement of devitalized tissue and hematoma by granulation tissue
- Increased myoblastic activity

Staging, Grading or Classification Criteria
- Grade 1 = localized edema within muscle, damage at microscopic level
- Grade 2 = partial tearing, perifascial edema
- Grade 3 = full thickness tearing, significant hematoma formation

CLINICAL ISSUES

Presentation
- Most common signs/symptoms
  - Pain (severe onset in acute rupture)
  - Weakness (weak internal rotation)
  - Deformity, especially on attempted contraction
  - Swelling
  - May present as a chest wall mass in elderly without significant history of trauma
- Clinical profile
  - Weightlifter most common
    - During humeral extension at the beginning of lift
    - Hematoma proximal medial arm or chest wall
    - Musculotendinous ruptures - chest wall hematoma
    - Tendinous avulsions from humerus - ecchymosis

Demographics
- Age: Young adult
- Gender: M > F

Natural History & Prognosis
- Complete tear usually retracts and fibrosis occurs with visible deformity of chest wall
- Loss of strength with conservative treatment
- Primary and delayed repair have > 90% restoration of strength and function

Treatment
- Conservative: RICE (rest, ice, compression, elevation)
- Surgical
  - Primary or delayed repair
  - Complete rupture = indication for repair
- Complications: Re-rupture, infection, heterotopic ossification

DIAGNOSTIC CHECKLIST

Consider
- Surgical repair in athletes in order to restore strength
- Anomalous anatomy may cause unexpected collateral injury (e.g., to median nerve)

Image Interpretation Pearls
- Coronal and axial FS PD FSE or STIR
- Axial images to include lateral lip of bicipital groove of proximal humeral diaphysis

SELECTED REFERENCES

1. Miller M: Surgical atlas of sports medicine. Treatment of suprascapular nerve entrapment. Philadelphia PA, Saunders, 341-6, 2003
2. Dodds SD et al: Injuries to the pectoralis major. Sports Med 32(14):945-52, 2002
3. Hanna CM et al: Pectoralis major tears: Comparison of surgical and conservative treatment. Br J Sports Med 35(3):202-6, 2001
4. Carrino JA et al: Pectoralis major muscle and tendon tears: Diagnosis and grading using magnetic resonance imaging. Skeletal Radiol 29(6):305-13, 2000
5. Anbari A et al: Delayed repair of a ruptured pectoralis major muscle. A case report. Am J Sports Med 28(2):254-6, 2000
6. Schepsis AA et al: Rupture of the pectoralis major muscle. Outcome after repair of acute and chronic injuries. Am J Sports Med 28(1):9-15, 2000
7. Connell DA et al: Injuries of the pectoralis major muscle: Evaluation with MR imaging. Radiology 210(3):785-9, 1999

PECTORALIS MAJOR TEAR

IMAGE GALLERY

Typical

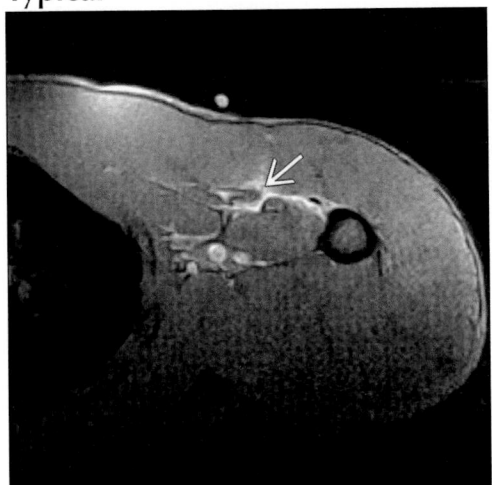
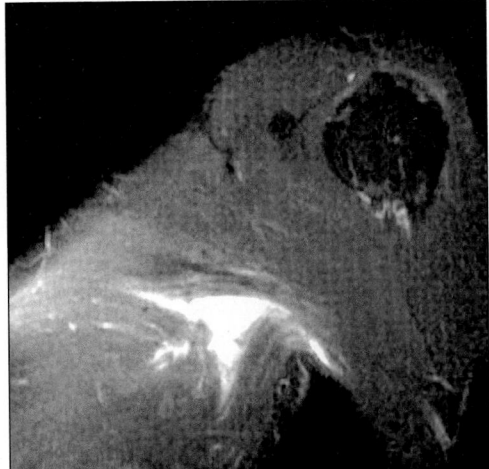

(Left) Axial T2* GRE MR of the left chest demonstrates a tear of the pectoralis major tendon with retraction (arrow). The retracted tendon edge is surrounded by hematoma. *(Right)* Coronal STIR MR shows a full thickness tear of the pectoralis tendon with an adjacent hematoma.

Typical

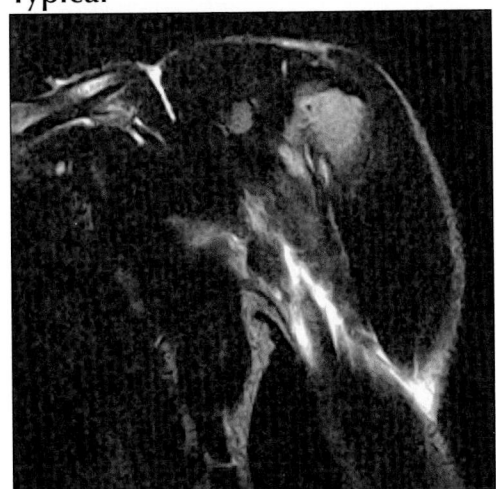
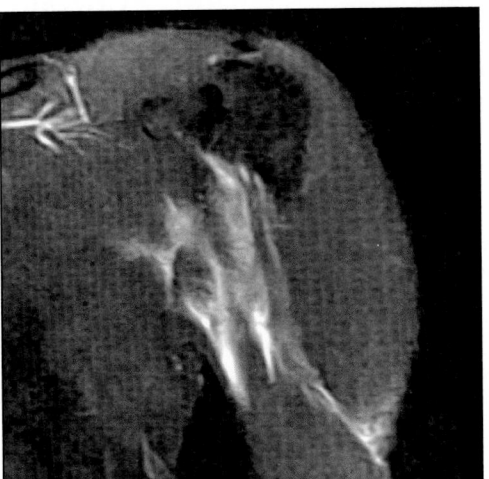

(Left) Coronal T2 FSE MR shows the frayed tendon edge retracted from the humerus and surrounded by hemorrhage. *(Right)* Coronal STIR MR shows a full thickness tear of the pectoralis tendon with retraction and hyperintense hematoma.

Typical

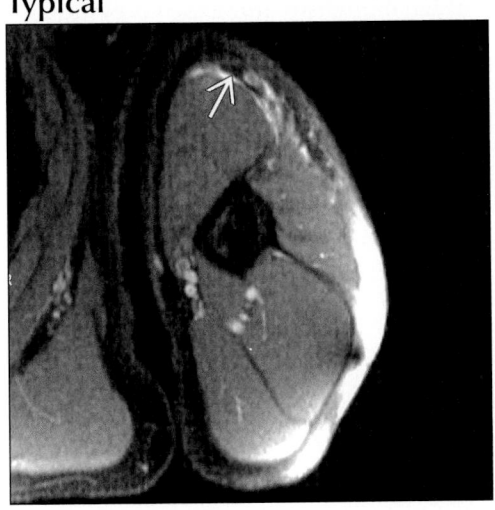
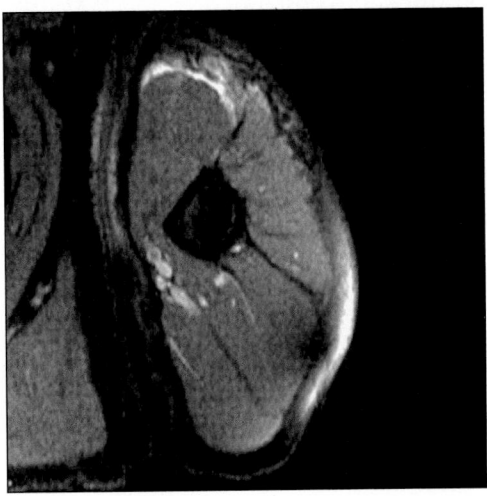

(Left) Axial STIR MR shows hemorrhage surrounding a myotendinous junction strain of the long head of the biceps tendon (arrow) sustained while weightlifting. *(Right)* Axial STIR MR of left upper arm demonstrates subcutaneous hemorrhage and partial tearing of the biceps tendon. This is also a common injury of weightlifting and may be associated with a pectoralis tear.

LABRAL CYST, SHOULDER

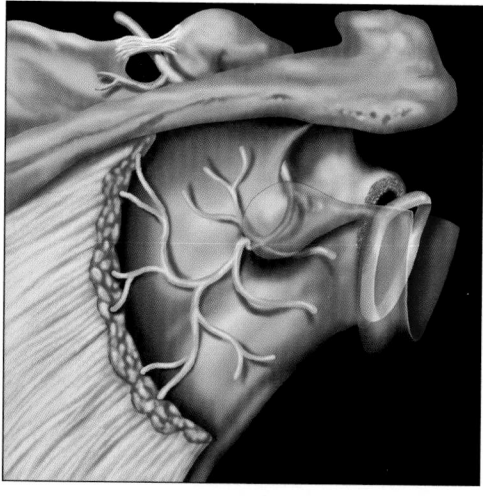

Coronal graphic demonstrates a labral cyst extending from a superior labral tear into the spinoglenoid notch compressing the suprascapular nerve.

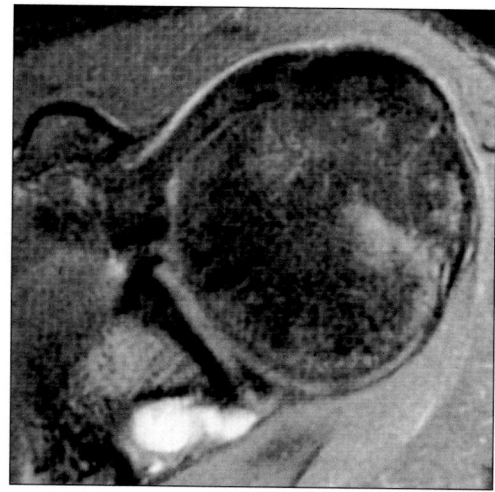

Axial FS PD FSE MR shows a large cyst in the spinoglenoid notch associated with a tear of the posterosuperior labrum and denervation changes of the infraspinatus.

TERMINOLOGY

Abbreviations and Synonyms
- Paralabral cysts, paralabral ganglion cysts

Definitions
- Cyst arising from labral tear, capsular tear

IMAGING FINDINGS

General Features
- Best diagnostic clue
  - Cystic mass extending from a labral and/or capsular tear
  - Hyperintense cystic mass on T2WI
  - Often multiloculated
- Location
  - Most commonly adjacent to posterosuperior labrum
    - Including superior labrum anterior to posterior (SLAP) tears
  - Multiple locations adjacent to labrum
  - Funneled between supraspinatus (SS) and infraspinatus (IS)
    - "Path of least resistance" to spinoglenoid notch or suprascapular notch to compress suprascapular nerve (SSN)

- Size: Varies from few mms to large dissecting cyst (several cms)
- Morphology
  - Flattened to round
  - +/- Loculations
  - Cyst within (intralabral) or adjacent to (paralabral) labrum in continuity with a labral tear
  - +/- Labral/capsular tear healed

MR Findings
- T1WI
  - Decreased signal intensity cystic mass
    - +/- Intraosseous cystic mass
  - Fatty atrophy of affected muscles with chronic denervation
- T2WI
  - Cystic-appearing mass arising from or immediately adjacent to labrum or capsule
    - Hyperintense
  - +/- Increased signal intensity intraosseous cystic mass
  - +/- Denervation - high signal and/or atrophy of affected muscles (supraspinatus ± infraspinatus)
    - FS PD FSE most sensitive for acute and subacute changes of muscle
  - Labral tear fluid signal extending through labrum (specific not sensitive)
  - Irregular intermediate signal granulation tissue, low signal fibrosis with healed tear

DDx: Labral Cyst, Shoulder

Hematoma	Normal Vessel	PSGI	Non Comm Cyst	Non Comm Cyst

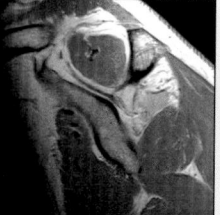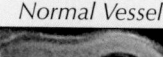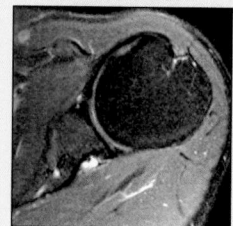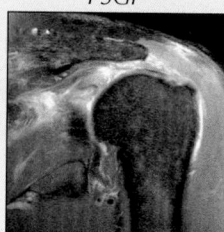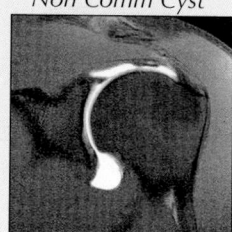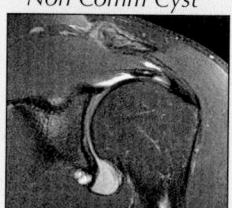

Sag PD FSE MR	Ax FS PD FSE MR	Cor FS PD FSE	Cor T1FS Arthro	Cor FS PD FSE

LABRAL CYST, SHOULDER

Key Facts

Terminology
- Cyst arising from labral tear, capsular tear

Imaging Findings
- Hyperintense cystic mass on T2WI
- Often multiloculated
- Most commonly adjacent to posterosuperior labrum
- +/- Cyst filled with contrast material

Top Differential Diagnoses
- Neoplasm
- Muscle Denervation
- Normal Blood Vessels
- Hematoma of Non Communicating Cyst
- Posterior Superior Glenoid Impingement (PSGI)

Pathology
- Cyst arises from break in integrity of joint: Labral tear, degeneration, capsular tear or capsular diverticulum
- Instability, especially if labral tear remains patent (nonhealed)

Clinical Issues
- Suprascapular nerve compression syndrome if cyst located posterosuperiorly
- Axillary nerve compression syndrome if cyst inferior and dissects into quadrilateral space

Diagnostic Checklist
- FS PD FSE for detection and characterization of all paralabral cysts

- STIR: Decreased spatial resolution, increased contrast resolution
- Labral tear = intermediate to increased signal at surface of labrum on short TE sequences
- MR arthrography
  - +/- Cyst filled with contrast material
    - Depends on if original tear has healed or not
  - Cysts, +/- communicate with joint (uncommon without communication)
    - +/- Visualization of cyst with T1WI (esp. with fat saturation)
    - T2WI (FS PD FSE) required if paralabral cyst does not fill with contrast

Ultrasonographic Findings
- Hypoechoic/anechoic cystic mass through transmission
- +/- Visualization with ultrasound, associated abnormalities not seen (e.g., labral tear)

Imaging Recommendations
- Best imaging tool: MRI - identifies associated labral pathology
- Protocol advice: FS PD FSE images to identify the smaller paralabral cysts

DIFFERENTIAL DIAGNOSIS

Neoplasm
- + Internal enhancement
- No association with labral or capsular tear
- Benign
  - Lipoma
- Malignant
  - Metastasis
  - Lymphoma, myeloma extension from scapula

Muscle Denervation
- Posttraumatic neurapraxia
- Parsonage-Turner syndrome
  - Idiopathic denervation of shoulder girdle muscles
  - Acute brachial neuritis
- No labrocapsular abnormality

- +/- Nerve distribution

Normal Blood Vessels
- Normal plexus in spinoglenoid notch, suprascapular notch
- +/- Varices
- +/- Mass effect on suprascapular nerve
- Enlarged with congestive heart failure

Hematoma of Non Communicating Cyst
- + History of trauma
- +/- Scapular fracture
- Hyperintense fluid signal intensity on T2WI
- Chronic cases: Blooming with T2* GRE
- One way valve mechanism in non communicating paralabral cyst

Posterior Superior Glenoid Impingement (PSGI)
- Internal impingement
- Undersurface posterior supraspinatus tendon tear
  - Partial tear most common
  - +/- Anterior infraspinatus tendon tear
- Triad
  - Undersurface cuff tear
  - Posterior superior labral fraying/tear
  - Humeral head chronic impaction injury
- Athletes
- Occupational
  - Overhead activities, (e.g., mechanic)

PATHOLOGY

General Features
- General path comments
  - +/- Compression neuropathy
  - +/- Asymptomatic
  - "Ball-valve" mechanism
  - Draining cyst without repairing labral tear leads to recurrence
- Etiology

- ○ Cyst arises from break in integrity of joint: Labral tear, degeneration, capsular tear or capsular diverticulum
- ○ Slow growing
- ○ Original tear may heal
- Epidemiology: 3-5% of labral tears associated with cyst
- Associated abnormalities
  - ○ Instability, especially if labral tear remains patent (nonhealed)
  - ○ SLAP (superior labrum anterior to posterior) lesion
    - ▪ Cyst posterosuperiorly, anterosuperiorly
    - ▪ Superior cyst diagnostic of SLAP lesion
  - ○ Denervation of supraspinatus and infraspinatus muscles = compression neuropathy
  - ○ Deltoid and teres minor denervation
    - ▪ Inferior cyst compressing axillary nerve
    - ▪ Athletes
  - ○ Bankart fracture (anteroinferior glenoid rim fx)
  - ○ Bankart lesion (anterior inferior labral tear)
  - ○ Bankart variation lesion
    - ▪ Perthes
    - ▪ Anterior labroligamentous periosteal sleeve avulsion lesion (ALPSA)
  - ○ Clinical instability
    - ▪ Anterior
    - ▪ Posterior
    - ▪ Multi directional
    - ▪ Microinstability

Gross Pathologic & Surgical Features
- Glistening mass: Various sizes usually adjacent to labrum

Microscopic Features
- Cyst with wall containing spindle-shaped cells
- Cyst contains mucoid material
- Fatty infiltration of muscle tissue in chronically denervated muscles

CLINICAL ISSUES

Presentation
- Most common signs/symptoms
  - ○ Suprascapular nerve compression syndrome
    - ▪ Pain, weakness of SS and IS
    - ▪ Proprioceptive change
    - ▪ Mimics rotator cuff tear
- Clinical profile
  - ○ Suprascapular nerve compression syndrome if cyst located posterosuperiorly
  - ○ Axillary nerve compression syndrome if cyst inferior and dissects into quadrilateral space
  - ○ Patient with instability history (labral tear)
  - ○ Patient with history suggesting SLAP lesion (superior labral tear)
  - ○ Pain and weakness of supraspinatus and infraspinatus and proprioceptive changes (suprascapular denervation)
  - ○ Weakness of deltoid and teres minor (axillary denervation)
  - ○ +/- Asymptomatic patient

Demographics
- Age
  - ○ Adolescent status post athletic injury
  - ○ Adult with gradual onset of SSN denervation syndrome
- Gender: M > F

Natural History & Prognosis
- If symptomatic + nerve compression (may lead to irreversible damage), drainage required to relieve compression
  - ○ Address labral damage to prevent recurrence
- Labral tear may heal and cyst remains or becomes asymptomatic
  - ○ Conservative treatment may be successful

Treatment
- Removal of cyst if symptomatic and repair of labral tear if present
- Arthroscopic approach

DIAGNOSTIC CHECKLIST

Consider
- Instability, SLAP lesion, other labral tear in association with SSN compression in setting of a cyst

Image Interpretation Pearls
- FS PD FSE for detection and characterization of all paralabral cysts
- T2* sensitive to intralabral signal in tears and less sensitive to small paralabral cysts
- Paralabral cysts communicate with a labral tear until proven otherwise

SELECTED REFERENCES

1. Grainger AJ et al: Direct MR arthrography: A review of current use. Clin Radiol 55(3):163-76, 2000
2. Tirman PF et al: A practical approach to imaging of the shoulder with emphasis on MR imaging, Orthop Clin North Am 28(4):483-515, 1997
3. Steiner E et al: Ganglia and cysts around joints. Radiol Clin North Am 34(2):395-425, 1996
4. Tirman PF et al: Association of glenoid labral cysts with labral tears and glenohumeral instability: Radiologic findings and clinical significance. Radiology 190(3):653-8, 1994
5. Fritz RC et al: Suprascapular nerve entrapment: Evaluation with MR imaging. Radiology 182(2):437-44, 1992

LABRAL CYST, SHOULDER

IMAGE GALLERY

Typical

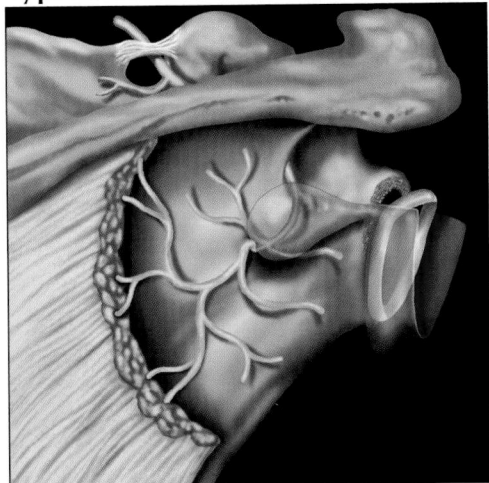
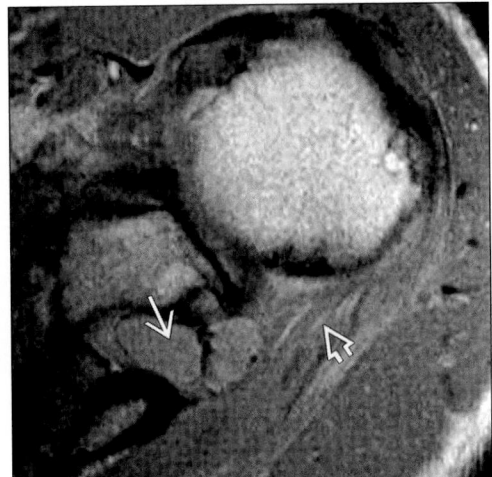

(Left) Coronal graphic shows a spinoglenoid notch cyst extending from a posterosuperior labral tear. The cyst courses between the supraspinatus and infraspinatus as the "path of least resistance". *(Right)* Axial PD FSE MR shows a large paralabral cyst (arrow) extending into the spinoglenoid notch, associated with bony erosion and intraosseous cyst formation. Note the infraspinatus denervation (open arrow).

Typical

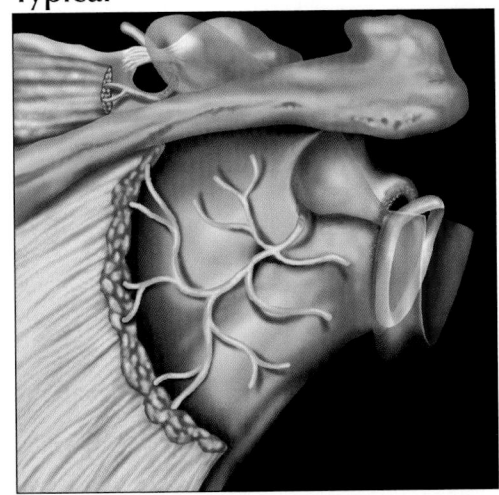
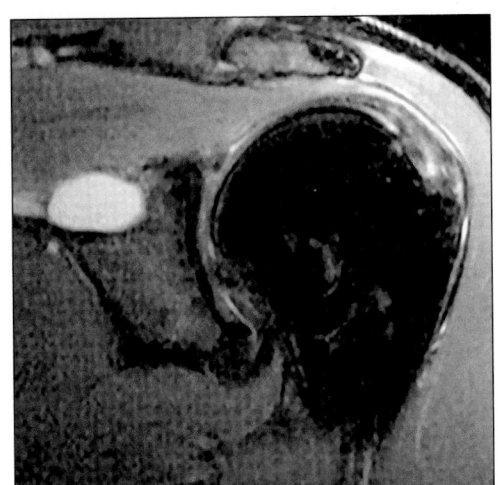

(Left) Coronal graphic shows a paralabral cyst extending from a superior labral tear into the suprascapular notch. *(Right)* Coronal FS PD FSE MR shows a large paralabral cyst within the suprascapular notch.

Typical

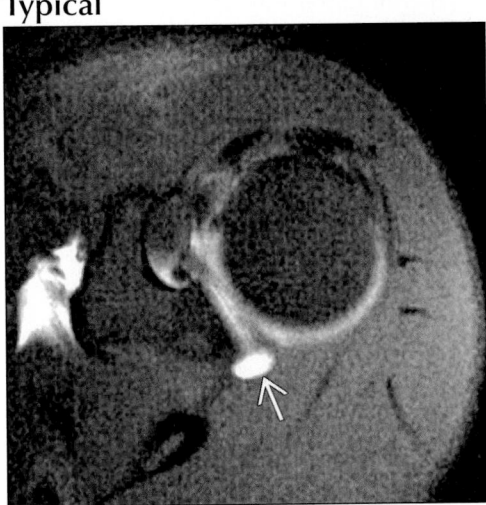
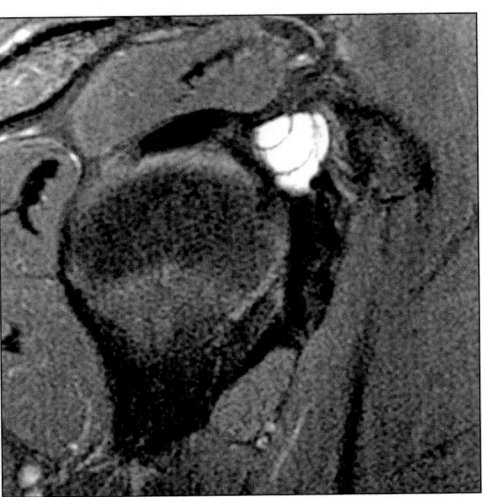

(Left) Axial T1 arthrogram shows filling of a posterior superior labral cyst (arrow), indicating a patent communicating labral tear. *(Right)* Sagittal FS PD FSE MR shows an anterior multiloculated cyst associated with an anterior superior labral tear.

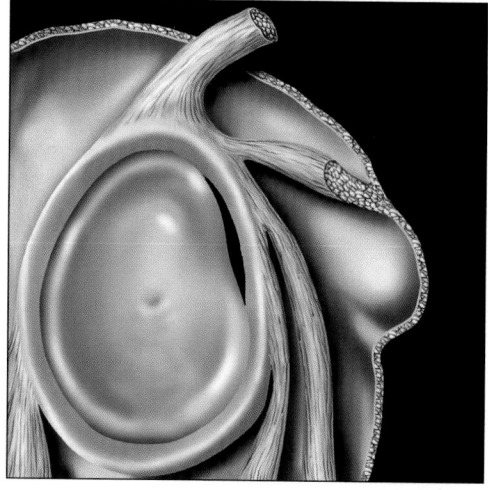

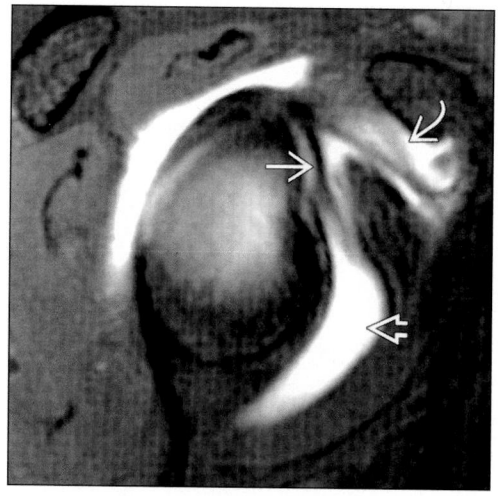

Sagittal graphic shows normal separation of the anterior superior labrum between the equator anteriorly and biceps anchor superiorly consistent with a sublabral foramen.

Sagittal T1 MR-arthrographic image demonstrates a sublabral foramen (arrow) in the anterosuperior quadrant. Foramen of Rouviere (open arrow) and Weitbrecht (curved arrow).

TERMINOLOGY

Abbreviations and Synonyms

- Sublabral foramen or sublabral hole (SH), Buford complex (BC), labral types, synovial recesses, cord-like middle glenohumeral ligament (MGHL/MGL)

Definitions

- Sublabral foramen
  - Relative lack of attachment of the anterior labrum to the glenoid rim in the anterior superior quadrant
- Buford complex
  - Cord-like MGL
  - MGL attaches directly to superior labrum anterior to biceps
  - Absent anterosuperior labrum
- Labral types
  - Superior wedge labrum
  - Posterior wedge labrum
  - Anterior wedge labrum
  - Superior and anterior wedge labrum
  - Meniscoid labrum
- Synovial recesses
  - Six anatomic types with respect to the glenohumeral ligaments
  - Cord-like MGL
    - Prominent - thickened middle glenohumeral ligament

IMAGING FINDINGS

General Features

- Best diagnostic clue
  - Sublabral foramen: Fluid undermining anterosuperior labrum on axial images
  - Buford complex: Thickened MGL in cross sectional diameter + absent anterosuperior labrum
  - Labral types
    - Labrum attached to glenoid in its periphery
    - Labrum mobile along its central border
    - Labrum secured to glenoid
  - Synovial recesses
    - Visualized on sagittal images as capsular variations relative to MGL
  - Cord-like MGL: Hypointense thick MGL on T1 and T2WI axial and sagittal images
- Location: Anterior superior quadrant
- Size: Anterior superior (anterosuperior) quadrant from equator (anterior indentation of glenoid rim as visualized on sagittal images) to biceps labral complex in a 12 o'clock position
- Morphology
  - Sublabral foramen
    - A gap or potential space between anterosuperior labrum and glenoid rim
    - Linear or slit-like morphology

DDx: Anterosuperior Variations, Shoulder

Ant Sup Tear	Ant Sup Tear	Bankart Lesion	Biceps Disloc	Type VII SLAP
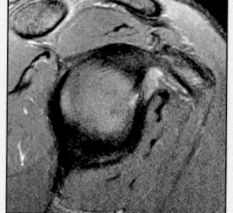	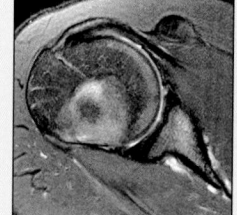	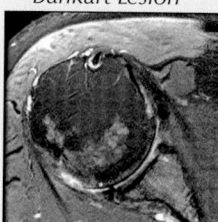	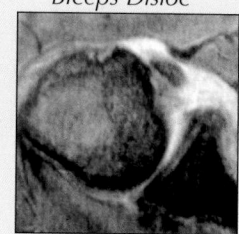	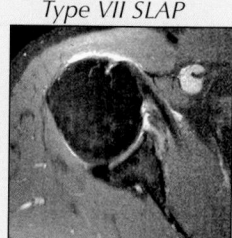
Sag FS PD FSE	Ax FS PD FSE	Ax FS PD FSE	Ax T2* GRE MR	Ax FS PD FSE MR

ANTEROSUPERIOR VARIATIONS, SHOULDER

Key Facts

Imaging Findings
- Sublabral foramen: Fluid undermining anterosuperior labrum on axial images
- Buford complex: Thickened MGL in cross sectional diameter + absent anterosuperior labrum
- Cord-like MGL: Hypointense thick MGL on T1 and T2WI axial and sagittal images

Top Differential Diagnoses
- Anterosuperior Labrum Tear
- Superior Labrum Anterior to Posterior (SLAP) Lesion
- Superior Dissection of Bankart Lesion
- Glenoid Labrum Articular Disruption (GLAD) Lesion
- Biceps Dislocation
- Subscapularis Tear

Pathology
- Congenital variation of anatomy
- May be developmental
- 5-30% of shoulder MRI

Clinical Issues
- Most common signs/symptoms: Asymptomatic
- Meniscoid labrum at risk for SLAP lesions
- Avoid tacking down cord-like MGHL arthroscopically as frozen shoulder may result

Diagnostic Checklist
- Normal variants exist in anterosuperior quadrant above or at level of the subscapularis
- The anterior labrum is firmly attached to the glenoid rim below the level of the subscapularis

---

- Focal up to contour of entire anterosuperior quadrant
  - Buford Complex
    - Direct attachment of cord-like MGL to superior labrum at biceps labral complex merging of superior glenohumeral (SGL), MGL, and superior labrum
  - Meniscoid labrum
    - Circumferential free central margin with symmetric anterior and posterior labral tissue
  - Synovial recesses
    - Type 1: One recess above MGL
    - Type 2: One recess below MGL
    - Type 3: Two recesses (superior subscapular recess above MGL & inferior subscapular recess below MGL)
    - Type 4: No MGL (one large recess above inferior glenohumeral ligament or IGL)
    - Type 5: MGL as two small synovial folds
    - Type 6: Complete absence of synovial recesses
  - Cord-like MGL
    - Cord-like compared to more normal sheet-like appearance of ligamentous tissue

MR Findings
- T1WI
  - Sublabral foramen
    - Difficult to visualize as fluid signal beneath anterosuperior labrum is hypointense
  - Buford complex
    - Complete absence of anterosuperior labrum above the level of the subscapularis
    - Thick cord-like MGL anterior to anterosuperior glenoid rim deep to subscapularis tendon
  - Labral types
    - Except for meniscoid labrum requires T2WI to appreciate fluid underneath labral free edge
    - Synovial recesses require the presence of fluid and/or FS PD FSE to identify capsular variations on sagittal images
  - Cord-like MGL

- Thick hypointense MGL may be mistaken for a detached anterior labrum above the epiphyseal line
- T2WI
  - Sublabral foramen
    - Hyperintense fluid signal which undermines anterosuperior labrum
    - Not to be confused with a SLAP lesion
    - Superior to anterior glenoid notch (above the equator or physeal line) representing superior third of anterior glenoid
    - The Bankart lesion in comparison exists below the physeal line
  - Buford complex
    - Hyperintense fluid signal surrounding hypointense MGL on axial and sagittal images
    - ± Remnant or hypoplastic anterosuperior labral tissue at level of subscapularis
    - Normal labral attachment in anteroinferior quadrant
  - Labral types
    - Hyperintense fluid beneath detached free edge (superior quadrant) of labrum overhanging articular cartilage + labrum, well attached peripherally
    - No fluid seen beneath central or peripheral attachment of labrum to articular cartilage
  - Synovial recesses
    - Hypointense MGL and IGL define recesses in contrast to adjacent hyperintense fluid
  - Cord-like MGL
    - Hyperintense fluid surrounding hypointense MGL on multiple axial images
    - MGL crosses superior border of subscapularis on sagittal images

Imaging Recommendations
- Best imaging tool: MRI
- Protocol advice: FS PD FSE (coronal, axial and sagittal), T2* GRE (axial plane), MR arthrography

ANTEROSUPERIOR VARIATIONS, SHOULDER

DIFFERENTIAL DIAGNOSIS

Anterosuperior Labrum Tear
- Labrum irregular and of high signal on T2WI
- +/- Throwing sports history
- Irregular labral morphology
- No anterior inferior instability
  - T1WI, T2* GRE WI, PD WI

Superior Labrum Anterior to Posterior (SLAP) Lesion
- Abduction/external rotation injury
- Torn superior labrum
- May propagate anteriorly, posteriorly, or involve MGHL
- +/- Microinstability
- +/- Superior labrum anterior cuff (SLAC) lesion

Superior Dissection of Bankart Lesion
- History of dislocation
- Abnormal anterior inferior quadrant abnormal
- +/- Type V SLAP lesion - inferior extension of a SLAP II
- +/- Bankart fracture
- +/- Hill-Sachs fracture

Glenoid Labrum Articular Disruption (GLAD) Lesion
- History of trauma
- Localized to anterior inferior quadrant
- Labral tear
- Chondral defect
- Forced adduction injury

Biceps Dislocation
- Mimics cord-like middle glenohumeral ligament
- +/- Subscapularis tear
  - +/- Partial tear
- +/- Predisposing hidden lesion
- +/- Biceps tendinosis

Subscapularis Tear
- +/- Impingement
- +/- Supraspinatus tear
- +/- Anterior dislocation
  - > 40 years old
- Hyperintense gap on T2WI
- +/- Hidden lesion

PATHOLOGY

General Features
- Etiology
  - Congenital variation of anatomy
  - May be developmental
- Epidemiology
  - Common
  - 5-30% of shoulder MRI

Gross Pathologic & Surgical Features
- Sublabral foramen normal communication between sublabral foramen and subscapularis bursa
- Buford complex
- Cord-like MGL + deficient anterior superior labrum (Buford) is less common than a cord-like MGL + sublabral foramen beneath a normal anterior superior labrum

Staging, Grading or Classification Criteria
- Six arrangements of synovial recesses
- Type A labrum
  - Unattached free edge
- Type B labrum
  - Attached to articular cartilage centrally
- Foramen of Weitbrecht
  - Normal foramen between MGL and superior glenohumeral ligament (SGL) creating a synovial recess
- Foramen of Rouviere
  - Normal foramen between MGL and IGL defining a synovial recess

CLINICAL ISSUES

Presentation
- Most common signs/symptoms: Asymptomatic

Demographics
- Age: Adolescents and adults
- Gender: M = F

Natural History & Prognosis
- Meniscoid labrum at risk for SLAP lesions

Treatment
- Avoid tacking down cord-like MGHL arthroscopically as frozen shoulder may result
- Sublabral foramen should not be reattached

DIAGNOSTIC CHECKLIST

Consider
- Normal variants exist in anterosuperior quadrant above or at level of the subscapularis
- The anterior labrum is firmly attached to the glenoid rim below the level of the subscapularis

SELECTED REFERENCES

1. Grigorian M et al: Magnetic resonance imaging of the glenoid labrum. Semin Roentgenol 35(3):277-85, 2000
2. Beltran JJ et al: MR arthrography of the shoulder: Variants and pitfalls. Radiographics 17(6):1403-12, 1997
3. Stoller DW: MR arthrography of the glenohumeral joint. Radiol Clin North Am 35(1):97-116, 1997

IMAGE GALLERY

Typical

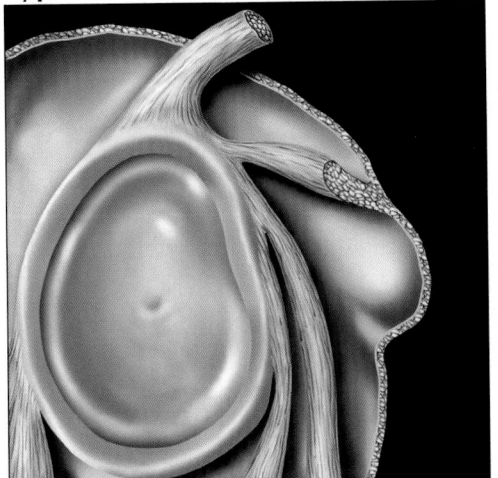 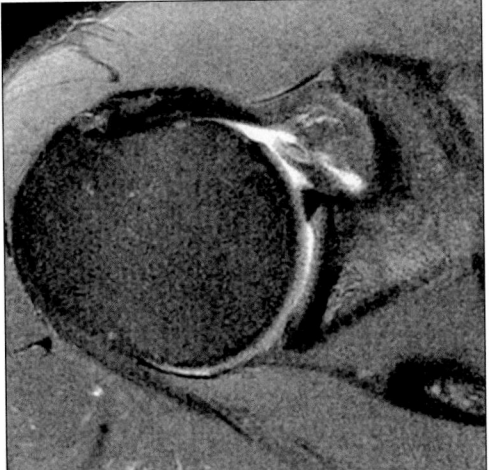

(Left) Sagittal graphic shows a firmly normal attached anterosuperior labrum. *(Right)* Axial FS PD FSE MR shows an anterosuperior labrum attached directly to the glenoid articular cartilage.

Typical

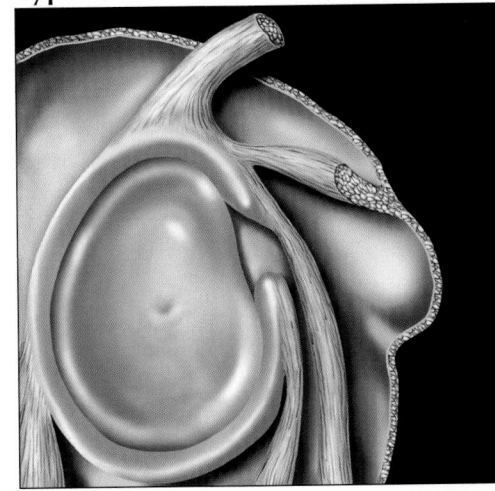 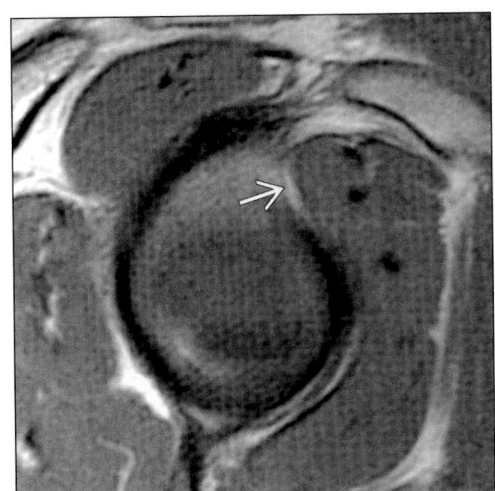

(Left) Sagittal graphic shows a Buford complex with absence of the anterosuperior labrum in association with a cord-like middle glenohumeral ligament. *(Right)* Sagittal PD FSE MR shows absence (arrow) of the anterosuperior labrum in a patient with a Buford complex.

Typical

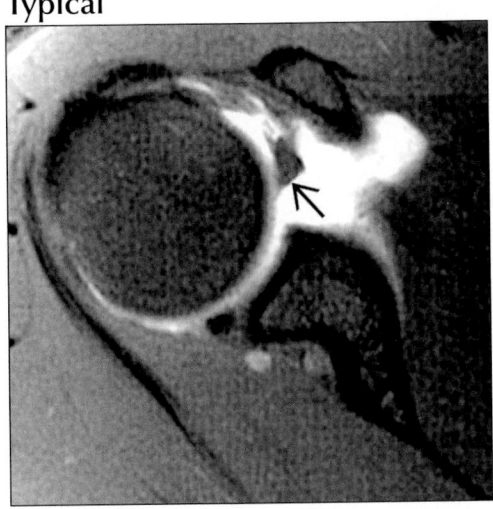 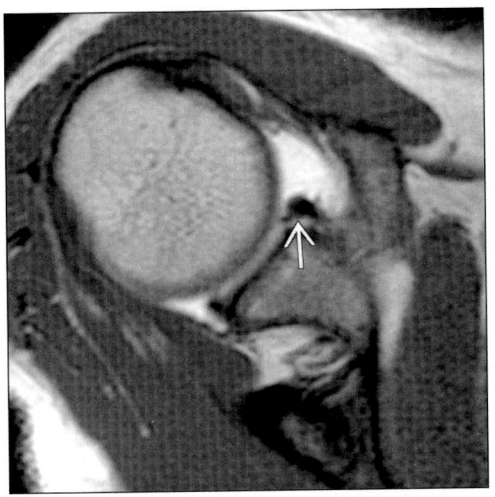

(Left) Axial FS PD FSE shows the absent anterosuperior labrum in association with cord-like middle glenohumeral ligament (arrow). Note absent anterosuperior labrum in associated Buford complex. This should not be mistaken for a labral tear. *(Right)* Axial MR arthrogram demonstrates a sublabral foramen (arrow) anterosuperiorly.

ADHESIVE CAPSULITIS, SHOULDER

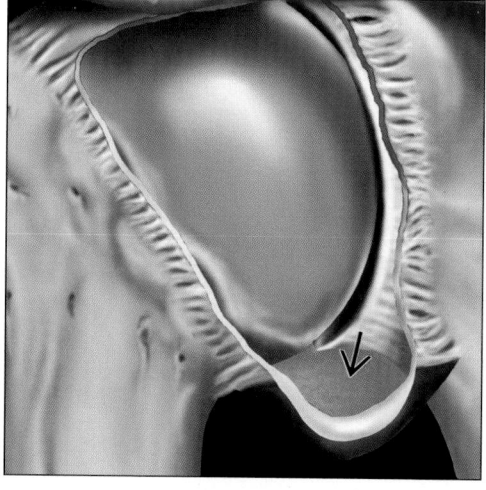

Coronal graphic shows thickening of the inferior capsule with synovitis (arrow) in a patient with limitation of shoulder movement.

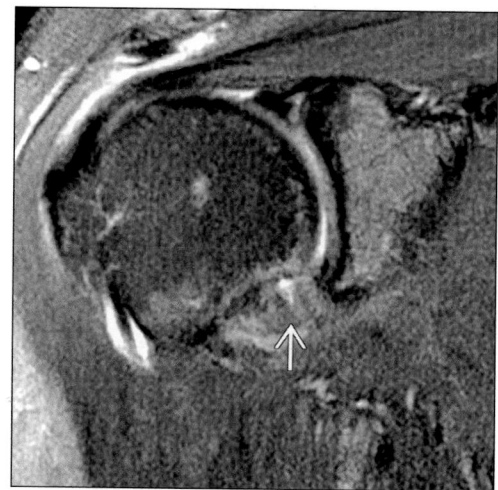

Coronal FS PD FSE MR shows thickening and edema (arrow) within the inferior aspect of the capsule (the axillary pouch of inferior glenohumeral ligament).

TERMINOLOGY

Abbreviations and Synonyms
- Frozen shoulder (FS), frozen shoulder syndrome (FSS)

Definitions
- Painful restriction of active and passive shoulder movement and scapulothoracic motion
  - Primary - no predisposing history or cause
  - Secondary - antecedent event such as trauma or previous surgery
- Duration: At least 1 month, stable vs. progression

IMAGING FINDINGS

General Features
- Best diagnostic clue: Indistinct edematous inferior capsule (axillary pouch) on T2WI, on coronal and axial image
- Location
  - Axillary pouch, synovium of rotator interval
  - Involvement of entire axillary pouch from inferior pole of glenoid to humeral head
  - Segmental involvement of IGL (inferior glenohumeral ligament)
    - Parahumeral portion
    - Paraglenoid portion

- Size: Thickened capsule measuring > 3 mm on coronal images
- Morphology
  - Edematous
  - Thickened
  - Indistinct inferior capsule
  - +/- Rotator interval synovitis

Radiographic Findings
- Arthrography
  - Contracted irregular capsule
  - +/- Decreased volume
  - Over injection leading to capsular rupture often therapeutic
    - Results in increased mobility

MR Findings
- T1WI
  - Thickened indistinct hypointense capsule
    - Diffuse
    - Adjacent to humerus
    - Adjacent to glenoid
  - Hypointense capsule measuring greater than 3 mm thick on coronal images
- T2WI
  - Thickening and increased signal on T2WI of the rotator interval
  - Thickening conspicuous on FS PD FSE, T2* GRE and STIR

DDx: Adhesive Capsulitis, Shoulder

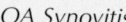

OA Synovitis	Capsule Sprain	2° Adhesive Caps	Capsule Rupture	Capsule Tear

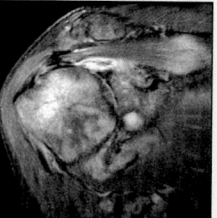 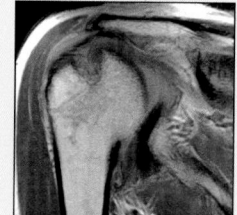 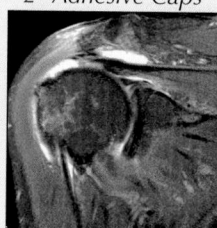 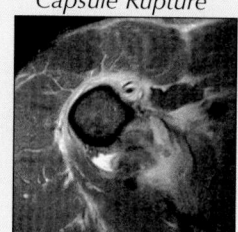 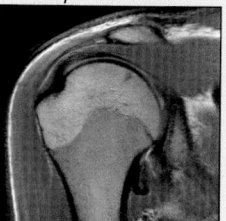

Cor FS PD FSE	Cor PD FSE MR	Cor FS PD FSE	Ax FS PD FSE	Cor PD FSE MR

ADHESIVE CAPSULITIS, SHOULDER

Key Facts

Terminology
- Painful restriction of active and passive shoulder movement and scapulothoracic motion
- Primary - no predisposing history or cause
- Secondary - antecedent event such as trauma or previous surgery

Imaging Findings
- Best diagnostic clue: Indistinct edematous inferior capsule (axillary pouch) on T2WI, on coronal and axial image

Top Differential Diagnoses
- Impingement Syndrome
- Neuromuscular Dysfunction
- Osteoarthritis (OA)
- Cervical Disease

- Capsular Injury
- Secondary Adhesive Capsulitis (2° Adhesive Caps)

Pathology
- Inflammation of the inferior shoulder capsule causing
- Limited range of motion
- Frozen shoulder
- 10-20% patients with diabetes

Clinical Issues
- +/- History of trauma
- Often considered rotator cuff disease clinically

Diagnostic Checklist
- Diffuse edema with indistinct appearance of IGL on coronal FS PD FSE

- ○ FS PD FSE sensitive to capsular edema and synovitis
- ○ Thickened indistinct hyperintense capsule
- ○ Loss of normal hypointense linear capsule
  - Coronal images to evaluate inferior capsule below glenohumeral osseous structures
  - Sagittal images helpful in evaluating rotator interval
- ○ Capsular scarring shown on PD FSE as intermediate signal fibrosis between IGL and inferior labrum
- ○ Intermediate signal in synovitis contained within the axillary pouch
- ○ +/- Effusion
  - Hyperintense on T2WI
  - +/- Capsular contraction
- STIR: Thickened indistinct hyperintense capsule
- MR arthrography
  - ○ Capsule enhances diffusely, acutely
  - ○ Restricted capsular volume

Imaging Recommendations
- Best imaging tool: MRI
- Protocol advice: FS PD FSE and PD FSE in coronal plane

DIFFERENTIAL DIAGNOSIS

Impingement Syndrome
- Impingement associated with painful shoulder movement mimicking adhesive capsulitis
- Capsular swelling associated with RTC (rotator cuff) disease as a secondary adhesive capsulitis
- Anterior shoulder pain with abduction
- +/- Thickening, increased signal of supraspinatus tendon on short and long TE sequences
- +/- Thickened coracoacromial ligament

Neuromuscular Dysfunction
- +/- History of nerve injury
- Specific muscle groups affected rather than global frozen shoulder
  - ○ Except in paresis
- +/- History of antecedent viral prodrome

- ○ Parsonage-Turner syndrome

Osteoarthritis (OA)
- +/- History of trauma
- +/- Limitation of movement
- Common findings of OA
  - ○ Chronic symptoms
  - ○ Subchondral cysts, edema, sclerosis
- Synovitis mimics adhesive capsulitis

Cervical Disease
- +/- Disc abnormality on MRI
- Radiating pain without global loss of movement
- +/- Neuromuscular dysfunction

Capsular Injury
- +/- Thickening of capsule secondary to injury and swelling
- Hyperintense on T2WI
- +/- Discrete tear
- + History of trauma
  - ○ Dislocation
  - ○ Abduction and external rotation injury
- +/- Complete rupture

Secondary Adhesive Capsulitis (2° Adhesive Caps)
- Trauma
- Surgery
- Regional abnormality
- Inflammatory disease
- Metabolic disease

PATHOLOGY

General Features
- General path comments
  - ○ Inflammation of the inferior shoulder capsule causing
    - Limited range of motion
    - Frozen shoulder
  - ○ Accompanying other shoulder disorders such as impingement (secondary adhesive capsulitis)

ADHESIVE CAPSULITIS, SHOULDER

- Etiology
  - Idiopathic
  - Secondary (known disorders)
    - Trauma
    - Surgery
    - Degenerative (acromioclavicular arthritis)
    - Intrinsic rotator cuff and biceps tendinitis/tear
    - Inflammatory disease
    - Metabolic disease (including diabetes mellitus)
  - Autoimmune theory proposed
    - Increased C-reactive protein and HLA-B27
- Epidemiology
  - Affects approximately 3% of general population
  - 10-20% patients with diabetes
    - 36% Insulin dependent diabetes

Gross Pathologic & Surgical Features

- Thickened, indurated inferior capsule (axillary pouch of IGL)
- Rotator interval involvement
- Capsule often contracted
- Effusion
- Arthroscopic
  - Proliferative synovitis
  - Capsular and intraarticular subscapularis tendon thickening
  - Fibrosis

Microscopic Features

- Influx of fibrosis and chronic inflammatory cells

Staging, Grading or Classification Criteria

- Adhesive capsulitis
  - Primary (idiopathic)
  - Secondary (known disorders)
    - Systemic (e.g., diabetes mellitus)
    - Extrinsic (e.g., humeral fractures)
    - Intrinsic (e.g., cuff tendinitis, tears and acromioclavicular arthritis)

CLINICAL ISSUES

Presentation

- Most common signs/symptoms
  - Adult patient with painful limited range of shoulder motion
  - Restricted active and passive motion with loss of anterior elevation, external and internal rotation
  - +/- History of trauma
  - Often considered rotator cuff disease clinically
- Clinical profile
  - Associated rotator cuff disease
  - Painful and restricted passive and active range of shoulder motion at physical examination

Demographics

- Age: 40-70 years
- Gender: F > M

Natural History & Prognosis

- Usually self limiting and effectively treated conservatively
- Small percentage ~ 10% have persistent symptoms

Treatment

- Conservative
  - Typically physical therapy
  - Passive stretching exercises
    - Overhead elevation
    - External rotation
    - 90 degrees of abduction
    - Internal rotation
  - NSAIDs, then possible corticosteroids
- Surgical
  - Injection of fluid into joint leading to capsular rupture often therapeutic
  - Brisement or distension arthrography
  - Manipulation under anesthesia
  - Surgical if failure of conservative management
  - Arthroscopic capsular release
- Complications
  - Biceps tendon sheath and subscapularis rupture reported with some conservative treatments

DIAGNOSTIC CHECKLIST

Consider

- Primary or secondary adhesive capsulitis when MRI findings of IGL involvement are demonstrated

Image Interpretation Pearls

- Diffuse edema with indistinct appearance of IGL on coronal FS PD FSE
- Synovitis is intermediate relative to hyperintense joint fluid within axillary pouch on FS PD FSE images
- Adhesive capsulitis and capsular sprain of the IGL have a similar appearance on MR

SELECTED REFERENCES

1. Hannafin JA et al: Adhesive capsulitis. A treatment approach. Clin Orthop 372:95-109, 2000
2. Carrillon Y et al. Magnetic resonance imaging findings in idiopathic adhesive capsulitis of the shoulder. Rev Rhum Engl Ed 66(4):201-6, 1999
3. Warner JJ: Frozen shoulder: Diagnosis and management. J Am Acad Orthop Surg 5(3):130-40, 1997
4. Warner JJ et al: Arthroscopic release for chronic, refractory adhesive capsulitis of the shoulder. J Bone Joint Surg 78(12):1808-16, 1996
5. Shaffer B et al: Frozen shoulder. A long-term follow-up. J Bone Joint Surg 74(5):738-46, 1992
6. Bigliani LU et al: Operative management of failed rotator cuff repairs. Orthop Trans 12:674, 1988
7. Bulgen DY et al: Immunological studies in frozen shoulder. J Rheumatol 9(6):893-8, 1982
8. DePalma AF: Loss of scapulohumeral motion (frozen shoulder). Ann Surg 135:193-204, 1952

ADHESIVE CAPSULITIS, SHOULDER

IMAGE GALLERY

Typical

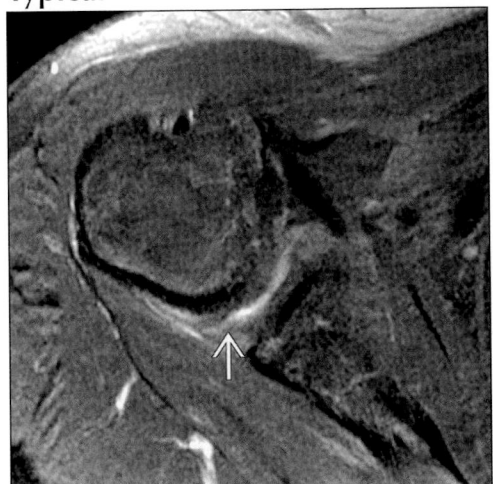 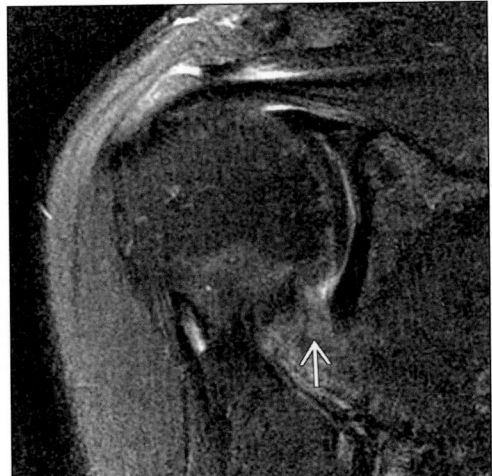

(Left) Axial FS PD FSE MR shows diffuse edema and an indistinct appearance (arrow) of the inferior capsule in a patient with limitation of motion, consistent with adhesive capsulitis. *(Right)* Coronal FS PD FSE MR shows diffuse edema and indistinctness of the inferior capsule (arrow), in adhesive capsulitis. Differential would include a capsular sprain.

Typical

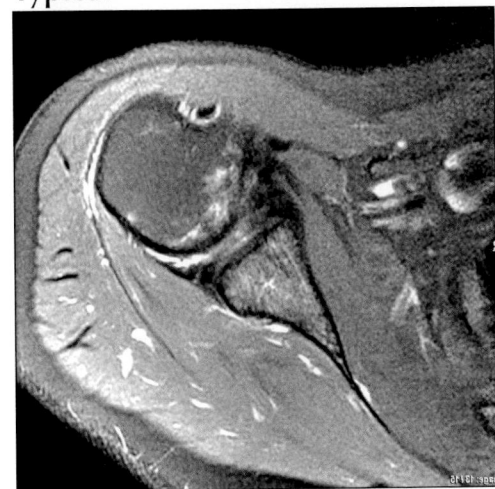 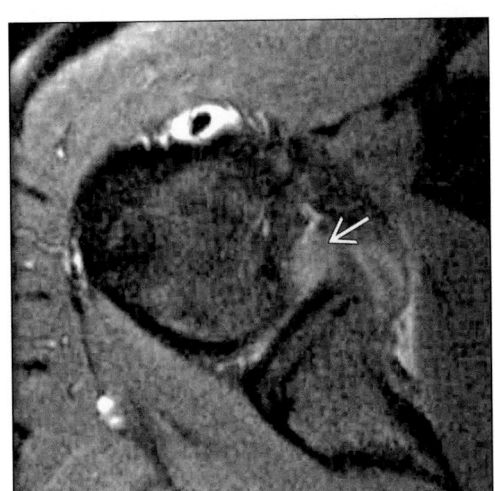

(Left) Axial FS PD FSE MR in a patient without clinical findings of adhesive capsulitis demonstrates normal decreased signal intensity of the capsule and labral complex. *(Right)* Axial FS PD FSE MR shows the poorly defined and thickened (synovitis) capsule (arrow) of adhesive capsulitis.

Typical

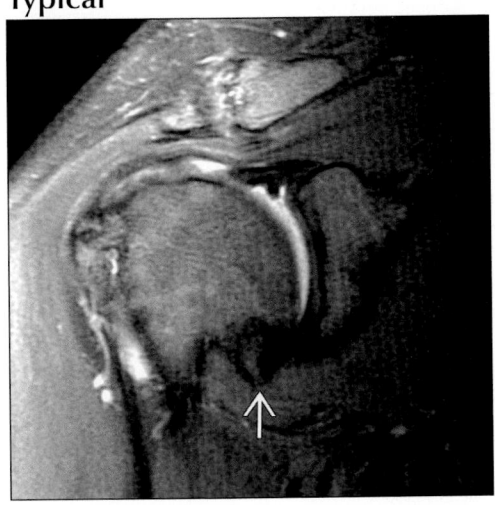 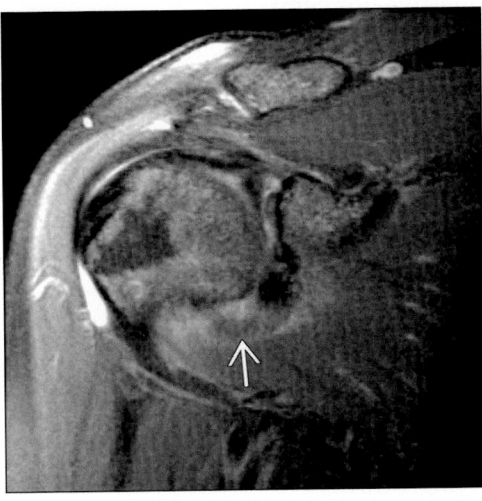

(Left) Coronal FS PD FSE MR shows the normal hypointense appearance of the axillary pouch (arrow). *(Right)* Coronal FS PD FSE MR shows the thickened, edematous and indistinct morphology of the axillary pouch of the IGL (arrow) in adhesive capsulitis.

BANKART LESION

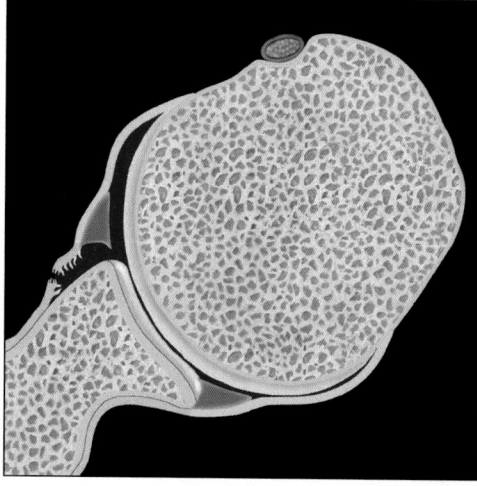

Axial graphic shows avulsion of the inferior glenohumeral labroligamentous attachment to the glenoid with disruption of the scapular periosteum.

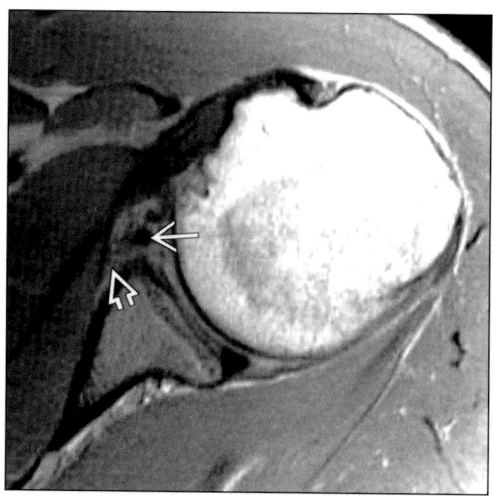

Axial PD shows avulsion of anteroinferior labrum (arrow) & ligament. Note disrupted scapular periosteum & deep surface of subscapularis tendon (open arrow).

TERMINOLOGY

Abbreviations and Synonyms
- Inferior glenohumeral ligament labral complex (IGHLC or IGLLC) avulsion, osseous Bankart, soft tissue Bankart

Definitions
- Detachment of the inferior glenohumeral ligament (IGHL) and labrum from the anterior glenoid after anterior dislocation
  - Periosteum ruptured
  - Bankart lesion encompasses both soft tissue Bankart lesions with an anterior inferior labral avulsion, and osseous or bony Bankart lesions with an associated fracture of the anteroinferior glenoid rim
  - Bankart variants encompass other anterior labral tears based on the type of detachment of the labrum and capsule from the anterior glenoid
    - Perthes lesion (intact scapular periosteum)
    - ALPSA (anterior labroligamentous periosteal sleeve avulsion)
    - Capsular & intraligamentous IGL (inferior glenoid ligament) tears associated +/- Bankart lesion
    - HAGL (humeral avulsion of the glenohumeral ligament) - may be associated with a Bankart lesion

IMAGING FINDINGS

General Features
- Best diagnostic clue
  - Detached IGHL/labrum from underlying glenoid, +/- fracture of adjacent glenoid
    - History of dislocation
- Location: Anterior inferior glenoid labrum
- Size
  - Varies from small discrete tear to displaced avulsions
    - Labral tear may extend superiorly to equator (level of subscapularis or BLC - biceps labral complex)
- Morphology: Varies from linear tear to frank avulsion

Radiographic Findings
- Radiography
  - +/- Glenoid rim fracture with variable amount of displacement/comminution
    - Subglenoid or subcoracoid dislocation

CT Findings
- CT arthrography
  - Contrast extending into anterior labral tear

MR Findings
- T1WI
  - Hypointense edema (acute) or sclerosis (chronic Bankart) in anteroinferior glenoid rim

DDx: Bankart Lesion

Perthes	ALPSA	IGL Sprain	Adhes. Capsul.	SLAP IX
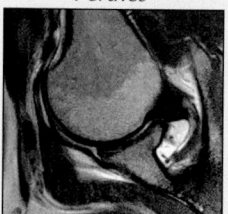	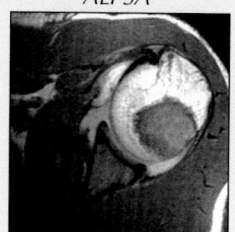	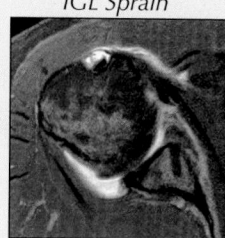	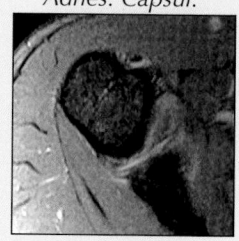	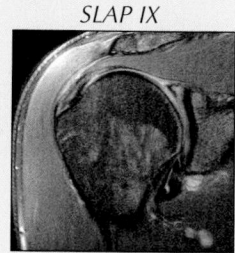
ABER PD FSE	Ax PD FSE MR	Ax FS PD FSE MR	Ax T2* GRE MR	Cor FS PD FSE

BANKART LESION

Key Facts

Terminology
- Detachment of the inferior glenohumeral ligament (IGHL) and labrum from the anterior glenoid after anterior dislocation

Imaging Findings
- Morphology: Varies from linear tear to frank avulsion
- +/- Fracture of the underlying glenoid (Bankart fx)

Top Differential Diagnoses
- ALPSA Lesion
- Partially Torn Non-Distracted Labrum after Subluxation
- Perthes Lesion
- HAGL Lesion
- IGL Tear
- Supraspinatus Tear
- Subscapularis Tear

Pathology
- Scapular periosteum is disrupted
- Etiology: Occurs after initial anterior dislocation of the shoulder of patient < 40 years old

Clinical Issues
- Results in recurrent instability if improper healing of initial lesion occurs

Diagnostic Checklist
- Bankart variation lesions if labrum displaced medially (ALPSA) or in normal position (Perthes) with intact scapular periosteum

---

- ○ Glenoid rim fracture visualized in contrast to adjacent marrow fat signal
  - ■ Axial
  - ■ Sagittal shows entire extent of anterior inferior glenoid quadrant
- T2WI
  - ○ +/- Fracture of the underlying glenoid (Bankart fx)
    - ■ Increased signal intensity and visible hypointense fracture line
  - ○ Hyperintense Hill-Sachs fracture (posterolateral humeral head)
  - ○ Thickened, hyperintense IGHLC - acute dislocation
  - ○ Hypointense - chronic osseous and capsular changes
    - ■ Fibrosis/healing of labrum
  - ○ Labrum - discretely torn with hyperintense fluid, within or undermining labrum
  - ○ ABER (abduction and external rotation) view demonstrates avulsion or absence of the anterior inferior labrum with associated tears of the IGL (inferior glenohumeral ligament)
    - ■ Use in conjunction with MR arthrography
  - ○ Scar tissue - intermediate signal intensity
- T2* GRE
  - ○ Demonstrates intralabral signal intensity with greater sensitivity than FS PD FSE or PD FSE images
  - ○ Osseous Bankart fx visualized with poor contrast on T2* GRE
- Avulsed, distracted labrum on coronal images at or medial to the inferior pole of the glenoid

Imaging Recommendations
- Best imaging tool: MRI and MR arthrography
- Protocol advice
  - ○ T2* GRE for intralabral signal/tears
  - ○ FS PD FSE to identify paralabral cysts and fluid undermining labral tears

DIFFERENTIAL DIAGNOSIS

ALPSA Lesion
- Bankart variant
- Intact periosteum
- IGHLC avulsion
- +/- Bankart fracture
- +/- Hill-Sachs lesion

Partially Torn Non-Distracted Labrum after Subluxation
- +/- Glenoid labrum articular disruption (GLAD) lesion
- History suggestive
- ABER (abduction external rotation) injury
- Labral tear = increased signal intensity on short TE sequence

Perthes Lesion
- Bankart variant
- No medial displacement
- No periosteal disruption
- ABER position used for diagnosis

HAGL Lesion
- Humeral capsular disruption
- Injury at humeral attachment of IGL
- Status post dislocation
- Hyperintense on T2WI (esp. FS PD FSE)
  - ○ Soft tissue edema (capsule)
  - ○ Effusion
  - ○ J-shaped axillary pouch of IGL

IGL Tear
- Discontinuous decreased signal capsule with interposed hyperintensity on T2WI
- Anterior dislocation/subluxation

Supraspinatus Tear
- Impingement related
- Status post anterior dislocation
  - ○ > 40 years old
  - ○ +/- Bankart fracture
  - ○ +/- Hill-Sachs lesion

Subscapularis Tear
- Status post anterior dislocation
  - ○ > 40 years old
  - ○ +/- Bankart fracture
  - ○ +/- Hill-Sachs lesion

BANKART LESION

1

60

- Posterior dislocation
  - +/- History of tonic-clonic seizure
  - Forward fall onto adducted internally rotated shoulder

Adhesive Capsulitis (Adhes Capsul)
- Thickened edematous capsule detected at the axillary pouch of the IGL
- Hyperintense capsule on T2WI
- Frozen shoulder

SLAP Lesion (Esp. Type V and IX)
- Superior labrum tear
- SLAP V (superior extension of a Bankart lesion) and IX (circumferential labral tear) involve the anterior inferior labrum
- Increased signal intensity linear abnormality on short TE sequences

PATHOLOGY

General Features
- General path comments
  - Scapular periosteum is disrupted
  - IGHLC "weak link" of static stabilizer in young shoulders
    - Ruptures after dislocation
- Etiology: Occurs after initial anterior dislocation of the shoulder of patient < 40 years old
- Epidemiology
  - 50% of all joint dislocations
  - Bankart lesion most common lesion in under 40 age group accounting for > 90% of lesions
- Associated abnormalities
  - Accompanied by osteochondral fracture (bony Bankart) in some cases
    - Glenoid deficiency = bony Bankart resulting in inverted pear appearance of glenoid (high recurrence rate)
  - Tears of the rotator interval lead to continued instability
  - Hill-Sachs fracture of posterolateral superior humeral head
    - Engaging = catching and click when moving in and out of ABER position
  - Partial or complete rotator cuff tears
  - Biceps tendon/anchor lesions in ~ 12% of patients post anterior dislocation
  - Brachial plexus injuries, posterior glenoid labral tear in up to 11% of patients post anterior dislocation

Gross Pathologic & Surgical Features
- Avulsion of IGHLC attachment to the glenoid after anterior dislocation of the shoulder
- Glenoid deficiency
- Posterolateral humeral head impaction fx

Microscopic Features
- Hemorrhagic, torn, fibrocartilaginous labrum with variable degrees of fibrosis depending on chronicity
- Ligamentous failure of IGL at glenoid insertion + capsular deformation or stretch with recurrent dislocation

CLINICAL ISSUES

Presentation
- Most common signs/symptoms
  - Status post anterior dislocation (single or multiple dislocations)
  - Pain and apprehension with abduction and external rotation
- Clinical profile: Positive apprehension (feeling of instability) test in patients with recurrent instability

Demographics
- Age: Younger patient (< 40 years)
- Gender: M > F

Natural History & Prognosis
- Results in recurrent instability if improper healing of initial lesion occurs
  - Medial displacement = ALPSA lesion, Bankart variation
  - Nondisplaced but with intact periosteum = Perthes lesion, Bankart variation

Treatment
- Conservative with a sling
- Surgical or arthroscopic repair for repeat dislocations
  - Glenoid deficiency = open repair
  - No deficiency - arthroscopic repair restoring normal anatomy
    - Place labrum on the "corner" of the glenoid

DIAGNOSTIC CHECKLIST

Consider
- Consider in younger patient with history of dislocation
- Does not occur spontaneously without dislocation

Image Interpretation Pearls
- Bankart variation lesions if labrum displaced medially (ALPSA) or in normal position (Perthes) with intact scapular periosteum
- Identify anterior inferior labral tears, scarring and tears of the IGL on coronal images at or medial to the inferior pole of the glenoid

SELECTED REFERENCES

1. DeBerardino TM et al: Prospective evaluation of arthroscopic stabilization of acute, initial anterior shoulder dislocations in young athletes. Two to five-year follow-up. Am J Sports Med 29(5):586-92, 2001
2. Gartsman GM et al: Arthroscopic treatment of anterior-inferior glenohumeral instability. Two to five-year follow-up. J Bone Joint Surg Am 82-A (7): 991-1003, 2000
3. Burkhart SS et al: Traumatic glenohumeral bone defects and their relationship to failure of arthroscopic Bankart repairs: Significance of the inverted-pear glenoid and the humeral engaging Hill-Sachs lesion. Arthroscopy 16(7): 677-94, 2000

IMAGE GALLERY

Typical

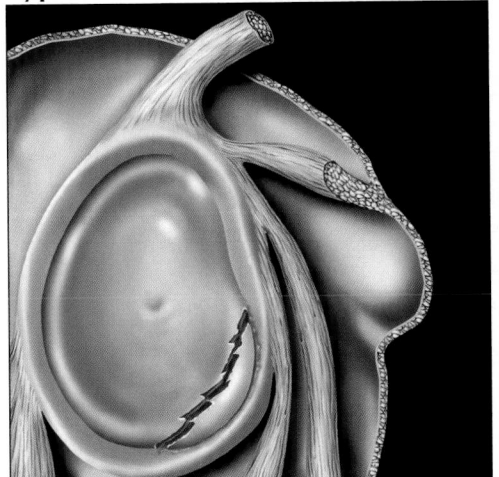
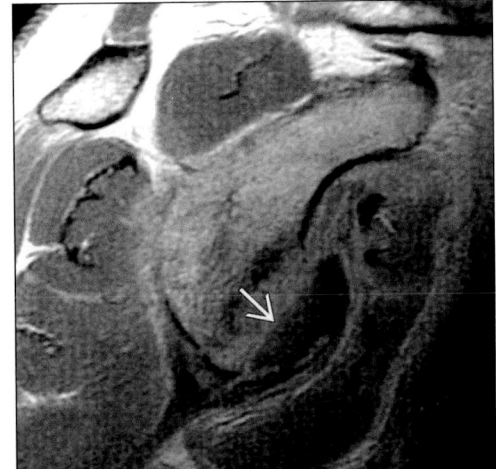

(Left) Sagittal graphic shows a fracture through the anteroinferior glenoid, consistent with a Bankart fracture. A large fracture results in glenoid deficiency and is treated with an open surgical procedure. *(Right)* Sagittal PD FSE MR shows fracture through the anteroinferior glenoid (arrow), representing an osseous Bankart lesion. The patient developed glenoid deficiency.

Typical

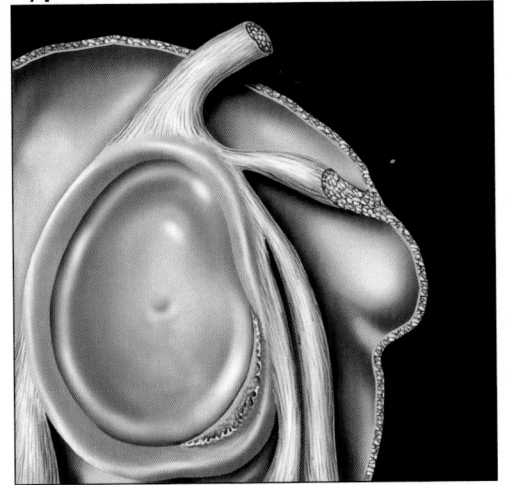
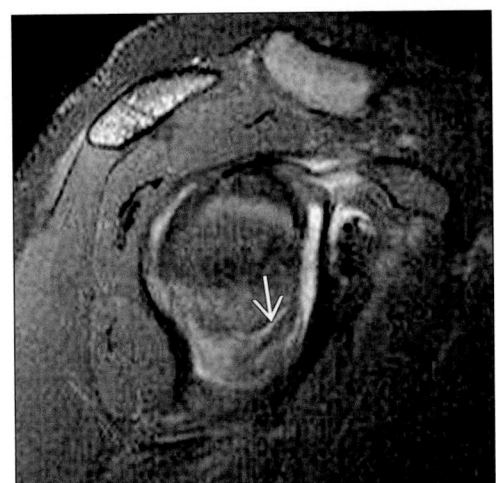

(Left) Sagittal graphic shows fibrocartilaginous Bankart (avulsion of the inferior glenohumeral labroligamentous attachment to the glenoid) as a result of anterior dislocation. *(Right)* Sagittal PD FSE MR shows a Bankart lesion (arrow) anteroinferiorly.

Typical

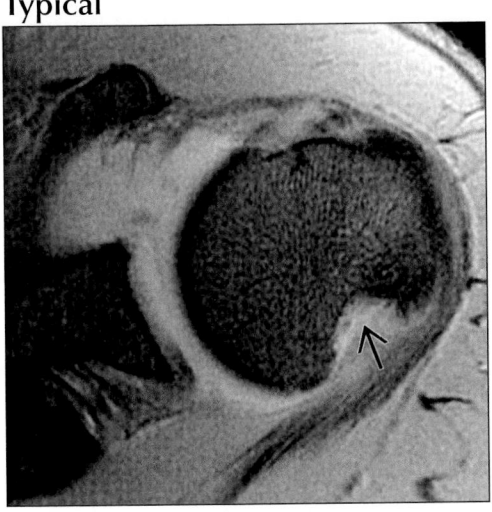
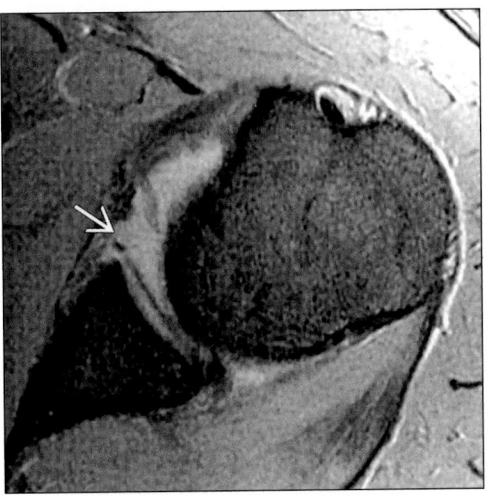

(Left) Axial T2* GRE MR in a patient after anterior dislocation shows a posterolateral Hill-Sachs fracture (arrow) involving the superior humeral head (engaging Hill-Sachs). Bankart lesion - anteriorly. *(Right)* Axial T2* GRE MR shows fragmentation and avulsion of the anterior inferior glenoid labrum (arrow).

PERTHES LESION

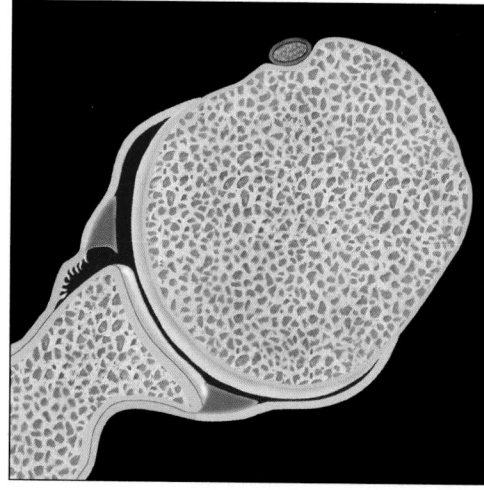

Axial graphic demonstrates an avulsion of the inferior glenohumeral labroligamentous attachment to the glenoid with an intact periosteum (Perthes lesion).

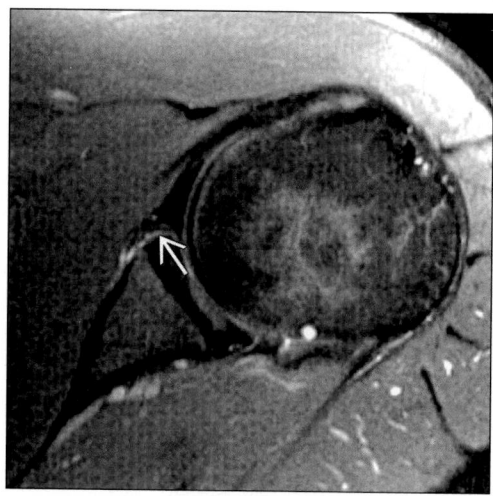

Axial FS PD FSE MR demonstrates linear increased signal intensity (arrow) beneath an avulsed labrum. The labrum is only minimally displaced and the scapular periosteum is intact.

TERMINOLOGY

Abbreviations and Synonyms
- Bankart variant

Definitions
- Detached inferior glenohumeral ligamentous complex (IGHLC or IGLLC) with intact scapular periosteum, which is stripped medially
- Nondisplaced with neutral positioning of the shoulder, labral attachment often incompetent

IMAGING FINDINGS

General Features
- Best diagnostic clue
  - Normal position of the inferior glenohumeral ligament and labrum relative to underlying glenoid
    - Accompanied by hemorrhage/edema of inferior glenohumeral ligament (IGL) attachment site
    - + Anterior dislocation/subluxation
- Location: Anterior inferior glenoid at insertion of IGL to labrum
- Size: Small tear at base of nondisplaced or mildly displaced IGHLC after anterior dislocation
- Morphology: Periosteum redundant/lax

Radiographic Findings
- Radiography
  - +/- Bankart fracture (anterior inferior glenoid fracture)
  - +/- Hill-Sachs deformity (posterolateral humeral head impaction)

CT Findings
- NECT
  - +/- Bankart fracture
  - +/- Hill-Sachs deformity
- CT arthrography
  - Nondisplaced IGHLC
  - +/- Extension of contrast underneath nondisplaced labrum and periosteum

MR Findings
- T1WI
  - Often normal (scapular periosteum intact)
  - Not recommended for primary diagnosis of Perthes lesion
- T2WI
  - Subtle linear increased signal intensity at base of usually nondisplaced labrum - sublabral hyperintensity
  - +/- Fracture (fx) of underlying glenoid
    - Increased signal intensity and visible hypointense fracture line at site of Bankart fx

DDx: Perthes Lesion

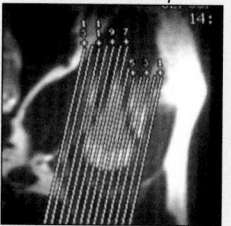

ABER Prescrip

Cor T1WI MR

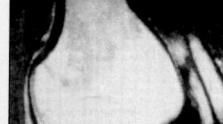

Normal ABER

T1 ABER

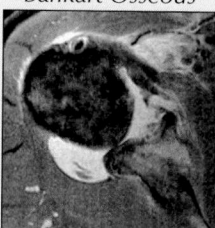

Bankart Osseous

Ax FS PD FSE MR

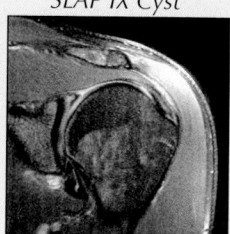

SLAP IX Cyst

Cor FS PD FSE

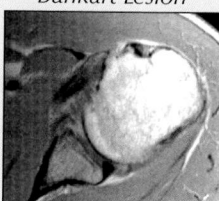

Bankart Lesion

Ax PD FSE MR

PERTHES LESION

Key Facts

Terminology
- Detached inferior glenohumeral ligamentous complex (IGHLC or IGLLC) with intact scapular periosteum, which is stripped medially

Imaging Findings
- Normal position of the inferior glenohumeral ligament and labrum relative to underlying glenoid
- Accompanied by hemorrhage/edema of inferior glenohumeral ligament (IGL) attachment site
- + Anterior dislocation/subluxation
- Morphology: Periosteum redundant/lax
- Subtle linear increased signal intensity at base of usually nondisplaced labrum - sublabral hyperintensity

Top Differential Diagnoses
- Bankart Lesion
- Subscapularis Rupture
- Anterior Labroligamentous Periosteal Sleeve Avulsion (ALPSA) Lesion
- Normal Labrum and Attachment
- SLAP Lesion (esp. Type V & IX)
- Adhesive Capsulitis
- Supraspinatus Tear

Clinical Issues
- Most common signs/symptoms: Status post anterior dislocation (single or multiple dislocations)

Diagnostic Checklist
- Intact hypointense scapular periosteum

- ■ +/- Distraction of fracture fragment
  - ○ Associated posterolateral superior humeral head Hill-Sachs fx
  - ○ Hypointense redundant periosteum
  - ○ Edema and hemorrhage: Increased signal in surrounding soft tissues in acute cases
  - ○ +/- Hyperintense edema/hemorrhage between intact periosteum and adjacent glenoid
  - ○ FS PD FSE
    - ■ Sensitive for edema and fluid
    - ■ Greater contrast compared to long TE (T2 FSE)
- PD/Intermediate
  - ○ High resolution PD good for anatomic delineation of IGHLC
  - ○ +/- Fracture of the underlying glenoid, posterosuperior humeral head
  - ○ Intermediate signal in resynovialized labrum
- STIR
  - ○ Hyperintense edema and hemorrhage in surrounding soft tissues
  - ○ Provides improved contrast resolution to visualize medially stripped scapular periosteum
  - ○ Sensitive to associated anterior inferior bony glenoid hyperintense edema and cystic changes
- Normal position of the inferior glenohumeral ligament and labrum
- Labrum may be normal in appearance
  - ○ Labrum maintains hypointensity on axial images (T1 & T2WI)
- In chronic Perthes the labrum is partially healed and fibrosed
  - ○ +/- Heterogeneous hypointense to intermediate signal intensity on all pulse sequences
- MRI arthrography
  - ○ Chronic cases with resynovialization and nondisplacement
  - ○ ABER position
    - ■ = Abduction external rotation (arm placed behind the head)
    - ■ Coronal localizer to prescribe axial images

Imaging Recommendations
- Best imaging tool: MRI, consider MR arthrography especially with ABER positioning
- Protocol advice
  - ○ FS PD FSE axial, coronal; high resolution PD axial; MR arthrography
    - ■ Abduction and external rotation (ABER) imaging to detect detached labrum

DIFFERENTIAL DIAGNOSIS

Bankart Lesion
- Includes soft tissue (labrum only) Bankart and osseous Bankart (fracture of anterior inferior glenoid rim)
- Disrupted scapular periosteum
- Fibrosis of disrupted scapular periosteum may mimic intact periosteum as seen in the Perthes lesion
- Most common lesion after anterior dislocation
  - ○ Under 40 years of age
- +/- Hill-Sachs lesion of posterolateral humeral head
- Labrum often fragmented of avulsed
- +/- Anterior distraction/displacement of labrum
- Hyperintense on T2WI (esp. FS PD FSE)
  - ○ Soft tissue edema and effusion
  - ○ Hyperintense labral tear

Subscapularis Rupture
- Status post anterior dislocation
  - ○ > 40 years
  - ○ +/- Bankart fracture
  - ○ +/- Hill-Sachs lesion
- Posterior dislocation
  - ○ +/- History of tonic-clonic seizure
  - ○ Forward fall onto adducted internally rotated shoulder
- Discontinuous decreased signal subscapularis tendon with interposed hyperintensity on T2WI
- Hyperintense edema T2WI, (FS PD FSE) surrounding edema

PERTHES LESION

Anterior Labroligamentous Periosteal Sleeve Avulsion (ALPSA) Lesion
- Medially and inferiorly displaced labrum and IGL
- Intact periosteum
- IGHLC avulsion
- A type of Bankart variant
- +/- Bankart fracture
- +/- Hill-Sachs fracture

Normal Labrum and Attachment
- No history of dislocation
- No sublabral hyperintensity on T2WI
- No signal abnormalities including base of labrum

SLAP Lesion (esp. Type V & IX)
- Superior labral tear
- SLAP V (superior extension of a Bankart) and IX (circumferential labral tear) involve anterior inferior labrum
- Increased linear signal intensity on short TE sequences

Adhesive Capsulitis
- Thickened edematous capsule
- Hyperintense T2WI
- Frozen shoulder

Supraspinatus Tear
- Impingement - most common cause
- Status post anterior dislocation
  - > 40 years of age
  - +/- Bankart fracture
  - +/- Hill-Sachs lesion
- Hyperintense signal at tear site on T2WI
- +/- Tendon retraction
- +/- Fatty atrophy of cuff muscles
- Tendon size measured on coronal and sagittal images in centimeters

PATHOLOGY

General Features
- General path comments: The scapular periosteum is intact
- Etiology
  - Occurs after anterior shoulder dislocation
    - Often after initial dislocation
- Epidemiology
  - Shoulder is the most common dislocated joint, 50% of all joint dislocations
    - Perthes is uncommon Bankart variation ~ 5-10%

Gross Pathologic & Surgical Features
- Avulsion of the inferior glenohumeral labral ligamentous attachment to the glenoid after anterior dislocation of the shoulder
- Fibrosis and resynovialization in chronic cases
- +/- Normal at arthroscopy especially in the chronic state
- +/- Osteochondral fracture

Microscopic Features
- Hemorrhagic, torn, fibrocartilaginous labrum with variable degrees of fibrosis depending on chronicity

CLINICAL ISSUES

Presentation
- Most common signs/symptoms: Status post anterior dislocation (single or multiple dislocations)

Demographics
- Age: Younger patient (< 40 years)
- Gender: M > F

Natural History & Prognosis
- Recurrent instability if improper healing of initial lesion

Treatment
- Mobilized surgically or arthroscopically
- Normal anatomy is reapproximated and then repaired
- Bone block procedure in case of glenoid deficiency (large Bankart fracture)

DIAGNOSTIC CHECKLIST

Consider
- Intact hypointense scapular periosteum
- Use fluid sensitive sequence (FS PD FSE) in the axial plane

SELECTED REFERENCES

1. Wischer TK et al: Perthes lesion (a variant of the Bankart lesion): MR imaging and MR arthrographic findings with surgical correlation. AJR 178(1):233-7, 2002
2. Burkhart SS et al: Traumatic glenohumeral bone defects and their relationship to failure of arthroscopic Bankart repairs: Significance of the inverted-pear glenoid and the humeral engaging Hill-Sachs lesion. Arthroscopy 16(7):677-94, 2000
3. Grainger AJ et al: Direct MR arthrography: A review of current use. Clin Radiol 55(3):163-76, 2000
4. Cvitanic OP et al: Using abduction and external rotation of the shoulder to increase the sensitivity of MR arthrography in revealing tears of the anterior glenoid labrum. AJR 169(3):837-44, 1997
5. Tirman PF et al: A practical approach to imaging of the shoulder with emphasis on MR imaging. Orthop Clin North Am 28(4):483-515, 1997
6. Neviaser TJ: The anterior labroligamentous periosteal sleeve avulsion lesion: A cause of anterior instability of the shoulder. Arthroscopy 9(1):17-21, 1993

PERTHES LESION

IMAGE GALLERY

Typical

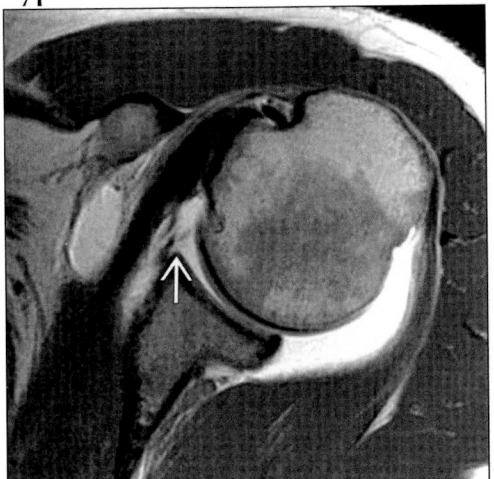

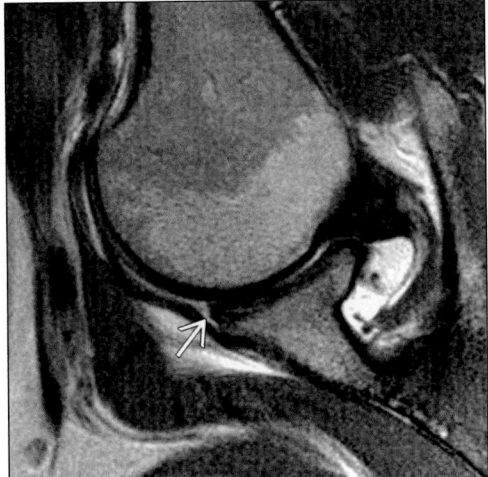

(Left) Axial T1 MR arthrogram image demonstrates tearing of the anterior labrum (arrow) at the mid glenoid level. *(Right)* Sagittal oblique post-arthrographic T1 ABER MR arthrogram image shows a Perthes lesion (arrow) with an intact scapular periosteum. The labrum was slightly fragmented but in relatively normal position at arthroscopy.

Typical

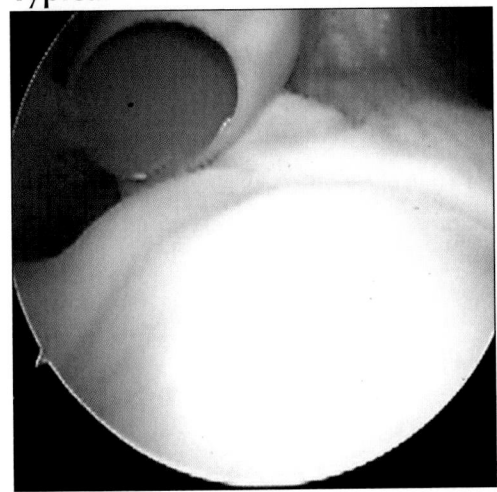

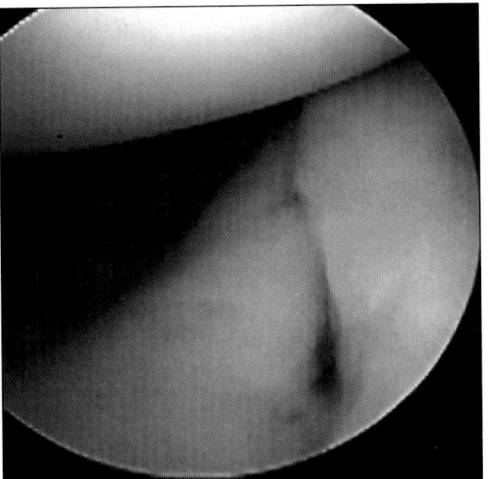

(Left) Sagittal oblique arthroscopic view shows a normal positioned labrum. The cannula is lifting the meniscoid edge of the labrum up. *(Right)* Axial oblique arthroscopic view demonstrates mobility of the labrum with traction, consistent with a Perthes lesion. At first inspection, the patient was considered normal and capsulorraphy was initially considered as a treatment option.

Typical

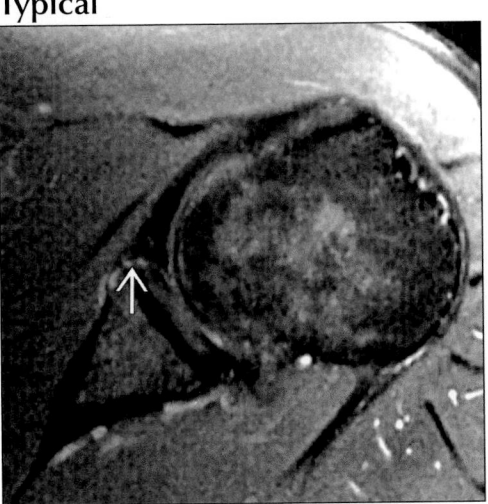

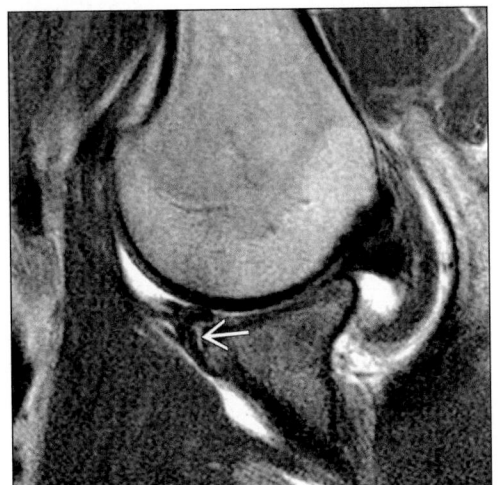

(Left) Axial FS PD FSE MR demonstrates increased signal intensity at the base of the labrum (arrow) in this patient after anterior dislocation. *(Right)* PD FSE MR ABER image in the same patient demonstrates a Perthes lesion with increased signal intensity (arrow) "rounding the corner" of the glenoid beneath the detached labrum.

ALPSA LESION

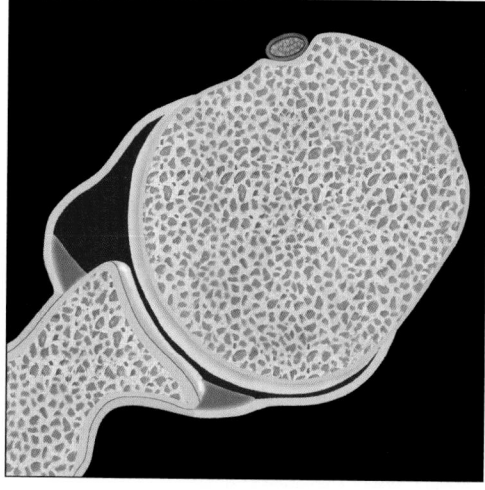

Axial graphic shows medial displacement and inferior rotation of the inferior glenohumeral labroligamentous attachment to the glenoid. This is the most important feature of an ALPSA lesion.

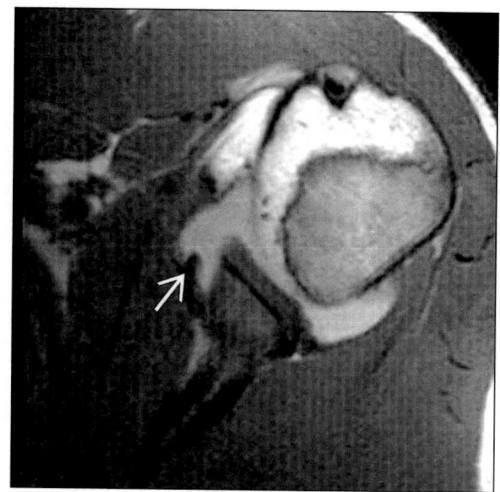

Axial T1 arthrogram of ALPSA lesion demonstrates medial displacement of the IGHLC (arrow) along the anterior neck of glenoid & surrounding hemorrhage.

TERMINOLOGY

Abbreviations and Synonyms

- Anterior labroligamentous periosteal sleeve avulsion (ALPSA) lesion

Definitions

- Avulsion of inferior glenohumeral labroligamentous complex (IGHLC or IGLLC) from anterior inferior glenoid with an intact scapular periosteum
- Medial displacement and inferior shifting of the IGHLC
- Bankart variation lesion (ALPSA has intact anterior scapular periosteum)
- Glenoid deficiency
  - Bankart fracture decreases inferior glenoid surface area resulting in continued instability

IMAGING FINDINGS

General Features

- Best diagnostic clue
  - Medial displacement of IGHLC on axial and coronal MR images in patient with history of anterior dislocation
    - Acute cases: Edema/hemorrhage

- Chronic cases: Variable degrees of fibrosis, fibrous mass
- Location: Anterior inferior shoulder
- Size
  - Varies from
    - Subtle medial displacement and inferior rotation
    - Displacement up to a few centimeters especially if associated with an underlying glenoid fracture
- Morphology
  - Irregular, often amorphous mass
    - Fibrotic IGHL complex
    - Medially displaced along scapular neck

Radiographic Findings

- Radiography
  - +/- Anterior inferior glenoid fracture = Bankart fracture
  - +/- Hill-Sachs impaction fracture (posterolateral superior humeral head)

CT Findings

- NECT
  - +/- Anterior inferior glenoid fracture = Bankart fracture
  - +/- Posterolateral superior humeral head (HH) fracture (Hill-Sachs)
- CT arthrography
  - Medial displacement of IGHLC

DDx: ALPSA Lesion

Bankart Lesion	Bankart Fx	Non Displ Tear	IGL Tear	Adhes Capsulitis
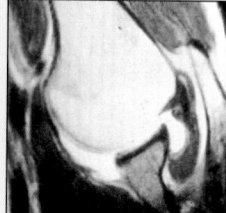	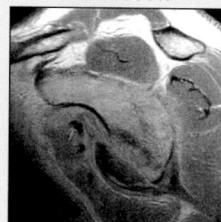	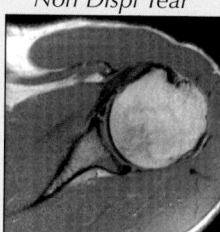	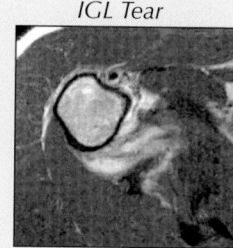	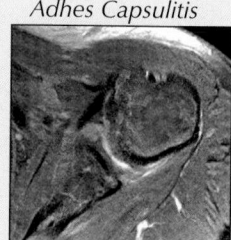
ABER T1 Arthro	Sag PD FSE MR	Ax PD FSE MR	Ax T1 Arthro.	Ax FS PD FSE

ALPSA LESION

Key Facts

Terminology
- Avulsion of inferior glenohumeral labroligamentous complex (IGHLC or IGLLC) from anterior inferior glenoid with an intact scapular periosteum
- Medial displacement and inferior shifting of the IGHLC

Imaging Findings
- Medial displacement of IGHLC on axial and coronal MR images in patient with history of anterior dislocation
- Acute cases: Edema/hemorrhage
- Chronic cases: Variable degrees of fibrosis, fibrous mass
- Medial and inferior displacement of labrum

Top Differential Diagnoses
- Bankart Lesion
- Perthes Lesion
- HAGL Lesion
- Subscapularis Tear
- Supraspinatus Tear
- IGL Tear

Clinical Issues
- Most common signs/symptoms: Status post anterior dislocation (single or multiple dislocations) - pain & apprehension with abduction and external rotation

Diagnostic Checklist
- Bankart lesion in differential diagnosis
- Identify medial or inferior labral displacement

MR Findings
- T1WI
  - Deformity of axillary pouch with medial displacement of anteroinferior labrum and IGL
  - Hypointense osseous edema associated with Bankart and Hill-Sachs fractures
- T2WI
  - Hyperintense edema and hemorrhage in joint capsule and surrounding soft tissues
  - +/- Fracture of the underlying glenoid
    - Increased signal intensity and visible hypointense fracture line
    - +/- Distraction of fracture fragment
    - = Bankart fracture
  - +/- Hill-Sachs fracture
  - Medial displacement of thickened/hyperintense IGHLC - acute
    - Hypointense - chronic
  - FS PD FSE/PD FSE sensitive for osseous and capsular edema
- PD/Intermediate
  - Less sensitive for osseous edema
  - Visualization of articular cartilage and labral tears
  - High resolution PD for anatomic delineation of IGHLC and fibrosis (chronic)
  - +/- Fracture of the underlying glenoid, posterosuperior humeral head
- STIR
  - Hyperintense edema and hemorrhage in surrounding soft tissues
  - Increased contrast resolution for hyperintense osseous edema
  - Improved visualization of axillary pouch displacement adjacent to hyperintense fluid and edema
- MR arthrography
  - Medial and inferior displacement of labrum
  - Chronic cases with resynovialization and minimal medial displacement
  - ABER (abduction external rotation) position helpful
  - Inferior ALPSA with medial and inferior displacement below inferior pole of glenoid

Imaging Recommendations
- Best imaging tool: MRI
- Protocol advice
  - High resolution PD, FS PD FSE in axial and coronal plane
  - MR arthrography helpful especially with ABER positioning

DIFFERENTIAL DIAGNOSIS

Bankart Lesion
- No medial displacement/inferior shift
- Most common lesion after anterior dislocation
  - < 40 years
- Periosteal disruption
- +/- Bankart fracture
  - +/- Glenoid deficiency
- +/- Hill-Sachs lesion
- Labrum often fragmented
- +/- Anterior distraction/displacement of labrum
- Hyperintense on T2WI (esp. FS PD FSE)
  - Soft tissue edema
  - Effusion

Perthes Lesion
- No medial displacement
- No periosteal disruption
- ABER position helpful
- A type of Bankart variant
- +/- Bankart fracture
- +/- Hill-Sachs lesion
- Hyperintense on T2WI (esp. FS PD FSE)
  - Soft tissue edema
  - Effusion

HAGL Lesion
- Humeral capsular disruption of IGL attachment
- Status post dislocation
- +/- Bankart fracture
- +/- Hill-Sachs lesion
- Hyperintense on T2WI (esp. FS PD FSE)
  - Soft tissue edema

○ Effusion
○ Injured capsule (J-shaped axillary pouch)

Subscapularis Tear
- Status post anterior dislocation
  ○ > 40 years; +/- Bankart fracture; +/- Hill-Sachs lesion
- Posterior dislocation
  ○ +/- History of tonic-clonic seizure
  ○ Forward fall onto adducted internally rotated shoulder
- Discontinuous decreased signal of subscapularis tendon with interposed hyperintensity on T2WI
- Surrounding edema - hyperintense on T2WI (esp. FS PD FSE)

Supraspinatus Tear
- Impingement
- Status post anterior dislocation
  ○ > 40 years old
  ○ +/- Bankart fracture
  ○ +/- Hill-Sachs lesion
- Thickened, increased signal intensity tendon on T2WI most common
  ○ Discontinuous tendon with interposed hyperintensity

IGL Tear
- Discontinuous decreased signal capsule with interposed hyperintensity on T2WI
- Status post anterior dislocation/subluxation
- +/- Bankart fracture
- +/- Hill-Sachs lesion

Adhesive Capsulitis (Adhes Capsulitis)
- Thickened edematous capsule
- Hyperintense on T2WI
- Frozen shoulder
- +/- Secondary to abduction external rotation injury or systemic disease (diabetes)

PATHOLOGY

General Features
- General path comments
  ○ Medial displacement of labroligamentous structures leads to healing of IGHLC medially on scapular neck
    ■ Decreases chances for stable healing
- Etiology: Anterior shoulder dislocation resulting in IGHLC avulsion with medial displacement of intact scapular periosteum and "rolling up" of IGHLC
- Epidemiology: Shoulder dislocations account for 50% of all joint dislocations
- Associated abnormalities
  ○ Glenoid fracture
  ○ Hill-Sachs fracture
  ○ Rotator interval tear
  ○ Superior labrum anterior-posterior (SLAP) lesion
  ○ Rotator cuff tear

Gross Pathologic & Surgical Features
- Avulsion of IGHLC attachment to glenoid with medial displacement after anterior dislocation of shoulder
- Glenoid deficiency requires open procedure (usually bone block)

- Fibrous tissue deposited in chronic ALPSA

Microscopic Features
- Hemorrhagic, torn, fibrocartilaginous labrum with variable degrees of fibrosis depending on chronicity

CLINICAL ISSUES

Presentation
- Most common signs/symptoms: Status post anterior dislocation (single or multiple dislocations) - pain & apprehension with abduction and external rotation
- Clinical profile: Positive apprehension test in patients with recurrent shoulder instability

Demographics
- Age: Typically younger patient (< 40 years)
- Gender: M > F

Natural History & Prognosis
- Recurrent shoulder instability if improper (in displaced position) healing of initial lesion
- IGL incompetence

Treatment
- Surgical
  ○ Dissection of ALPSA away from glenoid and conversion to Bankart (mobilize and disrupt scapular periosteum)
    ■ Place labrum on anterior lateral corner of glenoid back in anatomic location for treatment of recurrent instability
    ■ Correct IGL capsular stretch or injury

DIAGNOSTIC CHECKLIST

Consider
- Bankart lesion in differential diagnosis

Image Interpretation Pearls
- Identify medial or inferior labral displacement
- Do not confuse a cord-like middle glenohumeral ligament for an ALPSA lesion

SELECTED REFERENCES
1. Gartsman GM et al: Arthroscopic treatment of anterior-inferior glenohumeral instability. Two to five-year follow-up. J Bone Joint Surg 82-A(7):991-1003, 2000
2. Grainger AJ et al: Direct MR arthrography: A review of current use. Clin Radiol 55(3):163-76, 2000
3. Burkhart SS et al: Traumatic glenohumeral bone defects and their relationship to failure of arthroscopic Bankart repairs. Significance of the inverted-pear glenoid and the humeral engaging Hill-Sachs lesion. Arthroscopy 16(7):677-94, 2000
4. Tirman PF et al: A practical approach to imaging of the shoulder with emphasis on MR imaging, Orthop Clin North 28(4):483-515, 1997
5. Cvitanic O et al: Using abduction and external rotation of the shoulder to increase the sensitivity of MR arthrography in revealing tears of the anterior glenoid labrum. AJR 169(3):837-44, 1997

ALPSA LESION

IMAGE GALLERY

Typical

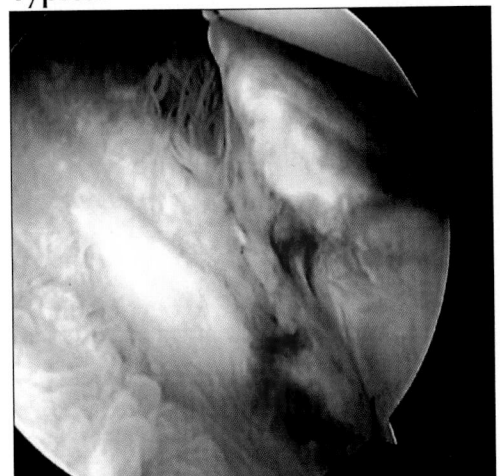
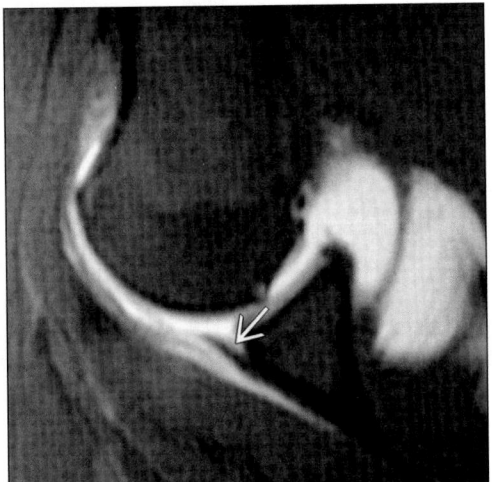

(Left) Axial oblique arthroscopic view of an ALPSA lesion demonstrates medial displacement of the IGHLC along the neck of the glenoid + surrounding hemorrhage. Face of glenoid is far right, humeral head is at the top right of the picture. *(Right)* ABER MR T1 arthrogram shows medial displacement of the IGHLC attachment (arrow) to the glenoid consistent with an ALPSA lesion.

Typical

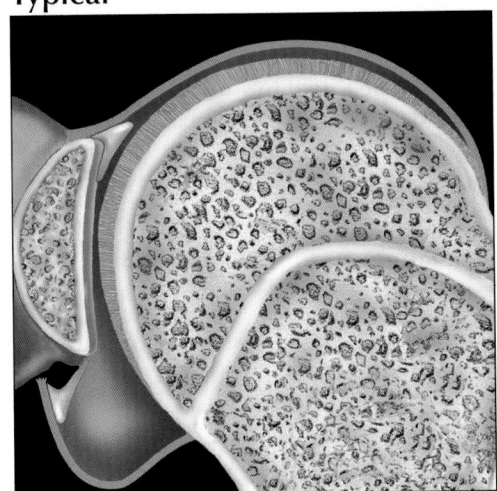
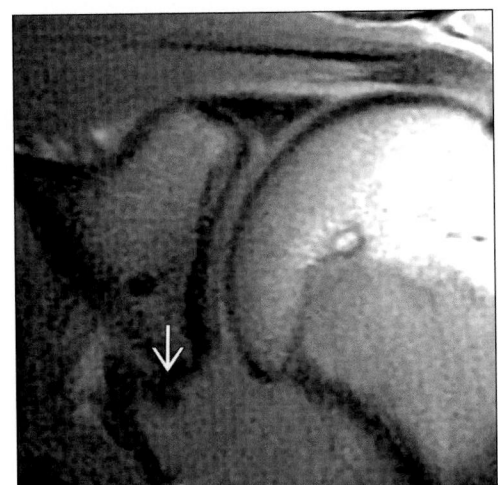

(Left) Coronal graphic shows medial and inferior labral ligamentous displacement along the inferior neck of the scapula. *(Right)* Coronal PD FSE MR image demonstrates medial displacement (arrow) along the scapular neck of the labroligamentous attachment, consistent with an ALPSA lesion.

Typical

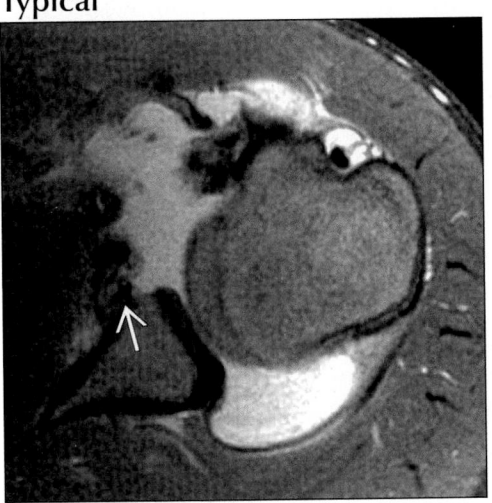
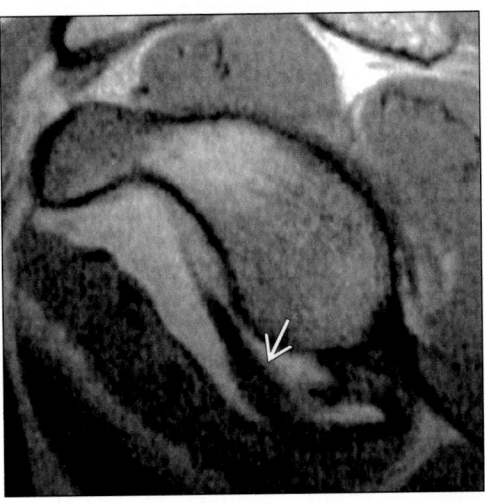

(Left) Axial FS PD FSE MR demonstrates medial displacement (arrow) of the labroligamentous attachment in association with disruption of the subscapularis tendon in this post-operative unstable patient. *(Right)* Sagittal T2 FSE MR demonstrates inferior and medial shifting of the labroligamentous attachment on the glenoid (arrow).

GLAD LESION

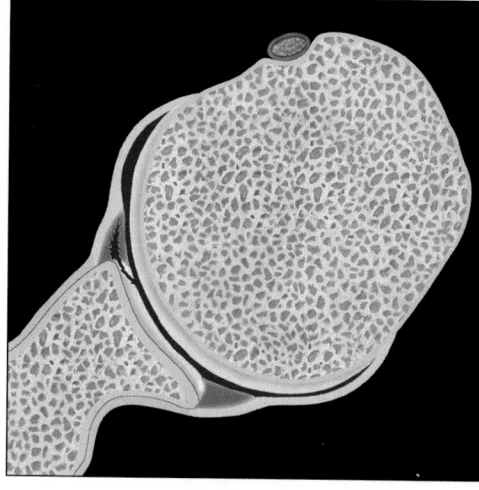

Axial graphic shows a flap tear of the anterior glenoid labrum and a small articular cartilage defect (chondral flap) adjacent to the labral tear.

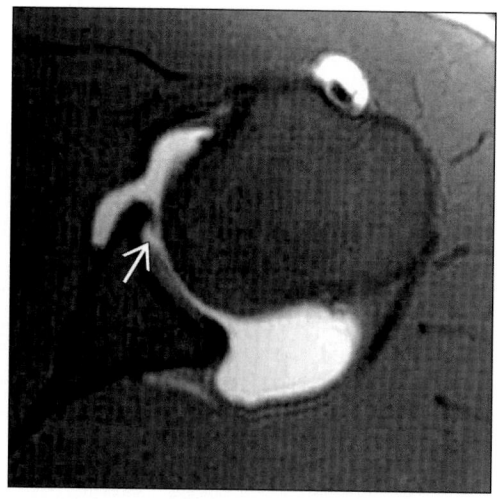

Axial FS T1 arthrogram shows a hyaline articular cartilage defect (arrow) with adjacent fraying/partial tearing of the base of the labrum in a clinically stable patient.

TERMINOLOGY

Abbreviations and Synonyms
- Glenoid labrum articular disruption (GLAD), glenoid articular rim divot (GARD)

Definitions
- Partial tear of the anterior glenoid labrum with adjacent articular cartilage chondral defect in clinically stable patient
- Labrum is not detached

IMAGING FINDINGS

General Features
- Best diagnostic clue: Irregular increased signal intensity on FS PD FSE/T2WI sequences within the anterior labrum and adjacent cartilage
- Location: Anterior glenoid rim and adjacent hyaline articular cartilage
- Size: Varies from small tear (1-2 mm) to approximately 1 centimeter
- Morphology
  - Irregular interface between fluid and/or granulation in tear and adjacent labrum
  - Larger tears +/- instability
  - Chondral lesion as flap tear or divot

MR Findings
- T1WI
  - Irregular intermediate signal in substance of the labrum or at interface with glenoid = tear, fraying
  - Labral irregularity and chondral lesion not well seen on T1WI
  - Hypointense subchondral sclerosis anterior inferior glenoid rim
  - Anterior inferior capsular thickening
  - Labral tear is typically non detached
  - +/- Underlying hypointense bone marrow edema
- T2WI
  - Irregular hyperintense signal in substance of labrum or at interface with glenoid
  - +/- Hyperintense fluid within the tear
  - Hyperintense chondral defect
    - Divot
    - Flap
  - +/- Underlying hyperintense bone marrow edema
  - Labral tear usually nondisplaced
  - FS PD FSE
    - Increased signal at labral attachment, or in substance of the labrum
    - Chondral defect visualized on FS PD FSE
    - Glenoid rim edema is hyperintense
  - T2 FSE
    - Chondral defect not well visualized
- PD/Intermediate

DDx: GLAD Lesion

SLAP Cyst	Bankart	Perthes Cyst	Reverse Bankart	ALPSA
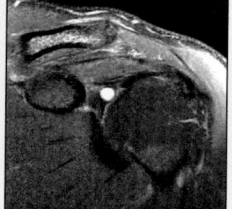	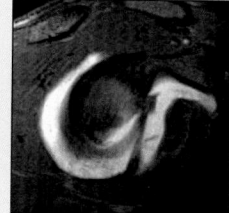	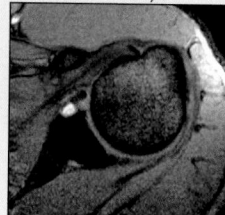	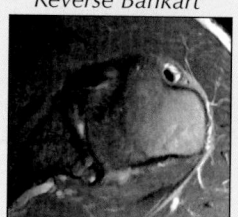	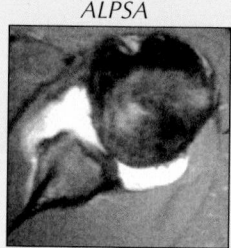
Cor FS PD FSE	Sag FS PD FSE	Ax T2* GRE MR	Ax FS PD FSE	Ax T2* GRE MR

GLAD LESION

Key Facts

Terminology
- Partial tear of the anterior glenoid labrum with adjacent articular cartilage chondral defect in clinically stable patient

Imaging Findings
- Best diagnostic clue: Irregular increased signal intensity on FS PD FSE/T2WI sequences within the anterior labrum and adjacent cartilage

Top Differential Diagnoses
- Bankart Lesion
- Loose Body
- Anterior Labroligamentous Periosteal Sleeve Avulsion (ALPSA) Lesion
- SLAP Lesion
- Posterior Labral Tear

- Perthes Lesion

Pathology
- Labral tear without associated capsular ligament disruption
- Forced adduction injury on abducted arm in external rotation
- Abduction external rotation injury in case of subluxation without dislocation

Clinical Issues
- Pain, especially with internal rotation or with adduction

Diagnostic Checklist
- Small anterior labral tear with adjacent chondral defect seen on FS PD FSE or PD FSE

  - o Intermediate to increased signal in labrum or at the interface with the glenoid = tear, fraying
    - Especially if fluid is found within the tear
    - PD high resolution images useful
    - +/- Intermediate signal intensity of underlying bone reactive changes (less sensitive compared to FS PD FSE)
- T2* GRE
  - o Labral tear hyperintense
  - o Cartilage defect not seen if joint fluid is isointense to hyaline cartilage
- T1 C+: Defect may enhance with intravenous contrast thus increasing it's conspicuity
- MR arthrography
  - o Contrast filling tear
  - o Contrast extends into chondral defect

Imaging Recommendations
- Best imaging tool: MRI
- Protocol advice
  - o FS PD FSE
  - o Arthrography in the ABER position demonstrates partial labral tear by placing stress on the capsular ligamentous attachments

DIFFERENTIAL DIAGNOSIS

Bankart Lesion
- Unstable patient
- Underlying fracture or chondral defect
- History of anterior dislocation (not seen in GLAD lesion)
- +/- Underlying Bankart fracture
- +/- Hill-Sachs fracture

Loose Body
- Clinical differential diagnosis in physical exam
- +/- Catching, locking, and/or clicking
- Absence of labral tear
- Round lesion of decreased signal intensity on all pulse sequences

Anterior Labroligamentous Periosteal Sleeve Avulsion (ALPSA) Lesion
- Intact scapular periosteum
- History of anterior dislocation
- +/- Underlying Bankart fracture
- +/- Hill-Sachs fracture
- Medial displacement of IGHLC (inferior glenohumeral labral ligament complex)

SLAP Lesion
- Superior labral biceps anchor tear
- Lesion propagates to
  - o Anterior labrum (type V)
  - o MGL (middle glenohumeral ligament) (type VII)
  - o Posterior labrum (type VIII)
  - o Circumferentially (type IX)
  - o +/- Flap labral component
- +/- Speed's (bicipital resistance) test, O'Brien's test (active compression test for SLAP lesions)
- +/- Traction injury
- Increased signal intensity abnormality on short TE sequences in biceps anchor
- +/- Hyperintense tear on T2WI
- +/- Paralabral cyst

Posterior Labral Tear
- History of posterior dislocation/subluxation
- Increased signal intensity on short TE sequences in posterior labrum
- +/- Underlying Bankart fracture
- +/- Hill-Sachs fracture
- Pain with adduction, internal rotation

Perthes Lesion
- Intact scapular periosteum
- History of anterior dislocation
- +/- Underlying Bankart fracture
- +/- Hill-Sachs fracture
- Cyst beneath periosteum
- Normal labral position

GLAD LESION

PATHOLOGY

General Features
- General path comments
  - Labral tear without associated capsular ligament disruption
    - Described initially in stable patients
- Etiology
  - Forced adduction injury on abducted arm in external rotation
  - Abduction external rotation injury in case of subluxation without dislocation
  - Impaction of humeral head against glenoid fossa
- Epidemiology: Uncommon injury
- Associated abnormalities: Underlying trabecular injury of glenoid may occur

Gross Pathologic & Surgical Features
- Torn labrum
  - Superficial anterior inferior labrum
  - Inferior flap-type labral tear
  - IGL firmly attached to labrum and glenoid rim
- Adjacent hyaline chondral defect
  - Anterior inferior quadrant of glenoid fossa
  - Fibrillation
  - Erosion
- Variable amounts of hemorrhage
- +/- Granulation
- +/- Fibrosis depending on chronicity of lesion

Microscopic Features
- Hemorrhagic, torn, fibrocartilaginous labrum with variable degrees of fibrosis depending on chronicity
- Articular cartilage defect
- +/- Infiltration of inflammatory cells
- +/- Inflamed synovium

CLINICAL ISSUES

Presentation
- Most common signs/symptoms
  - Pain, especially with internal rotation or with adduction
  - Clicking, locking

Demographics
- Age: Younger physically active patient
- Gender: M > F, due to injury during physical activity with extreme range of motion

Natural History & Prognosis
- Continued pain unless healing/resynovialization occurs
- Continued pain is indication for arthroscopic debridement
- Focal osteoarthritic change

Treatment
- Conservative
  - Physical therapy until healing
- Surgical
  - Arthroscopic debridement

DIAGNOSTIC CHECKLIST

Consider
- Bankart lesion in patient that has dislocated and/or is unstable

Image Interpretation Pearls
- Small anterior labral tear with adjacent chondral defect seen on FS PD FSE or PD FSE
- Accurate history important
- MR arthrography useful for the detection of the partial labral tear

SELECTED REFERENCES

1. Amrami KK et al: Radiologic case study. Glenolabral articular disruption (GLAD) lesion. Orthopedics 25(1):29, 95-6, 2002
2. Grainger AJ et al: Direct MR arthrography: A review of current use. Clin Radiol 55(3):163-76, 2000
3. Sanders TG et al: The glenolabral articular disruption lesion: MR arthrography with arthroscopic correlation. AJR 172(1):171-5, 1999
4. Neviaser TJ: The GLAD lesion: Another cause of anterior shoulder pain. Arthroscopy 9(1):22-3, 1993

GLAD LESION

IMAGE GALLERY

Typical

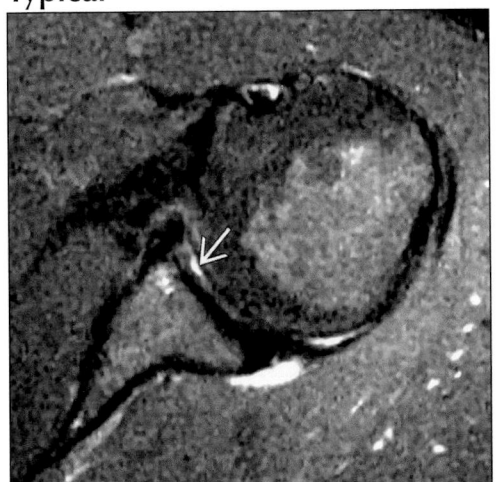
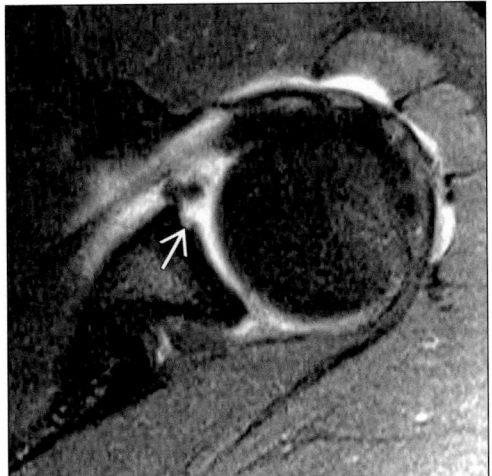

(Left) Axial FS PD FSE MR shows a small articular cartilage defect (arrow) with underlying reactive bone marrow edema. There is fraying at the base of the labrum. A small posterior paralabral cyst was associated with an old healed posterior tear. *(Right)* Axial FS PD FSE MR shows an articular cartilage defect (arrow) with adjacent torn labrum in a clinically stable patient.

Typical

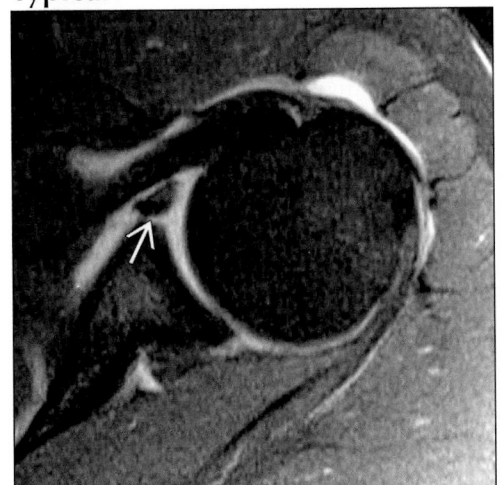
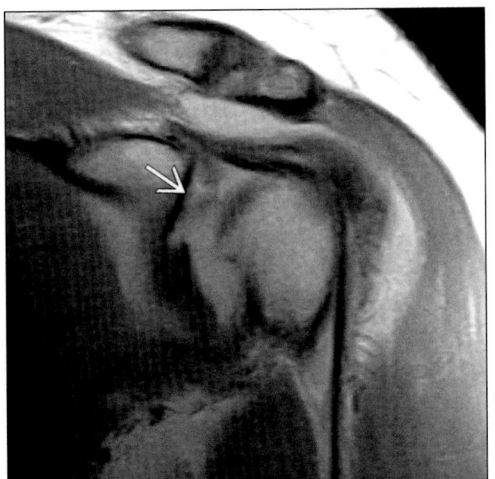

(Left) Axial FS PD FSE MR shows small corner fracture (arrow) of anterior glenoid with an adjacent tear of anterior labrum. Patient was stable clinically but experienced pain & a clunk with humeral rotation. Positive history of remote subluxation. *(Right)* Coronal PD FSE MR Shows the chondral defect (arrow).

Typical

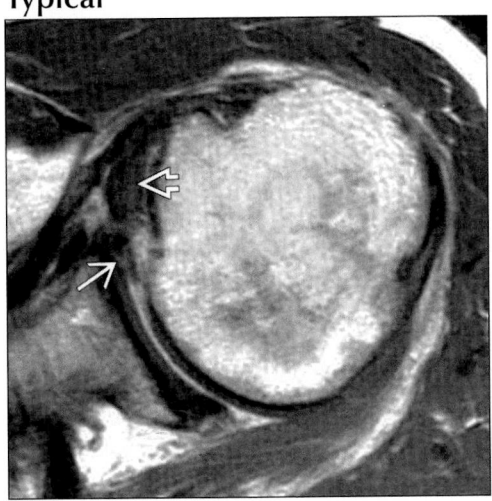
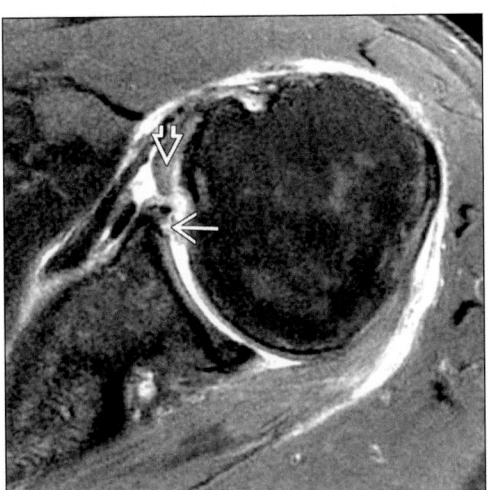

(Left) Axial PD FSE MR demonstrates a GLAD lesion (arrow) in this patient with a dislocated biceps tendon (open arrow) and extensive partial tearing of the subscapularis tendon. *(Right)* Axial FS PD FSE MR shows GLAD lesion (arrow) in addition to biceps instability (open arrow) resulting from chronic impingement and a rotator interval "hidden lesion".

HAGL LESION

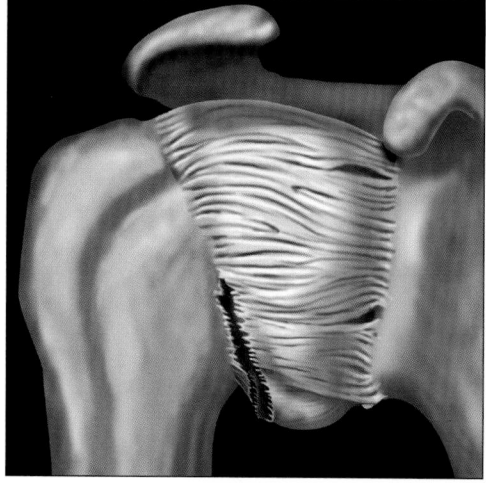

Coronal graphic shows a tear of inferior glenohumeral ligament at its humeral attachment, consistent with a HAGL lesion (humeral avulsion of the glenohumeral ligament).

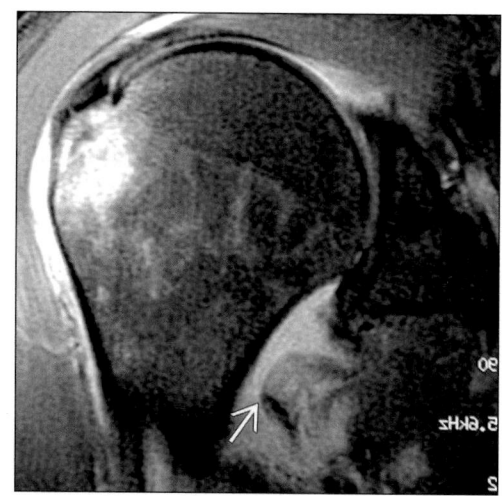

Coronal PD FSE MR shows a HAGL lesion (arrow) with the torn inferior axillary pouch retracted from its anatomic neck attachment.

TERMINOLOGY

Abbreviations and Synonyms
- Humeral avulsion of the glenohumeral ligament
- HAGL + humeral bone avulsion = BHAGL (bone humeral avulsion of glenohumeral ligament)

Definitions
- Tearing/avulsion of the inferior glenohumeral ligament (IGHL or IGL) attachment to the humerus after anterior dislocation/subluxation

IMAGING FINDINGS

General Features
- Best diagnostic clue
  - Discontinuous IGHL fibers at the humeral interface
    - Capsule assumes "J" shape on coronal images (normal axillary pouch has a U-shaped contour)
  - + Surrounding edema/hemorrhage seen best on coronal PD/T2 images
- Location: Humeral avulsion of the inferior glenohumeral ligament attachment site
- Size: Varies from a partial tear in capsule to large avulsion
- Morphology: Varies from discrete tear to edematous markedly irregular tear

Radiographic Findings
- Radiography
  - +/- Bankart fracture (anterior inferior glenoid fracture)
  - +/- Hill-Sachs deformity (posterolateral humeral head impaction)
  - +/- Avulsion of bone fragment of humeral neck/head = BHAGL

CT Findings
- NECT
  - +/- Bankart fracture (anterior inferior glenoid fracture)
  - +/- Hill-Sachs deformity - posterolateral humeral head impaction fracture
- CT arthrography
  - Extravasation of contrast through humeral interface defect into anterior parahumeral soft tissues

MR Findings
- T1WI
  - Decreased signal intensity at humeral interface of capsule
  - +/- Fat signal within bone fragment (marrow)
- T2WI
  - Discontinuous capsule at the humeral interface - anatomic neck attachment of IGL (inferior glenohumeral ligament)

DDx: HAGL Lesion

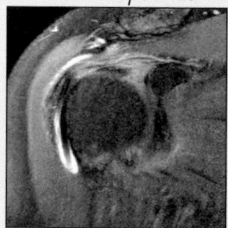
Adhes Capsulitis
Cor FS PD FSE

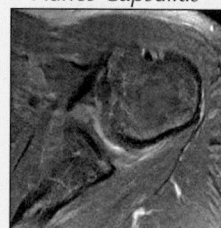
Adhes Capsulitis
Ax FS PD FSE

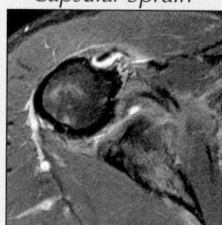
Capsular Sprain
Ax FS PD FSE

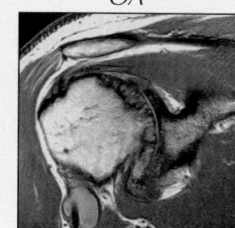
OA
Cor PD FSE MR

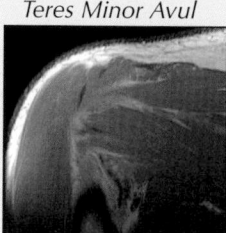
Teres Minor Avul
Cor PD FSE MR

HAGL LESION

Key Facts

Terminology
- Tearing/avulsion of the inferior glenohumeral ligament (IGHL or IGL) attachment to the humerus after anterior dislocation/subluxation

Imaging Findings
- Discontinuous IGHL fibers at the humeral interface
- Capsule assumes "J" shape on coronal images (normal axillary pouch has a U-shaped contour)

Top Differential Diagnoses
- Midcapsular Disruption (IGL Tear)
- Bankart Lesion
- Perthes Lesion
- ALPSA Lesion
- Adhesive Capsulitis (Adhes Capsulitis)
- Subscapularis Tear

- Synovitis
- Reverse HAGL

Pathology
- Humeral avulsion of the inferior glenohumeral ligament
- Torn capsule at the humeral attachment

Clinical Issues
- Most common signs/symptoms: Patient with recent anterior shoulder dislocation complaining of continued pain, with apprehension

Diagnostic Checklist
- High index of suspicion for capsular damage after anterior dislocation of the shoulder

---

- o Edema and hemorrhage at humeral interface on axial T2 images
  - ■ Hyperintensity
- o +/- Hill-Sachs lesion
  - ■ Hyperintense edema associated with fx
  - ■ +/- Depression or flattening posterolateral humeral head
- o Hyperintense supraspinatus tears/strains
  - ■ Fluid signal intensity filled gap (hyperintense)
- PD/Intermediate
  - o High resolution images show discontinuous capsule
  - o PD FSE sensitive to scarring of axillary pouch while FS PD FSE is sensitive to edema in acute stretching injuries or tears
- T2* GRE: Hemorrhage in chronic cases may "bloom"
- MR arthrography
  - o Extravasation of contrast through tear
    - ■ Contrast inferior to axillary pouch

Imaging Recommendations
- Best imaging tool: MRI
- Protocol advice: FS PD FSE, PD FSE coronal and axial images

DIFFERENTIAL DIAGNOSIS

Midcapsular Disruption (IGL Tear)
- Axillary pouch sprain
- Status post anterior dislocation/subluxation
- Discontinuous capsule
  - o Axillary pouch/IGHL
  - o Normally decreased in signal intensity
- Hyperintense on T2WI
- 1/3 lesions seen in cadaveric study on anterior dislocation lesions

Bankart Lesion
- Difficult to asses exact location of IGL in cases of extensive labral capsular trauma
- Most common lesion after anterior dislocation
- < 40 years old
- Periosteal disruption

- +/- Bankart fracture
  - o +/- Glenoid deficiency
- +/- Hill-Sachs lesion
- Labrum often fragmented
- +/- Anterior distraction/displacement of labrum

Perthes Lesion
- Intact periosteum
- Abduction with external rotation (ABER) imaging helpful
- A type of Bankart variant
- +/- Bankart fracture
- +/- Hill-Sachs lesion

ALPSA Lesion
- Medial displacement
- A type of Bankart variant
- +/- Bankart fracture
- +/- Hill-Sachs lesion
- ABER imaging helpful

Adhesive Capsulitis (Adhes Capsulitis)
- Thickened edematous capsule
- Hyperintense capsule on T2WI
- Frozen shoulder
- +/- Secondary to primary cause (e.g., rotator cuff disease)

Subscapularis Tear
- Status post anterior dislocation
  - o > 40 years old
  - o +/- Bankart fracture
  - o +/- Hill-Sachs lesion
- Posterior dislocation
  - o +/- History of tonic-clonic seizure
  - o Forward fall onto adducted and internally rotated shoulder
- Discontinuous decreased signal subscapularis tendon with interposed hyperintensity on T2WI
- Hyperintense on T2WI (esp. FS PD FSE) - surrounding edema

Synovitis
- Multiple causes

- +/- Osteoarthritis (OA)
- Thickened synovium
- Intermediate signal synovium on FS PD FSE
- Fluid is hyperintense on FS PD FSE
- Synovitis frequently seen in axillary pouch

Reverse HAGL
- Avulsion of posterior shoulder stabilizers
- +/- Teres minor tears
- Hyperintense edema at injury site on T2WI

PATHOLOGY

General Features
- General path comments
  - Humeral avulsion of the inferior glenohumeral ligament
  - Unusual compared to classic Bankart lesion after anterior dislocation
  - May be associated with small bone fragment from humerus
    - = BHAGL lesion
- Etiology: Anterior shoulder dislocation or severe subluxation
- Epidemiology
  - Anterior shoulder dislocation = 50% of all joint dislocations
  - Cadaveric study showed ~ 30% of experimental dislocations are associated with HAGL + subscapularis tendon tears
  - Isolated HAGL lesions uncommon
- Associated abnormalities
  - Tears of the rotator interval may lead to continued instability
  - Hill-Sachs fracture of posterosuperior humeral head
  - Partial or complete rotator cuff tears post anterior dislocation
  - Biceps tendon/anchor lesions in ~ 12% of patients post anterior dislocation
  - Brachial plexus injuries, posterior glenoid labral tear in up to 11% of patients post anterior dislocation

Gross Pathologic & Surgical Features
- Torn capsule at the humeral attachment
- Angled scope is often needed to visualize the defect

Microscopic Features
- Torn glenohumeral capsule
- + Variable amounts of hemorrhage
- + Inflammatory cells

Staging, Grading or Classification Criteria
- IGL labral complex (IGLLC) lesions
  - Bankart lesion = avulsion of IGLLC from the glenoid rim
    - Labral avulsion
    - Labral avulsion + anterior inferior glenoid rim fracture
  - Axillary pouch sprain = IGL complex tears at its mid portion
  - HAGL - IGL complex tears from its humeral insertion

CLINICAL ISSUES

Presentation
- Most common signs/symptoms: Patient with recent anterior shoulder dislocation complaining of continued pain, with apprehension
- Clinical profile: Positive apprehension test in patients with recurrent instability

Demographics
- Age: Adults
- Gender: M > F

Natural History & Prognosis
- Recurrent instability in selected cases
- +/- Healing with conservative treatment

Treatment
- Conservative treatment in selected cases
  - Small tears with surrounding hemorrhage allowing fibrinogenic/healing factors to accomplish healing
  - Physical therapy
- Surgical or arthroscopic repair if continued instability
- Need angled arthroscope for adequate visualization

DIAGNOSTIC CHECKLIST

Consider
- Associated Bankart lesion, rotator cuff tear, Hill-Sachs lesion

Image Interpretation Pearls
- Coronal and axial images helpful
- High index of suspicion for capsular damage after anterior dislocation of the shoulder
- Abnormal morphology of axillary pouch of IGL with "J" shaped configuration on coronal images

SELECTED REFERENCES
1. Bokor DJ et al: Anterior instability of the glenohumeral joint with humeral avulsion of the glenohumeral ligament. A review of 41 cases. J Bone Joint Surg Br 81(1):93-6, 1999
2. Stoller DW et al: The Shoulder. Magnetic resonance imaging in orthopaedics and sports medicine. vol 1. 2nd ed. Philadelphia PA, J.B. Lippincott, 597-742, 1997
3. Beltran J et al: Glenohumeral instability: Evaluation with MR arthrography. Radiographics 17(3):657-73, 1997
4. Tirman PF et al: A practical approach to imaging of the shoulder with emphasis on MR imaging. Orthop Clin North Am 28(4):483-515, 1997
5. Tirman PF et al: Humeral avulsion of the anterior shoulder stabilizing structures after anterior shoulder dislocation: Demonstration by MRI and MR arthrography. Skeletal Radiol 25(8):743-8, 1996
6. Wolf EM et al: Humeral avulsion of glenohumeral ligaments as a cause of anterior shoulder instability. Arthroscopy 11(5):600-7, 1995

HAGL LESION

IMAGE GALLERY

Typical

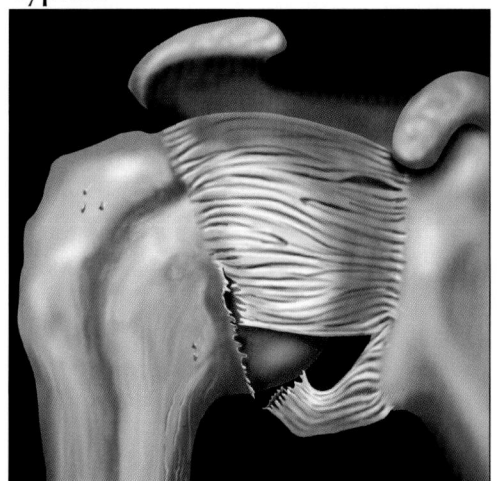
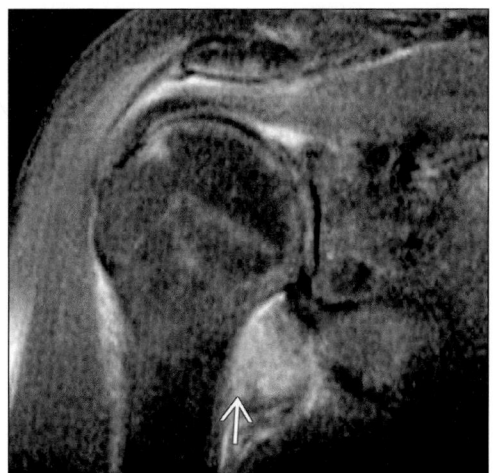

(Left) Coronal graphic shows HAGL lesion with tearing of the axillary pouch and extension into the mid inferior glenohumeral ligament. *(Right)* Coronal STIR MR shows a HAGL lesion (arrow) with the inferior capsule forming a "J" shape. The residual capsule is markedly edematous.

Typical

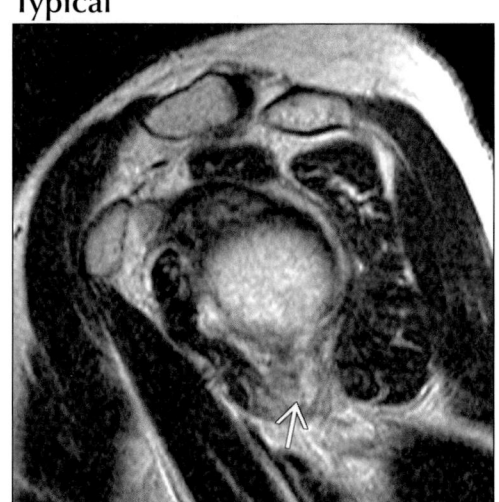
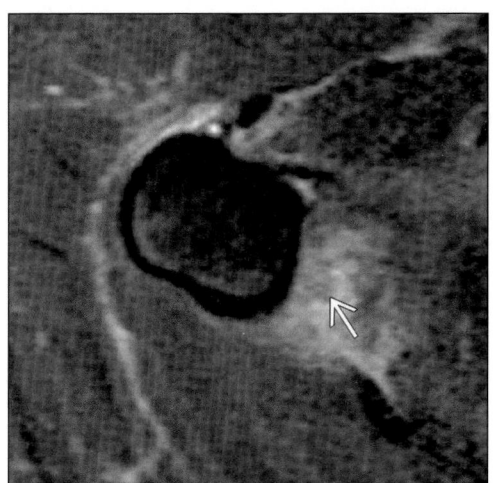

(Left) Sagittal T2 FSE MR shows a HAGL lesion (arrow) with retraction and edema of the inferior capsule (IGL). *(Right)* Axial FS PD FSE MR in a patient with a proven HAGL lesion. The inferior capsule is distorted and hyperintense (arrow).

Typical

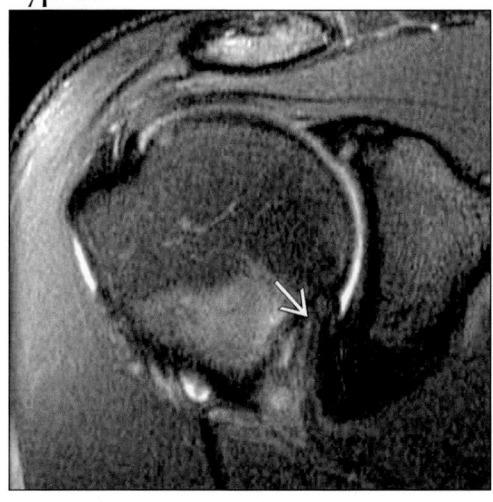
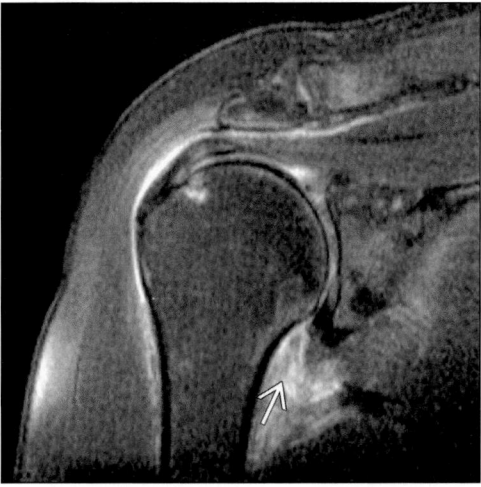

(Left) Coronal FS PD FSE MR shows a partial tear of the capsule attachment to the humerus (arrow), consistent with a HAGL lesion without retraction. *(Right)* Coronal STIR MR shows a blow out of the inferior capsule (arrow) which was described as a HAGL lesion at surgery. This is indistinguishable from a mid capsular rupture in this image.

IGL TEARS

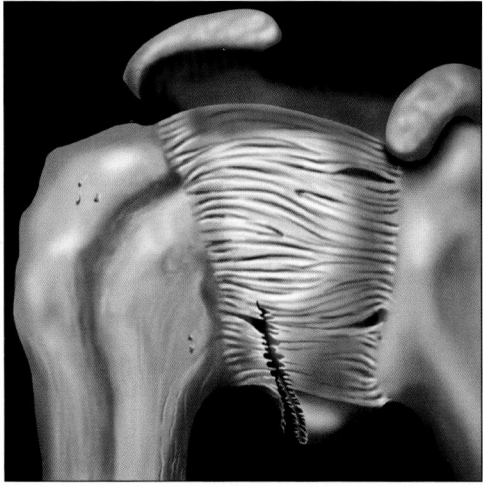

Coronal graphic shows a tear through the mid portion of the inferior glenohumeral ligament.

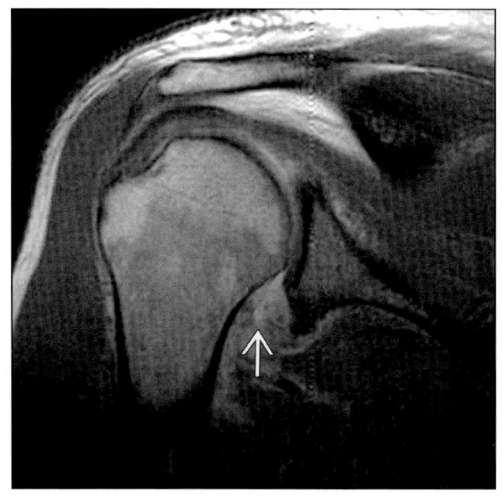

Coronal PD FSE MR shows a tear (arrow) of the mid aspect of the inferior glenohumeral ligament seen as distortion and disorganization of the ligament.

TERMINOLOGY

Abbreviations and Synonyms
- Inferior glenohumeral ligament (IGL) tears, IGL disruption

Definitions
- Ligament substance tears of IGL after anterior dislocation/severe subluxation (excluding Bankart and HAGL lesions)

IMAGING FINDINGS

General Features
- Best diagnostic clue: Discontinuous fibers of mid IGL (within the substance) on coronal images with surrounding edema/hemorrhage
- Location: Axillary pouch component of IGL
- Size: Varies from intrasubstance stretch injury to large tear
- Morphology: From discrete tear to diffuse edematous ligament

Radiographic Findings
- Radiography
  - +/- Bankart fracture (anterior inferior glenoid fracture)

- +/- Hill-Sachs deformity (posterolateral humeral head impaction)

CT Findings
- CT arthrography
  - Coronal reformatting
  - Extravasation of contrast material through the capsular tear
  - Single or double contrast (air)

MR Findings
- T1WI
  - Axillary pouch signal change from hypointense to intermediate
  - Axillary pouch IGL thickening
  - Increased laxity of IGL on coronal images
- T2WI
  - Hyperintense edema of thickened axillary pouch (coronal) on FS PD FSE
  - Edema (without impaction fx) or cystic change in posterolateral humeral head (same location as Hill-Sachs lesion)
  - +/- Associated Hill-Sachs/Bankart lesions
  - Chronic IGL scarring demonstrated with increased sensitivity on PD FSE as intermediate signal intensity
  - IGL edema may be asymmetric toward humeral or glenoid attachment site of axillary pouch
  - Associated hyperintense supraspinatus strains/tears

DDx: IGL Tears

Adhes. Capsulitis	Subscap. Tear	Subscap. Tear	Bankart	HAGL Lesion
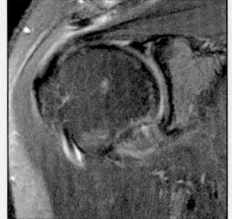	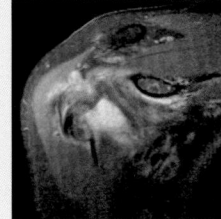	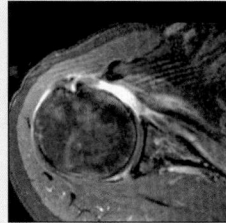	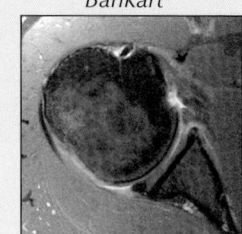	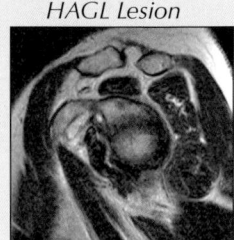
Cor FS PD FSE	Cor FS PD FSE	Ax FS PD FSE MR	Ax FS PD FSE MR	Sag T2 FSE MR

IGL TEARS

Key Facts

Imaging Findings
- Best diagnostic clue: Discontinuous fibers of mid IGL (within the substance) on coronal images with surrounding edema/hemorrhage
- Extravasation of contrast material through the capsular tear (extends inferior to axillary pouch)

Top Differential Diagnoses
- Bankart Lesion
- Humeral Avulsion of Inferior Glenohumeral Ligament (HAGL) Lesion
- Capsular Sprain without Disruption
- Subscapularis Tear (Subscap. Tear)
- Adhesive Capsulitis (Adhes Capsulitis)

Pathology
- General path comments: Mid ligament tear of the IGL less common than Bankart lesion and more common than HAGL

Clinical Issues
- Most common signs/symptoms: Patient with recent anterior shoulder dislocation presenting with joint pain, +/- instability
- Clinical profile: Positive apprehension test in patients with recurrent instability

Diagnostic Checklist
- Associated Bankart lesion, RTC tear, Hill-Sachs lesion
- Use PD FSE & FS PD FSE coronal images to evaluate morphology and signal changes in axillary pouch of IGL

- Fluid signal intensity filled gap
  - A GAGL (glenoid avulsion of glenohumeral ligament) lesion represents a tear of the axillary pouch (IGL) attachment to glenoid rim without avulsion of anterior inferior or inferior labrum
    - Hyperintense fluid signal or intermediate signal fibrosis between IGL and anterior inferior, inferior labrum or posteroinferior labrum
- MR arthrography
  - Extravasation of contrast material through the capsular tear (extends inferior to axillary pouch)
  - Sensitive in chronic cases where edema/hemorrhage is absent

Imaging Recommendations
- Best imaging tool
  - MRI and MR arthrography
    - MR arthrography in chronic cases
- Protocol advice: FS PD FSE and PD FSE in coronal and axial planes

DIFFERENTIAL DIAGNOSIS

Bankart Lesion
- Anterior dislocation
  - IGL labral complex failure from glenoid rim
- < 40 years old
- Periosteal disruption
- +/- Bankart fracture
  - +/- Glenoid deficiency
- +/- Hill-Sachs lesion
- Labrum fragmented or avulsed
  - +/- Anterior distraction/displacement of labrum

Humeral Avulsion of Inferior Glenohumeral Ligament (HAGL) Lesion
- Tear of IGHL at humeral interface
- +/- Bankart fracture
- +/- Hill-Sachs lesion
- Mimics IGL tear
- 1/3 of lesions associated with subscapularis tears

Capsular Sprain without Disruption
- Thickened edematous capsule with ligament failure
- Hyperintense on T2WI
- Mimics adhesive capsulitis
- +/- Bankart lesion
- +/- Hill-Sachs lesion

Subscapularis Tear (Subscap. Tear)
- Status post anterior dislocation
  - > 40 years old
  - +/- Bankart fracture
  - +/- Hill-Sachs lesion
- Posterior dislocation
  - +/- History of tonic-clonic seizure
  - Forward fall onto adducted internally rotated shoulder
- Discontinuous decreased signal subscapularis tendon with interposed hyperintensity on T2WI

Adhesive Capsulitis (Adhes Capsulitis)
- Thickened edematous capsule
- Hyperintense capsule on T2WI
- Frozen shoulder
  - Primary (idiopathic)
  - Secondary (e.g., diabetes, humerus fx, rotator cuff tendinosis/tears)

PATHOLOGY

General Features
- General path comments: Mid ligament tear of the IGL less common than Bankart lesion and more common than HAGL
- Etiology: Anterior shoulder dislocation or external rotation abduction injury
- Epidemiology
  - 50% of all joint dislocations
  - Cadaveric study showed ~ 35% of experimental dislocations of the shoulder involved mid ligament
    - Primarily older age group
  - Isolated HAGL lesions uncommon
- Associated abnormalities

IGL TEARS

- ○ Tears of the rotator interval
- ○ Hill-Sachs fracture of posterosuperior humeral head
- ○ Partial or complete rotator cuff tears after anterior dislocation
- ○ Biceps tendon/anchor lesions in ~ 12% of patients after anterior dislocation
- ○ Brachial plexus injuries, posterior glenoid labral tear in up to 11% of patients after anterior dislocation

Gross Pathologic & Surgical Features

- Torn capsule at its mid portion
- Angled scope to visualize the defect
- Torn glenohumeral capsule with variable amounts of hemorrhage

Microscopic Features

- Normal IGL complex
  - ○ Three layers of collagen fibers from glenoid to humerus + circumferential orientation
  - ○ Normal IGL complex thicker adjacent to glenoid compared to humerus
  - ○ Biomechanical failure including ligament lengthening when stretching forces exceed tensile properties of IGL

Staging, Grading or Classification Criteria

- IGL injuries
  - ○ Bankart - IGL labral avulsion from glenoid rim
  - ○ Mid ligament
    - ▪ GAGL - IGL tear without labral avulsion
  - ○ HAGL - humeral avulsion of glenohumeral ligament

CLINICAL ISSUES

Presentation

- Most common signs/symptoms: Patient with recent anterior shoulder dislocation presenting with joint pain, +/- instability
- Clinical profile: Positive apprehension test in patients with recurrent instability

Demographics

- Age: ≥ 40 years of age
- Gender: M > F

Natural History & Prognosis

- May heal with conservative treatment
- Recurrent instability in some cases

Treatment

- Conservative especially where instability is not clinically apparent
  - ○ Small tears with surrounding hemorrhage allowing fibrinogenic/healing factors to accomplish healing
  - ○ Physical therapy
- Surgical or arthroscopic repair if continued instability
- Angled arthroscope for adequate visualization in some cases

DIAGNOSTIC CHECKLIST

Consider

- Associated Bankart lesion, RTC tear, Hill-Sachs lesion

Image Interpretation Pearls

- Use PD FSE & FS PD FSE coronal images to evaluate morphology and signal changes in axillary pouch of IGL

SELECTED REFERENCES

1. Neviaser RJ et al: Concurrent rupture of the rotator cuff and anterior dislocation of the shoulder in the older patient. J Bone Joint Surg Am 70(9):1308-11, 1998
2. Tirman PF et al: A practical approach to imaging of the shoulder with emphasis on MR imaging, Orthop Clin North Am 28(4):483-515, 1997
3. Beltran J et al: Glenohumeral instability: Evaluation with MR arthrography. Radiographics 17(3):657-73, 1997
4. Tirman PF et al: Humeral avulsion of the anterior shoulder stabilizing structures after anterior shoulder dislocation: Demonstration by MRI and MR arthrography. Skeletal Radiol 25(8):743-8, 1996

IGL TEARS

IMAGE GALLERY

Typical

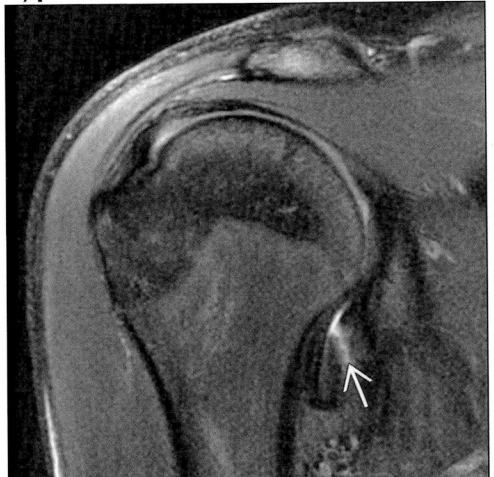 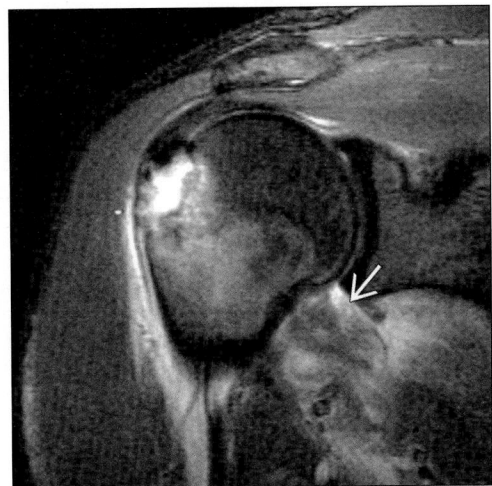

(Left) Coronal FS PD FSE MR shows a discrete tear of the inferior glenohumeral ligament (arrow) adjacent to the inferior labrum (GAGL lesion). This was a proven inferior glenohumeral ligament tear. (Right) Coronal FS PD FSE MR shows inferior glenohumeral tear involving the entire axillary pouch. There is ligament thickening, edema and disruption (arrow).

Typical

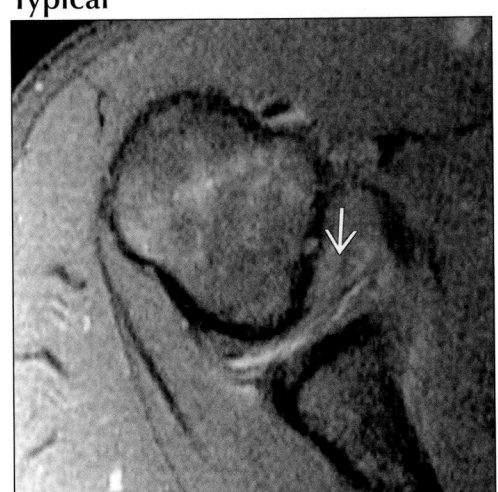 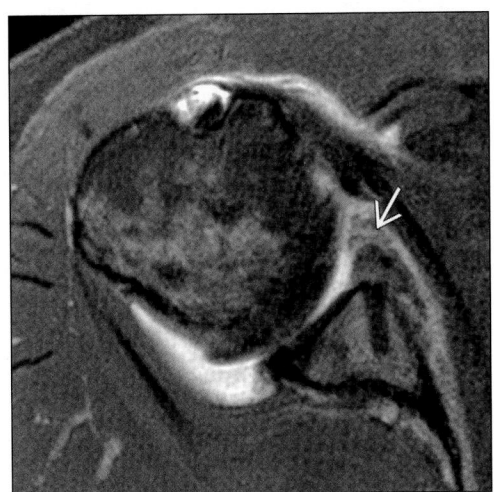

(Left) Axial FS PD FSE MR shows an inferior glenohumeral ligament sprain (arrow) after anterior dislocation. (Right) Axial FS PD FSE MR shows an inferior glenohumeral sprain with thickening of IGL (arrow) after a Bankart repair.

Typical

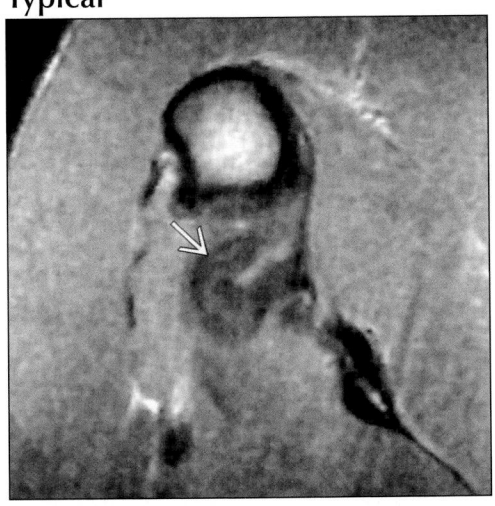 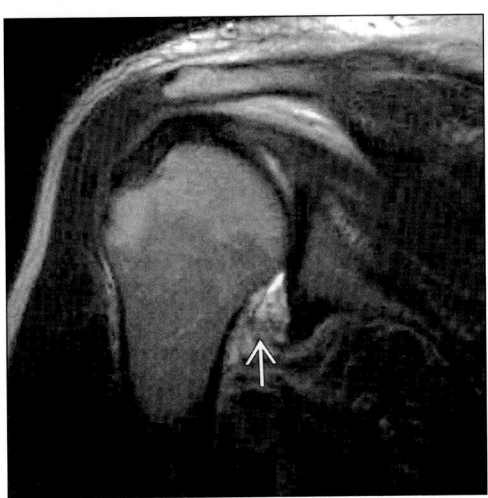

(Left) Axial PD FSE MR shows a sprain (arrow) of the inferior capsule in a patient after anterior dislocation. (Right) Coronal T2 FSE MR shows disruption (arrow) of the mid portion of the inferior glenohumeral ligament after anterior dislocation.

BENNETT LESION

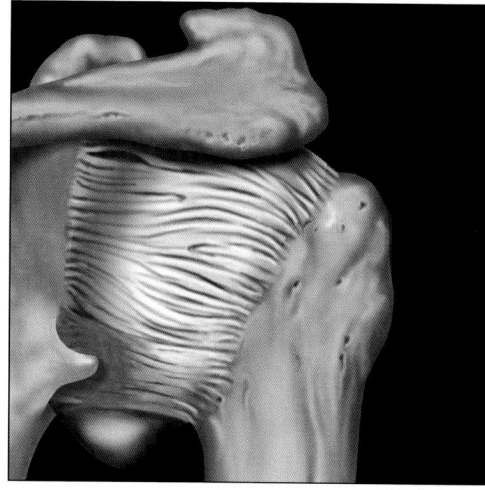

Coronal graphic shows heterotopic ossification posterior to posterior aspect of shoulder joint associated with capsular inflammatory changes and fibrosis.

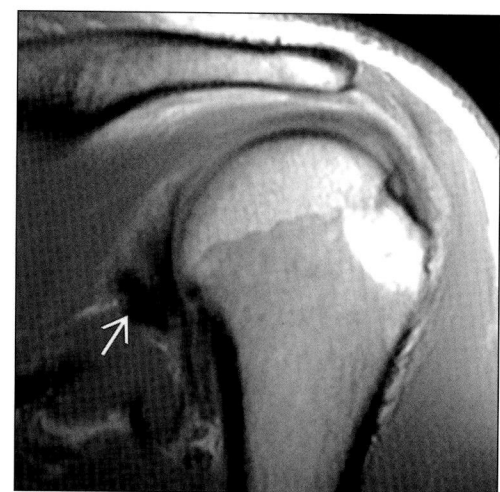

Coronal PD FSE MR shows identical findings with graphic: Heterotopic ossification (arrow) posterior to the glenohumeral joint with thickening of the posterior capsule.

TERMINOLOGY

Abbreviations and Synonyms
- Bennett lesion (BL)

Definitions
- Extraarticular, posterior ossification associated with posterior labral injury and posterior articular surface cuff pathology in throwing athletes

IMAGING FINDINGS

General Features
- Best diagnostic clue
  - Globular hypointense ossification on T1 & T2WI
  - Adjacent to torn or degenerated posterior labrum
- Location: Soft tissues adjacent to posterior/posteroinferior glenoid rim
- Size
  - Ossification several mms to > 1 cm
  - Labral tear focal to extensive
- Morphology
  - Ossification is crescentic
  - +/- Fragmentation
  - Labral tear is irregular and increased in signal on short TE sequences

- Short TE sequences = T1WI, PD/Intermediate WI, T2* GRE WI
  - +/- Thickened, scarred posterior capsule

Radiographic Findings
- Radiography
  - Mineralization adjacent to posterior glenoid on axillary view
  - Subchondral sclerosis - posterior glenoid
  - Subchondral lucencies representing cysts

CT Findings
- NECT
  - Ossification adjacent to posterior glenoid
  - Subchondral posterior glenoid rim sclerosis
  - Subchondral glenoid rim cysts
- CT arthrography
  - +/- Posterior labral tear with contrast extending into tear

MR Findings
- T1WI
  - Decreased signal intensity, globular to crescent-like ossification within posterior soft tissues
  - Subchondral decreased signal, sclerosis common
  - +/- Subchondral rounded hypointensity cysts
- T2WI
  - Hypointense crescent-shaped area of ossification posteroinferior glenoid rim

DDx: Bennett Lesion

Post. Labr. Tear	PSGI	Post. Caps. Tear	Scap. Stress Fx	Ca++ Tendinitis

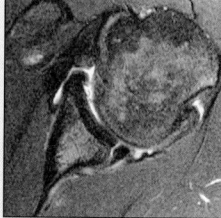 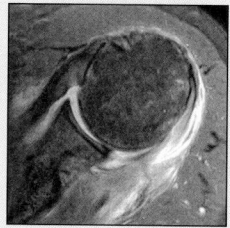 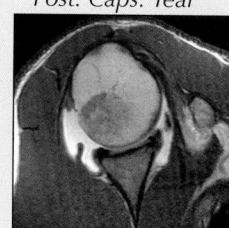 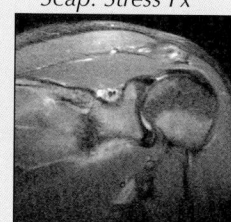 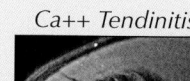 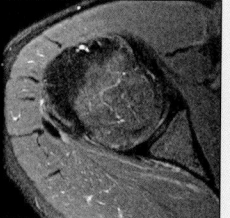

Ax FS PD FSE MR	Ax FS PD FSE MR	Ax T1 Arthro.	Cor FS PD FSE	Ax FS PD FSE MR

BENNETT LESION

Key Facts

Imaging Findings
- Globular hypointense ossification on T1 & T2WI
- Location: Soft tissues adjacent to posterior/posteroinferior glenoid rim
- Ossification several mms to > 1 cm
- Ossification adjacent to posterior glenoid
- Decreased signal intensity, globular to crescent-like ossification within posterior soft tissues
- T2* GRE: Calcium may "bloom", thus increasing sensitivity due to susceptibility

Top Differential Diagnoses
- Posterior Labral Tear
- Posterosuperior Glenoid Impingement (PSGI)
- Posterior Capsular Tear (Post. Caps Tear)

- Scapular Fracture, Scapular Stress Fracture (Scap Stress Fx)
- Calcific

Pathology
- Extraarticular posterior ossification associated with posterior labral injury
- Dystrophic/heterotopic ossification

Clinical Issues
- Posterior shoulder pain especially with throwing activities

Diagnostic Checklist
- PD, T2* GRE to identify images calcification or ossification
- CT confirmation for bone detail

  - At insertion of posterior joint capsule
  - Hypointense thickening of posterior capsule
  - Associated hyperintense joint effusion
  - Ossification (or calcification) may be segmental or uninterrupted
  - +/- Adjacent chondromalacia
    - Increased signal intensity within the hyaline articular cartilage
    - +/- Surface irregularity, ulceration, defect
  - FS PD FSE
    - Edema and hemorrhage in surrounding soft tissues: Increased signal
    - Labrum may be discretely torn or markedly heterogeneous
    - Hypointense ossification may blend in with capsule
    - Detection of chondral degeneration
- T2* GRE: Calcium may "bloom", thus increasing sensitivity due to susceptibility
- MR arthrography
  - Associated with posterior labral tear with contrast extending into tear

Nuclear Medicine Findings
- Bone Scan: Increased uptake if posterior glenoid rim is remodeled/damaged

Imaging Recommendations
- Best imaging tool: MRI for posterior labrum and articular sided cuff lesions
- Protocol advice
  - PD, FS PD FSE/T2 WI + T2* GRE
  - MR arthrography

DIFFERENTIAL DIAGNOSIS

Posterior Labral Tear
- Increased signal intensity on short TE sequences
- Status post posterior dislocation/subluxation
- +/- Distraction of labrum
- +/- Bony glenoid rim fracture
  - + Reverse Bankart

- +/- Lesser tuberosity fracture
  - = Reverse Hill-Sachs
- POLPSA (posterior labrocapsular periosteal sleeve avulsion)
  - Medial displacement of posterior capsule, labrum and posterior scapular periosteum

Posterosuperior Glenoid Impingement (PSGI)
- Throwing athletes
- Internal impingement
- Impingement of undersurface of posterior supraspinatus
  - Humeral head
  - Posterosuperior labrum
- Triad of findings
  - Partial tear of undersurface posterior supraspinatus/anterior infraspinatus
    - +/- Complete tear
  - Posterosuperior labral degeneration/tearing
  - Humeral head posterosuperior subcortical cystic changes

Posterior Capsular Tear (Post. Caps Tear)
- Posterior band of inferior glenohumeral ligament
- +/- Associated IGL (inferior glenohumeral ligament) tear at glenoid, humeral neck or axillary pouch segments
- Status post posterior dislocation/subluxation
- MR arthrography helpful

Scapular Fracture, Scapular Stress Fracture (Scap Stress Fx)
- Status post excessive throwing activity
- Baseball athletes
- Abnormal forces on normal bone
- +/- Decreased signal intensity callus/fracture line on all pulse sequences
- +/- Increased signal intensity edema on T2WI especially FS PD FSE

Calcific

- Calcium hydroxyapatite deposition in rotator cuff tendons
  - Hypointense hydroxyapatite deposits on T1 & T2WI
- May fragment
- Silent phase (subclinical): Limited to tendons
- Mechanical phase (clinical): +/- Subbursal and intrabursal rupture
- Hyperintense inflammatory fluid (T2WI)

PATHOLOGY

General Features

- General path comments
  - Extraarticular posterior ossification associated with posterior labral injury
  - Dystrophic/heterotopic ossification
- Etiology
  - Posterior capsular avulsion secondary to traction from the posterior band of the IGHL
  - Deceleration phase of pitching
    - Posterior subluxation during cocking of the arm
  - Described by Edward Bennett 1837-1907 (Irish surgeon)
    - Originally thought to be secondary to traction injury of the long head of the triceps brachii
- Epidemiology
  - Posterior capsule - 36% of posterior shoulder instability
  - Posterior labral injuries - 86% of posterior shoulder instability
- Associated abnormalities: Posterosuperior glenoid impingement

Gross Pathologic & Surgical Features

- Posterior labrum degeneration/tearing with surrounding hemorrhage
- Dystrophic/heterotopic calcification or ossification
- Associated posterior articular surface rotator cuff tear

Microscopic Features

- Hemorrhagic, torn, fibrocartilaginous posterior labrum with variable degrees of fibrosis depending on chronicity
- Ossification or calcification within variable degrees of soft tissue fibrosis +/- inflammatory cells

CLINICAL ISSUES

Presentation

- Most common signs/symptoms
  - Posterior shoulder pain especially with throwing activities
  - Tenderness at posterior inferior glenoid region
- Clinical profile
  - Young athlete
  - Common in baseball players

Demographics

- Age: Adolescent/young adult
- Gender: M > F

Natural History & Prognosis

- Pain may subside with cessation of throwing
- Arthroscopic debridement of posterior labral tear

Treatment

- Conservative: Physical therapy, NSAIDs
- Surgical: Arthroscopic debridement of soft tissue ossification

DIAGNOSTIC CHECKLIST

Consider

- Posterior labral tear/instability

Image Interpretation Pearls

- PD, T2* GRE to identify images calcification or ossification
- CT confirmation for bone detail

SELECTED REFERENCES

1. Miniaci A et al: Magnetic resonance imaging of the shoulder in asymptomatic professional baseball pitchers. Am J Sports Med 30(1):66-73, 2002
2. Yoneda M et al: Arthroscopic removal of symptomatic Bennett lesions in the shoulders of baseball players. Arthroscopic Bennett-plasty. Am J Sports Med 30(5):728-36, 2002
3. Yu JS et al: The POLPSA lesion: MR imaging findings with arthroscopic correlation in patients with posterior instability. Skeletal Radiol 31(7):396-9, 2002
4. Grainger AJ et al: Direct MR arthrography. A review of current use. Clin Radiol 55(3):163-76, 2000
5. De Maeseneer M et al: The Bennett lesion of the shoulder. J Comput Assist Tomogr 22(1):31-4, 1998
6. Tirman PF et al: A practical approach to imaging of the shoulder with emphasis on MR imaging. Orthop Clin North Am 28(4):483-515, 1997
7. Ferrari JD et al: Posterior ossification of the shoulder: The Bennett lesion. Etiology, diagnosis, and treatment. Am J Sports Med 22(2):171-5; discussion 175-6, 1994

BENNETT LESION

IMAGE GALLERY

Typical

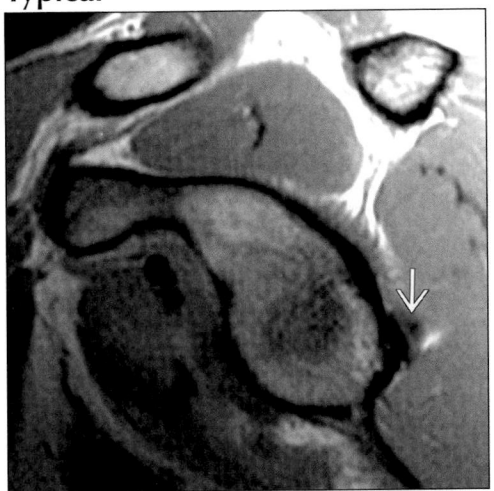 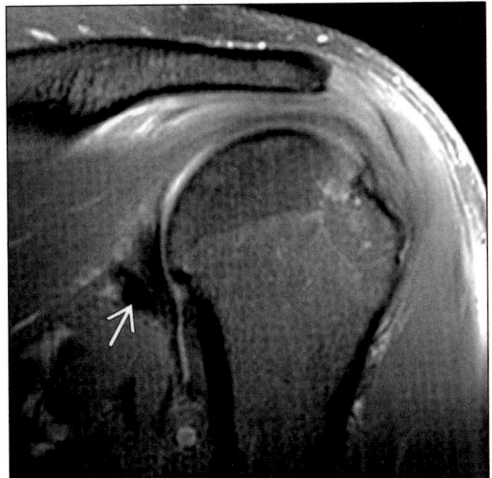

(Left) Sagittal PD FSE MR shows heterotopic ossification (arrow) posterior to the joint in a professional baseball pitcher, consistent with a Bennett lesion. *(Right)* Coronal FS PD FSE MR shows the irregular ossification adjacent to the posteroinferior glenoid. The patient was a professional baseball pitcher.

Typical

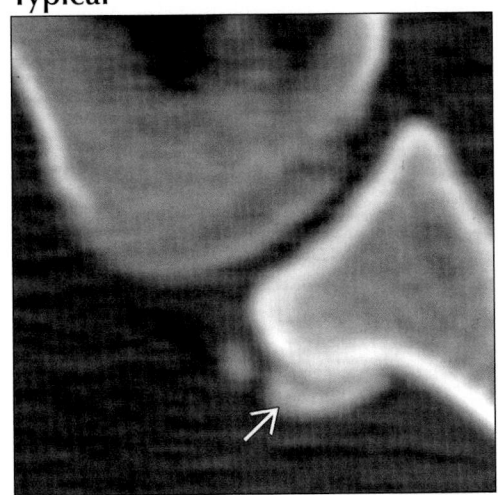 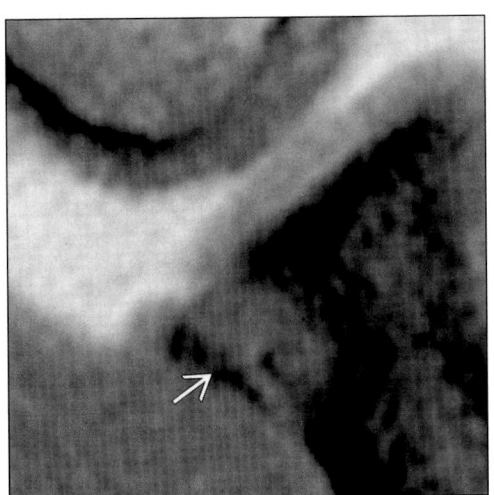

(Left) Axial NECT shows ossification (arrow) posterior to the joint in a throwing athlete consistent with a Bennett lesion. *(Right)* Axial T2* GRE MR shows heterotopic ossification (arrow) in a baseball pitcher. The posterior labrum was torn.

Typical

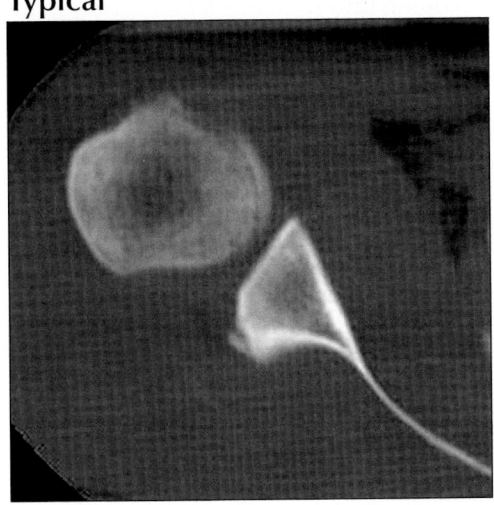 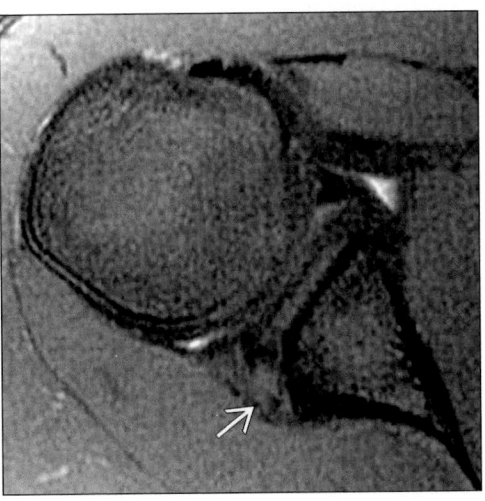

(Left) Axial NECT shows ossification posterior to the joint in a throwing athlete. *(Right)* Axial T2* GRE MR shows hypointense, heterotopic ossification (arrow) in a baseball pitcher posterior to the posteroinferior glenoid.

POSTERIOR LABRAL TEAR, SHOULDER

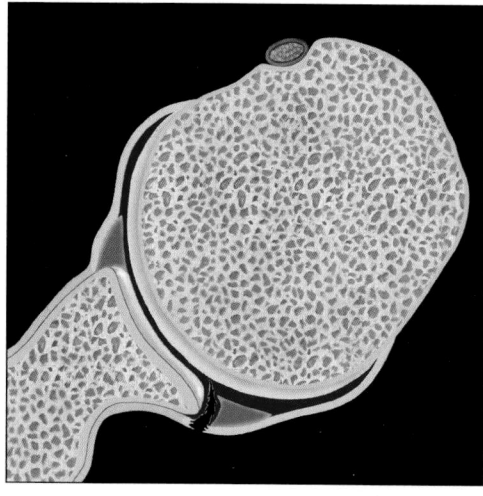

Axial graphic shows a tear at the base of the avulsed posterior labrum.

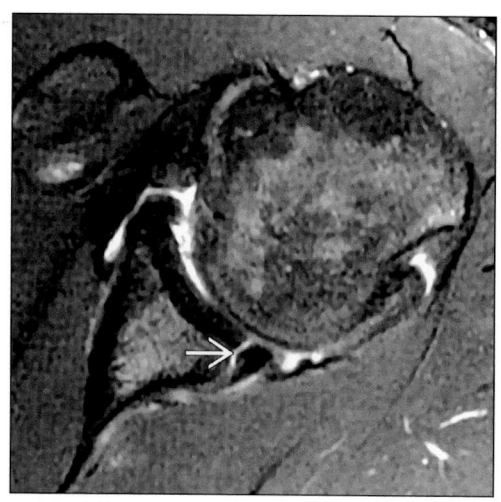

Axial FS PD FSE MR shows a hyperintense tear (arrow) at the base of the posterior labrum with mild posterior displacement after posterior dislocation.

TERMINOLOGY

Abbreviations and Synonyms
- Reverse Bankart (RB), posterior band inferior glenohumeral ligament (PBIGHL)

Definitions
- Posterior labral/capsular/glenoid rim injury secondary to posterior dislocation/subluxation

IMAGING FINDINGS

General Features
- Best diagnostic clue: Torn/detached posterior glenohumeral ligament/labrum from underlying glenoid, +/- fracture of glenoid
- Location: Posterior glenoid/labrum extending for variable distance anteriorly/inferiorly/superiorly
- Size: Discrete tear to large complete avulsion
- Morphology: Varies from discrete to irregular edematous tear

Radiographic Findings
- Radiography
  - +/- Posterior glenoid rim fracture with variable amount of displacement/comminution
  - Trough sign

- Deep reverse Hill-Sachs lesion appearing as a "trough" of the anterior humerus
  - Lesser tuberosity avulsion
    - Subscapularis intact
    - +/- History of seizures

CT Findings
- NECT
  - +/- Glenoid rim fracture with variable amount of displacement/comminution
  - Trough sign
    - Reverse Hill-Sachs lesion of the anterior humerus creating an anterior defect or "trough"
    - Coronal/sagittal reconstruction
  - Lesser tuberosity avulsion fracture
    - Subscapularis attached to bone
    - History of seizures common
  - +/- Glenoid version - hypoplasia
- CT arthrography
  - Contrast extending into posterior labral tear

MR Findings
- T1WI
  - Increased signal tear in substance of labrum
  - +/- Fracture of the underlying glenoid: Reverse Bankart
    - Hypointense fracture line
    - Hypointense surrounding edema

DDx: Posterior Labral Tear, Shoulder

Reverse HAGL	Folded Capsule	Post. Dislocation	Glenoid Version	Vascularity
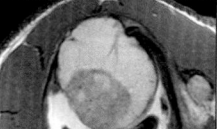	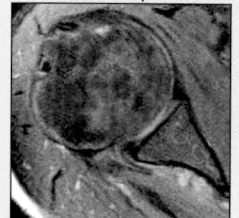	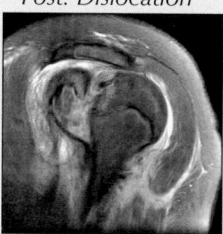	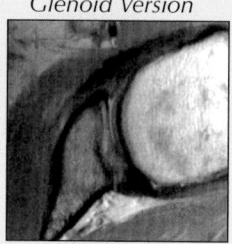	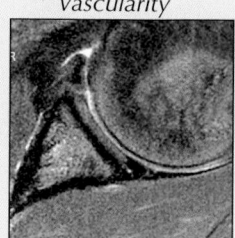
Ax T1 Arthro.	Ax FS PD FSE MR	Sag FS PD FSE	Ax PD FSE	Ax FS PD FSE MR

POSTERIOR LABRAL TEAR, SHOULDER

Key Facts

Imaging Findings
- Best diagnostic clue: Torn/detached posterior glenohumeral ligament/labrum from underlying glenoid, +/- fracture of glenoid

Top Differential Diagnoses
- Bennett Lesion
- Humeral Fracture
- Teres Minor Avulsion/Reverse HAGL
- Glenoid Version (Retroversion)
- Normal Vascularity/Anatomy

Pathology
- Posterior band of IGHLC "weak link" static stabilizer in most shoulders
- Posterior force on flexed, adducted internally rotated shoulder at risk

Epidemiology: 2-12% shoulder dislocations are posterior and result in posterior labral tear

Clinical Issues
- Pain after trauma
- Pain with activities that require flexion, adduction, and internal rotation
- Recurrent posterior subluxation more common than dislocation

Diagnostic Checklist
- Requires high index of suspicion
- Identify posterior labral tear, anterior humerus (lesser tuberosity) bone edema
- Indicators of posterior dislocation/subluxation

- Avulsion of lesser tuberosity fragment hyperintense - (contains bone marrow)
- T2WI
  - +/- Accompanied by a fracture of underlying glenoid
    - Reverse Bankart: Increased signal intensity edema with visible fracture line, +/- distraction
  - FS PD FSE
    - Sensitive for marrow edema in reverse Hill-Sachs and reverse Bankart lesions
    - Linear hyperintense fluid often visualized underneath labral attachment to glenoid rim in posterosuperior or posteroinferior quadrant on sagittal images
  - Avulsion of lesser tuberosity fragment
    - +/- Subscapularis tear or partial tear
    - Hyperintense edema/fluid in tear
    - Interrupted fibers
  - +/- Paralabral cyst - chronic cases
    - Focal
    - Dissect superiorly or inferiorly
  - +/- Glenoid version - hypoplasia
- PD/Intermediate
  - High resolution PD good for anatomic delineation of posterior band of inferior glenohumeral ligament complex
  - Increased signal tear within labrum
- MR arthrography
  - Contrast extending through posterior labral tear
  - Redundancy of posterior capsule and IGL stretching
- Labrum focally torn or with multiple linear tears and/or diffuse signal intensity
  - Axial images
- Chronic lesion partially healed and fibrosed
  - Heterogeneous but predominantly decreased signal intensity on all pulse sequences

Nuclear Medicine Findings
- Bone Scan: Increased uptake with reverse Bankart fracture

Imaging Recommendations
- Best imaging tool: MRI, consider MR arthrography
- Protocol advice: FS PD FSE axial, coronal and sagittal

DIFFERENTIAL DIAGNOSIS

Bennett Lesion
- Ossification adjacent to posterior labrum/glenoid injury
- Throwing athlete
- Baseball players
- Posterior contractures common

Humeral Fracture
- Distal to lesser tuberosity fracture indicating different mechanism
- Anatomic/surgical neck
  - +/- Comminution, distraction
- Radiographs/CT/MRI diagnostic

Teres Minor Avulsion/Reverse HAGL
- Results from posterior dislocation
- Avulsion from humerus
- Forced external rotation on internally rotated shoulder
- Direct trauma on anterior joint

Glenoid Version (Retroversion)
- Posteriorly angulated glenoid
- Congenitally small posterior glenoid (hypoplasia)
- Compensatory hypertrophy of hyaline cartilage to stabilize posterior glenoid
- Predisposes to posterior instability

Normal Vascularity/Anatomy
- Vessels may be found in and around posterior inferior labrum
- Capsule may fold, mimicking labral abnormality
  - Especially in external rotation

PATHOLOGY

General Features
- General path comments
  - Posterior band of IGHLC "weak link" static stabilizer in most shoulders
  - Injured after dislocation

○ Avulsion of posterior band IGHL +/- teres minor insertion = reverse HAGL lesion
- Etiology
  - ○ Posterior force on flexed, adducted internally rotated shoulder at risk
  - ○ Tonic-clonic seizure resulting in decerebrate rigidity + fall onto anterior shoulder
    - +/- Posterior dislocation
  - ○ Dislocation can occur after major injury, repetitive minor trauma, and atraumatic processes
- Epidemiology: 2-12% shoulder dislocations are posterior and result in posterior labral tear
- Associated abnormalities
  - ○ Lesser tuberosity humeral avulsion fracture
  - ○ Reverse Bankart fracture of posterior glenoid rim
  - ○ Reverse Hill-Sachs fracture (impaction) of anterior humerus (lesser tuberosity)
  - ○ +/- Subscapularis and teres minor tears
  - ○ Predisposing bony anatomy for posterior dislocation includes
    - Increased humeral retroversion
    - Glenoid retroversion (version)
    - Glenoid hypoplasia
  - ○ Posterior instability associated with labral tears
    - Capsular laxity
    - Rotator interval (coracohumeral and superior glenohumeral ligaments) laxity/incompetence
    - Superior glenohumeral ligament tear
  - ○ Microinstability with posterosuperior labral tears as a subtype of SLAP II
    - Posterior peelback lesion includes the posterior labral component of a SLAP II + partial articular surface tear of the posterior cuff (between the supraspinatus and infraspinatus)
    - Abnormal obligate translation as a result of posterior capsular contracture elevating humeral head as external rotation occurs
    - Seen in overhand throwing (late cocking phase)

Gross Pathologic & Surgical Features
- Avulsion of the inferior glenohumeral labral ligamentous attachment to the glenoid
- Posterior labrocapsular periosteal sleeve avulsion (POLPSA) with posterior capsular stripping of the labrum

Microscopic Features
- Hemorrhagic, torn, fibrocartilaginous labrum with variable degrees of fibrosis depending on chronicity

CLINICAL ISSUES

Presentation
- Most common signs/symptoms
  - ○ Pain after trauma
  - ○ Pain with activities that require flexion, adduction, and internal rotation
- Clinical profile
  - ○ Difficulty in performing activities of daily living, including hair combing, shaving, and eating
  - ○ Patients describing pain with
    - Throwing (follow through)
    - Bench press (lock out)

- Swimming (pull through)
- Rowing

Demographics
- Age: Typically younger patient
- Gender: M > F in athletics; seizures M = F

Natural History & Prognosis
- Pain and dysfunction may be insidious
- May resolve with conservative therapy
- Recurrence with atraumatic and traumatic posterior dislocations with humeral and glenoid osseous defects
  - ○ Recurrent posterior subluxation more common than dislocation
- Often requires surgery

Treatment
- Conservative treatment if associated with posterior dislocation: Attempt closed reduction
- Non dislocation: Physical therapy aimed at strengthening, NSAIDs
- Surgical: Correcting anatomic deformities, repair of labrum/capsule

DIAGNOSTIC CHECKLIST

Consider
- Isolated muscle damage, Bennett lesion

Image Interpretation Pearls
- Requires high index of suspicion
- Identify posterior labral tear, anterior humerus (lesser tuberosity) bone edema
  - ○ Indicators of posterior dislocation/subluxation

SELECTED REFERENCES

1. Wolf EM et al: Arthroscopic capsular plication for posterior shoulder instability. Arthroscopy 14(2):153-63, 1998
2. Tirman PF et al: A practical approach to imaging of the shoulder with emphasis on MR imaging. Orthop Clin North Am 28(4):483-515, 1997
3. Pollock RG et al: Recurrent posterior shoulder instability. Diagnosis and treatment. Clin Orthop (291):85-96, 1993
4. Matsen FA et al: Glenohumeral instability. The Shoulder. Philadeplphia PA, WB Saunders, 26-622, 1990
5. Neer CS: Fractures and dislocation of the shoulder.Fractures. Philadelphia PA, JB Lippincott, 686-7, 1975
6. Scott DJ Jr: Treatment of recurrent posterior dislocations of the shoulder by glenoplasty. Report of three cases. J Bone Joint Surg Am 49(3):471-6, 1967
7. Wilson JC et al: Traumatic posterior (retroglenoid) dislocation of the hyumerus. J Bone Joint Surg 31(A):160-72, 1949

IMAGE GALLERY

Typical

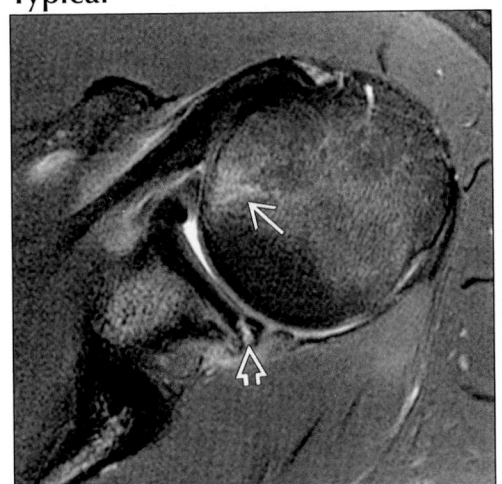 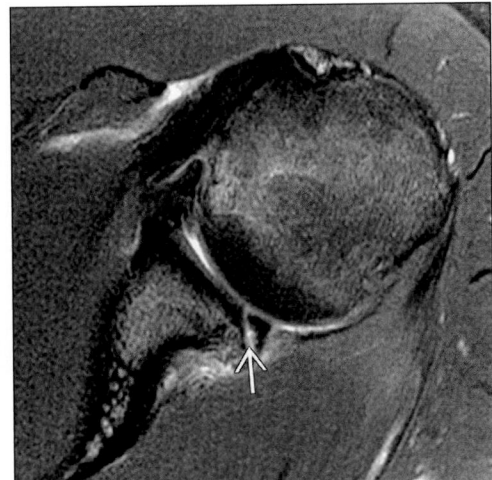

(Left) Axial FS PD FSE MR shows a reverse Bankart lesion (open arrow) and an anterior (reverse) Hill-Sachs bone trabecular injury (arrow). *(**Right**)* Axial FS PD FSE MR shows a reverse Bankart lesion (arrow) and a reverse Hill-Sachs lesion. Note the flattening of the posterior glenoid rim.

Typical

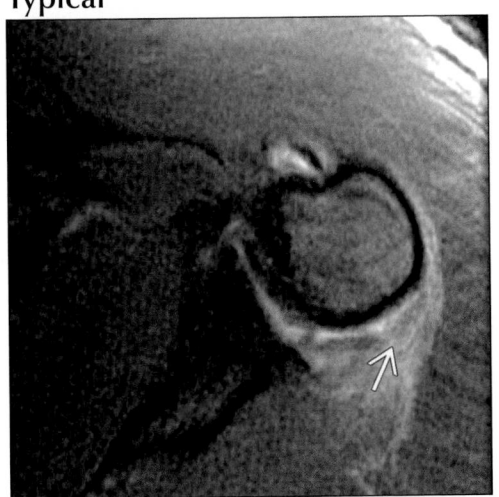 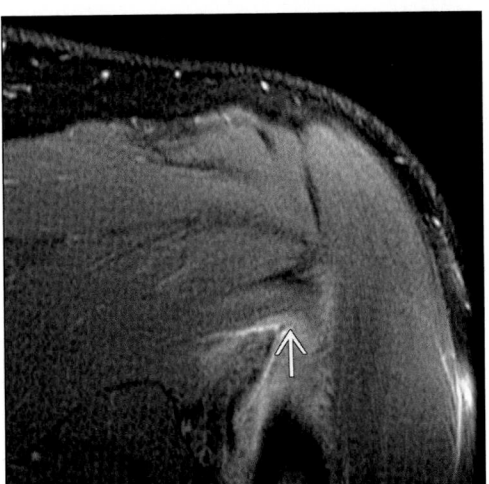

(Left) Axial FS PD FSE MR shows an avulsion of the teres minor muscle and the capsule from the humerus (arrow) indicating reverse HAGL lesion. *(**Right**)* Coronal FS PD FSE MR shows a reverse HAGL lesion (arrow).

Typical

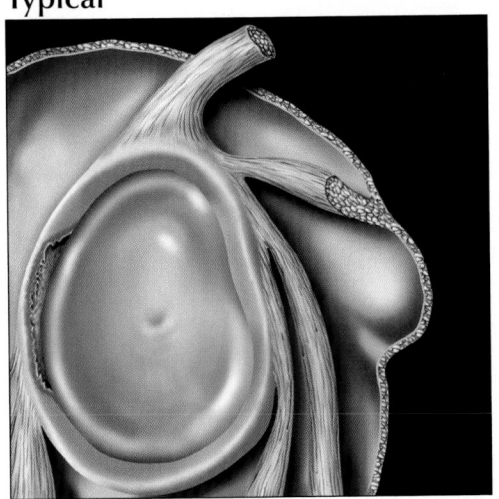 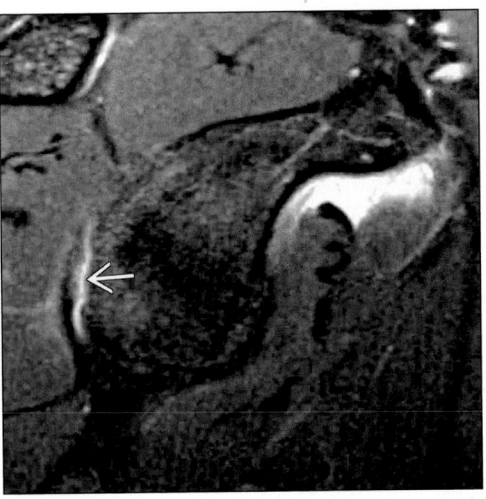

*(**Left**)* Sagittal graphic shows a posterior labral tear after a posterior dislocation. *(**Right**)* Sagittal FS PD FSE MR shows a posterior labral tear (arrow) with fluid signal between the labrum and glenoid rim.

HIDDEN LESION, SHOULDER

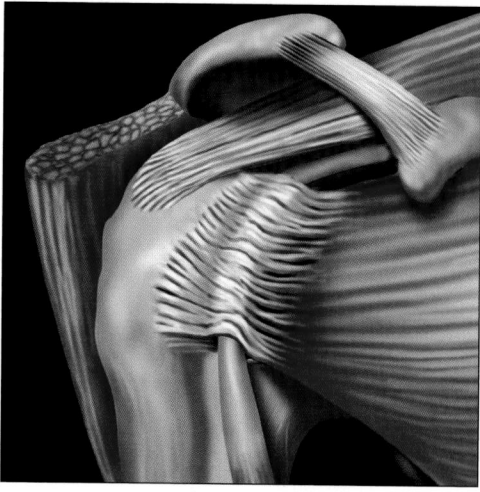

Coronal graphic shows subluxation of the biceps tendon medially indicating biceps instability - a hallmark of the hidden lesion.

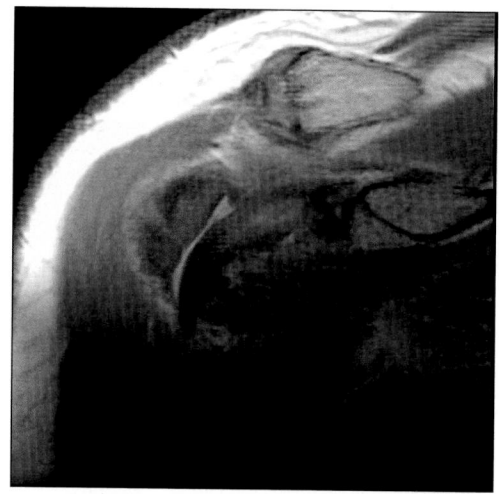

Coronal PD FSE MR shows biceps subluxation from the superior aspect of the bicipital groove (biceps instability).

TERMINOLOGY

Definitions

- Superolateral region of rotator interval receives insertions from
  ○ Superior glenohumeral ligament (SGHL)
  ○ Coracohumeral ligament (CHL)
  ○ Subscapularis tendon
- Hidden (difficult to visualize at arthroscopy) rotator interval lesions = lesions of SGHL/CHL complex

IMAGING FINDINGS

General Features

- Best diagnostic clue
  ○ Subluxation or dislocation of long head biceps tendon (LHBT) from the superior aspect of bicipital groove
    ▪ Distal subscapularis tearing
  ○ Tear of SGHL/CHL complex
- Location: Lateral aspect of the rotator interval (RI), medial wall of the bicipital sheath
- Size
  ○ Range
    ▪ Lax SGHL/CHL complex; small tear
    ▪ +/- Additional involvement of the subscapularis tendon insertion

- Morphology
  ○ Irregular thickened SGHL/MCHL complex (lax) to frank tear +/- subscapularis
  ○ Subscapularis tear, +/- SGHL/CHL complex

Radiographic Findings

- Radiography
  ○ Lesser tuberosity cystic degenerative changes
    ▪ +/- Clinical subcoracoid impingement
  ○ Secondary findings associated with subacromial impingement - predisposing factor
    ▪ Acromial spurs
    ▪ Type III acromion (hooked)
    ▪ Humeral head (HH) subcortical greater tuberosity cysts
    ▪ Superior HH migration - rotator cuff (RTC) full thickness tear

CT Findings

- NECT
  ○ Upper aspect of lesser tuberosity: Subcortical cystic (degenerative) changes
    ▪ +/- Clinical subcoracoid impingement
  ○ Secondary findings associated with subacromial impingement - predisposing
    ▪ Use coronal & sagittal reconstruction images to visualize
- CT arthrography
  ○ +/- Torn labrum, cuff, biceps subluxation/dislocation

DDx: Hidden Lesion, Shoulder

SLAC Lesion	Subcoracoid Imp.	SLAP Synovitis	Microinstability

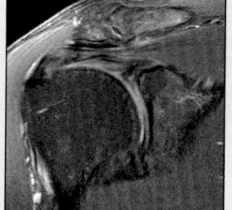
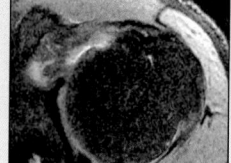
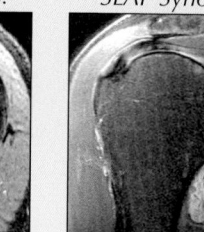
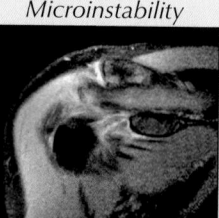

Cor FS PD FSE	Ax FS PD FSE MR	Cor FS PD FSE	Cor STIR MR

HIDDEN LESION, SHOULDER

Key Facts

Imaging Findings
- Subluxation or dislocation of long head biceps tendon (LHBT) from the superior aspect of bicipital groove
- Location: Lateral aspect of the rotator interval (RI), medial wall of the bicipital sheath
- Hyperintensity within distal subscapularis tendon
- Increased signal intensity/frank tear of SGHL/CHL complex
- +/- Biceps tendinosis

Top Differential Diagnoses
- Microinstability
- Superior Labrum Anterior Cuff (SLAC) Lesion
- Rotator Interval Tear
- Biceps Tendinosis

- Biceps Tendon Rupture
- SLAP Lesion
- Subcoracoid Impingement

Pathology
- Superior aspect of the bicipital groove and lateral aspect of the RI
- Subscapularis insertion
- Tears of SGHL/CHL complex and subscapularis

Clinical Issues
- Impingement pain with biceps symptoms
- Repair of torn structures

Diagnostic Checklist
- Axial images for detection of biceps subluxation

MR Findings
- T1WI
  - Frayed/tear of the anterior cuff, +/- intermediate signal
  - Anterior cuff as represented by anterior supraspinatus, subscapularis and rotator cuff interval
  - +/- Increased signal of biceps tendon = tendinosis
  - Biceps flattened if subluxed
- T2WI
  - Hyperintensity within distal subscapularis tendon
    - +/- Small interstitial tear (hyperintense fluid synovium in gap)
    - +/- Frank tear (hyperintense fluid synovium in gap)
  - Increased signal intensity/frank tear of SGHL/CHL complex
    - Sagittal images hyperintense focus in area of the SGHL/CHL complex
  - +/- Hyperintense tear of anterior rotator cuff with fluid signal filled gap
  - Subluxation/dislocation of biceps tendon
  - +/- Biceps tendinosis
    - Thickening
    - Hyperintensity
  - +/- Fluid filled subcoracoid bursa (hyperintense)
  - +/- Subchondral hyperintense cysts at lesser tuberosity
    - Subcoracoid impingement
- PD/Intermediate
  - High resolution image
    - Zip 512/interpolation
  - Tear of SGHL/CHL complex at insertion on humeral head
  - Thickened/hyperintense/lax SGHL/CHL complex
  - +/- Subscapularis partial or complete tear
    - Partial tear most common
  - +/- Supraspinatus anterior tear
- STIR
  - Less spatial resolution than FS PD FSE
  - SGHL/CHL complex difficult to visualize
- MR arthrography

  - +/- Extravasation of contrast material into subacromial bursa - complete RTC tears
  - +/- Torn, thickened SGHL/CHL complex

Imaging Recommendations
- Best imaging tool: MRI
- Protocol advice: FS PD FSE in axial and sagittal planes

DIFFERENTIAL DIAGNOSIS

Microinstability
- Hidden lesion is a component of microinstability
- Supraspinatus anterior undersurface partial tear
- Superior labrum/glenohumeral ligament dysfunction
- "Superior instability"

Superior Labrum Anterior Cuff (SLAC) Lesion
- +/- Microinstability
- Abnormal translation and chafing of cuff on glenoid rim
- Partial undersurface cuff tear
- +/- Unstable superior labrum anterior to posterior (SLAP) lesion
- SGHL/interval failure

Rotator Interval Tear
- Rarely isolated
- CHL = RI roof, torn
- +/- Subcoracoid bursitis
- +/- Subcoracoid impingement
- Extravasation of contrast into subacromial space with arthrography
  - +/- Supraspinatus tear

Biceps Tendinosis
- +/- Impingement
  - Impingement most common cause
- Thickened intermediate to hyperintense tendon
- Short TE sequences sensitive for tendon degeneration
  - T1WI, PD/Intermediate WI, T2* GRE WI

Biceps Tendon Rupture
- +/- Impingement: Most common cause
- Fluid signal intensity fills gap
  - Hyperintense on T2WI, STIR, T2* GRE

SLAP Lesion
- Biceps anchor tear
- +/- LHB tendon tear
- Propagate - extended SLAP lesion
- + Speed's test (bicipital resistance test)
- O'Brien's test (active compression test to entrap anterosuperior labrum)

Subcoracoid Impingement
- +/- Hidden lesion
- +/- Anterior RTC tear
- +/- Subcoracoid bursitis
  - Bursa anterior to subscapularis tendon
  - Bursa lateral to subscapularis joint recess
- +/- Hyperintense subcortical lesser tuberosity cysts (T2)
  - Subcoracoid impingement

PATHOLOGY

General Features
- General path comments
  - Superior aspect of the bicipital groove and lateral aspect of the RI
  - Subscapularis insertion
    - Anterior fibers of the subscapularis merge with CHL and transverse the bicipital groove
    - Deep fibers of subscapularis may tear without retraction of entire tendon
- Etiology
  - Lax or torn SGHL/CHL complex allows LHBT to sublux or dislocate
  - Subscapularis tear/partial tear allows subluxation of LHBT
    - Medial insertion of subscapularis may be disrupted without associated biceps instability if CHL intact laterally
  - The SGHL/CHL complex and the insertion of the subscapularis tendon must be torn to allow medial dislocation of the biceps tendon
  - Tears of SGHL/CHL complex and subscapularis
    - Chronic overuse; acute trauma
- Epidemiology
  - Subscapularis tears: 47% involve the SGHL/CHL complex
  - Incidence of SGHL/CHL lesions in 165 arthroscopically treated shoulder patients: 18%
- Associated abnormalities: Anterior instability; impingement

Gross Pathologic & Surgical Features
- Frayed, degenerated or frankly torn structures in superolateral & anterior aspect of the joint (lateral RI)
- CHL is a bursal structure and is not visualized from the articular side at arthroscopy

Microscopic Features
- Collagen degeneration without influx of inflammatory cells

- "Tendinosis" is preferred term over tendinitis
  - RTC degeneration/tear
- Inflammatory cells

CLINICAL ISSUES

Presentation
- Most common signs/symptoms
  - Impingement pain with biceps symptoms
    - Pain radiating down anterior arm
    - Pain with elbow flexion/supination
- Clinical profile
  - Impingement patient
  - Athletes or workers participating in overhead activities - common
  - Acute trauma
  - Associated with Bankart or Bankart variant

Demographics
- Age: > 40 years
- Gender: M > F

Natural History & Prognosis
- Improve with cessation of repetitive overhead motion
- Post trauma, +/- responds to conservative therapy

Treatment
- Conservative
  - Reduce pain and inflammation (NSAIDs), restore range of motion, strengthening (physical therapy)
- Surgical
  - Repair of torn structures
  - Arthroscopic treatment to repair nonresponsive RTC tear

DIAGNOSTIC CHECKLIST

Consider
- This lesion in setting of biceps subluxation/instability

Image Interpretation Pearls
- Axial images for detection of biceps subluxation
- Pseudosubluxation may be present above level of superior biceps groove where LHBT courses through RI
- Identify tears of distal subscapularis tendon on axial images

SELECTED REFERENCES

1. Bennett WF: Subscapularis, medial, and lateral head coracohumeral ligament insertion anatomy: Arthroscopic appearance and incidence of "hidden" rotator interval lesions. Arthroscopy 2173-80, 2001
2. Bennett WF: The specificity of the Speed's test. Arthroscopic evaluation of the biceps tendon at the level of the bicipital groove. Arthroscopy 14:789-96, 1998
3. Walch G et al: Subluxations and dislocations of the tendon of the long head of the biceps. J Shoulder Elbow Surg 7:100-8, 1998

HIDDEN LESION, SHOULDER

IMAGE GALLERY

Typical

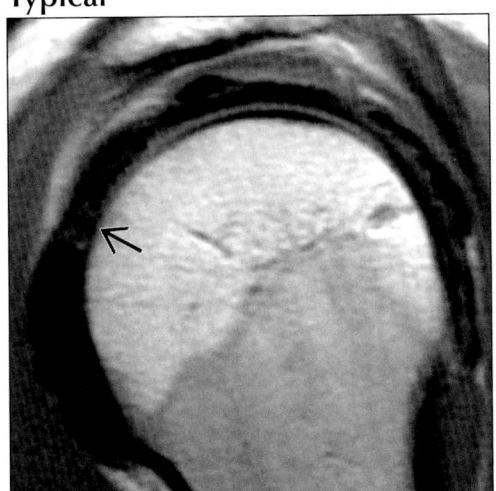 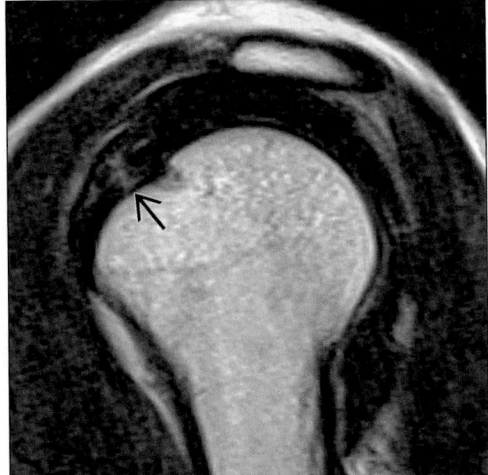

(Left) Sagittal PD FSE MR shows an intact superior glenohumeral ligament attachment (arrow) to the humerus adjacent to the biceps tendon. *(Right)* Sagittal T2 FSE MR shows a torn attachment (arrow) of the distal SGHL.

Typical

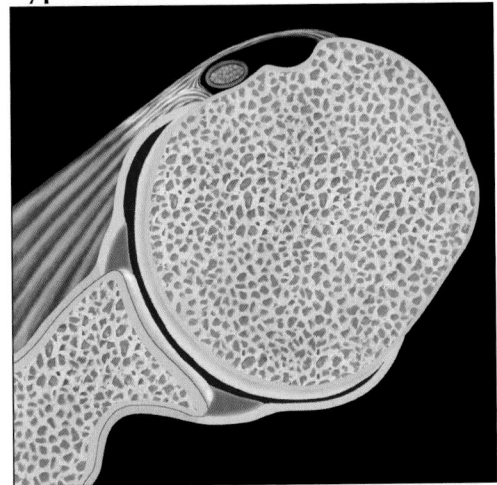 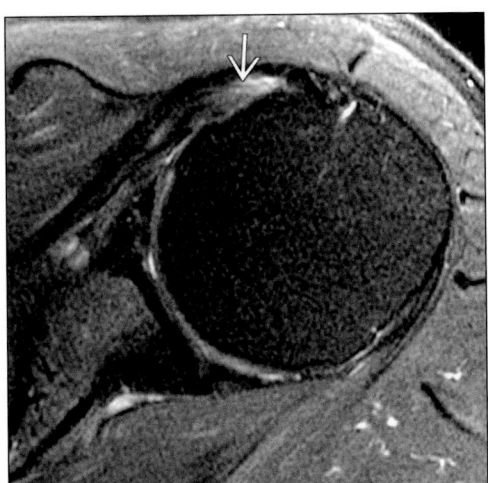

(Left) Axial graphic shows dislocation of the biceps tendon indicating instability in the presence of a hidden lesion. *(Right)* Axial FS PD FSE MR shows tearing (arrow) of the distal aspect of the subscapularis tendon just below the insertion site of the SGHL. There is minimal biceps subluxation.

Typical

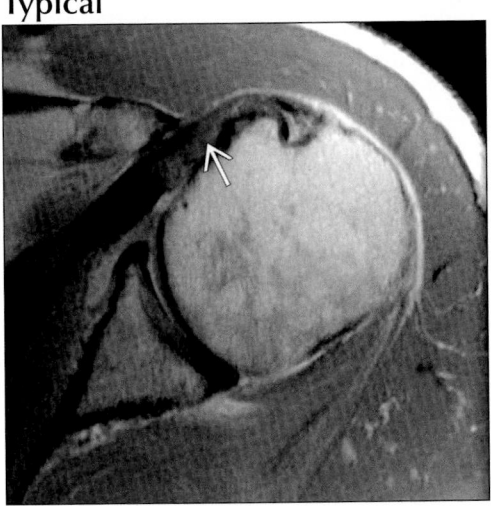 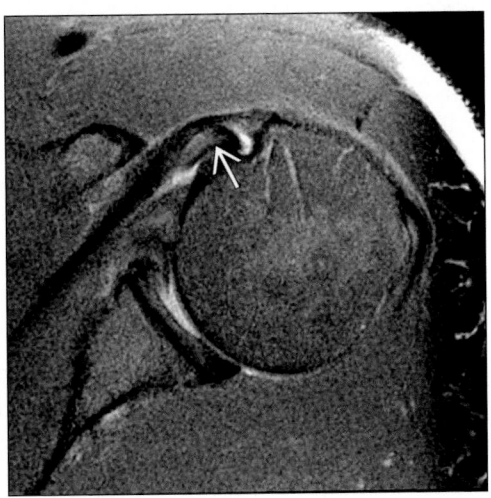

(Left) Axial PD FSE MR shows subluxation of the degenerated biceps because of the presence of a rotator interval hidden lesion. The partially torn subscapularis is demonstrated (arrow). *(Right)* Axial FS PD FSE MR shows subluxation and near-complete dislocation of the biceps tendon (arrow) indicating a hidden lesion.

BICEPS TENDINOSIS

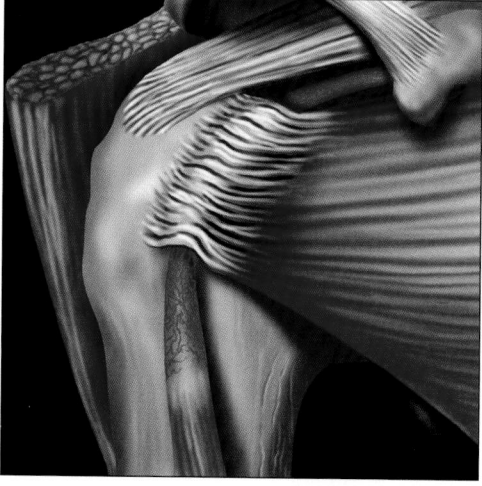

Coronal graphic shows an indurated, degenerated biceps tendon consistent with tendinosis.

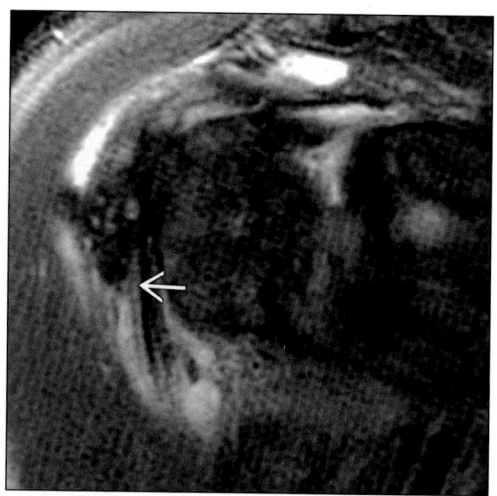

Coronal FS PD FSE MR shows thickening and longitudinal splitting (arrow) of the biceps tendon within the bicipital groove surrounded by inflamed biceps sheath.

TERMINOLOGY

Abbreviations and Synonyms
- Biceps tendinitis, biceps tendon degeneration

Definitions
- Degeneration of the long head biceps (LHB) as a result of chronic microtrauma or acute traumatic injury

IMAGING FINDINGS

General Features
- Best diagnostic clue: Thickening and increased signal intensity of LHB within rotator interval (RI) or bicipital groove on FS PD FSE and PD FSE images
- Location
  - LHBT originates on the supraglenoid tubercle/superior labrum
  - Passes through the anterosuperior joint to enter the humeral bicipital groove
- Size
  - Thickened enlarged tendon (> 5 mm)
    - +/- Thinned if chronically partially torn
- Morphology
  - Thickened, inhomogeneous tendon with visible surface fraying
  - Tendon torn or partially torn in advanced cases with fluid entering defect

Radiographic Findings
- Radiography
  - +/- Sclerosis of superior aspect bicipital groove
    - Chronic cases if accompanied by biceps instability
  - +/- Small associated subchondral cysts in chronic cases on either side of bicipital groove = degenerative change
  - +/- Acromial remodeling/sclerosis
  - +/- Acromial spurs (impingement)
  - Humeral head subchondral sclerosis/cysts

CT Findings
- NECT
  - Acromial spurs (impingement)
  - Acromial remodeling/sclerosis
  - Sagittal reconstruction
- CT arthrography
  - Thickened tendon - tendinosis
  - Small irregular tendon in RI or groove if frayed/partially torn

MR Findings
- T1WI
  - Thickened intermediate signal intensity tendon - tendinosis

DDx: Biceps Tendinosis

Type I BLC	Type II BLC	Type III BLC	Magic Angle	Magic Angle
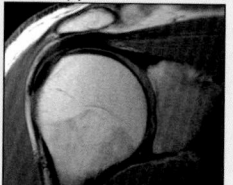	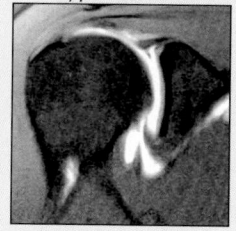	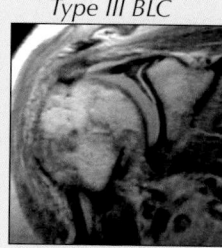	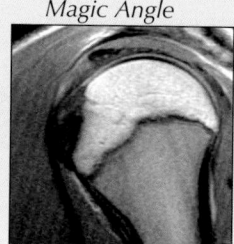	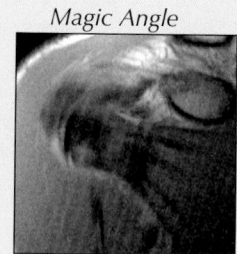
Cor PD FSE MR	Cor FS PD FSE	Cor PD FSE MR	Sag PD FSE MR	Cor PD FSE MR

BICEPS TENDINOSIS

Key Facts

Terminology
- Degeneration of the long head biceps (LHB) as a result of chronic microtrauma or acute traumatic injury

Imaging Findings
- Best diagnostic clue: Thickening and increased signal intensity of LHB within rotator interval (RI) or bicipital groove on FS PD FSE and PD FSE images
- FS PD FSE to show morphology and signal alterations

Top Differential Diagnoses
- SLAP Lesion (Superior Labrum Anterior to Posterior)
- Rotator Cuff Tear
- Subscapularis Tear
- Magic Angle
- Normal Biceps Labral Complex (BLC)

Pathology
- Accompanies rotator cuff disease, especially impingement

Clinical Issues
- Upper arm/shoulder pain often radiating into upper arm especially in overhead athletes
- Typical complaint of dull anterior shoulder pain, esp. with lifting, elevated pushing or pulling
- Pain with Yergason's, Speed's +/- O'Brien's tests

Diagnostic Checklist
- Sagittal images show thickened tendon in RI
- Magic angle produces pseudo hyperintensity of intraarticular biceps tendon on sagittal images

---

- Small, frayed/partially torn, irregular tendon in RI or groove
- +/- Supraspinatus tendinopathy
  - Thickened, intermediate signal intensity tendon
- Acromial spurs (impingement)
  - Spur with marrow fat signal
- T2WI
  - Thickened, irregular tendon frayed and increased in signal intensity
  - Attenuated biceps tendon in partial tear or longitudinal split
  - +/- Supraspinatus tendinopathy
    - FS PD FSE and PD FSE are sensitive to tendinosis while partial tearing or fraying usually requires confirmation of T2 FSE images
  - Acromial remodeling
    - Hypointense sclerosis
    - Impingement (predisposing)
- MR arthrography
  - Thickened filling defect = enlarged tendon/tendinosis
- Thinning of chronic partial tears
- Subluxation or dislocation with biceps instability
  - Flattened against bicipital groove/lesser tuberosity
- Sagittal images - thickened abnormal tendon in RI

Ultrasonographic Findings
- Thickened decreased attenuation tendon
- Tears often directly visible
- Advantage - allows dynamic evaluation with pain correlation

Imaging Recommendations
- Best imaging tool: MRI
- Protocol advice
  - FS PD FSE to show morphology and signal alterations
  - T2 FSE to distinguish between tendinosis and tears

DIFFERENTIAL DIAGNOSIS

SLAP Lesion (Superior Labrum Anterior to Posterior)
- At the level of biceps labral complex
- 9 types
- May extend to anterior, posterior labrum, middle glenohumeral ligament (MGHL)
- Traction injury

Rotator Cuff Tear
- Especially SLAC (superior labrum anterior cuff) lesion
  - SLAP lesion + undersurface anterior supraspinatus partial tear
- Thickened, increased signal intensity tendon with partial or full thickness gap (T2WI)
- Impingement common cause of tear and biceps tendinosis

Subscapularis Tear
- +/- Anterior dislocation in older patient
- +/- Posterior dislocation at any age
  - Especially after seizures
- Discontinuous tendon fibers
- Anterior extension of impingement tear

Magic Angle
- At curve between RI and bicipital groove
- 55 degrees to the external magnetic field
- Artifact
- Increased signal on short TE sequences
  - T1WI, PD/Intermediate WI, T2* GRE WI

Normal Biceps Labral Complex (BLC)
- Type I
  - No biceps labral sulcus
- Type II
  - Small biceps labral sulcus at superior pole of glenoid
- Type III
  - Meniscoid labrum
  - Deep biceps labral sulcus
  - Sulcus extends around the supraglenoid tubercle corner

BICEPS TENDINOSIS

○ Associated with SLAP lesions

PATHOLOGY

General Features
- General path comments
  - Accompanies rotator cuff disease, especially impingement
    - When anterior cuff is torn, biceps is impinged upon by exposure to acromion through rotator cuff tear gap
- Etiology
  - Chronic overuse leads to impingement syndrome
  - Biceps instability associated with impingement/hidden lesion
  - Overhead athletes, esp. baseball pitchers, tennis players, and swimmers - chronic microtrauma
- Epidemiology: Common with subacromial impingement, 20-60% association
- Associated abnormalities
  - Tears of medial head coracohumeral ligament and superior glenohumeral ligament (hidden lesion)
  - Rotator interval tear
  - Subacromial impingement syndrome
  - SLAP lesions
  - Biceps tenosynovitis

Gross Pathologic & Surgical Features
- Thickened, indurated tendon
- Loss of integrity in partially or completely torn tendons
- Synovitis biceps in proximal extraarticular course
- Osteophytes

Microscopic Features
- Collagen degeneration without influx of inflammatory cells: "Tendinosis" is preferred term over tendinitis
- Hypertrophy of tendon

Staging, Grading or Classification Criteria
- Biceps tendon lesions
  - Type A - impingement tendinitis
  - Type B - subluxation
  - Type C - attritional tendinitis
- Biceps tendinitis criteria for tenodesis
  - Reversible tendon change
    - < 25% partial thickness tear from a normal width tendon
    - Normal bicipital groove location
    - Normal tendon size
  - Irreversible tendon change
    - Partial thickness tear/fraying > 25% of normal tendon width
    - Subluxation
    - Disruption of bicipital groove osseous or ligamentous anatomy

CLINICAL ISSUES

Presentation
- Most common signs/symptoms
  - Upper arm/shoulder pain often radiating into upper arm especially in overhead athletes
  - Typical complaint of dull anterior shoulder pain, esp. with lifting, elevated pushing or pulling
  - Often positive impingement signs
  - Pain with Yergason's, Speed's +/- O'Brien's tests
    - Yergason's test - bicipital groove pain with resisted supination
    - Speed's test - bicipital resistance test
    - O'Brien's test - active compression test to entrap anterosuperior labrum (SLAP lesions)
- Clinical profile: Active athlete or patient with subacromial impingement

Demographics
- Age
  - Young athlete
  - Adult with impingement
- Gender: M = F

Natural History & Prognosis
- Rest and conservative treatment to allow healing

Treatment
- Conservative
  - NSAIDs
  - Physical therapy
- Surgical
  - Recalcitrant pain without tear
    - Release of transverse humeral ligament
    - Tenosynovectomy as in treating de Quervain's tenosynovitis
  - Biceps tenodesis in cases of partial or complete tears

DIAGNOSTIC CHECKLIST

Consider
- Associated with rotator cuff tear or SLAP lesion
  - Biceps tendinosis in conjunction with impingement syndrome

Image Interpretation Pearls
- Sagittal images show thickened tendon in RI
- Magic angle produces pseudo hyperintensity of intraarticular biceps tendon on sagittal images

SELECTED REFERENCES

1. Beall DB et al: Association of biceps tendon tears with rotator cuff abnormalities: Degree of correlation with tears of the anterior and superior portions of the rotator cuff. AJR 180(3):633-9, 2003
2. Beltran J et al: Shoulder: Labrum and bicipital tendon. Top Magn Reson Imaging 14(1):35-49, 2003
3. Patton WC et al: Biceps tendinitis and subluxation. Clin Sports Med 20(3):505-29, 2001
4. Gartsman GM et al: Arthroscopic biceps tenodesis: Operative technique. Arthroscopy 16(5):550-2, 2000
5. Iannotti JP et al: Disorders of the shoulder: diagnosis and management. Disorders of the bicpes tendon. Lippincott Williams & Willkins, Philadelphia PA, 159-90, 1999
6. Read JW et al: Shoulder ultrasound: Diagnostic accuracy for impingement syndrome, rotator cuff tear, and biceps tendon pathology. J Shoulder Elbow Surg 7(3):264-71, 1998
7. Beltran J et al: MR arthrography of the shoulder: Variants and pitfalls. Radiographics 17(6):1403-12; discussion 1412-5, 1997

BICEPS TENDINOSIS

IMAGE GALLERY

Typical

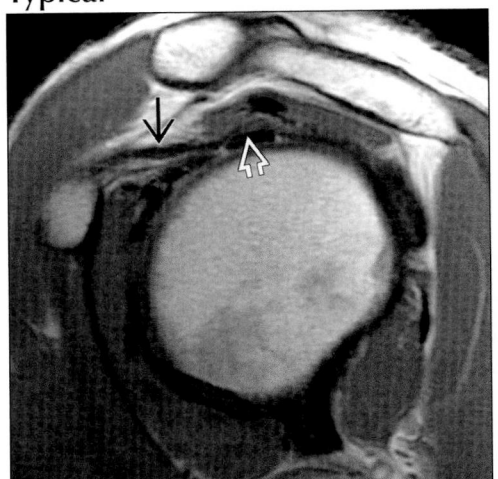

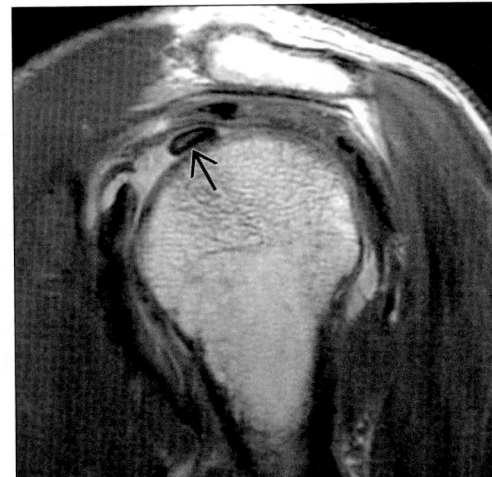

(Left) Sagittal PD FSE MR shows normal biceps tendon (open arrow) within the rotator interval. Note the coracohumeral ligament (arrow) extending from the coracoid to form the roof of the rotator interval. *(Right)* Sagittal PD FSE MR shows biceps tendinosis with thickening and increased signal intensity (arrow) in the tendon.

Typical

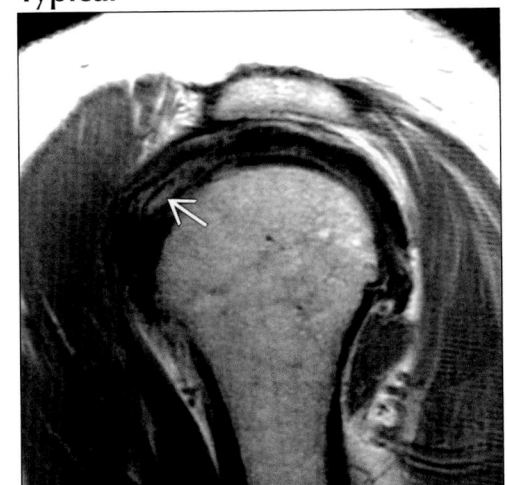

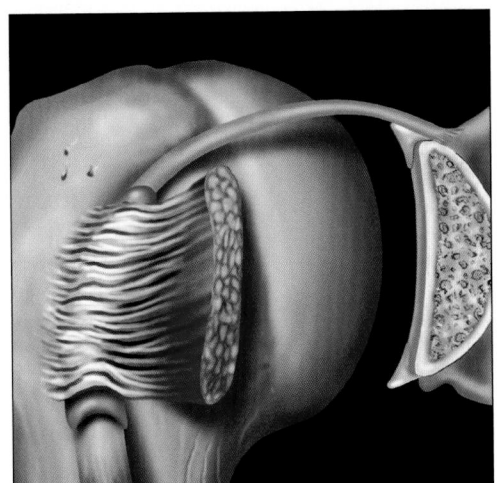

(Left) Sagittal PD FSE MR shows marked thickening and moderate increased signal intensity (arrow) in severe biceps tendinosis. *(Right)* Coronal graphic shows a type I biceps labral complex with labrum adherent to superior pole of glenoid.

Typical

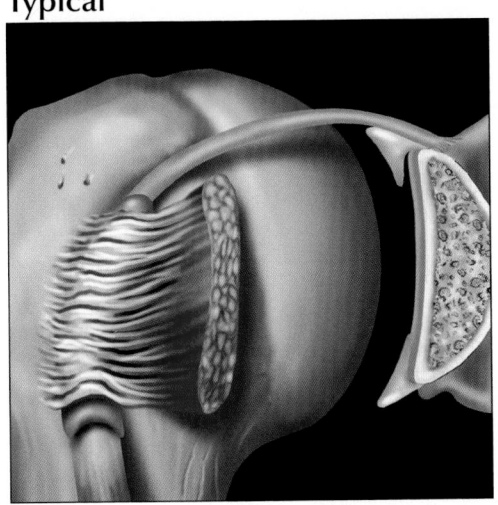

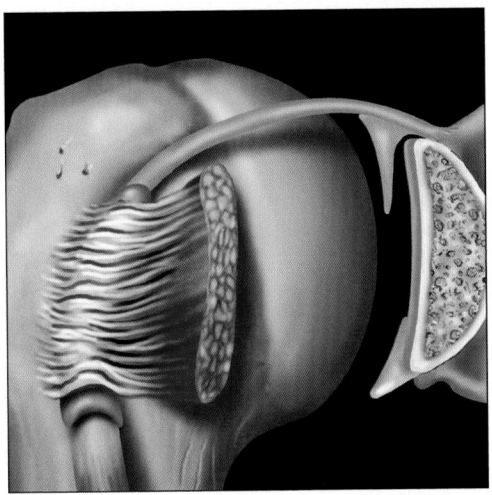

(Left) Coronal graphic shows a type II biceps labral complex with small sulcus. *(Right)* Coronal graphic shows a type III biceps labral complex with a meniscoid superior labrum and deep sulcus.

BICEPS TENDON TEAR

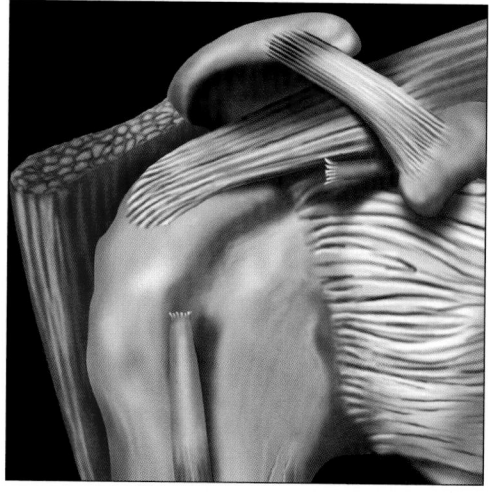

Coronal graphic shows a tear of the long head of the biceps tendon with retraction of the distal end into the mid bicipital groove.

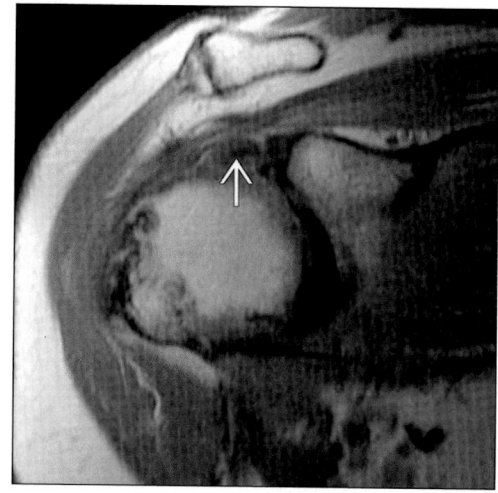

Coronal PD FSE MR shows biceps stump (arrow) in the superior aspect of the joint in a patient with a tear of the biceps tendon. Note the empty bicipital groove superiorly.

TERMINOLOGY

Definitions
- Rupture of long head biceps tendon (LHBT)

IMAGING FINDINGS

General Features
- Best diagnostic clue
  - Tear or gap in the biceps tendon, +/- retraction of tendon edges
    - Proximal stump is often extending from supraglenoid tubercle
- Location
  - Rotator interval (RI) most common
  - Adjacent to biceps anchor
- Size: Tear varies from millimeter range to extensive (several centimeters)
- Morphology
  - Gap in thickened, irregular increased signal intensity tendon on all pulse sequences
  - Thinned tendon = chronic partial tear

Radiographic Findings
- Radiography
  - Secondary findings associated with subacromial impingement - predisposing
    - Acromial spurs
    - Humeral head (HH) subchondral greater tuberosity cysts
    - Type III acromion (hooked)
    - Superior HH migration with rotator cuff (RTC) tears

CT Findings
- NECT
  - Secondary findings associated primarily with subacromial impingement
    - Subacromial spurs
    - HH subcortical degenerative cysts
    - Osteophytes, cysts at bicipital groove
- CT arthrography
  - Bicipital groove filled with contrast, lack of biceps "filling defect"
  - +/- Supraspinatus tendon tear with contrast extending through tear

MR Findings
- T1WI
  - Hypointense biceps stump visualized in superior aspect of the joint
    - Stump degenerated/frayed (intermediate signal intensity)
  - Superior labrum anterior-posterior (SLAP) lesions
    - SLAP IV bucket-handle tear of meniscoid labrum + biceps tendon extension

DDx: Biceps Tendon Tear

Biceps Tenodesis	Biceps Tendinosis	Biceps Tendinosis	RI Tear	Hidden Lesion
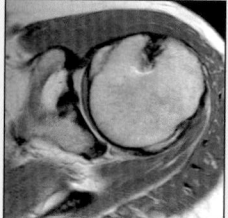	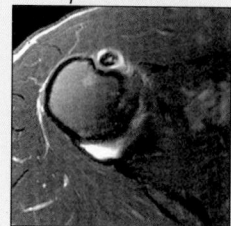	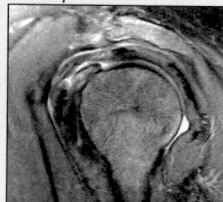	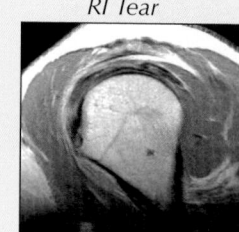	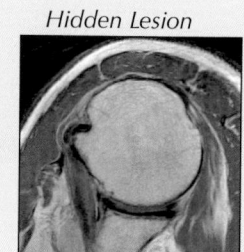
Ax PD FSE MR	Ax FS PD FSE MR	Sag FS PD FSE	Sag PD FSE MR	Ax PD FSE MR

BICEPS TENDON TEAR

Key Facts

Imaging Findings

- Tear or gap in the biceps tendon, +/- retraction of tendon edges
- Fluid signal intensity (hyperintense) filling gap in the tendon
- +/- Fluid (hyperintensity) within subacromial +/- subcoracoid bursae = reactive
- Irregular biceps stump visualized in superior aspect of the joint

Top Differential Diagnoses

- SLAP lesion
- Supraspinatus Impingement
- Greater Tuberosity Bone Trabecular Injury/Fracture
- Subcoracoid Impingement
- Biceps Tenodesis

- Rotator Interval Tear (RI Tear)
- Hidden Lesion

Pathology

- Seen with supraspinatus impingement/tear
- Distal tendon edge may retract into upper arm
- Predisposing tendinosis
- Subacromial impingement
- Subcoracoid impingement

Clinical Issues

- Asymmetrical pain over bicipital groove compared to contralateral shoulder

Diagnostic Checklist

- Check for empty bicipital groove in all three planes
- Identify biceps stump in RI

- ▪ Increased signal intensity within biceps anchor, +/- fragment
- ○ HH subchondral hypointense greater tuberosity cysts
- T2WI
  - ○ Fluid signal intensity (hyperintense) filling gap in the tendon
  - ○ +/- Rotator cuff tear
    - ▪ Fluid signal hyperintensity filling gap of torn tendon = complete tear
    - ▪ Fluid signal hyperintensity extending into partial gap of torn tendon = partial tear
  - ○ +/- Fluid (hyperintensity) within subacromial +/- subcoracoid bursae = reactive
  - ○ +/- Hyperintense effusion
  - ○ Irregular biceps stump visualized in superior aspect of the joint
    - ▪ Stump degenerated/frayed (intermediate to hyperintense)
  - ○ +/- SLAP lesion
  - ○ Hyperintense greater tuberosity cysts
- PD/Intermediate
  - ○ Gap in tendon
  - ○ + Synovitis
    - ▪ Thickened increased signal intensity synovial lining
    - ▪ Seen on PD/Intermediate
- Variable retraction and degeneration of the tendon edges
- Type III acromion (impingement): Visualized on sagittal images

Imaging Recommendations

- Best imaging tool: MRI
- Protocol advice
  - ○ FS PD FSE/T2WI
  - ○ T1/PD for tendinosis/pretear

DIFFERENTIAL DIAGNOSIS

SLAP lesion

- Tear of biceps anchor

- +/- Tendon tear
- May propagate into
  - ○ Anterior labrum, posterior labrum
  - ○ Middle glenohumeral ligament (MGHL/MGL)
  - ○ Circumferentially
- + Speed's test (bicipital resistance test)
- O'Brien's test (active compression test to entrap anterosuperior labrum)

Supraspinatus Impingement

- Pain anteriorly with abduction
- +/- Hyperintense fluid signal on T2WI extending into tear/partial tear
- +/- Thickening, increased signal of supraspinatus tendon on short and long TE sequences
- +/- Thickened coracoacromial ligament

Greater Tuberosity Bone Trabecular Injury/Fracture

- Hyperintense greater tuberosity on T2WI
- + History of trauma
- +/- Visualized fracture fragment
  - ○ Hypointense fracture line
  - ○ Hyperintense edema on T2WI
- +/- Anterior dislocation

Subcoracoid Impingement

- Impingement of coracoid on subscapularis/biceps at RI
- Pain with internal rotation
- +/- Hyperintense subchondral cysts on T2WI
- Predisposes to biceps tendinosis/instability
- Elongated coracoid predisposing
- +/- Rotator interval (coracohumeral ligament component) tear

Biceps Tenodesis

- Absent biceps in rotator interval
- + Micrometallic artifact
- + Surgical history

Rotator Interval Tear (RI Tear)

- Roof = coracohumeral ligament (CHL) and supraspinatus
- History of impingement

BICEPS TENDON TEAR

- +/- History of anterior dislocation
- +/- Subcoracoid impingement
- Leads to contrast extension into subacromial bursa at arthrography
- +/- Synovitis
- Hyperintense roof of RI - T2WI

Hidden Lesion
- Subcategory of RI lesion
- Deep fiber subscapularis + CHL dysfunction
- Biceps instability
- +/- Biceps tendon tear
- Hyperintensity, irregularity on T2WI

PATHOLOGY

General Features
- General path comments
  - Seen with supraspinatus impingement/tear
  - Distal tendon edge may retract into upper arm
  - Predisposing tendinosis
- Etiology
  - Chronic overuse/microtrauma
    - Subacromial impingement with tear "exposing" biceps tendon to repetitive trauma of acromion
  - Acute traction to shoulder
- Epidemiology
  - Shoulder pain in 7-25% Western general population
  - Biceps tear commonly accompanies impingement (rotator cuff disease)
- Associated abnormalities
  - Subacromial impingement
  - Subcoracoid impingement
  - SLAP lesions
  - Lesser tuberosity degenerative change, subcortical cysts
  - Biceps tenosynovitis

Gross Pathologic & Surgical Features
- Usually thickened, indurated tendon edges
- Disruption in integrity of tendon
- Muscle belly may retract
  - Less obvious than with distal biceps tear
  - Muscle edematous

Microscopic Features
- Preexisting collagen degeneration = tendinosis

Staging, Grading or Classification Criteria
- Biceps tendon lesions
  - Type A - impingement tendinitis
  - Type B - subluxation
  - Type C - attritional tendinitis
- Biceps tendinitis criteria for tenodesis
  - Reversible tendon change
    - < 25% partial thickness tear from a normal width tendon
    - Normal bicipital groove location
    - Normal tendon size
  - Irreversible tendon change
    - Partial thickness tear/fraying > 25% of normal tendon width
    - Subluxation

- Disruption of bicipital groove osseous or ligamentous anatomy

CLINICAL ISSUES

Presentation
- Most common signs/symptoms
  - Asymmetrical pain over bicipital groove compared to contralateral shoulder
  - Positive impingement signs
  - Pain with Yergason's, Speed's +/- O'Brien's tests
    - Yergason's test - bicipital pain with resisted supination
    - Speed's test - bicipital resistance
    - O'Brien's test - active compression test for SLAP lesions
  - Muscle belly may retract
    - Leads to "Popeye sign"
    - Less obvious than with distal biceps tear because of anchor of short head tendon preventing retraction
- Clinical profile: Impingement patient, athlete

Demographics
- Age: Adult with impingement, athletes
- Gender: M > F

Natural History & Prognosis
- Tenosynovitis and tendinosis without tear will often improve with conservative management
- Pain from full thickness tears and partial tears often progresses
  - Requires arthroscopic/surgical management

Treatment
- Conservative: Physical therapy and NSAIDs
- Partial full thickness tears - tenodesis

DIAGNOSTIC CHECKLIST

Consider
- Impingement syndrome

Image Interpretation Pearls
- Check for empty bicipital groove in all three planes
- Identify biceps stump in RI
- Distinguish between intraarticular or extraarticular tear
- Inspect biceps labral complex on coronal images for an intact biceps tendon

SELECTED REFERENCES

1. Beltran JM et al: Shoulder: Labrum and bicipital tendon. Top Magn Reson Imaging 14(1):35-49, 2003
2. Gartsman GM et al: Arthroscopic biceps tenodesis: Operative technique. Arthroscopy 16(5):550-2, 2001
3. Ken Yamaguchi et al: Disorders of the Shoulder. Disorders of the biceps tendon. Philadelphia PA, Lippincott Williams & Wilkins, 159-90, 1999
4. Tirman PF et al: A practical approach to imaging of the shoulder with emphasis on MR imaging. Orthop Clin North Am 28(4):483-515, 1997

BICEPS TENDON TEAR

IMAGE GALLERY

Typical

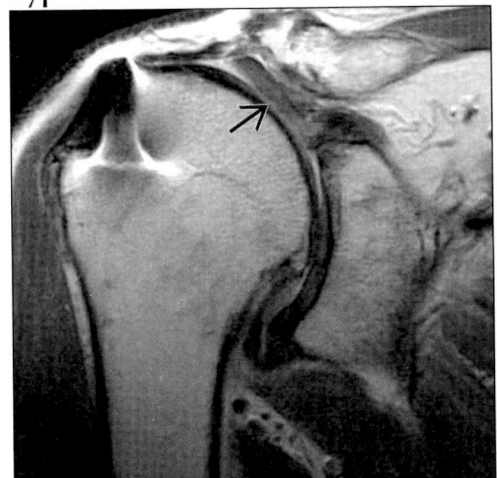 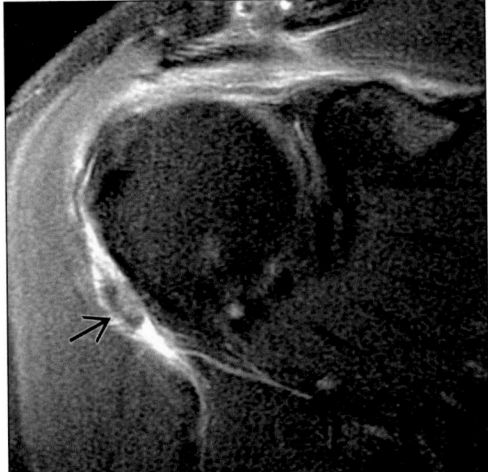

(Left) Coronal PD FSE MR shows the biceps stump (arrow) directed superiorly. *(Right)* Coronal FS PD FSE MR shows the distal stump (arrow) within the bicipital groove surrounded by edema and fluid in a patient with biceps rupture.

Typical

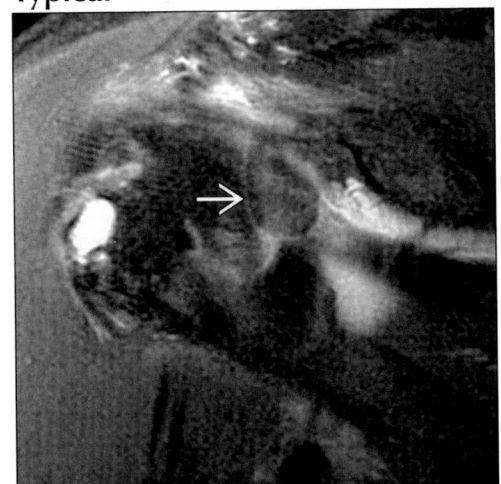 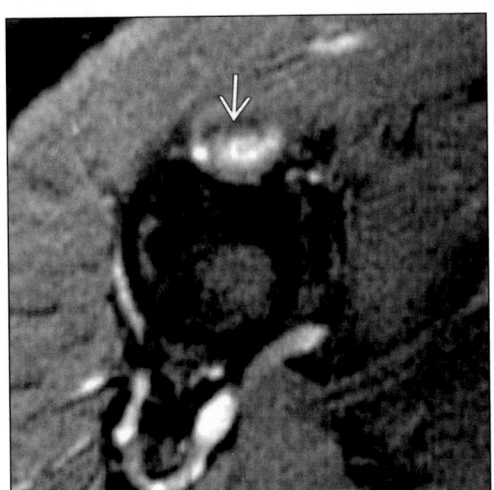

(Left) Coronal FS PD FSE MR shows stump (arrow) of the biceps anchor in the superior aspect of shoulder joint in a patient with biceps rupture. *(Right)* Axial STIR MR shows the top of the distal stump (arrow) of the biceps and an empty bicipital tendon sheath within the groove.

Typical

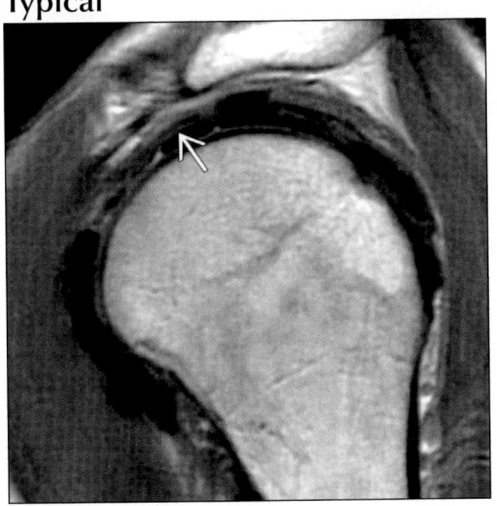 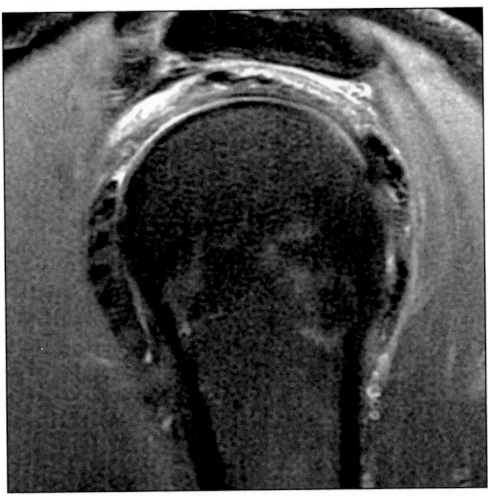

(Left) Sagittal PD FSE MR shows normal biceps tendon (arrow) in the rotator interval. *(Right)* Sagittal FS PD FSE MR shows an empty rotator interval in a patient with a biceps rupture.

SLAP LESIONS I-IV

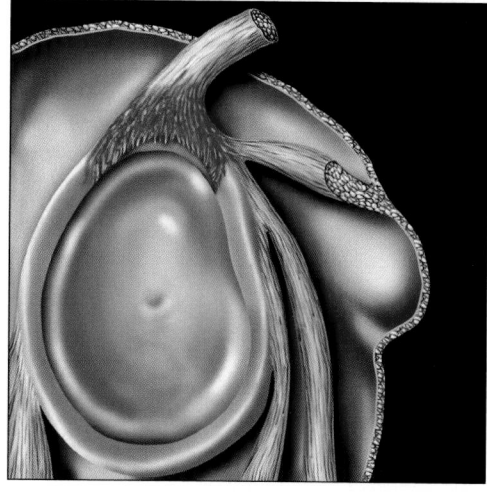

Sagittal graphic demonstrates detachment of the superior labrum extending from anterior to posterior in a type II SLAP lesion.

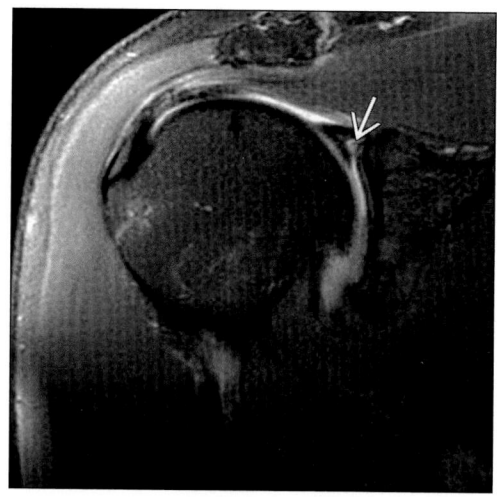

Coronal FS PD FSE MR demonstrates irregular increased signal intensity (arrow) within the superior labrum in a patient with a type II SLAP lesion.

TERMINOLOGY

Abbreviations and Synonyms
- Superior labrum from anterior-to-posterior (SLAP) lesions or tears

Definitions
- SLAP lesions I through IV vary from simple fraying and fragmentation of the biceps labral complex (BLC) to a bucket-handle tear +/- biceps extension
  - Extended SLAP lesions = types V through IX

IMAGING FINDINGS

General Features
- Best diagnostic clue: Hyperintense linear fluid signal within superior labrum on FS PD FSE coronal images
- Location
  - SLAP I - superior labrum
  - SLAP II - superior labrum and biceps anchor
  - SLAP III - superior labrum
  - SLAP IV - superior labrum + biceps tendon
  - SLAC (superior labral anterior cuff) - labral tear restricted to anterior aspect of superior labrum
    - Represents a subtype of SLAP II
    - Associated with anterior supraspinatus articular sided partial tear

- Posterior peelback - posterosuperior labrum + posterior undersurface cuff tear
    - Represents a subtype of SLAP II
- Size
  - Focal of frayed and degeneration labrum in SLAP I
  - Complete anterior to posterior extension in SLAP II-IV
- Morphology
  - SLAP I - indistinct margins vs. normal triangular shape with intrasubstance degeneration
    - Normal variant in degenerative shoulder
  - SLAP II
    - Detachment of superior labrum from superior pole of glenoid vs. linear labral tear from anterior-to-posterior
  - SLAP III
    - Bucket-handle tear of a meniscoid superior labrum
  - SLAP IV
    - Bucket-handle tear of superior meniscoid labrum
    - Extension into ± complete avulsion of biceps tendon

MR Findings
- T1WI
  - SLAP I
    - Intermediate signal within the boundaries of superior labrum at level of biceps labral complex
  - SLAP II-IV

DDx: SLAP Lesions I-IV

Biceps Rupture	Paralabral Cyst	Hidden Lesion	Micro-Insta/SLAC	Supraglen Cyst

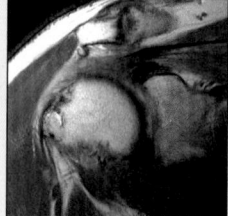 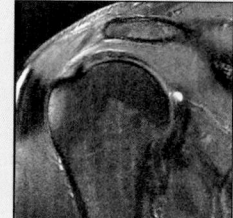 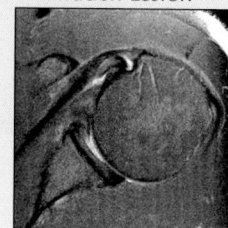 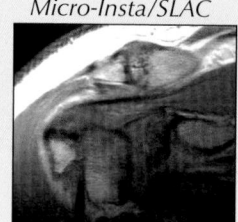 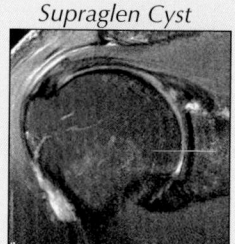

Cor PD FSE MR	Cor FS PD FSE	Ax FS PD FSE	Cor PD FSE MR	Cor FS PD FSE

SLAP LESIONS I-IV

Key Facts

Terminology
- SLAP lesions I through IV vary from simple fraying and fragmentation of the biceps labral complex (BLC) to a bucket-handle tear +/- biceps extension

Imaging Findings
- Best diagnostic clue: Hyperintense linear fluid signal within superior labrum on FS PD FSE coronal images
- Focal of frayed and degeneration labrum in SLAP I

Top Differential Diagnoses
- Impingement
- Sublabral Foramen (Hole)
- Buford Complex
- Rotator Cuff Tendinopathy/Partial Tear

Pathology
- Anterior rotator cuff tears
- Posterosuperior rotator cuff tears
- Paralabral cyst

Clinical Issues
- Patient status post traction injury (forced extension on flexed forearm), typically type II
- Patient status post fall on outstretched hand (31%), usually type III, IV or extended SLAP (type V with anterior labral extension)
- Patient status post anterior dislocation (16%), often extended SLAP (type V)

Diagnostic Checklist
- Age related degeneration in SLAP I as a normal finding

- Intermediate signal intensity within superior labrum visualized anterior and posterior to BLC where biceps tendon attaches to superior labrum
- T2WI
  - SLAP I
    - Intermediate to hyperintense labral degeneration without linear tear
  - SLAP II
    - Linear hyperintense tear along long axis of superior labrum (coronal plane)
    - Fluid signal between superior labrum and superior pole of glenoid creating a greater than 5 mm displacement of labrum and biceps anchor on coronal images
    - +/- Paralabral cyst
  - SLAP III
    - Identify fragmented superior labrum into two separate components on coronal & sagittal images through BLC
  - SLAP IV
    - Split of biceps tendon with hyperintense linear longitudinal tear vs. avulsion with absent intraarticular tendon
  - Associated anterior inferior, posterior inferior extension in extended SLAP lesions
  - Hyperintense signal on FS PD FSE and T2 FSE images in associated partial articular surface rotator cuff tears
    - SLAP II subtypes: Classic SLAP II, posterior peelback, SLAC lesion
  - Confusing terminology (not recommended) used in describing labral tract
    - GLOM (glenoid labrum ovoid mass) sign: Low signal intensity mass anterior to glenoid rim as sign of avulsed anterior labrum
    - "Cheerio" sign - displaced fragment of a bucket-handle SLAP tear
- MR arthrography
  - Contrast extension into SLAP lesion
  - +/- Communication with a paralabral cyst

Imaging Recommendations
- Best imaging tool: MRI, MR arthrography

- Protocol advice
  - FS PD FSE, PD FSE, T2* GRE
  - Coronal, axial and sagittal images of BLC

DIFFERENTIAL DIAGNOSIS

Impingement
- Clinical signs may mimic impingement as the long head of the biceps is involved in both processes
- Shoulder pain anteriorly with abduction
- +/- Thickening, increased signal of supraspinatus tendon (SST) on short and long TE sequences
- +/- Thickened coracoacromial ligament

Sublabral Foramen (Hole)
- Sublabral hole confined to anterior superior labrum
- No involvement of BLC

Buford Complex
- Buford complex confined to anterior superior labrum
- Absent anterior superior labrum above equator
- Cord-like glenohumeral ligament
  - Mimics displaced labral fragment

Rotator Cuff Tendinopathy/Partial Tear
- Seen with SLAC lesions
- +/- Thickening, increased signal of supraspinatus tendon on FS PD FSE images
- FS PD FSE and T2 FSE most sensitive
- Microinstability - associated
- Seen with posterior peelback lesions
- Evaluate for associated hidden lesion

PATHOLOGY

General Features
- General path comments
  - Normal anatomy of biceps labral complex (BLC)
  - Type 1: BLC firmly attached to superior pole of glenoid
  - Type 2: Biceps attached to superior labrum lateral to superior glenoid

- Fluid-filled sublabral sulcus formed at superior pole of glenoid
  - Type 3: Meniscoid labrum associated with a large sulcus
    - Should not be mistaken for a SLAP lesion
- Etiology
  - Eccentric overload of biceps during followthrough
  - Compression of superior glenoid rim
    - Fall on outstretched arm
  - Repetitive pull on long head of biceps tendon (LHBT) with overhead sports
  - Microinstability
- Epidemiology: Most common (40% of all SLAP lesions)
- Associated abnormalities
  - Anterior rotator cuff tears
    - Anterior cuff undersurface secondary to failure of the SGHL/CHL/RI (microinstability and abnormal translation of the cuff)
    - Results in "impingement"/chaffing of the cuff undersurface on the superior glenoid rim = SLAC lesion
    - SLAC as a SLAP type II subtype with anterior component of SLAP II
  - Posterosuperior rotator cuff tears
    - Posterior subtype SLAP type II lesion = posterior peelback lesion (posterosuperior component of a SLAP II tear)
    - Posterior capsular contractions lead to abnormal obligate translation
    - Undersurface posterior SST anterior infraspinatus tendon and posterior peelback lesion + HH chondral chaffing/impaction
  - Paralabral cyst
    - Often associated with SLAP lesion/labral tear especially (SLAP II)
    - Represents joint fluid extruded through tear

Gross Pathologic & Surgical Features
- Bare labral footprint
- > 5 mm sublabral sulcus
- Displaceable biceps root (rolls over glenoid)
- Effects of SLAP lesions
  - Biceps anchor disruption
  - Humeral head translation (microinstability)
  - Strain of humeral head restraints
  - Glenohumeral laxity/instability

Microscopic Features
- Fibrocartilaginous degeneration and/or tear of the superior labrum/biceps anchor
- Hemorrhagic synovium

Staging, Grading or Classification Criteria
- Type I: Degenerative fraying
- Type II: Detachment of the biceps anchor and superior labrum
  - Anterior variety = SLAC (superior labral anterior cuff) lesion
  - Anterior to posterior variety = classical type II SLAP
  - Posterior variety = posterior peelback lesion = internal impingement
- Type III: Bucket-handle tear of superior labrum leaving biceps intact still
- Type IV: Bucket-handle tear extending into biceps

CLINICAL ISSUES

Presentation
- Most common signs/symptoms
  - Patient status post traction injury (forced extension on flexed forearm), typically type II
  - Patient status post fall on outstretched hand (31%), usually type III, IV or extended SLAP (type V with anterior labral extension)
  - Patient status post anterior dislocation (16%), often extended SLAP (type V)
- Clinical profile
  - Posttraumatic patient
  - Only approximately one-third with symptoms referable to the biceps tendon
  - Rotator cuff pain common especially with type II lesions
  - Active compression and provocation tests

Demographics
- Age
  - Typically young patient for most SLAP lesions
  - Type I lesions (degenerative) seen in older patients
- Gender: M > F

Natural History & Prognosis
- Small tears/stable tears may heal but unstable tears require surgical stabilization

Treatment
- Conservative
  - Reducing pain and inflammation (NSAIDs), restoring range of motion, strengthening (physical therapy)
- Surgical
  - Type I - debridement
  - Type II - stabilize
    - Bioabsorbable tack
  - Type III - debride
  - Type IV - suture of biceps, reattachment of labrum
    - Biceps tenodesis

DIAGNOSTIC CHECKLIST

Consider
- Age related degeneration in SLAP I as a normal finding

Image Interpretation Pearls
- Fluid signal intensity within the substance of the labrum vs. detachment of the entire labrum at the BLC; characterize SLAP lesions

SELECTED REFERENCES

1. Beltran JM et al: Shoulder. Labrum and bicipital tendon. Top Magn Reson Imaging 14(1):35-49, 2003
2. Musgrave DS et al: SLAP lesions: Current concepts. Am J Orthop 30(1):29-38, 2001
3. Stoller DW et al: The shoulder. Magnetic resonance imaging in orthopaedics and sports medicine. vol 1. 2nd ed. Philadelphia PA, J.B. Lippincott, 597-742, 1997

SLAP LESIONS I-IV

IMAGE GALLERY

Typical

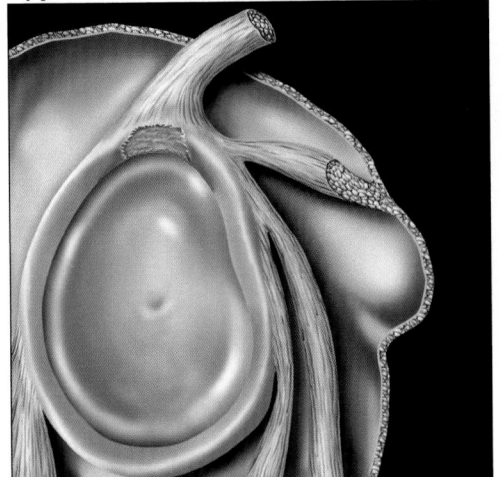
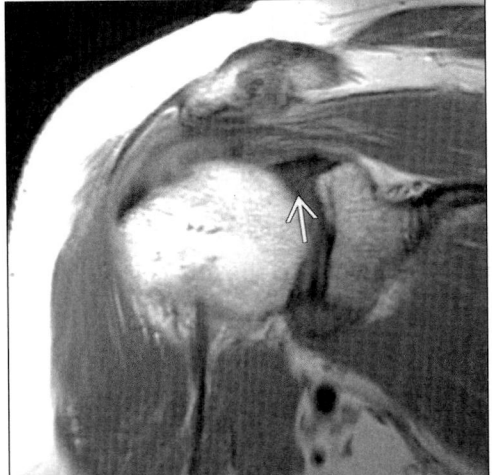

(Left) Sagittal graphic demonstrates a type I SLAP lesion as degenerative fraying and induration. *(Right)* Coronal PD FSE MR demonstrates diffuse increased signal intensity within the superior labrum (arrow) in a patient with a type I SLAP lesion.

Typical

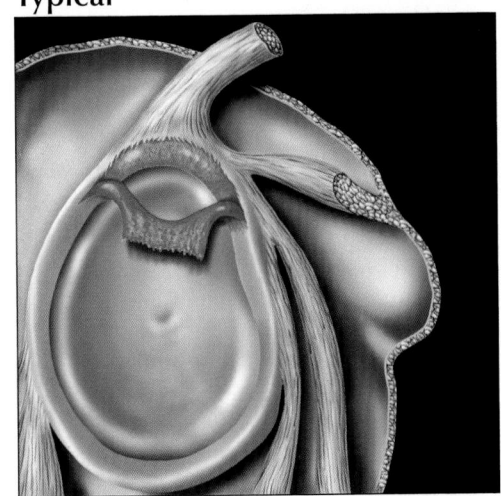
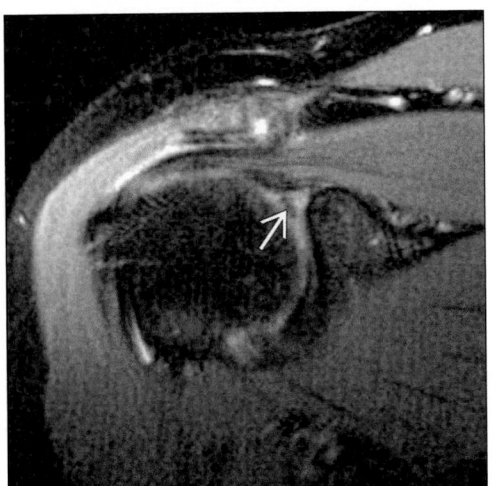

(Left) Sagittal graphic shows a type III SLAP lesion with bucket handle tear at the superior labrum/biceps anchor. *(Right)* Coronal STIR MR demonstrates a type III SLAP lesion with a bucket-handle fragment (arrow).

Typical

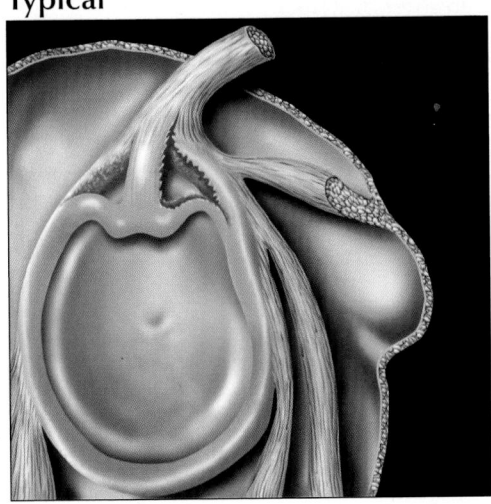
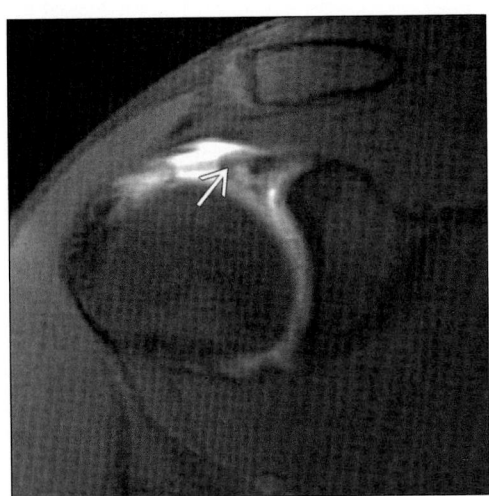

(Left) Sagittal graphic demonstrates a type IV SLAP lesion with the bucket handle tear extending into the biceps tendon itself. *(Right)* Coronal FS T1 arthrogram demonstrates a SLAP II lesion with extension into the biceps tendon (arrow). The superior labrum was divided into two fragments.

SLAP LESIONS V-IX

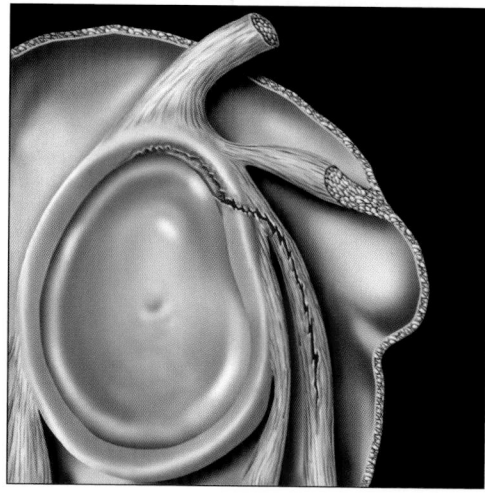

Sagittal graphic demonstrates a tear of the superior labrum (biceps labral complex) extending into the middle glenohumeral ligament (SLAP VII Lesion).

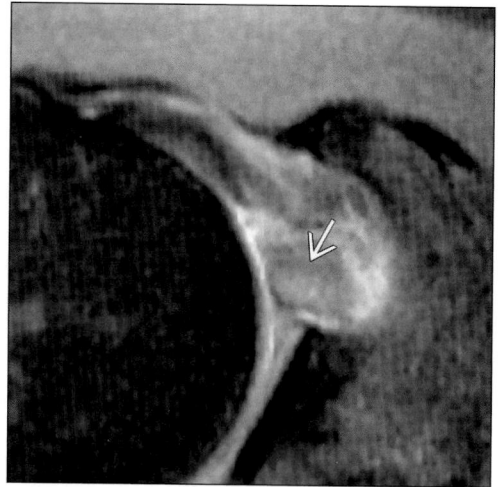

Axial FS PD FSE MR shows a type VII SLAP lesion extending into the middle glenohumeral ligament which is thickened and edematous (arrow).

TERMINOLOGY

Abbreviations and Synonyms
- Superior labrum anterior to posterior (SLAP) lesions

Definitions
- Tear of the superior labrum at the biceps labral complex
- Extension of the SLAP lesion into surrounding structures = extended SLAP lesions
  - Anterior labrum (type V)
  - Flap tear superior labrum (type VI)
  - MGHL (type VII)
  - Posterior labrum (type VIII)
  - Circumferential involvement (type IX)
- Classic SLAP II - a tear extending from the anterior aspect to the posterior aspect of the superior labrum

IMAGING FINDINGS

General Features
- Best diagnostic clue
  - Fluid signal intensity on T2WI (FS PD FSE) within the substance of the superior labrum of biceps labral complex (BLC)

- Signal may be linear and involve irregularity/tearing of: Anterior/posterior labrum ± inferior labrum, MGHL
- Location
  - Biceps labral complex
  - SLAP tears may be associated with
    - Bankart lesion (type V)
    - Reverse Bankart lesion (type VIII)
    - Middle glenohumeral ligament (type VII)
    - Circumferential labral involvement (type IX)
- Size: Up to all four quadrants of the glenoid rim
- Morphology: Tears vary from focal flap tear in type VI to complete labral detachment of anterior, posterior, superior and inferior labrum in type IX

MR Findings
- T1WI
  - SLAP V
    - Intermediate signal of tear with superior extension of an anteroinferior Bankart lesion
    - ± Bony Bankart fracture - anterior inferior glenoid rim
    - ± Hill-Sachs posterolateral impaction fracture (superior humeral head)
  - SLAP VI - IV
    - Difficult to visualize without FS PD FSE, PD FSE or T2* GRE
- T2WI
  - SLAP V

DDx: SLAP Lesions V-IX

Type V SLAP	Type V SLAP	Type VI SLAP	Type VII SLAP	Type VIII SLAP
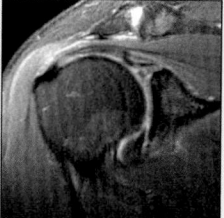	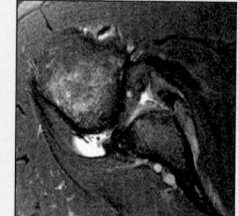	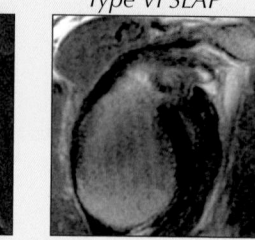	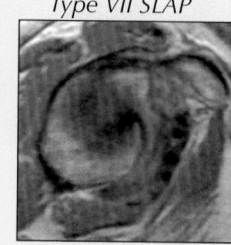	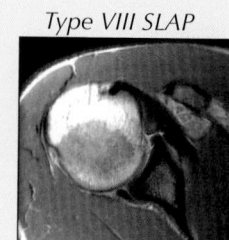
Cor FS PD FSE	Ax FS PD FSE	Sag PD FSE MR	Sag PD FSE MR	Ax PD FSE MR

SLAP LESIONS V-IX

Key Facts

Terminology
- Tear of the superior labrum at the biceps labral complex
- Extension of the SLAP lesion into surrounding structures = extended SLAP lesions
- Anterior labrum (type V)
- Flap tear superior labrum (type VI)
- MGHL (type VII)
- Posterior labrum (type VIII)
- Circumferential involvement (type IX)

Imaging Findings
- Fluid signal intensity on T2WI (FS PD FSE) within the substance of the superior labrum of biceps labral complex (BLC)

Top Differential Diagnoses
- Impingement
- Sublabral Foramen
- Buford Complex
- Rotator Cuff Tendinopathy/Partial tear

Pathology
- Eccentric overload of biceps during follow through

Clinical Issues
- Patient status post fall on outstretched hand (31%), usually type III, IV or V lesion

Diagnostic Checklist
- Evaluate all labral quadrants including BLC and inferior glenohumeral ligament labral complex

---

- Hyperintense fluid undermining anterior labrum from anterosuperior to anteroinferior quadrant + SLAP II findings (linear hyperintensity vs. detachment of superior labrum at BLC)
- SLAP VI
  - Hypointense anteroposterior labral flap tear + SLAP II surrounded by hyperintense joint fluid
  - Visualized on sagittal images with either superior or inferior displacement of unstable flap
- SLAP VII
  - Hypointense fluid within a split MGL secondary to anterior extension of a type II SLAP lesion
  - Thickened edematous MGL
- SLAP VIII
  - Fluid undermining posterior labrum
  - Posterosuperior to posteroinferior
  - Posterior instability
  - Reverse Hill-Sachs lesion (anteromedial impaction fracture humeral head)
  - Lesser tuberosity fracture in posterior dislocation
  - ± Subscapularis stretched or detached ± teres minor tendon tear
  - ± Posterior labrocapsular periosteal sleeve avulsion (POLPSA)
- SLAP IX
  - Avulsion ± fluid undermining the entire labrum circumferentially
  - BLC involved
  - IGL labral complex involved (lower two thirds of labrum)
  - Labrum ± severe degeneration & osseous glenoid cystic changes associated with the concentric labral avulsion
- PD/Intermediate
  - +/- Synovitis
    - Intermediate to increased signal intensity thickened synovium
    - Increased signal compared to joint fluid
- MR arthrography
  - Contrast extending into SLAP lesion
  - +/- Reverse Bankart lesion (SLAP VIII)
  - Contrast delineates avulsion
  - Define healed/partially healed resynovialized lesion

- ± Communication with a paralabral cyst
- Irregularity and/or widening of recess beneath the superior labrum

Imaging Recommendations
- Best imaging tool: MRI, MR arthrography
- Protocol advice: FS PD FSE/PD FSE , T2* GRE in coronal, axial, and sagittal planes at BLC

DIFFERENTIAL DIAGNOSIS

Impingement
- Clinical signs may mimic impingement (as the long head of the biceps is involved)
- Pain anteriorly with abduction
- +/- Thickening, increased signal of supraspinatus tendon on short and long TE sequences
- +/- Thickened coracoacromial ligament

Sublabral Foramen
- Anterior superior labrum involved without osseous glenoid attachment
- Sublabral hole confined to anterior superior quadrant
- Normal anatomical finding at imaging
- No involvement of BLC

Buford Complex
- Buford complex confined to anterior superior labrum
- Absent anterior superior labrum
- Above equator
- Cord-like MGHL
  - Mimics displaced labral fragment

Rotator Cuff Tendinopathy/Partial tear
- Microinstability
  - Includes both SLAP + rotator cuff tendinopathy
- +/- Thickening, increased signal of supraspinatus tendon on FS PD FSE (for tendinosis) and T2 FSE (for tear)
- Associated with SLAC lesion and posterior peel back lesions
- +/- Hidden lesion of internal

SLAP LESIONS V-IX

PATHOLOGY

General Features
- General path comments: With microinstability
- Etiology
  - Eccentric overload of biceps during follow through
  - Compression of superior glenoid rim
    - Fall on outstretched arm
  - Repetitive pull on long head of biceps tendon (LHBT) with overhead sports
- Epidemiology: 6% of shoulder arthroscopy
- Associated abnormalities
  - Microinstabilitiy
    - SGHL avulsion or laxity
    - MGHL/MGL avulsion (straight anterior laxity)
    - SLAC (superior labrum anterior cuff)
    - SLAP lesions I through IX
    - Posterior peelback SLAP
    - Interval tears

Gross Pathologic & Surgical Features
- Bare labral footprint
- > 5 mm sublabral sulcus
- Displaceable biceps (root rolls over glenoid)
- Effects of SLAP lesions
  - Biceps anchor disruption
  - Humeral head translation (microinstability)
  - Strain of humeral head restraints
  - Glenohumeral laxity/instability

Microscopic Features
- Fibrocartilaginous degeneration and/or tear of the superior labrum/biceps anchor
- Hemorrhagic synovium

Staging, Grading or Classification Criteria
- Type V, VI, VII, VIII, IX

CLINICAL ISSUES

Presentation
- Most common signs/symptoms
  - Patient status post fall on outstretched hand (31%), usually type III, IV or V lesion
  - Patient status post anterior dislocation (16%), often a type V
- Clinical profile
  - Posttraumatic patient
  - Approximately one-third have symptoms referable to the biceps tendon
  - Bicipital groove tenderness
    - Speed's test (resisted forward flexion of a supinated arm)
    - Yergason's test (resisted supination with the elbow flexed 90 degrees)
  - Crank or clunk test - pain +/- popping with compression and rotation
  - O'Brien's active compression test for SLAP lesions - pain with resisted elevation with forearm fully pronated

Demographics
- Age: Typically young patient for most SLAP lesion

- Gender: M > F

Natural History & Prognosis
- Small tears/stable tears may heal but unstable tears require surgical stabilization

Treatment
- Conservative
  - Reduction of pain and inflammation (NSAIDs), restoration of range of motion, strengthening (physical therapy)
- Surgical
  - Restoration of anatomy including MGHL/IGHLC
  - Stabilize and reattach labrum

DIAGNOSTIC CHECKLIST

Consider
- Anterior, posterior or inferior labral tears in association with a SLAP II lesion
- Identify subchondral glenoid erosions as a secondary finding of associated labral pathology

Image Interpretation Pearls
- Fluid signal intensity within substance of the labrum vs. complete avulsion with fluid signal at labral tear
- Evaluate all labral quadrants including BLC and inferior glenohumeral ligament labral complex

SELECTED REFERENCES

1. Beltran JM et al: Shoulder: Labrum and bicipital tendon. Top Magn Reson Imaging 14(1):35-49, 2003
2. Bencardino JT et al: Superior labrum anterior-posterior lesions: Diagnosis with MR arthrography of the shoulder. Radiology 214(1):267-71, 2001
3. Musgrave DS et al: SLAP lesions: Current concepts. Am J Orthop 30(1):29-38, 2001
4. Grainger AJ et al: Direct MR arthrography: A review of current use. Clin Radiol 55(3):163-76, 2000
5. Snyder SJ et al: SLAP lesions of the shoulder. Arthroscopy 6(4):274-9, 1990

IMAGE GALLERY

Typical

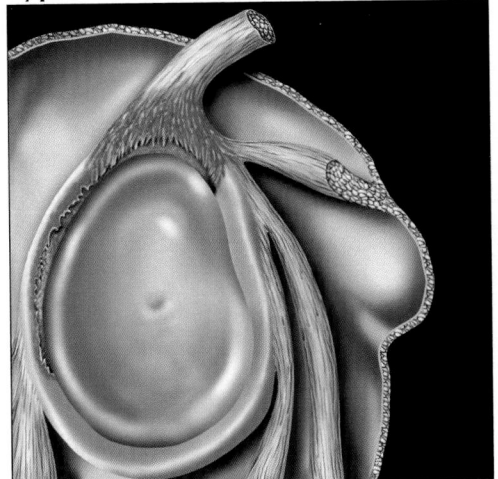 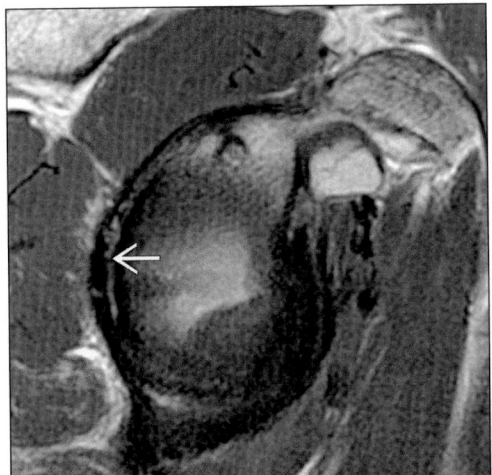

(Left) Sagittal graphic demonstrates a type VIII SLAP lesion with tearing and inflammation of the biceps anchor extending posteriorly to involve the posterior labrum. *(Right)* Sagittal PD FSE MR demonstrates a type VIII SLAP (arrow) with extension into the posterior labrum.

Typical

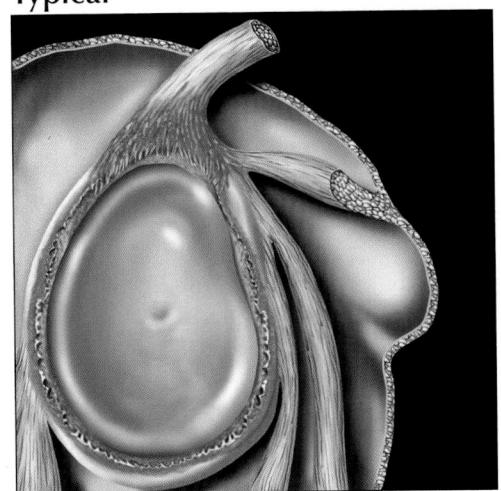 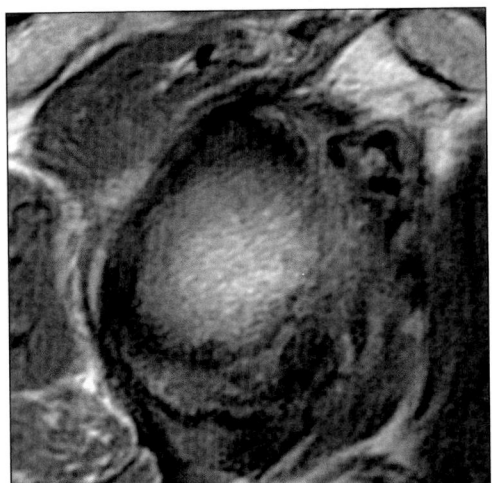

(Left) Sagittal graphic shows a type IX SLAP with tearing of the biceps anchor and circumferential labral tearing. *(Right)* Sagittal PD FSE MR demonstrates circumferential labral tearing in a patient with a type IX SLAP lesion.

Typical

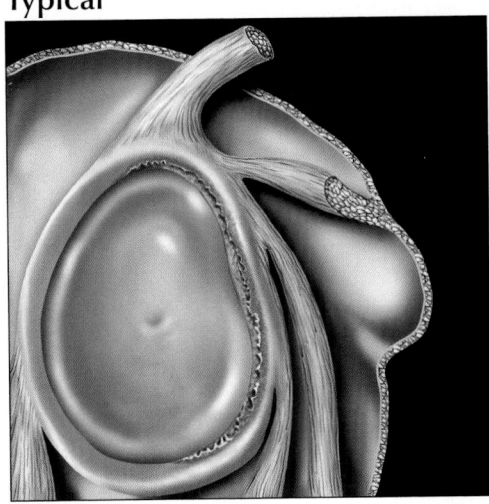 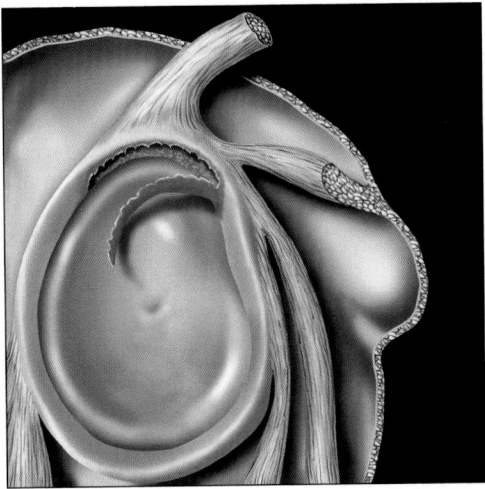

(Left) Sagittal graphic demonstrates a type V SLAP involving the biceps anchor in association with a Bankart lesion. *(Right)* Sagittal graphic demonstrates a type VI SLAP with a flap component displaced inferiorly with the anterior component attached.

BICEPS TENDON DISLOCATION

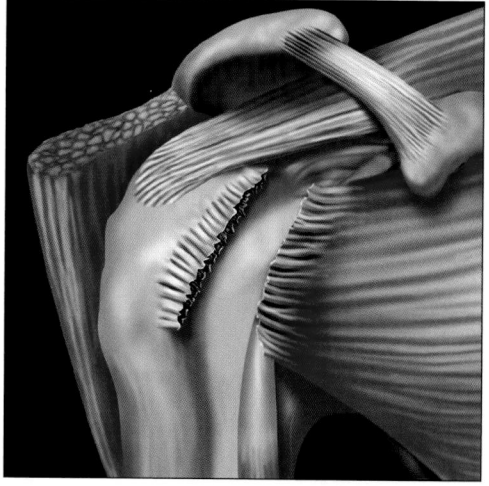

Coronal graphic shows a tear of the subscapularis tendon and a dislocation of the biceps from the bicipital groove.

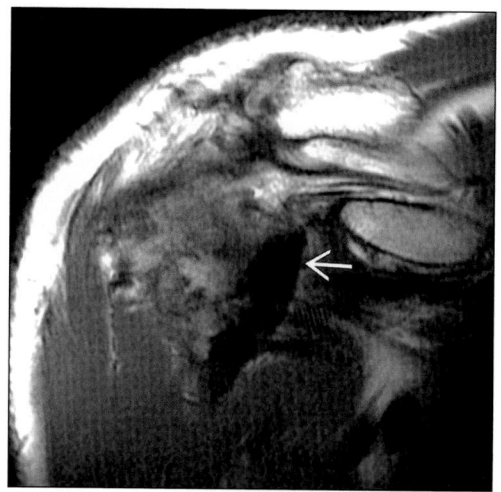

Coronal PD FSE MR shows torn subscapularis tendon and medial dislocation of the biceps (arrow). Irregular bicipital groove is lateral to the dislocated biceps tendon.

TERMINOLOGY

Abbreviations and Synonyms
- Biceps instability

Definitions
- Dislocation of the long head of biceps tendon (LHBT/LBT) from the bicipital groove
- Disruption of stabilizing ligaments including transverse ligament, coracohumeral ligament (CHL) and superior glenohumeral ligament (SGHL/SGL) & subscapularis tendon

IMAGING FINDINGS

General Features
- Best diagnostic clue: Empty bicipital groove with oval decreased signal structure outside the groove on all pulse sequences
- Location: Bicipital groove and rotator interval (RI)
- Size: Tendon flattened, enlarged or partially torn
- Morphology
  - Dislocated tendon
    - +/- Flattened/thickened due to preexisting tendinosis
  - Normal tendon: Oval shape, hypointense

Radiographic Findings
- Radiography
  - +/- Degenerative changes (degenerative cysts) surrounding bicipital groove of humerus
  - Acromial remodeling/sclerosis - impingement
  - Acromial spurs (impingement)

CT Findings
- NECT
  - +/- Degenerative changes of lesser and greater tuberosities
  - +/- Empty bicipital groove
- CT arthrography
  - Empty bicipital groove
  - Tendon sheath filled with contrast

MR Findings
- T1WI: Increased signal intensity fat fills bicipital groove
- T2WI
  - Decreased signal intensity fat within bicipital groove with FS
    - Hemorrhage hyperintense
    - Surrounding edema hyperintense
  - Increased signal intensity subchondral cysts of humerus at bicipital groove = degenerative change
    - +/- Adjacent bone marrow edema
    - Subcoracoid impingement

DDx: Biceps Tendon Dislocation

Ant. Lab. Tear	Subluxation	SLAP VII	Buford MGL	Air Bubble
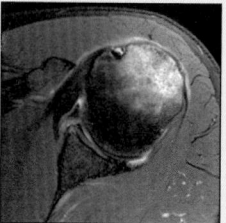	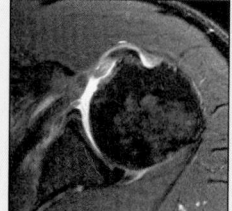	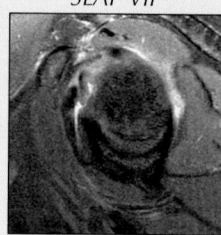	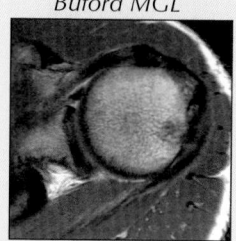	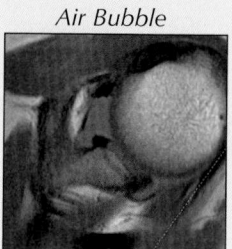
Ax FS PD FSE MR	Ax FS PD FSE MR	Sag FS PD FSE	Ax PD FSE MR	Ax PD FSE MR

BICEPS TENDON DISLOCATION

Key Facts

Terminology
- Dislocation of the long head of biceps tendon (LHBT/LBT) from the bicipital groove
- Disruption of stabilizing ligaments including transverse ligament, coracohumeral ligament (CHL) and superior glenohumeral ligament (SGHL/SGL) & subscapularis tendon

Imaging Findings
- Best diagnostic clue: Empty bicipital groove with oval decreased signal structure outside the groove on all pulse sequences

Top Differential Diagnoses
- Torn Detached Labrum
- Rotator Interval "Hidden Lesion"
- Biceps Tendinosis

- Biceps Rupture
- SLAP Lesion
- Subcoracoid Impingement

Pathology
- +/- Dislocation into joint deep to subscapularis
- +/- Dissection into subscapularis tendon
- Rarely dislocates superficial to tendon

Clinical Issues
- Upper arm/shoulder pain often radiating into upper arm

Diagnostic Checklist
- Identify empty bicipital groove
- Document biceps anterior, posterior or within torn subscapularis fibers on axial images

---

- ○ +/- Subscapularis tear or partial tear - hyperintense with discontinuous fibers
  - ▪ Subscapularis interstitial split with interposed dislocated tendon
  - ▪ Superficial fibers may be preserved with deep fibers torn
  - ▪ Rarely deep fibers preserved and superficial fibers + CHL torn, allowing superficial subluxation
- ○ Distal SGHL, CHL tear (hidden lesion) in association with biceps dislocation
  - ▪ Increased signal intensity replacing decreased signal intensity ligamentous structures
  - ▪ SGHL, CHL may be thickened and degenerated and lax without complete tear
- T2* GRE: Sensitive to visualization of hypointense fibers of biceps
- Tendon flattened against bicipital groove/lesser tuberosity - subluxation
- MR arthrography
  - ○ Empty bicipital groove
  - ○ Tendon sheath filled with contrast

Ultrasonographic Findings
- Dislocation of the biceps tendon with an empty bicipital groove

Imaging Recommendations
- Best imaging tool: MRI
- Protocol advice: Axial FS PD FSE + T2* GRE

DIFFERENTIAL DIAGNOSIS

Torn Detached Labrum
- Fall on abducted externally rotated arm
- Mimics dislocated biceps
- +/- Anterior dislocation/subluxation
- Detached fragment hypointense on all pulse sequences
- Follow on consecutive axial images to confirm structure is labrum not LHBT

Rotator Interval "Hidden Lesion"
- Common cause of LHBT dislocation
- SGHL/CHL dysfunction

- LHBT subluxation progresses to dislocation
- LHBT subluxation deep to subscapularis
- Irregular increased signal of SGHL/CHL on FS PD FSE at lateral aspect of joint

Biceps Tendinosis
- Thickened hyperintense tendon on all pulse sequences
- Short TE sequences most sensitive
- Associated with impingement
- +/- SLAP (superior labrum anterior to posterior) lesion

Biceps Rupture
- Discontinuous, irregular, frayed tendon on all pulse sequences
- +/- Impingement syndrome
- +/- Stump visualization in superior part of shoulder joint by supraglenoid tubercle
- Distal end may retract into upper arm
- Pain often relieved at time of rupture

SLAP Lesion
- At the level of biceps labral complex
- Involves tendon itself
- Propagates into
  - ○ Anterior labrum
  - ○ Posterior labrum (SLAP VIII)
  - ○ Middle glenohumeral ligament or MGL (SLAP VII)
  - ○ Circumferentially (SLAP IX)
- Positive Speed's test (bicipital resistance test)

Subcoracoid Impingement
- Impingement of coracoid on subscapularis/biceps
- Internal rotation
- +/- Hyperintense subcortical cysts on T2WI
- Predisposes to biceps tendinosis/instability
- Elongated coracoid (predisposing)

Anterosuperior Variations, Shoulder
- Buford complex
- Sublabral foramen
- Cord-like MGL may mimic dislocated biceps
- Above equator of glenoid
- 20% of general population
- Follow cord-like MGL to confirm its identity

BICEPS TENDON DISLOCATION

PATHOLOGY

General Features
- General path comments
  - Dislocates after loss of stabilizing structures
  - +/- Dislocation into joint deep to subscapularis
  - +/- Dissection into subscapularis tendon
  - Rarely dislocates superficial to tendon
  - Superficial fibers of subscapularis + inferior fibers of CHL continue as transverse bicipital ligament
    - Covers biceps groove
- Etiology
  - Torn rotator cuff leads to tear of stabilizing structures allowing dislocation of LHBT
  - Deep fibers of subscapularis must be torn
  - Shallow bicipital groove predisposes to dislocation
  - Rotator interval hidden lesion common cause of instability
    - Predisposes to subluxation/dislocation
  - Subscapularis tendon & coracohumeral ligament
    - Major restraints of biceps dislocation
  - Transverse ligament
    - Less important role in stabilizing LBT within groove
- Epidemiology: More common with impingement, up to 30% of impingement patients
- Associated abnormalities
  - Subscapularis rupture
    - Deep surface partial tear
    - Interstitial partial tear
    - Superficial fiber partial tear
  - Supraspinatus tear
    - Predisposes to LHBT tendinosis/dislocation
  - Subcoracoid impingement - predisposes

Gross Pathologic & Surgical Features
- Degenerated tendon dislocated out of bicipital groove
- Associated with torn subscapularis tendon
- Flattening, fraying, and degenerative changes at surgery

Microscopic Features
- Collagen degeneration without influx of inflammatory cells: "Tendinosis" is preferred term over tendinitis

Staging, Grading or Classification Criteria
- Two types of LBT dislocation
  - Type 1: Intact insertional fibers of subscapularis
    - LBT anterior to subscapularis
  - Type 2: Detached subscapularis tendon
    - LBT deep to subscapularis tendon

CLINICAL ISSUES

Presentation
- Most common signs/symptoms
  - Upper arm/shoulder pain often radiating into upper arm
  - Asymmetrical pain over the bicipital groove compared to contralateral shoulder
  - Pain with Yergason's, Speed's +/- O'Brien's tests

- Yergason's test - bicipital groove pain with resisted supination of forearm in 90 degrees of elbow flexion
- Speed's test - bicipital resistance test with bicipital groove pain in a flexed arm, forearm supination at 30 degrees of elbow flexion
- O'Brien's test - active compression test to entrap anterosuperior labrum (SLAP lesions) between humeral head and glenoid in 90 degrees of flexion and 20 degrees of cross-body adduction (downward force applied to internally rotated arm)
- Clinical profile: Common complaint of dull anterior shoulder pain (esp. with lifting, elevated pushing or pulling)

Demographics
- Age
  - Adult (impingement)
  - Athletes
- Gender: M > F

Natural History & Prognosis
- Continued pain with use of biceps
- Often requires surgical management

Treatment
- Conservative: Physical therapy, NSAIDs
- Tenodesis/tenotomy for recalcitrant cases of pain
- Rotator cuff/SGHL/CHL repair with LHBT reduction

DIAGNOSTIC CHECKLIST

Consider
- Torn labrum as differential diagnosis
- Evaluate subscapularis

Image Interpretation Pearls
- Identify empty bicipital groove
- Document biceps anterior, posterior or within torn subscapularis fibers on axial images
- Note medial location of biceps on anterior coronal images

SELECTED REFERENCES

1. Beltran JM et al: Shoulder: Labrum and bicipital tendon. Top Magn Reson Imaging 14(1):35-49, 2003
2. Beall DP et al: Association of biceps tendon tears with rotator cuff abnormalities: Degree of correlation with tears of the anterior and superior portions of the rotator cuff. AJR 180(3):633-9, 2003
3. Gartsman et al: Arthroscopic biceps tenodesis: Operative technique. Arthroscopy 16(5):550-2, 2000
4. Read JW et al: Shoulder ultrasound: Diagnostic accuracy for impingement syndrome, rotator cuff tear, and biceps tendon pathology. J Shoulder Elbow Surg 7(3):264-71, 1998
5. Sethi N et al: Disorders of the long head of the biceps tendon. J Shoulder Elbow Surg 8(6):644-54, 1998
6. Beltran J et al: MR arthrography of the shoulder: Variants and pitfalls. Radiographics 17(6):1403-12; discussion 1412-5, 1997

BICEPS TENDON DISLOCATION

IMAGE GALLERY

Typical

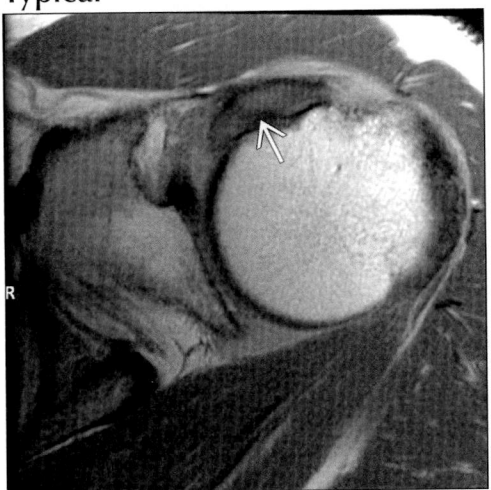 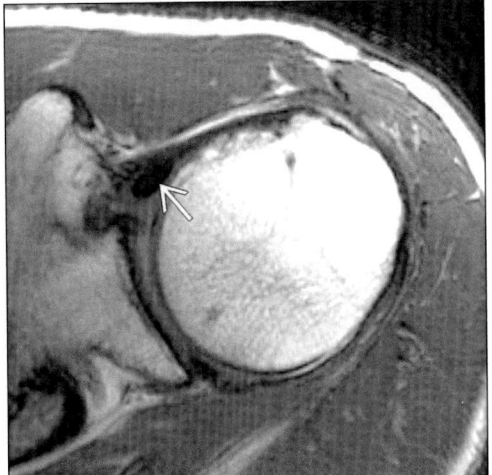

(Left) Axial PD FSE MR shows tendinosis within a dislocated biceps tendon adjacent to the lesser tuberosity (arrow). The superior aspect of the bicipital groove can be seen laterally in association with a tear of the coracohumeral ligament. *(Right)* Axial PD FSE MR shows dislocated biceps tendon in the anterosuperior aspect of the joint (arrow). This should not be mistaken for a middle glenohumeral ligament in association with a sublabral foramen or Buford complex.

Typical

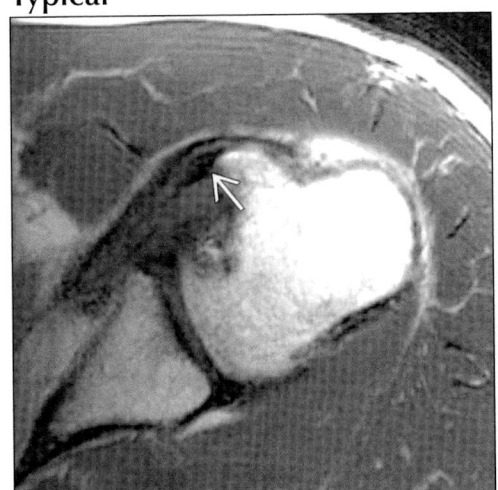 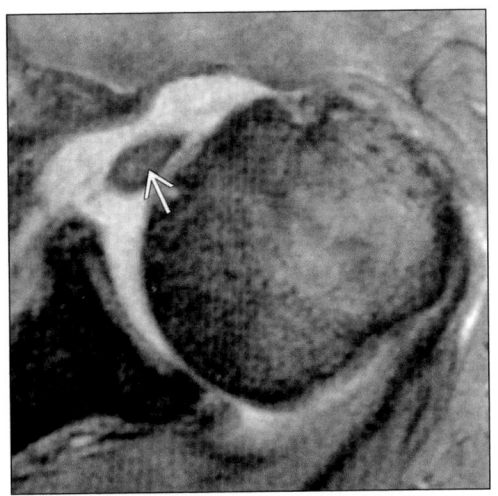

(Left) Axial PD FSE MR shows dislocation of the biceps tendon (arrow) through a partially torn subscapularis tendon and superior glenohumeral ligament. The superficial fibers of the subscapularis and coracohumeral ligament are intact. *(Right)* Axial T2* GRE MR shows complete dislocation of a degenerated biceps tendon (arrow) in association with a complete tear of the subscapularis tendon.

Typical

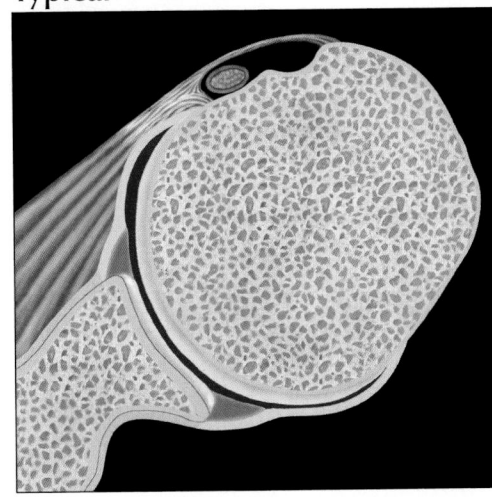 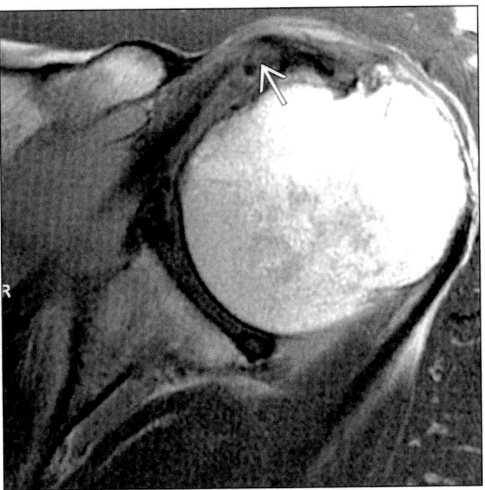

(Left) Axial graphic shows dislocation of the biceps tendon deep to the still intact superficial fibers of the subscapularis tendon and coracohumeral ligament. *(Right)* Axial PD FSE MR shows subluxation and near-complete dislocation of the biceps (arrow) secondary to partial tear of the subscapularis tendon and tear of the superior glenohumeral ligament.

SUBACROMIAL IMPINGEMENT

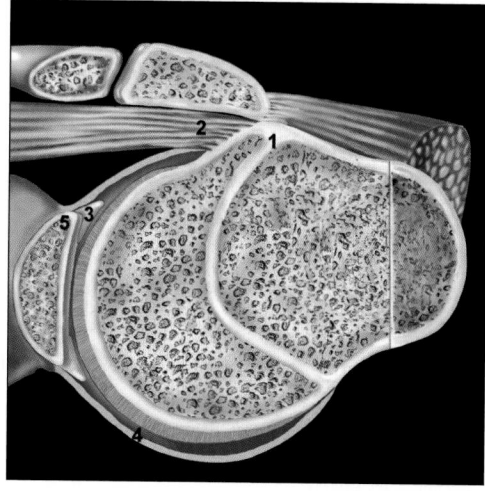

Coronal graphic shows impingement of the supraspinatus tendon on the acromion. (1. Lesser tub. 2. SST 3. LAB 4. Ant cap. 5. Glenoid)

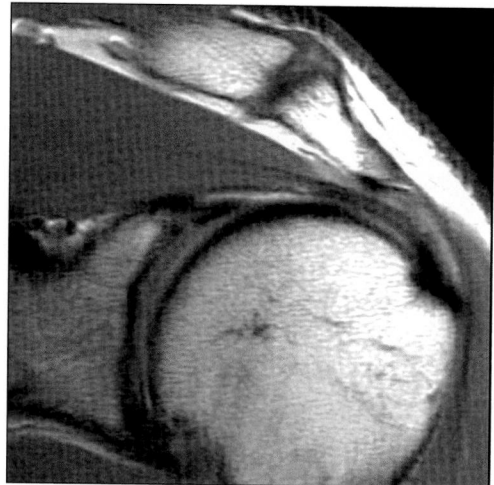

Coronal PD FSE MR shows marked lateral downsloping of the anterior acromion (type B) in a patient with subacromial impingement.

TERMINOLOGY

Abbreviations and Synonyms
- Primary extrinsic impingement, rotator cuff (RTC) impingement, subacromial impingement syndrome (SAIS), supraspinatus impingement

Definitions
- Progressively painful compression of supraspinatus tendon (SST) & subacromial bursa
  - Between humeral head and coracoacromial arch

IMAGING FINDINGS

General Features
- Best diagnostic clue
  - Hooked acromion on sagittal images with supraspinatus degeneration +/- tearing
    - +/- Reactive bursitis (bursal fluid)
- Location: Osseous acromial outlet and RTC
- Size
  - Diminished subacromial outlet
  - Subacromial space < 7 mm considered increased risk
- Morphology: Impingement risk depends on shape of acromion

Radiographic Findings
- Radiography

- Hooked acromion (type III acromion) on outlet view associated with increased risk
- Subacromial spurs
- +/- Acromioclavicular (AC) joint arthritis
  - Subchondral cysts, spurs

CT Findings
- NECT
  - Subacromial spurs
  - +/- AC sclerosis, hypertrophy
    - Cysts
    - Anterior inferior acromial spurs
  - Coronal, sagittal reconstruction
    - Sagittal reconstruction helpful for acromial shape
- CT arthrography
  - Contrast enters rotator cuff tear

MR Findings
- T1WI
  - Thickened tendon with intermediate signal intensity in impingement related tendinopathy
  - +/- Thick coracoacromial (CA) ligament (narrows subacromial space on sagittal images)
  - Hooked acromion on sagittal images
  - +/- Hypointense greater tuberosity cysts
- T2WI
  - Tendon degeneration
    - Thickened tendon with increased signal intensity
  - Full thickness, supraspinatus tear

DDx: Subacromial Impingement

Hidden Lesion	PSGI	PSGI	Subcoracoid Impin	Os Acromiale
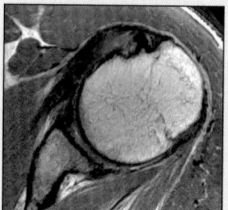	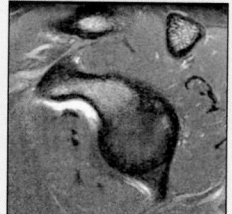	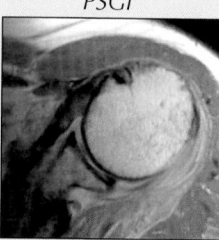	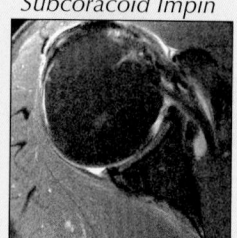	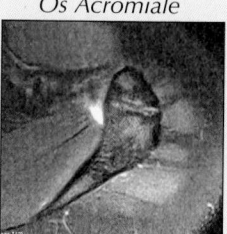
Ax PD FSE MR	Sag FS PD FSE	Ax PD FSE MR	Ax FS PD FSE	Ax FS PD FSE

SUBACROMIAL IMPINGEMENT

Key Facts

Terminology
- Progressively painful compression of supraspinatus tendon (SST) & subacromial bursa

Imaging Findings
- Hooked acromion on sagittal images with supraspinatus degeneration +/- tearing
- Morphology: Impingement risk depends on shape of acromion

Top Differential Diagnoses
- Internal Impingement (Posterosuperior Glenoid Impingement - PSGI)
- Suprascapular Denervation
- Adhesive Capsulitis
- Subcoracoid Impingement
- Hidden Lesion

Pathology
- Epidemiology: 95% of rotator cuff tears secondary to chronic impingement beneath coracoacromial arch

Clinical Issues
- Most common signs/symptoms: Insidious onset of shoulder pain especially with abduction and forward flexion
- Pain to palpation of the rotator cuff within the range of extension

Diagnostic Checklist
- Impingement syndrome = clinical diagnosis
- MR osseous and soft tissue findings are associated with clinical syndrome

---

  - Hyperintense fluid-filled gap
  - Partial tear
    - Hyperintensity undersurface
    - Hyperintensity bursal surface
    - Hyperintensity in interstitium
  - +/- Hyperintense greater tuberosity cysts
  - +/- Fluid signal intensity (hyperintense) in bursae
    - Subacromial
    - Subcoracoid
  - +/- Thickened coracoacromial ligament
- T1 C+
  - Partial tears, +/- enhancement
  - Full thickness tears, +/- enhancement
  - Bursitis - enhancement inflamed synovium
- MR arthrography
  - Tendon tear may be filled with contrast (partial and complete)
- Thickened heterogeneous tendon or torn tendon
- Type III acromion as a congenital variant or acquired osteophyte
- Type III (anterior inferiorly hooked) acromion process predisposes to subacromial impingement
- Acromion enthesophyte formation
  - Marrow containing
  - Marrow fat signal on T1WI
- Lateral downsloping predisposes to subacromial impingement
  - Coronal images

Imaging Recommendations
- Best imaging tool: MRI in all three planes
- Protocol advice
  - FS PD/T2 FSE in coronal plane for evaluation of RTC
  - Sagittal PD/T2 FSE or T2 FSE for evaluation of osseous acromial outlet

DIFFERENTIAL DIAGNOSIS

Internal Impingement (Posterosuperior Glenoid Impingement - PSGI)
- Throwing athletes
- Occupational

- Triad of findings
  - Posterosuperior humeral head impaction injury
  - Posterosuperior labrum fraying/frank tearing
  - Posterosuperior rotator cuff tearing (partial)
- Impingement inside shoulder joint
- Abduction with external rotation (ABER) MR arthrography used for the detection of partial undersurface tears

Acute Trauma
- Rotator cuff tear on acute traumatic basis
- +/- Preexisting impingement
- +/- Fracture of humerus, glenoid or both
- Hyperintense edema/hemorrhage on T2WI

Os Acromiale
- Degenerative changes may lead to pain with abduction
- Failure of fusion of normal ossification
- Preacromion (most distal type of os acromiale) - excised
  - Others surgically fused
- +/- Rotator cuff tear

Suprascapular Denervation
- Mimics impingement clinically
  - Weakness and pain of supraspinatus and infraspinatus
- Denervation hyperintense muscles on T2WI, STIR, FS PD FSE
- +/- Paralabral cyst - compression neuropathy

Adhesive Capsulitis
- Limitation in both active & passive range of motion
  - Impingement: Usually no limitation in passive range of motion
- Thickened hyperintense capsule on coronal images
  - Axillary pouch of inferior glenohumeral ligament (IGHL)
  - Rotator interval
- Frozen shoulder
- +/- Rotator cuff tear

SUBACROMIAL IMPINGEMENT

Subcoracoid Impingement
- +/- Subscapularis tendon tear
- +/- Hyperintense lesser tuberosity cysts - T2WI
- Pain with internal rotation
- +/- Hidden lesion

Hidden Lesion
- Biceps instability
- Superior glenohumeral ligament (SGHL)/coracohumeral ligament (CHL) abnormality
- +/- Subscapularis tear

PATHOLOGY

General Features
- General path comments: Physical impingement with repetitive microtrauma
- Etiology
  - Primary extrinsic (coracoacromial arch)
    - Subacromial spur
    - Acromioclavicular joint OA
    - Coracoacromial (CA) ligament
    - Variation in size and thickness
    - Calcification/ossification less common
  - Type III (hooked) acromion
  - Lateral downsloping of the anterior acromion
  - Os acromiale
    - Unfused apophysis of anterior acromion
  - Secondary extrinsic
    - Impingement associated with instability (glenohumeral)
    - Athletes in overhead throwing activities
    - No osseous abnormality of the coracoacromial arch
    - Continuum from instability to subluxation resulting in impingement
    - Anterior instability
- Epidemiology: 95% of rotator cuff tears secondary to chronic impingement beneath coracoacromial arch
- Associated abnormalities: Biceps tendinosis/tears

Gross Pathologic & Surgical Features
- Type III (anterior inferiorly hooked) acromion process
- Enthesophyte formation acromion
- Lateral downsloping of anterior acromion

Microscopic Features
- Collagen degeneration with apoptosis (cell death) of tendon cells
  - Increase in collagen type III, glycosaminoglycan, proteoglycan and smooth muscle actin (SMA)
- Hypertrophic & inflammatory bursitis
  - Inflammatory changes are peritendinous

Staging, Grading or Classification Criteria
- Clinical subacromial impingement
  - Stage I: Reversible edema & hemorrhage typically in active patient ≤ 25 years
  - Stage II: Fibrosis and tendinitis
  - Stage III: Degeneration & rupture often associated with osseous changes most commonly in patients > 40 years
- Acromial shape

- Type I: Flat undersurface - sagittal MR
- Type II: Curved undersurface - sagittal MR
- Type III: Anterior 1/3 hook - sagittal MR
  - Associated with impingement
- Type IV: Convex undersurface
  - Not associated with impingement
- Lateral downsloping of anterior acromion on coronal MR images
  - Type A: Mild or non lateral downsloping
  - Type B: Moderate to marked lateral downsloping

CLINICAL ISSUES

Presentation
- Most common signs/symptoms: Insidious onset of shoulder pain especially with abduction and forward flexion
- Clinical profile
  - Pain to palpation of the rotator cuff within the range of extension
  - Pain and weakness to supraspinatus testing
  - Younger athletes participating in sports requiring overhead arm movements
  - Range of motion often preserved
  - Painful range of motion

Demographics
- Age: Adult > 40 years
- Gender: M > F

Natural History & Prognosis
- Improves with cessation of inciting activities
- Subacromial decompression - recalcitrant cases

Treatment
- Initial treatment conservative: Physical therapy
- Steroid injections
- Recalcitrant cases: Subacromial decompression/acromioplasty

DIAGNOSTIC CHECKLIST

Image Interpretation Pearls
- Impingement syndrome = clinical diagnosis
- MR osseous and soft tissue findings are associated with clinical syndrome
- Acromial shape & slope
- AC joint osteophytes
- Anterior inferior acromial spur

SELECTED REFERENCES
1. Fritz RC et al: MR imaging of the rotator cuff. Magn Reson Imaging Clin N Am 5(4):735-54, 1997
2. Bigliani LU et al: Subacromial impingement syndrome. J Bone Joint Surg Am 79(12):1854-68, 1997
3. Bigliani LU et al: Arthroscopic resection of the distal clavicle. Orthop Clin North Am 24(1):133-41, 1993
4. Bigliani LU et al: Relationship of acromial architecture and diseases of the rotator cuff Orthopad 20(5):302-9, 1991

SUBACROMIAL IMPINGEMENT

IMAGE GALLERY

Typical

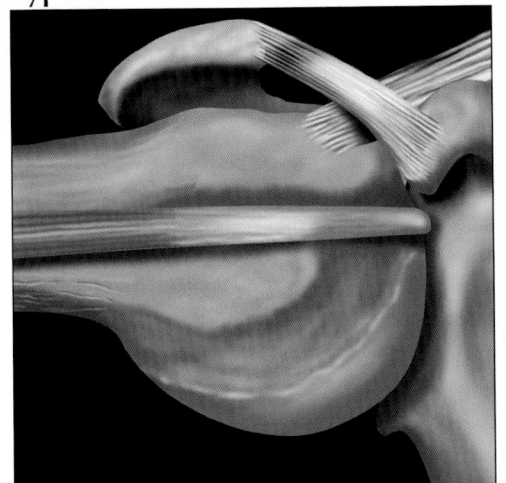

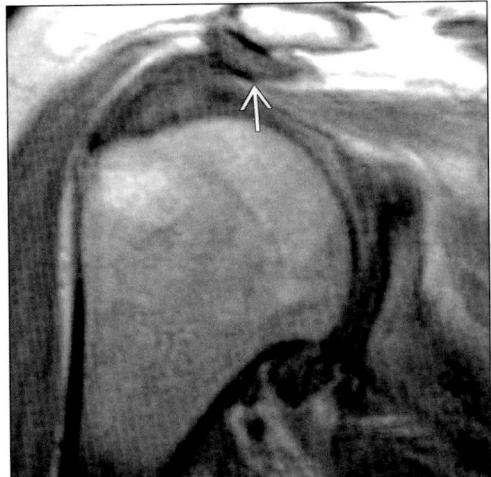

(Left) Coronal graphic in abduction and external rotation demonstrates approximation of the coracoacromial arch with the greater tuberosity. *(Right)* Coronal PD FSE MR shows marked thickening of the coracoacromial ligament (arrow) and moderate tendinosis with thickening of the supraspinatus tendon.

Typical

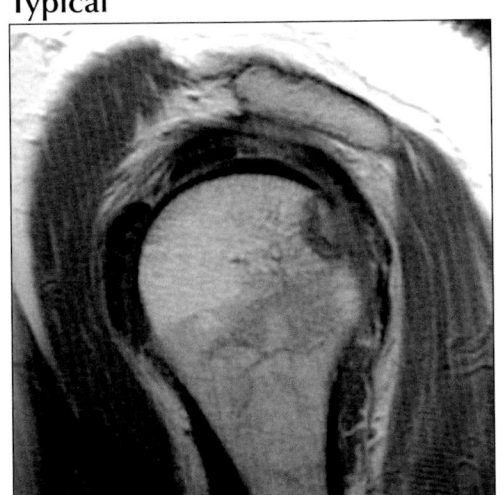

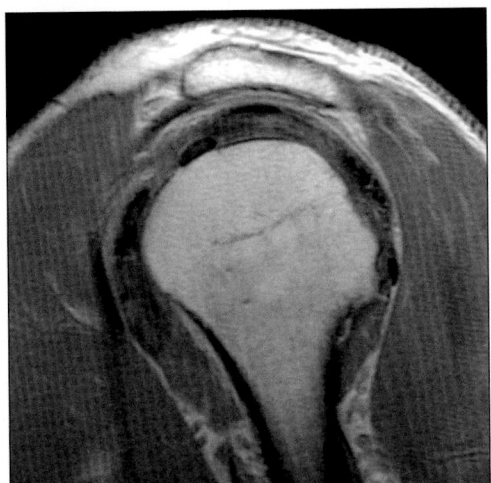

(Left) Sagittal T1 FSE MR shows type I acromion process. The patient has a rotator cuff tear and Hill-Sachs deformity secondary to trauma. *(Right)* Sagittal PD FSE MR shows type II acromion (lower association of cuff tears compared to type III) with thickened coracoacromial ligament.

Typical

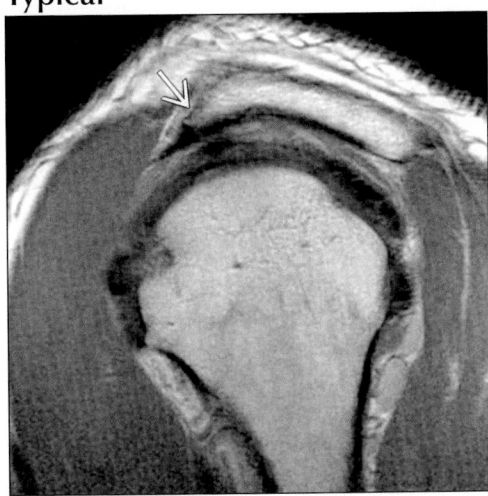

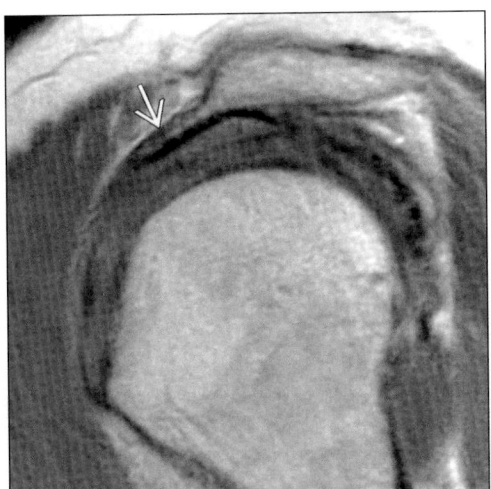

(Left) Sagittal PD FSE MR shows type III acromion (arrow) process with an anterior hook. *(Right)* Sagittal PD FSE MR shows a large enthesophyte of the anterior acromion at the insertion of the coracoacromial ligament (arrow).

OS ACROMIALE

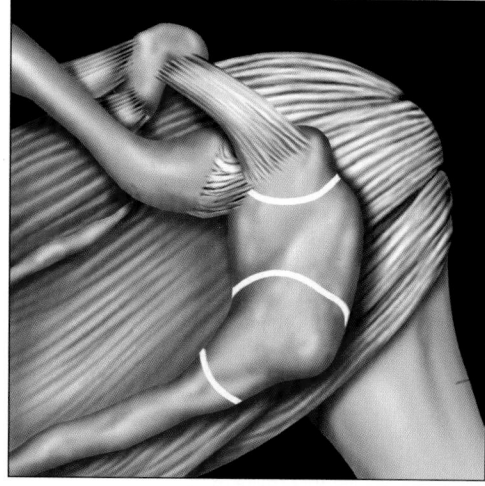

Coronal graphic shows the ossification centers of the acromion where an os acromiale may develop as a failure of fusion of the pre-, meso-, meta or basiacromion.

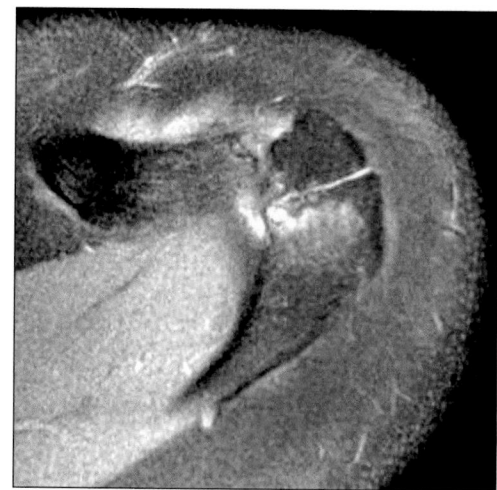

Axial FS PD FSE MR shows a meso os acromiale (most common) with degenerative changes at the synchondrosis. There are also mild degenerative changes of os acromiale clavicular joint.

TERMINOLOGY

Abbreviations and Synonyms
- Acromioclavicular (AC), usually in reference to the acromioclavicular joint, mesoacromion-preacromion (meso-pre) variety

Definitions
- Unfused acromial ossification center which normally fuses at approximately age 25-30
  - Relatively mobile with shoulder abduction causing impingement

IMAGING FINDINGS

General Features
- Best diagnostic clue: Separate articulation at the distal acromion separate from the AC joint
- Location
  - At one of three acromial ossification centers in patient older than 25-30 years
    - Basiacromion-metaacromion (most proximal)
    - Metaacromion-mesoacromion
    - Mesoacromion-preacromion (most distal)
- Size: 1-2 cm (size of secondary ossification center if meso-pre variation)
- Morphology

  - Disc shaped secondary ossification center
  - +/- Degenerative change

Radiographic Findings
- Radiography
  - Secondary ossification center of the acromion in one of three locations
    - Line of demarcation
    - Axillary view
  - +/- Degenerative changes
  - +/- Osteophyte formation
    - Medullary bone extends into osteophyte allowing identification
  - Patient ≥ 30 years

CT Findings
- NECT
  - Failure of fusion of secondary ossification center of the acromion
    - Line of demarcation = lucency
  - Degenerative changes common
    - Peri-synchondrosis sclerosis
    - +/- Lucencies (cysts)
  - Reconstruction in coronal, sagittal plane helpful

MR Findings
- T1WI

DDx: OS Acromiale

Clavicle Fx	Lymphoma	AC Sep	Subacrom. Veins	Subacrom. Vessels
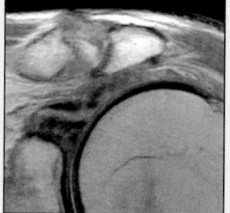	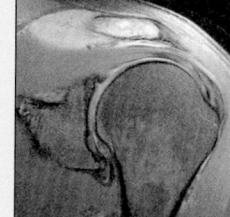	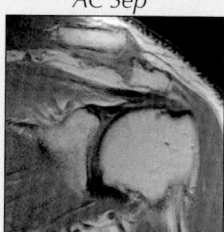	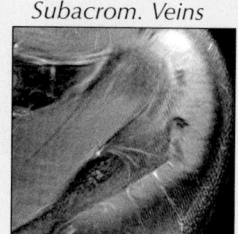	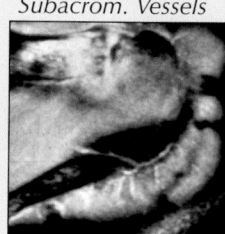
Cor PD FSE	Cor FS PD FSE	Cor PD FSE	Ax FS PD FSE	Ax STIR MR

OS ACROMIALE

Key Facts

Imaging Findings
- Best diagnostic clue: Separate articulation at the distal acromion separate from the AC joint
- At one of three acromial ossification centers in patient older than 25-30 years
- Basiacromion-metaacromion (most proximal)
- Metaacromion-mesoacromion
- Mesoacromion-preacromion (most distal)

Top Differential Diagnoses
- Acromial Fracture/Stress Response
- Normal Childhood/Adolescent Ossification Center
- Subacromial Vessel
- Acromioclavicular Joint Arthritis
- Impingement
- Clavicle Fracture

- Acromioclavicular Joint Separation

Pathology
- Failure of fusion of the normal acromial ossification center, +/- mobile distal acromion
- ± Impingement

Clinical Issues
- Insidious onset of shoulder pain
- Pain especially with abduction and forward flexion (impingement symptoms)

Diagnostic Checklist
- Use axial and sagittal images to identify "a second AC joint (pseudo - AC joint)" in os acromiale

---

- o Unfused secondary acromial ossification center with increased signal intensity (marrow) within the ossification
- o +/- Peri-synchondrosis sclerosis (hypointensity)
- o +/- Hypointense cysts
- o +/- Hypointense sclerosis throughout os acromion
- T2WI
  - o Pseudo-double AC joint appearance
  - o Corticated structure with marrow center
  - o +/- Edema (hyperintense)
    - Degenerative change
    - Stress response
  - o +/- Hyperintense cysts
  - o +/- Hypointense sclerosis
  - o +/- Supraspinatus tendinopathy
    - Thickening
    - Fluid signal (hyperintensity) fills gap
- PD/Intermediate: Corticated structure with marrow center
- T2* GRE
  - o Unfused ossification demarcation - hyperintense
  - o Bone marrow edema often obscured
    - Secondary to susceptibility
    - Not a marrow sensitive technique

Imaging Recommendations
- Best imaging tool: MRI
- Protocol advice
  - o Obtain axial MR images in superior location to include acromion
  - o FS PD FSE to visualize edema across articulation

DIFFERENTIAL DIAGNOSIS

Acromial Fracture/Stress Response
- History of trauma (direct impact)
- Hyperintensity on T2WI
- FS PD FSE sensitive for marrow edema
- Lymphoma of the scapular spine may mimic stress response (rare)

Normal Childhood/Adolescent Ossification Center
- Unfused ossification center normal < 25 years
- Normal structure mimics os acromiale
- Other ossification centers usually present allowing differentiation
  - o Acromion: One of last ossification centers to fuse
- No signal alterations
- Children have normal high signal hyaline articular cartilage on T2WI

Subacromial Vessel
- Mimics ossification center junction (synchondrosis)
- High signal intensity on T2WI
- Artery and/or vein
- +/- Misregistration artifact

Acromioclavicular Joint Arthritis
- Involves AC joint
- + Hyperintense edema T2WI
- + Hyperintense subchondral cysts T2WI
- + Hypointense subchondral sclerosis all pulse sequences
- Hyperintense synovitis PD, T2WI, T1WI

Impingement
- Anterior pain with abduction
- Lidocaine injection into AC joint/os acromiale to differentiate origin of pain
- +/- Thickening, increased signal of supraspinatus tendon on short and long TE sequences
- +/- Thickened coracoacromial ligament

Clavicle Fracture
- +/- AC separation
- + History of trauma
- Hypointense fracture line mimics os acromiale on all pulse sequences
- + Hyperintense edema on T2WI

Acromioclavicular Joint Separation
- Type I injuries - sprained but intact coracoclavicular (CC) and AC ligaments

- Type II injuries - complete disruption of the AC ligaments with sprained but intact CC ligament
- Type III injury - both CC and AC ligaments completely disrupted
- Type IV injuries - posterior displacement of the clavicle relative to the acromion + buttonholing through the trapezius muscle
- Type V injuries - clavicle markedly displaced superiorly - disruption of muscle attachments
- Type VI injuries - inferior displacement of distal clavicle below the acromion or the coracoid process
  - Rare
- Fracture line hypointense on all pulse sequences
- Perilesional hyperintense edema on T2WI

PATHOLOGY

General Features
- General path comments
  - Failure of fusion of the normal acromial ossification center, +/- mobile distal acromion
    - ± Impingement
  - Coracoacromial ligament inserts onto os acromiale
    - May lead to instability - impingement
  - Failure of recognition of os acromiale associated with ineffective acromioplasty
    - Cause of failed acromioplasty
- Etiology: Failure of fusion of the normal acromial ossification at one of three locations before age 25-30
- Epidemiology: 8.2% of general population over 25 years old
- Associated abnormalities: Rotator cuff (RTC) tears

Gross Pathologic & Surgical Features
- Mature bone with synchondrosis between the os acromiale and acromion

Microscopic Features
- Articulation with acromion
  - Fibrous tissue
  - Cartilage
  - Periosteum
  - Synovium

Staging, Grading or Classification Criteria
- Acromial ossification center failure of fusion
  - Basiacromion-metaacromion (type C)
  - Metaacromion-mesoacromion (type A)
  - Mesoacromion-preacromion (type B - most common)

CLINICAL ISSUES

Presentation
- Most common signs/symptoms
  - Insidious onset of shoulder pain
  - Pain especially with abduction and forward flexion (impingement symptoms)
  - Most common types are meso or metaacromial

Demographics
- Age
  - ≥ 30 years

- Impingement in older patients
- Not clear if os acromiale predisposes to earlier onset of impingement
  - Os acromiale represents normal ossification center before age 25-30
- Gender: M ≥ F

Natural History & Prognosis
- Improve with conservative treatment for impingement syndrome

Treatment
- Conservative: Physical therapy, NSAIDs
- Surgical treatment for recalcitrant cases
  - Excision of preacromion
  - Symptomatic meso-, meta-, or basiacromion may be stabilized and fixed to the remainder of the acromion

DIAGNOSTIC CHECKLIST

Image Interpretation Pearls
- Use axial and sagittal images to identify "a second AC joint (pseudo - AC joint)" in os acromiale

SELECTED REFERENCES

1. Gumina S et al: Relationship between os acromiale and acromioclavicular joint anatomic position. J Shoulder Elbow Surg 12(1):6-8, 2003
2. Carlson DW et al: Os acromiale. Am J Orthop 31(8):458, 2002
3. Sammarco VG: Os acromiale, Frequency, anatomy, and clinical implications. J Bone Joint Surg Am 82(3):394-400, 2000
4. Ryu RK et al: The treatment of symptomatic os acromiale. Orthopedics 22(3):325-8, 1999
5. Nicholson GP et al: The acromion: Morphologic condition and age-related changes. A study of 420 scapulas. J Shoulder Elbow Surg 5(1):1-11, 1996
6. Hutchinson MR et al: Arthroscopic decompression of shoulder impingement secondary to os acromiale. Arthroscopy 28-32, 1993
7. Edelson JG et al: Os acromiale. Anatomy and surgical implications. J Bone Joint Surg Br 75(4):551-5, 1993
8. MK Mudge et al: Rotator cuff tears associated with os acromiale. J Bone Joint Surg 427-9, 1984

OS ACROMIALE

IMAGE GALLERY

Typical

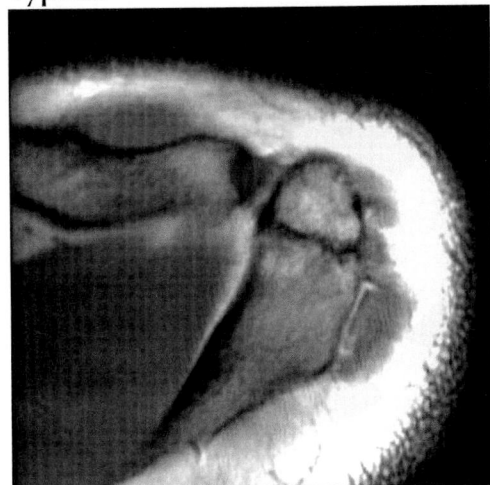 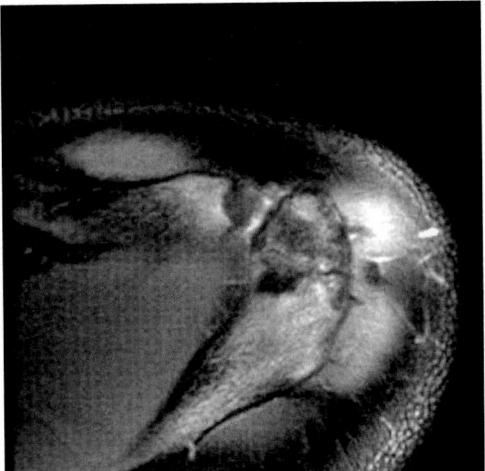

(Left) Axial PD/Intermediate MR through the superior aspect of the joint demonstrates failure of fusion of the mesoacromion ossification center resulting in an os acromiale. *(Right)* Axial STIR MR shows the meso os acromiale.

Typical

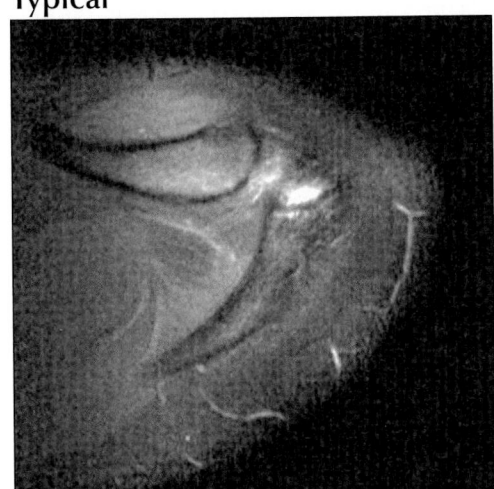 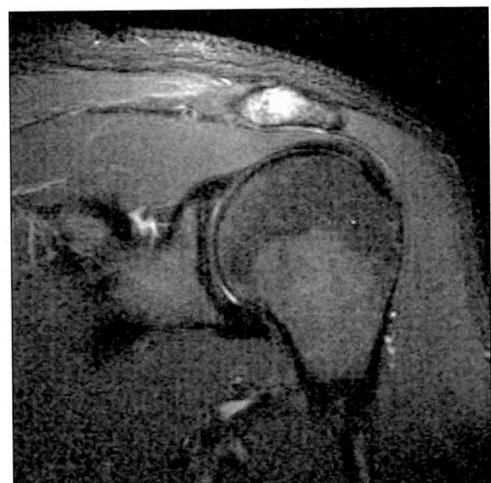

(Left) Axial STIR MR shows hyperintense stress response at the level of a symptomatic os acromiale. *(Right)* Coronal STIR MR shows the stress response at the junction of the acromion and os acromiale resulting in increased signal intensity.

Typical

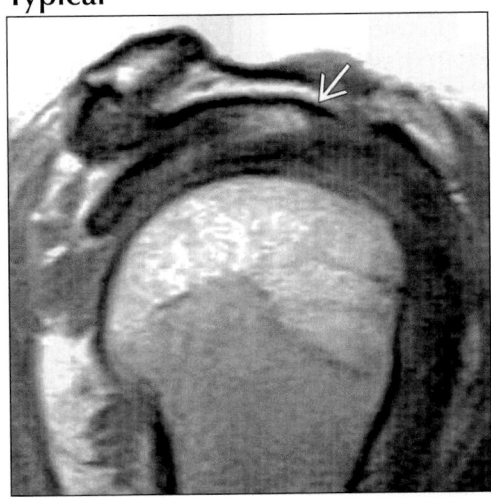 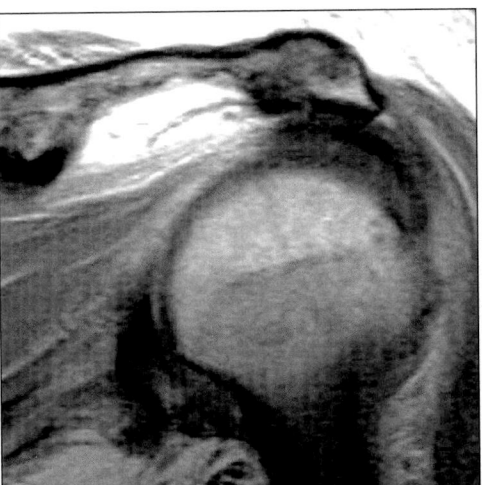

(Left) Sagittal PD FSE MR shows changes of an acromioplasty anteriorly (arrow) with the presence of an os acromiale posteriorly. The patient was symptomatic at the osseous acromion outlet. *(Right)* Coronal PD FSE MR shows degenerative changes of the more posteriorly located os acromiale formed between the meta- and mesoacromion.

ACROMIOCLAVICULAR JOINT ARTHRITIS

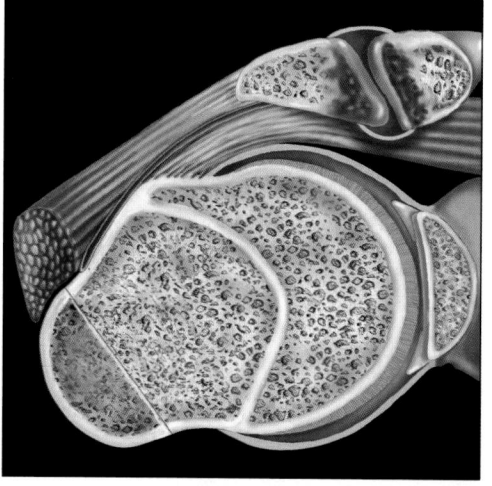

Coronal graphic shows osteoarthritic changes of the AC joint including mild chondromalacia, subchondral cyst formation, reactive bone changes, and effusion.

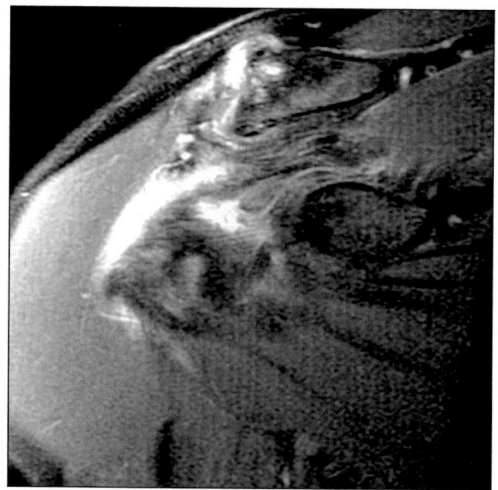

Coronal FS PD FSE MR shows osteoarthritic changes of the AC joint including minimal subchondral cyst formation of the distal clavicle, synovitis, and joint effusion.

TERMINOLOGY

Abbreviations and Synonyms
- Degenerative joint disease (DJD), osteoarthritis (OA), acromioclavicular (AC) joint arthrosis

Definitions
- Degenerative osteoarthritis of the acromioclavicular joint (AC joint)
- Primary: Gradual process of destruction & regeneration as a result of chronic microtrauma
  ○ Chronic "wear and tear"
- Secondary: Non-inflammatory degenerative joint disease
  ○ Secondary to
    ▪ Previous trauma
    ▪ Congenital deformity
    ▪ Infection
    ▪ Metabolic disorder

IMAGING FINDINGS

General Features
- Best diagnostic clue
  ○ Osteoarthritic changes including
    ▪ Chondromalacia
    ▪ Distal clavicular and/or proximal acromial cysts, edema
    ▪ Synovitis
    ▪ Subchondral sclerosis
    ▪ Periarticular edema
- Location: Articulation between the acromion and clavicle
- Size
  ○ Osteoarthritis (OA)
    ▪ +/- Alteration of morphology
    ▪ +/- Hypertrophic spur formation
    ▪ +/- Increase in size of joint (esp. with spurs)
- Morphology
  ○ Progressive loss of articular cartilage
    ▪ Associated new bone formation
    ▪ +/- Capsular fibrosis

Radiographic Findings
- Radiography
  ○ Views used
    ▪ Anterior and posterior
    ▪ Coracoacromial outlet "Y" view
    ▪ 15 degree cephalic tilt
  ○ Joint space narrowing
  ○ Subchondral sclerosis/eburnation
  ○ Subchondral cysts
  ○ Osteophyte formation
  ○ +/- Attrition/remodeling

DDx: Acromioclavicular Joint Arthritis

Normal CC Lig	AC Separation	Chronic AC Sep	Clavicle Fx	Os Acromiale

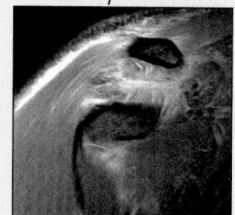 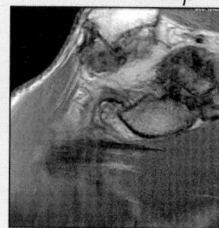 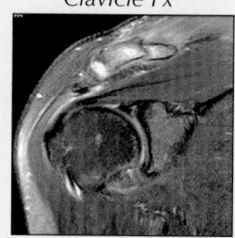 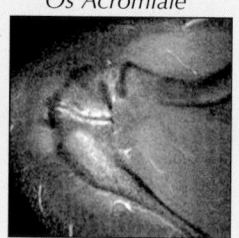

Cor PD FSE MR	Cor FS PD FSE	Cor PD FSE MR	Cor FS PD FSE	Ax FS PD FSE MR

ACROMIOCLAVICULAR JOINT ARTHRITIS

Key Facts

Terminology
- Degenerative osteoarthritis of the acromioclavicular joint (AC joint)
- Secondary: Non-inflammatory degenerative joint disease

Imaging Findings
- Location: Articulation between the acromion and clavicle
- Joint space narrowing
- Subchondral sclerosis/eburnation
- Subchondral cysts
- Osteophyte formation
- +/- Attrition/remodeling
- Hyperintensity in hyaline cartilage degeneration

Top Differential Diagnoses
- Posttraumatic Osteolysis
- Degenerative Changes of an Os Acromiale
- Subacromial Impingement
- AC Separation

Pathology
- Secondary to acromioclavicular separation or as typical degenerative change
- Joint instabilities may be predisposing

Clinical Issues
- Most common signs/symptoms: Anterosuperior shoulder pain
- Positive cross-body or horizontal adduction test
- Positive lidocaine injection test
- Associated rotator cuff disease in the elderly

CT Findings
- NECT
  - Tomographic imaging option
    - Characterization in cases of fragmentation/fx
  - Narrowing
  - Sclerosis
  - Cysts
  - Osteophytes
  - AC joint hypertrophy

MR Findings
- T1WI
  - Decreased signal intensity subchondral cysts
    - Decreased signal also visualized in sclerosis and/or degenerative edema
  - Marrow fat signal seen extending into osteophytes
    - Marrow extension into spur
    - Differentiation from hypointense ligament
- T2WI
  - Hyperintensity in hyaline cartilage degeneration
  - Subchondral bone marrow edema (hyperintense)
  - +/- Hyperintense effusion
  - Intermediate signal synovial thickening
    - +/- Irregularity/frond formation
  - FS PD FSE - edema demonstrated with fat saturation
    - Subchondral decreased signal indicating sclerosis
    - Subchondral cysts (hyperintense)
- PD/Intermediate
  - Cartilage seen on both FS PD FSE and PD FSE
  - Edema not as hyperintense compared to FS PD FSE or STIR
- T2* GRE: Cartilage abnormalities may be overlooked as both cartilage and fluid are of similar signal intensity
- T1 C+: Synovium enhances in case of synovitis

Nuclear Medicine Findings
- + Uptake

Imaging Recommendations
- Best imaging tool: MRI
- Protocol advice: FS PD FSE

DIFFERENTIAL DIAGNOSIS

Posttraumatic Osteolysis
- History of trauma, often weight lifting
- Edema and clavicular destruction
- FS PD FSE sensitive

Degenerative Changes of an Os Acromiale
- Occurs between os acromiale and remaining acromion
- Lateral and posterior to AC joint
- Common findings of OA
  - Chronic symptoms and characteristic radiographic and MRI findings
  - Synchondrosis irregularity
  - Subchondral cysts, edema, sclerosis

Subacromial Impingement
- Anterior shoulder pain with abduction
- Lidocaine injection into AC joint to differentiate AC vs. subacromial pathology
- +/- Thickening, increased signal of supraspinatus tendon on short and long TE sequences
- +/- Thickened coracoacromial ligament

AC Separation
- Posttraumatic
- Torn coracoclavicular ligament in more advanced cases
- +/- Fracture of clavicle

PATHOLOGY

General Features
- General path comments
  - Fatigue fracture of the collagen meshwork followed by increased hydration of the articular cartilage (as opposed to desiccated cartilage seen with aging) and loss of proteoglycans from the matrix into the synovial fluid
    - Secondary to instability of AC joint
    - Fibrillation of the cartilage follows + deep clefts and regeneration/proliferation of chondrocytes

ACROMIOCLAVICULAR JOINT ARTHRITIS

- Proliferative changes occur at the joint margins with formation of osteophytes
- Articular cartilage thins and is fissured in areas of maximum mechanical stress, underlying bone becomes sclerotic and subchondral cysts form
- Compression of weakened bone with variable degrees of collapse
- Loose bodies
- Synovial hypertrophy produces joint pain by nerve stimulation and weeping of synovial fluid producing increased intraarticular pressure thereby stretching joint lining
- Molecular changes in osteoarthritic cartilage include: Increased water, weakening of type II collagen network, shorter collagen chains and alteration of proteoglycans
- Increased levels of degrading enzymes including matrix metalloproteinase (MMPs or collagenase, gelatinase, and stromelysin)

- Etiology
  - Secondary to acromioclavicular separation or as typical degenerative change
  - Joint instabilities may be predisposing
- Epidemiology: Common abnormality (between 30-70% of population) especially > 50 years
- Associated abnormalities
  - Deformities occur
  - Subluxations
  - Coracoclavicular ligament fibrosis, heterotopic calcifications

Gross Pathologic & Surgical Features

- Osteoarthritic changes consisting of chondromalacia, synovitis, subchondral sclerosis, periarticular edema, and distal clavicular and/or proximal acromial cysts and edema
- Degraded cartilage with loss of sheen, fissured and/ or ulcerated cartilage surface, variable degrees of articular surface collapse
  - Subchondral geodes (cysts) containing variable degrees of debris
  - Buttressing osteophytes to increase surface area

Microscopic Features

- Degenerative arthritis with variable amounts of inflammatory cells, chondral degeneration, subarticular geodes, and subchondral osteocytic buildup (sclerosis)
  - Diminution of chondrocytes in superficial zones with chondrocyte swelling to variable degrees
  - Cartilage matrix loses its ability to stain for proteoglycans with Alcian blue or safranin-O
  - Matrix chondrocytes demonstrate proliferation in clusters (brood capsules)
  - Neovascularity penetrates layer of calcified cartilage and new chondrocytes extend up from deeper layers
  - Hypertrophied synovium becomes folded into villous folds with variable infiltration of plasma cells, and lymphocytes

CLINICAL ISSUES

Presentation

- Most common signs/symptoms: Anterosuperior shoulder pain
- Clinical profile
  - Pain includes top of shoulder, AC joint and upper arm (referred)
  - Positive cross-body or horizontal adduction test
  - Positive lidocaine injection test
  - Associated rotator cuff disease in the elderly
  - Clicking
  - Catching
- Clinical profile
  - Athlete
  - Middle aged to elderly active patient

Demographics

- Age: Adult
- Gender: M > F

Natural History & Prognosis

- Progressive debilitating disease without medical intervention

Treatment

- Non-steroidal antiinflammatory drugs, physical therapy
- Mumford procedure for advanced cases

DIAGNOSTIC CHECKLIST

Consider

- Posttraumatic osteolysis

Image Interpretation Pearls

- FS PD FSE images are sensitive to subchondral marrow edema and fluid within AC joint proper
- AC hypertrophy
- Association between moderate AC joint arthrosis (with edema of distal clavicle and acromion) and posterosuperior labral tears

SELECTED REFERENCES

1. Stein BE et al: Detection of acromioclavicular joint pathology in asymptomatic shoulders with magnetic resonance imaging. J Shoulder Elbow Surg 10(3):204-8, 2001
2. Clarke HD et al: Acromioclavicular joint injuries. Orthop Clin North Am 31(2):177-87, 2000
3. Shaffer BS: Painful conditions of the acromioclavicular joint. J Am Acad Orthop Surg 7(3):176-88, 1999
4. Fukuda K et al: Biomechanical study of the ligamentous system of the acromioclavicular joint J Bone Joint Surg 68(3):434-40, 1986
5. Cahill BR: Osteolysis of the distal part of the clavicle in male athletes. J Bone Joint Surg 64(7):1053-8, 1982

ACROMIOCLAVICULAR JOINT ARTHRITIS

IMAGE GALLERY

Typical

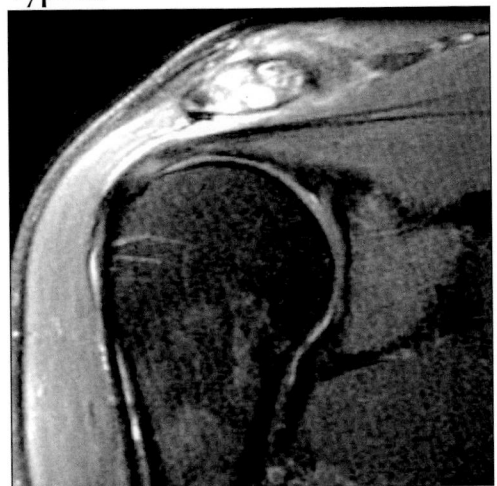 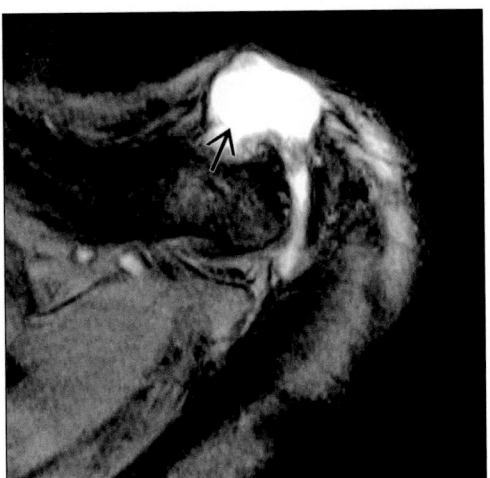

(Left) Coronal FS PD FSE MR shows hyperintense bone marrow edema within proximal aspect of acromion and surrounding soft tissue edema in a weight-lifter with distal clavicular posttraumatic osteolysis. (Right) Axial T2* GRE MR shows degenerative cyst (arrow) extending anteriorly & superiorly from the osteoarthritic AC joint.

Typical

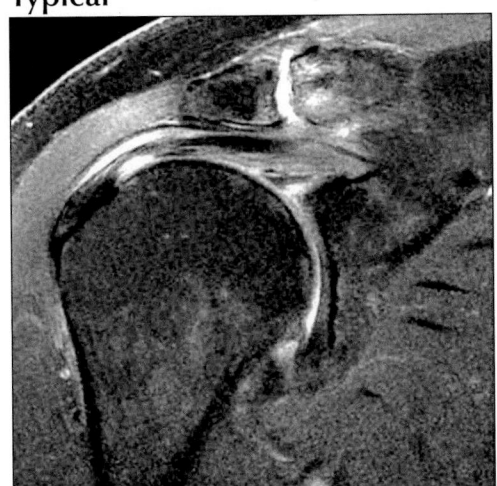 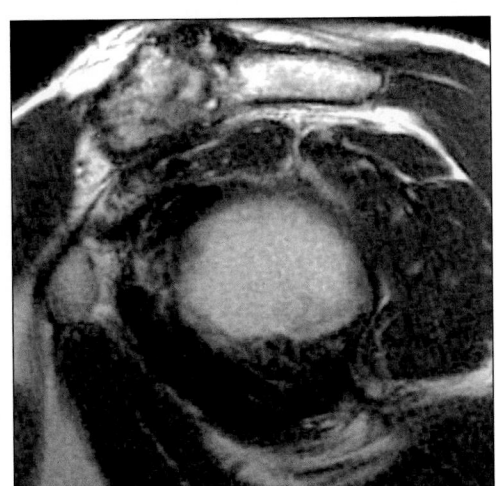

(Left) Coronal FS PD FSE MR shows AC degenerative disease as chondromalacia with underlying bone reactive change, synovitis, and joint effusion. (Right) Sagittal T2 FSE MR shows hypertrophic AC joint with narrowing of the supraspinatus outlet.

Typical

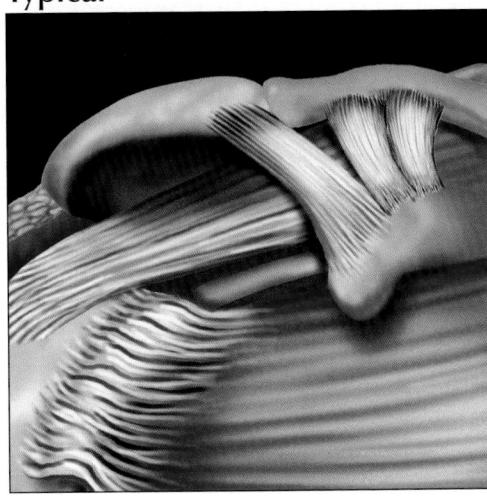 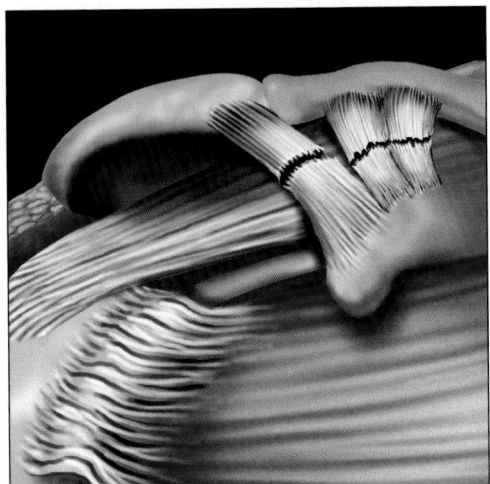

(Left) Coronal graphic shows normal coracoacromial ligament and the two components of the coracoclavicular ligament (trapezoid & conoid). (Right) Coronal graphic shows tear of the coracoacromial and coracoclavicular ligaments in an AC separation.

AVN, SHOULDER

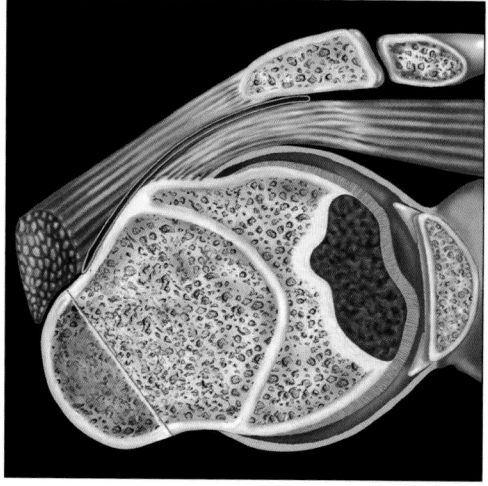

Coronal graphic shows avascular necrosis of the superomedial aspect of the humeral head with mild articular surface collapse.

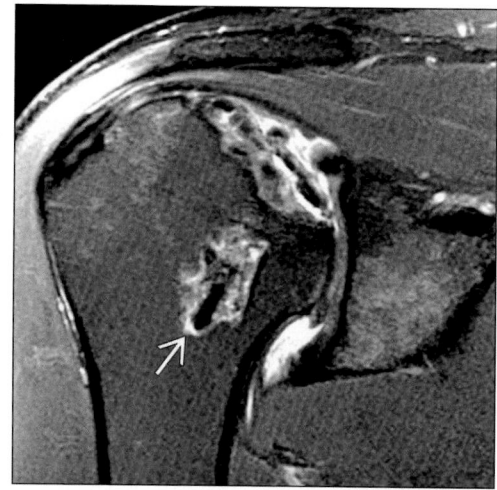

Coronal FS PD FSE MR shows avascular necrosis of the superomedial humeral head including "double line sign" (arrow).

TERMINOLOGY

Abbreviations and Synonyms
- Avascular necrosis (AVN)
  - Subchondral
- Bone infarct (BI), bone necrosis, bone death, bone infarction
- Osteonecrosis, aseptic necrosis, ischemic necrosis, ischemic bone death

Definitions
- AVN is ischemic death of the cellular elements of bone and marrow

IMAGING FINDINGS

General Features
- Best diagnostic clue
  - Serpiginous lines in subchondral cancellous marrow
  - "Double line sign": Decreased hypointense periphery lines with adjacent hyperintense inner border on T2WI
- Location: Superomedial aspect of humeral head most common
- Size: Varies from small to large areas of affected bone
- Morphology: Irregular serpiginous linear morphology of peripheral outline

Radiographic Findings
- Radiography
  - Arclike, subchondral, lucent lesion may be associated with areas of patchy loss of bone opacity with sclerotic areas and subchondral collapse
  - Eventually sclerotic +/- collapse
  - Radiographic findings may be delayed relative to initial clinical event

CT Findings
- NECT
  - Serpiginous outline
  - Interface of increased density

MR Findings
- T1WI
  - Edema: Moderate decrease in signal intensity
  - Predominately decreased signal intensity serpiginous lines
  - Central focus with marrow fat signal as most common appearance
- T2WI
  - Double line sign: Decreased signal intensity peripheral with adjacent increased signal intensity inner margin
  - Nonspecific area of edema within cancellous bone associated with AVN focus

DDx: AVN, Shoulder

Normal Physis	Normal Physis	Osteophyte OA	Osteoarthritis	Charcot Shoulder
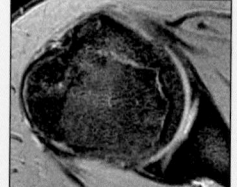	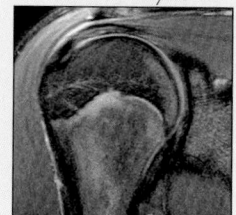	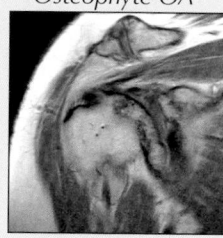	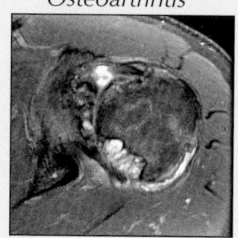	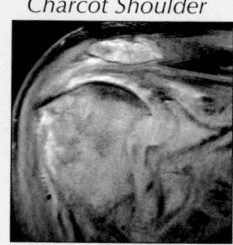
Ax T2* GRE MR	Cor FS PD FSE	Cor PD FSE MR	Ax FS PD FSE MR	Cor PD FSE MR

AVN, SHOULDER

Key Facts

Terminology
- AVN is ischemic death of the cellular elements of bone and marrow

Imaging Findings
- Serpiginous lines in subchondral cancellous marrow
- Size: Varies from small to large areas of affected bone
- Morphology: Irregular serpiginous linear morphology of peripheral outline
- Double line sign: Decreased signal intensity peripheral with adjacent increased signal intensity inner margin

Top Differential Diagnoses
- Osteoarthritis (OA)
- Marrow Tumor
- Bone Tumors & Metastases

- Osteochondral Injury

Pathology
- General path comments: Patient with predisposing factor - steroid use or underlying disease such as sickle cell anemia
- Steroid-induced osteonecrosis range from 2% to < 25%

Clinical Issues
- Clinical features of AVN depend on the stage of the disease, often asymptomatic
- Generalized shoulder pain

Diagnostic Checklist
- Evaluate for underlying abnormalities/disease

  - Collapse of subchondral surface in more advanced cases
  - Well-marginated cyst in cystic degeneration
  - FS PD FSE is sensitive to ischemic marrow related edema in acute AVN
- T2* GRE
  - Double line sign may be accentuated
  - Edema may be obscured because of susceptibility
- T1 C+: Granulation component of double line sign may enhance with contrast
- MR arthrography
  - Contrast extension underneath unstable devitalized bone

Nuclear Medicine Findings
- Bone Scan
  - "Cold spot": Absent uptake where blood supply has been disrupted preventing radiotracer from accumulating
  - Nonspecific uptake in acute cases where revascularization has occurred

Imaging Recommendations
- Best imaging tool: MRI (both T1 and T2 are diagnostic)
- Protocol advice: T1, FS PD FSE, T2WI and STIR

DIFFERENTIAL DIAGNOSIS

Osteoarthritis (OA)
- +/- History of antecedent trauma
- Subchondral changes but often with chronic symptoms and typical radiographic and MRI finding
  - Chondromalacia
  - Hyperintense subchondral cysts on T2WI
  - Hyperintense edema on T2WI
  - Hypointense sclerosis on all pulse sequences

Marrow Tumor
- Internal marrow replaced
- Lack of cortical disruption in AVN differentiates from malignant degeneration
- Well-marginated cyst differentiate cystic degeneration of infarct from malignant degeneration

- Vague areas of radiolucencies in infarct may mimic neoplastic processes

Bone Tumors & Metastases
- Enchondroma
  - Stippled hypointense calcifications
  - Chondroid matrix
  - Metaphyseal, diaphyseal or diametaphyseal
- Chondrosarcoma
  - Endosteal scalloping
- Myeloma
- Metastases

Osteochondral Injury
- History of trauma
- Affects chondral surface and subchondral bone
- Osteochondritis dissecans (OCD) +/- history of trauma
  - Young patient
  - Fracture unusual in humeral head epiphyseal area

PATHOLOGY

General Features
- General path comments: Patient with predisposing factor - steroid use or underlying disease such as sickle cell anemia
- Etiology
  - Conditions which disrupt blood supply to the bone
  - Intrinsic or extrinsic abnormality in the blood vessel supplying part of the bone may lead to infarct
  - Common predisposing factors
    - Trauma
    - Renal transplant
    - Steroids (endogenous and exogenous including Cushing syndrome)
    - Collagen vascular disease (lupus)
    - Pancreatitis
    - Alcoholism
    - Gaucher disease, Fabry's disease, sickle cell anemia, gout
    - Arteritis (radiation and other causes)
    - Idiopathic

- Epidemiology
  - Second most frequent (femoral head is most common) site of involvement for osteonecrosis
  - Steroid-induced osteonecrosis range from 2% to < 25%
  - Systemic lupus erythematosus (SLE) AVN incidence of 5-6% of patients
  - Alcohol intake and hyperuricemia account for up to 60% and 40% of cases of idiopathic bone infarct respectively
- Associated abnormalities
  - Signs and symptoms of underlying disease or physiologic state that led to infarct
  - Secondary osteoarthritis with associated complications

Gross Pathologic & Surgical Features

- Pale bone marrow with variable degrees of necrosis depending on age of infarct and duration of ischemia
- Secondary osteoarthritis develops after structural failure and collapse of articular surface
- Cystic degeneration in areas of bone infarction may occur

Microscopic Features

- Medullary necrosis appears yellowish with occasional flecks of calcium
- Serpiginous capsule of grayish glistening collagen surrounds area of necrosis
- Necrotic marrow fat in subchondral ischemia
- Bone trabeculae devoid of osteocytes
- Vascular granulation tissue or grayish glistening collagen separates dead tissue from underlying living bone contributing to increased signal of the double line sign

Staging, Grading or Classification Criteria

- Stage 0: Asymptomatic, normal radiograph, histology abnormal
- Stage 1: +/- Symptoms, radiographs normal, MRI shows abnormal signal, histology abnormal
- Stage 2: Symptomatic, radiographs show osteopenia, sclerosis, MRI characteristic (Chinese figures/double line sign)
- Stage 3: Symptomatic, subchondral lucency (crescent sign), subchondral collapse, articular shape preserved
- Stage 4: Articular surface collapse + superimposed osteoarthritic change

CLINICAL ISSUES

Presentation

- Most common signs/symptoms
  - Clinical features of AVN depend on the stage of the disease, often asymptomatic
  - Generalized shoulder pain
  - Presentation depends on underlying disease if present
- Clinical profile: Patients with underlying disease e.g., SLE

Demographics

- Age
  - Depends on underlying disease if present

- Patients with sickle cell anemia present with bone infarcts in the first few decades of life
- Gender: M:F = 8:1
- Ethnicity
  - Infarcts associated with sickle cell anemia
  - Bone infarcts associated with Gaucher's disease

Natural History & Prognosis

- Occurs suddenly and often heals well without residua unless progression of underlying disease influences infarct

Treatment

- Idiopathic lesions are treated conservatively (symptomatically)
- Treatment of underlying disease

DIAGNOSTIC CHECKLIST

Consider

- Evaluate for underlying abnormalities/disease

Image Interpretation Pearls

- AVN if double line on T2WI
  - Especially if superior medial humeral head affected
- Central marrow fat signal is the most common finding

SELECTED REFERENCES

1. Kim SK et al: Natural history and distribution of bone and bone marrow infarction in sickle hemoglobinopathies. J Nucl Med 43(7):896-900, 2002
2. Lau WF et al: Extensive bone infarct in myeloid leukemia correlation of bone scan and magnetic resonance imaging. Clin Nucl Med 26(2):165-6, 2001
3. Umans H et al: The diagnostic role of gadolinium enhanced MRI in distinguishing between acute medullary bone infarct and osteomyelitis. Magn Reson Imaging 18(3):255-62, 2000
4. Cerilli LA et al: Angiosarcoma arising in a bone infarct. Ann Diagn Pathol 3(6):370-3, 1999
5. Ahn BC et al: Intramedullary fat necrosis of multiple bones associated with pancreatitis. J Nucl Med 39(8):1401-4, 1998
6. Butt WP: MRI diagnosis of bone marrow infarction in the child with leukaemia. Clin Radiol 53(1):77, 1998
7. Stoller DW et al: The Shoulder. Magnetic resonance imaging in orthopaedics and sports medicine. vol 1. 2nd ed. Philadelphia PA, J.B. Lippincott, 597-742, 1997

AVN, SHOULDER

IMAGE GALLERY

Typical

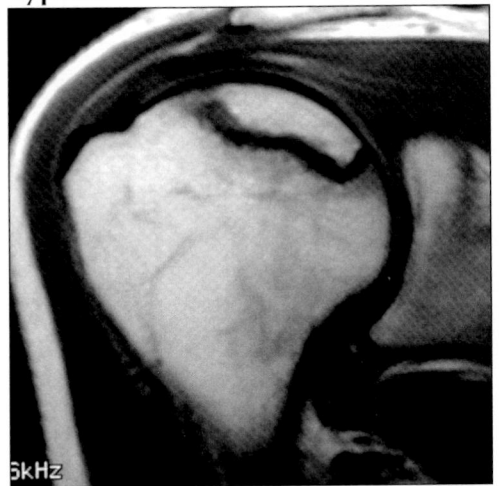 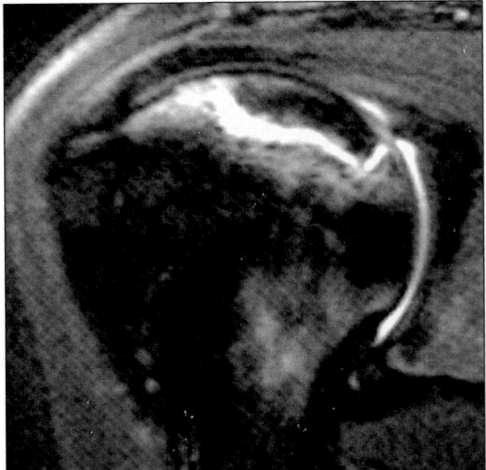

(Left) Coronal T1WI MR shows serpiginous linear decreased signal intensity line within the superomedial aspect of the humeral head, consistent with avascular necrosis. *(Right)* Coronal STIR MR subacute to chronic lesion of avascular necrosis with suppression of central marrow fat containing region.

Typical

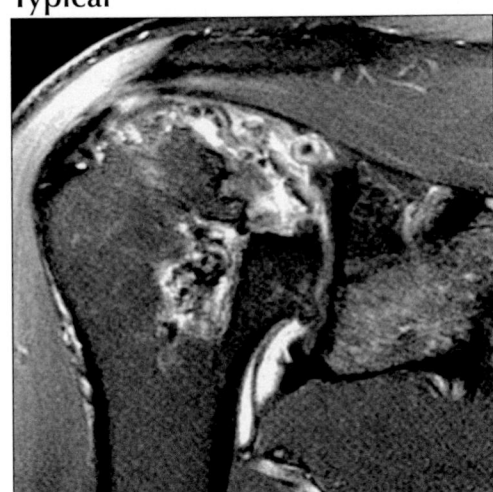 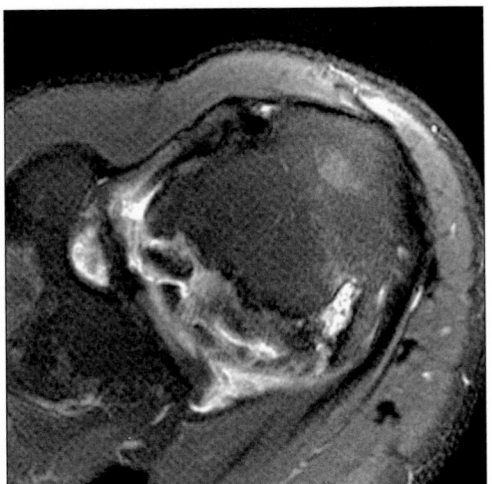

(Left) Coronal FS PD FSE MR shows fragmentation and loss of the spherical humeral head in a patient with advanced chronic AVN. *(Right)* Axial FS PD FSE MR shows fragmentation of the superomedial humeral head in image of the same patient.

Typical

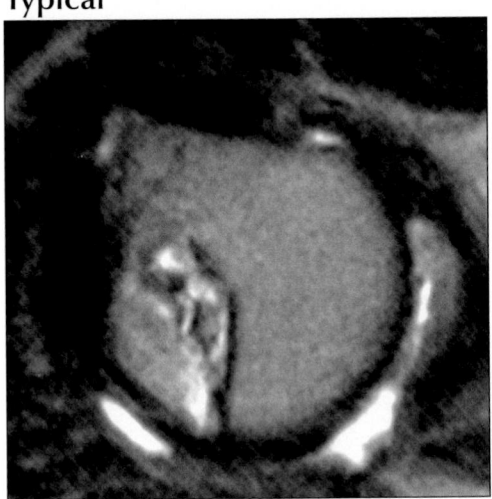 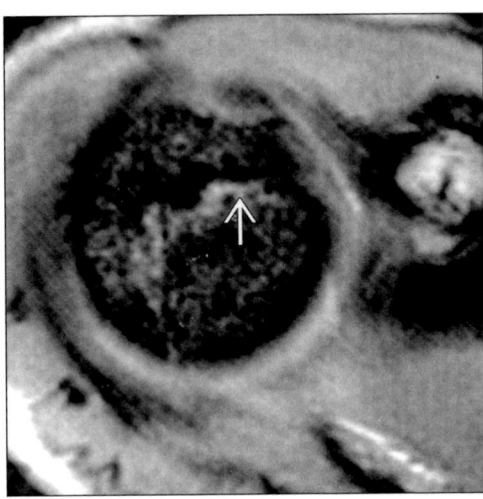

(Left) Axial T2 FSE MR shows the typical double line sign in a patient with chronic avascular necrosis of the humeral head. The patient had Caissons disease. *(Right)* Axial T2* GRE MR shows the double line sign (arrow) at humeral head.

OSTEOCHONDRAL INJURIES, SHOULDER

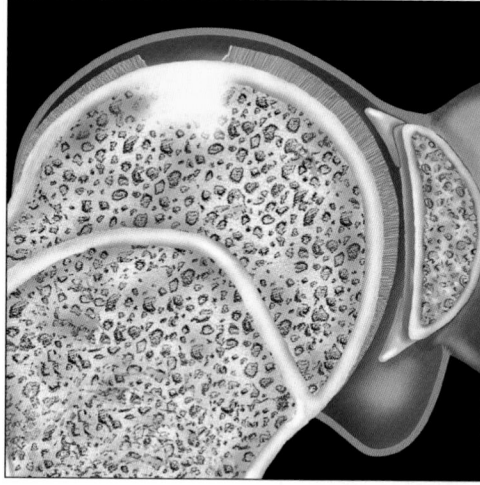

Coronal graphic shows a chondral defect involving the superior aspect of the humeral head with associated bone marrow edema.

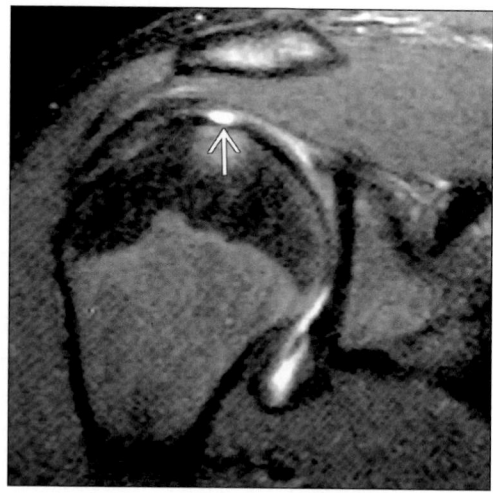

Coronal STIR MR shows a chondral defect of the superior aspect of the humeral head (arrow) with underlying bone marrow edema in a symptomatic young athlete.

TERMINOLOGY

Abbreviations and Synonyms
- Osteochondral injury (OCI)

Definitions
- Injury to articular cartilage +/- underlying bone fracture, bone trabecular injury or associated reactive stress response (edema)

IMAGING FINDINGS

General Features
- Best diagnostic clue: Alteration in contour and/or signal of hyaline articular cartilage with underlying bone changes
- Location
  - Glenoid, esp. anterior inferior after anterior dislocation
  - Other common sites of involvement
    - Posterosuperior humeral head (HH) - Hill-Sachs deformity after anterior dislocation
    - Posterior glenoid - reverse Bankart after posterior dislocation
    - Lesser tuberosity - reverse Hill-Sachs after posterior dislocation
    - HH - hyaline articular cartilage, superior aspect
    - Supraglenoid tubercle - associated with superior labrum anterior to posterior (SLAP) lesion
- Size: Varies from small chondral defect (millimeter) to large area of cartilage denudation
- Morphology
  - From defined chondral defect to irregular chondral lesion
    - Associated with underlying osseous changes

Radiographic Findings
- Radiography
  - +/- Fracture of humeral head/glenoid
  - +/- Subchondral sclerosis in chronic cases

CT Findings
- CT arthrography
  - Chondral defect filled with contrast
  - +/- Glenoid or humeral head fracture

MR Findings
- T1WI
  - Subchondral sclerosis (decreased signal intensity)
  - +/- Hypointense fracture
  - Hypointense subchondral edema
- T2WI
  - Increased signal intensity in hyaline articular cartilage, well defined or irregular chondral defect
  - Underling bone marrow edema - hyperintense signal (impaction)

DDx: Osteochondral Injuries, Shoulder

Lessr Tub Fx	Scapula Stress Fx	Surg. Neck Fx	Reactive Edema
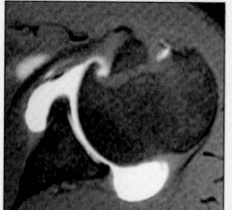	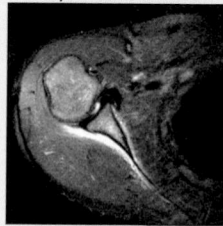	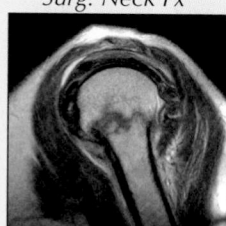	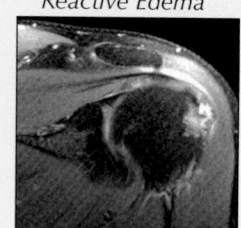
Ax T1 Arthro.	Ax STIR	Sag T2 FSE	Cor FS PD FSE

OSTEOCHONDRAL INJURIES, SHOULDER

Key Facts

Imaging Findings
- Best diagnostic clue: Alteration in contour and/or signal of hyaline articular cartilage with underlying bone changes
- Increased signal intensity in hyaline articular cartilage, well defined or irregular chondral defect
- Underling bone marrow edema - hyperintense signal (impaction)

Top Differential Diagnoses
- Osteoarthritis (OA)
- Bare Area of Humerus (Posterosuperior) or Glenoid (Central)
- Reactive Edema
- Humeral Head or Glenoid Fracture
- Surgical neck fracture

- Anatomic neck fracture
- Lesser tuberosity fracture
- Scapular stress fracture

Pathology
- Tidemark zone is weakest part of hyaline articular cartilage and most often disrupted

Clinical Issues
- Most common signs/symptoms: Intermittent locking, recurrent effusions, crepitus, and persistent pain
- Clinical profile: Active patient, often athlete
- Age: Younger active patient < 40 years old

Diagnostic Checklist
- Check for increased signal intensity or fluid in hyaline cartilage on FS PD FSE or PD FSE images

---

- FS PD FSE - increased signal intensity in hyaline articular cartilage
  - Well defined or irregular chondral defect evaluated with FS PD/T2 FSE
- PD/Intermediate: Edema is not well visualized without fat saturation
- STIR
  - Spatial resolution is decreased
  - Increased signal intensity in hyaline articular cartilage
  - Chondral defect, +/- filled with hyperintense fluid
  - +/- Underlying bone marrow edema (hyperintense)
- T2* GRE
  - Bone edema often obscured by susceptibility artifact
  - T2* GRE WI may show joint fluid isointense to cartilage
  - T2* only sensitive to larger chondral defects relative to FS PD FSE images
- T1 C+: Bone reactive changes (edema) may enhance following IV gadolinium administration
- MR arthrography
  - Contrast fills articular cartilage defect

Nuclear Medicine Findings
- Bone Scan: Increased uptake of radiotracer in bone involvement

Imaging Recommendations
- Best imaging tool: MRI
- Protocol advice: FS PD FSE or PD sequence in at least 2 planes

DIFFERENTIAL DIAGNOSIS

Osteoarthritis (OA)
- Gradual, insidious onset
- Osteochondral injury/defect
- Subchondral cysts
- Subchondral edema
- Subchondral sclerosis
- Older patient/post traumatic patient

Bare Area of Humerus (Posterosuperior) or Glenoid (Central)
- Cartilage thinning to absence
- Normal variant
- Posterosuperior humeral head
- Central glenoid

Reactive Edema
- Edematous changes in reaction to adjacent inflammatory process
  - Rotator cuff disease
  - Reactive osteitis
- Early OA
- Associated with bone trabecular injury

Humeral Head or Glenoid Fracture
- Surgical neck fracture
  - History of acute trauma
  - Edema
- Anatomic neck fracture
  - History of acute trauma
  - Edema mimics OCI
- Lesser tuberosity fracture
  - After seizure
  - +/- Subscapularis tear
- Scapular stress fracture
  - Athlete
  - Baseball
  - Hyperintense edema (T2)
  - +/- Fragmentation

Avascular Necrosis (AVN)
- Predisposing condition
  - Steroids
  - Alcoholism
- Double line sign
- +/- Synovitis
- +/- Articular surface collapse

OSTEOCHONDRAL INJURIES, SHOULDER

PATHOLOGY

General Features
- General path comments
  - Tidemark zone is weakest part of hyaline articular cartilage and most often disrupted
    - Between overlying cartilage and subchondral bone
  - Shearing injuries produce chondral injury rather than osteochondral injury
  - Mild fibrillation, fissuring, flap lesion, defect or osteochondral fracture
- Etiology
  - Rotational forces and direct trauma - injury to articular cartilage
  - Secondarily involve underlying bone
- Epidemiology: Young active patients most common
- Associated abnormalities: SLAP lesions, soft tissue injury, hematoma

Gross Pathologic & Surgical Features
- Mild lesion on MRI may show no discernible abnormality at gross inspection
- Fibrillation
- Cartilage softening
- Fissures and chondral flaps
- Partial and full thickness chondral defects
- Bone injuries ranging from bone trabecular injury to fracture

Microscopic Features
- Chondrocyte disruption followed by swelling
- If underlying bone involved, blood vessels are ruptured and hematoma is formed
- Cell death due to interrupted blood supply
- Avulsion of articular cartilage
  - Between deep calcified and juxta-articular noncalcified cartilage
- Subchondral compression and trabecular fractures
  - +/- Injury to articular cartilage

Staging, Grading or Classification Criteria
- Outerbridge classification for chondromalacia
  - Grade 0: Normal cartilage
  - Grade I: Chondral softening and swelling
    - MRI: Increased signal intensity FS PD FSE
  - Grade II: Partial thickness defect with fissures on the surface not reaching subchondral bone or not exceeding 1.5 cm in diameter
    - MRI: Surface irregularity
  - Grade III: Fissuring to the level of subchondral bone in area with a diameter more than 1.5 cm
    - MRI: Partial to small full thickness defect
  - Grade IV: Exposed bone
    - MRI: Cartilage loss down to bone

CLINICAL ISSUES

Presentation
- Most common signs/symptoms: Intermittent locking, recurrent effusions, crepitus, and persistent pain
- Clinical profile: Active patient, often athlete

Demographics
- Age: Younger active patient < 40 years old
- Gender: M > F

Natural History & Prognosis
- Heal or form isolated defect with underlying secondary arthritic change with increased symptoms

Treatment
- Conservative
  - Rest followed by physical therapy
  - NSAIDs
- Surgical
  - Chondral defects: Debridement, microfracture, mosaicplasty and other chondral resurfacing techniques depending on severity of lesion
  - Less experience with surgical treatments compared to knee

DIAGNOSTIC CHECKLIST

Consider
- In posttraumatic setting

Image Interpretation Pearls
- Underlying bone marrow edema associated with chondral injury
- Check for increased signal intensity or fluid in hyaline cartilage on FS PD FSE or PD FSE images

SELECTED REFERENCES

1. Farmer JM: Chondral and osteochondral injuries. Diagnosis and management. Clin Sports Med 20(2):299-320, 2001
2. Martinek V et al: Treatment of osteochondral injuries. Genetic engineering. Clin Sports Med 20(2):403-16, 2001
3. Bredella MA et al: Accuracy of T2-weighted fast spin-echo MR imaging with fat saturation in detecting cartilage defects in the knee: Comparison with arthroscopy in 130 patients. AJR 172(4):1073-80, 1999
4. Yu JS et al: Osteochondral defect of the glenoid fossa: Cross-sectional imaging features. Radiology 206:35-40, 1998

OSTEOCHONDRAL INJURIES, SHOULDER

IMAGE GALLERY

Typical

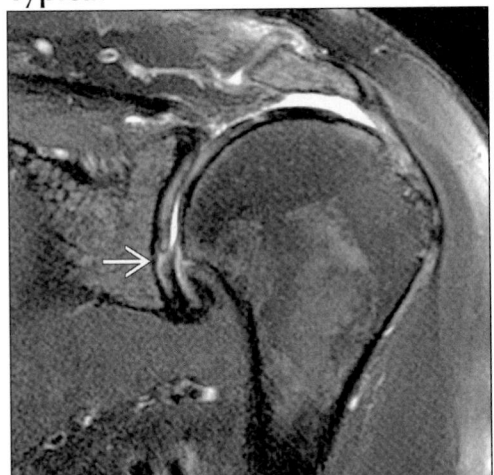 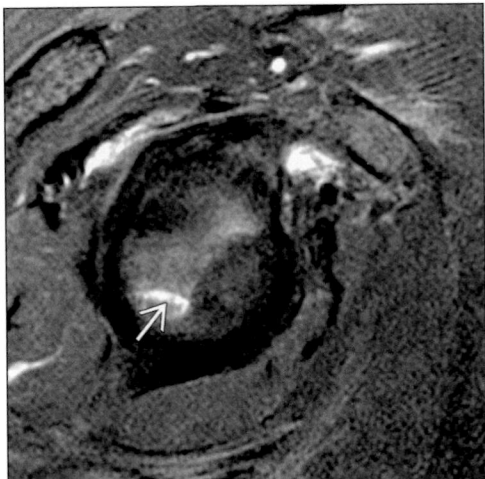

(Left) Coronal FS PD FSE MR shows a chondral flap lesion (arrow) involving the mid glenoid hyaline articular cartilage. There is a small chondral defect of the superior humeral head. (Right) Sagittal FS PD FSE MR shows the chondral flap lesion (arrow) involving the hyaline articular cartilage of the glenoid fossa.

Typical

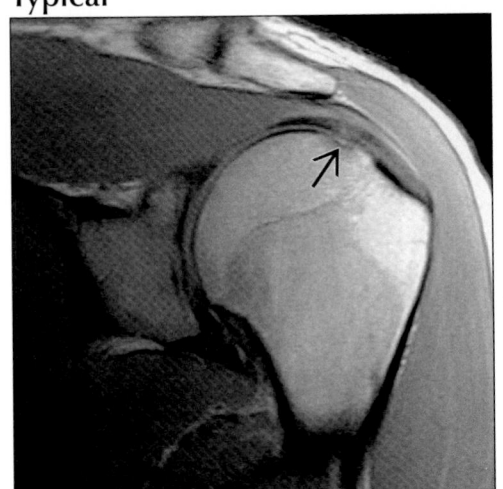 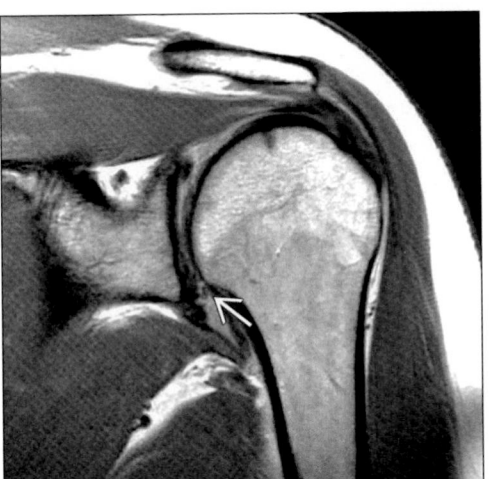

(Left) Coronal PD FSE MR shows a subtle osteochondral injury (arrow) of the superior aspect of the humeral head adjacent to a mild strain of the supraspinatus. (Right) Coronal PD FSE MR shows grade III-IV chondromalacia of the superomedial aspect of the humeral head. Note the small loose chondral fragment in the joint adjacent to the inferior labrum (arrow).

Typical

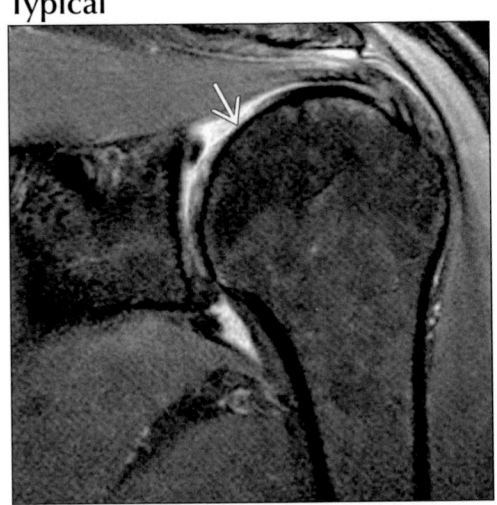 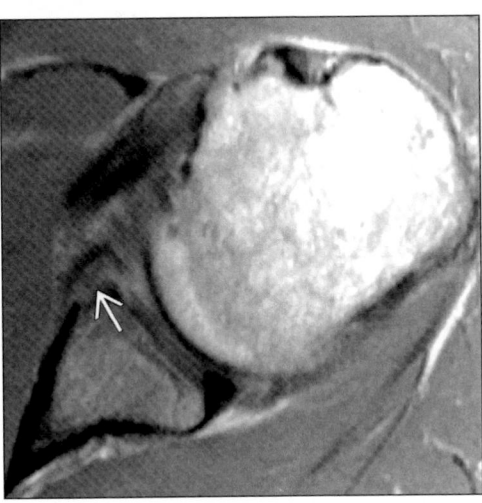

(Left) Coronal FS PD FSE MR shows chondromalacia of the superomedial HH (arrow). (Right) Axial PD FSE MR in a patient after anterior dislocation shows an osteochondral fracture of the anterior glenoid (arrow) – Bankart lesion.

GREATER TUBEROSITY FRACTURE

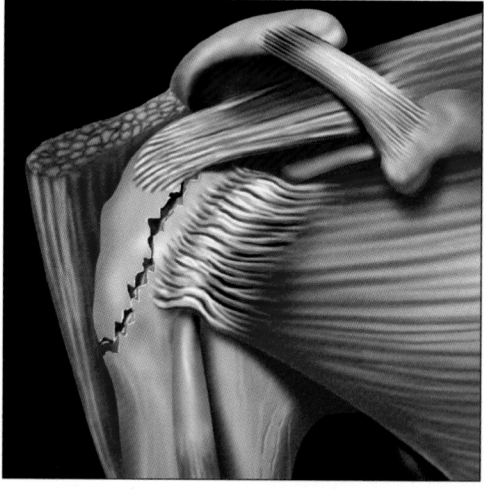

Coronal graphic shows a fracture of the greater tuberosity that is still attached to the supraspinatus tendon. There is mild fracture diastasis.

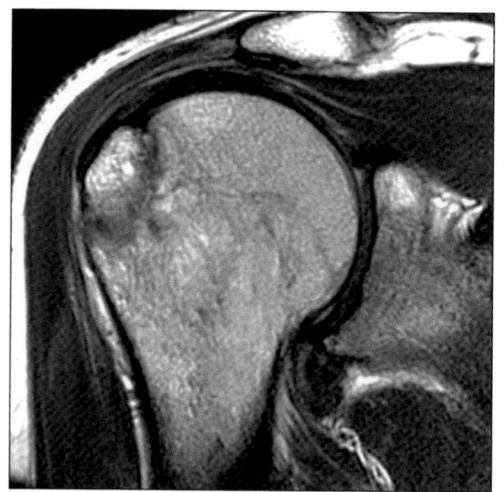

Coronal PD FSE MR shows a minimally displaced greater tuberosity fracture with an intact supraspinatus tendon.

TERMINOLOGY

Abbreviations and Synonyms
- Greater tuberosity fracture (GTFx)

Definitions
- Fracture of the greater tuberosity of the humerus after direct impact injury or anterior dislocation impact
  - Extended Hill-Sachs fracture in case of anterior dislocation

IMAGING FINDINGS

General Features
- Best diagnostic clue
  - Increased signal within the greater tuberosity on FS PD FSE
  - +/- Linear decreased signal intensity line on all pulse sequences
- Location: Greater tuberosity of the humerus
- Size: Nondisplaced trabecular injury to displaced comminuted fracture 2-5 cm in size
- Morphology: Nondisplaced fracture to comminuted fracture with distracted fragments

Radiographic Findings
- Radiography
  - Occult in case of trabecular injury

- = Bone contusion
  - Fracture line or comminuted fragment
  - Variable displacement
  - +/- Heal in displaced/malaligned position

CT Findings
- NECT
  - Subtle disruption of trabecular pattern
    - = Bone contusion
  - Fracture line or comminuted fragment
  - Characterization of fracture fragments
    - Displacement
    - Angulation
  - May heal in displaced/malaligned position
  - Reconstruction in coronal, sagittal plane

MR Findings
- T1WI
  - Decreased signal intensity
    - Perifracture edema
    - Bone trabecular injury without fracture line
  - Fracture line of decreased signal intensity
  - Displaced fragments seen as marrow containing
    - +/- Displacement
    - +/- Comminution
- T2WI
  - Increased signal at the fracture site
    - Perifracture hyperintense edema
    - Bone trabecular injury without fracture line

DDx: Greater Tuberosity Fracture

Surg Neck Fx	Anatomic Neck Fx	Degen Cysts	GT Avulsion	Failure FS

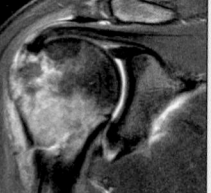
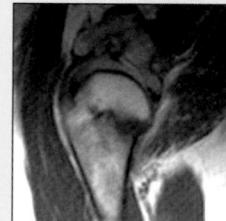
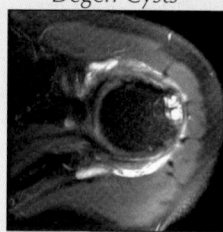
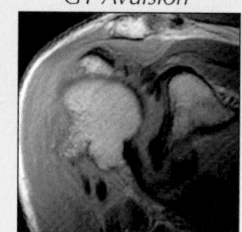
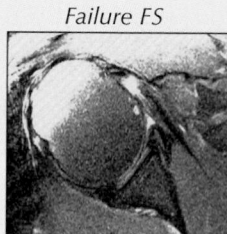

Cor FS PD FSE	Cor Oblq T1 WI	Ax FS PD FSE MR	Cor PD FSE MR	Ax FS PD FSE MR

GREATER TUBEROSITY FRACTURE

Key Facts

Imaging Findings
- Increased signal within the greater tuberosity on FS PD FSE
- +/- Linear decreased signal intensity line on all pulse sequences
- Occult in case of trabecular injury
- Increased signal at the fracture site
- Perifracture hyperintense edema
- Bone trabecular injury without fracture line
- FS PD FSE images sensitive

Top Differential Diagnoses
- Supraspinatus Tear
- Subscapularis Rupture
- Bankart Lesion
- Perthes Lesion
- Subcortical Degenerative Cystic Change
- Proximal Humeral fractures
- Failure of Fat Saturation (Failure FS)

Pathology
- Direct impact
- Greater tuberosity avulsion after anterior dislocation
- Occurs after anterior dislocation of the shoulder or direct impact

Clinical Issues
- Posttraumatic after anterior dislocation
- Association with anterior dislocation (5-33% of cases)

Diagnostic Checklist
- FS PD FSE or STIR coronals images are sensitive to associated marrow edema

---

- o Fracture line = decreased signal intensity +/- interposed hyperintensity fluid
- o +/- Increased signal rotator cuff strain
  - ▪ +/- Partial to complete tear
  - ▪ +/- Fluid-filled (hyperintense) gap
- o +/- Capsular sprain
  - ▪ Thickened hyperintense sprain
- o FS PD FSE images sensitive
  - ▪ Esp. with bone trabecular injury
  - ▪ Non FS images may not identify edema or fracture morphology
- PD/Intermediate
  - o Edema not well seen without FS
  - o Without FS perifracture reactive change is intermediate in signal intensity
  - o PD FSE useful for chondral evaluation
- STIR
  - o Increased signal at the fracture site
    - ▪ Perifracture edema
    - ▪ Bone trabecular contusion without fracture line
- T2* GRE
  - o Hypo or hyperintense fracture line easily visualized
  - o Edema often obscured by susceptibility artifact

Imaging Recommendations
- Best imaging tool: MRI
- Protocol advice: T1WI + FS PD FSE

DIFFERENTIAL DIAGNOSIS

Supraspinatus Tear
- +/- Impingement
- +/- Anterior dislocation
  - o > 40 years
- Hyperintense gap on T2WI
- +/- SLAP (superior labrum anterior posterior) lesion
  - o SLAC (superior labrum anterior cuff) lesion
- Associated bursitis

Subscapularis Rupture
- +/- Impingement
- +/- Anterior dislocation

- o > 40 years
- Hyperintense gap on T2WI in case of tear
- +/- Associated capsular tear
  - o Esp. with dislocation
- +/- Biceps instability
  - o Subluxation
  - o Dislocation

Bankart Lesion
- + Anterior dislocation
- Posttraumatic pain and decreased range of motion
- Disrupted scapular periosteum
- Hyperintensity on T2WI = edema
- Displacement of labrum

Perthes Lesion
- Intact periosteum
- A type of Bankart variation
- + Anterior dislocation, subluxation
- Hyperintensity on T2WI = edema
- Abduction with external reduction (ABER) imaging useful

Subcortical Degenerative Cystic Change
- Common finding in older age group
- Exaggerated with athletic activity
- No associated history of trauma
- Involves "bare area"
- Vascular perforation channels in some cases
- Filled with contrast at arthrography
- +/- Adjacent degenerative chondromalacia outside the "bare area"

Proximal Humeral fractures
- Anatomic neck
- Surgical neck
- Lesser tuberosity
- +/- Comminution
- +/- Displacement

Failure of Fat Saturation (Failure FS)
- Due to curved shoulder surface
- Susceptibility
- Frequency selective fat saturation

- o Usually not seen with STIR
- Paradoxical water saturation
  - o Leads to hypointense deltoid
  - o Due to shift of water precessional frequency into saturation frequency range
- Leads to bright signal in marrow containing humerus
- Mimics bone trabecular injury/nondisplaced fracture
- No fracture line identified
- T2* GRE or STIR sequence used when fat suppression fails with FS PD FSE

PATHOLOGY

General Features

- General path comments
  - o Direct impact
  - o Anterior dislocation with IGHLC (inferior glenohumeral ligament complex) or RTC (rotator cuff) abnormality
  - o Greater tuberosity avulsion after anterior dislocation
    - Supraspinatus tendon remains intact
- Etiology
  - o Occurs after anterior dislocation of the shoulder or direct impact
  - o Hill-Sachs fracture represents variant of greater tuberosity fracture
- Epidemiology
  - o Greater tuberosity fracture is common, especially after anterior dislocation
  - o Proximal humeral
    - 4-5% of all fractures in adult
    - < 1% of children's fractures
    - 40% involve greater tuberosity
- Associated abnormalities
  - o Dislocation findings
    - Bankart lesion
    - Perthes lesion
    - ALPSA lesion
    - Supraspinatus tear
    - Subscapularis tendon tear
    - Capsular sprain
    - Hill-Sachs deformity = variant of greater tuberosity fracture
  - o Rotator cuff strain
    - +/- Tear

Gross Pathologic & Surgical Features

- Fracture of greater tuberosity often involving chondral surface
- Nondisplaced, displaced or comminuted
- Displaced
  - o Superior - supraspinatus involved
  - o Posterior - infraspinatus or teres minor involved

Microscopic Features

- Disruption of trabeculae
- +/- Involving the subchondral endplate and hyaline cartilage
- Surrounding hemorrhage

Staging, Grading or Classification Criteria

- Modified Neer classification of proximal humeral fractures

  - o Type I - no displaced segment
  - o Type II to V - one segment is displaced
    - Type II - anatomic neck
    - Type III - surgical neck
    - Type IV - avulsion of greater tuberosity
    - Type V - avulsion of the lesser tuberosity
  - o Type VI - fracture dislocation

CLINICAL ISSUES

Presentation

- Most common signs/symptoms
  - o Posttraumatic after anterior dislocation
  - o Limited range of motion and pain
- Clinical profile
  - o Anterior dislocation
  - o +/- Direct trauma
  - o Common in sports
    - Snow skiing

Demographics

- Age: Proximal humerus fractures - 75% of fractures in patients older than 40 years
- Gender: After age 50 increase incidence in females

Natural History & Prognosis

- Typically heals after conservative therapy
- Association with anterior dislocation (5-33% of cases)

Treatment

- Conservative measures unless a large fragment with displacement is present

DIAGNOSTIC CHECKLIST

Consider

- In setting of direct trauma or anterior dislocation

Image Interpretation Pearls

- FS PD FSE or STIR coronals images are sensitive to associated marrow edema

SELECTED REFERENCES

1. Burkhart SS et al: Traumatic glenohumeral bone defects and their relationship to failure of arthroscopic Bankart repairs: Significance of the inverted-pear glenoid and the humeral engaging Hill-Sachs lesion. Arthroscopy 16(7):677-94, 2000
2. Kim SH et al: Arthroscopic treatment of symptomatic shoulders with minimally displaced greater tuberosity fracture. Arthroscopy 16(7):695-700, 2000
3. Reinus WR et al: Fractures of the greater tuberosity presenting as rotator cuff abnormality: Magnetic resonance demonstration. J Trauma 44(4):670-5, 1998
4. Tirman PF et al: A practical approach to imaging of the shoulder with emphasis on MR imaging. Orthop Clin North Am 28(4):483-515, 1997

GREATER TUBEROSITY FRACTURE

IMAGE GALLERY

Typical

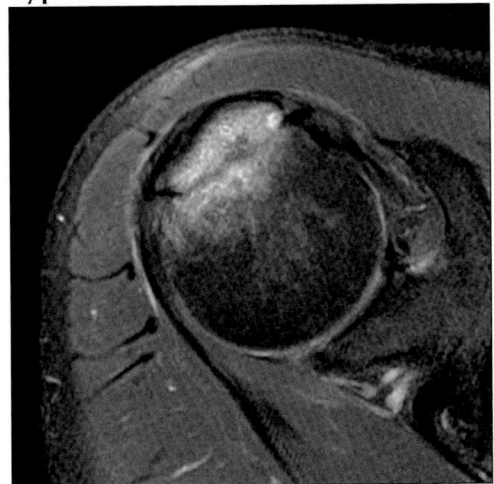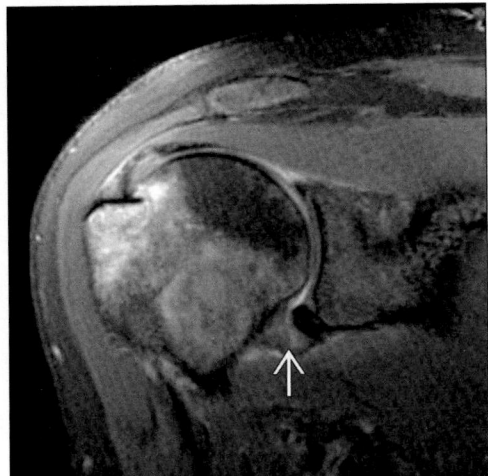

(Left) Axial FS PD FSE MR shows a nondisplaced greater tuberosity fracture with the fracture line seen as linear decreased signal intensity. There is surrounding edema. *(Right)* Coronal FS PD FSE MR shows a nondisplaced greater tuberosity fracture with rotator cuff strain. There is a capsular sprain (arrow) present in this patient status post anterior dislocation while skiing.

Typical

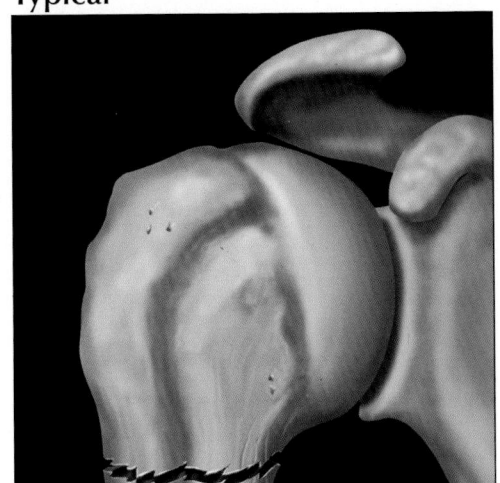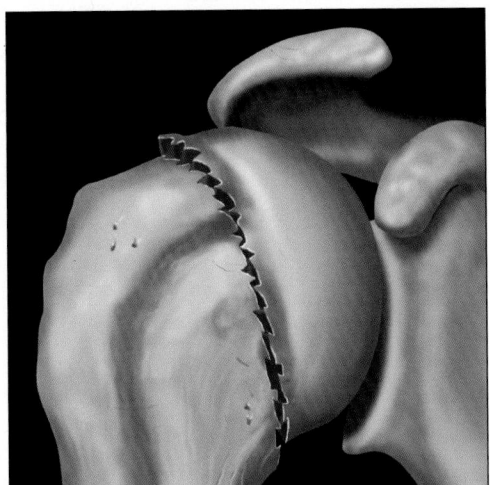

(Left) Coronal graphic shows a surgical neck transverse fracture. *(Right)* Coronal graphic shows an anatomic neck fracture with minimal displacement.

Typical

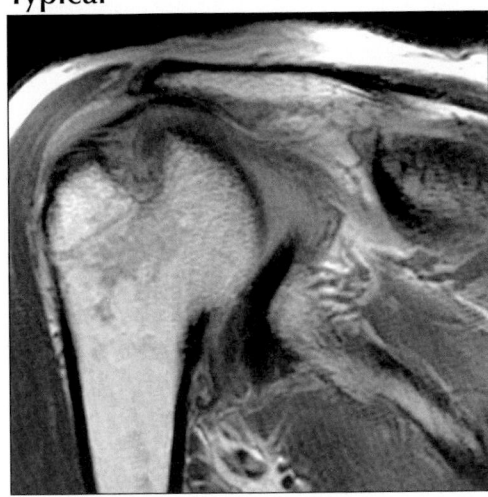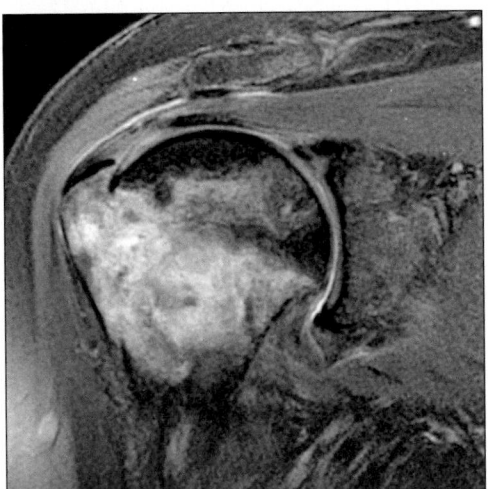

(Left) Coronal PD FSE MR shows a depressed Hill-Sachs fracture (greater tuberosity impaction fracture) in a patient post anterior dislocation. The rotator cuff is strained. *(Right)* Coronal FS PD FSE MR shows a slightly displaced fracture of the greater tuberosity with slight elevation, associated supraspinatus strain and hyperintense marrow edema.

OSTEOARTHRITIS, SHOULDER

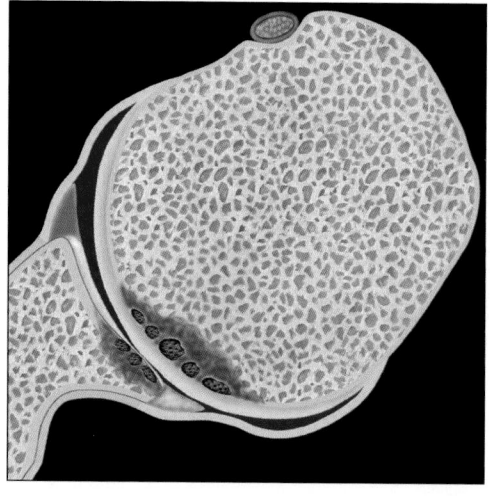

Axial graphic shows chondromalacia, subchondral cystic change & surrounding sclerosis of glenoid & humeral head. Note the asymmetric wear of the posterior glenoid.

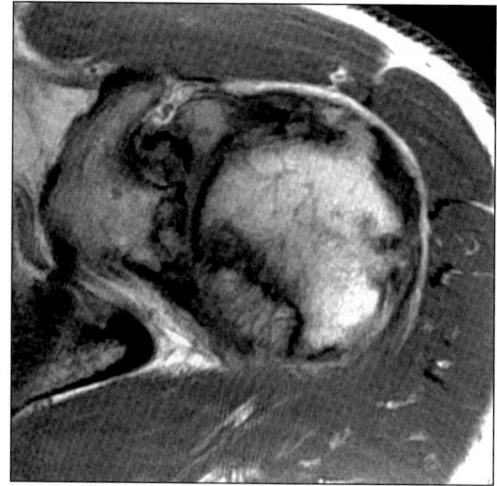

Axial PD FSE MR shows advanced osteoarthritic changes: Subchondral cyst formation with sclerosis of humeral head & glenoid. Osteophytes, loose bodies, and synovitis are associated.

TERMINOLOGY

Abbreviations and Synonyms
- Osteoarthritis (OA), degenerative joint disease (DJD)

Definitions
- Degenerative arthritis characterized by chondromalacia, osteophyte formation, subchondral cysts and synovitis
  - Primary: Gradual process of destruction & regeneration as a result of chronic microtrauma
  - Secondary: Non-inflammatory degenerative joint disease resulting from predisposing event such as previous trauma, congenital deformity, infection or a metabolic disorder

IMAGING FINDINGS

General Features
- Best diagnostic clue: Chondromalacia +/- subchondral sclerosis, subchondral cysts and/or edema, and osteophytes
- Location: Shoulder joint hyaline chondral surfaces and subchondral bone
- Size: Small localized area (typically post trauma) to entire glenohumeral joint
- Morphology

  - Progressive loss of articular cartilage with associated new bone formation and capsular fibrosis
  - Osteophytes prominent

Radiographic Findings
- Radiography
  - Joint space narrowing
  - Subchondral sclerosis/eburnation of increased density
  - Subchondral cysts
  - Osteophyte formation

MR Findings
- T1WI
  - Decreased signal intensity subchondral cysts
  - Marrow fat signal extends into osteophytes
  - Subchondral decreased signal indicating sclerosis and/or edema
  - Evaluate posterior glenoid version
- T2WI
  - Subarticular cysts seen as high signal rounded lesions
  - Hyperintensity in hyaline cartilage
  - Subchondral bone marrow edema (bright signal)
  - Subchondral decreased signal = sclerosis
  - General thinning of articular (hyaline) cartilage with occasional focal defects

DDx: Osteoarthritis, Shoulder

Diab. Arthropathy	HH OCD	PSGI	AVN	RA
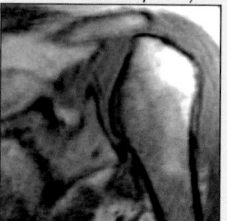	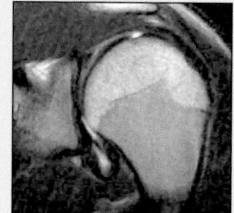	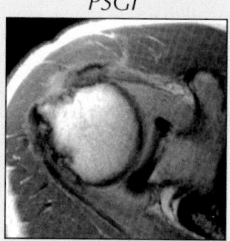	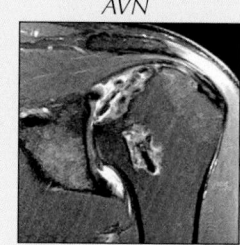	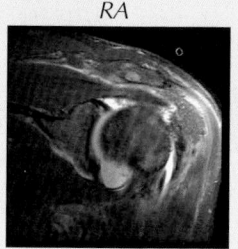
Cor PD FSE MR	Cor PD FSE MR	Ax PD FSE MR	Cor FS PD FSE	Cor FS PD FSE

OSTEOARTHRITIS, SHOULDER

Key Facts

Terminology
- Degenerative arthritis characterized by chondromalacia, osteophyte formation, subchondral cysts and synovitis

Imaging Findings
- Joint space narrowing
- Subchondral sclerosis/eburnation of increased density
- Subchondral cysts
- Osteophyte formation especially involving the humeral head
- Loose bodies
- Posterior glenoid wear leads to increased retroversion of the glenoid

Top Differential Diagnoses
- Inflammatory Arthritis

- Synovitis
- Septic Arthritis
- Neuropathic Arthritis

Pathology
- Begins as fatigue fracture of the collagen meshwork followed by increased hydration of the articular cartilage (as opposed to desiccated cartilage seen with aging) and loss of proteoglycans from the matrix into the synovial fluid

Clinical Issues
- Slowly progressive pain with utilization of the joint and variable degrees of swelling (effusion)

Diagnostic Checklist
- Utilize FS PD FSE to visualize chondral findings

- ○ FS PD FSE (more sensitive sequence than T2 FSE) shows hyperintensity in hyaline cartilage and subchondral bone marrow edema
- PD/Intermediate
  - ○ Synovitis seen as thickening of the synovium especially on proton density images
  - ○ PD FSE: Cartilage not as well seen
- T2* GRE: Subarticular cysts seen as high signal erosions on gradient echo images
- T1 C+: Synovium enhances with synovitis
- Osteophyte formation especially involving the humeral head
- Loose bodies
- Posterior glenoid wear leads to increased retroversion of the glenoid
- Asymmetric joint space narrowing

Imaging Recommendations
- Best imaging tool: MRI
- Protocol advice: FS PD FSE

DIFFERENTIAL DIAGNOSIS

Inflammatory Arthritis
- Polyarticular systemic disease (e.g., rheumatoid arthritis)
- +/- Serum indicators
- Synovitis +/- erosions

Synovitis
- Associated with prominent erosions that may mimic subarticular cysts
- +/- Polyarticular

Septic Arthritis
- Positive blood cultures
  - ○ White cell count of more than 75,000/mm³

Neuropathic Arthritis
- Secondary to loss of nerve supply
- Fragmentation, destruction
- Secondary to diabetes (diab. arthropathy)

Cuff Tear Arthropathy
- Secondary to long-standing chronic massive rotator cuff tear
- Considered form of osteoarthritic change in shoulder

Milwaukee Shoulder
- Secondary to hydroxyapatite crystal deposition disease
- Severe degenerative changes

Capsulorrhaphy Arthropathy
- Secondary to over tightening for instability
- Osteoarthritis changes may be focal depending on exact type of resulting disability

Avascular Necrosis (AVN)
- Double line sign may mimic subchondral cysts

Humeral Head Osteochondral Defect (HH OCD)
- Focal articular cartilage defect
- + History of trauma

Posterosuperior Glenoid Impingement (PSGI)
- Internal impingement
- Athletes
- Undersurface supraspinatus tear, posterosuperior labral fraying/tear, humeral head posterosuperior chronic impaction injury

PATHOLOGY

General Features
- General path comments
  - ○ Begins as fatigue fracture of the collagen meshwork followed by increased hydration of the articular cartilage (as opposed to desiccated cartilage seen with aging) and loss of proteoglycans from the matrix into the synovial fluid
    - ■ Shoulder predisposed to unique instabilities because of non weight-bearing anatomy

OSTEOARTHRITIS, SHOULDER

- Compression of weakened bone with subchondral collapse
- Loose bodies - fragmentation of osteochondral surfaces
- +/- Osteonecrosis
- Synovial hypertrophy - joint pain by nerve stimulation
- Synovial fluid - increased intraarticular pressure "stretching the joint lining" = pain
- Etiology
  - Post-operative instability patients (secondary arthritis)
  - Younger patient if posttraumatic or post-operative (secondary arthritis)
  - Leading theory - chronic microtrauma leading to disruption of the articular surface, fibrillation, eburnation, eventually subchondral cysts, and osteophytes
  - If asymmetric capsular contracture is present, premature obligate translation results in chondral damage/DJD
    - Obligate translation - movement of the humeral head in a direction opposite that of the tight capsule
  - Tendon ruptures/weakness of muscle group lead to eccentric loading of the joint = OA
- Epidemiology: Relatively uncommon compared to impingement
- Associated abnormalities
  - Rotator cuff tears
    - Often indication for MRI with known shoulder OA

Gross Pathologic & Surgical Features
- Chondromalacia, osteophyte formation, subchondral cysts, synovitis
- Degraded cartilage with loss of sheen, fissured and/or ulcerated cartilage surface, articular surface collapse
- Subchondral geodes (cysts) with debris
- Buttressing osteophytes to increase surface area
- Eccentric glenoid wear (posteriorly) contracture of anterior capsule and subscapularis

Microscopic Features
- Synovial infiltration with polymorphonuclear leukocytes (PMNs) (synovitis)
- Diminution of chondrocytes in superficial zones with chondrocyte swelling
- Cartilage matrix loses its ability to stain for proteoglycans with Alcian blue or safranin-O
- Matrix chondrocytes demonstrate proliferation in clusters (brood capsules)
- Neovascularity penetrates layer of calcified cartilage
- New chondrocytes extend up from the deeper layers
- Hypertrophied synovium becomes folded into villous folds with variable infiltration of plasma cells, and lymphocytes

CLINICAL ISSUES

Presentation
- Most common signs/symptoms

- Slowly progressive pain with utilization of the joint and variable degrees of swelling (effusion)
- Often antecedent traumatic history
- Decreased motion (external rotation loss > internal rotation loss)
- Crepitus

Demographics
- Age: Elderly patient or younger patient if posttraumatic or post-operative
- Gender: $M \geq F$

Natural History & Prognosis
- Progressively debilitating disease unless medical intervention

Treatment
- Usually conservative
  - Physical therapy
  - NSAIDs
- Total shoulder replacement in severe cases

DIAGNOSTIC CHECKLIST

Consider
- Secondary OA if findings are focal

Image Interpretation Pearls
- Utilize FS PD FSE to visualize chondral findings
- Asymmetrical wear of the posterior glenoid

SELECTED REFERENCES

1. Kelley MJ et al: Osteoarthritis and traumatic arthritis of the shoulder. J Hand Ther 13(2):148-62, 2000
2. Rockwood CA Jr et al: Disorders of the acromioclavicular joint. 2nd ed. Philadelphia PA, WB Saunders, 483-553, 1998
3. Stoller DW et al: Magnetic resonance imaging in orthopaedics and sports medicine. vol 1. 2nd ed. Philadelphia PA, J.B. Lippincott, 597-742, 1997
4. Matsen FA III: Early effectiveness of shoulder arthroplasty for patients who have primary glenohumeral degenerative joint disease. J Bone Joint Surg Am 78(2):260-4, 1996
5. Bigliani LU et al: Glenohumeral arthroplasty for arthritis after instability surgery. J Shoulder Elbow Surg 4(2):87-94, 1995
6. Matsen FA III et al: Practical evaluation and management of the shoulder. Philadelphia PA, WB Saunders, PAGE, 1994
7. Resnick D: Bone and Joint Imaging. 1st ed. Philadephia PA, WB Saunders, 1330, 1989

OSTEOARTHRITIS, SHOULDER

IMAGE GALLERY

Typical

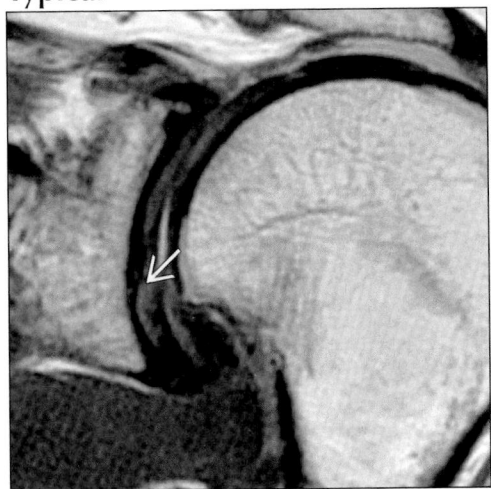 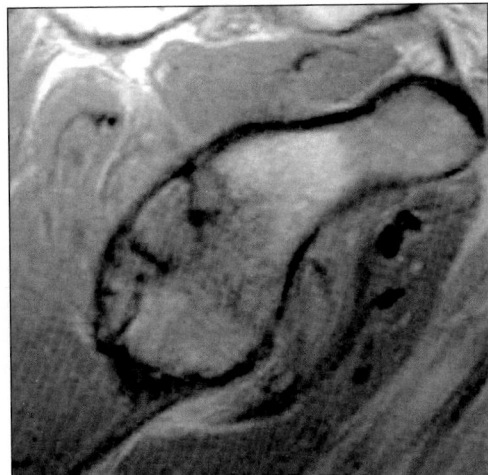

(Left) Coronal PD FSE MR shows a chondral flap lesion (arrow) of the glenoid in a patient with early manifestations of osteoarthritis. There is minimal chondromalacia of the humeral head and osteophyte formation. *(Right)* Sagittal PD FSE shows posterior glenoid subchondral cysts in this patient with chronic posterior instability and secondary osteoarthritis. Note the synovitis in the anterior joint.

Typical

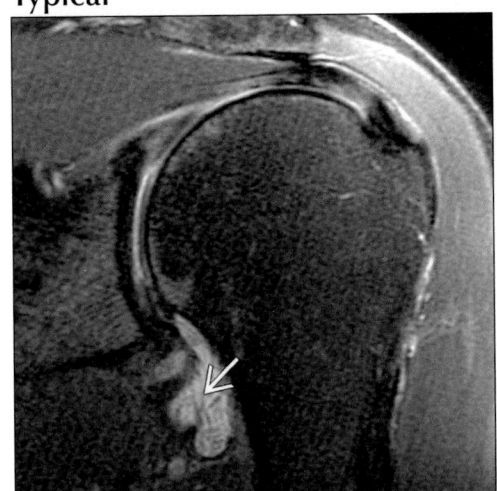 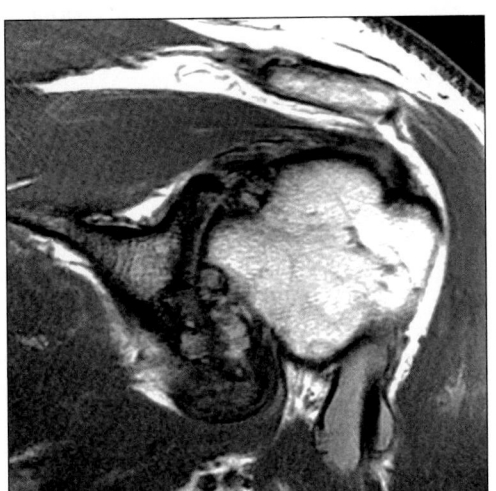

(Left) Coronal FS PD FSE MR shows marked synovitis with synovial fronds (arrow) visible in the axillary pouch. Humeral head chondromalacia with underlying bone marrow reactive edema is present. *(Right)* Coronal PD FSE MR shows advanced osteoarthritic change with some foci of osteonecrosis/subcortical cystic change, osteophyte formation, synovitis, and joint debris.

Typical

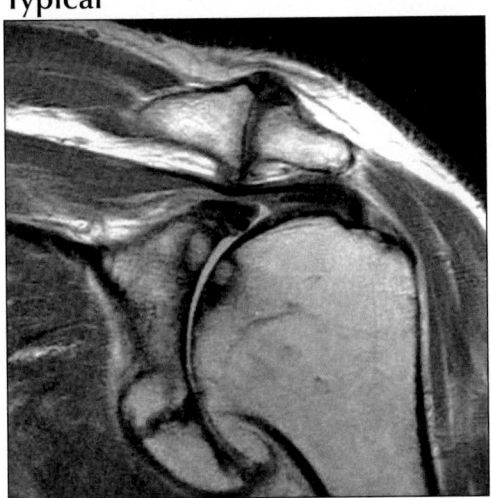 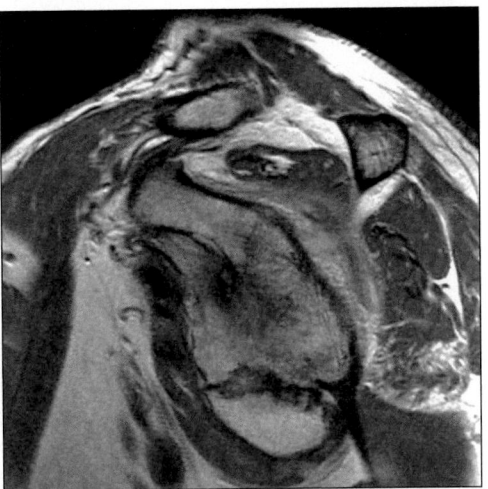

(Left) Coronal PD FSE MR shows advanced osteoarthritis changes including full thickness chondral loss, subcortical cyst formation, and large osteophytes. There is partial rotator cuff tearing. *(Right)* Sagittal PD FSE MR shows marked osteoarthritic change of the glenoid. A chronic fracture of the inferior glenoid is seen as transverse linear signal intensity.

RHEUMATOID ARTHRITIS, SHOULDER

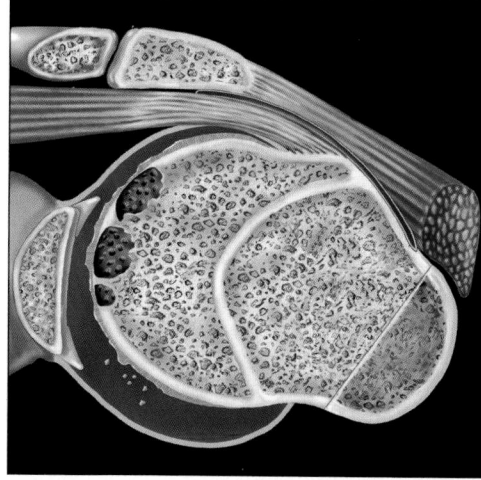

Axial graphic shows erosive changes, cartilage degradation and joint debris in a patient with rheumatoid arthritis.

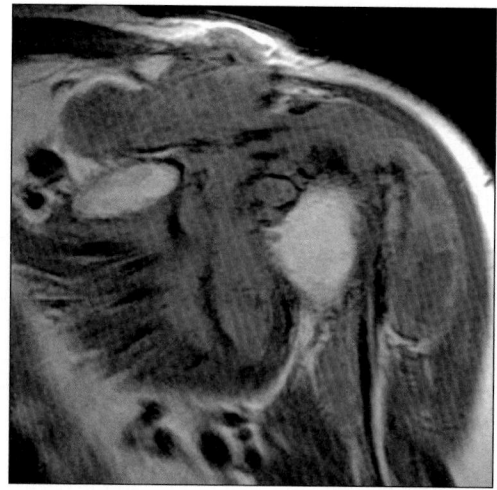

Coronal PD FSE MR shows severe synovitis within the shoulder joint as well as hypertrophic bursitis. There are erosive changes within the humeral head. The rotator cuff is torn.

TERMINOLOGY

Abbreviations and Synonyms
- Rheumatoid arthritis (RA)

Definitions
- Systemic inflammatory arthritic condition requiring the presence of 4 of the following 7 criteria for > 6 weeks
- Classification criteria for rheumatoid arthritis
  - Morning stiffness
  - Oligo or polyarthritis in three or more joints or several joint groups
  - Arthritis of either wrist, metacarpophalangeal joint or proximal interphalangeal joint
  - Symmetric arthritis
  - Rheumatoid nodules over bony prominences, extensor surfaces or juxta-articular
  - Abnormal amounts of serum rheumatoid factor
  - Radiographic changes including erosions and juxta-articular demineralization

IMAGING FINDINGS

General Features
- Best diagnostic clue

- Thickened edematous synovium with effusion in patient with chronic articular inflammation
  - Erosions common
- Location
  - Affects synovium first → secondary cartilage and bone destructive changes → deformity
  - Paraarticular nodules - in 20% of RA patients
    - Mixed signal intensity masses in the skin, synovium, tendons, sclera, viscera
  - Joint space, greater tuberosity and acromioclavicular joint
- Size: Usually diffuse involvement of synovium
- Morphology
  - Thickened irregular synovium usually in the presence of joint effusion
    - Synovitis followed by erosive/destructive changes

Radiographic Findings
- Radiography
  - Joint space narrowing
    - Flattening of glenoid fossa
  - Effusion and erosion
  - Occasional cyst formation (cystic rheumatoid)
  - +/- Joint destruction

CT Findings
- NECT: Joint space narrowing, effusion, occasional cyst formation (cystic rheumatoid) followed by destruction
- CECT: Inflamed synovium enhances

DDx: Rheumatoid Arthritis, Shoulder

OA	OA	Gr Tuberosity Fx	Charcot Joint	Hemangioma
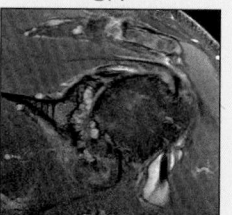	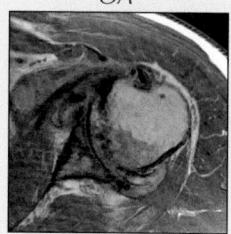	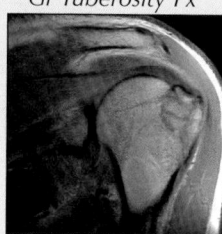	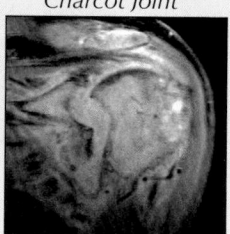	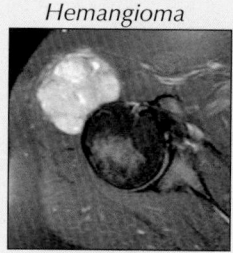
Cor FS PD FSE	Ax PD FSE MR	Cor PD FSE MR	Cor STIR MR	Ax FS PD FSE

RHEUMATOID ARTHRITIS, SHOULDER

Key Facts

Terminology
- Systemic inflammatory arthritic condition requiring the presence of 4 of the following 7 criteria for > 6 weeks

Imaging Findings
- Thickened edematous synovium with effusion in patient with chronic articular inflammation
- Affects synovium first → secondary cartilage and bone destructive changes → deformity
- Erosions and fluid are decreased in signal intensity

Top Differential Diagnoses
- Systemic Lupus Erythematosus
- Osteoarthritis (OA)
- Greater Tuberosity Fracture (Gr Tuberosity Fx)
- Neuropathic Joint (Charcot Joint)

- Extraarticular Mass

Pathology
- Pannus (granulation/synovium) tissue erodes cartilage & bone

Clinical Issues
- Pain, swelling, morning stiffness
- 10% improve after first attack of synovitis and up to 60% remissions
- Up to 10% disabled

Diagnostic Checklist
- Evaluate PD images for synovial thickening, effusions and erosions

MR Findings
- T1WI
  - Erosions and fluid are decreased in signal intensity
  - Elevation of humeral head
  - Distal clavicle resorption
- T2WI
  - Hyperintense joint effusion & subacromial-subdeltoid bursitis
  - Diffuse hyaline cartilage loss
  - Rice bodies - decreased signal masses within effusion
  - Erosions: Increased signal intensity defects in the subchondral bone (marginal, central)
  - FS PD FSE shows subchondral edema
  - Cuff atrophy
- PD/Intermediate: Demonstrates inflamed synovium as thickened increased signal intensity joint lining
- T2* GRE: Erosions visualized (less sensitive compared to FS PD FSE)
- T1 C+: Inflamed synovium will enhance

Nuclear Medicine Findings
- Bone Scan: Bone reactive change will demonstrate increased uptake

Imaging Recommendations
- Best imaging tool: MRI
- Protocol advice
  - T1 and FS PD FSE, +/- PD FSE
    - PD FSE & FS PD FSE demonstrates hypertrophied synovium and chondral erosions

DIFFERENTIAL DIAGNOSIS

Systemic Lupus Erythematosus
- Characteristic rash and other symptoms/signs
- Bone involvement different from RA
- Erosions uncommon
- +/- Subluxation

Psoriatic Arthritis
- Seronegative spondyloarthropathy
- Asymmetric, erosive, destructive articular process

- Proliferative osseous changes
- Primarily involves wrist/hands, feet, sacroiliac joint and spine

Osteoarthritis (OA)
- Primary vs. secondary: Secondary to trauma
- Subchondral cysts
- Osteophytes
- Not systemic disease

Greater Tuberosity Fracture (Gr Tuberosity Fx)
- + History of trauma
- Bone trabecular injury, comminuted fracture
- Hyperintense on T2WI of greater tuberosity
- FS PD FSE most sensitive
- Mimics erosion(s)

Neuropathic Joint (Charcot Joint)
- No neural supply to joint
- Fragmentation/disorganization
- Diabetes associated
- Mimics erosion(s)

Extraarticular Mass
- Mimics bursal effusion/enlargement
- Hemangioma/lipoma/metastatic disease
- Extraarticular
- Hyperintense on T2WI
  - Few exceptions (desmoid)
- Hypointense on T1WI
  - Exceptions (lipoma, fatty components of hemangioma)

PATHOLOGY

General Features
- General path comments
  - Rheumatoid factor (RF): IgM
  - Lab tests alone do not confirm the diagnosis of RA
    - RF present in normal individuals: Often low titers
    - Present in other diseases

RHEUMATOID ARTHRITIS, SHOULDER

- Genetics: HLA-D allele DR4 is associated with RA patients
- Etiology
  - Combination of genetic and environmental factors
  - The interaction of antigen presenting macrophages with T cells
    - Helper/inducer theory likely inciting event
  - Complexes of IgM & IgG rheumatoid factor can deposit in blood vessels and lead to vasculitis
    - Leads to vasculitis with secondary effects
  - Hepatitis B vaccine may be causative in a small number of patients
- Epidemiology: 2% of general population
- Associated abnormalities
  - Felty's syndrome characterized by splenomegaly and leukopenia
  - Still's disease characterized by fever, rash and splenomegaly
  - Sjögren syndrome characterized by decreased salivary and lacrimal gland secretion
    - Lymphoid proliferation
  - Extraarticular manifestations
    - Nodules, lymphadenopathy, splenomegaly, vasculitis, myopathy, sensory changes
    - Neuropathy
    - Direct compression of nerves/vessels from synovitis
    - Visceral changes including pericarditis, pulmonary fibrosis, nodules, and pleuritic pain

Gross Pathologic & Surgical Features

- Pannus (granulation/synovium) tissue erodes cartilage & bone
  - Direct extension of pannus occurs at the margins of the joint
  - Pannus +/- tendon sheaths
  - Rice bodies as detached fibrotic synovial villi
- Uniform joint space narrowing

Microscopic Features

- Vascular congestion and synovial cell proliferation
- Infiltration of subsynovial layers by PMNs, lymphocytes & plasma cells
- Synovial villous formation

Staging, Grading or Classification Criteria

- Stage I
  - No destructive changes - radiographic examination
  - +/- Radiographic evidence of osteoporosis
- Stage II
  - Radiographic evidence of periarticular osteoporosis +/- subchondral bone destruction
  - +/- Mild cartilage destruction
  - +/- Limited joint mobility
  - No joint deformities
  - + Muscle atrophy
  - +/- Extraarticular soft tissue lesions nodules, tenosynovitis
- Stage III
  - Radiographic evidence of cartilage and bone destruction + periarticular osteoporosis
  - Joint deformity (e.g., subluxation, ulnar deviation, hyperextension) without fibrous or bony ankylosis
- Stage IV

- + Criteria of stage III
- Fibrous or bony ankylosis
- Remission of RA - 5 or more of the following conditions present for at least 2 consecutive months
  - Duration of morning stiffness not exceeding 15 minutes
  - No fatigue
  - No joint pain
  - No joint tenderness or pain with motion
  - No soft tissue swelling in joints or tendon sheath

CLINICAL ISSUES

Presentation

- Most common signs/symptoms
  - Pain, swelling, morning stiffness
  - 7 inclusion criteria

Demographics

- Age: Adult for classical RA, variants (juvenile) affect younger patients
- Gender
  - Female - 3% of overall population
  - Male - 1% of overall population

Natural History & Prognosis

- 10% improve after first attack of synovitis and up to 60% remissions
- Up to 10% disabled
- Poor prognostic indicators include
  - High RF, periarticular erosions, rheumatoid nodules, muscle wasting, joint contractures

Treatment

- Conservative
  - Rest, physical therapy
  - Pyramid pharmaceutical approach including NSAIDs, antimalarials, disease modifying agents
    - MTX, sulfasalazine, gold, penicillamine, steroids and cytotoxic drugs
- Surgical
  - Synovectomy, arthroplasty, arthrodesis, osteotomy

DIAGNOSTIC CHECKLIST

Consider

- Other causes of synovitis
  - Clinical picture, are the findings monoarticular or polyarticular, etc.

Image Interpretation Pearls

- Evaluate PD images for synovial thickening, effusions and erosions

SELECTED REFERENCES

1. Gibbons CE et al: Long-term results of arthroscopic synovectomy for seropositive rheumatoid arthritis: 6-16 year review. Int Orthop 26(2):98-100, 2002
2. Matsuno H et al: Relationship between histological findings and clinical findings in rheumatoid arthritis. Pathol Int 52(8):527-33, 2002

IMAGE GALLERY

Typical

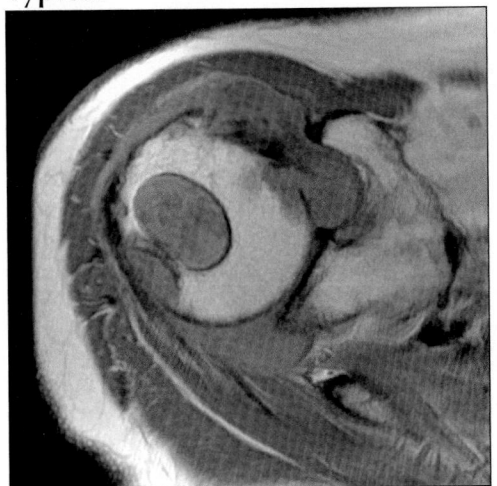 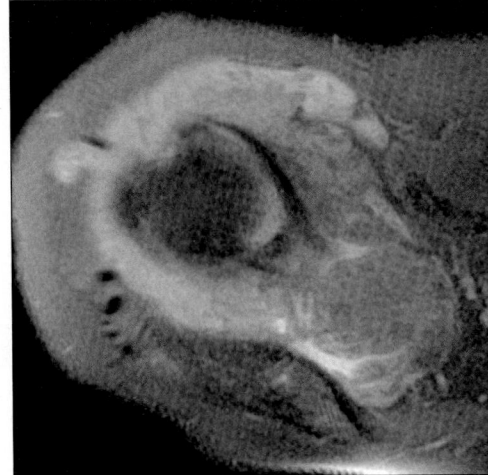

(Left) Axial PD FSE MR shows large erosions within the humeral head in a patient with rheumatoid arthritis. There is severe synovitis. *(Right)* Axial FS PD FSE MR shows the synovial pannus.

Typical

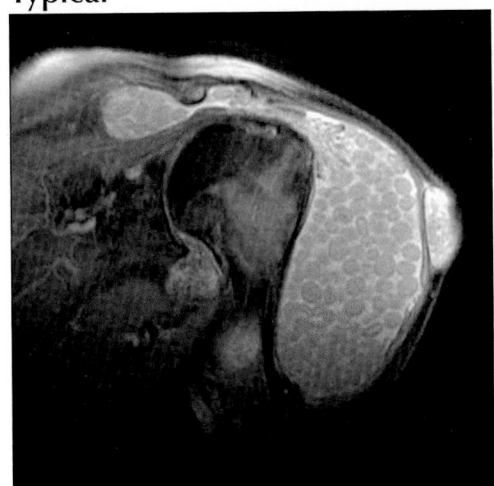 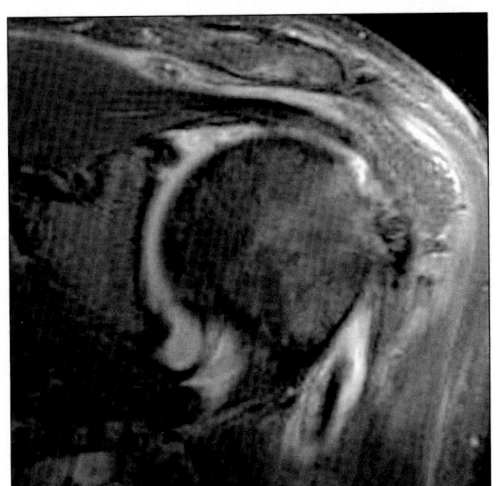

(Left) Coronal STIR MR shows numerous rice bodies within subacromial bursa in a patient with rheumatoid arthritis. The patient presented with a palpable mass which was initially diagnosed as soft tissue sarcoma. Note axillary pouch synovitis. *(Right)* Coronal STIR MR shows rice bodies and synovitis within the subacromial bursa in a patient with rheumatoid arthritis.

Typical

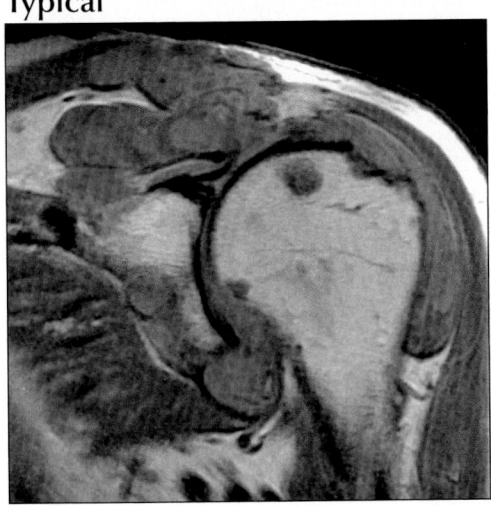 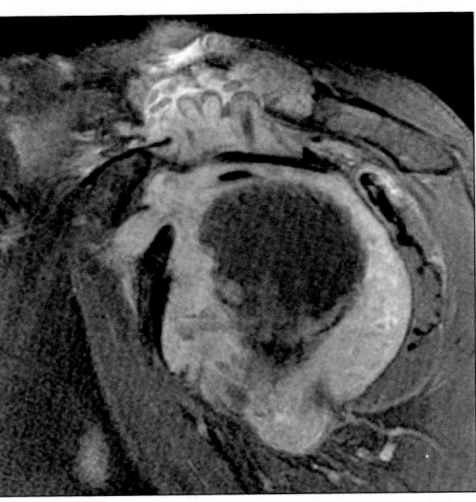

(Left) Coronal PD FSE MR shows rice bodies within the bursa and marked proliferative pannus. *(Right)* Sagittal FS PD FSE MR shows rice bodies within the subacromial bursa and marked synovitis and rice bodies within the joint.

QUADRILATERAL SPACE SYNDROME

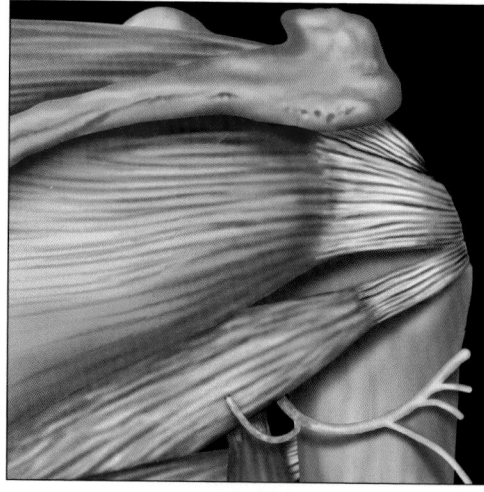

Coronal graphic shows an abnormal axillary nerve within the quadrilateral space. There are resulting denervation changes of the teres minor.

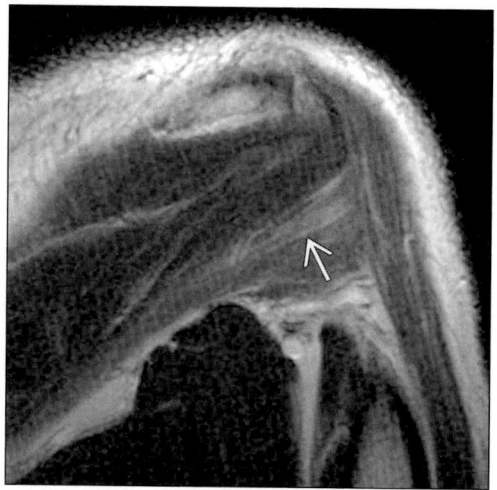

Coronal T2 FSE MR shows denervation within the deltoid and teres minor (arrow) muscles. These findings are consistent with axillary involvement.

TERMINOLOGY

Abbreviations and Synonyms
- Quadrilateral space syndrome (QSS)

Definitions
- Entrapment neuropathy (compression) of the axillary nerve (AN) in quadrilateral space

IMAGING FINDINGS

General Features
- Best diagnostic clue: Increased signal intensity within teres minor (TM) and deltoid muscle (DM) indicating denervation on FS PD FSE or STIR images
- Location: Humerus laterally, teres major (TMA) inferiorly, teres minor (TM) superiorly, long head of triceps medially
- Size
  - Mass: Variable size range - millimeters to centimeters
  - Fibrosis: Strands of variable size
- Morphology
  - Compression within boundaries of quadrilateral space
    - Mass
    - Fibrous band
        - Fracture
  - Fatty atrophy of deltoid or teres minor

Radiographic Findings
- Radiography
  - +/- Osseous changes associated with anterior/posterior dislocation if labral cyst responsible for QSS (mass compression)
    - +/- Bankart fracture (anterior inferior glenoid rim)
    - +/- Hill-Sachs deformity (posterolateral humeral head)
    - Cyst dissects from inferior labrum

CT Findings
- NECT
  - +/- Anterior/posterior dislocation findings as clue to cystic mass responsible for QSS
    - +/- Bankart fracture
    - +/- Hill-Sachs deformity
    - Cyst dissects from inferior labrum tear
    - Anterior dislocation cause of axillary neurapraxia
- CT arthrography
  - +/- Inferior labral tear/cyst
    - Contrast fills tear/cyst
    - Anteroinferior or posteroinferior

MR Findings
- T1WI
  - +/- Streaky decreased signal intensity = fibrosis

DDx: Quadrilateral Space Syndrome

Axillary Praxia	Axillary Praxia	Hematoma	Parsonage-Turner
Ax STIR MR	Cor T2 FSE MR	Cor FS PD FSE	Sag FS PD FSE

QUADRILATERAL SPACE SYNDROME

Key Facts

Imaging Findings

- Best diagnostic clue: Increased signal intensity within teres minor (TM) and deltoid muscle (DM) indicating denervation on FS PD FSE or STIR images
- +/- Streaky decreased signal intensity = fibrosis

Top Differential Diagnoses

- Anterior Shoulder Dislocation
- Proximal Humeral Fracture
- Brachial Neuritis
- Mass Lesion

Pathology

- Nerve & vessel damaged/occluded in QSS
- Distal branch of axillary nerve involved
- ± Involvement of posterior humeral circumflex artery

Clinical Issues

- Paresthesias, muscle weakness and tenderness on palpation of the quadrilateral space
- Paresthesias involve lateral shoulder and upper posterior arm
- Resolution with time in case of posttraumatic neurapraxia
- Progress if secondary to compressing mass

Diagnostic Checklist

- Posttraumatic axillary neurapraxia if patient presents with TM and DM increased signal after anterior dislocation on FS PD FSE or STIR
- FS PD FSE show demonstrates in muscle in acute and subacute phases, T1WI demonstrates fatty atrophy

- o +/- Decreased signal intensity mass - compressive neuropathy
- T2WI
  - o +/- Hypointense fibrosis - compression
  - o Increased signal intensity mass - compressive neuropathy (FS PD FSE - STIR)
    - ▪ +/- Cystic mass: Paralabral cyst extending into space
  - o Muscles atrophic + mildly increased in signal = chronic denervation
    - ▪ Decreased size
  - o Muscles increased in size + increased in signal intensity = acute + subacute denervation
    - ▪ Swelling
  - o T2 FSE less sensitive to edema
- PD/Intermediate: Masses of intermediate signal intensity
- T2* GRE
  - o Fatty atrophy of chronic denervation as decreased signal within the TM +/- DM
  - o Decreased muscle volume (mass) + hypointensity of fatty infiltration
- T1 C+
  - o Cystic mass may demonstrate rim enhancement
  - o Denervated muscles show enhancement in acute, subacute phase
- MR arthrography
  - o Inferior labral tear associated with inferiorly directed paralabral cyst

Ultrasonographic Findings

- +/- Cystic mass
  - o Anechoic
  - o Through transmission

Imaging Recommendations

- Best imaging tool: MRI
- Protocol advice
  - o T1/PD + FS PD FSE in all three planes
  - o Consider using intravenous contrast to differentiate cystic and solid soft tissue mass

DIFFERENTIAL DIAGNOSIS

Anterior Shoulder Dislocation

- +/- Axillary neurapraxia (axillary praxia)
- +/- Labral tear
  - o Bankart lesion
  - o Bankart variant lesion
  - o +/- Rotator cuff tear
- +/- Hill-Sachs fracture

Proximal Humeral Fracture

- History of trauma
- Anatomic neck, surgical neck
- +/- Comminution
- Shoulder pain with abduction

Brachial Neuritis

- +/- Parsonage-Turner syndrome (idiopathic brachial neuritis)
- Posttraumatic neurapraxia
- +/- Viral prodrome
- +/- History of trauma

Mass Lesion

- Benign
  - o Lipoma
  - o Hemangioma
- Metastasis
- Compression of nerve by mass effect
- Central fibrosis = neuroma
- + Contrast enhancement if solid tumor
- Rim enhancement of benign cystic mass

Hematoma

- History of trauma
- Compression of nerve by mass effect
- Hyperintense on T2WI
- +/- Blooming: Chronic on GRE
  - o Hemosiderin

QUADRILATERAL SPACE SYNDROME

PATHOLOGY

General Features
- General path comments
  - Nerve & vessel damaged/occluded in QSS
  - Distal branch of axillary nerve involved
    - ± Involvement of posterior humeral circumflex artery
- Etiology
  - Nerve +/- artery compressed with resulting denervation/ischemia
  - Compression
    - Proximal humeral and scapular fractures
    - Fibrous bands (posttraumatic)
    - Mass (including teres minor hypertrophy)
  - Axillary nerve innervates teres minor, deltoid muscles and posterolateral cutaneous area of upper arm/shoulder
- Epidemiology
  - Uncommon abnormality
  - > 3% patients presenting with shoulder pain/dysfunction
- Associated abnormalities
  - Inferior labral tears
  - TM, DM muscle denervation changes
  - Anterior instability if labral tear present
    - Bankart lesion
    - Perthes lesion
    - Anterior labroligamentous periosteal sleeve avulsion (ALPSA) lesion
    - Extended superior labrum anterior to posterior (SLAP) lesion (type V)

Gross Pathologic & Surgical Features
- Axillary nerve passes through quadrilateral space with posterior circumflex artery
- Denervation changes within the affected muscles
- Swollen muscle belly - early and subacute phase
- Fatty atrophy = chronic phase
  - Deltoid and teres minor

Microscopic Features
- Enlarged extracellular fluid space = early and subacute (phase)
- Fatty infiltration = chronic
- Myofibril atrophy → become small and angular with early denervation

Staging, Grading or Classification Criteria
- Early, subacute ~ 0-3 months
- Chronic - corresponds to fatty atrophy > 3 months
- Three stages of nerve injury
  - Neurapraxia: Transient episode of motor paralysis with little or no sensory or autonomic dysfunction
    - No disruption of the nerve or its sheath occurs
    - With removal of the compressing force, recovery should be complete
  - Axonotmesis: More severe nerve injury with disruption of the axon and myelin sheath with preservation of connective tissue
    - Motor, sensory, and autonomic paralysis results
    - Degeneration of axon distal to site of injury
    - Regeneration of axon is spontaneous
  - Neurotmesis: Nerve sheath and connective tissue elements are torn
    - Regeneration does not occur

CLINICAL ISSUES

Presentation
- Most common signs/symptoms
  - Paresthesias, muscle weakness and tenderness on palpation of the quadrilateral space
    - Paresthesias involve lateral shoulder and upper posterior arm
- Clinical profile
  - Athletes
  - Pain increased by abduction & external rotation of arm

Demographics
- Age: 22 to 35 years
- Gender: M > F

Natural History & Prognosis
- Resolution with time in case of posttraumatic neurapraxia
- Progress if secondary to compressing mass

Treatment
- Conservative in case of neurapraxia
- Relief of compression due to mass or fibrous bands may be necessary
- Surgical extirpation

DIAGNOSTIC CHECKLIST

Consider
- Posttraumatic axillary neurapraxia if patient presents with TM and DM increased signal after anterior dislocation on FS PD FSE or STIR

Image Interpretation Pearls
- FS PD FSE show demonstrates in muscle in acute and subacute phases, T1WI demonstrates fatty atrophy

SELECTED REFERENCES

1. DeLee J et al: Orthopaedic sports medicine. Basic science and injury of muscle, tendon and ligaments. vol 1. 2nd ed. Philadelphia PA, Saunders, 1-66, 2003
2. Sallomi D et al: Muscle denervation patterns in upper limb nerve injuries: MR imaging findings and anatomic basis. AJR 171(3):779-84, 1998
3. Helms CA et al: Acute brachial neuritis (Parsonage-Turner syndrome): MR imaging appearance--report of three cases. Radiology 207(1):255-9, 1998
4. Francel TJ: Quadrilateral space syndrome: Diagnosis and operative decompression technique. Plast Reconstr Surg 87:911-6, 1991
5. Cahill BR et al: Quadrilateral space syndrome. J Hand Surg 65-9, 1983

QUADRILATERAL SPACE SYNDROME

IMAGE GALLERY

Typical

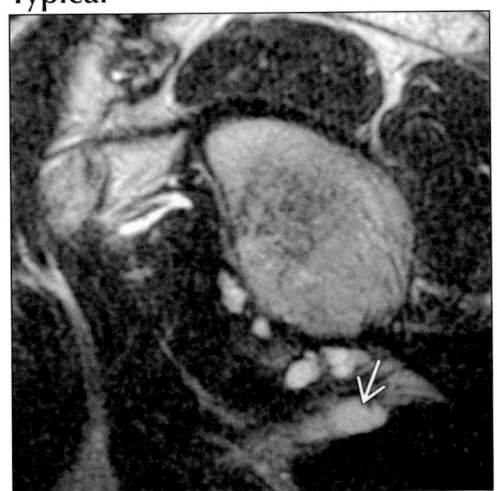
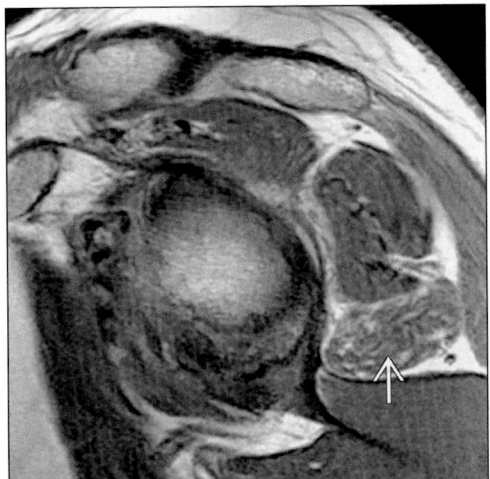

(Left) Sagittal PD FSE MR image in a patient with quadrilateral space syndrome shows an inferiorly dissecting paralabral cyst (arrow) in a professional football player. *(Right)* Sagittal PD FSE MR shows denervation atrophy of the teres minor (arrow). This is a manifestation of quadrilateral space syndrome.

Typical

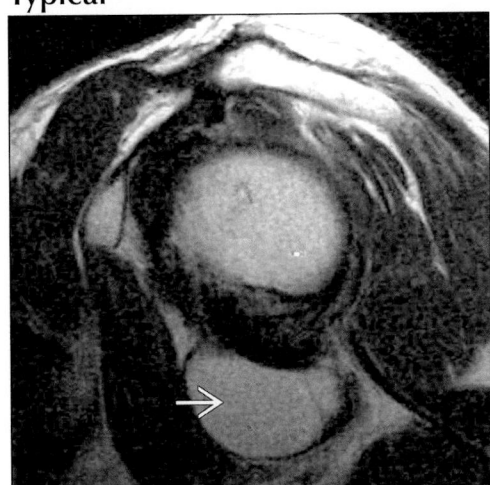
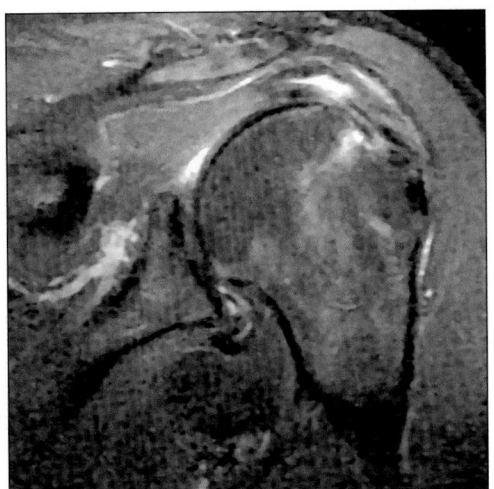

(Left) Sagittal PD FSE shows a large lipoma (arrow) within the quadrilateral space. It is difficult without fat saturation to differentiate between fat and a cyst. *(Right)* Coronal FS PD FSE MR in the same patient shows the mass in the quadrilateral space which represents a lipoma with suppression of fat signal.

Typical

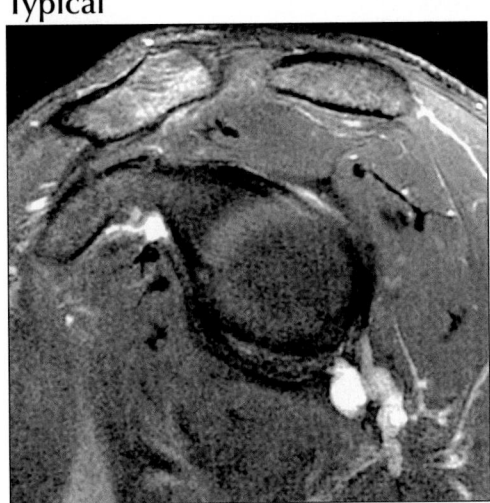
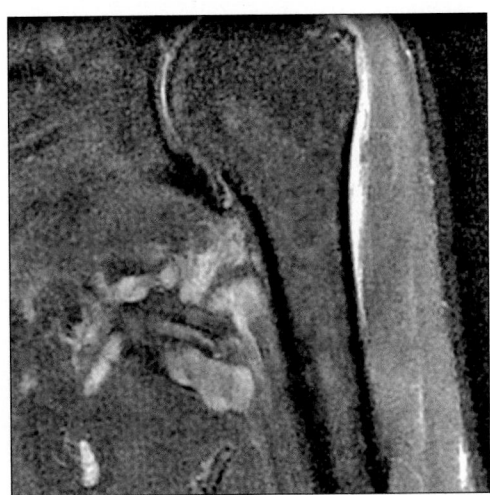

(Left) Sagittal FS PD FSE MR shows an inferiorly dissecting cyst into the quadrilateral space. *(Right)* Coronal STIR MR shows varices within the quadrilateral space as a cause of quadrilateral space syndrome. Deltoid muscle is hyperintense.

SUPRASCAPULAR, SPINOGLENOID NOTCH

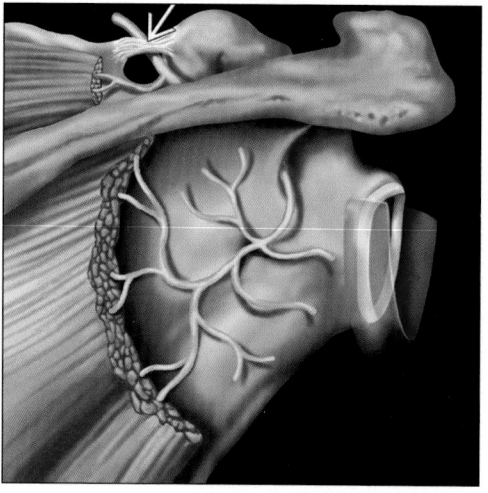

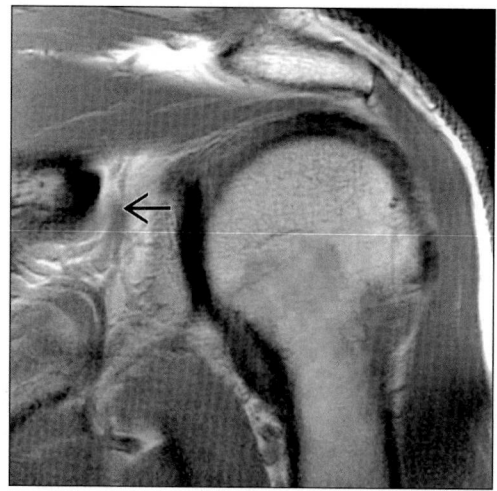

Coronal graphic shows suprascapular nerve extending beneath transverse scapular ligament (arrow) of the suprascapular notch & distributing terminal branches in spinoglenoid notch.

Coronal PD FSE MR shows the suprascapular nerve (arrow) within the suprascapular and spinoglenoid notch.

TERMINOLOGY

Abbreviations and Synonyms
- Suprascapular notch (SSN), spinoglenoid notch (SGN)

Definitions
- Impingement of the suprascapular nerve within the SSN or SGN

IMAGING FINDINGS

General Features
- Best diagnostic clue: Denervation as increased (T2WI) signal (acute/subacute) or atrophy (chronic) of supraspinatus (SS) and/or infraspinatus
- Location
  - SSN is at superior glenoid
  - SGN is at posterior glenoid
  - Suprascapular nerve exits brachial plexus
    - Traverses underneath the transverse scapular ligament to enter the SSN
    - Travels posteriorly/inferiorly to enter the SGN
- Size: Notches 1-3 cms in size
- Morphology: Fibroosseous tunnel at scapular notch and posterior concavity in spinoglenoid notch

Radiographic Findings
- Radiography

  - Subtle widening of the SGN on axillary view
    - Chronic cyst and erosion formation

CT Findings
- NECT
  - Widening of the SGN on axial view
    - Cyst and erosion
    - Coronal reformations
- CT arthrography
  - Labral tear associated with cyst causing denervation
    - Contrast extends through tear
    - Coronal reconstructions
    - Superior labrum anterior-posterior (SLAP) lesion most common

MR Findings
- T1WI
  - Fatty atrophy (increased signal of fat) of affected muscles with chronic denervation
    - Supraspinatus
    - Infraspinatus
  - Labral tear as intermediate signal extending through labrum or base of labrum
    - SLAP lesion most common
    - Posterosuperior labral tear
- T2WI
  - Denervation: High signal of affected muscles
    - +/- Atrophy (hypointense on FS PD FSE)

DDx: Suprascapular, Spinoglenoid Notch

Parsonage-Turner	Infraspinat Tear	Lipoma	Lipoma	Normal Vessels
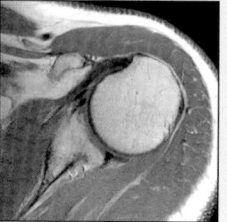	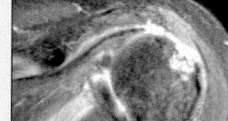	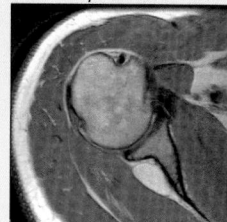	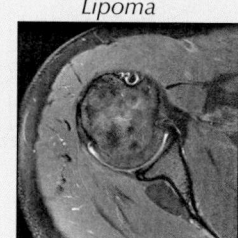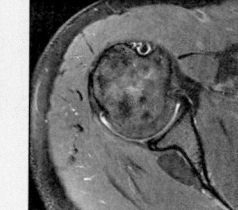	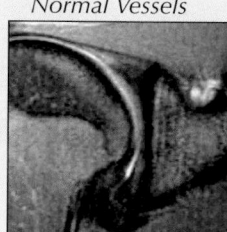
Ax PD FSE MR	Cor FS PD FSE	Ax PD FSE MR	Ax FS PD FSE	Cor FS PD FSE

SUPRASCAPULAR, SPINOGLENOID NOTCH

Key Facts

Imaging Findings
- Best diagnostic clue: Denervation as increased (T2WI) signal (acute/subacute) or atrophy (chronic) of supraspinatus (SS) and/or infraspinatus
- Suprascapular nerve exits brachial plexus
- Traverses underneath the transverse scapular ligament to enter the SSN
- Travels posteriorly/inferiorly to enter the SGN
- Denervation: High signal of affected muscles
- +/- Hyperintense cystic septated mass arising from or adjacent to labrum or capsule

Top Differential Diagnoses
- Mass Compression of Suprascapular Nerve
- Effect of Adjacent Trauma
- Parsonage-Turner Syndrome

- Cervical Spine Disease
- Infraspinatus Tear

Pathology
- Suprascapular nerve originates from brachial plexus (C5-C6)

Clinical Issues
- SSN compression syndrome
- Pain, weakness of SS and IS
- Proprioceptive change
- Mimics rotator cuff tear clinically

Diagnostic Checklist
- Assume paralabral cysts communicate with labral tears

- +/- Hyperintense cystic septated mass arising from or adjacent to labrum or capsule
- Labral tear as linear hyperintensity or avulsion
- FS PD FSE sensitive for showing acute and subacute changes of muscle edema (denervation)
- Intraosseous cyst
  - + Hyperintense bone reactive edema
  - Intraosseous extension of paralabral cyst

Imaging Recommendations
- Best imaging tool: MRI
- Protocol advice
  - FS PD FSE for denervation in acute/subacute phase
  - T1WI demonstrates chronic fatty atrophy

DIFFERENTIAL DIAGNOSIS

Mass Compression of Suprascapular Nerve
- Neoplasm
  - Extension from scapula
- Metastatic disease
- Varices
  - Compression neuropathy
  - Congestive heart failure (CHF)
- Lipoma

Effect of Adjacent Trauma
- Neurapraxia (failure of conduction)
- Callus from adjacent fracture
- +/- Hematoma
- Axonotmesis (disruption axon and myelin sheath)
- Direct neurotmesis (severance of nerve)

Parsonage-Turner Syndrome
- Shoulder girdle muscles
  - Supraspinatus
  - Infraspinatus
  - Deltoid
- +/- Viral prodrome
- Shoulder pain + weakness
- Self limiting

Cervical Spine Disease
- + Radiculitis
- Shoulder pain
- +/- Weakness
- +/- Disc herniation
- +/- Stenosis

Infraspinatus Tear
- Rare in isolation
- +/- Internal impingement
  - Throwing athletes
  - Occupational
  - Posterosuperior labrum tear
  - Posterosuperior cuff (supraspinatus/infraspinatus) partial articular surface tear
  - Posterosuperior humeral head - cystic erosions
- Discontinuous fibers + hyperintense edema/hemorrhage on T2WI

PATHOLOGY

General Features
- General path comments
  - Suprascapular nerve originates from brachial plexus (C5-C6)
  - Location of nerve compression
    - Proximal entrapment at scapular incisura
    - Distal entrapment at spinoglenoid notch
  - Cysts arising from posterosuperior aspect of the joint are "funneled" between the supraspinatus and infraspinatus
    - To SSN and SGN
    - Path of least resistance
- Etiology
  - Sling effect with contact between suprascapular nerve and transverse scapular ligament
  - Proximal entrapment - muscle denervation
    - Supraspinatus
    - Infraspinatus
  - Distal entrapment - muscle denervation
    - Infraspinatus

o Paralabral cysts (suprascapular or spinoglenoid notch)
o Stretch injury to nerve
o Scapular fractures
o Adduction and internal rotation - increased suprascapular nerve tension deep to spinoglenoid ligaments
o Hyperabduction + eccentric contraction of infraspinatus
o Overhead activities
  ▪ Volleyball and tennis
o Soft tissue masses
o Osseous tumors
o Vascular malformations
• Epidemiology
  o Most common cause: Compression by cyst
  o Spinoglenoid ligament in 50-80% of cases
• Associated abnormalities: Erosion of SGN in case of chronic cyst

Gross Pathologic & Surgical Features
• Anatomic fossa that transmits the SSN
• Compression may be by cyst, mass, varix or thickened transverse scapular ligament
• Spinoglenoid ligament (lateral to transverse scapular ligament)
  o Type I - thin fibrous band
  o Type II - distinct ligament
  o Inserts into posterior capsule
  o Tightens with adduction and internal rotation
  o Additional potential site of nerve injury
• Suprascapular notch
  o U-shaped morphology
  o Wide open to enclosed with bone

Microscopic Features
• Nerve undergoes Wallerian degeneration if compressed
• If compressed by cyst: Cyst with wall containing spindle-shaped cells
  o Cyst contains mucoid material
• Fatty infiltration of muscle tissue in chronically denervated muscles

Staging, Grading or Classification Criteria
• Three stages of nerve injury
  o Neurapraxia: Transient episode of motor paralysis with little or no sensory or autonomic dysfunction
    ▪ No disruption of the nerve or its sheath occurs
    ▪ With removal of the compressing force, recovery should be complete
  o Axonotmesis: More severe nerve injury with disruption of the axon and myelin sheath with preservation of connective tissue
    ▪ Motor, sensory, and autonomic paralysis results
    ▪ Degeneration of axon distal to site of injury
    ▪ Regeneration of axon is spontaneous
  o Neurotmesis: Nerve sheath and connective tissue elements are torn
    ▪ Regeneration does not occur

CLINICAL ISSUES

Presentation
• Most common signs/symptoms
  o SSN compression syndrome
    ▪ Pain, weakness of SS and IS
    ▪ Proprioceptive change
    ▪ Mimics rotator cuff tear clinically
• Clinical profile
  o Suprascapular nerve compression syndrome if located posterosuperiorly
  o Instability and/or SLAP lesion (labral tear)
  o Pain and weakness of supraspinatus and infraspinatus, proprioceptive changes (suprascapular denervation)
  o EMG
    ▪ Nerve conduction studies from Erb's point to supraspinatus

Demographics
• Age
  o Adult with gradual onset of SSN denervation syndrome
  o Occasionally teen athlete with labral tear
• Gender: M > F

Natural History & Prognosis
• Nerve compression may lead to irreversible damage and requires drainage to relieve compression
  o Address labral damage to prevent recurrence if caused by cyst
  o Treat neoplasm, metastatic lesion

Treatment
• Relief of mass compression

DIAGNOSTIC CHECKLIST

Consider
• Identify mass in SSN +/- SGN if increased signal in supraspinatus and infraspinatus muscle
• Assume paralabral cysts communicate with labral tears

SELECTED REFERENCES
1. DeLee J et al: Orthopaedic sports medicine. vol 1. 2nd ed. Philadelphia PA, Saunders, 1154-60, 2003
2. Tirman PF et al: A practical approach to imaging of the shoulder with emphasis on MR imaging. Orthop Clin North Am 28(4):483-515, 1997
3. Steiner E et al: Ganglia and cysts around joints. Radiol Clin North Am 34(2):395-425, 1996
4. Tirman PF et al: Association of glenoid labral cysts with labral tears and glenohumeral instability: Radiologic findings and clinical significance. Radiology 190(3):653-8, 1994
5. Fritz RC et al: Suprascapular nerve entrapment: Evaluation with MR imaging. Radiology 182(2):437-44, 1992

SUPRASCAPULAR, SPINOGLENOID NOTCH

IMAGE GALLERY

Typical

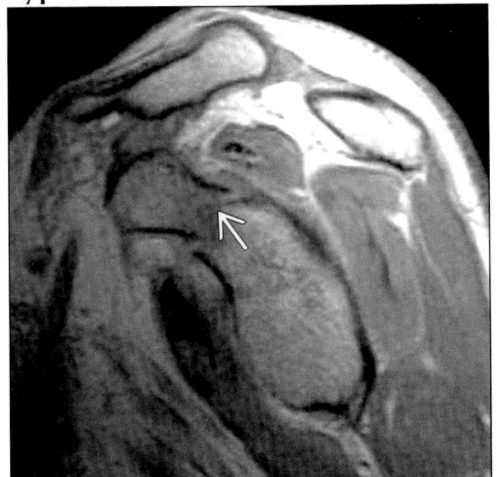 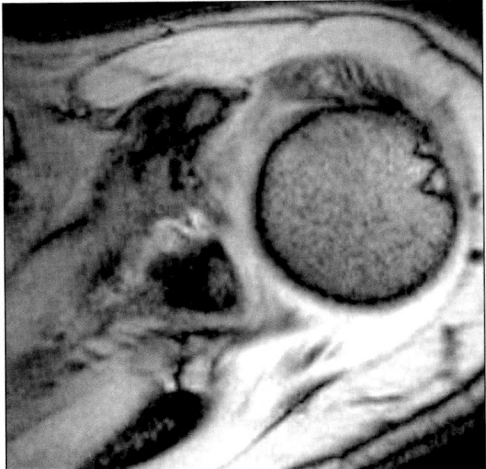

(Left) Sagittal PD FSE MR shows a fracture (arrow) through the base of the coracoid with surrounding callus. Subtle hyperintensity in the supraspinatus and infraspinatus muscles, consistent with suprascapular denervation. *(Right)* Axial T2* GRE MR shows a fracture through the base of the coracoid process and edema within the infraspinatus muscle.

Typical

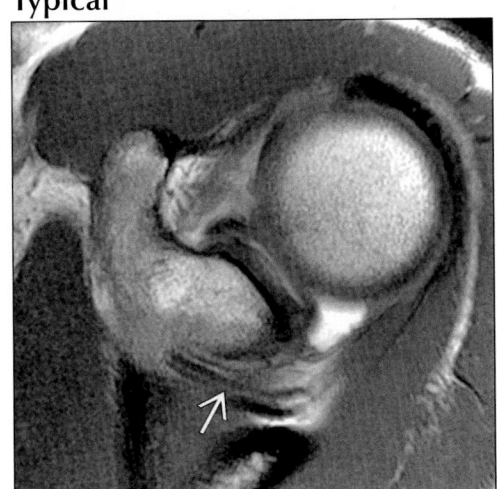 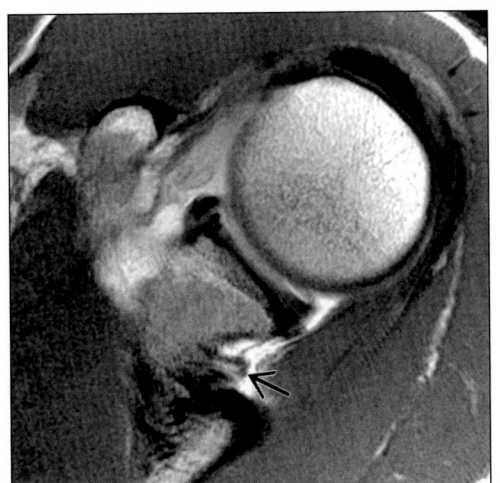

(Left) Axial PD FSE MR shows normal suprascapular neurovascular bundle (arrow) within the suprascapular and spinoglenoid notch. *(Right)* Axial PD FSE MR shows the suprascapular neurovascular bundle (arrow) within the spinoglenoid notch at the posterior aspect of the scapula.

Typical

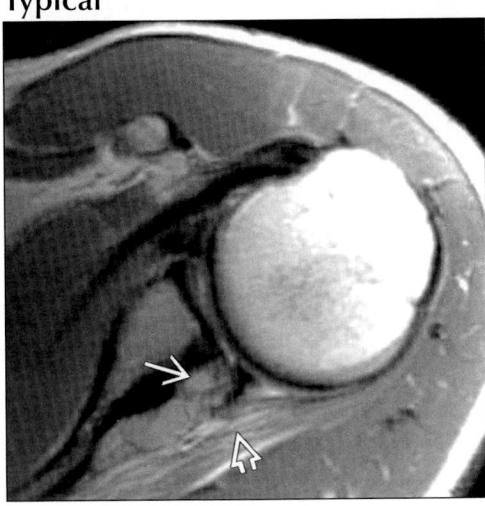 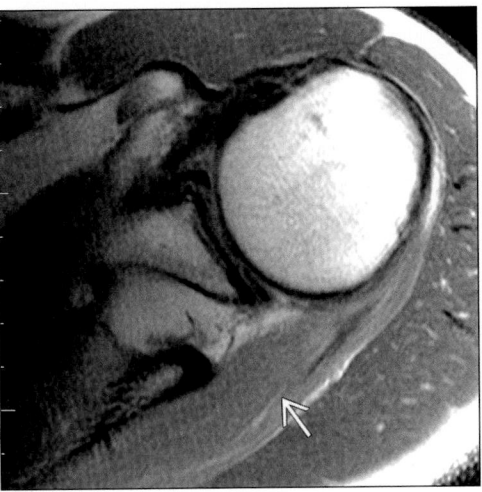

(Left) Axial PD FSE MR shows intraosseous (arrow) extension of a spinoglenoid notch cyst into the posterior glenoid rim. Chronic changes of infraspinatus atrophy (open arrow) are present. *(Right)* Axial PD FSE MR shows a cyst extending from a posterosuperior labral tear into the spinoglenoid notch with compression neuropathy involving the infraspinatus (arrow).

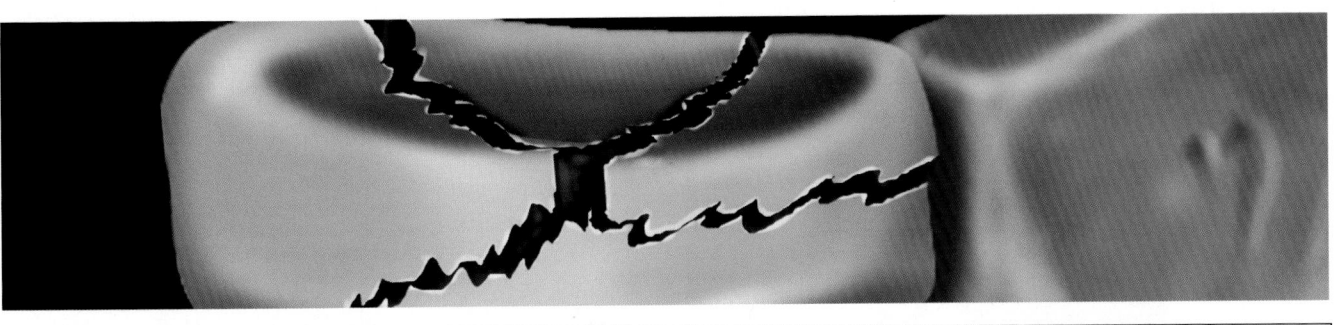

SECTION 2: Elbow

LATERAL EPICONDYLITIS

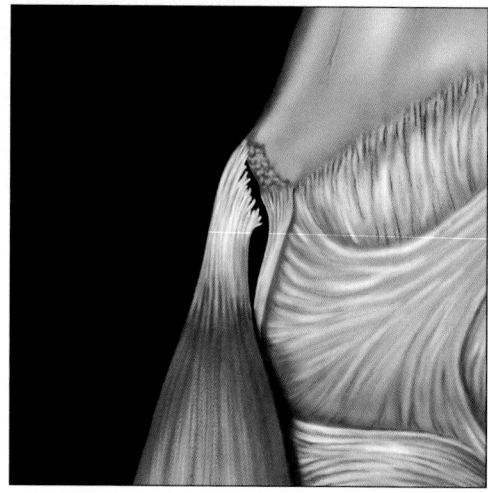

Coronal graphic shows degeneration and extensive partial tearing of the common extensor tendon origin from the lateral epicondyle. The ECRB is affected first.

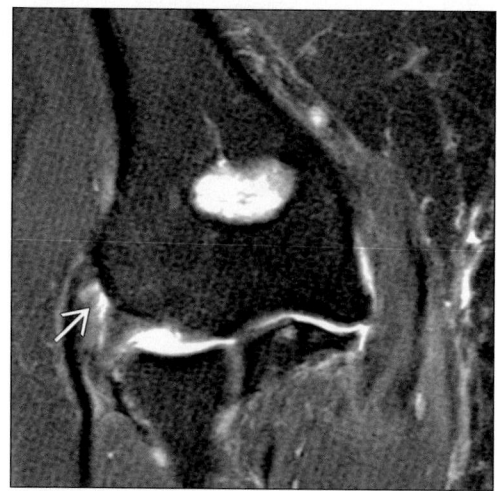

Coronal FS PD FSE MR shows an extensive partial tear of the common extensor tendon origin (arrow).

TERMINOLOGY

Abbreviations and Synonyms
- Tennis elbow, extensor carpi radialis brevis (ECRB) partial avulsion

Definitions
- Chronic microtrauma (overuse) injury of the extensor/tendons originating on the lateral epicondyle

IMAGING FINDINGS

General Features
- Best diagnostic clue: Thickening and increased signal intensity within the common extensor origin from the lateral epicondyle on all pulse sequence
- Location
  - Common extensor tendon origin from the lateral epicondyle
    - Extensor carpi radialis brevis (ECRB) usually affected first
  - +/- Degeneration, tear of the underlying lateral collateral ligamentous complex (especially the lateral ulnar collateral ligament)
- Size: Varies from tendon being subjectively thickened to small interstitial partial tear to complete avulsion including tear of underlying collateral ligaments

- Morphology
  - Varies from thickening and heterogenous appearance = tendinosis
  - +/- Discrete tear
  - +/- Large irregular tear

Radiographic Findings
- Radiography
  - +/- Lateral soft tissue swelling
  - +/- Fractures/bone trabecular injury if posterior dislocation trauma
    - Capitellum
    - Radial head/neck
    - Coronoid process
  - +/- Osteoarthritis (OA) if old trauma
    - Loose bodies
    - Osteophytes
    - Subchondral sclerosis
    - Subchondral cysts

CT Findings
- NECT
  - +/- Fractures/bone trabecular injury if posterior dislocation trauma
  - +/- OA if chronic trauma
- CT arthrography
  - Posterior capsular rupture with extravasation of contrast if post trauma

DDx: Lateral Epicondylitis

LUCL Tear	Radial Head Fx	Valgus Injury	Post Dislocation	Post Dislocation

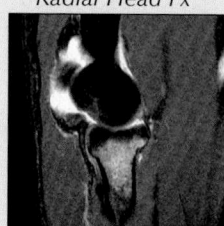 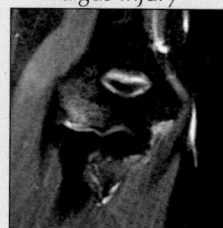 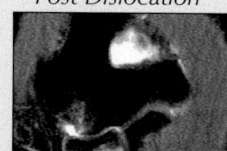 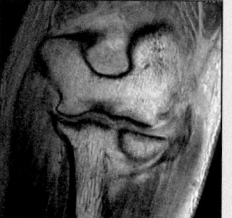

Cor PD FSE MR	Sag FS PD FSE	Cor STIR MR	Cor FS PD FSE	Cor PD FSE MR

LATERAL EPICONDYLITIS

Key Facts

Terminology
- Tennis elbow, extensor carpi radialis brevis (ECRB) partial avulsion

Imaging Findings
- Best diagnostic clue: Thickening and increased signal intensity within the common extensor origin from the lateral epicondyle on all pulse sequence

Top Differential Diagnoses
- Trauma and Fibrosis of the Radiohumeral Meniscus Synovial Fringe
- Radial Head/Neck Fracture
- Radial Neuropathy
- Capitellum Fracture
- Posterior Dislocation

Pathology
- Degeneration of the common extensor tendon secondary to chronic varus stress overload
- The ECRB muscle lies deep to the extensor carpi radialis longus muscle and superficial to the joint capsule
- Up to 50% of tennis players

Clinical Issues
- Adult patient with lateral elbow pain
- 90% of patients respond to conservative measures

Diagnostic Checklist
- Associated findings if posttraumatic tendon tear
- Coronal FS PD FSE or STIR to visualize common extensor origin

---

- o Through disrupted lateral ulnar collateral ligament/radial collateral ligament (RCL) if ligaments torn

MR Findings
- T1WI
  - o Increased signal intensity within the common extensor tendon origin at the lateral epicondyle
  - o Tendon often thickened
  - o Intermediate signal lateral ulnar collateral ligament (LUCL) in advanced cases = sprains +/- tear
  - o Decreased signal intensity loose bodies may be present
  - o Decreased signal intensity edema/fracture lines post trauma
- T2WI
  - o Increased signal/thickening of common extensor tendon with tendinosis
  - o Increased signal intensity within the tendon - partial tear to complete tears
    - ▪ Variable disruption of fibers
    - ▪ ECRB macroscopic tear, +/- tear of extensor digitorum communis
  - o Increase signal intensity within the common extensor muscle belly in case of muscle strain
  - o Strains and tears of the LUCL in advanced cases (increased signal, +/- discontinuous fibers)
  - o Osteochondral injuries
    - ▪ Increased signal intensity bone marrow with fracture/trabecular injury: Posterior dislocation
    - ▪ Capitellum
    - ▪ Humeral trochlea
    - ▪ Coronoid process
    - ▪ Radial head/neck
- PD/Intermediate
  - o Spatial resolution excellent
  - o Synovitis seen as intermediate to increased signal thickened synovium
- STIR
  - o Improved contrast resolution
  - o Lower spatial resolution
  - o Necessary at low field

Imaging Recommendations
- Best imaging tool: MRI
- Protocol advice: FS PD FSE or STIR coronal and axial images

DIFFERENTIAL DIAGNOSIS

Trauma and Fibrosis of the Radiohumeral Meniscus Synovial Fringe
- MRI can define the normal tendon/synovial fringe
- = Radiocapitellar meniscus
  - o Not true fibrocartilaginous meniscus
- +/- Inflammation, thickening
- Posterolateral joint

Radial Head/Neck Fracture
- Acute traumatic injury with positive X-rays/MRI
- +/- Posterior dislocation
- +/- Coronoid process fracture/other fractures
- Impaction injury due to axial overloading in a fall onto the outstretched arm
- Radial head injuries - rare in children
  - o Occur in the radial neck
- Most common elbow fracture in adults

Radial Neuropathy
- Tenderness located over the lateral epicondyle with epicondylitis
- Pain over arcade of Frohse/supinator muscle (upper border)
  - o Symptoms of radial tunnel syndrome
- Difficulty with writing
- +/- Humeral fracture
- Forearm pain common

Capitellum Fracture
- Shear injury due to transmitted axial overload from radial head in fall on outstretched arm
- Rare
  - o 6% of elbow fractures
  - o Rare in children < 10 years
- Coronal defect with variable anterior displacement

LATERAL EPICONDYLITIS

- Fracture occurs in coronal plane and is identified on sagittal images

Posterior Dislocation
- Fall on outstretched hand (FOOSH) injury
- +/- Capitellar fx
- Lateral ligamentous disruptions
  - LUCL
- +/- Common extensor tendon tear
- +/- Coronoid fx
- Sudden posterior force
- Osteoarthritis as a complication

PATHOLOGY

General Features
- General path comments
  - Relevant anatomy
    - Lateral epicondyle - orgin for extensor carpi radialis brevis, extensor digitorum communis, extensor carpi ulnaris
    - Posterior interosseous branch of the radial nerve (PIN) - innervation of dorsal compartment of forearm
    - PIN passes deep to the mobile wad (brachioradialis, extensor carpi radialis longus and extensor carpi radialis brevis) in entering dorsal compartment
    - PIN enters supinator (deep to ECRB) passing through arcade of Frohse
  - Degeneration of the common extensor tendon secondary to chronic varus stress overload
  - The ECRB muscle lies deep to the extensor carpi radialis longus muscle and superficial to the joint capsule
- Etiology
  - Overuse syndrome caused by chronic varus stress across the elbow
  - Overuse of wrist extension and/or supination
- Epidemiology
  - Up to 50% of tennis players
  - 95% of reported cases in general population other than tennis players
- Associated abnormalities
  - Loose bodies
  - Ulnohumeral osteophytes
  - Chondral lesions
  - Synovitis

Gross Pathologic & Surgical Features
- Thickening of the tendon, +/- macroscopic partial tearing (superficial or deep) or through-and-through tearing
  - ECRB tendon with grayish, gelatinous, and friable immature tissue, +/- tear of the LUCL

Microscopic Features
- Angiofibroblastic tendinosis with lack of inflammation
  - Microscopic tearing with formation of reparative tissue
  - Involves extensor carpi radialis brevis tendon

Staging, Grading or Classification Criteria
- Stage I: Reversible inflammatory changes
- Stage II: Nonreversible pathologic changes to origin of the ECRB muscle
- Stage III: Rupture of ECRB muscle origin
- Stage IV: Secondary changes such as fibrosis or calcification

CLINICAL ISSUES

Presentation
- Most common signs/symptoms
  - Adult patient with lateral elbow pain
  - Most common reason for visit to the doctor's office for elbow pain
- Clinical profile
  - Tennis player or other activity resulting in chronic, repeated varus stress
  - Tenderness to palpation over insertion of conjoined tendon just distal to lateral epicondyle vs. tenderness more distally over arcade of Frohse (radial tunnel syndrome)
  - Lateral epicondylitis pain aggravated by resisted wrist extension and passive flexion with full elbow extension

Demographics
- Age: Adults
- Gender: F = M depending on activities (equal among male and female tennis players)

Natural History & Prognosis
- Surgical treatment = 85% of patients with pain relief and return to full activity

Treatment
- Conservative
  - Physical therapy and steroid injection with decrease in physical activity
    - 90% of patients respond to conservative measures
- Surgical
  - Unhealthy amorphous tissue excised
  - Tendon repair
  - Tendon release

DIAGNOSTIC CHECKLIST

Consider
- Associated findings if posttraumatic tendon tear
  - Esp. posterior dislocation

Image Interpretation Pearls
- Coronal FS PD FSE or STIR to visualize common extensor origin
- Evaluate underlying ligaments

SELECTED REFERENCES

1. Miller M et al: Elbow arthroscopy. Surgical atlas of sports medicine. Philadelphia PA, Saunders, 53:375-85, 2003
2. Ciccotti MG et al: Epicondylitis in the athlete. Clin Sports Med 20(1):77-93, 2001

IMAGE GALLERY

Typical

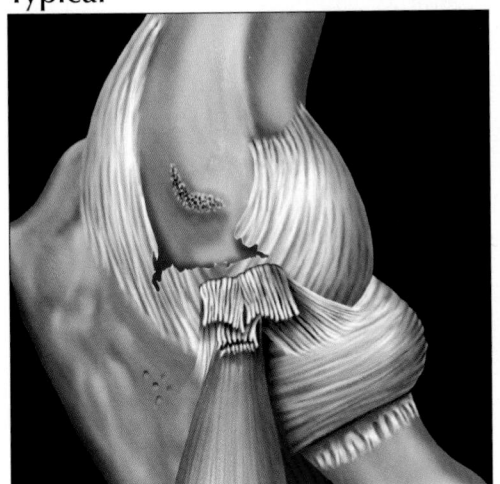 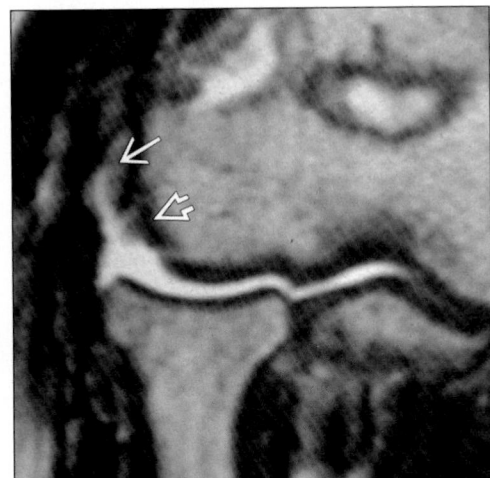

(Left) Sagittal graphic shows a complete tear of the common extensor tendon origin and the underlying lateral ulnar collateral ligament from the lateral epicondyle. *(Right)* Coronal T2 FSE MR shows a tear of the origin of the lateral ulnar collateral ligament (open arrow) with an extensively partially torn common extensor tendon origin (arrow).

Typical

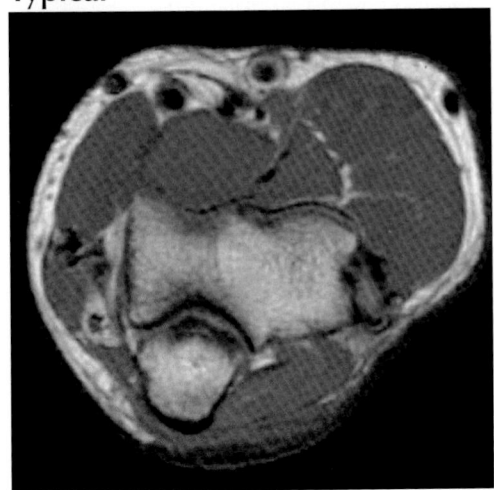 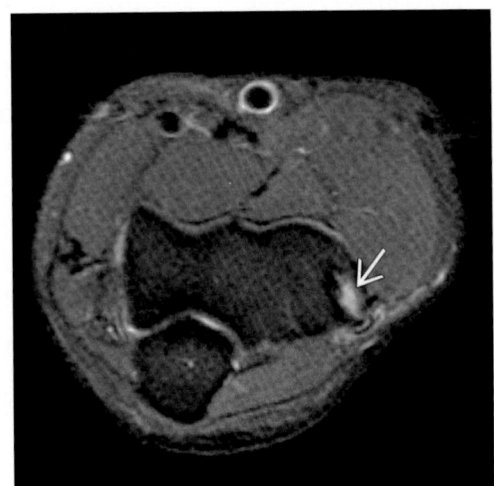

(Left) Axial PD FSE MR shows extensive partial tearing (intermediate signal) of the common extensor tendon origin from the lateral epicondyle. *(Right)* Axial FS PD FSE MR shows (hyperintense) extensive partial tearing of the common extensor tendon origin from the lateral epicondyle (arrow).

Typical

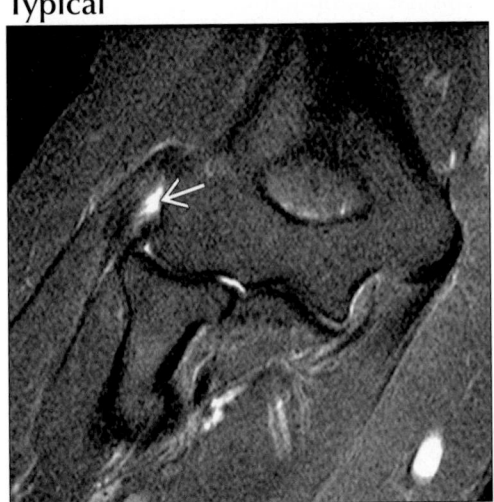 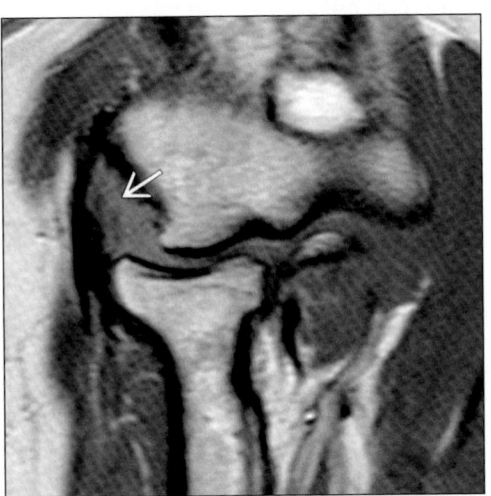

(Left) Coronal FS PD FSE shows partial tearing (arrow) with retraction of the extensor carpi radialis brevis portion of the common extensor tendon origin. The LUCL is intact but degenerated and frayed. *(Right)* Coronal PD FSE MR shows extensive partial tearing (arrow) of the common extensor tendon origin with a complete tear of the origin of the lateral ulnar collateral ligament.

MEDIAL EPICONDYLITIS

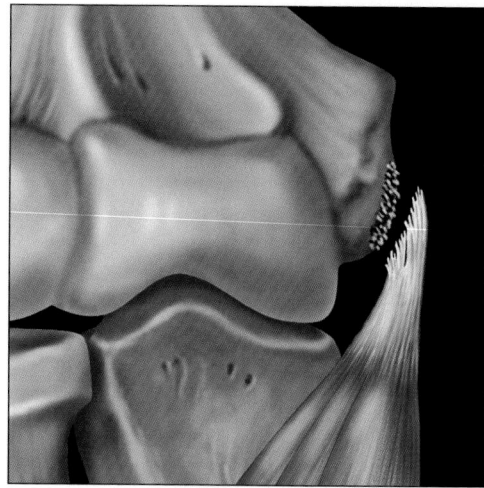

Coronal graphic shows a tear of the flexor pronator origin from the medial epicondyle. Typical patient suffers from acute repetitive valgus stress.

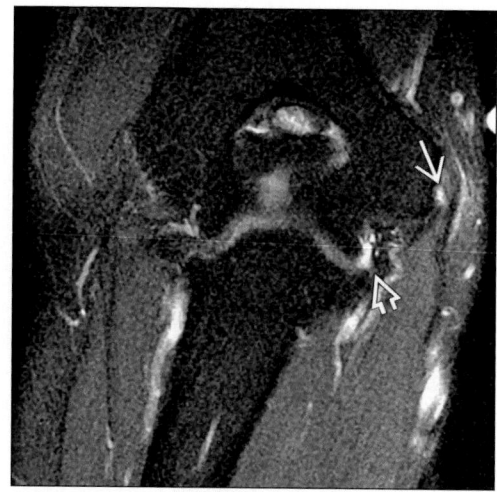

Coronal STIR shows partial tearing of flexor pronator origin medial epicondyle (arrow). Chronic thickening of medial collateral ligament with chronic repetitive valgus stress (open arrow).

TERMINOLOGY

Abbreviations and Synonyms
- Golfer's elbow, pitcher's elbow, medial tennis elbow

Definitions
- Overuse tendinopathy of flexor pronator group (FPG)
- Due to chronic valgus stress
  - Associated with dominant hand in golf
    - Golfer's elbow
  - Associated with throwing sports
    - Baseball
    - Thrower's elbow

IMAGING FINDINGS

General Features
- Best diagnostic clue: Thickening and increased signal intensity within flexor pronator group muscle, tendon at level of medial epicondyle
- Location: FPG origin from the medial epicondyle
- Size
  - Varies: Tendon thickened
  - Small interstitial partial tear
  - Complete avulsion
    - Including sprain/tear of underlying collateral ligaments

- Morphology: Varies from thickening and heterogenous appearance, discrete tear to large irregular tear

Radiographic Findings
- Radiography
  - +/- Medial soft tissue swelling
  - +/- Medial epicondyle avulsion (little leaguer's elbow - related)
  - +/- Sublime tubercle hypertrophy
    - Medial collateral ligament (MCL) chronic valgus stress
  - +/- Traction spur and calcification
  - Lateral impaction
    - Capitellar/radial head fx/osteoarthritis (fx rare)
    - +/- Loose bodies

CT Findings
- CT arthrography
  - +/- Medial capsular disruption
  - +/- MCL tear
    - Acute valgus stress

MR Findings
- T1WI
  - Intermediate signal intensity tendon
  - +/- Reactive hypointense epicondylar edema
  - Partial MCL tear
  - Lateral impaction

DDx: Medial Epicondylitis

Ulnar Neuritis	Coronoid OA	Chron Med Epi Av	Acute Little Leag	Post Disloc
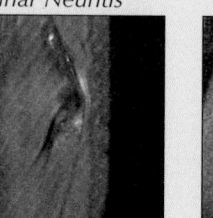	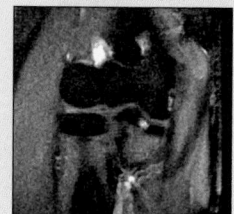	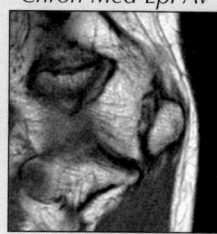	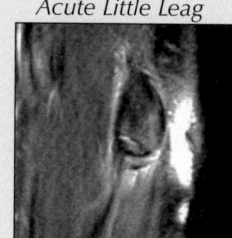	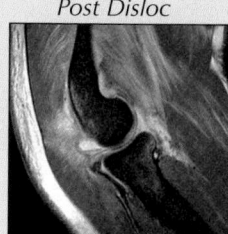
Sag FS PD FSE	Cor STIR MR	Cor PD FSE MR	Sag FS PD FSE	Sag FS PD FSE

MEDIAL EPICONDYLITIS

Key Facts

Terminology
- Overuse tendinopathy of flexor pronator group (FPG)
- Due to chronic valgus stress
- Associated with dominant hand in golf
- Associated with throwing sports

Imaging Findings
- Best diagnostic clue: Thickening and increased signal intensity within flexor pronator group muscle, tendon at level of medial epicondyle
- Fluid signal intensity within the tendon in the case of partial or complete tear
- Lateral compression

Top Differential Diagnoses
- MCL Strain without Tendon Disruption
- Medial Elbow Bone Injury
- Ulnar Neuritis
- Posterior Dislocation

Pathology
- Degeneration of the common flexor tendon secondary to overload caused by chronic valgus stress
- Most common site is interface between pronator teres and flexor carpi radialis origins
- Repeated valgus stress causing tendon degeneration

Clinical Issues
- Athlete participating in throwing sports with onset of medial elbow pain

Diagnostic Checklist
- Coronal FS PD FSE
- Hyperintense flexor pronator origin

- T2WI
  - Thickened increased signal intensity tendon
  - +/- Discontinuous fibers = tear
  - +/- Reactive hyperintense epicondylar edema
  - +/- Hyperintense MCL tear if acute
  - +/- Hyperintense (FS PD FSE & STIR) FPG muscle swelling/edema
  - Lateral impaction
    - Hyperintense capitellum when edematous
    - Hyperintense subchondral cysts (chronic)
    - Hypointense subchondral sclerosis
    - Hypointense loose bodies (osteoarthritis)
  - Ulnar neuritis
    - Hyperintensity and thickening of the nerve usually within the cubital tunnel
    - FS PD FSE or STIR
- PD/Intermediate
  - Synovitis intermediate to hyperintense relative to joint fluid
  - High spatial resolution and signal
- MR arthrography
  - +/- Medial capsular disruption/MCL
- Medial tension overload
  - Increased signal intensity within the common flexor tendon origin at the medial epicondyle, tendon often thickened
- Fluid signal intensity within the tendon in the case of partial or complete tear
- Increase signal intensity within the common flexor muscle belly in case of muscle strain
- Avulsion of medial epicondyle in skeletally immature individuals
- Strains and tears of the MCL
- Lateral compression
  - Osteochondral injuries of the humeral capitellum
    - Chondromalacia and underlying bone marrow edema or cysts
    - Loose bodies

Imaging Recommendations
- Best imaging tool: MRI
- Protocol advice
  - To detect increased signal intensity within the FPG
    - FS PD FSE or STIR images

DIFFERENTIAL DIAGNOSIS

MCL Strain without Tendon Disruption
- Coronal T2 images useful to distinguish between MCL tear and medial epicondylitis
- Discontinuous ligament fibers
- + Surrounding edema
  - Hyperintense on T2WI
- FS PD FSE sensitive
- Coronal, axial images

Medial Elbow Bone Injury
- MRI for diagnosis of bone contusion and fracture
- Acute traumatic event vs. chronic repetitive microtrauma
- Include epicondylar avulsion (Chronic Med Epi Av)
  - Acute or chronic
  - +/- Posttraumatic osteoarthritis (OA)
    - Coronoid/trochlea
- Acute and chronic little league (little leag)
- +/- Comminution
- Acute valgus stress or impact

Ulnar Neuritis
- Associated medial epicondylitis
- +/- Nerve swelling
- Neurapraxia often seen with MCL injury
- +/- Anconeus epitrochlearis
- +/- Cubital tunnel mass
- Hyperintense on T2WI (FS PD FSE)

Posterior Dislocation
- Fall on outstretched arm injury
- Lateral bone injuries
  - Mimics chronic impaction of medial epicondylitis
- +/- Lateral ulnar collateral ligament (LUCL) tear
- +/- Coronoid process fracture

MEDIAL EPICONDYLITIS

PATHOLOGY

General Features
- General path comments
  - Relevant anatomy
    - Medial epicondyle is origin for: Pronator teres, flexor carpi radialis, flexor digitorum superficialis, palmaris longus, flexor carpi ulnaris
    - Soft tissue lesion (medial epicondylitis): Interval between pronator teres & extensor carpi radialis
  - Degeneration of the common flexor tendon secondary to overload caused by chronic valgus stress
  - Bowlers, archers, and weightlifters
  - Little leaguer's elbow a traction apophysitis, requires different treatment
  - Most common site is interface between pronator teres and flexor carpi radialis origins
  - Valgus stress on medial elbow is high during late cocking and acceleration phases of the throw
    - Golfers - valgus stress - from top of the backswing to just before ball impact
- Etiology
  - Repeated valgus stress causing tendon degeneration
  - Early acceleration phase of throwing
  - Dominant elbow of a golfer
  - Tennis players who hit forehand with heavy topspin are at risk
- Epidemiology
  - 10-20% of reported epicondylitis
  - Less common than lateral epicondylitis
    - 10 to 20 times less frequent

Gross Pathologic & Surgical Features
- Thickening of the tendon
- +/- Macroscopic partial tearing of flexor pronator origin
- +/- Macroscopic through-and-through tearing
- Avulsed epicondyle in the case of some children
- +/- Tear of the medial collateral ligament

Microscopic Features
- Microscopic tendon degeneration
- Partial or complete tear
- Injury surrounded by hemorrhage and inflammation

CLINICAL ISSUES

Presentation
- Most common signs/symptoms
  - Athlete participating in throwing sports with onset of medial elbow pain
  - +/- Acute traumatic event
- Clinical profile
  - Overuse syndrome found in athletes participating in throwing sports
  - Tenderness (point tenderness) distal & anterior to medial epicondyle
    - Flexor carpi radialis
    - Pronator teres origin
  - Pain with resisted wrist flexion & forearm pronation with elbow extended
  - +/- Associated ulnar neuropathy
  - Clinical diagnosis confused with ulnar neuropathy or MCL instability
  - Limitation of elbow extension in severe cases
  - In children the injury is often to the medial epicondyle itself manifesting as a stress fracture or avulsion of the epicondyle

Demographics
- Age: 30 to 50 years old
- Gender
  - M = F
  - Most common in throwing athletes

Natural History & Prognosis
- Duration of symptoms is related to length of time prior to receiving treatment
- Athletes who delay treatment tend to have a slower recovery course

Treatment
- Conservative
  - Physical therapy and steroid injection with decrease in physical activity
- Surgical
  - Release of the common flexor origin and extirpation of pathologic surrounding tissue
  - Tendon repair
  - Ulnar neuritis + common flexor tendinosis
    - Transposition or decompression of ulnar nerve

DIAGNOSTIC CHECKLIST

Consider
- Chronic repetitive valgus stress on acute valgus trauma
  - Golf, baseball

Image Interpretation Pearls
- Coronal FS PD FSE
- Hyperintense flexor pronator origin

SELECTED REFERENCES

1. Miller MD et al: Surgical atlas of sports medicine. Philadelphia PA, Saunders, 375-442, 2003
2. Fitzgerald RH Jr. et al: Orthopaedics. St. Louis MO, Mosby, 1223-1331, 2002
3. Chen FS et al: Medial elbow problems in the overhead-throwing athlete. J Am Acad Orthop Surg. 9(2):99-113, 2001
4. Fritz RC: MR imaging of sports injuries of the elbow. Magn Reson Imaging Clin N Am 7(1):51-72, 1999
5. Ciccotti MG: Epicondylitis in the athlete. Instr Course Lect 48:375-81, 1999
6. Nirschl RP: Prevention and treatment of elbow and shoulder injuries in the tennis player. Clin Sports Med 7(2):289-308, 1998
7. Plancher KD et al: Medial and lateral epicondylitis in the athlete. Clin Sports Med 15(2):283-305, 1996
8. Hannah GA et al: The elbow in athletics. Sports Medicine Secrets. Philadelphia PA, Hanley & Belfus, 249-55, 1994

MEDIAL EPICONDYLITIS

IMAGE GALLERY

Typical

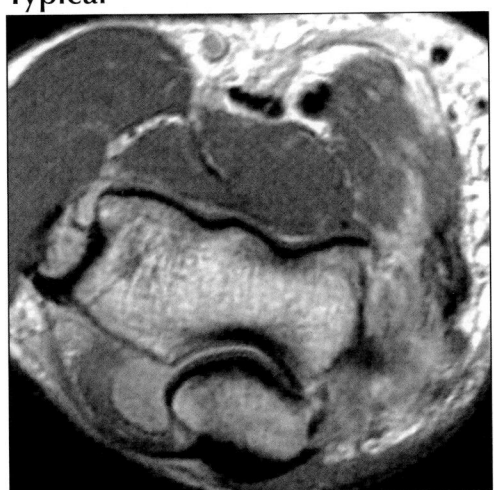
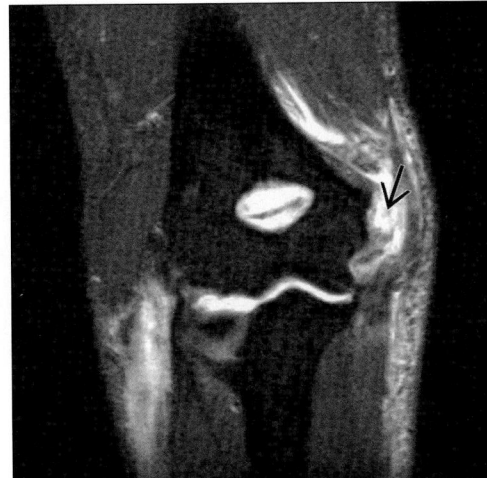

(Left) Axial PD FSE MR shows an acute valgus injury in a patient with an acute "medial joint blow out". This represents acute post-traumatic medial epicondylitis. *(Right)* Coronal STIR MR shows hyperintensity in an acute valgus injury with medial blow out of the conjoined tendon (arrow).

Variant

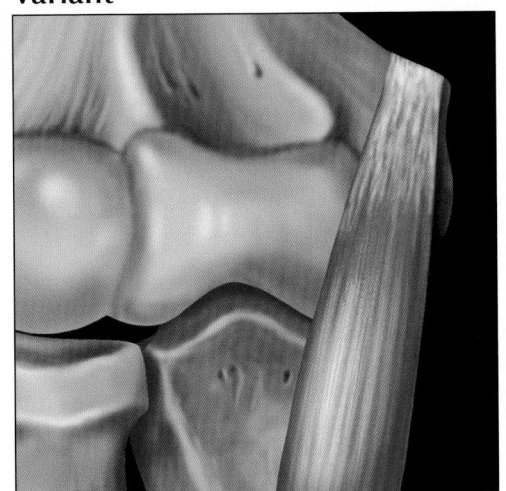
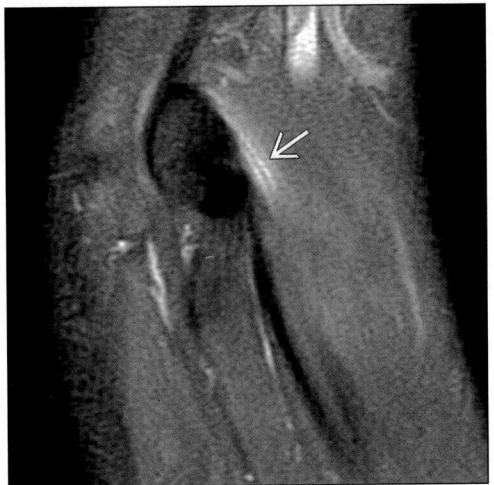

(Left) Coronal graphic shows inflammatory changes in the pronator teres humeral head origin which can be seen with an acute strain causing medial pain. *(Right)* Sagittal FS PD FSE MR shows an acute strain of the humeral head of the pronator teres with increased signal intensity (arrow) in a patient with medial epicondylar pain.

Typical

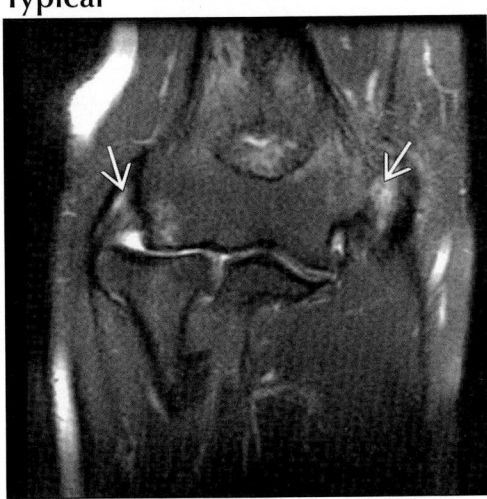
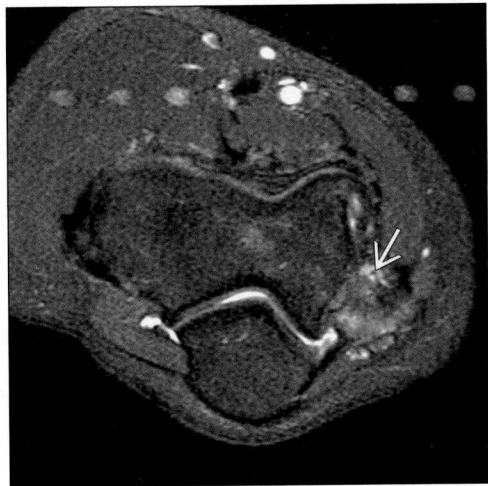

(Left) Coronal FS PD FSE MR shows both medial and lateral epicondylitis with partial tearing of both tendon origins (arrows). *(Right)* Axial FS PD FSE MR shows medial epicondylitis with tearing and thickening of the flexor pronator origin (arrow). Note the intact (hypointense) posterior band of the medial collateral ligament.

BICEPS TENDON RUPTURE

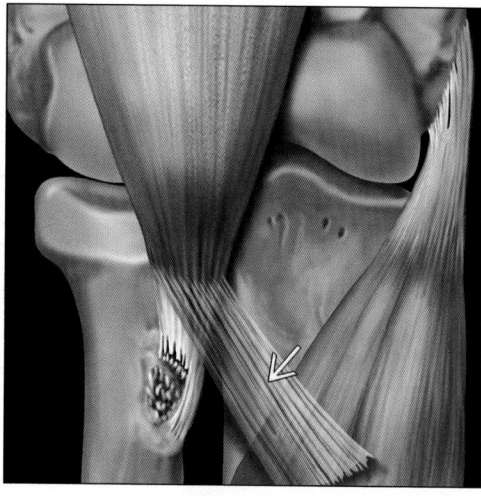

Coronal graphic shows a rupture of the biceps tendon from the radial tuberosity. Note the lacertus fibrosus (arrow) preventing retraction of the tendon.

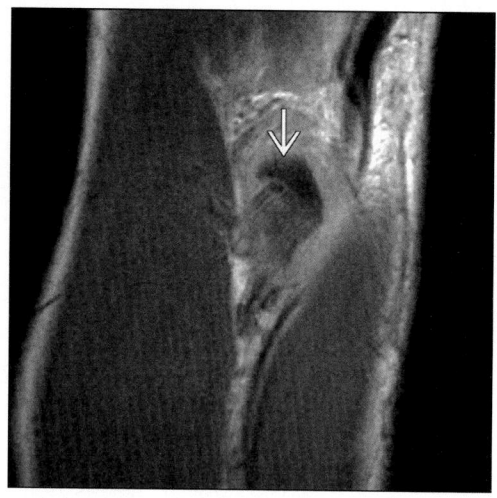

Coronal PD FSE MR ruptured segment of distal biceps tendon (arrow). Fibers of lacertus are still intact. Linear decreased signal intensity structure to right represents brachial vein.

TERMINOLOGY

Abbreviations and Synonyms
- Distal biceps avulsion, distal biceps tendon (DBT) rupture

Definitions
- Rupture of distal biceps tendon DBT from its insertion on the radial tuberosity

IMAGING FINDINGS

General Features
- Best diagnostic clue
  - Complete disruption of DBT from the radial tuberosity
  - +/- Retraction
  - Discontinuous decreased signal intensity tendon on all imaging sequences
- Location: Distal biceps tendon insertion on the radius represents site of rupture
- Size: Small, partial to complete tear, +/- large gap with retraction
- Morphology: Tendon thickened and retracted

Radiographic Findings
- Radiography
  - +/- Hypertrophy of the radial tuberosity

- +/- Antecubital swelling

CT Findings
- NECT
  - +/- Hypertrophy of radial tuberosity associated with chronic tendinosis
  - +/- Antecubital density = soft tissue swelling
  - Sagittal reconstruction for measuring tear gap

MR Findings
- T1WI
  - Decreased signal intensity fluid surrounds tendon
  - Hypointense tendon thickened and retracted
  - Distal tendon end frayed, hyperintense due to preexisting degeneration
  - +/- Hypertrophy of the radial tuberosity
  - +/- Hyperintense common extensor tendon origin
    - Lateral epicondylitis association
- T2WI
  - Increased signal intensity fluid surrounds the torn tendon
  - +/- Retraction of torn tendon
  - Fluid filled bicipital bursa (hyperintense)
  - Discontinuous decreased signal intensity tendon = tear
  - FS PD FSE sensitive to edema
  - +/- Hyperintense common extensor tendon origin
    - Lateral epicondylitis
    - +/- Lateral collateral ligament damage

DDx: Biceps Tendon Rupture

Radial Head Fx	Radial Neck Fx	Bursitis	Normal	Lipoma
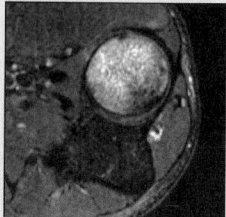	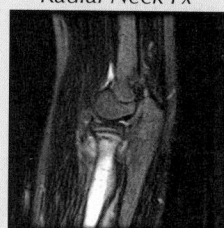	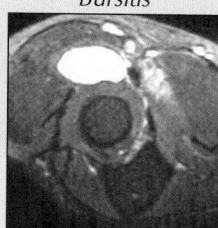	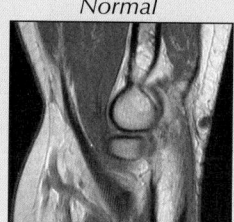	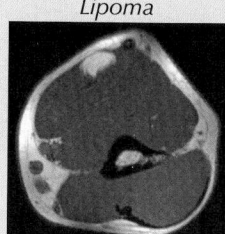
Ax FS PD FSE MR	Sag FS PD FSE	Ax FS PD FSE MR	Sag PD FSE MR	Ax T1WI MR

BICEPS TENDON RUPTURE

Key Facts

Terminology
- Rupture of distal biceps tendon DBT from its insertion on the radial tuberosity

Imaging Findings
- Complete disruption of DBT from the radial tuberosity
- Location: Distal biceps tendon insertion on the radius represents site of rupture
- +/- Hypertrophy of the radial tuberosity
- Increased signal intensity fluid surrounds the torn tendon
- +/- Retraction of torn tendon

Top Differential Diagnoses
- Bicipital Radial Bursitis

Pathology
- Aponeurosis is the lacertus fibrosus
- Eccentric contraction against resistance such as sudden forced extension of a flexed forearm

Clinical Issues
- Forced extension of a flexed forearm
- Biceps muscle belly "balls up" in proximal forearm
- +/- Retraction
- Body builders/weight lifters may present earlier

Diagnostic Checklist
- Measure retraction to help surgeon with planning
- Axial images must include radial tuberosity

- PD/Intermediate
  - Hyperintense hemorrhage adjacent to torn tendon
  - Visualization of lacertus
  - Fluid filled bicipital bursa intermediate to increased signal intensity
  - Discontinuous decreased signal intensity tendon fibers
  - +/- Synovitis
    - PD sensitive to synovial thickening
- STIR
  - Useful at low mid field or when fat suppression is inadequate at high field
  - Fluid filled bicipital bursa hyperintense
- Partial tears with fluid not completely through the tendon - uncommon
- Tendinosis: Increased signal intensity within a variably thickened tendon
- Measure retraction on sagittal images using internal anatomic reference for surgical planning

Ultrasonographic Findings
- Torn tendon edge can be localized and seen surrounded by hypoechoic fluid

Imaging Recommendations
- Best imaging tool: MRI
- Protocol advice: Sagittal FS PD FSE to identify torn tendon +/- retraction

DIFFERENTIAL DIAGNOSIS

Bicipital Radial Bursitis
- Fluid within the bursae of the antecubital fossa
- Intact biceps tendon seen on MRI
- Hyperintense on T2WI
- Cystic mass
- +/- Rim enhancement with I.V. Gadolinium

Brachialis Strain
- Inserts on coronoid process
- Musculocutaneous innervation
- Similar mechanism of injury
- Deep to biceps

Biceps Mass
- Lipoma may mimic myotendinous junction tear
- Fat saturation used for differentiation
  - FS PD FSE
  - STIR
- Malignancy (rare)
- Neuroma

Normal Biceps
- Biceps "spreads out" on sagittal images
  - Mimics tendinosis

PATHOLOGY

General Features
- General path comments
  - History of preexisting pain (chronic tendinosis)
  - May present suddenly without antecedent symptoms
  - Lacertus fibrosus may prevent retraction of completely torn tendon
    - +/- Preserves supination and forearm flexion
  - Aponeurosis is the lacertus fibrosus
    - Extends from the myotendinous junction to the medial deep fascia of the forearm
- Etiology
  - Eccentric contraction against resistance such as sudden forced extension of a flexed forearm
  - Heavy weightlifting
  - Traumatic fall
  - Sports activities
    - Snow boarding
    - Football
- Epidemiology
  - Increasing frequency esp. in 40-60 year olds
    - Typical patient - 50 years old
  - Rupture of proximal biceps tendon 90-97% of all biceps ruptures
    - Involves the long head
  - Most common tendon rupture in elbow region
- Associated abnormalities

BICEPS TENDON RUPTURE

○ +/- Lacertus fibrosus tear
  ▪ Intact tendon preserves some supination
○ +/- Lateral epicondylitis
  ▪ Seen with biceps tears
  ▪ Secondary instability may predispose
  ▪ Possible association of lateral epicondylitis and biceps tear
○ Bicipital bursitis
  ▪ Hemorrhage

Gross Pathologic & Surgical Features
• Disrupted tendon with variable degrees of retraction
• +/- Hypertrophic bicipital radial bursitis
• Tendinosis and macroscopic tear of the tendon

Microscopic Features
• Variable amounts of hemorrhage and inflammatory cells

CLINICAL ISSUES

Presentation
• Most common signs/symptoms
  ○ Forced extension of a flexed forearm
  ○ Dominant arm
• Clinical profile
  ○ Ecchymosis anterior to elbow
  ○ Limited elbow motion
    ▪ Acute inflammation and swelling
  ○ Partial rupture
    ▪ Palpable crepitus with pronation and supination
  ○ Biceps muscle belly "balls up" in proximal forearm
    ▪ "Popeye" sign
    ▪ Absence of biceps tendon with palpation of antecubital fossa
  ○ +/- Retraction
    ▪ Aponeurosis (intact lacertus limits retraction)

Demographics
• Age: Average age = 55 years
• Gender: M > F (rare in female patients)

Natural History & Prognosis
• Body builders/weight lifters may present earlier
• With retraction, tendon will not regain function
• Intact lacertus may preserve supination improving prognosis
• Complete rupture - deformity of the arm

Treatment
• Goal - restore supination and flexion
• Conservative
  ○ Mild strain/partial tear
    ▪ Rest, ice, immobilization, physical therapy, NSAIDs
• Surgical
  ○ Repair of complete tear
    ▪ Biceps tendon inserted to apex of tuberosity to maximize mechanical efficiency
  ○ MRI useful for presurgical planning - measuring gap using landmark reference
  ○ Tenodesis
• Complications (surgical)
  ○ Radial nerve palsy

○ Posterior interosseous nerve palsy
○ Heterotopic ossification
○ Radioulnar synostosis
○ Elbow flexion contracture

DIAGNOSTIC CHECKLIST

Consider
• Bursitis
  ○ Partial tear
  ○ Intact lacertus fibrosis

Image Interpretation Pearls
• Measure retraction to help surgeon with planning
• Axial images must include radial tuberosity

SELECTED REFERENCES

1. Morrison KD et al: Comparing and contrasting methods for tenodesis of the ruptured distal biceps tendon. Hand Clin 18(1):169-78, 2002
2. Toczylowski HM et al: Complete rupture of the distal biceps brachii tendon in female patients. A report of 2 cases. J Shoulder Elbow Surg 11(5):516-8, 2002
3. Gifuni P et al: Avulsion of the distal tendon of the biceps brachii. Reattachment to the radial tuberosity via 1-incision technique. Chir Organi Mov 86(1):29-35, 2001
4. Williams BD et al: Partial tears of the distal biceps tendon. MR appearance and associated clinical findings. Skeletal Radiol 30(10):560-4, 2001
5. Belli P et al: Sonographic diagnosis of distal biceps tendon rupture: a prospective study of 25 cases. J Ultrasound Med 20(6):587-95, 2001
6. Bell RH et al: Repair of distal biceps brachii tendon ruptures. J Shoulder Elbow Surg 9(3):223-6, 2000
7. Fritz RC: MR imaging of sports injuries of the elbow. Magn Reson Imaging Clin N Am 7(1):51-72, 1999
8. Le Huec JC et al: Distal rupture of the tendon of biceps brachii. Evaluation by MRI and the results of repair. J Bone Joint Surg Br 78(5):767-70, 1996

IMAGE GALLERY

Typical

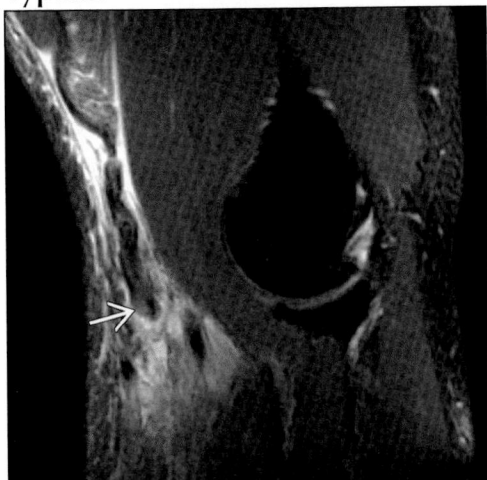 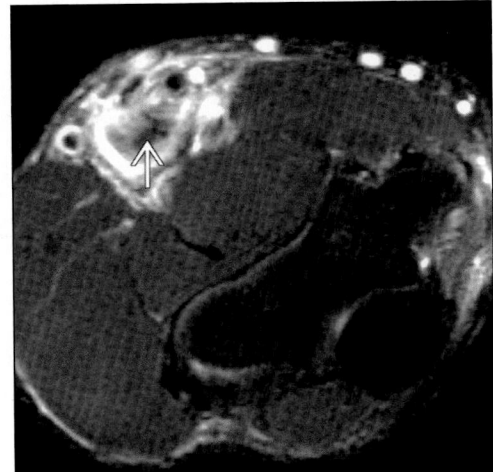

(Left) Sagittal FS PD FSE shows torn retracted distal biceps tendon (arrow) surrounded by hemorrhage. *(Right)* Axial FS PD FSE MR shows torn proximally retracted tendon (arrow) associated with hyperintense hemorrhage.

Typical

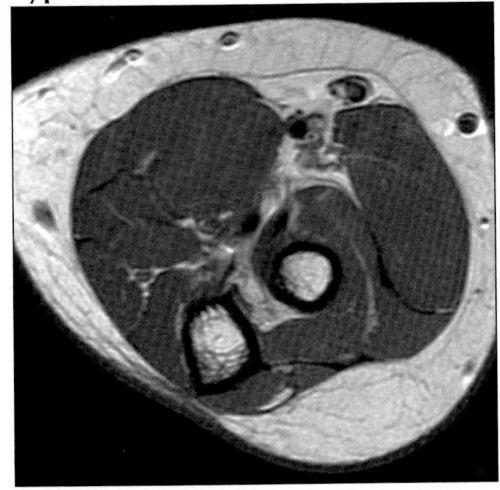 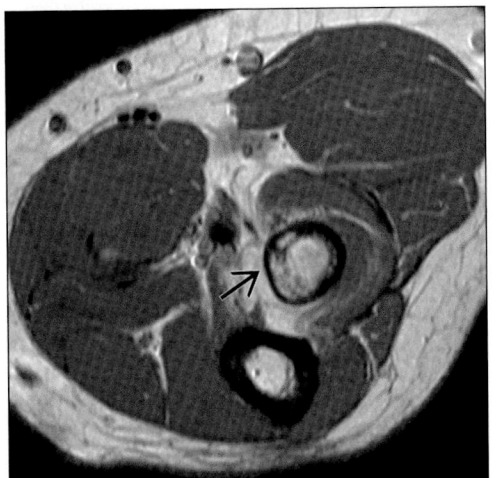

(Left) Axial PD FSE MR Shows a normal biceps insertion onto the radial tuberosity. *(Right)* Axial PD FSE MR shows a chronic biceps insertional rupture (arrow) with partial atrophy of the supinator muscle.

Typical

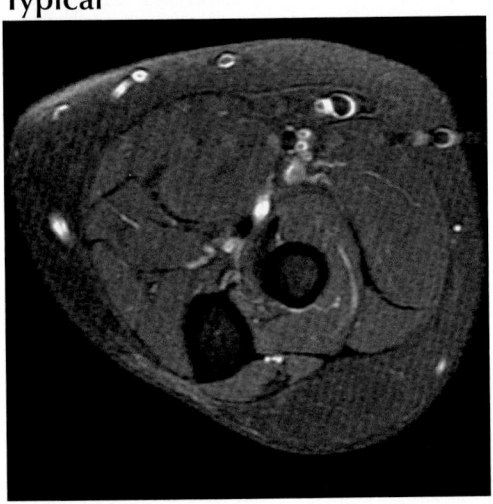 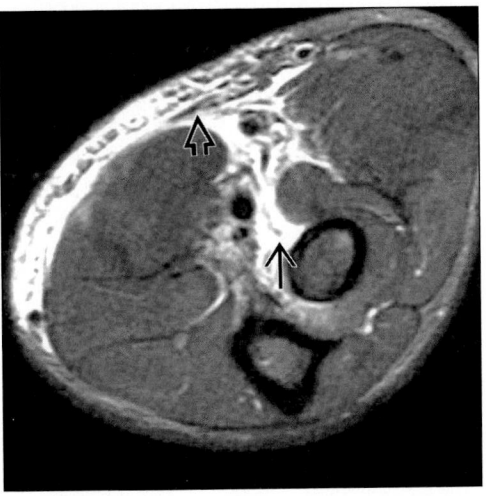

(Left) Axial FS PD FSE MR shows a normal insertion of the biceps tendons. Note the absence of edema. *(Right)* Axial T2 FSE MR shows an acute distal biceps rupture with hyperintense edema (arrow). Note the hemorrhage coursing along the lacertus fibrosus (open arrow) which is ruptured.

TRICEPS TENDON RUPTURE

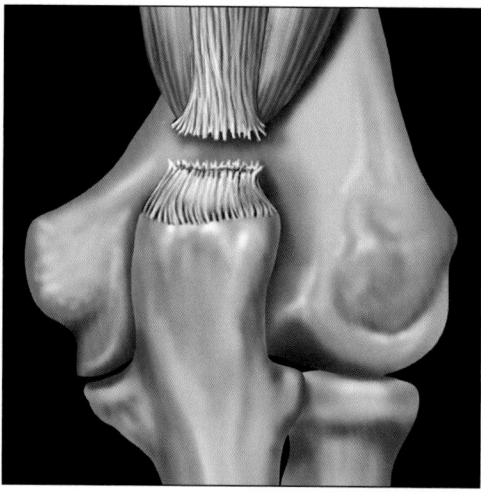

Coronal graphic shows a transverse tear through the distal aspect of the triceps tendon.

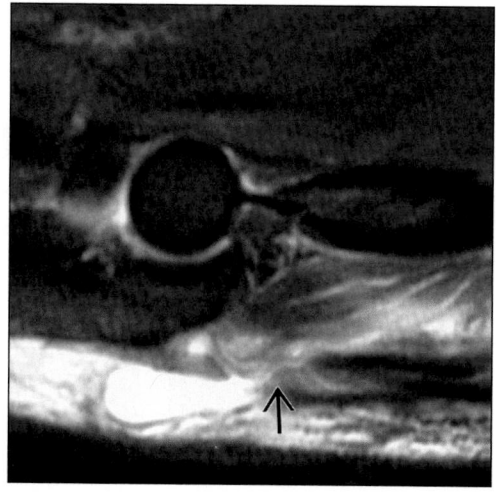

Sagittal FS PD FSE MR shows a complete tear of the distal aspect of the triceps tendon (arrow) in a patient who suffered direct trauma to an extended elbow.

TERMINOLOGY

Abbreviations and Synonyms
- Triceps rupture

Definitions
- Rupture of triceps tendon
- From the insertion site on the olecranon

IMAGING FINDINGS

General Features
- Best diagnostic clue
  - A tear or gap in the triceps tendon which can become filled with
    - Hemorrhage
    - Granulation tissue
- Location
  - Affects the distal portion of the triceps tendon
  - Mid tendon ruptures uncommon
  - Myotendinous ruptures uncommon (direct trauma)
- Size: Tear may vary from millimeter range to large (several centimeters)
- Morphology: Tear may vary from partial disruption to complete disruption with irregular gap

Radiographic Findings
- Radiography

  - Lateral radiograph - small avulsion of olecranon
  - Flecks of osseous tissue < 20% of patients
  - +/- Soft tissue swelling
    - Olecranon bursitis
  - +/- Olecranon destructive changes in late osteomyelitis

CT Findings
- NECT
  - +/- Olecranon destructive changes (osteomyelitis)
  - +/- Soft tissue swelling (bursitis)
  - +/- Small avulsion from olecranon
  - +/- Olecranon commonly fractured
    - Partial tears

MR Findings
- T1WI
  - Partial or complete disruption from the olecranon (interrupted fibers)
  - Discontinuous decreased signal intensity tendon
  - +/- Tendon retraction
  - Tendinosis is seen as increased signal intensity within a variably thickened tendon
  - Fluid (decreased) signal intensity gap
  - +/- Hypointense bursal fluid
    - Hemorrhagic bursitis
  - +/- Hypointense soft tissue fluid/edema
- T2WI
  - Increased signal intensity fluid gap in complete tear

DDx: Triceps Tendon Rupture

Olec Stress Fx	Tendon Xanthoma	Tendon Xanthoma	Synovitis	Olecranon Fx
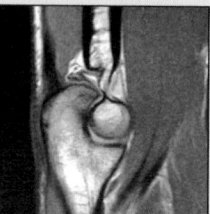	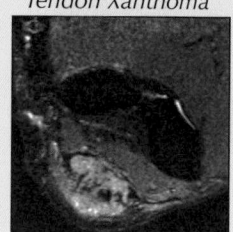	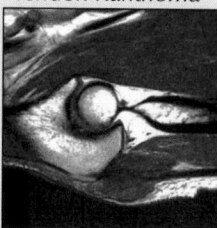	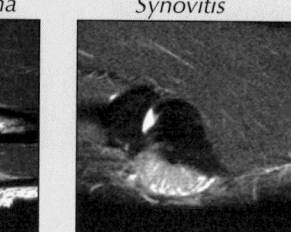	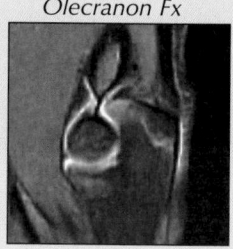
Sag PD FSE MR	Ax STIR MR	Sag PD FSE MR	Sag STIR MR	Sag FS T1C+ MR

TRICEPS TENDON RUPTURE

Key Facts

Terminology
- Rupture of triceps tendon
- From the insertion site on the olecranon

Imaging Findings
- Partial or complete disruption from the olecranon (interrupted fibers)
- +/- Tendon retraction
- Increased signal intensity fluid gap in complete tear

Top Differential Diagnoses
- Olecranon Bursitis
- Triceps Muscle Contusion/Hematoma
- Olecranon Fracture
- Mass
- Posterior Dislocation

Pathology
- Deceleration stress on a contracted triceps muscle
- Eccentric contraction against resistance
- Olecranon hemorrhagic bursitis
- Radial head fractures

Clinical Issues
- Pain at the posterior aspect of the elbow
- Age: Typically a middle-aged man who suffered forced flexion of an extended forearm

Diagnostic Checklist
- Sagittal FS PD FSE for tear detection

- ■ Tendo-osseous attachment - avulsion of insertion +/- osseous fleck/fragment
- ■ Musculotendinous tear less common
- ■ +/- Bursitis
- ■ Visualized on FS PD FSE
- ○ Partial tears - intermediate fluid signal intensity of anterior to posterior surface defect through the tendon
- ○ Tendinosis - intermediate signal intensity within a thickened tendon
- ○ +/- Reactive hyperintense hyperemia in olecranon
- ○ +/- Hyperemic bone trabecular injury/fracture
  - ■ Especially with trauma, partial triceps tear
- ○ +/- Hyperintense hemorrhage within muscle if myotendinous junction tear/muscle tear
  - ■ Direct trauma
- ○ T2* GRE used when fat suppression fails
- PD/Intermediate
  - ○ Excellent spatial resolution
  - ○ Delineate morphology of tendon edges
- STIR
  - ○ Useful at low field
    - ■ Esp. sagittal plane
  - ○ Less spatial resolution
  - ○ When frequency selective fat saturation is not available

Imaging Recommendations
- Best imaging tool: MRI
- Protocol advice: FS PD FSE - tears best seen on sagittal images

DIFFERENTIAL DIAGNOSIS

Olecranon Bursitis
- Adult men
- Dominant arm
- +/- Infection
- +/- Sports activity

Triceps Muscle Contusion/Hematoma
- + History of trauma

- Hyperintense on T2WI
- +/- Hematoma

Olecranon Fracture
- Fall on a flexed, supinated forearm
- Olecranon epiphysis fuses at 16-18 years
- Direct trauma
- Throwing injury (pitchers)
  - ○ +/- Stress response/fx
- Hyperintense edema on T2WI

Mass
- Tendon xanthoma
  - ○ Hyperlipidemia
- Lipoma
- Adjacent neuroma
- Adjacent synovitis
  - ○ In joint distending recess adjacent to triceps

Posterior Dislocation
- Fall on outstretched hand (FOOSH) injury
- +/- Capitellar fx
- Lateral ligamentous disruptions
  - ○ Lateral ulnar collateral ligament (LUCL)
- +/- Common extensor tendon tear
- +/- Coronoid fx
- Lateral, posterior pain

PATHOLOGY

General Features
- General path comments: Previous olecranon bursectomy - predisposing
- Etiology
  - ○ Deceleration stress on a contracted triceps muscle
  - ○ Eccentric contraction against resistance
    - ■ Sudden forced flexion of an extended forearm
    - ■ Direct trauma onto the tendon with muscle contracted and forearm extended
  - ○ Motorcycle accidents
  - ○ Football/soccer/rugby trauma
  - ○ Systemic disease process
    - ■ Hyperparathyroidism

- Steroid use of lupus erythematosus
- Epidemiology: Uncommon, < 1% of tendon tears at the elbow
- Associated abnormalities
  - Olecranon hemorrhagic bursitis
  - Radial head fractures

Gross Pathologic & Surgical Features
- Thickened indurated tendon edges
- Disruption of tendon
  - Variable retraction
- An intratendinous bursa +/- involved with tears of the triceps tendon

Microscopic Features
- Preexisting collagen degeneration without influx of inflammatory cells
- "Tendinosis" is preferred term over tendinitis
- Fatty infiltration of muscle tissue in chronically torn tendons
- Tendinosis and macroscopic tear of the tendon
- Variable amounts of hemorrhage and inflammatory cells

Staging, Grading or Classification Criteria
- Grade I - mild strain
- Grade II - intermediate partial tear
- Grade III - complete disruption

CLINICAL ISSUES

Presentation
- Most common signs/symptoms
  - Pain at the posterior aspect of the elbow
  - At the level of the olecranon insertion of the triceps tendon
- Clinical profile
  - Palpable depression proximal to olecranon
  - Swelling and posterior ecchymosis
  - Increased incidence in patients who have undergone a previous olecranon bursectomy
  - Traumatic event
  - Sports - football
  - Motorcycle accidents

Demographics
- Age: Typically a middle-aged man who suffered forced flexion of an extended forearm
- Gender: M > F

Natural History & Prognosis
- Complete ruptures need surgical repair
- Partial tears may heal with appropriate conservative measures

Treatment
- Conservative management: Partial tear
  - Rest, ice, temporary splinting
- Surgical management
  - Full tear - repair
  - Acute tear
    - Repair recommended
  - Delayed operative treatment

- Reconstruction: Periosteal flap, fascia flap, split triceps into reinforcing flap, rotation anconeus flap

DIAGNOSTIC CHECKLIST

Consider
- Olecranon bursitis
- Olecranon osteomyelitis

Image Interpretation Pearls
- Sagittal FS PD FSE for tear detection

SELECTED REFERENCES

1. Pina A et al: Traumatic avulsion of the triceps brachii. J Orthop Trauma 16(4):273-6, 2002
2. Dev S et al: Rupture of the triceps muscle at its attachments. Injury 30(1):70-1, 1999
3. Strauch RJ: Biceps and triceps injuries of the elbow. Orthop Clin North Am 30(1):95-107, 1999
4. Dev S et al: Rupture of the triceps muscle at its attachments. Injury 30(1):70-1, 1999
5. Strauch RJ: Biceps and triceps injuries of the elbow. Orthop Clin North Am 30(1):95-107, 1999
6. Fritz RC et al: The Elbow. Magnetic resonance imaging in orthopaedic and sports medicine. vol 1. 2nd ed. Philadelphia PA, J.B. Lippincott, 743-849, 1997

TRICEPS TENDON RUPTURE

IMAGE GALLERY

Typical

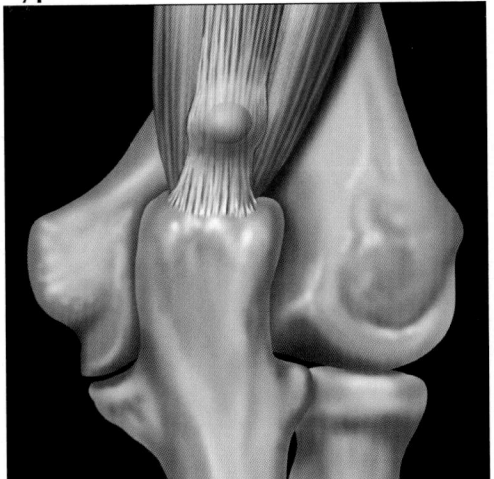
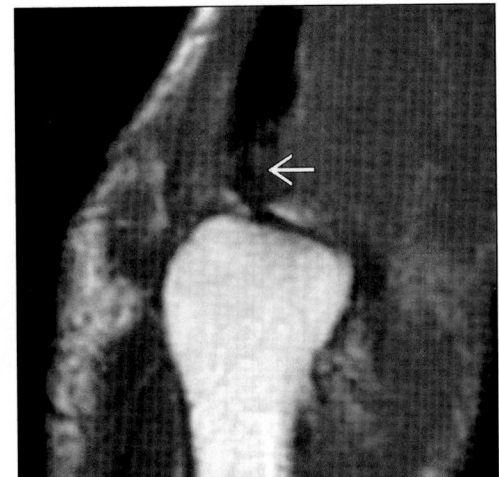

(Left) Coronal graphic shows tendinosis at the distal aspect of the triceps tendon. *(Right)* Coronal T1WI MR shows irregular increased signal intensity within a non-torn tendon, consistent with tendinosis (arrow).

Typical

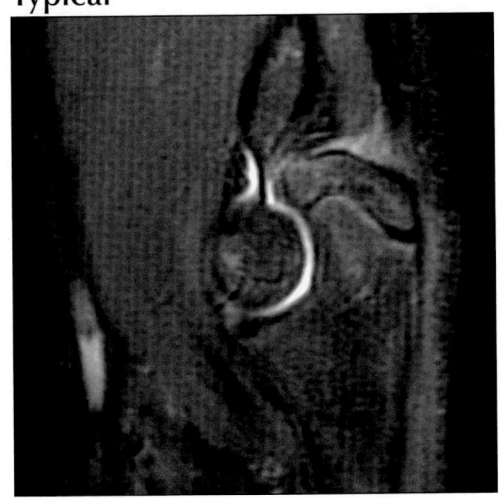
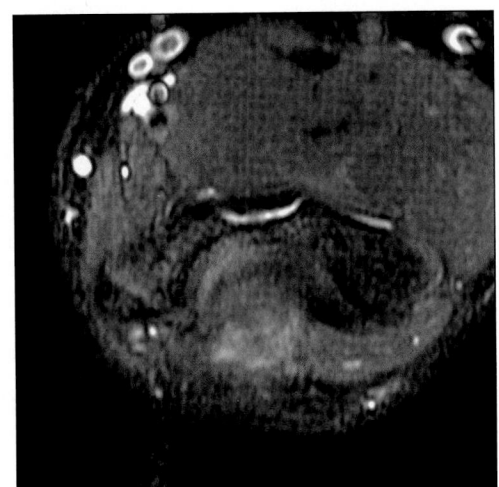

(Left) Sagittal FS PD FSE MR shows a strain of the triceps tendon with a trabecular injury of the olecranon. *(Right)* Axial FS PD FSE MR in the same patient shows the triceps tendon strain. The clinical impression was of a biceps strain (rare in adolescents) secondary to pain with flexion.

Typical

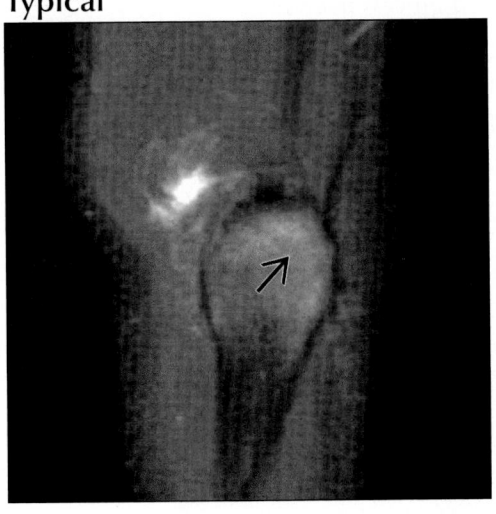
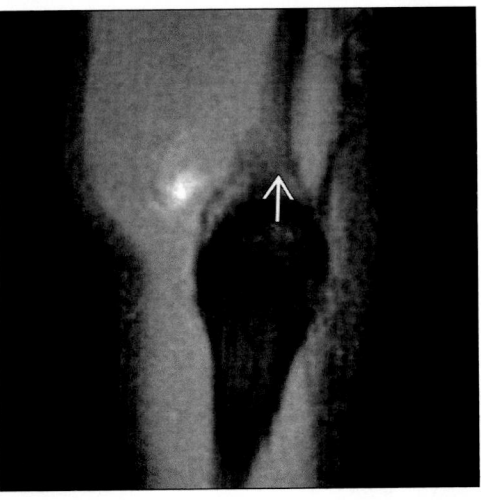

(Left) Coronal FS PD FSE MR shows a hyperintense partial muscle tear. There is a trabecular injury (arrow) of the olecranon. *(Right)* Coronal T2* GRE MR shows tendinosis (arrow) of the triceps and a hyperintense tear of the myotendinous junction involving the muscle belly itself.

LATERAL COLLATERAL LIGAMENT INJURY

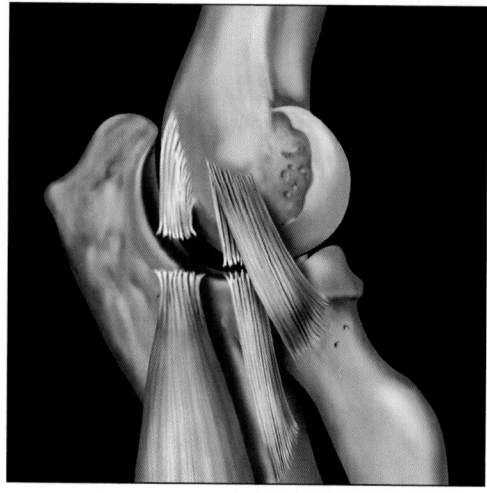

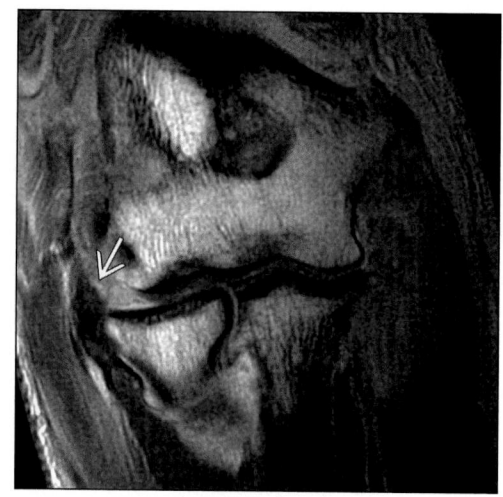

Sagittal graphic shows tear at lateral ulnar collateral ligament & extensor tendon origin. Injury to structures are associated with posterior dislocation or chronic lateral epicondylitis.

Coronal PD FSE MR shows a complete tear of the origin of LUCL (arrow) and common extensor tendon origin in this posterior dislocation patient.

TERMINOLOGY

Abbreviations and Synonyms
- Lateral ulnar collateral ligament (LUCL) injury, radial collateral ligament (RCL) injury, lateral collateral ligament (LCL) complex injury = LUCL + RCL, posterolateral rotatory instability (PLRI)

Definitions
- Elbow instability primarily from injury to the lateral collateral ligament complex
  - Posttraumatic - fall on an outstretched hand
  - LUCL tear +/- secondary to chronic lateral epicondylitis
- Progresses to subluxations, dislocation
- Component of PLRI as a result of axial compression, supination and valgus force
  - Lateral instability is spectrum of disease from PLRI to posterior dislocation

IMAGING FINDINGS

General Features
- Best diagnostic clue
  - Tears - disruption of the normal continuous decreased signal intensity ligament

- Irregularity and increased signal seen on T2-weighted MR images
- Location
  - RCL (also known as radial collateral ligament proper) - undersurface of lateral epicondyle (anterior aspect) to annular ligament holding radial head
  - LUCL - undersurface of lateral epicondyle (more posterior aspect) beneath radial neck to lateral ulnar diametaphysis
  - Tear usually occurs at humeral side
- Size: Tear may be small discrete or complete "blowout"
- Morphology: Disruption in the normal continuous linear ligament appearance

Radiographic Findings
- Radiography
  - Dislocation
  - Perched elbow
  - +/- Normal, if spontaneous reduction has occurred
  - +/- Coronoid process fracture
  - +/- Radial head/neck fracture
  - +/- Capitellar fracture
  - Intercondylar, medial condylar/lateral condylar fractures with posterior dislocation - unusual

CT Findings
- NECT
  - +/- Dislocation
  - +/- Perched elbow

DDx: Lateral Collateral Ligament Injury

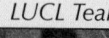
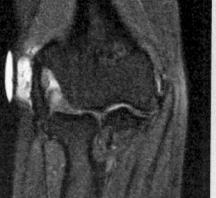

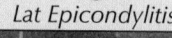
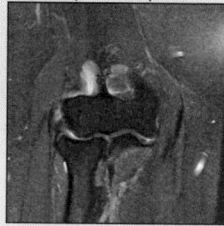

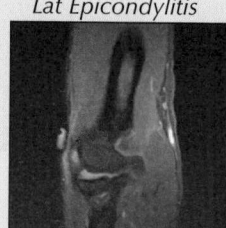

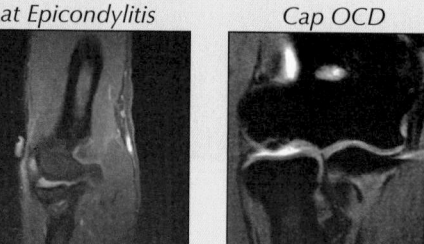

LUCL Tear	Lat Epicondylitis	Lat Epicondylitis	Cap OCD
Cor FS PD FSE	Cor FS PD FSE	Cor FS PD FSE	Cor STIR MR

LATERAL COLLATERAL LIGAMENT INJURY

Key Facts

Terminology
- Elbow instability primarily from injury to the lateral collateral ligament complex

Imaging Findings
- Tears - disruption of the normal continuous decreased signal intensity ligament
- Irregularity and increased signal seen on T2-weighted MR images
- Perched elbow

Top Differential Diagnoses
- Lateral Epicondylitis
- Capitellum Osteochondritis Dissecans (OCD)
- Lateral Epicondylar/Condylar Fracture
- Radial Head/Neck Fracture

Pathology
- General path comments: Ligament tear results in abnormal motion in which the radius and ulna move away from the humerus most often resulting in PLRI

Clinical Issues
- Elbow pain
- Pain with lateral pivot shift apprehension test
- Three stages of progressive instability beginning with subluxation and progressing to dislocation

Diagnostic Checklist
- Associated with LUCL tear of lateral ligament complex
- Coronal FS PD to evaluate the disruption of the LUCL deep to the common extensor (if intact) origin

---

- ○ +/- Coronoid process fracture
- ○ +/- Radial head/neck fracture
- ○ +/- Capitellar fracture
- ○ Intercondylar, medial condylar/lateral condylar fractures with posterior dislocation - unusual
- ○ Reconstructions helpful
- ○ +/- Loose bodies
- CT arthrography
  - ○ Contrast extends through lateral capsular defect when torn

MR Findings
- T1WI
  - ○ Tear of LUCL at origin on the humerus = discontinuous fibers
  - ○ Surrounding hypointense edema/hemorrhage
- T2WI
  - ○ Disruption of ligamentous fibers with fluid signal intensity
  - ○ Perched elbow
    - ▪ Coronoid perched on dorsal aspect of trochlea
    - ▪ Disruption of anterior and posterior capsule
    - ▪ High signal intensity (edema) around the injury
  - ○ Dislocation = PLRI, perched elbow
    - ▪ Complete dislocation of the radius and ulna
    - ▪ Progressive disruption of the medial collateral ligament
  - ○ Fractures common especially after elbow dislocation, hyperintense edema
    - ▪ Coronoid process
    - ▪ Capitellum
    - ▪ Radial head
    - ▪ Multiple
- STIR
  - ○ Useful at low, mid field
  - ○ Less spatial resolution

Imaging Recommendations
- Best imaging tool: MRI
- Protocol advice: FS PD FSE in all three planes

DIFFERENTIAL DIAGNOSIS

Lateral Epicondylitis
- Mimics PLRI
- Advanced cases may include disruption of the LUCL, therefore overlapping signs may develop

Clinically Swollen Tender Elbow
- Posttraumatic
- PLRI may be a diagnosis of exclusion
- MRI used for soft tissue discrimination

Capitellum Osteochondritis Dissecans (OCD)
- Necrosis of bone followed by healing response and reossification
- 12-16 year age group
  - ○ After ossification of capitellum
- 20% bilateral
- Chronic valgus stress with lateral impaction
- Seen in gymnasts and adolescent baseball pitchers

Lateral Epicondylar/Condylar Fracture
- Fall on an outstretched hand
  - ○ +/- Radial head impaction
- Varus stress with elbow flexed/supinated, avulsion by common extensor action
- 17% of distal humerus fractures
- Common in 5-10 year (peak = 6 years)
- Rotation of fracture fragment due to action of forearm extensors/supinators

Radial Head/Neck Fracture
- +/- Posterior dislocation
- +/- Coronoid process fracture/other fractures
- Impaction injury due to axial overloading in a fall on to the outstretched arm
- Radial head injuries are rare in children
  - ○ Occur in the radial neck
- Most common elbow fracture in adults

LATERAL COLLATERAL LIGAMENT INJURY

PATHOLOGY

General Features
- General path comments: Ligament tear results in abnormal motion in which the radius and ulna move away from the humerus most often resulting in PLRI
- Etiology
  - Oblique orientation of normal LUCL allows for lateral and posterior stabilization
  - Fall on outstretched hand
  - Chronic tennis elbow
  - Elbow instability spectrum of soft tissue and bone injury
    - From lateral to medial in three different stages: PLRI, perched elbow, dislocation
    - Instability progressing from lateral to medial encircling elbow = Horii circle
  - Most common cause of PLRI is elbow dislocation
- Epidemiology: Relatively uncommon
- Associated abnormalities: +/- Lateral epicondylitis (tendinosis and or tearing of the common extensor tendon origin)

Gross Pathologic & Surgical Features
- Tear at origin of LUCL with or without lateral epicondylitis for PLRI
- Dislocated ulna and radius in more advanced stages

Microscopic Features
- Microscopic and macroscopic tearing of the LUCL (early)
  - Followed by the anterior and posterior elbow joint capsule
  - Then medial ligamentous structures
- Variable amounts of hemorrhage and inflammatory cells

Staging, Grading or Classification Criteria
- Posterolateral instability
  - Stage I
    - PLRI: Posterolateral subluxation of the ulna and radius relative to the humerus
    - Tear of the LUCL
  - Stage II
    - Perched elbow: Coronoid perched on trochlea
  - Stage IIIA
    - Complete dislocation with tear of the posterior band of the ulnar (medial) collateral ligament
    - Elbow is stable to valgus stress
  - Stage IIIB
    - Complete dislocation with tear of the entire ulnar (medial) collateral ligament
    - Elbow is unstable in all directions
  - = Horii circle (progressive lateral to medial instability)

CLINICAL ISSUES

Presentation
- Most common signs/symptoms
  - Elbow pain
  - Pain with lateral pivot shift apprehension test
- Clinical profile
  - Swelling and pain after traumatic event
  - Patient is often guarding leading to difficult diagnosis at presentation
  - Rotational instability
  - Positive elbow pivot shift test
  - Supination/valgus added during flexion causing the radius and ulna to sublux posteriorly
  - + Lateral pivot shift test and posterolateral rotatory drawer test with examination under anesthesia
    - Subluxation of radiocapitellar joint with "dimple sign" during examination under anesthesia

Demographics
- Age: Recurrent complete dislocation occurs more frequently in children
- Gender: M ≥ F

Natural History & Prognosis
- Three stages of progressive instability beginning with subluxation and progressing to dislocation
- Develops insidiously after initial injury

Treatment
- Conservative
  - Mild sprain
    - Rest, ice, temporary splinting, physical therapy
- Surgical
  - LUCL isolated tear
    - Repair if PLRI
  - Post dislocation
    - Repair of tendon avulsions
    - Preservation of radial head if possible
    - Excision of interposed fracture fragments
    - Reconstruction of coronoid fracture
- Complications
  - Deformity
  - Laxity
  - Heterotopic calcification
  - Contracture
  - Neuropathy

DIAGNOSTIC CHECKLIST

Consider
- Associated with LUCL tear of lateral ligament complex

Image Interpretation Pearls
- Coronal FS PD to evaluate the disruption of the LUCL deep to the common extensor (if intact) origin

SELECTED REFERENCES

1. O'Driscoll SW: Elbow instability. Acta Orthop Belg 65(4):404-15, 1999
2. Bredella MA et al: MR imaging findings of lateral ulnar collateral ligament abnormalities in patients with lateral epicondylitis. AJR. 173(5):1379-82, 1999
3. Fritz RC: MR imaging of sports injuries of the elbow. Magn Reson Imaging Clin N Am 7(1):51-72, 1999
4. Putnam MD et al: Painful conditions around the elbow. Orthop Clin North Am 30(1):109-18, 1999
5. Potter HG et al: Posterolateral rotatory instability of the elbow: Usefulness of MR imaging in diagnosis. Radiology 204(1):185-9, 1997

IMAGE GALLERY

Typical

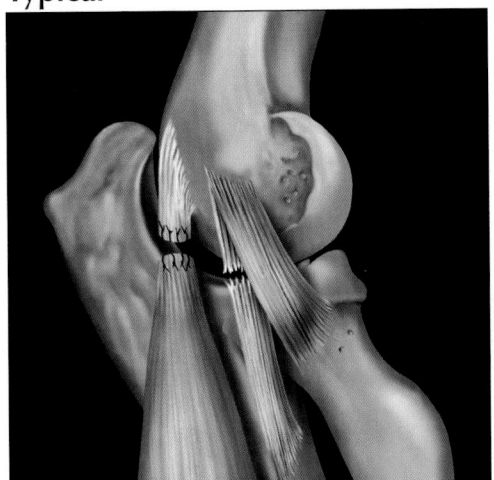
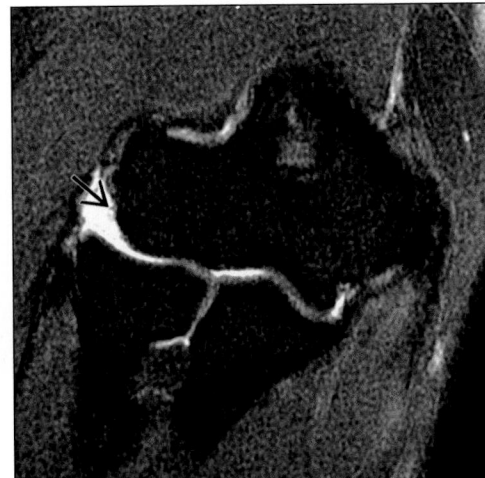

(Left) Sagittal graphic shows post-operative changes of the common extensor tendon origin with an over-aggressive release resulting in an iatrogenic disruption of the lateral ulnar collateral ligament. *(Right)* Coronal STIR MR shows a tear of the lateral ulnar collateral ligament (arrow) after common extensor tendon origin release. The ligament disruption may have been preexisting.

Typical

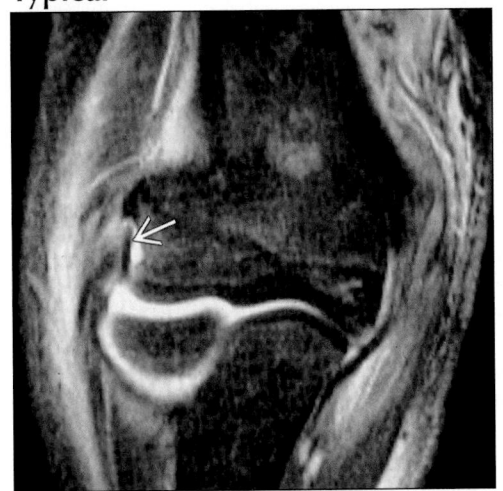
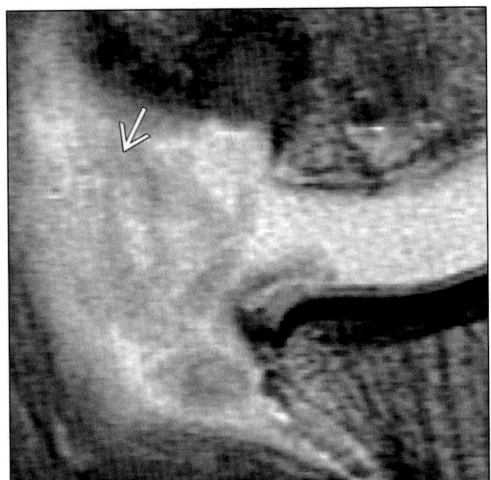

(Left) Coronal FS PD FSE MR shows an avulsion of the lateral epicondyle cortex (arrow) after posterior dislocation of the elbow. The majority of the lateral ulnar collateral ligament is intact. *(Right)* Coronal T1 arthrogram shows a complete blow out of lateral aspect of joint (arrow).

Typical

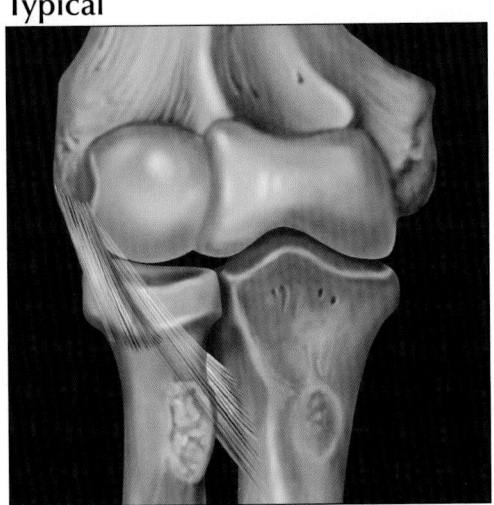
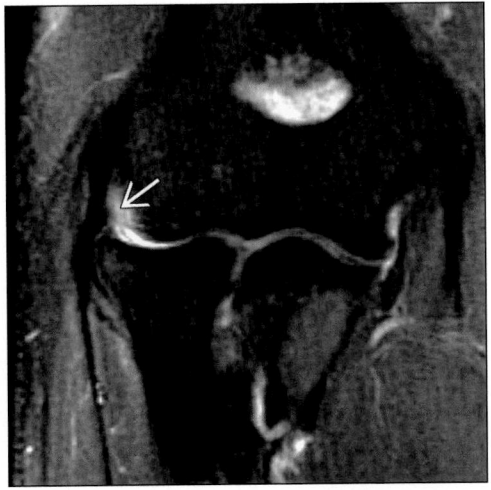

(Left) Coronal graphic shows the normal anatomy of the radial collateral ligament (laterally) and the lateral ulnar collateral ligament (deep to the radial head/neck). *(Right)* Coronal FS PD FSE shows tear of the origin of the lateral ulnar collateral ligament (arrow) adjacent to an intact common extensor tendon origin and a bone trabecular injury of the lateral aspect of the radial head.

POSTERIOR DISLOCATION, ELBOW

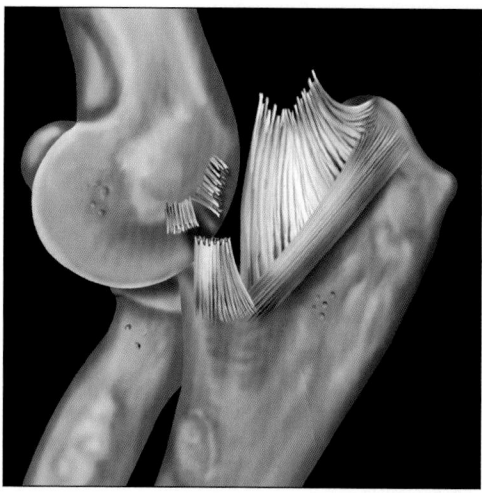

Sagittal graphic shows posterior dislocation of the olecranon and radius with tearing of the soft tissue constraints.

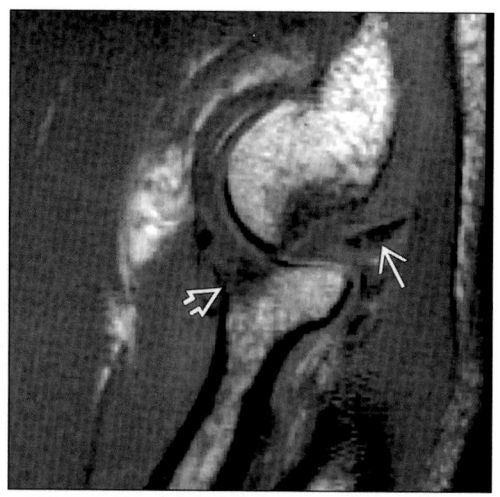

Sagittal PD FSE MR shows fracture pattern in posterior dislocation: Anterior radial head (open arrow) & posterior capitellum. There are loose fragments (arrow) from impaction fracture.

TERMINOLOGY

Abbreviations and Synonyms
- Elbow dislocation

Definitions
- In a posterior dislocation, the ulna is normally dislocated posteriorly to the humerus, with associated posterior displacement of the radius
- Posterior, posterolateral or posteromedial, open or closed, simple or complex types

IMAGING FINDINGS

General Features
- Best diagnostic clue
  - Empty semilunar notch on lateral radiograph
    - + Distal humerus aligned with radial head on 90 degree flexed view
  - Posterior displacement of ulna and radius on sagittal MR images
- Location: Typically in the humeroulnar joint +/- medial epicondylar injury
- Size
  - Size of the injury is related to associated bony and ligamentous injuries
  - +/- Delayed healing results in residual instability

- Morphology
  - Posterior, posteromedial or posterolateral dislocation
  - +/- Disrupted ligaments
  - +/- Impaction or avulsion fractures

Radiographic Findings
- Radiography
  - Lateral views - the humeral epicondyles will be aligned with the radial head
    - Anterior to the empty cup-shaped semilunar notch of the ulna
  - A horizontal lucency may be seen in the coronoid process of the ulna
    - +/- Displacement, indicating a fracture
  - Lucent lines and or distortion may also be seen in the radial head indicating fractures
  - On AP views, medial humeral epicondylar lucent lines may be seen in adults indicating fractures
  - Below 15 years of age, there may be increased distance between the medial condylar epiphysis and the humerus
    - = An epiphyseal (Salter type 1) fracture
  - Fat pad signs will not be reliable
    - Secondary to severe distortion of the anatomy and potential rupture of the joint capsule

CT Findings
- NECT

DDx: Posterior Dislocation, Elbow

LUCL Tear	MCL Sprain	Lat Epi LUCL Tear	Radial Fx	Old Post Disloc
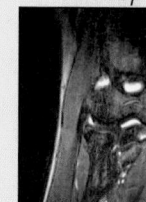	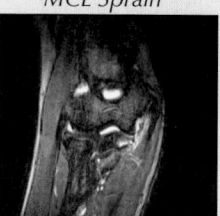	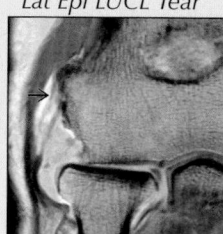	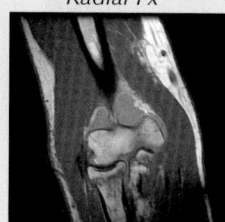	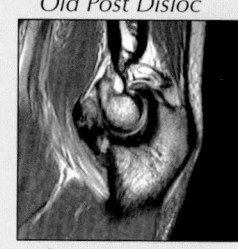
Cor STIR MR	Cor STIR MR	Cor T1 Arthro.	Cor PD FSE MR	Sag PD FSE MR

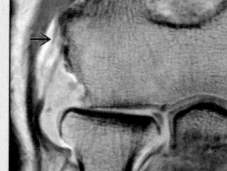

POSTERIOR DISLOCATION, ELBOW

Key Facts

Terminology
- In a posterior dislocation, the ulna is normally dislocated posteriorly to the humerus, with associated posterior displacement of the radius

Imaging Findings
- Empty semilunar notch on lateral radiograph
- Posterior displacement of ulna and radius on sagittal MR images
- Disruption of normal anatomy and low signal of medial collateral ligament (MCL) on coronal views

Top Differential Diagnoses
- Supracondylar Fracture
- Radial Head/Neck Fracture
- Lateral Ulnar Collateral Ligament Tear (LUCL Tear)
- Lateral Epicondylitis

- Medial Collateral Ligament Sprain

Pathology
- Commonly associated with ligamentous injury
- Etiology: Fall onto an outstretched hand
- Posterior dislocations are the most common type of elbow dislocation

Clinical Issues
- Most common signs/symptoms: Pain and swelling of posterior mass within palpable semilunar notch

Diagnostic Checklist
- Nerve damage, vascular damage, interposed epicondylar fractures
- Characteristic associated fractures (e.g., coronoid)

- ○ Linear lucencies in medial epicondyle, radial head or coronoid process indicating fractures
- ○ Fracture comminution and displacement assessed
  - ▪ Coronal, sagittal reconstructions helpful
- ○ Soft tissue swelling evident on soft tissue windows

MR Findings
- T1WI
  - ○ Decreased marrow signal indicating areas of bone stress
  - ○ Low signal joint effusion
  - ○ Disruption of normal anatomy and low signal of medial collateral ligament (MCL) on coronal views
  - ○ Low signal lines indicating fracture lines +/- bony displacement
- T2WI
  - ○ Increased marrow signal indicating edema
  - ○ FS PD FSE visualization improved
    - ▪ High signal joint effusion +/- periarticular leakage with capsular rupture
    - ▪ Disruption of MCL anatomy with high signal tears
    - ▪ High signal stress lesions at bony attachments of torn ligaments
    - ▪ Edema/disruption of neurovascular structures
    - ▪ Disruption of LCL anatomy with high signal tears: RCL, LUCL
    - ▪ +/- Medial epicondylar avulsion in children (+ hyperintense surrounding edema)
  - ○ Characteristic associated fxs
    - ▪ "Kissing" fxs of radial head, capitellum
    - ▪ Coronoid fx
- STIR
  - ○ Bright signal edema
  - ○ Alternative at low and midfield
- T2* GRE
  - ○ Coronal images show damage to articular cartilage for larger defects
  - ○ FS PD FSE is a more sensitive chondral imaging sequence

Imaging Recommendations
- Best imaging tool: MRI
- Protocol advice: FS PD FSE/T2 sagittal images

DIFFERENTIAL DIAGNOSIS

Supracondylar Fracture
- Fall on outstretched hand (FOOSH) injury
- Transverse lucency in metaphysis on AP or angled AP view
- Anterior humeral line displaced to anterior to mid third of capitellum in 94%
- Extraarticular in children but may be intraarticular in adults
- 60% of pediatric elbow fractures

Radial Head/Neck Fracture
- Radial head - adults, radial neck - children
- Most common elbow fracture in adults
- Fall on out stretched hand injury

Lateral Ulnar Collateral Ligament Tear (LUCL Tear)
- Predisposes to posterior dislocation
- Hyperintense edema and tear are demonstrated on FS PD FSE
- Best visualized on posterior coronal images

Lateral Epicondylitis
- Most commonly extensor carpi radialis brevis (ECRB) affected
- Tendon may tear with posterior dislocation
- +/- LUCL tear

Medial Collateral Ligament Sprain
- May tear with posterior dislocation
- Valgus stress
- Disrupted ligament + hyperintensity on T2WI

PATHOLOGY

General Features
- General path comments
  - ○ Commonly associated with ligamentous injury
  - ○ Endstage instability following posterolateral rotatory instability

- Perched elbow
- Frank dislocation
- +/- Single traumatic event without predisposing instability
- Etiology: Fall onto an outstretched hand
- Epidemiology
  - Incidence: 6 of every 100,000 individuals
  - Posterior dislocations are the most common type of elbow dislocation
  - More common in children; peak incidence is 11-15 years
- Associated abnormalities
  - The semilunar notch of the ulna may show variable morphology
    - A shallower notch or one with a reduced angle of circumference may predispose to dislocation
  - Ligament injuries and fractures associated with later onset of osteoarthritis
  - Associated fractures
    - Radial head (10% and most common)
    - Coronoid
    - Olecranon
    - Medial and lateral epicondyles
  - Neurapraxia may occur in up to 20% of cases involving ulnar nerve or anterior interosseus branch of the median nerve

Gross Pathologic & Surgical Features

- Dislocation of ulna and radius, +/- fractures with varying degrees of depression/displacement with surrounding hemorrhage and soft tissue injury

Microscopic Features

- Disruption of bone cortex and trabeculae with surrounding hemorrhage in acute cases

Staging, Grading or Classification Criteria

- Instability
  - Stage I: Posterolateral subluxation of ulna and radius + disruption of lateral ulnar collateral ligament
  - Stage II: Complete dislocation with coronoid perched on trochlea + disruption anterior and posterior joint capsule = perched elbow
  - Stage III: Complete posterior dislocation + disruption medial collateral complex

CLINICAL ISSUES

Presentation

- Most common signs/symptoms: Pain and swelling of posterior mass within palpable semilunar notch
- Clinical profile
  - In children - avulsion of the medial humeral epicondylar epiphysis (Salter type 1 injury) - common
  - In adults, fractures may occur to the radial head, coronoid process and medial epicondyle - common

Demographics

- Age: Usually young active patients (30 years = mean age)
- Gender: M:F = 2-2.5:1

Natural History & Prognosis

- In uncomplicated dislocations, 60% will have late symptoms of pain
- Pain on valgus stressing and flexion contracture
- Incomplete recovery more likely with fractures, posterolateral direction, delayed reduction and rigid immobilization
- Fractures associated with secondary osteoarthritis
- Duration of immobilization has negative association with later complications of reduced range of motion and flexion contractions
- Redislocation associated with poor outcome

Treatment

- Conservative
  - Reduction, bracing in pronation, protected mobilization
- Surgical
  - Repair of MCL, repair of tendon avulsions
  - Preservation of radial head if possible, excision of interposed soft tissue or osteochondral fragment within epicondylar fractures
  - Reconstruction of coronoid process
- Complications
  - Failed reduction may be due to entrapped medial epicondyle fracture fragment, inverted cartilaginous flap or osteochondral fragment
  - Late complications include MCL laxity, posterolateral instability, heterotopic ossification, flexion contracture, median and ulnar nerve palsy
  - Volkmann's ischemic contracture
  - Brachial artery injury

DIAGNOSTIC CHECKLIST

Consider

- Nerve damage, vascular damage, interposed epicondylar fractures

Image Interpretation Pearls

- Characteristic associated fractures (e.g., coronoid)

SELECTED REFERENCES

1. Ring D et al: Posterior dislocation of the elbow with fractures of the radial head and coronoid. J Bone Joint Surg Am 84-A(4):547-51, 2002
2. Kumar A et al: Closed reduction of posterior dislocation of the elbow. A simple technique. J Orthop Trauma 13(1):58-9, 1999
3. Limb D et al: Median nerve palsy after posterolateral elbow dislocation. J Bone Joint Surg Br 76(6):987-8, 1994
4. Josefsson PO et al: Dislocations of the elbow and intraarticular fractures. Clin-Orthop (246):126-30, 1989
5. Mehlhoff TL et al: Simple dislocation of the elbow in the adult. Results after closed treatment Div of Orthopedic Surgery. J Bone Joint Surg Am 70(2):244-9, 1988
6. Josefsson PO et al: Surgical versus non-surgical treatment of ligamentous injuries following dislocation of the elbow joint. A prospective randomized study. J Bone Joint Surg Am 69(4):605-8, 1987

IMAGE GALLERY

Typical

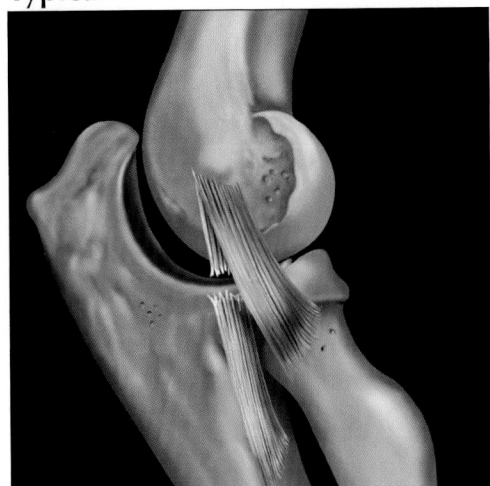 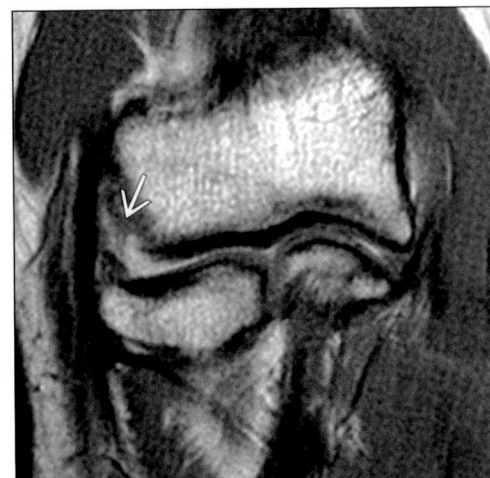

(Left) Sagittal graphic shows a tear of the lateral ulnar collateral ligament – the soft tissue findings of stage I instability (posterolateral rotatory instability). (Right) Coronal PD FSE MR shows a tear of the LUCL (arrow) in a patient with posterolateral rotatory instability (PLRI).

Typical

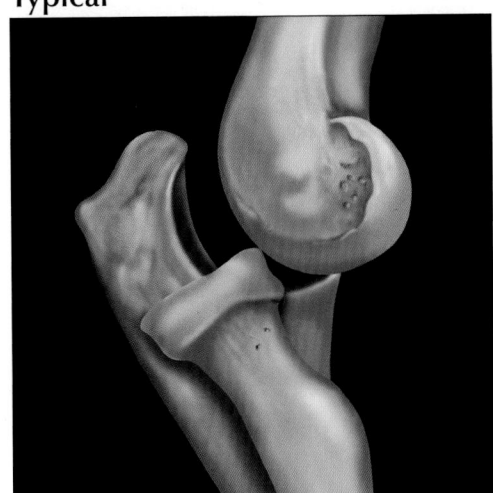 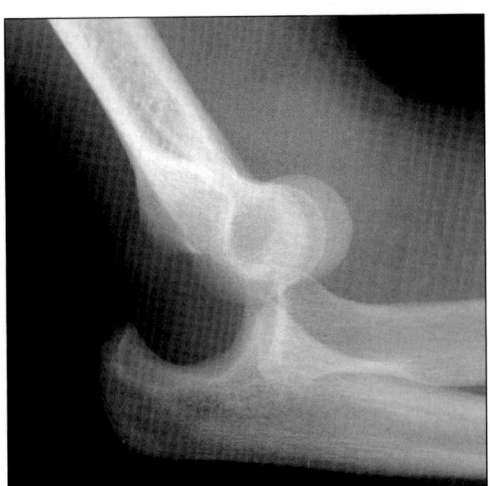

(Left) Sagittal graphic shows stage II lateral instability known as the perched elbow. (Right) Lateral radiography shows a perched elbow nearly dislocated.

Typical

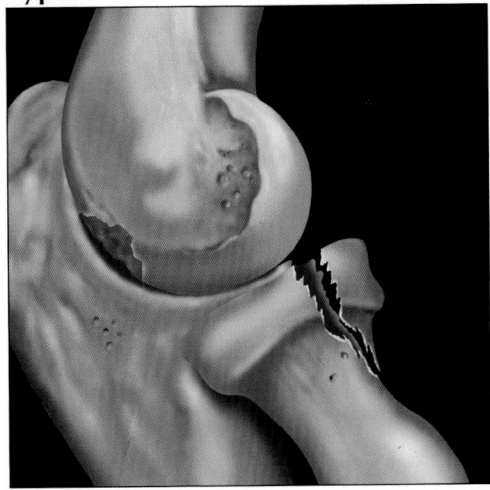 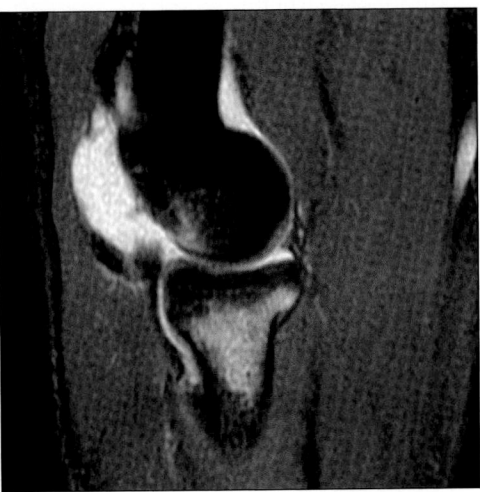

(Left) Sagittal graphic shows the bony injury seen with posterior dislocation including a fracture of the anterior aspect of the radial head and a posterior capitellar fracture. (Right) Sagittal STIR MR shows associated bony injuries of a recent posterior dislocation including the radial head and posterior capitellum.

MCL ELBOW INJURY

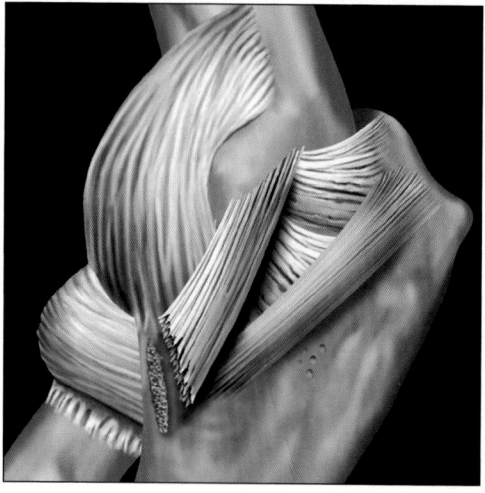

Sagittal graphic shows a complete tear of the distal aspect of the medial collateral ligament – anterior band.

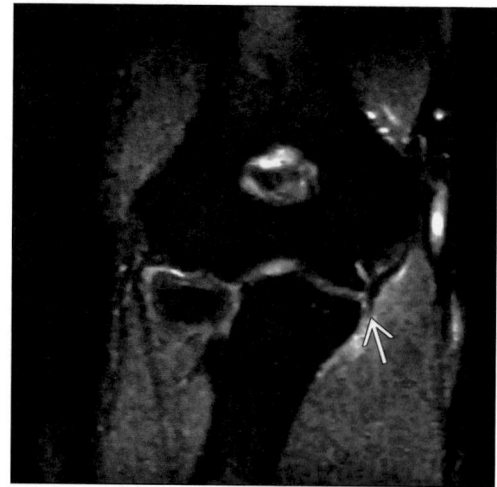

Coronal STIR MR shows a tear of the distal aspect of the medial collateral ligament (arrow) at its insertion on the sublime tubercle.

TERMINOLOGY

Abbreviations and Synonyms
- Medial collateral ligament (MCL) elbow injury

Definitions
- Injury to the medial collateral ligament (anterior band of MCL)
- Valgus stress, injury to the elbow

IMAGING FINDINGS

General Features
- Best diagnostic clue
  - Tears as disruption of the normally continuous hypointense MCL
  - + Irregularity and increased signal seen on T2 weighted MR images
  - Anterior band - most important medial structure injured
- Location
  - Undersurface of medial epicondyle to sublime tubercle of ulna
    - Proximal to distal
- Size: Tear may be small discrete or complete "blowout"
- Morphology

  - Disruption in the normal continuous linear ligament
  - +/- Thickening in chronic cases

Radiographic Findings
- Radiography
  - +/- Sublime tubercle hypertrophy
  - +/- Medial epicondyle avulsion
  - +/- Medial soft tissue swelling
  - +/- Traction spur

CT Findings
- NECT
  - +/- Sublime tubercle degenerative changes
  - +/- Avulsion of medial epicondyle
  - +/- Medial soft tissue edema
    - Streaky medium attenuation in paraarticular fat
  - +/- Traction spur
  - Lateral impaction injuries
    - Capitellar/radial head fx/osteoarthritis (OA)
- CT arthrography
  - +/- Medial capsular disruption
  - Contrast extends "around corner" of sublime tubercle in distal deep partial tear
  - Coronal reconstructions
  - "T" sign

MR Findings
- T1WI

DDx: MCL Elbow Injury

Ulnar Spur	Anc Epitrochlear	Prox Hyperintens.	Sublime Fx	Normal MCL
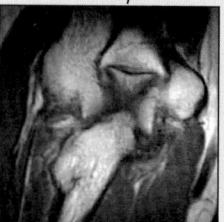	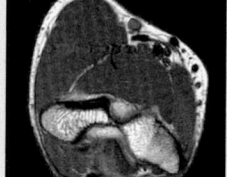	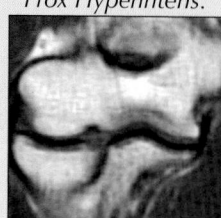	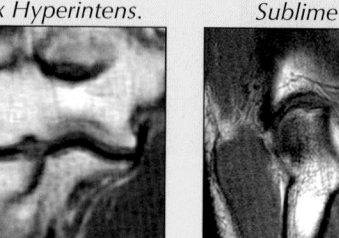	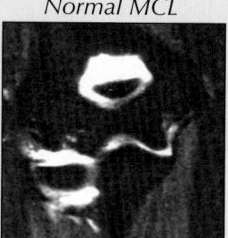
Cor PD FSE MR	Ax PD FSE MR	Cor PD FSE MR	Cor PD FSE MR	Cor T1 arth FS

MCL ELBOW INJURY

Key Facts

Imaging Findings
- Tears as disruption of the normally continuous hypointense MCL
- + Irregularity and increased signal seen on T2 weighted MR images
- Anterior band - most important medial structure injured
- Arthrography demonstrates "T" sign - distal partial tears that spare the superficial fibers

Top Differential Diagnoses
- Medial Epicondylitis with Intact MCL
- Little Leaguer's Elbow
- Ulnar Neuropathy
- Traction Spur of MCL
- Sublime Tubercle Fracture

- Normal MCL

Pathology
- Degeneration and tearing of the MCL caused by repetitive valgus stress

Clinical Issues
- Pain after valgus stress injury
- Medial pain especially at overhand throwing
- Usually acute episode superimposed on chronic repetitive valgus stress

Diagnostic Checklist
- Partial tear, flexor pronator group strain without ligamentous damage
- Coronal and axial FS PD FSE or STIR

- ○ +/- Heterotopic ossification
  - ▪ Increased signal = fat in bone marrow
- ○ Epicondylar avulsion
  - ▪ Corticated structure
  - ▪ Donor site on humerus
  - ▪ Surrounding hypointense edema
  - ▪ Little leaguer's elbow
- ○ +/- Thickened increased signal intensity ligament
  - ▪ Chronic cases
- ○ +/- Traction spur
  - ▪ Hyperintense if contains marrow
  - ▪ Hypointense if purely calcification
- ○ Lateral impaction injury
  - ▪ Hypointense capitellum when edematous
  - ▪ Hypointense subchondral cysts (chronic)
  - ▪ Hypointense subchondral sclerosis
  - ▪ Hypointense loose bodies (OA)
- • T2WI
  - ○ Increased signal within the ligament
    - ▪ Most commonly anterior band
  - ○ +/- Discontinuous fibers (through and through tear)
  - ○ Tear may be
    - ▪ Proximal
    - ▪ Mid substance
    - ▪ Distal
  - ○ +/- Sublime tubercle hyperintensity
    - ▪ Stress response/avulsive stress
  - ○ +/- Sublime tubercle hypertrophy
  - ○ +/- Hyperintense flexor pronator strain/tear
  - ○ Increased signal (stress response or fracture) at humeral origin site or attachment site on the ulnar coronoid
- • PD/Intermediate
  - ○ Heterotopic ossification or epicondylar avulsion: Increased signal (fat in bone marrow), corticated structure
  - ○ Synovitis hyperintense relative to joint fluid
- • STIR: Increased signal within the ligament, most commonly the anterior band
- • T1 C+
  - ○ Enhancement of inflamed/injured MCL
  - ○ FS used in conjunction with T1WI
- • MR arthrography

- ○ Extravasation of contrast in cases of complete ruptures
- ○ Contrast extends "around corner" of sublime tubercle in distal deep partial tear
- ○ Arthrography demonstrates "T" sign - distal partial tears that spare the superficial fibers
  - ▪ "T" sign: Contrast interposed between the partially torn ligament and the medial aspect of the coronoid
  - ▪ Seen on coronal images
- • Increased signal (stress response or fracture) at humeral origin site or attachment site on the ulnar coronoid

Imaging Recommendations
- Best imaging tool: MRI
- Protocol advice: FS PD FSE in coronal/axial plane

DIFFERENTIAL DIAGNOSIS

Medial Epicondylitis with Intact MCL
- MRI can differentiate
- Chronic valgus stress
- +/- Ulnar neuritis
- Thrower's/golfer's elbow
- Traction tendinosis

Little Leaguer's Elbow
- MCL sprain often accompanies little leaguer's elbow (component of little league elbow)
- Traction apophysitis
- Common in adolescent pitchers
- Valgus stress
- +/- Medial epicondyle avulsion

Ulnar Neuropathy
- Neurapraxia often seen with MCL injury
- +/- Anconeus epitrochlearis
- Traction neurapraxia
- +/- Cubital tunnel mass

Traction Spur of MCL
- Chronic valgus stress

MCL ELBOW INJURY

- +/- Visible marrow in calcification
- Throwers
- Rare

Sublime Tubercle Fracture
- Type of coronoid process fracture
- MCL avulsion
  - Unusual
- Hyperintense edema on T2WI

Normal MCL
- Thin decreased signal intensity ligament
- Spreads out at humeral origin (proximal hyperintensity)
- Oblique orientation from ventral to dorsal

PATHOLOGY

General Features
- General path comments
  - Relevant anatomy
    - Anterior band MCL = primary soft tissue restraint to valgus stress
    - Normal anterior band extends from medial epicondyle to the coronoid tubercle (sublime tubercle)
    - Osseous anatomy = primary source of stability
    - Posterior band - thickening of posterior capsule with insertion along margin of semilunar notch
    - Transverse ligament no role in elbow stability
  - Excessive valgus stress
  - At 90° of flexion, MCL provides 55% of the resistance to valgus stress at the elbow
  - In full extension, the MCL + bony architecture + anterior capsule maintain valgus stability
  - Anterior band inserts on sublime tubercle and provides major contribution to valgus stability
  - Acceleration phase overhead throw = most valgus stress to the elbow - risk of damage to MCL
  - Valgus force can overcome tensile strength of MCL - chronic microscopic tears or tear
- Etiology
  - Degeneration and tearing of the MCL caused by repetitive valgus stress
  - Athletes during the acceleration phase of throwing or as acute valgus injury
  - Mid substance ruptures most common followed by distal then proximal ruptures
- Epidemiology: Common in throwing athletes

Gross Pathologic & Surgical Features
- Thickened, partially torn or completely torn anterior band of the medial collateral ligament

Microscopic Features
- Degeneration, partial or complete rupture
- Variable amounts of hemorrhage and inflammatory cells

Staging, Grading or Classification Criteria
- Partial tear
  - Proximal, mid substance, distal
- Complete tear

CLINICAL ISSUES

Presentation
- Most common signs/symptoms
  - Pain after valgus stress injury
  - Medial pain especially at overhand throwing
- Clinical profile
  - 40% - symptoms of ulnar neuropathy
  - Acute "pop" - specific injury
  - Limited elbow extension
  - Crepitus with range of motion
  - Tinel's sign/tenderness along cubital tunnel
  - Palpation to distinguish flexor - pronator musculotendinous origin strain/tear from MCL tenderness
  - Pain with resisted wrist pronation/supination in musculotendinous unit injury

Demographics
- Age: Children (usually athletes) or adults
- Gender: M > F

Natural History & Prognosis
- Usually acute episode superimposed on chronic repetitive valgus stress
- Return to competitive throwing after successful rehabilitation and reconstruction when indicated
- Patients are often asymptomatic with a lax MCL since osseous anatomy is intact

Treatment
- Conservative management
  - Mild sprain
    - Rest, ice, temporary splinting, training modification
- Surgical
  - Repair or reconstruction of complete disruption in athletes
    - Bunnell suture technique to reattach ligament
    - Graft harvest - palmaris longus weaved in a figure-eight pattern
- Complications (surgical)
  - Nerve injury
    - Medial antebrachial cutaneous nerve branches
    - ulnar nerve

DIAGNOSTIC CHECKLIST

Consider
- Partial tear, flexor pronator group strain without ligamentous damage

Image Interpretation Pearls
- Coronal and axial FS PD FSE or STIR

SELECTED REFERENCES
1. Chen FS et al: Medial elbow problems in the overhead-throwing athlete. J Am Acad Orthop Surg 9(2):99-113, 2001
2. Maloney MD et al: Elbow injuries in the throwing athlete. Difficult diagnoses and surgical complications. Clin Sports Med 18(4):795-809, 1999

IMAGE GALLERY

Typical

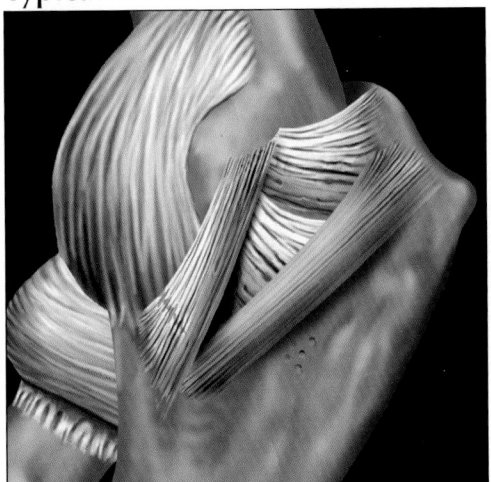

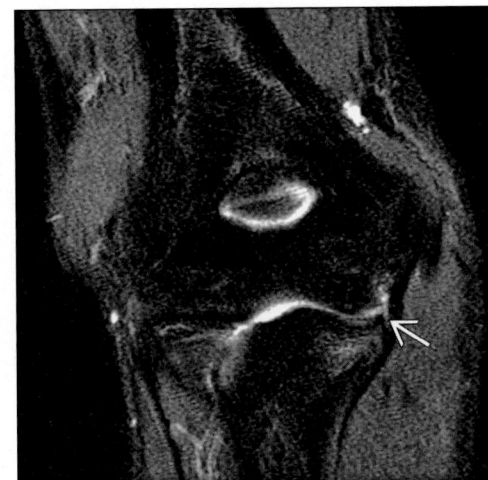

(Left) Sagittal graphic shows a partial tear of the anterior band of the medial collateral ligament at its insertion on the sublime tubercle. *(Right)* Coronal STIR MR shows a partial tear (arrow) with high signal going "around the corner" of the sublime tubercle with an adjacent bone trabecular injury.

Typical

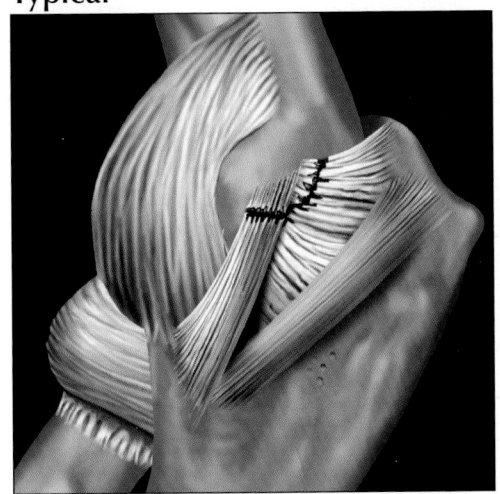

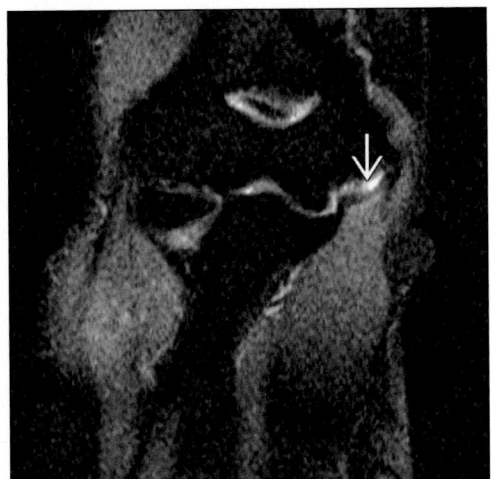

(Left) Sagittal graphic shows a proximal tear of the UCL. *(Right)* Coronal STIR MR shows a sprain of the proximal aspect of the medial collateral ligament (arrow) in this symptomatic patient.

Typical

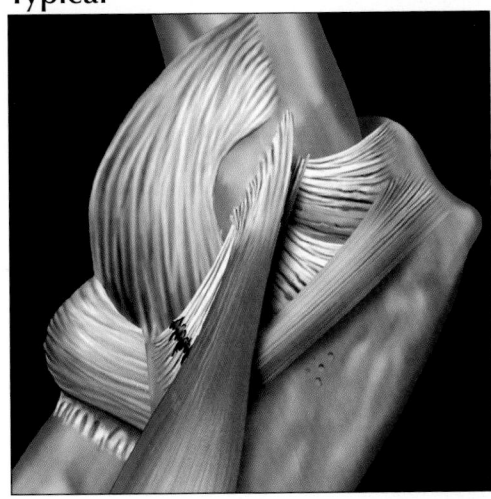

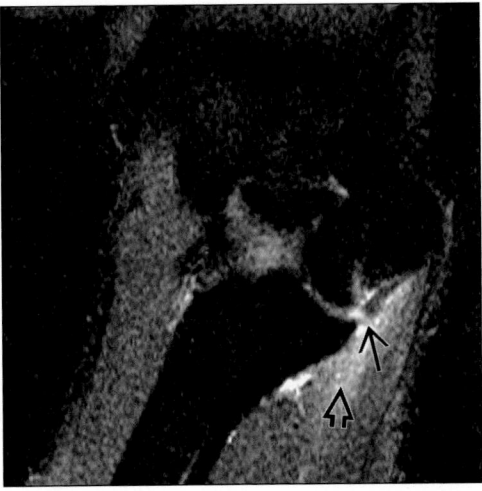

(Left) Sagittal graphic shows a tear of the medial collateral ligament with a strain of the flexor pronator origin. *(Right)* Coronal STIR MR shows a complete tear of the distal aspect of the medial collateral ligament anterior band (arrow) and an adjacent flexor pronator origin strain (open arrow).

LITTLE LEAGUER'S ELBOW

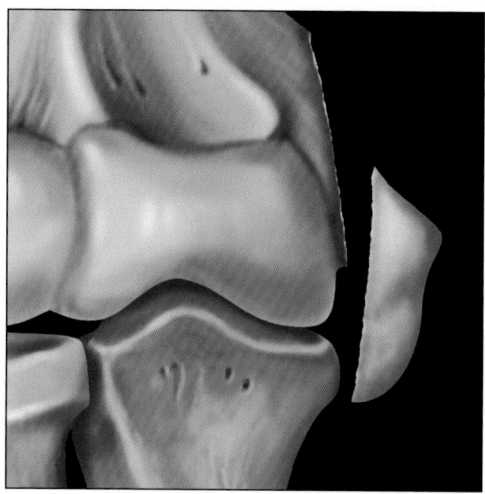

Coronal graphic shows an avulsion of the medial epicondyle, consistent with little leaguer's elbow.

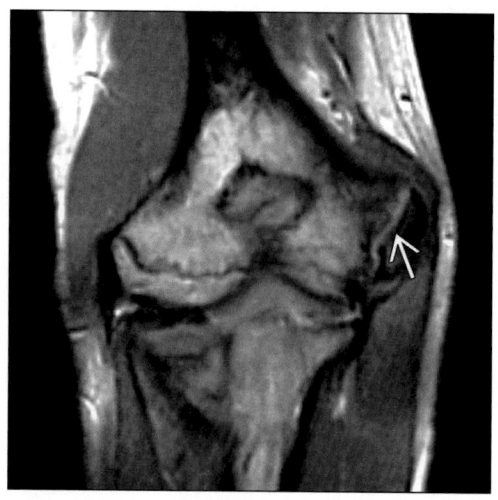

Coronal PD FSE MR shows slight distraction (arrow) of the medial epicondylar ossification center in a baseball pitcher. There is a strain of the flexor pronator origin.

TERMINOLOGY

Abbreviations and Synonyms
- Little leaguer's elbow, extension overload injury, medial epicondylar avulsion, medial epicondylitis
- Medial epicondyle apophysitis, thrower's elbow

Definitions
- Valgus stress injury
  - Results in tension injuries on the medial aspect of the elbow
  - Compressive injuries on the lateral aspect
- Traction apophysitis of medial epicondyle (stress fx, avulsion or delayed closure of medial epicondylar apophysis)

IMAGING FINDINGS

General Features
- Best diagnostic clue
  - Lucent line running through medial epicondyle on radiograph
  - Focal high signal on fluid sensitive MR sequences
- Location: Medial epicondyle of the distal humerus and attached soft tissues
- Size: 1-2 cm
- Morphology

  - Displaced ossific nucleus of medial epicondyle (child)
  - Crescentic avulsion of bony margin (adolescent)
  - Medial soft tissue swelling +/- calcification (adult)

Radiographic Findings
- Radiography
  - Fragmentation or widening of medial epicondyle apophysis
  - Early callus formation
  - Overgrowth of apophysis
  - Avulsion of medial epicondyle
    - May become entrapped within joint in children

CT Findings
- NECT
  - Lucent line indicating separation of epicondyle
  - Overgrowth of apophysis
  - Avulsion of medial epicondyle
- CT arthrography
  - +/- Medial capsular tear with extravasation of contrast
  - +/- Medial collateral ligament (MCL) tear

MR Findings
- T1WI
  - Low signal zone of separation through epicondylar region
  - +/- Hypointense epicondylar edema

DDx: Little Leaguer's Elbow

Med Epicondylitis	Ulnar Neuritis	Valgus Stress	Part Tear MCL	Muscle Strain
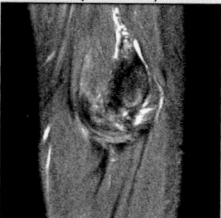	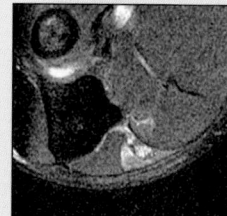	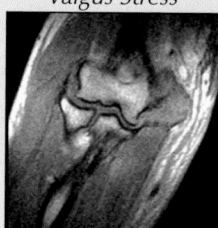	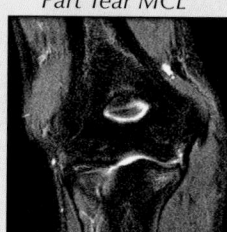	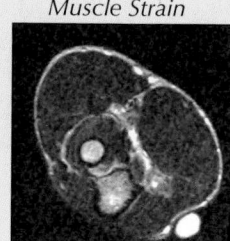
Sag FS PD FSE	Ax FS PD FSE	Cor PD FSE MR	Cor STIR MR	Ax T2 FSE MR

LITTLE LEAGUER'S ELBOW

Key Facts

Imaging Findings
- Variable signal within fragment depending on sclerosis
- Marrow edema in parent bone/humerus
- High signal fluid in medial collateral ligament (MCL) tears

Top Differential Diagnoses
- Capitellar Osteochondritis (OCD)
- Medial/Lateral Epicondylitis
- MCL Sprain
- Stress Fracture
- Ulnar Neuritis
- Muscle Strain

Pathology
- Excessive valgus stress

- Repetitive throwing motion
- Childhood injury pattern (pre-fusion) is microtrauma to apophysis and ossification center for medial epicondyle
- Adolescent pattern = avulsion of medial epicondyle +/- nonunion
- Adult pattern = ligament avulsions and muscle strains

Clinical Issues
- Pain localized to medial epicondyle
- Pain may also involve posterior and lateral aspects

Diagnostic Checklist
- Presence of lateral pathology (OCD)
- FS PD FSE to identify subchondral marrow edema and signal changes in the adjacent flexor pronator origin

---

- o +/- Discontinuous MCL = tear
- T2WI
  - o Variable signal within fragment depending on sclerosis
    - ▪ Sclerosis - hypointense
    - ▪ Edema - hyperintense
  - o Marrow edema in parent bone/humerus
  - o High signal fluid in medial collateral ligament (MCL) tears
    - ▪ Incomplete tear
    - ▪ Complete tear
- STIR
  - o High signal within the fragment and in parent bone
  - o High signal edema in MCL complex +/- defects
  - o High sensitivity for edema
  - o Lower spatial resolution

Ultrasonographic Findings
- Hypoechoic areas in soft tissues attaching to medial epicondyle
- Instability on valgus stressing with ligament injuries
- Hyperechoic separated fragments and soft tissue calcification

Imaging Recommendations
- Best imaging tool
  - o Acute phase: AP radiograph
  - o Static and dynamic ultrasound +/- therapeutic injection
  - o Full assessment = MR in coronal and axial planes
- Protocol advice: T1/PD + FS PD FSE in all three planes

DIFFERENTIAL DIAGNOSIS

Capitellar Osteochondritis (OCD)
- Necrosis of bone followed by healing response and reossification
- Lateral elbow
- 12-16 year age group (after ossification of capitellum)
- 20% bilateral
- Chronic valgus stress with lateral impaction seen in gymnasts and adolescent pitchers

Medial/Lateral Epicondylitis
- Overuse tendinopathy
- Medial epicondylitis often component of little league elbow
- Lateral epicondylitis = tennis elbow
- Failure of underlying collateral ligament
- Hyperintense tendons on T2WI

MCL Sprain
- Affects primarily anterior band of MCL
- Common with little league elbow
- +/- Acute valgus stress
  - o MCL + flexor pronator avulsion = medial blowout
- Often chronic repetitive microtrauma
- Proximal, mid-ligament or distal tears

Stress Fracture
- May affect different bones in elbow (esp. olecranon)
- Chronic repetitive microtrauma
- Abnormal stresses on normal bone
- Stress response - pre-fracture stress phenomenon

Ulnar Neuritis
- Often accompanies medial epicondylitis and little leaguer's elbow
- Traction/overuse neurapraxia in throwers
- +/- Anconeus epitrochlearis
- +/- Ulnar/humeral osteophytes
- Hyperintense on T2WI +/- swelling
  - o Normal ulnar nerve is intermediate on FS PD FSE signal

Muscle Strain
- Muscle fiber tearing
- Typically at myotendinous junction
- Hyperintense on T2WI
- +/- Intramuscular hematoma

PATHOLOGY

General Features
- General path comments

LITTLE LEAGUER'S ELBOW

- Relevant anatomy
  - Valgus stress is resisted by the medial collateral ligament complex
  - Anterior bundle - most important
  - Posterior bundle
  - Transverse ligament
  - Static support is given by the ulnohumeral joint and radial head
  - Excessive valgus stress
- Etiology
  - Repetitive throwing motion
    - Baseball pitch
    - Tennis serve
    - Javelin throw
    - Football pass
  - Acute valgus stress less common than repetitive throwing motion
- Epidemiology
  - Highest incidence in the 5-14 year age group
  - Overuse injuries 30-50% of all elbow injuries
  - Increased incidence with family history of osteochondritis
- Associated abnormalities
  - Capitellar osteochondritis
  - Radial head osteochondrosis
  - Olecranon apophysitis
  - MCL sprain
  - Ulnar hypertrophy
  - Olecranon osteophytosis

Gross Pathologic & Surgical Features
- Childhood injury pattern (pre-fusion) is microtrauma to apophysis and ossification center for medial epicondyle
- Adolescent pattern = avulsion of medial epicondyle +/- nonunion
- Adult pattern = ligament avulsions and muscle strains

Microscopic Features
- Irregular ossification of medial epicondyle apophysis
- Disruption of collagen fibrils in medial ligament complex and common flexor origin
- Increased number of fibroblasts
- Increased number of osteoblasts and osteoclasts

Staging, Grading or Classification Criteria
- Type 1 avulsions = entire apophysis separates and rotates
- Type 2 avulsions = smaller 'flake' avulsion in more mature bone

CLINICAL ISSUES

Presentation
- Most common signs/symptoms
  - Pain localized to medial epicondyle
  - Pain may also involve posterior and lateral aspects
  - Loss of range of motion
  - Flexion contracture
  - Recent change in activity patterns
- Clinical profile: Throwing athlete, often children

Demographics
- Age: Children through adults

- Gender: M:F = 6:1 (mainly reflects sports)

Natural History & Prognosis
- May heal with cessation of valgus stress overload (medial tension)
- Prognosis
  - Depends on expert rehabilitation
  - After rest, gradual build up of throwing activity over 3 weeks
    - Cessation if symptoms return
  - Most cases recover well
  - Late osteoarthritis (OA) and deformities occur in both under treated and appropriately treated cases

Treatment
- Conservative: Rest, ice, temporary splinting, training modification
- Surgical
  - Closed reduction or open repair with internal fixation
  - MCL injury (less common in young throwing athletes) is treated with reconstruction using a tendon graft with anterior submuscular transposition of the ulnar nerve
- Complications: Instability, early osteoarthritis, epicondylar under/overgrowth giving varus and valgus deformities

DIAGNOSTIC CHECKLIST

Consider
- Avulsion/entrapment of apophysis in unfused skeleton
- Presence of lateral pathology (OCD)
- Ulnar neuropathy
- Ligament damage

Image Interpretation Pearls
- AP radiograph
- MR
  - FS PD FSE to identify subchondral marrow edema and signal changes in the adjacent flexor pronator origin
  - Coronal images demonstrate the medial tension injury with widening and fragmentation of the medial epicondylar ossification center
- Static/dynamic ultrasound

SELECTED REFERENCES

1. Klingele KE et al: Little league elbow. Valgus overload injury in the paediatric athlete. Sports Med 32(15):1005-15, 2002
2. Sofka CM et al: Imaging of elbow injuries in the child and adult athlete. Radiol Clin North Am 40(2):251-65, 2002
3. Farsetti P et al: Long-term results of treatment of fractures of the medial humeral epicondyle in children. J Bone Joint Surg Am 83-A(9):1299-305, 2001
4. Grana W: Medial epicondylitis and cubital tunnel syndrome in the throwing athlete. Clin Sports Med 20(3:541-8, 2001

IMAGE GALLERY

Typical

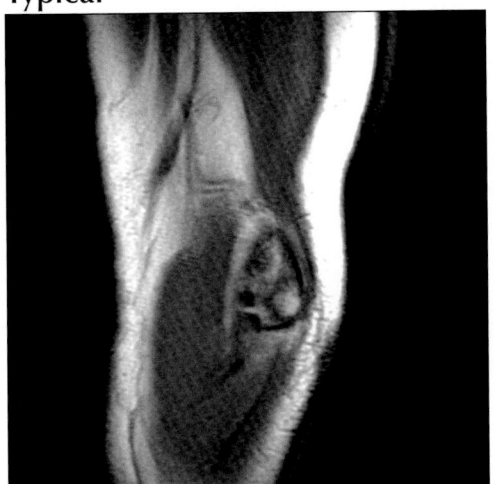 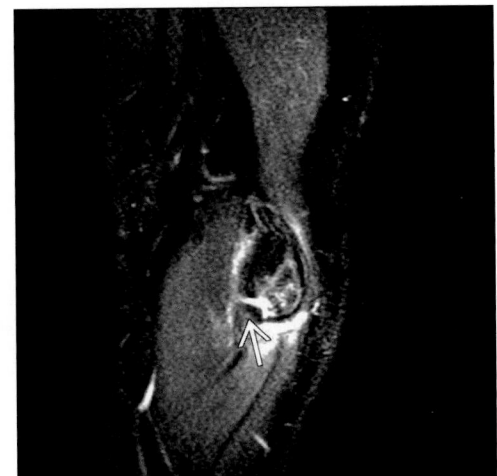

(Left) Sagittal PD FSE MR shows partial avulsion of the medial epicondyle in a symptomatic young baseball pitcher. *(Right)* Sagittal STIR MR shows avulsion of the medial epicondyle (arrow) with surrounding edema extending into the flexor pronator muscle origin.

Typical

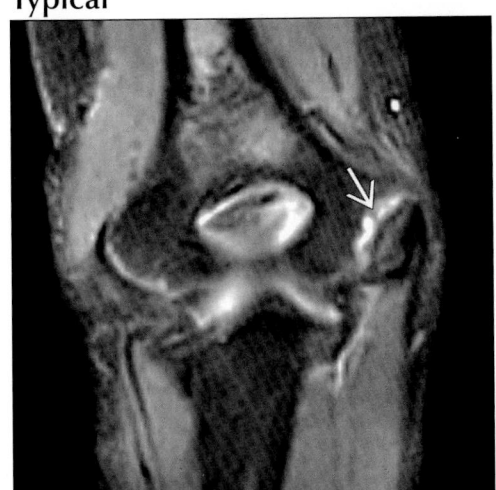 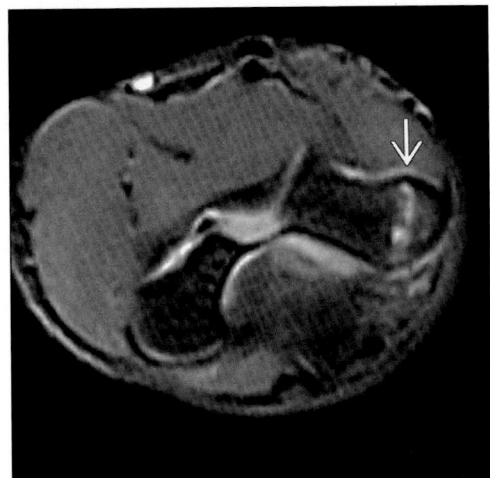

(Left) Coronal FS PD shows avulsion of the medial epicondyle (arrow) in a little league pitcher, consistent with little leaguer's elbow. *(Right)* Axial FS PD FSE MR shows increased signal intensity at the base of the medial epicondyle (arrow) representing a medial epicondylar epiphyseal stress fx.

Typical

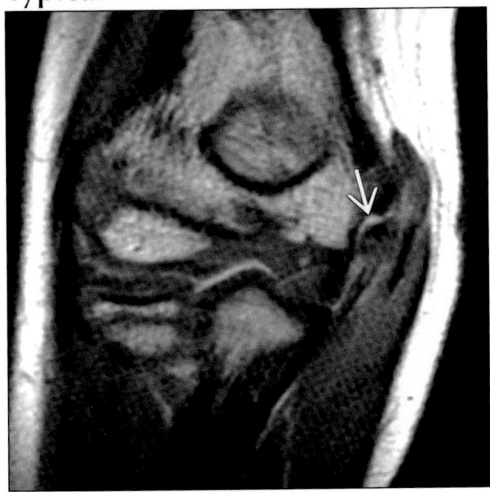 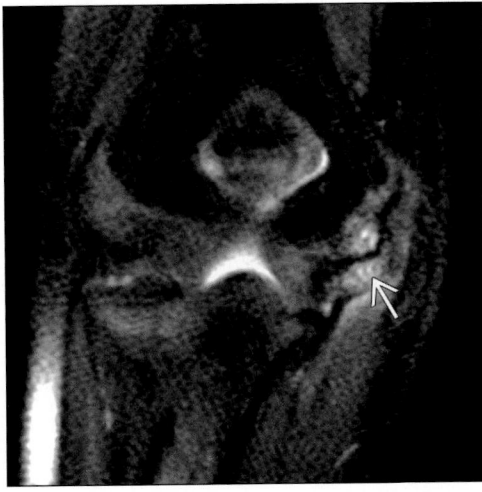

(Left) Coronal PD FSE MR shows partial avulsion of the medial epicondyle (arrow) with strain of the flexor pronator origin. *(Right)* Coronal STIR MR shows a tear of the proximal aspect of the medial collateral ligament (arrow) with surrounding edema and subchondral changes of the medial epicondyle in a patient with little leaguer's elbow.

ULNAR NEUROPATHY

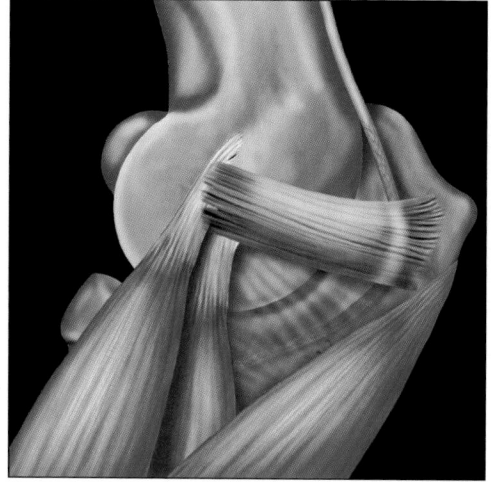

Sagittal graphic shows an inflamed ulnar nerve traversing deep to the cubital tunnel retinaculum.

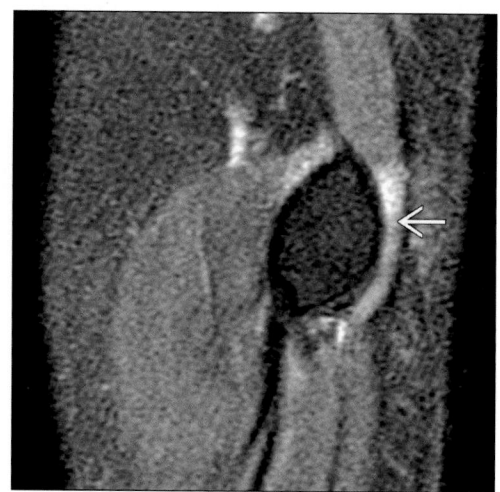

Sagittal FS PD FSE MR shows an inflamed hyperintense ulnar nerve (arrow) posteriorly in a patient with ulnar neuritis. The focal area of the signal abnormality indicates neuritis.

TERMINOLOGY

Abbreviations and Synonyms
- Cubital tunnel syndrome (CTS), cubital tunnel retinaculum (CTR)

Definitions
- Compression of the ulnar nerve within the cubital tunnel at the level of the elbow

IMAGING FINDINGS

General Features
- Best diagnostic clue
  - Thickening and increased signal intensity of the ulnar nerve
  - Patient with clinical evidence of ulnar neuropathy
- Location: Occurs most commonly at the level of the cubital tunnel of the elbow
- Size
  - The nerve is normally flattened to oval shaped and mildly increased in signal on FS PD FSE/T2WI
    - Asymptomatic
  - Neuropathy - nerve swollen, edematous, increased in size
- Morphology
  - +/- Swelling

- Nerve flattening: Mass compression
- Traumatic injury : +/- Severing, discontinuity

Radiographic Findings
- Radiography
  - +/- Soft tissue swelling at level of cubital tunnel
  - +/- Soft tissue mass
    - +/- Anconeus epitrochlearis

CT Findings
- NECT
  - Fatty atrophy of affected muscles in chronic cases
    - Decreased attenuation
  - +/- Soft tissue mass
  - +/- Anconeus epitrochlearis
- CECT
  - +/- Enhancement of nerve
  - +/- Synovial enhancement in cases of synovitis

MR Findings
- T1WI
  - Displacement, flattening, or thickening of the nerve
  - Thickened cubital tunnel retinaculum
  - +/- Anconeus epitrochlearis
    - Normal muscle signal intensity
  - +/- Hypointense mass
  - Osteophytes with marrow fat signal
  - +/- Intermediate to mildly hyperintense synovial mass/synovitis

---

DDx: Ulnar Neuropathy

Prom Med Triceps	Prom Med Triceps	Leprosy	Epicondylitis	UN Transposition
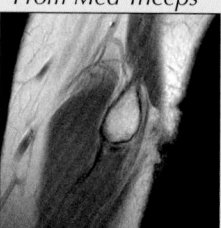	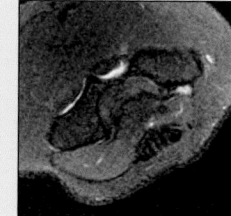	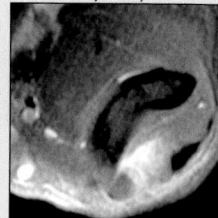	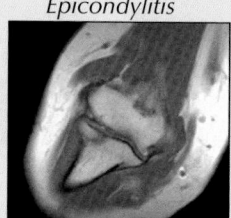	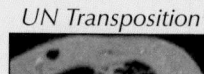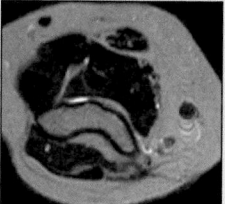
Sag PD FSE MR	Ax FS PD FSE MR	Ax FS T1C+ MR	Cor PD FSE MR	Ax T2 FSE MR

ULNAR NEUROPATHY

Key Facts

Terminology
- Compression of the ulnar nerve within the cubital tunnel at the level of the elbow

Imaging Findings
- Thickening and increased signal intensity of the ulnar nerve
- Location: Occurs most commonly at the level of the cubital tunnel of the elbow

Top Differential Diagnoses
- Enlarged Perineural Veins
- Increased Signal Intensity Nerve in Normal Cases
- Brachial Plexitis/Parsonage-Turner Syndrome
- Prominent Medial Head of Triceps
- Leprosy
- Medial Epicondylitis

Pathology
- Subject to entrapment and injury by a wide variety of causes
- Mass compression of the nerve or as the result of a posttraumatic neurapraxia

Clinical Issues
- Severe pain at elbow or wrist with radiation into hand or up into the shoulder and neck
- Athletes with medial epicondylitis and pain and paresthesias in ulnar nerve distribution
- Age: Most commonly seen in adults

Diagnostic Checklist
- Identify anconeus epitrochlearis or prominent medial head of triceps

- T2WI
  - Mass lesion with proximal swelling of the nerve
    - Fat saturated images (FS PD FSE)
  - Increased signal intensity of the nerve (FS PD FSE)
  - +/- Anconeus epitrochlearis
    - Muscle signal intensity on T2WI
  - +/- Hyperintense mass
  - Nerve enlarged with leprosy
- PD/Intermediate
  - Excellent spatial resolution
  - Visualize synovitis/synovial mass
    - Intermediate to hyperintense synovial thickening
    - Relative to hypointense fluid
- STIR
  - Similar contrast as FS PD FSE except less spatial resolution
  - Improved for low mid field
- T1 C+
  - +/- Enhancing nerve
  - +/- Enhancing compressing mass
  - +/- Perineural enhancement with inflammation

Imaging Recommendations
- Best imaging tool: MRI
- Protocol advice: FS PD FSE demonstrates signal abnormality of the nerve and associated compressing mass

DIFFERENTIAL DIAGNOSIS

Enlarged Perineural Veins
- Contain hypointense flow void
- Common in cubital tunnel
- Increased venous pressure

Increased Signal Intensity Nerve in Normal Cases
- Pathologic nerve is of greater increased signal intensity on T2WI
  - Fat saturated images (FS PD FSE) sensitive to neural edema
- +/- Thickening of pathologic nerve

Brachial Plexitis/Parsonage-Turner Syndrome
- Other nerves/muscles most often involved
- +/- Viral prodrome
- Pain followed by weakness
- Rare distal form: Shoulder girdle muscles

Prominent Medial Head of Triceps
- Cause of nerve compression
- Rare
- +/- Hyperintensity on T2WI: Stress myositis

Leprosy
- Hansen's bacillus
- Enlarged nerve
- +/- Calcification
- Distal wasting

Medial Epicondylitis
- Chronic valgus stress
- Throwers, golfer's elbow
- +/- MCL tear
- +/- Hyperintensity in flexor pronator muscle belly
- Chronic repetitive microtrauma

PATHOLOGY

General Features
- General path comments
  - Relevant anatomy
    - Ulnar nerve - in anterior compartment of proximal arm, along medial intermuscular septum
    - Ulnar nerve enters posterior compartment: Mid humerus, through medial intermuscular septum at arcade of Struthers
    - Ulnar nerve passes distally: Posterior aspect medial intermuscular septum, deep into Osborne's fascia, enters cubital tunnel
    - Distal to cubital tunnel - Ulnar nerve passes between two heads of flexor carpi ulnaris (FCU) muscle (most frequent site of compression)

ULNAR NEUROPATHY

- Cubital tunnel bordered: Anteriorly - medial epicondyle, laterally - olecranon process, posteriorly - Osborne's fascia
  - Subject to entrapment and injury by a wide variety of causes
  - Compression, traction, friction, or direct trauma
- Etiology
  - Mass compression of the nerve or as the result of a posttraumatic neurapraxia
  - Commonly caused by a thickened cubital tunnel retinaculum (Osborne's ligament)
    - Results in dynamic compression during flexion
  - Ulnar neurapraxia often secondary to repeated valgus stress injury and medial epicondylitis (athletes)
  - Throwing athletes
    - Chronic ulnar nerve traction injury
    - Increase ulnar nerve pressure with elbow flexion/wrist extension & with arm in the cocking position of a throw
    - Flexor carpi ulnaris generates compressive force
  - Other causes of compression
    - Intermuscular septum: Arcade of Struthers (musculofascial band 5-8 cms proximal to medial epicondyle)
    - Medial intermuscular septum
    - Fascia of FCU heads
    - Medial head of the triceps muscle
    - Malunion of condylar fracture, nonunion of condylar fracture, epiphyseal injury to the lateral side of the elbow may cause chronic neurapraxia
    - Congenitally shallow groove or dysfunctional or absent retinaculum +/- subluxation and dysfunction
- Epidemiology
  - 22% of population suffers from dynamic compression during flexion in association with a thickened cubital tunnel retinaculum
  - 10% of population suffers from static compression in association with an anomalous muscle, the anconeus epitrochlearis
  - Second most common entrapment neuropathy in the upper extremity (after median)
- Associated abnormalities: Anconeus epitrochlearis

Gross Pathologic & Surgical Features
- Edematous/indurated nerve often surrounded by fibrous stranding
- Heterotopic ossification or other mass may be found compressing the nerve
- Anconeus epitrochlearis may be found in place of the cubital tunnel retinaculum

Microscopic Features
- Edematous nerve with variable numbers of inflammatory cells

Staging, Grading or Classification Criteria
- Three stages of nerve injury
  - Neurapraxia: Transient (failure of conduction)
    - No disruption of the nerve or its sheath occurs
  - Axonotmesis: Disruption of axon and myelin sheath with preservation of connective tissues
    - Motor, sensory, and autonomic paralysis results

- Regeneration of axon
  - Neurotmesis: Nerve, myelin sheath and connective tissue elements are severed
    - Regeneration does not occur

CLINICAL ISSUES

Presentation
- Most common signs/symptoms
  - Ranges from transient paraesthesias in ring and small fingers to clawing of these digits and severe intrinsic muscle atrophy
  - Severe pain at elbow or wrist with radiation into hand or up into the shoulder and neck
- Clinical profile
  - Adult or child with pain and paresthesias in forearm in the ulnar nerve distribution
  - Athletes with medial epicondylitis and pain and paresthesias in ulnar nerve distribution

Demographics
- Age: Most commonly seen in adults
- Gender: F ≥ M

Natural History & Prognosis
- Return to normal function with adequate decompression
- Chronic compression associated with pain, muscle weakness, and/or atrophy, outcome favorable

Treatment
- Physical therapy
- Removal of osteophyte or anconeus if paresthesias present
- Decompression in situ - relief almost immediate but may not be as favorable prognosis
- Nerve transposition - favorable prognosis after healing of post operative swelling

DIAGNOSTIC CHECKLIST

Image Interpretation Pearls
- Identify anconeus epitrochlearis or prominent medial head of triceps

SELECTED REFERENCES

1. Miller MD et al: Surgical Atlas of Sports Medicine. Philadelphia PA, Saunders, 407-12, 2003
2. Chen FS et al: Medial elbow problems in the overhead-throwing athlete. J Am Acad Orthop Surg 9(2):99-113, 2001
3. Ciccotti MG: Medial collateral ligament instability and ulnar neuritis in the athlete's elbow. Instr Course Lect 48:383-91, 1999

ULNAR NEUROPATHY

IMAGE GALLERY

Typical

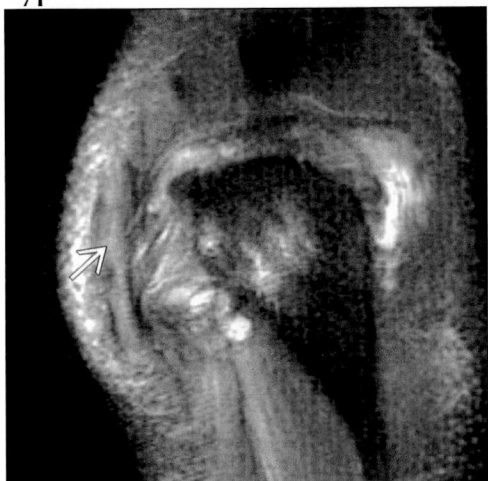 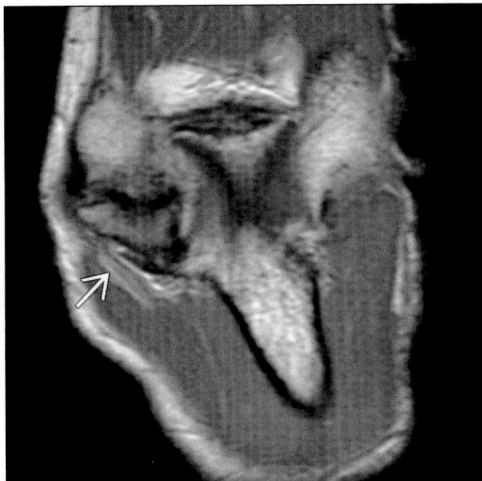

(Left) Coronal STIR MR shows an inflamed synovial mass posteromedially displacing an inflamed ulnar nerve medially (arrow). *(Right)* Coronal PD FSE shows a traction spur of the medial aspect of the ulna adjacent to a slightly displaced ulnar nerve (arrow) in a patient with clinical ulnar neuritis.

Typical

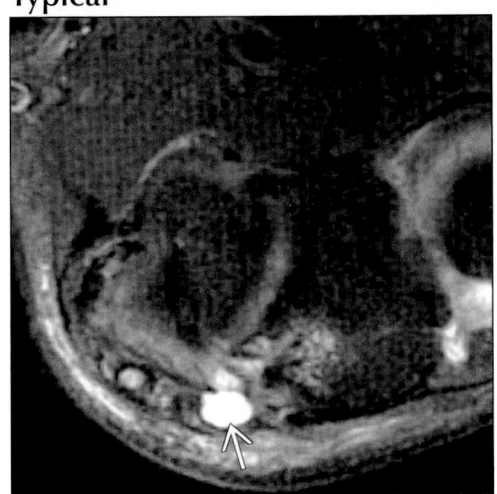 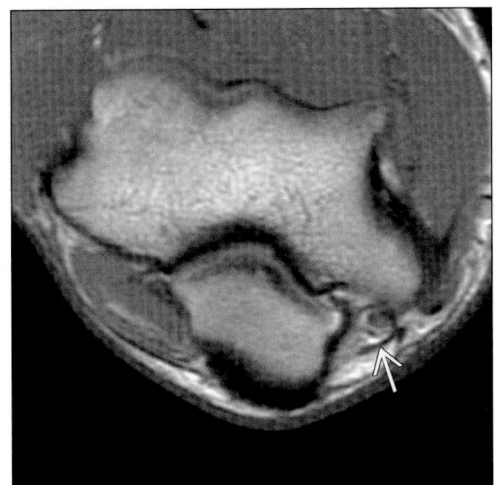

(Left) Axial FS PD FSE MR shows synovitis (arrow) in the posteromedial aspect of the joint in a patient with a chronic medial condylar fracture. There is mass effect on the nerve. *(Right)* Axial PD FSE MR shows scarring of the retinaculum (arrow) in a patient with clinical ulnar neuritis.

Typical

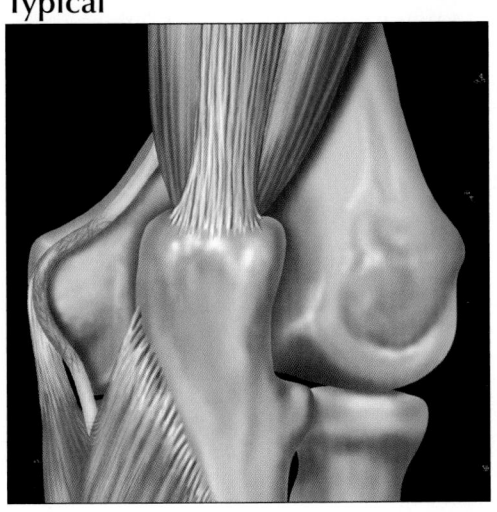 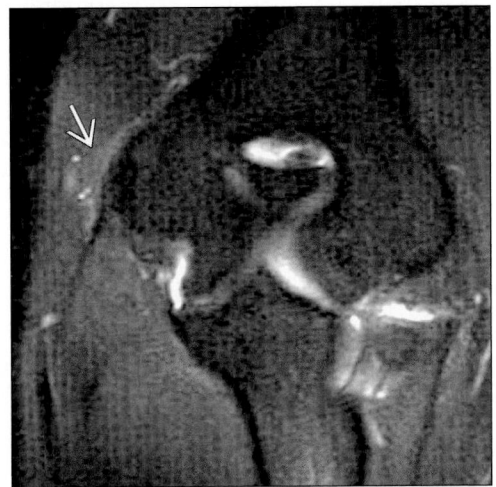

(Left) Coronal graphic shows subluxation of ulnar nerve with ulnar neuritis. These patients usually have an absent medial retinaculum. *(Right)* Coronal STIR MR shows an inflamed ulnar nerve (arrow) with subluxation to the peripheral aspect of the medial epicondyle.

RADIAL NEUROPATHY

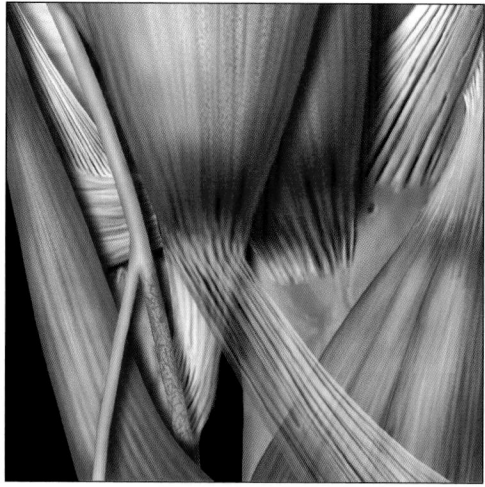

Coronal graphic shows inflamed radial N adjacent to biceps tendon. Deep branch pierces supinator, becomes posterior interosseous N. Fibrous arcade of Frohse = potential entrapment site.

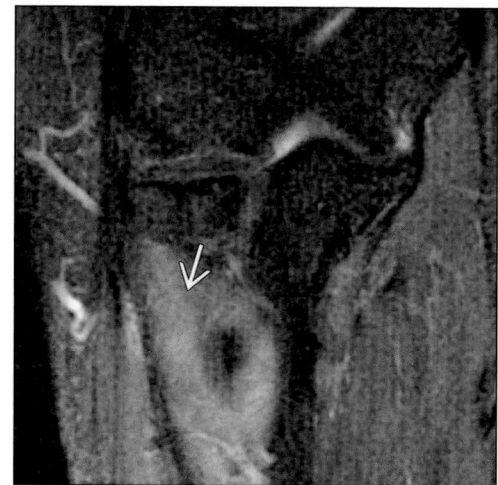

Coronal FS PD FSE MR shows increased signal intensity within the supinator muscle (arrow) and the proximal extensor muscle belly in a patient with proven high radial neuropathy.

TERMINOLOGY

Abbreviations and Synonyms
- Radial neuropathy (RN), RN entrapment syndrome, posterior interosseous nerve (PIN) syndrome

Definitions
- Compression syndrome of the radial nerve
  - Including the supinator, triceps, anconeus brachioradialis, extensor carpi radialis longus, extensor digitorum communis, extensor indicis, extensor digiti quinti (minimi), extensor carpi ulnaris, abductor pollicis longus and extensor pollicis brevis muscle bellies
  - Sensory disturbance of the dorsal and radial aspects of the wrist indicating the entrapment or compression occurred before the split into the superficial and deep components at the level of the supinator muscle
  - No sensory disturbance with posterior interosseous compression alone

IMAGING FINDINGS

General Features
- Best diagnostic clue

  - Denervation findings in all or some of the muscles supplied by the radial nerve
    - Diffuse increased signal intensity on T2 or proton density fat saturated images with or without atrophy changes
  - PIN syndrome - denervation findings in all or some of the muscles supplied by the posterior interosseous nerve
- Location
  - Entrapment neuropathy usually occurring proximal to the elbow most commonly by a fibrous arch of the long head of the triceps or the lateral head of the triceps
  - Entrapped by humeral fracture and callus formation (Holstein-Lewis fracture)
    - High radial lesion (before takeoff of PIN)
- Size: Affected muscles may be atrophic
- Morphology: Usually fibrous entrapment of the long head or the lateral head of the triceps, mass compression or traumatic injury to nerve less commonly

MR Findings
- T1WI: Fibrosis (streaky hypointense signal intensity on all pulse sequences) at the arcade of Frohse entrapment site
- T2WI

DDx: Radial Neuropathy

Lat Epicondylitis	AI Neuropathy	Pronator Syndrome	Pronator Syndrome	Ulnar Neuropathy

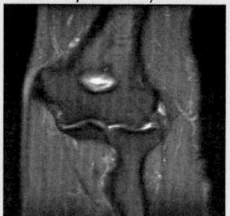 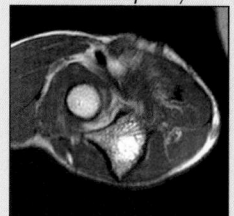 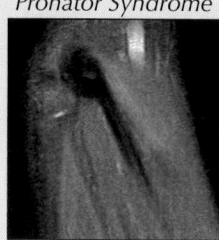 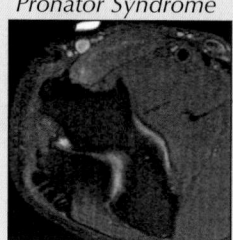 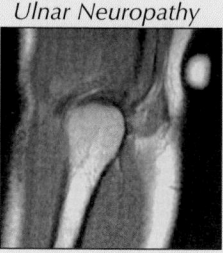

Cor FS PD FSE	Ax PD FSE MR	Sag FS PD FSE	Ax FS PD FSE	Cor PD FSE MR

RADIAL NEUROPATHY

Key Facts

Imaging Findings
- Denervation findings in all or some of the muscles supplied by the radial nerve
- Diffuse increased signal intensity on FS PD FSE in all or some of the muscles supplied by PIN (indicating denervation)
- Reduced muscle belly size +/- fatty infiltration indicating atrophy

Top Differential Diagnoses
- Nonspecific Myositis/Trauma
- Median Neuropathy
- Recalcitrant Lateral Epicondylitis

Pathology
- High radial lesion - entrapment neuropathy occurring proximal to the elbow

- Entrapment neuropathy occurring distal to elbow
- Epidemiology: Rare

Clinical Issues
- A high radial lesion will lead to functional loss of
- Accessory forearm supination (supinator), flexion (brachioradialis), wrist digital extension
- Radial: 2/3 dorsal sensation/abduction of thumb
- Clinical profile: After fracture or with muscle hypertrophy

Diagnostic Checklist
- In patient with abrupt weakness or total paralysis in distribution of PIN
- Identify muscle groups with high signal on FS PD FSE in distribution of radial nerve

---

- ○ Diffuse increased signal intensity on FS PD FSE in all or some of the muscles supplied by PIN (indicating denervation)
- ○ Reduced muscle belly size +/- fatty infiltration indicating atrophy
- STIR: Increased signal in muscle with denervation
- T1 C+: +/- Muscle enhancement with denervation

Imaging Recommendations
- Best imaging tool: MRI
- Protocol advice
  - ○ FS PD FSE shows the increased muscle signal to best advantage
  - ○ T1WI demonstrates the interstitial fatty tissues as fat signal intensity

DIFFERENTIAL DIAGNOSIS

Nonspecific Myositis/Trauma
- Muscle signal increase on FS PD FSE and muscle dysfunction
- Trauma with asymmetric muscle involvement

Median Neuropathy
- Anterior interosseous syndrome (AIN syndrome)
  - ○ Abrupt weakness or total paralysis of flexor pollicis longus and usually profundus tendon to index finger
  - ○ Median branch
- Pronator syndrome - little weakness or sensory loss

Recalcitrant Lateral Epicondylitis
- Tenderness located over the lateral epicondyle not radial nerve as in compression neuropathy
- Constant aching pain at the arcade of Frohse and difficulty with writing

Ulnar Neuropathy
- +/- Anconeus epitrochlearis
- Hyperintensity of nerve +/- increased diameter on FS PD FSE

PATHOLOGY

General Features
- General path comments
  - ○ Relevant anatomy (PIN & potential sites of compression)
    - Radial nerve (RN) between brachialis & brachioradialis at cubital fossa
    - RN divides in superficial & PIN branches at elbow
    - PIN enters radial tunnel proximal to radiocapitellar (RC) joint
    - Fascia superficial to PIN anterior to RC joint
    - Leash of Henry (radial recurrent artery & venae comitantes)
    - PIN deep to fibrous edge extensor carpi radialis brevis (ECRB)
    - PIN passes through arcade of Frohse (tendinous origin of supinator)
    - Fascial bands at exit from supinator distally
  - ○ Entrapment or neuritis
  - ○ Radial nerve splits at the level of the supinator muscle with the deep branch becoming the PIN
    - After exiting the muscle, the nerve passes beneath the fibrous arcade of Frohse where it can become entrapped
  - ○ PIN - compression after take off of the branches to the radial wrist extensors and the radial sensory nerve
    - Paralysis of digital extensors and dorsoradial deviation of the wrist due to paralysis of the ECU
  - ○ Compression of lateral branch
    - Paralysis of the abductor pollicis longus, extensor pollicis brevis, extensor pollicis longus, and extensor indicis
  - ○ Compression of medial branch
    - Paralysis of ECU, extensor digiti quinti, and extensor digitorum communis
  - ○ Radial tunnel syndrome - controversial, thought to be a result of overuse
    - May represent early posterior interosseous nerve syndrome
    - Diagnosis based on subjective symptoms

RADIAL NEUROPATHY

- Etiology
  - High radial lesion - entrapment neuropathy occurring proximal to the elbow
    - Most commonly by a fibrous arch of the long head or the lateral head of the triceps
    - Humeral diaphyseal fracture
    - Weakness of supination
  - Entrapment neuropathy occurring distal to elbow
    - Most commonly arcade of Frohse fibrous entrapment (PIN syndrome)
    - Exit from the supinator muscle
    - Fracture dislocation humeral shaft - Holstein-Lewis fracture
    - Fracture dislocation (especially Monteggia fx)
    - Mass (lipomas or ganglions)
- Epidemiology: Rare

Gross Pathologic & Surgical Features
- Swollen muscle belly - early and subacute

Microscopic Features
- Enlarged extracellular fluid space = early and subacute
- Fatty infiltration = chronic
- Myofibrils atrophy and become small and angular early denervation

Staging, Grading or Classification Criteria
- Two syndromes associated with PIN
  - Posterior interosseous nerve syndrome: Loss of motor function to muscles innervated by PIN (electrophysiologic studies usually diagnostic)
  - Radial tunnel syndrome (RTS): Vague forearm pain without motor function loss & associated with lateral epicondylitis (limited objective findings in radial tunnel syndrome in contrast to PIN syndrome)
- 3 Stages of nerve injury
  - Neurapraxia = transient episode of motor paralysis with little or no sensory or autonomic dysfunction
  - Axonotmesis = more severe nerve injury with disruption of the axon and myelin sheath but with preservation of connective tissues
  - Neurotmesis = nerve, myelin sheath, and connective tissue elements are severed

CLINICAL ISSUES

Presentation
- Most common signs/symptoms
  - A high radial lesion will lead to functional loss of
    - Accessory forearm supination (supinator), flexion (brachioradialis), wrist digital extension
    - Radial: 2/3 dorsal sensation/abduction of thumb
  - Radial tunnel syndrome - pain over the anterolateral proximal forearm in the region of the radial neck without weakness or sensory deficit
  - PINS - inability to extend the metacarpal phalangeal joints of the thumb and fingers + radial deviation of the wrist with extension
  - Wartenberg's syndrome - pain over distal radial forearm associated with paresthesias over dorsal radial hand

- Wrist movement or when tightly pinching the thumb and index digit may increase symptoms
  - Positive Tinel's sign over the radial sensory nerve + local tenderness
- Clinical profile: After fracture or with muscle hypertrophy

Demographics
- Age: Children/adults
- Gender: M > F

Natural History & Prognosis
- Surgical treatment of PIN syndrome more reliable than RTS
- Usually progressive and requires surgical decompression
- Excellent if signs of recovery occur within six months
- Good results in recalcitrant cases after surgery

Treatment
- Conservative
  - Typically surgical treatment is required
- Surgical
  - Vessels or fibrous bands at the arcade of Frohse are released and the arcade is divided if tight
  - Supinator tunnel may be widened if necessary
- Complications
  - Nerve injury, hematoma, other complications of surgery

DIAGNOSTIC CHECKLIST

Consider
- In patient with abrupt weakness or total paralysis in distribution of PIN

Image Interpretation Pearls
- Identify muscle groups with high signal on FS PD FSE in distribution of radial nerve

SELECTED REFERENCES

1. Miller MD et al: Surgical atlas of sports medicine. Philadelphia PA, Saunders, 407-12, 2003
2. Dickerman RD et al: Radial tunnel syndrome in an elite power athlete: A case of direct compressive neuropathy. J Peripher Nerv Syst 7(4):229-32, 2002
3. Chen WS et al: Posterior interosseous neuropathy associated with tuberculous arthritis of the elbow joint: Report of two cases. J Hand Surg Am 19(4):611-3, 1994

RADIAL NEUROPATHY

IMAGE GALLERY

Typical

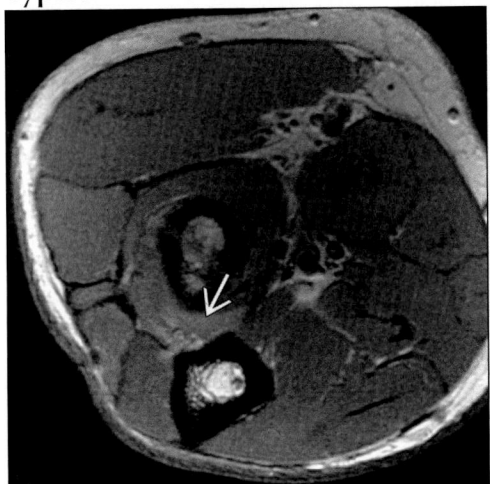 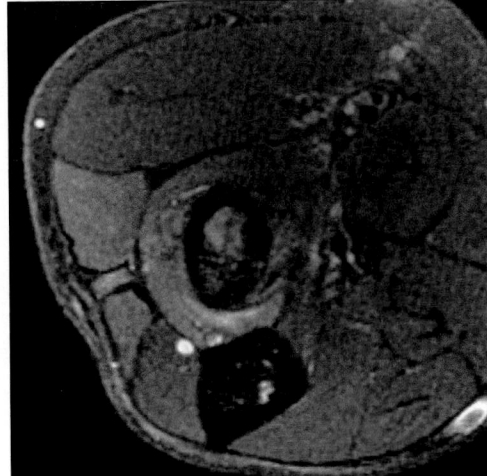

(**Left**) Axial PD FSE MR shows hyperintensity within the supinator and extensor muscle bellies (arrow) in a patient with post surgical radial neuropathy. There are post-surgical changes of biceps repair. (**Right**) Axial FS PD FSE in the same patient shows increased signal intensity within the denervated muscles. The neuropathy was post-surgical but the patient regained function.

Typical

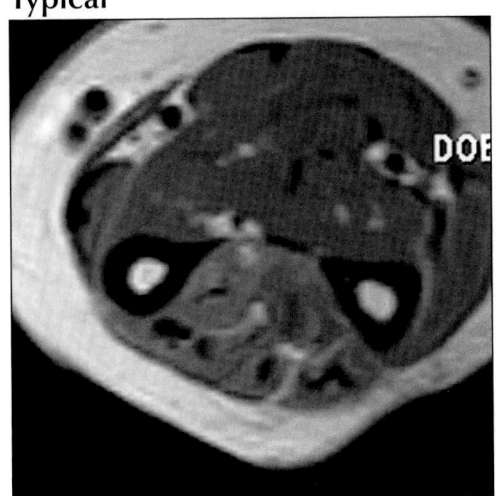 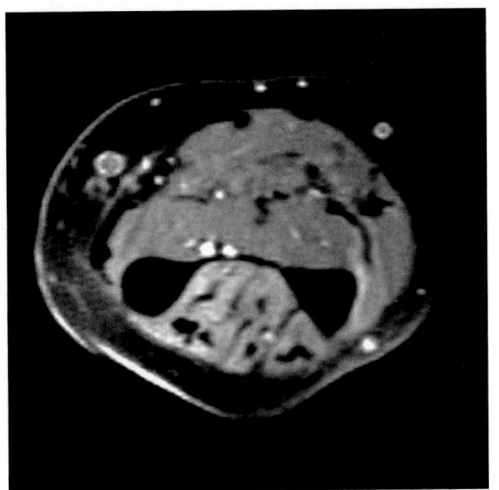

(**Left**) Axial PD FSE MR shows increased signal intensity within the extensor muscle bellies in a patient with posterior interosseous syndrome. (**Right**) Axial STIR MR of the same patient shows the denervation changes.

Typical

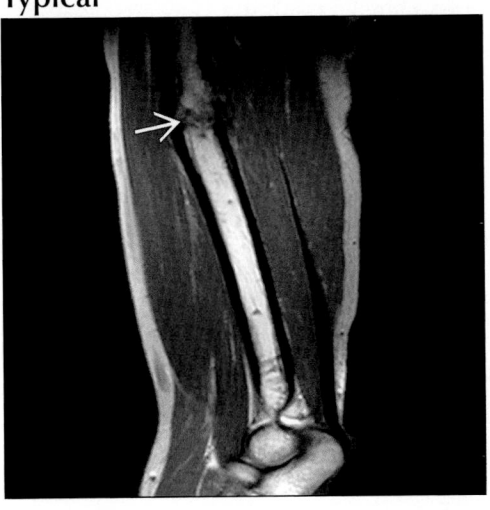 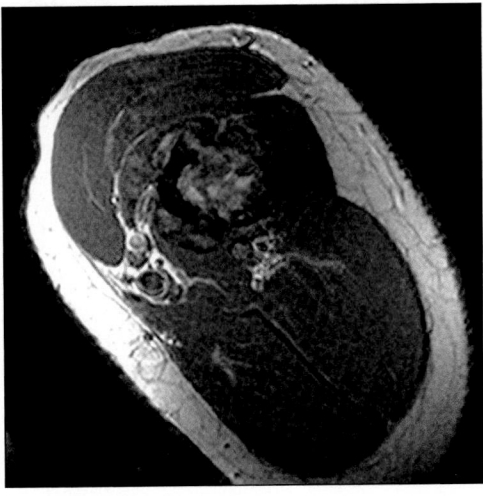

(**Left**) Sagittal PD/Intermediate MR shows a fracture (arrow) of the mid humerus with developing callus formation in a patient with radial neuropathy at the spiral groove level. (**Right**) Axial PD/Intermediate MR in the same patient shows the mass effect on area structures by the developing callus. This patient had radial neuropathy with paralysis of the hand extensors.

MEDIAN NEUROPATHY

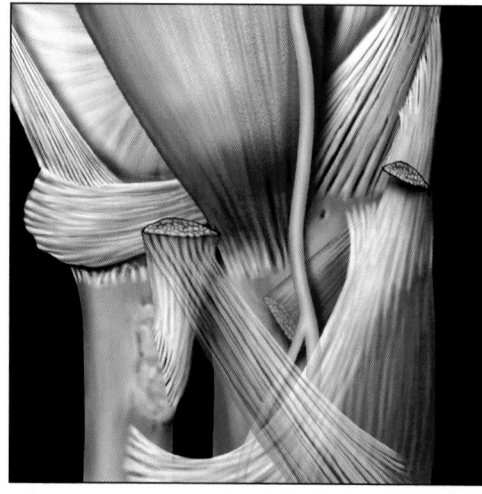

Coronal graphic shows median nerve passing through the antecubital fossa deep to the lacertus fibrosus adjacent to long head of the biceps tendon.

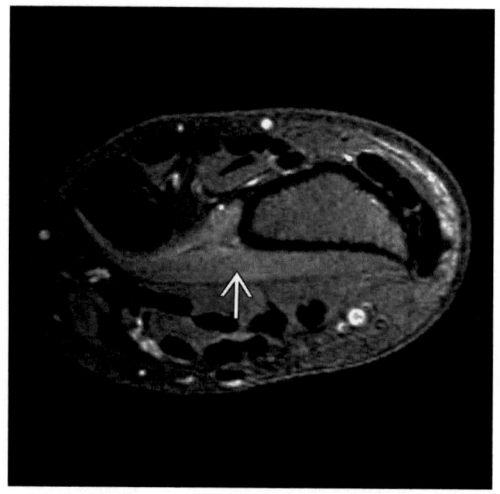

Axial FS PD FSE MR shows denervation changes within the pronator quadratus (arrow) muscle at the wrist. This often indicates anterior interosseous nerve syndrome.

TERMINOLOGY

Abbreviations and Synonyms
- Anterior interosseous nerve syndrome (AINS)
  - Kiloh-Nevin syndrome
- Pronator syndrome (PS)

Definitions
- AINS - denervation of flexor pollicis longus and profundus flexor to second and third digits
  - +/- Pronator quadratus muscle
- Pronator syndrome
  - Motor nerve involvement rare
  - Sensory symptoms +/- paresthesias in median nerve distribution

IMAGING FINDINGS

General Features
- Best diagnostic clue: Denervation findings in affected muscles
- Location
  - Compression/injury at
    - Level of the humeral shaft (Holstein-Lewis fracture)
    - Humeral supracondylar process/ligament of Struthers

- Pronator teres
- Size: Affected muscles may be atrophic
- Morphology
  - +/- Mass compression
    - Mass identified on MR, CT, ultrasound

Radiographic Findings
- Radiography
  - +/- Supracondylar process compression for proximal lesion
  - +/- Humeral fracture

CT Findings
- NECT
  - +/- Supracondylar process visualized on sagittal reconstruction
  - +/- Humeral fracture adjacent to nerve

MR Findings
- T1WI
  - Fatty atrophy of affected muscles - chronic cases
  - +/- Hypointense fracture of humerus
  - +/- Angulation/callus
- T2WI
  - Affected muscle shows diffuse increased signal intensity
  - Flexor pollicis longus and profundus flexor to index finger swelling/hyperintensity
  - +/- Findings in pronator quadratus

DDx: Median Neuropathy

PQ Strain	PQ Strain	Flexor Strain	High Radial Atrop	PIN Syndrome

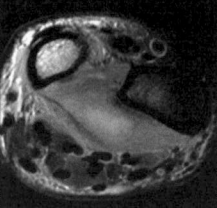 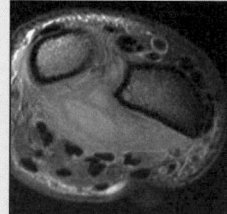 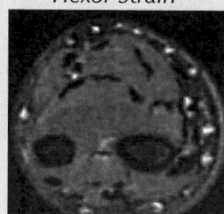 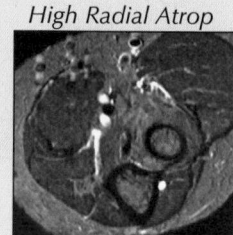 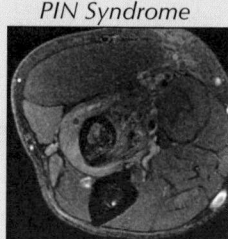

Ax FS PD FSE	Ax FS PD FSE MR	Ax STIR MR	Ax FS PD FSE	Ax FS PD FSE MR

MEDIAN NEUROPATHY

Key Facts

Terminology
- Anterior interosseous nerve syndrome (AINS)
- Pronator syndrome (PS)

Imaging Findings
- Affected muscle shows diffuse increased signal intensity
- Flexor pollicis longus and profundus flexor to index finger swelling/hyperintensity
- +/- Findings in pronator quadratus

Top Differential Diagnoses
- C6/7 Radiculopathy
- Flexor Superficialis Crossover Syndrome
- Brachial Neuritis/Parsonage-Turner Distal Form
- Radial Neuropathy
- Muscle Trauma

Pathology
- AINS: Motor loss without sensory loss
- Pronator syndrome: Entrapment syndrome of median nerve with similar etiology than AINS but different clinical picture
- Three types of median nerve compression (compression at elbow occurs as either AINS or PS)

Clinical Issues
- Pain along the course of median nerve

Diagnostic Checklist
- FS PD FSE or STIR are sensitive for muscle signal intensity changes; identify appropriate muscle involvement

---

- ▪ Indicating denervation
    - ○ +/- Ligament of Struthers: Compression site
    - ○ FS PD FSE
        - ▪ Variable amounts of hemorrhage - hyperintense
- STIR
    - ○ Muscle: Increased signal with denervation
    - ○ Effective at low field
- T1 C+
    - ○ +/- Muscle enhancement with denervation
    - ○ Portion of large muscle belly may be affected
    - ○ +/- Nerve enhancement
- Reduced muscle size with or without fatty infiltration indicating atrophy
- Fibrosis (streaky decreased signal intensity on all pulse sequences) in the entrapment region

Imaging Recommendations
- Best imaging tool: MRI
- Protocol advice: FS PD FSE/T2 for visualization of muscle changes

DIFFERENTIAL DIAGNOSIS

C6/7 Radiculopathy
- Check for dysfunction of contribution from radial nerve
    - ○ Radial nerve involvement = radiculopathy vs. compression neuropathy
- Cervical spine MRI findings
    - ○ Disc abnormalities, stenosis

Flexor Superficialis Crossover Syndrome
- Paresthesias in forearm & hand while pronating wrist
- Resisted flexion of flexor superficialis of 3rd finger
- Entrapment at pronator teres & flexor superficialis cross over - variant of pronator syndrome

Brachial Neuritis/Parsonage-Turner Distal Form
- Difficult to differentiate
- +/- Viral prodrome
- + Pain followed by weakness

- Self limiting

Radial Neuropathy
- Denervation of extensor muscles
- Posterior interosseous (PIN) syndrome
- High lesion - supinator atrophy (high radial atrop)

Muscle Trauma
- Strain
- Hyperintense on T2WI
- Mimics subacute denervation
- Stress response
- Acute trauma

PATHOLOGY

General Features
- General path comments
    - ○ AIN = largest branch of median nerve and is completely motor
        - ▪ Supplies fibers for deep pain and proprioception in the radiocarpal, radioulnar, intercarpal, and carpometacarpal joints
        - ▪ No cutaneous sensory involvement
        - ▪ Separates from superficial branch approximately 5-8 cm distal to lateral epicondyle
        - ▪ Supplies flexor pollicis longus, pronator quadratus and radial aspect of flexor digitorum profundus
    - ○ AINS: Motor loss without sensory loss
        - ▪ Compression with weakness of thumb and index fingers
        - ▪ Includes intrinsic hand weakness in the presence of a Martin-Gruber anastomosis
    - ○ Martin-Gruber anastomosis (15% of normal population) branches from median to ulnar nerve in forearm
        - ▪ Innervates: 1st dorsal interosseus, adductor pollicis, abductor digiti minimi
    - ○ Pronator syndrome: Entrapment syndrome of median nerve with similar etiology than AINS but different clinical picture
        - ▪ Negative Phalen's test and Tinel's sign

MEDIAN NEUROPATHY

- Absent specific weaknesses associated with AINS
- Negative EMG as opposed to positive findings with AINS
- Distal skin sensory changes in the distribution of the median nerve
- More proximal compression (often in muscular athletes) than AINS and includes sensory loss
- Etiology
  - Anterior interosseous nerve syndrome
    - Neuritis, brachial plexitis
    - Local fracture (supracondylar)
    - Soft tissue trauma to the forearm
    - Thrombosed vessels
    - Enlarged bursae
    - Aberrant fibrous bands
    - +/- Idiopathic
  - Pronator syndrome
    - Compression of median nerve: Ligament of Struthers and supracondylar process of humerus
    - Lacertus fibrosus (bicipital aponeurosis)
    - Heads of pronator muscle
    - Fibrous bands within pronator muscle
    - Tendinous origin of flexor digitorum superficialis
    - Aberrant median artery
    - Fibrous component of flexor carpi radialis muscle originating from ulna
    - Soft tissue trauma
    - Overuse (heavy use) of forearm muscle
    - +/- Occurs spontaneously
- Epidemiology
  - Median nerve compression in athletes (elbow)
  - Median nerve compression in the general population occurs at the wrist

Gross Pathologic & Surgical Features
- Swollen muscle belly - early and subacute
- Fatty atrophy = chronic
- Anterior interosseous nerve compression
  - Fibrous bands of deep head of pronator teres or flexor digitorum superficialis (FDS)
  - Aberrant or anomalous vessels
  - Anomalous muscles
    - Gantzer's muscle (anomalous slip of the origin of the flexor pollicis longus)
- Pronator syndrome compression
  - Ligament of Struthers
    - +/- Connects (1% of limbs) supracondylar process (anomalous ± osseous excrescence) from anteromedial distal humerus to medial epicondyle
  - Thickened lacertus fibrosus connection to pronator teres
  - Pronator teres hypertrophy
  - Thickened fibrous arch of FDS
  - Persistent median artery
  - Enlarged bursa

Microscopic Features
- Enlarged extracellular fluid space = early and subacute
- Myofibrils atrophy and become small and angular in early denervation

Staging, Grading or Classification Criteria
- Three types of median nerve compression (compression at elbow occurs as either AINS or PS)

- Carpal tunnel syndrome (CTS)
  - Intermittent pain, paresthesias and numbness
  - Median nerve distribution
  - Thenar atrophy and weakness
  - Permanent loss of median sensation in hand secondary to median nerve compression deep to transverse carpal ligament
- AINS
  - Palsy of flexor pollicis longus, flexor digitorum profundus of index finger and pronator quadratus
  - Spontaneous or posttraumatic onset
- PS
  - Pain proximal third forearm anteriorly
  - Intermittent median paresthesias
  - No motor symptoms
  - No permanent loss of sensation

CLINICAL ISSUES

Presentation
- Most common signs/symptoms
  - Pain along the course of median nerve
  - PS: No weakness or sensory loss +/- paresthesias
    - Aching pain in the proximal volar forearm
  - AINS: Abrupt weakness or total paralysis of flexor pollicis longus & profundus tendon to 2nd & 3rd digits - proximal forearm pain
- Clinical profile: Pronator syndrome: Exacerbated by practicing tennis serves or throwing actions which require forearm pronation and wrist flexion

Demographics
- Age: Children after fracture/adults - repetitive microtrauma
- Gender: F > M overall for median neuropathy (including carpal tunnel)

Natural History & Prognosis
- +/- Resolution with conservative therapy
- +/- Decompressive surgery for treatment

Treatment
- Rest, modify activities, NSAIDs, decompressive surgery

DIAGNOSTIC CHECKLIST

Image Interpretation Pearls
- FS PD FSE or STIR are sensitive for muscle signal intensity changes; identify appropriate muscle involvement

SELECTED REFERENCES
1. Fitzgerald RH et al: Orthopaedics. Hand and peripheral nerve soft-tissue and bone injuries. St. Louis MO, Mosby, 1936-40, 2003
2. Nicholas JA et al: The Upper Extremity in Sports Medicine. 2nd ed. St. Louis MO, Mosby, 1995

IMAGE GALLERY

Typical

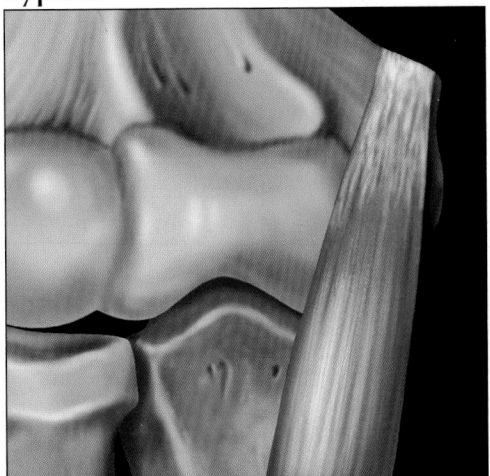
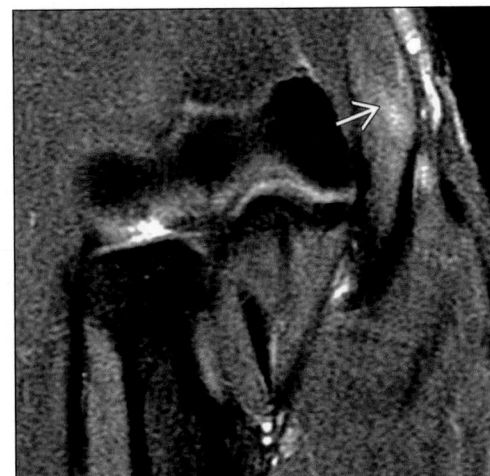

(Left) Coronal graphic shows inflammatory changes in the pronator teres muscle. The muscle can hypertrophy as a result of exercise and impinge upon the median nerve. (Right) Coronal FS PD FSE MR shows increased signal within the pronator teres muscle (arrow) indicative of strain.

Typical

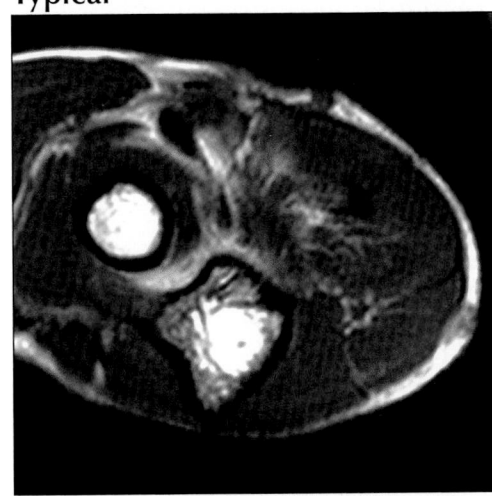
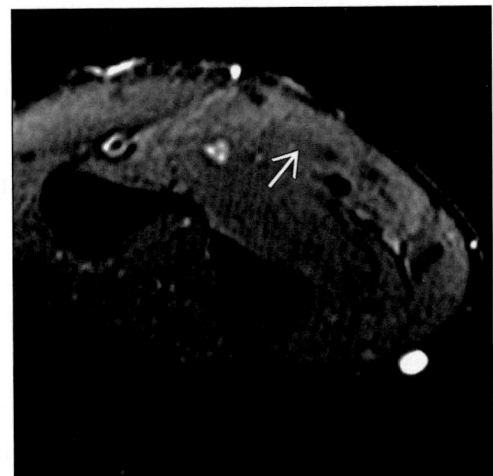

(Left) Axial PD FSE MR shows scarring within the antecubital fossa in a patient with clinical anterior interosseous nerve syndrome. (Right) Axial STIR MR image shows early denervation (arrow) of increased signal intensity within a flexor muscle belly in a patient with median neuropathy.

Typical

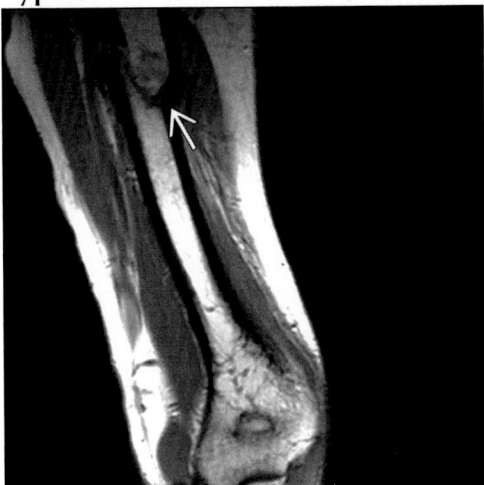
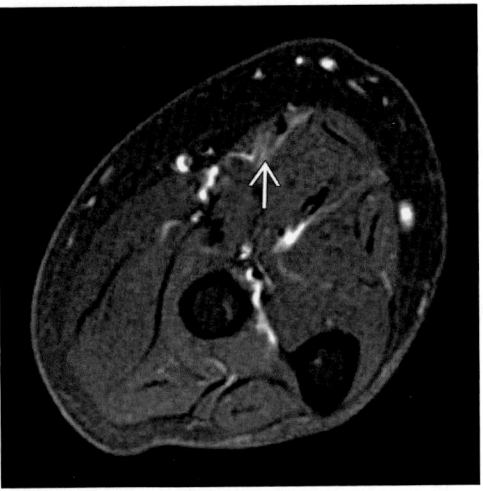

(Left) Coronal PD FSE MR using a large field of view shows a Holstein-Lewis fracture (arrow) which caused median neuropathy. (Right) Axial FS PD FSE MR shows increased signal intensity (arrow) within anterior fibers of the pronator teres in median neuropathy.

ANCONEUS EPITROCHLEARIS

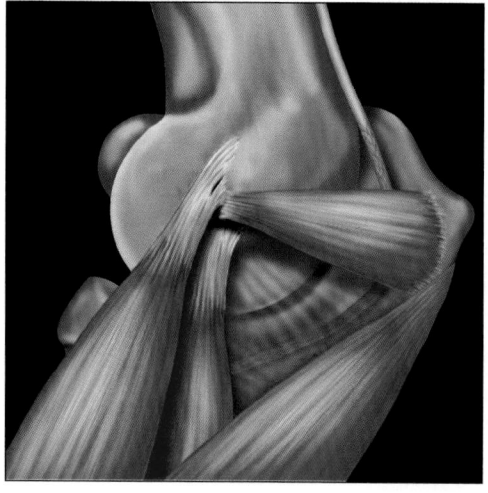

Sagittal graphic shows an anconeus epitrochlearis superficial to the ulnar nerve. The accessory muscle may exert mass effect upon the nerve causing ulnar neuropathy.

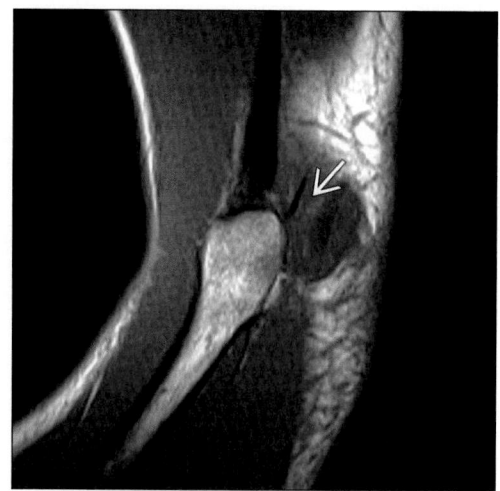

Sagittal PD FSE MR shows an anconeus epitrochlearis muscle belly (arrow) posterior to the medial epicondyle.

TERMINOLOGY

Abbreviations and Synonyms
- Anomalous muscle

Definitions
- Accessory/anomalous muscle replacing cubital tunnel retinaculum which may cause compression ulnar neuropathy

IMAGING FINDINGS

General Features
- Best diagnostic clue: Muscle covering cubital tunnel seen best on axial images (follows normal muscle signal intensity on all pulse sequences)
- Location: Roof of cubital tunnel
- Size: Varies from small thin to bulky muscle
- Morphology: Oval shaped muscle on axial images

CT Findings
- NECT: To identify muscle in correct location

MR Findings
- T1WI: Follows muscle signal intensity in correct anatomic location - intermediate signal
- T2WI: Normal hypointense muscle signal intensity covering cubital tunnel

- PD/Intermediate: Intermediate, normal muscle signal intensity surrounded by hyperintense fat
- STIR
  - Decreased normal signal intensity muscle
  - Less spatial resolution
- T1 C+: No enhancement unless inflammation/myositis

Imaging Recommendations
- Best imaging tool: MRI
- Protocol advice: T1, PD and FS PD FSE demonstrate this anomalous muscle

DIFFERENTIAL DIAGNOSIS

Hematoma
- Increased signal on T2WI
- History of trauma/contusion

Neuroma
- Increased signal on T2WI, variable amounts of fibrous tissue centrally
- Enhances diffusely

Synovial Mass
- Seen with inflammatory arthritides (rheumatoid-RA), inflammatory osteoarthritis (OA) and post trauma

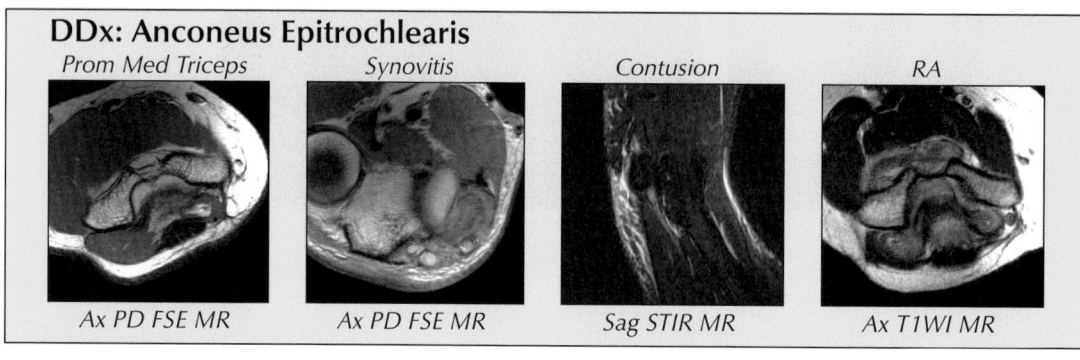

DDx: Anconeus Epitrochlearis

Prom Med Triceps	Synovitis	Contusion	RA
Ax PD FSE MR	Ax PD FSE MR	Sag STIR MR	Ax T1WI MR

ANCONEUS EPITROCHLEARIS

Key Facts

Terminology
- Accessory/anomalous muscle replacing cubital tunnel retinaculum which may cause compression ulnar neuropathy

Imaging Findings
- Best diagnostic clue: Muscle covering cubital tunnel seen best on axial images (follows normal muscle signal intensity on all pulse sequences)
- Location: Roof of cubital tunnel
- Best imaging tool: MRI
- Protocol advice: T1, PD and FS PD FSE demonstrate this anomalous muscle

Top Differential Diagnoses
- Hematoma
- Neuroma

- Synovial Mass

Pathology
- Etiology: Muscle compresses ulnar nerve causing neuropathy or produces relative vascular steal phenomenon

Clinical Issues
- Most common signs/symptoms: Ulnar neuritis if symptomatic
- Clinical profile: Athlete with ulnar neuritis

Diagnostic Checklist
- Other causes of ulnar neuritis
- Follows muscle signal intensity on all pulse sequences

Prominent Medial Head of Triceps Muscle
- Causes mass effect and compression of ulnar nerve
- Proximal to majority of cubital tunnel
- Hypertrophied component of triceps muscle

PATHOLOGY

General Features
- General path comments
  - Accessory muscle
  - Causes ulnar neuropathy
- Etiology: Muscle compresses ulnar nerve causing neuropathy or produces relative vascular steal phenomenon
- Epidemiology: 11% of general population
- Associated abnormalities: Ulnar neuritis

Gross Pathologic & Surgical Features
- Normal to inflamed muscle

Microscopic Features
- Normal to inflamed muscle with variable influx of inflammatory cells

CLINICAL ISSUES

Presentation
- Most common signs/symptoms: Ulnar neuritis if symptomatic
- Clinical profile: Athlete with ulnar neuritis

Demographics
- Age: Adolescent/adult
- Gender: M = F

Natural History & Prognosis
- May progress requiring extirpation of muscle for refractory ulnar neuritis

Treatment
- Physical therapy, NSAIDs, then surgery if nonresponsive to conservative measures

- Conservative
  - Rest, ice, NSAIDs - acute neuritis
- Surgical
  - Removal of muscle for chronic recalcitrant cases

DIAGNOSTIC CHECKLIST

Consider
- Other causes of ulnar neuritis

Image Interpretation Pearls
- Follows muscle signal intensity on all pulse sequences

SELECTED REFERENCES

1. Fritz RC et al: Magnetic resonance imaging of the musculoskeletal system: Part 3. The elbow. Clin Orthop (324):321-39, 1996
2. Masear VR et al: Ulnar compression neuropathy secondary to the anconeus epitrochlearis muscle. J Hand Surg 14(5):917-9, 1989

IMAGE GALLERY

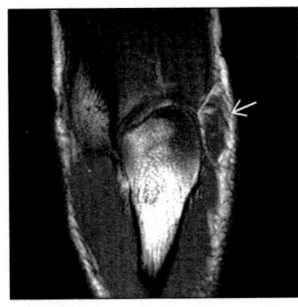 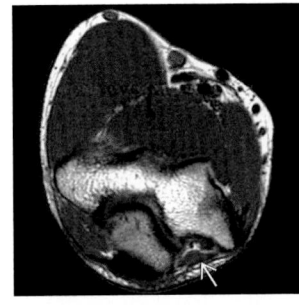

(Left) Coronal PD FSE MR shows an anconeus epitrochlearis (arrow) adjacent to the olecranon process. (Right) Axial PD FSE MR shows a small anconeus epitrochlearis covering the cubital tunnel (arrow).

CORONOID PROCESS FRACTURE

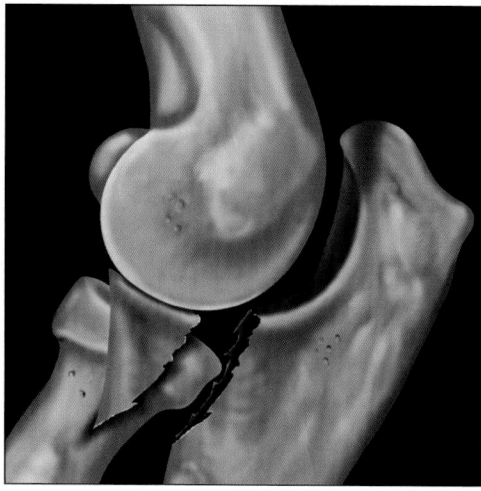
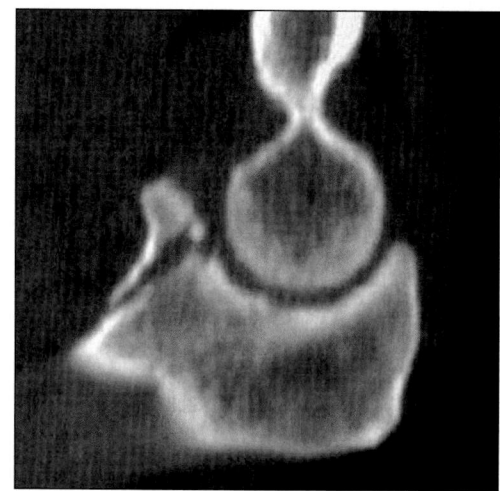

Sagittal graphic shows a fracture through base of coronoid process with distraction of fracture fragment centrally. The finding is usually diagnostic of posterior subluxation/dislocation.

Sagittal CT reconstruction image shows a comminuted fracture through the base of the coronoid process in a patient who is status post dislocation.

TERMINOLOGY

Abbreviations and Synonyms
- Regan/Morrey fracture, posterior elbow dislocation, terrible triad of the elbow, sublime tubercle fracture

Definitions
- A distraction injury due to bony avulsion of brachialis insertion by posterior dislocation of ulna
- Hyperextension or posterior dislocation

IMAGING FINDINGS

General Features
- Best diagnostic clue
  - Linear decreased signal intensity surrounded by edema on FS PD FSE/T2WI of the coronoid process
  - Lucent fracture line passing through coronoid process on lateral/angled lateral radiograph
- Location: Coronoid process on the anterior/cubital articular margin of the proximal ulna
- Size
  - Varies
    - Tip only
    - < 50% of process avulsed
    - > 50% of process avulsed
- Morphology
  - Transverse through tip
  - Oblique through anteromedial facet

Radiographic Findings
- Radiography
  - Linear lucency = fracture line with variable fragment size
    - Displacement on lateral or angled lateral views
  - Associated fractures of radius and distal humerus, esp. on radial head view
  - Associated posterior dislocation of elbow
  - Positive fat pad sign on lateral view

CT Findings
- NECT
  - Linear lucencies in coronoid process indicating fractures
  - Soft tissue swelling will be evident on soft tissue windows
  - Fracture comminution and displacement can be assessed
  - Sagittal reconstructions helpful

MR Findings
- T1WI
  - Decreased marrow signal indicating bone stress
  - Hypointense lines indicating fracture
  - +/- Bony displacement on sagittal views
  - Hypointense joint effusion

DDx: Coronoid Process Fracture

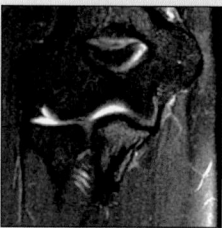
Normal Marrow
Cor FS PD FSE

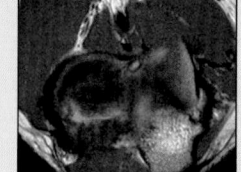
Loose Body
Ax PD FSE MR

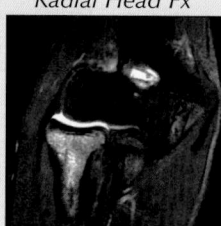
Radial Head Fx
Cor FS PD FSE

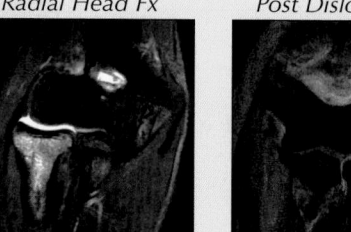
Post Dislocation
Cor FS PD FSE

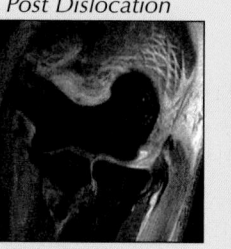

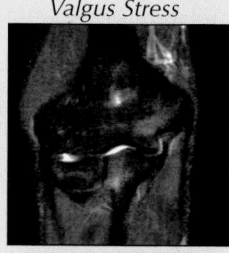
Valgus Stress
Cor FS PD FSE

CORONOID PROCESS FRACTURE

Key Facts

Terminology

- A distraction injury due to bony avulsion of brachialis insertion by posterior dislocation of ulna
- Hyperextension or posterior dislocation

Imaging Findings

- Associated fractures of radius and distal humerus, esp. on radial head view
- Associated posterior dislocation of elbow
- Linear lucencies in coronoid process indicating fractures
- Sagittal reconstructions helpful

Top Differential Diagnoses

- Supracondylar Fracture
- Medial Epicondylar Avulsion Fracture
- Radial Head/Neck Fracture

- Olecranon Fracture
- Posterior Dislocation (Post Dislocation)
- Valgus Stress
- Normal Marrow

Pathology

- Fall on an outstretched arm

Clinical Issues

- Pain and loss of function
- Swelling and discoloration
- Early mobilization important

Diagnostic Checklist

- The percentage size of avulsed fragment
- Fat sat/STIR MR for MCL assessment and marrow edema to show occult fractures

---

  - ○ Disruption of normal anatomy and signal of medial collateral ligament (MCL) on coronal views
- T2WI
  - ○ Increased marrow signal indicating edema
  - ○ Visualization improved by using FS sequence (FS PD FSE)
  - ○ FS PD FSE
    - ▪ Very sensitive for bony injury shown as high signal areas in marrow space
    - ▪ Graphic illustration of joint effusion/leakage
    - ▪ Most sensitive method for demonstrating MCL injury
  - ○ High signal joint effusion
  - ○ +/- Periarticular leakage with capsular rupture
  - ○ Low signal fracture lines
    - ▪ +/- Interposed fluid
  - ○ Disruption of MCL anatomy
    - ▪ High signal tears
    - ▪ Associated high signal stress lesions (marrow edema) at bony attachments
- STIR
  - ○ Less signal (decreased signal to noise ratio)
  - ○ Improved results for low field imaging
- T2* GRE
  - ○ Coronal images to show larger defects of articular cartilage
    - ▪ Deficiencies with subchondral low signal areas
    - ▪ Application useful when fat suppression techniques show inhomogeneous signal

Imaging Recommendations

- Best imaging tool: MRI
- Protocol advice: FS PD FSE/T2WI

DIFFERENTIAL DIAGNOSIS

Supracondylar Fracture

- Anterior humeral line displaced anterior to mid third of capitellum in 94%
- Often seen in children
- Fracture line may not be visible in up to 25%
- Hyperextension from fall onto extended forearm

- Accounts for about 60% of pediatric elbow fractures
- Rare in adults (< 3%)

Medial Epicondylar Avulsion Fracture

- Acute valgus stress
- Chronic repetitive valgus injury
- < 2% of elbow fractures in children
- 10% of elbow fractures in adolescence
- Associated with olecranon fracture

Radial Head/Neck Fracture

- Posterior dislocation
- +/- Coronoid process fracture
- An impaction injury due to axial overloading in a fall on to the outstretched arm
- Radial head injuries are rare in children and usually occur in the radial neck
- Is the most common elbow fracture in adults

Olecranon Fracture

- Acute flexion on extended forearm
- Clinical presentation similar
- Fall on a flexed, supinated forearm
- Throwing injury (pitchers)
- Accounts for about 20% of adult elbow fractures

Posterior Dislocation (Post Dislocation)

- Seen as overall picture with coronoid process fracture
- Fall on out stretched hand injury (FOOSH)
- +/- Capitellar fx
- Lateral ligamentous disruptions
  - ○ LUCL
- + Surrounding hemorrhage
- Associated with coronoid fracture
- +/- Radial head fracture

Valgus Stress

- Acute traumatic injury
- Chronic repetitive microtrauma
- Baseball pitchers are predisposed
- Medial epicondylitis
- +/- MCL tear

CORONOID PROCESS FRACTURE

Normal Marrow
- Relative increased signal of red marrow on T2WI
  - FS PD FSE and STIR
  - Red marrow hypointensity does not usually extend across the physeal scar
- Fat signal intensity on T1WI

PATHOLOGY

General Features
- Etiology
  - Fall on an outstretched arm
  - Hyperextension of elbow
- Epidemiology
  - Occurs in 10-15% of elbow dislocations
  - 40% are associated with elbow dislocation
- Associated abnormalities
  - Associated with other elbow fractures, esp. radial head
  - Posterior dislocation (in 15%)
  - Injury to anterior band of MCL and anterior capsule
  - Terrible triad - coronoid fx, radial head fx, MCL sprain

Gross Pathologic & Surgical Features
- Caused by humeral trochlea during posterior dislocation/subluxation
- Larger fragment size associated with injury to anterior band of medial collateral ligament

Microscopic Features
- Disruption of cortex and trabeculae
- Avulsion of osteo-tendinous complex of brachialis
- Hemorrhage with cellular infiltrate ranging from osteoblast and osteoclast to inflammatory cells depending on fracture age
- Avulsion of the osteo-ligamentous complex of the anterior band of the MCL

Staging, Grading or Classification Criteria
- Based on classification of Regan and Morrey
  - Type I: Avulsion of tip of coronoid process
  - Type II: Involves < 50% of coronoid process
  - Type III: Involves > 50% of coronoid process

CLINICAL ISSUES

Presentation
- Most common signs/symptoms
  - Pain and loss of function
  - Swelling and discoloration
  - Loss of joint stability (late)

Demographics
- Age: Usually young active patient
- Gender: M > F

Natural History & Prognosis
- Small fracture responds well with conservative therapy
- Delayed mobilization - failure to heal properly
- Prognosis worsened by presence of other fractures, especially radial head fractures
- Prognosis deteriorates with fracture complexity
- Improved by early mobilization
- Improved by maintaining integrity of radioulnar joint
- May be improved by repair of collateral ligaments

Treatment
- Conservative
  - Viable option if < 50% of coronoid is fractured and no other elbow fractures exist
  - Early mobilization important
- Surgical
  - If > 50% of coronoid is involved, other fractures exist or valgus instability is found
  - ORIF, external fixation or reconstruction with osteo-cartilaginous graft from olecranon
  - Coronoid fracture + olecranon fracture
    - Lag screw fixation from posterior during fixation of olecranon

DIAGNOSTIC CHECKLIST

Consider
- Presence of other fractures
- Presence of valgus instability
- The percentage size of avulsed fragment

Image Interpretation Pearls
- Lateral and angled lateral radiographs for judging size of fragment
- Fat sat/STIR MR for MCL assessment and marrow edema to show occult fractures

SELECTED REFERENCES

1. O'Driscoll SW et al: Difficult elbow fractures. Pearls and pitfalls. Instr Course Lect 52:113-34, 2003
2. Ring D et al: Posterior dislocation of the elbow with fractures of the radial head and coronoid. J Bone Joint Surg Am 84-A(4):547-51, 2002
3. Closkey RF et al: The role of the coronoid process in elbow stability. A biomechanical analysis of axial loading. J Bone Joint Surg Am 82-A(12):1749-53, 2000
4. Sonin A: Fractures of the elbow and forearm. Semin Musculoskelet Radiol 4(2) p171-91, 2000
5. Akagi M: Avulsion fracture of the sublime (coronoid) tubercle of the ulna in throwing athletes. Am J Roentgenol 173(3):849-50, 1999
6. Moritomo H et al: Reconstruction of the coronoid for chronic dislocation of the elbow. Use of a graft from the olecranon in two cases. J Bone Joint Surg Br 80(3):490-2, 1998

CORONOID PROCESS FRACTURE

IMAGE GALLERY

Typical

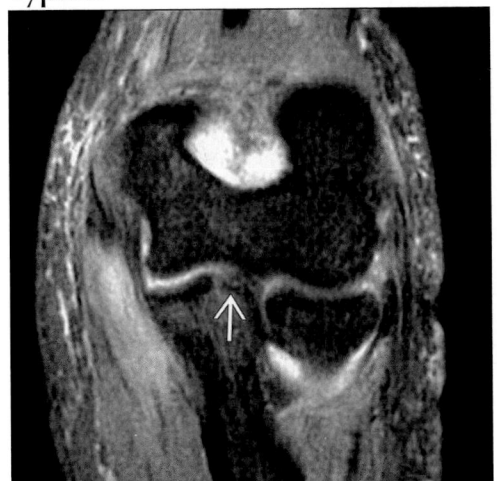
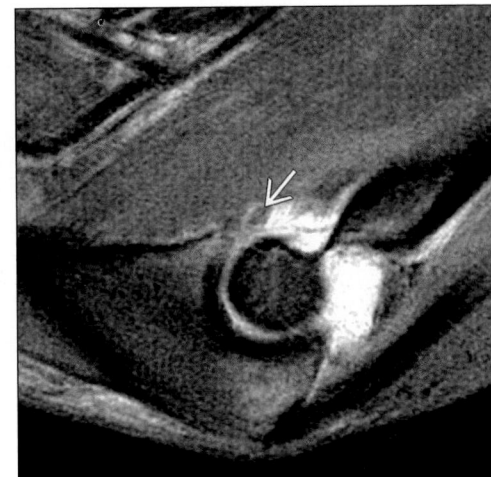

(Left) Coronal STIR MR shows an extensor bone trabecular injury of the coronoid process with a small fracture *(arrow)* involving the coronoid tip, nondisplaced. *(Right)* Sagittal STIR MR shows a fracture at the tip of the coronoid process *(arrow)* and a bone trabecular injury of the olecranon process after posterior dislocation.

Typical

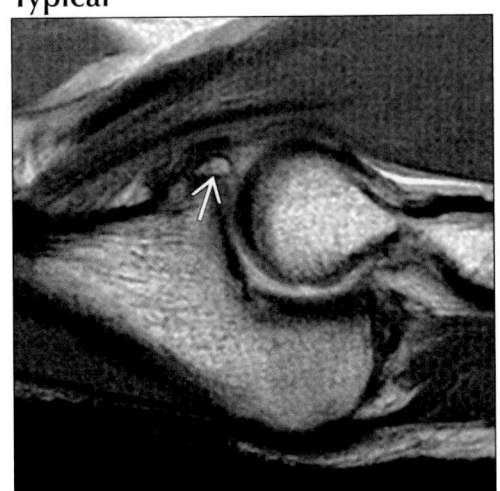
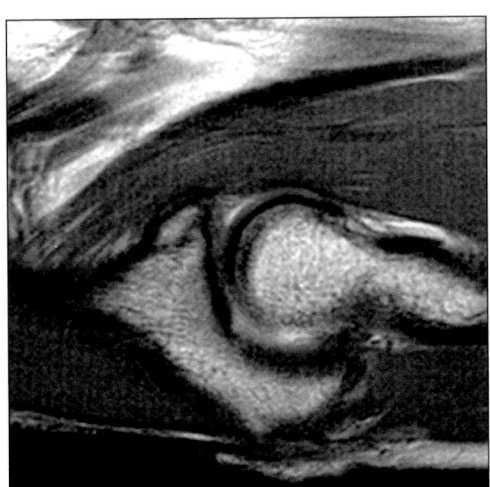

(Left) Sagittal PD FSE MR shows a small nondisplaced nonunited distal tip coronoid fracture *(arrow)* in a patient with a remote history of trauma. *(Right)* Sagittal PD FSE MR in the same patient demonstrates an irregular appearance of the coronoid tip that healed and united.

Typical

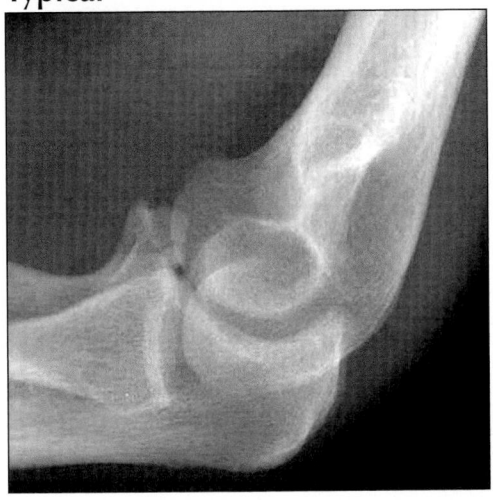
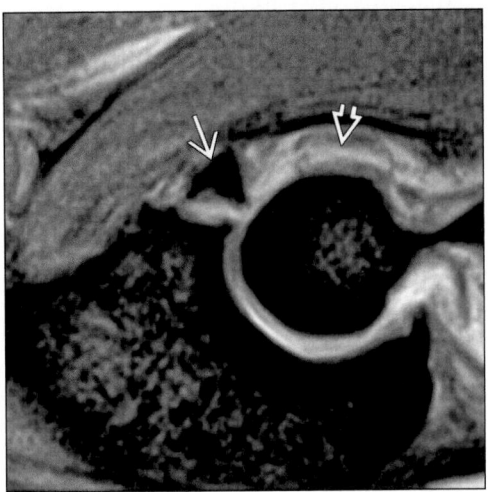

(Left) Lateral radiography shows fracture at the base of the coronoid process. *(Right)* Sagittal T2* GRE MR shows a fracture through the base of the coronoid process *(arrow)*. There is (intermediate signal intensity) synovitis *(open arrow)* in the anterior joint capsule.

CAPITELLAR OSTEOCHONDRITIS

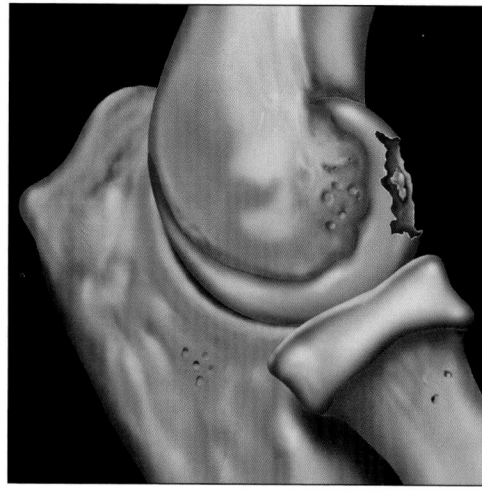

Sagittal graphic shows osteochondritis dissecans lesion of the anterior aspect of the capitellum with chondral fragmentation.

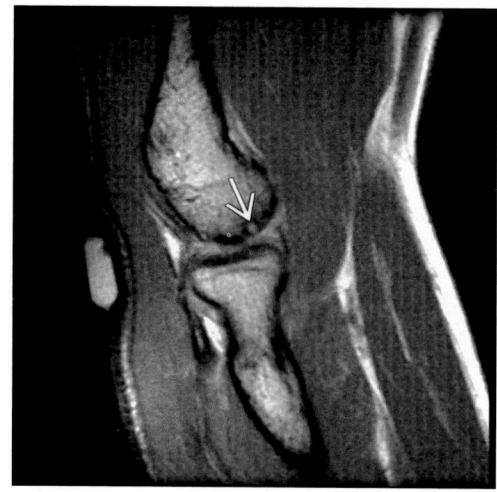

Sagittal PD FSE MR shows subchondral cystic change (arrow) in a patient with capitellar osteochondritis dissecans.

TERMINOLOGY

Abbreviations and Synonyms
- Osteochondritis dissecans (OCD)

Definitions
- Overuse of the elbow causing a subchondral reactive process of the humeral capitellum
- Resulting in the loosening of a fragment of cartilage and bone
- Osteocartilaginous osteochondritis dissecans fragment
  - Necrosis of bone followed by healing response and reossification

IMAGING FINDINGS

General Features
- Best diagnostic clue
  - Decreased or intermediate signal intensity within the capitellum
    - In contrast to normal marrow fat (increased signal intensity)
- Location: Anterior surface of the capitellum within the elbow joint
- Size: 1-2 cm affected area
- Morphology: Semilunar large fragment to multiple smaller fragments

Radiographic Findings
- Radiography
  - Flattening of capitellar profile - earliest sign
  - Enlarging lucent zone
  - Patchy sclerosis and fragmentation
  - Loose body formation
  - Radiohumeral degeneration

CT Findings
- NECT
  - Lucent zone surrounding an area of separating bone
  - Intraarticular loose bodies

MR Findings
- T1WI
  - Hypointense (low signal) zone of separation around developing fragment
  - Low signal within the fragment
  - +/- Intermediate signal intensity synovial thickening = synovitis
- T2WI
  - Variable signal within fragment depending on degree of sclerosis
  - Hyperintense fluid rim surrounding loose fragments
- STIR
  - High signal within the fragment and in deeper bone = edema
  - High signal rim signifies loose fragment

DDx: Capitellar Osteochondritis

Valgus Impaction	Pseudodefect	Psuedodefect	Posterior Cap OA	Old Trauma
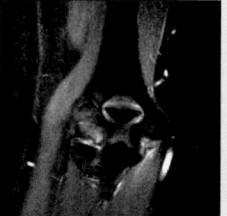	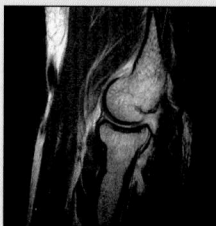	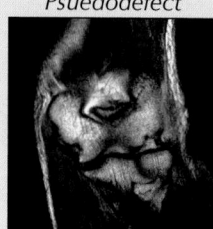	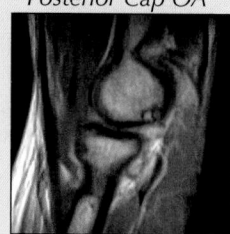	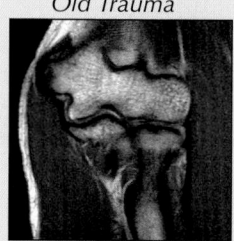
Cor STIR MR	Sag PD FSE MR	Cor PD FSE MR	Sag PD FSE MR	Cor PD FSE MR

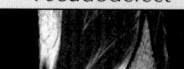

CAPITELLAR OSTEOCHONDRITIS

Key Facts

Terminology
- Overuse of the elbow causing a subchondral reactive process of the humeral capitellum

Imaging Findings
- Decreased or intermediate signal intensity within the capitellum
- In contrast to normal marrow fat (increased signal intensity)
- Location: Anterior surface of the capitellum within the elbow joint
- Hyperintense fluid rim surrounding loose fragments

Top Differential Diagnoses
- Panner's Disease
- Pseudodefect of the Capitellum
- Posterior Dislocation

- Valgus Impaction Fracture

Pathology
- Loose body formation and residual deformity often present
- Chronic valgus stress with lateral impaction - gymnasts and adolescent pitchers

Clinical Issues
- Often athletes with insidious onset of pain or history of trauma

Diagnostic Checklist
- Panner's disease in younger (5-11 years) patients
- 45 degree flexed AP view, FS T1 C+, MR arthrogram

- T2* GRE
  - Low signal fragment
  - Loose body detection
- T1 C+
  - IV gad will cause enhancement of granulation tissue in defect (not as hyperintense as joint fluid)
  - Enhancing synovium = synovitis
- MR arthrography
  - Evaluation of extension of fluid into subchondral bone
- Loose osteochondrotic fragment visualized
- Fluid between interface of fragment and donor site in capitellum in unstable lesions
- Cyst-like lesions in capitellum underneath the fragment in unstable lesions

Imaging Recommendations
- Best imaging tool: MRI
- Protocol advice: PD/FS PD FSE for lesion detection and characterization

DIFFERENTIAL DIAGNOSIS

Panner's Disease
- Seen in younger patients (5-11 year old patients)
- Loose body formation and residual deformity usually not seen in Panner's disease
- Probably avascular necrosis secondary to trauma
- Osteochondrosis of entire capitellum

Pseudodefect of the Capitellum
- Normal anatomy
- Posteriorly located

Capitellum Fracture
- Shear injury due to transmitted axial overload from radial head in fall on outstretched arm
- Rare
  - 6% of elbow fractures
  - Not in children < 10 years old
- Coronal defect with variable anterior displacement
- Fracture is in coronal plane (best seen on sagittal images)

Posterior Dislocation
- Fall on out stretched hand (FOOSH) injury
- +/- Capitellar fracture
- Lateral ligamentous disruptions
  - LUCL
- +/- Common extensor tendon tear
- +/- Coronoid fx
- Lateral pain
- Sudden posterior force
- ± Osteoarthritis (OA)
  - Sclerosis
  - Chondromalacia
  - Loose bodies

Posterolateral Rotatory Instability (PLRI)
- Spectrum of disease from PLRI to posterior dislocation
- Disruption of ligamentous fibers with hyperintense fluid signal intensity on T2WI
- Chronic tennis elbow
- Often fall on outstretched hand
- Tear of origin of LUCL with or without lateral epicondylitis

Valgus Impaction Fracture
- Acute valgus injury
- +/- Chronic repetitive trauma (valgus extension overload)
- Hyperintense bone marrow on T2WI
- FS PD FSE or STIR more sensitive to marrow edema
- Medial collateral ligament (MCL) sprain common

PATHOLOGY

General Features
- General path comments
  - Loose body formation and residual deformity often present
  - The capitellum has a relatively poor blood supply
    - End arteries are vulnerable
- Etiology
  - Chronic valgus stress with lateral impaction - gymnasts and adolescent pitchers

CAPITELLAR OSTEOCHONDRITIS

○ Increased rotary, compressive or axial loads - throwing athletes
○ Radiocapitellar compressive and shearing forces during acceleration and deceleration phases
○ Increased valgus forces (esp. if MCL is lax)
• Epidemiology
○ Occurs in the 12-16 year age group (after ossification of capitellum)
○ Accounts for 6% of all cases of OCD
○ 20% bilateral
○ Common in relatives of affected patients
• Associated abnormalities
○ Flexion contracture
○ OCD in other joints

Gross Pathologic & Surgical Features
• Necrotic desiccated bone fragment in unstable lesions
• Early features consist of flattening of the profile of the capitellum
• As condition progresses, attrition of hyaline cartilage occurs with similar features seen in radial head
• Trabecular shearing injuries with microtrauma response (hemorrhage) demarcates zone of stress overloading
• Zone of stress overloading fills with granulation tissue as fragment starts to separate and move
• Joint fluid penetrates along weakened zone of stress overloading and promotes separation

Microscopic Features
• Osteonecrosis with variable amounts of healing
• Initial changes consistent with avascular necrosis
• Development of osteochondral fragment
• Granulation tissue fills the zone of separation

Staging, Grading or Classification Criteria
• Stable lesions
○ Small size
○ No fluid between interface of humerus and osteochondritis fragment
• Unstable lesions
○ Large size (typically > 1 cm)
○ Cyst-like lesion beneath the osteochondrotic lesion
○ Contains loose granulation tissue
○ Loose fragment
○ Fluid insinuating beneath the fragment at arthrography
• Osteochondritis grading
○ Grade 1: Intact hyaline cartilage
○ Grade 2: Prominent zone of separation (which enhances), stable
○ Grade 3: Fluid fills zone of separation, unstable
○ Grade 4: Fragment has become loose intraarticular body

CLINICAL ISSUES

Presentation
• Most common signs/symptoms
○ Often athletes with insidious onset of pain or history of trauma
○ Poorly localized lateral pain with activity
○ Catching or locking

○ Flexion contracture

Demographics
• Age: 13-16 year children
• Gender: M:F = 6:1 (mainly reflects sports)

Natural History & Prognosis
• 50% of cases with radiographic change will progress to osteoarthritis
• Early arthroscopic debridement results in good response
• 50% of cases with loose body removal show poor outcome
• Poor prognosis
○ Advanced lesion
○ Large fragment
○ Established OA

Treatment
• Stable lesions treated with rest and splinting
• Unstable lesions often treated with abrasion chondroplasty or microfracture unless large, displaced fragment is found
• Conservative: Grade 1-2 - 50% will recover with rest
• Surgical: Grade 2-4 - drilling, microfracture, autologous chondrocyte transplantation, arthroscopic debridement, wiring and bone graft, wedge osteotomy
• Complications: Residual flattening of capitellum, arthrofibrosis, recurrent loose bodies

DIAGNOSTIC CHECKLIST

Consider
• Panner's disease in younger (5-11 years) patients

Image Interpretation Pearls
• 45 degree flexed AP view, FS T1 C+, MR arthrogram

SELECTED REFERENCES

1. Harada M et al: Fragment fixation with a bone graft and dynamic staples for osteochondritis dissecans of the humeral capitellum. J Shoulder Elbow Surg 11(4):368-72, 2002
2. Byrd JW et al: Arthroscopic surgery for isolated capitellar osteochondritis dissecans in adolescent baseball players. Minimum three-year follow-up. Am J Sports Med 30(4):474-8, 2002
3. Bradley JP et al: Osteochondritis dissecans of the humeral capitellum. Diagnosis and treatment. Clin Sports Med 20(3):565-90, 2001
4. Bowen RE et al: Osteochondral lesions of the capitellum in pediatric patients. Role of magnetic resonance imaging. J Pediatr Orthop 21(3):298-301, 2001
5. Kiyoshige Y et al: Closed-wedge osteotomy for osteochondritis dissecans of the capitellum. A 7- to 12-year follow-up. Am J Sports Med 28(4):534-7, 2000
6. Takahara M et al: Nonoperative treatment of osteochondritis dissecans of the humeral capitellum. Am J Sports Med 27(6):728-32, 1999
7. Takahara M et al: Long term outcome of osteochondritis dissecans of the humeral capitellum. Clin Orthop (363):108-15, 1999
8. Kaeding CC: Musculoskeletal injuries in adolescents. Prim Care 25(1):211-23, 1998

CAPITELLAR OSTEOCHONDRITIS

IMAGE GALLERY

Typical

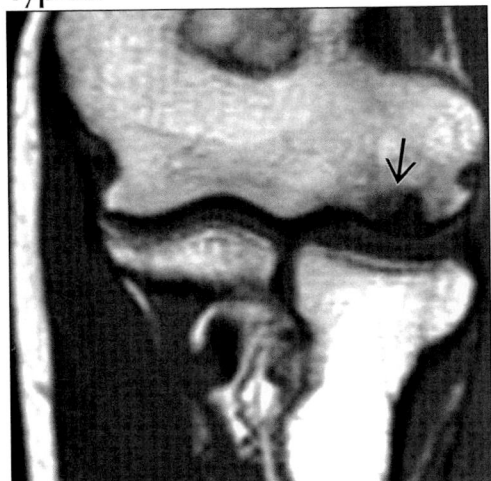
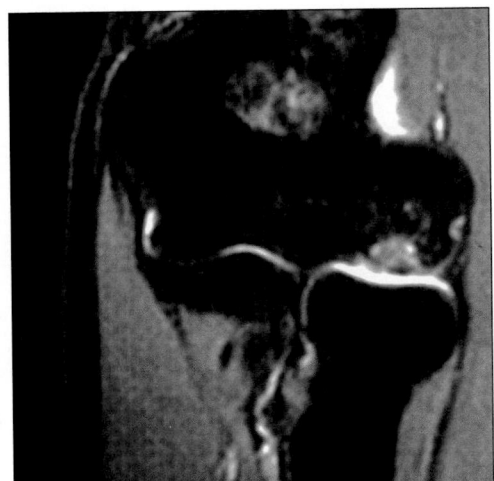

(Left) Coronal T1WI MR shows hypointense focus of osteochondritis dissecans (arrow) of the capitellum. No collapse of the articular surface is seen. *(Right)* Coronal STIR MR of the same patient demonstrates the OCD lesion as hyperintense. No loose fragment is seen.

Typical

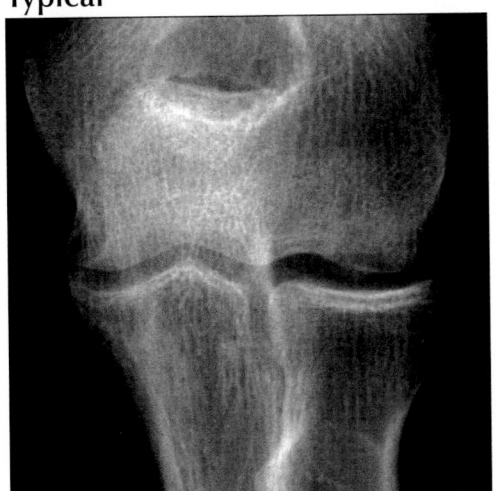
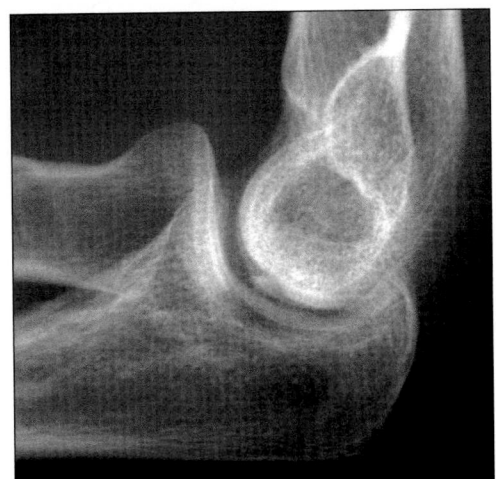

(Left) Anteroposterior radiography shows an osteochondritis dissecans lesion at the capitellum adjacent to the radial head. *(Right)* Lateral radiography shows the lesion involving the mid aspect of the capitellum.

Other

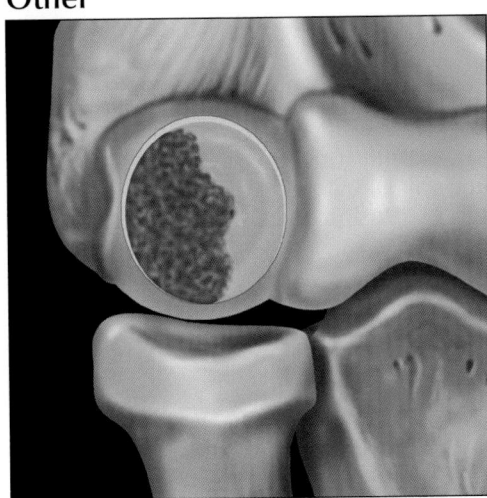
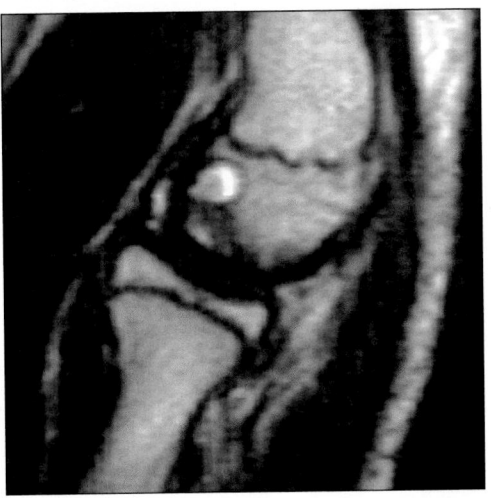

(Left) Coronal graphic shows capitellar osteochondrosis (Panner's disease) involving the lateral aspect of the capitellum. *(Right)* Sagittal T2 FSE MR shows subchondral cystic change of the anterior aspect of the capitellum in association with linear changes in a patient with Panner's disease – capitellar osteochondrosis.

RADIAL HEAD FRACTURE

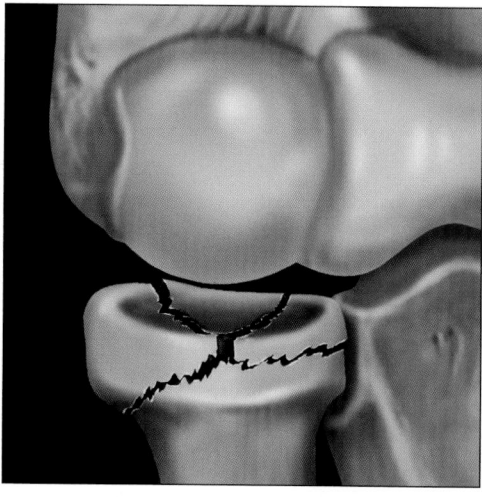

Coronal graphic shows a comminuted radial head fracture.

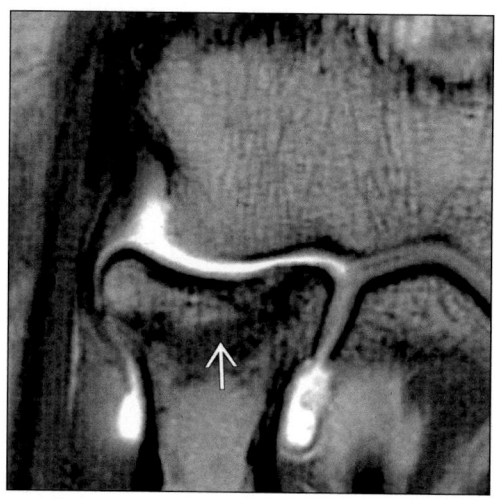

Coronal T1 arthrogram shows a nondisplaced radial head fracture (arrow).

TERMINOLOGY

Abbreviations and Synonyms
- Essex-Lopresti fracture, terrible triad of the elbow, lateral column fracture

Definitions
- Impaction injury due to axial overloading in a fall on to the outstretched arm

IMAGING FINDINGS

General Features
- Best diagnostic clue
  - Linear decreased signal intensity within the radial head surrounded by edema
  - Positive fat pad sign on radiographs in the absence of other findings is suggestive
- Location
  - Radial head
  - Anterolateral aspect of head more vulnerable because of lack of subchondral bone
- Size: Small nondisplaced to comminuted complex fracture
- Morphology
  - Nondisplaced cortical disruption
  - Severely comminuted/displaced

Radiographic Findings
- Radiography
  - Linear lucencies representing fracture lines
    - Variable fragment size and number on lateral or angled lateral views
  - Associated fractures of ulna and distal humerus, especially on lateral head view
  - +/- Associated posterior dislocation of elbow
  - Positive fat pad sign on lateral view

CT Findings
- NECT
  - Linear lucencies in radial head indicating fracture
  - Fracture comminution and displacement can be assessed
  - Soft tissue swelling evident on soft tissue windows
  - Assessment of occult coronoid fractures
  - Best method to detect osteochondral fragments (+/- arthrogram)

MR Findings
- T1WI
  - Decreased marrow signal indicating bone stress (contusion)
  - Low signal lines indicating fracture +/- bony displacement on axial views
  - Low signal joint effusion

DDx: Radial Head Fracture

Radial Neck Fx	Radial Neck Fx	OA	Post Disloc	Post Disloc

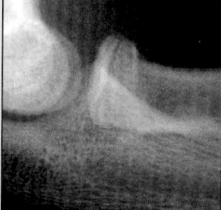 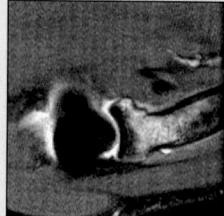 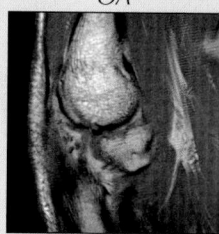 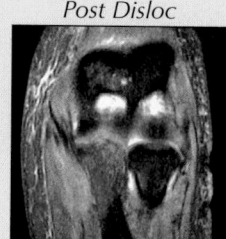 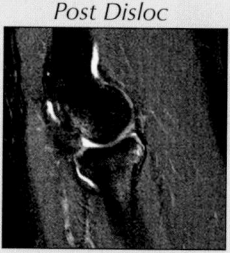

Lat Radiography	Sag STIR MR	Sag PD FSE MR	Cor STIR MR	Sag STIR MR

RADIAL HEAD FRACTURE

Key Facts

Imaging Findings
- Linear decreased signal intensity within the radial head surrounded by edema
- Positive fat pad sign on radiographs in the absence of other findings is suggestive
- Anterolateral aspect of head more vulnerable because of lack of subchondral bone
- Increased marrow signal indicating edema
- +/- Capitellar fx, coronoid fx in posterior dislocation

Top Differential Diagnoses
- Capitellar Fracture
- Olecranon Fracture
- Capitellum Osteochondritis Dissecans (OCD)
- Posterior Dislocation
- Osteoarthritis (OA)

- Radial Neck Fracture

Pathology
- Etiology: Fall on an outstretched arm (FOOSH)
- Accounts for about 30% of adult elbow fractures
- Posterior dislocation of elbow

Clinical Issues
- Pain and loss of function

Diagnostic Checklist
- Presence of other fractures, especially coronoid and scaphoid
- Presence of valgus instability
- Fat sat/STIR MR for MCL assessment and marrow edema to show occult fractures

---

- Disruption of normal anatomy and signal of collateral ligaments on coronal views
- T2WI
  - Increased marrow signal indicating edema
  - High signal joint effusion, +/- periarticular leakage of fluid or hemorrhage with capsular rupture
  - Low signal fracture line surrounded by high signal edema
  - Disruption of ligamentous anatomy
    - Hyperintense tears and associated high signal stress lesions at bony attachments
  - FS PD FSE: Visualization of edema improved with fat saturation
  - +/- Capitellar fx, coronoid fx in posterior dislocation
- PD/Intermediate
  - High resolution delineation of anatomy
  - Synovitis intermediate signal
  - Fracture lines hypointense
- STIR
  - Very sensitive for bony injury shown, as high signal areas in marrow space
  - Less spatial resolution than FS PD FSE/PD
- T2* GRE: Coronal images helpful for showing damage to articular cartilage, focal deficiencies with variable subchondral increased signal intensity

Imaging Recommendations
- Best imaging tool: MRI
- Protocol advice
  - FS PD FSE for edema and articular cartilage
  - T1WI for visualization of hypointense fracture line
  - Coronal, sagittal and axial planes for fracture morphology, displacement and angulation

DIFFERENTIAL DIAGNOSIS

Capitellar Fracture
- Uncommon
- Coronal plane
- Shear fracture
- Rare - 6% elbow fractures
- Rare in children < 10 years

Olecranon Fracture
- Fall on a flexed, supinated forearm
- Olecranon epiphysis fuses at 16-18 years
- Direct trauma
- Throwing injury (pitchers)
- Stress injury seen in throwing sports

Capitellum Osteochondritis Dissecans (OCD)
- Necrosis of bone followed by healing response and reossification
- 12-16 year age group (after ossification of capitellum)
  - Panner's disease younger (7-10 years old)
- 20% bilateral
- Chronic valgus stress with lateral impaction seen in gymnasts and adolescent pitchers

Posterior Dislocation
- +/- Lateral ligamentous damage
- +/- Fractures/trabecular injuries of posterior capitellum, anterior radial head
- Fall on outstretched hand (FOOSH) injury
- +/- Extensor tendon tear
- End stage instability

Osteoarthritis (OA)
- +/- Antecedent trauma
- +/- Subchondral cysts
- +/- Osteophytes
- +/- Loose bodies

Radial Neck Fracture
- Usually children/adolescents
- Essentially same lesion as radial head fracture
- Hyperintense edema on T2WI
- +/- Cortical buckle

PATHOLOGY

General Features
- Etiology: Fall on an outstretched arm (FOOSH)
- Epidemiology

RADIAL HEAD FRACTURE

- ○ Accounts for about 30% of adult elbow fractures
- ○ Most common elbow fracture in adults
- ○ Proximal radial injuries are rare in children and usually occur in the radial neck
- Associated abnormalities
  - ○ Posterior dislocation of elbow
  - ○ Capitellar fracture
  - ○ Disruption of anterior band of medial collateral ligament (MCL)
  - ○ Triceps tendon rupture
  - ○ Dislocation of the distal radioulnar joint (Essex Lopresti Fx)
  - ○ Scaphoid fracture
  - ○ Terrible triad = radial head and coronoid fractures + MCL tear

Gross Pathologic & Surgical Features

- Disruption of radial head with variable bone fragment size and number
- Osteochondral injury to adjacent capitellum
- Osteochondral free fragments
- Avulsion of insertion of anterior band of MCL

Microscopic Features

- Break of cortex and trabeculae
- Hemorrhage with cellular infiltrate
- Osteoblasts, osteoclasts, and inflammatory cells
  - ○ Depending on fracture age
- Avulsion of the osteo-ligamentous complex of the anterior band of the MCL
- Flap-tearing, fissuring or fibrillation of articular cartilage on capitellum

Staging, Grading or Classification Criteria

- Based on classification by Mason
  - ○ Type I = displacement < 2 mm
  - ○ Type II = displacement > 2 mm
  - ○ Type III = comminuted
  - ○ Type IV = comminution + dislocation

CLINICAL ISSUES

Presentation

- Most common signs/symptoms
  - ○ Pain and loss of function
  - ○ Swelling and discoloration
  - ○ Point tenderness over radial head
  - ○ Crepitus if fracture is displaced
  - ○ Associated wrist tenderness
  - ○ Loss of joint stability (late)
- Clinical profile: FOOSH injury

Demographics

- Age: Young to adult
- Gender: M > F

Natural History & Prognosis

- Prognosis decreased by
  - ○ Delayed mobilization
  - ○ Presence of other fractures, especially coronoid fractures
  - ○ Deteriorates with increase in grade of fracture
  - ○ Potentially decreased by radial head excision
- Improved by

- ○ early mobilization
- ○ Maintaining integrity of radioulnar joint
- ○ Repair of collateral ligaments

Treatment

- Conservative
  - ○ NSAIDs, physical therapy
- Surgical
  - ○ Fixation or excision in extreme cases

DIAGNOSTIC CHECKLIST

Consider

- Presence of other fractures, especially coronoid and scaphoid
- Presence of valgus instability
- Extent of fracture comminution

Image Interpretation Pearls

- Lateral and angled lateral radiographs (radial head view)
- NECT for associated coronoid fracture
- Fat sat/STIR MR for MCL assessment and marrow edema to show occult fractures

SELECTED REFERENCES

1. O'Driscoll SW et al: Difficult elbow fractures. Pearls and pitfalls. Instr Course Lect 52:113-34, 2003
2. Ring D et al: Open reduction and internal fixation of fractures of the radial head. J Bone Joint Surg Am 84-A(10):1811-5, 2002
3. Ring D et al: Posterior dislocation of the elbow with fractures of the radial head and coronoid. J Bone Joint Surg Am 84-A(4):547-51, 2002
4. Wildin CJ et al: The incidence of simultaneous fractures of the scaphoid and radial head. J Hand Surg Br 26(1):25-7, 2001
5. Van Glabbeek F et al: Current concepts in the treatment of radial head fractures in the adult. A clinical and biomechanical approach. Acta Orthop Belg 67(5):430-41, 2001
6. Sonin A: Fractures of the elbow and forearm. Semin Musculoskelet Radiol 4(2):171-91, 2000
7. Heim U: Combined fractures of the radius and the ulna at the elbow level in the adult. Analysis of 120 cases after more than 1 year. Rev Chir Orthop 84(2):142-53, 1998
8. Janssen RP et al: Resection of the radial head after Mason type-III fractures of the elbow. Follow-up at 16 to 30 years. J Bone Joint Surg Br 80(2):231-3, 1998

RADIAL HEAD FRACTURE

IMAGE GALLERY

Typical

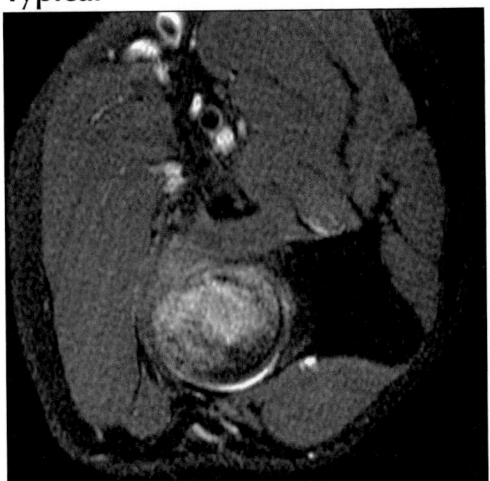 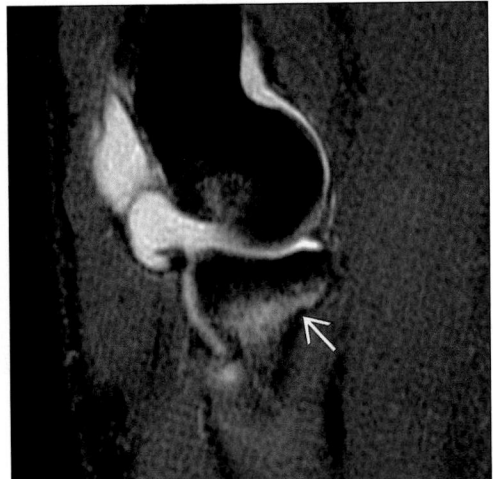

(Left) Axial STIR MR shows mildly impacted central radial head fracture. Note the fracture line of linear decreased signal intensity and associated hyperintense marrow edema. *(Right)* Sagittal STIR MR shows a radial neck fracture (arrow) as the result of a recent posterior dislocation.

Typical

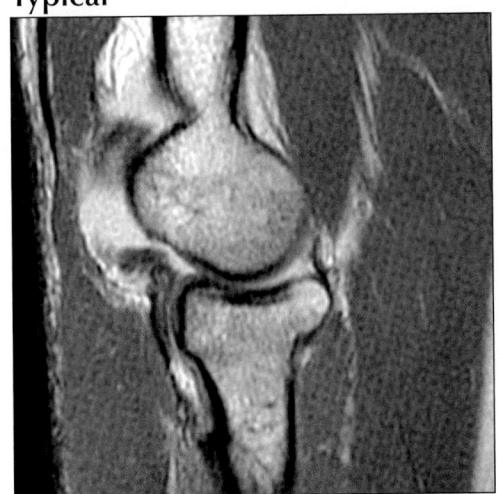 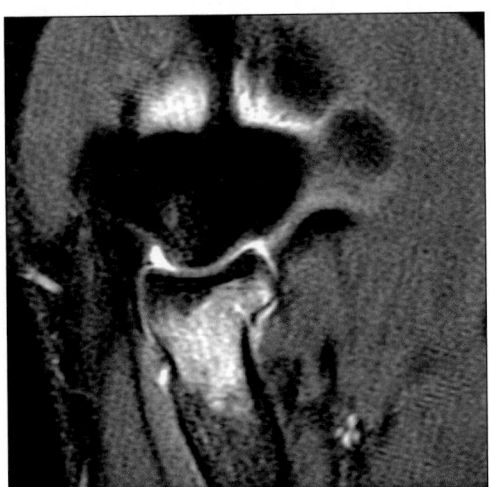

(Left) Sagittal PD FSE MR shows the slightly angulated radial neck fracture at the junction of the head and neck and a posterior capsular blow out in a patient who is status post posterior dislocation. *(Right)* Coronal STIR MR shows a fracture at the base of the radial head with discontinuity of hypointense cortex.

Variant

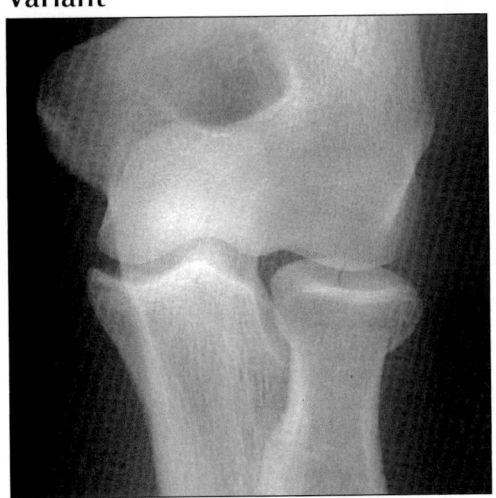 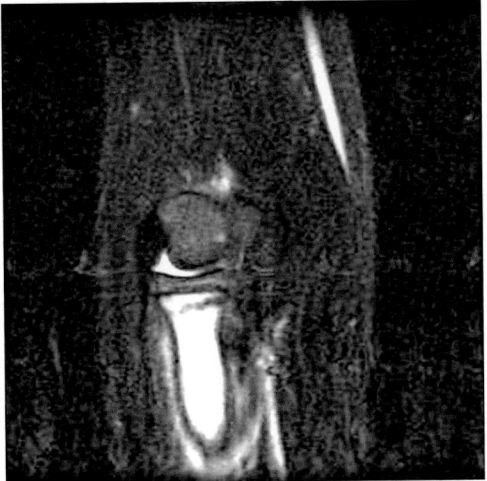

(Left) Anteroposterior radiography shows a comminuted radial head fracture which also involves radial head and neck junction – a common finding. *(Right)* Coronal STIR MR shows hyperintense bone marrow edema and surrounding periostitis and soft tissue edema with a radial head/neck fracture just proximal to the physis.

LOOSE BODIES AND OS SUPRATROCHLEARE

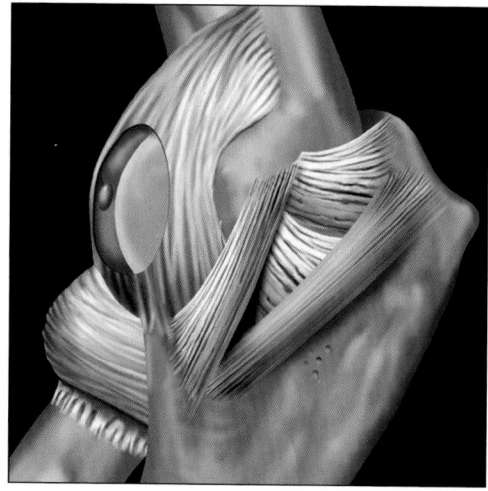

Sagittal graphic shows loose body within the anterior aspect of the joint.

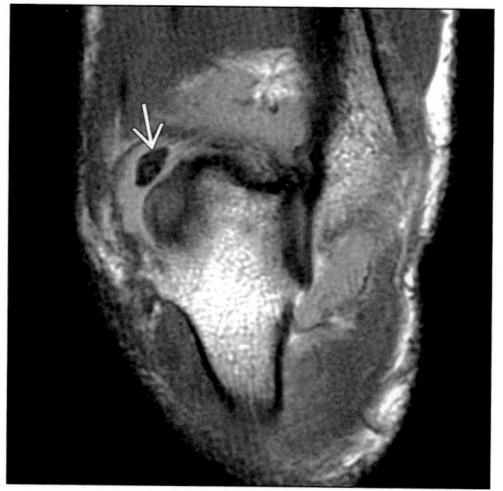

Coronal PD FSE MR shows loose body (arrow) within the posterior aspect of the joint adjacent to the olecranon process. There is synovitis present.

TERMINOLOGY

Abbreviations and Synonyms
- Os supratrochleare dorsale (OSD), loose bodies (LB)

Definitions
- Loose bodies are osteochondral fragments within the joint capsule
- Accessory ossicles are developmental variations of normal ossification of a joint, often in relation to a tendon

IMAGING FINDINGS

General Features
- Best diagnostic clue: Corticated rounded opacity intimately related to the joint
- Location
  ○ Loose bodies are most common anteriorly but are also found in the bare area of the ulnar trochlear notch
    ▪ Also seen in olecranon fossa (esp. in throwing athletes)
  ○ Os supratrochleare is found in olecranon fossa
- Size
  ○ Loose bodies may be minute to several millimeters
  ○ Os supratrochleare typically 1-2 cm

- Morphology
  ○ Loose bodies are laminated, rounded osteochondral particles
    ▪ Usually calcified but may be purely cartilaginous
  ○ Os supratrochleare is a thickly corticated, ovoid bony structure

Radiographic Findings
- Radiography
  ○ Rounded opacities of varying size and location
  ○ Non-calcified forms will be invisible
  ○ May vary location or remain fixed indicating synovial attachment
  ○ Os supratrochleare shows dense cortication +/- remodeling of olecranon fossa
  ○ Fragmentation/sclerosis suggests increasing impingement

CT Findings
- NECT: To confirm presence and location of loose bodies, especially when small
- CT arthrogram
  ○ To show synovial attachment and differentiate from periarticular calcification/osteophytes

MR Findings
- T1WI
  ○ Low signal round structures with variable internal high signal equivalent to fat (marrow)

DDx: Loose Bodies and Os Supratrochleare

Com Troch Fx	Lat Condyle Fx	Chondromatosis
Cor PD FSE MR	Cor PD FSE MR	Ax PD FSE MR

LOOSE BODIES AND OS SUPRATROCHLEARE

Key Facts

Imaging Findings
- Best diagnostic clue: Corticated rounded opacity intimately related to the joint
- Remodeling of olecranon fossa on sagittal images with os supratrochleare

Top Differential Diagnoses
- Osteochondritis Dissecans
- Panner's Disease (Osteochondrosis of Capitellum)
- Synovial Osteochondromatosis (Chondromatosis)
- Fracture

Pathology
- The trochlear notch is an area devoid of articular cartilage in the mid portion of the ulnar articulating surface
- Acts as a trap for loose bodies

- Elbow is second most common location for loose bodies
- Os supratrochleare is more common in males and usually found in dominant arm

Clinical Issues
- Presentation: Reduced range of motion
- Extension only in the case of os supratrochleare
- Elbow joint pain
- +/- Grating
- True locking and catching

Diagnostic Checklist
- Presence of other injuries in traumatic origin
- Possibility of osteochondritises or synovial chondromatosis
- AP/Lateral radiographs

- ○ Adjacent moderate signal synovial thickening
- ○ Remodeling of olecranon fossa on sagittal images with os supratrochleare
- T2WI
  - ○ High signal joint effusion
  - ○ Low signal loose bodies and synovial folds/hypertrophy
  - ○ FS PD FSE for chondral (intermediate signal) fragment visualization
- STIR: May show increased signal within loose bodies/os and adjacent bone in impingement
- T2* GRE: Useful for showing calcified loose bodies
- MR arthrography
  - ○ Demonstrates loose bodies
  - ○ Air bubbles (hypointense) may mimic loose bodies

Ultrasonographic Findings
- Rounded highly reflective intraarticular structures of variable size
- Free mobility within the joint or local attachment to synovium
- Dynamic imaging may demonstrate joint locking

Imaging Recommendations
- Best imaging tool
  - ○ Plain films, 30% sensitive
  - ○ MR +/- arthrogram
    - ▪ MR superior for chondral fragments
  - ○ NECT for presence of very small loose bodies
  - ○ Ultrasound popular where access to expertise exists
- Protocol advice: CT, MR with T1; FS PD FSE +/- T2* GRE

DIFFERENTIAL DIAGNOSIS

Osteochondritis Dissecans
- Typical presentation
- Most commonly affects humeral capitellum
- May produce loose bodies
- 20% bilateral
- Chronic valgus stress with lateral impaction seen in gymnasts and adolescent pitchers

- Necrosis of bone followed by healing response and reossification
- 13-16 year olds

Panner's Disease (Osteochondrosis of Capitellum)
- Typical age group
  - ○ 5-11 year old patients
- Usually heals
- Residual deformity usually not seen in Panner's disease
- Loose body formation usually not seen in Panner's disease
- Probably avascular necrosis secondary to trauma

Synovial Osteochondromatosis (Chondromatosis)
- May be indistinguishable
- Chondral bodies often calcify
- Synovial metaplasia
- Hypointense bodies in joint

Fracture
- Especially comminuted
- +/- Displaced
- Avulsion of epicondyle extraarticular
  - ○ Little leaguer's elbow
- Hyperintense edema on T2WI
- +/- Posterior dislocation

PATHOLOGY

General Features
- General path comments
  - ○ The trochlear notch is an area devoid of articular cartilage in the mid portion of the ulnar articulating surface
    - ▪ Should not be mistaken for osteochondral defect
    - ▪ Acts as a trap for loose bodies
    - ▪ +/- A bony ridge
  - ○ The os supratrochleare is intraarticular and may therefore grow through synovial nutrition
- Etiology

LOOSE BODIES AND OS SUPRATROCHLEARE

- o Os supratrochleare is an accessory bone of developmental origin
- o Loose bodies arise from osteochondral injuries or degeneration
- Epidemiology
  - o Elbow is second most common location for loose bodies
  - o Os supratrochleare is more common in males and usually found in dominant arm
- Associated abnormalities
  - o Articular cartilage defects
  - o Synovial hypertrophy
  - o Remodeling of olecranon fossa by os supratrochleare

Gross Pathologic & Surgical Features
- Variable number of intraarticular osteochondral fragments
- Articular cartilage attrition, fraying or defect
- Synovial hypertrophy and hyperemia

Microscopic Features
- Laminated articular cartilage
- Variable attachment to locally hypervascular synovium
- Variable matrix calcification/ossification
- Inflammatory infiltrate may be seen if acute impingement occurring

CLINICAL ISSUES

Presentation
- Most common signs/symptoms
  - o Presentation: Reduced range of motion
    - ▪ Extension only in the case of os supratrochleare
  - o Elbow joint pain
  - o +/- Grating
  - o True locking and catching

Demographics
- Age: Children/adults
- Gender: M > F

Natural History & Prognosis
- Premature arthritis if loose bodies left untreated
- Altered elbow function from growing os supratrochleare
- Generally excellent results from arthroscopic removal

Treatment
- Conservative: Direct blow to previously asymptomatic os supratrochleare may settle with rest
- Surgical: Arthroscopic removal or limited arthrotomy for very large os supratrochleare
- Complications: Infection, neurovascular damage, hematoma, contractures, arthrofibrosis

DIAGNOSTIC CHECKLIST

Consider
- Presence of other injuries in traumatic origin
- Possibility of osteochondritises or synovial chondromatosis

Image Interpretation Pearls
- AP/Lateral radiographs
- MR for lesion location and characterization
  - o T1WI for detection of loose bodies containing non-sclerotic marrow fat
  - o FS PD FSE for articular cartilage fragments adjacent to hyperintense joint fluid

SELECTED REFERENCES

1. Clasper JC et al: Arthroscopy of the elbow for loose bodies. Ann R Coll Surg 83(1):34-6, 2001
2. Miller JH et al: Detection of intraarticular bodies of the elbow with saline arthrosonography. Clin Radiol 56(3):231-4, 2001
3. Kelly EW et al: Complications of elbow arthroscopy J Bone Joint Surg 83A:25-34, 2001
4. Bianchi S et al: Detection of loose bodies in joints. Radiol Clin North Am 37(4):679-90, 1999
5. Hsu HC et al: Os supratrochleare dorsale of the elbow. A report of two cases. Zhonghua Yi Xue Za Zhi 61(11):667-72, 1998
6. Quinn SFet al: Evaluation of loose bodies in the elbow with MR imaging. J Magn Reson Imaging 4(2):169-72, 1994
7. Ogilvie-Harris DJ et al: Arthroscopy of the elbow for removal of loose bodies. Arthroscopy 9(1):5-8, 1993

LOOSE BODIES AND OS SUPRATROCHLEARE

IMAGE GALLERY

Typical

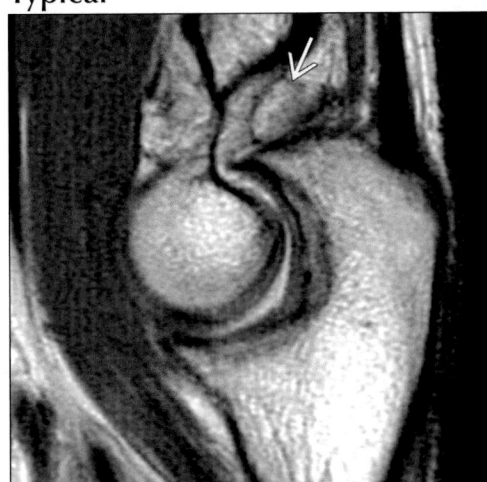

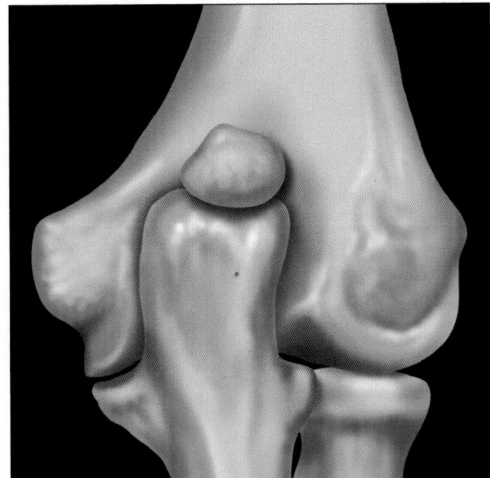

(Left) Sagittal PD FSE MR shows a loose body within the olecranon fossa adjacent to the olecranon tip (arrow). This mimics an os supratrochlear dorsale. *(Right)* Coronal graphic shows an supertrochleare dorsale at the proximal aspect of the olecranon process.

Typical

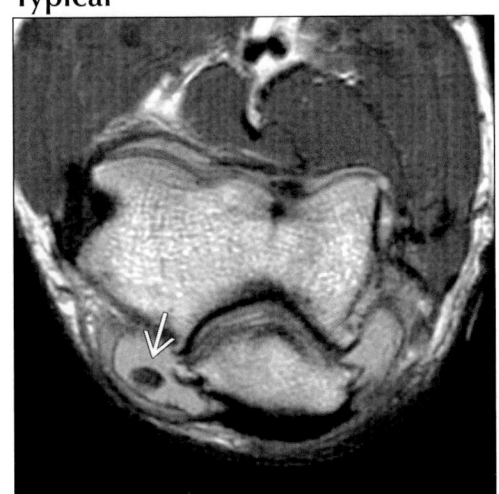

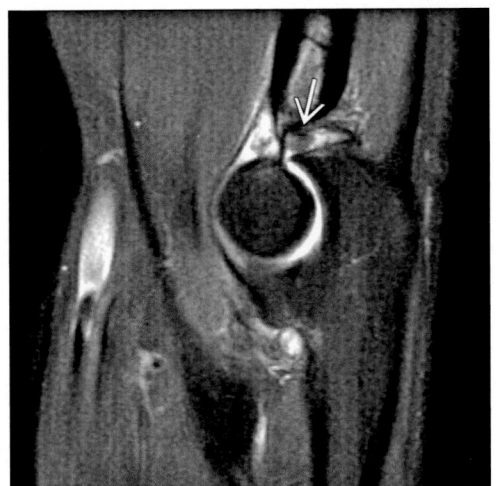

(Left) Axial PD FSE MR shows a hypointense sclerotic loose body within the posterior lateral aspect of the joint (arrow). *(Right)* Sagittal FS PD FSE MR shows a loose body within the olecranon fossa adjacent to the olecranon tip (arrow), and a small loose body within the anterior coronoid fossa.

Variant

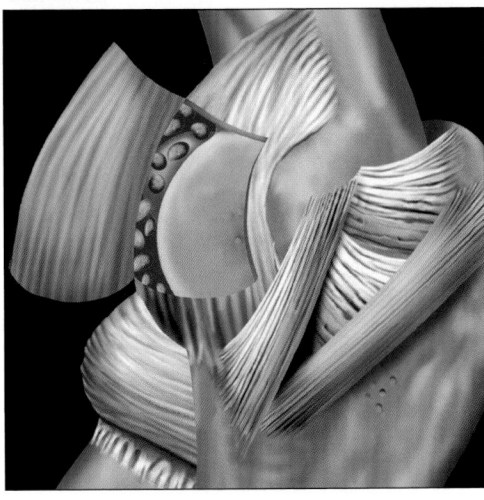

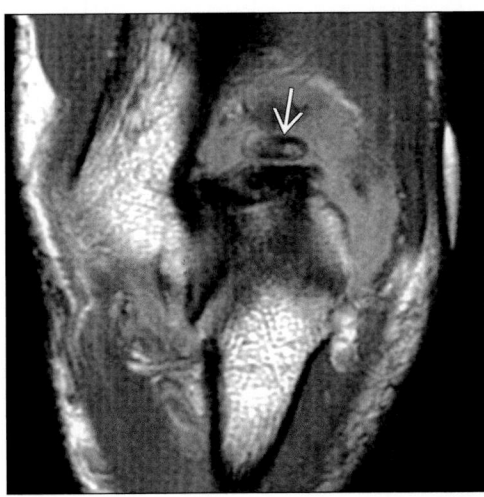

(Left) Sagittal graphic shows multiple loose bodies in elbow joint capsule synovial osteochondromatosis. *(Right)* Coronal PD FSE MR shows a loose body adjacent to the olecranon tip (arrow).

OLECRANON FRACTURE

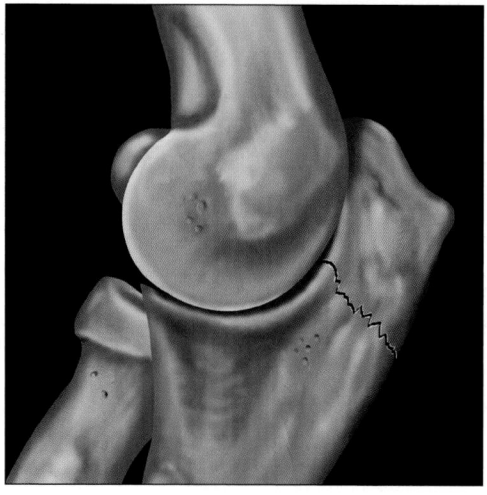

Sagittal graphic shows a transverse fracture through the olecranon process.

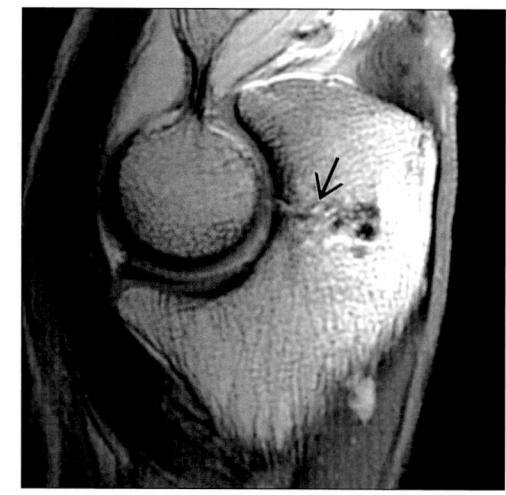

Sagittal PD FSE shows a nondisplaced fracture through the olecranon process (arrow).

TERMINOLOGY

Definitions
- Distraction injury due to resisted triceps contraction
  - Forced flexion on an extended forearm
  - High energy direct impact injury

IMAGING FINDINGS

General Features
- Best diagnostic clue
  - Proximal displacement of olecranon fragment, positive fat pad sign - radiographs
  - Linear decreased signal intensity surrounded by edema of olecranon on FSE PD/T2WI
- Location: Olecranon process of the proximal ulna
- Size
  - Varies from a flake to complete involvement
  - Usually isolated injury
- Morphology
  - Nondisplaced cortical disruption
  - Small "flake" avulsion
  - Transverse oblique defect near base

Radiographic Findings
- Radiography
  - Linear lucency representing fracture line

- Variable fragment size and displacement on lateral view
  - Positive fat pad sign on lateral view

CT Findings
- NECT
  - Linear lucencies in olecranon indicating fractures
  - Fracture comminution and displacement can be assessed
  - Soft tissue swelling evident on soft tissue windows
  - Sagittal reconstruction for best assessment

MR Findings
- T1WI
  - Decreased marrow signal indicating bone stress
  - Low signal lines indicating fracture lines, +/- bony displacement on sagittal/coronal views
  - Low signal joint effusion
  - Disruption of normal anatomy and signal of triceps tendon on sagittal views
- T2WI
  - Increased marrow signal indicating edema
  - Low signal fracture lines
    - +/- High signal hemorrhage interposed between fracture lines
  - FS PD FSE visualization improved by using FS
  - High signal joint effusion

DDx: Olecranon Fracture

Cortical Notch	Cortical Notch	Oss Centers	Ulnar Stress Fx
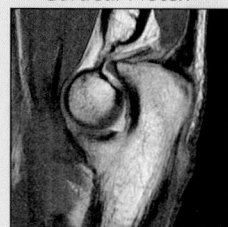	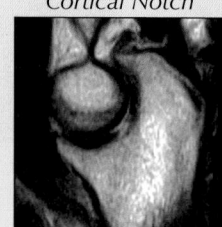	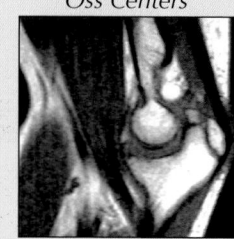	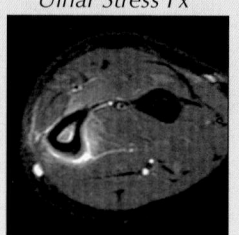
Sag PD FSE MR	Sag PD FSE MR	Sag T1WI MR	Ax STIR MR

OLECRANON FRACTURE

Key Facts

Terminology
- Distraction injury due to resisted triceps contraction
- Forced flexion on an extended forearm
- High energy direct impact injury

Imaging Findings
- Proximal displacement of olecranon fragment, positive fat pad sign - radiographs
- Linear decreased signal intensity surrounded by edema of olecranon on FSE PD/T2WI

Top Differential Diagnoses
- Posterior Dislocation
- Radial Head/Neck Fractures
- Cortical Notch
- Ulnar Stress Fracture
- Normal Ossification Center/Variation

Pathology
- Olecranon epiphysis fuses at 16-18 years
- Fall on a flexed, supinated forearm

Clinical Issues
- Pain and loss of function
- Swelling and hemorrhagic effusion

Diagnostic Checklist
- Always ensure there is not a concomitant fracture of coronoid process
- Identify location of fracture with respect to midpoint of trochlear notch
- Lateral radiograph, FS PD FSE/STIR MR for occult fractures and triceps status

---

- o Disruption of triceps tendon anatomy with high signal tears and associated high signal stress lesions at bony attachments
- STIR
  - o Very sensitive for bony injury, shown as high signal areas in marrow space
  - o Especially at low field
  - o Less spatial resolution than FS PD FSE

Imaging Recommendations
- Best imaging tool: Radiographs, MRI
- Protocol advice: FS PD FSE/T2WI

DIFFERENTIAL DIAGNOSIS

Posterior Dislocation
- Fall on outstretched hand injury (FOOSH)
- +/- Capitellar fx
- Lateral ligamentous disruptions
- +/- Common extensor tendon tear
- +/- Coronoid fx

Radial Head/Neck Fractures
- Essex-Lopresti fracture
- May accompany posterior dislocation
- +/- Coronoid process fracture/other fractures
- Impaction injury due to axial overloading in a fall on to the outstretched arm
- Radial head injuries are rare in children
  - o Usually occur in the radial neck
- Most common elbow fracture in adults

Cortical Notch
- Normal variation
- "Bare area"
- Mimics osteochondral defect

Ulnar Stress Fracture
- Abnormal stresses on normal bone
- Increased signal intensity on T2WI
- Fat suppression sequences sensitive (FS PD FSE)
- +/- Periostitis

Normal Ossification Center/Variation
- Normal childhood development
- May mimic fractures
- Absent edema in adjacent ossified bone
- Normally fuses at 16-18 years
- Failure of fusion = os supratrochleare dorsale
- Bipartite olecranon
- Patella cubiti

PATHOLOGY

General Features
- General path comments
  - o Olecranon epiphysis fuses at 16-18 years
  - o Midpoint of trochlear notch critical in determining stability of healing
- Etiology
  - o Fall on a flexed, supinated forearm
  - o Direct trauma (direct blow to olecranon in flexed position)
  - o Hyperextension
  - o Throwing injury (pitchers)
- Epidemiology
  - o Accounts for about 20% of adult elbow fractures
  - o Approximately 6% of childhood elbow injuries
- Associated abnormalities
  - o High velocity injuries, +/- other upper limb fractures
  - o Hyperextension injuries, +/- fractures of radial head or lateral epicondyle due to varus/valgus loads with olecranon locked into olecranon fossa

Gross Pathologic & Surgical Features
- Transverse disruption of olecranon typically with one fragment
  - o Most common pattern
- Most fractures are intraarticular
- Avulsion of insertion of triceps
- Tearing of fibrous sheath formed from capsule, lateral ligaments, triceps tendon and periosteum
- 2-31% will be open fractures

OLECRANON FRACTURE

Microscopic Features
- Disruption of cortex and trabeculae
- Hemorrhage with cellular infiltrate ranging from osteoblast and osteoclast to inflammatory cells depending on fracture age
- Separation of collagen bundles of triceps aponeurosis

Staging, Grading or Classification Criteria
- Colton's classification for displacement & pattern of fracture
  - Type I: Nondisplaced (< 2 mm) and stable
  - Type II: Displaced
    - A - avulsion
    - B - transverse
    - C - comminuted
    - D - fracture/dislocations
- Number of fractures, displacement and location will determine management
- 80% will have little (< 2 mm) or no displacement
- Displacement of > 2 mm is usual indication for ORIF
- Displacement of > 1.5 cm is unusual
- Olecranon stress fracture
  - Pain during acceleration phase of throwing
  - Also seen in adults

CLINICAL ISSUES

Presentation
- Most common signs/symptoms
  - Pain and loss of function
  - Swelling and hemorrhagic effusion
  - Point tenderness over olecranon
  - Inability to extend against gravity
  - Ulnar neuropathy
    - Pain with extension and flexion
- Clinical profile
  - Athlete
  - After severe trauma
    - Direct impact to extended elbow

Demographics
- Age: Children/adults
- Gender: M > F

Natural History & Prognosis
- Best outcome seen in minimally/nondisplaced fractures
- Degenerative changes seen in < 20%
- > 80% of patients have good outcome

Treatment
- Conservative: For nondisplaced fractures, 3 weeks cast in 90 degrees flexion
  - Acceptable for displaced fractures in elderly patients with concomitant illness
- Surgical: Tension band wiring for fractures proximal to midpoint of trochlear notch, plate fixation for fractures distal to midpoint
  - Locking nails and screws are also used
  - Severe comminution or poor bone quality may require excision and triceps advancement
  - Percutaneous techniques
- Complications

- Loss of extension
- Nonunion
- Ulnar nerve palsies
- Heterotopic bone formation
- Ulna-humeral arthrosis
- Painful hardware

DIAGNOSTIC CHECKLIST

Consider
- Presence of other fractures, especially coronoid
- Always ensure there is not a concomitant fracture of coronoid process
- Identify location of fracture with respect to midpoint of trochlear notch
- In high velocity injury, exclude injuries elsewhere
- In low velocity, consider general medical condition of patient

Image Interpretation Pearls
- Lateral radiograph, FS PD FSE/STIR MR for occult fractures and triceps status

SELECTED REFERENCES

1. O'Driscoll SW et al: Difficult elbow fractures: Pearls and pitfalls. Instr Course Lect 52:113-34, 2003
2. Gicquel P et al: Biomechanical analysis of olecranon fracture fixation in children. J Pediatr Orthop 22(1):17-21, 2002
3. Caterini R et al: Fractures of the olecranon in children. Long-term follow-up of 39 cases. J Pediatr Orthop B 11(4):320-8, 2002
4. Karlsson MK et al: Fractures of the olecranon: A 15- to 25-year followup of 73 patients. Clin Orthop (403):205-12, 2002
5. Akman S et al: Long-term results of olecranon fractures treated with tension-band wiring technique. Acta Orthop Traumatol Turc 36(5):401-7, 2002
6. Bailey CS et al: Outcome of plate fixation of olecranon fractures. J Orthop Trauma 15(8):542-8, 2001
7. Sonin A: Fractures of the elbow and forearm. Semin Musculoskelet Radiol 4(2):171-9, 2000

OLECRANON FRACTURE

IMAGE GALLERY

Typical

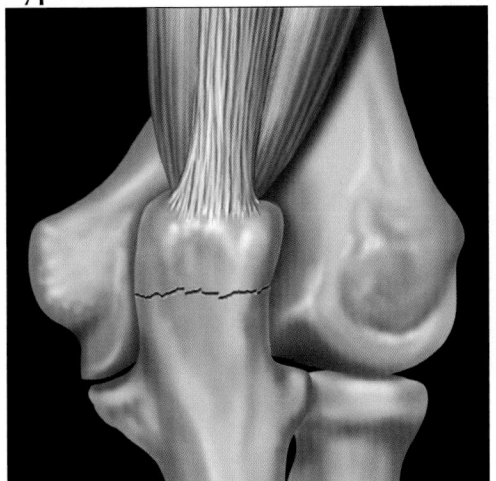 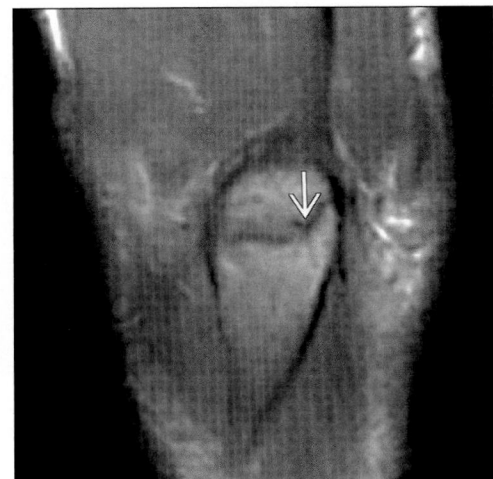

(Left) Coronal graphic shows a nondisplaced fracture of the olecranon process. *(Right)* Coronal PD FSE MR shows a hypointense nondisplaced fracture of the olecranon process (arrow).

Typical

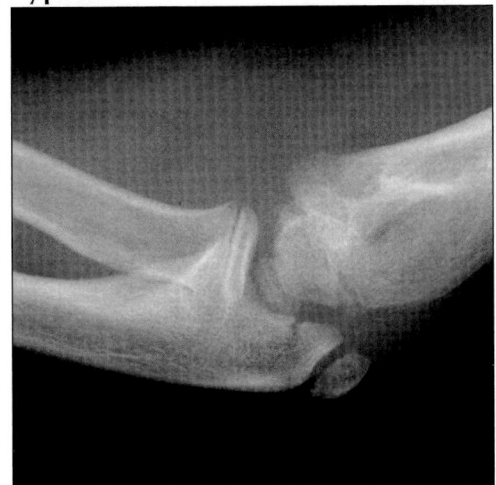 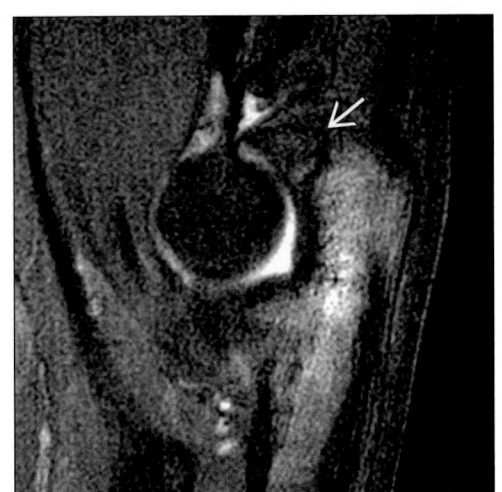

(Left) Lateral radiography shows an olecranon fracture and an olecranon ossification center. *(Right)* Sagittal STIR MR shows a stress fracture (arrow) line surrounded by adjacent hyperintense edema.

Typical

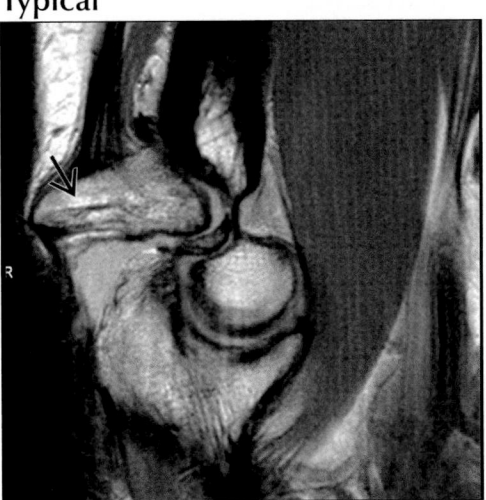 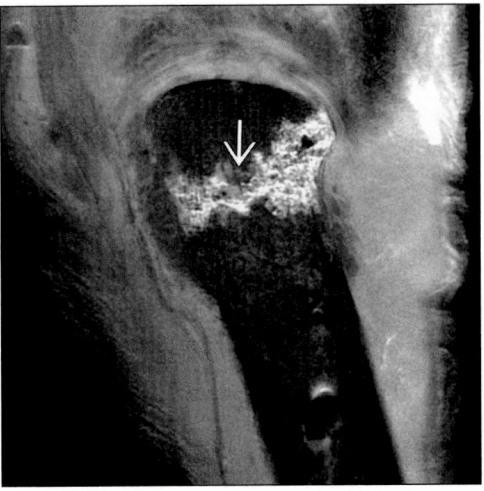

(Left) Sagittal PD FSE MR shows an old ununited olecranon fracture (arrow) still attached to the triceps tendon. There is also a loose body in the olecranon fossa. *(Right)* Coronal FS PD FSE MR shows a nondisplaced olecranon fracture (arrow) obscured by hyperintense trabecular edema.

LATERAL CONDYLAR FRACTURE

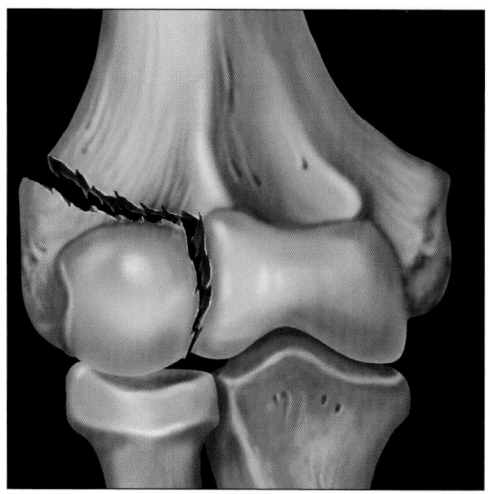

Coronal graphic shows a lateral condylar fracture. The lateral condylar fragment is slightly displaced.

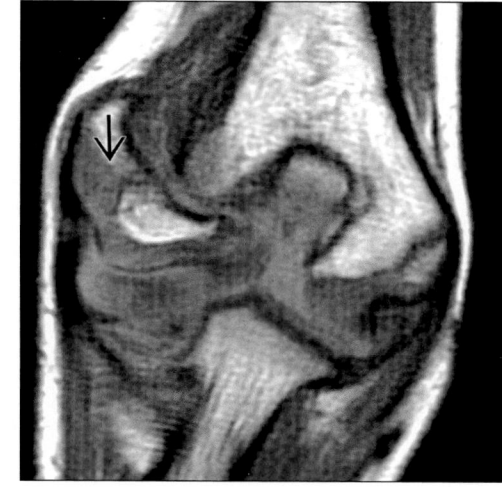

Coronal PD FSE MR shows a lateral condylar fracture (arrow) with rotation and slight distraction of the lateral condylar fragment still attached to the common extensor tendon origin.

TERMINOLOGY

Abbreviations and Synonyms
- Lateral condylar fx, lateral condyle fracture

Definitions
- An avulsion injury caused by contraction of forearm extensor/supinator muscles
  - Fall on to an out stretched hand (FOOSH)
  - Impaction injury caused by transmitted load through the radial head
  - Intraarticular extension

IMAGING FINDINGS

General Features
- Best diagnostic clue
  - + Posterior fat pad sign on radiography
  - Lucent fracture line, +/- displacement seen on NECT
  - Linear decreased signal intensity fracture with surrounding edema on MRI
- Location
  - Lateral column of distal humerus
    - Between lateral metaphysis and articular surface
  - Through medial trochlear notch or capitellotrochlear groove
- Size
  - Varies from a subtle crack to an extensively displaced lesion
  - Difficult to detect in immature skeleton
- Morphology
  - Undisplaced cortical/physeal disruption
  - Postero-inferiorly displaced fragment

Radiographic Findings
- Radiography
  - Linear lucency representing fracture line with variable fragment size and displacement on AP view
  - Associated fractures of radial head on lateral view
  - Widening of intercondylar distance on AP view
  - Posterior fat pad sign is reliable indicator of injury
  - Oblique views may be needed to show posteriorly displaced fragment

CT Findings
- NECT
  - Linear lucency in condyle
  - Fracture comminution and displacement can be assessed
  - Soft tissue swelling evident on soft tissue windows

MR Findings
- T1WI
  - Decreased marrow signal indicating bone stress
  - Hypointense fracture lines, +/- bony displacement on axial views

DDx: Lateral Condylar Fracture

Post Dislocation	Post Dislocation	Capitellum OCD	Rad Head/Neck Fx	Rad Head/Neck Fx

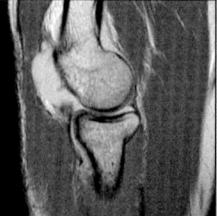 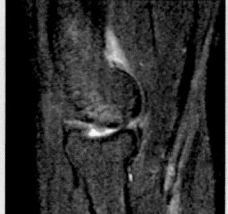 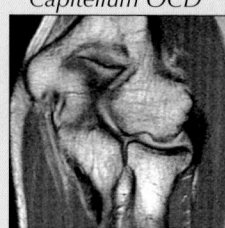 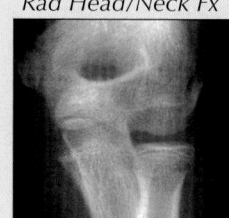 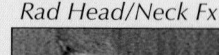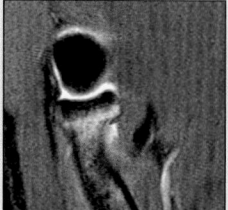

Sag PD FSE MR	Sag STIR MR	Cor PD FSE MR	AP Radiography	Cor STIR MR

LATERAL CONDYLAR FRACTURE

Key Facts

Terminology
- An avulsion injury caused by contraction of forearm extensor/supinator muscles
- Fall on to an out stretched hand (FOOSH)
- Impaction injury caused by transmitted load through the radial head

Imaging Findings
- Linear lucency representing fracture line with variable fragment size and displacement on AP view
- Associated fractures of radial head on lateral view
- Increased marrow signal indicating edema

Top Differential Diagnoses
- Supracondylar Fracture
- Radial Head/Neck Fracture (Rad Head/Neck Fx)

- Capitellum Osteochondritis Dissecans (Capitellum OCD)
- Olecranon Fracture
- Posterior Dislocation

Pathology
- Associated with delayed complications

Clinical Issues
- Pain and loss of function
- Swelling and discoloration

Diagnostic Checklist
- Presence of neurovascular complications
- Presence of other injuries in elbow and upper limb
- Fat sat/STIR MR for assessment of physeal injury, articular cartilage and common extensor origin

---

- o Hypointense joint effusion
- T2WI
  - o Increased marrow signal indicating edema
  - o Fracture lines through condylar and physis
  - o Surrounded by hyperintense edema
  - o Fx visualization improved by using FS PD FSE
  - o Hyperintense joint effusion
- STIR
  - o Sensitive for bony marrow edema
  - o Hyperintense areas in marrow space

Nuclear Medicine Findings
- Bone Scan: + Uptake after 24-72 hours

Imaging Recommendations
- Best imaging tool: CT/MRI
- Protocol advice
  - o Acute phase: Lateral and AP radiograph +/- oblique view
  - o Late phase: Axial and coronal MR to evaluate presence of physeal and ligamentous/capsular injuries plus status of articular cartilage

DIFFERENTIAL DIAGNOSIS

Supracondylar Fracture
- Fall on outstretched hand (FOOSH) injury
- Transverse lucency in metaphysis on AP or angled AP view
- Anterior humeral line displaced anterior to mid third of capitellum in 94%
- Extraarticular in children but may be intraarticular in adults
- 60% of pediatric elbow fractures
- Rare in adults (< 3%)

Radial Head/Neck Fracture (Rad Head/Neck Fx)
- Associated posterior dislocation
- Associated with coronoid process fracture/other fractures

- An impaction injury due to axial overloading in a fall on to the outstretched arm
- Radial head injuries are rare in children
  - o Usually occur in the neck of radius
- Most common elbow fracture in adults

Capitellum Osteochondritis Dissecans (Capitellum OCD)
- Necrosis of bone followed by healing response and reossification
- 12-16 year age group
  - o After ossification of capitellum
- Panner's disease (osteochondrosis)
  - o 7-10 years
  - o Degeneration/necrosis capitellum + regeneration and recalcification
- 20% bilateral
- Chronic valgus stress with lateral impaction
- Seen in gymnasts and adolescent baseball pitchers

Olecranon Fracture
- Acute flexion on extended forearm
- Clinical presentation similar
- Fall on a flexed, supinated forearm
- Throwing injury (pitchers)
- Accounts for about 20% of adult elbow fractures

Posterior Dislocation
- Fall on outstretched hand injury
- +/- Capitellar fx/coronoid fx
- Lateral ligamentous disruptions
  - o LUCL
- + Surrounding hemorrhage
- +/- Capsular disruption

PATHOLOGY

General Features
- General path comments
  - o Associated with delayed complications
    - ■ Deformity
    - ■ Nonunion

LATERAL CONDYLAR FRACTURE

- Complications result of inadequate fixation at the time of fracture
- Etiology
  - Fall on an outstretched hand, with impaction of radial head
  - Varus stress with elbow flexed/supinated, avulsion by common extensor action
- Epidemiology
  - 18% of distal humerus fractures
  - Common in 5-10 year age (peak = 6 years)
  - Second most common elbow fx
- Associated abnormalities: Olecranon fractures

Gross Pathologic & Surgical Features

- Rotation of fracture fragment due to action of forearm extensors/supinators
- Disruption of blood supply if significant soft tissue injury occurs
- Articular cartilage may remain intact and preserve stability

Microscopic Features

- Disruption of cortex and trabeculae
- Hemorrhage with cellular infiltrate ranging from osteoblast and osteoclast to inflammatory cells depending on fracture age
- Avulsion of the osteo-tendinous complex of the common extensor origin

Staging, Grading or Classification Criteria

- Classification of Milch for unicondylar humeral fractures
  - Milch type I fx: Lateral trochlear ridge intact - preserved medio-lateral stability (Salter Harris type II)
  - Milch type II fx: Fracture line medial to trochlear groove so lateral trochlear ridge is part of fragment
    - Unstable (Salter Harris type IV), more common
    - Stability may be preserved by articular cartilage hinge even with complete physeal injury
- Jakob classification based on displacement
  - Type 1: Incomplete & nondisplaced
  - Type 2: Extends through epiphysis - fragment laterally displaced
  - Type 3: Lateral condyle rotates or is completely displaced

CLINICAL ISSUES

Presentation

- Most common signs/symptoms
  - Pain and loss of function
  - Swelling and discoloration
  - Point tenderness lateral condyle
  - Crepitus
- Clinical profile: Trauma patient

Demographics

- Age: Child/adult
- Gender: M > F

Natural History & Prognosis

- Poor prognosis associated with comminution, delayed reduction and unstable fixation
- Undisplaced type I injuries have excellent outcome (98% asymptomatic)
- Delayed reduction has worse outcome
- Aggressive dissection (iatrogenic soft tissue stripping) or the injury itself associated with AVN

Treatment

- Conservative: Undisplaced Milch type I - splint or percutaneous pinning
- Surgical: Displaced (> 3 mm) Milch type I + type II = ORIF with K-wires or screws
- Complications: Seen in 33%, loss of flexion/extension, nonunion and malunion, cubitus varus (lateral spur formation), AVN, valgus angulation, ulnar nerve palsy, myositis ossificans

DIAGNOSTIC CHECKLIST

Consider

- Displacement of fragment
- Stability of fracture
- Presence of neurovascular complications
- Presence of other injuries in elbow and upper limb

Image Interpretation Pearls

- Lateral and AP radiographs
- Fat sat/STIR MR for assessment of physeal injury, articular cartilage and common extensor origin
- T2* GRE also visualizes physis and provides visualization of epiphyseal cartilage (thick in a child)

SELECTED REFERENCES

1. O'Driscoll SW et al: Difficult elbow fractures. Pearls and pitfalls. Instr Course Lect 52:113-34, 2003
2. Fitzgerald RH Jr. et al: Orthopaedics. St. Louis MO, Mosby, 286-95, 2002
3. Horn BD et al: Fractures of the lateral humeral condyle. Role of the cartilage hinge in fracture stability. J Pediatr Orthop 22(1):8-11, 2002
4. Toh S et al: Long-standing nonunion of fractures of the lateral humeral condyle. J Bone Joint Surg Am 84-A(4):593-8, 2002
5. Vocke-Hell AK et al: Sonographic differentiation of stable and unstable lateral condyle fractures of the humerus in children. J Pediatr Orthop B 10(2):138-41, 2001
6. Sonin A: Fractures of the elbow and forearm. Semin Musculoskelet Radiol 4(2):171-91, 2000
7. Kamegaya M et al: Assessment of stability in children's minimally displaced lateral humeral condyle fracture by magnetic resonance imaging. J Pediatr Orthop 19(5):570-2, 1999
8. Bast SC et al: Nonoperative treatment for minimally and nondisplaced lateral humeral condyle fractures in children. J Pediatr Orthop 18(4):448-50, 1998

LATERAL CONDYLAR FRACTURE

IMAGE GALLERY

Typical

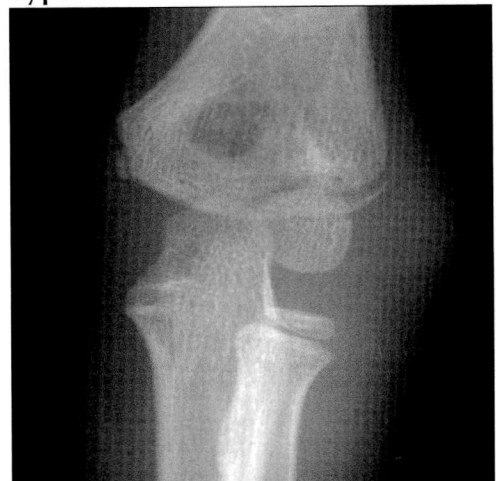 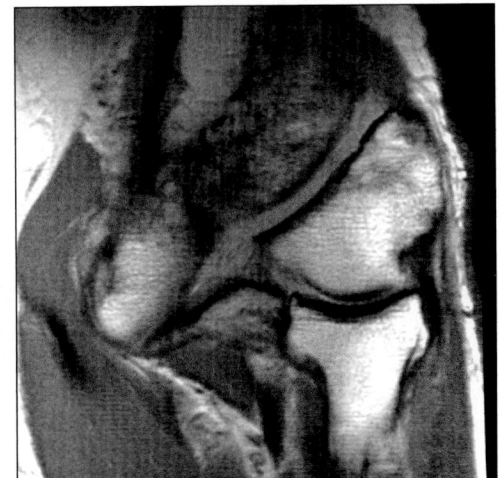

(Left) Anteroposterior radiography shows a lateral condylar fracture with marked lateral soft tissue swelling. *(Right)* Coronal PD FSE MR shows a chronic lateral condylar fracture in a 57 year old patient who suffered the fracture at age 10.

Typical

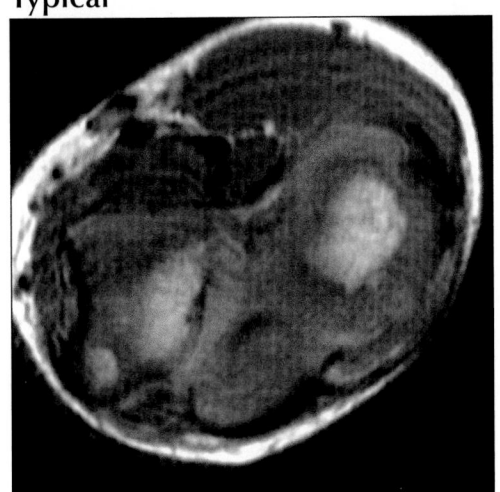 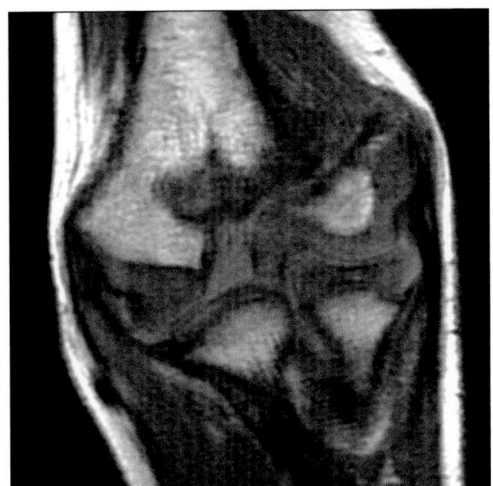

(Left) Axial PD FSE MR shows the lateral condylar fracture with slight distraction and separation of the condylar fragment. *(Right)* Coronal PD FSE MR shows lateral condylar fracture with slight rotation of the fracture fragment in an adolescent.

Typical

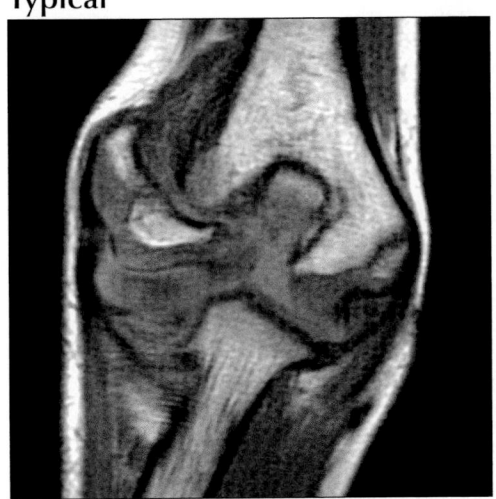 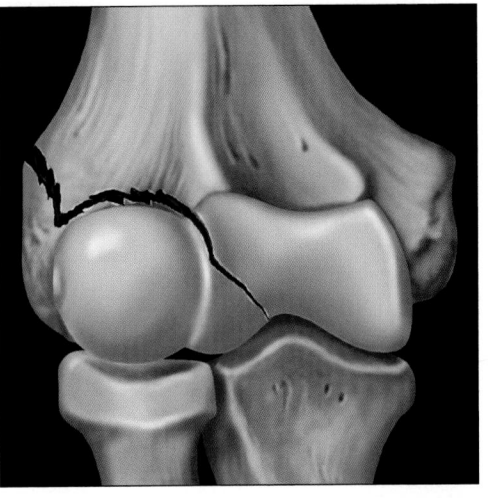

(Left) Coronal PD FSE MR shows slight rotation of a lateral condylar fracture and intraarticular synovitis. *(Right)* Coronal graphic shows a lateral condylar fracture with distal extension into the lateral aspect of the trochlea (type II fx).

CAPITELLUM FRACTURE

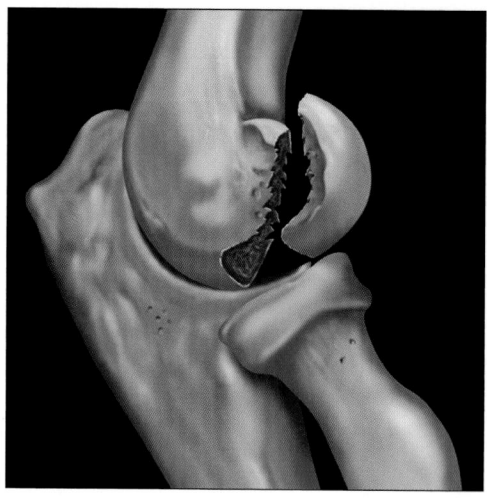

Coronal graphic shows fracture through humeral capitellum oriented in coronal plane. Other elbow fractures commonly associated, esp. radial head (20%). Also seen with posterior dislocation.

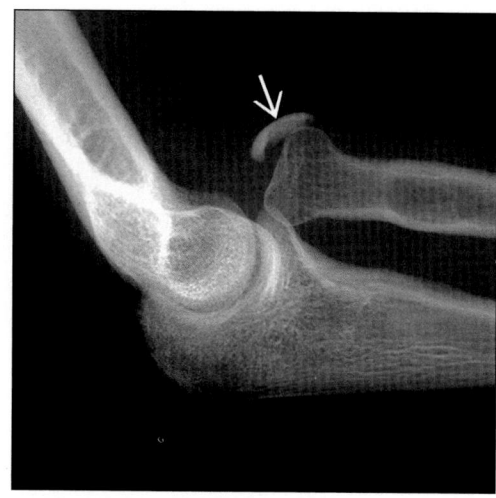

Lateral radiography shows coronally oriented displaced rotated capitellar fracture (arrow). Fractures occur coronal plane. Radial head is dislocated anteriorly indicating capsular rupture.

TERMINOLOGY

Abbreviations and Synonyms
- Hahn-Steinthal, Kocher-Lorenz, Broberg-Morrey, McKee, coronal shear fracture

Definitions
- Shear injury due to transmitted axial overload from radial head in fall on out stretched arm

IMAGING FINDINGS

General Features
- Best diagnostic clue: Fracture line seen on NECT, or linear decreased signal intensity fracture with surrounding edema on MRI
- Location: Distal end of lateral column of the humerus, osseous or articular cartilage, in coronal plane
- Size: Nondisplaced cortical break to anteriorly displaced fragment
- Morphology: Nondisplaced cortical disruption, sleeve avulsion of articular cartilage, comminuted and displaced

Radiographic Findings
- Radiography: Linear lucency fracture line - seen best on lateral view with positive fat pad sign

CT Findings
- NECT: Linear lucency (lucencies if comminuted) indicating fractures

MR Findings
- T1WI: Decreased marrow signal indicating edema with low signal lines indicating fracture lines
- T2WI: Increased marrow signal indicating edema and effusion, +/- displaced fragment

Imaging Recommendations
- Best imaging tool: Radiographs in acute phase = lateral, angled lateral, MRI
- Protocol advice: FS PD FSE

DIFFERENTIAL DIAGNOSIS

Pseudodefect
- Posterior normal variation

Capitellar Osteochondritis (OCD)
- Usually insidious in onset

Capitellum Bone Injury from Posterior Dislocation
- Posterior aspect secondary to radial head impaction

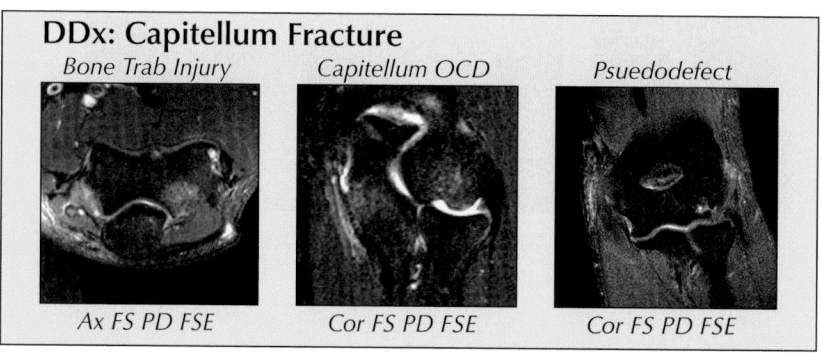

DDx: Capitellum Fracture

Bone Trab Injury — Ax FS PD FSE

Capitellum OCD — Cor FS PD FSE

Psuedodefect — Cor FS PD FSE

CAPITELLUM FRACTURE

Key Facts

Terminology
- Hahn-Steinthal, Kocher-Lorenz, Broberg-Morrey, McKee, coronal shear fracture

Imaging Findings
- Best diagnostic clue: Fracture line seen on NECT, or linear decreased signal intensity fracture with surrounding edema on MRI
- Location: Distal end of lateral column of the humerus, osseous or articular cartilage, in coronal plane
- Size: Nondisplaced cortical break to anteriorly displaced fragment
- Morphology: Nondisplaced cortical disruption, sleeve avulsion of articular cartilage, comminuted and displaced

- Radiography: Linear lucency fracture line - seen best on lateral view with positive fat pad sign
- T2WI: Increased marrow signal indicating edema and effusion, +/- displaced fragment

Top Differential Diagnoses
- Pseudodefect
- Capitellar Osteochondritis (OCD)
- Capitellum Bone Injury from Posterior Dislocation

Clinical Issues
- Most common signs/symptoms: Pain and swelling after fall on outstretch arm

Diagnostic Checklist
- Fracture is in coronal plane and best visualized on sagittal images

PATHOLOGY

General Features
- Etiology: Fall on an out stretched arm or direct blow to elbow
- Epidemiology: Rare - 6% of elbow fractures (not usually seen in children < 10 years old)

Gross Pathologic & Surgical Features
- Coronal defect with variable anterior displacement

Microscopic Features
- Disruption of cortex and trabeculae

Staging, Grading or Classification Criteria
- Type I: Hahn-Steinthal - coronal fracture of capitellum with no extension to trochlea
- Type II: Kocher-Lorenz - sleeve avulsion of articular cartilage
- Type III: Broberg and Morrey - comminuted
- Type IV: McKee - type III + extension to trochlea

CLINICAL ISSUES

Presentation
- Most common signs/symptoms: Pain and swelling after fall on outstretch arm

Demographics
- Age: Adolescents, adults
- Gender: F > M

Natural History & Prognosis
- Delayed mobilization and presence of other fractures complicates recovery

Treatment
- Conservative
  - Type I: Closed reduction, sling in flexion; early mobilization important
- Surgical
  - Type I: Wire or screw fixation, type II: Excision, type III/IV: Cancellous lag/Acutrac screws

DIAGNOSTIC CHECKLIST

Consider
- Presence of other fractures, especially radial head

Image Interpretation Pearls
- Fracture is in coronal plane and best visualized on sagittal images

SELECTED REFERENCES

1. Ring D et al: Articular fractures of the distal part of the humerus. J Bone Joint Surg Am 85-A(2):232-8, 2003
2. Mehdian H et al: Fractures of capitellum and trochlea. Orthop Clin North Am 31(1):115-27, 2000
3. Tomas FJ et al: Modified radial head--capitellum projection in elbow trauma. Br J Radiol 71(841):74-5, 1998

IMAGE GALLERY

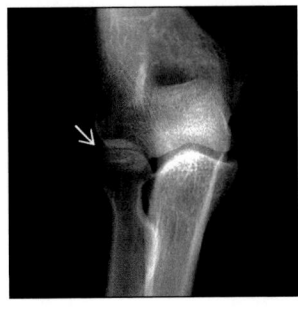 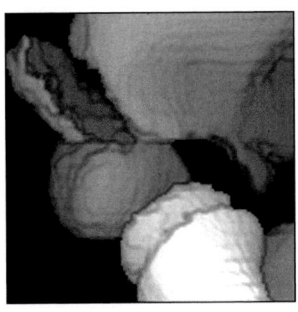

(Left) Anteroposterior radiography shows a coronal shear fracture (arrow) of the capitellum with displacement. The center of rotation at the radiocapitellar joint is anterior to axis of humeral shaft, predisposing to shear injuries. *(Right)* Coronal NECT demonstrates a shear fracture of the capitellum with displacement in this patient who is status post posterior dislocation.

SUPRACONDYLAR FRACTURE

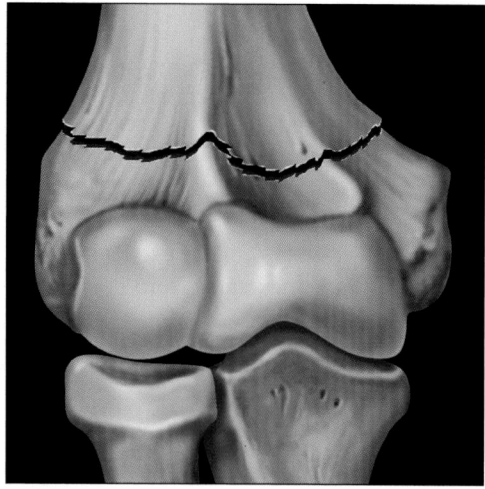

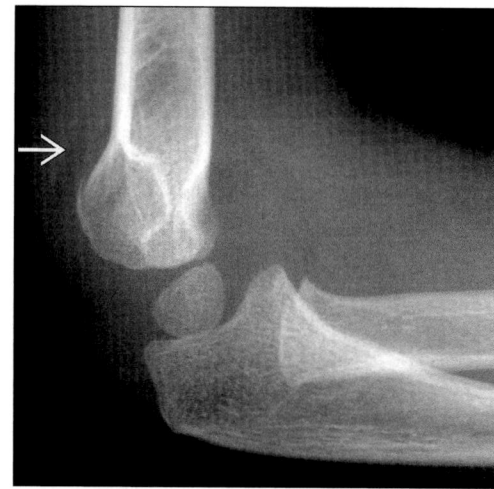

Coronal graphic shows a supracondylar fracture. Fracture line may not be visible on radiographs requiring utilization of the anterior humeral line sign.

Lateral radiography shows a posteriorly displaced distal humerus (anterior humeral line displaced) and a positive fat pad sign (arrow) in this young patient with a supracondylar fracture.

TERMINOLOGY

Abbreviations and Synonyms
- Gartland fracture

Definitions
- Transverse fracture of the distal humerus from a bending force in hyperextension
- Transmitted posterior force in flexion of elbow

IMAGING FINDINGS

General Features
- Best diagnostic clue
  - Radiographs
    - Positive fat pad sign
    - Transverse metaphyseal lucency
    - Disruption of anterior humeral line
  - Linear decreased signal intensity surrounded by edema on PD FSE/T2WI of supracondylar humerus
- Location
  - Thin distal humerus at risk between the olecranon and coronoid fossae
  - Extraarticular in children
- Size: Involves entire distal humerus above condylar epiphyses
- Morphology

- Plastic deformity of distal humerus
- Posterior angulation/displacement
- Fracture line angles from anterior distal to posterior proximal

Radiographic Findings
- Radiography
  - Transverse lucency in metaphysis on AP or angled AP view
  - Fracture line may not be visible in up to 25%
  - Positive fat pad sign on lateral view
  - Anterior humeral line displaced anterior to mid third of capitellum in 94%

CT Findings
- NECT: Linear lucencies in distal humeral metaphysis indicating fracture
- CTA: CT angiography to assess vascular injury

MR Findings
- T1WI
  - Decreased marrow signal indicating bone edema
  - Low signal line indicating fracture line
    - +/- Fragment rotation/displacement on sagittal views
  - Low signal joint effusion
- T2WI
  - Increased marrow signal indicating edema
  - FS PD FSE - visualization improved by using FS

DDx: Supracondylar Fracture

Post Dislocation	Post Dislocation	Lat Condylar Fx	Olecranon Fx	Olecranon Fx
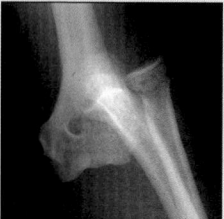	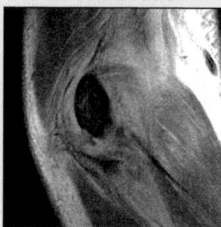	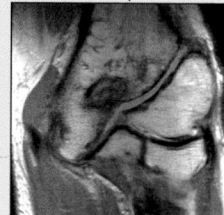	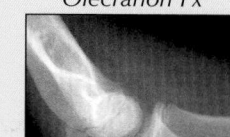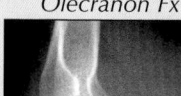	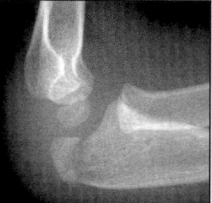
AP Radiography	Sag FS PD FSE	Cor PD FSE MR	Lat Radiography	Lat Radiography

SUPRACONDYLAR FRACTURE

Key Facts

Terminology
- Gartland fracture
- Transverse fracture of the distal humerus from a bending force in hyperextension

Imaging Findings
- Disruption of anterior humeral line
- Transverse lucency in metaphysis on AP or angled AP view
- Fracture line may not be visible in up to 25%
- Positive fat pad sign on lateral view
- Anterior humeral line displaced anterior to mid third of capitellum in 94%

Top Differential Diagnoses
- Lateral Condylar Fracture

Pathology
- Extension injury more common (95% of cases) than flexion type
- Type I: Nondisplaced fracture (30%)
- Type II: Displaced but intact posterior cortex (24%)
- Type III: Displaced plus complete cortical disruption (45%)

Clinical Issues
- Clinical profile: Typically active child

Diagnostic Checklist
- Presence of other fractures, especially olecranon and medial epicondyle
- Associated vascular and neural injuries
- T1W and FS PD FSE sagittal and coronal views for assessment of occult bony and soft tissue injuries

---

- o High signal joint effusion
  - +/- Periarticular extension of fluid with capsular rupture and vascular injury
  - o Low signal fracture lines surrounded by edema
- STIR
  - o Very sensitive for bony injury shown as high signal areas in marrow space
  - o Especially useful at mid and low-field
- T2* GRE
  - o Thin slice capability useful for detailed analysis of fragment and adjacent soft tissues
  - o Susceptibility decreases utility for detection of edema in bone

Imaging Recommendations
- Best imaging tool: Radiographs, CT, MRI
- Protocol advice
  - o FS PD FSE, T1
  - o CT to assess for comminution

DIFFERENTIAL DIAGNOSIS

Lateral Condylar Fracture
- Fall on an outstretched hand, with impaction of radial head
- Varus stress with elbow flexed/supinated, avulsion by common extensor action
- 17% of distal humerus fractures
- Common in 5-10 year (peak = 6 years)

Other Distal Humerus Fractures
- Medial epicondyle
  - o Varus force on extended arm
- Medial condyle
  - o Uncommon
  - o Avulsion with forced varus and direct impact on flexed elbow
- T-condylar and lateral epicondyle fractures
  - o Less common distal humerus fractures
  - o T-condylar = supracondylar with intraarticular extension

Olecranon Fracture
- Fall on a flexed, supinated forearm
- Olecranon epiphysis fuses at 16-18 years
- Direct trauma
- Throwing injury (pitchers)

Valgus Injury
- Throwing activities
- Includes trabecular injury
- +/- Bone trabecular injury of the capitellum
- +/- MCL tear

Capitellum Osteochondritis Dissecans
- Necrosis of the bone followed by healing response and reossification
- 12-16 year age group (after ossification of capitellum)
- 20% bilateral
- Chronic valgus stress with lateral impaction seen in gymnasts and adolescent pitchers
- Panner's disease (ages 7-10 years) as a osteochondrosis

Posterior Dislocation
- Ulna and radius displaced proximally
- +/- Extensor tendon tear
- +/- Fractures
  - o Coronoid, radial head, posterior capitellum
- Lateral ulnar collateral ligament (LUCL) tear common
- LUCL tear, posterolateral rotating instability (PLRI) predisposing
- Supracondylar fx associated

PATHOLOGY

General Features
- General path comments
  - o Extension injury more common (95% of cases) than flexion type
  - o Is extraarticular in children but may be intraarticular in adults
  - o Brachial artery and median nerve are vulnerable to traction over angulated fracture fragment
- Etiology

SUPRACONDYLAR FRACTURE

- ○ Hyperextension form - fall onto extended forearm
- ○ Flexion type - fall onto point of elbow
- Epidemiology
  - ○ Accounts for about 60% of pediatric elbow fractures
    - Most common pediatric elbow fracture
  - ○ Rare in adults (< 3%)
  - ○ Common in nondominant side (1.5:1)
- Associated abnormalities
  - ○ Other elbow fractures, esp. olecranon and medial condylar
  - ○ Distal radial fracture (5-6%)
  - ○ Olecranon avulsion fracture
  - ○ Medial condyle impaction
  - ○ Traction injuries to brachial artery (0.5%) and anterior interosseous branch of median nerve (4%)
  - ○ Median neuropathy

Gross Pathologic & Surgical Features

- Oblique transverse fracture through thin aspect of distal humerus between medial and lateral pillars
- Failure of anterior cortex (tensile side)
- Plastic deformity of posterior cortex (compression side)
- Posterior rotation +/- varus malalignment

Microscopic Features

- Disruption of cortex and trabeculae
- Hemorrhage with cellular infiltrate ranging from osteoblast and osteoclast to inflammatory cells
  - ○ Depends on fracture age

Staging, Grading or Classification Criteria

- Flexion or extension fracture (extension = 96% of fractures)
- Based on classification of Gartland (for extension injuries)
  - ○ Type I: Nondisplaced fracture (30%)
  - ○ Type II: Displaced but intact posterior cortex (24%)
  - ○ Type III: Displaced plus complete cortical disruption (45%)

CLINICAL ISSUES

Presentation

- Most common signs/symptoms
  - ○ Pain and loss of function
  - ○ Swelling and discoloration
  - ○ Decreased distal pulse
- Clinical profile: Typically active child

Demographics

- Age
  - ○ Common in children < 10 years old
  - ○ Median age of incidence = 6 years
- Gender: M > F

Natural History & Prognosis

- Return of function in over 90%
- Temporary nerve impairment in 10-16% but most recover
- Return of range of motion (ROM) may take a year
- Neurovascular injuries in displaced supracondylar fractures
  - ○ Anterior interosseous branch of median nerve

- ○ Radial nerve
- ○ Brachial artery
- Use of crossed pins may increase incidence of nerve injury
- Olecranon osteotomy reduces functional outcome compared to triceps splitting approach to open reduction with internal fixation (ORIF)

Treatment

- Conservative
  - ○ Type I, splinting in 90 degrees flexion
- Surgical
  - ○ Type II and III = percutaneous lateral pin fixation or ORIF with cross pinning
    - ORIF may be needed in up to 20%
- Complications
  - ○ Failure of reduction
  - ○ Vascular injury (rare)
  - ○ Median nerve injury (traumatic and iatrogenic – up to 5%)
  - ○ Volkmann's contracture secondary to unrecognized untreated acute vascular injury
  - ○ Cubitus varus as most common complication (Baumann angle 2-5 degrees greater than unaffected side)
  - ○ Loss of function

DIAGNOSTIC CHECKLIST

Consider

- Presence of other fractures, especially olecranon and medial epicondyle
- Associated vascular and neural injuries

Image Interpretation Pearls

- T1W and FS PD FSE sagittal and coronal views for assessment of occult bony and soft tissue injuries

SELECTED REFERENCES

1. O'Driscoll SW et al: Difficult elbow fractures. Pearls and pitfalls. Instr Course Lect 52:113-34, 2003
2. Gosens T et al: Neurovascular complications and functional outcome in displaced supracondylar fractures of the humerus in children. Injury 34(4):267-73, 2003
3. Skaggs DL et al: Operative treatment of supracondylar fractures of the humerus in children. The consequences of pin placement. J Bone Joint Surg Am 83-A(5):735-40, 2001
4. Cheng JC et al: Epidemiological features of supracondylar fractures of the humerus in Chinese children. J Pediatr Orthop B 10(1):63-7, 2001
5. O'Hara LJ et al: Displaced supracondylar fractures of the humerus in children. Audit changes practice. J Bone Joint Surg Br 82(2):204-10, 2000
6. Sonin A: Fractures of the elbow and forearm. Semin Musculoskelet Radiol 4(2):171-91, 2000
7. McKee MD et al: Functional outcome after open supracondylar fractures of the humerus. The effect of the surgical approach. J Bone Joint Surg Br 82(5):646-51, 2000
8. Fleuriau-Chateau P et al: An analysis of open reduction of irreducible supracondylar fractures of the humerus in children. Can J Surg 41(2):112-8, 1998

SUPRACONDYLAR FRACTURE

IMAGE GALLERY

Typical

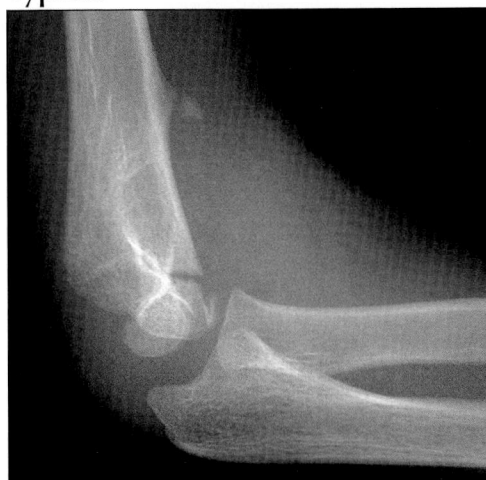
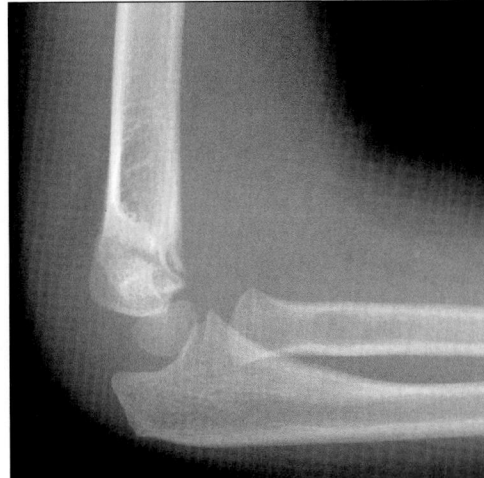

(Left) Lateral radiography shows a supracondylar fracture and fracture of a supracondylar process. Note the supracondylar fracture line seen as a linear lucency. *(Right)* Lateral radiography shows supracondylar fracture with a visible lucency.

Typical

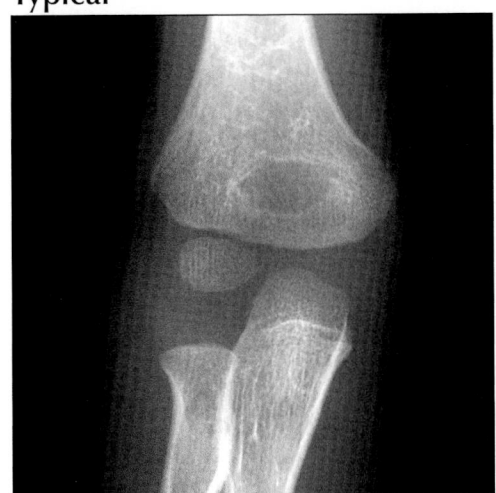
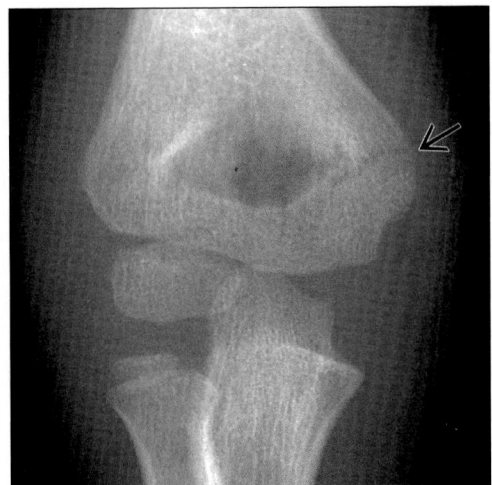

(Left) Anteroposterior radiography shows no visible fracture lines in this patient with a supracondylar fracture. *(Right)* Anteroposterior radiography shows medial lucency (arrow) in a patient with supracondylar fracture. AP radiography is not as sensitive as lateral radiography for the detection of supracondylar fractures.

Typical

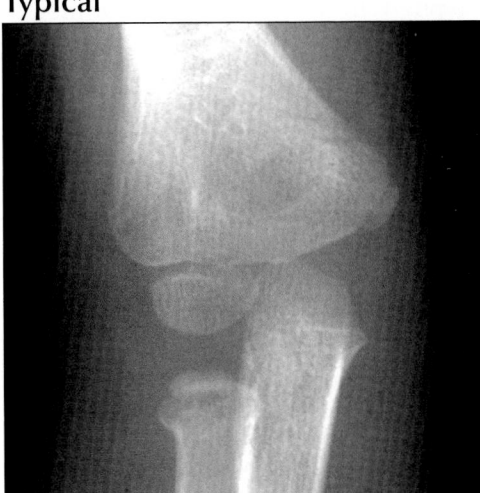
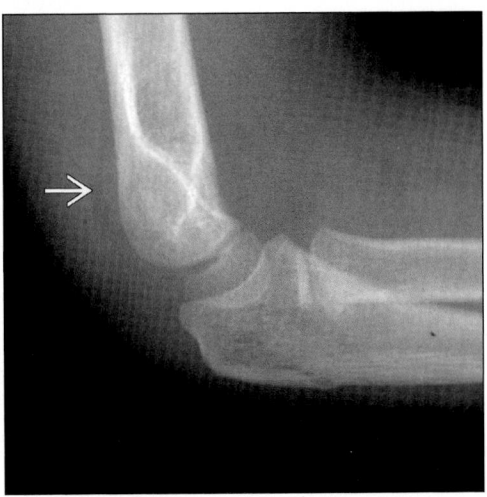

(Left) Anteroposterior radiography shows a visible fracture line medially in this patient with supracondylar fracture. *(Right)* Lateral radiography shows the supracondylar fracture and associated olecranon fracture. Note the soft tissue swelling and positive posterior fat pad sign (arrow).

MEDIAL CONDYLAR FRACTURE

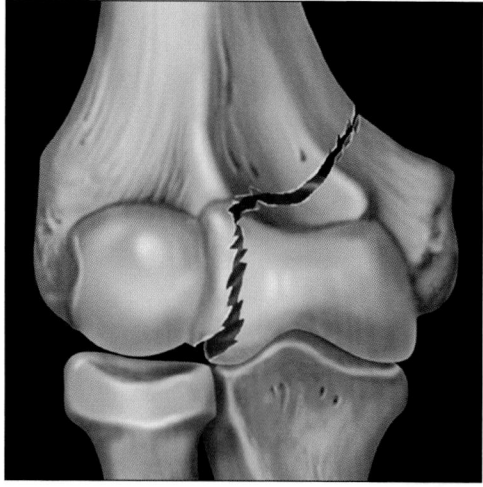

Coronal graphic shows a fracture extending through the humeral trochlea and separating the medial condyle, consistent with a medial condylar fracture.

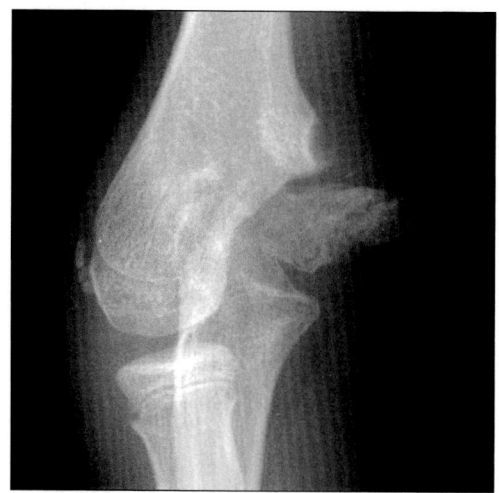

Lateral radiography shows a chronic medial condylar fracture with rotation and separation of the medial condylar fragment.

TERMINOLOGY

Abbreviations and Synonyms
- Medial condyle (MC) fracture, medial sided injuries

Definitions
- An avulsion injury caused by varus & direct impact on flexed elbow
  ○ Contraction of forearm flexor muscles in a fall on to the outstretched arm
  ○ Impaction injury by transmitted load through the olecranon process in a fall onto olecranon
- Fracture line includes the trochlear articular surface
  ○ Epicondylar injury remains extraarticular not affecting the trochlea

IMAGING FINDINGS

General Features
- Best diagnostic clue
  ○ Lucent fracture line, +/- displacement
    ■ Fracture line extends to and includes the trochlear articular surface isolating medial condyle
  ○ Decreased signal intensity fracture line surrounded by edema on T2WI
- Location
  ○ The articular portion of the medial column of the distal humerus
    ■ Medial epicondyle injuries are purely extraarticular and not referred to as medial condylar fractures
- Size
  ○ Varies from a subtle crack to an extensively displaced lesion
  ○ Difficult to detect in immature skeleton
- Morphology
  ○ Nondisplaced cortical disruption
  ○ Antero-inferiorly displaced fragment

Radiographic Findings
- Radiography
  ○ Linear lucency representing fracture line with variable fragment size and displacement on AP view
  ○ Associated fractures of olecranon on lateral view
  ○ Widening of intercondylar distance on AP view
  ○ Displaced epiphysis in children before ossification of trochlea
  ○ Fat pad sign is variable depending upon extension to articular surface
  ○ Wide separation of fragment in children - unstable fracture

CT Findings
- NECT
  ○ Linear lucency in condyle

DDx: Medial Condylar Fracture

Lateral Con Fx	Post Disloc	Valgus Injury	Valgus Injury	Capit OCD
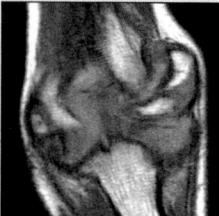	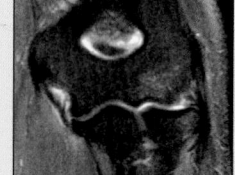	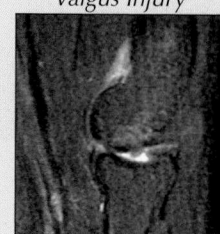	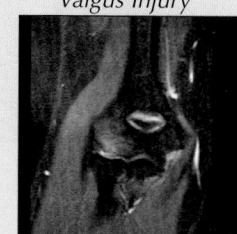	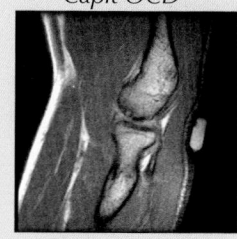
Cor PD FSE MR	Cor FS PD FSE	Sag FS PD FSE	Cor STIR MR	Sag PD FSE MR

MEDIAL CONDYLAR FRACTURE

Key Facts

Terminology
- An avulsion injury caused by varus & direct impact on flexed elbow
- Contraction of forearm flexor muscles in a fall on to the outstretched arm
- Impaction injury by transmitted load through the olecranon process in a fall onto olecranon

Imaging Findings
- Lucent fracture line, +/- displacement
- Fracture line extends to and includes the trochlear articular surface isolating medial condyle
- Decreased signal intensity fracture line surrounded by edema on T2WI

Top Differential Diagnoses
- Supracondylar Fracture

- Olecranon Fracture
- Lateral Condylar Fracture

Pathology
- Olecranon fracture
- Ulnar nerve damage - forms base of cubital tunnel

Clinical Issues
- Pain and loss of function
- Swelling and discoloration

Diagnostic Checklist
- Ulnar nerve injury
- Forearm compartment syndrome
- Fat sat/STIR MR for assessment of ulnar nerve, physeal fracture, forearm muscles and common flexor origin

---

  - Fracture comminution and displacement can be assessed
  - Soft tissue swelling will be evident on soft tissue windows

MR Findings
- T1WI
  - Decreased marrow signal indicating bone stress
  - Hypointense fx lines +/- bony displacement on axial views
  - Hypointense joint effusion
- T2WI
  - Increased marrow signal indicating edema
  - High signal joint effusion
  - Low signal fracture line in bone and high signal fracture line cartilage
  - Alteration of signal within ulnar nerve + surrounding edema
  - FS PD FSE provides superior contrast & spatial resolution
- STIR
  - Very sensitive for bony injury shown as high signal areas in marrow space
  - Critical at low field

Imaging Recommendations
- Best imaging tool: Radiographs, MRI
- Protocol advice
  - Axial and coronal MR
    - Especially to evaluate ulnar nerve (T1 and FS PD FSE or STIR)
    - Physeal injury in children and ligamentous/capsular injuries

DIFFERENTIAL DIAGNOSIS

Supracondylar Fracture
- Fall on outstretched hand (FOOSH) injury
- Transverse lucency in metaphysis on AP or angled AP view
- Anterior humeral line displaced anterior to mid third of capitellum in 94%

- Extraarticular in children but may be intraarticular in adults
- 60% of pediatric elbow fractures
- Rare in adults (< 3%)

Olecranon Fracture
- Fall on a flexed, supinated forearm
- Olecranon epiphysis fuses at 16-18 years
- Direct trauma
- Throwing injury (pitchers)

Lateral Condylar Fracture
- Fall on an outstretched hand, with impaction of radial head
- Varus stress with elbow flexed/supinated, avulsion by common extensor action
- 17% of distal humerus fractures
- Common in 5-10 year (peak = 6 years)

Valgus Injury
- Throwing activities
- Includes trabecular injury
- +/- Bone trabecular injury of the capitellum
- +/- MCL tear

Capitellum Osteochondritis Dissecans (OCD)
- Necrosis of bone followed by healing response and reossification
- 12-16 year age group (after ossification of capitellum)
- 20% bilateral
- Chronic valgus stress with lateral impaction seen in gymnasts and adolescent pitchers
- Panner's disease (ages 7-10 years) as an osteochondrosis

Posterior Dislocation
- +/- Lateral ligamentous damage
- +/- Fractures/trabecular injuries of posterior capitellum, anterior radial head
- FOOSH injury
- +/- Extensor tendon tear
- End stage instability

MEDIAL CONDYLAR FRACTURE

PATHOLOGY

General Features
- General path comments
  - Developmental appearances
  - Diagnosis may be difficult before ossification of trochlea
  - Ossification mnemonic = CRITOL
    - C = capitellum at 1-2 years
    - R = radial head at 2-4 years
    - I = internal (medial) epicondyle at 4-6 years
    - T = trochlea at 8-11 years
    - O= olecranon at 9-11 years
    - L = lateral epicondyle at 10-11 years
- Etiology
  - Fall on an outstretched arm, with avulsion from contraction of forearm flexor muscles
  - Fall onto point of elbow in flexion, with impact of olecranon
- Epidemiology
  - < 2% of elbow fractures in children
  - 10% of elbow fractures in adolescence
  - < 5% of elbow fractures in adults
- Associated abnormalities
  - Olecranon fracture
  - Ulnar nerve damage - forms base of cubital tunnel

Gross Pathologic & Surgical Features
- Epiphysis may become trapped within the joint in children
- Rotation of fracture fragment due to action of forearm flexors
- Disruption of blood supply if significant soft tissue injury occurs

Microscopic Features
- Disruption of cortex and trabeculae
- Hemorrhage with cellular infiltrate ranging from osteoblast and osteoclast to inflammatory cells depending on fracture age
- Avulsion of the osteo-tendinous complex of the common flexor origin
- Avulsion of osteo-ligamentous complex of medial collateral ligament

Staging, Grading or Classification Criteria
- Based on classification of Milch for unicondylar fracture
  - Type I: Lateral trochlear ridge intact, preserved medio-lateral stability (Salter Harris type II)
  - Type II: Originates in capitotrochlear sulcus so lateral trochlear ridge is part of fragment
    - Unstable (Salter Harris type IV)
- Kilfoyle classification (similar to Jakob of lateral condyle fx)
  - Type I: Incomplete & nondisplaced
  - Type II: Through epiphysis
  - Type III: Lateral condyle rotates or displaced

CLINICAL ISSUES

Presentation
- Most common signs/symptoms

- Pain and loss of function
- Swelling and discoloration
- Point tenderness medial condyle
- Ulnar nerve palsy
- Forearm compartment syndrome
- Clinical profile: Post trauma patient

Demographics
- Age: Children/adults
- Gender: M > F

Natural History & Prognosis
- Poor prognosis if comminution, failed reduction and unstable fixation
- Nondisplaced Milch type I injuries have excellent outcome
- Incarcerated fragments in children may be missed and result in poor outcome, mainly due to ulnar nerve dysfunction

Treatment
- Conservative: Nondisplaced Milch type I; splint in elbow + wrist flexion to reduce tension of forearm flexors
- Surgical: Displaced (> 3 mm) Milch type I + type II = ORIF with reconstruction plates +/- anterior transposition of ulnar nerve; excision of fragment has variable outcomes
- Complications: Seen in 33%
  - Loss of flexion/extension, nonunion and pseudoarthrosis, cubitus varus (undergrowth of trochlea) or valgus (overgrowth of medial condyle), AVN, ulnohumeral arthrosis, myositis ossificans

DIAGNOSTIC CHECKLIST

Consider
- Ulnar nerve injury
- Forearm compartment syndrome
- Extent of fracture displacement
- Incarceration of fracture fragment

Image Interpretation Pearls
- Lateral and AP radiographs
- Fat sat/STIR MR for assessment of ulnar nerve, physeal fracture, forearm muscles and common flexor origin

SELECTED REFERENCES

1. O'Driscoll SW et al: Difficult elbow fractures. Pearls and pitfalls. Instr Course Lect 52:113-34, 2003
2. Leet AI et al: Medial condyle fractures of the humerus in children. J Pediatr Orthop 22(1):2-7, 2002
3. Farsetti P et al: Long-term results of treatment of fractures of the medial humeral epicondyle in children. J Bone Joint Surg Am 83-A(9):1299-305, 2001
4. Nagi ON et al: Fractures of the medial humeral condyle in adults. Singapore Med J 41(7):347-51, 2000
5. Sonin A: Fractures of the elbow and forearm. Semin Musculoskelet Radiol 4(2):171-91, 2000

MEDIAL CONDYLAR FRACTURE

IMAGE GALLERY

Variant

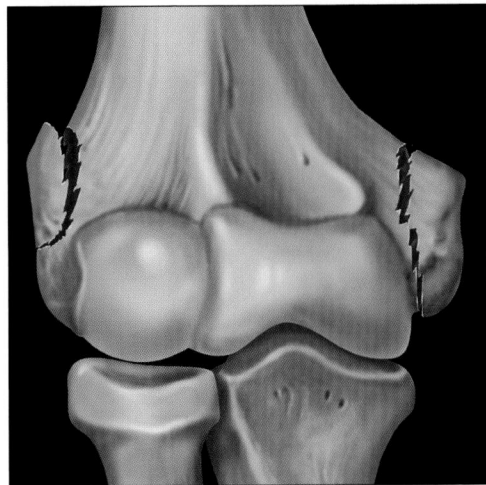

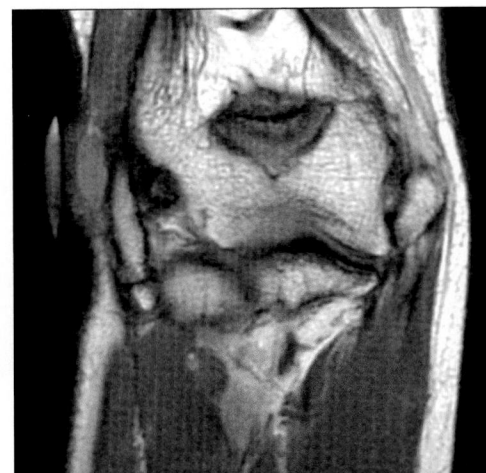

(Left) Coronal graphic shows a chronic medial and lateral epicondylar fracture. This is an unusual injury. *(Right)* Coronal PD FSE MR shows chronic medial and lateral epicondylar fractures with hypointense fracture lines. There is osteophyte formation on the lateral aspect of the joint.

Variant

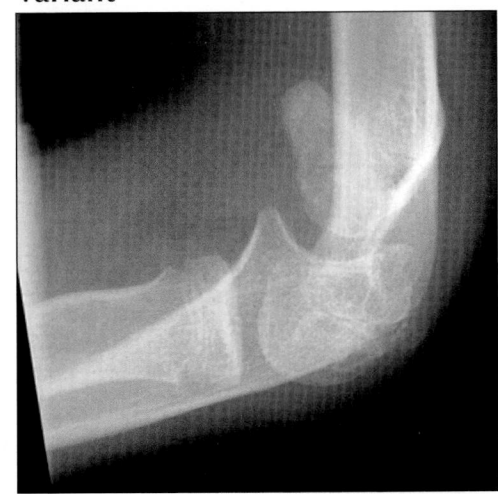

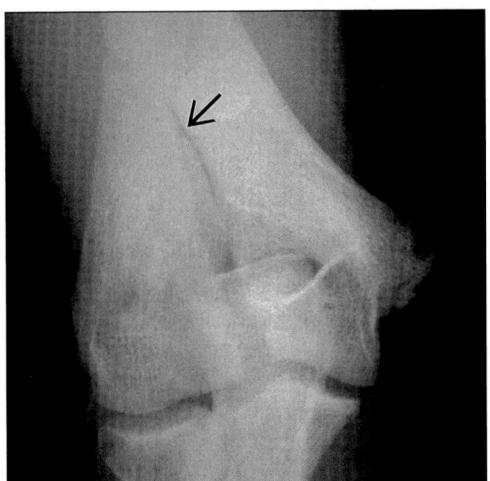

(Left) Lateral radiography shows a chronic medial condylar fracture with rotation and slight proximal migration of the medial condylar fragment still articulating with the ulna. *(Right)* Anteroposterior radiography shows an intercondylar fracture (arrow) extending from the lateral aspect of the trochlea up to the lateral diametaphysis.

Variant

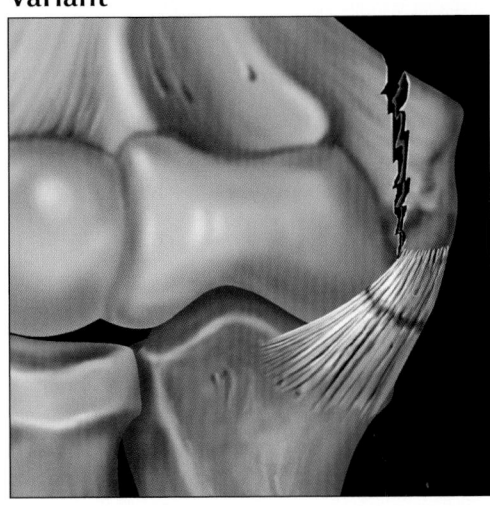

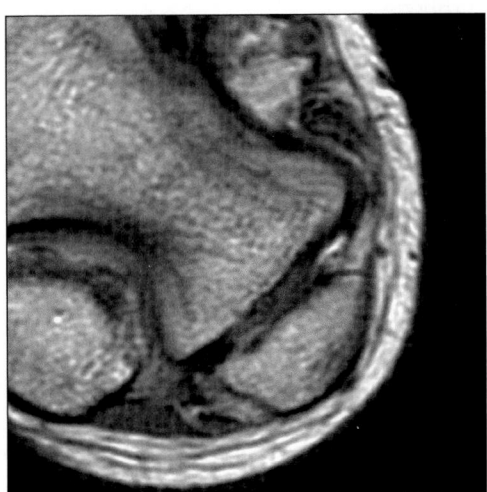

(Left) Coronal graphic shows an avulsion of the medial condyle/epicondyle in a patient after closure of the physis analogous to a little leaguer's elbow in a pre-adolescent patient. *(Right)* Axial PD FSE MR shows chronic avulsion of the medial epicondyle in a patient who suffered a fracture in childhood with resulting fibrous union.

BICIPITAL RADIAL BURSITIS

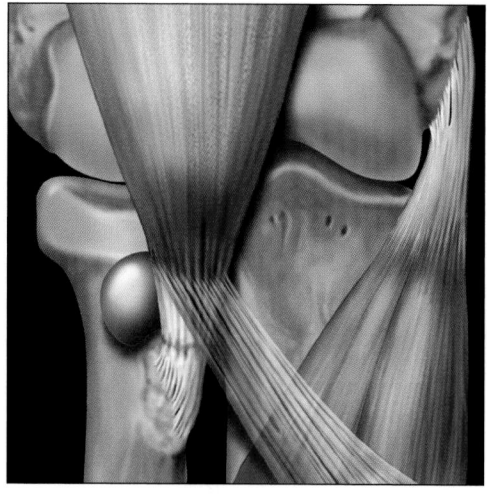

Coronal graphic shows a distended bicipital radial bursa adjacent to the distal biceps tendon.

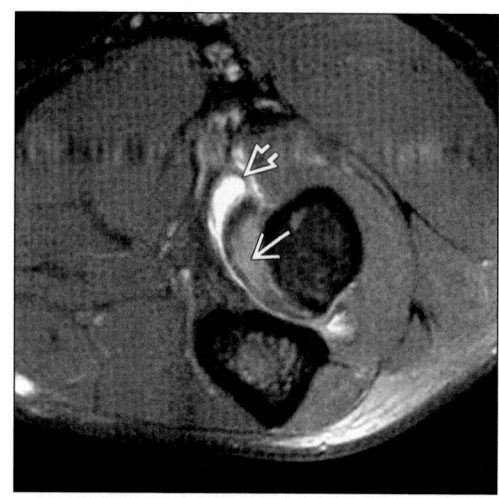

Axial FS PD FSE MR shows marked tendinosis (arrow) of the distal biceps insertion with surrounding distal bicipital radial bursitis (cubital bursitis) (open arrow).

TERMINOLOGY

Abbreviations and Synonyms
- Cubital bursitis, antecubital bursitis, distal bicipital radial bursitis

Definitions
- Inflammation of the bicipital radial bursa
- Sac-like cavities/potential cavity containing synovial fluid at frictional sites
  - Tendons/muscles pass over bone prominence

IMAGING FINDINGS

General Features
- Best diagnostic clue: High signal, fluid intensity mass
- Location
  - Interposed between distal biceps tendon and anterior aspect of the radial tuberosity
  - +/- Communication with the elbow joint below the annular ligament
- Size: Varies from a few mms to several cms depending on the amount of fluid contained
- Morphology
  - Flattened synovial sac not visualized on MRI unless distended with fluid
  - Variable amounts of internal debris

Radiographic Findings
- Radiography
  - Nonspecific soft tissue swelling
  - +/- Antecubital mass

CT Findings
- NECT
  - +/- Antecubital mass
  - Fluid attenuation
- CECT
  - +/- Rim enhancement
  - Smooth border

MR Findings
- T1WI
  - Homogeneous decreased signal intensity mass in characteristic location
  - +/- Associated tendinosis of biceps tendon
    - Thickening and intermediate signal intensity at insertion
  - Decreased signal in adjacent bone - reactive edema
  - Thick intermediate intensity lining in case of chronic bursitis
- T2WI
  - Increased signal intensity fluid on FS PD FSE
  - Hyperintense flattened, oval, or round shaped cystic appearing mass

DDx: Bicipital Radial Bursitis

Biceps Rupture	Biceps Rupture	Normal Vessels	Hemorrhage	Post Dislocation
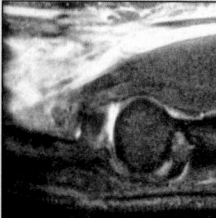	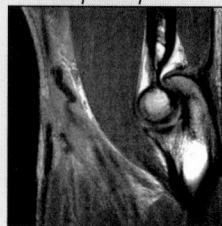	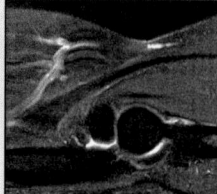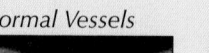	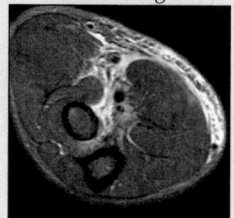	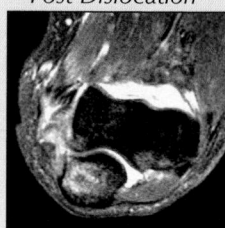
Sag FS PD FSE	Sag PD FSE MR	Sag FS PD FSE	Ax FS PD FSE	Ax FS PD FSE

BICIPITAL RADIAL BURSITIS

Key Facts

Terminology
- Inflammation of the bicipital radial bursa

Imaging Findings
- Best diagnostic clue: High signal, fluid intensity mass
- Interposed between distal biceps tendon and anterior aspect of the radial tuberosity
- +/- Communication with the elbow joint below the annular ligament
- Increased signal intensity fluid on FS PD FSE
- Hyperintense flattened, oval, or round shaped cystic appearing mass

Top Differential Diagnoses
- Biceps Tendinosis or Partial Tear
- Capitellum Osteochondritis Dissecans
- Posterior Dislocation
- Radial Head Fracture
- Normal Structures

Pathology
- May fill with fluid and present as mass on antecubital fossa

Clinical Issues
- Antecubital mass (if large) or pain associated with supination
- Clinical profile: History of biceps pain
- May present insidiously: Found after athletic activity

Diagnostic Checklist
- FS PD FSE most sensitive for hyperintense fluid detection
- Axial imaging plane recommended

  - Fluid signal intensity on all pulse sequences unless containing inflammatory debris or calcification
    - Decreased signal structures if calcified
    - Intermediate signal if contains inflammatory, hemorrhagic or exudative debris
    - +/- Rice bodies in patients with rheumatoid arthritis
- STIR
  - Similar contrast as FS PD FSE
  - Less spatial resolution
  - More homogeneous fat saturation
- T2* GRE
  - Hypointense rim/debris if chronic hemorrhage
  - Hyperintense mass
- T1 C+
  - May demonstrate thin rim enhancement after gadolinium administration
  - Homogeneous decreased signal intensity center - simple cyst
  - +/- Thickened rind, enhancing - previous inflammation

Ultrasonographic Findings
- Typically hypo or anechoic mass with through transmission

Imaging Recommendations
- Best imaging tool: MRI
- Protocol advice
  - FS PD FSE demonstrates fluid filled bursa
    - T2* GRE if fat suppression inadequate in axial plane

DIFFERENTIAL DIAGNOSIS

Biceps Tendinosis or Partial Tear
- Tendinopathy on MR images
- May coexist
- Forced extension on flexed forearm
  - Tear
- Chronic repetitive microtrauma
  - Tendinosis

- +/- Hypertrophy of radial tubercle

Antecubital Mass
- Neoplastic
  - Diffuse enhancement
  - In contrast to rim enhancement with bursitis
- Benign
  - Neuroma
  - Lipoma
    - Fat signal on T1WI
    - Saturates with fat suppression
  - Hematoma
    - + History of trauma

Capitellum Osteochondritis Dissecans
- Overuse syndrome of the elbow
- Subchondral reactive process of the humeral capitellum
- Flattening of capitellar profile is earliest sign
- Necrosis of bone followed by healing response and reossification
- Chronic valgus stress with lateral impaction seen in gymnasts and adolescent pitchers
- Increased rotary, compressive or axial loads seen in throwing athletes
- Occurs in the 12-16 year age group
  - After ossification of capitellum
- Lateral pain

Posterior Dislocation
- Fall on out stretched hand (FOOSH)
- +/- Capitellar fx
- +/- Radial head fx
- Lateral ligamentous disruptions
  - Lateral ulnar collateral ligament injury (LUCL)
- + Surrounding hemorrhage
- +/- Coronoid fracture
- Lateral pain

Radial Head Fracture
- Fall on outstretched hand injury (FOOSH)
- Accounts for 30% of adult elbow fractures
- Most common elbow fracture in adults
- Proximal radial injuries rare in children

BICIPITAL RADIAL BURSITIS

- o Usually occur in the radial neck
- Osteochondral injury to adjacent capitellum common
- +/- Osteochondral free fragments

Normal Structures
- Blood vessels
  - o Hyperintense on T2WI, STIR

PATHOLOGY

General Features
- General path comments
  - o May fill with fluid and present as mass on antecubital fossa
    - Often mistaken for neoplasm
- Etiology
  - o Inflammation of the bursa with variable amounts of fluid
    - Friction of tendon with supination/pronation leads to inflammation of bursa
    - Radial tuberosity hypertrophy predisposing
- Epidemiology: Relatively uncommon
- Associated abnormalities
  - o Associated with biceps tendinopathy/tear
    - Radial tuberosity hypertrophy

Gross Pathologic & Surgical Features
- Indurated, fluid-filled bursa of variable size

Microscopic Features
- Hypertrophied bursal synovial lining with infiltration of inflammatory cells
- Fibrosis and granulation tissue

CLINICAL ISSUES

Presentation
- Most common signs/symptoms
  - o Antecubital mass (if large) or pain associated with supination
  - o Acute bursitis
    - Pain
    - Tenderness
    - Limited motion
    - +/- Swelling/redness
  - o Chronic bursitis
    - Recurrent bursitis
    - Limited motion
- Clinical profile: History of biceps pain

Demographics
- Age: Typically adult patient
- Gender: Most likely M > F due to higher incidence of biceps disease in males

Natural History & Prognosis
- May present insidiously: Found after athletic activity
- +/- Resolution with cessation of predisposing activities
- Conservative treatment leads to resolution

Treatment
- Acute bursitis
  - o Rest immobilization

- o High pose NSAIDs
- o +/- Narcotic analgesics
- o Aspiration, steroid injection after anesthetic
- o Systemic corticosteroid for resistant acute cases
  - After rule out infection, gout
- Chronic bursitis
  - o Splinting/rest less helpful
  - o Remove calcium if present

DIAGNOSTIC CHECKLIST

Consider
- In the setting of overuse

Image Interpretation Pearls
- FS PD FSE most sensitive for hyperintense fluid detection
- Axial imaging plane recommended

SELECTED REFERENCES

1. Bond JR et al: Radiologic case study. Partial tear of the distal biceps tendon with mass-like bicipitoradial bursitis and associated hyperostosis of the radial tuberosity. Orthopedics 26(4):376, 448-50, 2003
2. Yamamoto T et al: Bicipital radial bursitis. CT and MR appearance. Comput Med Imaging Graph 25(6):531-3, 2001
3. Ramsey ML: Distal biceps tendon injuries. Diagnosis and management. J Am Acad Orthop Surg 7(3):199-207, 1999
4. Brinker MR et al: The adult elbow. Fundamentals of Orthopaedics. Philadelphia PA, WB Saunders, 153-64, 1999
5. Chen WS et al: Recalcitrant bicipital radial bursitis. Arch Orthop Trauma Surg 119(1-2):105-8, 1999
6. Fritz RC et al: MR imaging of the elbow. An update. Radiol Clin North Am 35(1):117-44, 1997
7. Fritz RC et al: The Elbow. Magnetic resonance imaging in orthopedica and sports medicine. vol 1. 2nd ed. Philadelphia PA, J.B. Lippincott, 743-849, 1997

BICIPITAL RADIAL BURSITIS

IMAGE GALLERY

Typical

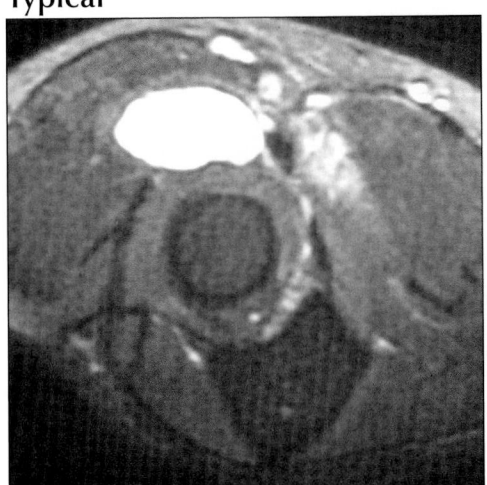 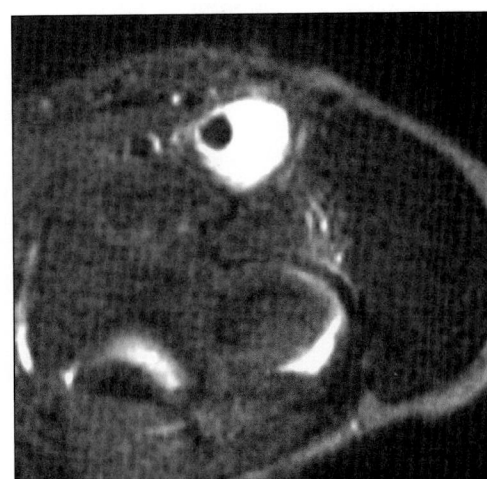

(Left) Axial FS PD FSE MR shows a distended cubital bursa consistent with bicipital radial bursitis. *(Right)* Axial T2 FSE MR shows a distended bursa surrounding the biceps tendon. This mimics a tenosynovium. The distal biceps tendon is invested by paratenon, not tenosynovium.

Typical

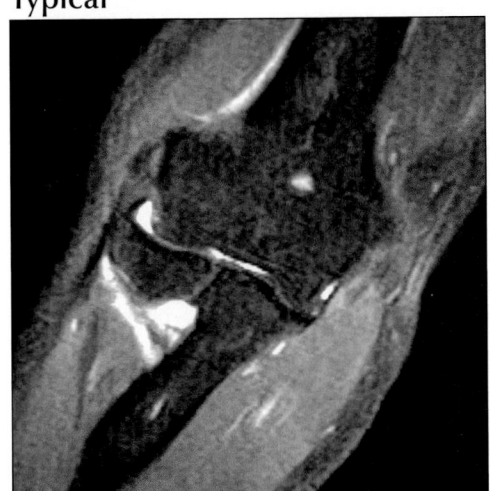 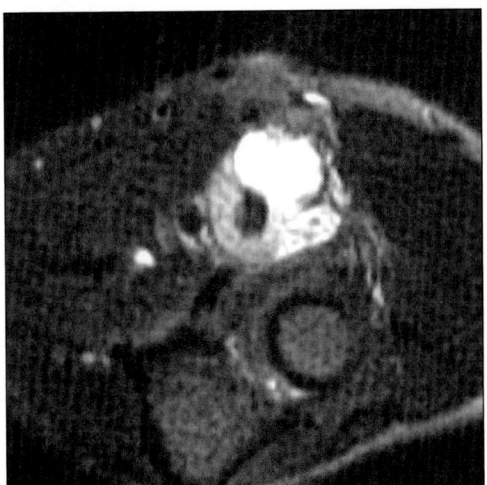

(Left) Coronal STIR MR shows fluid surrounding the distal biceps insertion consistent with bicipital radial bursitis. *(Right)* Axial T2 FSE MR shows a distended distal bicipital radial bursa surrounding the biceps tendon. There is hypertrophic synovitis present within the bursa which may mimic a neoplasm.

Typical

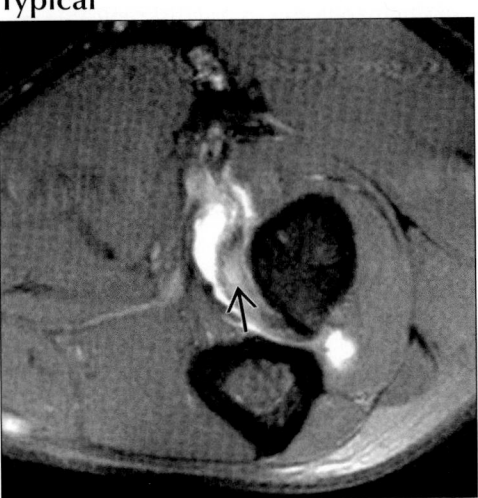 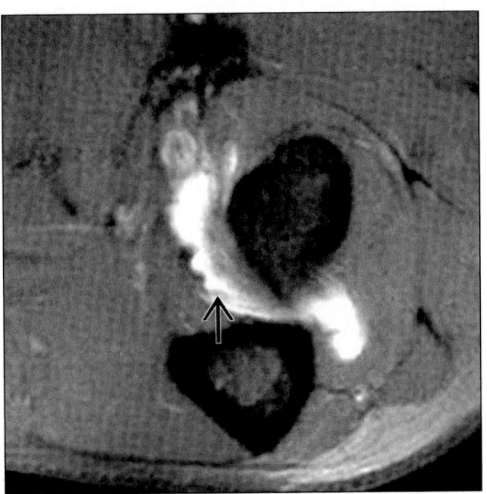

(Left) Axial FS PD FSE shows tendinosis (arrow) of the insertion of the biceps on the radius with surrounding distal radial bursitis. *(Right)* Axial FS PD FSE MR shows the distended bursa (arrow) indicating inflammatory change (same patient as the image on the left).

OLECRANON BURSITIS

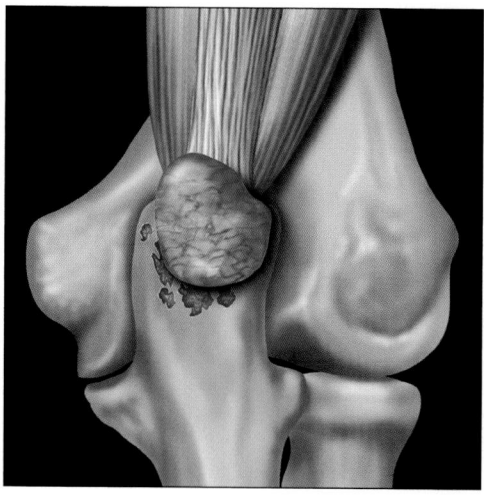

Coronal graphic shows a distended olecranon bursa in a patient with olecranon bursitis.

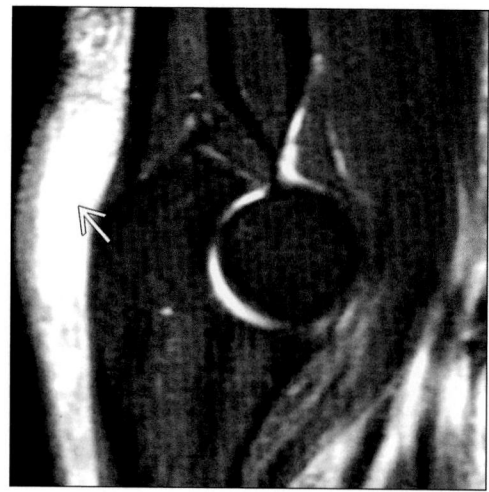

Sagittal STIR MR shows hyperintense fluid-filled olecranon bursa (arrow) in a patient with clinical olecranon bursitis.

TERMINOLOGY

Abbreviations and Synonyms
- Miner's elbow, student's elbow, draftsman's elbow

Definitions
- Inflammation of the bursa overlying the olecranon process at the proximal aspect of the ulna

IMAGING FINDINGS

General Features
- Best diagnostic clue: Fluid containing mass (fluid signal intensity) in olecranon bursa in symptomatic patient
- Location: Superficial bursa between integument and olecranon, intratendinous bursa, and subtendinous bursa between the triceps and tip of the olecranon
- Size: Varies from a few mms to several cms depending on the amount of fluid contained within
- Morphology: The olecranon bursa is a flattened synovial sacs not usually visualized on MRI unless distended with fluid

MR Findings
- T2WI: High-signal, fluid intensity mass in superficial soft tissues adjacent to the olecranon process and triceps insertion
- T1 C+: +/- Rim enhancement
- Variable amounts of internal, typically hemorrhagic debris
- Osteomyelitis rare

Ultrasonographic Findings
- Typically hypo or anechoic mass with through transmission

Imaging Recommendations
- Best imaging tool: MRI
- Protocol advice: FS PD FSE demonstrates bursal fluid

DIFFERENTIAL DIAGNOSIS

Triceps Tendinosis or Partial Tear
- Tendinopathy on MR images, +/- edema

Mass/Nonspecific Edema
- In area of bursa - hemangioma, synovitis, neuroma

PATHOLOGY

General Features
- General path comments: Inflammation of the olecranon bursa with variable amounts of fluid
- Etiology

DDx: Olecranon Bursitis

Edema	Hemangioma	Hemangioma	Triceps Tear	Synovitis
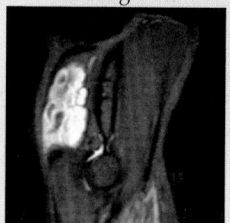	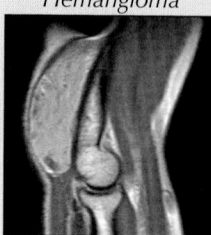	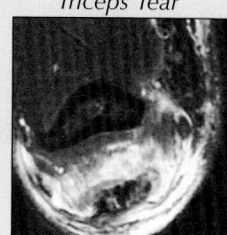	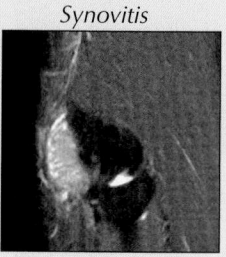	
Sag FS PD FSE	Sag FS PD FSE	Sag PD FSE MR	Ax FS PD FSE	Sag STIR MR

OLECRANON BURSITIS

Key Facts

Terminology
- Miner's elbow, student's elbow, draftsman's elbow
- Inflammation of the bursa overlying the olecranon process at the proximal aspect of the ulna

Imaging Findings
- Best diagnostic clue: Fluid containing mass (fluid signal intensity) in olecranon bursa in symptomatic patient
- Location: Superficial bursa between integument and olecranon, intratendinous bursa, and subtendinous bursa between the triceps and tip of the olecranon
- T2WI: High-signal, fluid intensity mass in superficial soft tissues adjacent to the olecranon process and triceps insertion
- Protocol advice: FS PD FSE demonstrates bursal fluid

Top Differential Diagnoses
- Triceps Tendinosis or Partial Tear
- Mass/Nonspecific Edema

Pathology
- General path comments: Inflammation of the olecranon bursa with variable amounts of fluid
- Associated abnormalities: Associated with triceps tendinopathy and tears

Clinical Issues
- Clinical profile: May be seen in patients with underlying systemic disease

Diagnostic Checklist
- FS PD FSE sensitive for demonstrating fluid

- Secondary to acute or repetitive trauma or systemic disease
  - Traumatic bursitis commonly a football injury associated with artificial turf
  - Ice hockey
- Epidemiology: Relatively common
- Associated abnormalities: Associated with triceps tendinopathy and tears

Gross Pathologic & Surgical Features
- Indurated, fluid-filled bursa of variable size
  - Subcutaneous bursa

Microscopic Features
- Hypertrophied bursal synovial lining with infiltration of inflammatory cells +/- fibrosis
- May be infected
  - Staphylococcus aureus common

CLINICAL ISSUES

Presentation
- Most common signs/symptoms
  - Acute - painless distention after direct blow
  - Chronic - recurrent traumatic episodes - large rubbery mass +/- pain
- Clinical profile: May be seen in patients with underlying systemic disease

Demographics
- Age: Adolescent or adult patient
- Gender: M = F

Natural History & Prognosis
- Will subside with cessation of causative activities and anti-inflammatory drugs in most cases

Treatment
- Conservative treatment unless extensive
  - Antibiotics for infected bursitis
- Extensive cases require bursectomy

DIAGNOSTIC CHECKLIST

Consider
- In case of fluid, pain and swelling in the superficial soft tissues adjacent to the olecranon process

Image Interpretation Pearls
- FS PD FSE sensitive for demonstrating fluid

SELECTED REFERENCES

1. Brinker MR et al : The adult elbow. Fundamentals of Orthopaedics. Philadelphia PA, WB Saunders Co, 153-64, 1999
2. Fritz RC et al: MR imaging of the elbow. An update. Radiol Clin North Am 35(1):117-44, 1997
3. Steiner E et al: Ganglia and cysts around joints. Radiol Clin North Am 34(2):395-425, 1996
4. Olsen NK et al: Bursal injections. Physiatric Procedures in Clinical Practice. Philadelphia PA, Hanley & Belfus, 36-43, 1995

IMAGE GALLERY

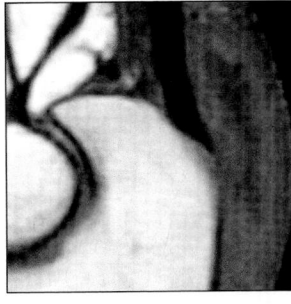 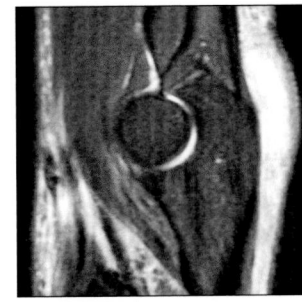

(Left) Sagittal T1WI MR shows decreased signal intensity fluid within the olecranon bursa and thickened synovial lining in a patient with a bursal infection. *(Right)* Sagittal STIR MR shows the distended infected olecranon bursa.

SYNOVIAL FRINGE, ELBOW

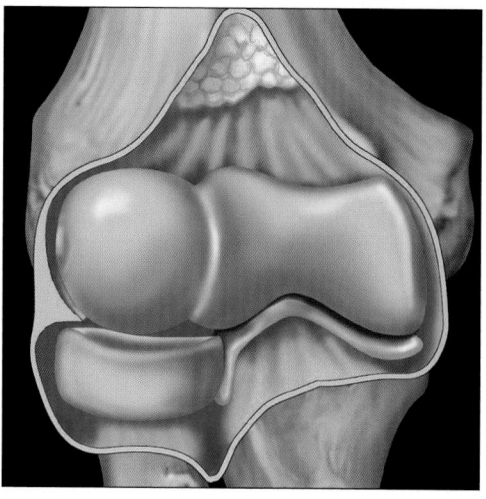

Coronal graphic shows the folding of the lateral capsule between the capitellum and radius known as the synovial fringe or radiocapitellar labrum. This is not a true labrum or meniscus.

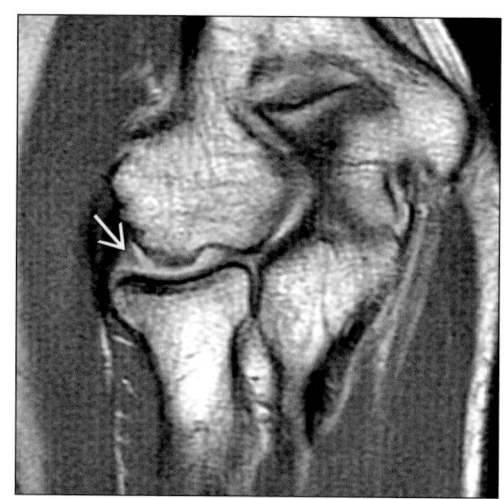

Coronal PD FSE MR shows the fold of synovium known as the synovial fringe (arrow) laterally. This synovial plica is triangular shaped.

TERMINOLOGY

Abbreviations and Synonyms
- Synovial fold, synovial plica, radiohumeral meniscus, radiocapitellar labrum

Definitions
- A thickened fold or fibrotic fringe of synovial tissue at the lateral margin of the radiocapitellar joint

IMAGING FINDINGS

General Features
- Best diagnostic clue: Synovial fold projecting into the joint (directed medially) from posterior/lateral fat pad on MR arthrography
- Location: Lateral capsule of radiohumeral joint
- Size: Length 1-5 cm, width 1-10 mm, thickness 1-4 mm
- Morphology: Rigid fibrous meniscoid fold - pliable thin band, no fibromyxoid components, therefore not a meniscus

Radiographic Findings
- Radiography: Areas of lucency and/or sclerosis on radial head and capitellum indicating chondromalacia

CT Findings
- NECT: Shows areas of lucency and/or sclerosis in radial head and capitellum indicating chondromalacia

MR Findings
- T2WI: High signal in capitellum, radial head = chondromalacia
- PD/Intermediate: +/- Synovitis - thickening hyperintensity relative to fluid
- MR arthrography
  - Coronal images - synovial fold, articular cartilage damage and lateral soft tissue damage

Ultrasonographic Findings
- Localized thickening of lateral joint capsule, detection increased with saline sonoarthrography

Imaging Recommendations
- Best imaging tool: MRI
- Protocol advice: FS PD FSE/T2WI

DIFFERENTIAL DIAGNOSIS

Osteoarthritis (OA)/Loose Bodies
- +/- Synovitis

Synovitis
- May be mass like (posterolateral aspect of joint)

DDx: Synovial Fringe, Elbow

OA	Synovitis	Bifid Fringe	Loose Body
Sag PD FSE MR	Ax T2 FSE MR	Cor T1 FS Arthr	Ax FS PD FSE MR

2

88

SYNOVIAL FRINGE, ELBOW

Key Facts

Terminology
- Synovial fold, synovial plica, radiohumeral meniscus, radiocapitellar labrum

Imaging Findings
- Best diagnostic clue: Synovial fold projecting into the joint (directed medially) from posterior/lateral fat pad on MR arthrography
- Location: Lateral capsule of radiohumeral joint
- Size: Length 1-5 cm, width 1-10 mm, thickness 1-4 mm
- Morphology: Rigid fibrous meniscoid fold - pliable thin band, no fibromyxoid components, therefore not a meniscus
- T2WI: High signal in capitellum, radial head = chondromalacia

- PD/Intermediate: +/- Synovitis - thickening hyperintensity relative to fluid

Top Differential Diagnoses
- Osteoarthritis (OA)/Loose Bodies
- Synovitis

Pathology
- Etiology: Chronic repetitive trauma in pronation/supination
- Symptomatic folds show hypertrophy and increase in number of nerve fibers

Diagnostic Checklist
- MR arthrography will effectively characterize the lesion

Normal Variant
- Bifid synovial fringe

PATHOLOGY

General Features
- Etiology: Chronic repetitive trauma in pronation/supination
- Epidemiology: Up to 50% of elbows

Gross Pathologic & Surgical Features
- Thin membrane with fibrillar free edge and rigid shelf with triangular profile attached to capsule
- Originate from synovium adjacent to posterior fat pad

Microscopic Features
- Two synovial layers separated by thin fatty stroma with villous free edge - tough fibrous core projecting from capsule with synovial covering
- Symptomatic folds show hypertrophy and increase in number of nerve fibers

CLINICAL ISSUES

Presentation
- Most common signs/symptoms: Pain on lateral joint line +/- locking, snapping elbow (flexion/pronation test), over radial head

Demographics
- Age: Adult (mid life)
- Gender: M = F

Natural History & Prognosis
- Excellent outcome after resection

Treatment
- Conservative: If symptoms are mild and rest is possible
- Surgical: Arthroscopic resection

DIAGNOSTIC CHECKLIST

Consider
- Loose bodies, lateral epicondylitis

Image Interpretation Pearls
- MR arthrography will effectively characterize the lesion

SELECTED REFERENCES

1. Duparc F et al: The synovial fold of the humeroradial joint: Anatomical and histological features, and clinical relevance in lateral epicondylalgia of the elbow. Surg Radiol Anat 24(5):302-7, 2002
2. Antuna SA et al: Snapping plicae associated with radiocapitellar chondromalacia. Arthroscopy 17(5):491-5, 2001
3. Awaya H et al: Synovial fold syndrome. MR imaging findings. Am J Roentgenol 177(6):1377-81, 2001

IMAGE GALLERY

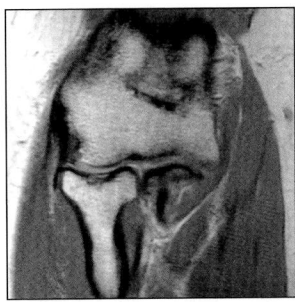 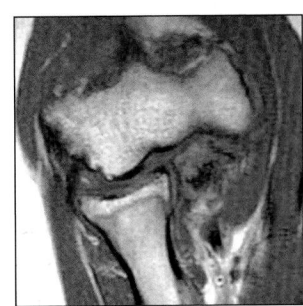

(Left) Coronal PD FSE MR shows a slightly irregular synovial fringe with central radial chondromalacia. *(Right)* Coronal PD FSE MR shows heterotopic ossification within the synovial fringe.

OSTEOARTHRITIS, ELBOW

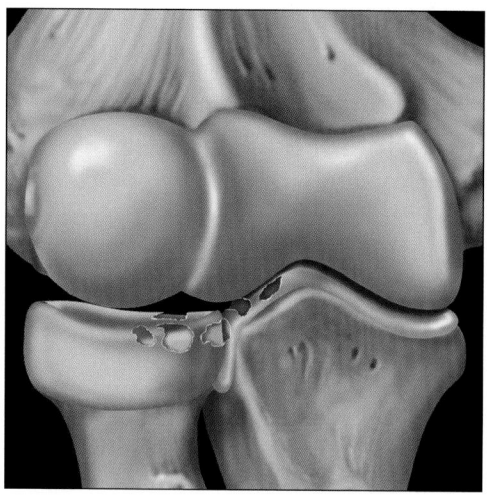

Coronal graphic demonstrates early findings of OA including erosions of the ulna and radial head.

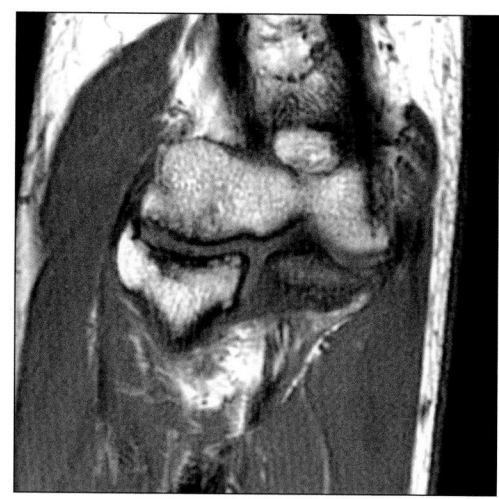

Coronal PD FSE MR demonstrates arthrosis of the capitellum and radius with osteophyte formation, subchondral sclerosis and loss of articular cartilage.

TERMINOLOGY

Abbreviations and Synonyms
- Osteoarthritis (OA), degenerative joint disease (DJD)

Definitions
- Degenerative arthritis characterized by chondromalacia, osteophyte formation, subchondral cysts and synovitis
- Primary - gradual process of destruction & regeneration as a result of chronic microtrauma
- Secondary - non-inflammatory DJD
  - Previous trauma, congenital deformity, infection or metabolic disorder

IMAGING FINDINGS

General Features
- Best diagnostic clue: Chondromalacia, +/- subchondral sclerosis, subchondral cysts and/or edema, and osteophytes
- Location: Hyaline chondral surfaces of the elbow
- Size: Small localized area (typically post trauma), compartment or whole elbow
- Morphology: Progressive loss of articular cartilage with associated new bone formation and capsular fibrosis

Radiographic Findings
- Radiography
  - Joint space narrowing
  - Subchondral sclerosis/eburnation: Increased density
  - Subchondral cyst lucencies
  - Osteophyte formation

CT Findings
- CT arthrography: Loose bodies as filling defects

MR Findings
- T1WI
  - Decreased signal intensity subchondral cysts: High signal marrow extends into osteophytes
  - Subchondral decreased signal indicates sclerosis and/or edema
- T2WI
  - FS PD FSE hyperintensity in hyaline cartilage and subchondral bone marrow edema
    - Thinning of articular (hyaline) cartilage with occasional focal defects
    - Edema well demonstrated with fat saturation
    - Subchondral decreased signal indicating sclerosis (sclerosis best visualized on T1WI)
    - Subchondral cysts (increased signal), and osteophytes
- PD/Intermediate
  - PD FSE cartilage can be visualized

DDx: Osteoarthritis, Elbow

RA	Trauma	Psuedodefect	Cortical Notch
Sag FS PD FSE	Sag FS PD FSE	Cor FS PD FSE	Sag PD FSE MR

OSTEOARTHRITIS, ELBOW

Key Facts

Terminology
- Primary - gradual process of destruction & regeneration as a result of chronic microtrauma
- Secondary - non-inflammatory DJD

Imaging Findings
- Best diagnostic clue: Chondromalacia, +/- subchondral sclerosis, subchondral cysts and/or edema, and osteophytes

Top Differential Diagnoses
- Inflammatory Arthritis
- Crystal Deposition Disease
- Osteochondral Defects in Acute Trauma
- Osteochondromatosis
- Normal Elbow Anatomy

Pathology
- Affects up to 90% of older individuals
- Elbow is affected less commonly than weight bearing joint such as the knee and hip
- Loose bodies: Cause catching and locking
- Deformities
- Subluxations
- Ankylosis

Clinical Issues
- Pain with utilization of the joint
- +/- Swelling (effusion)

Diagnostic Checklist
- Secondary OA in cases where the findings are focal
- Utilize FS PD FSE to visualize the chondral erosions

- Synovial thickening seen well
  - Edema may not be quite as bright on PD relative to FS PD FSE
- T2* GRE: With fat suppression, cartilage abnormalities - decreased signal areas on T1 weighted GRE images
- T1 C+: Synovium enhances in cases of synovitis

Nuclear Medicine Findings
- Bone Scan: Increased tracer uptake with subchondral fractures or cysts or general sclerosis

Imaging Recommendations
- Best imaging tool: MRI
- Protocol advice
  - FS PD FSE MRI
  - T1WI & T2* GRE to identify loose bodies

- Hyperintense edema on T2WI
- +/- Synovitis

Osteochondromatosis
- Loose bodies
- Synovial metaplasia
- +/- Calcifications
- T2* GRE images to detect osteochondral loose bodies

Normal Elbow Anatomy
- Posterolateral pseudodefect (Pseudodefect)
  - Between capitellum and lateral epicondyle
  - Mimics OA and OCD
- Cortical Notch
  - Ulna "bare area"
  - Mimics chondromalacia

DIFFERENTIAL DIAGNOSIS

Inflammatory Arthritis
- Polyarticular systemic disease
- Rheumatoid arthritis (RA) affects elbow frequently
- +/- RA factor
- Synovitis common
- +/- Erosions

Crystal Deposition Disease
- Polyarticular arthritis
- Calcium pyrophosphate dihydrate
  - Chondrocalcinosis
  - Pseudogout
  - Pyrophosphate arthropathy
- Calcium hydroxyapatite
  - Asymptomatic calcification
  - Calcific tendonitis, bursitis & periarthritis
  - Chronic, destructive joint disease
- Monosodium urate monohydrate
  - Hyperuricemia
  - Gouty arthritis
  - Tophaceous gout

Osteochondral Defects in Acute Trauma
- +/- Hypointense fracture line

PATHOLOGY

General Features
- General path comments
  - Begins as fatigue fracture of the collagen meshwork followed by increased hydration of the articular cartilage and loss of proteoglycans from the matrix into the synovial fluid
    - Fibrillation of the cartilage follows with deep clefts appearing and regeneration/proliferation of chondrocytes
    - Proliferative changes occur at the joint margins with formation of osteophytes
    - Loose bodies - fragmentation of osteochondral surfaces follows
    - Synovial hypertrophy produces joint pain by nerve stimulation and weeping of synovial fluid produces increased intraarticular pressure thereby "stretching" the joint lining = pain
    - Increased levels of degrading enzymes including matrix metalloproteinase
    - Increased intraarticular levels of collagenase, neutral proteases and degradative products of proteoglycans
    - Desicated cartilage seen early with aging

OSTEOARTHRITIS, ELBOW

- Etiology
  - Multiple theories - chronic microtrauma (primary) leading to disruption of the articular surface
    - Fibrillation, eburnation, subchondral cysts, and osteophytes form
    - Secondary OA results from healing of major trauma or other predisposing events
    - Joint instability may be predisposing
- Epidemiology
  - Affects up to 90% of older individuals
  - Elbow is affected less commonly than weight bearing joint such as the knee and hip
- Associated abnormalities
  - Loose bodies: Cause catching and locking
  - Deformities
  - Subluxations
  - Ankylosis

Gross Pathologic & Surgical Features
- Degraded cartilage with loss of sheen
  - Subchondral geodes (cysts) containing variable degrees of debris
  - Buttressing osteophytes to increase surface area
- Fissured and/or ulcerated cartilage surface
- Articular surface collapse

Microscopic Features
- Diminution of chondrocytes in superficial zones with chondrocyte swelling to variable degrees
- Cartilage matrix loses its ability to stain for proteoglycans with Alcian blue or safranin-O
- Matrix chondrocytes demonstrate proliferation in clusters (brood capsules)
- Neovascularity penetrates layer of calcified cartilage & new chondrocytes extend up from deeper layers
- Hypertrophied synovium becomes folded into villous folds with variable infiltration of plasma cells, and lymphocytes

Staging, Grading or Classification Criteria
- Cartilage damage
  - Fissuring
  - Abnormal matrix calcification
  - Osteocyte formation
  - Osteoarthritis
- Posttraumatic & valgus extension overload injury as two common groups of degenerative arthritis

CLINICAL ISSUES

Presentation
- Most common signs/symptoms
  - Pain with utilization of the joint
  - +/- Swelling (effusion)
- Clinical profile
  - Primary osteoarthritis
    - Posttraumatic
    - Usually affects men
    - Ulnar neuropathy findings are rare
    - Arthrosis changes are more global - osteophytes in anterior & posterior compartments
    - Limited flexion & extension

- Limitation of forearm rotation - radial head osteophytes
  - Chronic posterior elbow impingement
    - Valgus extension overload
    - Progressive posterior elbow pain
    - Limited elbow extension
    - Younger group than posttraumatic arthritis
    - Associated neuropathy (ulnar nerve) - numbness/tingling in ring & small fingers
    - Posterior fossa impingement pain relieved with local anesthetic injection
    - Integrity of medial collateral ligament - chronic laxity associated with radiocapitellar arthritis, with pain aggravated by valgus load & forearm rotation

Demographics
- Age
  - Typically older patients (over 50 years) unless history of trauma
    - Posttraumatic - 4th to 6th decades
    - Chronic posterior impingement ≤ 40 years
- Gender: M > F

Natural History & Prognosis
- Progressively debilitating disease without medical intervention

Treatment
- Conservative
  - Physical therapy (PT); NSAIDs for pain management; hyaluronic acid injections, glucosamine & chondroitin supplements
- Surgical
  - Indicated for patients with persistent symptoms and pain
  - Arthroscopy (debridement)
  - Arthroplasty
  - Total joint replacement

DIAGNOSTIC CHECKLIST

Consider
- Secondary OA in cases where the findings are focal
  - Instability is predisposing

Image Interpretation Pearls
- Utilize FS PD FSE to visualize the chondral erosions

SELECTED REFERENCES
1. Miller MD et al: Surgical atlas of sports medicine. Philadelphia PA, Saunders, 436-42, 2003
2. Bredella MA et al: Accuracy of T2-weighted fast spin-echo MR imaging with fat saturation in detecting cartilage defects in the knee. Comparison with arthroscopy in 130 patients. AJR 172(4):1073-80, 1999
3. Fritz RC et al: The elbow. Magnetic resonance imaging in orthopedics and sports medicine. vol 1. 2nd ed. J.B. Lippincott 743-849, 1997
4. Fritz RC et al: MR imaging of the elbow. An update. Radiol Clin North Am 35(1):117-44, 1997

IMAGE GALLERY

Typical

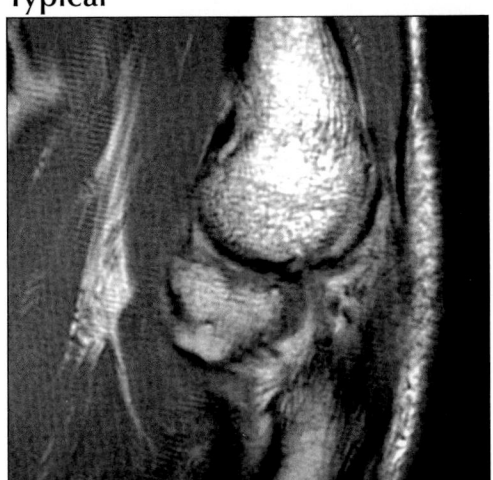
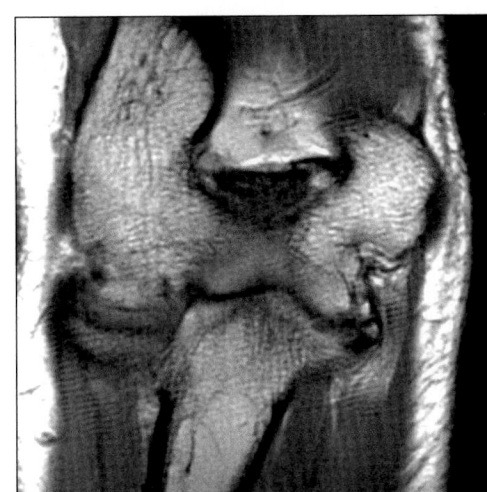

(Left) Sagittal PD FSE MR shows osteoarthritic changes of the radiocapitellar joint including post traumatic bone deformities, chondral erosions, and osteophyte formation. *(Right)* Coronal PD FSE MR shows osteoarthritic changes medially including osteophyte formation in an old ununited sublime tubercle fracture and adjacent trochlear osteophyte formation.

Typical

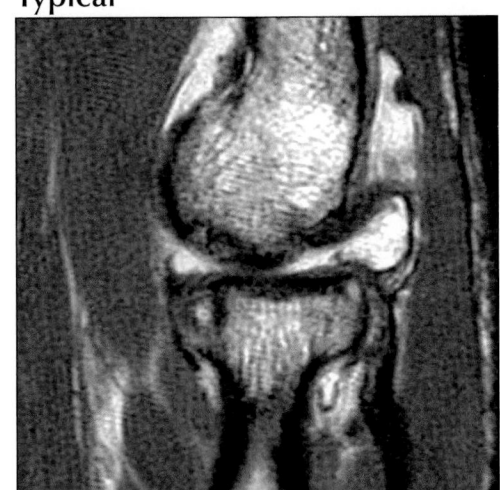
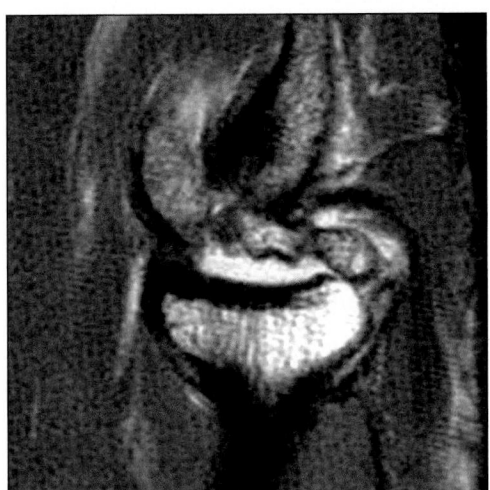

(Left) Sagittal PD FSE MR shows findings of osteoarthritis including chondral loss, subchondral cyst formation, subchondral sclerosis, synovitis, and joint debris. *(Right)* Sagittal PD FSE MR shows loose body formation in the posterolateral recess.

Variant

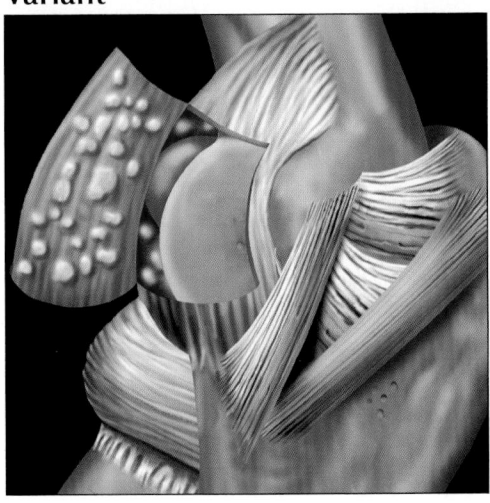
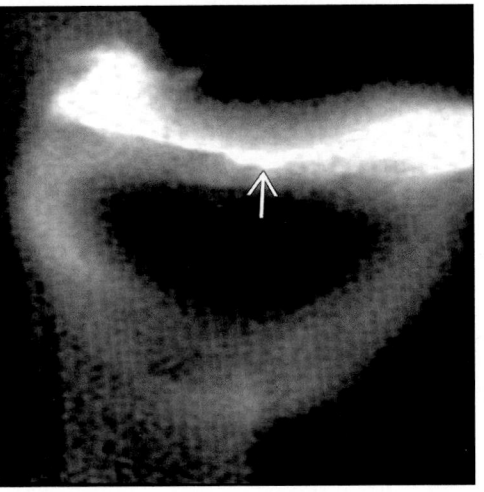

(Left) Sagittal graphic shows chondroid metaplasia and chondral body formation in a patient with synovial chondromatosis. These bodies would be intermediate on PD and T2WI. *(Right)* Coronal FS T1 MR high resolution arthrogram shows superficial chondral erosions of the radial head (arrow) without joint space narrowing.

RHEUMATOID ARTHRITIS, ELBOW

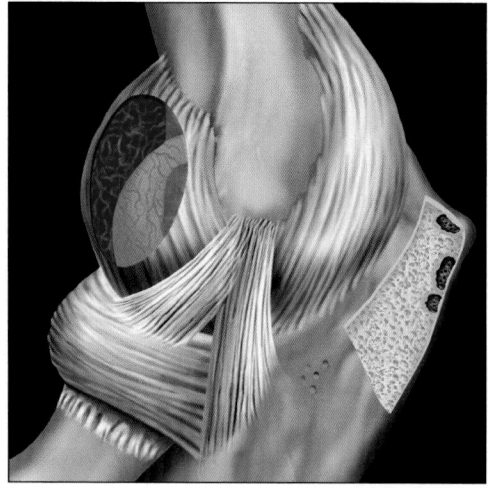

Sagittal graphic shows inflamed synovium within the joint and erosive changes within the posterior aspect of the olecranon. This patient has olecranon rheumatoid bursitis.

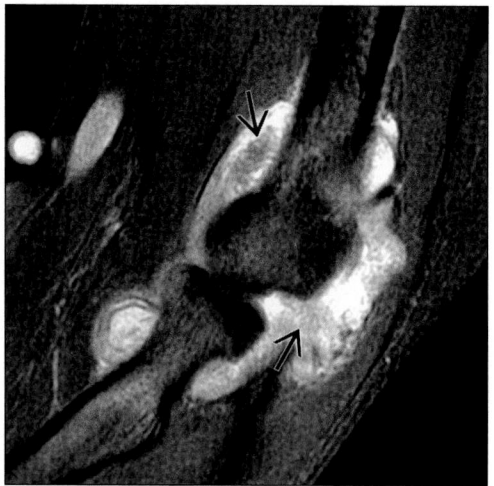

Sagittal FS PD FSE shows marked synovial changes (arrows) and reactive bone marrow edema in a patient with rheumatoid arthritis.

TERMINOLOGY

Abbreviations and Synonyms

- Rheumatoid arthritis (RA), degenerative joint disease (DJD)

Definitions

- Systemic inflammatory arthritic condition requiring the presence of 4 out of the following 7 criteria for > 6 weeks
  - Classification criteria for rheumatoid arthritis
    - Morning stiffness
    - Oligo or polyarthritis in three or more joints or several joint groups
    - Arthritis of either wrist, metacarpophalangeal joint or proximal interphalangeal joint
    - Symmetric arthritis
    - Rheumatoid nodules over boney prominences, extensor surfaces or juxta-articular
    - Abnormal amounts of serum rheumatoid factor
    - Radiographic changes including erosions and juxta-articular demineralization

IMAGING FINDINGS

General Features

- Best diagnostic clue

  - Thickened edematous synovium in association with effusion in patient with suggestive clinical symptomatology
  - Erosions common
- Location
  - Synovium of elbow joint
  - Affects synovium first then secondarily cartilage and bone leading to deformity
  - Nodules - in 20% of RA patients as mixed signal intensity masses in the skin, synovium, tendons, sclera, viscera
- Size: Usually diffuse involvement of synovium or tenosynovium
- Morphology
  - Thickened irregular synovium in the presence of a joint effusion
    - Synovitis followed by erosive/destructive changes

Radiographic Findings

- Radiography: Joint space narrowing, effusion, occasional cyst formation (cystic rheumatoid) followed by destruction

CT Findings

- NECT: Joint space narrowing, effusion, occasional cyst formation (cystic rheumatoid) followed by destruction
- CECT: Enhancement of inflamed synovium (pannus)

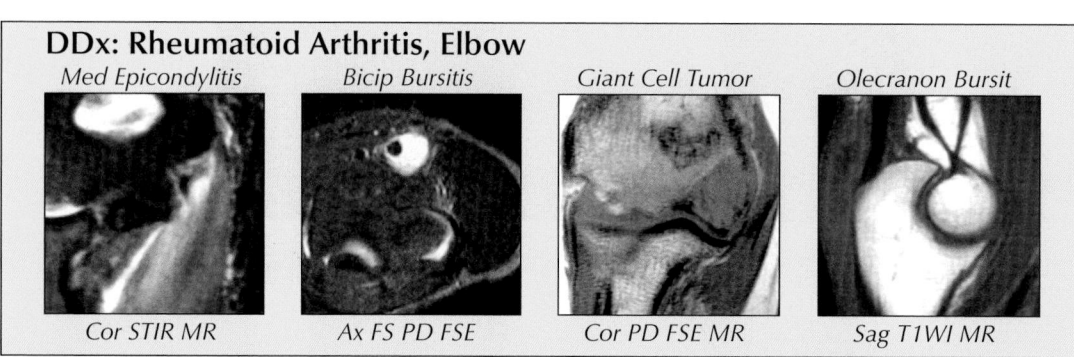

DDx: Rheumatoid Arthritis, Elbow

Med Epicondylitis	Bicip Bursitis	Giant Cell Tumor	Olecranon Bursit
Cor STIR MR	Ax FS PD FSE	Cor PD FSE MR	Sag T1WI MR

RHEUMATOID ARTHRITIS, ELBOW

Key Facts

Imaging Findings
- Thickened edematous synovium in association with effusion in patient with suggestive clinical symptomatology
- Best imaging tool: MRI

Top Differential Diagnoses
- Synovitis
- Other Inflammatory/Crystal Deposition Arthritis
- Osteoarthritis (OA)
- Medial Epicondylitis (Med Epicondylitis)
- Olecranon Bursitis (Olecranon Bursit)
- Bicipital Radial Bursitis (Bicip Bursitis)
- Tumor

Pathology
- Rheumatoid factor (RF) against Fc portion of autologous IgG
- Lab tests alone do not confirm the diagnosis of RA
- RF can be present (usually low titers) in normal individuals and other disease states

Clinical Issues
- Most common signs/symptoms: Elbow stiffness, pain and swelling
- Age: Adult for classical RA; variants (juvenile) - younger patients

Diagnostic Checklist
- Evaluate PD or FS PD FSE images for synovial thickening

MR Findings
- T1WI
  - Erosions, effusions are decreased in signal intensity
  - FS T1 shows thickened edematous synovium as a relative increase in signal intensity
- T2WI
  - Joint effusion - hyperintense fluid
  - Hyperintense olecranon bursitis
  - Narrowed hyaline articular cartilage
  - Erosions - increased signal intensity defects in the subchondral bone at the joint edges
  - FS PD FSE sensitive to edema
    - Hyperintense ulnar nerve associated with impingement related to synovitis, articular destruction and instability
- PD/Intermediate: Demonstrates inflamed synovium as thickened increased signal intensity joint lining
- STIR
  - Generally less effective because of low signal (standard STIR) and blurriness (FSE STIR)
  - Used at low and mid field more commonly
- T2* GRE
  - Less sensitive to chondral erosions or subchondral edema
  - Sensitive for loose body identification
  - Rheumatoid nodules (intermediated signal) on extensor surface of elbow
- T1 C+: Enhancement of synovium especially with fat saturation

Nuclear Medicine Findings
- Bone Scan: Bone reactive change will demonstrate increased uptake

Imaging Recommendations
- Best imaging tool: MRI
- Protocol advice
  - PD FSE with and without FS
  - PD & FS PD FSE images show thickened synovium or cartilage loss

DIFFERENTIAL DIAGNOSIS

Synovitis
- Characteristic symptoms/signs especially bone involvement different from RA
  - Subchondral edema and chondral erosions unusual
- PD demonstrates synovitis
  - Hyperintense compared to relatively hypointense fluid

Other Inflammatory/Crystal Deposition Arthritis
- Calcium pyrophosphate dihydrate crystal deposition disease (CPDD)
- +/- Tophi - gout - uric acid crystals
- Pseudogout - gout like pain attacks
- Chondrocalcinosis - asymptomatic

Osteoarthritis (OA)
- +/- Antecedent trauma
- +/- Subchondral cysts
- +/- Monoarticular
- +/- Osteophytes

Medial Epicondylitis (Med Epicondylitis)
- Valgus stress injury
- Usually chronic repetitive microtrauma
- Thrower's, golfer's elbow

Olecranon Bursitis (Olecranon Bursit)
- Without RA
- Fluid signal intensity on T2WI
- +/- Infection
- +/- Olecranon osteomyelitis

Bicipital Radial Bursitis (Bicip Bursitis)
- Without RA
- Fluid signal intensity on T2WI
- +/- Biceps tendinosis
- +/- Biceps tear

Tumor
- Bone destruction may mimic erosion
- Giant cell tumor

RHEUMATOID ARTHRITIS, ELBOW

- +/- Synovitis

PATHOLOGY

General Features
- General path comments
  - Rheumatoid factor (RF) against Fc portion of autologous IgG
    - Most RF = IgM
    - RF may also be IgG, IgA or IgE
    - All types of RF form immune complexes with autologous IgG
  - Lab tests alone do not confirm the diagnosis of RA
    - RF can be present (usually low titers) in normal individuals and other disease states
- Genetics: HLA-D allele DR4 is associated with RA patients
- Etiology
  - Combination of genetic and environmental factors
  - Interaction of antigen presenting macrophages with T cells (helper/inducer theory) likely inciting event
  - Complexes of IgG rheumatoid factor can deposit in blood vessels and lead to vasculitis causing secondary effects
  - Hepatitis B vaccine may be causative in a small number of patients
- Epidemiology: 3% of women & 1% of men overall
- Associated abnormalities
  - Extraarticular manifestations
    - Nodules, lymphadenopathy, splenomegaly, vasculitis, myopathy, sensory changes from neuropathy or direct compression from synovitis
    - Visceral changes including pericarditis, pulmonary fibrosis, nodules, and pleuritic pain
  - Elbow entrapment neuropathies caused by pannus
    - Anterior interosseous syndrome reported

Gross Pathologic & Surgical Features
- Pannus (granulation/synovium) tissue erodes cartilage & bone
  - Direct extension of pannus occurs at the margins of the joint
  - Tendon sheaths can be involved with pannus

Microscopic Features
- Vascular congestion and synovial cell proliferation occurs
- Infiltration of subsynovial layers by PMNs, lymphocytes & plasma cells
- Synovial villous formation is seen

Staging, Grading or Classification Criteria
- Inclusion classification criteria (as described in definition above)
- Progression of RA
  - Polypoid fibrovascular thickening of synovium + synoviocyte hyperplasia = pannus eroding into articular cartilage
  - Pannus growth + chondral erosions = subchondral extension + cyst formation
  - Ankylosis of joint

CLINICAL ISSUES

Presentation
- Most common signs/symptoms: Elbow stiffness, pain and swelling

Demographics
- Age: Adult for classical RA; variants (juvenile) - younger patients
- Gender: Female 3% of overall population, male 1%

Natural History & Prognosis
- 10% improve after first attack of synovitis and up to 60% can have remissions
- Up to 10% can become disabled
- Poor prognostic indicators include
  - High rheumatoid factor, periarticular erosions, rheumatoid nodules, muscle wasting, joint contractures

Treatment
- Conservative
  - Rest
  - Pharmaceutical approach including NSAIDs, antimalarials, disease modifying agents (MTX, sulphasalazine, gold, penicillamine), steroids and cytotoxic drugs
  - Physical therapy
- Surgical
  - Synovectomy
  - Arthroplasty, arthrodesis, osteotomy

DIAGNOSTIC CHECKLIST

Consider
- Synovitis
  - Etiologies monoarticular or polyarticular

Image Interpretation Pearls
- Evaluate PD or FS PD FSE images for synovial thickening
- Subchondral marrow edema, synovitis (pannus) + pancompartmental chondral erosions are characteristic of rheumatoid arthritis
- Effusions often distend joint capsule

SELECTED REFERENCES
1. Kauffman JI et al: Surgical management of the rheumatoid elbow. J Am Acad Orthop Surg 11(2):100-8, 2003
2. Murphy MS: Management of inflammatory arthritis around the elbow. Hand Clin 18(1):161-8, 2002
3. Rahme H: The Kudo elbow prosthesis in rheumatoid arthritis. A consecutive series of 26 elbow replacements in 24 patients followed prospectively for a mean of 5 years. Acta Orthop Scand 73(3):251-6, 2002
4. Matsuno h et al: Relationship between histological findings and clinical findings in rheumatoid arthritis. Pathol Int 52(8):527-33, 2002
5. Fink B et al: Results of elbow endoprostheses in patients with rheumatoid arthritis in correlation with previous operations. J Shoulder Elbow Surg 11(4):360-7, 2000

RHEUMATOID ARTHRITIS, ELBOW

IMAGE GALLERY

Typical

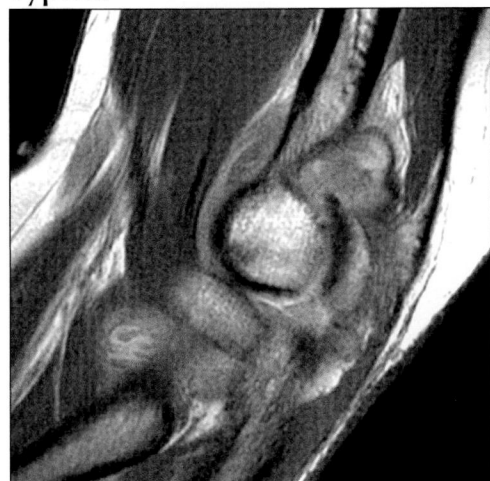 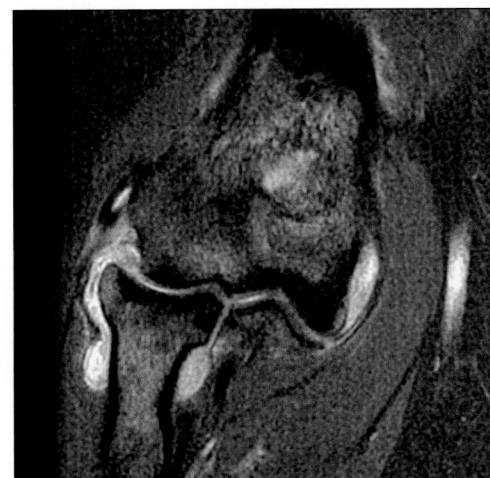

(Left) Sagittal PD FSE MR shows marked synovial proliferation in a patient with rheumatoid arthritis. *(Right)* Coronal FS PD FSE MR shows marked synovial proliferation in a patient with rheumatoid arthritis. The patient also has lateral epicondylitis with tearing of the common extensor tendon origin.

Typical

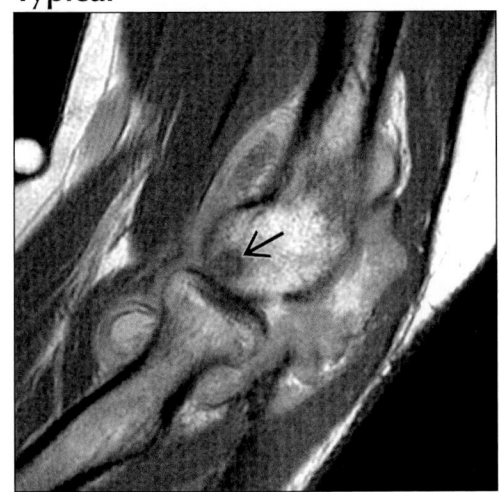 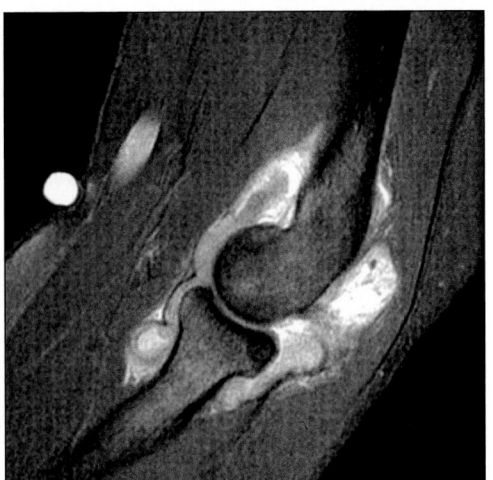

(Left) Sagittal PD FSE MR shows an erosion (arrow) of the capitellum in association with synovial proliferation in a patient with RA. *(Right)* Sagittal FS PD FSE MR shows synovial thickening in a patient with antecubital pain.

Typical

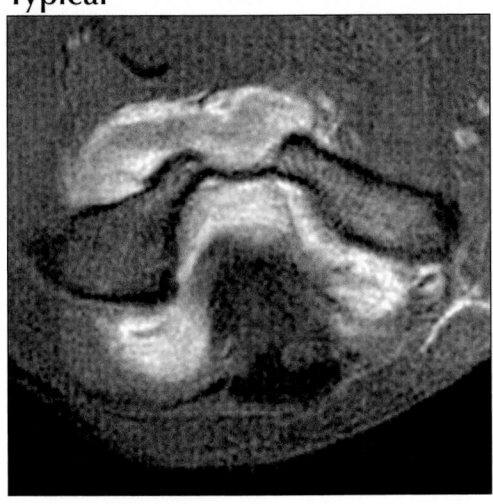 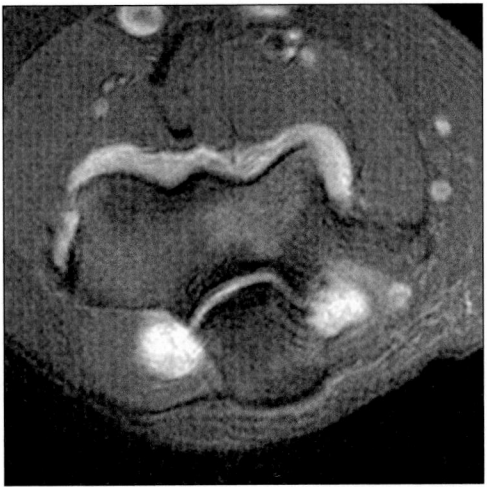

(Left) Axial FS PD FSE MR shows the thickened increased signal intensity synovium. *(Right)* Axial FS PD FSE MR shows markedly thickened synovium and bone reactive edema.

OSTEOMYELITIS, ELBOW

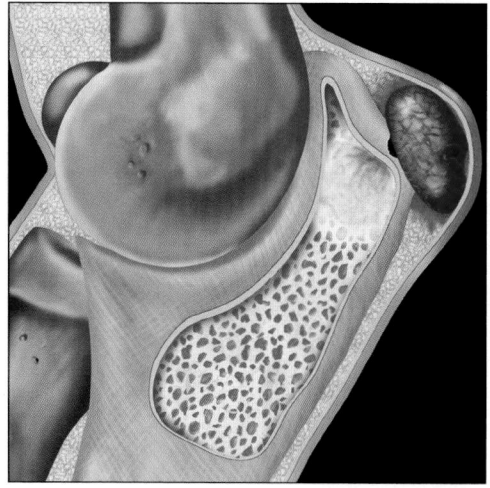

Sagittal graphic shows infected olecranon bursitis with adjacent olecranon cortical destruction and medullary osteomyelitis.

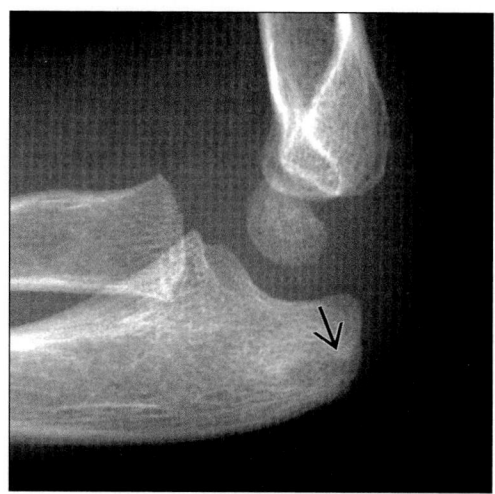

Lateral radiography shows bone destruction (arrow) on the olecranon and bursal soft tissue swelling in this pediatric patient with osteomyelitis.

TERMINOLOGY

Abbreviations and Synonyms
- Acute hematogenous osteomyelitis, chronic osteomyelitis

Definitions
- Acute hematogenous osteomyelitis in pediatric patient
- Chronic posttraumatic osteomyelitis in adult patient
- Often due to adjacent infectious bursitis in adult

IMAGING FINDINGS

General Features
- Best diagnostic clue
  - Bone marrow hyperintensity on T2WI
  - Osseous erosion + sinus tract identified on T2WI
  - Bone destructive change with cortical irregularity identified on T1WI
- Location
  - Bone marrow in hematogenous osteomyelitis
  - Osteitis ± marrow involvement in secondary (trauma or surgery) osteomyelitis
- Size: Variable from epiphyseal involvement to diaphyseal + soft tissue involvement
- Morphology: Focal, Brodie abscess or larger area of medullary or cortical destruction

Radiographic Findings
- Radiography
  - Insensitive for early osteomyelitis
  - Changes delayed 10-14 days after onset of fever
  - Soft tissue edema/swelling
  - Focal lucency to frank destruction of bone
  - Periosteal elevation + underlying lucency (subperiosteal abscess)
  - Intramedullary abscess - focal lucency ± tract to cortical surface
  - Sequestration (necrotic fragments) + involucrum (periosteal bone) as parosteal ossification
  - Joint effusion

CT Findings
- NECT
  - Early bone destruction
  - Cortical + trabecular bone detail
  - Periosteal elevation, cortical destruction, intramedullary abscess + sinus tracts
  - Joint effusions = hypodense
- CECT
  - Infected regions enhance
  - Soft tissue findings: Abscesses enhance peripherally, sinus tracts enhance

MR Findings
- T1WI

DDx: Osteomyelitis, Elbow

Stress Fracture	Stress Response	Humeral Fracture	Olecranon Fx	Olecranon Burs.
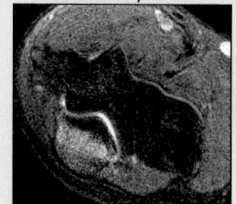	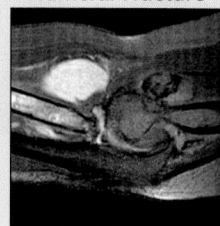	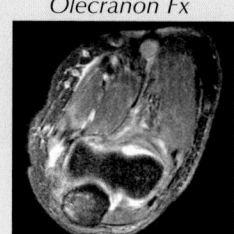	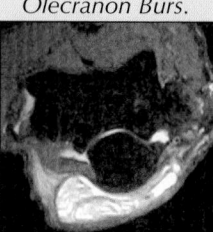	
Sag STIR MR	Ax STIR MR	Sag FS PD FSE	Ax FS PD FSE	Ax STIR MR

OSTEOMYELITIS, ELBOW

Key Facts

Imaging Findings

- Bone marrow hyperintensity on T2WI
- Osseous erosion + sinus tract identified on T2WI
- Bone destructive change with cortical irregularity identified on T1WI

Top Differential Diagnoses

- Cellulitis
- Septic Arthritis
- Elbow Fracture
- Osteoid Osteoma
- Other Bone Tumors
- Panner's Disease
- Olecranon Bursitis without Osteomyelitis (Olec Bursitis)

Pathology

- Staphylococcus aureus = most common infecting organism in all age groups
- Chronic osteomyelitis = most common form of osteomyelitis in adult & 2° to trauma
- Hematogenous seeding
- Direct contamination
- Contiguous spread

Clinical Issues

- Most common signs/symptoms: Pain
- Fever

Diagnostic Checklist

- Identify association of marrow edema with disruption/erosion of cortex + soft tissue sinus tract

- o Hypointense marrow edema + cortical destruction
- o Hypointense reactive joint effusion
- o Soft tissue hypointense abscess
- o Tract from skin to cortex
- o Hypointense to intermediate signal in metaphysis/diametaphysis in child
- T2WI
  - o Hyperintense marrow involvement
  - o Hyperintense intraosseous abscess
  - o Cortical destruction: Intermediate to hyperintense
  - o Cloaca (periosteal opening): Focal hyperintensity in hypointense periosteum
  - o Sinus tract: Intermediate to hyperintense
  - o Brodie abscess (round abscess cavity due to chronic pyogenic infection): Hyperintense + hypointense sclerotic rim
  - o Cellulitis: Reticulated subcutaneous hyperintensity
  - o Myositis: Hyperintense muscle + enlargement
- T1 C+
  - o Enhancement
    - ▪ Bone marrow - inflammation
    - ▪ Abscess - peripheral enhancement of adjacent infected soft tissue (thick wall)
    - ▪ Sequestrum - enhancement peripheral to sequestrum
    - ▪ Cortical erosion/destruction - ± enhancement
    - ▪ Sinus tract - peripheral enhancement
- Sequestrum: Hypointense on T1 + T2WI
- Involucrum (periosteal reaction): Hypointense on T1 & T2WI

Nuclear Medicine Findings

- Bone Scan: Increased uptake with bone destructive changes of osteomyelitis

Imaging Recommendations

- Best imaging tool: MR sensitive to marrow edema & soft tissue involvement
- Protocol advice: T1 + FS PD FSE or STIR axial, coronal & sagittal

DIFFERENTIAL DIAGNOSIS

Cellulitis

- Subcutaneous fat involvement
- Hypointense on T1, hyperintense on T2
- Reticulated pattern on T1 & T2
- Underlying muscle or deep fascial planes intact

Septic Arthritis

- Large hyperintense (T2WI) joint effusion with capsular distension, ± scalloping of capsule (synovitis)
- Diabetes, steroids, intravenous drug use = predisposing factors

Crystal Induced Arthropathies

- Requires T2* gradient echo for visualization of susceptibility
- Effusion
- Degenerative findings including labral tears
- Chondral - hyaline cartilage degeneration

Elbow Fracture

- Hypo or hyperintense fracture line
- Adjacent hyperintensity of soft tissue without sinus tract or osseous erosion
- Olecranon fracture may mimic osteomyelitis
- Radiographs often helpful for differentiation
- History of trauma

Eosinophilic Granuloma

- Proliferating histiocytes
- Punched-out calvarial lesions + button sequestrum
- Tubular bones - osteolytic destruction ± lamellar periosteal reaction

Osteoid Osteoma

- Lesion < 2 cm
- Painful lesion
- Requires FS PD, T2 or STIR to demonstrate hyperintensity of lesion & edema

Other Bone Tumors

- Ewing sarcoma
- Osteosarcoma

- Solid lesion = central enhancement & peritumoral edema

Myositis Ossificans
- Mass of calcified or ossified granulation tissue
- ± Reactive hyperintense soft tissue edema on T2WI adjacent to ossification

Panner's Disease
- Osteochondrosis seen in 5-11 years old
- Bone destruction without clinical picture of infection
- Unusual location for infection

Olecranon Bursitis without Osteomyelitis (Olec Bursitis)
- Hyperintense mass on T2WI
- Cystic appearing
- +/- Rim enhancement
- No bone changes without osteomyelitis

PATHOLOGY

General Features
- General path comments
  - Relevant anatomy for infection
    - Periosteum (periostitis)
    - Cortex (osteitis)
    - Marrow (osteomyelitis)
    - Metaphysis: > 1 year to skeletal maturity
    - Metaphysis/epiphysis - hematogenous involvement in infants
    - Subcutaneous fat (cellulitis)
- Etiology
  - Staphylococcus aureus = most common infecting organism in all age groups
  - Common organisms = Streptococcus, Pseudomonas, Haemophilus, Enterobacter
- Epidemiology
  - Chronic osteomyelitis = most common form of osteomyelitis in adult & 2° to trauma
  - Staphylococcus aureus = 80-90%

Gross Pathologic & Surgical Features
- Hematogenous seeding
  - Children
  - Via vasculature
  - Vascular metaphyseal bone
- Direct contamination
  - Penetrating trauma
  - Post-surgical
- Contiguous spread
  - Soft tissue infection
  - Septic arthritis

Microscopic Features
- Leukocytic infiltration of marrow
- Vascular compression
- Necrosis, abscesses + sequestra

Staging, Grading or Classification Criteria
- Acute/subacute & chronic hematogenous osteomyelitis
- Brodie abscess
- Chronic recurrent multifocal osteomyelitis (CRMO)

- Posttraumatic osteomyelitis

CLINICAL ISSUES

Presentation
- Most common signs/symptoms: Pain
- Clinical profile
  - Fever
  - Restricted motion + point tenderness
  - Elevated sedimentation rate, C-reactive protein & WBC count
  - Soft tissue swelling + erythema + sinus tract

Demographics
- Age
  - Young children most commonly affected
  - Adults with direct contamination (trauma, post-op)
- Gender: M = F

Natural History & Prognosis
- Osseous destruction will reoccur if untreated
- Prognosis good if treated early
- Develop into chronic infection
- Intramedullary, subperiosteal abscesses
- Soft tissue extension

Treatment
- Conservative
  - IV antibiotics
- Surgical
  - Debridement & antibiotic-impregnated beads

DIAGNOSTIC CHECKLIST

Consider
- Identify association of marrow edema with disruption/erosion of cortex + soft tissue sinus tract
- Axial images to identify hypointense sequestrum

SELECTED REFERENCES

1. Van Holsbeeck MT et al: Musculoskeletal Ultrasound. 2nd ed. Philadelphia PA, Mosby, 265-8, 2001
2. Greenspan A: Osteomyelitis, infectious arthritis, and soft-tissue infections. Orthopaedic Radiol 3rd ed. 753-84, 2000
3. Mettler FA et al: Skeletal System. Essentials of Nuclear Medicine Imaging. 4th ed. Philadelphia PA, WB Saunders, 285-333, 1998
4. Resnick D: Pelvis and Hip. Internal Derangements of joints. 1st ed. Philadelphia PA, WB Saunders, 473-554, 1997

IMAGE GALLERY

Typical

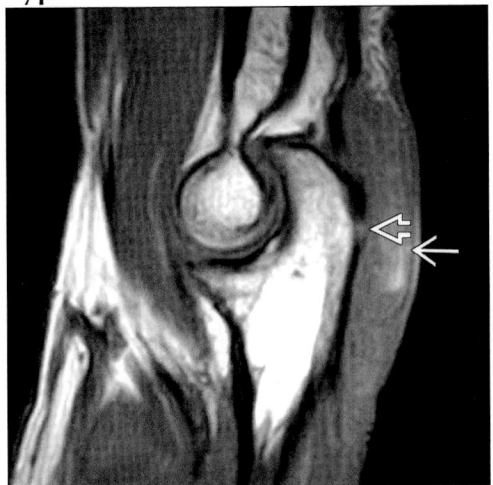
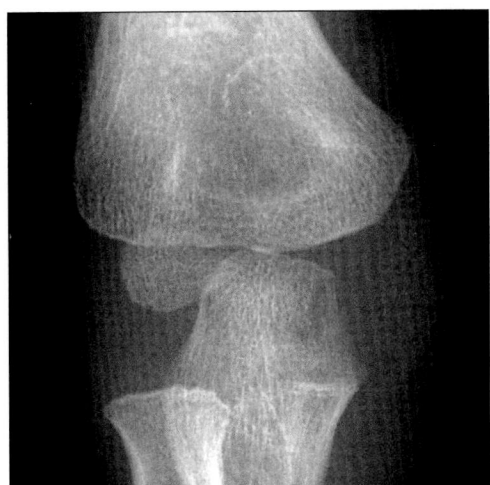

(Left) Sagittal T1WI MR shows infected olecranon bursitis (arrow). Note the early olecranon cortical (open arrow) erosion without associated hypointense bone marrow edema. No osteomyelitis developed. *(Right)* Anteroposterior radiography shows bone destructive change in the olecranon in this 4 year old with proven osteomyelitis.

Typical

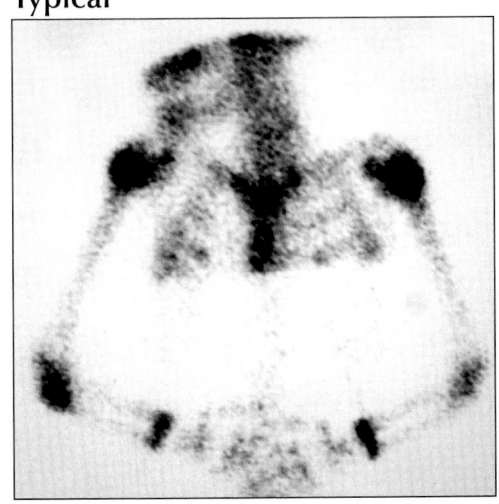
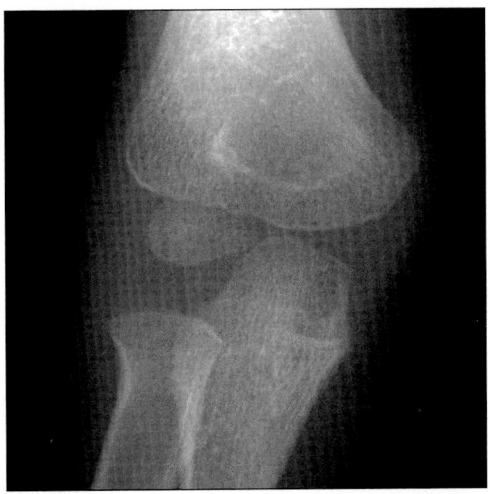

(Left) Bone scan from posterior projection shows increased tracer activity in the right olecranon in this pediatric patient with olecranon osteomyelitis. *(Right)* Anteroposterior radiography shows lucency of the olecranon at presentation in this room with pain and an increased white blood cell count.

Typical

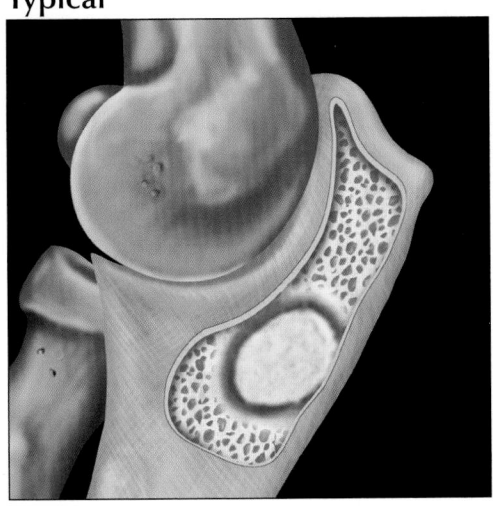
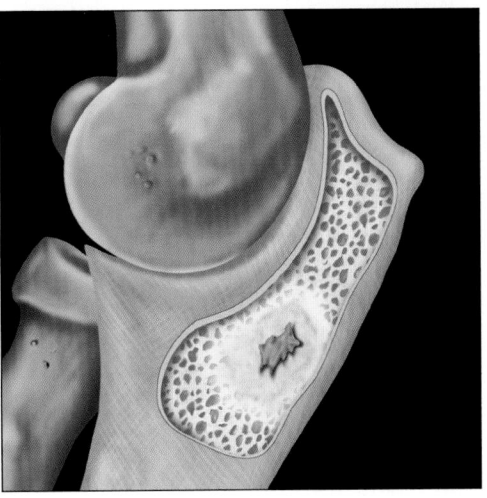

(Left) Sagittal graphic shows an intramedullary abscess. Osseous related changes are hyperintense on T2WI, especially FS PD FSE. *(Right)* Sagittal graphic shows a sequestrum in the olecranon in this patient with chronic osteomyelitis. A sequestrum is hypointense on T1 & T2WI.

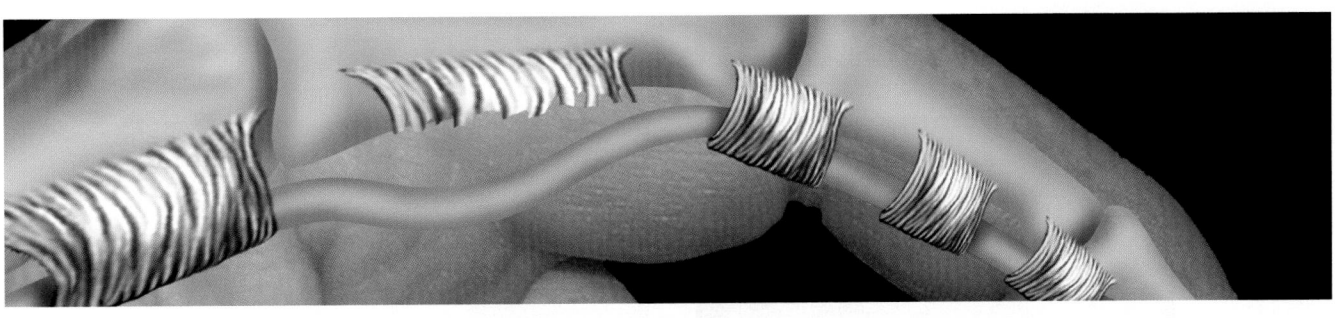

SECTION 3: Wrist and Hand

SCAPHOLUNATE LIGAMENT TEAR

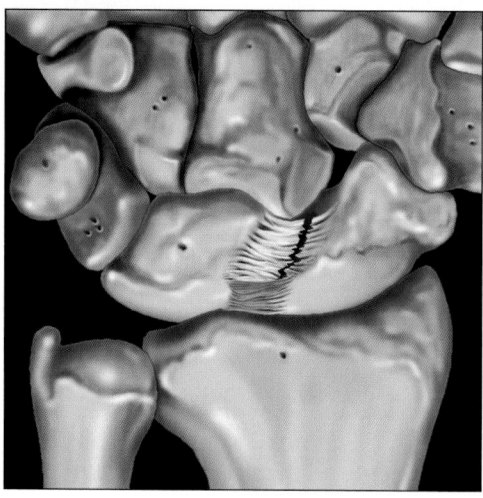

Coronal graphic shows tear of the volar component of the scapholunate ligament. Intact membranous component is seen proximally.

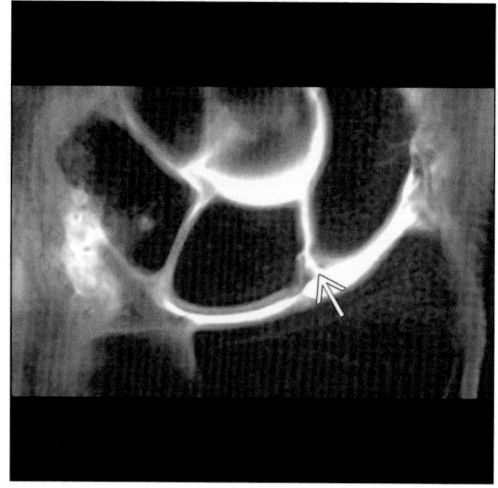

Coronal T1 C+ MR (intraarticular contrast) shows complete dissociation (arrow) between scaphoid and lunate. Hyperintense fluid extends across the membranous and volar scapholunate ligament.

TERMINOLOGY

Abbreviations and Synonyms
- SL or scapholunate instability, stage I perilunate instability

Definitions
- Dissociation = ligamentous disruption between scaphoid + lunate
- Instability = inability to withstand normal loading
- Rotatory subluxation - abnormal radiographic alignment of dissociated scaphoid

IMAGING FINDINGS

General Features
- Best diagnostic clue: Discontinuity of the scapholunate ligament
- Location
  - Intrinsic scapholunate ligament complex = scapholunate interosseous ligament
    - Dorsal component (important key stabilizer)
    - Membranous component
    - Volar component
  - Extrinsic SL ligament complex
    - Radioscaphocapitate (RSC)
    - Long radiolunate (radiolunotriquetral) (RLT)
    - Short radiolunate
    - Radioscapholunate (RSL) (ligament of Testut)
  - Scaphotrapeziotrapezoid ligament complex
- Size
  - Variable based on associated osseous vs. ligamentous disruption of major carpal links
    - Scaphotrapeziotrapezoid (STT) = radial link
    - Triquetrohamate (TH) = ulnar link
- Morphology
  - Scapholunate interosseous ligament
    - Dorsal component = trapezoidal
    - Membranous = wedge-shaped
    - Volar = thin slightly oblique fibers

Radiographic Findings
- Radiography
  - Anteroposterior view - signs of unstable injuries
    - Loss of scapholunate articular parallelism
    - Scapholunate interval diastasis > 3 mm
    - Decreased scaphoid cortical ring-to-pole interval (> 4 mm asymmetry or absolute value < 7 mm)
    - Asymmetric radioscaphoid interval (normal = 4 mm)
    - Lunate extension
    - Degenerative arthritis
  - Lateral view - signs of unstable injuries
    - Radioscaphoid angle > 80°
    - Capitolunate angle > 20°
    - SL angle > 70°

DDx: Scapholunate Ligament Tear

Dorsal Ganglion	Scaphoid Fracture	Radius Fracture
Cor FS PD MR	Cor T1WI MR	Cor T1WI MR

SCAPHOLUNATE LIGAMENT TEAR

Key Facts

Imaging Findings
- Best diagnostic clue: Discontinuity of the scapholunate ligament
- Intrinsic scapholunate ligament complex = scapholunate interosseous ligament
- Scapholunate interval diastasis > 3 mm
- Key structure = disruption of dorsal component of SL ligament

Top Differential Diagnoses
- Dorsal Wrist Ganglion
- De Quervain's Stenosing Tenosynovitis
- Scaphoid Fracture
- Radius Fracture
- Avascular Necrosis of Scaphoid

Pathology
- SL dissociation requires injury to both SL intrinsic ligament + the extrinsic RSC ligament
- Scapholunate advanced collapse (SLAC) wrist = progressive proximal capitate migration, radioscaphoid & capitolunate arthrosis in untreated SL dissociation

Clinical Issues
- Most common signs/symptoms: Pain & soft tissue swelling involving dorsoradial wrist
- Watson test (scaphoid shift test) for SL instability = pain on ulnar to radial deviation
- Audible click at SL interval

Diagnostic Checklist
- Evaluate all three components of SL ligament

- - Dorsal intercalated segment instability (DISI) deformity

MR Findings
- T1WI
  - Scapholunate gap increased to > 3 mm (equivalent of the Terry Thomas sign on radiography) = dissociation
  - Volar or palmar flexion of scaphoid on sagittal images
  - DISI with dorsal tilting of lunate, increased capitolunate angle to > 30° & increased scapholunate angle > 80°
- T2WI
  - Hyperintense linear signal in partial or complete tear
  - Complete ligamentous disruption with hyperintense fluid-filled gap
  - Hyperintense synovial fluid communication between radiocarpal & midcarpal compartment
  - Key structure = disruption of dorsal component of SL ligament
  - Associated synovitis of extrinsic volar radiocarpal ligaments
  - Degenerative perforations may exist in membranous portion with intact volar + dorsal components
- T1 C+
  - MR arthrography
    - Flap tears
    - Perforations
    - Integrity of dorsal component SL ligament

Imaging Recommendations
- Best imaging tool: MR to identify separate components of SL interosseous ligament + associated scaphoid or distal radius fractures
- Protocol advice
  - T1 or PD + FS PD FSE coronal & axial plane
  - FS PD FSE sagittal

DIFFERENTIAL DIAGNOSIS

Dorsal Wrist Ganglion
- Most common soft tissue mass in wrist
- From capsule over SL joint
- Painless mass associated with injuries to SL ligament
- ± Weakness of grip, pain or paresthesias from nerve compression or irritation

De Quervain's Stenosing Tenosynovitis
- Radial sided wrist pain
- Inability to abduct thumb + swelling, crepitus and pain on radial side of wrist
- Affects abductor pollicis longus (APL) + extensor pollicis brevis (EPB) tendons

Scaphoid Fracture
- Tuberosity
- Distal pole
- Waist
- Proximal pole
- Fracture line = horizontal oblique, vertical oblique or transverse
- Hypointense fracture line + variable edema of subchondral marrow on T2WI

Radius Fracture
- Low energy metaphyseal injuries → Colles' fx
- Articular injuries - violent injuries, frequently comminuted + unstable
- Identify components of articular fractures: Metaphyseal or shaft, radial styloid, dorsal medial/palmar medial articular fragments

Avascular Necrosis of Scaphoid
- 2° to proximal pole or waist fractures
- Necrotic bone hypointense on T1 + hyperintense on FS PD FSE or STIR in acute + subacute stages
- Reactive marrow edema of distal pole may not represent necrosis

Kienböck's Disease
- Avascular necrosis lunate
- Related to ulnar + lunar negative variance

SCAPHOLUNATE LIGAMENT TEAR

- Lunate marrow hypointense on T1WI + hyperintense on FS PD or T2 FSE images in early stages
- Hypointense lunate on all pulse sequences in advanced degenerative arthrosis

PATHOLOGY

General Features
- General path comments
  - Relevant anatomy
    - Scapholunate ligament complex = intrinsic + extrinsic ligaments
    - Extrinsic ligaments = gross stability
    - Intrinsic = fine tuning of stability
    - Scaphotrapeziotrapezoid (STT) ligament complex = significant volar constraint
- Etiology
  - Axial compression/hyperextension + intercarpal supination
  - Ulnar deviation
  - Forward fall onto outstretched hand, or backward on a pronated hand
  - SL dissociation requires injury to both SL intrinsic ligament + the extrinsic RSC ligament
- Epidemiology
  - Most common type of carpal instability
  - Residual of perilunate injury or as isolated injury
  - Association with scaphoid + distal radial fractures

Gross Pathologic & Surgical Features
- Classification
  - Acute (< 6 weeks)
    - Stable - partial ligament disruption
    - Unstable (dynamic or static) - complete ligament disruption
  - Chronic
    - Stable, unstable, fixed
    - Pancarpal arthrosis
    - Scapholunate advanced collapse (SLAC) wrist = progressive proximal capitate migration, radioscaphoid & capitolunate arthrosis in untreated SL dissociation
    - DISI deformity with midcarpal collapse

Microscopic Features
- Scaphoid attachment of SL ligament has fewer Sharpey's fibers than lunate attachment (more susceptible to tear)
- Histology of ligaments = collagen fibers, connective tissue with fat, vessels + elastic fibers

Staging, Grading or Classification Criteria
- Arthroscopic
  - Grade I & II = partial tear SL ligament
  - Grade III & IV = complete disruption
- Perilunar instability (PLI)
  - Stage I PLI: Scapholunate failure
  - Stage II PLI: Capitolunate failure
  - Stage III PLI: Triquetrolunate failure
  - Stage IV PLI: Dorsal radiocarpal ligament failure with volar rotation of the lunate

CLINICAL ISSUES

Presentation
- Most common signs/symptoms: Pain & soft tissue swelling involving dorsoradial wrist
- Clinical profile
  - Pain & tenderness anatomic snuffbox
  - Watson test (scaphoid shift test) for SL instability = pain on ulnar to radial deviation
  - Audible click at SL interval

Demographics
- Age: Adult population
- Gender: No bias
- Association with sports that place dorsal stress on carpus (loading wrist in palmar flexion)

Natural History & Prognosis
- Secondary changes in chronic SL injuries
  - Capsular contractures
  - Intercarpal collapse
  - Scaphoid + midcarpal fixation
  - Degenerative arthritis
  - SLAC

Treatment
- Conservative
  - Cast immobilization
- Surgical - acute
  - Close reduction + internal fixation
  - Open reduction + 1° repair or reconstruction
- Surgical - chronic
  - Open reduction + reconstruction
  - Arthrodesis

DIAGNOSTIC CHECKLIST

Consider
- Evaluate all three components of SL ligament
- Dorsal component SL ligament tears are more symptomatic

SELECTED REFERENCES
1. Theumann NH et al: Extrinsic carpal ligaments: Normal MR arthrographic appearance in cadavers. Radiol 226(1):171-9, 2003
2. Szabo RM et al: Dorsal intercarpal ligament capsulodesis for chronic, stable scapholunate dissociation: Clinical results. J Hand Surg 27(6):978-84, 2002
3. Totterman SM et al: MRI findings of scapholunate instabilities in coronal images: A short communication. Semin Musculoskelet Radiol 5(3):251-6, 2001
4. Lewis DM et al: Scapholunate instability in athletes. Clin Sports Med 20(1):131-40, 2001
5. Blatt G et al: The wrist and its disorders. Scapholunate injuries. 2nd ed. Philadelphia Pennsylvania, W.B. Saunders, (15):268-306, 1997
6. Larsen CF et al: Analysis of carpal instability. Description of the scheme. J Hand Surg 20A:757-64, 1995
7. Dobyns JH et al: Carpal instability - nondissociative. J Hand Surg 19B:763-73, 1994
8. Berger RA et al: Magnetic resource imaging of anterior radiocarpal ligament. J Hand Surg 19A:295-303, 1994

SCAPHOLUNATE LIGAMENT TEAR

IMAGE GALLERY

Typical

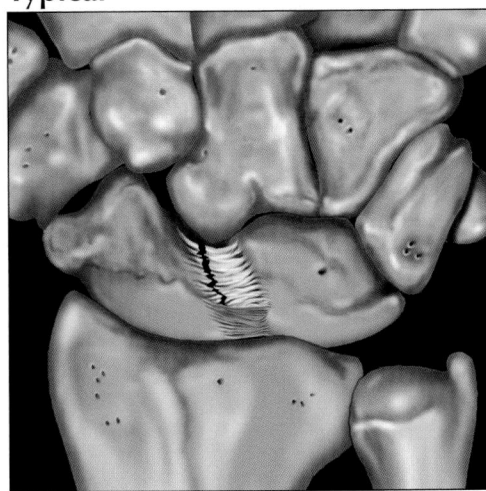
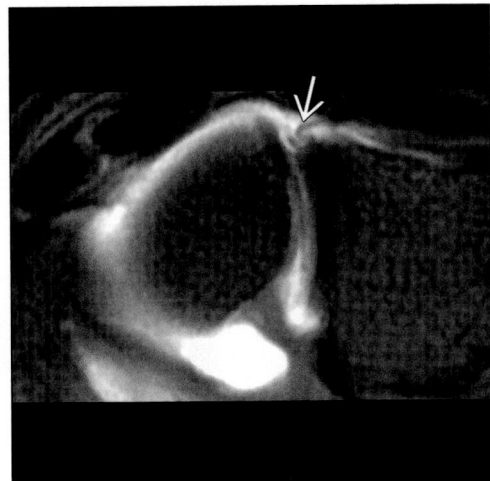

(Left) Coronal graphic shows tear of the dorsal component of the scapholunate interosseous ligament. The dorsal component of the SL ligament is biomechanically the strongest. *(Right)* Axial T1 C+ (MR arthrogram) shows absence of the dorsal component (arrow) of the scapholunate ligament in scapholunate instability (scaphoid on the left, lunate is on the right, dorsal is superior).

Typical

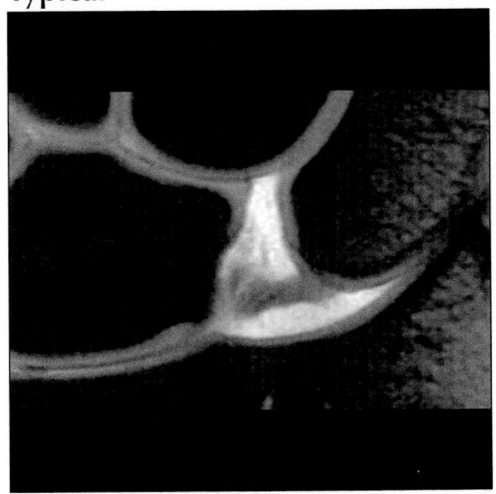
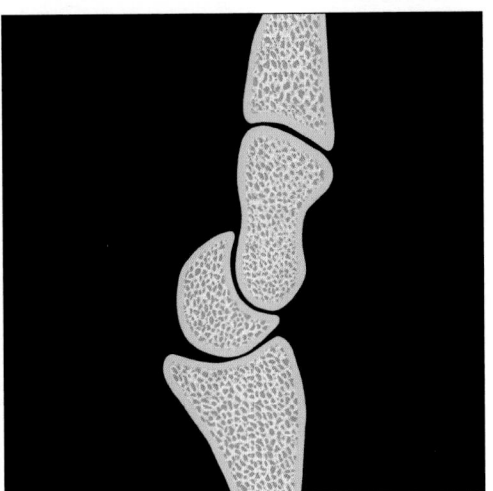

(Left) Coronal T1 C+ MR (intraarticular contrast) shows scapholunate diastasis between scaphoid and lunate in complete scapholunate ligament disruption. The remnant of the membranous component of SL ligament is shown. *(Right)* Sagittal graphic shows dorsal tilting of the lunate in DISI deformity. The capitate lunate angle is > 30 degrees.

Typical

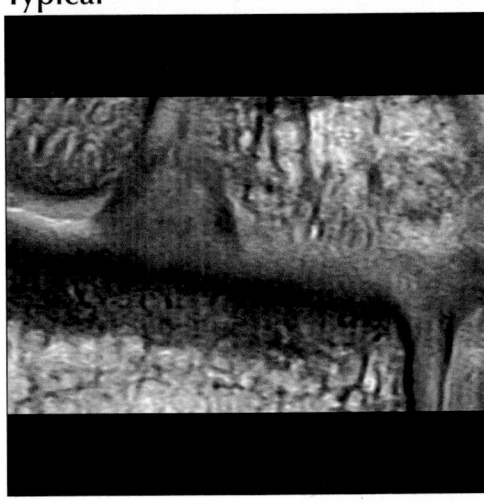
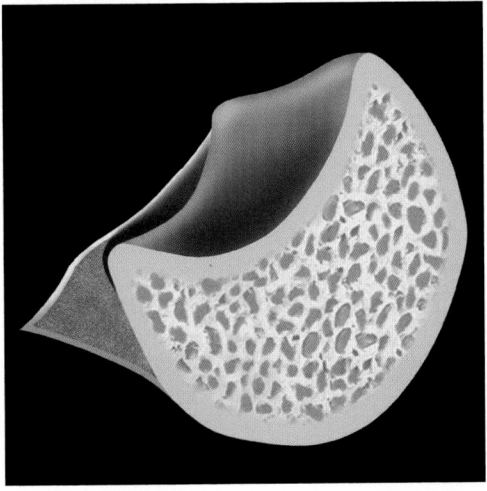

(Left) Coronal T1WI MR shows triangular shaped membranous component of scapholunate ligament with direct attachment to articular cartilage surfaces of scaphoid and lunate (scaphoid on left, lunate on right). *(Right)* Coronal graphic through triangular shaped membranous component of SL ligament. The apex of the triangle is directed distally. The membranous component of SL ligament is the weakest structure of SL complex (lunate shown).

LUNOTRIQUETRAL INSTABILITY

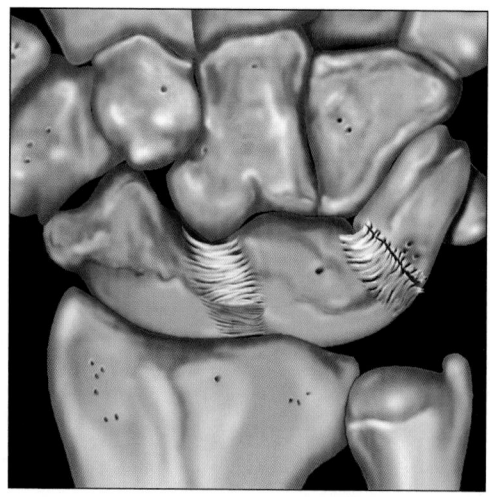

Coronal graphic shows tear of volar and membranous components of LT ligament. The volar fibers of LT ligament are biomechanically the strongest.

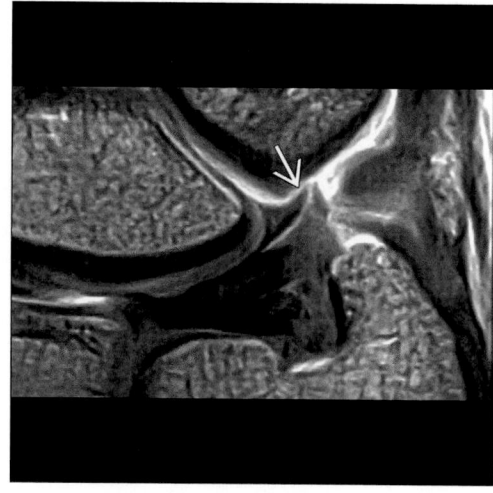

Coronal T1 MR arthrography shows flap tear (arrow) of lunate attachment of membranous component of LT ligament. Fluid extends across LT interval. Meniscus homologue & TFC are present.

TERMINOLOGY

Abbreviations and Synonyms
- LT ligament sprain or tear, lunotriquetral ligament sprain, lunotriquetral ligament tear

Definitions
- Partial or complete tear of lunotriquetral ligament

IMAGING FINDINGS

General Features
- Best diagnostic clue: Discontinuity of normally hypointense LT ligament across LT interval
- Location
  - LT ligament components
    - Dorsal
    - Membranous
    - Volar
- Size
  - Variable based on associated injuries
    - Distal radioulnar joint (DRUJ) subluxation + arthritis
    - Chondromalacia distal ulna
    - Triangular fibrocartilage complex (TFCC) injury
    - Triquetrohamate instability
- Morphology

  - Flap tears or complete absence of ligament
  - Focal membranous injuries with ulnocarpal impaction - positive ulnar variance

Radiographic Findings
- Radiography
  - Disruption of normal convex arc (Gilula's lines) proximal carpal row
    - Step off between lunate & triquetrum

MR Findings
- T1WI
  - Delta-shaped or linear ligament best visualized on coronal images
  - Absence of hypointense horseshoe-shaped structure
  - Loss of normal smooth convexity of proximal carpal row
  - Disruption of LT interval is pronounced with ulnar deviation
  - ± Dorsiflexion of triquetrum relative to lunate on sagittal images
- T2WI
  - Normal LT ligament does not extend into interval
  - Axial images to separate volar, membranous & dorsal components of ligament
  - Separate components more difficult to appreciate on coronal images
  - FS PD FSE or MR arthrography for insertional site tears or perforations

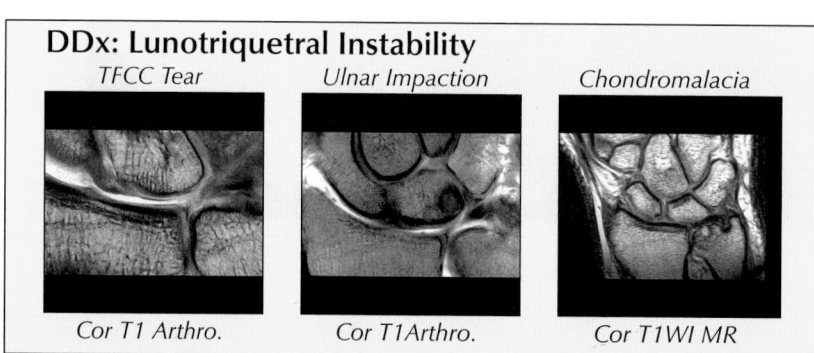

DDx: Lunotriquetral Instability

TFCC Tear	Ulnar Impaction	Chondromalacia
Cor T1 Arthro.	Cor T1Arthro.	Cor T1WI MR

LUNOTRIQUETRAL INSTABILITY

Key Facts

Imaging Findings

- Best diagnostic clue: Discontinuity of normally hypointense LT ligament across LT interval
- Flap tears or complete absence of ligament
- Focal membranous injuries with ulnocarpal impaction - positive ulnar variance

Top Differential Diagnoses

- TFCC Tear
- Subluxation or Dislocation DRUJ
- Subluxation Extensor Carpi Ulnaris (ECU)
- Midcarpal Instability
- Ulnar Impaction Syndrome

Pathology

- LT injury = stage III PLI (triquetral dislocation + radiotriquetral ligament failure)

- Isolated LT sprain 2° to ulnar sided injury = more common pattern of injury (than concomitant radial injury)
- LT injury associated with increased load transmission across ulnar side wrist + ulnar positive variance

Clinical Issues

- Most common signs/symptoms: Pain on ulnar aspect of wrist
- ± Painful wrist click in radial or ulnar deviation
- Traumatic event = fall on outstretched hand or twisting/rotatory injury
- Eventual VISI deformity

Diagnostic Checklist

- Identify associated ulnocarpal impaction syndrome

- ± Triquetral offset distal relative to lunate convexity on coronal images
- ± Flap tears at triquetral attachment
- Hyperintense linear fluid communicating between radiocarpal & midcarpal compartments through LT space
- Less common - increased distance between lunate & triquetrum
- Extension of hyperintense fluid possible with membranous degeneration but intact dorsal & volar LT components
- ± Volar intercalated segment instability (VISI) pattern on sagittal MR (LT dissociation)
  - Scapholunate angle < 30 or 40 degrees
  - Capitolunate angle > 10 degrees
- T1 C+
  - MR arthrography
    - Identification of flap tears
    - Separation of LT components
    - Improved visualization of radiocarpal & midcarpal communication
    - Associated chondral lesions of proximal lunate, triquetrum & distal ulna in cases of positive ulnar variance
    - Increased sensitivity for associated TFCC lesions

Imaging Recommendations

- Best imaging tool
  - MR superior to conventional arthrography, motion studies & cineradiography
  - MR for LT morphology & fluid extension
  - MR arthrography increases sensitivity & specificity of conventional MR
- Protocol advice: T1 or PD & FS PD FSE coronal, sagittal & axial images

DIFFERENTIAL DIAGNOSIS

TFCC Tear

- Traumatic vs. degenerative
- Centrum of TFCC is thin & most common site of tear
- Ulnar-sided wrist pain

Subluxation or Dislocation DRUJ

- Tear of dorsal or volar margins TFCC + centrum (disc) = DRUJ instability
- Compare supination & pronation on axial images at level of sigmoid notch of distal radius

Subluxation Extensor Carpi Ulnaris (ECU)

- Ulnar to fovea on axial images
- Associated with hyperintense fluid on T2WI
- ± Inhomogeneous boggy synovial thickening

Midcarpal Instability

- "Catch-up clunk" with movement from radial to ulnar deviation
- Proximal row snaps (clunks) into extension in delayed movement with ulnar deviation
- Associated with VISI

Ulnar Impaction Syndrome

- Triad of LT, TFCC tear, chondromalacia of proximal ulnar lunate & proximal radial aspect triquetrum

Ulnar Head Chondromalacia

- Subchondral sclerosis (hypointense) distal ulna
- ± Cystic changes
- Attenuation of subchondral plate

Partial LT Coalition

- More symptomatic than complete coalition
- ± Associated subchondral sclerosis & degenerative marrow edema

PATHOLOGY

General Features

- General path comments
  - Relevant anatomy
    - LT ligament: Dorsal, volar + membranous (fibrocartilaginous membrane) components
    - Other palmar or volar constraints to ulnar carpal bones = palmar radiocarpal, ulnocarpal + midcarpal ligaments

LUNOTRIQUETRAL INSTABILITY

- Dorsal constraints = dorsal scaphotriquetral & radiotriquetral ligaments
- Lunate & triquetrum stabilized by intrinsic & extrinsic carpal ligaments
- Proximal carpal row = intercalated segment between radius & distal row
- Etiology
  - PLI (progressive perilunar injury/instability) - palmar radial force with dorsiflexion + ulnar deviation
  - LT injury = stage III PLI (triquetral dislocation + radiotriquetral ligament failure)
  - LT injury occurs after SL injury or fx (stage I PLI) & lunocapitate dissociation (stage II PLI)
  - Perilunar instability results in DISI unless SL ligament heals, then VISI pattern predominates (forme fruste of stage III PLI)
  - Perilunar pattern - intercarpal supination with injury from radial to ulnar direction
  - Isolated LT sprain 2° to ulnar sided injury = more common pattern of injury (than concomitant radial injury)
  - Reverse perilunar injury originating on ulnar side of wrist instead of radial side
  - Reverse perilunar pattern - intracarpal pronation + radial deviation forces capitate into LT joint
  - Isolated LT injury also seen with wrist palmar flexed mechanism
  - Combined SL dissociation + LT injury = less common
  - Inflammatory arthritis - LT lesions
  - Ulnar positive variance associated with degenerative LT membranous tears
  - LT injury associated with increased load transmission across ulnar side wrist + ulnar positive variance
  - Ulnar positive variance
    - Ulnar & triquetral chondromalacia
    - TFCC tear
    - LT instability
- Epidemiology
  - Less common relative to SL injuries
  - Part of perilunar injury pattern
  - Membranous perforations in 13% of individuals > 40 yrs.

Gross Pathologic & Surgical Features
- LT ligament partial to complete tear
- Palmar flexion lunate
- ± Fx of radial styloid or scaphoid, disruption of SL joint as part of stage III PLI

Microscopic Features
- Synovitis
- Joint wear/degeneration
- Abnormal ligament tension
- Variable amounts of collagen fibers, connective tissue + elastic fibers

Staging, Grading or Classification Criteria
- Static VISI = palmar flexion of lunate
- Static VISI = ligament injuries
  - Dorsal radiotriquetral
  - Scaphotriquetral
  - Lunotriquetral

CLINICAL ISSUES

Presentation
- Most common signs/symptoms: Pain on ulnar aspect of wrist
- Clinical profile
  - Symptoms related to partial vs. complete tears
  - ± Painful wrist click in radial or ulnar deviation
  - Stiffness, weakness, instability
  - Traumatic event = fall on outstretched hand or twisting/rotatory injury
  - Complete LT dissociation = static carpal collapse
  - Stress tests - for LT mobility, pain & crepitus
    - Ulnar-side compression test
    - LT ballottement test
    - Dorsal-palmar shear test

Demographics
- Age: Adult population
- Gender: No bias

Natural History & Prognosis
- Progression from minimal symptoms to ulnar wrist pain
- Sensation of instability
- Ulnar nerve paresthesias
- Eventual VISI deformity

Treatment
- Conservative
  - Immobilization
  - Anti-inflammatory agents
  - Wrist splint for acute injuries
- Surgical
  - Chronic symptoms not responsive to immobilization
  - Acute LT dissociation with static deformity
  - Arthroscopic debridement + pinning
  - Ligament repair vs. reconstruction with free tendon graft vs. arthrodesis

DIAGNOSTIC CHECKLIST

Consider
- Identify associated ulnocarpal impaction syndrome
- Assess carpal arc offset between triquetrum & lunate

SELECTED REFERENCES

1. Weiss LE et al: Lunotriquetral injuries in the athlete. Hand Clin 16(3):170-9, 2000
2. Shin AY et al: Lunotriquetral instability: Diagnosis and treatment. J Am Acad Orthop Surg 8(3):170-9, 2000
3. Bishop AT et al: The wrist. Diagnosis and operative treatment. Lunotriquetral sprains. St. Louis Missouri, Mosby, 527-49, 1998
4. Alexander CE et al: The wrist and it's disorders. Triquetrolunate instability. 2nd ed. Philadelphia Pennsylvania, W.B. Saunders, 307-15, 1997

LUNOTRIQUETRAL INSTABILITY

IMAGE GALLERY

Typical

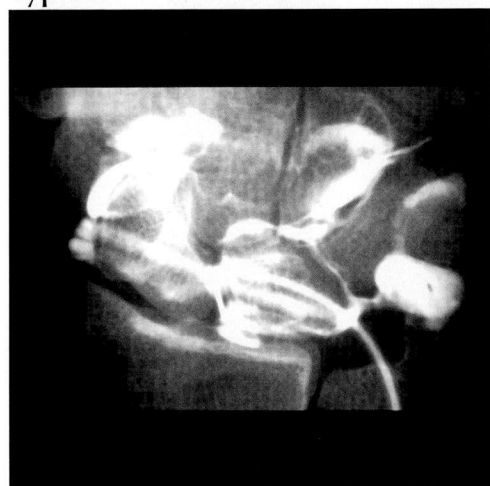

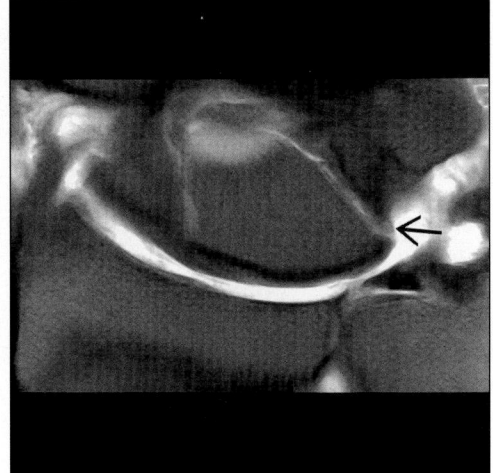

(Left) Anteroposterior radiography (arthrogram) shows contrast communicating across LT interval into midcarpal space in the presence of a LT ligament tear. *(Right)* Coronal T1 C+ MR (MR arthrogram) shows subtle offset (arrow) of LT convexity in association with LT ligament tear (lunate on left, triquetrum on right).

Typical

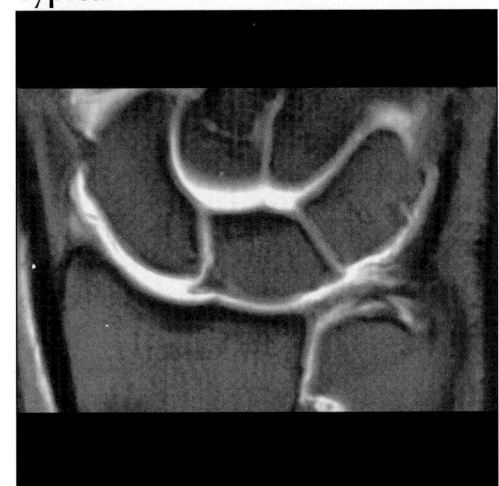

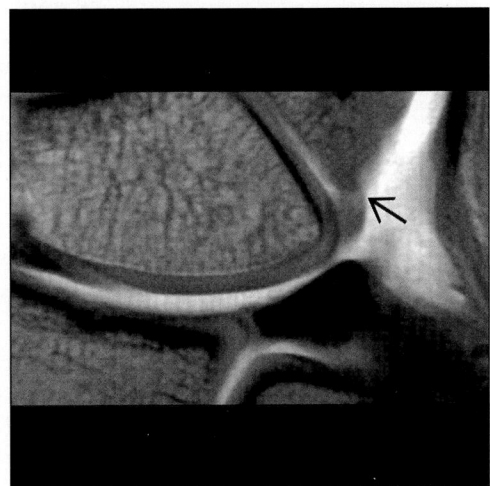

(Left) Coronal T1 C+ MR (MR arthrogram) shows the combination of both SL and LT ligament tears. There is loss of normal smooth convexity of the proximal carpal row. *(Right)* Coronal T1 C+ MR (MR arthrogram) shows mild distal offset of (arrow) the triquetrum (right) relative to lunate (left) in torn volar and membranous components of LT ligament.

Typical

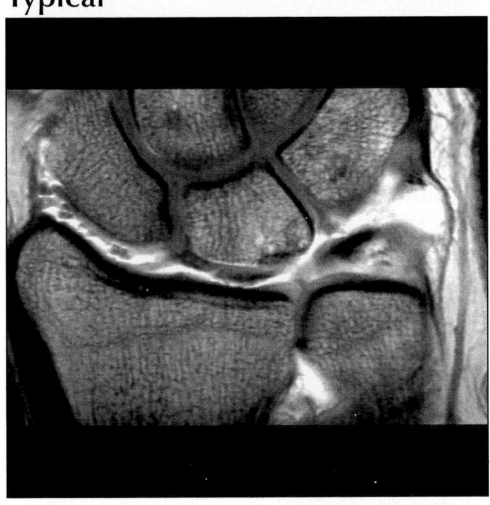

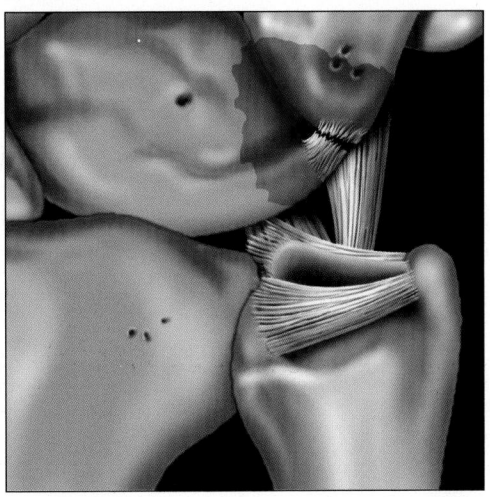

(Left) Coronal T1 C+ MR (MR arthrogram) shows ulnar impaction syndrome with the triad of findings including LT ligament tear, TFC tear, and chondromalacia of the proximal ulnar aspect of lunate. *(Right)* Coronal graphic shows ulnar impaction syndrome with disruption of the LT ligament. Chondromalacia of the lunate and triquetral surfaces are shown in red. The central disk of TFC is torn.

MID CARPAL INSTABILITY

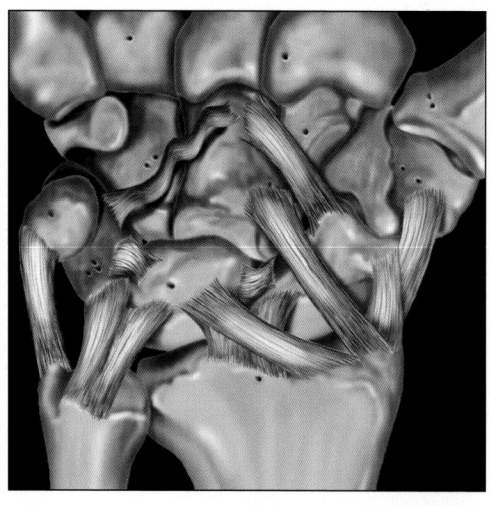

Coronal graphic shows palmar MCI with laxity of ulnar arm of arcuate ligament. Palmar MCI is also associated with laxity of dorsal radiolunotriquetral ligament.

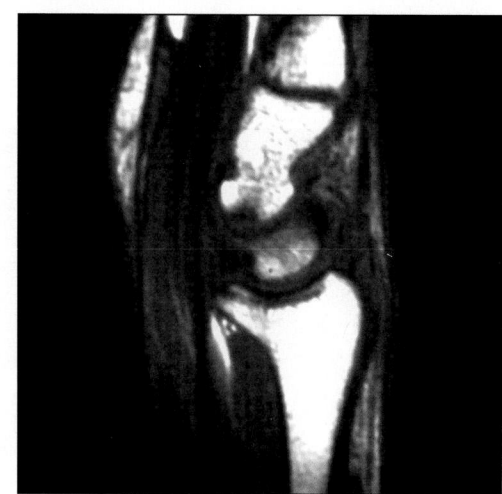

Sagittal T1WI MR shows static VISI with subchondral sclerosis of the distal lunate and proximal capitate.

TERMINOLOGY

Abbreviations and Synonyms
- MCI, PMCI = palmar MCI, DMCI=dorsal MCI, carpal instability nondissociative

Definitions
- Lack of support of the proximal carpal row & midcarpal joint

IMAGING FINDINGS

General Features
- Best diagnostic clue: Volar intercalated segmental instability (VISI) on sagittal MR images
- Location: Loss of normal joint forces between proximal & distal carpal rows
- Size: Varies based on etiology and classification
- Morphology
  - Palmar
  - Dorsal
  - Extrinsic: 2° to distal radius malunion

Radiographic Findings
- Radiography
  - Normal
  - PMCI = dynamic condition
  - Lateral radiography in neutral radioulnar deviation

    - ± VISI
    - ± Mild palmar translation of distal carpal row
  - Videofluoroscopy in posteroanterior (PA) + lateral planes with wrist from radial to ulnar deviation

CT Findings
- NECT
  - VISI pattern posterior with volar tilt of lunate + palmar translocation of distal row
  - Sclerosis between distal lunate and proximal capitate

MR Findings
- T1WI
  - VISI pattern with volar tilt of lunate + palmar translocation of distal row
  - VISI = palmar flexion instability
    - Scapholunate < 30°
    - Capitolunate angle ≥ 30°
    - Scaphoid & lunate both tilt volarly
    - Lunate translates dorsally
    - Distal pole capitate tilts dorsally
    - Proximal pole (head) capitate tilts volarly
  - Hypointense sclerosis between distal lunate and proximal capitate
- T2WI
  - Attenuated or disrupted lunotriquetral ligament
  - Hyperintense fluid extension across LT or SL (scapholunate) interval

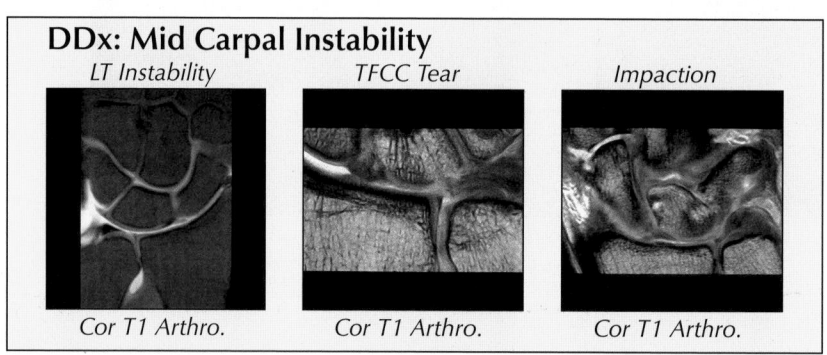

DDx: Mid Carpal Instability

LT Instability	TFCC Tear	Impaction
Cor T1 Arthro.	Cor T1 Arthro.	Cor T1 Arthro.

MID CARPAL INSTABILITY

Key Facts

Imaging Findings
- Best diagnostic clue: Volar intercalated segmental instability (VISI) on sagittal MR images
- VISI pattern with volar tilt of lunate + palmar translocation of distal row
- Hypointense sclerosis between distal lunate and proximal capitate

Top Differential Diagnoses
- Lunotriquetral (LT) Instability
- Distal Radioulnar Joint (DRUJ) Instability
- Triangular Fibrocartilage Complex (TFCC) Tears
- Ulnocarpal Impaction Syndrome
- Extensor Carpi Ulnaris (ECU) Subluxation

Pathology
- Injury to ulnar arm arcuate ligament

- Dorsiflexion - injury
- PMCI = most common pattern of MCI
- Palmar MCI = ulnar midcarpal instability or carpal instability nondissociative (CIND)

Clinical Issues
- Most common signs/symptoms: Painful clunk ulnar side of carpus
- Clunk with ulnar deviation with forearm in pronation ("catch-up clunk")
- Tenderness over ulnar carpus & triquetrohamate joint
- Positive midcarpal shift test - painful clunk with passive ulnar deviation

Diagnostic Checklist
- Associated capitolunate sclerosis or VISI

- ○ ± Hyperintense synovitis vs. ligament attenuation associated with ulnar arm of arcuate ligament + dorsal radiotriquetral ligament (palmar MCI)
- ○ ± Ulnar minus variance
- T1 C+
  - ○ MR arthrography
    - ▪ Associated extension of contrast directly communicating across SL or LT interval

Imaging Recommendations
- Best imaging tool
  - ○ Videofluoroscopy in PA + lateral planes if available
  - ○ Static VISI + ligamentous abnormalities best identified on MR
  - ○ Chronic ligamentous laxity difficult to visualize
- Protocol advice: T1 or PD + FS PD FSE coronal, sagittal and axial images

DIFFERENTIAL DIAGNOSIS

Lunotriquetral (LT) Instability
- Dissociation between triquetrum + lunate
- Volar flexion of lunate
- Absence or flap tear of normal delta-shaped or linear ligament on coronal images

Distal Radioulnar Joint (DRUJ) Instability
- Dorsal or volar radioulnar ligament involvement + TFCC centrum tear
- Fracture of sigmoid notch of distal radius
- Axial MR in full supination + pronation to document ulnar subluxation relative to sigmoid notch of distal radius
- Volar margin tears = dorsal subluxation
- Dorsal tears = volar subluxation

Triangular Fibrocartilage Complex (TFCC) Tears
- Traumatic
- Degenerative
- Tear of dorsal or volar margins of TFCC + centrum (disc) = DRUJ instability

- Ulnar-sided wrist pain
- Associated with positive ulnar variance

Ulnocarpal Impaction Syndrome
- Positive ulnar variance
- TFCC tear
- LT tear
- Chondromalacia proximal lunate + triquetrum
- Eccentric sclerosis proximal ulnar lunate
- Painful compression between distal ulna & lunate

Extensor Carpi Ulnaris (ECU) Subluxation
- Normal ECU is ulnar to ulnar styloid
- Recurrent subluxation = sudden palpable snap in forearm with active supination & wrist flexion + ulnar deviation
- ± Thickened synovial tendon sheath

PATHOLOGY

General Features
- General path comments
  - ○ Arcuate ligament complex = major stabilizer of midcarpal joint
  - ○ Triquetrohamatocapite ligament = ulnar arm of arcuate ligament
  - ○ Radial arm arcuate extends from distal aspect of radioscaphocapitate (RSC) ligament
  - ○ Space of Poirier = weak area between capitate & lunate
- Etiology
  - ○ Injury to ulnar arm arcuate ligament
  - ○ Dorsal radiotriquetral (RLT) = check-rein to prevent flexion of proximal row (laxity may be present in PMCI)
  - ○ Dorsiflexion - injury
  - ○ Also flexion, compression, rotation & distraction injuries
  - ○ 50% - minimal trauma history
- Epidemiology
  - ○ MCI incidence < scapholunate dissociation
  - ○ MCI incidence ≥ lunotriquetral instability

MID CARPAL INSTABILITY

○ PMCI = most common pattern of MCI

Gross Pathologic & Surgical Features
- Palmar MCI
  ○ Laxity ulnar arm arcuate ligament
  ○ Laxity dorsal radiolunotriquetral ligament
- Dorsal MCI
  ○ Laxity palmar radioscaphocapitate ligament
- Extrinsic MCI
  ○ Dorsal displacement & angulation of distal radius
  ○ Adaptive Z-deformity of carpus

Microscopic Features
- Stretching of collagen & elastic fibers of affected ligaments

Staging, Grading or Classification Criteria
- Palmar MCI = ulnar midcarpal instability or carpal instability nondissociative (CIND)
- Dorsal MCI = capitolunate instability pattern (CLIP) or chronic capitolunate instability
- Extrinsic MCI = associated with distal radius malunion

CLINICAL ISSUES

Presentation
- Most common signs/symptoms: Painful clunk ulnar side of carpus
- Clinical profile
  ○ Clunk with ulnar deviation with forearm in pronation ("catch-up clunk")
  ○ ± History of trauma
  ○ Asymptomatic phase prior to presentation
  ○ ± Bilateral presentation
  ○ Palmar sag of ulnar side of carpus
  ○ Prominent ulnar head with wrist in neutral deviation
  ○ Localized synovitis
  ○ Tenderness over ulnar carpus & triquetrohamate joint
  ○ Reproduce clunk - active ulnar deviation of pronated wrist
  ○ With extreme ulnar deviation (after clunk) the volar sag of ulnar carpus is absent
  ○ Positive midcarpal shift test - painful clunk with passive ulnar deviation

Demographics
- Age: Adult population
- Gender: F = M

Natural History & Prognosis
- Dynamic becomes fixed VISI
- Loss of normal physiologic VISI to DISI with radial to ulnar deviation
- Proximal carpal row remains flexed & distal row palmarly subluxed until extreme ulnar deviation
- With ulnar deviation of wrist distal row abruptly reduces & proximal row snaps into extension = "catch-up clunk"

Treatment
- Conservative
  ○ Activity modification for milder cases of PMCI
  ○ Nonsteroidal anti-inflammatory medications
  ○ Steroid injections
  ○ Wrist immobilization
  ○ Dorsally directed pressure on pisiform with splint = reduces ulnar carpal sag & VISI
  ○ Activating hypothenar muscles + extensor carpi ulnaris + flexor carpi ulnaris = reset midcarpal position
- Surgical
  ○ Ligament reconstruction
  ○ Capsular tightening
  ○ Limited midcarpal arthrodesis

DIAGNOSTIC CHECKLIST

Consider
- Clinical exam of characteristic clunk as well as symptoms must be assessed in combination with MRI findings
- Associated capitolunate sclerosis or VISI
- Clunking of the carpus may be present in asymptomatic wrists

SELECTED REFERENCES

1. Lichtman DM et al: The wrist and its disorders. Midcarpal and proximal carpal instabilities. 2nd ed. Philadelphia Pennsylvania, W.B.Saunders, (17):316-328, 1997
2. Wright TW et al: The wrist and its disorders. Carpal instability nondissociative. 2nd ed. Philadelphia Pennsylvania, W.B. Saunders, (23):550-68, 1997
3. Viegas SF et al: Extrinsic wrist ligaments in the pathomechanics of ulnar translocation instability. J Hand Surg 20A:312-8, 1995
4. Sennwald GR et al: Kinematics of the wrist and its ligaments. J Hand Surg 18:805-14, 1993
5. Ambrose L et al: Lunate-triquetral and midcarpal joint instability. Han Clin 8:653-68, 1992
6. Trumble T et al: Kinematics of the ulnar carpus related to the volar intercalated segment instability pattern. J Hand Surg 15A:364-92, 1990
7. Viegas SF et al: Ulnar sided perilunate instability: An anatomic and biomechanic study. J Hand Surg 15A:268-77, 1990
8. Lichtman DM et al: The ulnar arcuate ligament complex: Its anatomy and functional significance. Presented at the 43rd Annual Meeting of the Am Society for Surg of the Hand, 1988
9. Brown DE et al: Midcarpal instability. Hand Clin 3:135-40, 1987
10. Louis DS et al: Central carpal instability-capitate lunate instability pattern: Diagnosis by dynamic displacement. Orthopedics 7:1693-6, 1984
11. Mayfield JK: Patterns of injury to carpal ligaments. Clin Orthop 187:36-42, 1984
12. Johnston RP et al: Chronic capitolunate instability. J Bone Joint Surg 68A:1164-76, 1980
13. Mayfield JK et al: Carpal dislocations: Pathomechanics and progressive perilunar instability. J Hand Surg 5:226-41, 1980

IMAGE GALLERY

Typical

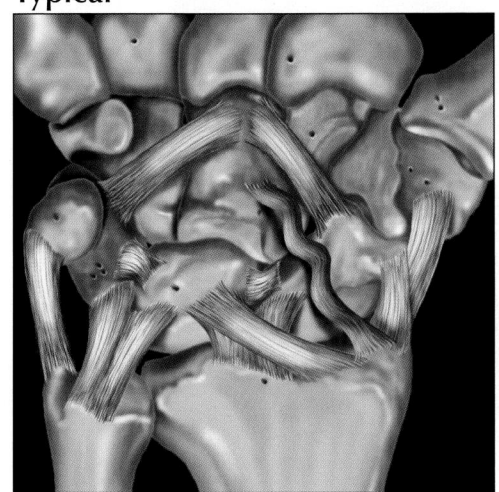 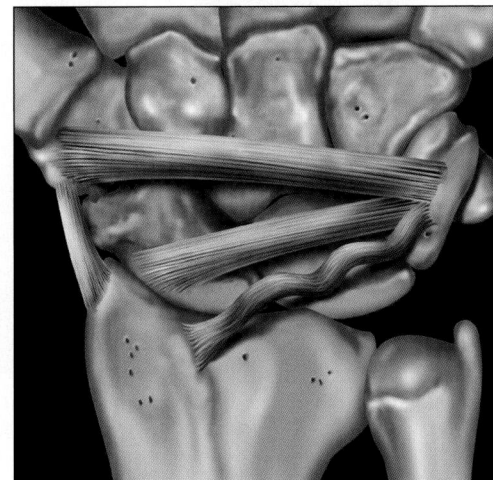

(Left) Coronal graphic shows dorsal MCI with laxity of palmar radioscaphocapitate ligament. *(Right)* Coronal graphic shows palmar MCI with laxity of radiotriquetral ligament.

Typical

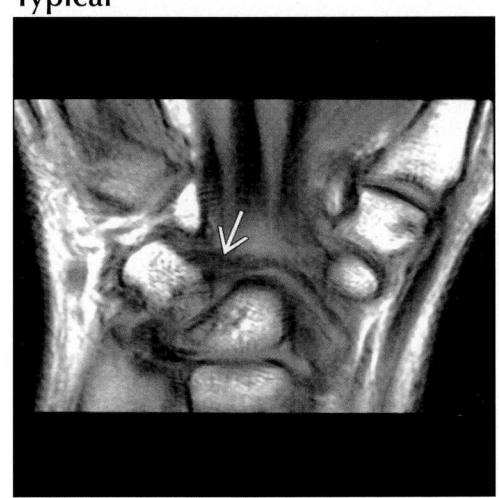 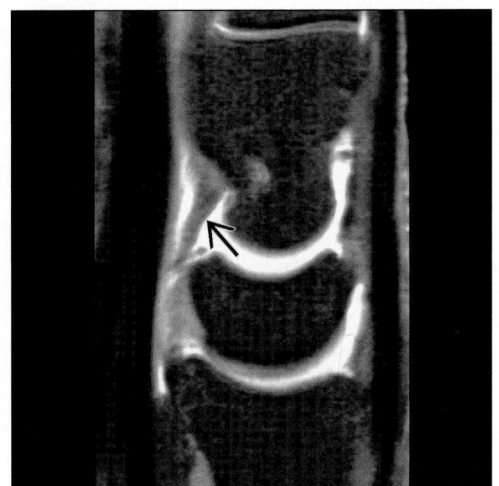

(Left) Coronal T1WI MR of the volar wrist shows normal orientation of the V or deltoid shaped arcuate ligament. The ulnar arm *(arrow)* is shown on the left. The arcuate ligament complex represents the major stabilizer of the midcarpal joint. *(Right)* Sagittal T1 C+ MR (MR arthrogram) shows ulnar arm of *(arrow)* arcuate ligament volar to capitate and lunate. This ligament is also know as the triquetrohamatocapitate ligament.

Typical

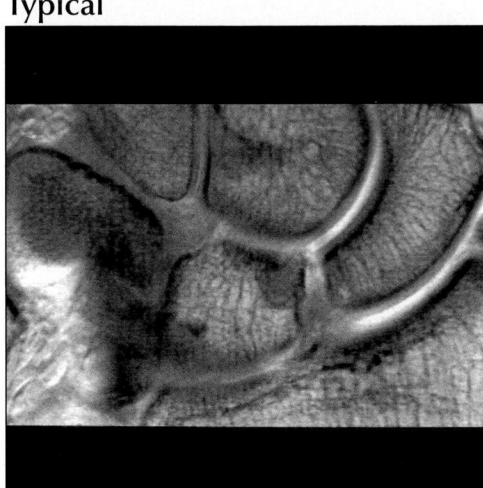 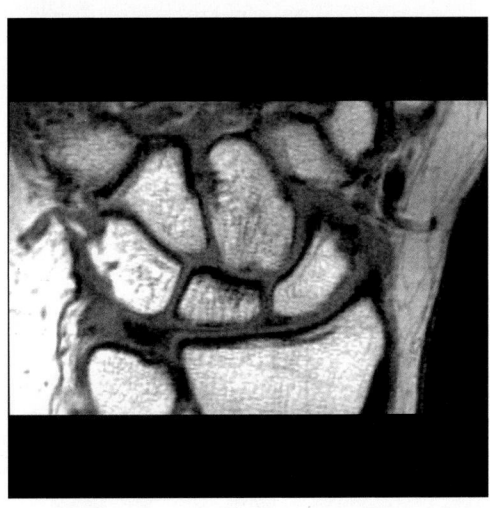

(Left) Coronal T1 C+ MR (MR arthrogram) shows subchondral sclerosis at the capitolunate articulation as a representation of the clinical diagnosis of MCI. *(Right)* Coronal T1WI MR shows capitolunate arthritis as an advanced manifestation of MCI.

ULNOCARPAL ABUTMENT

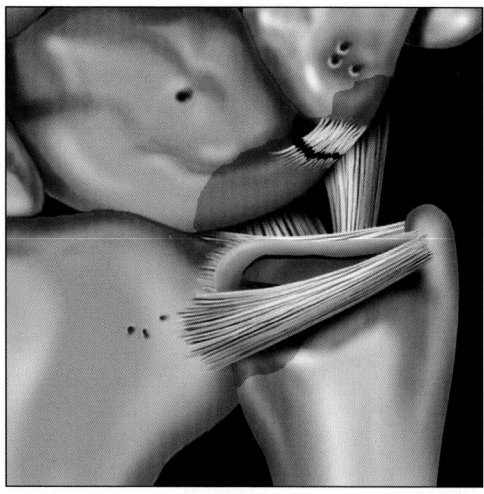

Coronal graphic shows chondromalacia of the distal ulna, proximal lunate and triquetrum. With tear of the LT ligament and central TFC, ulnar positive variance is not required.

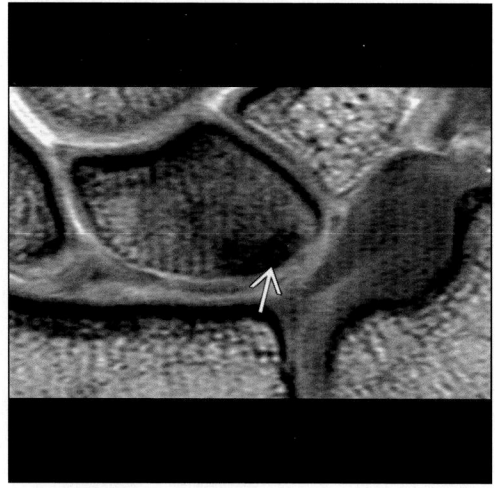

Coronal T1 C+ MR (MR arthrogram) shows hypointense eccentric sclerosis (arrow) of the proximal ulnar aspect of the lunate opposite the TFC tear. The LT ligament is disrupted.

TERMINOLOGY

Abbreviations and Synonyms
- Ulnar impaction syndrome, ulnolunate abutment, ulnolunate impaction syndrome, ulnar impaction, ulnocarpal loading

Definitions
- Degenerative condition caused by excessive load-bearing across the ulnar aspect of the wrist

IMAGING FINDINGS

General Features
- Best diagnostic clue: Eccentric sclerosis proximal ulnar lunate
- Location
  - Lunate
  - Triquetrum
  - Triangular fibrocartilage (TFC)
  - Distal ulna
  - Lunotriquetral (LT) ligament
- Size: Lunate sclerosis restricted to proximal ulnar lunate usually < 40% subchondral area
- Morphology: Positive ulnar variance is associated

Radiographic Findings
- Radiography

  - Posteroanterior (PA) + lateral view
  - Ulnar plus or ulnar neutral position
  - Lunate subchondral sclerosis
  - Triquetral sclerosis more difficult to identify
  - ± Cyst formation in ulnar head, lunate or triquetrum

MR Findings
- T1WI
  - Hypointense eccentric sclerosis proximal ulnar aspect lunate & proximal radial aspect triquetrum
  - Area of subchondral sclerosis in lunate > triquetrum
  - Normal marrow fat signal identified distal & radial to sclerosis in lunate
  - Triquetral sclerosis may not be present
  - Neutral or positive ulnar variance
  - Less commonly negative ulnar variance
  - ± Hypointense cystic change lunate > triquetrum > distal ulna
  - ± Associated trauma
    - Distal radius
    - Ulnar styloid
- T2WI
  - Hyperintense central perforation TFC (FS PD FSE)
  - Eccentric sclerosis either hypointense or hyperintense - based on degenerative marrow edema
  - Hyperintense cystic change > in proximal ulnar aspect lunate
  - Chondromalacia in normally intermediate signal intensity articular cartilage of distal ulna

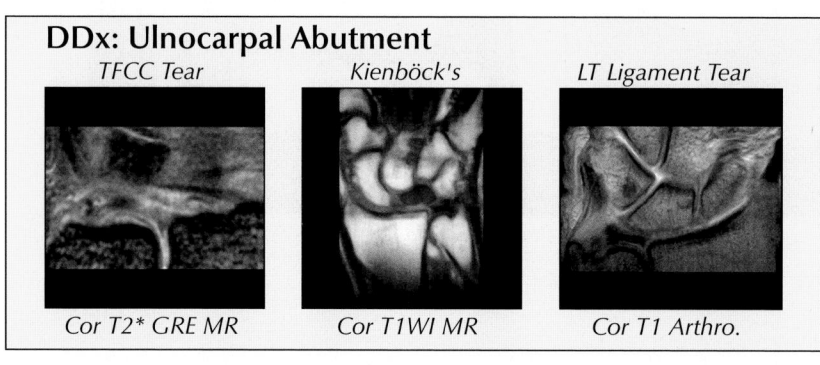

DDx: Ulnocarpal Abutment

TFCC Tear	Kienböck's	LT Ligament Tear
Cor T2* GRE MR	Cor T1WI MR	Cor T1 Arthro.

ULNOCARPAL ABUTMENT

Key Facts

Imaging Findings
- Best diagnostic clue: Eccentric sclerosis proximal ulnar lunate
- Morphology: Positive ulnar variance is associated
- Area of subchondral sclerosis in lunate > triquetrum
- Hyperintense central perforation TFC (FS PD FSE)

Top Differential Diagnoses
- Traumatic Triangular Fibrocartilage Complex (TFCC) Abnormalities
- Kienböck's Disease
- Ulnar Impingement
- Distal Radioulnar Joint (DRUJ) Instability

Pathology
- Increase ulnar length = increased forces across ulnocarpal articulation

- Chondromalacia distal ulna, proximal lunate & triquetrum
- Palmer class 2 degenerative lesions of TFCC = ulnocarpal abutment

Clinical Issues
- Most common signs/symptoms: Pain over DRUJ
- Chronic or subacute dorsal pain/discomfort
- Pain increased with extremes of rotation + ulnar deviation
- Tenderness between ulnar head & triquetrum/lunate
- In contrast to DRUJ pathology, pain not present throughout entire range of pronation to supination

Diagnostic Checklist
- Positive ulnar variance not required

- ○ Hyperintense fluid across torn LT ligament on FS PD FSE
- ○ Lunate-triquetrum proximal arc offset associated with LT ligament tear
- ○ Attenuated centrum of TFC

Imaging Recommendations
- Best imaging tool: MR to identify sclerosis, ligament disruption, cystic change and chondromalacia
- Protocol advice
  - ○ T1 & FS PD FSE coronal, axial & sagittal
  - ○ T1 = improved visualization of sclerosis compared with proton density (PD)
  - ○ FS PD FSE = hyperintensity associated with sclerosis or cystic change

DIFFERENTIAL DIAGNOSIS

Traumatic Triangular Fibrocartilage Complex (TFCC) Abnormalities
- Central perforations
- Ulnar avulsion
- Distal avulsion
- Radial avulsion
- Without associated lunate, triquetral or ulnar chondromalacia

Kienböck's Disease
- Avascular necrosis lunate
- Related to trauma + ulnar negative variance
- Centralized lunate sclerosis
- ± Visualized lunate fracture

Ulnar Impingement
- Ulnar negative (minus) variance
- Scalloped concavity of ulnar aspect distal radius
- Convergence of ulna toward distal radius
- Pain with pronation & supination

Distal Radioulnar Joint (DRUJ) Instability
- Subluxation
- Dislocation
- Fractured ulnar head or sigmoid notch

- Ligament insufficiency (radioulnar)
- Pain throughout range of pronation - supination
- Intercarpal pathology
- Lunotriquetral instability
- Midcarpal instability
- ± LT ligament tear & volar intercalated segment instability (VISI)

PATHOLOGY

General Features
- General path comments
  - ○ TFC = articular disk (centrum) + dorsal & volar radioulnar ligaments
  - ○ TFCC = TFC, meniscus homologue (ulnocarpal meniscus), ulnar collateral ligament, sheath of extensor carpi ulnaris + ulnolunate & ulnotriquetral ligaments
  - ○ Ulnar variance = level of distal ulna relative to radius
  - ○ Positive variance = ulna is too long
  - ○ Pronation causes relative ulnar lengthening
  - ○ Lunate articulates with lunate facet of distal radius & TFC
- Etiology
  - ○ Acquired - trauma
    - Distal radius fractures with shortening + angulation
    - Fractures with ligamentous injuries of DRUJ (e.g., Galeazzi & Essex-Lopresti)
  - ○ Congenital
    - Madelung's deformity (dyschondroplasia)
    - Ulnar plus variance
    - Increase ulnar length = increased forces across ulnocarpal articulation
- Epidemiology
  - ○ TFC perforations - 40% prevalence by end of 5th decade
  - ○ 73% of wrists with TFC perforation, ulna + lunate erosions have positive or neutral ulnar variance

Gross Pathologic & Surgical Features
- TFCC degeneration/tear

ULNOCARPAL ABUTMENT

- Chondromalacia distal ulna, proximal lunate & triquetrum
- LT ligament disruption
- Central TFC attenuated in positive ulnar variance
- Degeneration of avascular central articular disc of TFC

Microscopic Features
- Degeneration TFC
- Chondral fibrillation, fraying, erosions
- Subchondral sclerosis
- Central zone of avascularity in TFC

Staging, Grading or Classification Criteria
- Palmer class 2 degenerative lesions of TFCC = ulnocarpal abutment
  - A = TFCC wear
  - B = TFCC wear + lunate, triquetrum ± ulnar chondromalacia
  - C = TFCC perforation + lunate, triquetrum ± ulnar chondromalacia
  - D = TFCC perforation + lunate, triquetrum ± ulnar chondromalacia & LT ligament perforation
  - E = TFCC perforation + lunate, triquetrum ± ulnar chondromalacia, LT perforation & ulnocarpal arthritis

CLINICAL ISSUES

Presentation
- Most common signs/symptoms: Pain over DRUJ
- Clinical profile
  - Chronic or subacute dorsal pain/discomfort
  - Pain increased with extremes of rotation + ulnar deviation
  - Intermittent clicking
  - Swelling
  - Decreased strength & motion
  - ± History of trauma
  - Positive ulnar variance
  - Tenderness between ulnar head & triquetrum/lunate
  - Pain exacerbated with ulnar deviation + forearm pronation (ulnar head displaced volar)
  - Ballottement distal ulna + ulnar deviation increases pain
  - LT ligament disruption - discomfort with loading of LT joint
  - In contrast to DRUJ pathology, pain not present throughout entire range of pronation to supination

Demographics
- Age: 50 years or above
- Gender: No bias

Natural History & Prognosis
- Increased load transmission through ulna = progression
- Address malunion of distal radial fractures, physeal arrest or Essex-Lopresti injury, positive ulnar variance
  - Essex-Lopresti: Fx/dislocation radial head + dislocation DRUJ

Treatment
- Conservative
  - Activity modification
  - Anti-inflammatory medication
- Surgical = unloading distal ulna
  - Debridement - TFCC
  - Wafer procedure (resect distal ulna beneath TFC)
  - Hemiresection distal ulna
  - Ulnar shortening osteotomy
  - Arthroscopic treatment (except for ulnar shortening osteotomy)
  - Fusion of DRUJ - Sauvé-Kapandji procedure
  - Ulnar recession (shortening) = procedure of choice
- Complications
  - Weakness + instability post Darrach procedure (resection of distal ulna)
  - Hemiresection → impingement
  - Sauvé-Kapandji → instability

DIAGNOSTIC CHECKLIST

Consider
- Eccentric lunate sclerosis (ulnar sided) associated with ulnocarpal abutment
- Positive ulnar variance not required

SELECTED REFERENCES

1. Sofka CM et al: Magnetic resonance imaging of the wrist. Semin Musculoskelet Radiol 5(3):217-26, 2001
2. Moy OJ et al: The wrist. Diagnosis and operative treatment. Ulnocarpal abutment. St. Louis MO, Mosby, 773-87, 1998
3. Loftus JB et al: The wrist and it's disorders: Disorders of the distal radioulnar joint and triangular fibrocartilage complex. 2nd ed. Philadelphia Pennsylvania, Saunders 385-414, 1997
4. Escobedo EM et al: MR imaging of ulnar impaction. Skeletal Radiol 24(2):85-90, 1995
5. Chun S et al: The ulnar impaction syndrome: Follow-up of ulnar shortening osteotomy. J Hand Surg 18:46-53, 1993
6. Uchiyama S et al: Radiographic changes in wrists with ulnar plus variance observed over a ten-year period. J Hand Surg 16:45-48, 1991
7. Boulas HJ et al: Ulnar shortening for tears of the triangular fibrocartilaginous complex. J Hand Surg 15:415-20, 1990
8. Palmer AK: Triangular fibrocartilage disorders: Injury patterns and treatment. Arthroscopy 6:125-32, 1990
9. Watson HK et al: Ulnar impingement syndrome after Darrach procedure: Treatment by advancement lengthening osteotomy of the ulna. J Hand Surg 14:302-6, 1989
10. Czitrom AA et al: Ulnar variance in carpal instability. J Hand Surg 12:205-8, 1987
11. Linscheid RL: Ulnar lengthening and shortening. Hand Clin 3:69-79, 1987
12. Viegas SF et al: Attritional lesions of the wrist joint. J Hand Surg 12:1025-29, 1987
13. Bell MJ et al: Ulnar impingement syndrome. J Bone Joint Surg Br 67:126-9, 1985
14. Palmer AK: Relationship between ulnar variance and triangular fibrocartilage complex of the wrist – anatomy and function. J Hand Surg 6:153-62, 1981

Typical

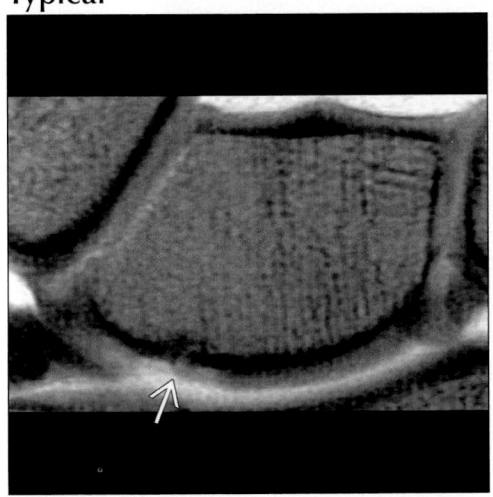
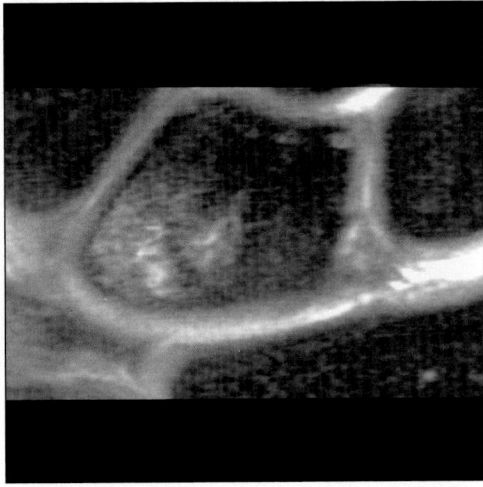

(Left) Coronal T1 C+ MR (MR arthrogram) shows chondral erosion (arrow) of the proximal ulnar aspect of the lunate with disruption of the TFC. (Right) Coronal FS PD FSE MR shows degenerative subchondral marrow edema of the proximal lunate in association with LT ligament degeneration. Ulnolunate impaction does not require positive ulnar variance.

Typical

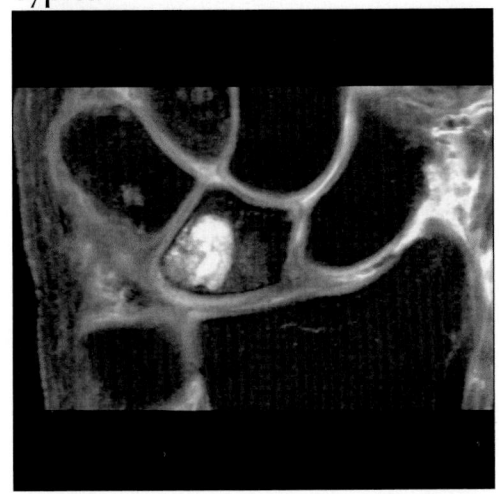
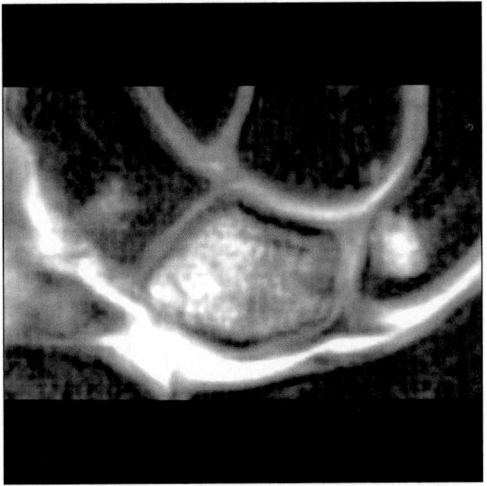

(Left) Coronal FS PD FSE MR shows large osseous cyst of the lunate in response to the stress of ulnolunate abutment syndrome. (Right) Coronal FS PD FSE MR shows a more diffuse pattern of lunate marrow edema which should not be confused with Kienböck's disease. The greatest stress is located on the ulnar aspect of the lunate. There is complete disruption of the TFC.

Other

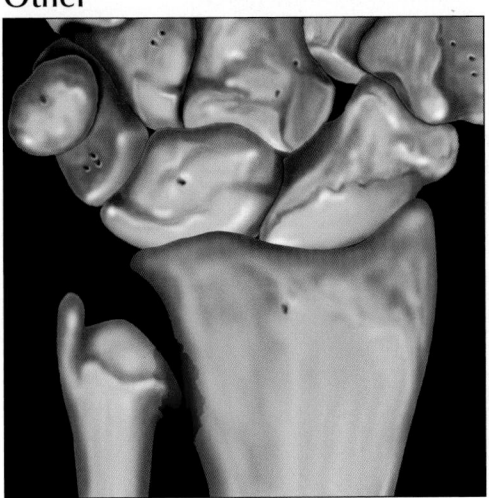
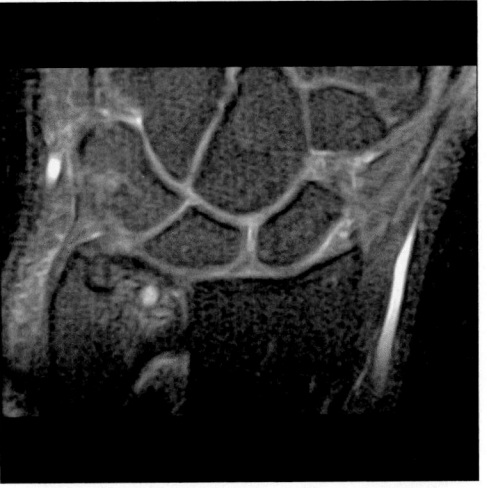

(Left) Coronal graphic shows ulnar impingement syndrome associated with degenerative changes of the distal ulna and negative ulnar variance. This is often confused with the diagnosis of ulnolunate abutment syndrome. (Right) Coronal FS PD FSE MR shows chondromalacia of the distal ulna without changes of the lunate in ulnar impingement syndrome.

DISTAL RADIOULNAR JOINT INSTABILITY

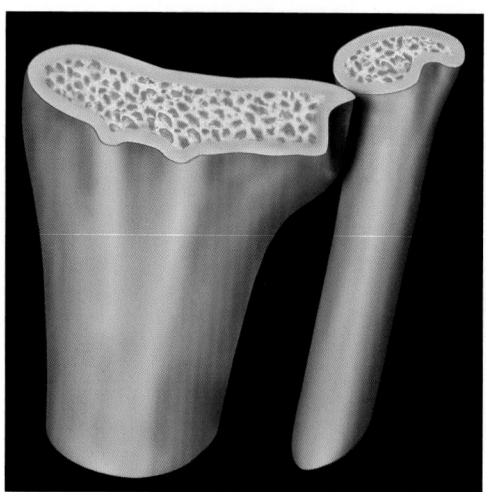

Axial graphic shows palmar dislocation of ulnar head relative to the sigmoid notch of distal radius.

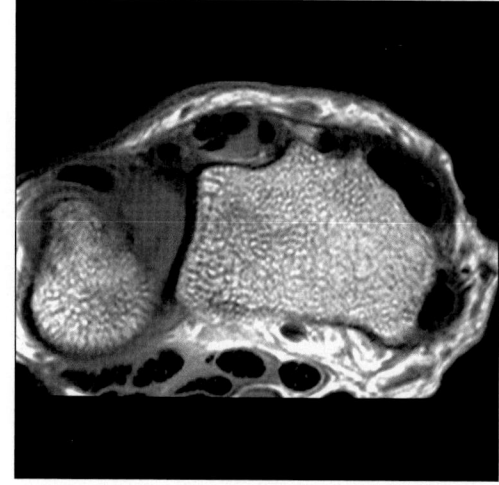

Axial T1WI MR shows DRUJ with volar subluxation of distal ulna secondary to disruption of dorsal DRUJ.

TERMINOLOGY

Abbreviations and Synonyms
- DRUJ instability, dislocation or subluxation of the DRUJ, sprained wrist

Definitions
- Loss of normal anatomic or kinematic relationship between distal radius + ulna with carpus

IMAGING FINDINGS

General Features
- Best diagnostic clue: Dorsal or volar displacement of distal ulna relative to sigmoid notch of distal radius
- Location: DRUJ, including articular surfaces & soft tissue constraints
- Size: Variable based on subluxation, dislocation & fractures of the distal radius
- Morphology: Ulnar dorsal or ulnar palmar dislocation

Radiographic Findings
- Radiography
  - Difficult to diagnose
  - True lateral - dorsal or volar displacement of ulna
  - Posteroanterior view
    - Increased gap between ulnar head & radius with dorsal subluxation of ulna
    - Ulna/radius superimposition in ulnar palmar dislocation
    - False negative rate - 60%

CT Findings
- NECT
  - Assess sigmoid notch morphology on axial images (e.g., abnormal convex or shallow arch post distal radius fracture)
  - Trace radioulnar lines (criterion of Mino) to establish ulnar head lies between dorsal & palmar borders of the radius

MR Findings
- T1WI
  - Dorsal or volar (palmar) subluxation of ulnar head relative to sigmoid notch on axial images
  - Dorsal prominence of ulna (ulna-dorsal) on sagittal images
  - Flattened or shallow sigmoid notch
  - Distal radioulnar joint diastasis on coronal images in ulnar dorsal subluxation
  - Massive disruption of stabilizing capsuloligamentous structures (e.g., Galeazzi fracture)
  - Subluxation or interposition of extensor carpi ulnaris (ECU tendon)
  - ± Intercalated segment instability pattern (VISI = volar, DISI = dorsal)
- T2WI

DDx: Distal Radioulnar Joint Instability

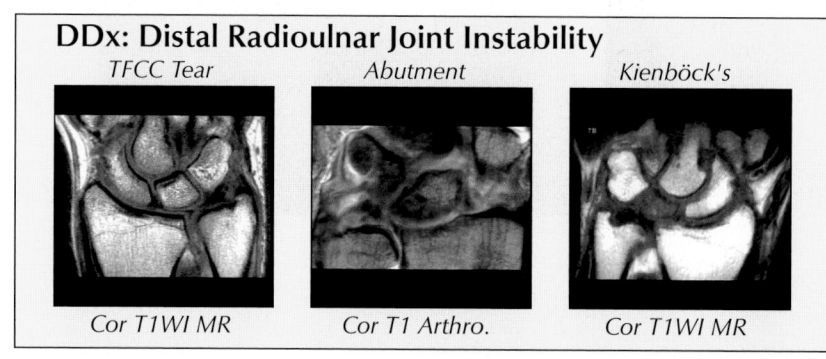

TFCC Tear	Abutment	Kienböck's
Cor T1WI MR	Cor T1 Arthro.	Cor T1WI MR

DISTAL RADIOULNAR JOINT INSTABILITY

Key Facts

Imaging Findings

- Best diagnostic clue: Dorsal or volar displacement of distal ulna relative to sigmoid notch of distal radius
- Flattened or shallow sigmoid notch
- Palmar (volar) distal radioulnar ligament (DRUL) disruption associated with ulnar dorsal dislocation
- Disruption of dorsal DRUL associated with ulnar palmar dislocation

Top Differential Diagnoses

- Traumatic Triangular Fibrocartilage Complex (TFCC) Abnormalities
- Ulnocarpal Abutment Syndrome
- Kienböck's Disease
- Subluxation of Extensor Carpi Ulnaris (ECU)
- Intercarpal Pathology

Pathology

- Fall on outstretched hand
- High energy hyperextension - rotation = radius or ulna fx + ligament disruption
- Majority of injuries = combination of osseous + ligamentous damage with DRUJ instability

Clinical Issues

- Most common signs/symptoms: Pain ulnar aspect wrist
- Increased symptoms in pronosupination

Diagnostic Checklist

- Use axial images in full pronation & supination to identify location of ulna relative to sigmoid notch

- o Palmar (volar) distal radioulnar ligament (DRUL) disruption associated with ulnar dorsal dislocation
- o Disruption of dorsal DRUL associated with ulnar palmar dislocation
- o Ulnocarpal ligamentous (ULC) complex hyperintensity: Tear associated with ulnar dorsal pattern
- o Tear dorsal infratendinous extensor retinaculum (subsheath of ECU seen in ulnar dorsal dislocation)
- o Pronator quadratus + distal interosseous membrane (IOM) hyperintensity as part of forced hypersupination & ulnar palmar dislocation

Imaging Recommendations

- Best imaging tool: MR identifies soft tissue (muscle, tendon & ligamentous) associated injuries
- Protocol advice
  - o T1 or PD & FS PD FSE MR coronal, axial & sagittal
  - o Axial images (PD or FS PD FSE) in full pronation & supination to establish location of ulna in sigmoid notch

DIFFERENTIAL DIAGNOSIS

Traumatic Triangular Fibrocartilage Complex (TFCC) Abnormalities

- Central perforation
- Ulnar, radial, or distal avulsion

Ulnocarpal Abutment Syndrome

- TFCC degeneration/perforation
- Lunate, triquetral & ulnar chondromalacia
- Lunotriquetral ligament perforation/tear
- Ulnocarpal arthritis

Kienböck's Disease

- Avascular necrosis of lunate
- Related to trauma + ulnar negative variance
- Centralized lunate sclerosis
- ± Visualized lunate fracture

Subluxation of Extensor Carpi Ulnaris (ECU)

- Palpable snap with forearm supination + wrist ulnar deviation
- ± Thickened tendon sheath
- ± Tenosynovitis

Intercarpal Pathology

- Lunotriquetral instability ± LT ligament tear & VISI
- Midcarpal instability

PATHOLOGY

General Features

- General path comments
  - o Relevant anatomy
    - DRUJ = diarthrodial trochoid articulation between head of ulna & sigmoid cavity of distal radius
    - TFC = articular disc + dorsal & palmar (volar) distal radioulnar ligaments
    - Palmar (volar) DRUL taut in supination
    - Dorsal DRUL taut in pronation
    - Ulnocarpal ligamentous (UCL) complex
    - Infratendinous extensor retinaculum (ECU subsheath)
    - Pronator quadratus muscle
    - Interosseous membrane (IOM)
- Etiology
  - o Palmar & dorsal DRUL tension exists at both extremes of rotation (pronation & supination)
  - o Rotational injury with forced pronation/supination + hyperextension
  - o Fall on outstretched hand
  - o High energy hyperextension - rotation = radius or ulna fx + ligament disruption
- Epidemiology
  - o Traumatic DRUJ dislocations or subluxations - common
  - o Majority of injuries = combination of osseous + ligamentous damage with DRUJ instability
  - o DRUJ instability without associated fracture usually misdiagnosed

DISTAL RADIOULNAR JOINT INSTABILITY

Gross Pathologic & Surgical Features
- Distal radius + carpal bones undergoes abnormal displacement relative to ulna
- Ulna is not the mobile bone dislocating from radius
- Physiologic radius translation dorsally in supination
- Physiologic radius translation in palmar direction in pronation
- Disruption of sigmoid notch congruity (e.g., displaced by fracture)
- Palmar & dorsal DRUL must be intact to maintain DRUJ stability in full range of forearm rotation
- Dorsal DRUL tear + tightening UCL complex = destabilizing effect = ulnar palmar DRUJ
- Disruption of infratendinous extensor retinaculum (ECU subsheath) with subluxation of ECU tendon in ulnar dorsal dislocation
- Essex Lopresti = IOM injury, dislocation or fracture of proximal radial head, distal ulna dorsally & longitudinally displaced
- Ulnar dorsal dislocation in hyperpronation
  - Disruption of palmar DRUL
  - UCL complex injury
  - Dorsal infratendinous extensor retinaculum tear
- Ulnopalmar dislocation in hypersupination
  - Disruption of dorsal DRUL
  - Stretching of pronator quadratus
  - Distal IOM tear

Microscopic Features
- Failure of tensile ligament restraint
- Tear of collagen fibers + interstitial connective tissue in ligament injury

Staging, Grading or Classification Criteria
- DRUJ dislocations in acute trauma divided into three groups
  - Type I: Dislocation DRUJ 2° to disruption of primary soft tissue structures or osseous injury (ulnar styloid fracture)
  - Type II: Intraarticular DRUJ fracture dislocations
  - Type III: Extraarticular DRUJ fracture dislocations

CLINICAL ISSUES

Presentation
- Most common signs/symptoms: Pain ulnar aspect wrist
- Clinical profile
  - Increased symptoms in pronosupination
  - Swelling & tenderness
  - Decrease/loss of wrist motion
  - Grip weakness
  - Piano key sign = prominent distal ulna in dorsal dislocations
  - Ulnar nerve dysesthesias
  - Audible snap

Demographics
- Age
  - Includes age ranges of Colles', Smith's, Galeazzi's & Essex Lopresti's injury
  - Young individuals - trauma
  - Elderly in association with osteoporosis fracture

- Gender: No bias

Natural History & Prognosis
- Delayed diagnosis common
- Recurrent DRUJ instability
- Limited range of rotation (forearm)
- Degenerative arthritis
- Complications
  - Malunion distal radius + distal/dorsal subluxation of distal ulna in type II injuries
  - Galeazzi fracture dislocation - malunion radius + residual DRUJ subluxation

Treatment
- Conservative
  - Type I: True DRUJ dislocations = reduction + immobilization
  - Type II: Intraarticular DRUJ fx dislocation = reduction + cast
- Surgical
  - Type I: Interposition of soft tissue (TFCC, ECU entrapment, osteochondral) = open reduction + K-wire fixation
  - Type II: Percutaneous K-wire fixation or external fixation vs. open repair to achieve anatomic reduction vs. osteotomy vs. hemiresection arthroplasty
  - Type III: Extraarticular DRUJ fx dislocation - reduction + internal fixation

DIAGNOSTIC CHECKLIST

Consider
- Use axial images in full pronation & supination to identify location of ulna relative to sigmoid notch
- Evaluate dorsal & volar (palmar) radioulnar ligaments of TFC on coronal, axial + sagittal images

SELECTED REFERENCES

1. May MM et al: Ulnar styloid fractures associated with distal radius fractures: Incidence and implications for distal radioulnar joint instability. J Hand Surg 27(6):965-71, 2002
2. Adams BD et al: An anatomic reconstruction of the distal radioulnar ligaments for posttraumatic distal radioulnar joint instability. J Hand Surg 27(2):243-51, 2002
3. Garcia-Elias M et al: The wrist. Diagnosis and operative treatment. Dorsal and palmar dislocations of the distal radioulnar joint. St. Louis Missouri, Mosby, 758-72, 1998
4. Bowers WH et al: The wrist and it's disorders. Treatment of chronic disorders of the distal radioulnar joint. 2nd ed. Philadelphia Pennsylvania, WB Saunders, 429-42, 1997
5. Aulicino PL et al: Acute injuries of the distal radioulnar joint. Hand Clin 7:283-93, 1991
6. Bowers WH: Instability of the distal radioulnar articulation. Hand Clin 7:311-27, 1991
7. Nathan R et al: Classification of distal radioulnar joint disorders. Hand Clin 7:239-47, 1991
8. Schuind F et al: The distal radioulnar ligaments: A biomechanical study. J Hand Surg 16:1106-14, 1991
9. Mino DE et al: Radiography and computerized tomography in the diagnosis of incongruity of the distal radio-ulnar joint. A prospective study. J Bone Joint Surg 67:247-52, 1985

IMAGE GALLERY

Typical

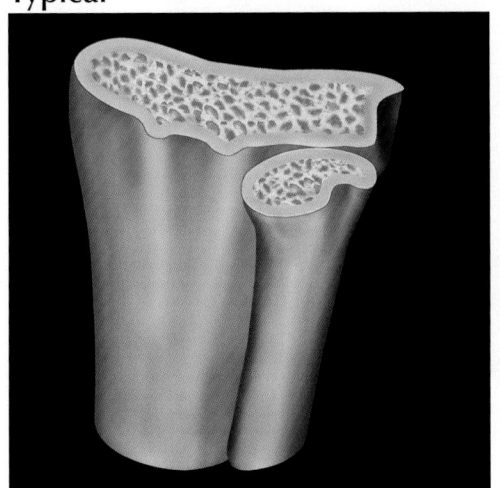

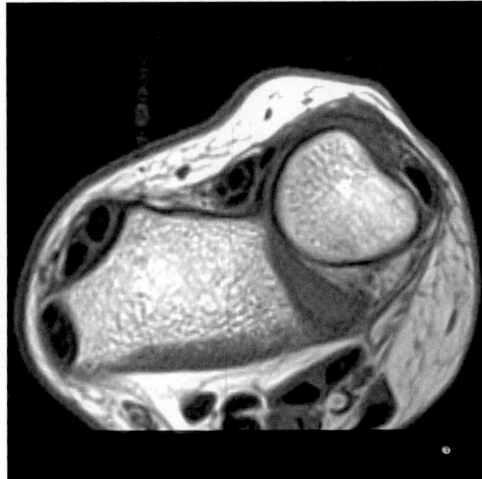

(Left) Axial graphic shows ulnar dorsal DRUJ instability with disruption of the palmar DRUL. Ulnar dorsal dislocation occurs in hyperpronation while ulnar palmar dislocation occurs in hypersupination. *(Right)* Axial T1WI MR shows a dorsally perched distal ulna. There is complete absence of palmar DRUL. Ulnar dorsal dislocation is also associated with injuries to the UCL complex and extensor retinaculum.

Typical

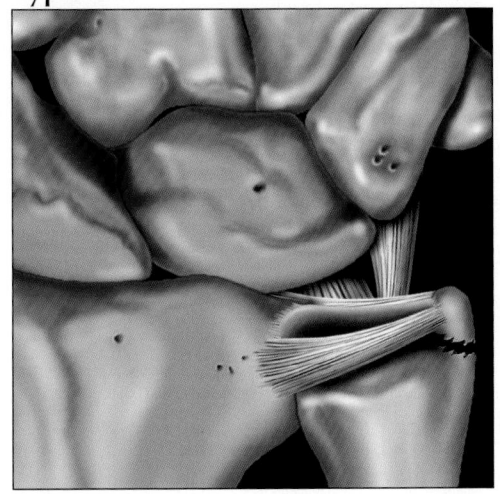

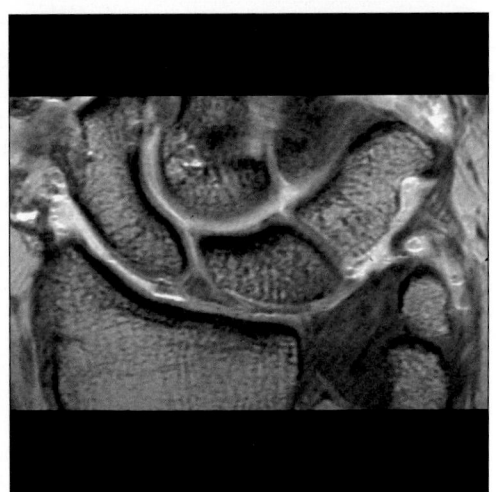

(Left) Coronal graphic shows DRUJ instability associated with a proximal fracture of the base of ulnar styloid. *(Right)* Coronal T1 C+ MR (MR arthrogram) shows the destabilizing effect of proximal ulnar styloid fracture with attached margins of TFCC.

Typical

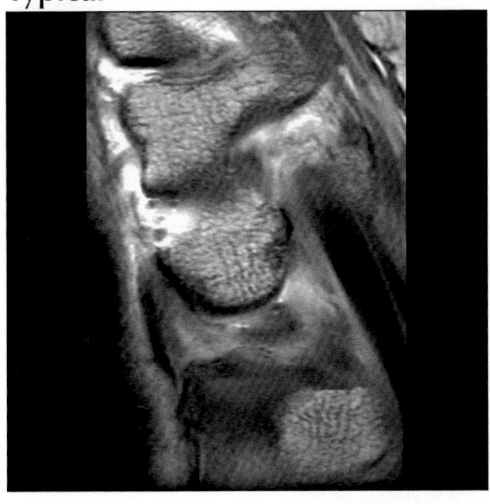

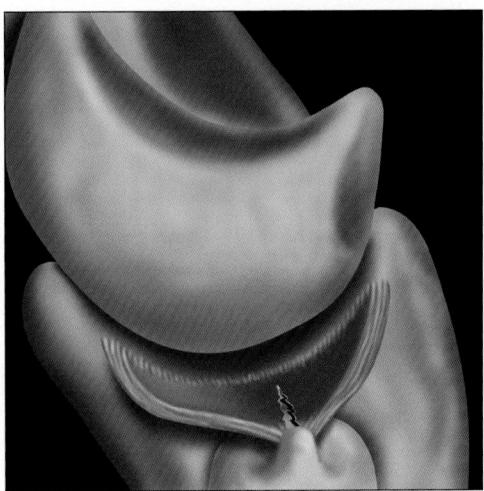

(Left) Sagittal T1 C+ MR (MR arthrogram) shows abnormal palmar translation of distal ulna relative to TFC and carpus in ulnar palmar dislocation (ulna is at lower right). *(Right)* Sagittal graphic shows tear of the centrum (or central disk) of TFC. The palmar and dorsal DRUL must be intact in order to maintain DRUJ stability. The DRULs represent volar and dorsal margins of TFC.

TRIANGULAR FIBROCARTILAGE TEAR

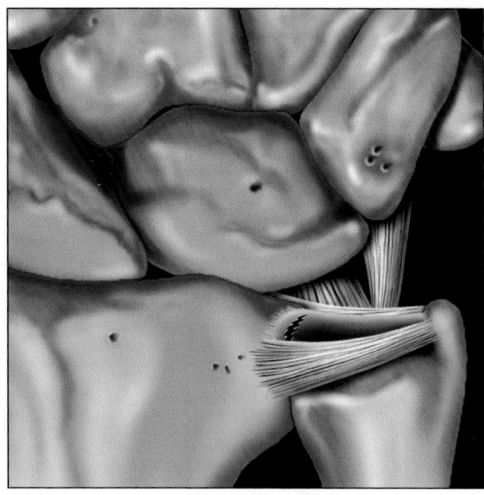

Coronal graphic shows traumatic (class 1) tear of the radial aspect of the TFC.

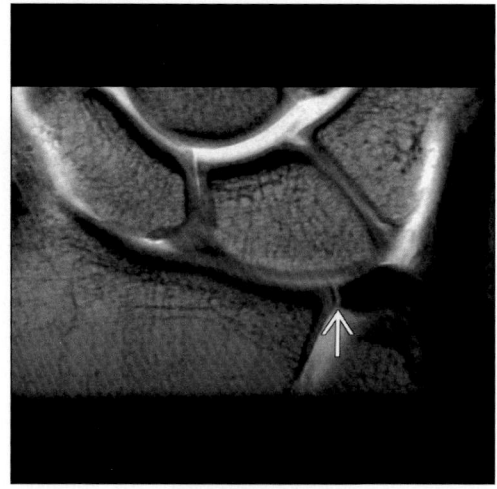

Coronal T1 C+ MR (MR arthrogram) shows focal tear (arrow) of the radial aspect of TFC disk.

TERMINOLOGY

Abbreviations and Synonyms
- TFC tears, TFC complex (TFCC) lesions, tears of the TFC

Definitions
- Tear of the TFC including central (disc) & peripheral margins

IMAGING FINDINGS

General Features
- Best diagnostic clue: Direct extension of fluid across TFC
- Location
  - TFC
    - Articular disk
    - Dorsal radioulnar ligament
    - Volar (palmar) radioulnar ligament
- Size: Variable from perforation, linear tear, to frank disruption
- Morphology
  - Circular perforation
  - Linear vertical or horizontal tear
  - Attenuation + tear
  - Gross disruption with gap
  - Absent fibrocartilaginous disk

Radiographic Findings
- Radiography
  - Not useful
  - Associated with ulnar styloid fractures
  - Positive ulnar variance
  - Conventional arthrography cannot characterize TFC morphology or differentiate normal communications from tears

MR Findings
- T1WI
  - Normal TFC = biconcave disk
  - Intermediate signal intensity intrasubstance degeneration
  - Volar margin tears associated with dorsal subluxation of ulna relative to radius
  - Dorsal tears associated with volar subluxation of ulna
  - Volar instability seen on supination in axial plane
  - Dorsal instability seen on pronation in axial plane
  - Radial sided tears: Dorsal to volar orientation
  - Ulnar avulsion ± ulnar styloid fracture
  - Radial avulsion ± sigmoid notch fractures
  - Hypointense sclerosis lunate, triquetrum & distal ulna in ulnolunate abutment syndrome
- T2WI
  - Traumatic lesions - perforation or avulsion

DDx: Triangular Fibrocartilage Tear

Abutment	Kienböck's	LT Ligament Tear
Cor T1 Arthro.	Cor T1WI MR	Cor T1 Arthro.

TRIANGULAR FIBROCARTILAGE TEAR

Key Facts

Imaging Findings
- Best diagnostic clue: Direct extension of fluid across TFC
- Traumatic lesions - perforation or avulsion
- Degenerative lesions = spectrum of ulnocarpal abutment (impaction) syndrome

Top Differential Diagnoses
- Ulnocarpal Abutment
- Kienböck's Disease
- Lunotriquetral (LT) Dissociation
- Extensor Carpi Ulnaris Tendinitis
- Instability of the Distal Radioulnar Joint (DRUJ)

Pathology
- Hyperextension of wrist + rotational load
- Degenerative = ulnocarpal abutment syndrome

- Palmer class 1 - traumatic
- Palmer class 2 - degenerative (ulnocarpal abutment syndrome)

Clinical Issues
- Most common signs/symptoms: Ulnar wrist pain
- Painful DRUJ rotation
- Pain with stress loading of DRUJ in pronation & supination
- Traumatic tears more common < 40 yrs
- Degenerative tears more common > 40 yrs

Diagnostic Checklist
- Coronal images using T1 or T2* gradient echo for intrasubstance degeneration & FS PD FSE for contour irregularities

---

  - Degenerative lesions = spectrum of ulnocarpal abutment (impaction) syndrome
  - FS PD FSE - improved definition of proximal & distal surfaces
  - Partial tears = contour irregularity of proximal (undersurface) or distal surfaces
  - Primary sign of TFC tear = hyperintense fluid extension across articular disk or discontinuity
  - Intermediate to hyperintense synovitis
  - Chondromalacia of proximal lunate, triquetrum & ulna - loss of normal intermediate signal intensity articular cartilage
- T2* GRE: Improved visualization of intrasubstance degeneration & tears
- T1 C+
  - Intravenous contrast ± improved conspicuity of partial tears
  - MR arthrography
    - Differentiate severe degeneration from partial tear
    - Performed with radiocarpal injection

Imaging Recommendations
- Best imaging tool: MR highly sensitive & specific for fluid extension, TFC morphology/tear pattern + chondromalacia of ulnar side of wrist
- Protocol advice
  - T1/PD + FS PD FSE coronal, axial & sagittal
  - T2* = additional value in augmenting intrasubstance degeneration
  - MR arthrography - not routinely required

DIFFERENTIAL DIAGNOSIS

Ulnocarpal Abutment
- TFCC degeneration/perforation
- Lunate, triquetral & ulnar chondromalacia
- Lunotriquetral ligament perforation/tear
- Ulnocarpal arthritis

Kienböck's Disease
- Avascular necrosis lunate
- Related to trauma + ulnar negative variance

- Centralized lunate sclerosis
- ± Visualized lunate fracture

Lunotriquetral (LT) Dissociation
- Dissociation between lunate & triquetrum
- Volar flexion lunate (VISI)
- Absence of horseshoe-shaped ligament
- Degenerative etiology vs. ulnar-sided trauma on outstretched hand

Extensor Carpi Ulnaris Tendinitis
- Dorsal ulnar-sided pain
- Thickened tendon sheath
- Hyperintense fluid (T2WI) surrounding tendon
- Synovial thickening intermediate signal (T2WI)
- ± Associated subchondral marrow edema distal ulna

Instability of the Distal Radioulnar Joint (DRUJ)
- Ulnar dorsal dislocation in hyperpronation
- Ulnar palmar dislocation in hypersupination
- Rotational injury with forced pronation/supination + hyperextension

PATHOLOGY

General Features
- General path comments
  - Relevant anatomy
    - TFC = articular disc, palmar (volar) radioulnar + dorsal radioulnar ligaments
    - TFCC = TFC, ulnolunate & ulnotriquetral ligaments, meniscus homologue, extensor carpi ulnaris tendon subsheath
- Etiology
  - Forearm pronation
  - Hyperextension of wrist + rotational load
  - Degenerative = ulnocarpal abutment syndrome
- Epidemiology
  - TFC tears associated with positive ulnar variance

- o Higher incidence of radial-sided lesions, except ulnar-sided tears seen more commonly in younger patients
- o Asymptomatic perforations common after age 40

Gross Pathologic & Surgical Features

- Palmer class 1 - traumatic
  - o A = central perforation
  - o B = ulnar avulsion + distal ulnar fracture
  - o C = distal avulsion
  - o D = radial avulsion + sigmoid notch fracture
- Palmer class 2 - degenerative (ulnocarpal abutment syndrome)
  - o A = TFCC wear (degeneration)
  - o B = TFCC wear + lunate, triquetral +/- ulnar chondromalacia
  - o C = TFCC perforation + lunate, triquetral, ulnar chondromalacia
  - o D = TFCC perforation + lunate, triquetral, ulnar chondromalacia & LT ligament perforations
  - o E = TFCC perforation + lunate, triquetral, ulnar chondromalacia, LT ligament tear & ulnocarpal arthritis

Microscopic Features

- TFC microstructure
  - o Short collagen fibers in central region in response to compression loads
  - o Superficial & deep layer (less organized) within articular disk
  - o Radial border = avascular
  - o Central disk = avascular
  - o Mucinous or myxoid degeneration in degenerative tears

Staging, Grading or Classification Criteria

- Palmer classification (1 = traumatic tears, 2 = degenerative tears)
- Bowers = classification of disorders of DRUJ & TFC
- Mayo classification = treatment and location based for traumatic & degenerative tear types

CLINICAL ISSUES

Presentation

- Most common signs/symptoms: Ulnar wrist pain
- Clinical profile
  - o Loss of strength
  - o Painful DRUJ rotation
  - o Catching or snapping
  - o Tenderness & pain over TFC
  - o Pain with stress loading of DRUJ in pronation & supination
  - o Dorsal-palmar ballottement of distal ulna = stress test (piano-key sign)
  - o Associated fractures (Colles', Galeazzi's & Essex Lopresti)

Demographics

- Age
  - o Traumatic tears more common < 40 yrs
  - o Degenerative tears more common > 40 yrs
- Gender: No bias

Natural History & Prognosis

- Attenuated central disc = communications, perforations & tears
- Increased perforation rate with excessive loading of TFC in setting of positive ulnar variance & ulnocarpal abutment syndrome
- Congenital perforations documented in infants & asymptomatic adults + degenerative wrists
- Traumatic tears may be associated with injuries to ECU tendon sheath & LT ligament
- Peripheral tears at ulnar fovea or radius result in reduced TFC tension with loss of suspensory trampoline effect

Treatment

- Conservative
  - o Relieve overloading of distal ulna
  - o Activity modification & anti-inflammatory medications
- Surgical
  - o Debride/repair tear
  - o Resection + debridement of flap tear
  - o Augmentation if repair not possible
  - o Reconstruction - better long term results than resection
  - o Triquetral impingement of ulnar styloid - limited ulnar styloidectomy

DIAGNOSTIC CHECKLIST

Consider

- Coronal images using T1 or T2* gradient echo for intrasubstance degeneration & FS PD FSE for contour irregularities
- Evaluate distal radioulnar ligaments (volar & dorsal margins of TFC)

SELECTED REFERENCES

1. Haims AH et al: Limitations of MR imaging in the diagnosis of peripheral tears of the triangular fibrocartilage of the wrist. AJR 178(2):419-22, 2002
2. Cooney WP: The wrist. Diagnosis and operative treatment. Tears of the triangular fibrocartilage of the wrist. vol 1. St. Louis Missouri, Mosby, (30):710-42, 1998
3. Loftus JB et al: The wrist and it's disorders. Disorders of the distal radioulnar joint and triangular fibrocartilage complex. 2nd ed. Philadelphia Pennsylvania, W.B. Saunders, (21):385-414, 1997
4. Totterman SMS et al: Lesions of the triangular fibrocartilage complex: MR findings with a three-dimensional gradient-recalled-echo sequence. Radiology 199:277-32, 1996
5. Totterman SMS et al: Triangular fibrocartilage complex: Normal appearance on coronal three-dimensional gradient-recalled-echo MR images. Radiology 195:521-7, 1995
6. Rettig ME et al: Clinical applications of MR imaging in hand and wrist surgery-magnetic resonance imaging. Magn Reson Imaging Clin North Am 3:361-8, 1995
7. Sugimoto H et al: Triangular fibrocartilage in asymptomatic subjects: Investigation of abnormal MR signal intensity. Radiology 191:193-7, 1994

TRIANGULAR FIBROCARTILAGE TEAR

IMAGE GALLERY

Typical

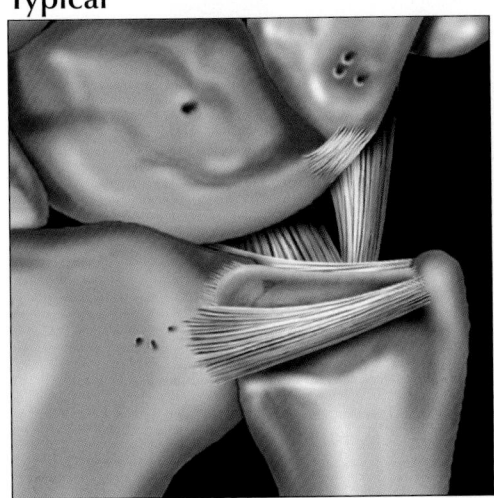

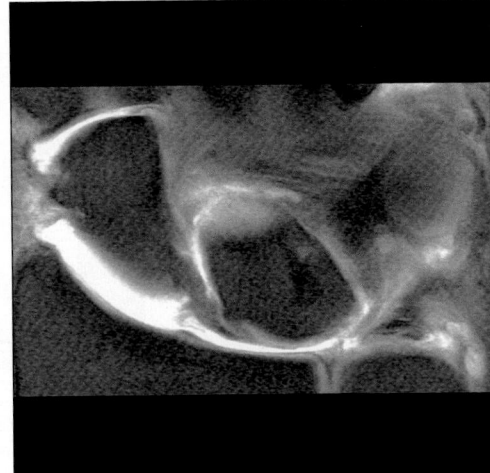

(Left) Coronal graphic shows degenerative (class 2) tear of the TFCC. Class 2 lesions of the TFCC represent part of the spectrum of ulnocarpal abutment syndrome. *(Right)* Coronal T1 C+ MR (MR arthrogram) shows degenerative (class 2) tear of the TFC.

Typical

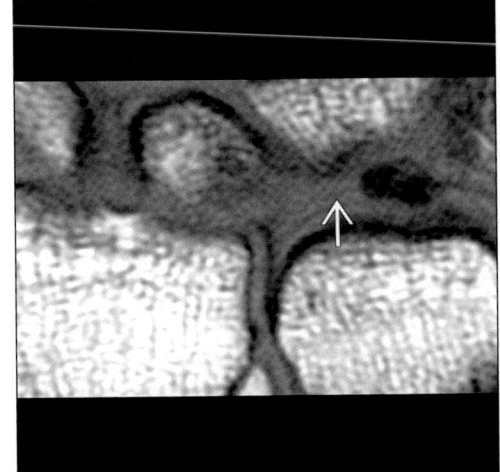

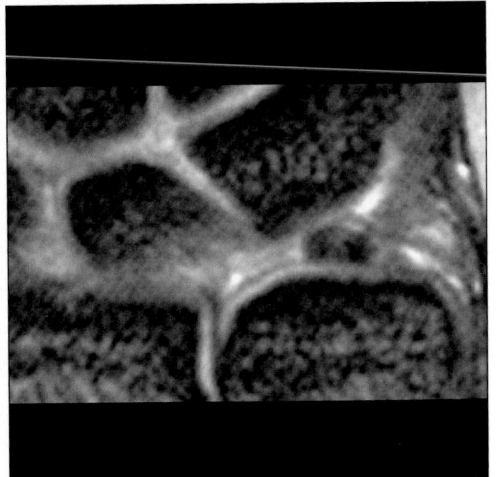

(Left) Coronal T1WI MR shows traumatic (class 1) tear (arrow) of the TFC associated with clinical DRUJ instability. *(Right)* Coronal FS PD FSE MR shows hyperintense central defect of the TFCC at the junction of the disk and dorsal radioulnar ligament (dorsal margin of the TFC).

Other

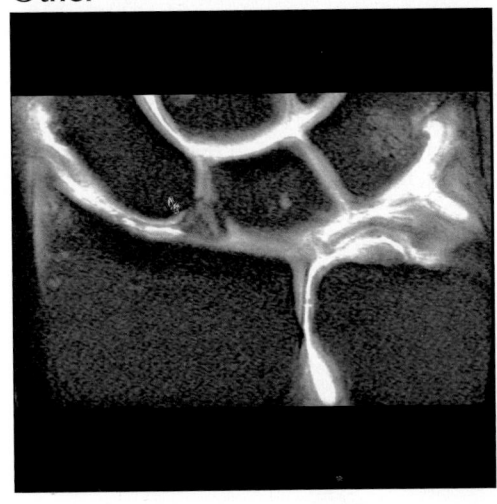

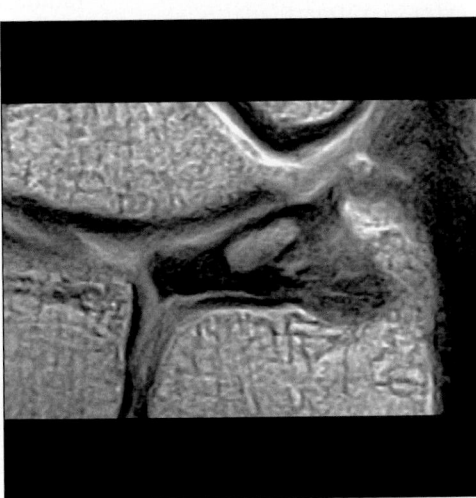

(Left) Coronal T1 C+ MR (MR arthrogram) shows degenerative TFC lesion with horizontal tear and chondromalacia of the distal ulna, lunate, and triquetrum. *(Right)* Coronal T1 C+ MR (MR arthrogram) shows normal foveal and styloid attachments of the TFC.

DISTAL RADIUS FRACTURES

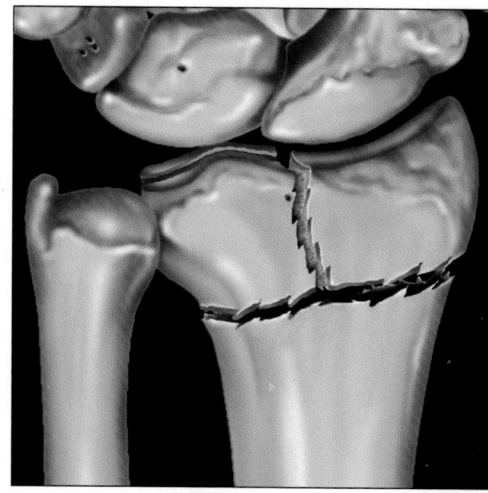

Coronal graphic shows intraarticular distal radius fracture with involvement of lunate fossa. The fractured lunate fossa is divided into a palmar and a dorsal medial component.

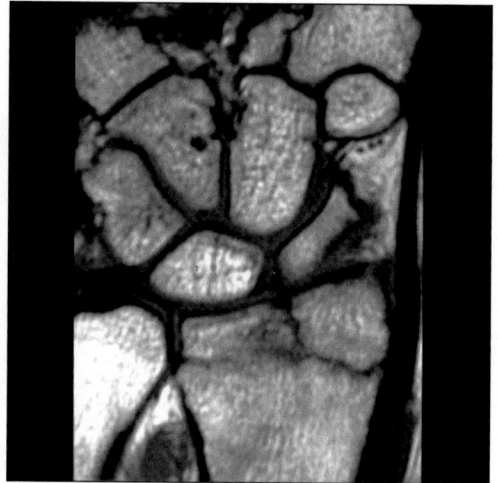

Coronal T1WI MR shows transverse distal radius fracture with secondary extension into radiocarpal joint & distal radioulnar joint. There is congruity of the distal radial articular surface.

TERMINOLOGY

Abbreviations and Synonyms
- Distal radius fractures, Colles' fracture, Smith's fracture

Definitions
- Extraarticular & intraarticular fractures of distal radius

IMAGING FINDINGS

General Features
- Best diagnostic clue: Linear fx line involving distal radius
- Location
  - Scaphoid fossa (SF)
  - Lunate fossa (LF)
  - Sigmoid notch (SN) - at distal radioulnar joint (DRUJ)
- Size: Variable with respect to extra vs. intraarticular & displacement of fragments
- Morphology
  - Colles' fracture: Distal metaphysis with dorsal displacement, angulation (silver fork deformity), radial angulation & radial shortening
  - Smith's fracture (reverse Colles'): Palmarly angulated fracture (garden spade deformity)
  - Barton's fracture: Intraarticular fracture-dislocation or subluxation (palmar vs. dorsal fracture) with displacement of carpus
  - Melone classification: 5 fracture types based on 4 fracture components

Radiographic Findings
- Radiography
  - Extraarticular nondisplaced & displaced
  - Intraarticular nondisplaced & displaced
  - Lateral radiography - useful for dorsal + volar displacement

CT Findings
- NECT
  - Bone technique with coronal & sagittal reformations
  - 3-D rendering for surgical planning
  - Identify displacement of key medial fragments (ulnar aspect of distal radius) & disruption of radiocarpal + distal radioulnar joints (DRUJ)

MR Findings
- T1WI
  - Fracture diastasis directly measured on coronal, axial or sagittal images
  - Scaphoid + lunate fossa evaluated on coronal images
  - Hypointense fracture line(s) extension to distal radius
  - Articular involvement

DDx: Distal Radius Fracture

TFC Tear	Abutment	SL Ligament Tear
Cor T1WI MR	Cor T1 Arthro.	Cor T1 Arthro.

DISTAL RADIUS FRACTURES

Key Facts

Imaging Findings
- Best diagnostic clue: Linear fx line involving distal radius
- Melone classification: 5 fracture types based on 4 fracture components

Top Differential Diagnoses
- Traumatic Triangular Fibrocartilage Complex (TFCC) Abnormalities
- Ulnocarpal Abutment Syndrome
- Kienböck's Disease
- Instability of Distal Radioulnar Joint (DRUJ)
- Intrinsic Ligament Pathology

Pathology
- Fall onto outstretched hand

- Weaker dorsal cortex associated with extraarticular metaphyseal fracture in elderly
- Greater longitudinal compression force in younger patient = intraarticular fracture + displacement

Clinical Issues
- Most common signs/symptoms: Pain at distal radius
- Deformity over distal radius
- Displacement of hand dorsally in Colles' fracture or palmarly in Smith fracture
- Swelling dorsum of hand & wrist with ecchymosis
- Radiocarpal arthrosis - associated with > 2 mm incongruity of articular surface

Diagnostic Checklist
- Characterize lunate fossa involvement into dorsal & palmar medial components on sagittal images

---

      - Radial shaft & styloid
- T2WI
  - Hypo to hyperintense fracture line
  - Hyperintense marrow edema & joint effusion
  - Intermediate to hyperintense synovitis + subcutaneus edema
  - Disruption of intermediate signal intensity chondral surfaces
  - Associated partial or complete ligament tears
  - Hyperintense edema of associated carpal fractures

Imaging Recommendations
- Best imaging tool: MR for osseous + soft tissue injury
- Protocol advice
  - Coronal, axial & sagittal T1, FS PD FSE
  - T2* GRE
    - Helpful in identifying fragments if subchondral edema is severe and obscures fracture detail

DIFFERENTIAL DIAGNOSIS

Traumatic Triangular Fibrocartilage Complex (TFCC) Abnormalities
- Central perforation
- Ulnar avulsion
- Distal avulsion
- Radial avulsion

Ulnocarpal Abutment Syndrome
- TFCC degeneration/perforation
- Lunate, triquetral & ulnar chondromalacia
- Lunotriquetral ligament perforation/tear

Kienböck's Disease
- Avascular necrosis of lunate
- Related to trauma + ulnar negative variance
- Centralized lunate sclerosis
- ± Visualized lunate fracture

Instability of Distal Radioulnar Joint (DRUJ)
- Ulnar dorsal dislocation in hyperpronation
- Ulna palmar dislocation in hypersupination

- Rotational injury with forced pronation/supination + hyperextension

Intrinsic Ligament Pathology
- Lunotriquetral dissociation with volar flexion of lunate & discontinuity of hypointense ligament
- Scapholunate dissociation with scaphoid flexion, ligamentous tear ± scapholunate interval diastasis

PATHOLOGY

General Features
- General path comments
  - Relevant anatomy = medial (ulnar) complex
    - Ulnar styloid
    - Triquetrum
    - Lunate and lunate fossa
    - TFC
    - Ulnocarpal meniscus
    - Ulnolunate ligament
    - Radiocarpal ligaments
- Etiology
  - Fall onto outstretched hand
  - Osteoporotic elderly woman - low energy injuries
  - Dorsiflexion hyperextension
  - Tension along palmar surface of wrist
  - Compression + comminution dorsal surface
  - Weaker dorsal cortex associated with extraarticular metaphyseal fracture in elderly
  - Greater longitudinal compression force in younger patient = intraarticular fracture + displacement
- Epidemiology
  - Distal radius fracture = one of the most common skeletal injuries
  - One-sixth of all fractures seen in acute setting
  - Majority = articular with disruption of radiocarpal & distal radioulnar joints

Gross Pathologic & Surgical Features
- Colles' fracture
  - Distal metaphysis radius
  - Dorsally displaced & angulated

DISTAL RADIUS FRACTURES

- Within 2 cm of articular surface
- ± Distal radiocarpal or radioulnar joint
- Radial angulation & shortening
- Smith's fracture
  - Reverse Colles'
  - Palmarly angulated fracture
  - Hand & wrist displaced palmarly
  - Extra or intraarticular
- Barton's fracture
  - Fracture dislocation of distal radius
  - Intraarticular (rim) fracture
  - Displaced dorsally or palmarly with carpus
  - Dislocation = primary feature
- Intraarticular fracture
  - Melone classification (attention to medial complex at level of lunate fossa) - 4 fracture components: Radial shaft, radial styloid, dorsal-medial, and volar-medial fragments
    - Type I: Minimally displaced
    - Type IIA: Dorsally displaced (most common) vs. volar displacement
    - Type IIB: Die-punch fracture with lunate impaction, most commonly on dorsal medial component
    - Type III: Addition of spike fragment from volar metaphysis
    - Type IV: Separation or rotation of dorsal & palmar medial fragments & disruption of distal radius articulations
    - Type V: Explosion fracture with comminution from articular surfaces to diaphysis

Microscopic Features

- Fracture histology - failure of trabecular & cortical bone
- Ligament histology
  - Capsular - collagen bundles or fascicles
  - Intraarticular - lined by synoviocytes
  - Mesocapsular - synovial capsular structure

Staging, Grading or Classification Criteria

- Frykman classification - intra or extraarticular fxs (including involvement of DRUJ) +/- ulnar styloid fx
- Universal classification - replaced Frykman classification including treatment algorithm
- Melone classification - based on degree & direction of displaced articular fragments + indications for open reduction
- Mayo classification - scaphoid, lunate, sigmoid notch as separate articulations with involvement of one or more articular fossae

CLINICAL ISSUES

Presentation

- Most common signs/symptoms: Pain at distal radius
- Clinical profile
  - Deformity over distal radius
  - Displacement of hand dorsally in Colles' fracture or palmarly in Smith fracture
  - Swelling dorsum of hand & wrist with ecchymosis

Demographics

- Age: Young to elderly
- Gender
  - High energy injuries in young male
  - Low energy in elderly female with osteoporosis

Natural History & Prognosis

- Stable vs. unstable reduction
- DRUJ instability
- Median nerve dysfunction & carpal tunnel syndrome
- Tendon injury & carpal injury
- Radiocarpal arthrosis - associated with > 2 mm incongruity of articular surface

Treatment

- Conservative
  - Melone type I: Stable
- Surgical
  - Melone type IIA: Unstable (dorsal or volar displacement), treatment with reduction + external fixation
  - Melone type IIB: Irreducible by closed techniques
  - Melone type III: Volar spike fragment from metaphysis places adjacent nerves & tendons at risk
  - Melone type IV
    - Arthroscopic percutaneous reduction & pinning
    - Open reduction and internal fixation (type IIB, III, IV)

DIAGNOSTIC CHECKLIST

Consider

- Associated involvement of radial styloid & ulnar styloid
- Characterize lunate fossa involvement into dorsal & palmar medial components on sagittal images

SELECTED REFERENCES

1. Freeland AE et al: The arthroscopic management of intra-articular distal radius fractures. Hand Surg 5(2):93-102, 2000
2. Trumble TE et al: Intra-articular fractures of the distal aspect of the radius. Instr Course Lect 48:465-80, 1999
3. Cooney WP: The wrist. Diagnosis and operative treatment. Fractures of the distal radius. Philadelphia PA, WB Saunders, (30):310-55, 1998
4. Rettig ME et al: The wrist and it's disorders: Fractures of the distal radius. 2nd ed. Philadelphia PA, WB Saunders, 347-72, 1997
5. Pruitt DL et al: Computed tomography scanning with image reconstruction in evaluation of distal radius fractures. J Hand Surg 19A:720, 1994
6. Leibovic SJ et al: Treatment of complex intraarticular distal radius fractures. Orthop Clin North Am 25:685, 1994
7. Metz VM et al: Imaging techniques for distal radius fractures and related injuries. Orthop Clin North Am 24:217, 1993
8. Johnston GHF et al: Computerized tomographic evaluation of acute distal radial fractures. J Hand Surg 17A:738, 1992
9. Bartosh RA et al: Intraarticular fractures of the distal radius: A cadaveric study to determine if ligamentotaxis restores radiopalmar tilt. J Hand Surg 15A:18, 1990

DISTAL RADIUS FRACTURES

IMAGE GALLERY

Typical

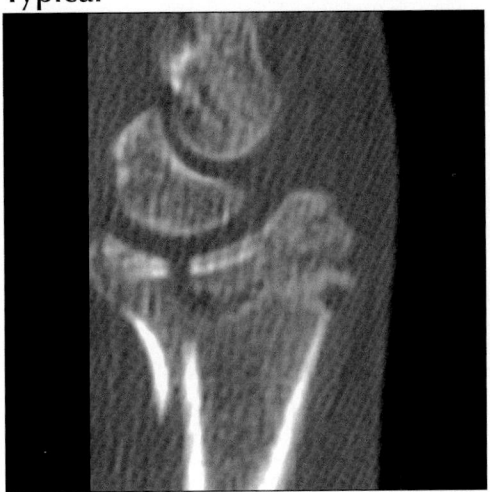

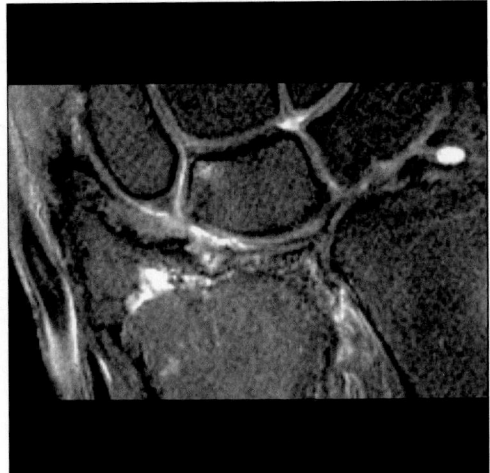

(Left) Sagittal NECT shows Melone type II fracture secondary to a die-punch mechanism of injury. The lunate has impacted the palmar medial fragment of the distal radius. *(Right)* Coronal FS PD FSE MR shows intraarticular distal radius fracture with die-punch mechanism of injury. Degenerative changes are shown between the lunate and lunate fossa of the distal radius.

Typical

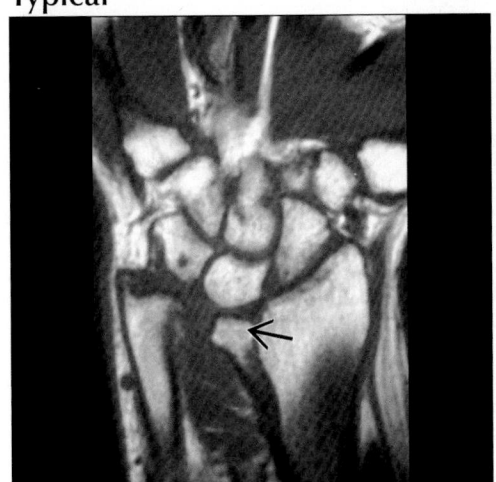

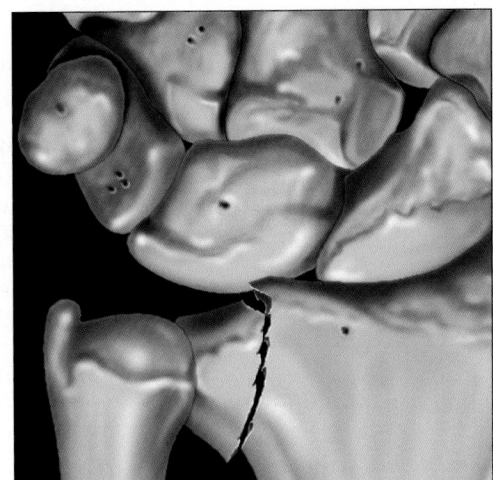

(Left) Coronal T1WI MR shows depressed lunate fossa (arrow) and diastasis of the distal radioulnar joint secondary to an unstable die-punch compression force. *(Right)* Coronal graphic shows depressed lunate fossa in an unstable type II fracture. In a double die-punch there would be the additional impaction of the scaphoid on distal radius.

Typical

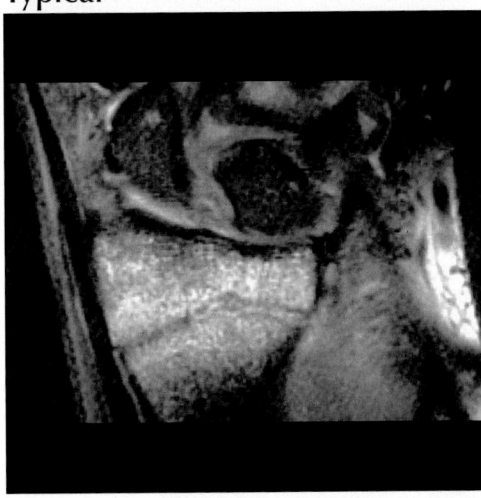

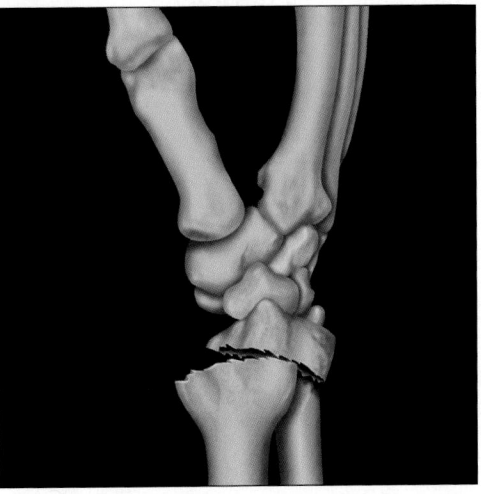

(Left) Coronal FS PD FSE MR shows hyperintense marrow edema associated with a transverse Colles' fracture of distal radius. *(Right)* Sagittal graphic shows Colles' fracture (extraarticular) with dorsal displacement of distal fragment.

DIE PUNCH FRACTURE, DISTAL RADIUS

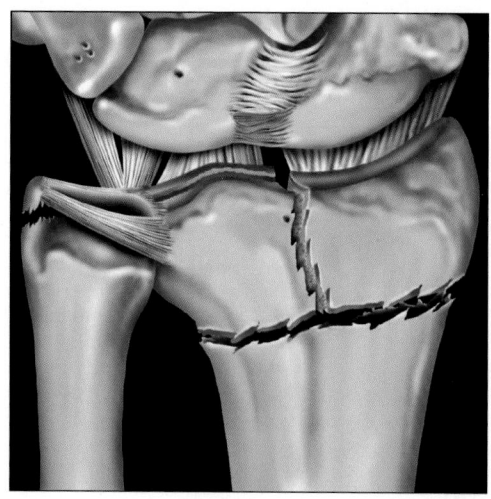

Coronal graphic shows articular injury with associated ulnar styloid fracture and involvement of the lunate fossa of distal radius (dorsal perspective).

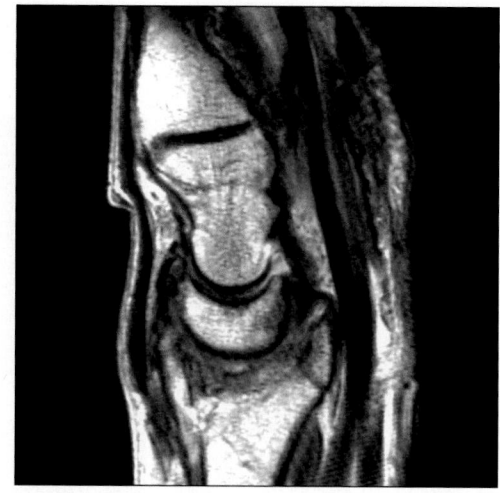

Sagittal T1WI MR shows unstable Melone type II fracture with lunate impaction on the dorsal medial fragment.

TERMINOLOGY

Abbreviations and Synonyms
- Lunate load fx, medial cuneiform fx

Definitions
- Intraarticular comminuted distal radius fx occurring 2° to lunate impaction of distal radius, splitting the distal radius in both coronal and sagittal planes

IMAGING FINDINGS

General Features
- Best diagnostic clue: Fracture that extends to involve lunate fossa of distal radius
- Location: Lunate fossa (dorsal medial or palmar medial)
- Size: Variable based on displacement of fragments
- Morphology: Dorsal displacement of articular surfaces vs. volar displacement

Radiographic Findings
- Radiography
  - Initial exam - anteroposterior (AP) and lateral views of wrist
  - ± Diagnostic
  - Typically 4 main fx fragments identified (Melone classification)
    - Metaphyseal
    - Radial styloid
    - Dorsal medial
    - Palmar medial

CT Findings
- NECT
  - Excellent bony detail
  - Better definition of fx fragments & patterns
  - Multiplanar reconstruction
    - Define fx displacement in 3-dimensions
    - Pre-operative planning
  - Accurate measurements
    - Articular step-off
    - Fragment displacement
    - Shortening

MR Findings
- T1WI
  - Fracture diastasis directly measured on coronal, axial or sagittal images
  - Scaphoid + lunate fossa evaluated on coronal images
  - Articular fractures
  - Radial shaft & styloid
  - Lunate fossa, dorsal medial & palmar medial fragments
- T2WI
  - Hypointense to hyperintense fracture line
  - Hyperintense marrow edema & joint effusion

DDx: Die Punch Fracture, Distal Radius

TFCC Tear	Abutment	Kienböck's	SL Ligament Tear
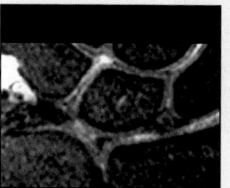	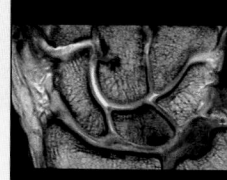	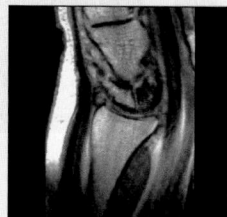	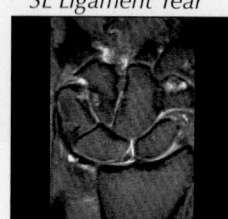
Cor FS PD MR	*Cor T1 Arthro.*	*Sag T1WI MR*	*Cor FS PD MR*

DIE PUNCH FRACTURE, DISTAL RADIUS

Key Facts

Imaging Findings

- Best diagnostic clue: Fracture that extends to involve lunate fossa of distal radius
- Fracture diastasis directly measured on coronal, axial or sagittal images
- Scaphoid + lunate fossa evaluated on coronal images
- Hypointense fracture line(s) extension to distal radius (T1 & T2WI)

Top Differential Diagnoses

- Traumatic Triangular Fibrocartilage Complex (TFCC) Abnormalities
- Ulnocarpal Abutment Syndrome
- Kienböck's Disease
- Instability of Distal Radioulnar Joint (DRUJ)
- Intrinsic Ligament Pathology

Pathology

- Etiology: Occurs primarily 2° to axial compression with lunate driven proximally, impacting dorsal medial aspect of distal radius
- Lunate impaction on dorsal medial component of lunate fossa with dorsal displacement

Clinical Issues

- Most common signs/symptoms: Fx secondary to fall on outstretched hand

Diagnostic Checklist

- Characterize lunate fossa into dorsal medial & palmar medial components of die punch fracture on sagittal images

- o Intermediate to hyperintense synovitis + subcutaneous edema
- o Disruption of intermediate signal intensity of chondral surfaces
- o Discontinuity of associated ligament tears
- o Hyperintense edema of associated carpal fractures
- T2* GRE: Helpful in identifying fragments if subchondral edema is severe & obscures fracture detail
- Hypointense fracture line(s) extension to distal radius (T1 & T2WI)

Imaging Recommendations

- Best imaging tool: MR for osseous + soft tissue injury
- Protocol advice: T1, FS PD FSE MR coronal, axial & sagittal

DIFFERENTIAL DIAGNOSIS

Traumatic Triangular Fibrocartilage Complex (TFCC) Abnormalities

- Central perforation
- Ulnar avulsion
- Distal avulsion
- Radial avulsion

Ulnocarpal Abutment Syndrome

- TFCC degeneration/perforation
- Lunate, triquetral & ulnar chondromalacia
- Lunotriquetral ligament perforation/tear

Kienböck's Disease

- Avascular necrosis of lunate
- Related to trauma - ulnar negative variance
- Centralized lunate sclerosis
- ± Visualized lunate fractures

Instability of Distal Radioulnar Joint (DRUJ)

- Ulnar dorsal dislocation in hyperpronation
- Ulnar palmar dislocation in hypersupination
- Rotational injury with forced pronation/supination + hyperextension

Intrinsic Ligament Pathology

- Lunotriquetral dissociation with volar flexion of lunate & discontinuity of hypointense ligament
- Scapholunate (SL) dissociation with scaphoid flexion, ligamentous tear ± interval diastasis

PATHOLOGY

General Features

- General path comments
  - o Relevant anatomy
    - Ulnar styloid
    - Lunate fossa
    - Triquetrum
    - Lunate
    - TFC
    - Ulnocarpal meniscus
    - Ulnolunate ligament
    - Radiocarpal ligament
- Etiology: Occurs primarily 2° to axial compression with lunate driven proximally, impacting dorsal medial aspect of distal radius
- Epidemiology
  - o Distal radius fracture = one of the most common skeletal injuries
  - o One-sixth of all fractures presenting acutely
  - o Majority = articular with disruption of radiocarpal & distal radioulnar joints

Gross Pathologic & Surgical Features

- Lunate impaction on dorsal medial component of lunate fossa with dorsal displacement
- Comminution of dorsal metaphysis
- Dorsal tilting
- Shortening of the radius
- Less common is lunate impaction on palmar medial fragment with volar displacement
- Double die punch = scaphoid & lunate impaction of distal radius articular surface

DIE PUNCH FRACTURE, DISTAL RADIUS

Microscopic Features
- Fracture histology = failure of trabecular & cortical bone
- Ligament histology
  - Capsular - collagen bundles or fascicles
  - Intraarticular - lined by synoviocytes
  - Mesocapsular - synovial capsular structure

Staging, Grading or Classification Criteria
- Fracture patterns
  - Type I - no significant displacement or angulation
  - Type IIa - classic die punch fx; unstable fx with dorsal displacement of dorsal medial fragment, dorsal tilt, shortening of radius
  - Type IIb - lunate impaction of palmar medial component of distal radius resulting in greater comminution and volar tilt
  - Type III - similar to type II fx with extra comminuted "spike" fragment displaced volarly
  - Type IV - wide separation of dorsal and palmar medial fragments
  - Type V - severely comminuted fx with severe disruption of distal radius articulations
- Melone fracture classification - four primary fx fragments
  - Metaphyseal
  - Radial styloid
  - Dorsal medial
  - Palmar medial

CLINICAL ISSUES

Presentation
- Most common signs/symptoms: Fx secondary to fall on outstretched hand
- Clinical profile
  - Pain
  - Swelling
  - Deformity
  - Decreased range of motion
  - Winter months > summer months

Demographics
- Age: Adults (60-80 years most common)
- Gender: F > M

Natural History & Prognosis
- Dependent upon severity of comminution
- Dependent upon amount of articular step-off
- Degree of displacement + ability to achieve anatomic reduction
- Type I fx - best prognosis
- Type IIb, III, IV fx - worst prognosis
- Complications
  - Chondral injury - eventual degenerative arthrosis
  - TFCC, SL, LT + extrinsic ligament tears
  - Tendinous disruptions 2° to lacerations by fx fragments
  - Nerve injuries (ulnar, radial, or median nerves)
  - Arterial injuries
  - Reflex sympathetic dystrophy

Treatment
- Conservative
  - Type I fx - treated with closed reduction
- Surgical
  - Type IIa, b, III + IV - open reduction almost always necessary
    - Internal and external fixation often used
  - Indications for open reduction
    - Persistent articular step-off > 2 mm
    - Radial shortening exceeding 3-5 mm
    - Dorsal tilt in excess of 10°

DIAGNOSTIC CHECKLIST

Consider
- Associated involvement of radial styloid & ulnar styloid
- Characterize lunate fossa into dorsal medial & palmar medial components of die punch fracture on sagittal images

SELECTED REFERENCES

1. Putman MD et al: Rockwood and Green's fractures in adults. Fractures of the distal radius. Philadelphia Pennsylvania, Lippincott Williams & Wilkins Publishers, 815-67, 2001
2. Fernandez DL et al: Green's operative hand surgery. Fractures of the distal radius. Philadelphia Pennsylvania, Churchill Livingstone, 934-5, 1999
3. Stoller DW: Magnetic resonance imaging in orthopaedics and sports medicine. 2nd ed. Philadelphia Pennsylvania, Lippincott Williams & Wilkins, 934-5, 1997
4. Leibovic SJ et al: Treatment of complex intra-articular distal radius fractures. Orthop Clin North Am 25:685, 1994
5. Pruitt DL et al: Computed tomography scanning with image reconstruction in evaluation of distal radius fractures. J Hand Surg 19A:720, 1994
6. Melone Jr. CP: Distal radius fractures: Patterns of articular fragmentation. Ortho Clin of N Am 24(2):239-53, 1993
7. Metz VM et al: Imaging techniques for distal radius fractures and related injuries. Orthop Clin North Am 24:217, 1993
8. Johnson GHF et al: Computerized tomographic evaluation of acute distal radial fractures. J Hand Surg 17A:738, 1992
9. Cooney WE et al: Symposium: Management of intra-articular fractures of the distal radius. Contemp Ortho 21:71, 1990
10. Xelrod TS et al: Open reduction and internal fixation of comminuted, intra-articular fractures of the distal radius. J Hand Surg 15A:1, 1990
11. Axelrod T et al: Limited open reduction of the lunate facet in comminuted intra-articular fractures of the distal radius. J Hand Surg 13A:38, 1988
12. Bartosh RA et al: Intraarticular fractures of the distal radius: A cadaveric study to determine if ligamentotaxis restores radiopalmar tilt. J Hand Surg 15A:18, 1990
13. Bassett RL: Displaced intraarticular fractures of the distal radius. Clin Ortho 214:148, 1987
14. Melone CP Jr: Open treatment for displaced articular fractures of the distal radius. Clin Orthop 202:103, 1986
15. Melone CP Jr: Articular fractures of the distal radius. Orthop Clin North Am 15:217, 1984

DIE PUNCH FRACTURE, DISTAL RADIUS

IMAGE GALLERY

Typical

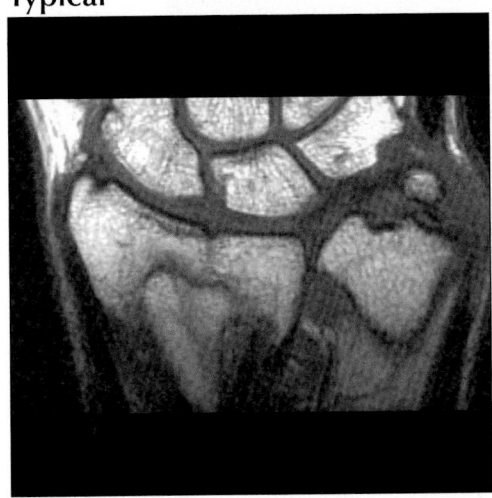 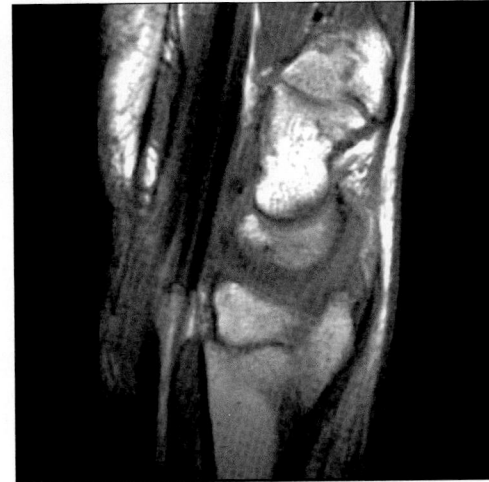

(Left) Coronal T1WI MR shows distal radius fracture involving ulnar styloid and lunate fossa without depression or displacement of dorsal or medial components of lunate fossa. *(Right)* Sagittal T1WI MR shows lunate impaction of the dorsal medial fragment resulting in dorsal displacement (type II fx).

Typical

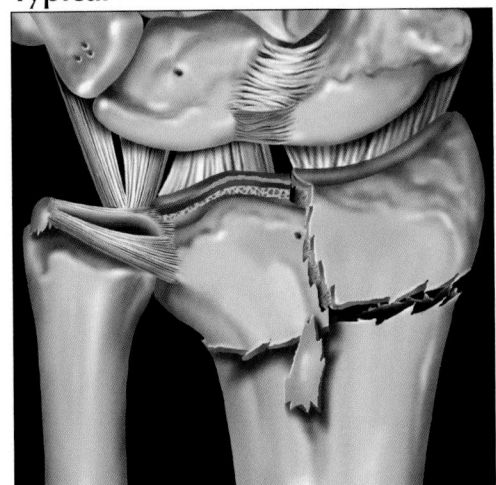 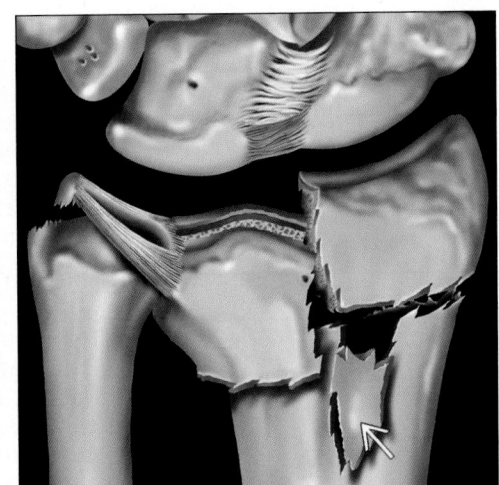

(Left) Coronal graphic (dorsal view) shows type II articular fracture with dorsal displacement of the dorsal medial fragment. *(Right)* Coronal graphic (volar view) shows an unstable type III fracture with additional metaphyseal spike fragment (arrow).

Typical

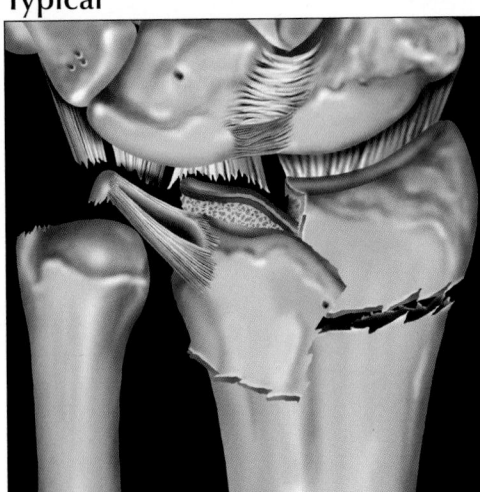 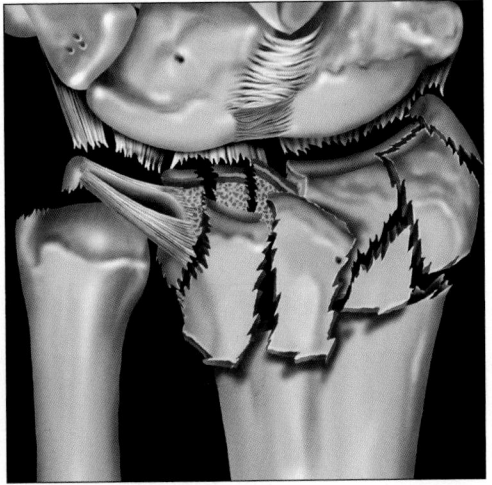

(Left) Coronal graphic (dorsal view) shows unstable type IV distal radius fracture with wide separation of the dorsal and palmar medial fragments. *(Right)* Coronal graphic (dorsal view) shows type V explosion fracture of the distal radius with severe comminution.

ULNAR STYLOID FRACTURE

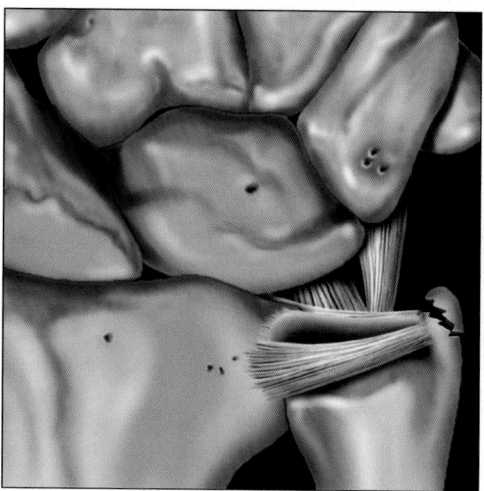

Coronal graphic shows distal ulnar styloid fracture without displacement of the TFCC attachments.

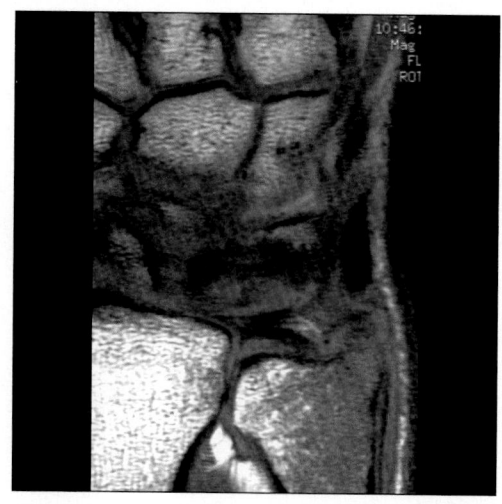

Coronal T1WI MR shows hypointense marrow edema associated with a nondisplaced ulnar styloid fracture.

TERMINOLOGY

Abbreviations and Synonyms
- Fracture of the ulnar styloid, avulsion fracture of ulnar styloid

Definitions
- Distal avulsion fractures or ulnar base fractures

IMAGING FINDINGS

General Features
- Best diagnostic clue: Transverse fracture line of ulnar styloid
- Location
  - Base
  - Mid styloid
  - Tip
- Size: Medial to lateral extent of base or less
- Morphology: Transverse fracture orientation

Radiographic Findings
- Radiography
  - Anteroposterior, lateral views
  - ± Associated distal radius fracture
  - Transverse fx of ulnar styloid
  - ± Fracture displacement

CT Findings
- NECT
  - Usually not performed for simple ulnar styloid fractures
  - To evaluate associated complex distal radius fractures
  - Accurate measurements for displaced fragments
  - Assess healing, callus formation, non-union

MR Findings
- T1WI
  - Hypointense fracture line
  - Hypointense marrow edema proximal & distal to fracture site
  - ± Displacement of fragments
  - Associated traumatic avulsion of triangular fibrocartilage (TFC) at its insertion at base of ulnar styloid
  - ± Distal radioulnar joint instability
- T2WI
  - Hypointense fracture line
  - Acute injuries with subchondral hyperintense marrow edema
  - Fluid & edema - hyperintense
  - Distal radioulnar joint (DRUJ) instability
    - Greatest risk with base fractures
    - Interosseous membrane hyperintensity (tears)

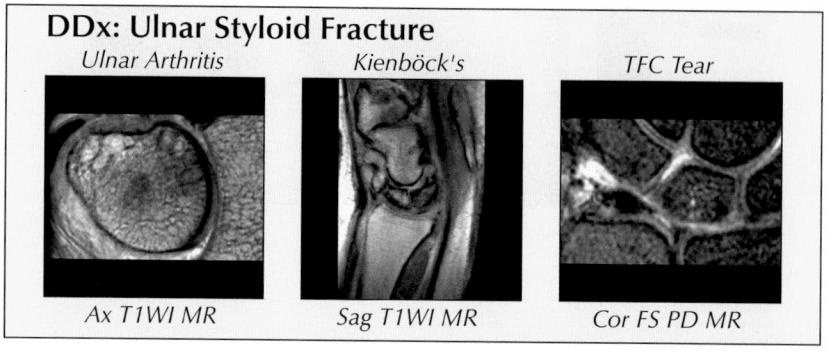

DDx: Ulnar Styloid Fracture

Ulnar Arthritis   *Kienböck's*   *TFC Tear*

Ax T1WI MR   *Sag T1WI MR*   *Cor FS PD MR*

ULNAR STYLOID FRACTURE

Key Facts

Imaging Findings
- Best diagnostic clue: Transverse fracture line of ulnar styloid
- Base
- Mid styloid
- Tip

Top Differential Diagnoses
- Ulnocarpal Abutment
- Kienböck's Disease
- Lunotriquetral Dissociation
- Extensor Carpi Ulnaris Tendinitis
- Instability of DRUJ

Pathology
- Fall on outstretched hand
- Isolated vs. in association with distal radius fractures

- Class I traumatic ulnar avulsion injuries of TFCC

Clinical Issues
- Most common signs/symptoms: Ulnar pain
- Point tenderness
- Swelling
- Associated wrist instability with base fxs
- Associated with Colles' fxs
- Associated with Essex-Lopresti (fx or fx-dislocation radial head + interosseous membrane disruption + dislocation DRUJ)
- Rate of non-union = 26%
- Nondisplaced base fx + unstable DRUJ = open repair

Diagnostic Checklist
- Identify base vs. distal ulnar styloid fractures & TFCC attachments

- Hyperintense fluid interposed between triangular fibrocartilage (TFC) & attachment to styloid base
  - Associated distal radius articular fractures
    - Ulnar styloid as part of the medial complex
  - Soft tissue injury
    - Ulnar collateral ligament of wrist
    - TFCC
    - Tendon injuries (e.g., extensor carpi ulnaris)

Imaging Recommendations
- Best imaging tool
  - MR for nondisplaced fractures & associated TFCC traumatic lesions
  - Articular fracture (distal radius) classification
- Protocol advice: T1/PD & FS PD FSE coronal, axial & sagittal images

DIFFERENTIAL DIAGNOSIS

Ulnocarpal Abutment
- TFCC degeneration/perforation
- Lunate, triquetral & ulna chondromalacia
- Lunotriquetral ligament perforation/tear
- Ulnocarpal arthritis

Kienböck's Disease
- Avascular necrosis lunate
- Related to trauma + ulnar negative variance
- Centralized lunate sclerosis
- ± Visualized lunate fracture

Lunotriquetral Dissociation
- Dissociation between lunate & triquetrum
- Volar flexion lunate (volar intercalated segment instability - VISI)
- Absence of horseshoe-shaped ligament
- Degenerative tear vs. ulnar-sided trauma on outstretched hand

Extensor Carpi Ulnaris Tendinitis
- Dorsal ulnar-sided pain
- Thickened tendon sheath
- Hyperintense fluid (T2WI) surrounding tendon

- Synovial thickening intermediate signal (T2WI)
- ± Associated subchondral marrow edema distal ulna

Instability of DRUJ
- Ulnar dorsal dislocation in hyperpronation
- Ulna palmar dislocation in hypersupination
- Rotational injury with forced pronation/supination + hyperextension

PATHOLOGY

General Features
- General path comments
  - Relevant anatomy = the medial complex
    - Ulnar styloid
    - Triangular fibrocartilage
    - Dorsal medial component (lunate fossa)
    - Palmar medial component (lunate fossa)
    - Triquetrum
    - Lunate
    - Ulnocarpal meniscus
    - Ulnolunate ligament
    - Radiolunate ligament
- Etiology
  - Fall on outstretched hand
  - Isolated vs. in association with distal radius fractures
    - Articular fractures
  - Tip of ulnar styloid
    - Avulsion by ulnar collateral ligament complex
  - Class I traumatic ulnar avulsion injuries of TFCC
- Epidemiology
  - Distal radius fractures - one of most common (74% of forearm fxs) skeletal injuries
    - Associated ulnar styloid fx in 61%
  - Subtype of traumatic TFCC tears
  - Association with Colles' fx > 50%

Gross Pathologic & Surgical Features
- Disruption of TFC medially (ulnar aspect)
- Styloid fracture
  - Tip
  - Midway from base to tip

ULNAR STYLOID FRACTURE

○ Base
- Fracture of tip
  ○ Styloid-carpal impaction
  ○ Avulsion may be associated with intact periosteal sleeve
- Fracture of base
  ○ Avulsion of TFC styloid attachment
  ○ Avulsion of foveal attachment (proximal to styloid tip)
  ○ Destabilizes ulnar attachment of TFC complex
- Distal radius articular fractures
- Extensor carpi ulnaris subsheath avulsion or stripped adjacent to styloid

Microscopic Features
- Fracture histology - failure of trabecular & cortical bone
- TFC histology
  ○ Disruption of collagen fibers

Staging, Grading or Classification Criteria
- Class 1 traumatic TFCC abnormalities (not associated with class 2 degenerative tears)
  ○ A: Central perforation
  ○ B: Ulnar avulsion
    ▪ ± Distal ulnar fracture
  ○ C: Distal avulsion
  ○ D: Radial avulsion
    ▪ ± Sigmoid notch fracture
- Melone distal radius articular fractures
  ○ Components = radial shaft, radial styloid, dorsal medial fragment, palmar medial fragment & ulnar styloid + ligamentous attachments to carpus (medially)
    ▪ Type I: Minimally displaced
    ▪ Type II: Die punch fracture with dorsal vs. volar displacement (medial fragment)
    ▪ Type IIa: Minimal/mild separation of fragments
    ▪ Type IIb: Comminution & displacement of medial fragments (dorsally) + double die punch (scaphoid + lunate)
    ▪ Type III: Addition of a spike fragment from volar metaphysis
    ▪ Type IV: Separation or rotation of dorsal & palmar medial fragment + disruption distal radius articulations
    ▪ Type V: Explosion fracture with severe comminution
- Ulnar styloid non-unions
  ○ Type 1: Distal styloid fx
  ○ Type 2: Base of styloid fx

CLINICAL ISSUES

Presentation
- Most common signs/symptoms: Ulnar pain
- Clinical profile
  ○ Point tenderness
  ○ Swelling
  ○ Restricted range of motion
  ○ Associated wrist instability with base fxs
    ▪ Radiocarpal
    ▪ DRUJ (fx displacement > 3 mm)

○ Associated with Colles' fxs
○ Associated with Essex-Lopresti (fx or fx-dislocation radial head + interosseous membrane disruption + dislocation DRUJ)

Demographics
- Age
  ○ Older adult women
  ○ Peak age (60-80 years)
  ○ Ulnar-sided TFC lesions more common in younger population
- Gender: F > M

Natural History & Prognosis
- Isolated ulnar styloid tip fxs clinically insignificant
- Displaced fractures of ulnar styloid base
  ○ Associated with ligamentous & TFC tears
  ○ DRUJ instability
  ○ Non-union risk
- Non-union of ulnar styloid
  ○ Type 1 associated with stable DRUJ (TFC insertion intact)
  ○ Type 2 associated with unstable DRUJ
  ○ Rate of non-union = 26%

Treatment
- Conservative
  ○ Isolated ulnar styloid tip fractures = closed reduction/immobilization
  ○ Nondisplaced fx base of styloid + stable DRUJ = immobilization
- Surgical
  ○ Nondisplaced base fx + unstable DRUJ = open repair
  ○ Base fx > 2 mm displacement or associated severe ligamentous or TFC injuries = open reduction

DIAGNOSTIC CHECKLIST

Consider
- Identify base vs. distal ulnar styloid fractures & TFCC attachments
- Associated with distal radius fractures

SELECTED REFERENCES

1. May MM et al: Ulnar styloid fractures associated with distal radius fractures: Incidence and implications for distal radioulnar joint instability. J Hand Surg 27(6):965-71, 2002
2. Kiyono Y et al: Ulnar-styloid nonunion and partial rupture of extensor carpi ulnaris tendon: Two case reports and review of the literature. J Orthop Trauma 16(9):674-7, 2002
3. Yanagida H et al: Radiologic evaluation of the ulnar styloid. J Hand Surg 27(1):49-56, 2002
4. Linscheid RL: The Wrist. Diagnosis and operative treatment. Disorders of the distal radioulnar joint. St. Louis Missouri, Mosby, 819-69, 1998
5. Hauck RM et al: Classification and treatment of ulnar styloid non-union. J Hand Surg 21A:418-22, 1996
6. Mann FA et al: Radiographic evaluation of the wrist: What does the hand surgeon want to know? Radiology 184:15-24, 1992
7. Melone CP et al: Traumatic disruption of the triangular fibrocartilage complex: Pathoanatomy. Clin Orthop 275:65-73, 1992

IMAGE GALLERY

Typical

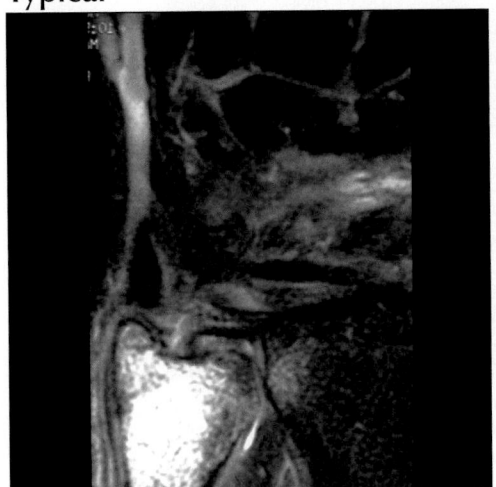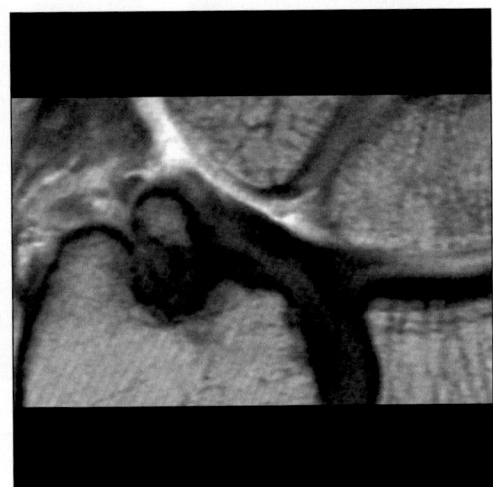

(*Left*) Coronal FS PD FSE MR shows hyperintense marrow edema associated with distal styloid fracture. (*Right*) Coronal T1 C+ MR (MR arthrogram) shows displaced ulnar styloid fracture with attachment of the ulnar margin of the TFCC.

Typical

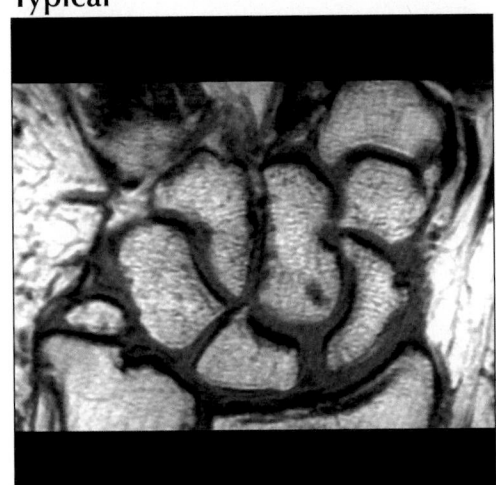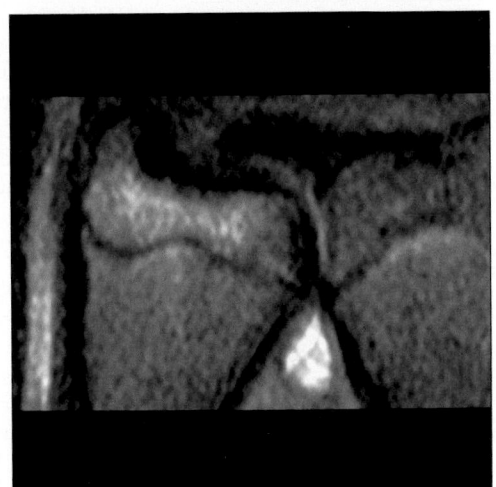

(*Left*) Coronal T1WI MR shows ulnar styloid fracture with impingement of the ulnotriquetral articulation. (*Right*) Coronal FS PD FSE MR shows hyperintense marrow edema of the distal ulnar epiphysis in trabecular microfracture.

Typical

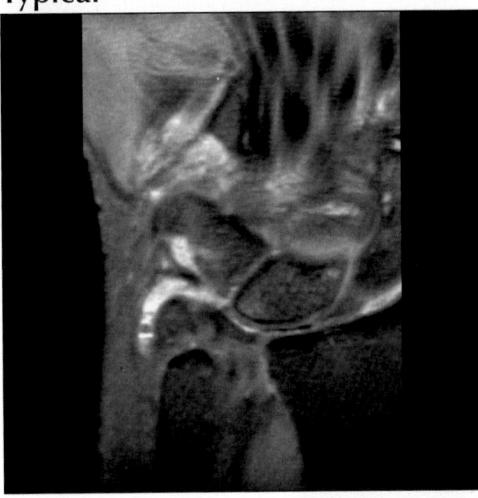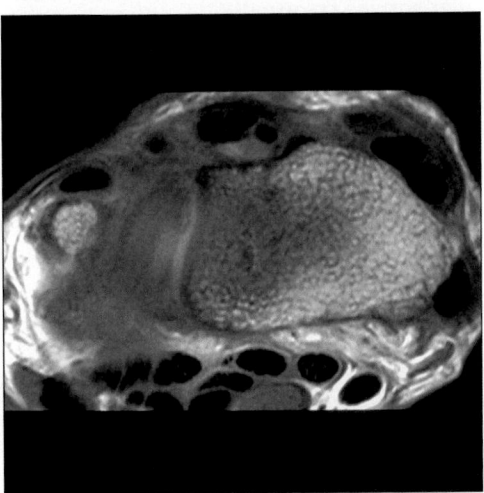

(*Left*) Coronal FS PD FSE MR shows hypointense chronic ulnar styloid fracture fragment. There is relative distal displacement of the TFCC as measured from the distal articular surface of the ulna. (*Right*) Axial T1WI MR shows the distal displacement of the ulnar styloid relative to the radiocarpal joint. The TFC articular disk is located to the right of styloid.

SCAPHOID FRACTURES

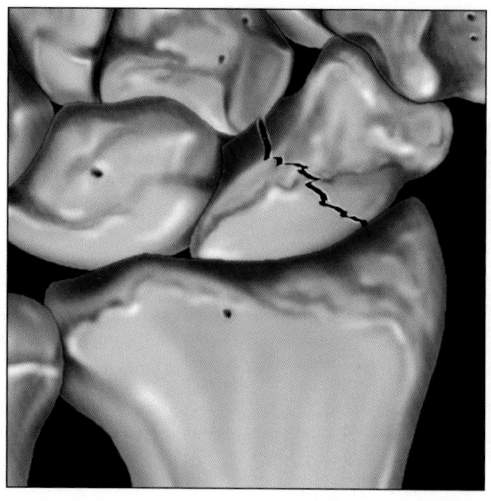

Coronal graphic shows transverse fracture of the middle third or waist of the scaphoid.

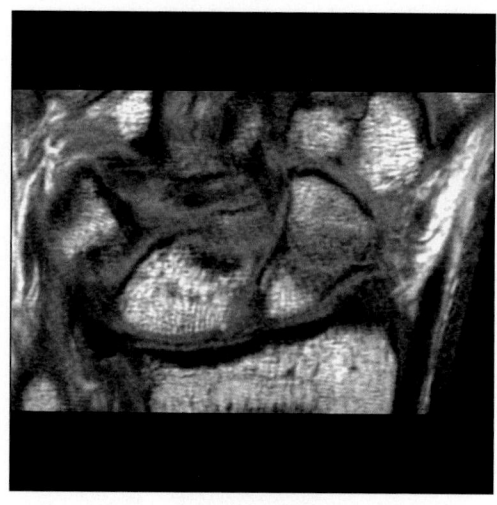

Coronal T1WI MR shows hypointense fracture line and adjacent marrow edema in fracture of middle third of the scaphoid.

TERMINOLOGY

Abbreviations and Synonyms
- Fractures of the scaphoid, navicular fracture

Definitions
- Disruption of scaphoid trabecular and/or cortical bone

IMAGING FINDINGS

General Features
- Best diagnostic clue: Transverse fracture line most commonly seen in middle third or waist of scaphoid
- Location
  - Tuberosity (distal volar prominence)
  - Distal third
  - Waist (middle third)
  - Proximal pole
- Size: Tuberosity & distal articular surface fxs usually smaller than distal third, middle third or proximal pole fxs
- Morphology
  - Horizontal oblique
  - Vertical oblique
  - Transverse

Radiographic Findings
- Radiography

- Absence or displacement of navicular fat stripe (NFS)
- Four radiographic views
  - 20° supination
  - 20° pronation
  - Neutral posteroanterior & lateral
- Distal tilt view for transverse fractures
- Scaphoid profile maximal in oblique views while making a fist + ulnar deviation
- Nondisplaced fractures - difficult to visualize

CT Findings
- NECT
  - Identify fractures when conventional radiographs negative
  - Bone technique ≤ 1 mm slice thickness + coronal & sagittal reformations
  - 3-D rendering for complex fractures ± dislocations
  - Most commonly used to assess fracture healing

MR Findings
- T1WI
  - Hypointense fracture line
  - ± Scaphoid flexion (humpback deformity) on sagittal images
  - Fracture extension to cortex differentiates acute from chronic fractures (intact cortex implies chronic)
  - Displacement (implies instability)
  - Angulation

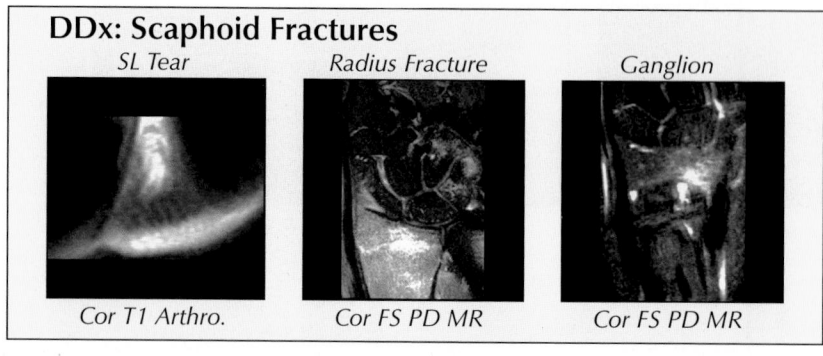

DDx: Scaphoid Fractures

SL Tear	Radius Fracture	Ganglion
Cor T1 Arthro.	Cor FS PD MR	Cor FS PD MR

SCAPHOID FRACTURES

Key Facts

Imaging Findings
- Best diagnostic clue: Transverse fracture line most commonly seen in middle third or waist of scaphoid
- ± Scaphoid flexion (humpback deformity) on sagittal images
- Evaluate for proximal pole hypointensity (avascular necrosis)
- Early scapholunate advanced collapse (SLAC) with chondral loss between distal pole scaphoid & distal radius (styloid)

Top Differential Diagnoses
- Scapholunate Ligament Tear
- Distal Radius Fractures
- Dorsal Wrist Ganglion
- De Quervain's Stenosing Tenosynovitis

Pathology
- Dorsiflexion secondary to fall
- Tensile fractures = transverse & begin in palmar cortex
- 80% in waist (middle third)
- 10% proximal pole
- 10% tuberosity or distal pole osteochondral injuries

Clinical Issues
- Most common signs/symptoms: Pain over anatomic snuffbox
- Limited range of motion
- Decreased grip strength
- Proximal third fx AVN = 14 to 39%

Diagnostic Checklist
- Evaluate scaphoid flexion deformity

- ○ Intercarpal instability - dorsal intercalated segment instability (DISI)
- ○ Displaced and unstable = > 1 mm step-off or increased capitolunate angle (> 30°)
- T2WI
  - ○ Hypo to hyperintense fracture line
  - ○ Hyperintense subchondral marrow edema adjacent to or on both sides of fracture
  - ○ Less common - diffuse scaphoid hyperintense marrow edema within scaphoid
  - ○ FS PD FSE or STIR sensitive to proximal pole edema
  - ○ Hyperintense signal associated with injury to scapholunate ligament + volar capsule (radioscaphocapitate & radiolunotriquetral ligaments)
  - ○ Evaluate for proximal pole hypointensity (avascular necrosis)
  - ○ Early scapholunate advanced collapse (SLAC) with chondral loss between distal pole scaphoid & distal radius (styloid)
- T2* GRE: Identifies loss of normal trabecular pattern (marrow edema is diminished relative to fx line)
- T1 C+: Document viability of proximal pole with enhancement

Imaging Recommendations
- Best imaging tool
  - ○ MR more sensitive & specific than radiography or CT
  - ○ CT best for chip fxs, tuberosity or articular surface + post op healing
- Protocol advice: T1, FS PD FSE coronal, axial & sagittal images

DIFFERENTIAL DIAGNOSIS

Scapholunate Ligament Tear
- Dissociation between scaphoid & lunate
- Scaphoid flexion relative to lunate
- Scapholunate (SL) angle > 70 degrees
- Associated with dorsal intercalated segment instability (DISI) & avulsion fracture

Distal Radius Fractures
- Low energy metaphyseal injuries (Colles')
- Violent (high energy) articular injuries ± comminuted & unstable
- Four components of articular fxs: Metaphyseal or shaft, radial styloid, dorsal medial & palmar medial components

Dorsal Wrist Ganglion
- Most common soft tissue mass in wrist
- Dorsal to SL interval
- 3rd to 5th decades
- Painless mass ± weakness of grip, pain or paresthesias

De Quervain's Stenosing Tenosynovitis
- Radial sided wrist pain
- Racquet sports, golf, occupational overuse
- Inability to abduct thumb, radial sided swelling, crepitus & pain
- Affects abductor pollicis longus (APL) + extensor pollicis brevis (EPR)

Capitate Fracture
- Isolated
- Fx + perilunate dislocation (scaphocapitate syndrome)
- Direct trauma
- Dorsiflexion mechanism
- Avascular necrosis & non-union

PATHOLOGY

General Features
- General path comments
  - ○ Relevant anatomy = scaphoid
    - Largest + most radial in proximal row
    - Proximal surface is biconvex for articulation with radius
    - Distal surface convex for articulation with trapezium & trapezoid
    - Dorsal surface = attachment of dorsal radiocarpal & radial collateral ligaments

SCAPHOID FRACTURES

- Palmar (volar) surface concavity containing radioscaphocapitate (RSC) ligament
- Flexor retinaculum attaches to scaphoid tubercle
- Medial - semilunar surface for lunate articulation
- Medial - large concavity for capitate articulation
- Vascular supply (radial artery): Dorsal ridge vessels supply proximal 70 to 80% of scaphoid; scaphoid tubercle branches distal 20 to 30%
- Absence of separate proximal pole blood supply = propensity for delayed healing & AVN of proximal pole
- Etiology
  - Dorsiflexion secondary to fall
  - Protective maneuver with outstretched arm
  - Forceful extension (hyperextension) + radial deviation - maximize forces across scaphoid
  - Tensile fractures = transverse & begin in palmar cortex
- Epidemiology: 79% of carpal fractures

Gross Pathologic & Surgical Features
- 80% in waist (middle third)
- 10% proximal pole
- 10% tuberosity or distal pole osteochondral injuries
- Waist fxs stable if noncomminuted & perpendicular to long axis of scaphoid
- Increased obliquity, dorsal comminution & displacement = instability
- Distal osteochondral fracture = flake of bone

Microscopic Features
- Internal vascularity
  - Dorsal scaphoid branch of radial artery
  - Volar scaphoid branch of radial artery
  - Nutrient vessels entering dorsal ridge
  - Bone failure initiated at palmar (volar) cortex

CLINICAL ISSUES

Presentation
- Most common signs/symptoms: Pain over anatomic snuffbox
- Clinical profile
  - Weakness
  - History of contact sport, fall or accident
  - Delayed diagnosis common
  - Limited range of motion
  - Pain with radial deviation & flexion
  - Decreased grip strength

Demographics
- Age
  - Young & elderly
  - Most common in adolescents & young athletes
- Gender: M > F

Natural History & Prognosis
- Uncomplicated fx = union rate up to 95%
- Associated injuries
  - SL dissociation
  - Capitate head shear fx & triquetral fx
  - Proximal pole fx - delayed healing
  - Tuberosity fx - good healing
- Complications

- Nonunion
- Malunion
- Degenerative changes
- Proximal pole AVN
- DISI
- Humpback deformity

Treatment
- Conservative
  - Immobilization & cast application
- Surgical
  - Internal fixation for displaced fxs
  - Herbert screws - interfragmentary compression = 92% success rate (Kirschner wires)
- Complications
  - Proximal third fx AVN = 14 to 39%
  - Middle third non-union = 20%
  - Pseudoarthrosis at fracture site

DIAGNOSTIC CHECKLIST

Consider
- Trabecular fracture line may persist with intact radial/ulnar cortices in healing phase
- Evaluate scaphoid flexion deformity
- Assess presence of SLAC arthritis
- Fracture line may be obscured on PD or conventional T2WI vs. T1 & FS PD FSE MR

SELECTED REFERENCES

1. Brydie A et al: Early MRI in the management of clinical scaphoid fracture. Br J Radiol 76(905):296-300, 2003
2. Cooney WP: Scaphoid fractures: Current treatments and techniques. Instr Course Lect 52:197-208, 2003
3. Rennie WJ et al: Posttraumatic cyst-like defects of the scaphoid: Late sign of occult microfracture and useful indicator of delayed union. AJR 180(3):655-8, 2003
4. McCallister WV et al: Central placement of the screw in simulated fractures of the scaphoid waist: A biomechanical study. J Bone Joint Surg Am 85A(1):72-7, 2003
5. Wu WC: Percutaneous cannulated screw fixation of acute scaphoid fractures. Hand Surg 7(2):271-8, 2002
6. Akahane M et al: Static scapholunate dissociation diagnosed by scapholunate gap view in wrists with or without distal radius fractures. Hand Surg 7(2):191-5, 2002
7. McGrory BJ et al: The wrist. Diagnosis and operative treatment. Malunion of the distal radius. vol 1. St. Louis Missouri, Mosby, 385-430, 1998
8. Markiewitz AD et al: The wrist and it's disorders. Carpal fractures and dislocations. 2nd ed. Philadelphia Pennsylvania, W.B. Saunders, 189-233, 1997
9. Duppe H et al: Long term results of fracture of the scaphoid. J Bone Joint Surg 76A:249-52, 1994
10. Adams BD et al: Treatment of scaphoid non-union with casting and pulse electromagnetic fields. A study continuation. J Hand Surg 17A:910-14, 1992
11. Diao G et al: Anatomic scaphoid classification: An algorithm for management of scaphoid fractures. Presented at the Am Soc for Surg of the Hand, 1992
12. Cope JR: Rotatory subluxation of the scaphoid. Clin Radiol 35:495-501, 1984

SCAPHOID FRACTURES

IMAGE GALLERY

Typical

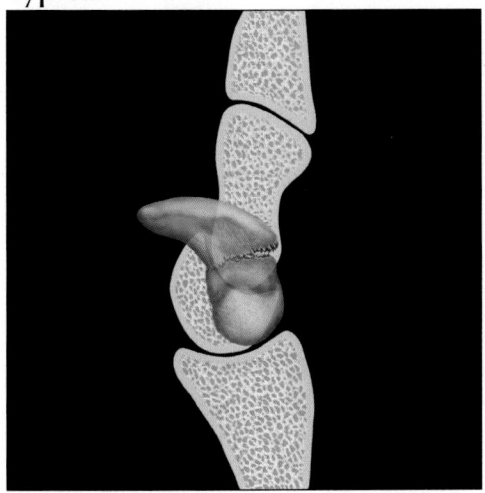

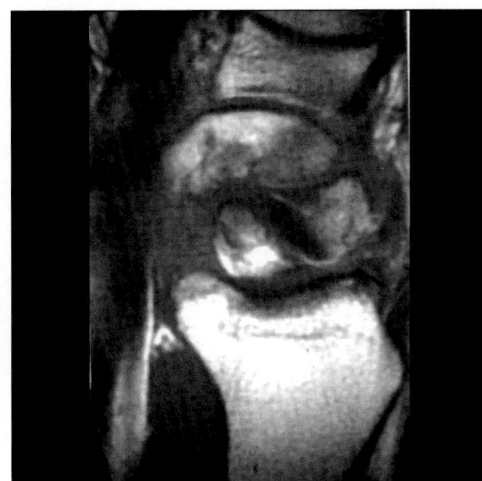

(Left) Sagittal graphic shows scaphoid flexion with humpback deformity resulting in foreshortening of the carpus. *(Right)* Sagittal T1WI MR shows humpback deformity of the scaphoid post internal fixation with a Herbert screw. This flexion deformity is associated with a DISI pattern even in the absence of a SL ligament tear.

Typical

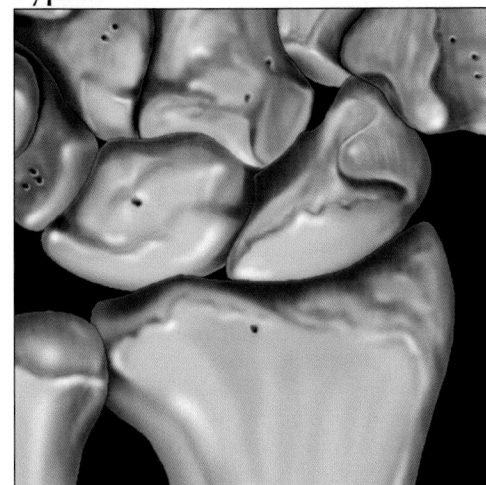

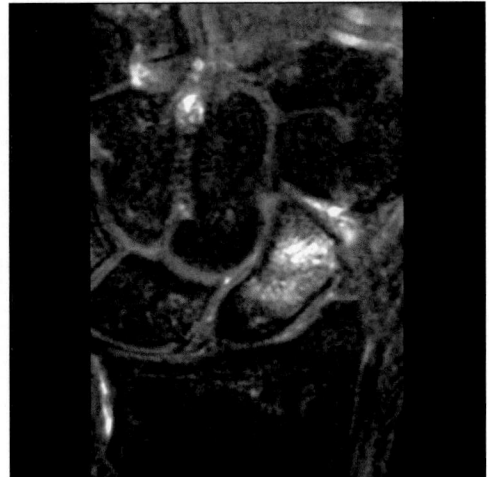

(Left) Coronal graphic shows flexion of the scaphoid with mild rotation in rotatory instability. *(Right)* Coronal FS PD FSE MR shows hyperintense marrow edema both proximal and distal to the scaphoid fracture site.

Typical

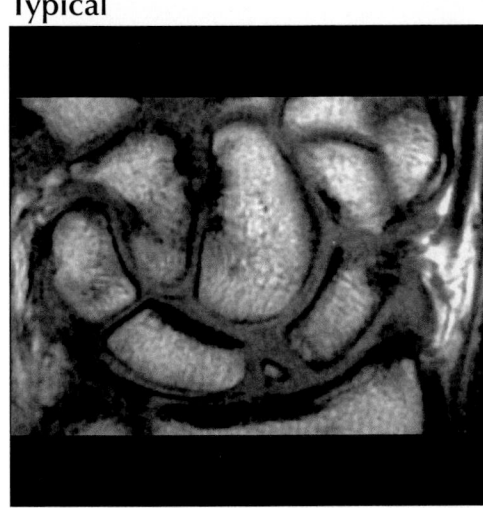

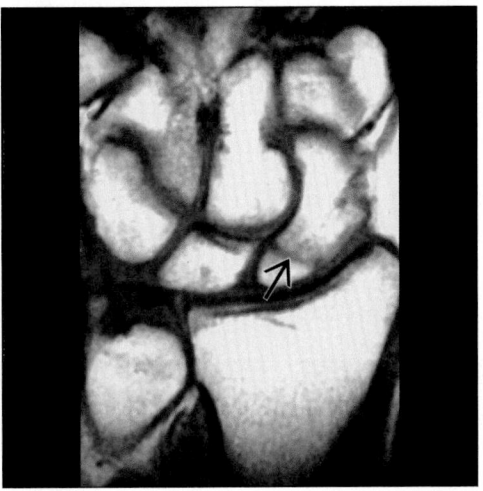

(Left) Coronal T1WI MR shows selective avulsion fracture from the scaphoid attachment of the SL ligament. *(Right)* Coronal T1WI MR shows persistent hypointense fracture line (arrow) across the proximal pole of the scaphoid despite intact radial and ulnar cortical margins in a healing scaphoid fracture. Radiographs were normal.

HAMATE FRACTURES

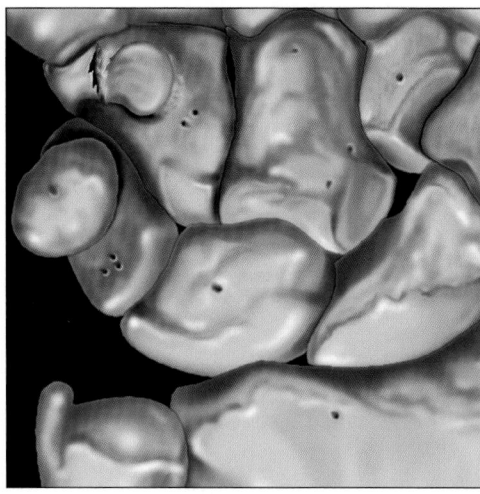

Coronal graphic shows hook of the hamate fracture with mild diastasis.

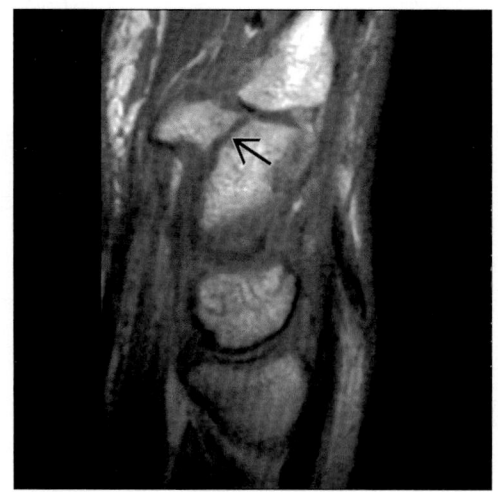

Sagittal T1WI MR shows nondisplaced hook of hamate fracture (arrow).

TERMINOLOGY

Abbreviations and Synonyms
- Fractures of the hamate, hamulus (hook of hamate) fracture, carpometacarpal fracture dislocation

Definitions
- Cortical & trabecular fracture involving the body or the hook of hamate

IMAGING FINDINGS

General Features
- Best diagnostic clue: Fracture line in hamate on direct axial images
- Location
  - Body - across articular surfaces
  - Hook
  - Proximal pole
- Size
  - Variable
  - Hook fx: ± Diastasis
  - Body fx: Nondisplaced vs. fracture dislocation
- Morphology
  - Usually transverse
  - ± Oblique or comminuted in body fractures

Radiographic Findings
- Radiography
  - Not diagnosed early
  - Carpal tunnel view = unreliable
  - 20° supination oblique = unreliable
  - 30° lateral & flexion/extension views often helpful
  - Loss of normal dense "C" (hook) on posteroanterior view

CT Findings
- NECT
  - Bone technique, ≤ 1 mm slice thickness
  - Coronal & sagittal reformations or direct acquisition
  - Cortical disruption
  - Lucent fracture line ± displacement
  - Loss of normal osseous concavity of hook
  - Have option of 3-D renderings for surgical planning

MR Findings
- T1WI
  - Hypointense fracture line
  - Hook fractures transverse on axial & vertical on sagittal images
  - Hypointense marrow edema of hook or body in acute injury
  - Subacute to chronic hook fxs may be missed on coronal images
  - ± Displacement of hook fxs (axial or sagittal plane)

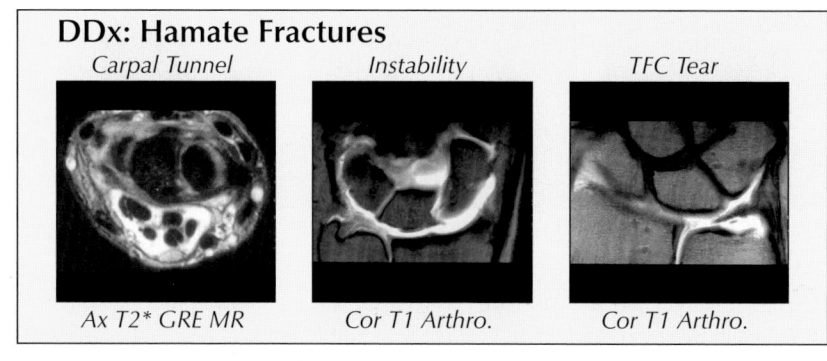

DDx: Hamate Fractures

Carpal Tunnel	Instability	TFC Tear
Ax T2* GRE MR	Cor T1 Arthro.	Cor T1 Arthro.

HAMATE FRACTURES

Key Facts

Imaging Findings
- Best diagnostic clue: Fracture line in hamate on direct axial images
- Body - across articular surfaces
- Hook
- Proximal pole

Top Differential Diagnoses
- Ulnar Tunnel Syndrome
- Carpal Tunnel Syndrome
- Ligament Sprain/Carpal Instability
- Flexor Tenosynovitis/Tendinitis
- Triangular Fibrocartilage (TFC) Tear

Pathology
- Fall on outstretched wrist (dorsiflexion)
- Direct trauma
- Fall or direct blow on flexed + ulnarly deviated fist
- Impaction against lunate articular surface (wrist in dorsiflexion & ulnar deviation)

Clinical Issues
- Most common signs/symptoms: Soreness in palm
- Distribution - ulnar aspect wrist
- ± Ulnar nerve palsy
- Decrease in grip strength
- Painful finger flexion
- ± Carpal tunnel syndrome
- Hook fxs at risk for non-union if involvement is palmar & not base

Diagnostic Checklist
- Always evaluate axial & sagittal images before excluding a fracture

- T2WI
  - Hypointense fracture line
  - Hyperintense marrow edema with body or hook fractures (hook or body edema)
  - Requires FS PD FSE or STIR to appreciate acute/subacute marrow edema
  - ± Displaced articular fx
  - ± Osteochondral fx
  - ± Dislocations
  - Effacement of ulnar aspect carpal tunnel
    - Level of ulnar sided flexor digitorum profundus tendons

Imaging Recommendations
- Best imaging tool
  - MR or CT
  - MR identifies subchondral marrow edema + associated chondral/soft tissue abnormalities
- Protocol advice: T1 (for edema & sclerosis detection) & FS PD FSE coronal, axial & sagittal

DIFFERENTIAL DIAGNOSIS

Ulnar Tunnel Syndrome
- Irritation of ulnar nerve in Guyon's canal
- Numbness or paresthesias
- Distribution = 5th finger & ulnar side of ring finger

Carpal Tunnel Syndrome
- Compromised motor/sensory function of median nerve at level of carpal tunnel
- Trauma + repetitive wrist activities
- Hemorrhage
- Infection
- Infiltrative disease
- Pain & numbness at thumb, index, middle fingers & radial ½ ring finger

Ligament Sprain/Carpal Instability
- Interosseous ligament sprain: Scapholunate, lunotriquetral
- Palmar carpal ligament
- Pisohamate ligament
- Palmar carpometacarpal ligament
- Dorsal carpometacarpal ligament

Flexor Tenosynovitis/Tendinitis
- Ulnar profundus tendons
- Single traumatic event or repetitive use
- Repair response: Inflammation, proliferation & maturation
- Hyperintensity of sheath (fluid) on T2WI

Triangular Fibrocartilage (TFC) Tear
- Traumatic vs. degenerative
- Centrum or disk = communication or perforation
- Tearing of dorsal or volar margins (radioulnar ligaments) + centrum = distal radioulnar joint (DRUJ) instability
- Primary sign = fluid extension across articular disk or discontinuity

Ulnar Styloid Fracture
- Complex distal radioulnar joint (DRUJ) dislocations
- Distal radial fxs - commonly associated
- TFCC injuries
  - Ulnar styloid avulsion at base destabilizes DRUJ

PATHOLOGY

General Features
- General path comments
  - Relevant anatomy = hamate or related structures
    - Pisohamate ligament - connects pisiform to hook of hamate (distally)
    - Hamate - supports 4th & 5th metacarpal bases
    - Most ulnar bone in distal row
    - Hook - projects from palmar surface
    - Distal surface articulates with 4th & 5th metacarpals by two facets with dividing anteroposterior ridge
    - Dorsal surface = triangular + roughened for ligamentous attachment
    - Palmar surface - pronounced hook

HAMATE FRACTURES

- Hook serves as ulnar attachment to distal flexor retinaculum + origins of flexor digiti minimi (FDM) & opponens digiti minimi (ODM)
- Palmar surface - insertion of flexor carpi ulnaris via pisohamate ligament
- Radial surface concavity = pulley mechanism for flexor tendons
- Ulnar surface articulates with triquetrum
- Triquetrohamate joint has spiral orientation - influences motion between carpal rows
- Etiology
  - Hook fracture
    - Fall on outstretched wrist (dorsiflexion)
    - Tension applied through transverse carpal & pisohamate ligament
    - Direct trauma
    - Catching a ball
    - Bat, hockey stick or golf club related
    - Dominant hand in racquet sports
    - Nondominant hand in other causes
  - Distal hamate - displaced articular fracture
    - Force propagated along 5th metacarpal shaft
    - Fall or direct blow on flexed + ulnarly deviated fist
  - Proximal pole osteochondral fracture
    - Impaction against lunate articular surface (wrist in dorsiflexion & ulnar deviation)
  - Osteochondral fractures of triquetral articular surface
    - Shearing injury or impaction against lunate
  - Bony fractures & dislocations
    - Direct crushing injuries
    - Punch-press accidents
    - Fall on hyperdorsiflexed & ulnar deviated wrist
    - Posterior dislocation or subluxation of 4th/5th metacarpals
- Epidemiology: 1.5% of carpal fxs

Gross Pathologic & Surgical Features
- Fx body - involvement of articular surfaces
- Intraarticular fracture involvement
  - Capitohamate
  - Triquetrohamate
  - Hamatometacarpal
- Base fxs of hook = good blood supply
- Palmar fxs of hook (towards tip) = greater displacement and risk of nonunion

Microscopic Features
- Palmar hook non-union
  - Inadequate fracture site callus
  - Osseous resorption
  - Decreased cancellous vascularity

Staging, Grading or Classification Criteria
- Body fractures (described relative to hook)
  - Medial (ulnar)
  - Lateral (radial)

CLINICAL ISSUES

Presentation
- Most common signs/symptoms: Soreness in palm
- Clinical profile

- Acute or chronic pain & tenderness
- Distribution - ulnar aspect wrist
- ± Ulnar nerve palsy
- Decrease in grip strength
- Painful finger flexion
- ± Carpal tunnel syndrome

Demographics
- Age: Young, active patients, especially athletes
- Gender: M > F, as a function of participation in baseball, hockey, golf & tennis

Natural History & Prognosis
- Majority of body fxs heal with immobilization
- Hook fxs at risk for non-union if involvement is palmar & not base

Treatment
- Conservative
  - Cast or splint immobilization
  - Nondisplaced hook fxs
- Surgical
  - Excision of displaced comminuted fx or non-union
  - Distal articular body fxs + dislocation of 4th & 5th metacarpals require open reduction and internal fixation (ORIF)
- Complications
  - Non-union

DIAGNOSTIC CHECKLIST

Consider
- A bipartite hook or os hamuli proprium (incomplete fusion of ossification center of hook) may mimic a fracture
- Always evaluate axial & sagittal images before excluding a fracture

SELECTED REFERENCES

1. David TS et al: Symptomatic, partial union of the hook of the hamate fracture in athletes. Am J Sports Med 31(1):106-200, 2003
2. Guha AR et al: Stress fracture of the hook of the hamate. Br J Sports Med 36(3):224-5, 2002
3. DeSchrijver F et al: Fracture of the hook of the hamate, often misdiagnosed as "wrist sprain". J Emerg Med 20(1):57-60, 2000
4. Akahane M et al: Fracture of hamate hook - diagnosis by the hamate hook lateral view 5(2):131-7, 2000
5. Cooney WP: The wrist. Diagnosis and operative treatment. Isolated carpal fractures. vol 1. St. Louis Missouri, Mosby, (19):474-89, 1998
6. Markiewit AD et al: The wrist and it's disorders. Carpal fractures and dislocations. 2nd ed. Philadelphia Pennsylvania, W.B. Saunders, (13):189-233, 1997

HAMATE FRACTURES

IMAGE GALLERY

Typical

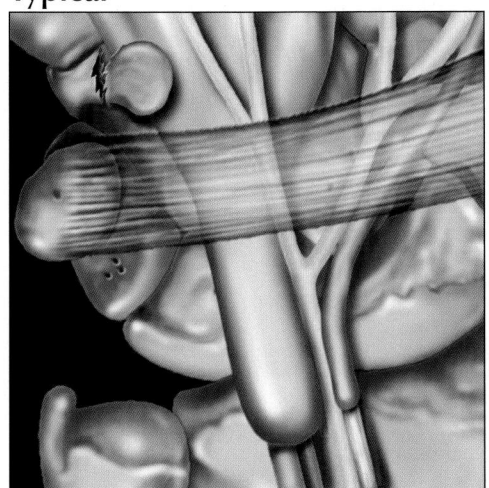

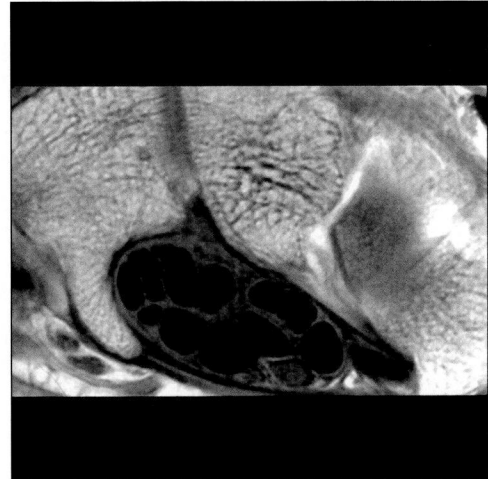

(Left) Coronal graphic shows hook of the hamate fracture with adjacent ulnar nerve (yellow) and flexor carpi ulnaris tendon sheath (blue, ulnar side). The flexor retinaculum is superficial to tendon sheath. *(Right)* Axial T1WI MR shows normal relationship of hook of the hamate to ulnar aspect of the carpal tunnel.

Typical

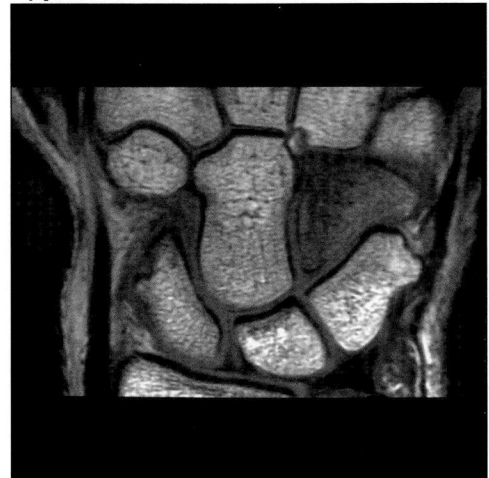

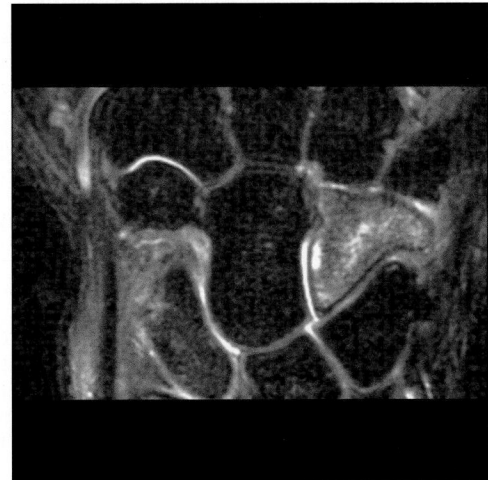

(Left) Coronal T1WI MR shows marrow edema in a nondisplaced fracture of body of the hamate. *(Right)* Coronal FS PD FSE MR shows hyperintense marrow edema of the hamate body. Hamate body edema may be seen with both hook and body fractures.

Typical

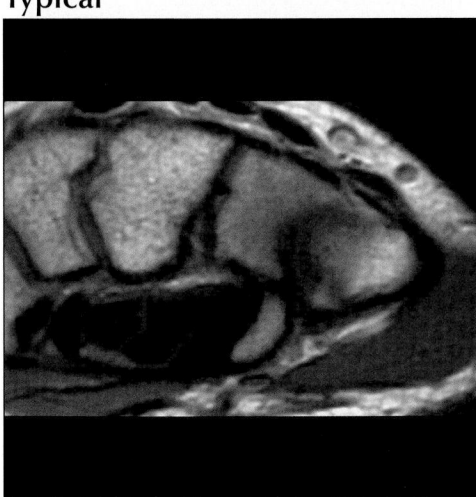

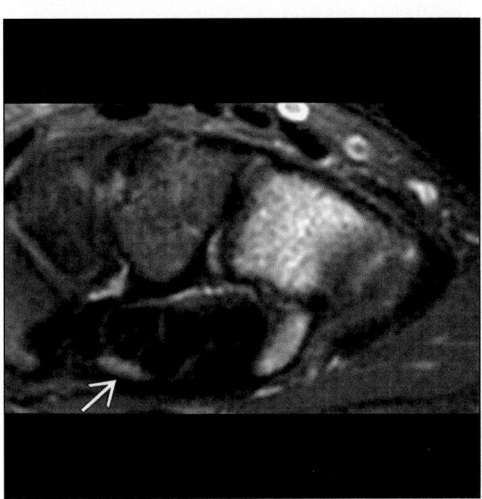

(Left) Axial T1WI MR shows impingement on the ulnar aspect of the carpal tunnel secondary to a hook fracture. *(Right)* Axial FS PD FSE MR shows hyperintensity of the median nerve (arrow) in association with effacement (flattening) of ulnar aspect of the carpal tunnel. There is marrow edema in both hook and body of the hamate.

SCAPHOID NON-UNION

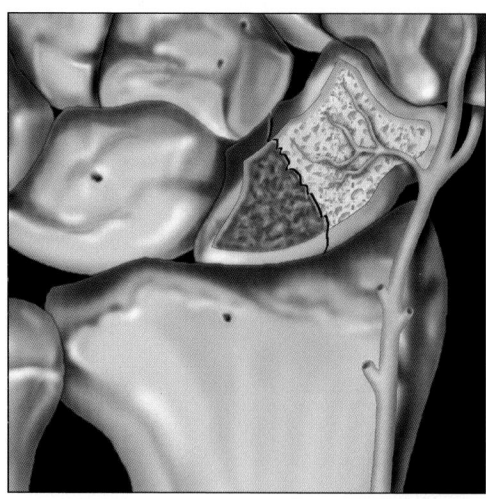

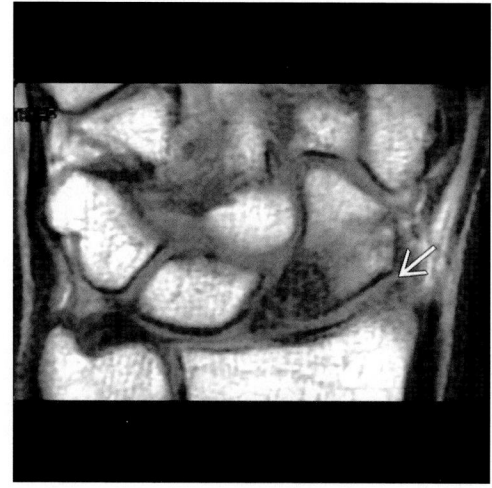

Coronal graphic shows fracture of proximal pole of scaphoid with avascular necrosis. The vascular supply via the radial artery is received from the distal pole.

Coronal T1WI MR shows hypointense AVN secondary to proximal pole fracture. Radioscaphoid sclerosis (arrow) represents stage I SLAC. SNAC represents SLAC and scaphoid non-union.

TERMINOLOGY

Abbreviations and Synonyms
- Non-union, non-union of scaphoid, scaphoid pseudoarthrosis

Definitions
- Scaphoid fracture fails to unite within 6 months of injury

IMAGING FINDINGS

General Features
- Best diagnostic clue: Absence of bridging trabecular bone on coronal or sagittal images
- Location
  - Proximal third fracture
  - Vertical oblique fracture middle third
- Size: Bridging radial to ulnar (lateral to medial cortex)
- Morphology: Non-union defect prismatic in shape with quadrilateral base

Radiographic Findings
- Radiography
  - Posteroanterior (PA), lateral & oblique
  - Fracture pattern
  - Location + displacement
  - Carpal instability
  - Arthritic change
  - Obtain grip compression PA in ulnar deviation if scapholunate (SL) angle < 70° with positive degenerative changes
  - PA-ulnar deviation: Fragment separation = unstable non-union = pseudoarthrosis
  - Assessment of healing inferior to CT or MRI

CT Findings
- NECT
  - Bone technique
  - ≤ 1 mm sections
  - Direct coronal images or coronal & sagittal reformations
  - Assessment of healing + detection of pseudoarthrosis

MR Findings
- T1WI
  - Hypointensity across fracture site
  - Displacement - cortical offset ≥ 1 mm
    - Dorsal intercalated segment instability (DISI) on sagittal images
    - Dorsal gap on sagittal images through scaphoid
    - Non-union = loss of coaptation
  - Instability
    - Between proximal & distal carpal rows
    - Increased scapholunate & capitolunate angles on sagittal images
    - DISI (sagittal plane)

DDx: Scaphoid Non-Union

Scaphoid Fracture	SL Ligament Tear	Radius Fracture

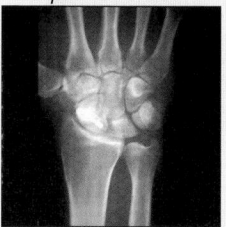

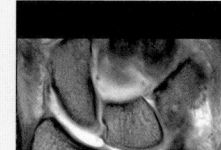

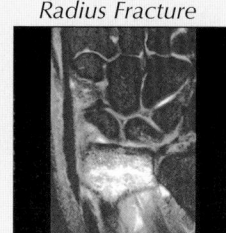

AP Radiography   *Cor T1 Arthro.*   *Cor FS PD MR*

SCAPHOID NON-UNION

Key Facts

Imaging Findings

- Best diagnostic clue: Absence of bridging trabecular bone on coronal or sagittal images
- Proximal third fracture
- Vertical oblique fracture middle third
- Morphology: Non-union defect prismatic in shape with quadrilateral base

Top Differential Diagnoses

- Scaphoid Fractures
- Scapholunate Ligament Tear
- Distal Radius Fractures
- De Quervain's Stenosing Tenosynovitis

Pathology

- DISI
- Loss of proximal fragment blood supply

Epidemiology

- Epidemiology: Non-union rate up to 12%
- Fragmentation & collapse proximal pole = late stage

Clinical Issues

- Most common signs/symptoms: Wrist pain
- Weakness of grip
- Loss of dorsiflexion
- Initially symptomatic post injury vs. delayed onset symptoms until degenerative changes or re-injury
- Displaced non-union more severe symptoms than nondisplaced non-union
- SNAC = greater arc injury (scaphoid non-union)
- 97% with arthritis in non-union ≥ 5 years in duration

Diagnostic Checklist

- Identify degenerative changes of SNAC

- Trabecular erosion - volar defect at fx site
  - Avascular necrosis (AVN)
    - Hypointense proximal pole AVN
    - Predisposed fx pattern & location = proximal third, vertical oblique middle third
- T2WI
  - Displacement
    - Offset + interruption of intermediate signal articular cartilage
    - Non-union site with persistent intermediate signal intensity
    - Hypointense - intermediate signal in pseudoarthrosis
  - Instability
    - ± Hyperintensity in prismatic volar defect associated with scaphoid angulation
    - Degenerative loss of joint space (chondral loss) radioscaphoid, scaphocapitate & capitolunate joints
    - Scaphoid non-union advanced collapse (SNAC)
  - Avascular necrosis
    - Hypointensity in chronic phase with nonviable marrow
    - Hyperintensity in acute/subacute phase with viable marrow
    - Diffuse marrow hyperintensity may represent proximal pole ischemia + reactive edema of distal pole
- T1 C+
  - Define non-union site
  - Enhancement of viable proximal pole marrow

Imaging Recommendations

- Best imaging tool
  - MR defines marrow changes in AVN + associated instability
  - CT for best detection of fracture healing & pseudoarthrosis

DIFFERENTIAL DIAGNOSIS

Scaphoid Fractures

- Most common fracture of carpus
- Associated dorsiflexion loading & radial deviation mechanism
- 70 to 80% involve middle third (scaphoid waist)
- Waist and proximal pole fractures at risk for delayed union & AVN
- Pain over anatomic snuffbox

Scapholunate Ligament Tear

- Dissociation between scaphoid & lunate
- Scaphoid flexion
- Scapholunate angle > 70 degrees
- Associated with DISI & avulsion fracture

Distal Radius Fractures

- Low energy metaphyseal injuries (Colles')
- Violent (high energy) articular injuries ± comminuted & unstable
- Articular fxs

De Quervain's Stenosing Tenosynovitis

- Radial sided wrist pain
- Racquet sports, golf, occupational overuse
- Inability to abduct thumb, radial sided swelling, crepitus & pain
- Affects abductor pollicis longus (APL) + extensor pollicis brevis (EPB)

PATHOLOGY

General Features

- General path comments
  - Relevant anatomy
    - Normal intact scaphoid exerts a flexion moment on radial side of the proximal row balanced by extension moment on ulnar side
- Etiology
  - Etiology of non-union
    - Severity of injury

SCAPHOID NON-UNION

- Fracture pattern (vertical oblique fracture)
- Location (proximal third)
- Displacement of fragments
- Ligamentous injury
- DISI
- Loss of proximal fragment blood supply
- Smaller diameter proximal pole - at risk
- Delayed diagnosis
- Ineffective immobilization
- Epidemiology: Non-union rate up to 12%

Gross Pathologic & Surgical Features
- Fx proximal thirds vs. vertical oblique fx middle third
- Cortical offset ≥ 1 mm
- Stage 1 perilunar instability (triquetrum, lunate & proximal fragment of scaphoid slide volarly into extension)
- Volar defect - trabecular erosion
- Fragmentation & collapse proximal pole = late stage

Microscopic Features
- Inadequate fracture site trabeculation
- Osseous resorption
- Interruption of blood supply with decreased cancellous vascularity

Staging, Grading or Classification Criteria
- Type 1: Simple non-union
  - Nondisplaced & no degenerative change
- Type 2: Unstable non-union
  - Displacement (> 1 mm) or DISI (SL angle > 70°), no degenerative change
- Type 3: Early arthritic non-union
  - Radioscaphoid arthritis
- Type 4: Scaphoid non-union advanced collapse (SNAC wrist)
- Type 5: Scaphoid non-union advanced collapse-plus (SNAC plus)
  - Arthritis throughout wrist

CLINICAL ISSUES

Presentation
- Most common signs/symptoms: Wrist pain
- Clinical profile
  - Weakness of grip
  - Loss of dorsiflexion
  - Initially symptomatic post injury vs. delayed onset symptoms until degenerative changes or re-injury
  - Displaced non-union more severe symptoms than nondisplaced non-union
  - SNAC = greater arc injury (scaphoid non-union)

Demographics
- Age: 2nd or 3rd decade most common
- Gender: M > F

Natural History & Prognosis
- 97% with arthritis in non-union ≥ 5 years in duration
- Degenerative arthritis sequence
  - Radioscaphoid (first)
  - Scaphocapitate (second)
  - Capitolunate (third)

- Degenerative change in nondisplaced non-unions confined to radioscaphoid joint
- Sparing of radiolunate joint
- SNAC
  - Late degenerative change with DISI
  - Stage 1 perilunar instability like SLAC
  - SNAC = greater arc injury (scaphoid non-union)
  - SLAC = lesser arc injury (scapholunate dissociation)

Treatment
- Conservative
  - Non displaced fxs < 6 months from injury - immobilization
  - Electrical stimulation
- Surgical
  - Symptomatic non-union in young patient
  - Type I simple = inlay bone graft
  - Type 2 unstable = volar wedge graft
  - Type 3 early = wedge graft, ORIF & styloidectomy
  - Type 4 SNAC = midcarpal fusion with scaphoid excision
  - Type 5 SNAC-plus = arthrodesis

DIAGNOSTIC CHECKLIST

Consider
- Identify degenerative changes of SNAC
- Evaluate for AVN or small fragment size of proximal pole (poor candidates for bone grafting)

SELECTED REFERENCES

1. Linscheid RL et al: The wrist. Diagnosis and operative treatment: Scaphoid fractures and nonunion. St. Louis MO, Mosby, (17):385-430, 1998
2. Kerluke L et al: Nonunion of the scaphoid: A critical analysis of recent natural history studies. J Hand Surg 18A:1-3, 1993
3. Kirschenbaum D et al: Scaphoid excision and capitolunate arthrodesis for radioscaphoid arthritis. J Hand Surg 18A:780-85, 1993
4. Jirenek WA et al: Long-term results after Russe bone-grafting: The effect of malunion of the scaphoid. J Bone Joint Surg 74A:1217-27, 1992
5. Krimmer VA et al: Advanced carpal collapse in scaphoid nonunion: Partial mediocarpal fusion as a therapeutic concept. Handchir Mikrochir Plas Chir 24:191-8, 1992
6. Lundstrom G et al: Natural history of scaphoid non-union, with special reference to "asymptomatic" cases. J Hand Surg 17B:697-700, 1992
7. Barton NJ: Twenty questions about scaphoid fractures. J Hand Surg 17B:289-310, 1992
8. Balsole RJ et al: Computed analyses of the pathomechanics of scaphoid waist non-unions. J Hand Surg 16A:899-908, 1991
9. Nakamura R et al: Analysis of scaphoid fractures displacement by three-dimensional computed tomography. J Hand Surg 16:485-92, 1991
10. Dias JJ et al: Patterns of union in fractures of the waist of the scaphoid. J Bone Joint Surg 71B:307-310, 1989
11. Amadio PC et al: Scaphoid malunion. J Hand Surg 14A:679-87, 1989

3

48

IMAGE GALLERY

Typical

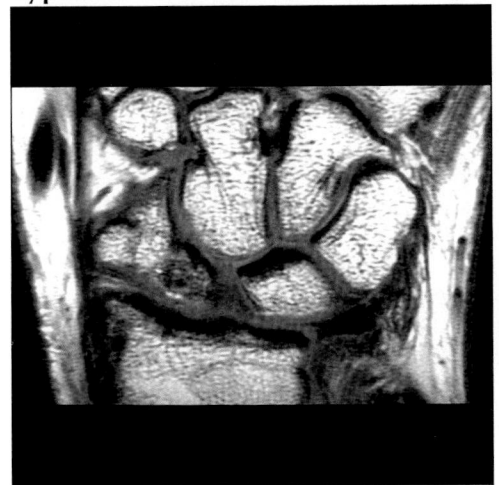
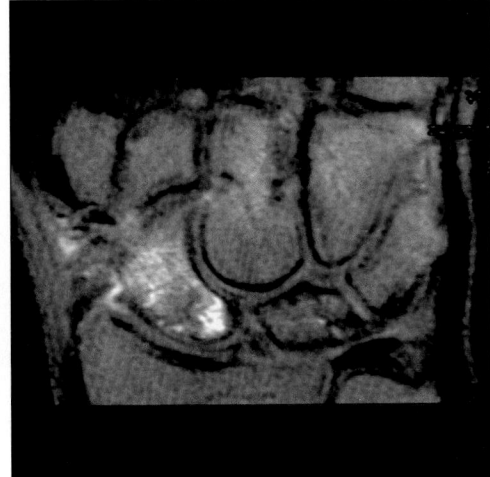

(Left) Coronal T1WI MR shows proximal pole AVN. (Right) Coronal FS PD FSE MR shows hyperintense marrow edema corresponding to intact scaphoid vascularity. Proximal pole shows greater hyperintensity compared to the distal two thirds of the scaphoid.

Typical

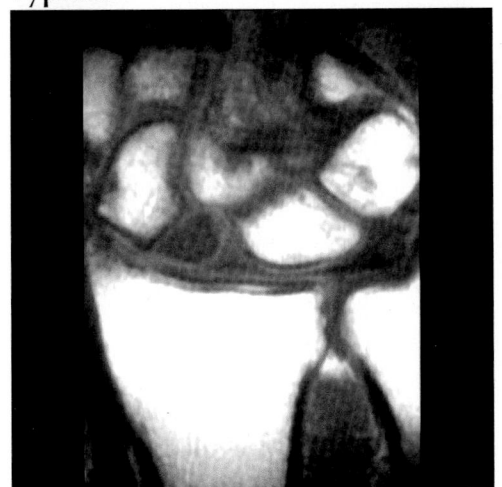
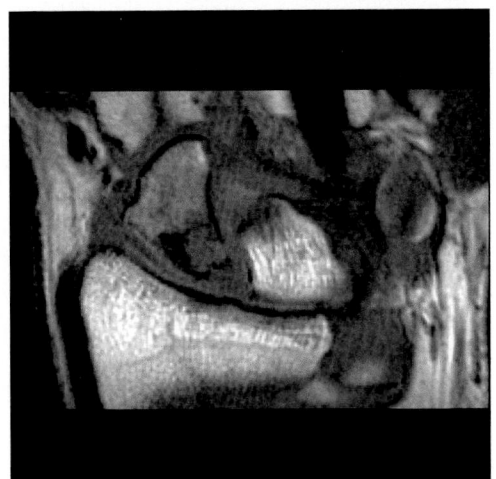

(Left) Coronal T1WI MR shows SNAC as a greater arc injury representing scaphoid non-union with the complication of AVN. Radial styloid-scaphoid sclerosis is present. (Right) Coronal T1WI MR shows AVN with fragmentation of the proximal pole.

Typical

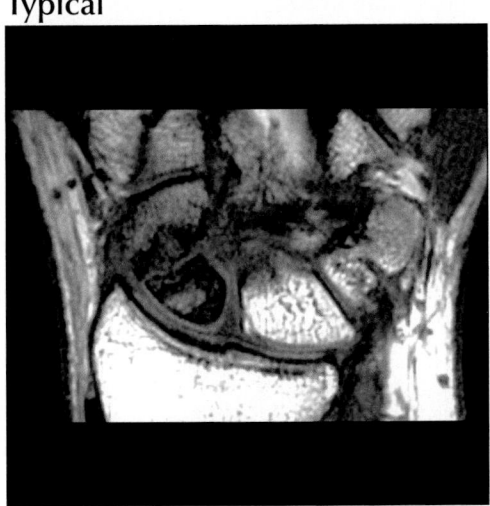
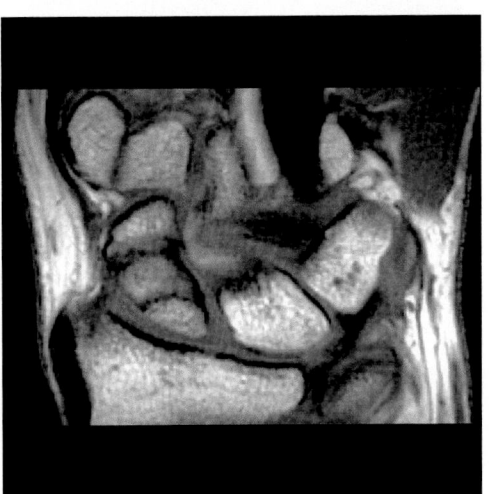

(Left) Coronal T1WI MR shows non-union with AVN of the proximal pole and fracture diastasis. (Right) Coronal T1WI MR shows non-union with a double fracture pattern of both the proximal and distal poles of the scaphoid. This pattern has a greater risk for instability.

KIENBOCK'S DISEASE

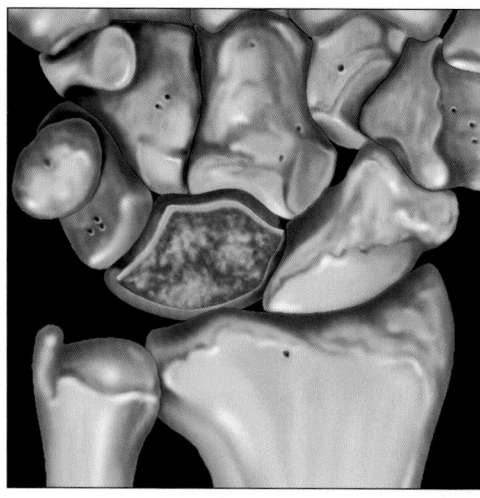

Coronal graphic shows AVN of the lunate with diffuse marrow ischemia.

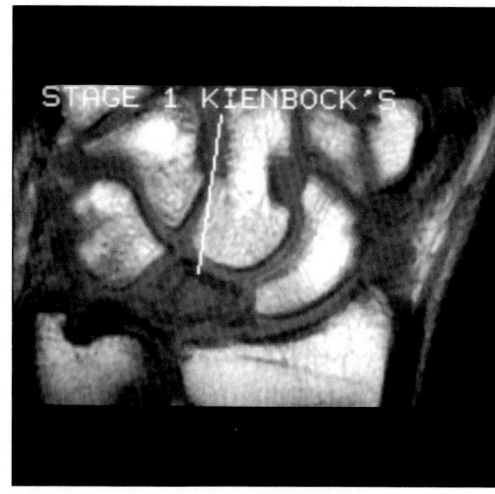

Coronal T1WI MR shows stage I Kienböck's with uniform hypointense sclerosis/edema.

TERMINOLOGY

Abbreviations and Synonyms
- Lunatomalacia, aseptic necrosis, avascular necrosis, osteochondritis, traumatic osteoporosis, osteitis

Definitions
- Avascular necrosis of lunate

IMAGING FINDINGS

General Features
- Best diagnostic clue: Hypointense lunate on T1WI
- Location
  - Lunate
  - Centralized or diffuse (sclerosis not eccentric)
- Size: Fracture to complete lunate collapse + degenerative changes at carpus
- Morphology
  - Fracture - linear (transverse) or compression
  - Marrow involvement centralized to diffuse involvement of lunate

Radiographic Findings
- Radiography
  - Increased density of lunate (early) or normal
  - ± Visualization of a fracture
  - Severe disease
    - Lunate collapse
    - Proximal migration capitate
    - Widening proximal carpal row
    - Rotation of scaphoid with foreshortening on anteroposterior (AP) views = "ring" sign

CT Findings
- NECT
  - Bone technique
  - 1 mm sections
  - Coronal & sagittal reformations or direct coronal + sagittal
  - Identify linear fracture or sclerosis

MR Findings
- T1WI
  - Hypointense transverse fracture line (stage I)
  - Centralized to diffuse marrow hypointensity (stage II)
  - Intact shape of lunate in (stage II)
  - Subtle collapse (stage II) of lunate on radial border (coronal images)
  - Lunate collapse + proximal migration of capitate (stage III)
  - Hypointense sclerosis + osteophyte formation (stage IV)
- T2WI
  - Stage I
    - Marrow hyperintensity

DDx: Kienböck's Disease

Acute Fracture	Impaction	Rheumatoid
Cor FS PD MR	Cor T1WI MR	Ax FS PD MR

KIENBOCK'S DISEASE

Key Facts

Imaging Findings
- Best diagnostic clue: Hypointense lunate on T1WI
- Size: Fracture to complete lunate collapse + degenerative changes at carpus
- Fracture - linear (transverse) or compression
- Marrow involvement centralized to diffuse involvement of lunate

Top Differential Diagnoses
- Carpal Instability
- Ulnar Impaction Syndrome
- Rheumatoid Arthritis
- Inflammatory Arthritis (Non-Rheumatoid)

Pathology
- Acute trauma
- Repeated minor trauma - 2° to excessive shear force

- Mechanism - interruption of blood supply to anatomically susceptible lunate
- Susceptible lunate = lunate with single nutrient vessel or compromised intraosseous blood supply

Clinical Issues
- Most common signs/symptoms: Dorsal tenderness about lunate
- Limited motion
- Diffuse swelling, localized synovitis
- Grip weakness
- Unilateral presentation (bilateral incidence low)

Diagnostic Checklist
- Sclerosis/marrow edema is typically central (not ulnar-sided or eccentric)

- Hypointense to hyperintense fracture (transverse)
- Microtrabecular compression fractures more common than well-defined transverse fracture
- Intermediate signal intensity synovitis
  - Stage II
    - ± Fracture lines usually hypointense if present
    - Viable marrow hyperintense on FS PD FSE or STIR
    - Use coronal & sagittal images to identify decreased height of radial aspect of lunate
  - Stage III
    - Lunate collapse in coronal plane
    - Anteroposterior elongation of lunate in sagittal plane
    - Proximal migration of capitate on coronal images
    - ± Scapholunate (SL) dissociation with hyperintensity of SL ligament
  - Stage IV
    - Hypointense sclerosis with areas of reactive marrow hyperintensity (degenerative)
    - Loss of intermediate signal intensity articular cartilage in radiocarpal & midcarpal articulations
- T1 C+: Enhancement of viable marrow (use intravenous contrast with fat suppression)

Imaging Recommendations
- Best imaging tool
  - MR superior in early detection of stage I changes including identification of fracture & marrow edema/sclerosis
  - MR - also used to follow outcome of radial shortening for revascularization of lunate

DIFFERENTIAL DIAGNOSIS

Acute Lunate Fracture
- 1.1 to 6.5% of carpal fxs
- Unusual as most fxs associated with Kienböck's disease
- Volar pole fractures - most common
- Treatment - cast immobilization

Carpal Instability
- Scapholunate

- Lunotriquetral
- Midcarpal

Ulnar Impaction Syndrome
- Triangular fibrocartilage (TFC) tear
- Chondromalacia proximal ulnar lunate & triquetrum

Rheumatoid Arthritis
- Polyarticular & symmetric
- Wrist & hand joints
- Active synovitis
- Median nerve compression 2° to volar tenosynovitis
- Fibrous or bony ankylosis

Inflammatory Arthritis (Non-Rheumatoid)
- Systemic lupus erythematosus (SLE)
- Progressive systemic sclerosis
- Psoriatic arthritis
- Gout, pseudogout

PATHOLOGY

General Features
- General path comments
  - Relevant anatomy
    - 80% lunates - both palmar and dorsal nutrient vessels
    - 20% lunates - single palmar vessel provides sole blood supply
    - There are three patterns of intraosseous blood supply to the lunate: Y pattern (59%), I pattern (31%), X pattern (10%)
- Etiology
  - Acute trauma
  - Repeated minor trauma - 2° to excessive shear force
  - Mechanism - interruption of blood supply to anatomically susceptible lunate
  - Susceptible lunate = lunate with single nutrient vessel or compromised intraosseous blood supply
  - Risk factors
    - Negative ulnar variance (ulnar minus)
    - Susceptible lunate geometry (oblong or square)
    - Vulnerable lunate vascularity

- ■ TFCC compliance (thicker TFCC in negative variance)
- Epidemiology: Incidence of 2.5% (stage III or IV disease)

Gross Pathologic & Surgical Features
- Fracture
- Cystic changes
- Fragmentation & collapse
- Radiocarpal or midcarpal arthritis

Microscopic Features
- Venous stasis
- Necrosis of bone
- Inflammatory response

Staging, Grading or Classification Criteria
- Stahl's classification based on clinical and radiographic criteria
- Decoulx = modified Stahl's (presence of fracture not required in early stages)
- Lichtman
  - ○ Stage I: Normal radiographs ± fracture
  - ○ Stage II: Sclerosis without collapse
  - ○ Stage III: Fragmentation + collapse
    - ■ IIIA = no instability
    - ■ IIIB = instability
  - ○ Stage IV: Perilunate arthritis
- MR classification based on Lichtman stage II
  - ○ A: Focal central hypointense T1, hyperintense T2
  - ○ B: Focal central hypointense T1 & T2
  - ○ C: Generalized hypointense T1 & hyperintense T2
  - ○ D: Generalized hypointense T1 & T2

CLINICAL ISSUES

Presentation
- Most common signs/symptoms: Dorsal tenderness about lunate
- Clinical profile
  - ○ Limited motion
  - ○ Diffuse swelling, localized synovitis
  - ○ Grip weakness
  - ○ Unilateral presentation (bilateral incidence low)

Demographics
- Age: 20 to 40 yrs.
- Gender: M:F = 2:1

Natural History & Prognosis
- Chronic wrist pain
- ± Associated flexor tendon or ligamentous tear
- Arthrosis of radiocarpal or midcarpal joints after lunate collapse

Treatment
- Conservative
  - ○ Immobilization to differentiate transient ischemia from Kienböck's disease
- Surgical
  - ○ Revascularization
  - ○ Radial wedge osteotomy
  - ○ Scaphoid-trapezium-trapezoid or scaphocapitate fusion

- ○ Salvage (proximal row carpectomy, arthrodesis)

DIAGNOSTIC CHECKLIST

Consider
- Sclerosis/marrow edema is typically central (not ulnar-sided or eccentric)
- More common pattern is without a defined transverse fx in early stages
- FS PD FSE or STIR to identify viable marrow

SELECTED REFERENCES
1. Palmer AK et al: The wrist. Diagnosis and operative treatment. Lunate fractures: Kienböck's disease. vol 1. St. Louis Missouri, Mosby, (18):431-739, 1998
2. Alexander CE et al: The wrist and it's disorders. Kienböck's disease and idiopathic necrosis of carpal bones. 2nd ed. Philadelphia Pennsylvania, W.B. Saunders, (18):329-46, 1997
3. Golimbu CN et al: Avascular necrosis of carpal bones. Magn Reson Imaging Clin N Am 3:281-303, 1995
4. Williams CS et al: Vascularity of the lunate. Hand Clin 9:391, 1993
5. Desser TS et al: Scaphoid fractures and Kienböck's disease of the lunate: MR imaging with histopathologic correlation. Magn Reson Imaging 8:357-61, 1995
6. Trumble TE et al: Histologic and magnetic resonance imaging correlations in Kienböck's disease. J Hand Surg 15:879-84, 1990
7. Sowa DT et al: Application of magnetic resonance imaging to ischemic necrosis of lunate. J Hand Surg 14A:1008-16, 1989
8. Amido PC et al: The genesis of Kienböck's disease: Evaluation of a case by magnetic resonance imaging. J Hand Surg Am 12:1044, 1987
9. Kristensen SS et al: Ulnar variance in Kienböck's disease. J Hand Surg Br 11:258, 1986
10. Gelberman RH et al: Kienböck's disease. Orthop Clin North Am 15:355-67, 1984
11. Kinnard P et al: Radial shortening for Kienböck's disease. Can J Surg 3:261-2, 1983
12. Morgan RF et al: Bilateral Kienböck's disease. J Hand Surg 8:928-32, 1983
13. Armistead RB et al: Ulnar lengthening in the treatment of Kienböck's disease. J Bone Joint Surg 6A:170-78, 1982
14. Eiken O et al: Radius shortening in malacia of the lunate. Scand J Plast Reconstr Surg 14:191-6, 1980
15. Gelberman RH et al: Ulnar variance in Kienböck's disease. J Bone Joint Surg 57A:674-6, 1975
16. Stahl F: On lunatomalacia (Kienböck's disease), a clinical and roentgenological study, especially on its pathogenesis and the late results of immobilization treatment. Acta Chir Scand 126:1-133, 1947

KIENBOCK'S DISEASE

IMAGE GALLERY

Typical

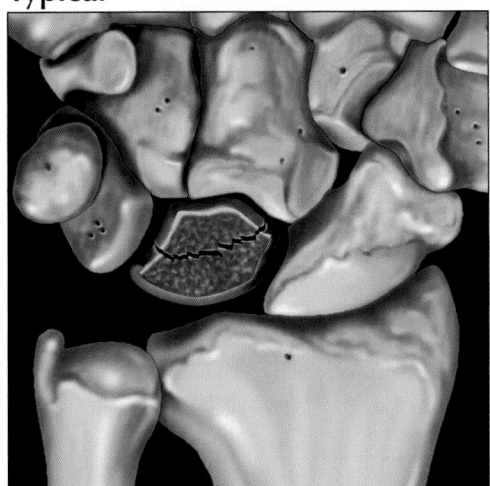

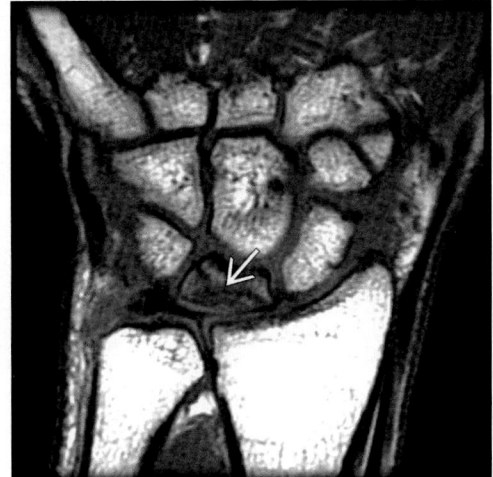

(Left) Coronal graphic shows transverse fracture of the lunate in stage I Kienböck's. *(Right)* Coronal T1WI MR shows transverse fracture (arrow) pattern with early lunate collapse. Kienböck's disease may present either with a discrete fracture or trabecular microfracture with diffuse marrow changes.

Typical

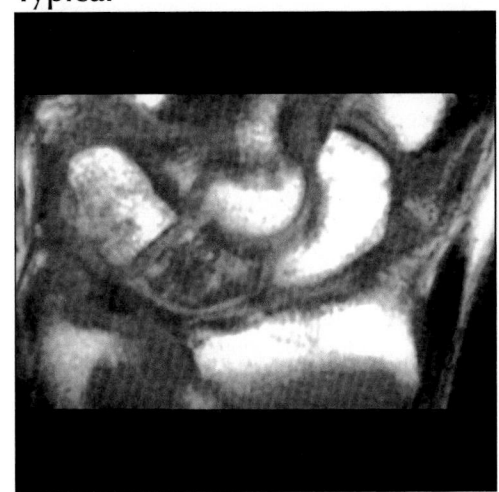

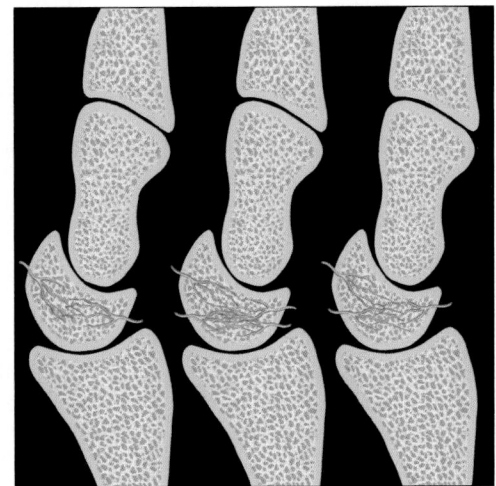

(Left) Coronal T1WI MR shows hypointense marrow edema with marrow fat inhomogeneity in stage I Kienböck's. *(Right)* Sagittal graphic shows the three common patterns of lunate's intraosseous vascular supply.

Typical

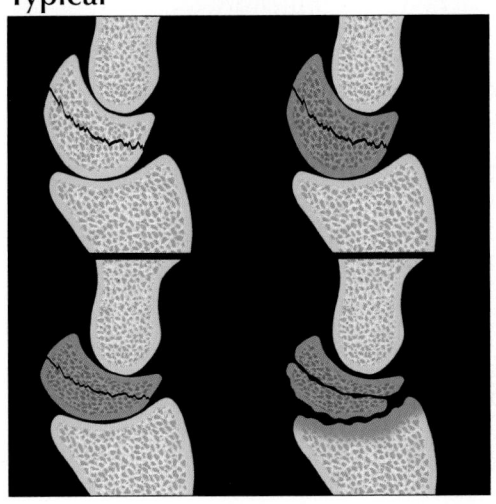

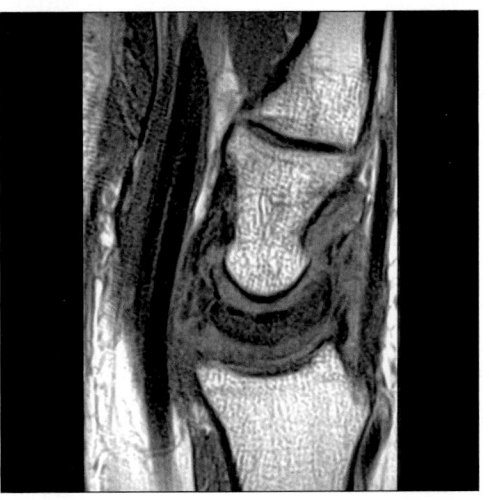

(Left) Sagittal graphic shows the progressive stages of lunate collapse. *(Right)* Sagittal T1WI MR shows elongation of the anteroposterior dimension of lunate collapse in stage III Kienböck's.

CARPAL TUNNEL SYNDROME

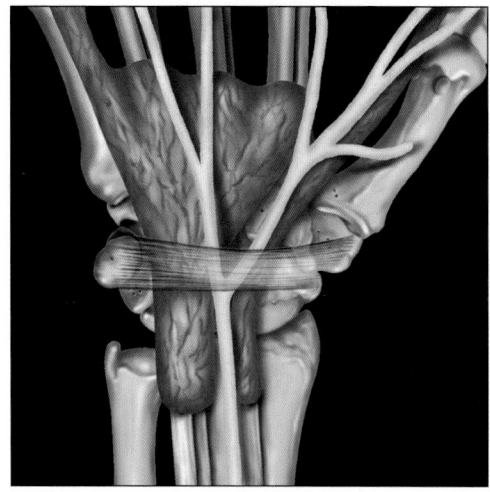

Coronal graphic shows inflammatory tenosynovitis of flexor tendons with compression of median nerve. Connective tissue degeneration is a more common cause of carpal tunnel syndrome.

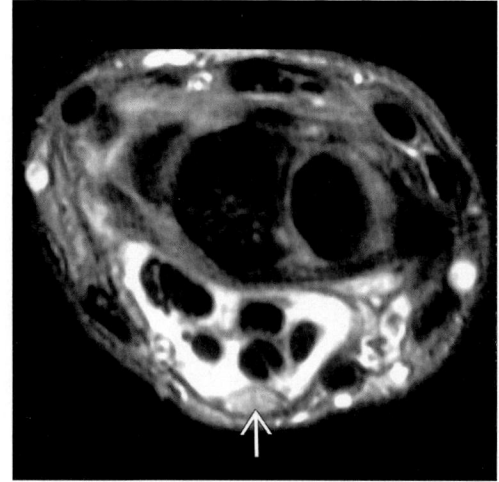

Axial T2* GRE MR shows edema surrounding the flexor tendons with hyperintensity within an enlarged medial nerve (arrow).

TERMINOLOGY

Abbreviations and Synonyms
- CTS

Definitions
- Clinical symptom complex secondary to compression of the median nerve at carpal tunnel

IMAGING FINDINGS

General Features
- Best diagnostic clue: Cross sectional enlargement & hyperintensity (FS PD FSE or STIR) of median nerve
- Location: Deep to flexor retinaculum (transverse carpal ligament)
- Size: Variable based on course of increased pressure on median nerve
- Morphology
  - Swelling or segmental enlargement of median nerve at level of pisiform
  - Flattening of median nerve at level of hamate

Radiographic Findings
- Radiography
  - Not diagnostic
  - Displaced capitate fracture
  - Visible deposits of amyloid

MR Findings
- T1WI
  - Intermediate signal intensity in swelling or segmental enlargement of median nerve at level of pisiform
    - Flattening of median nerve (level of hamate)
    - Palmar bowing of hypointense flexor retinaculum at level of hamate
    - Displaced proximal half of capitate fracture
    - Impingement in perilunar dislocation
    - Fracture of radius: Colles' or Smith's
- T2WI
  - Hyperintensity (diffuse or involving specific fascicles) of enlarged median nerve identified on axial cross section
  - FS PD FSE or STIR = improved sensitivity for nerve edema over non-fat suppression images
  - Incomplete release of flexor retinaculum associated with residual nerve hyperintensity
  - Pseudoneuroma - swelling of median nerve proximal to carpal tunnel
  - Hyperintense ganglions (e.g., triscaphe origin) which project deep to carpal tunnel & compress canal
  - Intermediate to hyperintense thickening of tenosynovium of flexor tendons
- T1 C+: Enhancement of synovium
- Fibrosis of median nerve = hypointense on T1 & T2WI

DDx: Carpal Tunnel Syndrome

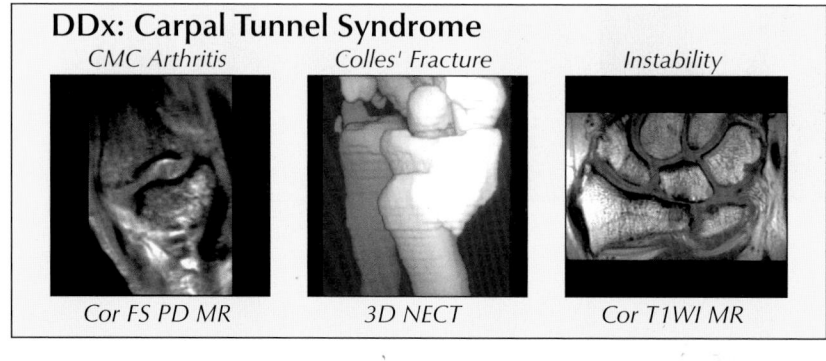

CMC Arthritis	Colles' Fracture	Instability
Cor FS PD MR	3D NECT	Cor T1WI MR

CARPAL TUNNEL SYNDROME

Key Facts

Imaging Findings
- Best diagnostic clue: Cross sectional enlargement & hyperintensity (FS PD FSE or STIR) of median nerve
- Swelling or segmental enlargement of median nerve at level of pisiform
- Flattening of median nerve at level of hamate
- FS PD FSE or STIR = improved sensitivity for nerve edema over non-fat suppression images

Top Differential Diagnoses
- De Quervain's Tenosynovitis
- Carpometacarpal (CMC) Arthritis
- Fractures of the Distal Radius
- Carpal Instabilities

Pathology
- Idiopathic - most common (associated with aging)

- Colles' fracture
- Inflammatory processes
- Median nerve tumors
- Tumors extrinsic to median nerve (space-occupying)

Clinical Issues
- Most common signs/symptoms: Numbness & tingling (median nerve distribution)
- Thumb, index, middle fingers + radial half of ring finger commonly affected
- Sensory findings minimal, hypesthesia to complete anesthesia
- Muscle atrophy & loss of function late findings

Diagnostic Checklist
- Thenar muscle hyperintensity (T2) in association with median nerve findings

Imaging Recommendations
- Best imaging tool: MR for nerve size, morphology & signal intensity and changes in carpal tunnel size or volume
- Protocol advice
  - T1 or PD + FS PD FSE or STIR axial, coronal & sagittal
  - Axial plane is essential
  - Intravenous contrast optional to enhance synovium

DIFFERENTIAL DIAGNOSIS

Cervical Radiculopathy
- Disc protrusion/extrusion
- Osteophytes
- Central canal or foraminal stenosis
- C5-C6 commonly simulates symptoms

Pronator Teres Syndrome
- Findings overlap with CTS
- ± Signal changes in median nerve distribution on FS PD FSE or STIR

Thoracic Outlet Syndrome
- Findings overlap with CTS
- ± Cervical rib, fibrous fascial bands - compression of brachial plexus

De Quervain's Tenosynovitis
- Radial-sided wrist pain
- Inability to abduct thumb
- Swelling, crepitus & pain on radial side
- Affects abductor pollicis longus (APL) & extensor pollicis brevis (EPB)

Carpometacarpal (CMC) Arthritis
- Sclerosis between trapezium & proximal 1st metacarpal
- 1st CMC subluxation
- Stretch of opponens pollicis muscle mimicking atrophy

Fractures of the Distal Radius
- Colles' fracture
- Median nerve involvement in 0.2 to 12%
- Laceration or contusion of nerve
- Comminuted fractures
- Melone type III (volar spike fragment) = greater incidence of median nerve involvement
- Edema and hematoma contribute to mass effect
- Callus or bony deformity

Carpal Instabilities
- Degenerative changes - hypertrophic bone
- Dorsal intercalated segment instability (DISI)
  - Lunate displaced toward proximal carpal canal
  - Scaphoid palmar flexes & contributes to decrease volume of carpal tunnel

PATHOLOGY

General Features
- General path comments
  - Relevant anatomy
    - Flexor retinaculum = transverse carpal ligament (TCL)
    - Proximal & distal margins of carpal tunnel = proximal & distal borders of flexor retinaculum
    - TCL radial attachment: Scaphoid, trapezium & fascia of thenar muscles
    - TCL ulnar attachment: Fascia proximal to pisiform + hook of hamate & distally to fascia of hypothenar muscles
- Etiology
  - Idiopathic - most common (associated with aging)
  - Colles' fracture
    - Decreased volume of carpal tunnel or direct nerve trauma
  - Inflammatory processes
    - Rheumatoid arthritis
    - Gout & pseudogout
    - Amyloid
  - Median nerve tumors

- Neurilemmomas (schwannomas)
- Fibromas
- Hamartomas
  - Tumors extrinsic to median nerve (space-occupying)
    - Ganglion, lipoma & hemangioma
- Epidemiology
  - \> 50% incidence during lifetime
  - Up to 100% incidence with repetitive motion activity

Gross Pathologic & Surgical Features
- Inflammation present in only 10%
- Edema present in 85%
- Vascular sclerosis in 98%
- Tenosynovitis: Uncommon
- Connective tissue degeneration: Common

Microscopic Features
- Increased pressure
- Impairment of intraneural microcirculation
- Ischemia correlates with symptoms
- Thin afferent nerve fibers most susceptible to pressure
- Fibrosynovial non-inflammatory synovium (response to chronic frictional/mechanical stresses)

Staging, Grading or Classification Criteria
- No widely used grading scheme
- Can be classified as mild, moderate, severe based on electrodiagnostic data (e.g., motor nerve conduction velocity) or by severity of clinical symptoms (sensory early, motor late)

CLINICAL ISSUES

Presentation
- Most common signs/symptoms: Numbness & tingling (median nerve distribution)
- Clinical profile
  - Thumb, index, middle fingers + radial half of ring finger commonly affected
  - Increased nocturnal pain ± burning
  - Sensory findings minimal, hypesthesia to complete anesthesia
  - Muscle atrophy & loss of function late findings
    - Opponens weakness: Earlier finding
    - Atrophy of opponens: Late finding
  - Abductor pollicis brevis muscle - early involvement
  - Positive Tinel's sign - paresthesias reproduced by tapping over nerve
  - Phalen's test: Symptoms in 30 seconds with wrist in forced palmar flexion
  - Carpal tunnel compression test - most accurate sign: Manual compression with wrist in flexion
  - Sensory threshold tests
    - Semmes-Weinstein monofilament test with wrist in both neutral & flexed positions
    - Tests for early CTS
  - Electrodiagnostic tests of median nerve conduction
    - Distal sensory latency
    - Midpalmar latency
    - Distal motor latency for advanced CTS
    - Kimura inching technique & ring finger differential measurements for early CTS

Demographics
- Age: Peak - 5th or 6th decade
- Gender: F > M

Natural History & Prognosis
- Progression of pain with paresthesias
- Numbness from intermittent to constant
- Thumb weakness with chronic compression

Treatment
- Conservative
  - Neutral position wrist splint
  - Avoid prolonged palmar flexion or extension activities
  - Steroid injections into carpal canal
- Surgical
  - History of increasing symptoms (years) + increase in distal sensory latency of median nerve (> 8.0 milliseconds)
  - Transverse carpal ligament release - open vs. endoscopic

DIAGNOSTIC CHECKLIST

Consider
- Thenar muscle hyperintensity (T2) in association with median nerve findings
- Partial to complete involvement of median nerve fascicles
- FS PD FSE, STIR or T1 C+ to enhance synovium

SELECTED REFERENCES

1. Bland JD: Carpal tunnel syndrome. Br J Gen Pract 53(487):149-50, 2003
2. Ruess L et al: Carpal tunnel syndrome and cubital tunnel syndrome: Work-related musculoskeletal disorders in four symptomatic radiologists. AJR 181(1):37-42, 2003
3. Beckenbaugh RD: The wrist. Diagnosis and operative treatment. Carpal tunnel syndrome. St. Louis Missouri, Mosby, (51):1197-1239, 1998
4. Relton H: The wrist and it's disorders. Nerve injuries associated with wrist trauma and entrapment. 2nd ed. Philadelphia Pennsylvania, W.B. Saunders, (27):473-86, 1997
5. Plancher KD et al: Compressive neuropathies and tendinopathies in the athlete elbow and wrist. Clin Sports Med 15:331-72, 1996
6. Ikeda K et al: Correlative MR-anatomic study of the median nerve. AJR 167:1233-36, 1996
7. Palmer DH et al: Endoscopic carpal tunnel release: A comparison of the two techniques with open release. Arthroscopy 9:498-508, 1993
8. Murphy RX et al: Magnetic resonance imaging in the evaluation of persistent carpal tunnel syndrome. J Hand Surg 18:113-20, 1993
9. Binkovitz LA et al: Masses of the hand and wrist: Detection and characterization with MR imaging. AJR 154:323-326, 1990
10. Mesgarzadeh M et al: Carpal tunnel: MR imaging I: Normal anatomy. Radiology 171:743-48, 1989

CARPAL TUNNEL SYNDROME

IMAGE GALLERY

Typical

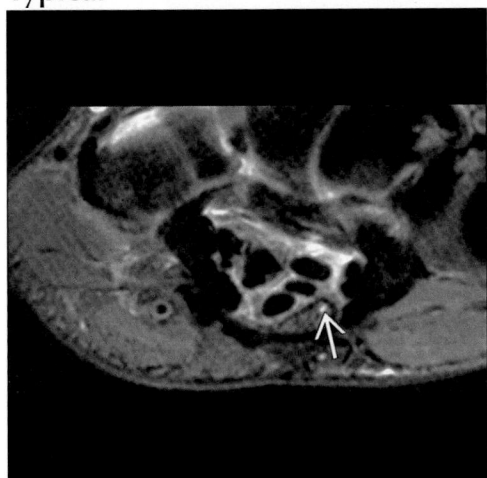
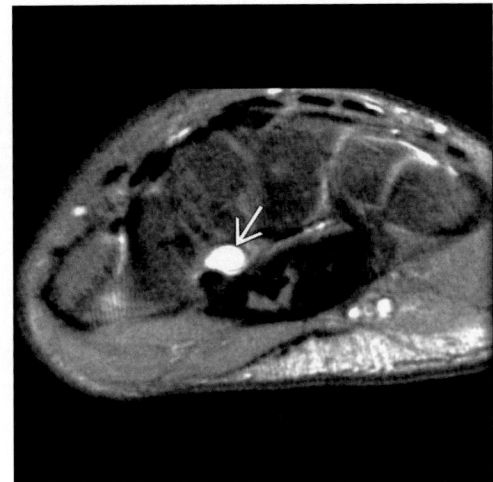

*(**Left**) Axial FS PD FSE MR shows carpal tunnel hyperintensity with discrete focus of median nerve edema (arrow). (**Right**) Axial FS PD FSE MR shows hyperintense volar ganglion (arrow) compressing the deep surface of the carpal tunnel in a patient with clinical carpal tunnel syndrome.*

Typical

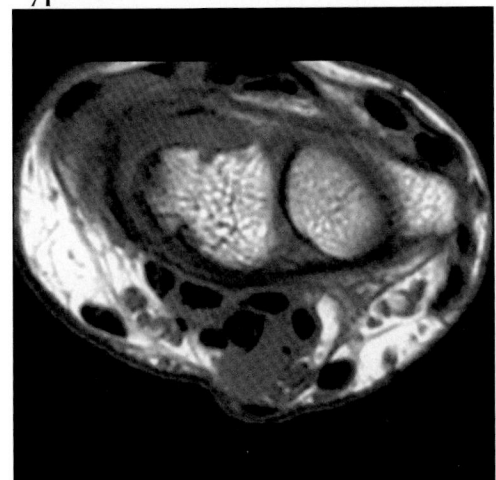
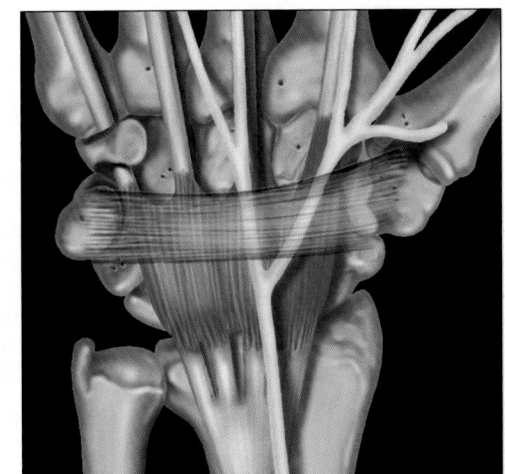

*(**Left**) Axial T1WI MR shows accessory superficialis muscle resulting in median nerve compression. (**Right**) Coronal graphic shows anomalous muscle belly of the flexor digitorum superficialis diminishing the carpal tunnel volume.*

Typical

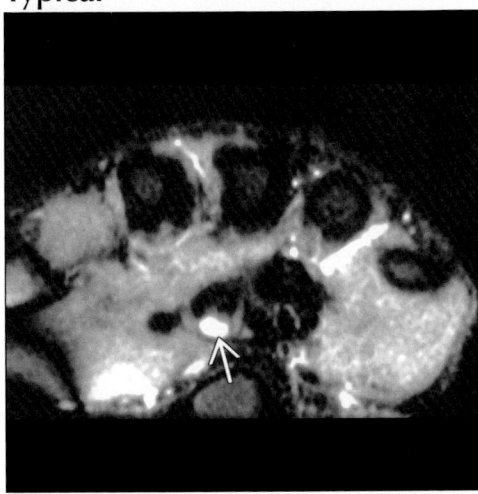
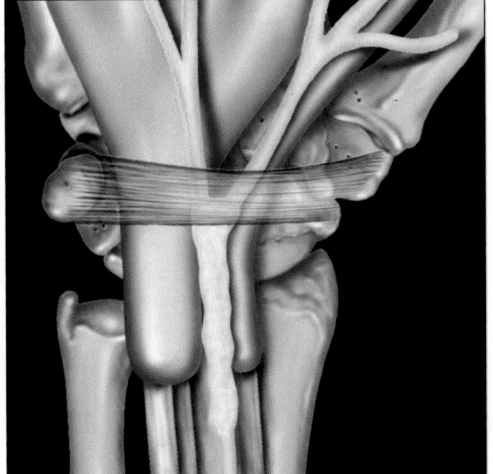

*(**Left**) Axial STIR MR shows benign peripheral nerve sheath tumor with hyperintensity of the median nerve (arrow) and subtle hyperintense changes of thenar muscle denervation. (**Right**) Coronal graphic shows edematous median nerve in carpal tunnel syndrome. Impairment of intraneural microcirculation leads to nerve ischemia.*

ULNAR TUNNEL SYNDROME

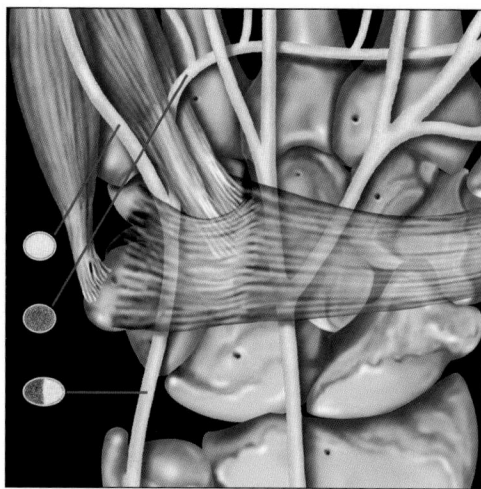

Coronal graphic shows potential sites of ulnar nerve involvement. Yellow represents sensory fibers, brown represents motor branch, and mixed yellow-brown represents both.

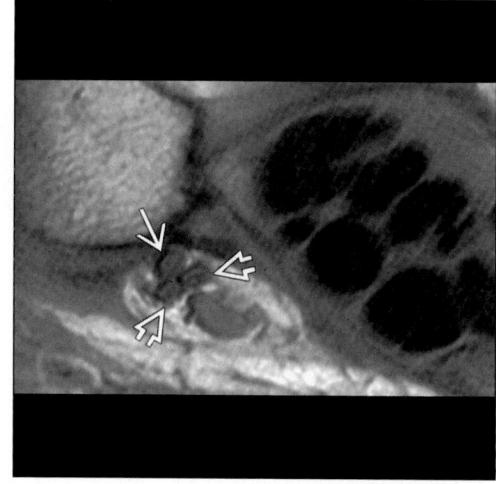

Axial T1WI MR shows normal division of the ulnar nerve into one motor (arrow) branch (deep) and two sensory (open arrows) branches (superficial) between the pisiform and ulnar artery.

TERMINOLOGY

Abbreviations and Synonyms
- Ulnar neuropathy, Guyon's canal syndrome

Definitions
- Numbness & tingling 5th (little) finger + ulnar side 4th (ring) finger palmar surface from irritation of ulnar nerve in Guyon's canal

IMAGING FINDINGS

General Features
- Best diagnostic clue: Compression of ulnar nerve in Guyon's canal
- Location: Guyon's canal
- Size: Variable, usually < 1 cm length of involvement
- Morphology: Round to ovoid mass

Radiographic Findings
- Radiography
  - Hamate hook fx
    - Impingement on ulnar nerve
  - Intercarpal arthritis ± spurring
  - Joint space narrowing ± soft tissue calcifications

CT Findings
- NECT: Sensitive to identifying fx fragment

MR Findings
- T1WI
  - Diffuse swelling (intermediate signal)
  - Enlargement of ulnar nerve
- T2WI
  - Hyperintense signal within ulnar nerve best demonstrated on axial FS PD FSE or STIR
  - May identify mass (usually with hyperintense signal)
    - Ganglion cyst
    - Aneurysm
    - Fracture
    - Anomalous muscle
- T2* GRE: Helpful to visualize increased neural edema

Imaging Recommendations
- Best imaging tool: MR identifies ulnar nerve edema, ganglion cyst formation & other compressive etiologies
- Protocol advice: T1/PD & FS PD FSE axial, coronal & sagittal images

DIFFERENTIAL DIAGNOSIS

Carpal Tunnel Syndrome
- Compressive neuropathy
- Infrequent in athletic population

DDx: Ulnar Tunnel Syndrome

Carpal Tunnel	Cubital Tunnel	Hamate Fracture
Ax FS PD MR	Cor T1 Arthro.	Ax T1WI MR

ULNAR TUNNEL SYNDROME

Key Facts

Imaging Findings
- Best diagnostic clue: Compression of ulnar nerve in Guyon's canal
- Enlargement of ulnar nerve
- Hyperintense signal within ulnar nerve best demonstrated on axial FS PD FSE or STIR

Top Differential Diagnoses
- Carpal Tunnel Syndrome
- Cubital Tunnel Syndrome
- Cervical Radiculopathy/Thoracic Outlet Syndrome
- Hamate Fracture

Pathology
- Soft tissue tumors
- Ganglion cysts
- Ulnar artery thrombosis or aneurysm

- Carpal fractures - hook of hamate most common
- Anomalous muscle belly

Clinical Issues
- Most common signs/symptoms: Paresthesias followed by decreased sensation at 4th & 5th fingers
- Hand weakness may develop
- Sensory and/or motor changes may be present based on pressure point
- Positive Tinel's sign over ulnar nerve
- Positive Phalen's test with paresthesias in 4th & 5th fingers

Diagnostic Checklist
- Axial FS PD FSE to visualize ulnar nerve edema

- Median nerve compression in osteofibrous canal (transverse carpal ligament & carpal bones)
- Result of direct trauma, repetitive use or anatomic anomalies

Cubital Tunnel Syndrome
- Weakness of wrist flexors
- Weakness flexors 4th & 5th digits
- Ulnar neuropathy at wrist produces a sensory deficit of the 5th digit and ulnar half of 4th digit
- With compression at the elbow (high ulnar lesion) - get additional sensory deficit of dorsal ulnar hand
- Electromyogram (EMG) may be needed to distinguish ulnar neuropathy at elbow vs. wrist

Cervical Radiculopathy/Thoracic Outlet Syndrome
- Disc protrusion/extrusion
- Osteophytes
- Central canal or foraminal stenosis
- Compression of brachial plexus by cervical rib, fascial slip, clavicle fx

Hamate Fracture
- Hook, body, proximal pole
- Soreness in palm
- ± Ulnar nerve palsy
- Ulnar sided pain + tenderness
- Bat, hockey stick, golf club or racquet sports related

PATHOLOGY

General Features
- General path comments
  - Relevant anatomy
    - Guyon's canal = tunnel formed by pisiform and hamate bones
    - Ulnar nerve passes deep to palmar carpal ligament and superficial to flexor retinaculum
    - Ulnar nerve divides into superficial and deep branches

    - Deep ulnar nerve = motor to hypothenar, interosseous, 3rd & 4th lumbricales & adductor pollicis muscles
    - Superficial ulnar nerve = sensory to skin of hypothenar eminence + 4th & 5th digits & motor function to palmaris brevis
- Etiology
  - Soft tissue tumors
  - Ganglion cysts
  - Scar tissue
  - Ulnar artery thrombosis or aneurysm
    - Chronic repetitive trauma (hypothenar hammer syndrome)
  - Carpal fractures - hook of hamate most common
  - Synovitis
  - Anomalous muscle belly
  - Arthritic changes
- Epidemiology
  - Less common than median nerve compression
  - Less common than ulnar nerve entrapment at elbow
  - Cyclists at risk from intermittent impaction
  - Golfers and baseball players at risk
  - Repetitive flexion/extension of wrist
  - Vibrating hand tools against hypothenar eminence

Gross Pathologic & Surgical Features
- Compression of ulnar nerve
  - Entrance to ulnar tunnel
  - Superficial branch (sensory)
  - Deep branch (motor)
- Hamate fx
- Distal radius fx
- Anomalous muscle
- Lipoma
- Ganglion
- Ulnar artery aneurysm or thrombosis
- Compression at level of elbow rarely associated with median nerve findings of fixed motor deficits in the hand
- Martin Gruber anastomosis (15% of population)
  - Anomalous motor & sensory findings
  - Ulnar-to-median anastomosis
- Riche-Cannieu anastomosis

ULNAR TUNNEL SYNDROME

○ Deep branch of ulnar nerve & median nerve in the hand

Microscopic Features
- Increased pressure
- Impairment of intraneural microcirculation
- Ischemia

Staging, Grading or Classification Criteria
- Three distinct zones within Guyon's canal
  ○ Zone 1 = proximal to bifurcation of deep (motor) branch and superficial (sensor) branch
    - Compression produces motor and sensory deficits
    - Commonly caused by ganglion cysts or hamate hook fx
  ○ Zone 2 = deep branch producing motor deficit
    - Often caused by ganglion cyst or fx hook hamate
  ○ Zone 3 = superficial branch producing sensory deficit
    - Related to ulnar artery aneurysm or thrombosis

CLINICAL ISSUES

Presentation
- Most common signs/symptoms: Paresthesias followed by decreased sensation at 4th & 5th fingers
- Clinical profile
  ○ Hand weakness may develop
  ○ Symptoms develop gradually
    - Leads to difficulty opening jars, holding objects, coordinating fingers while typing/playing musical instruments
  ○ Sensory and/or motor changes may be present based on pressure point
  ○ Positive Tinel's sign over ulnar nerve
  ○ Positive Phalen's test with paresthesias in 4th & 5th fingers
  ○ EMG's (± positive)
    - Denervation potentials in interosseous muscle
    - Motor nerve latency prolongation to 1st dorsal interossei
  ○ Compression at or proximal to origin of dorsal sensory branch ulnar nerve in distal third of forearm
    - Sensory deficit of dorsoulnar aspect of hand
  ○ Compression at elbow
    - Median nerve involvement possible
    - Fixed motor deficits
    - Ulnar clawhand (unopposed extensor digitorum communis & flexor digitorum profundus)

Demographics
- Age: Young to middle age adult in sports injuries
- Gender: No predilection

Natural History & Prognosis
- Recovery several months to years
  ○ Longer for older patients
  ○ With severe compression recovery may be incomplete

Treatment
- Conservative
  ○ Wrist splint
  ○ Anti-inflammatory medications
- Surgical
  ○ Mass in ulnar tunnel must be treated surgically
    - Resection of cysts, scar tissue results in improved sensation + decreased symptoms
  ○ Resection ligament that forms roof of Guyon's canal (palmar carpal ligament) to relieve pressure
- Complications
  ○ Nerve regrowth may be associated with pain
    - May last > 6 weeks and require additional medication, massage, therapy
  ○ Resection of ligament forming roof of Guyon's canal causes scar tissue formation and may result in recurring symptoms

DIAGNOSTIC CHECKLIST

Consider
- Eliminate injuries to forearm and upper neck ("double crush" injuries) when evaluating injuries to nerves of the hand/wrist
- Axial FS PD FSE to visualize ulnar nerve edema

SELECTED REFERENCES

1. Miller MD et al: Surgical atlas of sports medicine. Treatment of Guyan's canal syndrome (ulnar nerve compression at the wrist). Philadelphia Pennsylvania, Saunders, (66):477-89, 2003
2. McCue FC III et al: DeLee & Drez's orthopaedic sports medicine. The wrist in the adult. Philadelphia Pennsylvania, Saunders, (24):1337-63, 2003
3. Konig PSA et al: Variations of the ulnar nerve and ulnar artery in Guyon's canal: A cadaveric study. J Hand Surg 19:617, 1994
4. Beltran J et al: Diagnosis of compressive and entrapment neuropathies of the upper extremity. Value of MR imaging. AJR 163:525, 1994
5. Zeiss J et al: The ulnar tunnel at the wrist (Guyon's canal): Normal MR anatomy and variants. AJR 158:1081, 1992
6. Gross MS et al: The anatomy of the distal ulnar tunnel. Clin Orthop 196:238-47, 1985
7. Stern PJ et al: Compression of the deep branch of the ulnar nerve. A case report. J Hand Surg 8:72-4, 1983
8. Shea JD et al: Ulnar nerve compression syndromes at and below the wrists. J Bone Joint Surg 51:1095-1103, 1969
9. Thompson WAL et al: Peripheral entrapment neuropathies of the upper extremities. N Eng J Med 260:1261, 1959
10. Grundberg AB: Ulnar tunnel syndrome. Hand 9:72, 1934

ULNAR TUNNEL SYNDROME

IMAGE GALLERY

Typical

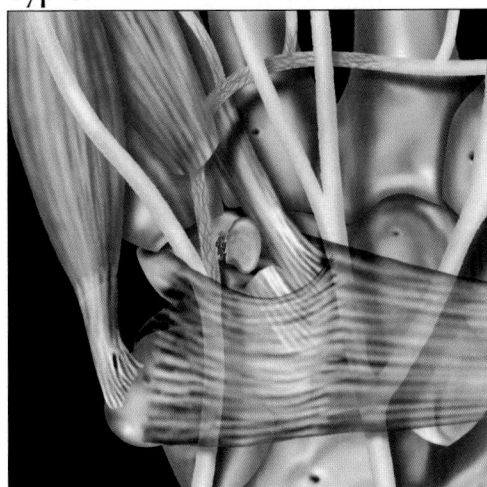

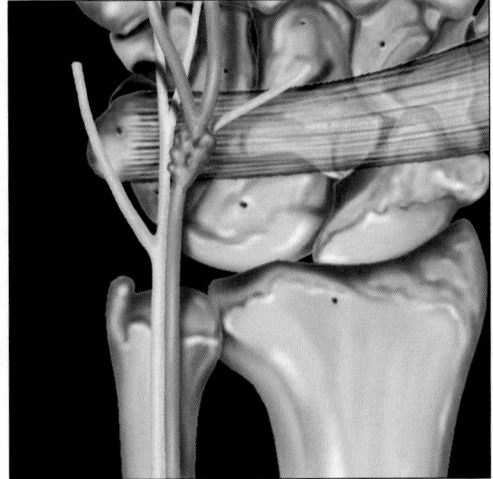

(Left) Coronal graphic shows edema of the motor branch of the ulnar nerve. *(Right)* Coronal graphic shows ulnar artery aneurysm with compression of the ulnar nerve.

Typical

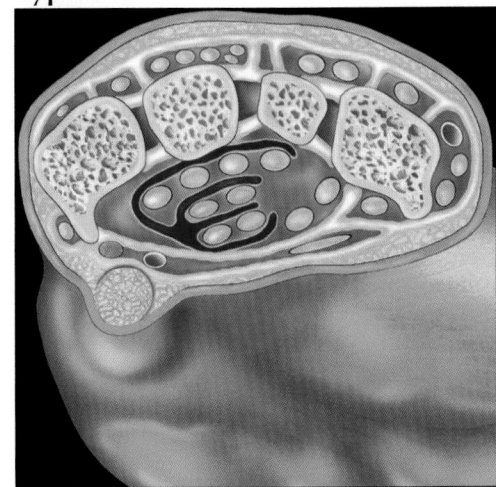

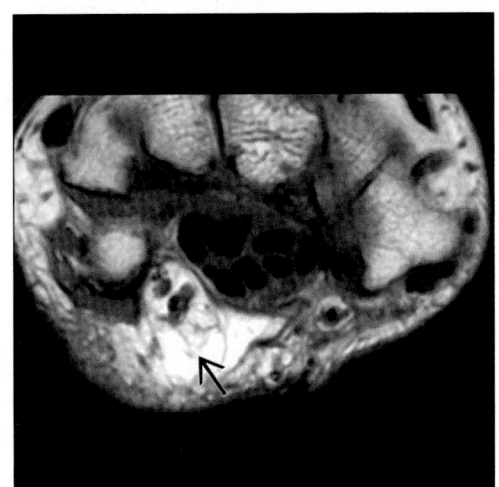

(Left) Axial graphic shows extrinsic compression of the ulnar tunnel secondary to a palmar lipoma. The ischemic ulnar nerve is located between the hook of the hamate and the lipoma. *(Right)* Axial T1WI MR shows lipomatous mass (arrow) occupying the ulnar tunnel.

Typical

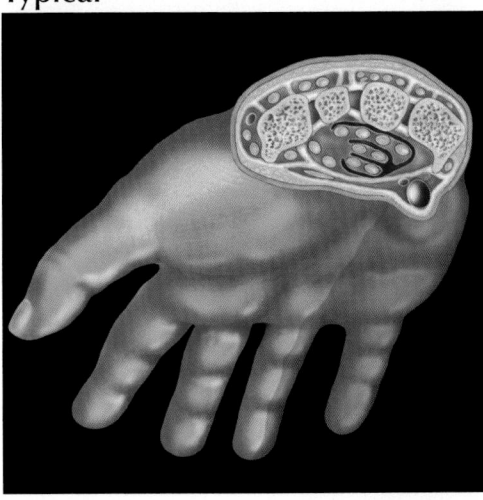

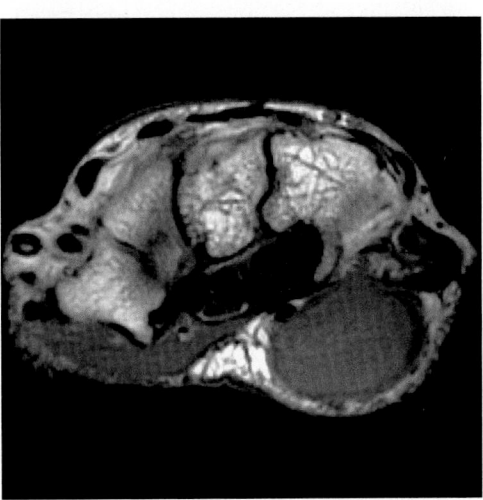

(Left) Axial graphic shows ganglion as a space occupying lesion within the ulnar tunnel. *(Right)* Axial T1WI MR shows hemorrhagic soft tissue mass superficial to the hook of the hamate with secondary compression of the ulnar nerve.

DEGENERATIVE ARTHRITIS, WRIST

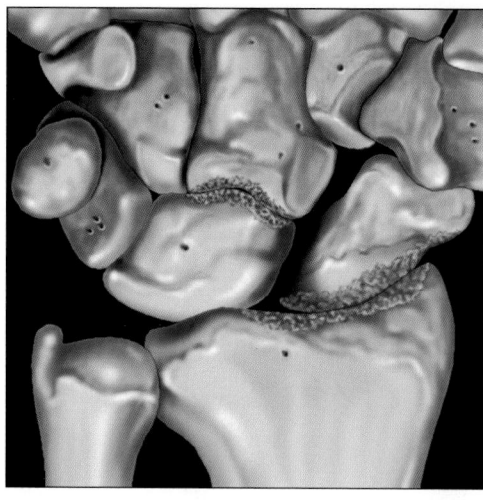

Coronal graphic shows stage III SLAC with arthrosis of the radioscaphoid and capitolunate articulations.

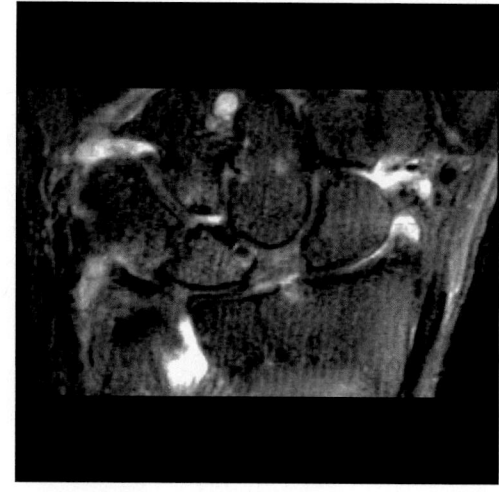

Coronal FS PD FSE MR shows widening of the scapholunate interval and proximal migration of the capitate in SLAC arthritis.

TERMINOLOGY

Abbreviations and Synonyms
- SLAC wrist, scapholunate advanced collapse, triscaphe arthritis

Definitions
- Carpal degeneration involving scaphoid occurring in three separate patterns

IMAGING FINDINGS

General Features
- Best diagnostic clue: Scaphoradial joint space narrowing in SLAC & sclerosis of triscaphe articulation
- Location
  - SLAC
    - Scaphoradial (SR)
    - Capitolunate (CL)
    - Scaphocapitate (SC)
  - Triscaphe
    - Scaphotrapezial
    - Scaphotrapezoidal
    - Trapeziotrapezoidal
- Size: SLAC - from isolated scaphoradial articulation to SR, CL, SC & hamate-lunate involvement
- Morphology

- Rotatory subluxation progression
- SLAC = radioscaphoid narrowing & proximal migration of capitate
- Narrowing of triscaphe articulations

Radiographic Findings
- Radiography
  - SLAC
    - SR, CL, SC narrowing + sclerosis
    - Foreshortening of scaphoid
    - Scapholunate gap
    - Scaphoid ring sign (anteroposterior view)
    - Dorsal intercalated segment instability (DISI) on lateral view
    - Degenerative changes between radius & distal scaphoid fragment in non-union of scaphoid
  - Triscaphe arthritis
    - Sclerosis & narrowing between scaphoid, trapezium & trapezoid

MR Findings
- T1WI
  - SLAC
    - Hypointense sclerosis, narrowing with chondral loss between radial styloid & scaphoid articulation
    - Narrowing + hypointense sclerosis involving entire radioscaphoid articulation
    - Hypointense sclerosis + narrowing capitolunate joint

DDx: Degenerative Arthritis, Wrist

SL Instability	Kienböck's	Scaphoid Fracture
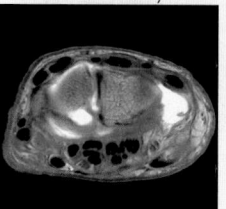	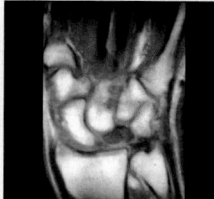	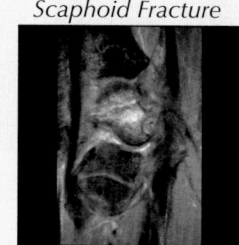
Ax T1 Arthro.	Cor T1WI MR	Sag FS PD MR

DEGENERATIVE ARTHRITIS, WRIST

Key Facts

Imaging Findings

- Best diagnostic clue: Scaphoradial joint space narrowing in SLAC & sclerosis of triscaphe articulation
- Size: SLAC - from isolated scaphoradial articulation to SR, CL, SC & hamate-lunate involvement
- SLAC = radioscaphoid narrowing & proximal migration of capitate

Top Differential Diagnoses

- Scapholunate Instability
- Kienböck's Disease
- Scaphoid Fracture
- Scaphoid Non-Union
- Ulnocarpal Impaction (Abutment)

Pathology

- High shear stresses over small contact surfaces
- Rotary subluxation scaphoid (RSS)
- Progression to radioscaphoid/SLAC or triscaphe arthrosis
- SLAC wrist = most common pattern comprising 55% of degenerative arthritis of wrist

Clinical Issues

- Most common signs/symptoms: Wrist pain with activity
- Stiffness with dorsiflexion & radial deviation

Diagnostic Checklist

- SLAC changes identified early by observing radial styloid sclerosis

○ Triscaphe
- Subchondral hypointense sclerosis (scaphotrapeziotrapezoid arthrosis)
- T2WI
  ○ SLAC
    - Loss of intermediate signal articular cartilage between radial styloid & dorsal pole scaphoid (in setting of scaphoid non-union)
    - Hypointense sclerosis or subchondral degenerative edema across entire radioscaphoid articulation
    - Intermediate signal chondral loss in capitolunate joint
    - Hyperintense fluid-filled gap between scaphoid & lunate
    - Discontinuity of scapholunate ligament
    - Sparing of scapholunate articulation
    - ± Degenerative hyperintense cyst within scaphoid, capitate or distal radius
  ○ Triscaphe
    - Hypointense sclerosis with intermediate signal intensity chondral loss
    - Hyperintense degenerative marrow edema - late

Imaging Recommendations

- Best imaging tool: MR identifies early SLAC changes at radioscaphoid joint + triscaphe sclerosis prior to narrowing
- Protocol advice: T1 (for sclerosis) & FS PD FSE coronal, axial & sagittal images

DIFFERENTIAL DIAGNOSIS

Scapholunate Instability

- Ligamentous disruption between scaphoid & lunate
- Scaphoid flexed relative to lunate
- Increased scapholunate angle
- DISI

Kienböck's Disease

- Avascular necrosis lunate
- Related to trauma & ulnar negative variance
- Lunate sclerosis

- ± Visualized lunate fracture

Scaphoid Fracture

- Most common fracture of the carpus
- Dorsiflexion loading + radial deviation
- 70-80% middle third of scaphoid
- Proximal pole & waist fxs at risk for delayed union & AVN

Scaphoid Non-Union

- Absence of bridging trabecular bone
- Proximal third fx at risk
- Vertical oblique fx middle third
- Volar non-union defect = prismatic shape

Ulnocarpal Impaction (Abutment)

- Positive ulnar variance
- TFCC tear
- Chondromalacia proximal lunate + triquetrum
- Eccentric sclerosis proximal ulnar lunate
- Lunotriquetral (LT) ligament tear

PATHOLOGY

General Features

- General path comments
  ○ Relevant anatomy
    - Scaphoradial
    - Capitolunate
    - Scaphocapitate
    - Hamate-lunate
    - Scaphotrapezial
    - Scaphotrapezoidal
    - Trapeziotrapezoidal
- Etiology
  ○ High shear stresses over small contact surfaces
  ○ SLAC wrist
    - Rotary subluxation scaphoid (RSS)
    - Scapholunate or periscaphoid dissociation
    - Predynamic to dynamic to static RSS
    - Progression to radioscaphoid/SLAC or triscaphe arthrosis

DEGENERATIVE ARTHRITIS, WRIST

- ▪ SLAC also caused by abnormal articular loading in scaphoid fx, non-union, Kienböck's & carpal fxs
  - ○ Triscaphe arthrosis
    - ▪ Load changes and articular pathology analogous to SLAC wrist
    - ▪ Disruption in ligamentous support of scaphoid distally
- Epidemiology
  - ○ Degenerative arthrosis in 5% of wrists
  - ○ SLAC wrist = most common pattern comprising 55% of degenerative arthritis of wrist
  - ○ Triscaphe arthritis = 20% degenerative wrist arthritis
  - ○ Both SLAC wrist + triscaphe arthritis = 10% of wrist degenerative arthritis

Gross Pathologic & Surgical Features

- SLAC stage I
  - ○ Arthrosis limited to radial styloid - scaphoid articulation
- SLAC stage II
  - ○ Arthrosis of the entire radioscaphoid articulation
- SLAC stage III
  - ○ Capitolunate arthrosis
- Additional destruction of scaphocapitate articulation with capitate impingement (proximal migration on radius)
- ± Secondary hamate-lunate joint narrowing
- Triscaphe
  - ○ Scaphotrapezial involvement twice as common as isolated scaphotrapezoidal
  - ○ Trapezium & trapezoid migrate proximally
- Ulnolunate & lunotriquetral arthritis related to ulnocarpal impaction syndrome

Microscopic Features

- Weakening of ligamentous collagen fibers, connective tissue & elastic fibers
- Trabecular stress loading with sclerosis
- Chondral & subchondral degeneration (fibrillation, fraying, erosions)

Staging, Grading or Classification Criteria

- SLAC arthritis involvement
  - ○ Stage I: Distal radius (radial-styloid) & distal radial aspect of scaphoid
  - ○ Stage IIa: Entire radioscaphoid joint
  - ○ Stage IIb: Radioscaphoid & secondary involvement STT joint
  - ○ Stage III: Periscaphoid arthritis with radioscaphoid & capitolunate joints
- Scaphotrapeziotrapezoid (STT) arthritis
  - ○ Involvement in either stage I, II or III SLAC
- Scaphoid non-union advanced collapse arthritis
  - ○ Stage I: Distal scaphoid & radial styloid
  - ○ Stage II: Addition of scaphocapitate with capitolunate preservation
  - ○ Stage III: Periscaphoid arthritis with radiostyloid distal scaphoid, scaphocapitate, & capitolunate (proximal scaphoid & lunate preserved)

CLINICAL ISSUES

Presentation

- Most common signs/symptoms: Wrist pain with activity
- Clinical profile
  - ○ Decreased grip strength in SLAC
  - ○ Stiffness with dorsiflexion & radial deviation
  - ○ Asymptomatic subgroup = older patients
  - ○ Localized tenderness
  - ○ STT arthritis associated with carpal tunnel syndrome, radiopalmar ganglion & de Quervain's

Demographics

- Age
  - ○ Middle-aged for symptomatic patients
  - ○ Older age group for asymptomatic patients
- Gender: M > F

Natural History & Prognosis

- Progression of post-traumatic arthritis with degenerative arthritis & ligament attenuation

Treatment

- Conservative
  - ○ Immobilization
  - ○ Anti-inflammatory medications
- Surgical
  - ○ SLAC wrist reconstruction
  - ○ Triscaphe arthrodesis

DIAGNOSTIC CHECKLIST

Consider

- SLAC changes identified early by observing radial styloid sclerosis
- SLAC & triscaphe arthritis may coexist

SELECTED REFERENCES

1. Sauerbier M et al: Midcarpal arthrodesis with complete scaphoid excision an interposition bone graft in the treatment of advanced carpal collapse. (SNAC/SLAC wrist): Operative technique and outcome assessment. J Hand Surg 25(4):341-5, 2000
2. Schweitzer AF et al: Frequency and spectrum of abnormalities in the bone marrow of the wrist: MR imaging findings. Skeletal Radiol 28(6):312-7, 1999
3. Cooney WP: The wrist. Diagnosis and operative treatment. Post-traumatic arthritis of the wrist. St. Louis MO, Mosby, (25):588-631, 1998
4. Watson HK et al: The wrist and it's disorders. Degenerative disorder of the carpus. 2nd ed. Philadelphia Pennsylvania, WB Saunders, (32):583-91, 1997
5. Krakauer JD et al: Surgical treatment of scapholunate advanced collapse. J Hand Surg 19(5):751-9, 1994
6. Fassler PR: Asymptomatic SLAC wrist: Does it exist? J Hand Surg 18(4):682-6, 1993

DEGENERATIVE ARTHRITIS, WRIST

IMAGE GALLERY

Typical

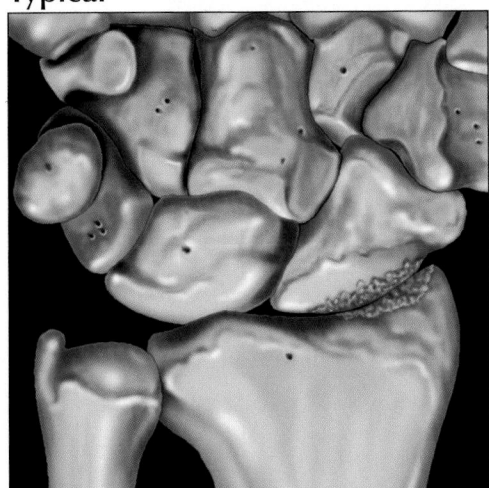 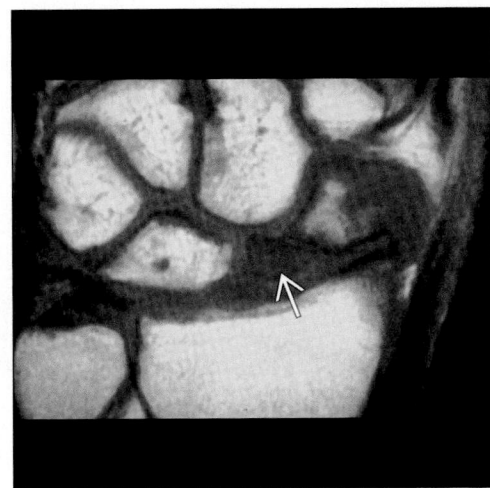

(Left) Coronal graphic shows stage I SLAC with arthrosis limited to the radial styloid-scaphoid articulation. The entire radioscaphoid articulation is involved in the progression to stage II SLAC. (Right) Coronal T1WI MR shows SLAC with scaphoid non-union (scaphoid non-union advanced collapse). Sclerosis (arrow) is shown in AVN of proximal pole of the scaphoid. Radial styloid-scaphoid arthritis is present.

Typical

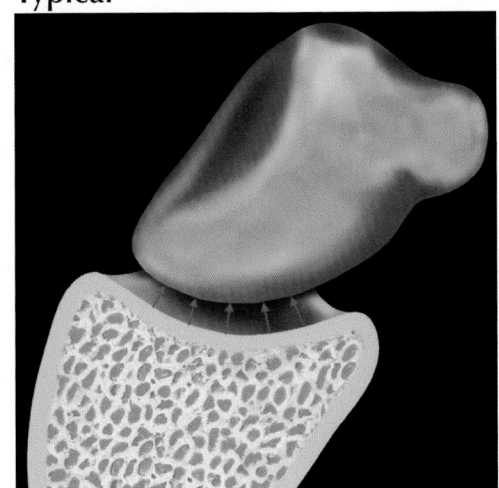 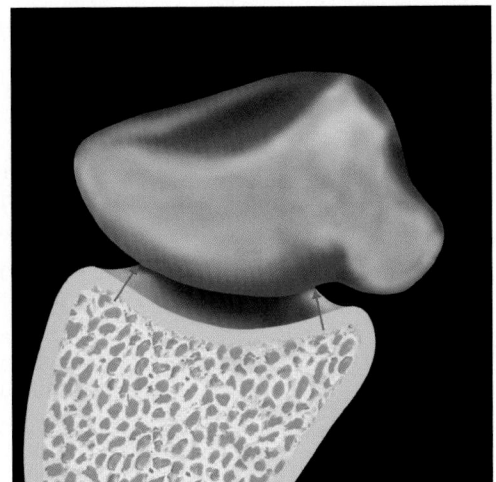

(Left) Sagittal graphic shows normal radioscaphoid congruous joint surfaces. (Right) Sagittal graphic shows rotational instability secondary to rotatory subluxation of scaphoid with abnormal load transfer to the volar and dorsal margins of distal radius.

Typical

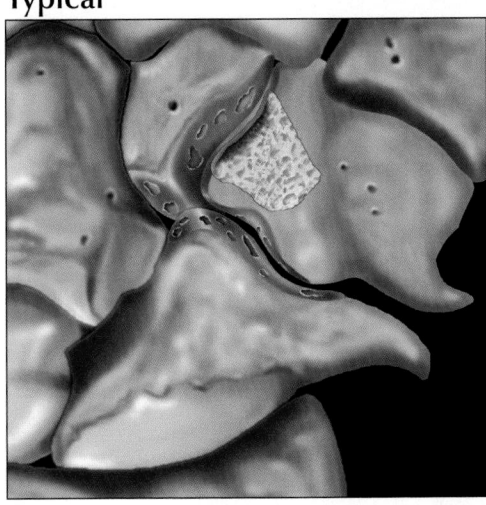 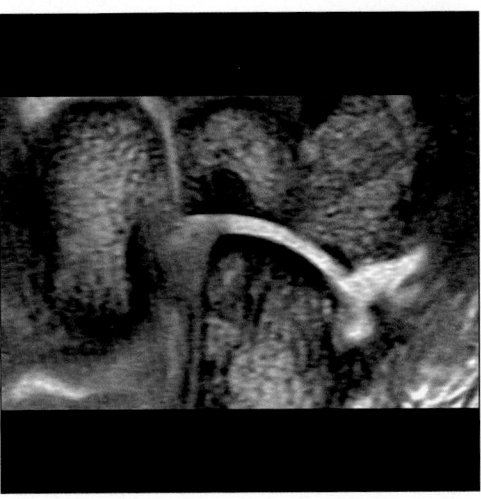

(Left) Coronal graphic shows triscaphe arthritis with degeneration of the scaphotrapeziotrapezoid articulation. (Right) Coronal T1 C+ MR (MR arthrogram) shows hypointense sclerosis with loss of articular cartilage in the triscaphe joint.

HAMATO-LUNATE IMPINGEMENT

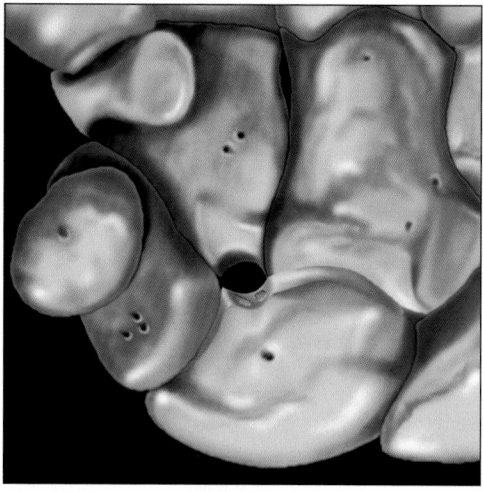

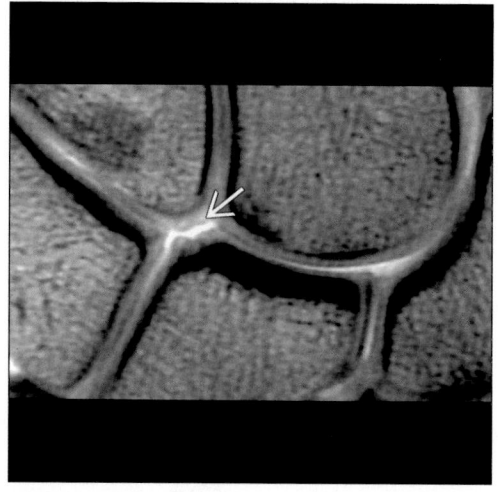

Coronal graphic shows type II lunate or medial lunate facet with subchondral erosion of proximal pole of hamate and accessory lunate facet.

Coronal T1 C+ MR (MR arthrogram) shows early chondral erosions (arrow) between the medial lunate facet and the proximal pole of hamate.

TERMINOLOGY

Abbreviations and Synonyms
- Type II lunate, chondromalacia of the hamate, medial lunate facet; hamate facet

Definitions
- Degenerative arthritis between a type II lunate with an extra facet and proximal hamate, a type I lunate has no extra or medial facet

IMAGING FINDINGS

General Features
- Best diagnostic clue: Chondral erosions between the medial lunate facet & proximal pole of the hamate
- Location: Between accessory lunate facet (medial) & proximal pole hamate
- Size: Accessory facet - 1 to 6 mm
- Morphology: Blunted to convex

Radiographic Findings
- Radiography
  - Difficult to visualize a small medial lunate facet (radiography is inaccurate)
    - Sclerosis proximal pole hamate
    - Demonstrates advanced changes

CT Findings
- NECT
  - Bone technique
  - 1 mm sections + reformations or direct coronal plane
  - Excellent bone detail (edge)
  - Poor articular cartilage visualization
  - Subchondral trabecular sclerosis

MR Findings
- T1WI
  - Extra medial lunate facet
  - Subchondral sclerosis proximal hamate or medial lunate facet = advanced finding
  - ± Associated capitolunate arthrosis
  - Hypointense subchondral edema of hamate = uncommon finding
  - Narrowing of hamate-lunate joint space
- T2WI
  - Inhomogeneity of intermediate intensity chondral surfaces of medial lunate facet & proximal hamate
  - Surface fibrillation, fraying or full thickness chondral defects
  - Four corner arthritis = chondral degeneration proximal hamate, proximal capitate, radial distal triquetrum & medial lunate facet
  - Hyperintense hamate or lunate marrow edema = unusual finding

DDx: Hamato-Lunate Impingement

Hamate Fracture	Kienböck's	Capitate Fracture	Triquetral Fx

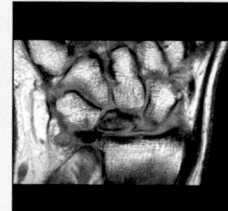
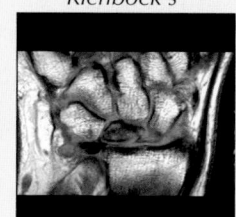
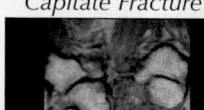
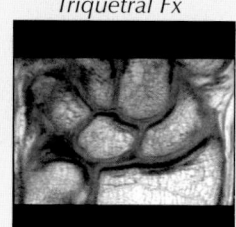

Ax T1WI MR	Cor T1WI MR	Cor T1WI MR	Cor T1WI MR

HAMATO-LUNATE IMPINGEMENT

Key Facts

Imaging Findings

- Best diagnostic clue: Chondral erosions between the medial lunate facet & proximal pole of the hamate
- Extra medial lunate facet
- Narrowing of hamate-lunate joint space
- Surface fibrillation, fraying or full thickness chondral defects

Top Differential Diagnoses

- Hamate Fracture
- Kienböck's Disease
- Capitate Fracture
- Lunotriquetral Ligament Tear
- Triquetral Fracture

Pathology

- Type II lunate = alteration of normal uniform loading

- Altered biomechanics leads to chondromalacia
- Increased pressure at lunate fossa in wrist extension & ulnar deviation
- Full ulnar deviation: Hamate & lunate impinge at articulation
- Chondromalacia secondary to impingement & abrasion of hamate & lunate

Clinical Issues

- Most common signs/symptoms: Ulnar-sided wrist pain
- Pain on radial & ulnar deviation of wrist
- Forced ulnar deviation intensifies pain
- LT instability

Diagnostic Checklist

- FS PD FSE to identify early cartilage erosions

- o ± Small subchondral cystic changes proximal pole hamate (intermediate to hyperintense)
- o Subchondral bone loss proximal pole hamate & medial lunate facet
- o ± Association with lunotriquetral (LT) ligament tears

Imaging Recommendations

- Best imaging tool: MR to detect size, apposition & early chondral degeneration
- Protocol advice: T1 (for sclerosis detection), FS PD FSE coronal, sagittal & axial images

DIFFERENTIAL DIAGNOSIS

Hamate Fracture

- Body or hook
- Hook fractures - most common
- Falls, direct trauma, use of a racquet or club
- Pain distal to pisiform, painful grip & pain over hook

Kienböck's Disease

- Avascular necrosis lunate
- Related to trauma & ulnar negative variance
- Dorsal tenderness lunate
- Synovitis

Capitate Fracture

- Direct trauma to dorsum wrist
- Dorsiflexion in neutral or ulnar deviation
- Dorsiflexion in radial deviation
- At risk for avascular necrosis & non-union of proximal pole in proximal fxs

Lunotriquetral Ligament Tear

- Dissociation between triquetrum & lunate
- Volar flexion lunate
- Flap morphology or absence of normal delta-shaped or linear ligament
- Volar intercalated segment instability

Triquetral Fracture

- Dorsal aspect - small fractures
- Hyperextension injury

- Secondary to ulnar styloid impingement on dorsal proximal aspect of bone
- Shear pattern of fx 2° to impingement
- Forced dorsiflexion & ulnar deviation
- Body fractures
  - o ± Displaced & associated with perilunate dislocations, crush trauma
  - o Volar intercalated segment instability (VISI)

PATHOLOGY

General Features

- General path comments
  - o Relevant anatomy of lunate
    - Between scaphoid radially & triquetrum medially (ulnarly)
    - Deep concave distal surface = articulation with head of capitate
    - Convex proximally with lunate facet of distal radius & triangular fibrocartilage
    - Medially = large flattened facet for articulation with triquetrum
    - Medial lunate facet seen in type II lunate for articulation with hamate
    - Radially - flattened facet for articulation with proximal (medial) end of scaphoid
    - Distal articular surface narrower than proximal (lunate = wedge-shaped)
    - Lunate narrower dorsally
    - Articular cartilage covers most of lunate
    - Articulation with radius, capitate, hamate, scaphoid & triquetrum
  - o Relevant anatomy of hamate
    - Most medial bone in distal row
    - Proximal surface = narrow, convex & smooth for lunate articulation
    - Distal surface articulates with forth & fifth metacarpals via two facets
    - Dorsal surface = triangular
    - Palmar surface = hook
    - Lateral surface = concavity of body & hook
    - Ulnar surface articulates with triquetrum

HAMATO-LUNATE IMPINGEMENT

- Spiral orientation of triquetrohamate joint facilitates motion between proximal and distal carpal rows
- Etiology
  - Type II lunate = alteration of normal uniform loading
  - Altered biomechanics leads to chondromalacia
  - Increased pressure at lunate fossa in wrist extension & ulnar deviation
  - Full ulnar deviation: Hamate & lunate impinge at articulation
  - Chondromalacia secondary to impingement & abrasion of hamate & lunate
- Epidemiology: Prevalence of type II lunates = 57%

Gross Pathologic & Surgical Features
- Cartilage erosion
- Exposed bone
- Chondromalacia in medial lunate facet & proximal pole hamate
- LT ligament disruption
- Scapholunate dissociation less common than LT ligament disruption
- Facet size 10-50% of distal aspect lunate

Microscopic Features
- Cartilage edema
- Fragmentation & fibrillation
- Cartilage denudation
- Synovitis
- Marrow edema
- Microhemorrhage
- Microfracture
- Hyperemia
- Cellular infiltration
- Fibrovascular tissue proliferation
- Subchondral cysts
  - Fluid
  - Myxoid
  - Fibrous
  - Cartilaginous
- Cartilage repair
  - Chondrocyte hypertrophy & increased nuclei
  - Irregular

Staging, Grading or Classification Criteria
- Type I lunate = conventional morphology (no lunate facet)
- Type II lunate = medial or hamate facet of lunate present

CLINICAL ISSUES

Presentation
- Most common signs/symptoms: Ulnar-sided wrist pain
- Clinical profile
  - Pain on radial & ulnar deviation of wrist
  - Ulnar-sided tenderness
  - Forced ulnar deviation intensifies pain
  - LT instability
  - Bilateral & symmetric
  - Ranges from asymptomatic to focally tender over proximal pole hamate

Demographics
- Age: Hamato-lunate impingement most common between 30 and 60 years (2° to medial lunate facet)
- Gender: M = F

Natural History & Prognosis
- Slow progression
- Good response to resection of head of the hamate

Treatment
- Conservative
  - Rest, activity modification
  - Anti-inflammatory medications
- Surgical
  - Resection of head of hamate for hamato-lunate impingement
  - Open vs. arthroscopic procedure
  - Relief of symptoms typical

DIAGNOSTIC CHECKLIST

Consider
- FS PD FSE to identify early cartilage erosions
- Medial lunate facet may be prominent with concave surface or small flattened corner

SELECTED REFERENCES

1. Thurston AJ et al: Hamato-lunate impingement: An uncommon cause of ulnar-sided wrist pain. Arthro Assn N Am 540-4, 2000
2. Malik AM et al: MR imaging of the type II lunate bone: Frequency, extent, and associated findings. AJR 335-8, 1999
3. Sagerman SD et al: Lunate morphology: Can it be predicted with routine X-ray films? J Hand Surg 20A:38-41, 1995
4. Green DP: Operative hand surgery. Carpal dislocations and instabilities. 3rd ed. New York NY, Churchill Livingstone, 1993
5. Viegas SF et al: The medial (hamate) facet of the lunate. J Hand Surg 15A:564-71, 1990
6. Burgess RC: Anatomic variations of the midcarpal joint. J Hand Surg 15A:129-31, 1990
7. Viegas SF: The lunato-hamate articulation of the midcarpal joint. Arthroscopy 6:5-10, 1990
8. Cantor RM et al: Diagnosis of dorsal and palmar rotation of the lunate on a frontal radiograph. J Hand Surg 13A:1897-93, 1989
9. Gilula La: Carpal injuries. Analytic approach and case exercises. AJR 133:503-17, 1979
10. Warwick R et al: Gray's anatomy, 35th Br ed. Philadelphia PA, WB Saunders 336-41,1973

HAMATO-LUNATE IMPINGEMENT

IMAGE GALLERY

Typical

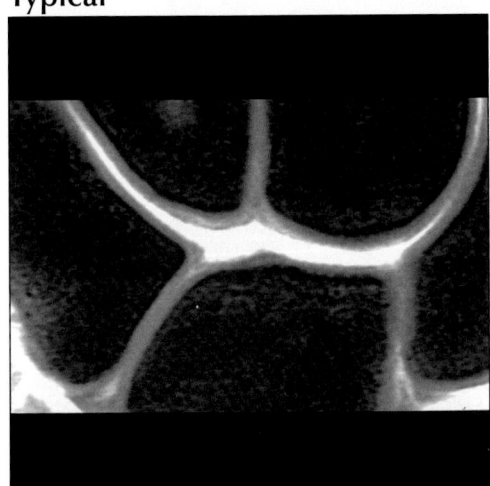

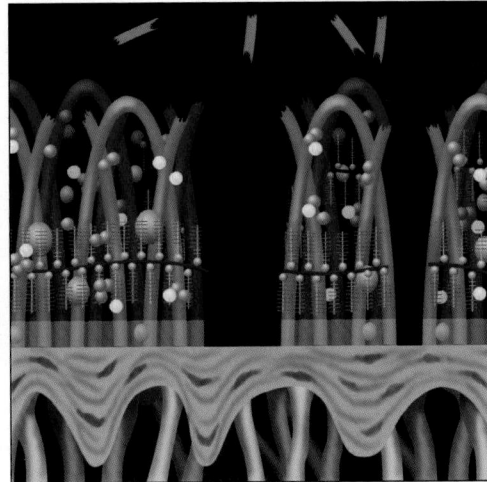

(Left) Coronal T1 C+ MR (MR arthrogram) shows early chondral loss of medial lunate facet and fibrillation of proximal pole of hamate (proximal pole scaphoid is to the right in all images). *(Right)* Coronal graphic shows histology of chondral degeneration with release of chondral debris into joint space. There is pronounced subchondral sclerosis in association with decreased proteoglycan aggregates.

Typical

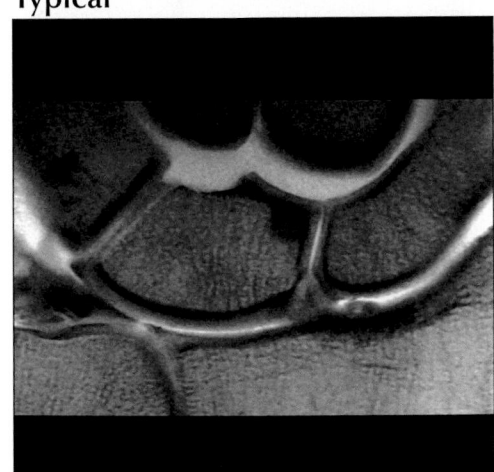

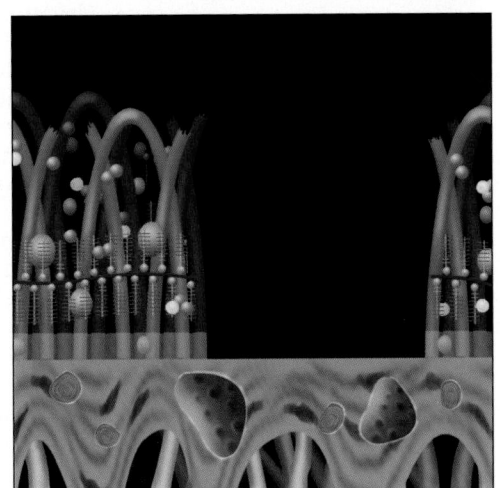

(Left) Coronal T1 C+ MR (MR arthrogram) shows full thickness chondral loss of medial lunate facet with subchondral sclerosis of proximal pole of hamate. *(Right)* Coronal graphic shows exposed surface of subchondral bone with full thickness chondral loss. Subchondral cyst formation is present.

Typical

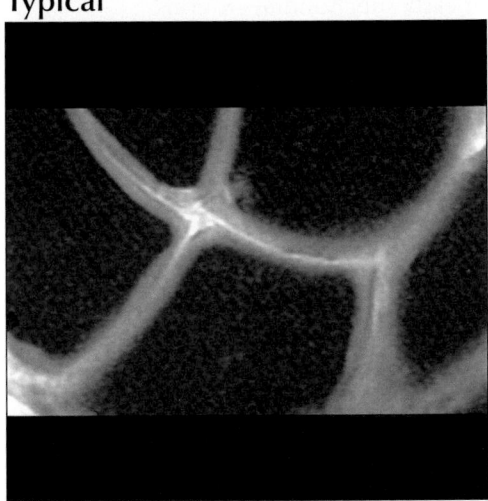

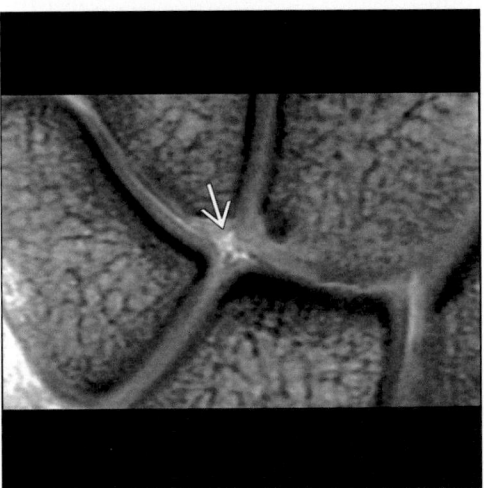

(Left) Coronal T1 C+ MR (MR arthrogram) shows hamato-lunate impingement with a small medial lunate facet. *(Right)* Coronal T1 C+ MR (MR arthrogram) shows superficial chondral degeneration of medial lunate facet and proximal pole of hamate (arrow) with subchondral sclerosis of adjacent capitate.

RHEUMATOID ARTHRITIS, WRIST AND HAND

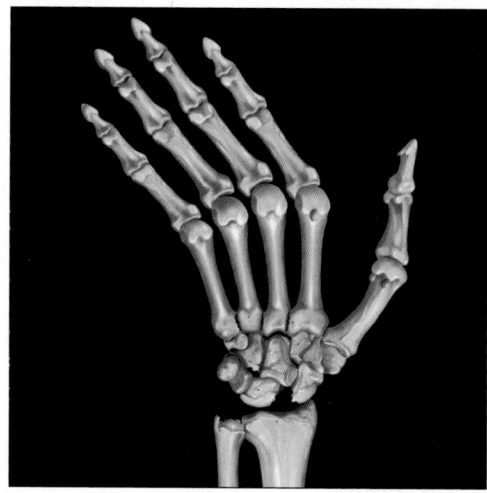

Coronal graphic shows ulnar deviation of the metacarpal phalangeal joints, proximal migration of the capitate, SL dissociation with ulnar and carpal erosions.

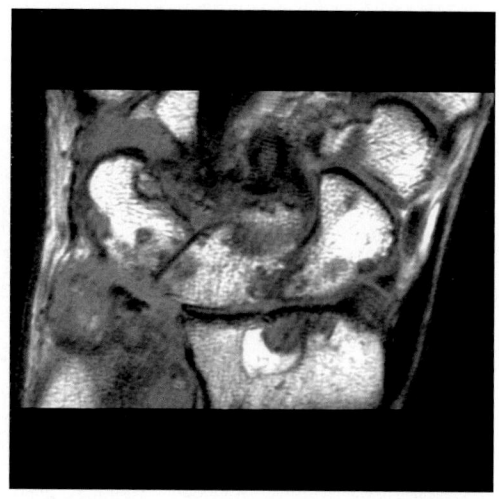

Coronal T1WI MR shows multiple carpal erosions with distal ulnar erosive changes and TFC destruction. Pannus tissue is intermediate in signal intensity.

TERMINOLOGY

Abbreviations and Synonyms
- RA, chronic polyarthritis

Definitions
- Systemic autoimmune inflammatory disorder of unknown etiology, primarily affecting synovial membranes and articular surfaces

IMAGING FINDINGS

General Features
- Best diagnostic clue: Inflammatory synovial/pannus tissue
- Location
  - Distal radioulnar joint
  - Ulnar & radial styloid
  - Scaphoid, triquetrum, pisiform
  - Radiocarpal, midcarpal, carpometacarpal
  - Metacarpal phalangeal, proximal interphalangeal
- Size: Variable from localized synovitis to involvement of the entire carpus (pancompartmental)
- Morphology: Erosions, joint space narrowing, soft tissue swelling & ulnar translocation

Radiographic Findings
- Radiography

- Negative in early stages of disease
- Soft tissue swelling visible - early stages
- First radiographic evidence of disease - ulnar styloid tip erosion
- Erosions are common at distal radius & ulna
- Triquetrum and pisiform - in early stages
- Marginal erosion at radial aspect trapezium common
- Juxta-articular osteopenia
- Pan-carpal progressive chondral loss
  - Gradual joint space narrowing
  - Joint obliteration
- Bony ankylosis - most common in midcarpal compartment in late stages
- Zig-zag deformity - radial deviation at radiocarpal joint & ulnar deviation at MCP joints
- Dorsal subluxation of ulna - common finding

CT Findings
- NECT
  - Sensitive for early subchondral erosions
  - Hypodense joint effusion
  - Joint space narrowing
  - Insensitive for early chondral loss
  - Superimposed osteoarthritic change visualized - sclerosis, osteophytosis
  - Bony ankylosis - late complication
- CECT: Pannus demonstrates vigorous enhancement

DDx: Rheumatoid Arthritis, Wrist and Hand

SLAC Wrist	Triscaphe	CPPD	Sudeck's
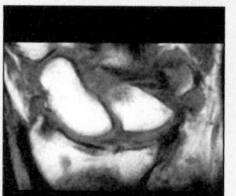	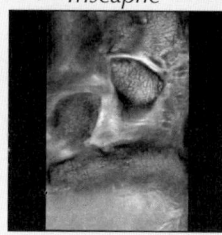	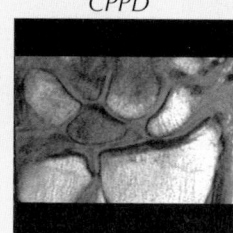	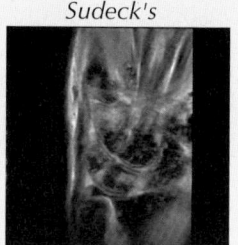
Cor T1WI MR	Cor T1 Arthro.	Cor T1WI MR	Cor FS PD MR

RHEUMATOID ARTHRITIS, WRIST AND HAND

Key Facts

Imaging Findings

- Best diagnostic clue: Inflammatory synovial/pannus tissue
- Morphology: Erosions, joint space narrowing, soft tissue swelling & ulnar translocation

Top Differential Diagnoses

- Osteoarthritis
- Autoimmune Chronic Polyarthritis
- Psoriatic Arthritis
- Infectious Arthritis
- Juvenile Chronic Arthritis
- Crystal Deposition Disease
- Reflex Sympathic Dystrophy (Sudeck's)

Pathology

- Characterized by bilateral, symmetrical joint involvement
- Characteristically involves carpal joints, MCP joints, PIP joints
- Hyperplasia of synovial cells

Clinical Issues

- Most common signs/symptoms: Insidious onset typical
- Joint swelling
- Bilateral involvement

Diagnostic Checklist

- 30% patients are rheumatoid factor negative

MR Findings

- T1WI
  - Hypointense subchondral sclerosis
  - Early erosions can be easily seen with reactive hypointense marrow edema
  - Early joint effusions - hypointense
  - Hypointense debris
  - Hypertrophied synovium
  - Tenosynovitis - hypointense
- T2WI
  - Hyperintense marrow edema visualized
  - Early joint effusions - hyperintense
  - Tenosynovitis - hyperintense
  - Partial tendon tears - hyperintense
  - Intermediate to hyperintense pannus
- T1 C+: Pannus will vigorously enhance

Ultrasonographic Findings

- Sonography
  - Hypoechoic joint effusion = common finding
  - Synovitis/precipitated fibrin - tiny floating hyperechoic foci = common finding
  - Thickened hypoechoic synovium (normal synovium not visualized by sonography)
  - Pannus - hypoechoic synovial masses
  - Tenosynovitis - hyperechoic
  - Tendon rupture - can be directly visualized
  - Synovial cysts - hypoechoic
  - Rheumatoid nodules - homogeneous hypoechoic masses

Nuclear Medicine Findings

- Skeletal scintigraphy
  - Limited due to lack of specificity
  - Increased nonspecific radiotracer accumulation in joint-centered distribution
  - Bilateral, symmetrical
  - May reveal extent of disease

Imaging Recommendations

- Best imaging tool: MR for synovium, articular cartilage & marrow
- Protocol advice

  - T1, FS PD FSE coronal, axial & sagittal
  - T1C+ with fat suppression for pannus

DIFFERENTIAL DIAGNOSIS

Osteoarthritis

- Scapholunate advanced collapse pattern (SLAC wrist)
- Triscaphe arthritis
- Combination of SLAC wrist & triscaphe arthritis

Autoimmune Chronic Polyarthritis

- Scleroderma (soft tissue calcification + tuft resorption)
- Systemic lupus erythematosus (no erosions)
- Dermatomyositis (intermuscular calcification)

Psoriatic Arthritis

- 2% of patients with psoriasis
- Polyarthritis with distal interphalangeal involvement
- Asymmetric oligoarthritis
- Arthritis mutilans

Infectious Arthritis

- Synovitis, soft tissue swelling, and effusion
- Juxta-articular osteoporosis

Juvenile Chronic Arthritis

- Effusion
- Metacarpophalangeal & interphalangeal joints
- Contracted tendons
- Capsular laxity

Crystal Deposition Disease

- Calcium pyrophosphate dihydrate crystal deposition disease (CPPD)
- Inflammatory arthritis
- Joint space loss (uniform)
- SLAC wrist

Reflex Sympathic Dystrophy (Sudeck's)

- Response to trauma
- Pain, vasomotor disturbance, decreased function & trophic changes
- Inhomogeneous marrow - patchy on FS PD FSE

RHEUMATOID ARTHRITIS, WRIST AND HAND

PATHOLOGY

General Features
- General path comments
  - Relevant anatomy
    - Synovium
- Etiology: Unknown etiology
- Epidemiology
  - RA incidence = 1% of population
  - Serum antinuclear antibodies (ANA) found in approximately 30% of patients

Gross Pathologic & Surgical Features
- Characterized by bilateral, symmetrical joint involvement
- Characteristically involves carpal joints, MCP joints, PIP joints
- Pannus: Synovial mass which results in marginal erosions at junction of articular cartilage & bare area of bone
- Chronic synovial-based inflammation can permanently damage tendons
- Chronic synovitis/inflammation may lead to capsular & ligamentous laxity
- Chronic synovitis leads to destruction of TFCC
- Tenosynovitis/swelling may lead to compression of median or ulnar nerves resulting in neuropathies
- Caput ulnar syndrome
  - Synovitis results in stretching of ulnar carpal ligaments
  - Pain, decreased range of motion, dorsal subluxation of ulna
  - Subluxed ulna may contact extensor tendons resulting in attrition & tearing

Microscopic Features
- Extensive synovial inflammation
  - Hyperplasia of synovial cells
  - Lymphocytes & plasma cells infiltrate synovial membrane
  - Fibrinous exudates
- Rheumatoid factor
  - Serum IgM antibody found in approximately 70% of patients
  - Directed against Fc fragment of IgG
  - High titers of RH factors are associated with severe disease

CLINICAL ISSUES

Presentation
- Most common signs/symptoms: Insidious onset typical
- Clinical profile
  - 4 of 7 criteria must be met for diagnosis
    - Morning stiffness lasting more than 1 hour
    - Arthritis of 3 or more joints
    - Arthritis of hand joints
    - Symmetric arthritis
    - Positive serum rheumatoid factor
    - Rheumatoid nodules
    - Radiographic changes
  - Other common signs/symptoms

- Malaise
- Weakness
- Weight loss
- Myalgias
- Fever of unknown origin
  - Physical exam
    - Joint swelling
    - Bilateral involvement
    - Erythema
    - Pain with active/passive range of motion
    - Tenderness to palpation
    - Joint malalignment
    - Neuropathy in median/ulnar nerve distribution

Demographics
- Age
  - 25-60 years most common
  - 40-60 years - peak incidence
- Gender: F:M = 3:1

Natural History & Prognosis
- Typically patients have slowly progressive disease with intermittent "flare-ups"
- Slowly, progressive joint destruction is typical
- Complications
  - Joint effusions → capsular distention → pain
  - Large synovial cysts
  - Tendinous tears/disruptions
  - Cartilaginous & bony destruction
  - Median and ulnar nerve neuropathies

Treatment
- Conservative
  - Decrease inflammation → delay joint effusion → preserve function
  - Pharmacotherapy
  - Physical therapy
- Surgical
  - Synovectomy & tenosynovectomy
  - Tendon ruptures
    - Attachment to adjoining tendon preferable to segmental grafting
  - Arthroplasty or arthrodesis

DIAGNOSTIC CHECKLIST

Consider
- 30% patients are rheumatoid factor negative

SELECTED REFERENCES

1. Nakahara N et al: Gadolinium-enhanced MR imaging of the wrist in rheumatoid arthritis: Value of fat suppression pulse sequences. Skeletal Radiol 25:639, 1996
2. Adolfsson L et al: Arthroscopic synovectomy of the rheumatoid wrist. J Hand Surg 18B:92-6, 1993
3. Taleisnik J: Rheumatoid arthritis of the wrist. Hand Clin 5:257-78, 1989
4. Ertel AN et al: Flexor tendon ruptures in patients with rheumatoid arthritis. J Hand Surg 13A:860-6, 1988
5. Abernathy PJ et al: Decompression of the extensor tendons at the wrist in rheumatoid arthritis. J Bone Joint Surg 61B:64, 1979

RHEUMATOID ARTHRITIS, WRIST AND HAND

IMAGE GALLERY

Typical

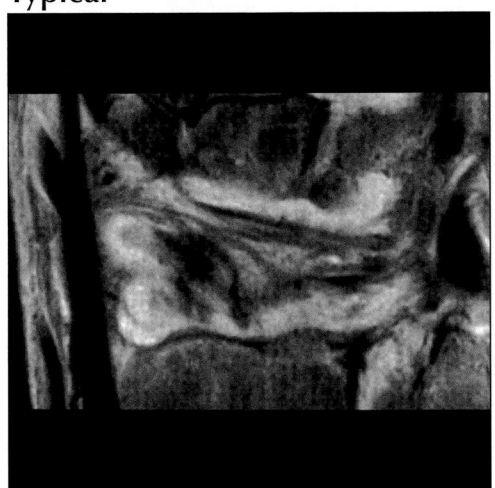
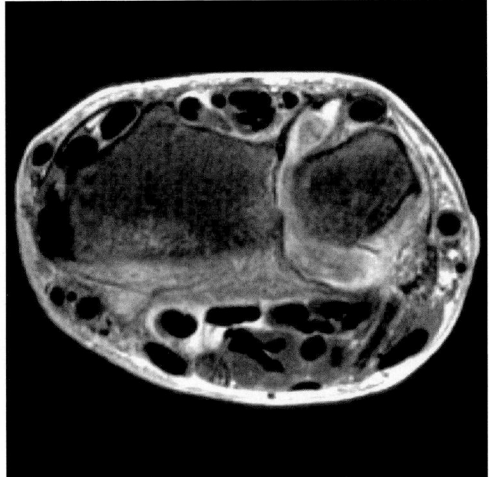

(Left) Coronal FS PD FSE MR shows dorsal pannus tissue with intermediate signal intensity of hypertrophied synovium. *(Right)* Axial FS PD FSE MR shows synovitis of distal radioulnar joint with heterogenous signal.

Typical

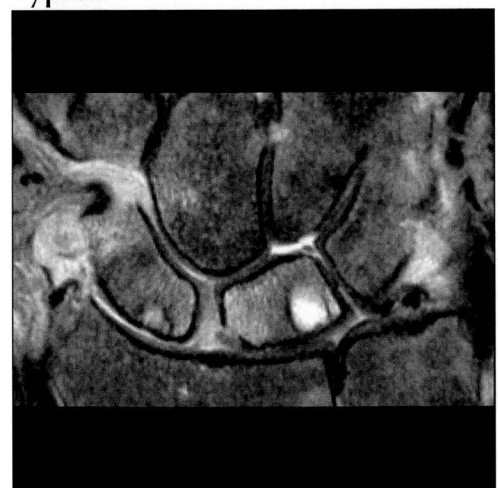
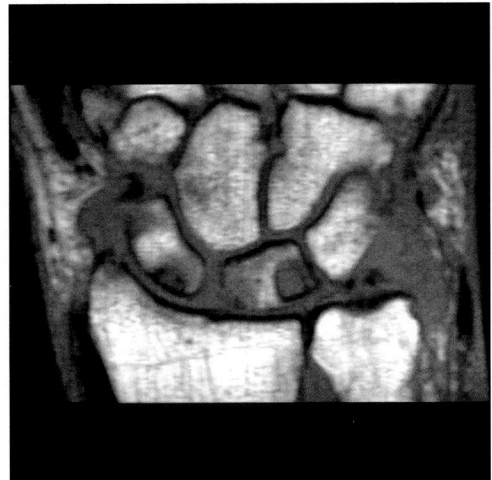

(Left) Coronal FS PD FSE MR shows scapholunate dissociation with carpal erosions and marrow edema. *(Right)* Coronal T1WI MR shows hypointense subchondral erosions and carpal cysts.

Variant

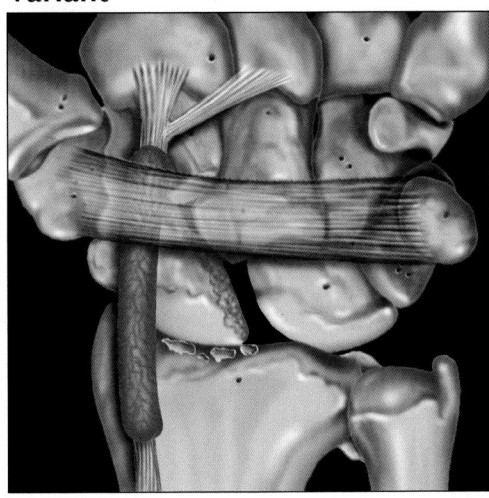
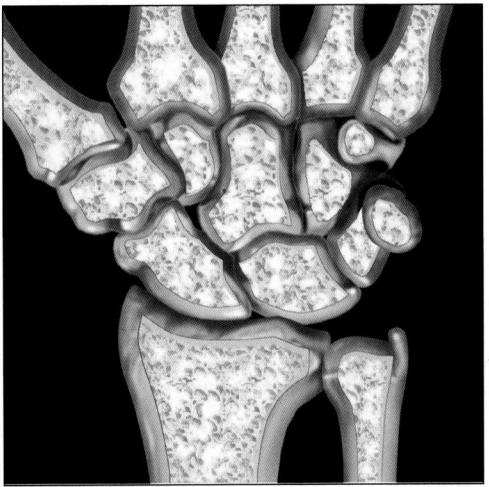

(Left) Coronal graphic shows tenosynovitis of flexor carpi radialis in association with scapholunate dissociation. These changes may also be seen in psoriatic arthritis, especially with isolated tendon involvement. *(Right)* Coronal graphic shows osteopenia of carpus in association with rheumatoid disease. Inflammatory arthritis usually demonstrates juxta-articular osteopenia similar to Sudeck's atrophy.

MADELUNG'S DEFORMITY

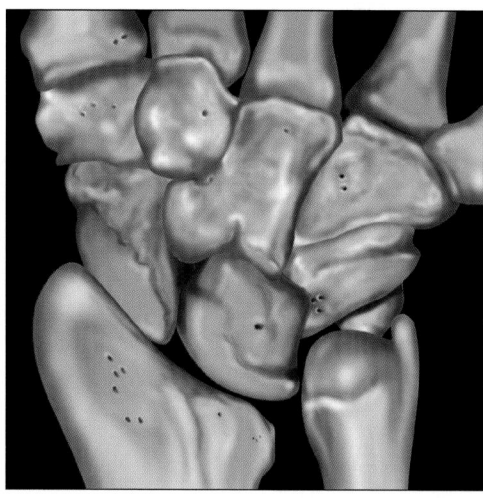

Coronal graphic shows Madelung's deformity with medial angulation of the distal radial articular surface and triangulation of the carpus.

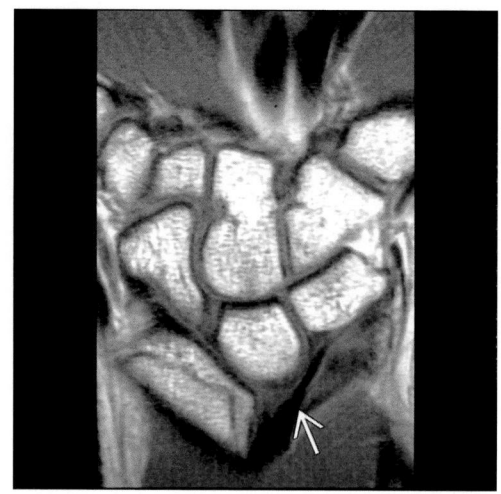

Coronal T1WI MR shows the hypointense thickened radiolunate ligament (arrow) extending to the medial aspect of the distal radial metaphysis (area of metaphyseal bone spike).

TERMINOLOGY

Abbreviations and Synonyms
- Dysplasia, dyschondrosteosis

Definitions
- Developmental growth disturbance of distal radial physis

IMAGING FINDINGS

General Features
- Best diagnostic clue: Distal radius epiphysis is triangular & medially tilted
- Location: Distal radial epiphysis
- Size: Involvement can range from changes in the distal radius & ulna to changes in carpal morphology
- Morphology: Distal radius epiphysis is triangular and medially beaked

Radiographic Findings
- Radiography
  - Radius short + dorsolateral curvature
  - Radial distal articular surface - excessive volar & ulnar inclination
  - Distal radial epiphysis - triangular & medially tilted
  - Lucent area in ulnar aspect distal radius + osteophytes
  - Premature closure of anteromedial quadrant of distal radius physis
  - Distal ulna is long & shows dorsal subluxation
  - Ulnar head enlarged & deformed
  - Distal ulnar physis - radially inclined
  - Carpus - triangular shape
  - Lunate - wedged in widened distal radioulnar interosseous space
  - Dorsal curvature carpus + radial bowing of lateral column
  - Reverse Madelung's deformity
    - Radius with volar convexity
    - Distal radial articular surface inclined dorsally

MR Findings
- T1WI
  - Ulnar angulation distal radial articular surface
  - Ulnar head - dorsoulnar configuration (dorsally prominent ulnar head)
  - Radius bowed
  - Physeal lesion - palmar ulnar aspect of distal radial physis
  - Triangulation of carpus
  - Groove & osseous spike develops at ulnar aspect of metaphyseal-diaphyseal junction from tethering effect of radiolunate ligament (hypointense & thick ligament)
  - Oblique radial triangular fibrocartilage (TFC) attachment

---

DDx: Madelung's Deformity

Radius Fracture	Die punch Fx	Impingement	DRUJ Instability
Sag FS PD MR	Cor FS PD MR	Cor T1 Arthro.	Ax T1WI MR

MADELUNG'S DEFORMITY

Key Facts

Imaging Findings
- Best diagnostic clue: Distal radius epiphysis is triangular & medially tilted
- Distal ulna is long & shows dorsal subluxation
- Distal ulnar physis - radially inclined
- Lunate - wedged in widened distal radioulnar interosseous space

Top Differential Diagnoses
- Distal Radius Fracture
- Die punch Fracture
- Osteochondroma
- Ulna Impingement Syndrome
- Distal Radioulnar Joint (DRUJ) Instability

Pathology
- Focal dysplasia distal radial physis

- Dyschondrosteosis form of mesomelic dwarfism
- Localized lesion = ulnopalmar zone distal radius
- Chevron carpus = osseous lesion midway between Madelung's & reverse Madelung's deformity
- Metaphyseal groove & spike at radiolunate ligament attachment to area of growth retardation

Clinical Issues
- Most common signs/symptoms: Wrist pain
- Deformity at infancy or adolescence
- Loss of motion
- Derangement of DRUJ
- Loss of supination

Diagnostic Checklist
- Identify radiolunate ligament on coronal images

- ○ ± Ischemic changes of lunate (hypointensity)
- T2WI
  - ○ Hypointense radiolunate ligament (palmar location)
  - ○ Physis - hyperintense
  - ○ Chevron carpus = mid-ulnar zone dyschondrosteosis
  - ○ Advanced dyschondrosteosis
    - ▪ Lack of proximal lunate support by radius
  - ○ Thick hypointense radiolunate ligament attached to distal radial physis

Imaging Recommendations
- Best imaging tool
  - ○ MR identifies soft tissue contributions (radiolunate ligament) in addition to marrow & chondral changes
  - ○ Monitoring of children
- Protocol advice
  - ○ T1 & FS PD FSE coronal, axial & sagittal
  - ○ T2* gradient echo = improved visualization of physis (hyperintense)

DIFFERENTIAL DIAGNOSIS

Distal Radius Fracture
- Intra- vs. extraarticular
- Articular components
  - ○ Metaphyseal
  - ○ Radial styloid
  - ○ Dorsal medial/palmar medial articular surface

Die punch Fracture
- Lunate load fracture
- Lunate impaction on lunate fossa of distal radius
- Dorsal displacement (dorsal medial fragment)
- Volar displacement (palmar medial fragment)

Osteochondroma
- Endochondral growth disorder
- Osteocartilaginous tumors
- Metaphyseal remodeling
- Multiple hereditary exostosis
- Osteochondroma in distal radius & ulna

- Spectrum: Asymmetric beaking of metaphyseal cortex to pedunculated metaphyseal osteochondromas

Ulna Impingement Syndrome
- Pain during pronation & supination
- Ulnar minus (negative) variance
- Scalloped concavity distal radius
- Ulnar convergence to distal radius
- ± Osteophytes
- ± Chondromalacia distal ulna

Distal Radioulnar Joint (DRUJ) Instability
- Dorsal or volar displacement of distal ulna
- Ulnar dorsal vs. ulnar palmar
- Rotational injury - fall on outstretched hand
- Injury to palmar or dorsal distal radioulnar ligaments (margins of TFC)
- Ulnar-sided wrist pain

PATHOLOGY

General Features
- General path comments
  - ○ Relevant anatomy
    - ▪ Distal radial physis
    - ▪ Radiolunate ligament = volar structure
    - ▪ Triangular fibrocartilage
    - ▪ Distal radioulnar joint
- Genetics
  - ○ Dominant, familial deformity
  - ○ Incomplete penetrance
  - ○ Bilateral occurrence documented
  - ○ Familial dysplasia profile
    - ▪ Hypoplasia of radius
    - ▪ Mesomelic dwarfism
- Etiology
  - ○ Focal dysplasia distal radial physis
  - ○ Dyschondrosteosis form of mesomelic dwarfism
  - ○ Primary or idiopathic form - nonheritable
  - ○ Bony lesions = dyschondrosteosis
- Epidemiology
  - ○ Rare in occurrence

MADELUNG'S DEFORMITY

○ Increased incidence in West Indies

Gross Pathologic & Surgical Features
- Ulnar head - dorsoulnar prominence
- Hand displaced radiopalmarly
- Tilting & bowing distal radius
- Variable forearm shortening
- Reverse Madelung's deformity
  - ○ Ulnar head palmar
  - ○ Wrist arched dorsally
- Extreme manifestation - hypoplasia entire radius
- Localized lesion = ulnopalmar zone distal radius
- Medial radial epiphysis deformity (tethering of epiphysis proximally)
- Chevron carpus = osseous lesion midway between Madelung's & reverse Madelung's deformity
- Metaphyseal groove & spike at radiolunate ligament attachment to area of growth retardation
- Oblique radial attachment TFC

Microscopic Features
- Normal chondrocytes
- Abnormally arranged cell columns
- Cambium layer cells of periosteum stream from periphery of physis
  - ○ Zone of Ranvier

Staging, Grading or Classification Criteria
- Madelung's
- Reverse Madelung's
- Chevron carpus
  - ○ Clinical deformity absent
  - ○ Triangulation of carpus, wedged between radius & ulna

CLINICAL ISSUES

Presentation
- Most common signs/symptoms: Wrist pain
- Clinical profile
  - ○ Deformity at infancy or adolescence
  - ○ Loss of motion
  - ○ Weakness
  - ○ Ligamentous stretching + carpal translation
  - ○ Derangement of DRUJ
  - ○ Poor correlation between symptoms & imaging findings
  - ○ Extensor tendon attrition over deformed ulnar head in adults
  - ○ Marked obliquity of carpal tunnel associated with susceptibility to median neuropathy in trauma
  - ○ Midcarpal joint involved 2° to triangular morphology of carpus
  - ○ Loss of supination
  - ○ Dorsiflexion, radial deviation also restricted

Demographics
- Age: Clinical manifestation during adolescence
- Gender: Female predominance

Natural History & Prognosis
- Progressive radiologic deterioration
- Bracing used to control symptoms
- End stage

○ Distal radius turned in ulnar + palmar direction
○ Carpus & hand appear volar to forearm while ulna shows dorsal subluxation

Treatment
- Conservative
  - ○ Bracing
- Surgical
  - ○ Indications: Persistent pain, loss of normal anatomy, grip weakness & severe deformity
  - ○ Resection of distal ulna
    - Darrach procedure
  - ○ Sauve-Kapandji procedure: DRUJ fusion and ulnar osteotomy
  - ○ Open or closed wedge osteotomy of radius
  - ○ External fixators
  - ○ Epiphysiodesis (distal ulna or radius)
  - ○ Radiocarpal & total wrist fusion
  - ○ Prophylactic excision of physeal bar in symptomatic adolescents

DIAGNOSTIC CHECKLIST

Consider
- Symptoms & imaging findings may not correlate
- Identify radiolunate ligament on coronal images

SELECTED REFERENCES

1. Vickers D: The wrist. Diagnosis and operative treatment. Madelung's deformity. vol 1. St. Louis Missouri, Mosby, (41):966-81, 1998
2. Rao, SB et al: The wrist and it's disorders. Congenital and developmental wrist disorders in children. 2nd ed. Philadelphia PA, W.B. Saunders, (29):509-39, 1997
3. Murphy MS et al: Radial opening wedge osteotomy in Madelung's deformity. J Hand Surg 21:1035-44, 1996
4. Watson HK et al: Madelung's deformity: A surgical technique. J Hand Surg 18:601-5, 1993
5. Langenskiold A et al: Specific collagen mRNAs elucidate the histogentic relationship between the growth plate, the tissue in the ossification groove of Ranvier, and the cambium layer of the adjacent periosteum. A preliminary report. Clin Orthop 297:51-4, 1993
6. Vickers D et al: Madelung deformity: Surgical prophylaxis (physiolysis) during the late growth period by resection of the dyschondrosteosis lesion. J Hand Surg 17:401-7, 1992
7. Fagg PS: Wrist pain in the Madelung's deformity of dyschondrosteosis. J Hand Surg 13:11-15, 1988
8. Nielson JB: Madelung's deformity: A follow-up study of 256 cases and a review of the literature. Acta Orthop Scand 48:379-84, 1977.
9. Golding JS et al: Madelung's disease of the wrist and dyschondrosteosis. J Bone Joint Surg 58:350-2, 1976
10. Langenskiold A: An operation for partial closure of an epiphyseal plate in children, and its experimental basis. J Bone Joint Surg 57:325-30, 1975

MADELUNG'S DEFORMITY

IMAGE GALLERY

Typical

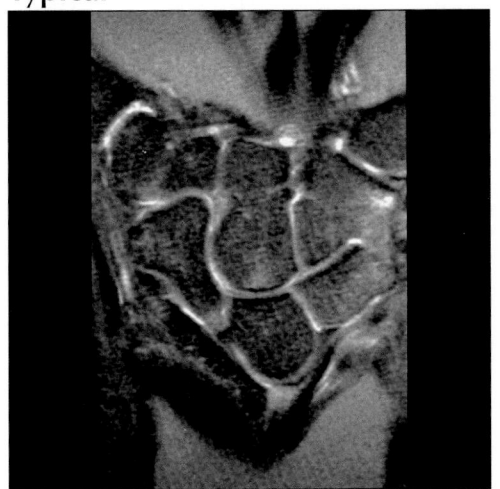
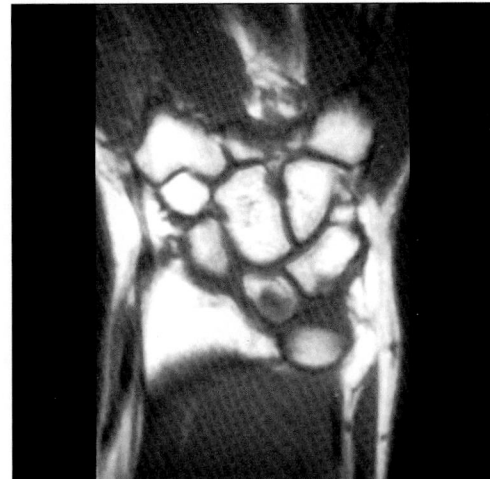

(Left) Coronal FS PD FSE MR shows Madelung's deformity with proximal migration of the lunate (triangulation of the carpus), medial angulation of the distal radius and oblique orientation of the TFC. *(Right)* Coronal T1WI MR shows Madelung's deformity complicated by lunate ischemia.

Typical

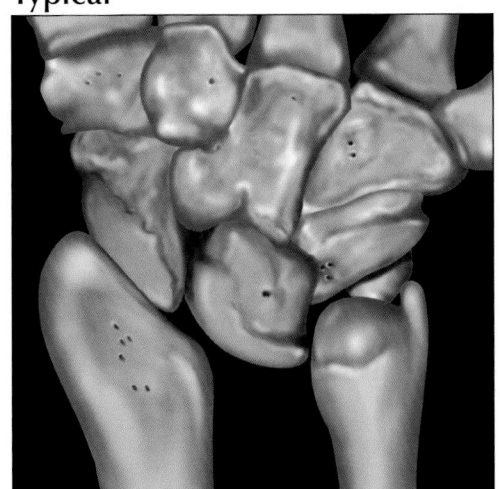
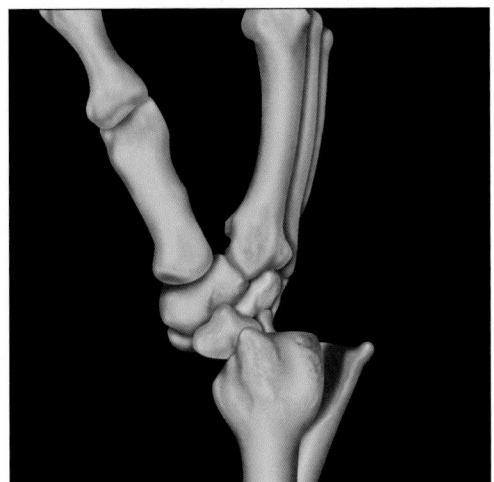

(Left) Coronal graphic shows advanced changes of Madelung's deformity with complete lack of a lunate fossa. The lunate is suspended without osseous support and is impinged between the radius and ulna. *(Right)* Sagittal graphic shows Madelung's deformity with dorsoulnar prominence of the ulnar head.

Typical

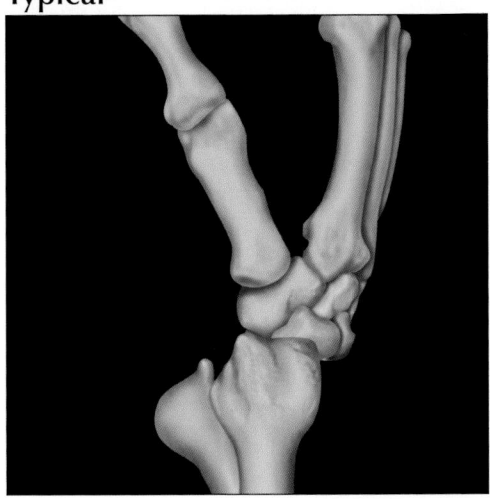
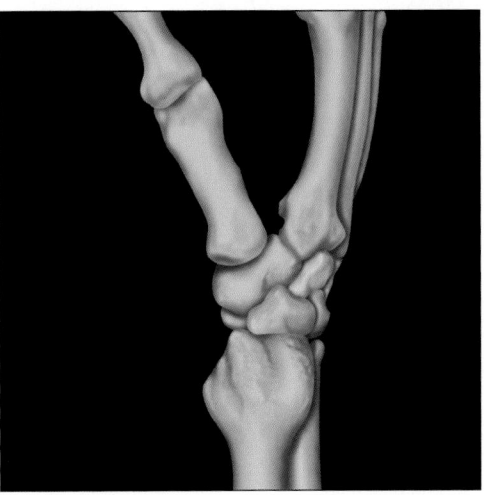

(Left) Sagittal graphic shows reverse Madelung's deformity with the ulnar head displaced in a palmar direction. *(Right)* Sagittal graphic shows Chevron carpus without displacement of distal ulna (no clinical deformity) despite triangulation of the carpus and wedging between the radius and ulna.

GANGLION CYST, WRIST

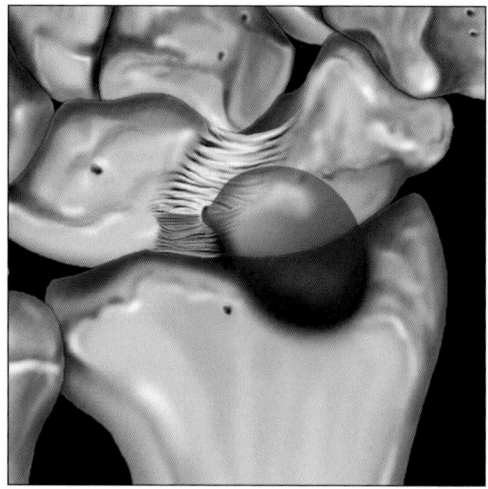

Coronal graphic shows dorsal ganglion cyst in communication with the dorsal and membranous fibers of the scapholunate ligament.

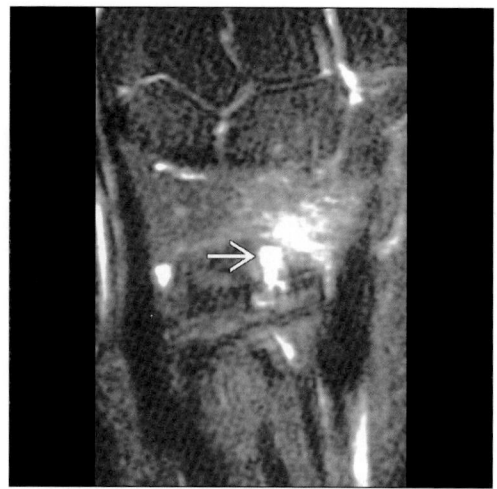

Coronal FS PD FSE MR shows dorsal ganglion (arrow) originating from dorsal component of the scapholunate ligament. This is adjacent to the dorsal interosseous nerve branch.

TERMINOLOGY

Abbreviations and Synonyms
- Ganglion, ganglia, carpal ganglion, dorsal wrist ganglion, dorsal ganglions, palmar wrist ganglion

Definitions
- Cystic mucinous soft tissue masses occurring about the wrist & hand in predictable locations

IMAGING FINDINGS

General Features
- Best diagnostic clue: Homogeneous fluid-filled mass in communication with the scapholunate interval
- Location
  - Dorsal scapholunate (SL) interval
  - Volar (palmar) radiocarpal joint
  - Dorsal retinaculum of 1st extensor component
  - Carpal tunnel
  - Guyon's canal
  - Triscaphe joint
  - Ulnocarpal
  - 2nd metacarpal-trapezial joint
- Size
  - Varies (usually 5 mm to 2 cm)
  - Size increases with activity

- Morphology: Oval with narrow stalk extending from origin

Radiographic Findings
- Radiography
  - Usually normal
  - Scapholunate (SL) dissociation with interval gap
  - Osteoarthritis
  - Intraosseous carpal ganglion
  - ± Soft tissue density

MR Findings
- T1WI
  - Hypointense to intermediate signal intensity mass
  - Normal adjacent subcutaneous tissue
  - Arthrosis scaphotrapezial or radioscaphoid
  - SL diastasis on coronal images
  - Stalk difficult to visualized on T1WI
- T2WI
  - Uniformly hyperintense soft tissue cystic mass
  - Unilocular or multiloculated
  - ± Hypointense capsule
  - Inhomogeneity of cyst related to mucin content
  - Narrow hyperintense stalk in communication with main cyst
  - Stalk extension through joint capsule
  - Stalk with elongated pedicle allows cyst presentation away from origin (e.g., cysts originating from SL interval maybe ulnar to extensor tendons)

DDx: Ganglion Cyst

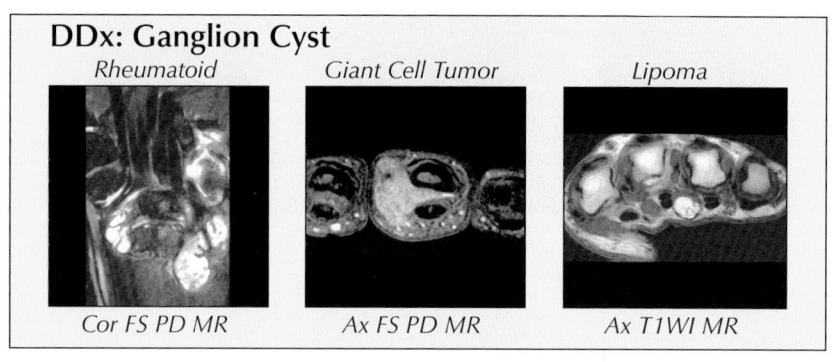

Rheumatoid	Giant Cell Tumor	Lipoma
Cor FS PD MR	Ax FS PD MR	Ax T1WI MR

GANGLION CYST, WRIST

Key Facts

Imaging Findings

- Best diagnostic clue: Homogeneous fluid-filled mass in communication with the scapholunate interval
- Dorsal scapholunate (SL) interval
- Volar (palmar) radiocarpal joint
- Morphology: Oval with narrow stalk extending from origin

Top Differential Diagnoses

- Rheumatoid Arthritis
- Synovitis
- Tenosynovitis
- Giant Cell Tumor of Tendon Sheath
- Benign Tumors

Pathology

- SL ligament - membranous & dorsal component origin
- Weakness in dorsal capsule
- Dorsal location where dorsal interosseous nerve approaches joint capsule

Clinical Issues

- Most common signs/symptoms: Localized soft tissue mass
- Localized pain + weakness (pain with dorsiflexion)
- ± Associated intraosseous carpal ganglion
- Recurrence rate with conservative treatment: 14-74%

Diagnostic Checklist

- Extension from SL joint = typical origin of ganglion which presents dorsally

---

- ○ Small hyperintense carpal tunnel ganglions frequently traced to scaphotrapeziotrapezoid (STT) joint
  - ■ 2° compression of median nerve
- ○ Cyst communication with adjacent tendon sheath
- ○ Intraosseous carpal ganglions - hyperintense
- T1 C+: To confirm cystic contents (peripheral enhancement) vs. soft tissue neoplasm

Imaging Recommendations

- Best imaging tool: MR identifies cyst vs. solid tumor, location, morphology, proximity to neurovascular structures, joint or tendon sheath communication
- Protocol advice: T1, PD, FS PD FSE or STIR coronal, axial & sagittal images (coronal & axial planes required)

DIFFERENTIAL DIAGNOSIS

Rheumatoid Arthritis

- Synovitis
- Articular cartilage destruction
- Ligamentous laxity, joint subluxations/dislocations
- Reactive subchondral edema (carpus)
- Tenosynovitis
- Rheumatoid nodule

Synovitis

- Inflammatory response - variety of stimuli
- Intermediate signal on T1WI
- Intermediate + hyperintensity on FS PD FSE
- Enhancement with T1C+

Tenosynovitis

- Trauma vs. repetitive use
- Hyperintensity on T2WI within tendon sheath
- Pain with activity
- Locking/triggering - sheath constriction or stenosing

Giant Cell Tumor of Tendon Sheath

- Benign fibrous histiocytoma originating from tendon sheath or joint capsule
- Soft tissue mass

- Inhomogeneous hypo to intermediate signal intensity on FS PD FSE images

Benign Tumors

- Lipoma
- Xanthoma
- Fibroma
- Hemangioma
- Osteochondroma
- Lymphangioma

Malignant Tumors

- Malignant fibrous histiocytoma
- Synovial sarcoma
- Chondrosarcoma

Infection

- Mycobacterial (TB)
- Fungal
- Pyogenic abscess

Vascular

- Aneurysm
- Arteriovenous malformation

PATHOLOGY

General Features

- General path comments
  - ○ Relevant anatomy
    - ■ SL interval
    - ■ Radiocarpal joint
    - ■ Guyon's canal
    - ■ Dorsal interosseous nerve branch
- Etiology
  - ○ SL ligament - membranous & dorsal component origin
  - ○ Stress forces epicentered between scaphoid & lunate
  - ○ Joint fluid pumped (one way valve) between collagen bundles
  - ○ Weakness in dorsal capsule
  - ○ Palmar radiocarpal ganglion near origin of radiocarpal ligament from triscaphe joints

GANGLION CYST, WRIST

- Epidemiology
  - Most common soft tissue mass of wrist
  - 50-70% of all soft tissue masses of wrist/hand
  - Dorsal SL origin incidence: 60-70% of all ganglions
  - Palmar radiocarpal incidence: 18-20%

Gross Pathologic & Surgical Features
- Cystic mucinous joint fluid in pseudocapsule
- Ganglion protrusion through SL ligament ± confined deep to radiocarpal ligament
- Protrusion through dorsal wrist capsule
- Palpable, firm & smooth
- ± Multilobular mass
- Dorsal location where dorsal interosseous nerve approaches joint capsule
- Cyst connects to joint capsule or tendon sheath via narrow stalk
- Palmar radiocarpal ganglion protrudes along flexor carpi radialis tendon sheath
- Retinacular ganglions associated with hypertrophic retinaculum superficial to stenosing tenosynovitis (de Quervain's)
- Guyon's canal ganglion from weak region in pisohamate ligament

Microscopic Features
- Collagen fiber break-down products
- Intercellular mucin
- Microscopic mucinous pools
  - Coalesce
  - Expand
- Dissection through subcutaneous tissue
- Compacted fibrous tissue = pseudocapsule
- Capsule lining
  - Compressed collagen fibers
  - Flat nonendothelial cells (nonsynovial)

CLINICAL ISSUES

Presentation
- Most common signs/symptoms: Localized soft tissue mass
- Clinical profile
  - Localized pain + weakness (pain with dorsiflexion)
  - Neurologic findings only with carpal tunnel or Guyon's canal involvement
  - Ganglion soft to firm
  - Does not move with adjacent tendon
  - ± Associated intraosseous carpal ganglion
  - Size & symptoms may increase after activity
  - Allen's test + doppler to confirm patency of radial artery

Demographics
- Age
  - Dorsal ganglion = 2nd, 3rd, 4th decades
  - Radiocarpal palmar ganglions: 5th, 6th & 7th decades
- Gender: F > M

Natural History & Prognosis
- Varying size & discomfort
- Resolution without treatment: 38-58%
- Recurrence rate with conservative treatment: 14-74%

- Palmar ganglion = highest rate of recurrence post aspiration & steroid injection

Treatment
- Conservative
  - Manual rupture
  - Cyst wall puncture
  - Aspiration & steroid injection
- Surgical
  - Excision including stalk

DIAGNOSTIC CHECKLIST

Consider
- Extension from SL joint = typical origin of ganglion which presents dorsally
- Intravenous contrast required for diagnosis when there is inhomogeneity of ganglion signal on FS PD FSE or STIR

SELECTED REFERENCES

1. Kozin SH et al: The wrist. Diagnosis and operative treatment. Soft-tissue problems and neoplasms. vol 1. St. Louis Missouri, Mosby, (49):1166-80, 1998
2. Bogumill GP: The wrist and it's disorders. Tumors of the wrist. 2nd ed. Philadelphia Pennsylvania, W.B. Saunders, (31):563-82, 1997
3. Vo P et al: Evaluating dorsal wrist pain: MRI diagnosis of occult dorsal wrist ganglion. J Hand Surg 20:667, 1995
4. Bianchi S et al: Ultrasonographic evaluation of wrist ganglia. Skel Radiol 23:201, 1994
5. Cardinal E et al: Occult dorsal carpal ganglion: Comparison of US and MR imaging. Radiolog 193:259, 1994
6. Greendyke SD et al: Anterior wrist ganglia from the scaphotrapezial joint. J Hand Surg 17:487-90, 1992
7. Jacobs LG et al: The volar wrist ganglion: Just a simple cyst? J Hand Surg 15:342-6, 1990
8. Hollister AM et al: The use of MRI in the diagnosis of an occult wrist ganglion cyst. Orthop Rev 18:1210-2, 1989
9. DeVilliers CM et al: Dorsal ganglion of the wrist – pathogenesis and biomechanics. Operative vs. conservative treatment. S Afr Med J 75:214-6, 1989
10. Harvey FJ et al: Carpal tunnel syndrome caused by a simple ganglion. Hand 13:164-6, 1981
11. Bowers WH et al: An intraarticular-intraosseous carpal ganglion. J Hand Surg 4:375-7, 1979
12. Dellon AL et al: Anatomic dissections relating the posterior interosseous nerve to the carpus, and the etiology of dorsal wrist ganglion pain. J Hand Surg 3:326-32, 1978

GANGLION CYST, WRIST

IMAGE GALLERY

Typical

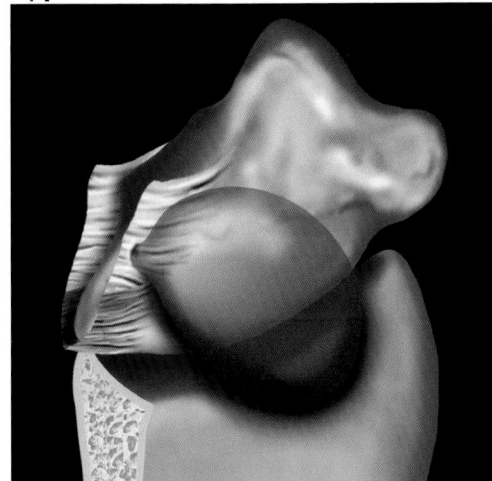
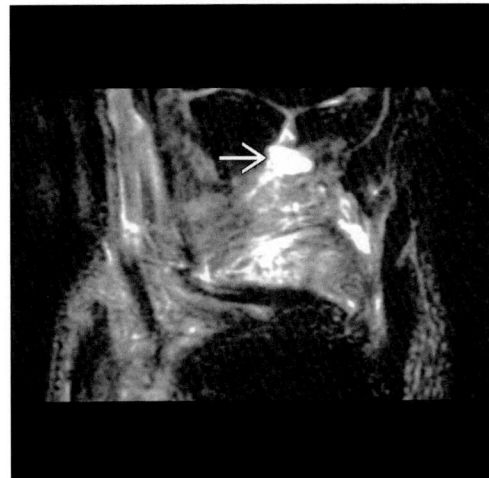

(Left) Coronal graphic shows the narrow stalk extending from scapholunate origin of this dorsal ganglion. Joint fluid extends through a one way valve mechanism in a dorsal capsule defect. *(Right)* Coronal FS PD FSE MR shows distal extension of a dorsal scapholunate ligament ganglion *(arrow)* between the capitate and trapezoid adjacent to the dorsal intercarpal ligament.

Typical

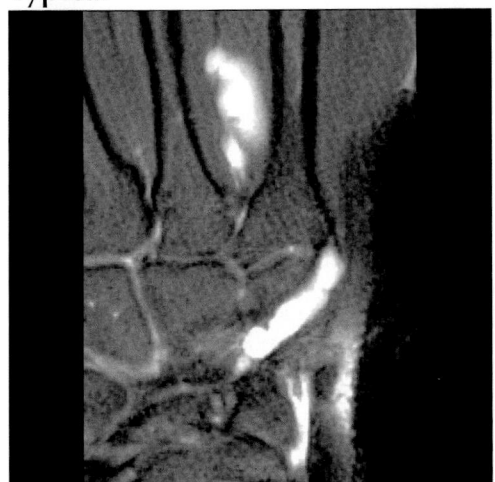
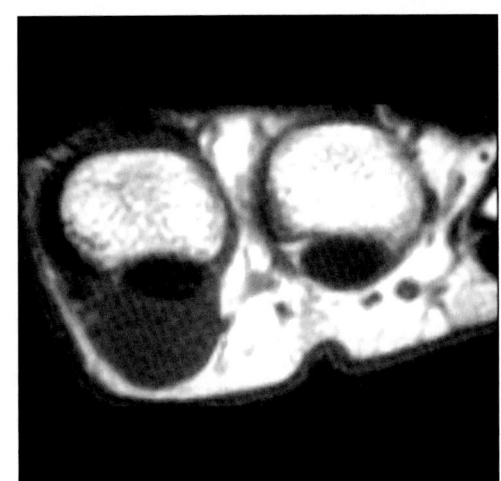

(Left) Coronal FS PD FSE MR shows radial and distal extension of a scapholunate ligament ganglion. This dorsal ganglion extends between the 2nd and 3rd metacarpals. *(Right)* Axial T1WI MR shows hypointense ganglion adjacent to the flexor tendon sheath of the 2nd digit.

Typical

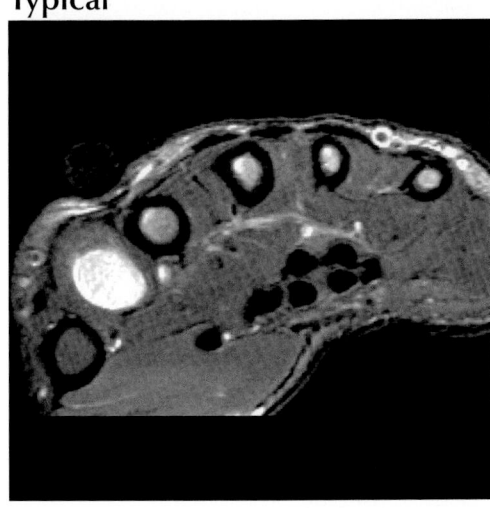
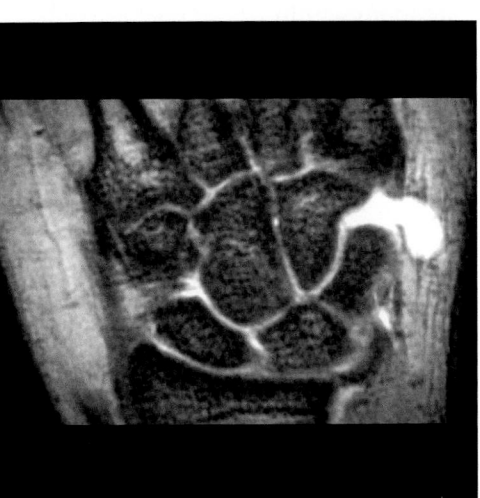

(Left) Axial FS PD FSE MR shows hyperintense ganglion dissecting into the 1st web space. The origin of this ganglion was the scapholunate interval. *(Right)* Coronal T2* GRE MR shows cystic ganglion communicating with the hamate triquetral joint.

DE QUERVAIN'S TENOSYNOVITIS

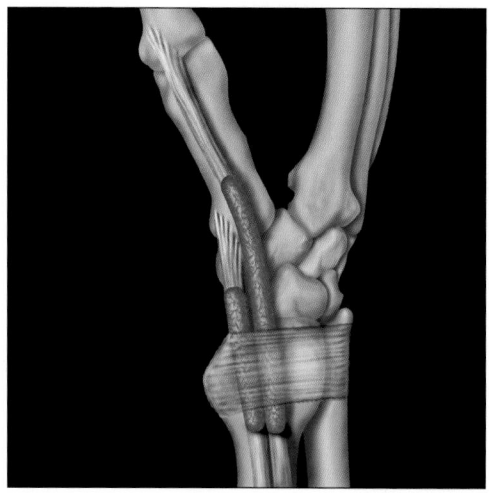

Sagittal graphic shows edema of the first extensor compartment tendons in de Quervain's tenosynovitis. The APL is located volar to the EPB at the level of radial styloid.

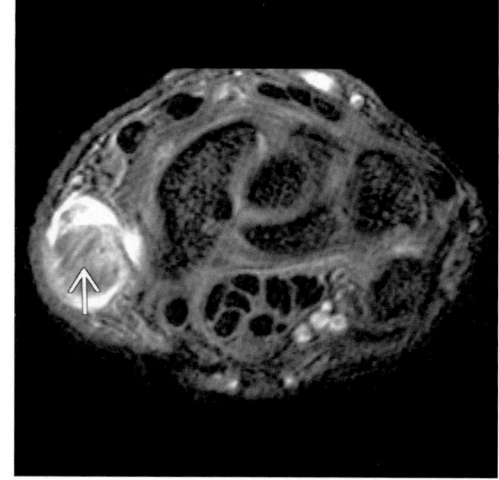

Axial FS PD FSE MR shows hyperintense tenosynovitis and tendon enlargement. The APL demonstrates a striated appearance secondary to enlargement of multiple slips (arrow).

TERMINOLOGY

Abbreviations and Synonyms
- Washer woman's sprain, stenosing tenosynovitis

Definitions
- Tenosynovitis & tendonitis of first dorsal extensor compartment

IMAGING FINDINGS

General Features
- Best diagnostic clue: Edema/fluid associated with first extensor compartment
- Location
  - Abductor pollicis longus (APL)
  - Extensor pollicis brevis (EPB)
  - Level of radial styloid
- Size: Variable - enlargement of tendons within fibroosseous tunnel
- Morphology: Cross sectional enlargement

Radiographic Findings
- Radiography
  - Rarely positive
  - ± Soft tissue swelling
  - Exclude other pathology
    - Fractures
    - Carpometacarpal (CMC) arthritis

CT Findings
- NECT
  - Limited usefulness due to limited soft tissue detail
  - Insensitive for intratendinous pathology
  - Tendon thickening
    - Surrounding hypodense fluid
    - Tenosynovitis
  - Multi-detector thin section CT + 3-D reformatted images
    - Emerging technique to evaluate tendon pathology
    - Promising results in evaluation of skeletally mature patients

MR Findings
- T1WI
  - Tenosynovitis
    - Hypo to intermediate signal intensity of fluid in distended sheath
    - Debris within sheath = intermediate signal
    - Hypointense effacement of subcutaneous fat radial to EPB & APL
  - Tendonitis/tendinosis
    - Hypointense with central/eccentric intermediate signal in grossly enlarged tendons (EPB & APL)
    - Enlargement from medial to lateral on coronal images & cross sectional on axial images

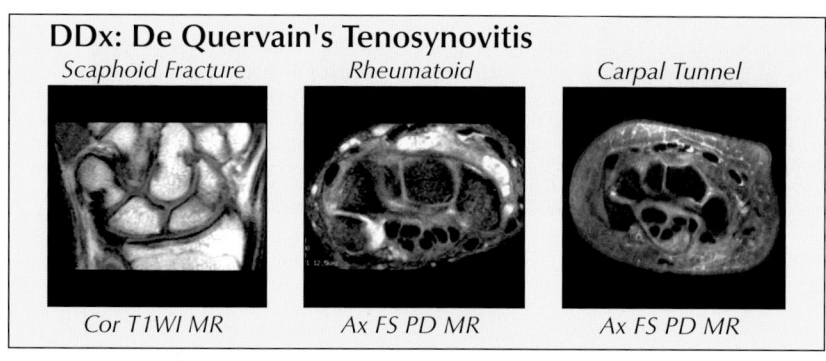

DDx: De Quervain's Tenosynovitis

Scaphoid Fracture	Rheumatoid	Carpal Tunnel
Cor T1WI MR	Ax FS PD MR	Ax FS PD MR

DE QUERVAIN'S TENOSYNOVITIS

Key Facts

Imaging Findings
- Best diagnostic clue: Edema/fluid associated with first extensor compartment
- Abductor pollicis longus (APL)
- Extensor pollicis brevis (EPB)
- Morphology: Cross sectional enlargement

Top Differential Diagnoses
- Scaphoid Fracture
- First Carpometacarpal Arthritis
- Inflammatory Arthropathies
- Carpal Tunnel Syndrome
- Dorsal Ganglion

Pathology
- Repetitive activities (chronic micro-overuse) leading to increased friction & inflammation

- Wringing
- Forceful grasp + repetitive use of thumb in ulnar deviation
- Tendons undergo stretch
- Epidemiology: Most common stenosing tenosynovitis in athletes

Clinical Issues
- Most common signs/symptoms: Pain at radial styloid
- Pain increased with wrist & thumb motion
- Swelling
- ± Tender nodule over radial styloid
- Point tenderness over 1st dorsal compartment
- ± Triggering or crepitus

Diagnostic Checklist
- Assess tendon enlargement at level of radial styloid

- - Maximum enlargement at and immediately distal to radial styloid
  - Longitudinal split - intermediate signal intensity
- T2WI
  - Tenosynovitis
    - Intermediate to hyperintense fluid surrounding EPB & APL
    - Adjacent subcutaneous fat - hyperintense
    - Chronic changes - intermediate signal
  - Tendinitis/tendinosis
    - Hypo to intermediate signal intensity
    - Medial & lateral convexity to tendon margins on coronal images
    - Tendon degeneration - tendinosis intermediate unless associated with hyperintense longitudinal split
    - ± Hypointense septum between tendons (subcompartment for EPB)
    - Striated APL related to enlargement of multiple slips
    - Longitudinal splitting more common in APL

Imaging Recommendations
- Best imaging tool: MR sensitive & specific for tenosynovitis + tendinosis
- Protocol advice
  - T1 or PD and FS PD FSE coronal, sagittal & axial
  - T2* optional for intratendinous degeneration

DIFFERENTIAL DIAGNOSIS

Scaphoid Fracture
- Most common fracture of carpus
- Dorsiflexion loading & radial deviation mechanism
- 70 to 80% involve middle third (waist)
- Pain over anatomic snuffbox
- Scaphoid flexion = humpback deformity

First Carpometacarpal Arthritis
- Sclerosis, hypertrophic bone, chondral loss
- Associated with triscaphe arthritis

Inflammatory Arthropathies
- Rheumatoid arthritis (RA) - hypertrophic synovium + erosions
- Systemic lupus erythematosus - deformities similar to RA
- Psoriatic - distal interphalangeal joints, selective tenosynovitis, arthritis mutilans
- Gout & pseudogout (gout - multiarticular, pseudogout - polyarticular)

Carpal Tunnel Syndrome
- Compromise of motion/sensory function of median nerve
- Trauma + repetitive activities: Hemorrhage, infection & infiltrative disease
- Swelling - median nerve at level of pisiform
- Partial to complete cross sectional hyperintensity on T2WI

Dorsal Ganglion
- Cystic mucinous mass
- Related to scapholunate interval
- Hyperintense, unilocular or multiloculated on T2WI
- Narrow stalk
- Weakness in dorsal capsule

Flexor Carpi Radialis (FCR) Tenosynovitis
- Repetitive wrist motion
- Pain with wrist flexion - radiates along FCR course
- FCR tendon - tight fit in tunnel

Intersection Syndrome
- Pain dorsal radial wrist 5 cm proximal to Lister's tubercle - where APL & EPB cross over 2nd extensor compartment
- Repetitive wrist motion & trauma
- Swelling, tenderness and crepitus

Wartenberg's Syndrome
- Irritation of superficial branch of radial nerve
- Extrinsic compression (wrist bands)
- Intrinsic pressure (dorsal fascia of brachioradialis muscle)

DE QUERVAIN'S TENOSYNOVITIS

- Pain with ulnar deviation
- Tenderness & Tinel's sign over superficial radial nerve

PATHOLOGY

General Features
- General path comments
  - Relevant anatomy
    - First extensor compartment - directly over radial styloid process
    - Fibroosseous tunnel = tubular passageway 2.5 cm in length formed by groove in radial styloid & overlying extensor retinaculum
    - Large APL & small EPB pass through fibroosseous tunnel - represents radial side of anatomic snuff box
    - Anatomic variations: Complete compartmentalization of EPB & multiple slips of APL
    - First dorsal compartment - serves as a pulley to align tendons with dorsum of thumb proximal to 1st metacarpal (APL) & proximal phalanx (EPB) insertions
    - Superficial radial nerve branch overlies first dorsal extensor compartment
- Etiology
  - Repetitive activities (chronic micro-overuse) leading to increased friction & inflammation
    - Grasping
    - Pinching
    - Wringing
  - Trauma = scarring with friction & inflammation
    - Direct blow
    - Fall onto thumb
  - Athletes at risk
    - Forceful grasp + repetitive use of thumb in ulnar deviation
    - Racquet sports
    - Golf - hyperabduction during golf swing
    - Fly fishing
    - Javelin & discus throwing
  - Tendons undergo stretch
    - Tunnel approach angle increases with ulnar deviation
- Epidemiology: Most common stenosing tenosynovitis in athletes

Gross Pathologic & Surgical Features
- Tendon inflammation
- Tendon enlargement
- Longitudinal septum divides APL & EPB in 20 to 30% of patients

Microscopic Features
- Inflammatory cells infiltrate common tendon sheath
- Tenosynovitis originates at tendon sheath or tenosynovium

CLINICAL ISSUES

Presentation
- Most common signs/symptoms: Pain at radial styloid

- Clinical profile
  - Pain increased with wrist & thumb motion
  - Radiation of pain to radial side of forearm
  - Swelling
  - ± Tender nodule over radial styloid
  - Point tenderness over 1st dorsal compartment
  - Positive Finkelstein test - not pathognomonic
    - Passive ulnar deviation reproduces pain
  - ± Triggering or crepitus

Demographics
- Age: 35 - 55 years
- Gender: F: M = 8 - 10:1

Natural History & Prognosis
- Majority (80%) improve with conservative treatment
- Surgery for recalcitrant cases
- Fibrosis develops within tendon sheath without treatment
  - Trigger finger with limited motion

Treatment
- Conservative
  - Anti-inflammatory medications
  - Rest, ceasing aggravating activities
  - Splinting (thumb spica splint)
  - Steroid injections: Excellent results
  - Physical therapy
- Surgical
  - Failure of conservative care
  - Decompression of common tendon sheath
  - Lysis of dividing septum if present
- Complications
  - Perineural fibrosis of superficial radial nerve
  - Inadequate decompression - tendon instability & adherence to scar tissue

DIAGNOSTIC CHECKLIST

Consider
- Assess tendon enlargement at level of radial styloid

SELECTED REFERENCES

1. Miller MD et al: Surgical atlas of sports medicine. Treatment of Guyan's canal syndrome (ulnar nerve compression at the wrist). Philadelphia Pennsylvania, W.B. Saunders, (66):477-89, 2003
2. Topper SM et al: The wrist. Diagnosis and operative treatment. Athletic injuries of the wrist. vol 1. St. Louis Missouri, Mosby, (45):1031-75, 1998
3. Novotny SR et al: The wrist and it's disorders. Occupational and sports injuries of the wrist. 2nd ed. Philadelphia Pennsylvania, W.B. Saunders, (28):487-508, 1997
4. Plancher KD et al: Compressive neuropathies and tendinopathies in the athletic elbow and wrist. Clin Sports Med 15:331-71, 1996

DE QUERVAIN'S TENOSYNOVITIS

IMAGE GALLERY

Typical

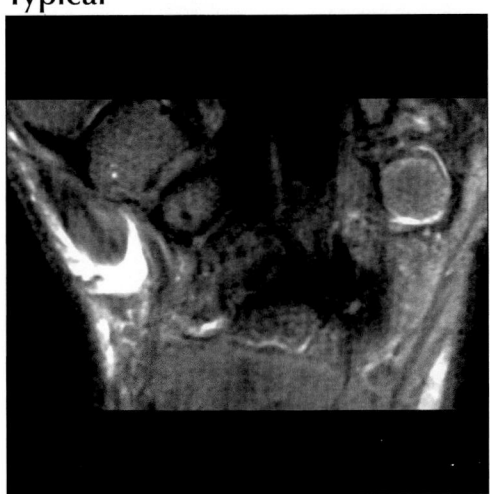 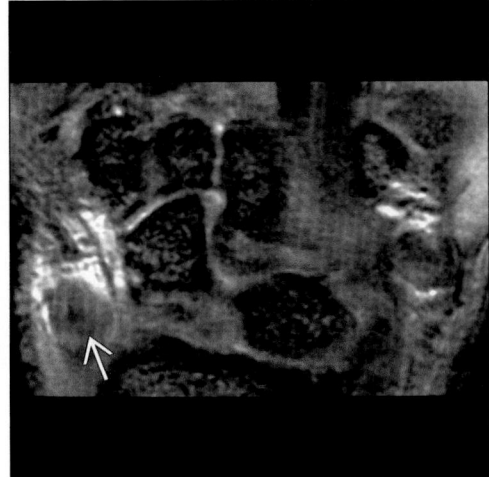

(Left) Coronal FS PD FSE MR shows hyperintense fluid associated with tenosynovitis and tendon degeneration of EPB and APL. *(Right)* Coronal FS PD FSE MR shows increased transverse dimension of the first extensor compartment (arrow).

Typical

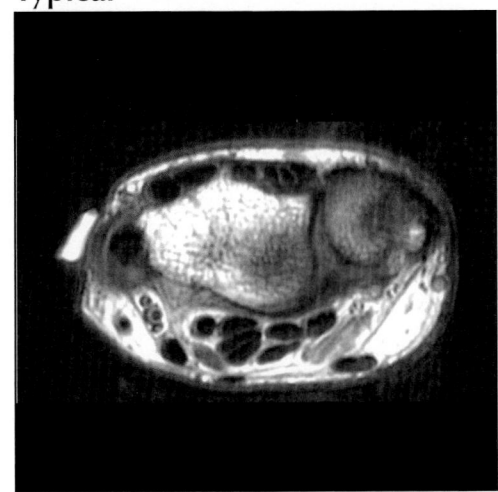 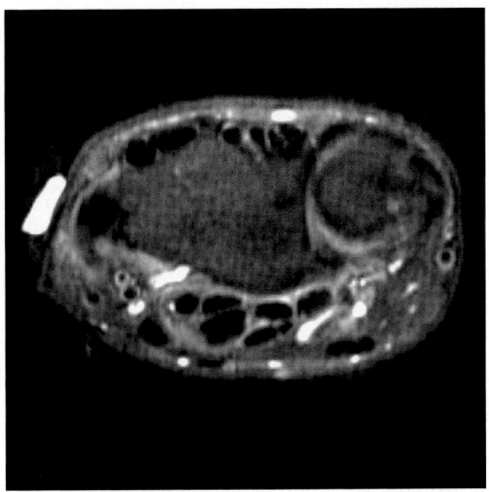

(Left) Axial T1WI MR shows hypointense fluid and effacement of subcutaneous fat along the radial aspect of EPB and APL. *(Right)* Axial FS PD FSE MR shows intermediate signal intensity in chronic changes of EPB and APL tendon inflammation.

Other

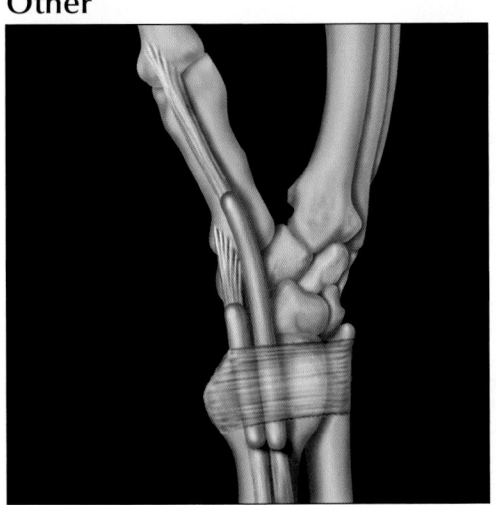 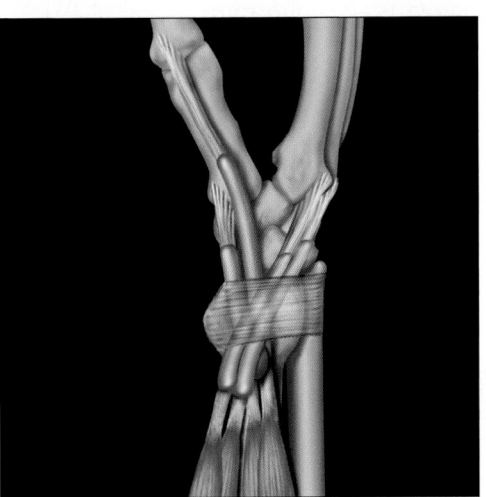

(Left) Sagittal graphic shows normal tendons of the first extensor compartment at level of the radial styloid. The EPB is associated with a separate subcompartment. *(Right)* Sagittal graphic shows intersection syndrome which also involves APL and EPB. In this syndrome there is inflammation as the first compartment tendons cross over the wrist extensors (second compartment).

EXTENSOR CARPI ULNARIS TENDINITIS

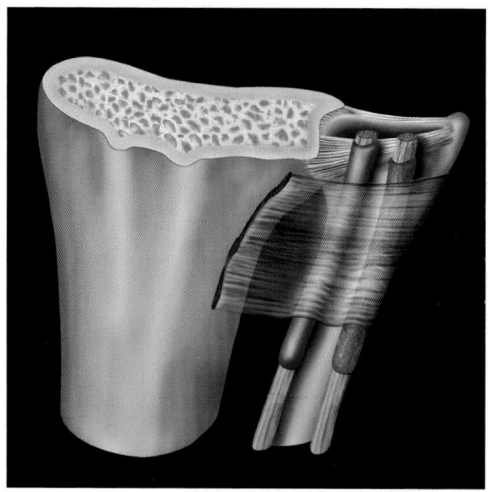

Coronal graphic shows ECU tenosynovitis with inflammation (red) of ECU tendon sheath ulnar to the extensor digiti minimi tendon (to the left).

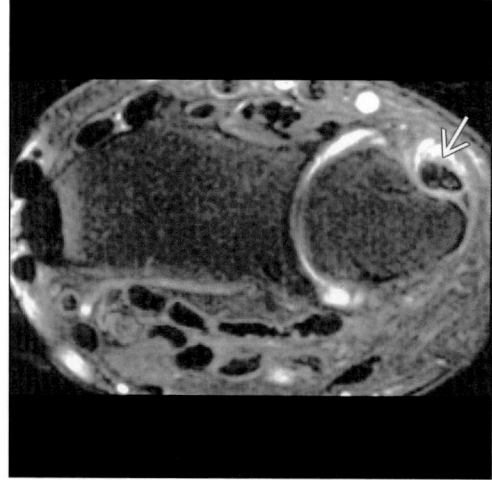

Axial FS PD FSE MR shows intermediate to hyperintense signal (arrow) in chronic ECU tenosynovitis.

TERMINOLOGY

Abbreviations and Synonyms
- ECU tendinitis or tendinosis

Definitions
- Inflammation of the synovial lining of extensor carpi ulnaris (ECU) tendon sheath from chronic strenuous use

IMAGING FINDINGS

General Features
- Best diagnostic clue: Distention of tendon sheath with fluid
- Location
  - Dorsal ulnar aspect of wrist
  - Sixth extensor compartment
- Size: Variable extent of tenosynovitis +/- subluxation & dislocation
- Morphology: Fluid in thickened sheath

Radiographic Findings
- Radiography
  - Usually negative
  - Osteoarthritis
  - Calcific tendinitis

MR Findings
- T1WI
  - Hypo to intermediate signal intensity fluid within sixth extensor compartment tendon sheath
  - Thickening - hypo to intermediate signal intensity of tendon sheath
  - Increased cross sectional diameter of ECU tendon
  - ± Fraying of tendon margins
  - Tendon degeneration with intermediate signal intensity
  - ECU subluxation or dislocation
- T2WI
  - Hyperintense fluid within ECU tendon sheath
  - Intermediate signal intensity of fluid - chronic tenosynovitis
  - Intermediate signal tendinosis - degeneration
  - Longitudinal splitting of tendon - hyperintense
  - Complete ECU rupture = replacement by hyperintense signal fluid
  - Hypointense foci = calcifications
- T1 C+: Intravenous contrast to enhance inflamed synovium

Imaging Recommendations
- Best imaging tool: MR evaluates sixth extensor compartment for fluid, tendon integrity & subluxation
- Protocol advice: T1, FS PD FSE axial, coronal & sagittal images

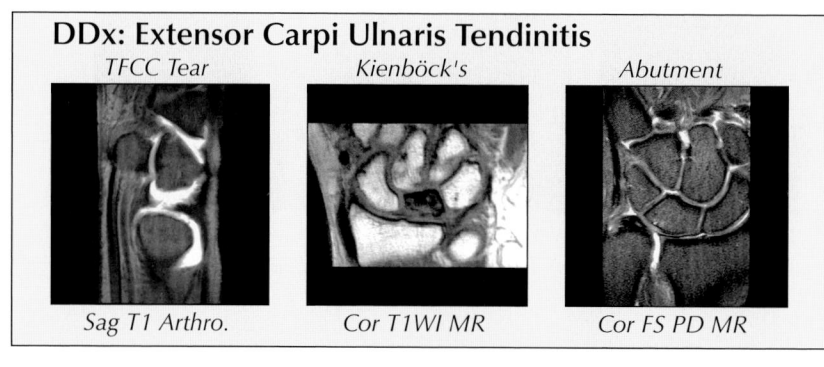

DDx: Extensor Carpi Ulnaris Tendinitis

TFCC Tear	Kienböck's	Abutment
Sag T1 Arthro.	*Cor T1WI MR*	*Cor FS PD MR*

EXTENSOR CARPI ULNARIS TENDINITIS

Key Facts

Imaging Findings
- Best diagnostic clue: Distention of tendon sheath with fluid
- Sixth extensor compartment
- Size: Variable extent of tenosynovitis +/- subluxation & dislocation
- Increased cross sectional diameter of ECU tendon

Top Differential Diagnoses
- Traumatic TFCC Abnormalities
- Kienböck's Disease
- DRUJ Instability
- Ulnocarpal Abutment Syndrome

Pathology
- Repetitive activities using ulnar deviation
- Reactive ECU tenosynovitis

- Primary ECU tenosynovitis
- Epidemiology: Second most frequent site of stenosing tenosynovitis in upper extremity
- Supination & ulnar deviation reproduces ECU instability

Clinical Issues
- Most common signs/symptoms: Pain dorsally at distal ulna
- Traumatic rupture of ECU subsheath = painful subluxation syndrome
- ECU subsheath rupture + extensor retinaculum disruption = chronic dislocation

Diagnostic Checklist
- Axial images in full pronation & supination to identify tendon subluxation

DIFFERENTIAL DIAGNOSIS

Traumatic TFCC Abnormalities
- Central perforations
- Ulnar avulsion
- Distal avulsion
- Radial avulsion
- Without associated lunate, triquetral or ulnar chondromalacia

Kienböck's Disease
- Avascular necrosis of lunate
- Related to trauma + ulnar negative variance
- Centralized lunate sclerosis
- ± Visualized lunate fracture

DRUJ Instability
- Subluxation
- Dislocation
- Fracture ulnar head in sigmoid notch
- Ligament insufficiency (radioulnar)
- Pain throughout range of pronation - supination
- Intercarpal pathology
- Lunotriquetral instability
- Midcarpal instability
- ± Lunotriquetral tear & volar intercalated segment instability (VISI)

Ulnocarpal Abutment Syndrome
- TFCC degeneration/perforation
- Lunate, triquetral & ulnar chondromalacia
- Lunotriquetral ligament perforation/tear
- Ulnocarpal arthritis

Intercarpal Pathology
- Lunotriquetral instability
- Midcarpal instability
- ± LT ligament tear and VISI

PATHOLOGY

General Features
- General path comments

- Relevant anatomy = sixth extensor compartment
  - Contains ECU tendon and sheath
  - Contributes to stability of ulnar aspect of wrist
  - Separate subsheath forms fibro-osseous tunnel
  - Subsheath attachments to ulnar styloid & head
  - Fibro-osseous tunnel maintains ECU position during rotation
  - Septum anchors fibro-osseous tunnel to radius dorsally
  - Retinaculum attaches to volar aspect of pisiform & triquetrum
  - Subsheath merges with capsule of distal radioulnar joint (DRUJ) proximally & triangular fibrocartilage complex (TFCC) distally
- Etiology
  - Repetitive activities using ulnar deviation
  - Reactive ECU tenosynovitis
    - Recurrent subluxation
    - Loss of sixth compartment integrity
  - Primary ECU tenosynovitis
    - Acute trauma
    - Repetitive wrist motion
    - Ulnar styloid non-union with roughened surface
- Epidemiology: Second most frequent site of stenosing tenosynovitis in upper extremity

Gross Pathologic & Surgical Features
- Supination
  - ECU tendon in dorsal position (normal)
- Pronation
  - ECU tendon in ulnar position (normal)
- ECU subluxation
- ECU dislocation
- Supination & ulnar deviation reproduces ECU instability
- ECU relocation
  - Pronation & radial deviation - relocates ECU tendon

Microscopic Features
- Tendon degeneration
  - Decreased collagen content
  - Loss of collagen cross linking = tendon stiffness
  - ± Decreased resistance to shear forces

EXTENSOR CARPI ULNARIS TENDINITIS

Staging, Grading or Classification Criteria
- Tenosynovitis - primary or reactive
- Tendinosis
- Longitudinal splitting
- Rupture

CLINICAL ISSUES

Presentation
- Most common signs/symptoms: Pain dorsally at distal ulna
- Clinical profile
  - Swelling
  - ± Crepitus
  - Traumatic rupture of ECU subsheath = painful subluxation syndrome
    - Painful snap with pronation & supination
  - ECU subsheath rupture + extensor retinaculum disruption = chronic dislocation
    - Forced supination
    - Palmar flexion
    - Ulnar deviation

Demographics
- Age
  - Athlete population
    - Racquet sports
    - Baseball
    - Golf
  - Association with rheumatoid arthritis (synovial cysts, subluxation/dislocation)
- Gender: No bias

Natural History & Prognosis
- Return to sports
  - Range of motion = 70% of opposite extremity
- Prognosis
  - Good with early & adequate treatment
  - Modification of racquet weight & biomechanics of swing patterns

Treatment
- Conservative (ECU tendinitis)
  - Diagnostic & therapeutic injection of lidocaine & cortisone
  - Splinting
  - Non-steroidal anti-inflammatories
  - Rest, ice, compression, elevation
- Conservative (ECU rupture)
  - Acute injury - long-arm cast in full supination & neutral wrist flexion/extension
- Surgical (ECU tendinitis)
  - Progressive fibrosis of sixth compartment requires release
- Surgical (traumatic rupture of ECU)
  - Chronic or non-responsive to conservative treatment = surgical reconstruction of retinaculum

DIAGNOSTIC CHECKLIST

Consider
- FS PD FSE or STIR to visualize tenosynovitis

- T2* gradient echo if fat-suppression inadequate
- Axial images in full pronation & supination to identify tendon subluxation

SELECTED REFERENCES

1. Kozin SH et al: The wrist. Tendinitis of the wrist. Diagnosis and operative treatment. vol 1. St. Louis Missouri, Mosby, (50):1181-96, 1998
2. Novotny SR et al: The wrist and it's disorders. Occupational and sports injuries of the wrist. 2nd ed. Philadelphia Pennsylvania, W.B. Saunders, (28):487-508, 1997
3. Thorson E et al: Common tendinitis problems in the hand and forearm. Orthop Clin North Am 23:65-74, 1992
4. Pitner MA: Pathophysiology of overuse injuries in the hand and wrist. Hand Clin 6:355-64, 1990
5. Stern PJ: Tendinitis, overuse syndromes and tendon injuries. Hand Clin 6:467-76, 1990
6. Osterman AL et al: Soft tissue injuries of the hand and wrist in racquet sports. Clin Sports Med 7:329-48, 1988
7. Herring SA et al: Introduction to overuse injuries. Clin Sports Med 6:255-39, 1987
8. Rowland SA: Acute traumatic subluxation of the extensor carpi ulnaris tendon at the wrist. J Hand Surg 11A:809-11, 1986
9. Haji AA et al: Stenosing tenosynovitis of the extensor carpi ulnaris. J Hand Surg 11A:515-20, 1986
10. Wood MD et al: Sports related extra-articular wrist syndrome. Clin Orthop 2020:93-102, 1986
11. Rayan GM: Recurrent dislocation of the extensor carpi ulnaris in athletes. Am J Sports Med 11:183-4, 1983
12. Burkhart SS et al: Post-traumatic recurrent subluxation of the extensor carpi ulnaris tendon. J Hand Surg 7A:1-3, 1982
13. Eckhardt WA et al: Recurrent dislocation of the extensor carpi ulnaris tendon. J Hand Surg 61:629-31, 1981
14. Dobyns JH et al: Sports stress syndromes of the hand and wrist. Am J Sports Med 6:236-54, 1978
15. Spinner M et al: Extensor carpi ulnaris: Its relationship to the stability of the distal radioulnar joint. Clin Orthop 68:124-9, 1970

EXTENSOR CARPI ULNARIS TENDINITIS

IMAGE GALLERY

Typical

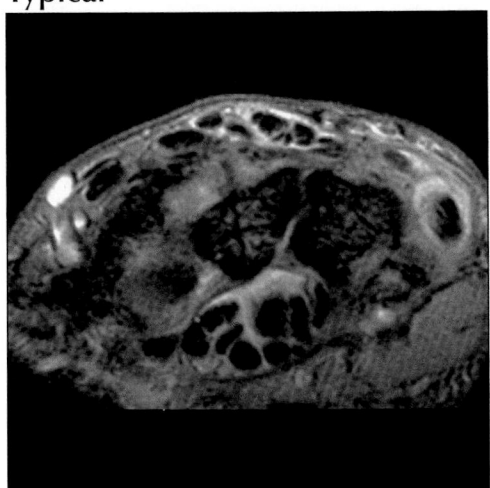 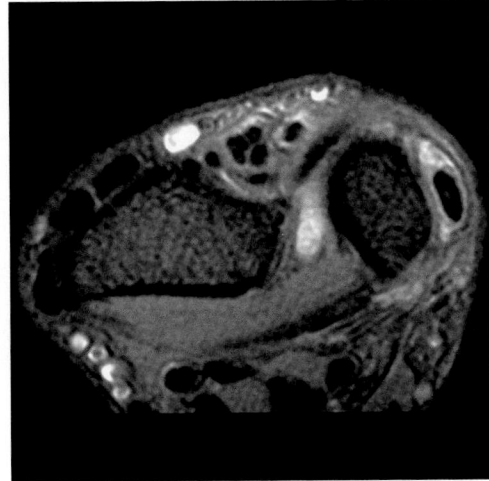

(Left) Axial FS PD FSE MR shows tenosynovitis and intrinsic tendon degeneration of the ECU. (Right) Axial FS PD FSE MR shows intermediate signal intensity synovial thickening in ECU tenosynovitis. Tendon sheath fluid is hyperintense.

Typical

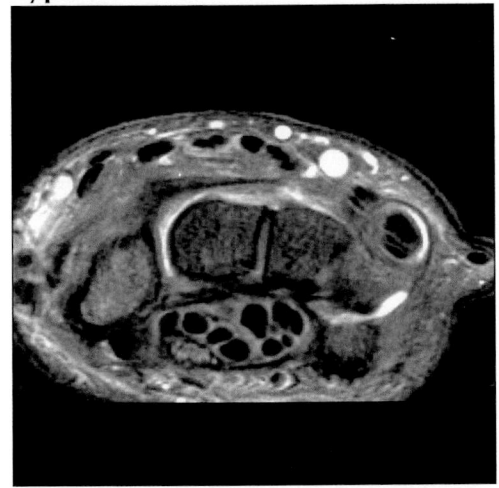 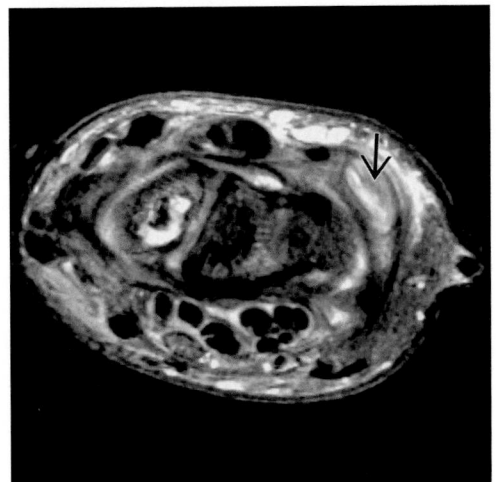

(Left) Axial FS PD FSE MR shows gross enlargement of the ECU tendon with intra-tendinous split. (Right) Axial FS PD FSE MR shows rupture with discontinuity (arrow) of ECU tendon at level of the proximal carpal row.

Typical

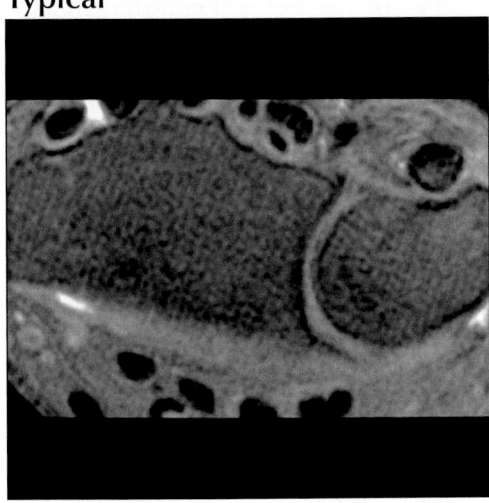 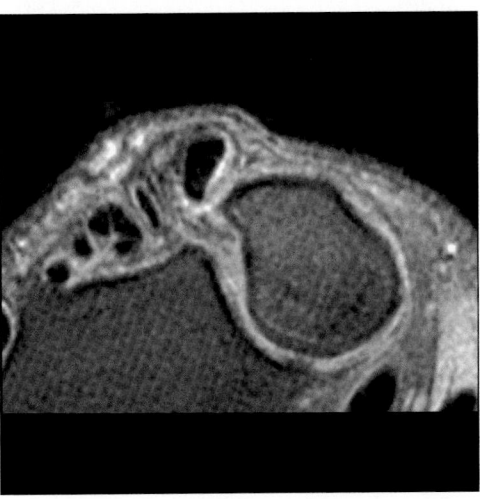

(Left) Axial FS PD FSE MR shows normal location of the ECU in partial supination. (Right) Axial FS PD FSE MR shows dislocation of ECU tendon in the position of maximal supination. Supination and ulnar deviation reproduce ECU instability.

GIANT CELL TUMOR TENDON SHEATH

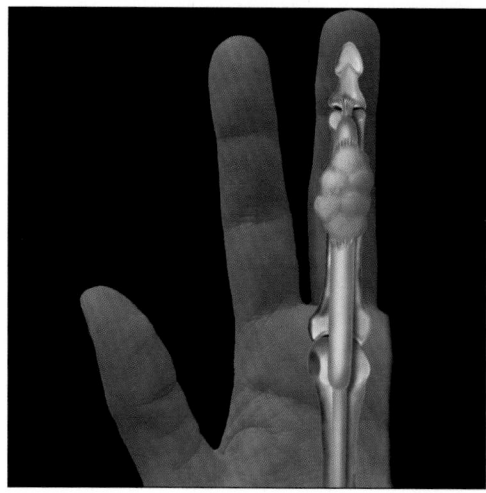

Coronal graphic shows giant cell tumor of the flexor tendon sheath of 3rd digit. Characteristic lobulations are present.

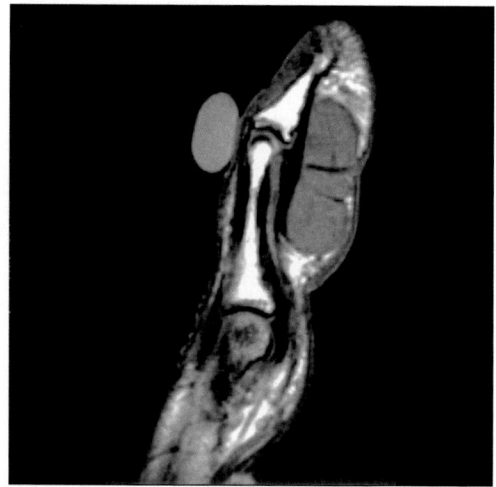

Sagittal T1WI MR shows hypointense to intermediate signal intensity volar soft tissue giant cell tumor with hypointense septations.

TERMINOLOGY

Abbreviations and Synonyms
- Extraarticular pigmented villonodular synovitis, GCTTS, histiocytoma, benign synovioma

Definitions
- Non-neoplastic benign tumor of giant cells in vicinity of joints, most commonly the hand, closely related to pigmented villonodular synovitis

IMAGING FINDINGS

General Features
- Best diagnostic clue: Intermediate signal intensity soft tissue mass on T1 & T2WIs
- Location
  - Volar aspect of hand and fingers adjacent to distal interphalangeal (DIP) joint
  - Two-thirds of masses located volar aspect of fingers - index and long finger most common
  - Slight predominance for right hand
- Size: Usually small (0.5-5 cm)
- Morphology: Well-circumscribed fibrous mass

Radiographic Findings
- Radiography
  - Adjacent cortical erosion due to pressure effect

- Intra-tumoral calcification occasionally present

MR Findings
- T1WI
  - Hypointense to intermediate signal intensity
  - Hypointense septations
  - Lobulations
  - Signal: ± Inhomogeneous
  - Convex bowing/bulge toward skin from tendon sheath
  - Flexor or extensor tendon related
  - Extension in transverse and longitudinal planes
  - Less common origin deep to tendon (between tendon & bone)
- T2WI
  - Low to intermediate signal intensity
  - Inhomogeneous
  - Hypointense hemosiderin foci
  - Hemosiderin distribution
    - Peripheral hypointense foci (± clumped)
    - Small hypointense foci throughout lesion
  - Fibrous septations - hypointense
  - Sharply defined interface without reactive edema of adjacent subcutaneous tissue
  - Adjacent osseous erosion - unusual but can occur
  - Greater long axis growth common
  - Minimal associated fluid
- T1 C+: Intense enhancement with intravenous contrast ± inhomogeneity

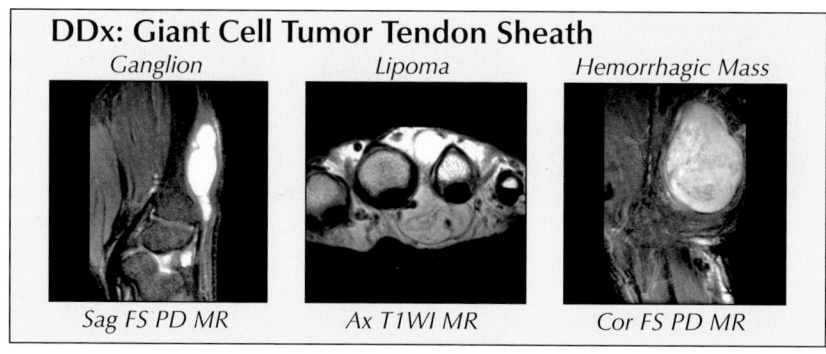

DDx: Giant Cell Tumor Tendon Sheath

Ganglion	Lipoma	Hemorrhagic Mass
Sag FS PD MR	Ax T1WI MR	Cor FS PD MR

GIANT CELL TUMOR TENDON SHEATH

Key Facts

Imaging Findings

- Best diagnostic clue: Intermediate signal intensity soft tissue mass on T1 & T2WIs
- Two-thirds of masses located volar aspect of fingers - index and long finger most common
- Morphology: Well-circumscribed fibrous mass
- Fibrous septations - hypointense
- Sharply defined interface without reactive edema of adjacent subcutaneous tissue

Top Differential Diagnoses

- Ganglion Cyst
- Lipomas
- Hemangiomas
- Foreign Bodies
- Synovial Sarcoma

Pathology

- Accepted theory - reactive or regenerative hyperplasia associated with inflammatory process
- 2nd most common mass of hand behind ganglions
- High rate of recurrence
- Firm, well-circumscribed lobulated mass

Clinical Issues

- Most common signs/symptoms: Painless slow growing mass present for weeks to years
- May cause limited function of digit due to size of lesion
- Osseous erosions related to lesion hypervascularity

Diagnostic Checklist

- T2* gradient echo to document hemosiderin

Imaging Recommendations

- Best imaging tool
  - MR to document size, morphology, location
  - MR diagnosis is sensitive & specific
- Protocol advice
  - T1, PD, FS PD FSE, STIR & T2* gradient echo in axial plane
  - FS PD FSE or T2* in coronal & sagittal plane
  - T1C+ for enhancement optional

DIFFERENTIAL DIAGNOSIS

Ganglion Cyst

- Thin-walled
- Mucinous fluid
- Related to trauma
- Hypointense on T1WI, hyperintense on FS PD FSE or STIR
- Nonenhancing except peripherally

Lipomas

- Fat signal on T1WI
- Suppressed signal on FS T2 FSE or STIR
- ± Fibrous bands
- Lobulations & septations
- Enhancement in areas of malignant change

Hemangiomas

- Cavernous
- Capillary
- Intramuscular
- Noncircumscribed
- Low to intermediate signal on T1WI
- Hyperintense serpiginous vessels on FS PD FSE
- Hypointense foci secondary to hemosiderin

Foreign Bodies

- Intermediate signal intensity of granulomatous reaction (T1 & T2WI)
- Adjacent subcutaneous tissue edema
- Inflammatory reaction
- ± Peripheral rim-like enhancement

- Gradient echo to emphasize susceptibility artifacts from metallic foreign bodies

Synovial Sarcoma

- Multipotential mesenchymal cell origin
- 15-35 years of age
- Close proximity to joints, however most are extraarticular in location
- Spotty calcification - 15%
- Aggressive tracking along tendons possible
- Thick septations are unusual
- ± Central necrosis

PATHOLOGY

General Features

- General path comments
  - Relevant anatomy
    - Synovial tissue of joints
    - Tendon sheaths
- Etiology
  - Accepted theory - reactive or regenerative hyperplasia associated with inflammatory process
  - Other theories
    - Trauma
    - Disturbed lipid metabolism
    - Osteoclastic proliferation
    - Infection
    - Vascular disturbances
    - Immune mechanisms
    - Inflammation
    - Neoplasia
    - Metabolic disturbances
- Epidemiology
  - 2nd most common mass of hand behind ganglions
  - High rate of recurrence

Gross Pathologic & Surgical Features

- Firm, well-circumscribed lobulated mass
- Tumors have mottled appearance
- Vary in color from grayish-brown to yellow-orange
- Nodular & villous morphology

GIANT CELL TUMOR TENDON SHEATH

Microscopic Features

- Mononuclear rounded or polygonal cells - lipid-laden histiocytes & multinucleated giant cells
- Variable number of giant cells present
- Hemosiderin-containing xanthoma cells in periphery of lesion

Staging, Grading or Classification Criteria

- Localized type and rare diffuse type
  - Rare diffuse form is soft tissue counterpart of pigmented villonodular synovitis (PVNS)

CLINICAL ISSUES

Presentation

- Most common signs/symptoms: Painless slow growing mass present for weeks to years
- Clinical profile
  - May cause occasional distal numbness
  - May cause limited function of digit due to size of lesion
  - Mass is non-transilluminating

Demographics

- Age
  - 30 to 50 years, peak 40-50
    - Rare < 10 or > 60 years
- Gender: F:M = 3:2

Natural History & Prognosis

- Progressive slow growth
- Late stage = exuberant, heavily pigmented villous synovial overgrowth
- Osseous erosions related to lesion hypervascularity

Treatment

- Surgical
  - Marginal excision
  - Complete excision - difficult
  - Bony debridement may be necessary
- Complications
  - Satellite lesions are common - incomplete resection
  - Puncturing lesions may result in seeding of operative bed
  - Tendon reconstruction may be necessary
  - Even with careful dissection, recurrence rates are 9-44%
  - No malignant degeneration reported

DIAGNOSTIC CHECKLIST

Consider

- True bone invasion is not typical and is suggestive of an aggressive neoplasm
- Reactive soft tissue edema is atypical
- T2* gradient echo to document hemosiderin

SELECTED REFERENCES

1. Hitora T et al: Multicentric localized giant cell tumour of the tendon sheath: Two separate lesions at different sites in a finger. Br J Dermatol 147(2):403-5, 2002
2. Al-Qattan MM: Giant cell tumours of tendon sheath: Classification and recurrence rate. J Hand Surg 26(1):72-5, 2001
3. Daniel JN et al: Giant cell tumor of the middle phalanx. Orthopedics 10:1097-9, 2000
4. Galliani I et al: Giant cell tumor of tendon sheath: A light and electron microscopic study. J Submicrosc Cytol Pathol 32 (1):69-76, 2000
5. Bogumill GP: The wrist and it's disorders. Tumors of the wrist. 2nd ed. Philadelphia Pennsylvania, Saunders, (31):563-82, 1997
6. Hughes TH et al: Pigmented villonodular synovitis: MRI characteristics. Skeletal Radiol 24:7-13, 1995
7. Miller TT et al: Benign soft tissue masses of the wrist and hand: MRI appearances. Skeletal Radiol 23:327-32, 1994
8. Jelinek J et al: Giant cell tumor of the tendon sheath: MR findings in nine cases. AJR 162:919-22, 1994
9. Kransdorf MJ et al: Fat containing soft-tissue masses of the extremities. Radiographics 11:81-106, 1991
10. Binkovitz LA et al: Masses of the hand and wrist: Detection and characterization with MR imaging. AJR 154:323-6, 1990
11. Poletti SC et al: The use of magnetic resonance imaging in the diagnosis of pigmented villonodular synovitis. Orthopedics 13:185-90, 1990
12. Jelinek JS et al: Imaging of pigmented villonodular synovitis with emphasis on MR imaging. AJR 152:337-42, 1989
13. Kottal RA et al: Pigmented villonodular synovitis: A report of imaging in two cases. Radiology 163:551-3, 1987
14. Patel MR et al: Pigmented villonodular synovitis of the writ invading bone – report of a case. J Hand Surg 9:854-58, 1984.

GIANT CELL TUMOR TENDON SHEATH

IMAGE GALLERY

Typical

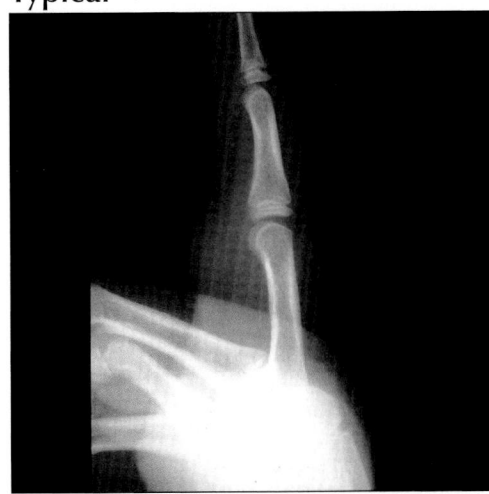
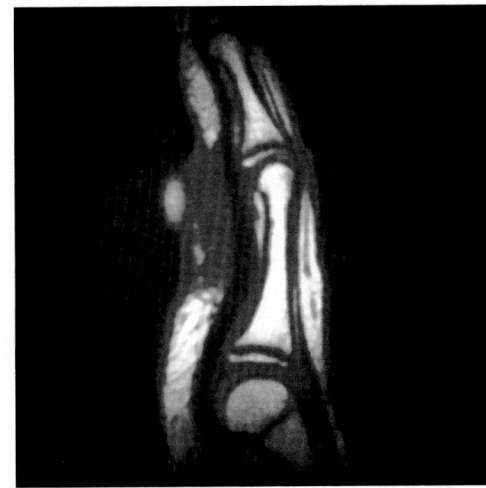

(Left) Lateral radiography shows volar soft tissue density adjacent to the proximal interphalangeal joint. *(Right)* Sagittal T1WI MR shows hypointense giant cell tumor associated with flexor tendon. The lesion bulges toward the skin from the tendon sheath.

Typical

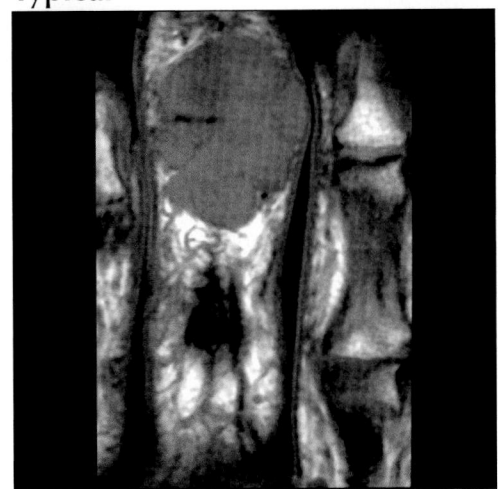
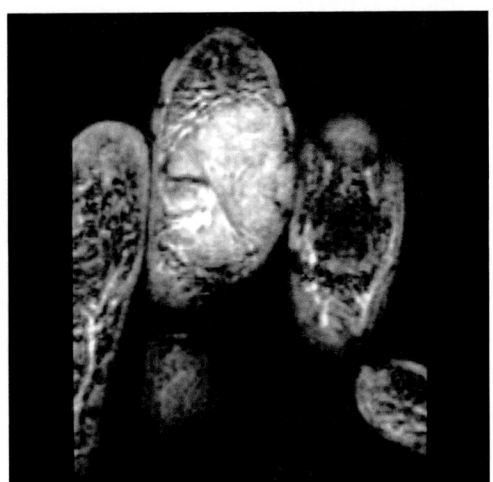

(Left) Coronal T1WI MR shows volar giant cell tumor with septations and lobulations. *(Right)* Coronal FS PD FSE MR shows characteristic intermediate signal with septations, lobulations, and hemosiderin foci.

Typical

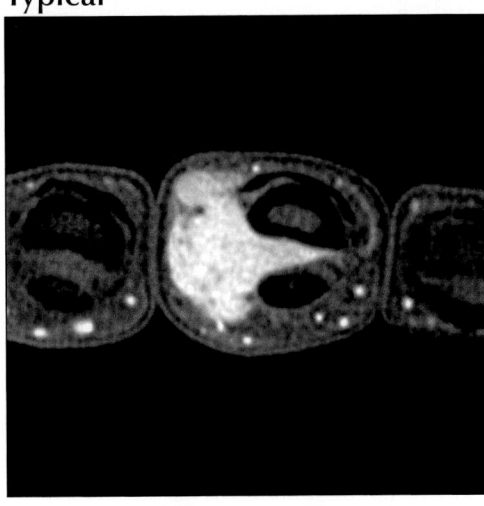
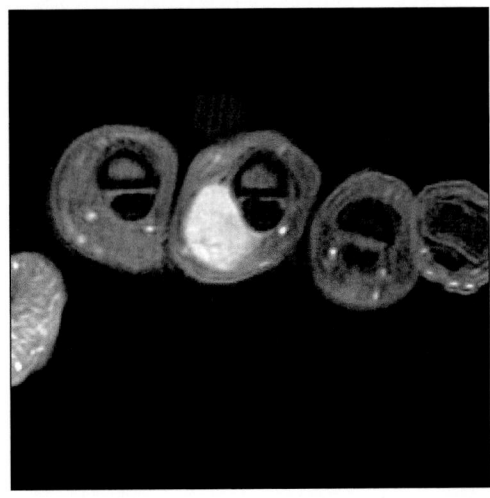

(Left) Axial T1 C+ MR shows intense enhancement with origin of the giant cell tumor between the tendon and bone. This is a less common presentation (deep to tendon). *(Right)* Axial T1 C+ MR shows inhomogeneous enhancement with the more typical pattern of giant cell tumor origin form superficial surface of the tendon sheath.

ULNAR COLLATERAL LIGAMENT TEAR, THUMB

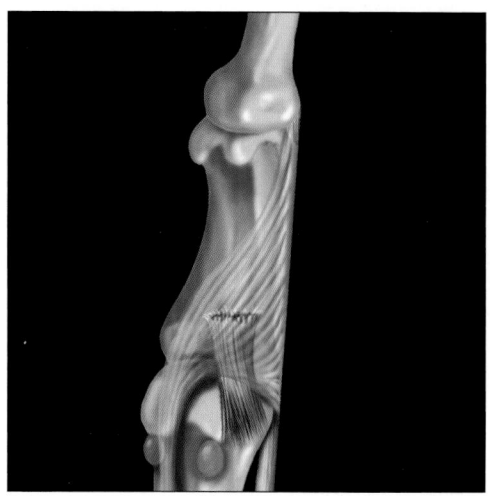

Sagittal graphic shows UCL tear without displacement or retraction. This represents gamekeeper's thumb.

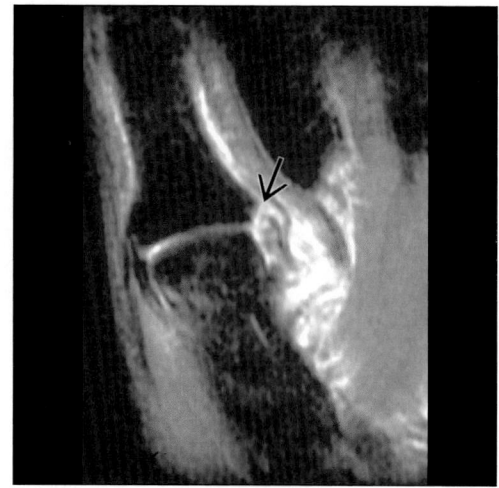

Coronal FS PD FSE MR shows gamekeeper's thumb with rupture of the distal attachment (arrow) of the UCL. The torn UCL remains deep to the overlying adductor aponeurosis.

TERMINOLOGY

Abbreviations and Synonyms
- UCL rupture, gamekeeper's thumb, ulnar collateral ligament rupture, skier's thumb

Definitions
- Disruption of the ulnar collateral ligament of the thumb

IMAGING FINDINGS

General Features
- Best diagnostic clue: Discontinuity of ulnar collateral ligament attachment to proximal phalanx
- Location: 1st metacarpophalangeal (MCP) joint
- Size: Variable based on UCL retraction deep to or superficial (Stener lesion) to adductor aponeurosis
- Morphology
  ○ Thickened, foreshortened UCL with proximal retraction
  ○ Mass-like tissue vs. horizontally directed UCL in Stener lesion

Radiographic Findings
- Radiography
  ○ Prior to stressing the MCP joint

  ○ Nondisplaced to minimal displacement (< 2 mm) avulsion fracture of proximal phalanx base = UCL avulsion without Stener lesion
  ○ Roberts' view = hyperpronated anteroposterior view
  ○ Arthrogram: Extravasation of contrast = capsular rupture
    ■ Adductor muscle
    ■ Sheath of extensor pollicis brevis
    ■ Sheath of extensor pollicis longus
    ■ UCL disruption - contrast outlines ruptured ligament

MR Findings
- T1WI
  ○ Incomplete rupture or complete rupture without a Stener lesion
    ■ Hypo to intermediate signal intensity UCL remains deep to overlying hypointense adductor aponeurosis
    ■ UCL thickening
    ■ Discontinuity at UCL attachment to proximal aspect proximal phalanx (thumb)
    ■ Intermediate signal intensity edema & fluid superficial & deep to UCL
    ■ Ulnar displacement of UCL & adductor aponeurosis
    ■ UCL orientation remains along long axis of 1st ray (thumb)
  ○ Complete rupture with a Stener lesion

DDx: Ulnar Collateral Ligament Tear, Thumb

UCL Sprain	MCP Dislocation	Thenar Sprain	FPL Tear
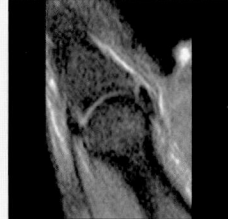	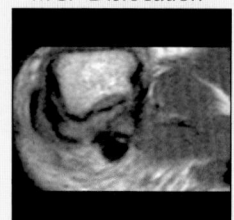	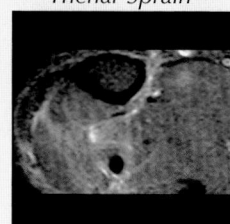	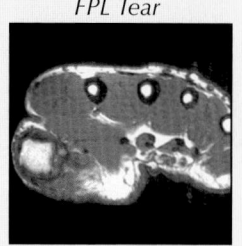
Cor FS PD MR	Ax T1WI MR	Ax FS PD MR	Ax T1WI MR

ULNAR COLLATERAL LIGAMENT TEAR, THUMB

Key Facts

Imaging Findings

- Best diagnostic clue: Discontinuity of ulnar collateral ligament attachment to proximal phalanx
- Size: Variable based on UCL retraction deep to or superficial (Stener lesion) to adductor aponeurosis
- Thickened, foreshortened UCL with proximal retraction
- Mass-like tissue vs. horizontally directed UCL in Stener lesion

Top Differential Diagnoses

- MCP Joint Capsular Trauma
- Degenerative Arthritis
- MCP Joint Dislocations
- Carpal Metacarpal (CMC) Joint Fractures/Dislocations

Pathology

- Gamekeeper's thumb = chronic injury to UCL (vs. acute trauma of skier's thumb)
- Displaced UCL = Stener lesion with proximal retraction (ligament folding) proximal to MCP joint

Clinical Issues

- Most common signs/symptoms: MCP joint pain
- Pain greatest on ulnar side of MCP joint
- Mass = displaced UCL stump on ulnar side of MCP joint or proximal to MCP joint

Diagnostic Checklist

- Identify retracted UCL with folded or horizontally directed fibers

---

- Intermediate signal intensity in retracted mass of UCL
- UCL trapped beneath adductor aponeurosis
- UCL directed superficial to linear adductor aponeurosis
- T2WI
    - Incomplete or complete rupture without Stener lesion
        - Thickened hypointense UCL with central signal inhomogeneity (focal hyperintense areas of edema)
        - Hyperintense fluid interposed between base of proximal phalanx & retracted ligament
        - Hyperintense fluid plane between distal ulnar aspect of 1st metacarpal & UCL + UCL & adductor aponeurosis
        - Hyperintense soft tissue edema superficial to adductor aponeurosis
        - Hyperintense subchondral edema ± osseous avulsion at UCL distal attachment to proximal phalanx
    - Complete rupture with Stener lesion
        - Gross displacement of UCL medial to adductor aponeurosis
        - Hypo to intermediate signal UCL retracted proximal to MCP
        - Trapped UCL either completely superficial to or intersecting the overlying adductor aponeurosis
        - UCL directional vector with increased horizontal orientation (no longer parallel to long axis of 1st digit)
        - "Yo-yo on a string" appearance of Stener lesion = retracted & balled-up UCL (yo-yo) with the more proximal linear adductor aponeurosis (the string)

Imaging Recommendations

- Best imaging tool: MR identifies UCL morphology, location, retraction, & position relative to adductor aponeurosis
- Protocol advice
    - T1, PD & FS PD FSE (vs. STIR or T2* gradient echo) in true coronal orthogonal plane through MCP joint
    - Axial images next most important plane

- Sagittal - may document retracted UCL & mass-like effect on ulnar-sided images

DIFFERENTIAL DIAGNOSIS

MCP Joint Capsular Trauma

- Capsule
    - Proper radial & UCL's (UCL sprain)
- Volar (palmar) plate = anterior or glenoid ligament
    - Two asymmetric checkrein ligaments
    - Origin = volar distal thumb metacarpal
    - Insertion = palmar edge proximal phalanx
    - Two sesamoid bones associated
    - Thickening of volar capsule
    - Edema & disruption of capsule in trauma

Degenerative Arthritis

- Sclerosis, osteophytosis, joint space narrowing, subluxation
- ± Reactive subchondral marrow edema

MCP Joint Dislocations

- Hyperextension
- Dorsal subluxation or dislocation = hyperextended position of proximal phalanx
- Associated palmar (volar plate) injury and thenar sprain

Carpal Metacarpal (CMC) Joint Fractures/Dislocations

- Occur at base of thumb not MCP joint
- Bennett's fx/dislocation
- Rolando's y-shaped fracture
- Extraarticular transverse vs. oblique fx
- Epiphyseal - Salter-Harris type III - V

PATHOLOGY

General Features

- General path comments
    - Relevant anatomy = MCP joint of the thumb

ULNAR COLLATERAL LIGAMENT TEAR, THUMB

- Capsule - reinforced by volar plate, collateral ligaments, & extensor pollicis brevis tendon
- Adductor aponeurosis = adductor pollicis aponeurosis
- Etiology
  - Forceful abduction of thumb
  - Hyperextension stress to UCL of thumb
  - Fall (skier's thumb) with hyperextension + abduction = UCL tear
  - Gamekeeper's thumb = chronic injury to UCL (vs. acute trauma of skier's thumb)
- Epidemiology
  - UCL injury of thumb MCP joint is common
  - UCL rupture - majority occur distally
  - Stener lesion - 50 to 70% of complete tears
  - Increased incidence of Stener lesions in skiers (80%)

Gross Pathologic & Surgical Features
- Partial tears UCL
- Complete rupture UCL: Distal > midsubstance
- Complete rupture + Stener
- ± Avulsed bone fragment (not required for Stener lesion)
- ± Volar subluxation proximal phalanx
- Nondisplaced UCL tear = discontinuity without retraction + intact adductor aponeurosis covering distal UCL
- Displaced UCL = Stener lesion with proximal retraction (ligament folding) proximal to MCP joint
- Proximal margin of adductor aponeurosis intersects or abuts folded UCL in Stener lesion
- Distal UCL end turned 180 degrees & directed proximally in Stener lesion

Microscopic Features
- Collagen, elastin & connective tissue failure
- Hemorrhagic & inflammatory cellular response
- Fracture healing

Staging, Grading or Classification Criteria
- Partial tears
  - Grade I - stretching
  - Grade II - incomplete but discrete tear
- Complete rupture
  - Grade III (with or without Stener lesion)

CLINICAL ISSUES

Presentation
- Most common signs/symptoms: MCP joint pain
- Clinical profile
  - Swelling
  - Tenderness MCP joint
  - Weakness in pinch
  - Pain greatest on ulnar side of MCP joint
  - Pain radiates from metacarpal head to proximal phalanx
  - Mass = displaced UCL stump on ulnar side of MCP joint or proximal to MCP joint
  - Abnormal thumb rotation (rotation of proximal phalanx on intact axis of radial collateral ligament)
  - Absent endpoint on joint stress test = complete tear UCL

- Instability in MCP flexion = proper collateral ligament tear with intact accessory collateral + volar plate
- Instability in flexion & extension = complete ulnar complex disruption
- Stability ≤ 10 degrees of opening
- Instability ≥ 30 degrees abduction arc on stress relative to contralateral side

Demographics
- Age
  - Young to middle aged adults
  - Activity related age groups
    - Football, hockey, wrestling, basketball & ski injuries
- Gender
  - M > F
  - Activity related

Natural History & Prognosis
- Partial tears & complete without Stener lesion may heal without surgery
- Fibrosis & granulation tissue in complete tears may delay or preclude ligament reattachment

Treatment
- Conservative
  - Partial tears (grade I & II)
  - Thumb spica cast vs. custom splint
  - Complete rupture without Stener lesion
- Surgical
  - Complete rupture with Stener lesion
  - Volar subluxation proximal phalanx
  - Primary repair of torn UCL - acute/subacute injuries
  - Reconstruction of chronic complete UCL ruptures
- Complications
  - Superficial branch of radial nerve injury
  - Failure of UCL repair
  - Loss of joint motion

DIAGNOSTIC CHECKLIST

Consider
- Evaluation of UCL tears & Stener lesions require coronal images through MCP parallel to the collateral ligament plane
- Identify retracted UCL with folded or horizontally directed fibers

SELECTED REFERENCES

1. Miller MD et al: Surgical atlas of sports medicine. Treatment of skier's/gamekeeper's thumb. Philadelphia Pennsylvania, WB Saunders, (67): 491-6, 2003
2. Graham TJ et al: DeLee & Drez's orthopaedic sports medicine. Athletic injuries of the adult hand. vol 2. 2nd ed. Philadelphia Pennsylvania, WB Saunders, (24):1381-1430, 2002
3. Plancher KD et al: Role of MR imaging in the management of skier's thumb injuries. MRI Clin North Am 7:73-84, 1999
4. Heyman T et al: Injuries of the ulnar collateral ligament of the thumb metacarpophalangeal joint. Biomechanical and prospective clinical studies on the usefulness of valgus stress testing. Clin Orthop 292:15-71, 1993

ULNAR COLLATERAL LIGAMENT TEAR, THUMB

Typical

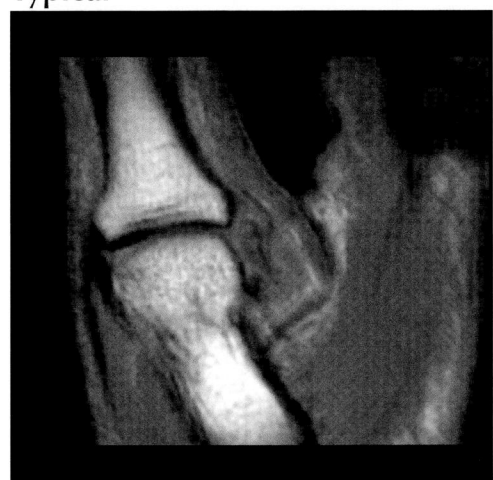
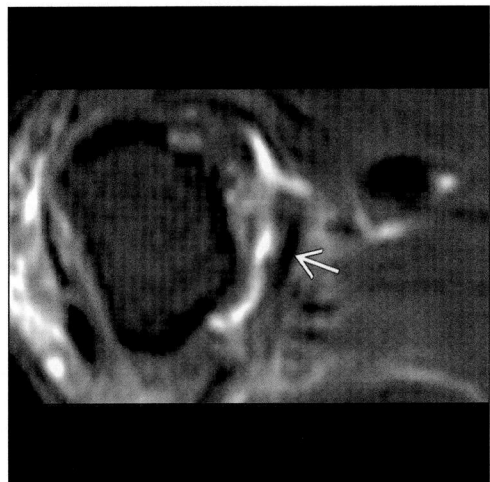

(Left) Coronal T1WI MR shows gamekeeper's thumb with thickening and partial retraction of the torn UCL. The UCL is still located deep to the adductor aponeurosis. *(Right)* Axial FS PD FSE MR shows displacement of the thickened UCL (arrow) superficial to the adductor aponeurosis in a Stener lesion.

Typical

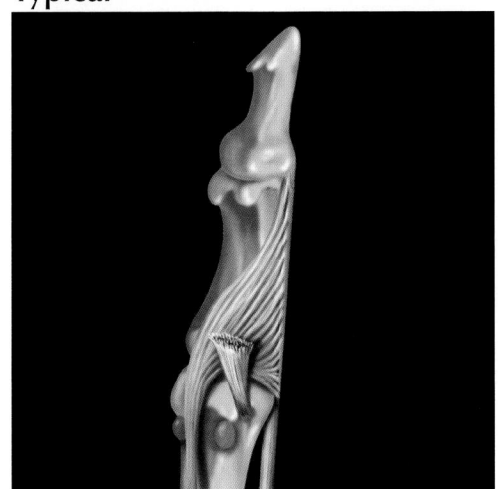
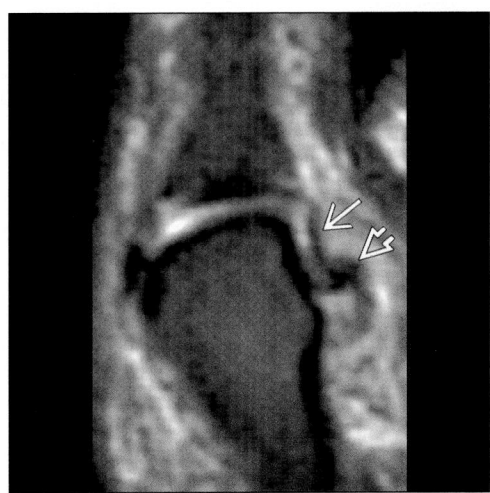

(Left) Sagittal graphic shows displacement of the retracted UCL superficial to the overlying adductor aponeurosis in a Stener lesion. *(Right)* Coronal FS PD FSE MR shows proximal retraction of the trapped UCL (open arrow) intersecting the overlying adductor aponeurosis (arrow) mimics yo-yo on a string.

Typical

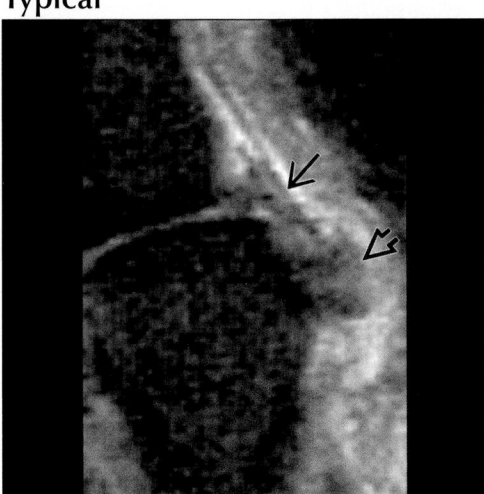
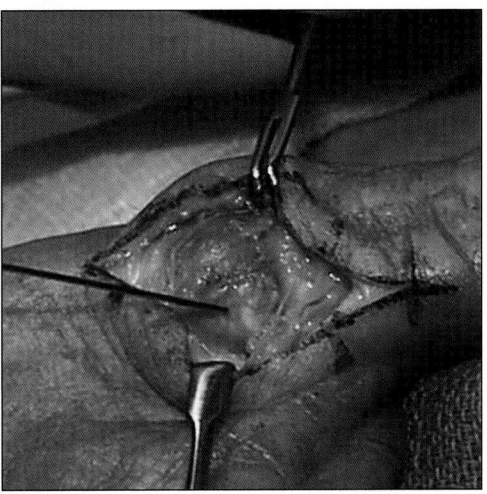

(Left) Coronal STIR MR shows retracted mass (open arrow) of the UCL (proximal to the MCP) intersecting the linear adductor aponeurosis (arrow) in a Stener lesion (skier's thumb). *(Right)* Intra-operative photograph shows Stener lesion at the level of the metacarpophalangeal joint.

FLEXOR ANNULAR PULLEY TEARS

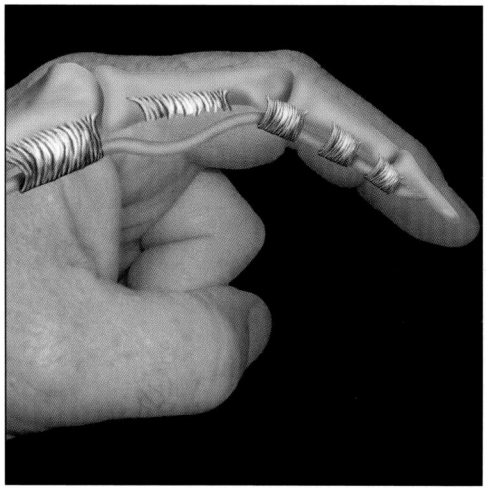

Sagittal graphic shows disruption of the A2 pulley with palmar bowing of the flexor tendon.

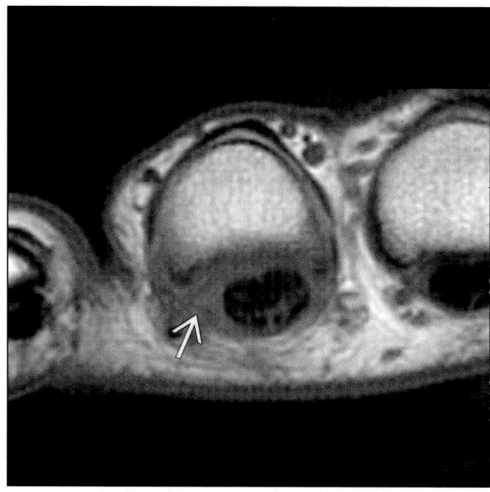

Axial T1WI MR shows discontinuity of the A2 pulley (arrow) with mild subluxation of the flexor tendon of the ring finger.

TERMINOLOGY

Abbreviations and Synonyms
- Digital annular pulley (DAP) tears, flexor pulley tears

Definitions
- Lesion of fibro-osseous theca or flexor tendon sheath

IMAGING FINDINGS

General Features
- Best diagnostic clue: Attenuation or rupture of flexor tendon sheath pulley on axial images
- Location
  - Long finger (baseball) & ring finger
  - A4 pulley (annular)
  - Interval between A2 & A4 pulley
  - A5 pulley
  - First two cruciate pulleys
- Size: Attenuation to frank disruption
- Morphology: Severe injury = overt bowstringing

Radiographic Findings
- Radiography
  - Not diagnostic
  - Nonspecific soft tissue swelling
  - No evidence of fracture or cortical avulsion

MR Findings
- T1WI
  - Bowstringing from proximal interphalangeal joint (PIP) to base of proximal phalanx on sagittal images = complete rupture of A2 pulley
  - Bowstringing from PIP - not reaching base of proximal phalanx = incomplete rupture of A2 pulley
  - Bowstringing at level of proximal phalanx to region distal to PIP joint = A2 + A3 rupture
  - Bowstringing at level of middle phalanx = A4 rupture
  - Hypointense to intermediate signal fluid associated with affected pulley
  - Hypointense cysts
  - Hypo to intermediate signal intensity fibrous tissue
- T2WI
  - Hyperintense fluid associated with affected tendon pulley
  - Discontinuity of pulley on axial images
  - Tendon displacement
    - Anterior displacement relative to proximal aspect proximal phalanx in A2 pulley area
    - Anterior displacement relative to middle phalanx in A4 pulley area
    - ± Medial or lateral subluxation
    - Hypointense fibrous scar tissue
  - Hyperintense

DDx: Flexor Annular Pulley Tears

Ex. Tenosynovitis	FlexTenosynovitis	FDP Tear	Rheumatoid
Ax FS PD MR	Cor FS PD MR	Ax FS PD MR	Ax T1 C+ MR

FLEXOR ANNULAR PULLEY TEARS

Key Facts

Imaging Findings
- Best diagnostic clue: Attenuation or rupture of flexor tendon sheath pulley on axial images
- Long finger (baseball) & ring finger
- Morphology: Severe injury = overt bowstringing

Top Differential Diagnoses
- Tenosynovitis
- Flexor Tendon Tear
- Degenerative Arthritis
- Inflammatory Arthritis
- Joint Trauma

Pathology
- Forcible contraction flexor digitorum profundus (FDP) against extreme force
- Professional baseball injury - pitching

- Rock climbing injury
- Pulley tears = 50% of lesions in elite climbers
- Ring & middle finger affected in climbing vs. middle finger in baseball pitchers
- Bowstringing of flexor tendon
- Failure A4 pulley
- Disruption of interval between A2 & A4
- A5 pulley & first 2 cruciate pulleys involved

Clinical Issues
- Most common signs/symptoms: Pain & tenderness over palmar (volar) & lateral aspects of flexor tendon
- ± DIP flexion with discomfort
- Restricted range of motion

Diagnostic Checklist
- Evaluate flexor tendon bowing on sagittal images

- PIP or distal interphalangeal joints (DIP) joint fluid
- Tenosynovitis
- Tendon sheath cyst

Ultrasonographic Findings
- Dynamic studies
- Scan with resisted flexion
- Measurement of flexor tendon bowstringing
  - Flexor tendon - phalanx (TP) distance > 1.0 mm = pulley injury
  - TP measurement (with forced flexion) > 3.0 mm = complete rupture of A2 pulley
  - TP distance (with forced flexion) > 5 mm = rupture A2 & A3 pulley
  - TP distance ≥ 2.5 mm at middle phalanx = complete rupture A4 pulley
- Assessment of tendon gliding (superficialis, profundus & sheaths)

Imaging Recommendations
- Best imaging tool
  - MR and dynamic ultrasound
  - MR resolution allows direct pulley visualization
- Protocol advice
  - T1, FS PD FSE, T2* gradient echo axial images
  - T1 & FS PD FSE sagittal and coronal images

DIFFERENTIAL DIAGNOSIS

Tenosynovitis
- Inflammation of tendon sheath
- Fluid within tendon sheath (hyperintense on T2WI)
- ± Thickened sheath
- ± Associated tendon degeneration
- ± Tendon fraying
- Fluid intermediate on T2WI with chronic changes

Flexor Tendon Tear
- Avulsion of flexor digitorum profundus
  - Type I - retracts to palm
  - Type II - retracts to PIP joint
  - Type III - osseous avulsion + retraction to A4 pulley

Degenerative Arthritis
- Sclerosis
- Osteophytosis
- Joint space narrowing
- Subluxation
- Reactive subchondral marrow edema
- DIP or PIP joints most common

Inflammatory Arthritis
- Rheumatoid
- Rheumatoid variants
- Tenosynovitis + intermediate signal intensity synovial hypertrophy on T2WI (FS PD FSE)

Joint Trauma
- Dislocations of metacarpophalangeal (MCP) joint (± avulsion fracture)
  - Lateral (coronal plane) injury
  - Dorsal MCP dislocations
  - Volar MCP dislocations
- Proximal interphalangeal joint dislocation
  - Coach's finger = jammed finger
  - Collateral ligaments - accessory & proper
  - Dorsal & volar dislocation
- Pilon fractures
  - Middle phalanx
  - Axial loading
  - Intraarticular comminution & displacement
- Distal interphalangeal dislocations
  - Ball-handling & contact sports
  - Dorsal dislocation

PATHOLOGY

General Features
- General path comments
  - Relevant anatomy = fibrous portion of fibroosseous flexion tunnel
    - Five digital annular pulleys (DAP) (condensations of transversely oriented fibrous bands)
    - Annular pulleys A1 to A5
    - Cruciate pulleys C1 to C3

- A2 (proximal aspect proximal phalanx) & A4 (mid aspect middle phalanx) = most important function of DAP
- DAP - stabilizes flexor tendons during flexion & resist ulnar/radial displacement as well as palmar bowing
- Etiology
  - Forcible contraction flexor digitorum profundus (FDP) against extreme force
  - Professional baseball injury - pitching
    - Distal tip of long finger for control
    - Increased angular velocity in throwing mechanism
  - Rock climbing injury
    - Support of body weight with DIP joint in flexion
    - High stress
    - Repetitive microtrauma
    - Local trauma varies with grip techniques (loads up to 700N)
    - Crimped technique - MCP joint extension, PIP flexion & DIP extension = excessive forces on A2 & A3 DAP
- Epidemiology
  - Pulley tears = 50% of lesions in elite climbers
  - Ring & middle finger affected in climbing vs. middle finger in baseball pitchers
  - 30% of finger injuries

Gross Pathologic & Surgical Features
- Bowstringing of flexor tendon
  - Failure A4 pulley
  - Disruption of interval between A2 & A4
  - A5 pulley & first 2 cruciate pulleys involved
- Less common - combined injury of A2 & A4 pulleys
- Partial tears - no tendon bowstringing
- Volar subluxation of tendon = DAP tear
- Associated tenosynovitis
- Fibrous tissue
- A2 & A3 pulley injuries (proximal phalanx) vs. A2 pulley rupture - requires forced flexion to differentiate

Microscopic Features
- Inflammatory infiltrate
- Fibrous tissue
- Tendons - low resistance to shear forces
- Tendon failure at end of linear portion of load-deformation relationship
- Collagen breakdown

CLINICAL ISSUES

Presentation
- Most common signs/symptoms: Pain & tenderness over palmar (volar) & lateral aspects of flexor tendon
- Clinical profile
  - Increased tenderness associated with inflammation
  - Tendon fullness - fluid or hemorrhage
  - ± DIP flexion with discomfort
  - Weakness
  - Pitcher - decreased velocity of pitches
  - Tendon bowstringing
  - Soft tissue swelling
  - Restricted range of motion

Demographics
- Age
  - Young adult
  - At risk age groups includes professional baseball pitchers (20-30 years) & rock climbers (20-40 years)
- Gender: M > F (related to activities with forcible contraction of FDP)

Natural History & Prognosis
- Delayed diagnosis = fixed contractures of PIP joint
- Fibrosis/scar tissue
- Weakness
- Tenosynovitis or partial tear of DAP - treated conservatively

Treatment
- Conservative
  - Immobilization
  - Anti-inflammatory medication
  - ± Steroid injection if strong inflammatory component (may alter healing process)
  - Indicated in absence of bowstringing
- Surgical
  - Complete rupture of flexor pulley system = reconstruction

DIAGNOSTIC CHECKLIST

Consider
- Evaluate flexor tendon bowing on sagittal images
- Evaluate pulley integrity directly on axial images

SELECTED REFERENCES

1. Klauser A et al: Finger pulley injuries in extreme rock climbers: Depiction with dynamic US. Musculoskeletal Imag 3:755-761, 2002
2. McCue FC III et al: The wrist in the adult. Orthopaedic sports medicine. vol 1. 2nd ed. Philadelphia PA, Saunders, (24):1337-63, 2002
3. Martinoli C et al: Sonographic evaluation of digital annular pulley tears. Skeletal Radiol 29:387-91, 2000
4. Hauger O et al: Pulley system in the fingers: Normal anatomy and simulated lesions in cadavers at MR imaging, CT, and US with and without contrast material distension of the tendon sheath. Radiol 217:201-12, 2000
5. Klauser A et al: Finger injuries in extreme rock climbers: Assessment of high resolution ultrasonography. Am J Sports Med 27:733-37, 1999
6. Gabl M et al: Disruption of the finger flexor pulley system in elite rock climbers. Am J Sports Med 26:651-55, 1998
7. Marco RA et al: Pathomechanics of closed rupture of the flexor tendon pulleys in rock climbers. J Bone Joint Surg 80:1012-9, 1998
8. Parellada JA et al: Bowstring injury of the flexor tendon pulley system: MR imaging. AJR 167:347-9, 1996
9. LeViet D et al: Diagnosis of digital pulley rupture by computed tomography. J Hand Surg 21:245-8, 1996
10. Rooks MD et al: Injury patterns in recreational climbers. Am J Sports Med 23:683-5, 1995
11. Bollen SR: Injury to the A2 pulley in rock climbers. J Hand Surg 12:268-70, 1990

IMAGE GALLERY

Typical

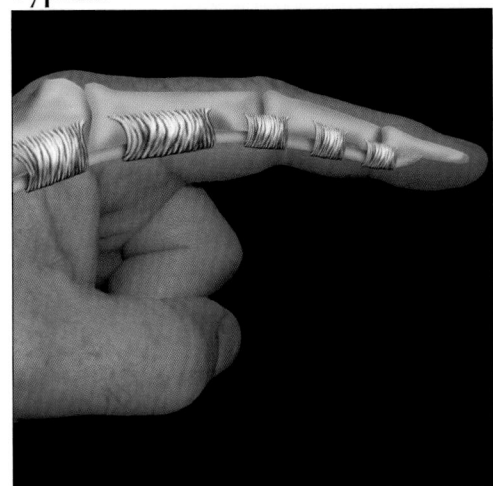

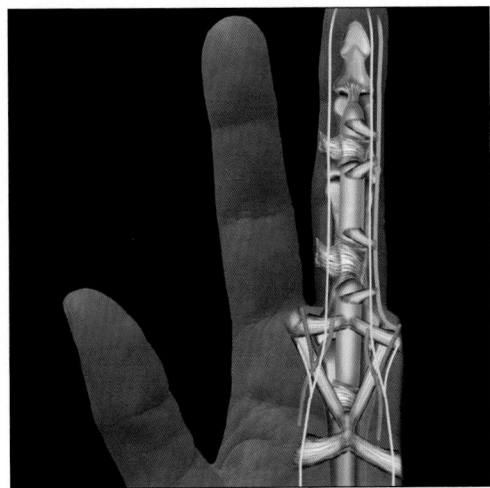

(Left) Sagittal graphic shows normal intact annular pulley system of the finger. *(Right)* Coronal graphic shows normal palmar digital fascial anatomy with intact cruciate and annular pulleys.

Typical

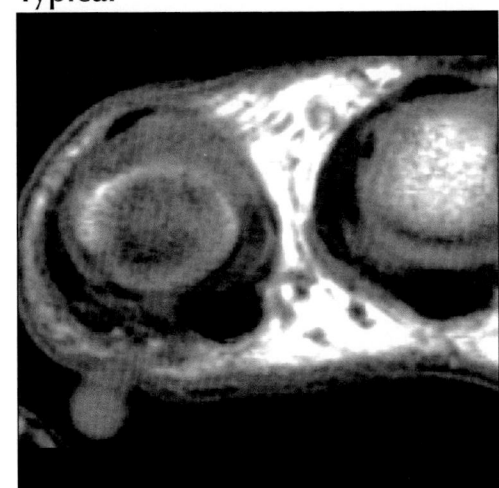

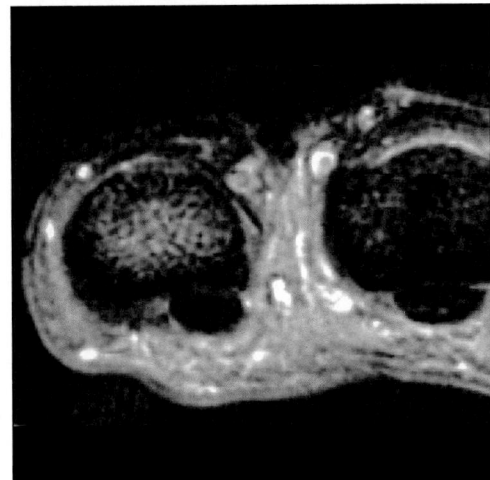

(Left) Axial T1WI MR shows ulnar subluxation of the flexor tendon in association with an A1 pulley tear. *(Right)* Axial FS PD FSE MR shows discontinuity of the annular ligament on the radial side of the flexor tendon.

Typical

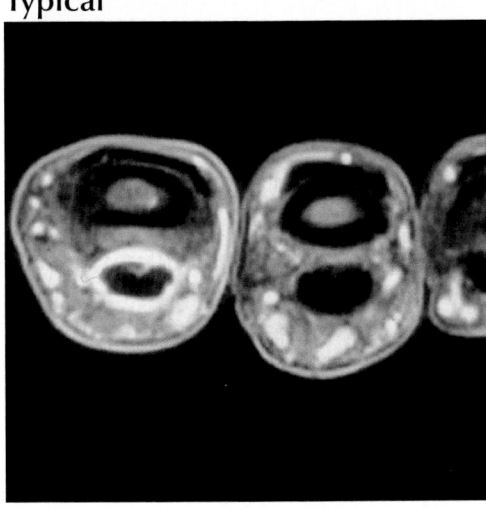

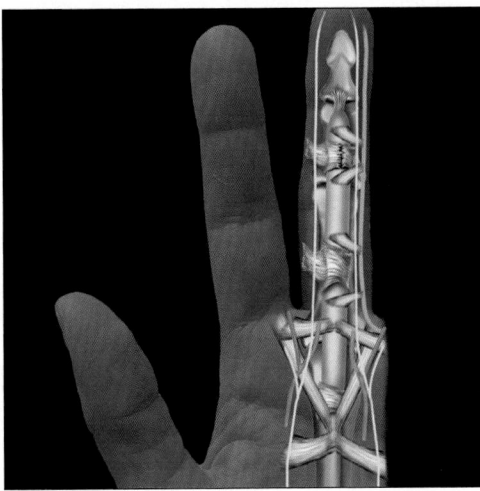

(Left) Axial T1 C+ MR shows tenosynovitis associated with an annular pulley sprain. *(Right)* Coronal graphic shows disruption of the A4 pulley at the level of the middle phalanx. The A2 and A4 pulleys are considered critical pulleys for finger flexion.

FLEXOR DIGITORUM PROFUNDUS AVULSIONS

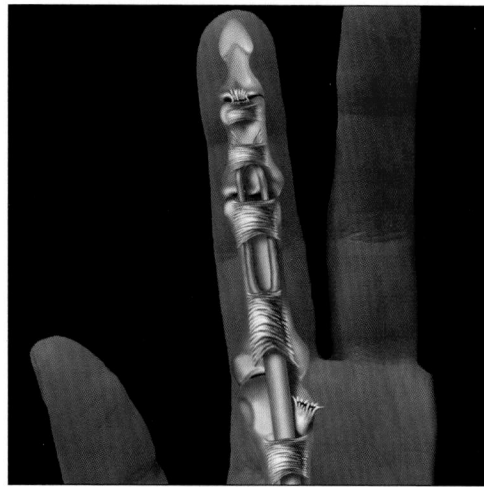

Coronal graphic shows type I avulsion of the FDP with tendon retraction into the palm.

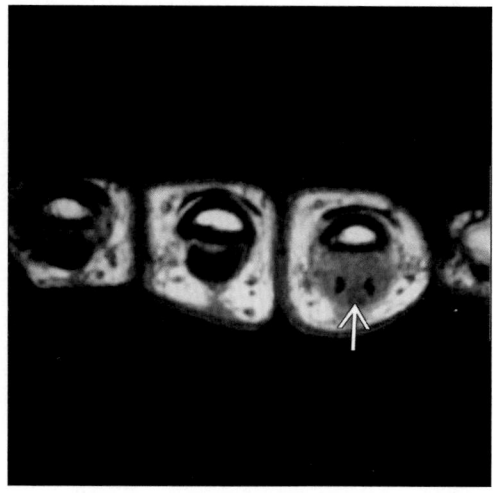

Axial T1WI MR shows absence (arrow) of the FDP tendon between the two slips of the flexor digitorum superficialis.

TERMINOLOGY

Abbreviations and Synonyms
- Avulsion of the flexor digitorum profundus (FDP), jersey finger

Definitions
- Avulsion of the FDP tendon

IMAGING FINDINGS

General Features
- Best diagnostic clue: Absent/retracted FDP tendon on axial or sagittal MR images
- Location
  ○ Insertion on distal phalanx
  ○ Ring finger = most frequently involved
- Size: Tendon retraction to palm, proximal interphalangeal (PIP) joint or A4 annular pulley (osseous avulsions are caught at level of A4 pulley)
- Morphology
  ○ Distal interphalangeal (DIP) joint in position of full extension after FDP avulsion
  ○ Retracted FDP thickened

Radiographic Findings
- Radiography
  ○ Often normal

○ Soft tissue swelling
○ Avulsion fracture at volar aspect of base of distal phalanx
○ Avulsed fragment + tendon retraction

CT Findings
- NECT
  ○ Limited soft tissue detail
  ○ Excellent osseous detail - avulsion fracture
  ○ 3-D multi-detector technique useful in evaluating tendinous injuries

MR Findings
- T1WI
  ○ Soft tissue detail
  ○ Discontinuity = complete disruption
  ○ Retracted tendons easily visualized on sagittal images
  ○ Hypointense marrow edema at site of avulsion fx
  ○ Profundus tendon in area between divisions of the flexor digitorum superficialis (FDS) tendon
  ○ Hypointense to intermediate signal intensity fluid along course of retracted FDP
- T2WI
  ○ Intermediate signal tendinosis
  ○ Hyperintense tenosynovitis
  ○ Hyperintense partial tendon tear
  ○ Hyperintense marrow edema at site of fx

DDx: Flexor Digiturum Profundus Avulsions

Distal Phalanx Fx	PIP Dislocation	Tenosynovitis
Sag T2* GRE MR	Cor T2* GRE MR	Ax T1 C+ MR

FLEXOR DIGITORUM PROFUNDUS AVULSIONS

Key Facts

Imaging Findings
- Best diagnostic clue: Absent/retracted FDP tendon on axial or sagittal MR images
- Ring finger = most frequently involved
- Size: Tendon retraction to palm, proximal interphalangeal (PIP) joint or A4 annular pulley (osseous avulsions are caught at level of A4 pulley)

Top Differential Diagnoses
- Fractures of the Distal Phalanx
- Flexor Pulley System Injury
- Dislocations of the Metacarpophalangeal (MCP) Joint
- Proximal Interphalangeal Joint Dislocation
- Tenosynovitis of Flexor Compartments

Pathology
- Traumatic disruptions

- Forced extension of flexed distal interphalangeal joint (DIP)
- Ring finger at highest risk
- FDP avulsions = unique to athletes

Clinical Issues
- Most common signs/symptoms: Tenderness along FDP
- Inability to flex DIP joint
- Local tenderness greatest at FDP stump site (PIP level at A4 pulley or distal palm)

Diagnostic Checklist
- T2* gradient echo images in axial plane may provide improved tendon contrast

○ Hyperintense fluid surrounding FDS slips (divisions) & centrally (within FDP tendon gap) on axial images
- Normal tendons = homogeneous hypointensity on T1 & T2WI

Imaging Recommendations
- Best imaging tool: MR to document FDP vs. FDS, site of avulsion & extent of retraction
- Protocol advice: Axial T1 or PD, FS PD FSE & T2* (gradient echo technique provides excellent tendon visualization)

DIFFERENTIAL DIAGNOSIS

Fractures of the Distal Phalanx
- Longitudinal - nondisplaced
- Transverse - often angulated
- Tuft - comminuted
- Distal phalanx of long finger most common

Flexor Pulley System Injury
- Fibro-osseous theca or flexor sheath
- Baseball pitchers & rock climbers - attenuation or rupture
- Forcible contraction of FDP
- Tenderness at volar & lateral aspects of middle phalanx

Dislocations of the Metacarpophalangeal (MCP) Joint
- Lateral or coronal plane injury (pain in collateral area)
- Dorsal MCP dislocations
- Volar MCP dislocations

Proximal Interphalangeal Joint Dislocation
- Coach's finger
- Jammed finger
- Collateral ligaments (accessory & proper) + volar plate = resistance to lateral deviation
- Swelling
- Tenderness (volar, lateral or dorsal)

Tenosynovitis of Flexor Compartments
- Flexor carpi ulnaris (FCU) tenosynovitis (at wrist and insertion)
- Flexor carpi radialis tenosynovitis (pain, swelling, tenderness over palmar radial wrist)
- Restrictive thumb-index tenosynovitis (Linburg's syndrome) at anatomic (variant) interconnection between flexor pollicis longus & index FDP
- Nonspecific trauma or inflammatory tenosynovitis of FDP or FDS tendons
  ○ Hypointense fluid on T1WI, hyperintense on T2WI
  ○ Single traumatic event
  ○ Repetitive use
  ○ Repair response

PATHOLOGY

General Features
- General path comments
  ○ Relevant anatomy (flexor tendon sheath pulley system)
    ▪ Critical A2 & A4 pulleys (for maximal finger flexion) originate from bone
    ▪ Annular pulleys: A1-A5 (thick, well defined)
    ▪ Cruciate pulleys: C1-C3 (thin, collapse in flexion)
    ▪ Palmar aponeurosis
    ▪ Short & long vincula - dorsal mesotenon that carries blood supply
- Etiology
  ○ Traumatic disruptions
    ▪ Athlete grasps the jersey of another athlete: Soccer, football (tight-ends, defensive players)
    ▪ Basketball - catching a finger on a basketball rim during a slam dunk
  ○ Forced extension of flexed distal interphalangeal joint (DIP)
  ○ Ring finger at highest risk
    ▪ Common muscle belly of long, middle & ring finger
    ▪ FDP insertion has low threshold for disruption

- Ring finger more prominent during grip relative to long finger + tethered by bipennate lumbrical muscles
- Epidemiology
  - FDP avulsions = unique to athletes
  - Ring finger in 75% of cases

Gross Pathologic & Surgical Features

- 3 types of FDP avulsion injuries
  - Type I
    - Tendon retraction into palm
    - Blood supply disruption
    - Tendon sheath scar
  - Type II
    - Tendon retracts to proximal interphalangeal (PIP) joint
    - FDP caught at chiasm of FDS
  - Type III
    - FDP avulsion + large osseous fragment
    - Bony fragment lodged at distal edge of A4 pulley

Microscopic Features

- Tendon histology
  - Collagen - fibers parallel to long axis
  - Endotenon- binds collagen
  - Epitenon - similar to synovium
  - Paratenon - surrounds epitenon & contains elastic fibers = tenosynovium of wrist flexors
  - Collagen failure/disruption in tears
    - Type I collagen in tendons
  - Elastin - small amount in tendon
  - Ground substance provides viscoelastic properties of tendon (proteoglycans, glycosaminoglycans, plasma proteins)

Staging, Grading or Classification Criteria

- Tendon disruptions are classified according to 5 zones
  - Zone 1 - From fingertip to midportion of middle phalanx
  - Zone 2 - From midportion middle phalanx to distal palmar crease
  - Zone 3 - From distal palmar crease to distal edge of carpal tunnel
  - Zone 4 - In carpal tunnel
  - Zone 5 - Proximal to carpal tunnel
- FDP disruptions (avulsion injuries)
  - Type I - FDP retracts to palm
  - Type II - Vincula vessels intact & tether retracting FDP
  - Type III - Large fragment of bone catches on A4 or A5 pulley
  - Type IV - Fx at FDP insertion, retraction permitted by separation of tendon from bone

CLINICAL ISSUES

Presentation

- Most common signs/symptoms: Tenderness along FDP
- Clinical profile
  - Inability to flex DIP joint
  - Swelling
  - Ecchymosis

- Local tenderness greatest at FDP stump site (PIP level at A4 pulley or distal palm)

Demographics

- Age: Young athletes most commonly affected
- Gender: Differences related to activity (M > F)

Natural History & Prognosis

- Untreated - deformity & loss of function
- Delay in treatment - tendon degradation by inflammatory cells making operative repair difficult

Treatment

- Conservative
  - No role with delayed treatment
- Surgical
  - Gold standard = primary repair
  - Reinsertion into base of distal phalanx
  - Reconstruction

DIAGNOSTIC CHECKLIST

Consider

- T2* gradient echo images in axial plane may provide improved tendon contrast
- Use T1WI sagittal images to identify osseous fragment

SELECTED REFERENCES

1. Sunagawa T et al: Three-dimensional CT imaging of the flexor tendon ruptures in the hand and wrist. J of Comp Assisted Tomog 27(2):169-74, 2003
2. Wright II PE: Arthritic hand. Cambell's operative orthopaedics. St. Louis MO, Mosby, 3707, 2003
3. Miller MD et al: Treatment of flexor digitorum profundus avulsions. Surgical atlas of sports medicine. Philadelphia PA, WB Saunders, (67):481-6, 2003
4. Graham TJ et al: Athletic injuries of the adult hand. Orthopaedic sports medicine. vol 1. 2nd ed. Philadelphia PA, WB Saunders, (24):1381-1430, 2002
5. Henry M: Fractures and dislocations of the hand. Rockwood and Green's fractures in adults. 3rd ed. Philadelphia PA, Lippincott Williams and Wilkins, 670, 2001
6. Perron AD et al: Orthopedic pitfalls in the emergency department. J of Emerg Med 19(1):76-80, 2001
7. VanHolsbeeck MT et al: Musculoskeletal ultrasound. 2nd ed. St. Louis MO, Mosby 541-7, 2001
8. Strickland JW: Flexor tendons – acute injuries. Green's operative hand surgery. 4th ed. Philadelphia PA, Elsevier Science, 1851-97, 1999
9. Schneider LH: Flexor tendons – late reconstruction. Green's operative hand surgery. 4th ed. Philadelphia PA, Elsevier Science, 1898-1949, 1999
10. Strickland JW: Flexor tendon-acute injuries. Green's operative hand surgery 4th ed. Philadelphia PA, Elsevier Science, 1866-8, 1999
11. Stoller DW. Magnetic resonance imaging. Orthopaedics and sports medicine. vol 1. 2nd ed. Philadelphia PA, Saunders, 987-90, 1997
12. Smith JH: Avulsion of the profundus tendon and simultaneous intraarticular fracture of the distal phalanx. J Hand Surg 6:600-1, 1981
13. Leddy JP et al: Avulsion of the profundus tendon insertion in athletes. J Hand Surg 2:66-9, 1977

FLEXOR DIGITORUM PROFUNDUS AVULSIONS

IMAGE GALLERY

Typical

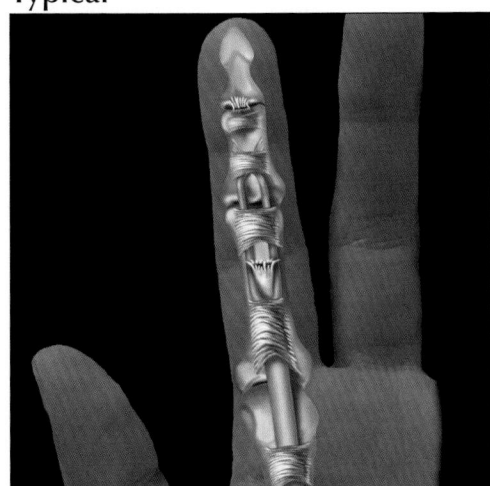 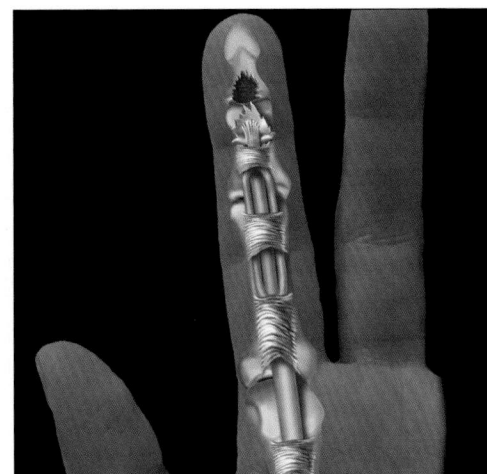

(Left) Coronal graphic shows type II FDP avulsion with tendon retraction to level of the PIP joint. The retracted tendon is caught at chiasm of the flexor digitorum superficialis. *(Right)* Coronal graphic shows type III FDP avulsion associated with a large bony fragment lodged at the level of distal A4 pulley.

Typical

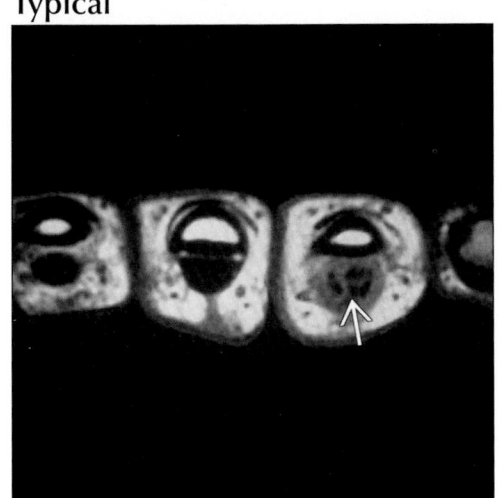 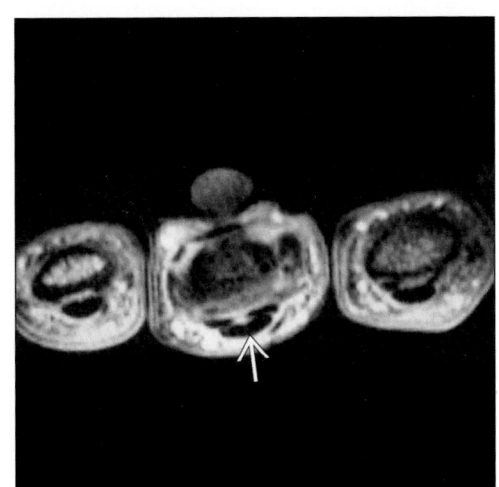

(Left) Axial T1WI MR shows abnormal morphology (arrow) of the retracted FDP tendon between the flexor digitorum superficialis slips. *(Right)* Axial T2* GRE MR shows normal position of the FDP tendon (arrow) superficial to the slips of the flexor digitorum superficialis tendon. This is at the level of the proximal aspect of the middle phalanx.

Typical

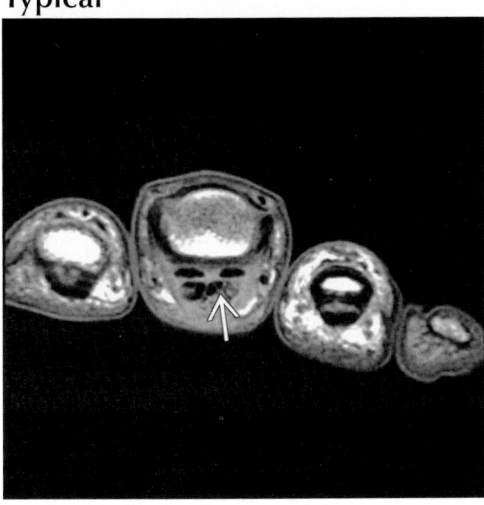 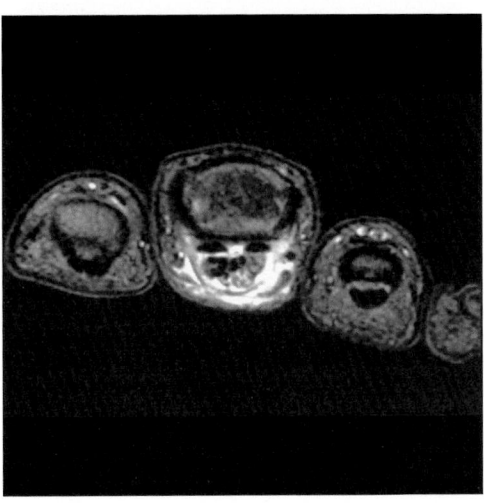

(Left) Axial T1WI MR shows high grade tearing (arrow) of the FDP tendon superficial to flexor digitorum superficialis slips. *(Right)* Axial FS PD FSE MR shows hyperintense edema surrounding the retracted torn fibers of FDP tendon.

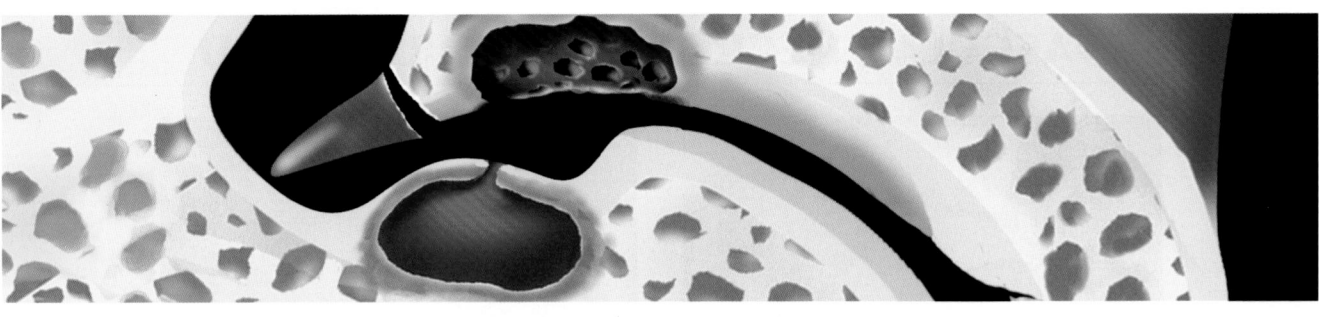

SECTION 4: Hip

Osteonecrosis

Marrow

Dysplasia

Overuse Syndromes and Muscle Trauma

Osseous Trauma

Labrum

Arthritis

Infection

AVASCULAR NECROSIS, FEMORAL HEAD

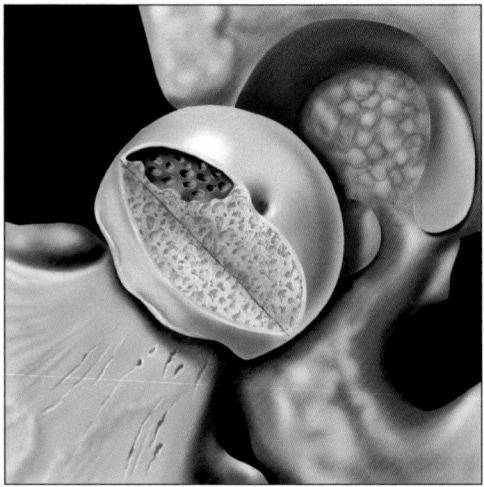

Coronal graphic shows anterolateral subchondral ischemic focus in early stage AVN. The overlying articular cartilage and subchondral plate are normal.

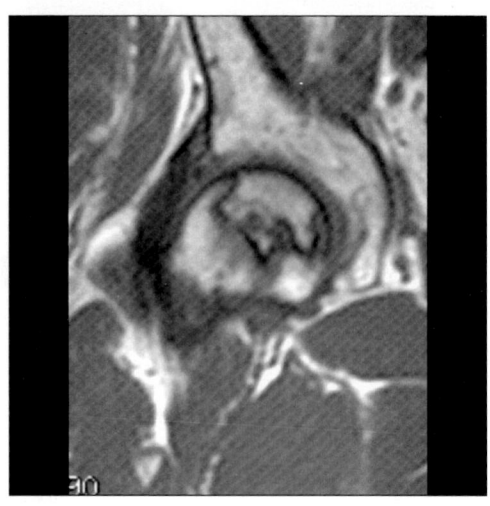

Coronal T1WI MR shows wedge-shaped subchondral ischemic focus with central marrow fat signal intensity. Hypointense peripheral band represents the reactive interface.

TERMINOLOGY

Abbreviations and Synonyms
- AVN, aseptic necrosis, osteonecrosis of the femoral head, ischemic necrosis

Definitions
- Region of dead trabecular bone + marrow extending to subchondral plate of femoral head

IMAGING FINDINGS

General Features
- Best diagnostic clue: Wedge-shaped subchondral ischemic focus
- Location: Anterolateral weightbearing femoral head most common
- Size: Variable from < 15% (mild) to > 30% (severe) involvement of femoral head
- Morphology: Linear to wedge-shaped subchondral necrotic focus

Radiographic Findings
- Radiography
  - Anteroposterior (AP) + frog lateral
  - Used in staging (not sensitive to stage 0 and I AVN)
  - Involvement of femoral head greater than involvement of joint space narrowing or acetabular findings
  - Femoral head sclerosis
  - Subchondral collapse = advanced sign
  - Ficat classification (stage 0 - IV)
  - Steinberg staging based on radiographs, bone scan + MRI

CT Findings
- NECT
  - More accurate than conventional radiographs for staging (extent of disease at stages II and higher)
  - Less sensitive relative to MR
  - Osteoporosis = first sign
  - Sclerosis + distortion of central bony asterisk (normal thickening of trabeculae in center of femoral head)

MR Findings
- T1WI
  - Hypointense peripheral band outlining central region of bone marrow = reactive interface between necrotic + reparative zones
  - ± Hypointense bone marrow edema of head + neck
  - Sagittal images to assess femoral head morphology for cortical flattening (supplemental to routine imaging with coronal + axial images)
  - ± Hypointense joint effusion

DDx: Avascular Necrosis, Femoral Head

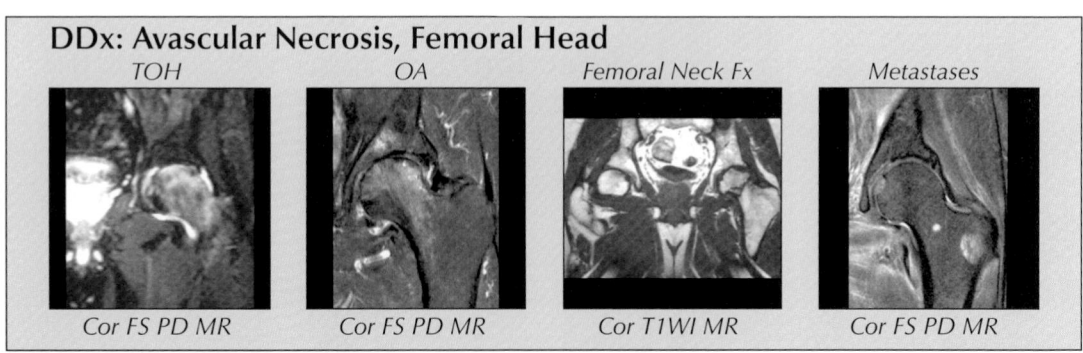

TOH	OA	Femoral Neck Fx	Metastases
Cor FS PD MR	Cor FS PD MR	Cor T1WI MR	Cor FS PD MR

AVASCULAR NECROSIS, FEMORAL HEAD

Key Facts

Imaging Findings
- Best diagnostic clue: Wedge-shaped subchondral ischemic focus
- Location: Anterolateral weightbearing femoral head most common
- Double line sign in 80% (hyperintense inner border parallel to hypointense periphery)

Top Differential Diagnoses
- Transient Osteoporosis of Hip (TOH)
- Degenerative Arthrosis
- Fracture (Fx)

Pathology
- Traumatic AVN - 10% non-displaced femoral neck fxs + 15-30% displaced fxs + 10% dislocations

- Corticosteroid use = 5-25% of cases of atraumatic AVN
- Double line sign = inflammatory response with granulation tissue inside reactive bone interface

Clinical Issues
- Most common signs/symptoms: Hip, groin or gluteal pain ± referred thigh or knee pain
- Increased risk of contralateral AVN
- Endstage = destruction of femoral head + joint osteoarthritis
- Core decompression for stage I & II: Best results with < 25% involvement of weight-bearing surface of femoral head

Diagnostic Checklist
- Early femoral head collapse requires sagittal images

- Wedge-shaped subchondral infarct
- T2WI
  - Double line sign in 80% (hyperintense inner border parallel to hypointense periphery)
  - Hypointense peripheral border more difficult to visualize on FS PD or T2 FSE images
  - Hypointense periphery = reparative tissue interface with necrotic region
  - ± Hyperintense femoral head + hyperintense neck edema + effusion
  - Staging Ficat + Arlet
    - Stage 1: Trabeculae normal to porotic ± double line sign
    - Stage 2: Sclerosis of trabeculae
    - Stage 3: Loss of spherical shape of femoral head
    - Stage 4: Collapse of femoral head, articular cartilage destruction + joint space narrowing
  - Mitchell MR classification
    - Qualitative assessment of alterations in MR signal in central region of osteonecrotic focus
- T1 C+
  - Decreased enhancement with gadolinium in early AVN
  - Nonviable trabeculae + marrow = no enhancement
  - Enhancement corresponds to reparative zone of hypointense band

Nuclear Medicine Findings
- Bone Scan
  - Earlier detection than conventional radiographs (less sensitive relative to MR)
  - Technetium labeled phosphate analogues + sulfur colloid

Imaging Recommendations
- Best imaging tool: MR more sensitive than CT or bone scintigraphy
- Protocol advice
  - T1 + FS PD FSE or STIR coronal + axials
  - Small FOV coronal
  - Sagittal T1 or FS PD FSE for evaluating femoral head sphericity (for early subchondral collapse)

DIFFERENTIAL DIAGNOSIS

Transient Osteoporosis of Hip (TOH)
- Osteoporosis femoral head + neck
- Resolves over a 10-12 month period
- ± Involvement of acetabular + femoral sides of the joint

Degenerative Arthrosis
- Articular cartilage degeneration
- Acetabular changes usually first
- Femoroacetabular impingement = osteoarthritis (OA) in a younger patient with a non-dysplastic hip

Fracture (Fx)
- Subchondral insufficiency fractures may mimic AVN-related subchondral capsule
- Capital + femoral neck stress fractures

Metastatic Disease
- Hypointense to hyperintense lesion not centered in subchondral femoral head
- Gross trabecular destruction as confirmed by CT

Infection
- Hyperintense marrow edema on both sides of joint
- Adjacent soft tissue hyperintense edema ± fluid
- Joint synovitis prominent

Osseous Contusion
- Localized subchondral marrow edema without fracture segment

---

PATHOLOGY

General Features
- General path comments
  - Relevant anatomy
    - Blood supply to femoral head = medial + lateral circumflex branches of the profunda femoral artery
- Etiology
  - Traumatic (most common)

AVASCULAR NECROSIS, FEMORAL HEAD

- Fracture of femoral head or neck
- Hip dislocation
- Disrupted vascular supply at time of injury
  - Atraumatic
    - Corticosteroid use and alcohol abuse = most common
    - Idiopathic
    - Sickle-cell anemia, Gaucher's disease, lupus, coagulopathies, hyperlipidemia, organ transplantation, Caisson's disease + thyroid disease
- Epidemiology
  - AVN responsible for 10% of total hip replacements
  - Traumatic AVN - 10% non-displaced femoral neck fxs + 15-30% displaced fxs + 10% dislocations
  - Corticosteroid use = 5-25% of cases of atraumatic AVN

Gross Pathologic & Surgical Features
- Cancellous bone - yellow necrosis extending to subarticular region
- Softening within necrotic cancellous bone at interface with viable bone = resorption of necrotic focus
- Collapse of femoral head load-bearing segment
- Collapse of femoral head + articular cartilage destruction + loose bodies + marginal osteophytes

Microscopic Features
- Central region of hyperintensity = necrosis of bone + marrow prior to capillary mesenchymal ingrowth
- Hypointense peripheral band = sclerotic margin of reactive tissue at necrotic + viable bone interface
- Double line sign = inflammatory response with granulation tissue inside reactive bone interface

Staging, Grading or Classification Criteria
- International classification
  - Stage 0 : Bone biopsy = osteonecrosis; normal imaging
  - Stage I: Positive bone scan ± MR
  - Stage II: Mottled femoral head with sclerosis/cyst/osteopenia on radiographs + no collapse + positive bone scan & MR
  - Stage III: Crescent sign lesions + depression femoral head articular surface
  - Stage IV: Flattening articular surface + joint space narrowing + secondary acetabular changes

CLINICAL ISSUES

Presentation
- Most common signs/symptoms: Hip, groin or gluteal pain ± referred thigh or knee pain
- Clinical profile
  - Decreased hip rotation + range of motion (worse in presence of a joint effusion)
  - Increased risk of contralateral AVN
  - Pain = deep + throbbing + worse with ambulation
  - ± Catching or popping sensation
  - ± History of trauma, steroid use, alcohol use or abuse
  - Trendelenburg gait

Demographics
- Age: Third to sixth decades most common
- Gender: M:F = 4:1

Natural History & Prognosis
- Endstage = destruction of femoral head + joint osteoarthritis
- Early identification + intervention may not alter result
- Disease progression greater with non-surgical treatment

Treatment
- Conservative = limited utility
  - Observation + protected weight-bearing
- Surgical
  - Core decompression ± bone grafts, osteotomy + electrical stimulation
  - Core decompression for stage I & II: Best results with < 25% involvement of weight-bearing surface of femoral head
  - Arthroplasty

DIAGNOSTIC CHECKLIST

Consider
- Identify subchondral fracture using high resolution coronal or sagittal images
- Early femoral head collapse requires sagittal images

SELECTED REFERENCES

1. Newberg AH et al: Imaging of the painful hip. Clin Orthop 406:19-28 Review, 2003
2. Cherian SF et al: Quantifying the extent of femoral head involvement in osteonecrosis. J Bone Joint Surg AM 85-A(2):309-15, 2003
3. Tsuji T et al: Evaluation of femoral perfusion in a non-traumatic rabbi osteonecrosis model with T2*-weighted dynamic MRI. J Orthop Res 21(2):341-51, 2003
4. May DA et al: Screening for avascular necrosis of the hip with rapid MRI: Preliminary experience. J Comput Assis Tomogr 24(2):284-7, 2000
5. Staudenherz A et al: Diagnostic patterns for bone marrow oedema syndrome and avascular necrosis of the femoral head in dynamic bone scintigraphy. Nucl Med Commun 18(12):1178-88, 1997
6. Mulliken BD et al: Prevalence of previously undetected osteonecrosis of the femoral head in renal transplant recipients. Radiology 192:831-4, 1994
7. Chang CC et al: Osteonecrosis: Current perspectives on pathogenesis and treatment. Semin Arthritis Theum 23:47-69, 1993
8. Tervonen O et al: Clinically occult avascular necrosis of the hip: Prevalence in an asymptomatic population at risk. Radiology 182:845-7, 1992
9. Beltran J et al: Core decompression for avascular necrosis of the femoral head: Correlation between long-term results and preoperative MR staging. Radiology 175:533-6, 1990
10. Meyers MH: Osteonecrosis of the femoral head: Pathogenesis and long-term results of treatment. Clin Orthop 231:51-61, 1988
11. Ficat RP: Idiopathic bone necrosis of the femoral head. J Bone Joint Surg Br 67B:3-9, 1985

4

4

IMAGE GALLERY

Typical

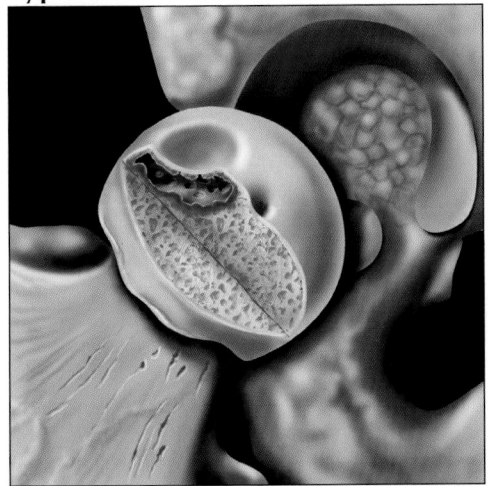

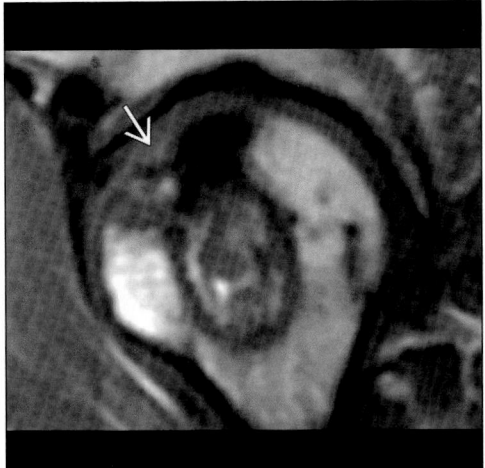

(Left) Coronal graphic shows subchondral fracture and collapse in a more advanced stage of AVN. *(Right)* Sagittal T1WI MR shows loss of the normal spherical shape of the femoral head secondary to subchondral collapse (arrow). This would represent the equivalent of a Ficat stage 3.

Typical

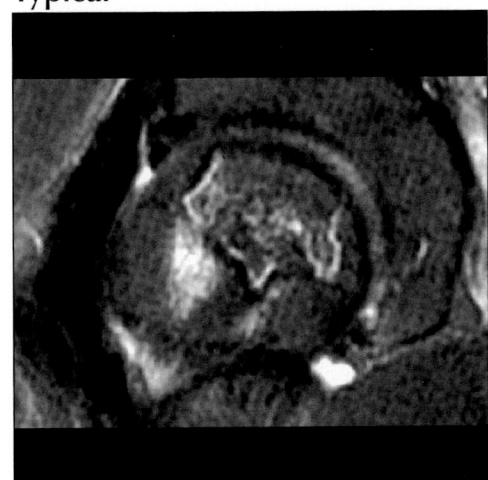

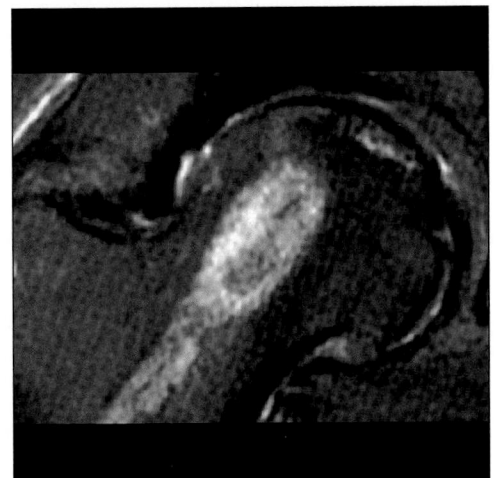

(Left) Coronal FS PD FSE MR shows AVN with characteristic double line sign. There is a hypointense peripheral border surrounding a hyperintense inner margin. *(Right)* Coronal FS PD FSE MR shows AVN subsequent to surgical core decompression. The decompression tract is hyperintense.

Typical

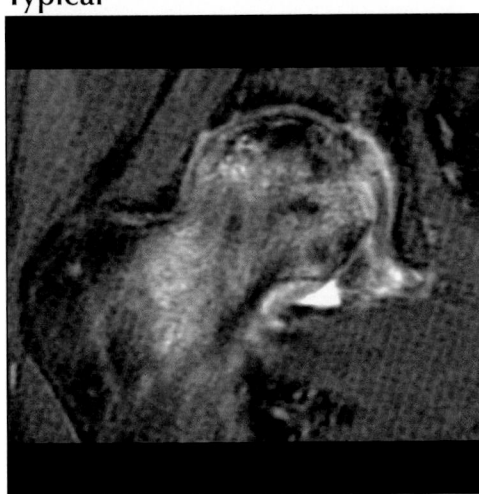

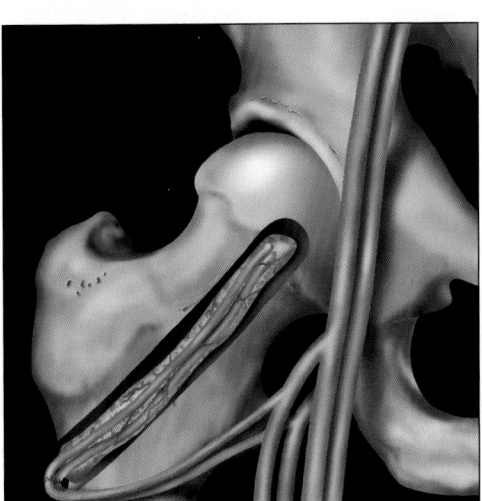

(Left) Coronal FS PD FSE MR shows extended hyperintense bone marrow edema pattern in the femoral head and neck associated with AVN. *(Right)* Coronal graphic shows treatment of AVN with vascularized free fibular graft.

LEGG-CALVE-PERTHES

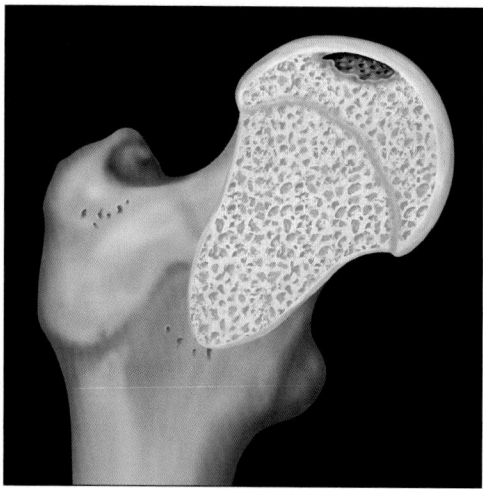

Coronal graphic shows subchondral necrosis in the proximal femoral epiphysis in early Legg-Calvé-Perthes.

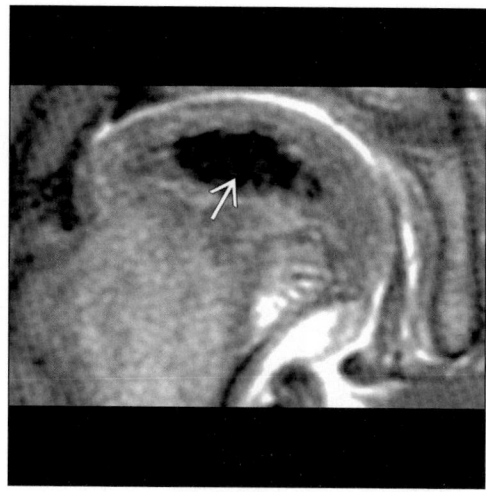

Coronal FS PD FSE MR shows hypointense ischemic focus (arrow) of the capital epiphysis associated with medial hyperintense metaphyseal irregularity. Joint effusion is hyperintense.

TERMINOLOGY

Abbreviations and Synonyms
- Perthes', avascular or ischemic necrosis of the proximal femoral epiphysis, Legg-Perthes disease, osteochondritis coxae juvenilis, coxa plana

Definitions
- Necrosis of osseous epiphysis of femoral head classified as an osteochondrosis

IMAGING FINDINGS

General Features
- Best diagnostic clue: Hypointensity of capital epiphysis on coronal MR images (T1 or T2)
- Location: Proximal femoral epiphysis
- Size: Variable size from peripheral irregularity of epiphyseal ossification center to complete replacement of normal marrow fat
- Morphology
  - Initially confined to epiphysis
  - Late remodeling = coxa plana & coxa magna

Radiographic Findings
- Radiography
  - Effusion, fragmentation + flattening of sclerotic capital epiphysis
  - Metaphyseal irregularity (rarefaction of lateral + medial metaphysis + cystic changes)
  - Joint space (inferomedial) widening + intact subchondral plate
  - Catterall classification (group I-IV) estimates amount of femoral head involvement
  - Waldenström's radiographic staging
    - Initial stage = increased head-socket distance, subchondral plate thinning + dense epiphysis
    - Fragmentation stage = subchondral fracture, inhomogeneous dense epiphysis + porous appearance + metaphyseal cysts
    - Reparative stage = normal bone in areas of resorption + removal of sclerotic bone + more homogeneous epiphysis
    - Growth stage = approaches normal femoral shape
    - Definite stage = final shape (joint congruency vs. incongruency)

MR Findings
- T1WI
  - Hypointense intraarticular effusion
  - Hypointense irregularity along periphery of ossific nucleus
  - Linear hypointensity traversing femoral ossification center in early stages
  - Revascularization of necrotic epiphysis = replacement of hypointense focus with marrow fat signal intensity

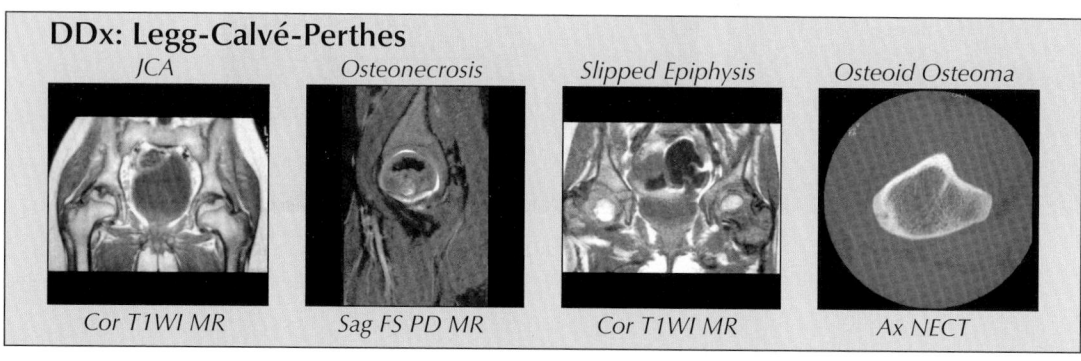

DDx: Legg-Calvé-Perthes

JCA	Osteonecrosis	Slipped Epiphysis	Osteoid Osteoma
Cor T1WI MR	Sag FS PD MR	Cor T1WI MR	Ax NECT

LEGG-CALVE-PERTHES

Key Facts

Imaging Findings

- Best diagnostic clue: Hypointensity of capital epiphysis on coronal MR images (T1 or T2)
- Size: Variable size from peripheral irregularity of epiphyseal ossification center to complete replacement of normal marrow fat
- Late remodeling = coxa plana & coxa magna
- Hypointense epiphyseal marrow center on T1 + T2WI

Top Differential Diagnoses

- Toxic Synovitis
- Septic Hip
- Juvenile Chronic Arthritis (JCA)
- Juvenile Osteonecrosis

Pathology

- Insufficiency of capital epiphyseal blood supply with physis acting as a barrier
- Ischemia may be arterial or venous-based leading to intraepiphyseal infarction
- 15 to 20% with bilateral involvement

Clinical Issues

- Most common signs/symptoms: Limp + groin, thigh or knee pain (referred)
- 3-12 years
- Gender: M:F = 4-5:1

Diagnostic Checklist

- Use coronal T1WI to detect subtle peripheral or linear areas of epiphyseal marrow hypointensity

4

7

  - ○ Coxa plana + coxa magna = late remodeling
- T2WI
  - ○ FS PD or T2 FSE images to assess articular cartilage thickness + chondral irregularities
  - ○ Physeal cartilage ± hyperintense on T2WI - in early stage disease
  - ○ Loss of femoral head containment in acetabulum
    - ■ Intermediate signal hypertrophied synovium in iliopsoas recess
    - ■ Thickening of intermediate signal epiphyseal cartilage
  - ○ Hyperintense joint effusion
- Hypointense epiphyseal marrow center on T1 + T2WI
- Sagittal T1 + T2WI also useful to display acetabular + femoral head cartilage

Nuclear Medicine Findings

- Bone scintigraphy
  - ○ Early decrease secondary to interruption of blood supply
  - ○ Increased uptake late - with secondary revascularization + repair + degenerative arthritis

Imaging Recommendations

- Best imaging tool: MR for early detection of epiphyseal ossification center irregularity
- Protocol advice
  - ○ Coronal T1, FS PD FSE + T2*
  - ○ Axial T1, PD + FS PD FSE
  - ○ Sagittal FS PD FSE

DIFFERENTIAL DIAGNOSIS

Toxic Synovitis

- Self-limiting acute synovitis (3 to 10 days)
- Boys < 4 years
- Minimal thigh atrophy
- Improves in < 5 days with bedrest + anti-inflammatory medications
- Significant effusion + capsular distension

Septic Hip

- Acutely ill + fever

- Increased white blood cell count + sedimentation rate
- Hips held in flexion, abduction + external rotation vs. hip adduction in Perthes'
- Joint effusion +/- joint debris +/- reactive marrow edema

Juvenile Chronic Arthritis (JCA)

- Limp + hip pain
- Chronicity + thigh atrophy
- Fever + rash + positive antinuclear antibody
- Epiphyseal erosions

Juvenile Osteonecrosis

- Distinction = identifiable etiology
- Sickle cell + thalassemia
- Idiopathic thrombocytopenia purpura
- Hip dislocation

Slipped Capital Femoral Epiphysis

- Posterior-inferior displacement of proximal femoral epiphysis
- Pain + limp
- Limitation of internal rotation + abduction

Osteoid Osteoma

- Local pain worse at night, decreased by salicylates
- Local swelling + point tenderness
- Extensive marrow edema on FS PD FSE or STIR

PATHOLOGY

General Features

- General path comments: Capital femoral epiphysis at risk
- Etiology
  - ○ Insufficiency of capital epiphyseal blood supply with physis acting as a barrier
  - ○ Overgrowth of articular cartilage medially + laterally
  - ○ Infarction - trabecular fracture with decreased epiphyseal height
  - ○ Disease progressive
  - ○ Ischemia may be arterial or venous-based leading to intraepiphyseal infarction

LEGG-CALVE-PERTHES

- Epidemiology
  - 15 to 20% with bilateral involvement
  - One in 1200 children < 15 years affected

Gross Pathologic & Surgical Features
- Initial stage
  - Necrosis of epiphyseal bone + marrow
  - Vascular invasion of dead bone
  - Epiphyseal cartilage hypertrophy
- Fragmentation
  - Dead bone resorbed
  - Unossified physeal cartilage in metaphysis develops cysts
  - Cartilage hypertrophy
- Reparative
  - Replacement of dead bone

Microscopic Features
- Epiphyseal cartilage
  - Disordered collagen fibrosis
  - Increased proteoglycan concentration
  - Decrease in structural glycoproteins
- Infarction
  - Necrosis of epiphyseal bone + marrow
  - New blood vessels invade
  - Resorption of dead bone + new bone formation

Staging, Grading or Classification Criteria
- Catterall - distribution of epiphyseal abnormalities based on anteroposterior + lateral radiographs
  - Group I: < ¼ epiphysis involved
  - Group II : < ½ epiphysis involved
  - Group III: Most of epiphysis involved
  - Group IV: Total epiphysis involved
  - Risk factors = lateral subluxation, calcification lateral to epiphysis, Gage's sign (radiolucent V in lateral epiphysis) + a horizontal physis
- Salter - Thompson: Extent + location of subchondral fracture
  - A = fracture < 50% span of epiphysis
  - B = fracture > 50% span of epiphysis
- Herring system: Based on lateral pillar involvement (lateral 15 to 30% of epiphysis = lateral pillar)
  - A = uninvolved lateral pillar
  - B = < 50% involvement of lateral pillar
  - C = > 50%

CLINICAL ISSUES

Presentation
- Most common signs/symptoms: Limp + groin, thigh or knee pain (referred)
- Clinical profile
  - No specific history of trauma
  - Decreased range of motion (internal rotation + abduction) + painful gait & muscle atrophy

Demographics
- Age
  - 3-12 years
  - Median = 7 years
- Gender: M:F = 4-5:1

Natural History & Prognosis
- Leg length inequality
- Thigh atrophy
- Epiphyseal changes + metaphyseal changes associated with poor prognosis
- Younger age of presentation = better prognosis
- > 8 years old = poor prognosis
- Classification post skeletal maturity
  - Mose - evaluate shape of femoral head
  - Stulberg - predicts long-term performance
  - Coxa plana, coxa magna
  - Arthritis = patients with Mose "fair" to "poor" outcomes
    - Defined by a 2 mm or > deviation of spherical femoral head compared to a circular template
  - > 20% epiphyseal extrusion or > 50% femoral head involvement = poor prognosis

Treatment
- Conservative
  - 50% improve with no treatment
  - Bed rest + abduction stretching & bracing
- Surgical
  - Femoral/pelvic osteotomies to contain hip

DIAGNOSTIC CHECKLIST

Consider
- Use coronal T1WI to detect subtle peripheral or linear areas of epiphyseal marrow hypointensity

SELECTED REFERENCES

1. Fitzgerald RH et al: Orthopaedics. Legg-Calvé-Perthes. St. Louis MO, Mosby, Sect 9 (9-19):1420-32, 2002
2. Cho TJ et al: Femoral head deformity in Catterall groups III and IV Legg-Calve-Perthes disease: Magnetic resonance imaging analysis in coronal and sagittal planes. J Pediatr Orthop 22(5):601-6, 2002
3. De Sanctis N et al: Prognostic evaluation of Legg-Calve-Perthes disease by MRI. Part I: The role of physeal involvement. J Pediatr Orthop 20(4):455-62, 2000
4. De Sanctis N et al: Legg-Calve-Perthes disease by MRI. Part II: Pathomorphologenesis and new classification. J Pediatr Orthop 20(4):463-70, 2000
5. Gabriel H et al: MR imaging of hip disorders. Radiographics 14:763-81, 1994
6. Bos CFA et al: Sequential magnetic resonance imaging in Perthes' disease. J Bone Joint Surg 73:219-24, 1991
7. Egund N et al: Legg-Calve-Perthes disease: Imaging with MR. Radiology 179:89-93, 1991
8. Rush BH et al: Legg-Calve-Perthes disease: Detection of cartilaginous and synovial changes with MR imaging. Radiology 167:473-6, 1988
9. Thompson GH et al: Legg-Calve-Perthes disease: Current concepts and controversies. Orthop Clin North Am 18:617, 1987
10. Toby EB et al: Magnetic resonance imaging of pediatric hip disorders. J Pediatr Orthop 5:665-71, 1985

IMAGE GALLERY

Typical

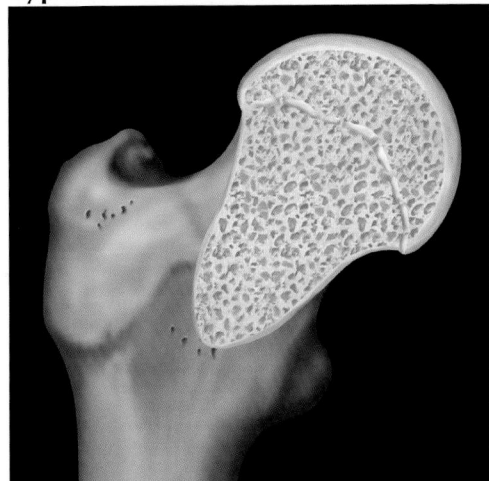 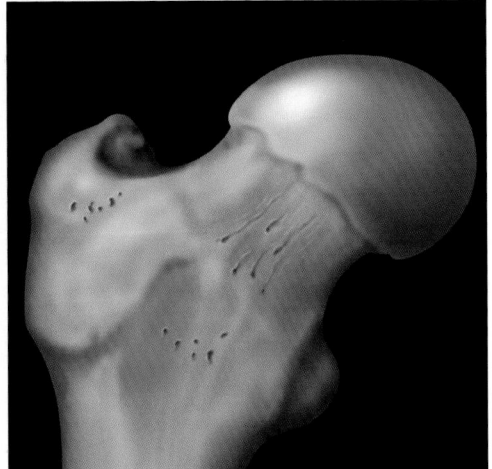

(Left) Coronal graphic shows ischemic injury to the physis leading to disorganization and bridging of the cartilage. *(Right)* Coronal graphic shows abnormal growth of the proximal femur as a late change of Legg-Calvé-Perthes (coxa magna, coxa plana).

Typical

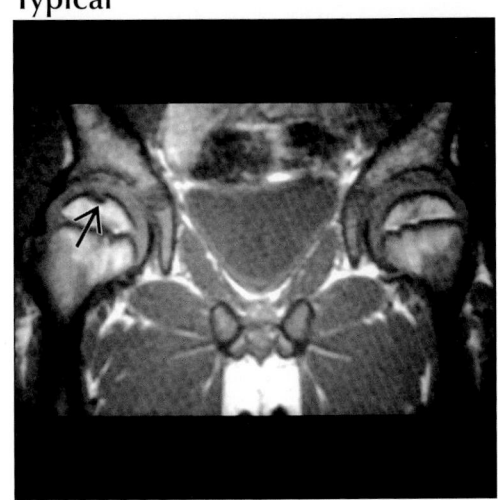 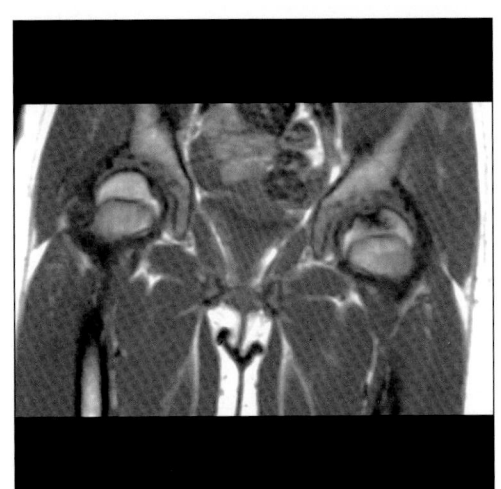

(Left) Coronal T1WI MR shows early Legg-Calvé-Perthes with hypointense ischemic change in the superior aspect of the right capital epiphysis (arrow). Bilateral physeal irregularity is present. *(Right)* Coronal T1WI MR shows left Legg-Calvé-Perthes with subchondral collapse associated with DDH.

Typical

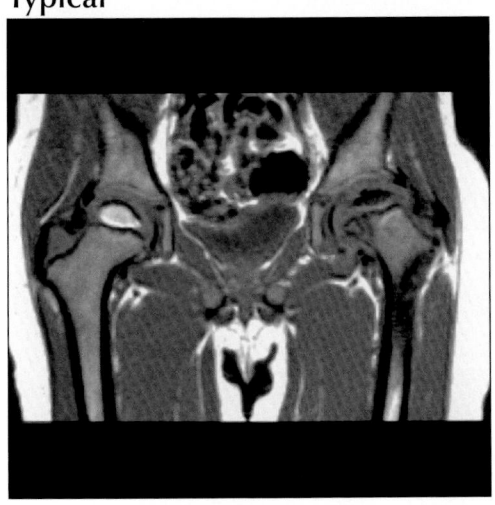 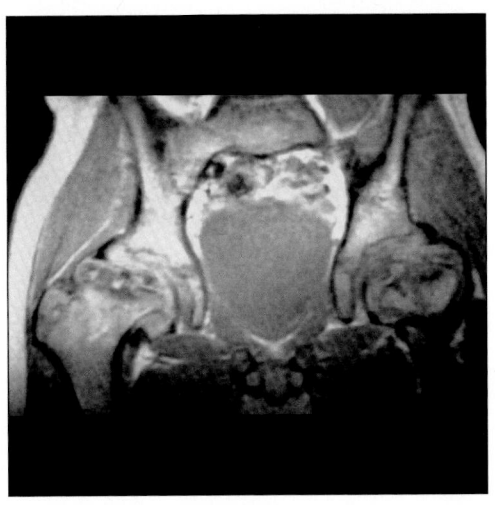

(Left) Coronal T1WI MR shows left ischemic capital epiphysis and medial metaphyseal sclerosis/cystic change. *(Right)* Coronal T1WI MR shows bilateral advanced remodeling with coxa plana and coxa magna deformity of the femoral heads.

TRANSIENT OSTEOPOROSIS OF THE HIP

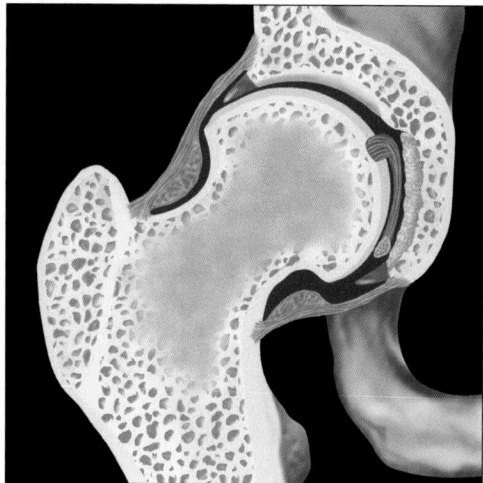

Coronal graphic shows transient osteoporosis of the hip with diffuse extension of marrow edema into the femoral head and neck.

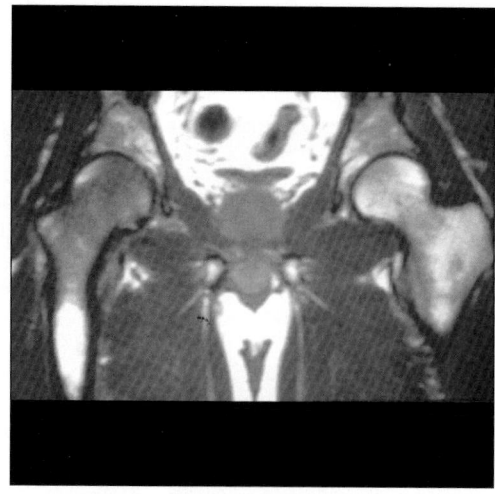

Coronal T1WI MR shows hypointense marrow edema involving right femoral head, neck and distal intertrochanteric region with partial sparing of the greater trochanter and lateral femoral head.

TERMINOLOGY

Abbreviations and Synonyms
- TOH, transient osteoporosis, transient osteonecrosis, algodystrophy

Definitions
- Self-limited diffuse bone marrow edema of femoral head and neck

IMAGING FINDINGS

General Features
- Best diagnostic clue: Hyperintense marrow signal in femoral head + neck on T2WI
- Location: Femoral head + extension to femoral neck
- Size: Diffuse involvement of majority of femoral head + variable extension into neck to intertrochanteric region
- Morphology
  - Variable within confines of femoral head + neck
    - Homogeneous
    - Partial marrow sparing may exist (greater trochanter)

Radiographic Findings
- Radiography
  - Initial radiographs = normal first few days
  - Osteopenia with decreased bone density = radiolucency + indistinct trabeculae + cortex
  - Osteopenia may be diffuse vs. patchy ± band-like
  - Demineralization of subchondral plate
  - Preservation of joint space
  - Remineralization within 10 months

CT Findings
- NECT
  - Decreased bone density with intact trabeculae
  - Attenuated subchondral plate
  - Normal joint space - view on coronal reformations

MR Findings
- T1WI
  - Hypointensity (large areas or diffusely) within femoral head, neck ± intertrochanteric region ± acetabulum
  - Edema pattern homogenous + well-marginated
  - ± Hypointense joint effusion
  - May see marrow sparing in medial + lateral-most margins of femoral head + greater trochanter 2° to greater concentration of fat marrow
  - Resolution associated with web-like or reticular areas of hypointensity
- T2WI
  - Hyperintensity femoral head + neck
  - Hyperintensity most conspicuous on T2 fat-suppression or STIR techniques

DDx: Transient Osteoporosis of the Hip

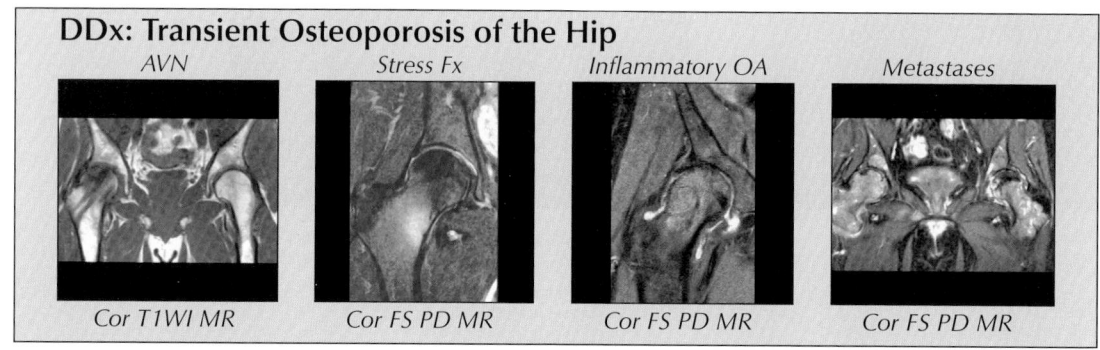

AVN	Stress Fx	Inflammatory OA	Metastases
Cor T1WI MR	Cor FS PD MR	Cor FS PD MR	Cor FS PD MR

TRANSIENT OSTEOPOROSIS OF THE HIP

Key Facts

Imaging Findings

- Best diagnostic clue: Hyperintense marrow signal in femoral head + neck on T2WI
- Size: Diffuse involvement of majority of femoral head + variable extension into neck to intertrochanteric region
- Hyperintensity most conspicuous on T2 fat-suppression or STIR techniques
- Contrast enhancement prominent

Top Differential Diagnoses

- Osteonecrosis
- Stress Fracture
- Inflammatory Osteoarthritis (OA)
- Osseous Contusion
- Osteomyelitis
- Infiltrative Neoplasm

Pathology

- Self-limited + unknown etiology
- Healthy middle-aged men affected
- Elevation of pressure within bone marrow
- Hydroxyapatite shift - reduced mineral content

Clinical Issues

- Most common signs/symptoms: Progressive hip pain
- Resolution of symptoms 6 to 10 months post onset
- Age: Third + fourth decades most common

Diagnostic Checklist

- Small FOV T1 + FS PD FSE to document marrow edema in the absence of a subchondral fracture

---

- ○ MR sensitive to marrow edema within 48 hours of onset of clinical symptoms
- ○ Less common association of acetabular hyperintensity
- ○ Hyperintensity may spare marrow within anterior, posterior, medial or lateral aspect femoral head
- ○ Marrow hyperintensity may show variability of anatomic distribution on sequential studies
- ○ Edema interface well-defined without a demarcating hypointense line or band (no double-line sign)
- ○ Normal cortex + subchondral plate
- ○ Normal adjacent soft tissues
- ○ Small to moderate hyperintense joint effusion
- T1 C+
  - ○ Contrast enhancement prominent
  - ○ Heterogenous

Imaging Recommendations

- Best imaging tool: MR sensitive + specific for bone marrow edema (sensitive to influx of free water)
- Protocol advice
  - ○ T1 (not PD) to show hypointense marrow edema in contrast to normal marrow fat signal
  - ○ Coronal FS PD FSE or STIR required (axial + sagittal are secondary planes of choice)

DIFFERENTIAL DIAGNOSIS

Osteonecrosis

- Early phase with subtle subchondral hypointense fracture on high resolution images + hyperintense marrow edema pattern on T2WI

Stress Fracture

- Hyperintense (T2WI) marrow centered within calcar
- Hypointense fracture line or medial cortical thickening of femoral neck

Inflammatory Osteoarthritis (OA)

- Synovitis + effusion
  - ○ Intermediate to hyperintense on T2WI
- Joint space narrowing, sclerosis + osteophytes

Osseous Contusion

- Femoral head ± neck marrow edema hypointense on T1 + hyperintense on T2WI without stress fracture
- +/- Trauma history

Osteomyelitis

- Hyperintense marrow edema adjacent to hyperintense soft tissue edema ± fluid + sinus tract
- +/- Suggestive clinical/laboratory findings

Infiltrative Neoplasm

- Replacement of normal trabecula ± aggressive features of cortical destruction + soft tissue extension

Normal Weight-Bearing Trabeculae

- Forms boundaries of Ward's triangle
- Band-like areas of hypointensity on T1WI
- No increased signal intensity on T2WI

Regional Migratory Osteoporosis

- Multiple anatomic sites involved sequentially - typically foot, knee, or hip
- Middle-aged men
- Localized pain + swelling in one joint
- Resolution < 12 months
- Large joints lower extremity
- Recovery associated with development of new site either ipsilateral or contralateral in location
- Synchronous involvement unusual
- May be closely related to TOH

Transient Bone Marrow Edema Syndrome

- Normal radiographic findings (no osteopenia)
- MR finding identical to transient osteoporosis of the hip
- May represent an earlier stage of TOH

Reflex Sympathetic Dystrophy

- More patchy + subarticular signal changes
- Prolonged clinical course
- Favors lower extremity joints other than hip

TRANSIENT OSTEOPOROSIS OF THE HIP

PATHOLOGY

General Features
- General path comments
  - Relevant anatomy
    - Femoral head = multiaxial, synovial ball-and-socket joint
    - Acetabulum = 40% bony coverage of femoral head
    - Femoral head forms two-thirds of a sphere with proximal transition into the femoral neck
    - Calcar femorale = weight-bearing bone in femur from inferomedial femoral neck cortex to lesser trochanter
    - Weight-bearing stress trabeculae - form the boundaries of Ward's triangle in femoral neck + head
    - 95% of femoral neck = intracapsular
- Etiology
  - Self-limited + unknown etiology
  - Women in third trimester (original description) with predilection for left hip
  - Healthy middle-aged men affected
  - Progressive demineralization
- Epidemiology: May represent an early stage of osteonecrosis

Gross Pathologic & Surgical Features
- Elevation of pressure within bone marrow
- Normal appearance of articular cartilage, cortex & subchondral bone
- Small joint effusion
- Synovial inflammation

Microscopic Features
- ± Necrotic fat cells
- Fibrovascular regenerative tissue
- Increased osteoid
- Edema: Difficult to document increased free water on histologic study
- Hydroxyapatite shift - reduced mineral content

CLINICAL ISSUES

Presentation
- Most common signs/symptoms: Progressive hip pain
- Clinical profile
  - Acute onset
  - Groin pain
  - Pain exacerbated by weight-bearing
  - Decreased range of motion + limp
  - Absence of infection or trauma
  - Involvement of one joint
  - Resolution of symptoms 6 to 10 months post onset

Demographics
- Age: Third + fourth decades most common
- Gender
  - More common in males
  - Also reported in pregnant women in third trimester

Natural History & Prognosis
- Self-limited

- Resolution of symptoms + radiographic + MR findings < 10 months
- Decreased joint effusion with resolution of symptoms
- No double-line sign develops

Treatment
- Conservative = clinical observation
  - Serial MR to document resolution
- Surgical
  - Core decompression - may produce rapid decrease in pain + shortened resolution time

DIAGNOSTIC CHECKLIST

Consider
- Small FOV T1 + FS PD FSE to document marrow edema in the absence of a subchondral fracture

SELECTED REFERENCES

1. Koo KH et al: Increased perfusion of the femoral head in transient bone marrow edema syndrome. Clin Orthop 402:171-5, 2002
2. Papadopoulos EC et al: Bone marrow edema syndrome. Orthopedics 24(1):69-73 Review, 2001
3. Bohndorf K et al: Musculoskeletal imaging: A concise multimodality approach. Germany, Thieme, 230-1, 2001
4. Kim YM et al: The pattern of bone marrow oedema on MRI in osteonecrosis of the femoral head. J Bone Joint Surg Br 82(6):837-41, 2000
5. Calvo E et al: Core decompression shortens the duration of pain in bone marrow oedema syndrome. Int Orthop 24(2):88-91, 2000
6. Koo KH et al: Borderline necrosis of the femoral head. Clin Orthop 358:158-65, 1999
7. Deutsch A et al: MRI of the musculoskeletal system: A teaching file. 2nd ed. Philadelphia PA, Lippincott Williams & Wilkins, (4):197-272, 1997
8. Doury P: Bone-marrow oedema, transient osteoporosis, and algodystrophy. J Bone Joint Surg Br 76:993, 1994
9. Richardson ML: Can MR imaging distinguishing transient osteoporosis of the femoral head and osteonecrosis? AJR 162:1244, 1994
10. Hayes CW et al: MR imaging of bone marrow edema pattern: Transient osteoporosis, transient bone marrow edema syndrome, or osteonecrosis. Radiographics 13:1001-11, 1993
11. Hofman S et al: Bone marrow oedema syndrome and transient osteoporosis of the hip: An MRI-controlled study of treatment by core decompression. J Bone Joint Surg Br 75:210, 1993
12. Potter H et al: Magnetic resonance imaging in diagnosis of transient osteoporosis of the hip. Clin Orthop 280:233-9, 1992
13. Schapira D: Transient osteoporosis of the hip. Semin Arthritis Rheum 22:98-105, 1992
14. Daniel WW et al: The early diagnosis of transient osteoporosis by magnetic resonance imaging. J Bone Joint Surg 74:1262-4, 1992
15. Hauzeur J et al: Study of magnetic resonance imaging in transient osteoporosis of the hip. J Rheumatol 18:1211-7, 1991
16. Wilson AJ et al: Transient osteoporosis: Transient bone marrow edema? Radiology 167:757, 1988
17. Curtiss PH Jr et al: Transient demineralization of the hip in pregnancy: A report of three cases. J Bone Joint Surg AM 41:1327, 1959

TRANSIENT OSTEOPOROSIS OF THE HIP

IMAGE GALLERY

Typical

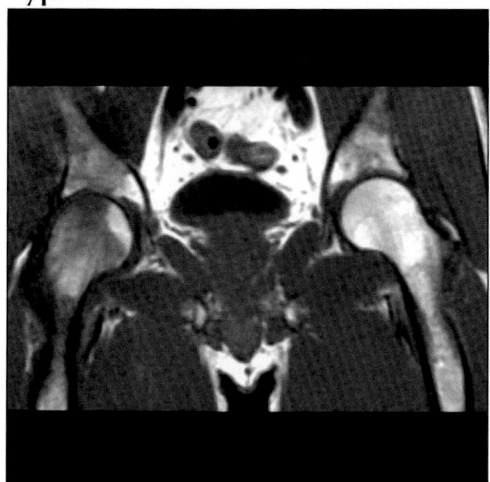
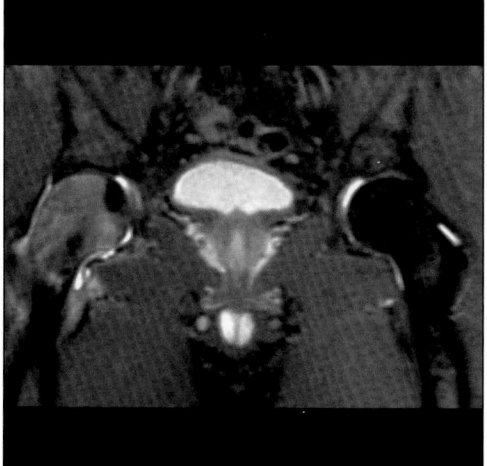

(Left) Coronal T1WI MR shows homogeneously hypointense marrow with medial sparing of the right femoral head. *(Right)* Coronal FS PD FSE MR shows uniform hyperintensity with associated joint effusion on the right. No ischemic focus is identified in TOH.

Variant

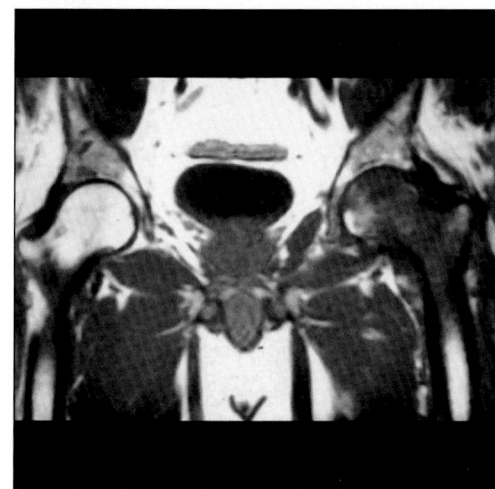
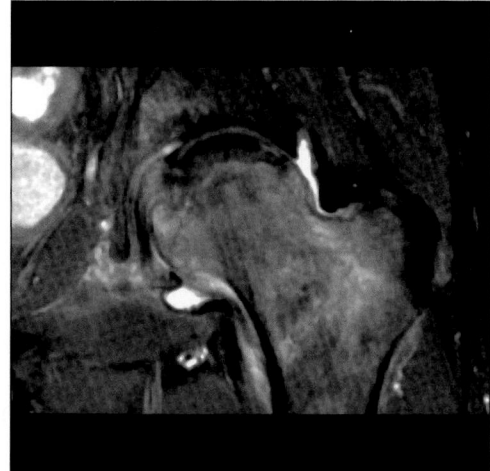

(Left) Coronal T1WI MR shows extended marrow edema pattern distal to the intertrochanteric area on the left. Note partial marrow sparing in the greater trochanter and medial femoral head (TOH). *(Right)* Coronal FS PD FSE MR shows hyperintense marrow edema of the acetabulum and femoral head/neck associated with early ischemic change mimicking TOH.

Variant

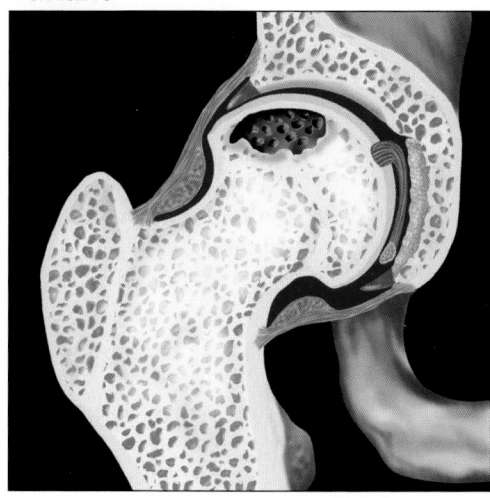
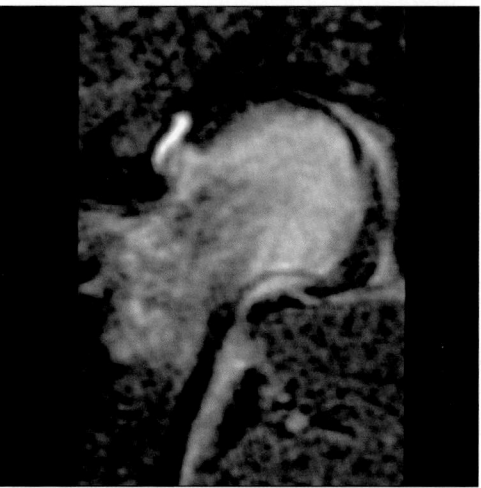

(Left) Coronal graphic shows extended marrow edema pattern of AVN simulating the changes of TOH. *(Right)* Coronal FS PD FSE MR shows hyperintense marrow edema associated with early femoral head ischemia. High resolution images are required to identify the AVN focus or subchondral fracture in early osteonecrosis.

DEVELOPMENTAL DYSPLASIA OF THE HIP

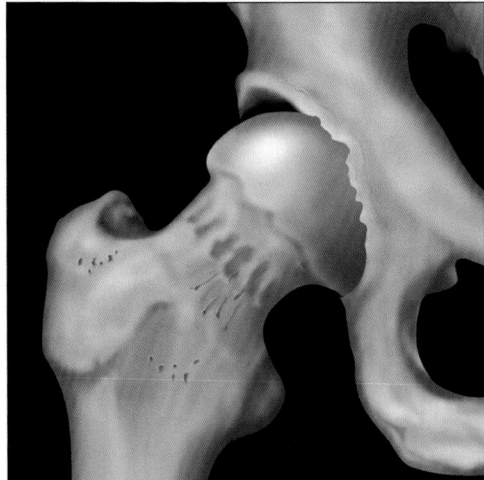

Coronal graphic shows shallow acetabulum characteristic of DDH.

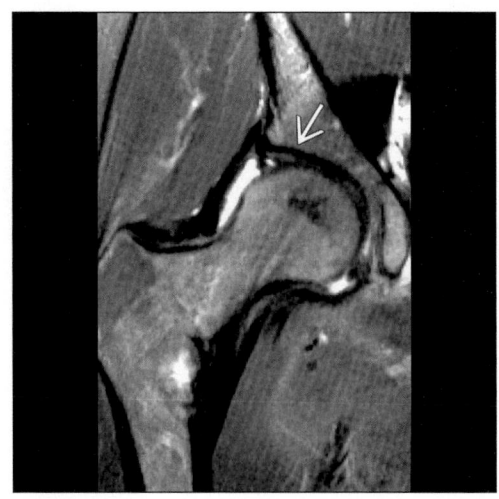

Coronal FS PD FSE MR shows shallow acetabulum (arrow) in an adult associated with an acetabular labral tear. Adult DDH is best identified on anterior coronal images.

TERMINOLOGY

Abbreviations and Synonyms
- Developmental dysplasia of the hip (DDH), congenital dysplasia of the hip (CDH), congenital hip dysplasia

Definitions
- Shallow (dysplastic) acetabular fossa ± superolateral migration of the femoral head

IMAGING FINDINGS

General Features
- Best diagnostic clue: Shallow acetabulum + subluxation of the femoral head
- Location
  - Left hip involvement: Up to 60%
  - Bilateral involvement: 20%
- Size: Subluxation to complete dislocation of femoral head
- Morphology: Shallow to false acetabulum in complete dislocation + acetabular labral deformity

Radiographic Findings
- Radiography
  - False negative diagnosis < six months
  - Femoral capital epiphysis in inner lower quadrant
  - Hilgenreiner's line through triradiate cartilage
  - Perkin's line (perpendicular to Hilgenreiner's) through lateral acetabular rim
  - Lateral subluxation of capital epiphysis = 2 mm or > from teardrop to metaphysis
  - Superior subluxation - delta of 2 mm or > from Hilgenreiner's line to metaphysis compared with normal side
  - Disruption of Shenton's curved line: Formed by inferior aspect of superior pubic ramus
  - Center edge angle < 25°: Associated with instability
  - Secondary signs
    - Excessive femoral head anteversion
    - Delayed ossification of femoral capital epiphysis

CT Findings
- NECT
  - Use coronal + axial CT images or reformations
  - Sector angle for acetabular coverage (capital epiphysis to acetabular rim relative to the horizontal axis)

MR Findings
- T1WI
  - Epiphyseal articular cartilage - intermediate signal (T1WI)
  - Coronal + axial planes to identify position of capital epiphysis
  - Can visualize ossific nucleus (hypoplastic) when not visible on conventional radiographs or CT

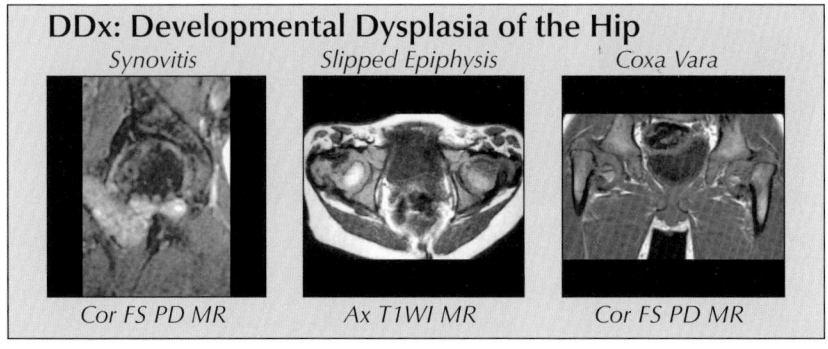

DDx: Developmental Dysplasia of the Hip

Synovitis	Slipped Epiphysis	Coxa Vara
Cor FS PD MR	Ax T1WI MR	Cor FS PD MR

DEVELOPMENTAL DYSPLASIA OF THE HIP

Key Facts

Imaging Findings
- Best diagnostic clue: Shallow acetabulum + subluxation of the femoral head
- Epiphyseal articular cartilage - intermediate signal (T1WI)

Top Differential Diagnoses
- Synovitis
- Septic Arthritis
- Slipped Capital Femoral Epiphysis
- Congenital Coxa Vara

Pathology
- First 6 postnatal weeks - acetabulum susceptible to remodeling
- Hourglass joint capsule: Compression between limbus + ligamentum teres

- Deficient superior + posterior acetabular rim

Clinical Issues
- Most common signs/symptoms: Palpable click or clunk using Ortolani & Barlow stress maneuvers
- Age: Newborns
- Gender: F:M = 6:1
- Positive family history, breech presentation, torticollis, scoliosis + metatarsus adductus
- Decreased range of motion
- Degenerative changes

Diagnostic Checklist
- Anterior coronal images to identify dysplastic acetabulum in adult

---

- ○ Hypointense joint effusions
- ○ Superolateral dislocation - use coronal plane
- ○ Anteroposterior (AP) relationship + dysplasia of acetabulum - use axial images
- ○ Mild acetabular dysplasia shown on anterior coronal images
- ○ Pulvinar - hyperintense signal of fat
- T2WI
  - ○ Epiphyseal articular cartilage intermediate on FS PD FSE
  - ○ Effusions hyperintense on T2WI
  - ○ Failure to reduce dislocated hip
    - Hourglass acetabulum, hypointense inverted labrum
    - Hypointense interposed iliopsoas tendon (seen on coronal, axial + sagittal images)
    - Direct visualization of fat suppressed pulvinar fibrofatty tissue
    - Hypertrophy of hypointense ligamentum teres
    - Acetabular labral coverage lateral to dysplastic acetabulum visualized on coronal images
    - Deformed labral limbus = horizontal slope vs. normal downward lateral slope
    - Inverted limbus of acetabular roof = inferomedial displacement with long axis superoinferior orientation on coronal images
  - ○ Serial follow-up studies for position of femoral head + acetabular morphology + labral coverage
  - ○ Acetabular index calculation from coronal MR (Hilgenreiner's line through triradiate cartilage + tangent through acetabular roof: > 30°)
- T2* GRE: Epiphyseal articular cartilage: Hyperintense
- Associated ischemic necrosis hypointense on T1WI + T2WI

Ultrasonographic Findings
- Up to 6 months: Application of ultrasound
- Visualized iliac bone, acetabulum, labrum, + femoral capital epiphysis
- Evaluate subluxation, dislocation, pulvinar, inverted labrum, hypoplastic ossific nucleus, acetabular dysplasia + ossification

Imaging Recommendations
- Best imaging tool
  - ○ Ultrasound dynamic exam diagnostic up to 6 months but operator dependent
  - ○ MR: Best visualization of deformed or inverted labrum + cartilaginous components of acetabular roof + capital epiphysis
- Protocol advice: T1, FS PD FSE + T2* gradient echo coronal images to identify acetabular concavity, decentralized femoral head + deformed/inverted labrum

DIFFERENTIAL DIAGNOSIS

Synovitis
- Intermediate signal synovium
- Hyperintense fluid + capsular distension on T2WI

Septic Arthritis
- Nonuniform hyperintense fluid on T2WI
- Reactive marrow edema + soft tissue edema
- Clinical signs of infection

Slipped Capital Femoral Epiphysis
- Posterior-inferior displacement of proximal femoral epiphysis
- Vertical growth plate + retroversion femoral neck
- Capital epiphysis retains acetabular coverage

Congenital Coxa Vara
- Decrease of femoral neck/shaft angle (< 120°)
- Limb bud insult

Hip Dislocations
- Post-traumatic with joint hemorrhage, osseous contusions + acetabular column fracture

Proximal Focal Femoral Deficiency
- Congenital hypoplasia or aplasia of proximal femur
- Acetabular dysplasia

DEVELOPMENTAL DYSPLASIA OF THE HIP

PATHOLOGY

General Features
- General path comments
  - Relevant anatomy
    - Triradiate or Y cartilage: Center of acetabulum - separates the ilium, ischium + pubis
- Genetics
  - Multifactorial
  - Increased joint laxity = dominant pattern
  - Acetabular dysplasia = polygenic
- Etiology
  - Laxity of joint capsule ligaments
  - Mechanical versus physiologic (elevated maternal estrogen levels)
  - First 6 postnatal weeks - acetabulum susceptible to remodeling
  - Inadequate contact between acetabulum + femoral head
- Epidemiology: Incidence: 1.5% of neonates

Gross Pathologic & Surgical Features
- Hourglass joint capsule: Compression between limbus + ligamentum teres
- Thick + tight transverse ligament
- Femoral head flattened medially
- Deficient superior + posterior acetabular rim

Microscopic Features
- Hyperplastic ligamentum teres
- Hypertrophic pulvinar

Staging, Grading or Classification Criteria
- Modified Graf staging
  - Type 1 = mature hip - alpha (acetabular roof) angle > 60° (alpha is geometric complement of acetabular index angle)
  - Type 2a = physiologic immaturity < 3 months with alpha 50-59°
  - Type 2b = immature > 3 months with alpha 50-59°
  - Type 2c = critical hip, subluxation - alpha 43-49°
  - Type 3 = eccentric head, dislocation - alpha < 43°
  - Type 4 = severe dysplasia, inverted labrum, alpha < 43°

CLINICAL ISSUES

Presentation
- Most common signs/symptoms: Palpable click or clunk using Ortolani & Barlow stress maneuvers
- Clinical profile
  - Ortolani's test: Hip abduction at 90° flexion + anteriorly directed pressure relocates femoral head
  - Barlow's test: Unstable femoral had dislocated by posteriorly directed pressure

Demographics
- Age: Newborns
- Gender: F:M = 6:1
- Risk factors
  - Positive family history, breech presentation, torticollis, scoliosis + metatarsus adductus

Natural History & Prognosis
- Limb shortening
- Decreased range of motion
- Degenerative changes
- Avascular necrosis
- Prognosis
  - Delayed diagnosis/treatment = irreversible dysplasia
  - Early diagnosis = good result with harness or splint

Treatment
- Conservative
  - Closed reduction + harness/spica cast
- Surgical
  - Adductor tenotomy + release of iliopsoas
  - Open reduction
  - Varus (derotational) vs. reconstructive osteotomy (Salter opening wedge, triple innominate, Chiari-medialization of femoral head)

DIAGNOSTIC CHECKLIST

Consider
- T2* gradient echo coronal images defines hypointense deformed limbus + displays articular cartilage as hyperintense
- Anterior coronal images to identify dysplastic acetabulum in adult

SELECTED REFERENCES

1. Murray KA et al: Radiographic imaging for treatment and follow-up of developmental dysplasia of the hip. Semin Ultrasound CT MR 22(4):306-40, 2001
2. Laor T et al: Limited magnetic resonance imaging examination after surgical reduction of developmental dysplasia of the hip. J Pediatr Orthop 20(5):572-4, 2000
3. Bassett GS et al: Fate of the psoas muscle after open reduction for developmental dislocation of the hip (DDH). J Pediatr Orthop 19(4):425-32, 1999
4. McNally EG et al: MRI after operative reduction for developmental dysplasia of the hip. J Bone Joint Surg Br 79(5):724-6, 1997
5. Gabriel H et al: MR imaging of hip disorders. Radiographics 14:763-81, 1994
6. Guidera KJ et al: Magnetic resonance imaging evaluation of congenital dislocation of the hips. Clin Orthop 261:96-101, 1990
7. Harcke HT et al: Preforming dynamic sonography of the infant hip. AJR 155:837-44, 1990
8. Johnson DN et al: MR imaging anatomy of the infant hip. AJR 153:127-33, 1989
9. Johnson ND et al: Complex infantile and congenital hip dislocation: Assessment with MR imaging. Radiology 168:151-6, 1988
10. Hensinger RN: Congenital dislocation of the hip: Treatment in infancy to walking age. Orthop Clin North Am 18:597, 1987

DEVELOPMENTAL DYSPLASIA OF THE HIP

Typical

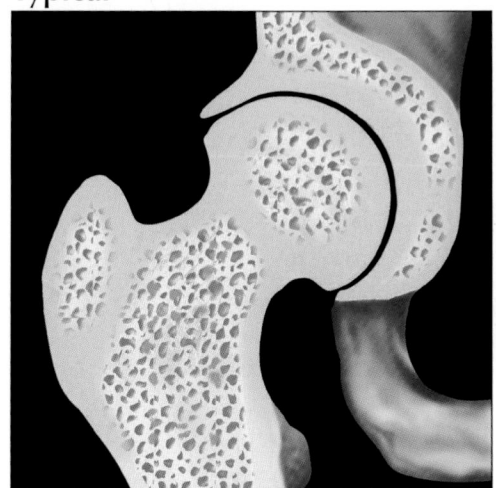

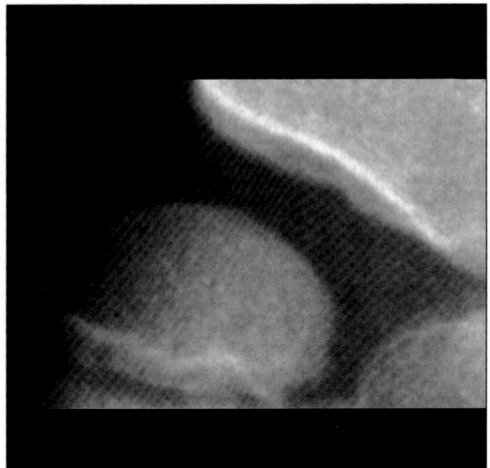

(Left) Coronal graphic shows normal acetabular and labral coverage of the femoral head in a non dysplastic hip. *(Right)* Anteroposterior radiography shows uncovered capital epiphysis with shallow acetabulum in DDH.

Typical

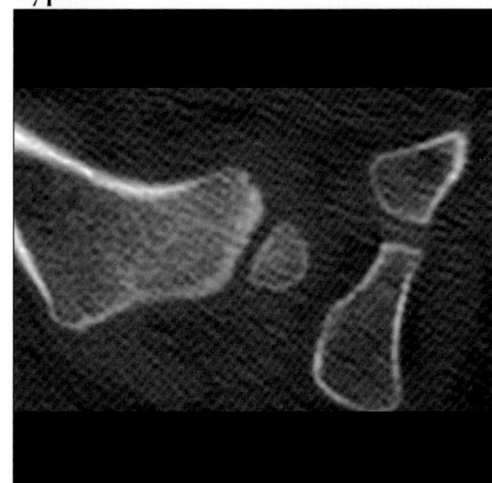

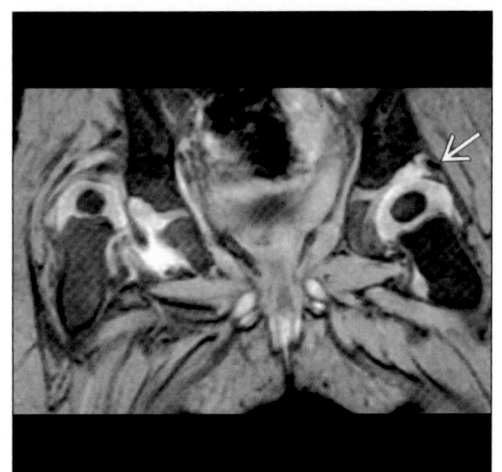

(Left) Axial NECT fails to show the superolateral position of the capital epiphysis. There is posterior subluxation of the capital epiphysis. *(Right)* Coronal T2* GRE MR shows superolateral dislocation of the right capital epiphysis with a false acetabulum and acetabular labral deformity (arrow). The left acetabulum is shallow.

Typical

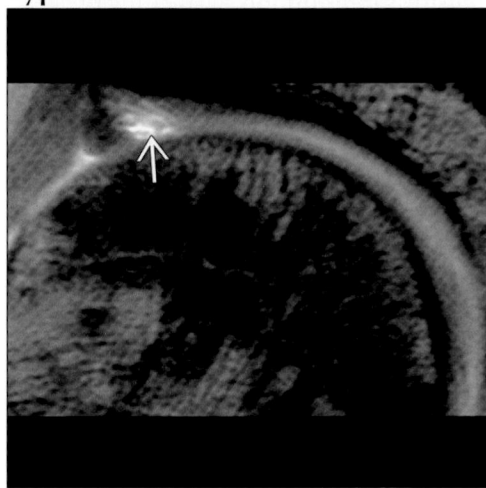

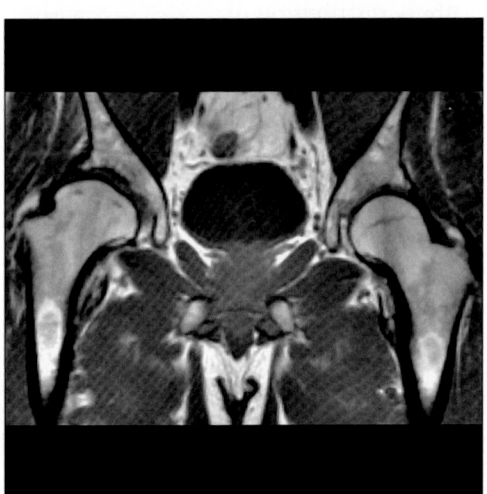

(Left) Coronal FS PD FSE MR shows chondral degeneration (arrow) as an early sign of osteoarthritis or lateral acetabular rim syndrome. Lateral acetabular rim syndrome in DDH is equivalent to femoroacetabular impingement in non dysplastic hips. *(Right)* Coronal T1WI MR shows remodeling of right femoral head and neck as a chronic complication of DDH.

MUSCLE STRAIN, HIP

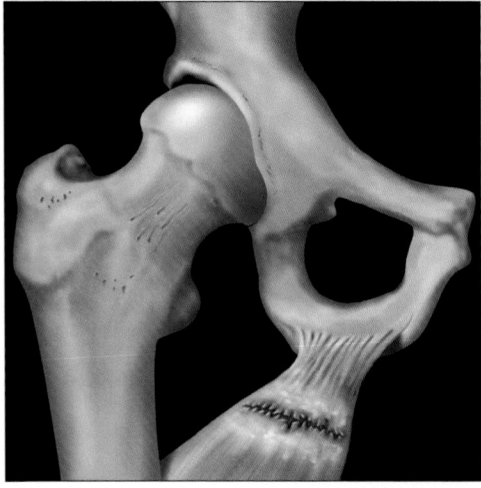

Coronal graphic shows partial tear of the adductor magnus muscle with associated edema.

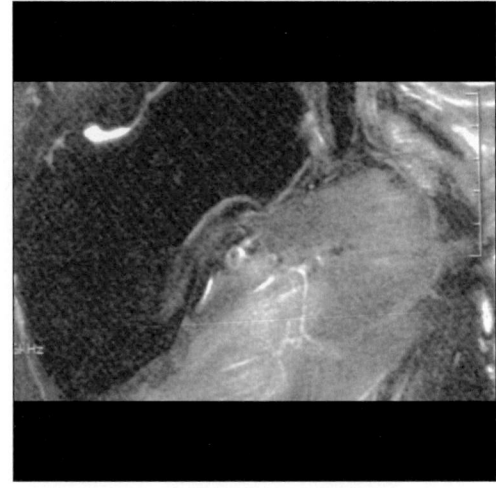

Coronal FS PD FSE MR shows adductor muscle group edema in grade I strain.

TERMINOLOGY

Abbreviations and Synonyms
- Muscle-tendon-unit (MTU) injuries, stretch-induced injuries, stretch injury, muscle ruptures

Definitions
- Stretch-induced injury to muscle fibers

IMAGING FINDINGS

General Features
- Best diagnostic clue: Hyperintense edema ± hemorrhage within affected muscle group on T2WI
- Location: Rectus femoris, hamstring, adductor longus + magnus involved
- Size: Variable with stretch-induced injuries involving distal junction of muscle-tendon-unit
- Morphology: Variable from feathery distribution of edema, to focal hemorrhage, to frank muscle disruption

MR Findings
- T1WI
  - No abnormality
  - Blurring of muscle fiber striations
  - Hypointense to hyperintense hemorrhagic fluid collection
  - Hypointense subcutaneous tissue edema
- T2WI
  - Grade I strain
    - Hyperintense edema ± hemorrhage with preservation of muscle morphology
    - Edema pattern = interstitial hyperintensity + feathery distribution on FS PD or T2 FSE + STIR images
    - Hyperintense subcutaneous tissue edema + intermuscular fluid
  - Grade II strain
    - Hyperintense hemorrhage with tearing of up to 50% of muscle fibers
    - Interstitial hyperintensity with focal hyperintensity representing hemorrhage in muscle belly ± intramuscular fluid
    - Hyperintense focal defect + partial retraction of muscle fibers
    - Associated myotendinous + tendinous injuries
    - Hyperintensity + interruption ± widening of muscle-tendon-unit
  - Grade III strain
    - Complete tearing ± muscle retraction
    - Hyperintense fluid filled gap = hyperintense on FS PD FSE + STIR
    - Associated adjacent hyperintense interstitial muscle changes

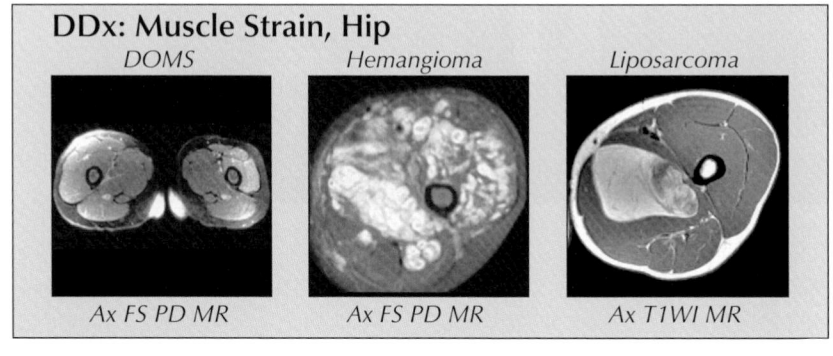

DDx: Muscle Strain, Hip

DOMS	Hemangioma	Liposarcoma
Ax FS PD MR	Ax FS PD MR	Ax T1WI MR

MUSCLE STRAIN, HIP

Key Facts

Imaging Findings
- Best diagnostic clue: Hyperintense edema ± hemorrhage within affected muscle group on T2WI
- Location: Rectus femoris, hamstring, adductor longus + magnus involved
- Morphology: Variable from feathery distribution of edema, to focal hemorrhage, to frank muscle disruption

Top Differential Diagnoses
- Delayed Onset Muscle Soreness (DOMS)
- Muscle Contusion
- Hemangioma
- Soft Tissue Tumor

Pathology
- Indirect injury secondary to excessive stretch

- Eccentric loading
- Muscles at risk cross multiple joints or have complex architecture

Clinical Issues
- Most common signs/symptoms: Muscle pain
- Weakness absent in primary (grade I) strain - no myofascial disruption
- Secondary strain: Weakness associated with separation of muscle from tendon or fascia
- Third-degree strain: Loss of function with complete myofascial separation
- Proximal hamstring injury most frequent site of involvement

Diagnostic Checklist
- Axial FS PD FSE or STIR to identify muscle edema

    ■ Retracted muscle fibers: Atrophy ± hypertrophic appearance 2° to retraction

Imaging Recommendations
- Best imaging tool: MR to document edema, hemorrhage + muscle/MTU tears
- Protocol advice
  ○ Axial FS PD, T2 FSE or STIR + T1
  ○ Coronal or sagittal FS PD FSE for longitudinal extent

DIFFERENTIAL DIAGNOSIS

Delayed Onset Muscle Soreness (DOMS)
- Non-acute injury
- Painful symptoms increase first 24 hours post exertion + peak 24 to 72 hours then subside
- Denervation - diffuse muscle group involvement + hyperintense signal on STIR or FS PD FSE
- Interstitial hemorrhage + hematoma
- Associated with muscle injury ± increased muscle size
- Grade I strain & DOMS = similar MR signal intensity changes

Muscle Contusion
- Compressive or concussive direct trauma
- Direct trauma - hematoma in blunt injuries + lacerations from penetrating injuries
- Fluid collections - swelling + weakness
- Muscle contracture + rhabdomyolysis
- Associated with metabolic disorders
- Muscle edema, atrophy + fatty infiltration = myopathic or neurogenic association

Infection
- Hyperintense/intermediate fluid on FS PD/T2 FSE or STIR images
- Focal involvement ± superficial tract
- Extensive subcutaneous tissue edema

Hemangioma
- Soft tissue intramuscular hemangioma
  ○ Non-circumscribed with predilection for thigh muscles of young adults

○ Pain = presenting symptom

Deep Venous Thrombosis
- Enlarged thrombosed popliteal vein
- Watershed hyperintensity in gastrocnemius/soleus muscle complex on T2WI
- Venous collateral development

Soft Tissue Tumor
- Lipoma
- Desmoid
- Malignant fibrous histiocytoma
- Liposarcoma
- Synovial sarcoma

PATHOLOGY

General Features
- General path comments
  ○ Relevant anatomy
    ■ Contractile element of muscle fibers = Z-lines
    ■ Muscle-tendon-unit - distal junction at risk
- Etiology
  ○ Indirect injury secondary to excessive stretch
  ○ Overuse - microtrauma
  ○ Muscle + myotendinous tears
  ○ Eccentric loading
  ○ Strains involve muscles with highest proportion of fast-twitch type II muscle fibers (e.g., rectus femoris, biceps femoris + medial head gastrocnemius)
  ○ Muscle-tendon-unit (MTU) = weakest biomechanical link → site of muscle failure
  ○ Muscles at risk cross multiple joints or have complex architecture
  ○ Risk factors include improper warm-up, fatigue, previous orthopedic injury
- Epidemiology: Muscle strains = 30% of sports-related injuries

Gross Pathologic & Surgical Features
- Irregular thinning myotendinous junction
- Hematoma
- Partial tear MTU

MUSCLE STRAIN, HIP

- Complete tear MTU
- Avulsion fracture

Microscopic Features
- Hemorrhagic response at injured fibers
- Muscle fiber necrosis
- Edema + macrophages
- Inflammatory cells + fibroblastic activity
- Random disruptions of Z-lines = damage to contractile elements of muscle

Staging, Grading or Classification Criteria
- Muscle strain
  - Grade I = minimal disruption musculotendinous junction
  - Grade II = partial tear with intact musculotendinous fibers present
  - Grade III = complete rupture of musculotendinous unit
  - Grade IIIB = avulsion fracture tendon origin or insertion

CLINICAL ISSUES

Presentation
- Most common signs/symptoms: Muscle pain
- Clinical profile
  - Weakness absent in primary (grade I) strain - no myofascial disruption
  - Edema + swelling
  - Secondary strain: Weakness associated with separation of muscle from tendon or fascia
  - Third-degree strain: Loss of function with complete myofascial separation
  - Proximal hamstring injury most frequent site of involvement

Demographics
- Age: Usually young athletes - speed athletes (especially sprinters), football, basketball, soccer
- Gender: Increased male incidence due to participation in sports requiring highly eccentric muscle activities

Natural History & Prognosis
- Incomplete to complete extension of injury
- Fibrous replacement
- Fatty replacement
- Muscle ossification
- Compartment syndrome
- Up to 25% recurrence rate for hamstring injuries

Treatment
- Conservative
  - Small fascial or tendinous tears
  - RICE protocol (rest, ice, compression, elevation)
  - Nonsteroidal antiinflammatory drugs
  - Protective exercises + passive stretching to prevent stiffness, atrophy, weakness
  - Isometric to isotonic exercises
  - Recovery period from two weeks (grade I) to > 2 months (grade II)
- Surgical
  - Rupture of muscle = possible surgical management

- Rupture of musculotendinous complex from origin or insertion
- Repair for avulsions with > 2 to 3 cm displacement of bone fragment
- Complications
  - Fibrosis + retraction of muscle
  - Reinjury
  - Myositis ossificans
  - Malunion or nonunion of osseous avulsions

DIAGNOSTIC CHECKLIST

Consider
- Axial FS PD FSE or STIR to identify muscle edema
- T1WI to visualize fatty atrophy
- Sagittal + coronal images to show longitudinal extent

SELECTED REFERENCES

1. DeLee JC et al: Orthopaedic sports medicine. Principles and practice. vol 2. 2nd ed. Philadelphia PA, WB Saunders, (26):1481-1504, 2003
2. Fitzgerald RH et al: Orthopaedics. St. Lois MO, Mosby, Sect 4(4-4):544-50, 2002
3. Sallay PI et al: Hamstring injuries among water skiers: Functional outcome and prevention. Am J Sports Med 24:130, 1996
4. Best T et al: Hamstring injuries: Expediting return to play. The Physician and Sportsmedicine 24:8, 1996
5. Clarkson PM et al: Associations between muscle soreness, damage and fatigue. Adv Exp Med Biol 384:457, 1995
6. Pomeranz SJ et al: MR imaging in the prognostication of hamstring injury. Radiology 189:897-900, 1993
7. Taylor DC et al: Experimental muscle strain injury: Early functional and structural deficits and the increased risk for reinjury. Am J Sports Med 21:190, 1993
8. Friden J et al: Structural and mechanical basis of exercise-induced muscle injury. Med Sci Sports Exerc 24:521, 1992
9. Taylor DC et al: Viscoelastic properties of muscle-tendon untis: The biomechanical effects of stretching. Am J Sports Med 18:300, 1990
10. DeSmet AA et al: Magnetic resonance imaging of muscle tears. Skel Radiol 19:283-6, 1990
11. Garrett WE JR: Muscle strain injuries: Clinical and basic aspects. Med Sci Sports Exerc 22:436, 1990
12. Garrett WE et al: Computed tomography of hamstring muscle strains. Med Sci Sports Exerc 21(5):506-14, 1989
13. Fleckenstein JL et al: Sports-related muscle injuries: evaluation with MR imaging. Radiology 172:793-8, 1989
14. Stauber WT: Eccentric action of muscles: Physiology, injury and adaptation. Exerc Sports Sci Rev 17:157, 1989
15. Garrett WE JR et al: Biomechanics of muscle tears and stretching injuries. Trans Orthop Res Soc 9:384, 1984
16. Zarins B et al: Acute muscle and tendon injuries in athletes. Clin Sports Med 2(1):167-82, 1983
17. Glick JM: Muscle strains: Prevention and treatment. Phys Sports Med 8:73, 1980

MUSCLE STRAIN, HIP

IMAGE GALLERY

Typical

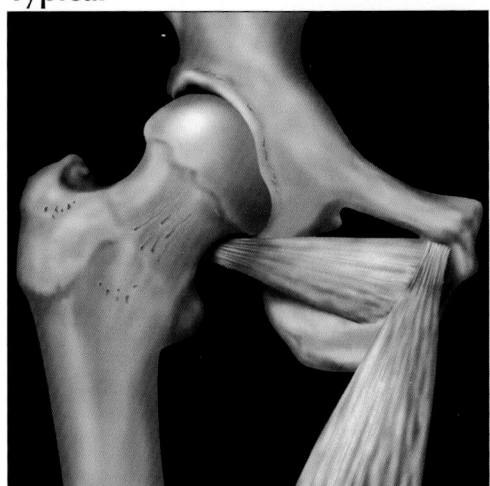

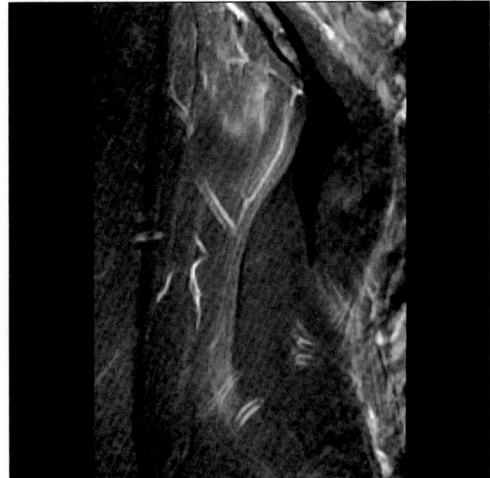

(Left) Coronal graphic shows grade I muscle strain with edema of the obturator externus (horizontally oriented) and adductor longus muscle (vertically oriented). Interstitial hyperintensity without muscle fiber discontinuity is shown. *(Right)* Coronal FS PD FSE MR shows interstitial muscle edema in a grade I muscle strain of proximal rectus femoris. The straight head originates from anterior inferior iliac spine and reflected head originates from upper acetabular rim.

Typical

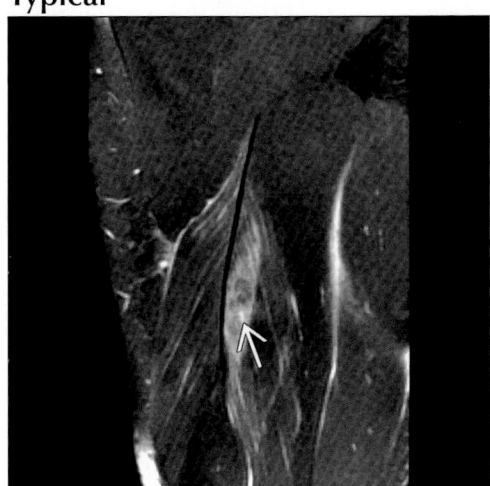

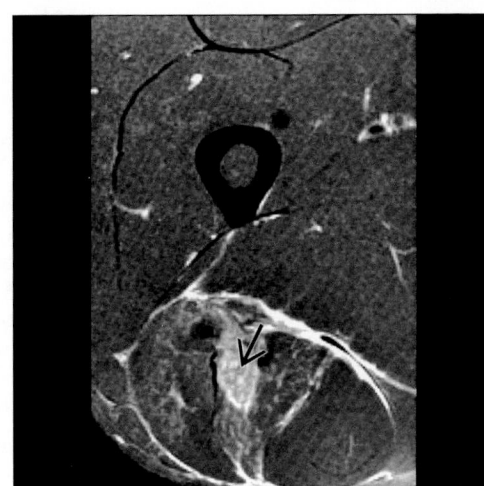

(Left) Coronal FS PD FSE MR shows focal hemorrhage (arrow) in a grade II strain of the biceps femoris muscle. Adjacent areas of grade I strain are seen with feathery distribution of edema. *(Right)* Axial FS PD FSE MR shows partial muscle tearing of the biceps femoris (arrow) at the myotendinous junction.

Typical

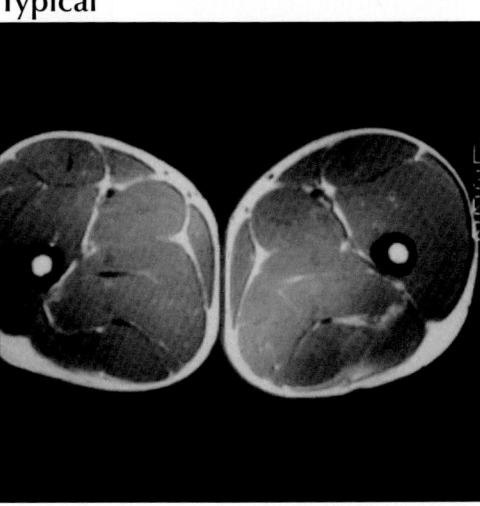

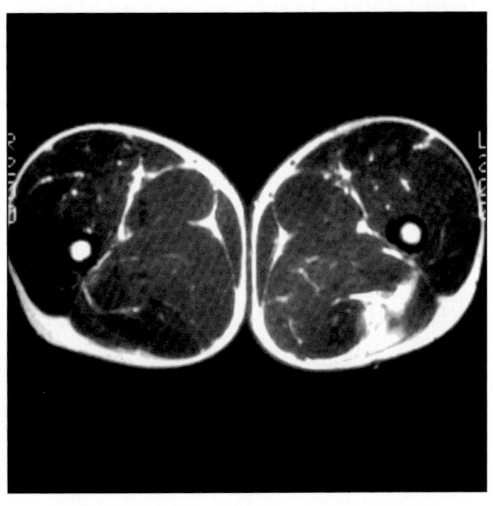

(Left) Axial PD/Intermediate MR shows grade I muscle strain of the left semitendinosus and medial aspect of the biceps femoris muscle in an olympic sprinter. There is normal muscle morphology. *(Right)* Axial T2WI MR shows hyperintense edema and muscle hemorrhage of left semitendinosus and medial biceps femoris muscle. The biceps femoris muscle is at risk for strain because of a higher proportion of fast-twitch muscle fibers.

4

21

RECTUS FEMORIS MUSCLE STRAIN

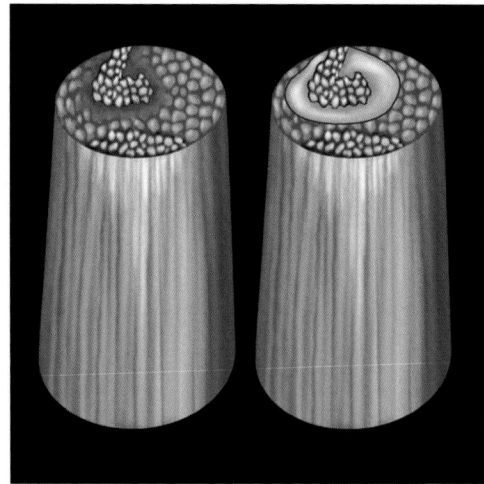

Axial graphic shows acute muscle strain involving deep tendon of the indirect head with surrounding hemorrhage in red. Chronic fibrous encasement and fluid are shown in blue.

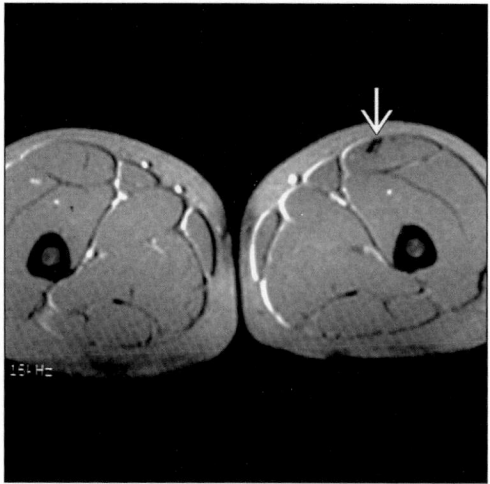

Axial T2* GRE MR shows focal hypointensity (arrow) secondary to trauma to deep intramuscular tendon of indirect head of left rectus femoris. The hypointensity represents fibrous encasement.

TERMINOLOGY

Abbreviations and Synonyms
- Muscle pull, Charlie horse, quadriceps strain

Definitions
- Stretch injury of rectus femoris during eccentric contraction

IMAGING FINDINGS

General Features
- Best diagnostic clue: Hyperintensity of affected muscle on T2WI
- Location
  - Distal musculotendinous junction (most common)
  - Midsubstance - strain of deep tendon of indirect (reflected) head
- Size: From focal hemorrhage to distal retraction of muscle fibers
- Morphology: Acute strain involving deep intramuscular tendon with associated local hemorrhage +/- edema leading to chronic pseudocyst

Radiographic Findings
- Radiography
  - Normal in mild strains

- ± Soft tissue mass in mid-substance strains 2° to hemorrhage + deranged architecture
- Complete rupture of distal musculotendinous junction + high riding patella (patella alta)

CT Findings
- NECT
  - Unreliable for mild strains
  - Low attenuation 2° to edema
  - Hyperdense regions 2° to hemorrhage
  - Affected muscle acutely enlarged compared to contralateral side
  - Soft tissue mass may be identified in mid-substance strains
- CECT: ± Enhancement

MR Findings
- T1WI
  - Low to intermediate signal intensity hemorrhage
  - ± Hyperintense subacute hemorrhage
  - Peripheral hypointense hemosiderin
  - Loss of normal muscle/fat striations
- T2WI
  - Hyperintense edema in affected muscle
  - Inhomogeneous signal intensity mass in mid-substance strains
  - Hypointense to intermediate signal = more organized central component of hematoma
  - Subacute injury = hyperintense edema + atrophy

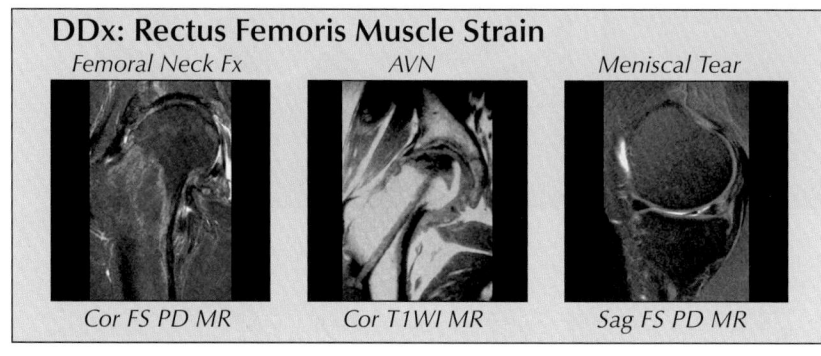

DDx: Rectus Femoris Muscle Strain
Femoral Neck Fx	AVN	Meniscal Tear
Cor FS PD MR	Cor T1WI MR	Sag FS PD MR

RECTUS FEMORIS MUSCLE STRAIN

Key Facts

Imaging Findings
- Best diagnostic clue: Hyperintensity of affected muscle on T2WI
- Distal musculotendinous junction (most common)
- Morphology: Acute strain involving deep intramuscular tendon with associated local hemorrhage +/- edema leading to chronic pseudocyst
- Hypointense signal with fibrous encasement of deep tendon + scar tissue on T2WI

Top Differential Diagnoses
- Fracture
- Radiculopathy
- Intrinsic Hip Pathology

Pathology
- Overuse/repetitive overload

- Rectus femoris = most frequently injured quadriceps muscle
- Injury to deep intramuscular tendon indirect head: Tear → fibrosis → pseudocyst formation

Clinical Issues
- Most common signs/symptoms: Groin or anterior thigh pain
- Common in sprinting or kicking sports - track and field, soccer, martial arts
- Mid-substance strains may present as anterior thigh soft tissue mass

Diagnostic Checklist
- Hypointense scar involving deep intramuscular tendon of indirect head

- ○ Adjacent hyperintense fluid signal
- ○ Hypointense signal with fibrous encasement of deep tendon + scar tissue on T2WI
- ○ Tendon of indirect head = cylindrical shape
- T2* GRE: Demonstrates susceptibility artifact 2° to hemorrhage
- T1 C+
  - ○ Variable synovial ± peripheral enhancement of hemorrhagic focus or muscle disruption
  - ○ "Bulls eye lesion" - peripherally enhancing muscular component of a mid-substance strain

Imaging Recommendations
- Best imaging tool
  - ○ MR to identify grade + anatomic extent of injury
  - ○ Origin vs. insertion injuries
  - ○ MR required for complete tears
- Protocol advice: T1 + FS PD FSE or STIR in axial ± coronal, sagittal planes

DIFFERENTIAL DIAGNOSIS

Fracture
- Avulsion: Anterior superior iliac spine, anterior inferior iliac spine, lesser trochanter
- Stress fracture - pelvic + femoral neck

Radiculopathy
- Lateral vs. central disk protrusion
- Neurologic exam
  - ○ Motor and sensory of lower extremities
  - ○ Reflex testing knees + ankles
- Associated low back pain

Intrinsic Hip Pathology
- Hip dislocation - traumatic dislocation = posterior
- Acetabular labral tears - trauma vs. degenerative disease (catching or clicking + pain)
- Avascular necrosis (AVN) of femoral head

Intrinsic Knee Pathology
- Meniscal tear
- Patellar trauma

- Retinacular injury
- Osseous contusion + osteochondral fracture

Sarcoma
- May mimic mid-substance strain + palpable mass
- Sarcomas - demonstrate central enhancement not seen in hemorrhage
- Disruption or gross invasion of muscle
- Neovascularity

PATHOLOGY

General Features
- General path comments
  - ○ Relevant anatomy
    - ▪ Quadriceps converge through a conjoined tendon to insert on superior aspect patella
    - ▪ Rectus femoris - origin crosses hip joint = knee extension + hip flexion
    - ▪ Quadriceps muscle fibers = type II (rapid forceful activity)
- Etiology
  - ○ Overuse/repetitive overload
  - ○ Inadequate stretching & warm-up exercises predisposes to strain
  - ○ Violent eccentric contraction
- Epidemiology
  - ○ Rectus femoris = most frequently injured quadriceps muscle
  - ○ Muscle strains = 30% of sports-related injuries
  - ○ Track & field, football, soccer, basketball
  - ○ Soccer has highest association with deep intramuscular tendon injuries of indirect head (requires sudden acceleration and bursts of speed)

Gross Pathologic & Surgical Features
- Musculotendinous junction
- Intrasubstance tear at muscle-tendon junction involving indirect head
- Injury to deep intramuscular tendon indirect head: Tear → fibrosis → pseudocyst formation

RECTUS FEMORIS MUSCLE STRAIN

Microscopic Features
- Hemorrhagic response
- Muscle fiber necrotic change
- Edema + macrophages
- Inflammatory cells + fibroblastic activity

Staging, Grading or Classification Criteria
- First-degree - small area muscle involvement without loss of function
- Second-degree - partial tear musculotendinous unit ± mass or hematoma
- Third-degree - complete tear musculotendinous unit ± mass or palpable defect ± retraction of mass or detached muscle segment

CLINICAL ISSUES

Presentation
- Most common signs/symptoms: Groin or anterior thigh pain
- Clinical profile
  - Common in sprinting or kicking sports - track and field, soccer, martial arts
  - Localized swelling
  - Loss of knee extension
  - Mid-substance strains may present as anterior thigh soft tissue mass
  - Chronic mid-substance strains - intramuscular fibrosis + recurrent hemorrhage
  - Tender to palpation
  - Thigh asymmetry in partial or complete tears
  - Complete rupture = palpable defect with retracted mass

Demographics
- Age: Young athletes
- Gender: As a function of participation in sports associated with powerful eccentric contraction of the quadriceps

Natural History & Prognosis
- Majority of cases improve with conservative treatment
- Surgery indicated for compartment syndrome, chronic strains + complete tears
- Compartment syndrome - occurs with severe strains, partial/full-thickness tears
- Full thickness tendon ruptures associated with renal failure, diabetes + rheumatoid arthritis

Treatment
- Conservative
  - RICE (rest, ice, compression, elevation)
  - Physical therapy = stretching + exercises
  - NSAIDs
  - Gradual return to activity
- Surgical
  - Decompression for compartment syndrome
  - Hematoma evacuation
  - Complete rupture: Repair
  - Resection of fibrosis in chronic strains

DIAGNOSTIC CHECKLIST

Consider
- Hypointense scar involving deep intramuscular tendon of indirect head

SELECTED REFERENCES

1. DeLee JC et al: Orthopaedic sports medicine. Principles and practice. vol 1. 2nd ed. Philadelphia PA, Saunders, 26(A):1481-505, 2003
2. Van Holsbeeck MT et al: Musculoskeletal ultrasound. 2nd ed. Philadelphia PA, WB Saunders, 30-7, 578-81, 2001
3. Temple HT et al: Rectus femoris muscle tear appearing as a pseudotumor. Am Jour Sports Med 26:544-8, 1998
4. Stoller DW: Magnetic resonance imaging in orthopaedics and sports med. vol 1. 2nd ed. Philadelphia PA, Saunders, 158-64, 1997
5. Garrett WE Jr: Muscle strain injuries. Am Jour Sports Med 24:S2-8, 1996
6. Sallay PI et al: Hamstring injuries among water skiers: Functional outcome and prevention. Am J Sports Med 24:130, 1996
7. Hughes C IV et al: Incomplete, intrasubstance strain injuries of the rectus femoris muscle. Am Jour Sports Med 23:500-6, 1995
8. Hasselman CT et al: An explanation for various rectus femoris strain injuries using previously undescribed muscle architecture. Am Jour Sports Med (23):493-99, 1995
9. Clarkson PM: Associations between muscle soreness, damage, and fatigue. Adv Exp Med Biol 384:457, 1995
10. Speer KP et al: Radiographic imaging of muscle strain injury. Am Jour Sports Med 21:89-96, 1993
11. Taylor DC et al: Experimental muscle strain injury: Early functional and structural deficits and the increased risk for reinjury. Am J Sports Med 21:190, 1993
12. Friden J et al: Structural and mechanical basis of exercise-induced muscle injury. Med Sci Sports Exerc 24:521, 1992
13. Taylor DC et al: Viscoelastic properties of muscle-tendon units: The biomechanical effects of stretching. Am J Sports Med 18:300, 1990
14. Garrett WE Jr: Muscle strain injuries: Clinical and basic aspects. Med Sci Sports Exerc 22:436, 1990
15. Stauber WT: Eccentric action of muscles: Physiology, injury and adaptation. Exerc Sports Sci Rev 17:157, 1989
16. Garrett WE Jr et al: The effect of muscle architecture on the biomechanical failure properties of skeletal muscle under passive extension. Am J Sports Med 16:7, 1988
17. Garrett WE Jr et al: Biomechanics of muscle tears and stretching injuries. Trans Orthop Res Soc 9:384, 1984
18. Zarins B et al: Acute muscle and tendon injuries in athletes. Clin Sports Med 2:167, 1983
19. Glick JM: Muscle strains: Prevention and treatment. Phys Sports Med 8:73, 1980

RECTUS FEMORIS MUSCLE STRAIN

Typical

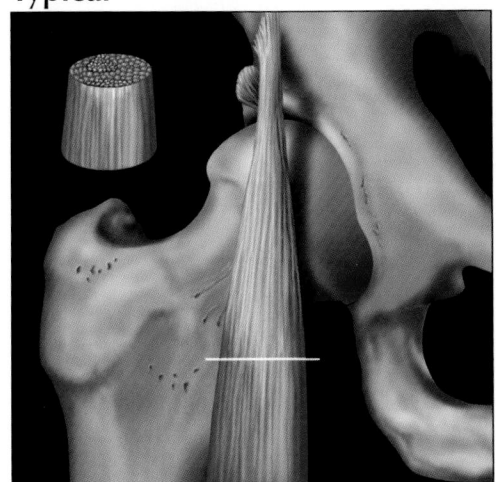
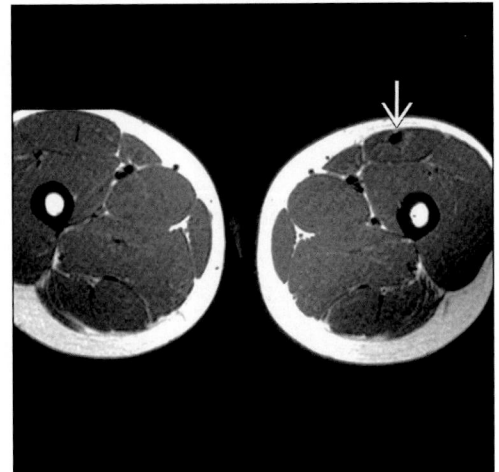

(Left) Coronal graphic shows normal anatomy of the rectus femoris muscle and tendons. The direct (anterior) and indirect (posterior) tendons are shown in axial cross-section. (Right) Axial T1WI MR shows hypointense fibrous scar (arrow) corresponding to the indirect tendon of the left thigh.

Typical

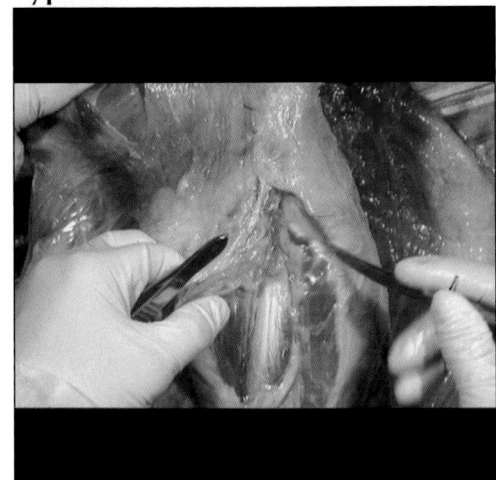
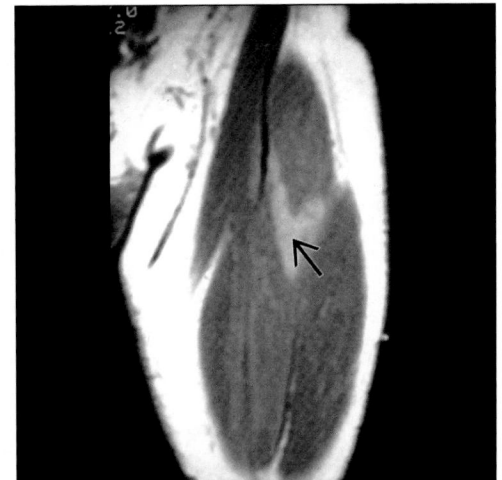

(Left) Surgical pathology shows gross dissection of the spindle-shaped (bipenniform) morphology of the rectus femoris muscle and associated tendon (white). (Right) Coronal PD/Intermediate MR shows tear (arrow) of the rectus femoris muscle belly with associated hemorrhagic fluid collection.

Typical

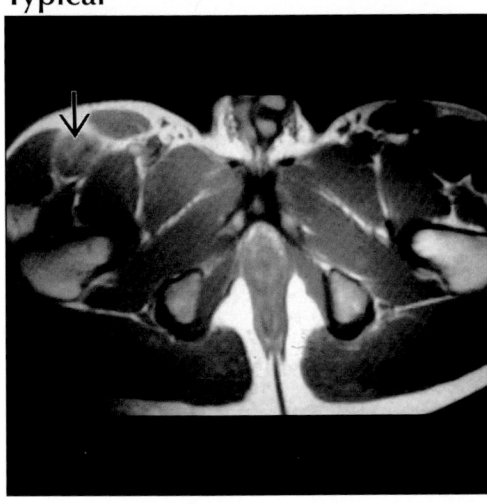
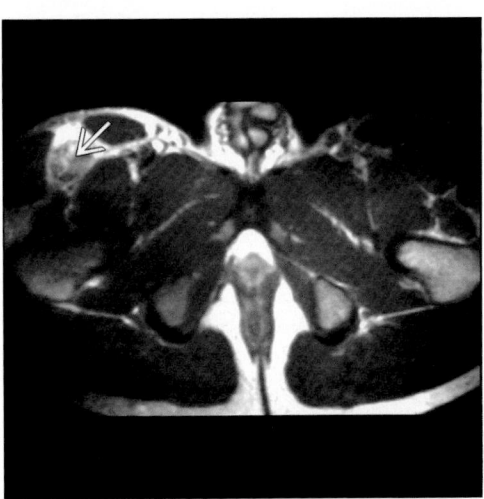

(Left) Axial PD/Intermediate MR shows right rectus femoris muscle atrophy (arrow) secondary to subacute basketball injury. (Right) Axial T2WI MR shows hyperintense edema (arrow) associated with muscle atrophy caused by violent eccentric contraction of right rectus femoris.

GLUTEUS MEDIUS MUSCLE STRAIN

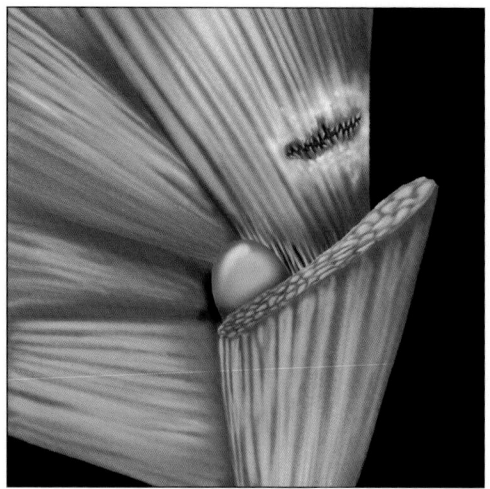

Coronal graphic shows partial tear of the gluteus medius muscle with surrounding edema.

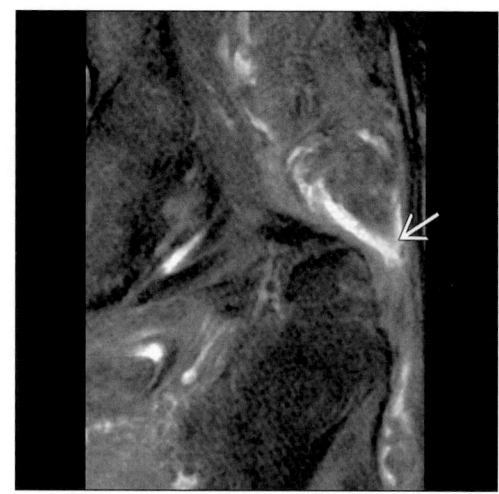

Coronal FS PD FSE MR shows partial tear (arrow) of gluteus medius muscle-tendon unit. Edema is hyperintense.

TERMINOLOGY

Abbreviations and Synonyms
- Muscle pull, "Charlie horse", greater trochanter pain syndrome

Definitions
- Indirect injury secondary to repetitive microtrauma, excessive force or stretch

IMAGING FINDINGS

General Features
- Best diagnostic clue: Muscle with hyperintense edema on T2WI (FS PD FSE)
- Location: Gluteus medius - anterior, middle + posterior parts muscle + tendon
- Size: Usually involves distal 1/3 of muscle (muscle-tendon unit)
- Morphology: Edema directed along long axis of muscle fibers + thickening of tendon

Radiographic Findings
- Radiography
  - Usually normal
  - Helpful to exclude other diagnoses
  - Intramuscular calcification or metaplastic bone + cartilage (myositis ossificans)

CT Findings
- NECT
  - Intramuscular edema = hypodense
  - Acute hemorrhage = hyperdense
  - Affected muscle is enlarged
  - Disruption of muscle architecture in partial/full thickness tears + fluid-filled gap

MR Findings
- T1WI
  - Intramuscular edema - blurring of muscle fibers
  - Hypointense intramuscular fluid
  - Focal muscular defects with retraction or tendon laxity
  - Thickening with intermediate signal in tendinous/myotendinous injuries
  - Subacute hemorrhage (methemoglobin) hyperintense on T1WI
- T2WI
  - Mild strains: Intramuscular edema/hemorrhage (increased T2 signal)
  - Preservation of muscle morphology
  - Hyperintense subcutaneous edema + intramuscular fluid
  - Hyperintense fluid/hemorrhage in disrupted muscle fibers or gaps
  - Variable increased signal in tendinous + myotendinous degeneration or tearing

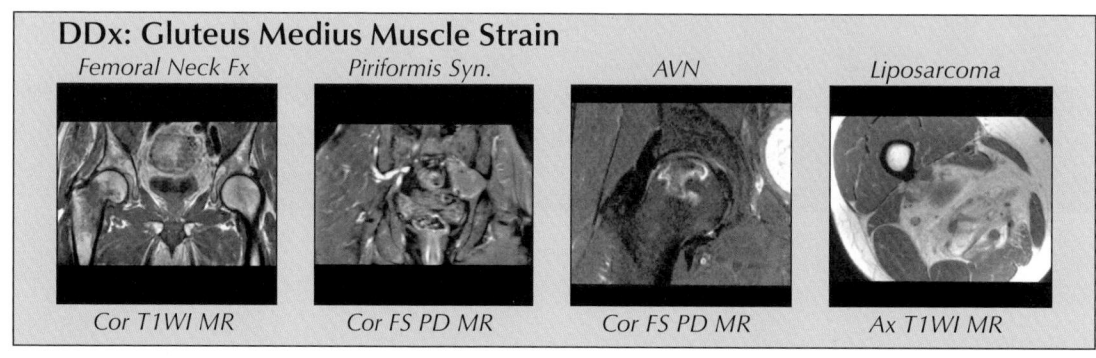

DDx: Gluteus Medius Muscle Strain

Femoral Neck Fx	Piriformis Syn.	AVN	Liposarcoma
Cor T1WI MR	Cor FS PD MR	Cor FS PD MR	Ax T1WI MR

GLUTEUS MEDIUS MUSCLE STRAIN

Key Facts

Imaging Findings

- Best diagnostic clue: Muscle with hyperintense edema on T2WI (FS PD FSE)
- Size: Usually involves distal 1/3 of muscle (muscle-tendon unit)
- Morphology: Edema directed along long axis of muscle fibers + thickening of tendon

Top Differential Diagnoses

- Fracture/Stress Fracture
- Greater Trochanteric Bursitis
- Intrinsic Hip Pathology
- Piriformis Syndrome
- Gluteal Tendon Avulsion

Pathology

- Overuse

- Microtrauma
- Stretch injury
- Occasionally in athletes - football, swimming, ice hockey

Clinical Issues

- Most common signs/symptoms: Lateral hip pain
- Pain radiating to the groin
- Trochanteric bursitis
- Pain at greater trochanter
- Altered gait
- Swelling - muscle enlargement

Diagnostic Checklist

- Associated with greater trochanteric bursitis ± muscle-tendon injuries of gluteus minimus

---

- ○ Tears - more localized hyperintense hemorrhage
- ○ Chronic hematomas demonstrate hypointense peripheral rim
- ○ Hypointense scar/fibrosis = chronic injury

Imaging Recommendations

- Best imaging tool: MR superior for soft tissue/muscle signal changes + differentiation of medius, minimus vs. maximus involvement
- Protocol advice
  - ○ T1 or PD + FS PD FSE or STIR in the coronal + axial plane
  - ○ ± Sagittal plane with FS PD FSE

DIFFERENTIAL DIAGNOSIS

Fracture/Stress Fracture

- Femoral neck = overuse vs. insufficiency in osteoporosis
- Calcar hyperintensity on FS PD FSE MR
- Frank cortical disruption
- Cortical sclerosis

Greater Trochanteric Bursitis

- Lateral aspect hip
- History of repetitive hip flexion
- Hypo to intermediate signal adjacent to greater trochanter on T1WI
- Hyperintense fluid parallel to lateral aspect of greater trochanter on T2WI

Intrinsic Hip Pathology

- Labral tears - traumatic vs. degenerative + painful catching or clicking
- Avascular necrosis of the femoral head - necrotic segment typically with double line sign (associated history of femoral neck fracture, dislocations or corticosteroid use)
- Osteoarthritis +/- femoroacetabular impingement

Piriformis Syndrome

- Sciatic nerve variations = increased risk for compression

- Hypertrophy of piriformis
- Trauma to gluteal region
- Fibrosis following trauma
- Piriformis muscle spasm

Lumbar Radiculopathy

- Disc protrusion - central, paracentral or lateral
- Disc extrusion
- Central + neural foraminal stenosis
- Spondylolisthesis

Gluteal Tendon Avulsion

- Muscle-tendon unit injury
- Hyperintense edema at insertion site on T2WI
- Associated with hyperintense trochanteric bursitis

Soft Tissue Tumor of the Hip + Pelvis

- Lipoma - fat signal
- Desmoid - hypointense fibrous bands on T1 & T2WI
- Malignant fibrous histiocytoma - inhomogeneous signal on T2WI
- Liposarcoma - variable fat + malignant foci
  - ○ Hypointense on T1WI + hyperintense on T2WI
- Synovial cell sarcoma - variable hyperintensity on T2WI (may mimic fluid but solid component is appreciated if window/level is adjusted correctly)

PATHOLOGY

General Features

- General path comments
  - ○ Relevant anatomy = gluteus medius
    - Anterior fibers: Active in hip flexion + internal rotation
    - Posterior fibers: Active in extension + external rotation
    - Entire muscle contributes to hip abduction
    - Gluteus minimus + medius + piriformis attach to greater trochanter
    - Bursa deep to gluteus medius is larger than bursa deep to gluteus minimus
- Etiology
  - ○ Overuse

GLUTEUS MEDIUS MUSCLE STRAIN

○ Microtrauma
○ Stretch injury
• Epidemiology
  ○ Occasionally in athletes - football, swimming, ice hockey
  ○ Subset of muscular + musculotendinous injuries (MTU injuries most frequent athletic related condition of hip + pelvis)

Gross Pathologic & Surgical Features
• Strains
• Tendinosis
• Tendonitis
• Tendon tears
• Avulsions
• Trochanteric bursitis

Microscopic Features
• Hemorrhagic elements
• Lack of inflammatory cells
• Fibrous tissue
• Tendinosis - degeneration similar to tendinosis of rotator cuff

Staging, Grading or Classification Criteria
• Grade I: Edema, hemorrhage + preservation of muscle morphology
• Grade II: Strain or tear involving up to 50% of muscle
• Grade III: Complete tear ± muscle retraction

CLINICAL ISSUES

Presentation
• Most common signs/symptoms: Lateral hip pain
• Clinical profile
  ○ Pain radiating to the groin
  ○ Trochanteric bursitis
  ○ Tenderness to palpation
  ○ Pain at greater trochanter
  ○ Altered gait
  ○ Pain with resisted extension/external rotation
  ○ Edema
  ○ Swelling - muscle enlargement
  ○ Palpable mass in complete tear + retraction

Demographics
• Age
  ○ Elderly population at greatest risk
  ○ Occasionally high-level athletes
• Gender: Females > males

Natural History & Prognosis
• Majority show improvement with conservative treatment
• Surgery for tendon avulsions or complete ruptures

Treatment
• Conservative
  ○ Rest, ice, compression, elevation (RICE)
  ○ Physical therapy
  ○ Steroid injections
• Surgical
  ○ Hematoma evacuation
  ○ Primary repair of complete ruptures

○ Reattachment of avulsed tendon

DIAGNOSTIC CHECKLIST

Consider
• Associated with greater trochanteric bursitis ± muscle-tendon injuries of gluteus minimus
• Coronal FS PD FSE or STIR images required to demonstrate muscle + muscle/tendon hyperintensity

SELECTED REFERENCES

1. Van Holsbeeck MT et al: Musculoskeletal ultrasound. 2nd ed. St. Louis MO, Mosby, 30-7:578-81, 2001
2. Kingzett-Taylor A et al: Tendinosis and tears of gluteus medius and minimus muscles as a cause of hip pain: MR imaging findings. Am J Roentg 173:1123-26, 1999
3. Chung CB et al: Gluteus medius tendon tears and avulsive injuries in elderly women: Imaging findings in six patients. Am J Roentg 173:351-53, 1999
4. Stoller DW: Magnetic resonance imaging in orthopaedics and sports medicine. 2nd ed. Philadelphia PA, Lippincott Williams & Wilkins, 158-64, 1347-56, 1997
5. Garrett WE Jr.: Muscle strain injuries. Am J Sports Med 24:S2-8, 1996
6. Sallay PI et al: Hamstring injuries among water skiers: Functional outcome and prevention. Am J Sports Med 24:130, 1996
7. Nicholas JA et al: The lower extremity and spine in sports medicine. 2nd ed. St. Louis MO, Mosby, 1042, 1995
8. Hughes C et al: Incomplete, intrasubstance strain injuries of the rectus femoris. Am J Sports Med 23:500, 1995
9. Speer KP et al: Radiographic imaging of muscle strain injury. Am J Sports Med 21:889-96, 1993
10. Taylor DC et al: Experimental muscle strain injury: Early functional and structural deficits and the increased risk for reinjury. Am J Sports Med 21:190, 1993
11. Friden J et al: Structural and mechanical basis of exercise-induced muscle injury. Med Sci Sports Exerc 24:521, 1992
12. Garrett WE Jr: Muscle strain injuries: Clinical and basic aspects. Med Sci Sports Exerc 22:436, 1990
13. Taylor DC et al: Viscoelastic properties of muscle-tendon units: The biomechanical effects of stretching. Am J Sports Med 18:300, 1990
14. Stauber WT: Eccentric action of muscles: Physiology, injury and adaptation. Exerc Sports Sci Rev 17:157, 1989
15. Garrett WE Jr et al: The effect of muscle architecture on the biomechanical failure properties of skeletal muscle under passive extension. Am J Sports Med 16:7, 1988
16. Garrett WE Jr et al: Biomechanics of muscle tears and stretching injuries. Trans Orthop Res Soc 9:384, 1984
17. Zarins B et al: Acute muscle and tendon injuries in athletes. Clin Sports Med 2:167, 1983
18. Glick JM: Muscle strains: Prevention and treatment. Phys Sports Med 8:73, 1980

IMAGE GALLERY

Typical

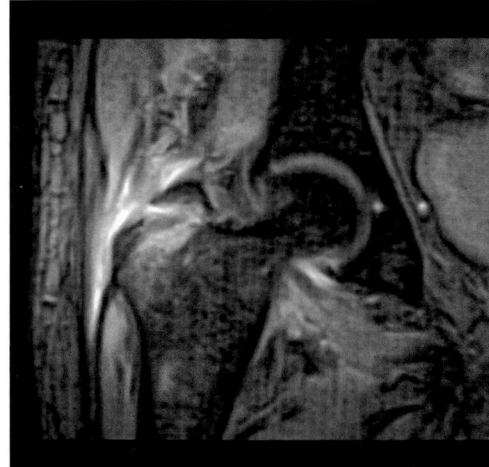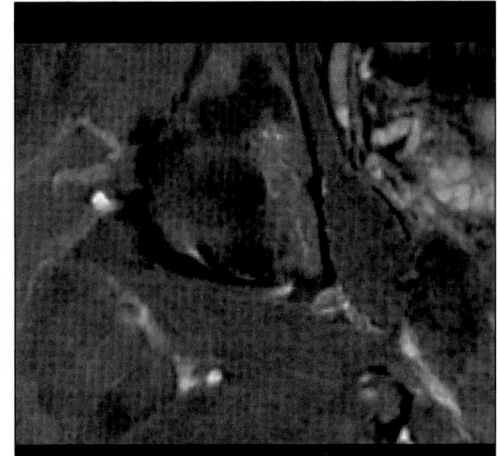

(Left) Coronal FS PD FSE MR shows gluteus medius strain associated with a greater trochanter fracture. *(Right)* Coronal FS PD FSE MR shows subtle hyperintense grade I gluteus medius muscle strain.

Typical

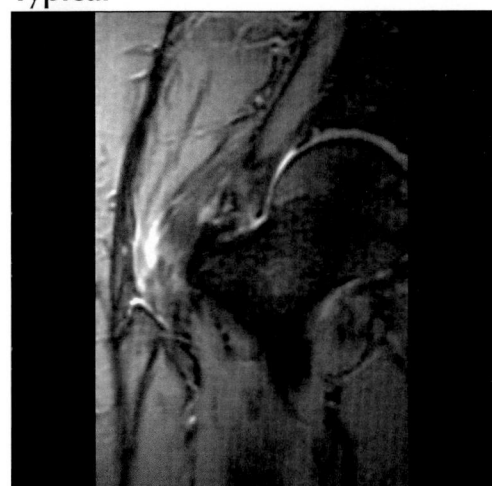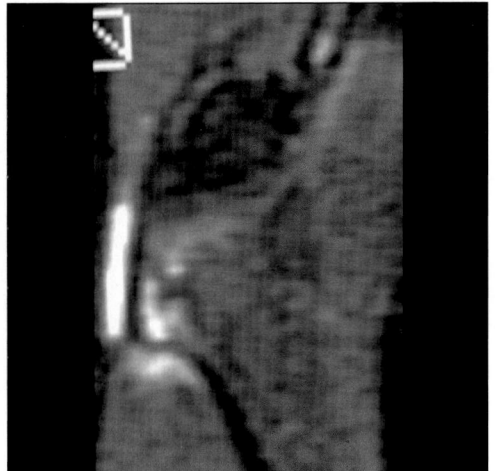

(Left) Coronal FS PD FSE MR shows musculotendinous unit hyperintensity in gluteus medius tendinosis. *(Right)* Coronal FS PD FSE MR shows greater trochanteric bursitis and adjacent subchondral edema. This often is often associated with gluteus medius strain.

Typical

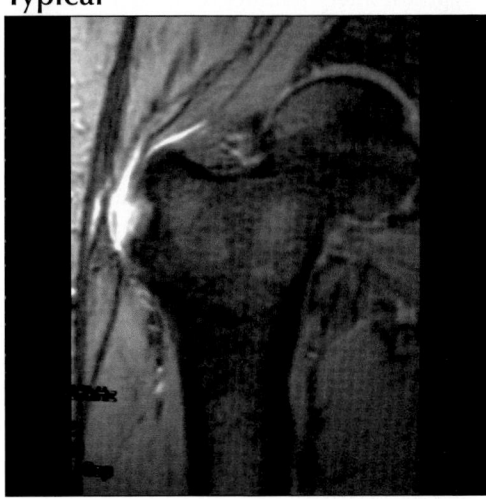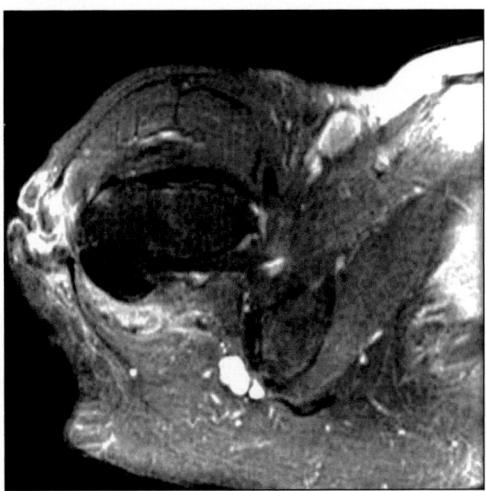

(Left) Coronal T2* GRE MR shows tear of the gluteus medius insertion from the lateral aspect of the greater trochanter. *(Right)* Axial FS PD FSE MR shows grade I strain of the gluteus medius muscle posterior to the lesser trochanter.

4

29

HAMSTRING TENDINOSIS

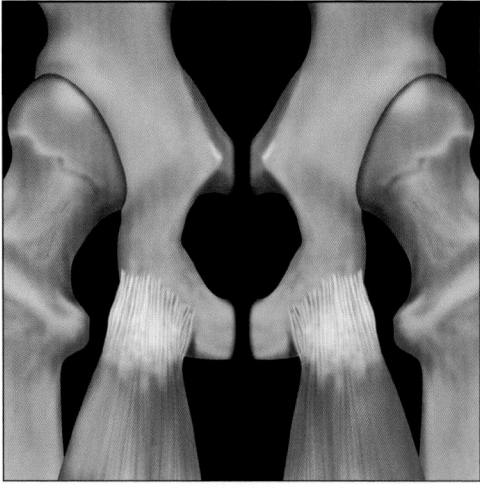

Coronal graphic shows edema and thickening of the common hamstring tendon, bilaterally. The semimembranosus, semitendinosus, and biceps femoris contributions are affected.

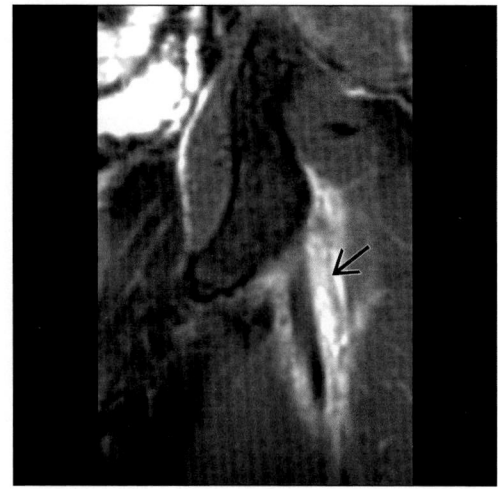

Coronal FS PD FSE MR shows hyperintense edema (arrow) surrounding a thickened common hamstring tendon. The attachment to the ischial tuberosity is intact.

TERMINOLOGY

Abbreviations and Synonyms
- Hamstring strains

Definitions
- Collagenous degeneration of the conjoined tendon of the hamstring muscles

IMAGING FINDINGS

General Features
- Best diagnostic clue: Hyperintensity associated with proximal conjoined tendon of common hamstring attachment on FS PD FSE MR
- Location
  - Ischial tuberosity
  - Proximal tendon
- Size: Proximal 1/3 (or less) of common hamstring tendon
- Morphology: Thickening of involved tendon segment ± splaying of proximal tendon attachment

Radiographic Findings
- Radiography
  - Usually normal
  - To exclude bony avulsion injury

CT Findings
- NECT
  - Limited soft tissue detail
  - ± Visualization of thickened conjoined tendon

MR Findings
- T1WI
  - Intermediate signal intensity in thickened hypointense tendon
  - Partial detachment of hamstring tendon from ischial tuberosity
  - Small osseous avulsion ± hypointense edema ischial tuberosity
  - Complete avulsion with distal retraction of common hamstring tendon
- T2WI
  - Intermediate to hyperintense signal within thickened proximal hamstring tendon
  - Soft tissue hyperintensity parallel to medial + lateral margins of common hamstring tendon
  - Localized hyperintense fluid adjacent to tendon degeneration
  - Adjacent hyperintense subchondral edema of ischial tuberosity
  - Hyperintense fluid influx in area of partial tear
  - Asymmetric involvement of hamstring tendons is a common finding

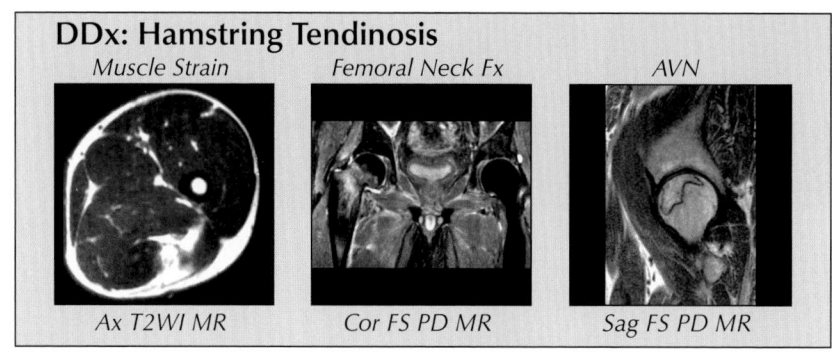

DDx: Hamstring Tendinosis

Muscle Strain	Femoral Neck Fx	AVN
Ax T2WI MR	Cor FS PD MR	Sag FS PD MR

HAMSTRING TENDINOSIS

Key Facts

Imaging Findings

- Best diagnostic clue: Hyperintensity associated with proximal conjoined tendon of common hamstring attachment on FS PD FSE MR
- Morphology: Thickening of involved tendon segment ± splaying of proximal tendon attachment

Top Differential Diagnoses

- Hamstring Muscle Strain/Tear
- Hip Stress Fractures
- Sacral Stress Fracture
- Intrinsic (Internal) Hip Pathology

Pathology

- Hip hyperflexion + knee extension
- Chronic repetitive microtrauma
- Ballistic stretching of hamstring

Clinical Issues

- Most common signs/symptoms: Gluteal pain + point tenderness
- Pain + tightness with forward kicking motion or dynamic hamstring stretch
- Painful static stretch of hamstring group
- Ecchymosis or palpable knot uncommon in proximal tendinosis
- Common in sports requiring bursts of speed, and repetitive hip stretch

Diagnostic Checklist

- Visualize proximal hamstring tendon origin on FS PD FSE or STIR posterior coronal images

---

- T1 C+: Synovial enhancement ± partial enhancement of degenerative foci within proximal hamstring tendons

Imaging Recommendations

- Best imaging tool: MR sensitive + specific for tendon thickening + signal changes
- Protocol advice: T1 + FS PD FSE or STIR coronal + axial images

DIFFERENTIAL DIAGNOSIS

Hamstring Muscle Strain/Tear

- Biceps femoris, semimembranous + semitendinosus
- Any location along course of musculotendinous junction
- Spectrum of grade I to grade III strains
- Local tenderness + palpation of injured site
- Ecchymosis
- Transient sciatica - in acute grade III hamstring strain

Hip Stress Fractures

- Femoral neck - with overuse + repetitive stress + insufficiency fractures in osteoporosis
- Hyperintense marrow (T2WI) + localized cortical thickening
- Extensive edema may obscure fracture line in acetabular stress fractures

Sacral Stress Fracture

- Disproportionate edema with sacral alar stress fxs relative to insufficiency fractures

Intrinsic (Internal) Hip Pathology

- Loose bodies
- Acetabular roof edema
- Labral tear
- AVN
- Femoral head erosion

Sacroiliitis

- Bilateral in ankylosing spondylitis or inflammatory bowel disease-associated arthritis

- Unilateral in most spondyloarthropathies
- Peripheral joint involvement in psoriatic, reactive + inflammatory bowel-associated arthritis
- Sacroiliitis with marrow edema + osseous erosions

Avascular Necrosis of Hip

- Wedge-shaped subchondral bone infarct
- Double line sign in 80%

PATHOLOGY

General Features

- General path comments
  - Relevant anatomy
    - Hamstring group = biceps femoris, semimembranosus + semitendinosus
    - Except short head of biceps all muscles of hamstring group cross hip and knee joint
    - Hamstring origin = ischial tuberosity
    - Hamstring insertion = proximal tibia
    - Short head of biceps femoris has origin from linea aspera + posterior femur
    - Musculotendinous junctions of biceps femoris extends along entire length of muscle (overlap)
    - Short head innervated by peroneal branch sciatic nerve; tibial branch for rest of hamstring group
- Etiology
  - Hip hyperflexion + knee extension
  - Chronic repetitive microtrauma
  - Medial hamstrings at risk during swing segment of recovery phase of running
    - Follow-through, forward swing, foot descent
  - Lateral hamstring at risk in take off segment of support phase
    - Foot strike, midsupport, take off
  - Inadequate warmup
  - Inflexibility
  - Fatigue
  - Hamstring-to-hamstring & hamstring-to-quadriceps imbalances
  - Ballistic stretching of hamstring

HAMSTRING TENDINOSIS

- Epidemiology: Hamstring strains = most common strain-related injury

Gross Pathologic & Surgical Features
- Partial disruption musculotendinous junction
- Partial tear
- Complete tear
- Avulsion fractures
- Thickened proximal tendon + degenerative origin

Microscopic Features
- Collagenous degeneration
- Increased intratendon ground substance
- Proliferation of fibroblasts/myofibroblasts
- Inflammatory cells absent

Staging, Grading or Classification Criteria
- Grade I: Small disruption musculotendinous junction
- Grade II: Partial tear
- Grade IIIa: Complete rupture
- Grade IIIb: Avulsion fracture origin or insertion of tendon

CLINICAL ISSUES

Presentation
- Most common signs/symptoms: Gluteal pain + point tenderness
- Clinical profile
  - Painful when sitting
  - Pain + tightness with forward kicking motion or dynamic hamstring stretch
  - Painful static stretch of hamstring group
  - Ecchymosis or palpable knot uncommon in proximal tendinosis
  - Common in sports requiring bursts of speed, and repetitive hip stretch
  - Feeling of impending "pull" of muscle

Demographics
- Age: Young athletes
- Gender: M ≥ F as a function of activity in football, soccer, basketball, sprinting, rowing, kickboxing

Natural History & Prognosis
- Improvement with conservative treatment
- Recovery process lengthy - up to 6 months
- Advanced tendinosis - untreated leads to tendon tears

Treatment
- Conservative
  - RICE (rest, ice, compression, elevation)
  - Reduce inflammatory process
  - Gradually progressive muscle strength + stretching program
  - Steroid injections = controversial + may result in tendon weakening + tear
- Surgical
  - Limited role in tendinosis
  - Debridement of involved tissue
  - Does not promote collagen synthesis
  - For treatment of tendon tears/avulsions

DIAGNOSTIC CHECKLIST

Consider
- Visualize proximal hamstring tendon origin on FS PD FSE or STIR posterior coronal images
- Identify associated muscle edema

SELECTED REFERENCES

1. DeLee JC et al: Orthopaedic sports medicine. Principles and practice. vol 1. 2nd ed. Philadelphia PA, Saunders 26(A):1481-504, 2003
2. Palmer WE et al: MR imaging of myotendinous strain. AJR 173:703-9, 1999
3. Clanton TO: Hamstring strains in athletes: Diagnosis and treatment. J Am Acad Orthop Surg 6:237-48, 1998
4. Orchard J: Preseason hamstring muscle weakness associated with hamstring muscle injury in Australian footballers. Am J Sports Med 25:81-5, 1997
5. El-Khoury GY et al: Imaging of muscle injuries. Skeletal Radiol 25:3-11, 1996
6. Orava S et al: Rupture of the ischial origin of the hamstring muscles. Am J Sports Med 23:702-5, 1995
7. Garrett WE et al: Computed tomography of the hamstrings muscle strain. J Med Sci Sports Exerc 21:508-14, 1989
8. Cross MJ et al: Surgical repair of chronic complete hamstring tendon rupture in the adult patient. Am J Sports Med 26:785-88, 1988
9. Oh I et al: Proximal strain distribution in the loaded femur. J Bone Joint Surg Am 60:75-85, 1988
10. Safran MR et al: The role of warmup in muscular injury and prevention. AM J Sports Med 16:123, 1988
11. Garrett WE et al: Biomechanical comparison of stimulated and nonstimulated skeletal muscle pulled to failure. Am J Sports Med 15:448-54, 1987
12. Garrett WE et al: Biomechanical comparison of stimulated and nonstimulated muscle pulled to failure. Am J Sports Med 15:448, 1987
13. Sim FH et al: Injuries of the pelvis and hip in athletes: The lower extremity and spine in sports medicine. St. Louis MO, CV Mosby, 1986
14. Metzmaker JN et al: Avulsion fractures of the pelvis. Am J Sports Med 13:349, 1985
15. Heiser TM et al: Prophylaxis and management of hamstring muscle injuries in intercollegiate football players. Am J Sports Med 12:368-70, 1984
16. Garrett WE et al: Histochemical correlates of hamstring injuries. Am J Sports Med 12:98-103, 1984
17. Casperson PC: Groin and hamstring injuries. J Athlet Train 17:43-5, 1982
18. Burkett LN: Investigation into hamstring strains: The case of the hybrid muscle. J Sports Med 3:228-31, 1976
19. Burkett LN: Causative factors in hamstring strain. Med Sci Sports Exerc 2:39-42, 1970
20. McMaster PE: Tendon and muscle ruptures: Clinical and experimental studies on the causes and location of subcutaneous ruptures. J Bone Joint Surg 15:705, 1933

HAMSTRING TENDINOSIS

IMAGE GALLERY

Typical

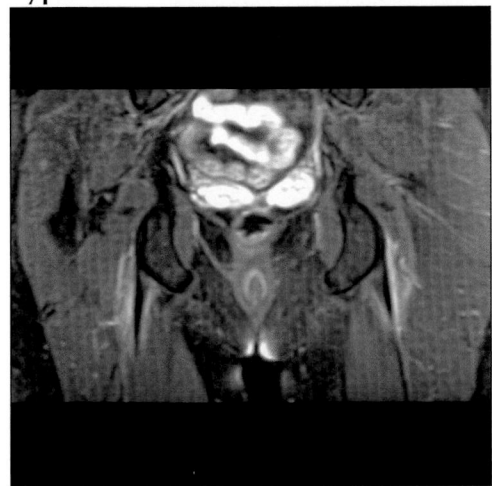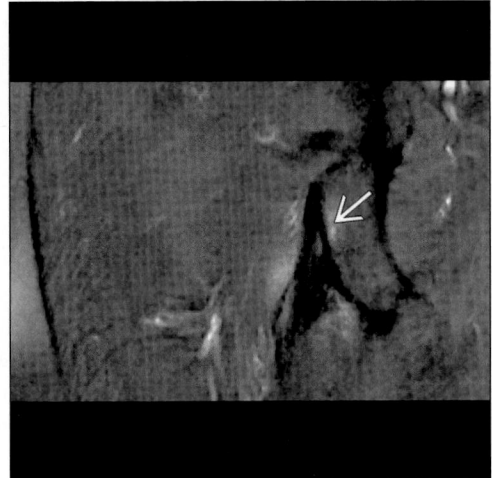

(Left) Coronal FS PD FSE MR shows bilateral common hamstring tendinosis with hyperintense edema adjacent to the thickened ischial tuberosity attachments. This injury was secondary to ballistic overstretching. (Right) Coronal FS PD FSE MR shows common hamstring tendinosis with adjacent reactive subchondral bone marrow edema (arrow) involving the ischial tuberosity. Interstitial tearing of the common hamstring tendon is present.

Typical

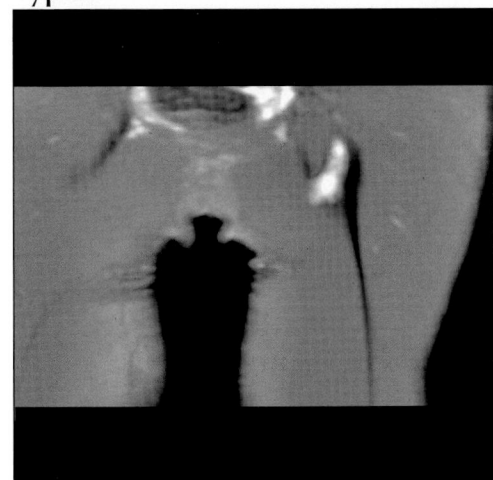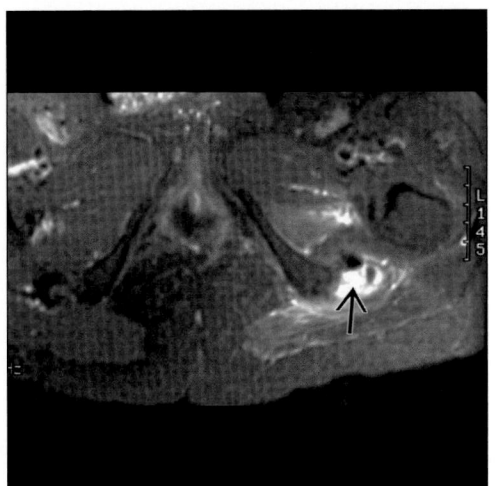

(Left) Coronal FS PD FSE MR shows high grade partial detachment of left common hamstring tendon. (Right) Axial FS PD FSE MR shows complete avulsion (arrow) of left hamstring tendon origin.

Typical

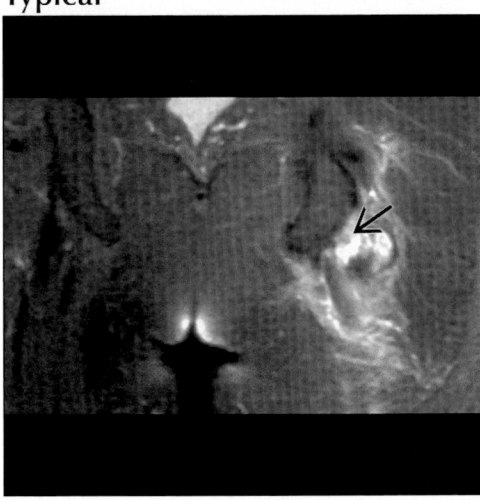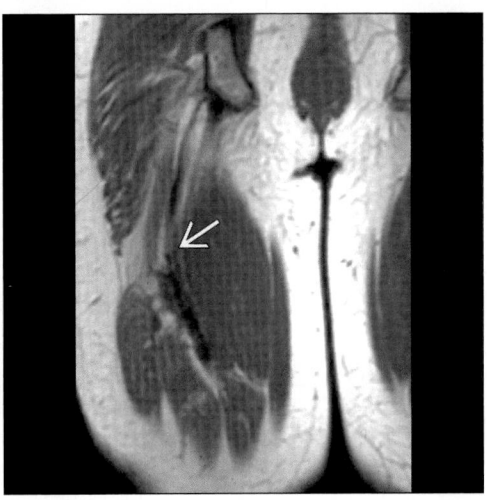

(Left) Coronal FS PD FSE MR shows focal hemorrhage (arrow) in left common hamstring tendon avulsion. (Right) Coronal T1WI MR shows distal retraction (arrow) of right common hamstring tendon avulsion.

PIRIFORMIS SYNDROME

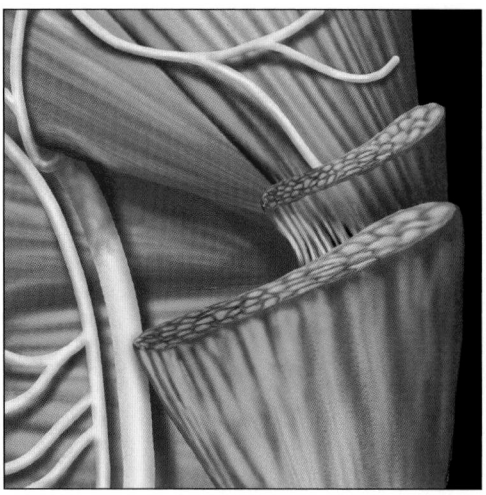

Coronal graphic shows entrapment (red) of sciatic nerve secondary to piriformis muscle hypertrophy (posterior to sciatic nerve). The nerve is involved as it passes through the sciatic notch.

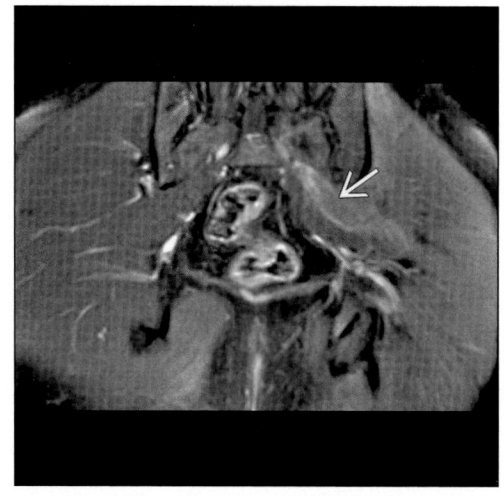

Coronal FS PD FSE MR shows hyperintense edema (arrow) of the left piriformis muscle.

TERMINOLOGY

Abbreviations and Synonyms
- Pseudosciatica, wallet sciatica, hip socket neuropathy, deep gluteal syndrome

Definitions
- Neuritis of proximal sciatic nerve secondary to irritation or compression by the piriformis muscle

IMAGING FINDINGS

General Features
- Best diagnostic clue: Piriformis hypertrophy
- Location: Piriformis - emerges from greater sciatic foramen + inserts on upper border greater trochanter
- Size: Variable piriformis hypertrophy - conforming to muscle boundaries
- Morphology
  - Variable based on presence of muscle hypertrophy
  - Piriformis = pyramid-shaped

Radiographic Findings
- Radiography
  - Usually normal
  - Intrinsic abnormality (of myositis ossificans, tumor with calcification)

CT Findings
- NECT
  - Hypertrophy of piriformis
  - Infiltrative tumor or space occupying lesion
  - Inflammation

MR Findings
- T1WI
  - Piriformis hypertrophy
  - Effacement of fat in greater sciatic foramen with muscle signal intensity
  - Loss of longitudinal muscle striations
  - Mass effect resulting in displacement of muscle from anterior to posterior
- T2WI
  - Diffuse muscle edema with hyperintensity on T2WI
  - Edema associated with tumor, abscess or hematoma
  - Hypointense fibrosis 2° to previous trauma
  - Normal gluteus minimus, medius + tensor fascia lata muscles
  - ± Signal changes within gluteus maximus
  - ± Gluteal atrophy with suppression of fat signal intensity (with fat suppression or STIR)

Imaging Recommendations
- Best imaging tool: MR to evaluate muscle asymmetry + signal intensity changes

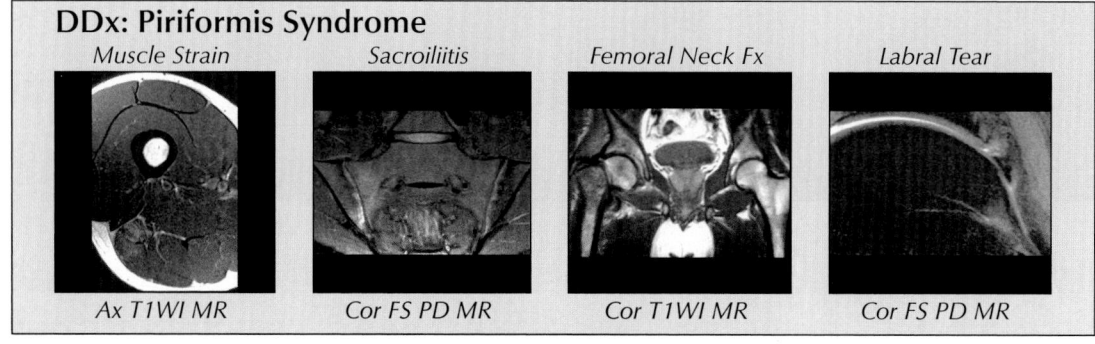

DDx: Piriformis Syndrome

Muscle Strain	Sacroiliitis	Femoral Neck Fx	Labral Tear
Ax T1WI MR	Cor FS PD MR	Cor T1WI MR	Cor FS PD MR

4

34

PIRIFORMIS SYNDROME

Key Facts

Imaging Findings
- Best diagnostic clue: Piriformis hypertrophy
- Size: Variable piriformis hypertrophy - conforming to muscle boundaries
- Diffuse muscle edema with hyperintensity on T2WI

Top Differential Diagnoses
- Hamstring Muscle Injury
- Lumbar Radiculopathy/Discogenic Pain/Facet Arthropathy
- Sacroiliitis or Sacroiliac Joint Injury
- Gluteal Muscle Strains
- Ischial Tuberosity Bursitis

Pathology
- Trauma to gluteal region = most common cause
- Overuse (high performance athletes)

- Anatomic variations include divisions of sciatic nerve splitting piriformis = predisposing to nerve compression
- Tumor compression
- Prolonged sitting = bilateral piriformis syndrome

Clinical Issues
- Most common signs/symptoms: Chronic gluteal pain which radiates into lower extremity similar to L5-S1 radiculopathy
- Pain with hip adduction + internal rotation

Diagnostic Checklist
- Evaluate morphology + signal intensity changes in piriformis muscle

---

- Protocol advice: T1 + FS PD FSE or STIR in the axial + coronal planes

- Avascular necrosis
- Loose bodies

DIFFERENTIAL DIAGNOSIS

Hamstring Muscle Injury
- Hamstring muscle edema
- Common hamstring tendon degeneration at origin
- Focal tear with fiber retraction

Lumbar Radiculopathy/Discogenic Pain/Facet Arthropathy
- Central, paracentral or lateral protrusion
- Facet hypertrophy + degenerative spondylolisthesis
- Paraspinal muscle strain
- Central vs. neural foraminal stenosis

Sacroiliitis or Sacroiliac Joint Injury
- Sclerosis on T1WI
- Hyperintensity on FS PD FSE or STIR
- Erosions in sacroiliitis
- Sacral alar fracture

Gluteal Muscle Strains
- Secondary to blunt trauma
- Edema vs. hematoma formation

Ischial Tuberosity Bursitis
- Hyperintensity (T2WI) on posterior coronal images
- ± Association with common hamstring tendon degeneration

Trochanteric Bursitis
- Curvilinear hyperintensity conforming to greater trochanter
- ± Effacement of adjacent subcutaneous tissue

Stress Fractures of Hip or Pelvis
- Acetabular hypointensity on T1WI + hyperintensity on T2WI

Intrinsic Hip Pathology
- Labral tears
- Chondral erosions of acetabulum + femoral head

PATHOLOGY

General Features
- General path comments
  - Relevant anatomy = piriformis
    - Origin - anterior to S2-S4 vertebrae + sacrotuberous ligament + upper margin greater sciatic foramen
    - Passes through greater sciatic notch
    - Inserts superior aspect of greater trochanter
    - Function: External rotation with hip extended
    - Hip abductor with hip in flexion
    - Innervated by L5, S1 + S2 nerve roots
    - Developmental variations exist in anatomic relationship between sciatic nerve + piriformis
- Etiology
  - Trauma to gluteal region = most common cause
  - Overuse (high performance athletes)
  - Compensatory contraction of hip external rotators in foot instability secondary to Morton's foot with prominent 2nd metatarsal head
  - Spinal stenosis
  - Anatomic variations include divisions of sciatic nerve splitting piriformis = predisposing to nerve compression
  - Intrinsic piriformis strain
  - Myositis
  - Tumor compression
  - Irritation of piriformis by sacroiliitis
  - Prolonged sitting = bilateral piriformis syndrome
  - Pseudoaneurysm of inferior gluteal artery
- Epidemiology: Up to 6% of sciatica cases

Gross Pathologic & Surgical Features
- Hypertrophy of piriformis
- Compression of sciatic nerve
- Myositis ossificans
- Associated mass lesion/entrapment (tumor, abscess or hematoma)

PIRIFORMIS SYNDROME

- Piriformis split by sciatic nerve

Microscopic Features
- Inflammation
- Interstitial myofibrositis
  - Extravasation of blood
  - Serotonin release from platelets
  - Prostaglandin E
  - Bradykinin
  - Histamine release
  - Neuritis
  - Fibrosis

Staging, Grading or Classification Criteria
- 6 cardinal features
  - Positive Laséque sign (pain at greater sciatic notch in knee extension + hip flexion)
  - Sausage-shaped mass - piriformis muscle
  - Gluteal atrophy - chronic
  - Trauma
  - Sacroiliac joint, gluteal muscle or greater sciatic notch pain
  - Pain increased by lifting the extremity + decreased by traction on involved extremity

CLINICAL ISSUES

Presentation
- Most common signs/symptoms: Chronic gluteal pain which radiates into lower extremity similar to L5-S1 radiculopathy
- Clinical profile
  - Pain with hip adduction + internal rotation
  - Tenderness of piriformis on digital rectal examination + external palpation
  - Pain with passive hip flexion + internal rotation (Freiberg's sign)
  - Pain with resisted abduction + external rotation (Pace's sign)
  - Laséque sign
  - Sacroiliac joint/greater sciatic notch pain
  - Pain with Valsalva maneuver
  - Dyspareunia; pain radiating to genitals

Demographics
- Age: 18-55 years (overlap with age range for low back pain)
- Gender: F:M = 6:1

Natural History & Prognosis
- Progression is typical without treatment
- Most cases improve with conservative treatment
- Surgery for refractory cases
- Functional biomechanical deficits
  - Tight piriformis muscle
  - Contraction and tightness of external rotators + adductors
  - Lumbosacral spine dysfunction
  - Sacroiliac joint hypomobility

Treatment
- Conservative
  - Rest
  - Physical therapy/stretching
  - Local injections with steroid/local anesthetic
  - Anti-inflammatories
  - Botox injections
- Surgical
  - Release of piriformis from greater tuberosity insertion
  - Lysis of adhesions/fibrosis surrounding piriformis or sciatic nerve

DIAGNOSTIC CHECKLIST

Consider
- Piriformis syndrome = absence of neurologic deficit (unlike typical sciatic pain)
- Evaluate morphology + signal intensity changes in piriformis muscle

SELECTED REFERENCES

1. Dezawa A et al: Arthroscopic release of the piriformis muscle under local anesthesia for piriformis syndrome. Arthroscopy 19(5):554-7, 2003
2. Nakamura H et al: Piriformis syndrome diagnosed by cauda equina action potentials: Report of two cases. Spine 15:28(2):E37-40, 2003
3. Fishman LM et al: BOTOX and physical therapy in the treatment of piriformis syndrome. Am J Phys Med Rehabil 81(12):936-42, 2002
4. Foster MR: Piriformis syndrome. Orthopedics 25(8):821-5, 2002
5. Fishman LM et al: Piriformis syndrome: Diagnosis, treatment, and outcome - a 10-year study. Arch Phys Med Rehabil 83(3):295-301, 2002
6. Reat MT: The piriformis syndrome - math or reality? Br J Sports Med 36(1):76, 2002
7. Rossi P et al: Magnetic resonance imaging findings in piriformis syndrome: A case report. Arch Phys Med Rehabil 82(4):519-21, 2001
8. Levin SM: Piriformis syndrome. Orthopaedics 23(3):183-4, 2000
9. Benson ER et al: Post-traumatic piriformis syndrome: Diagnosis and results of operative treatment. J Bone Surg Am 81:941, 1999
10. Fishman L et al: Electrophysiologic evidence of piriformis syndrome. Arch Phys Med Rehabil 73:359, 1992
11. Vandertop W et al: The piriformis syndrome. J Bone Joint Surg Am 73:1095, 1991
12. Silver JK: Piriformis syndrome: Assessment of current practice and literature review. Orthopaedics 21:1133, 1988
13. Pavlov H et al: Stress fractures of the pubic ramus. J Bone Surg Am 64:1020, 1982
14. Robinson DR: Piriformis syndrome in relation to sciatic pain. AM J Surge 73:355, 1947

IMAGE GALLERY

Typical

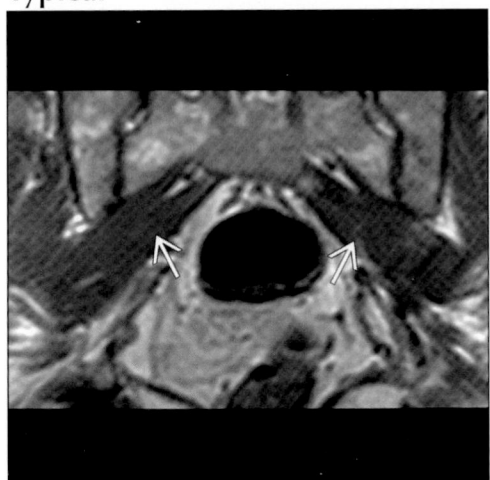 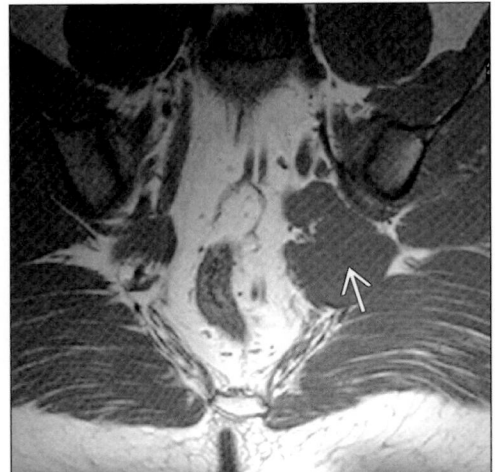

(Left) Coronal FS PD FSE MR shows normal anatomy of the piriformis muscle (arrows). The piriformis originates from the sacrum, greater sciatic foramen, and sacrotuberous ligament and inserts on the greater trochanter of the femur. *(Right)* Coronal T1WI MR shows asymmetric hypertrophy (arrow) of the left piriformis muscle (wallet sciatica) in a fighter pilot who carried his money in his left back pocket.

Typical

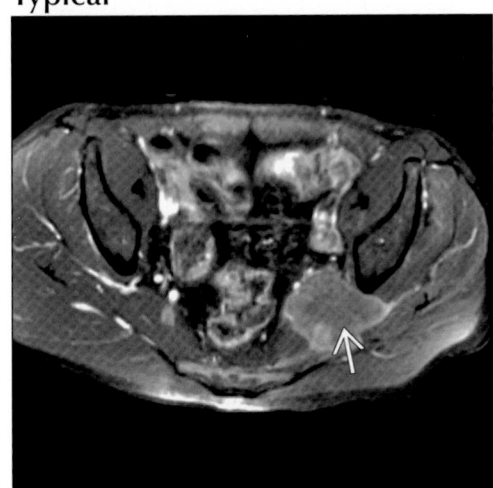 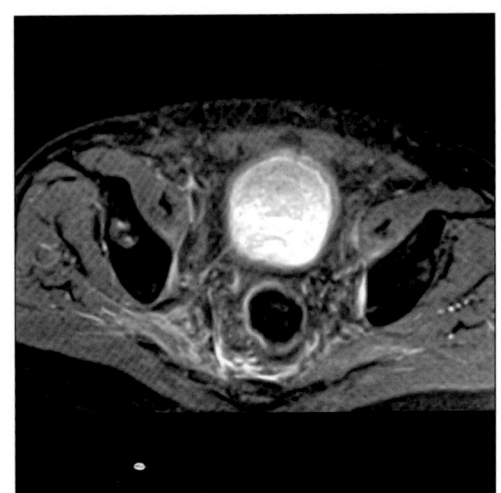

(Left) Axial FS PD FSE MR shows lymphoma (arrow) compressing and displacing left sciatic nerve. *(Right)* Axial FS PD FSE MR shows edema of the right piriformis muscle and adjacent sciatic nerve, which abuts its anterior margin.

Typical

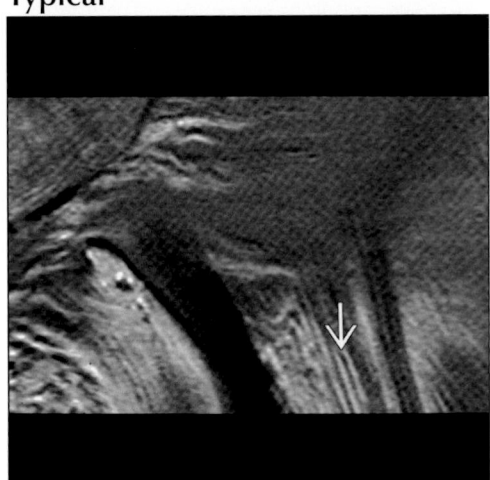 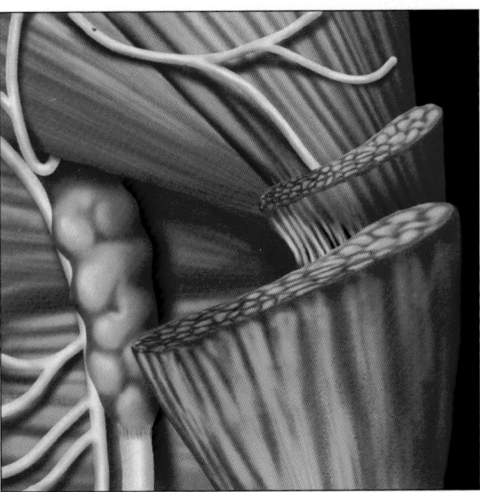

(Left) Coronal T1WI MR shows the course of the sciatic nerve (arrow) directly lateral and parallel to the hypointense semimembranosus tendon. *(Right)* Coronal graphic (posterior view) shows benign peripheral nerve sheath tumor of the sciatic nerve mimicking piriformis syndrome.

4

37

ILIOPSOAS BURSITIS

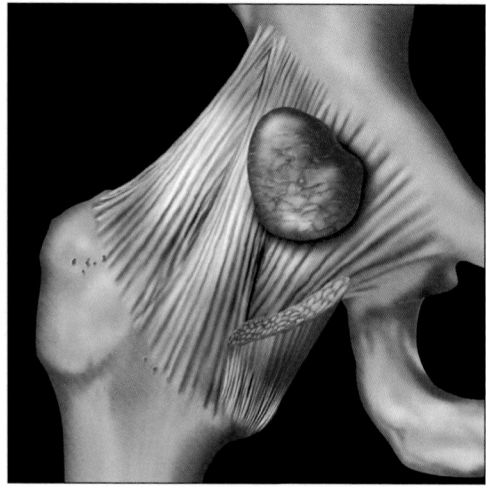

Coronal graphic shows distension of the iliopsoas bursa anterior to the joint capsule.

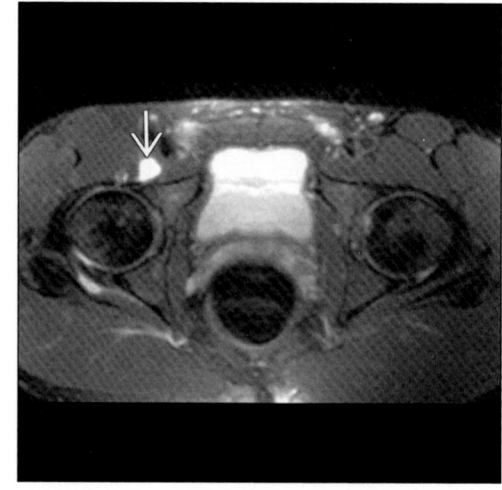

Axial FS PD FSE MR shows hyperintense iliopsoas bursal (arrow) distension medial to the right iliopsoas tendon. Note the anterior convexity and tear-drop morphology.

TERMINOLOGY

Abbreviations and Synonyms
- Iliopectineal bursitis, iliofemoral bursitis, sub-psoas bursitis, iliopsoas syndrome

Definitions
- Inflammation of the iliopsoas bursa

IMAGING FINDINGS

General Features
- Best diagnostic clue: Hyperintense fluid collection medial to iliopsoas muscle on T2WI
- Location: Bursa between anterior hip capsule + iliopsoas muscle
- Size: Variable (1 to 3 cm most common)
- Morphology: ± Tear-drop shaped on axial with anterior convexity + posterior communication with bursa

Radiographic Findings
- Radiography
  - Usually normal
  - Rarely a soft tissue mass is visualized
  - Concomitant disease of the hip may be identified
  - Bursography - incidentally filled during hip arthrography

CT Findings
- NECT
  - Thin-walled fluid density mass
  - Thickened wall in synovial proliferative process (rheumatoid)
- CECT: Wall ± enhancement

MR Findings
- T1WI
  - Hypointense to intermediate signal intensity mass
  - Displacement of adjacent iliopsoas tendon laterally
- T2WI
  - Hyperintensity with bursal distension
  - Usually uniformly increased signal
  - Less commonly heterogeneous signal = hemorrhage or proteinaceous debris
  - Axial images to show direct communication with hip = tail-like extension tapering medial to iliopsoas tendon
  - Well marginated borders
  - Long axis oriented superior to inferior on coronal images
  - Bursal fluid > volume than hip joint fluid
- T1 C+
  - Peripheral enhancement with intravenous contrast (bursal lining)
  - Fluid - no enhancement unless complicated by synovial proliferation

DDx: Iliopsoas Bursitis

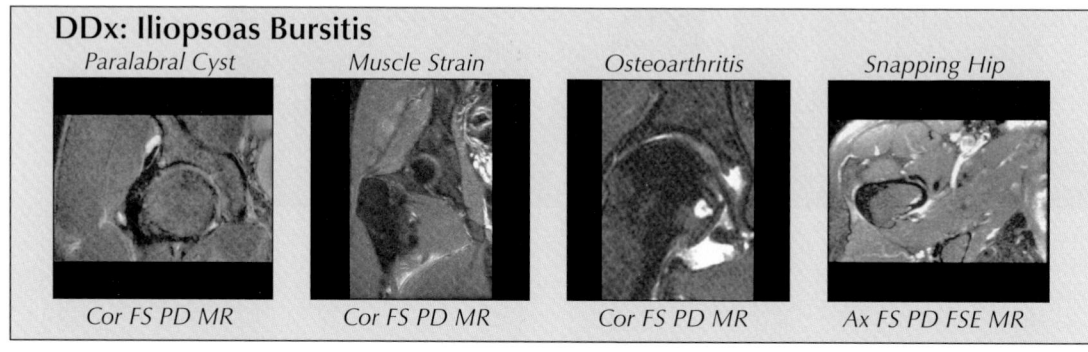

Paralabral Cyst	Muscle Strain	Osteoarthritis	Snapping Hip
Cor FS PD MR	Cor FS PD MR	Cor FS PD MR	Ax FS PD FSE MR

4

38

ILIOPSOAS BURSITIS

Key Facts

Imaging Findings
- Best diagnostic clue: Hyperintense fluid collection medial to iliopsoas muscle on T2WI
- Location: Bursa between anterior hip capsule + iliopsoas muscle
- Morphology: ± Tear-drop shaped on axial with anterior convexity + posterior communication with bursa

Top Differential Diagnoses
- Paralabral Cyst
- Muscle Strain
- Osteoarthritis
- Snapping Hip Syndrome

Pathology
- Overuse

- Rheumatoid arthritis: Synovial proliferation
- ± Snapping hip syndrome
- Discrete soft tissue cystic mass adjacent to femoral neurovascular bundle

Clinical Issues
- Most common signs/symptoms: Anterior groin mass
- Tender to palpation in femoral triangle
- Pain with activity progressing to pain at rest
- Delay in diagnosis common
- Improvement with conservative measures

Diagnostic Checklist
- FS PD FSE or STIR to document bursal origin

Ultrasonographic Findings
- Anechoic to hypoechoic fluid
- Well circumscribed fluid collection
- Hyperechoic if hemorrhage present

Imaging Recommendations
- Best imaging tool
  - Ultrasound = most cost-effective diagnostic test
  - MR = superior for soft tissue contrast + specificity (e.g., distinguishing from paralabral cyst or abscess)
- Protocol advice: FS PD FSE axial and coronal required ± T1 C+ (fat suppression)

DIFFERENTIAL DIAGNOSIS

Paralabral Cyst
- Associated with acetabular labral tears
- May project anteriorly

Muscle Strain
- Anterior muscle edema (e.g., rectus femoris)
- Not associated with bursal fluid distension

Osteoarthritis
- Joint effusion
- Synovitis
- Capsular distension
- Subchondral cysts

Snapping Hip Syndrome
- Iliotibial band irritation of greater trochanteric bursa with flexion + extension + internal rotation
- Sensation of hip dislocation
- Responds to conservative therapy

Effusion
- Capsular distension
- Scalloping of capsule with synovitis

Malignancy
- Malignant fibrous histiocytoma
- Liposarcoma
- Synovial cell sarcoma

- Metastatic lesions

Inflammatory Arthritides
- Rheumatoid - symmetrical + bilateral + uniform axial joint space narrowing
- Pannus + effusion + subchondral edema ± cysts

PATHOLOGY

General Features
- General path comments
  - Relevant anatomy = iliopsoas bursa
    - Largest bursa of hip & body
    - Bordered medially by iliopectineal muscle
    - Bordered laterally by anterior inferior iliac spine
  - Iliopsoas tendon crosses inferior aspect hip joint capsule
  - Psoas major origin = T12-L5 transverse processes + bodies
  - Iliacus origin = iliac wing
  - Psoas major + iliacus forms iliopsoas with insertion on lesser trochanter of femur
- Etiology
  - Overuse
    - Repetitive/strenuous hip flexion + extension
  - Rheumatoid arthritis: Synovial proliferation
  - Trauma
  - Degenerative + inflammatory component
  - Associated tendonitis/tenosynovitis
  - ± Snapping hip syndrome
  - Associated intraarticular pathology (e.g., avascular necrosis)
- Epidemiology: Iliopsoas bursal communication with hip in 15% of healthy individuals & 30% individuals with hip pathology

Gross Pathologic & Surgical Features
- Discrete soft tissue cystic mass adjacent to femoral neurovascular bundle
- ± Hemorrhage
- ± Communication with hip joint

ILIOPSOAS BURSITIS

Microscopic Features
- Synovial cells inflamed + hypertrophied
- Fibrosis
- Fibrin

CLINICAL ISSUES

Presentation
- Most common signs/symptoms: Anterior groin mass
- Clinical profile
  - Tender to palpation in femoral triangle
  - ± Pulsatile secondary to adjacent femoral vessels
  - ± Presentation as a pelvic mass from cephalad extension + compression of intrapelvic contents (colon, bladder, etc.)
  - Pain ± radiation distally to anterior thigh & knee
  - Exacerbating movements
    - Flexion
    - Abduction
    - External rotation
  - Pain with activity progressing to pain at rest
  - Delay in diagnosis common

Demographics
- Age: Young active adults
- Gender: Females slightly > males

Natural History & Prognosis
- Improvement with conservative measures
- Associated with snapping hip syndrome

Treatment
- Conservative
  - Anti-inflammatory medications
  - Hip abduction + external rotation stretching exercises
  - Deep heat
  - Ultrasound therapy
  - Steroid injection
- Surgical
  - Iliopsoas tendon release (rarely required)

DIAGNOSTIC CHECKLIST

Consider
- FS PD FSE or STIR to document bursal origin
- T1 C+ to exclude soft tissue malignant tumor

SELECTED REFERENCES

1. DeLee JC et al: Orthopaedic sports medicine. Principles and practice. vol 2. 2nd ed. Philadelphia PA, Saunders, (25):1443-62, 2003
2. Boutin FJ Sr: Bursitis: Operative orthopaedics. vol 4. 4th ed. Philadelphia PA, JB Lippincott Company, 3019-375, 2002
3. Wunderbaldinger P et al: Imaging features of iliopsoas bursitis. Eur Radiol 12(2):409-15, 2002
4. Morelli V et al: Groin injuries in athletes. Am Family Physician (8):1405-14, 2001
5. Van Holsbeeck MT et al: Musculoskeletal ultrasound. 2nd ed. St. Louis MO, Mosby, 576-7, 2001
6. Ruddy S et al: Kelley's textbook of rheumatology. 6th ed. Philadelphia PA, Saunders, 541-2, 2001
7. Pfirrmann CW et al: Greater trochanter of the hip: Attachment of the abductor mechanism and a complex of three bursae-MR imaging and MR bursography in cadavers and MR imaging in asymptomatic volunteers. Radiology 221(2):469-77, 2001
8. Chung CB et al: Gluteus medius tendon tears and avulsive injuries in elderly women: Imaging findings in six patients. AJR 173(2):351-3, 1999
9. Johnston CA et al: Iliopsoas bursitis and tendinitis. A review. Sports Med 25(4):271-83, 1998
10. Kozlov DB et al: Iliopsoas bursitis: Diagnosis by MRI. J Computer Assisted Tomog 22(4):625-8, 1998
11. Amrar-Vennier F et al: Subcutaneous trochanteric bursitis: An unrecognized cause of peritrochanteric pain revealed by imaging. J Radiol 79(6):557-62, 1998
12. Stoller DW: Magnetic resonance imaging in orthopaedics and sports medicine. vol 1. 2nd ed. Philadelphia PA, Saunders, 164-7, 1997
13. Fortin L et al: Bursitis of the iliopsoas: Four cases with pain as the only clinical indicator. J Rheumatol 22(10):1971-3, 1995
14. Toohey AK et al: Iliopsoas bursitis: Clinical features, radiographic findings, and disease associations. Semin Arthritis Rheum 20(1):41-7, 1990
15. Underwood PL et al: The varied clinical manifestations of iliopsoas bursitis. J of Rheum 15(11):1683-5, 1988
16. Weinreb JC et al: Iliopsoas muscles: MR study of normal anatomy and disease. Radiology 156(2):435-40, 1985
17. Sartoris DJ et al: Synovial cyst of the hip joint and iliopsoas bursitis: A spectrum of imaging abnormalities. Skeletal Radiol 14(2):85-94, 1985
18. Steinbach LS et al: Bursae and abscess cavities communicating with the hip. Diagnosis using arthrography and CT. Radiology 156(2):303-7, 1985
19. Penkava RR: Iliopsoas bursitis demonstrated by computed tomography. Am J of Roentg 153(1):175-6, 1980
20. Armstrong P et al: Iliopsoas bursa. Br J Radiol 45(535):493-5, 1972

4

40

ILIOPSOAS BURSITIS

IMAGE GALLERY

Typical

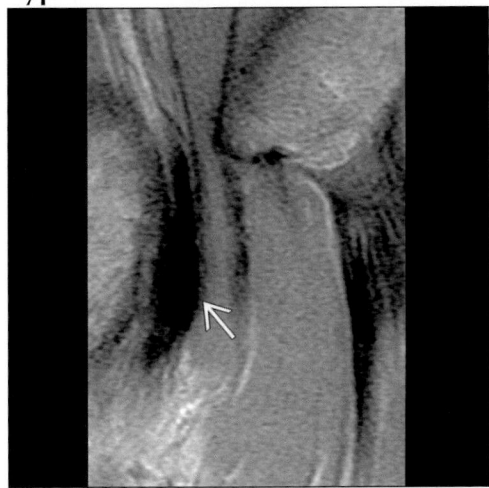
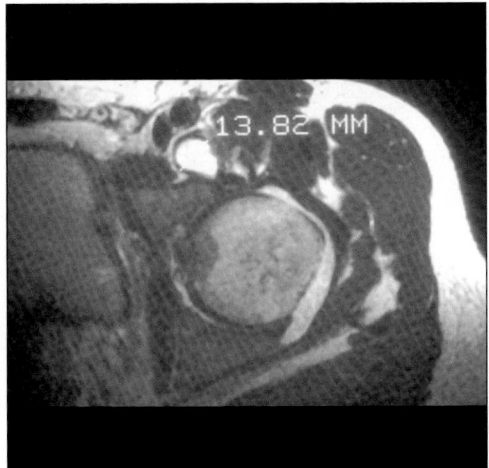

(Left) Coronal FS PD FSE MR shows anterior location of iliopsoas muscle and tendon (arrow). Tendon is hypointense relative to muscle. (Right) Axial T2WI MR shows hyperintense iliopsoas bursal fluid in communication with the hip joint. Patient presented with clicking of the hip.

Typical

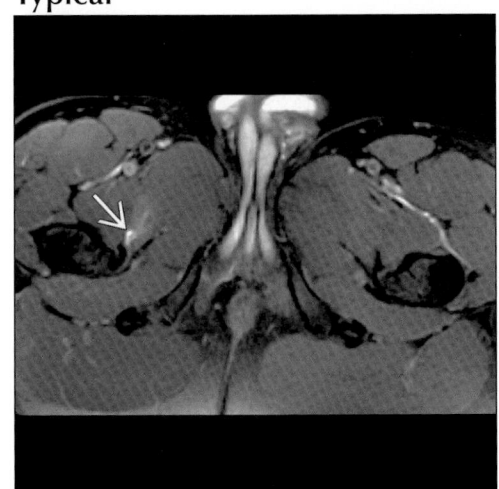
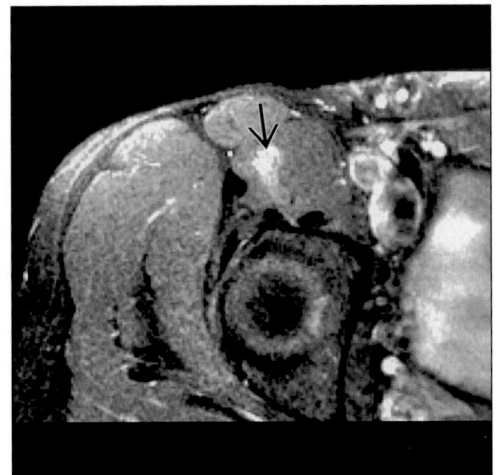

(Left) Axial FS PD FSE MR shows hyperintense fluid (arrow) associated with the insertion of right iliopsoas. This was associated with a more proximal bursal fluid collection in a patient presenting with snapping hip syndrome. (Right) Axial FS PD FSE MR shows dissection of bursal fluid into the iliopsoas muscle (arrow).

Typical

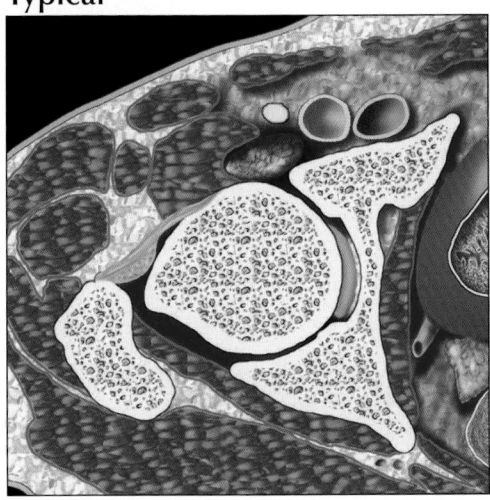
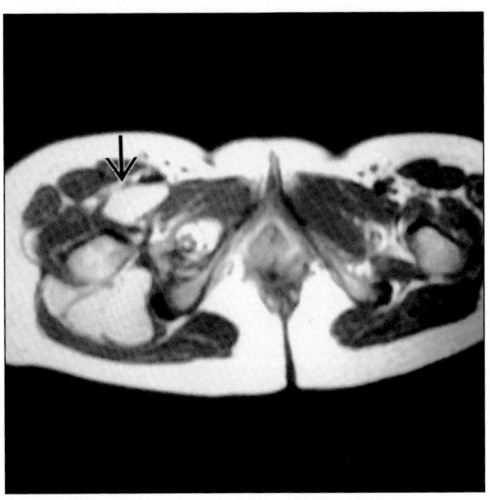

(Left) Axial graphic shows iliopsoas bursa medial to the iliopsoas muscle and anterior to the hip joint. (Right) Axial T2WI MR shows synovial fluid distension of right iliopsoas bursa (arrow), trochanteric and ischiotrochanteric bursa in a patient with rheumatoid arthritis.

SNAPPING HIP SYNDROME

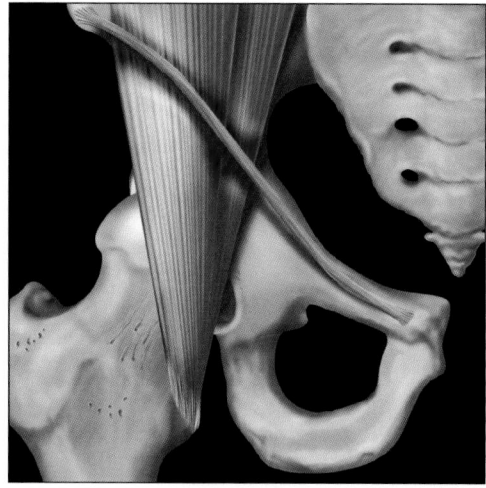

Coronal graphic shows iliopsoas impingement on the iliopectineal eminence during extension of the leg.

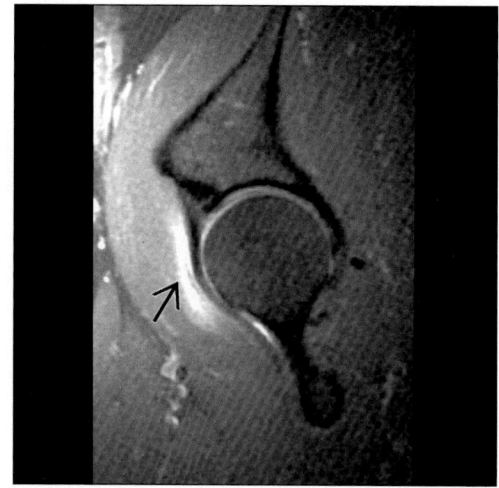

Sagittal FS PD FSE MR shows hyperintense edema parallel and anterior to the iliopsoas tendon (arrow).

TERMINOLOGY

Abbreviations and Synonyms
- Snapping hip, coxa saltans

Definitions
- Snapping or clicking sensation upon movement of hip

IMAGING FINDINGS

General Features
- Best diagnostic clue: Hyperintense inflammation of the greater trochanteric bursa or thickened iliotibial band on T2WI (external type)
- Location
  - External: Iliotibial tract
  - Internal : Iliopsoas tendon
  - Intraarticular: Loose bodies within hip joint
- Size
  - Variable based on causative factor
    - Iliotibial band, greater trochanteric bursa, anterior border gluteus maximus, femoral head, iliopectineal ridge, iliopectineal bursa, + lesser trochanter
- Morphology: Medial to lateral thickening of iliotibial band = snapping over greater trochanter

Radiographic Findings
- Radiography
  - Rarely helpful in internal or external etiologies
  - ± Identification for intraarticular etiologies (loose bodies, etc.)
  - Bursography: Injection of iliopsoas bursa with contrast during hip motion to assess iliopsoas muscle motion (rapid or jerky)

CT Findings
- NECT
  - ± Intraarticular etiology
  - Loose bodies + osteochondromatosis

MR Findings
- T1WI
  - External
    - Hypointense thickening of posterior iliotibial tract
    - Intermediate signal intensity thickening of greater trochanteric bursa
  - Internal
    - Iliopsoas bursa fluid (hypointense) distension medial to tendon
    - Marrow-containing (vs. cortical) exostosis projecting from lesser trochanter
  - Intraarticular
    - Hypointense, intermediate, or marrow fat signal intensity in loose bodies

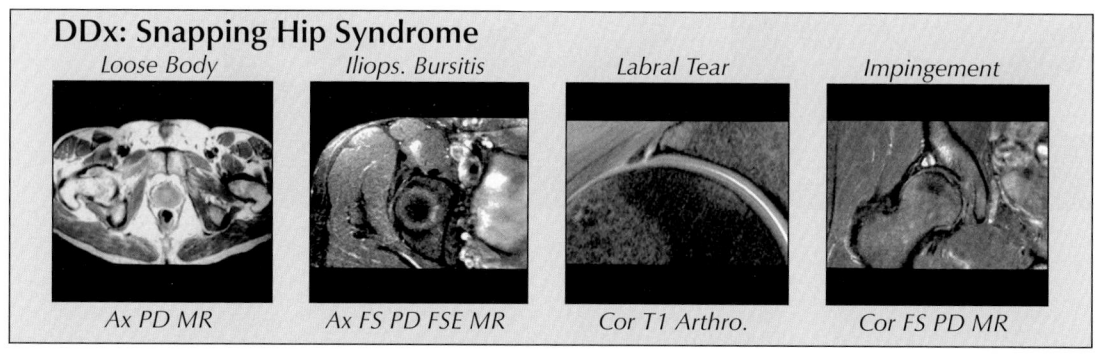

DDx: Snapping Hip Syndrome

Loose Body	Iliops. Bursitis	Labral Tear	Impingement
Ax PD MR	Ax FS PD FSE MR	Cor T1 Arthro.	Cor FS PD MR

SNAPPING HIP SYNDROME

Key Facts

Imaging Findings

- Best diagnostic clue: Hyperintense inflammation of the greater trochanteric bursa or thickened iliotibial band on T2WI (external type)
- Morphology: Medial to lateral thickening of iliotibial band = snapping over greater trochanter
- Hyperintense iliopsoas bursa fluid vs. tenosynovitis on T2WI

Top Differential Diagnoses

- Loose Bodies
- Iliopsoas Bursitis
- Labral Tears
- Synovial Chondromatosis
- Greater Trochanteric Bursitis

Pathology

- Intraarticular - labral or chondral fragments
- Epidemiology: Internal + external - individuals in dancing or athletics with no specific history of trauma
- Tight or thickened iliotibial band
- Tight iliopsoas

Clinical Issues

- Most common signs/symptoms: Palpable snap during hip flexion and extension
- Click (not snap) > intraarticular causes
- Pain with intraarticular etiologies

Diagnostic Checklist

- History + physical: Internal, external or intraarticular?

- T2WI
  - External
    - Hypointense to hyperintense iliotibial band + anterior border gluteus maximus
    - Hyperintense greater trochanteric bursa
  - Internal
    - Hyperintense iliopsoas bursa fluid vs. tenosynovitis on T2WI
  - Intraarticular
    - Hypointense to intermediate signal intensity of loose bodies adjacent to hyperintense joint fluid
- T1 C+: MR arthrography for labral tears + other intraarticular etiologies

Ultrasonographic Findings

- Real-time imaging during hip movement
- Sudden, abnormal movement of iliotibial band or gluteus maximus over greater trochanter
- Iliopsoas muscle movement over iliopectineal eminence, femoral head or lesser trochanter

Imaging Recommendations

- Best imaging tool
  - MR excellent for all etiologies
  - Ultrasound quick, non-invasive, but operator dependent
- Protocol advice: T1 + FS PD FSE in coronal, axial, + sagittal planes

DIFFERENTIAL DIAGNOSIS

Loose Bodies

- Cartilaginous or osteocartilaginous bodies in capsule or acetabular fossa
- Best visualized in contrast to adjacent hyperintense joint fluid on T2WI

Iliopsoas Bursitis

- Medial to iliopsoas tendon
- Enlargement of bursa with anterior convexity
- Uniform hyperintensity - most common appearance

Labral Tears

- Anterosuperior + posterosuperior tears most common
- Associated paralabral cysts

Synovial Chondromatosis

- Multiple intermediate signal intensity defects in joint fluid
- Morphology similar to synovial hyperplasia

Greater Trochanteric Bursitis

- Hyperintense thickening of bursa adjacent to greater trochanter on T2WI
- Frequently bilateral

Femoroacetabular Impingement

- Osteoarthritis in patients < 50 years
- Preferential acetabular chondral disease + labral tear prior to femoral head disease
- Non-dysplastic hips

PATHOLOGY

General Features

- General path comments
  - Relevant anatomy
    - Proximal iliotibial tract
    - Greater trochanter
    - Anterior margin gluteus maximus
    - Lesser trochanter
    - Iliopsoas tendon
    - Iliopectineal ridge
    - Iliopectineal bursa
    - Acetabulum
    - Femoral head
- Etiology
  - External - proximal iliotibial band slides over greater trochanter as hip extends from flexed position
  - Internal - iliopsoas tendon snaps over iliopectineal eminence
  - Intraarticular - labral or chondral fragments
  - Often related to tight tendons (taut iliotibial band)
  - Bursitis associated

SNAPPING HIP SYNDROME

○ Overuse
- Epidemiology: Internal + external - individuals in dancing or athletics with no specific history of trauma

Gross Pathologic & Surgical Features
- External
  ○ Tight or thickened iliotibial band
  ○ Bursitis or tendonitis
  ○ Gluteus maximus as causative structure associated with bursitis/tendonitis
- Internal
  ○ Tight iliopsoas
  ○ Associated bursitis/tendonitis
- Intraarticular
  ○ Loose bodies
  ○ Labral tear
  ○ Chondral lesions

Microscopic Features
- Inflammatory cells
- Synovial cells
- Fibrin/hemorrhage
- Fibrosis

CLINICAL ISSUES

Presentation
- Most common signs/symptoms: Palpable snap during hip flexion and extension
- Clinical profile
  ○ Pressure applied to greater trochanter will stop snapping with hip motion in external etiologies (iliotibial band reduced posterior to trochanter)
  ○ Snapping eliminated with internal etiologies by applying pressure over iliopsoas tendon at level of femoral head
  ○ Painful
  ○ Audible snap
  ○ Click (not snap) > intraarticular causes
  ○ Pain with intraarticular etiologies

Demographics
- Age: Young adults 15-40 years most common
- Gender: Females with slight predilection (depending on type of activity)
- At risk
  ○ Ballet dancers

Natural History & Prognosis
- Most cases mildly symptomatic
- Intraarticular pathology may show continued progression of pathology and symptoms (e.g., chondral degeneration)
- Improvement with conservative measures including activity modification

Treatment
- Conservative
  ○ Decrease causative activity
  ○ Anti-inflammatory medications
  ○ Steroid injections
  ○ Physical therapy
- Surgical
  ○ Partial tendon + bursa resection

○ Tendon lengthening procedures
○ Arthroscopy for intraarticular lesions (e.g., loose body removal, debridement of chondral lesions)

DIAGNOSTIC CHECKLIST

Consider
- History + physical: Internal, external or intraarticular?
- MRI excellent for intraarticular evaluation
- Sonography to evaluate iliotibial band, gluteus maximus or iliopsoas

SELECTED REFERENCES

1. DeLee JC et al: Orthopaedic sports medicine. Principles and practice. vol 2. 2nd ed. Philadelphia PA, Saunders, (25 A):1443-62, 2003
2. Bellabarba C et al: Idiopathic hip instability. An unrecognized cause of coxa saltans in the adult. Clin Orthop 355:261, 1998
3. Cardinal E et al: Ultrasound of the snapping iliopsoas tendon. Radiology 198:521, 1996
4. Janzen DL et al: The snapping hip: Clinical and imaging findings in the transient subluxation of the iliopsoas tendon. Can Assoc Radiol J 47:202, 1996
5. Allen WC et al: Coxa saltans: The snapping hip syndrome. J Am Acad Orthop Surg 3:303, 1995
6. Taylor GR et al: Surgical release of the "snapping iliopsoas tendon." J Bone Joint Surg Br 77:881, 1995
7. Vaccaro JP et al: Iliopsoas bursa imaging: Efficacy in snapping hip syndrome. Radiology 197:853, 1995
8. Brignall CG et al: The snapping hip syndrome: Treatment by Z-plasty. J Bone Joint Surg Br 73:253, 1991
9. Jacobson T et al: Surgical correction of the snapping iliopsoas tendon. Am J Sports Med 18:470, 1990
10. Silver SF et al: Case report 550. Skel Radiol 18:327, 1989
11. Glick JM: Hip arthroscopy using the lateral approach. Instr Course Lect 37:223, 1988
12. Staple TW et al: Snapping tendon syndrome: Hip tenography with fluoroscopic monitoring. Radiology 166:873, 1988
13. Harper MC et al: Primary iliopsoas bursography in the diagnosis of disorders of the hip. Clin Orthop 221:238, 1987
14. Scharberg JE et al: The snapping hip syndrome. Am J Sprots Med 12:361, 1984
15. Lyons JC et al: The snapping iliopsoas tendon. Mayo Clin Proc 59:327, 1984
16. House AJG: Orthopaedists and ballet. Clin Orthop 89:52, 1972

SNAPPING HIP SYNDROME

IMAGE GALLERY

Typical

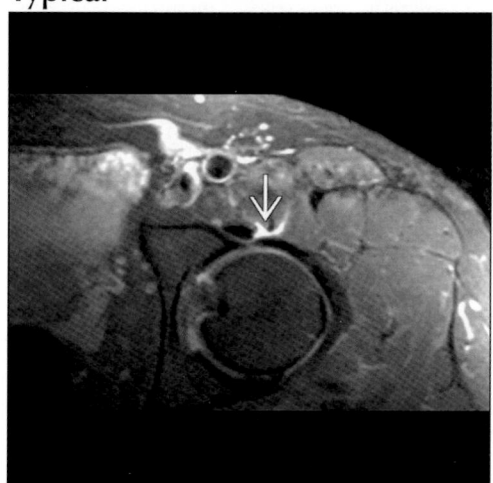
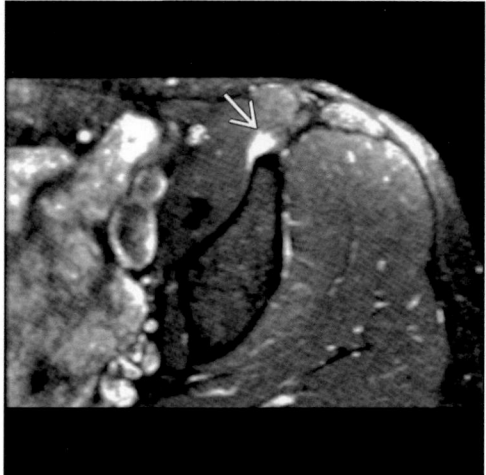

(Left) Axial FS PD FSE MR shows focal hyperintensity *(arrow)* adjacent and lateral to the iliopsoas tendon *(hypointense structure abutting anterior acetabulum)*. *(Right)* Axial FS PD FSE MR shows hyperintense fluid collection *(arrow)* deep to the iliopsoas muscle and adjacent to the anterior inferior iliac spine.

Typical

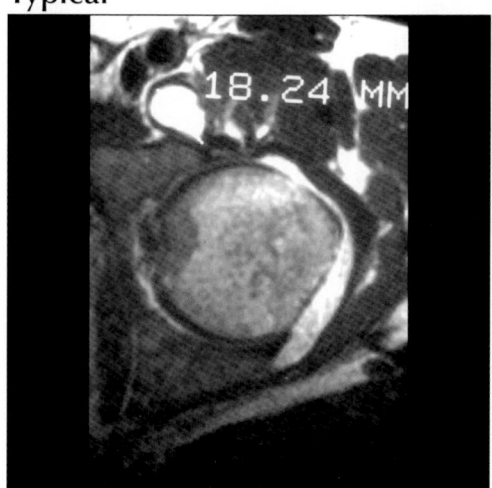
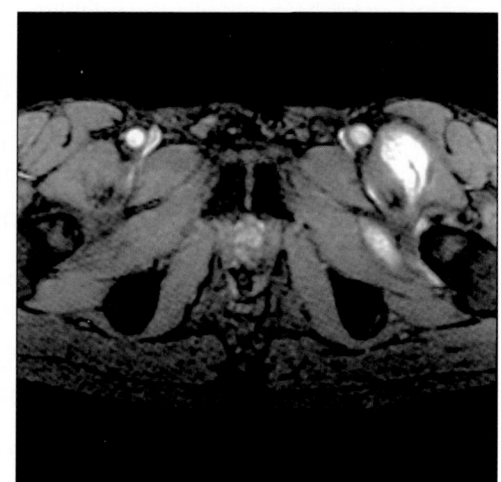

(Left) Axial T2WI MR shows an iliopsoas bursal fluid collection which was treated conservatively in a patient with snapping hip syndrome. *(Right)* Axial FS PD FSE MR shows anterior intramuscular extension of left iliopsoas bursa.

Typical

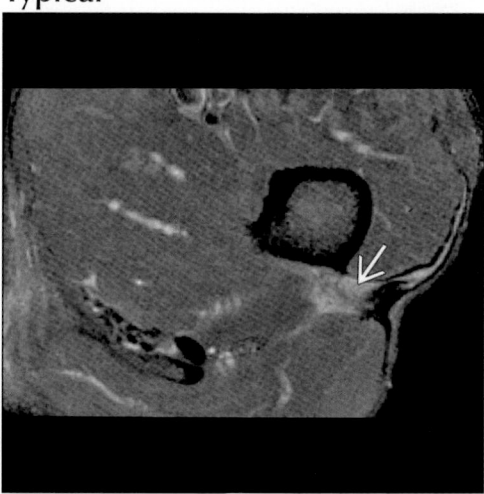
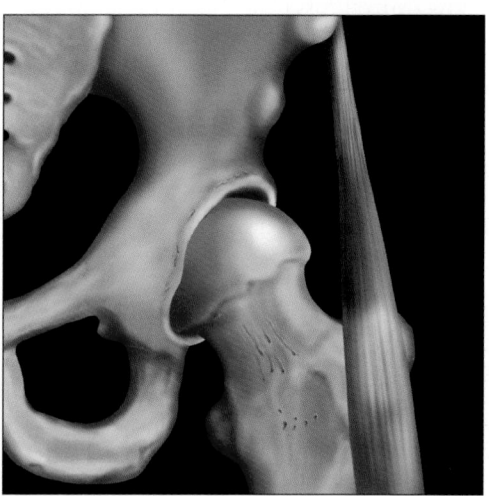

(Left) Axial FS PD FSE MR of the left hip shows posttraumatic hyperintense edema *(arrow)* medial to the iliotibial band. *(Right)* Coronal graphic of thickened iliotibial band in contact with greater trochanter.

FEMORAL HEAD FRACTURES

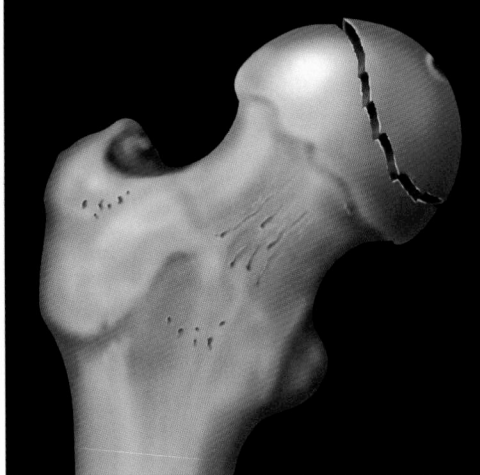

Coronal graphic shows nondisplaced femoral head fracture.

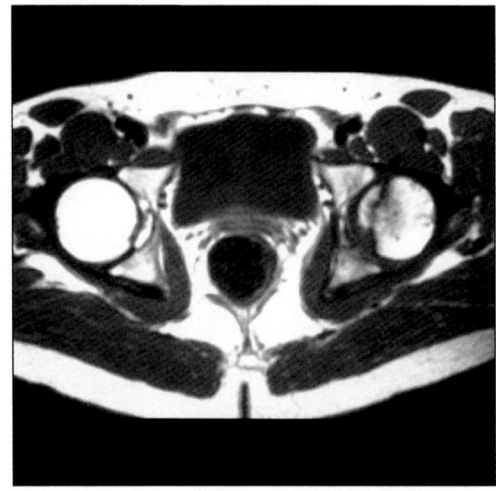

Axial T1WI MR shows medial capital fracture on the left with complete anterior to posterior extension.

TERMINOLOGY

Abbreviations and Synonyms
- Fractures of femoral head, capital fracture

Definitions
- Fracture (fx) of femoral head, usually associated with posterior hip dislocation

IMAGING FINDINGS

General Features
- Best diagnostic clue: Oblique fx femoral head relative to long axis of femoral neck
- Location: Femoral head
- Size
  - Fracture size increases if involves central fossa (fovea)
  - Smaller fractures located below central fossa
- Morphology: Oblique to vertical as viewed in coronal plane - most common

Radiographic Findings
- Radiography
  - Initial diagnostic examination
  - Anteroposterior view usually diagnostic
  - Lateral view - location of femoral head + fracture fragments
  - Oblique view (Judet views)
    - Fracture evaluation + acetabular evaluation

CT Findings
- NECT
  - Intraarticular fragments visualized
  - Multiplanar capability - for surgical planning

MR Findings
- T1WI
  - Hypointense fracture line
  - Localized to more diffuse hypointense femoral head edema
  - Hypointense to intermediate signal intensity hemorrhagic effusion
- T2WI
  - Hyperintense femoral head edema + effusions on T2WI
  - Evaluate complications
    - Muscle strains/tears - hyperintense
    - Labral tears: ± Hyperintense paralabral cysts
    - Chondral injuries - interruption of intermediate signal chondral surface
    - Avascular necrosis

Imaging Recommendations
- Best imaging tool
  - CT used for hip dislocations with fracture of the femoral head

---

DDx: Femoral Head Fractures

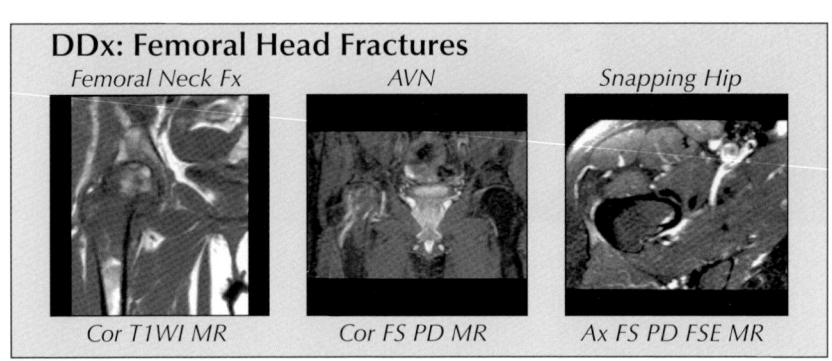

Femoral Neck Fx	AVN	Snapping Hip
Cor T1WI MR	Cor FS PD MR	Ax FS PD FSE MR

4

46

FEMORAL HEAD FRACTURES

Key Facts

Imaging Findings
- Best diagnostic clue: Oblique fx femoral head relative to long axis of femoral neck
- Fracture size increases if involves central fossa (fovea)
- Hyperintense femoral head edema + effusions on T2WI

Top Differential Diagnoses
- Femoral Neck Fracture
- Acetabular Fracture
- Pelvic Fracture
- Femoral Head Avascular Necrosis (AVN)

Pathology
- Shearing force from dislocation of hip
- Most commonly with posterior dislocation 2° motor vehicle accident (MVA)

- High energy injuries
- Associated sciatic nerve compression in posterior dislocation
- Pipkin classification for femoral head fracture dislocations

Clinical Issues
- Most common signs/symptoms: Pain in hip area
- Reduce hip ASAP - risk of AVN increases > 6 hrs
- Associated morbidity/mortality 2° to associated head, abdominal + pelvic trauma
- Age: Young adults - high-energy trauma victims (< 35 years) + trauma 2° to fall (> 65 years)

Diagnostic Checklist
- Association of femoral head fractures with posterior hip dislocations

---

- ○ MR used as primary exam in isolated capital fractures
- Protocol advice
  - ○ 1 mm thin section CT through acetabulum + femoral head
    - ▪ Coronal & sagittal reformations
  - ○ MR: Coronal, axial & sagittal T1 + FS PD FSE

DIFFERENTIAL DIAGNOSIS

Femoral Neck Fracture
- Subcortical
- Stress - groin, anterior thigh or knee pain (transverse + compression)
- Pauwels' classification - based on angulation of fracture line to the horizontal plane
- Garden classification - based on displacement of fragments

Acetabular Fracture
- Blunt high energy injuries
- Judet-Letournel classification of five elementary fractures based on column & wall involvement
- Complications = heterotropic ossification

Pelvic Fracture
- High energy pelvic fractures associated with hemorrhage
- Benign avulsion to massive pelvic disruptions
- Stable, rotationally unstable/vertically stable to rationally & vertically unstable

Femoral Head Avascular Necrosis (AVN)
- Necrotic segment → collapse anterosuperior aspect femoral head
- Traumatic vs. non-traumatic
- Associated with displaced fracture femoral neck + hip dislocation
- Groin or hip pain

Stress Fracture
- Pelvic stress fractures

- Pubic bone stress fractures - associated with long-distance running
- Sacrum - runners at risk; bilateral stress fractures with "H" sign on MRI

Snapping Hip Syndrome
- Painful, audible snap in hip flexion + extension
- External, internal or intraarticular etiologies
- Iliotibial band = external cause (sliding over greater trochanter), internal type = iliopsoas tendon catching

Slipped Capital Femoral Epiphysis
- Posterior inferior displacement proximal femoral epiphysis
- Childhood disorder
- Slip - in zone of hypertrophy in growth plate
- Pain + limp

PATHOLOGY

General Features
- General path comments
  - ○ Relevant anatomy
    - ▪ Vascular supply to head + neck originates from medial + lateral femoral circumflex arteries
    - ▪ Extracapsular vascular ring - cervical arteries
    - ▪ Ligamentum teres vascular supply to head insignificant in adult
    - ▪ Femoral head = multiaxial, synovial ball-and-socket joint
- Etiology
  - ○ Shearing force from dislocation of hip
  - ○ Most commonly with posterior dislocation 2° motor vehicle accident (MVA)
  - ○ High energy injuries
- Epidemiology
  - ○ Fractures of femoral head associated with posterior dislocations
  - ○ Rare relative to incidence of dislocations

Gross Pathologic & Surgical Features
- ± Fragmentation of surrounding osseous + cartilaginous structures

FEMORAL HEAD FRACTURES

- Entrapped fragments in joint
- Associated sciatic nerve compression in posterior dislocation
- Pipkin classification for femoral head fracture dislocations
  - I: Fracture caudad (below) central fovea + disrupted ligamentum teres
  - II: Fracture cephalad to fovea + ligamentum teres remains attached to fracture fragment
  - III: Femoral head fracture (Pipkin I or II) associated femoral neck fracture (± due to over aggressive closed reduction)
  - IV: Femoral head fracture (Pipkin I or II) + superoposterior acetabular rim fracture
- ± Impaction fracture
- Adolescents may shear off capital femoral epiphysis

Microscopic Features
- Fracture - vascular disruption
  - Hematoma
  - Revascularization
  - Callus vs. primary bone repair

Staging, Grading or Classification Criteria
- Pipkin classification for femoral head fracture
  - I: Below ligamentum teres - no associated injuries
  - II: Above ligamentum teres - no associated injuries
  - III: Either below or above - femoral neck fracture associated
  - IV: Either below or above - acetabular fracture

CLINICAL ISSUES

Presentation
- Most common signs/symptoms: Pain in hip area
- Clinical profile
  - Dislocated hip = 1st concern
  - Reduce hip ASAP - risk of AVN increases > 6 hrs
  - Maximum 2-3 attempts at closed reduction due to risk of AVN + iatrogenic injury
  - Associated morbidity/mortality 2° to associated head, abdominal + pelvic trauma

Demographics
- Age: Young adults - high-energy trauma victims (< 35 years) + trauma 2° to fall (> 65 years)
- Gender: Young males most common

Natural History & Prognosis
- Anatomic/near anatomic fracture alignment essential in younger patients
  - Preserve function and avoid complications (AVN, osteoarthritis)
- Outcome dependent on
  - Femoral head fracture type
  - ± Associated fractures (acetabular, femoral neck, pelvic ring)
  - Length of time until reduction
- Pipkin I & II - better prognosis than III & IV
- Open reduction indications
  - Failed closed reduction
  - Femoral neck fracture
  - Incongruent reduction
  - Intraarticular fragments

- Fracture repair

Treatment
- Conservative = Pipkin I
  - Closed reduction preferred
  - Displaced inferior fragment acceptable if does not involve weight bearing portion
  - Pipkin II - closed reduction only if fracture fragments congruent
- Surgical
  - Pipkin II - open reduction with internal fixation (ORIF) for displaced/unstable fracture fragments
  - Pipkin III - ORIF for younger patients (rigid pinning) & hemiprosthesis for older patients
  - Pipkin IV - ORIF for displaced/unstable acetabular fracture in younger patient + total arthroplasty in older individuals
  - Impacted femoral head fractures - surgically elevate & graft
  - Post reduction treatment - traction, minimal weight bearing, physical therapy
- Complications
  - AVN
  - Post-traumatic arthritis
  - Recurrent dislocation
  - Sciatic nerve injury

DIAGNOSTIC CHECKLIST

Consider
- Association of femoral head fractures with posterior hip dislocations
- Identify femoral head fracture orientation relative to fovea

SELECTED REFERENCES

1. LaVelle DG: Campbell's operative orthopaedics. vol 4. 10th ed. Philadelphia PA, Elsevier Science, 2922-8, 2003
2. Fitzgerald RH et al: Orthopaedics. St. Louis MO, Mosby, (3-13):346-88, 2002
3. Mostafa MM: Femoral head fractures. International Orthop 25:51-4, 2001
4. Bucholz RW et al: Rockwood and Green's fractures in adults. 5th ed. Philadelphia PA, Lippincott Williams & Wilkins, 1547-78, 2001
5. Harris JH Jr: Pelvis, acetabulum and hips. The radiology of emergency medicine. 4th ed. Philadelphia PA, Lippincott Williams & Wilkins, 796-97, 2000
6. Dreinhofer KE et al: Isolated traumatic dislocation of the hip: Long-term results in 50 patients. J Bone Joint Surg Br 76:6, 1994
7. Levin PE: Hip dislocations: Skeletal Trauma. vol 2. Philadelphia PA, WB Saunders, 1992
8. Epstein HC: Traumatic dislocation of the hip. Baltimore MA, Williams & Wilkins, 1980

FEMORAL HEAD FRACTURES

IMAGE GALLERY

Typical

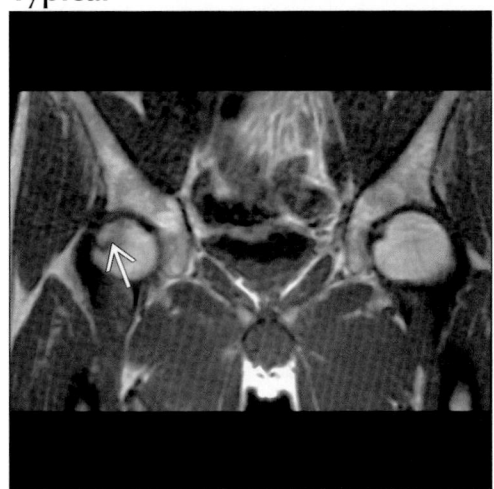 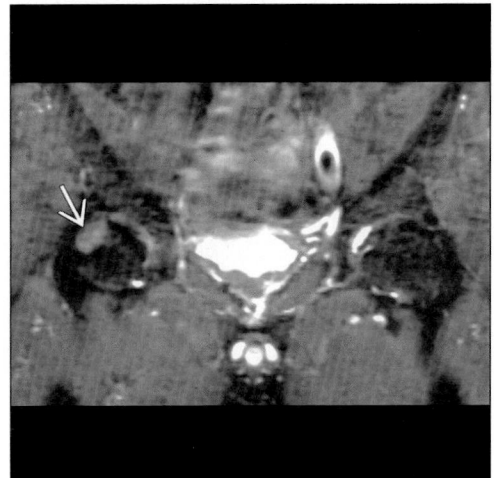

(Left) Coronal T1WI MR shows right nondisplaced fracture (arrow) of anterosuperior femoral head with hypointense fracture line. *(Right)* Coronal FS PD FSE MR shows hyperintense marrow edema (arrow) in a nondisplaced capital fracture involving the right hip.

Typical

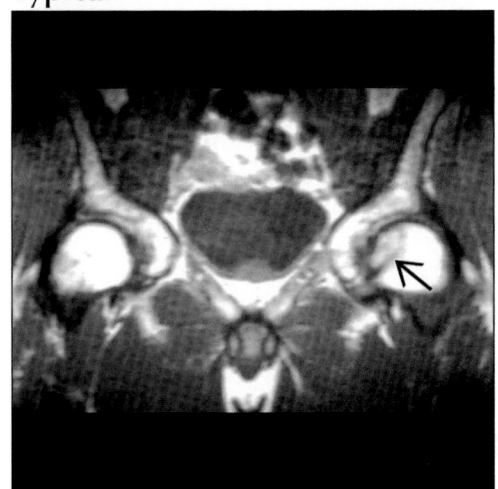 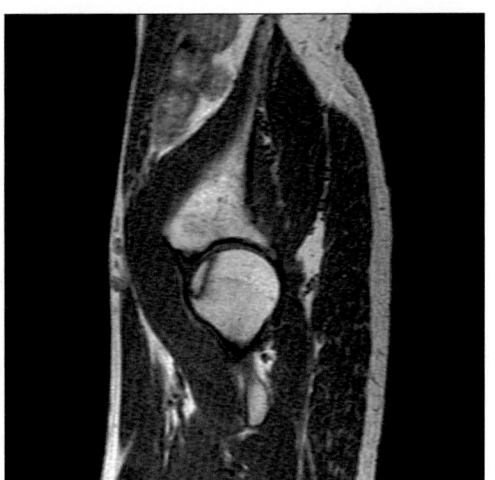

(Left) Coronal T1WI MR shows left medial capital fracture (arrow). *(Right)* Sagittal T1WI MR shows anterior capital fracture.

Typical

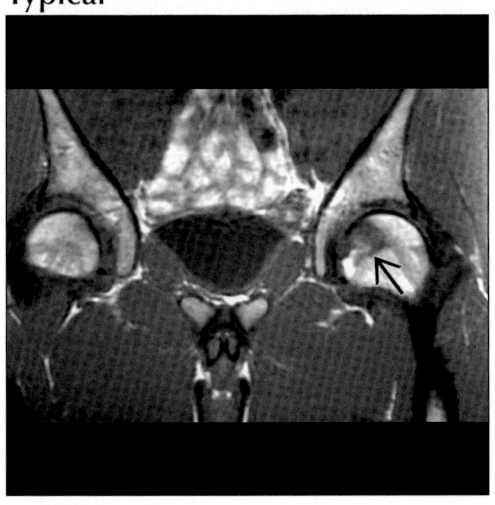 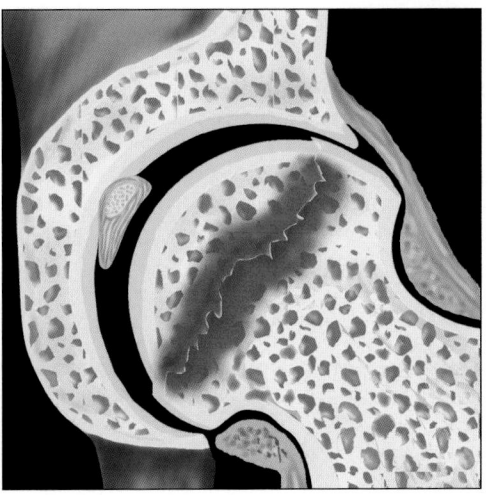

(Left) Coronal T1WI MR shows left osseous contusion with linear trabecular fracture (arrow) line parallel to physeal scar. *(Right)* Coronal graphic shows nondisplaced capital fracture with reactive marrow edema (red). Fracture line extends to the chondral surfaces.

FEMORAL NECK FRACTURES

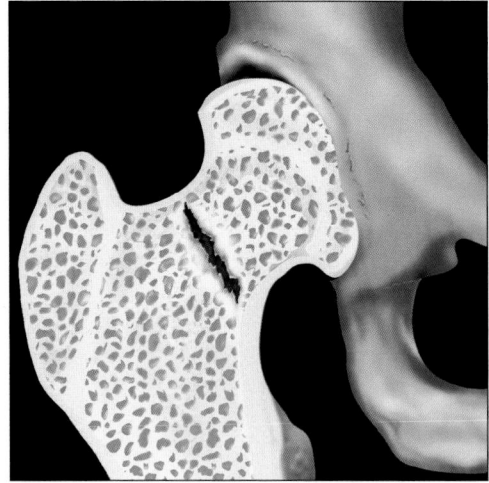

Coronal graphic shows stress fracture perpendicular to the long axis of the femoral neck.

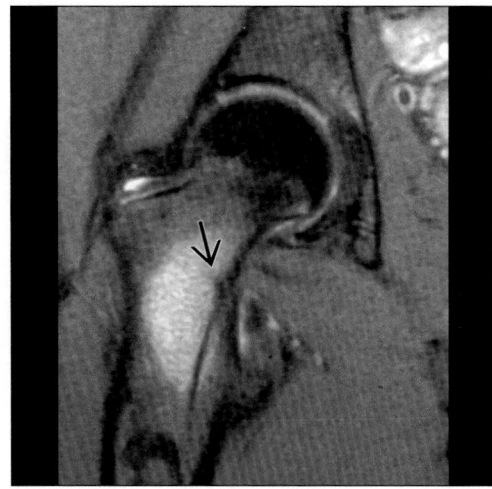

Coronal FS PD FSE MR shows medial femoral neck stress fracture (arrow) with associated subchondral hyperintense marrow edema.

TERMINOLOGY

Abbreviations and Synonyms
- Fracture of the proximal femur, subcapital femoral neck fracture, stress fracture, insufficiency fracture (fx)

Definitions
- Intracapsular femoral neck fractures = subcapital (common), transcervical (uncommon) or basicervical (uncommon)

IMAGING FINDINGS

General Features
- Best diagnostic clue: Medial femoral neck hyperintensity on FS PD FSE or STIR images
- Location
  - Subcapital
  - Transcervical
  - Basicervical
- Size
  - Incomplete to complete traversing femoral neck
  - Subchondral edema ↑ extensive than associated fx
- Morphology
  - Focal involvement of medial cortex
  - Fracture plane obliquity ranges from 30 degrees or less to > than 70 degrees (from horizontal)
  - Transverse vs. compression (medial) stress fractures

Radiographic Findings
- Radiography
  - Subcapital fracture
    - Pauwels classification based on direction of fracture angle from 0 to > 70 degrees
    - Garden classification based on displacement of fracture fragments

CT Findings
- NECT
  - Coronal reformations
  - Assess fracture obliquity (more vertical fractures are less stable) + displacement

MR Findings
- T1WI
  - Hypointense signal medial femoral neck in stress fracture
  - Discrete well-defined hypointense fracture line ± complete extension across femoral neck
  - Microtrabecular stress fracture with intact medial + lateral cortices
  - Hypointense joint effusion/hemorrhage ± synovitis
  - Early detection of hypointense sclerosis in avascular necrosis (AVN)
- T2WI
  - Hyperintense marrow edema on T2WI

DDx: Femoral Neck Fractures

AVN	Osteoarthritis	TOH	Cyst	Metastases
Sag T1WI MR	Cor T1WI MR	Cor T1WI MR	Cor FS PD MR	Cor T1WI MR

FEMORAL NECK FRACTURES

Key Facts

Imaging Findings

- Best diagnostic clue: Medial femoral neck hyperintensity on FS PD FSE or STIR images
- Incomplete to complete traversing femoral neck
- Subchondral edema ↑ extensive than associated fx
- Hyperintense marrow edema on T2WI

Top Differential Diagnoses

- Contusion
- AVN of the Femoral Head
- Osteoarthritis
- Transient Osteoporosis of Hip (TOH)
- Osseous Lesions

Pathology

- Fall with impact on greater trochanter + lateral rotation of femur

- Cyclic loading + microfracture + torsional force

Clinical Issues

- Most common signs/symptoms: Pain in groin, anterior thigh or knee
- Pain increased with weight-bearing or exertion
- Limitation of hip motion (internal rotation)
- Pain with axial compression or greater trochanter percussion
- Transverse stress fractures - risk for displacement
- Compression stress fractures - low risk for displacement

Diagnostic Checklist

- MR evaluation of contralateral side to evaluate for bilateral stress fractures

- Hypointense fracture line on T2WI - common
- Pathologic fractures associated with marrow replacement + trabecular destruction
- Direct visualization of associated chondral lesions in acetabulum + femoral head
- ± Associated hyperintense acetabulum & edema in trabecular microfracture
- Adjacent soft tissue edema + hemorrhage demonstrates hyperintensity
- T1 C+: Assess femoral head perfusion: Uniform increased signal intensity with intact perfusion

Imaging Recommendations

- Best imaging tool
  - MR identifies stress fracture, microtrabecular fracture + edema
  - Nondisplaced femoral neck fractures may not be visualized on conventional radiographs
- Protocol advice
  - Coronal T1 (for marrow fat signal contrast) + FS PD FSE or STIR
  - Secondary use of axial + sagittal planes

DIFFERENTIAL DIAGNOSIS

Contusion

- Hyperintense trabecular edema without fracture line or cortical irregularity on T2WI
- Symptoms may mimic stress fracture
- Pre-stress fracture stage

AVN of the Femoral Head

- Wedge-shaped subchondral bone infarct
- Double-line sign in 80%
- Articular cartilage intact initially

Osteoarthritis

- Loss of joint space with loss of articular cartilage
- Hypointense thickened stress trabeculae (calcar buttressing) on T1 + T2WI
- Ring of osteophytes
- Superolateral migration of femoral head

Transient Osteoporosis of Hip (TOH)

- Self-limiting
- Middle-aged males > pregnant females
- Progressive demineralization of femoral head
- Joint space preserved
- Diffuse hyperintensity femoral head + neck

Piriformis Syndrome

- Piriformis hypertrophy
- Muscle edema on FS PD FSE MR
- Fibrosis

Snapping Hip Syndrome

- Audible snap during hip flexion + extension
- External, internal or intraarticular etiologies
- External = iliotibial tract contact with greater trochanter
- Internal = iliopsoas tendon catching on structures posterior to it

Osseous Lesions

- Cyst - hypointense on T1WI, hyperintense on T2WI
- Metastatic disease - e.g., breast, prostate + lung
- Cystic erosion 2° to synovial inflammatory process

Greater Trochanteric Bursitis

- Tenderness over greater trochanter
- Symptoms increased with hip external rotation + adduction
- Irritation by iliotibial band
- Hyperintense edema or fluid adjacent + parallel to greater trochanter on FS PD FSE MR

PATHOLOGY

General Features

- General path comments
  - Relevant anatomy
    - Calcar femorale = weight-bearing bone of femur from inferomedial femoral neck cortex toward lesser trochanter

FEMORAL NECK FRACTURES

- Blood supply to femoral head - via femoral neck from branches of circumflex arteries
- Etiology
  - Fall with impact on greater trochanter + lateral rotation of femur
  - Cyclic loading + microfracture + torsional force
  - Direct trauma
  - Training errors, improper footwear + uneven running surfaces (stress fxs)
  - Coxa vara = predisposes athlete to risk of fracture
- Epidemiology
  - 15% of runners develop a stress fracture
    - 5-10% of stress fractures involve femoral neck

Gross Pathologic & Surgical Features
- Pauwels classification of femoral neck fractures
  - Pauwels I: Fracture line 0-30 degrees to horizontal
  - Pauwels II: Fracture line 30 to 70 degrees to horizontal
  - Pauwels III: Fracture line > 70 degrees to horizontal
- Garden classification of femoral neck fractures
  - Garden I: Incomplete or impacted
  - Garden II: Complete nondisplaced
  - Garden III: Complete with partial displacement
  - Garden IV: Complete fracture with total displacement
- Stress fracture - Blickenstaff & Morris classification
  - Type I: Endosteal or periosteal callus without fracture line
  - Type II: Fracture line
  - Type III: Displaced

Microscopic Features
- Vascular disruption of bone
- Hematoma
- Revascularization
- Resorption of devascularized bone
- Healing with callus vs. primary bone repair

Staging, Grading or Classification Criteria
- Blickenstaff/Morris classification for stress fractures
- Pauwels & Garden classification for femoral neck fractures

CLINICAL ISSUES

Presentation
- Most common signs/symptoms: Pain in groin, anterior thigh or knee
- Clinical profile
  - Pain increased with weight-bearing or exertion
  - Limitation of hip motion (internal rotation)
  - Pain with axial compression or greater trochanter percussion

Demographics
- Age
  - Transverse stress fractures (typically insufficiency fxs) = common in older patients (involves superior cortex of neck)
  - Compression stress fractures = common in younger patients (50% of fractures < 60 years)
- Gender

- Military population - male trainees with increased body mass index + poor fitness
- Female athletes - at risk with eating disorder, amenorrhea, premature osteoporosis

Natural History & Prognosis
- Transverse stress fractures - risk for displacement
- Compression stress fractures - low risk for displacement
- Surgical treatment for distraction injuries
- Early diagnosis + aggressive treatment required
- Healing: 6-12 months
- Complications: Delayed union, non-union, AVN (10-30%), secondary degenerative osteoarthritis

Treatment
- Conservative
  - Pre-fracture stress reaction = non weight-bearing until pain free → progressive weight-bearing
  - Compression stress fractures (medial) if nondisplaced = non weight-bearing
- Surgical
  - Tension-transverse stress fractures = immediate internal fixation regardless of the degree of displacement
  - Displaced = anatomic reduction + internal fixation
  - Knowles pinning
  - Endoprosthesis

DIAGNOSTIC CHECKLIST

Consider
- MR evaluation of contralateral side to evaluate for bilateral stress fractures
- Hyperintense bone marrow edema (T2WI) in the absence of a fracture line - document cortical + trabecular integrity with CT

SELECTED REFERENCES

1. DeLee JC et al: Orthopaedic sports medicine. Principles and practice. vol 2. 2nd ed. Philadelphia PA, Saunders, (25):1443-62, 2003
2. Spitz DJ et al: Imaging of stress fractures in the athlete. Radiol Clin North Am 40(2):313-31, 2002
3. Jackson M et al: The treatment of non-union after intracapsular fracture of the proximal femur. Clin Orthop 399:119-28, 2002
4. Bailie DS et al: Bilateral femoral neck stress fractures in a adolescent male runner. A case report. Am J Sports Med 29(6):811-3, 2001
5. Bosch E et al: Difficult-to-detect osseous injuries. Physician Sportsmed 21:116-22, 1993
6. Daffner RH et al: Stress fractures: Current concepts. AJR 159:245-52, 1992
7. Meaney JEM et al: Femoral stress fractures in children. Skeletal Radiol 21:173-6, 1992
8. Mink JH et al: Occult cartilage and bone injuries of the knee: Detection, classification, and assessment with MR. Radiology 170:823-9, 1989
9. Lee JK et al: Stress fractures: MR imaging. Radiology 169:217-20, 1988
10. Stafford SA et al: MRI in stress fracture. AJR 147:553-6, 1986

IMAGE GALLERY

Typical

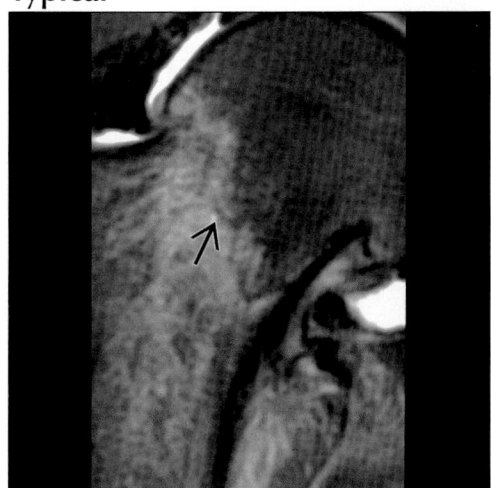 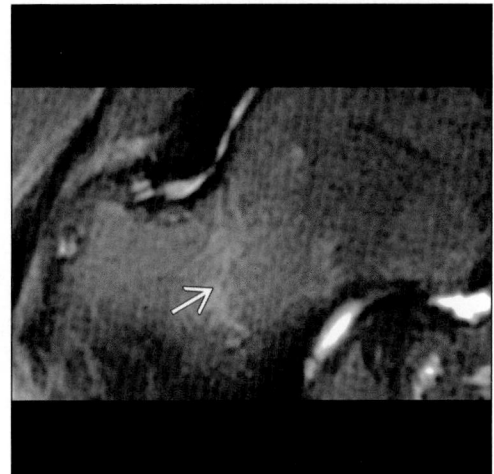

(Left) Coronal FS PD FSE MR shows hyperintense edema associated with acute femoral neck stress fracture (arrow). Note the more vertical orientation of the fracture. (Right) Coronal FS PD FSE MR shows early or pre-stress fracture stage with subtle trabecular linear hyperintensity (arrow). The medial and lateral cortices are intact.

Typical

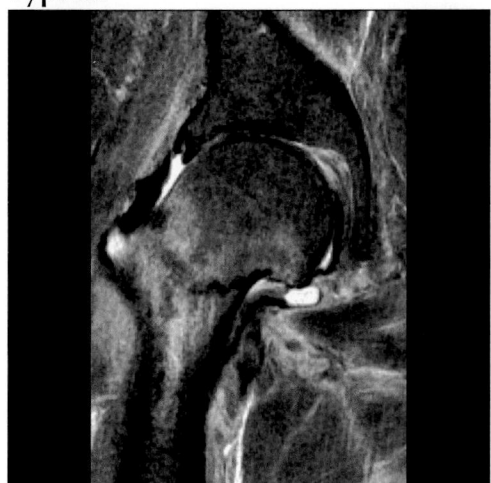 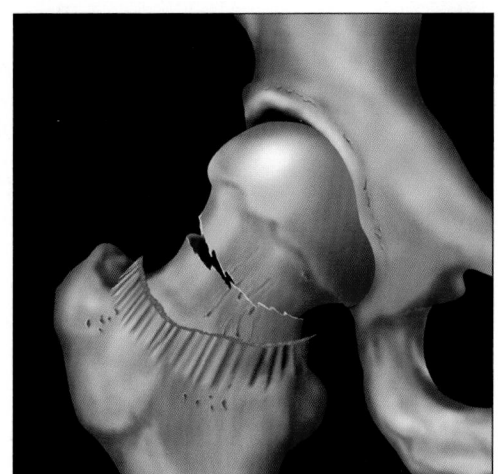

(Left) Coronal FS PD FSE MR shows complete transverse femoral neck fracture. (Right) Coronal graphic shows complete femoral neck fracture with displacement.

Variant

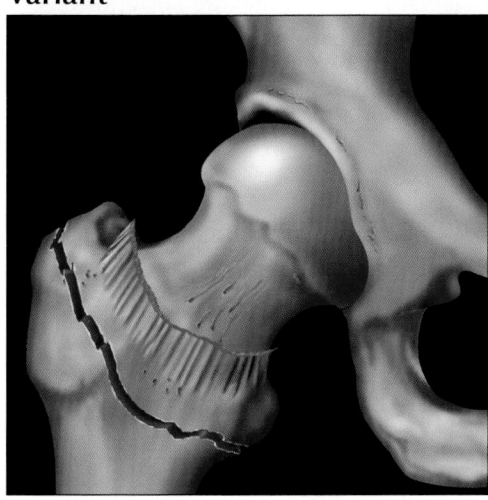 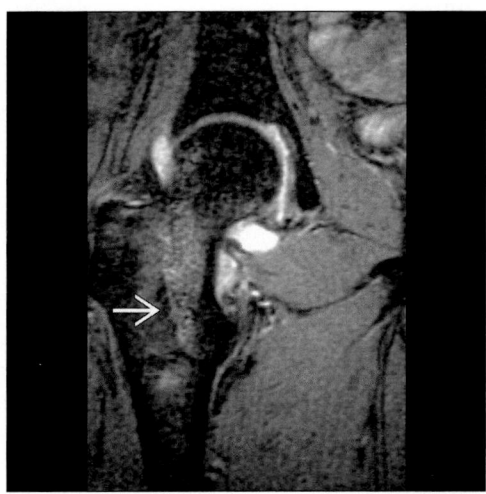

(Left) Coronal graphic shows intertrochanteric fracture extending from the greater to the lesser trochanter. (Right) Coronal T2* GRE MR shows hyperintense edema associated with hypointense fracture line (arrow) in an acute intertrochanteric fracture.

ACETABULAR FRACTURES

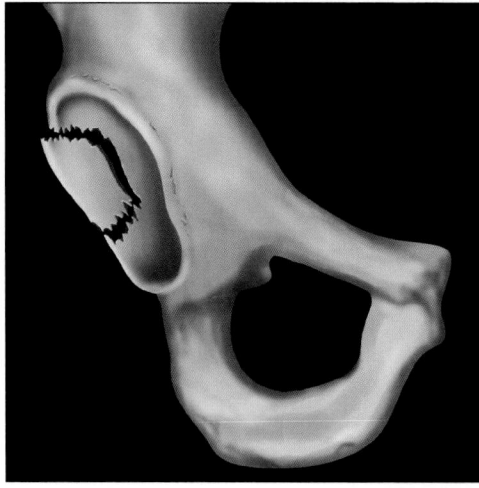

Coronal graphic shows posterior wall acetabular fracture.

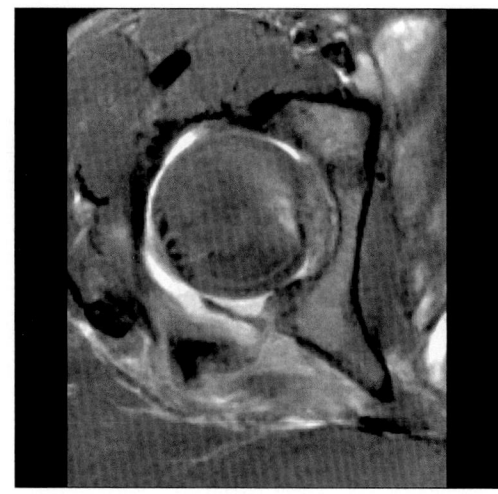

Axial FS PD FSE MR shows posterior wall fracture after posterior dislocation of the hip.

TERMINOLOGY

Abbreviations and Synonyms
- Acetabular trauma, fractures of the acetabulum

Definitions
- Fracture of the acetabulum of the hip, usually secondary to significant trauma

IMAGING FINDINGS

General Features
- Best diagnostic clue: Interruption of acetabular osseous column cortices
- Location
  - Anterior (iliopubic/iliopectineal) column
  - Posterior (ilioischial) column
  - Anterior/posterior (transverse)
  - Complex (T-shaped or stellate)
- Size: Variable based on simple vs. combination fracture types
- Morphology
  - Simple
    - Posterior wall
    - Anterior wall
    - Transverse
    - Anterior column

- Posterior column
  - Combination
    - Posterior column + posterior wall
    - Transverse + posterior wall
    - Complete (both column) = anterior + posterior columns
    - T-shaped
    - Anterior column + posterior hemitransverse

Radiographic Findings
- Radiography
  - Anteroposterior (AP) view pelvis
  - Oblique views (Judet views)
    - Iliac oblique view = 45° external oblique for evaluation of posterior column + anterior wall
    - Obturator oblique view = 45° internal oblique for evaluation of anterior column + posterior wall
  - Iliopectineal or iliopubic line: Disruption = fracture anterior column
  - Ilioischial line: Disruption = fracture posterior column
  - Pelvic inlet/outlet views: Pelvic ring fractures
  - Radiographs may underestimate fracture complexity & intraarticular fragments

CT Findings
- NECT
  - Intraarticular fragment visualization

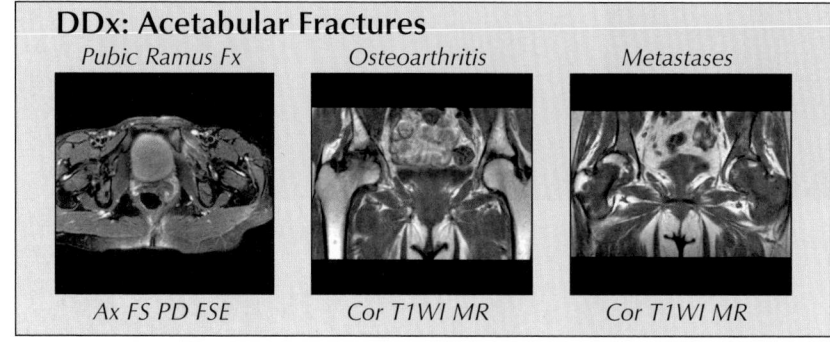

DDx: Acetabular Fractures

Pubic Ramus Fx	Osteoarthritis	Metastases
Ax FS PD FSE	*Cor T1WI MR*	*Cor T1WI MR*

ACETABULAR FRACTURES

Imaging Findings

- Best diagnostic clue: Interruption of acetabular osseous column cortices
- Anterior (iliopubic/iliopectineal) column
- Posterior (ilioischial) column
- Anterior/posterior (transverse)
- Complex (T-shaped or stellate)

Top Differential Diagnoses

- Hip Dislocations
- Avulsion Fractures
- Pelvic Ring Fractures
- Stress Fractures

Pathology

- Significant (high-energy) trauma

Key Facts

- Position of femur determines type of acetabular fractures
- Hip flexion + internal rotation = posterior wall + column injuries
- Hip extension + external rotation = anterior wall + column injuries
- Common (> 20%) = both columns, transverse + posterior wall, posterior wall

Clinical Issues

- Most common signs/symptoms: Pain at fracture site
- Pelvic ring fracture + associated bladder rupture

Diagnostic Checklist

- CT for displaced fragments or communition

- o Associated pelvic ring, soft tissue injuries +/or hematoma
- o Improved visualization of weight bearing dome of joint (not detected on conventional radiographs)
- o Femoral head fracture detection
- o 3-dimensional reformation delineates fracture pattern for surgical planning

MR Findings

- T1WI
  - o Hypointense fracture line + associated subchondral edema
  - o 3 orthogonal plane visualization of fracture with direct coronal, sagittal and axial images
  - o Intraarticular fragments: Marrow fat signal or sclerotic - hypointense
  - o Coronal & axial pelvic ring fracture detection
- T2WI
  - o Hyperintense marrow edema adjacent to fracture site
  - o Associated fracture detection of pelvic ring + femoral head
  - o Hypointense free fragments
  - o Improved visualization of medial wall acetabular fossa
  - o Disruption of intermediate signal intensity chondral surfaces
  - o Muscle trauma - hyperintense edema + hemorrhage on FS PD FSE

Imaging Recommendations

- Best imaging tool
  - o CT superior for osseous detail + spatial relationships for complex fractures + 3-D capability
  - o MRI - also helpful to appreciate 3 plane orthogonal anatomy, chondral + soft tissue pathology
- Protocol advice
  - o 1 mm thin section CT + reformation coronal + sagittal + 3-D rendering
  - o MR: Coronal, axial + sagittal T1 + FS PD FSE

DIFFERENTIAL DIAGNOSIS

Hip Dislocations

- Dislocation without acetabular fracture - severe trauma
- Dislocation with femoral head fracture - typically with posterior hip dislocation

Avulsion Fractures

- Anterior superior iliac spine (ASIS)
- Anterior inferior iliac spine (AIIS)
- Ischial apophysis

Pelvic Ring Fractures

- Stable = avulsion, Duverney's fracture (iliac wing), sacral (transverse) + ischiopubic rami
- Unstable = Malgaigne (unilateral ischiopubic rami), Straddle (obturator rings), bucket-handle (unilateral ischiopubic rami + contralateral sacroiliac joint) + dislocation (unilateral vs. bilateral)

Stress Fractures

- Pelvic - pubic ramus & sacrum (hyperintensity on FS PD FSE or STIR)
- Femoral neck stress - hypointense fracture line + hyperintense edema on T2WI (FS PD FSE or STIR)
- Groin, anterior thigh or knee pain

Intraarticular Derangements

- Avascular necrosis of the femoral head
- Hip osteoarthritis
- Acetabular labral tears

Osseous Lesions

- Cysts
- Metastatic trabecular destruction

PATHOLOGY

General Features

- General path comments
  - o Relevant anatomy
    - Acetabulum = contributions of ilium, ischium & pubic bone (form innominate bone)

ACETABULAR FRACTURES

- Superior gluteal artery + sciatic nerve exits pelvis at greater sciatic notch
- Etiology
  - Significant (high-energy) trauma
    - Femoral force transmitted to acetabulum
  - Position of femur determines type of acetabular fractures
  - Motor vehicle accident or fall from a height
  - Osteoporosis - low energy fractures in elderly (fall directly onto hip)
  - Hip flexion + internal rotation = posterior wall + column injuries
  - Hip extension + external rotation = anterior wall + column injuries
- Epidemiology
  - Common (> 20%) = both columns, transverse + posterior wall, posterior wall
  - Uncommon (< 10%) = T-shaped, transverse, anterior column, anterior column + posterior hemitransverse, posterior column + wall, anterior wall

Gross Pathologic & Surgical Features
- Anterior column fracture
  - Anterior column (larger of the two columns) extends from iliac wing to anterior acetabulum to superior pubic ramus
- Posterior column fractures
  - Posterior column - extends from sciatic notch to posterior acetabulum to ischium
- Acetabular wall fracture
  - Medial wall (quadrilateral plate)
  - Anterior wall
  - Posterior wall
  - Dome (superior, most weight-bearing surface of acetabulum)

Microscopic Features
- Vascular disruption of bone
- Hematoma
- Revascularization
- Devascularized bone ends resorbed
- Callus vs. primary bone repair

Staging, Grading or Classification Criteria
- Judet and Letournel
  - Simple or elementary fractures with single fracture plane
  - Combination fractures = consist of > 1 elementary type fractures
- Matta
  - Acetabular roof arcs
  - Force per unit area (pressure on acetabulum)
  - Nonoperative treatment for fracture lines outside roof arc measurements & femoral head congruent to roof in 3 projections

CLINICAL ISSUES

Presentation
- Most common signs/symptoms: Pain at fracture site
- Clinical profile
  - Pelvic ring fracture + associated bladder rupture

- Hip dislocations + femoral head/neck fractures
- Severe hemorrhage
- Solid organ injuries
- Head, thoracic + abdominal injuries

Demographics
- Age: Elderly patients + osteoporosis population at risk
- Gender: M > F
- Activity at risk
  - Motor vehicle collisions

Natural History & Prognosis
- Most injuries treated surgically
- Non-displaced or minimally displaced fractures treated conservatively
- Complications
  - Heterotropic ossification
  - Infection
  - Avascular necrosis
  - Post-traumatic arthritis
  - Deep venous thrombosis (DVT)
    - Deep pelvis + lower extremity veins
  - Nerve damage - sciatic, superior gluteal, femoral
  - Morel-Lavellee lesion
    - Internal degloving injury associated with crush or shearing component to hip girdle (local + regional hemorrhage)

Treatment
- Conservative
  - Bed rest
  - Femoral traction
  - Non-weight bearing with crutches
- Surgical
  - ORIF (open reduction with internal fixation)
  - Total hip arthroplasty

DIAGNOSTIC CHECKLIST

Consider
- CT for displaced fragments or communition

SELECTED REFERENCES

1. Guyton J et al: Cambell's operative orthopaedics. vol 1. 10th ed. St. Louis MO, Mosby, 2948-61, 2003
2. Fitzgerald RH et al: Orthopaedics. St. Louis MO, Mosby, 3:338-46, 2002
3. Bohndorf K et al: Musculoskeletal imaging: A concise multimodality approach. Germany, Thieme, Sect 1:58-9, 2001
4. Erb RE: Current concepts in imaging the adult hip. Clin in Sports Med 20(4):661-96, 2001
5. Saks BJ: Normal acetabular anatomy for acetabular fracture assessment: CT and plain film correlation. Radiology 159:139-45, 1986
6. Letournel E: Acetabular fracture classification and management. Clin Orthop 151:81-106, 1980

4

56

IMAGE GALLERY

Typical

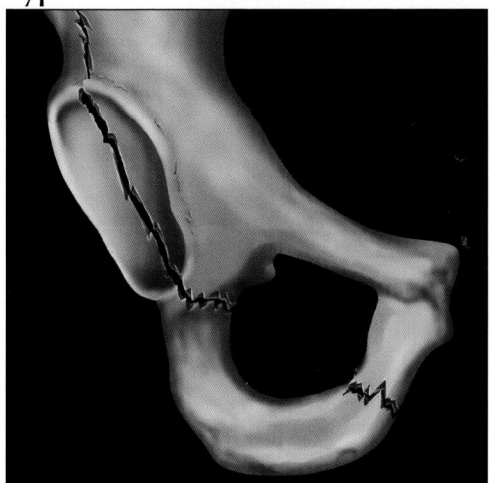 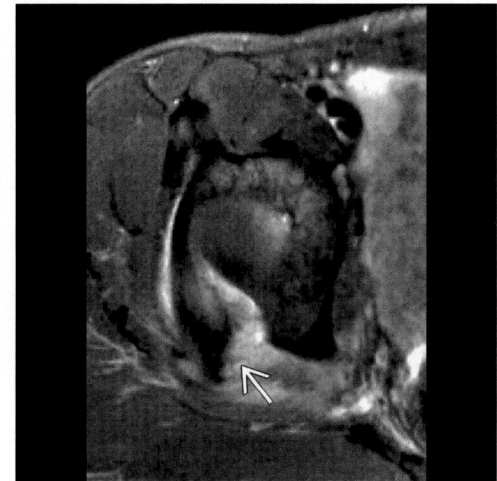

(Left) Coronal graphic shows posterior column fracture. *(Right)* Axial FS PD FSE MR shows displaced osseous fragment (arrow) in posterior column fracture.

Typical

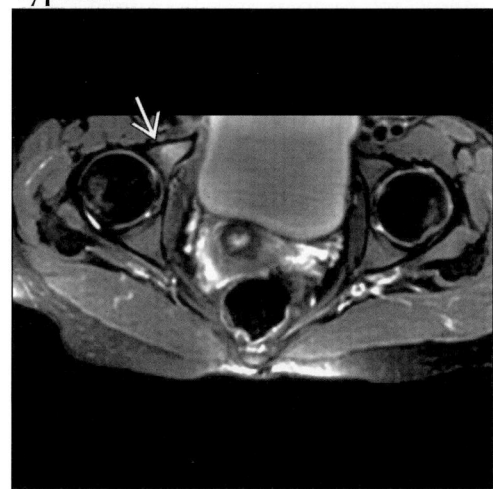 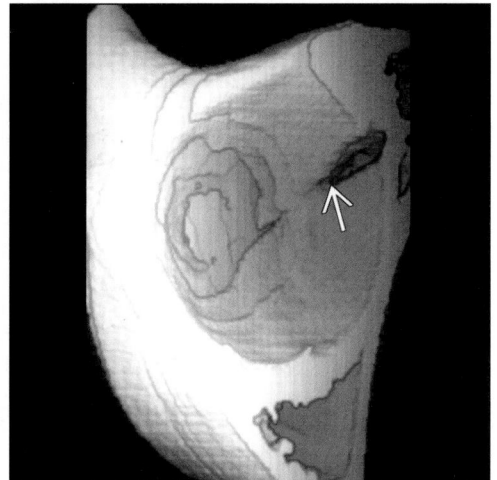

(Left) Axial FS PD FSE MR shows bone marrow edema of right anterior column (arrow) secondary to a non displaced fracture. *(Right)* Axial NECT (three dimensional rendering) shows acetabular roof fracture (arrow).

Typical

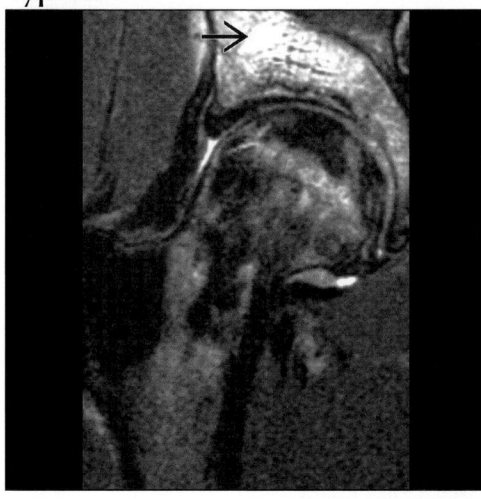 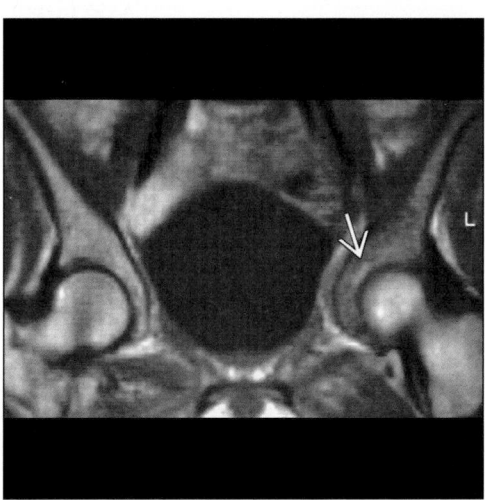

(Left) Coronal FS PD FSE MR shows hyperintense edema (arrow) in acetabular insufficiency fracture. The fracture line may not be seen in acetabular trabecular injuries. *(Right)* Coronal T1WI MR shows medial bowing of the left acetabulum with hypointense (arrow) bone marrow signal associated with osteoporotic acetabular insufficiency fractures.

4

57

HIP DISLOCATIONS

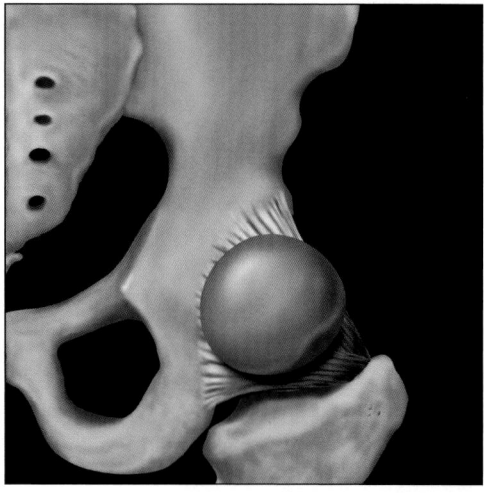

Coronal graphic shows posterior dislocation of the hip. The femoral head overlaps the posterior margin of the acetabulum.

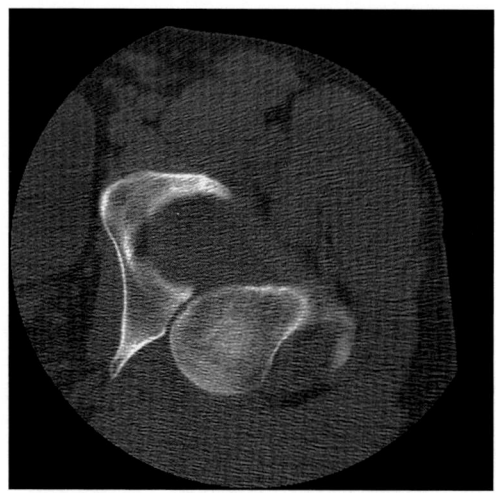

Axial NECT shows posterior dislocation after rollover MVA.

TERMINOLOGY

Abbreviations and Synonyms
- Dislocation of the hip, traumatic hip dislocation, dislocation of the femoral head

Definitions
- Disarticulation of femoral head from acetabulum of the hip

IMAGING FINDINGS

General Features
- Best diagnostic clue: Most common dislocation = posterior dislocation with femoral internal rotation + adduction placing femoral head lateral & superior to acetabulum
- Location: Anterior, posterior, central (medial)
- Size
  - Variable based on associated osseous, cartilage, joint space, muscle + ligament injuries
  - Femoral head fractures associated with posterior hip dislocation
- Morphology
  - Anterior dislocations - femoral head displaced into obturator, pubic or iliac region
  - Posterior dislocation - femoral head lies lateral + superior to acetabulum
  - Central - femoral head protrudes into pelvic cavity

Radiographic Findings
- Radiography
  - Initial diagnostic examination
  - Anteroposterior (AP) view is usually diagnostic
  - Lateral view - dislocated hip anterior or posterior to acetabulum
  - Oblique views (Judet views)
    - Iliac oblique view - 45° external oblique
    - Obturator oblique view - 45° internal oblique
  - Inlet/outlet views

CT Findings
- NECT
  - Intraarticular fragments
  - Associated fractures + pelvic soft tissue injury

MR Findings
- T1WI
  - Evaluate complications
    - Avascular necrosis (AVN) - hypointense subchondral fracture ± central marrow fat
    - Loose bodies ± central marrow
    - Labral tears - intermediate signal
    - Chondral injuries
    - Occult fractures

DDx: Hip Dislocations

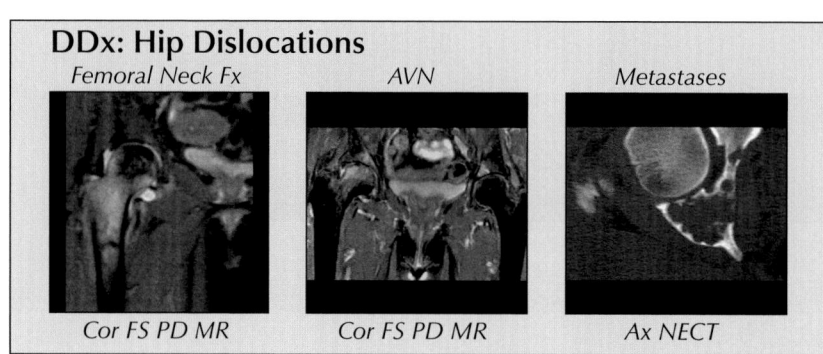

Femoral Neck Fx   *AVN*   *Metastases*

Cor FS PD MR   *Cor FS PD MR*   *Ax NECT*

HIP DISLOCATIONS

Key Facts

Imaging Findings
- Best diagnostic clue: Most common dislocation = posterior dislocation with femoral internal rotation + adduction placing femoral head lateral & superior to acetabulum
- Femoral head fractures associated with posterior hip dislocation
- Posterior dislocation - femoral head lies lateral + superior to acetabulum

Top Differential Diagnoses
- Femoral Neck Fracture (Fx)
- Femoral Head Fracture
- Acetabular Fracture
- Pelvic Fracture
- Femoral Head Avascular Necrosis (AVN)

Pathology
- High level of force required to dislocate hip
- Posterior dislocations - 90% of hip dislocations
- Anterior dislocations & central fractures/dislocations < 10% of hip dislocations
- 70% of all hip dislocations 2° to motor vehicle accidents (e.g., dashboard mechanism)

Clinical Issues
- Most common signs/symptoms: Pain, characteristic deformity

Diagnostic Checklist
- Evaluate for associated fracture of femoral head + acetabulum

- T2WI
  - Hyperintense marrow edema anterior or posterior acetabular rim
  - ± Anteroinferior fragment off femoral head with posterior displacement

Imaging Recommendations
- Best imaging tool
  - CT superior for fracture fragment location + spatial relationships of femoral head with 3D-CT
  - MR also excellent for 3 orthogonal plane visualization + complications including AVN
- Protocol advice
  - Thin section CT bone algorithm with coronal and sagittal reformations
  - MR with coronal, axial FS PD FSE or STIR

DIFFERENTIAL DIAGNOSIS

Femoral Neck Fracture (Fx)
- Stress - pain in groin, anterior thigh or knee (transverse vs. compression)

Femoral Head Fracture
- Capital fractures = uncommon
- Linear hypointense fracture line
- Hyperintense marrow edema

Acetabular Fracture
- Blunt high energy injuries
- Judet - Letournel classification of five elementary fractures based on column & wall involvement

Pelvic Fracture
- High energy pelvic fractures associated with hemorrhage
- Benign avulsion to massive pelvic disruptions

Femoral Head Avascular Necrosis (AVN)
- Necrotic segment collapse anterosuperior aspect femoral head
- Associated with displaced fractures femoral neck & hip dislocations

- Groin or hip pain

Stress Fracture
- Pubic stress fracture - associated with long distance running
- Sacrum - runners at risk; bilateral stress fractures with "H" sign on MRI

Snapping Hip Syndrome
- Painful, audible snap in hip flexion + extension
- External, internal or intraarticular etiologies

Slipped Capital Femoral Epiphysis
- Posterior-inferior displacement proximal femoral epiphysis
- Childhood disorder

Acetabular Tumor
- Primary or metastatic

PATHOLOGY

General Features
- General path comments
  - Relevant anatomy
    - Iliofemoral, pubofemoral, ischiofemoral, transverse + femoral head ligaments maintain femur in acetabulum
- Etiology
  - High level of force required to dislocate hip
  - Posterior dislocation
    - Most common type (90%)
    - Force to flexed knee transmitted to hip with dislocation of femoral head posteriorly
- Epidemiology
  - Posterior dislocations - 90% of hip dislocations
  - Anterior dislocations & central fractures/dislocations < 10% of hip dislocations
  - 70% of all hip dislocations 2° to motor vehicle accidents (e.g., dashboard mechanism)

Gross Pathologic & Surgical Features
- Osseous fragments

HIP DISLOCATIONS

- Joint space widening
- Posterior dislocation - associated sciatic nerve injury 2° to compression or laceration ± local hematoma
- Anterior dislocation - ± injury to femoral nerve + artery

Microscopic Features
- Fracture - vascular disruption

Staging, Grading or Classification Criteria
- Hip dislocation with fracture of femoral head using Pipkin classification
  - Pipkin I: Fx femoral head below central fossa
  - Pipkin II: Fx femoral head involving central fossa
  - Pipkin III: Fx femoral head + neck
  - Pipkin IV: Fx femoral head + superoposterior acetabular rim

CLINICAL ISSUES

Presentation
- Most common signs/symptoms: Pain, characteristic deformity
- Clinical profile
  - Posterior dislocation
    - Hip + gluteal pain
    - Lower extremity shortened, adducted, internally rotated and flexed
    - Lack of range of motion, inability to bear weight
    - Sciatic nerve injury with loss of sensation posterior leg/foot + inability to dorsiflex/plantar flex
    - Hematoma/soft tissue swelling
  - Anterior dislocation
    - Hip, gluteal, groin pain
    - Hip externally rotated, abducted, extended
    - Inability to walk/bear weight
    - Femoral nerve/artery injury with pain, pallor, pulselessness, loss of motor function & absent reflexes
  - Central dislocation
    - Shortened affected limb
    - Abducted/adducted or internally/externally rotated
    - Intra-pelvic soft tissue injury + hemorrhage

Demographics
- Age
  - Traumatic injuries motor vehicle accidents (MVA) < 35 years most common
  - Trauma 2° to falls > 65 years
- Gender
  - More common in young males
  - Associated with MVAs & sports injuries

Natural History & Prognosis
- Orthopaedic emergency
  - High incidence of AVN with prolonged dislocation
  - Reduce as soon as possible
- High morbidity/mortality
  - 2° to significant trauma
  - Severe intra-abdominal, intra-pelvic & head injuries
  - Pelvic ring fractures - severe hemorrhage

- Uncomplicated cases - closed reduction successful (76-93%)
- Poorer prognosis when fractures present
- Recurrent dislocations - ligamentous support disrupted
- Complications
  - AVN
  - Osteoarthritis
  - Sciatic nerve injuries
  - Femoral nerve/artery injuries
  - Deep venous thrombosis

Treatment
- Conservative
  - Closed reduction
  - Maneuvers recreated deforming force + applied longitudinal traction
  - Posterior dislocation - flexion, adduction, internal rotation/Stimson maneuver (prone)/Allis maneuver (supine)
  - Anterior dislocation - abduction, external rotation, extension
- Surgical
  - Open reduction for failed closed reduction, intra-articular loose bodies, interposed soft tissue, concomitant femoral head/neck fractures

DIAGNOSTIC CHECKLIST

Consider
- Evaluate for associated fracture of femoral head + acetabulum
- May require follow-up MR to exclude complication of AVN of femoral head

SELECTED REFERENCES

1. DeLee JC et al: Orthopaedic sports medicine. Principles and practice. Hip and pelvis. vol 2. 2nd ed. Philadelphia PA, Saunders, (25):1443-62, 2003
2. Brooks RA et al: Diagnosis and imaging studies of traumatic hip dislocations in the adult. Clin Orthop 377:15-23, 2000
3. Yang EC et al: Initial treatment of traumatic hip dislocations in the adult. Clin Orthop 377:24-31, 2000
4. Walden PD et al: Whistler technique used to reduce traumatic dislocation of the hip in the emergency department setting. J Emerg Med 17(3):441-4, 1999
5. Conway WF et al: CT and MR imaging of the hip. Radiology 198(2):297-307, 1996
6. Dreinhofer KE et al: Isolated traumatic dislocation of the hip: Long-term results in 50 patients. J Bone Joint Surg Br 76:6, 1994
7. Levin PE: Hip dislocations: Skeletal Trauma. vol 2. Philadelphia PA, WB Saunders, 1992
8. Epstein HC: Traumatic Dislocation of the Hip. Clin Orthop 92:116-42, 1973

HIP DISLOCATIONS

IMAGE GALLERY

Typical

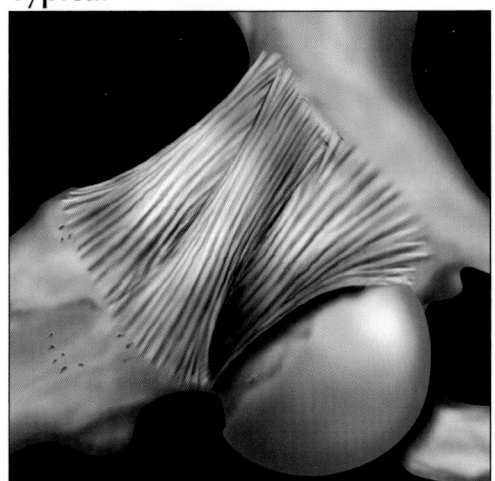 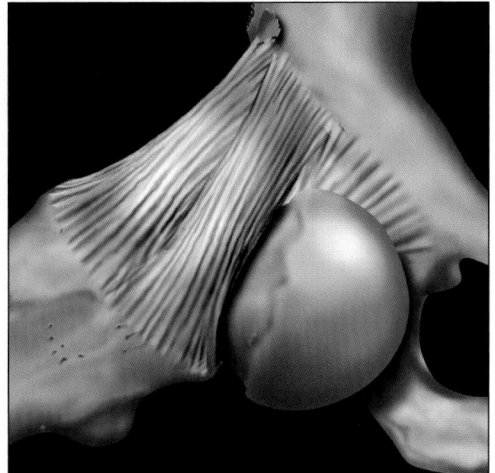

(Left) Coronal graphic shows anterior-inferior dislocation of the hip below the iliofemoral (lateral) and pubofemoral (medial) ligaments. *(Right)* Coronal graphic shows anterior dislocation with the femoral head anterior to the pubofemoral ligament.

Typical

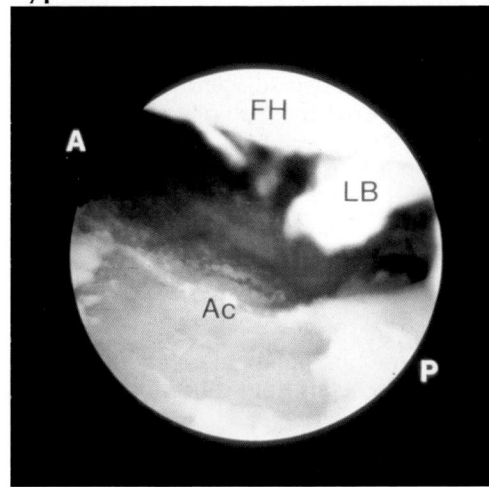 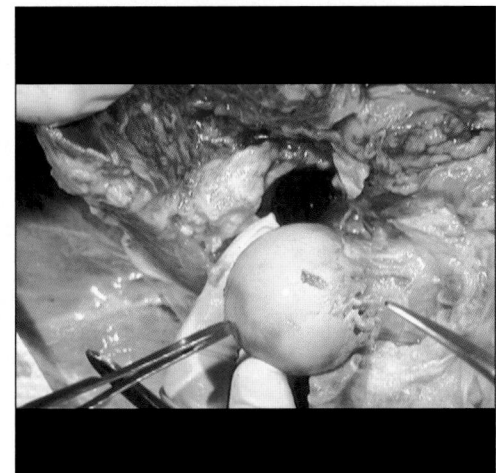

(Left) Arthroscopic view shows acetabular (Ac) chondral fracture with associated loose body (LB) secondary to a posterior hip dislocation. Femoral head (FH) is shown superiorly. *(Right)* Surgical pathology shows surgical dislocation of the femoral head.

Typical

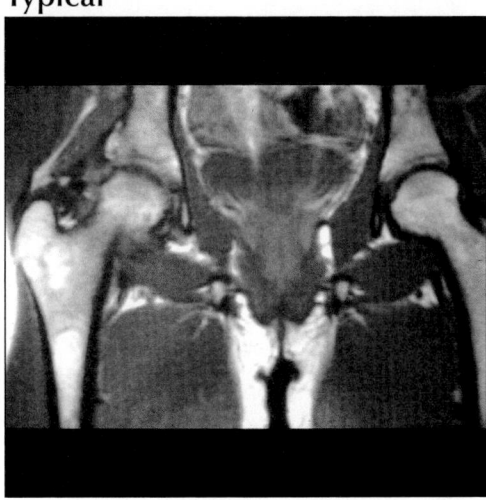 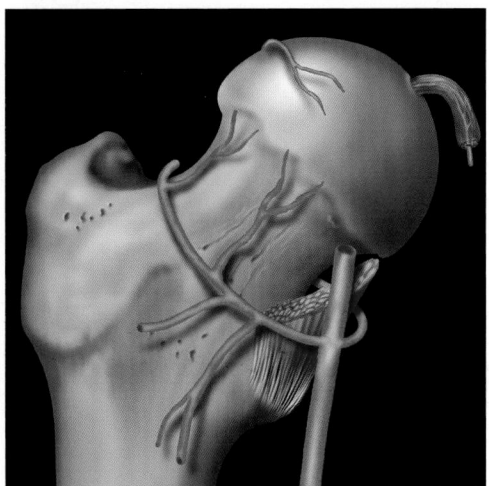

(Left) Coronal PD/Intermediate MR shows right posterior hip dislocation after reduction with osseous contusion of the femoral head, joint effusion, loose bodies, and acetabular rim fracture. *(Right)* Coronal graphic shows normal vascular supply of the proximal femur. The profunda femoral artery is shown medially. The medial and lateral circumflex branches encircle the femoral neck.

AVULSION FRACTURE

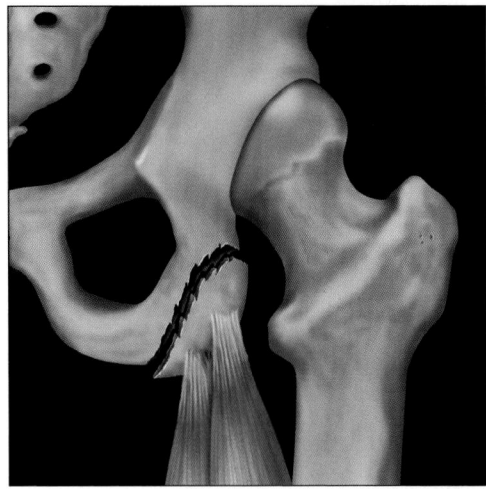

Coronal graphic shows osseous avulsion of the hamstring tendon attachment to the ischial tuberosity.

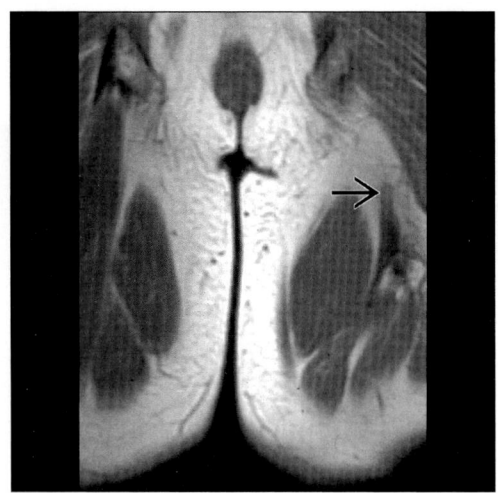

Coronal T1WI MR shows avulsed and retracted (arrow) left common hamstring tendon.

TERMINOLOGY

Abbreviations and Synonyms
- Avulsion injury, tug injury, tug lesion, pelvic avulsions

Definitions
- Bony or cartilaginous failure resulting in fracture 2° to a force applied by a musculotendinous unit

IMAGING FINDINGS

General Features
- Best diagnostic clue: Hyperintense marrow edema (T2WI) at avulsion fracture donor site
- Location
  - Anterior superior iliac spine (ASIS)
  - Anterior inferior iliac spine (AIIS)
  - Ischial apophysis
  - Iliac crest
  - Lesser trochanter
- Size
  - Variable based on location
  - Along course of apophyseal physis
- Morphology
  - Slight displacement ASIS
  - Displacement of AIIS fragment distally
  - Displaced fragment ischial tuberosity

Radiographic Findings
- Radiography
  - Osseous fragment identified adjacent to donor site
  - Contralateral views to distinguish open apophysis from avulsion fracture
  - Normal if apophysis not yet calcified
  - Exuberant callus
  - Changes may appear aggressive - mimicking primary or metastatic bone tumors

CT Findings
- NECT
  - Osseous detail of fracture fragment and donor site
  - Hematoma (heterogeneous fluid collection) at site of injury
  - Callus visualized ± simulating aggressive lesions

MR Findings
- T1WI
  - Contralateral side - MR to distinguish avulsed fragment from normal, open apophysis
  - Osseous avulsion may be difficult to visualize in bed of soft tissue + hematoma
  - Involved tendon often lax (redundant morphology)
  - ASIS
    - Mild displacement
    - ± Hypointense edema of adjacent marrow
    - ± Fluid adjacent to sartorius origin

DDx: Avulsion Fracture

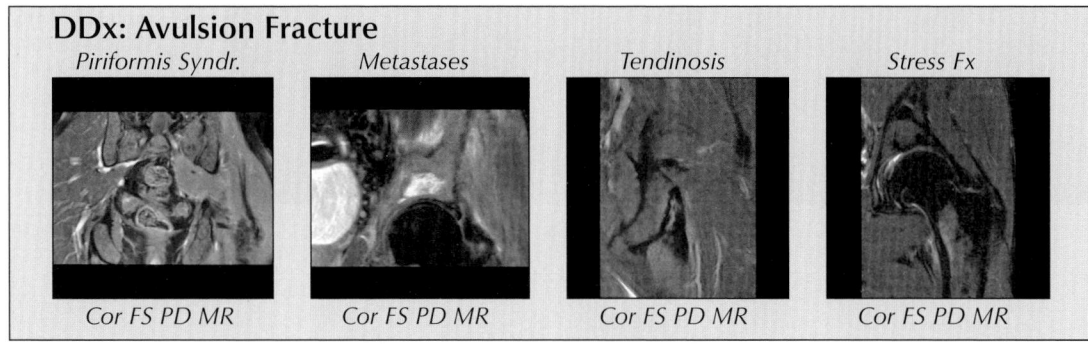

Piriformis Syndr.	Metastases	Tendinosis	Stress Fx
Cor FS PD MR	Cor FS PD MR	Cor FS PD MR	Cor FS PD MR

AVULSION FRACTURE

Key Facts

Imaging Findings
- Best diagnostic clue: Hyperintense marrow edema (T2WI) at avulsion fracture donor site
- Anterior superior iliac spine (ASIS)
- Anterior inferior iliac spine (AIIS)
- Ischial apophysis

Top Differential Diagnoses
- Piriformis Syndrome
- Primary or Metastatic Bone Lesion
- Sacroiliac Sprain
- Muscle Strain
- Tendinosis

Pathology
- Adolescents - traction on unfused apophysis

Key Facts
- Fracture 2° forceful concentric or eccentric muscle contraction
- Fractures 2° extreme passive stretch (dancers & gymnasts)

Clinical Issues
- Most common signs/symptoms: Local pain
- Iliac crest avulsion: ± RLQ pain mimicking appendicitis
- Point tenderness
- Altered gait

Diagnostic Checklist
- T1 to show avulsed fragment vs. FS PD FSE for donor site edema

- ○ AIIS
  - ▪ Distal fragment displacement
  - ▪ Laxity straight head rectus femoris
- ○ Ischial apophysis
  - ▪ Displaced fragment ± hypointense edema at donor site
- T2WI
  - ○ Hyperintense marrow edema at donor site
  - ○ Hyperintense fluid, soft tissue edema + hemorrhage at site of avulsion
  - ○ Associated muscle strain - hyperintense signal on FS PD FSE or STIR
  - ○ Hyperintense edema of iliopsoas adjacent to lesser trochanter
- Avulsed osseous fragment often hypointense on T1, FS PD FSE or STIR

Imaging Recommendations
- Best imaging tool
  - ○ MR to document status of musculotendinous unit + donor site marrow edema
  - ○ CT to identify subtle avulsion fragment with fleck or shell-like morphology
- Protocol advice
  - ○ T1 (to optimize fat marrow signal) + FS PD FSE in coronal & axial planes
  - ○ Sagittal plane helpful for rectus femoris injuries of straight head (AIIS) + reflected head (upper rim acetabulum)

DIFFERENTIAL DIAGNOSIS

Piriformis Syndrome
- Compression of sciatic nerve
- History of blunt trauma
- Lower sacroiliac joint, greater sciatic notch + piriformis pain
- Hypertrophy of piriformis ± palpable mass
- Muscle hyperintensity on T2WI

Primary or Metastatic Bone Lesion
- Malignant fibrous histiocytoma: Inhomogeneous on T2WI
- Liposarcoma: Variable fat content + areas of hyperintensity on T2WI
- Synovial cell sarcoma: Increased signal on T2WI
- Metastatic prostate: May be hypointense on T2WI
- Metastatic breast: May be hypo or hyperintense on T2WI

Sacroiliac Sprain
- Anterior + posterior sacroiliac ligament injury
- Interosseous sacroiliac ligament injury
- Sacrotuberous ligament injury
- Violent contraction of the hamstrings or abdominal muscles
- Torsion vs. direct trauma
- Forceful extension of flexed hip

Muscle Strain
- Musculotendinous injuries
- Abdominal muscle insertion on iliac wing
- Origin of gluteals from ilium + insertion on proximal femur
- Adductor origin from pubis
- Insertion of iliopsoas on lesser trochanter
- Hyperintense edema on FS PD FSE

Tendinosis
- Thickening of tendon origin + insertions
- Intermediate signal on T1 + T2WI
- Common hamstring tendinosis
- Gluteus medius tendinosis

Tendon Tear
- Common hamstring retraction with proximal tear
- Gluteus medius tear lateral surface greater trochanter
- Adductor injuries = "pulled groin"

Stress Fracture
- Repetitive stress
- Pubic ramus - long distance runners & joggers
- Sacral stress fractures - insufficiency vs. stress (runners)

AVULSION FRACTURE

PATHOLOGY

General Features
- General path comments
  - Relevant anatomy
    - Sartorius: Origin = ASIS + upper half iliac notch; insertion = medial surface proximal tibia
    - Rectus femoris: Origin = AIIS (straight head) + upper acetabular rim (reflected head); insertion = superior patella + patellar tendon to tibial tuberosity
    - Biceps femoris, semitendinosus + semimembranosus origin = ischial tuberosity
- Etiology
  - Adolescents - traction on unfused apophysis
  - Fracture 2° forceful concentric or eccentric muscle contraction
  - Fractures 2° extreme passive stretch (dancers & gymnasts)
  - Less common - avulsions 2° to chronic repetitive microtrauma
- Epidemiology: Avulsion fractures = 13.4% of children's pelvic fractures

Gross Pathologic & Surgical Features
- Displacement of ASIS limited by fascia lata + lateral inguinal ligament
- Displacement of AIIS limited by dual insertion of straight head of rectus + reflected head
- Ischial apophysis displacement limited by sacrotuberous ligament

Microscopic Features
- Hematoma
- Revascularization + resorption of devascularized bone fragment
- Callus + fibrous scar tissue

Staging, Grading or Classification Criteria
- By location
  - ASIS
  - AIIS
  - Ischial tuberosity

CLINICAL ISSUES

Presentation
- Most common signs/symptoms: Local pain
- Clinical profile
  - Swelling after activity
  - Limitation of activity
  - Iliac crest avulsion: ± RLQ pain mimicking appendicitis
  - Point tenderness
  - Discoloration 2° to hematoma
  - Altered gait
  - Pain + weakness - involved muscle placed under stress
  - Most commonly 2° to athletic-type injury
  - If no history of trauma - exclude infection + tumor
  - Atraumatic avulsion in adult - exclude metastatic + metabolic bone disease

- Biopsy may show mitoses in healing bone - mistaken for high-grade malignancy
- Less common avulsion sites
  - Greater trochanter (gluteus min./med.)
  - Pubic bone (gracilis + adductors)
  - Iliac crest (abdominal musculature)

Demographics
- Age: 14-25 years = most common
- Gender: Males > females
- Related activity
  - ASIS - forceful contraction of sartorius in kicking sports, jumping or running
  - AIIS - rectus femoris in kicking sports
  - Ischial tuberosity - hamstring in dancers, gymnasts, sprinting (hurdling) + football

Natural History & Prognosis
- Most injuries heal with conservative treatment
- Poor healing - chronic pain 2° to repetitive micromotion
- Surgery - for recalcitrant pain or severely displaced fragments

Treatment
- Conservative
  - Recovery slow: Average 4-8 weeks up to 4 months
  - Initial bedrest to non-weight bearing + crutches
  - Ice, anti-inflammatories
  - Physical therapy - gradual strengthening + progressive weight bearing
  - Re-injury if return to high level activity prematurely
- Surgical
  - Re-attachment of severely displaced avulsed fragment
  - Chronic pain: Resection of weak bony union + surgical reattachment

DIAGNOSTIC CHECKLIST

Consider
- T1 to show avulsed fragment vs. FS PD FSE for donor site edema

SELECTED REFERENCES

1. DeLee JC et al: Orthopaedic sports medicine. Principles and practice. vol 2. 2nd ed. Philadelphia PA, Saunders, (25):1443-62, 2003
2. Bui-Mansfield LT et al: Nontraumatic avulsion of the pelvis. Am J of Roentg 178:423-27, 2002
3. Bencardino JT et al: Imaging of hip disorders in athletes. Rad Clin of North Am 40(2):277-80, 2002
4. Van Holsbeeck MT et al: Musculoskeletal ultrasound. 2nd ed. St. Louis MO, Mosby, 190, 2001
5. Metzmaker JN et al: Avulsion fractures of the pelvis. Am J Sports Med 13:349, 1985
6. Kane WJ: Fractures of the pelvis: Fractures in adults. vol 2. Philadelphia PA, JB Lippincott, 1094-1196, 1984
7. Key JA et al: Management of fractures, dislocations, and sprains. St. Louis, MO, CV Mosby, 1951

AVULSION FRACTURE

IMAGE GALLERY

Typical

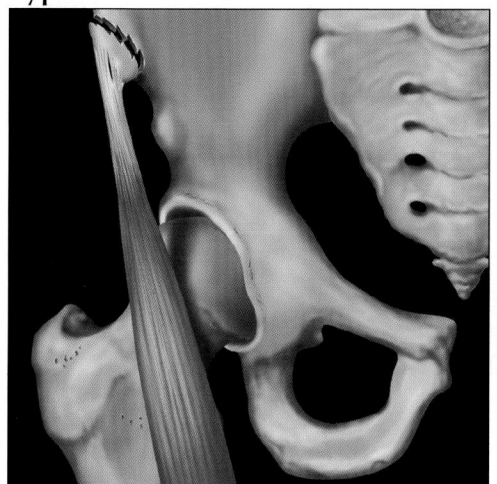
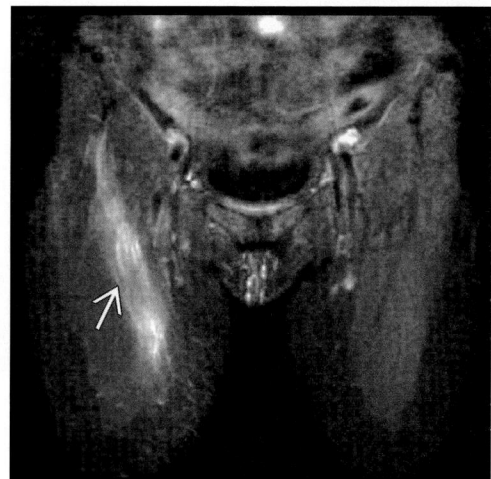

(Left) Coronal graphic shows avulsion of the anterior superior iliac spine at the sartorius origin. *(Right)* Coronal FS PD FSE MR shows hyperintense edema (arrow) of right sartorius muscle in association with a more proximal avulsion.

Typical

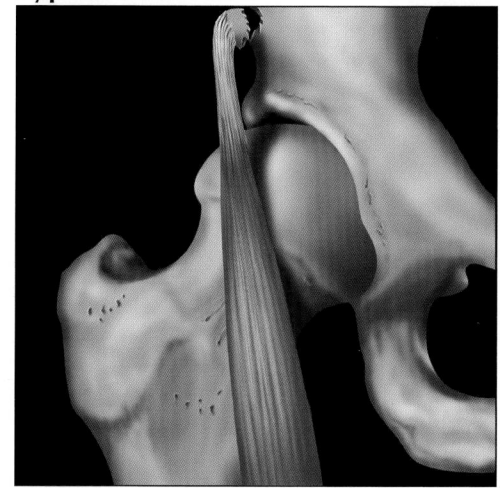
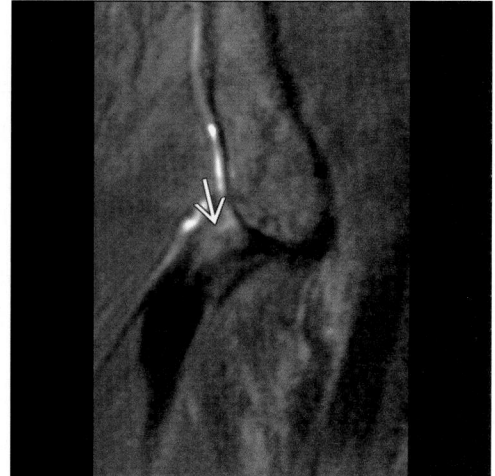

(Left) Coronal graphic shows avulsion of the anterior inferior iliac spine with origin of the straight head of the rectus femoris. *(Right)* Coronal FS PD FSE MR shows strain (arrow) of the straight head (rectus femoris) attachment to the anterior inferior iliac spine.

Typical

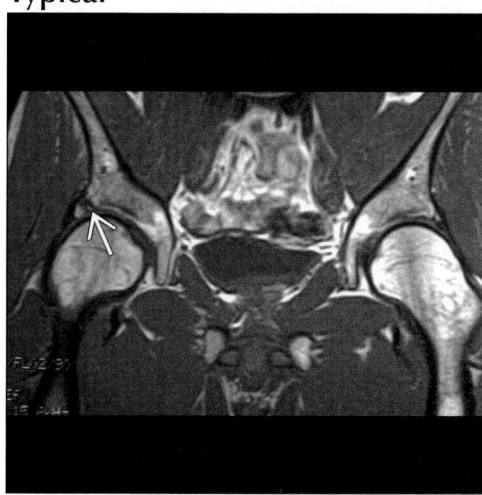
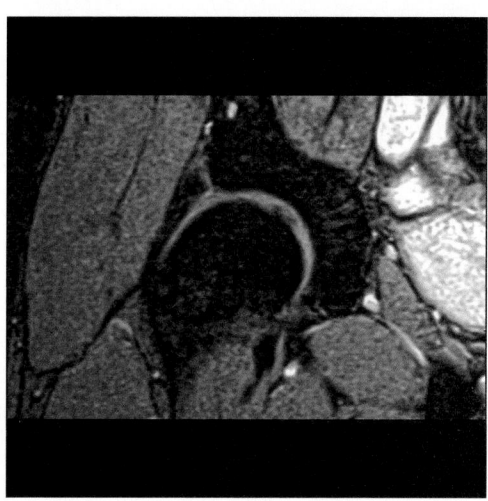

(Left) Coronal T1WI MR shows chronic lateral acetabular avulsion injury (arrow) from the reflected head of right rectus femoris attachment. *(Right)* Coronal FS PD FSE MR shows lateral acetabular rim avulsion.

PUBIC RAMI STRESS FRACTURES

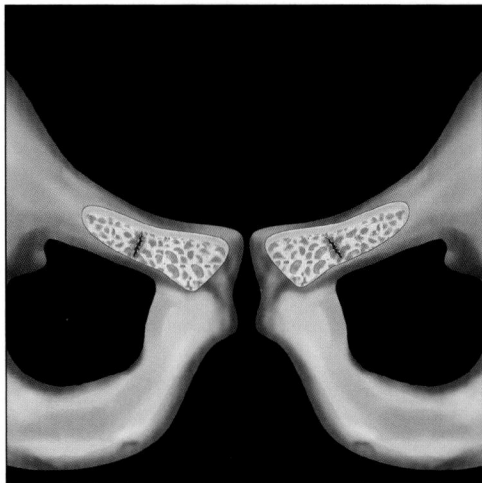

Coronal graphic shows bilateral pubic rami stress fractures.

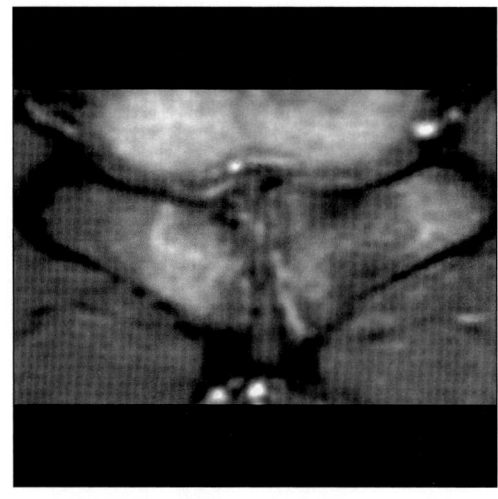

Coronal FS PD FSE MR shows hyperintense marrow edema associated with microtrabecular stress injuries to both superior pubic rami.

TERMINOLOGY

Abbreviations and Synonyms
- Stress fracture (fx), pubic rami, pelvic stress fx

Definitions
- Incomplete or complete fx of pubic ramus, 2° repetitive loading

IMAGING FINDINGS

General Features
- Best diagnostic clue: Hyperintense subchondral edema on FS PD FSE ± fx line
- Location: Superior + inferior pubic rami adjacent to pubic symphysis
- Size: Variable - unilateral or bilateral involvement
- Morphology: Stress fx perpendicular to cortices + diffuse medullary edema pattern

Radiographic Findings
- Radiography
  - Often negative, especially early
  - Sclerosis
  - Callus formation in healing stages
  - Fx ± visualized as linear lucency
  - Anteroposterior (AP) view: Usually diagnostic if radiographic signs present

- Oblique view may be useful
  - Oblique view - 45 degree anterior oblique
- If radiograph negative consider MR or bone scintigraphy

CT Findings
- NECT
  - Sclerosis
  - Trabecular or cortical fx
  - No trabecular destruction
  - Surrounding callus formation - healing stage

MR Findings
- T1WI
  - Hypointense marrow edema on T1WI
  - Unilateral vs. bilateral
  - Fx line ± visualized
  - ± Hypointense edema or soft tissue thickening
- T2WI
  - Hyperintense marrow edema
  - ± Fx visualization usually as single fx line perpendicular to long axis of superior pubic ramus
  - ± Thickened cortex - hypointense
  - ± Hyperintense edema parallel to superior/inferior border pubic ramus
  - Requires FS PD FSE or STIR

Nuclear Medicine Findings
- Bone Scan

DDx: Pubic Rami Stress Fractures

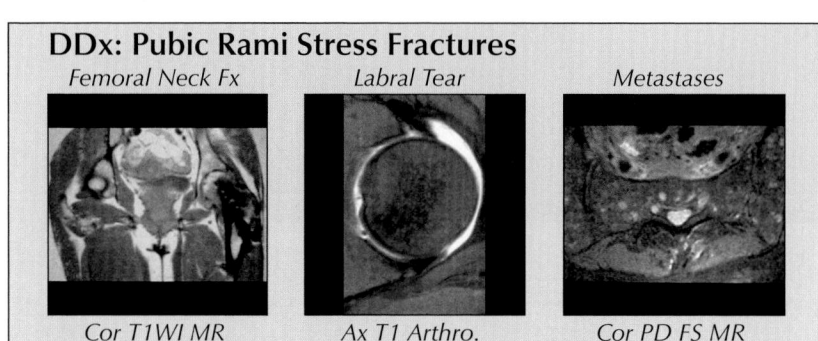

Femoral Neck Fx	Labral Tear	Metastases
Cor T1WI MR	*Ax T1 Arthro.*	*Cor PD FS MR*

PUBIC RAMI STRESS FRACTURES

Key Facts

Imaging Findings
- Best diagnostic clue: Hyperintense subchondral edema on FS PD FSE ± fx line
- Location: Superior + inferior pubic rami adjacent to pubic symphysis
- Morphology: Stress fx perpendicular to cortices + diffuse medullary edema pattern
- Hypointense marrow edema on T1WI

Top Differential Diagnoses
- Muscle Strain/Tear
- Femoral Neck Stress Fx
- Delayed Onset Muscle Soreness (DOMS)
- Osteomyelitis

Pathology
- Fatigue fx - repetitive loading normal bone

- Insufficiency fx - normal forces applied to abnormal or weakened bone
- Bone failure 2° cyclic, repetitive muscle contraction
- Female runners + military recruits

Clinical Issues
- Most common signs/symptoms: Groin pain
- Point tenderness inferior pubic ramus
- Painful abduction + resisted adduction
- Painful external hip rotation

Diagnostic Checklist
- Marrow edema without visible fx requires CT evaluation

○ Sensitive
○ ± Positive before onset of symptoms
○ Positive 2-3 wks before radiographic changes evident
○ Diagnostic if increased uptake on 3rd phase of bone scan
○ Tumor & osteomyelitis also demonstrate increased uptake on 3rd phase
○ Increased uptake persists for months in healing fractures

Imaging Recommendations
- Best imaging tool
  ○ MR superior in defining pubic ramus with associated edema of marrow + adjacent muscle
  ○ Bone scintigraphy nonspecific
- Protocol advice: T1 + FS PD FSE in coronal + axial planes

DIFFERENTIAL DIAGNOSIS

Muscle Strain/Tear
- Muscle belly + musculotendinous
- Violent muscular contraction
- Hyperintense edema FS PD FSE or STIR
- Inter + intramuscular hemorrhage

Femoral Neck Stress Fx
- Military recruits + runners
- Insufficiency fractures in osteoporosis
- Hyperintense marrow edema on FS PD FSE or STIR
- Calcar fx hypointense on T1 + T2WI

Intrinsic Hip Pathology
- Hip dislocation ± associated fx
- Acetabular labral tears - femoroacetabular impingement or osteoarthritis
- Avascular necrosis
- Osteoarthritis - superior joint space narrowing

Delayed Onset Muscle Soreness (DOMS)
- Nonacute injury
- Painful symptoms peak 24-72 hrs. post exertion

- Denervation - muscle group involvement - hyperintense on STIR + FS PD FSE
- Grade I (partial tearing of muscle fibers with no loss of function) strain & DOMS overlap in MR signal intensity changes

Osteomyelitis
- Erosions
- Hyperintense marrow edema - FS PD FSE + STIR
- Adjacent soft tissue mass
- Subcutaneous tissue edema

Metastatic Disease
- Cortical + trabecular destruction
- Reactive muscle edema
- Pathologic fx
- Prostate & breast may be hypointense on T1 & T2WI

PATHOLOGY

General Features
- General path comments
  ○ Relevant anatomy
    - Gracilis origin = lower half pubic symphysis + upper half pubic arch
    - Pectineus origin = pectineal line, pubis between iliopectineal eminence + pubic tubercle
    - Adductor longus origin = anterior pubis angle between crest + symphysis
    - Adductor brevis origin = outer surface inferior ramus pubis
    - Adductor magnus origin = ischial tuberosity, rami of ischium & pubis
    - Obturator externus orgin = outer margin obturator foramen
- Etiology
  ○ Fatigue fx - repetitive loading normal bone
  ○ Insufficiency fx - normal forces applied to abnormal or weakened bone
  ○ Bone failure 2° cyclic, repetitive muscle contraction
    - Insufficient repair time

- Osteoclastic resorption > osteoblastic bone formation
- Female runners + military recruits
  - Female vs. male pelvic geometry
  - Increased stride (gait) length to height ratio relative to taller male recruits
  - Decreased muscle bulk subjecting bones to greater force
- Post hip arthroplasty
  - Increased activity with new prosthesis-stress fx
- Insufficiency fx
  - Older women
  - Post menopausal osteoporosis
  - ± Secondary to sacral insufficiency fx - increased forces to pubic arch
- Tensile stress - generated by muscle mass originating from pubic ramus
- Excessive repetition of muscle contractions
- Malgaigne fx
  - Post traumatic ischiopubic rami fx associated with ipsilateral sacroillic joint disruption may mimic a pubic rami stress fx
- Epidemiology: Insufficiency fx - 1% females > 55 years

Gross Pathologic & Surgical Features
- Fx - unilateral or bilateral parasymphyseal
- Callus
- Absent soft tissue mass

Microscopic Features
- Osteoclastic resorption
- Lamellated bone filling osteoclastic cavities
- New periosteal + endosteal bone
- Periosteal reaction

CLINICAL ISSUES

Presentation
- Most common signs/symptoms: Groin pain
- Clinical profile
  - Gluteal + thigh pain
  - Point tenderness inferior pubic ramus
  - Painful abduction + resisted adduction
  - Painful external hip rotation
  - Antalgic gait
  - Athletes: Fx associated with intensified training
  - Pain relieved by rest
  - Pain inguinal, perineal or adductor
  - Standing sign: Unable to stand unsupported with affected leg

Demographics
- Age
  - Young adult: Stress fx
  - Older population (> 55 years): Insufficiency fx
- Gender: F > M
- Activity at risk
  - Military recruits

Natural History & Prognosis
- Most fxs heal with rest
- Cease training or causative activity
- Improper treatment or failure to rest = fx non-union
- Healing process slow: 4-12 wks up to 5 months

Treatment
- Conservative
  - Rest
  - Cessation of training regimen
  - Analgesics
  - Physical therapy
  - Stretching
  - Range-of-motion activity
  - Muscle strengthening
  - Non-union - most heal with rest
- Surgical
  - Rare except non-union or displaced fx

DIAGNOSTIC CHECKLIST

Consider
- Document fx in trabecular or cortical bone
- Marrow edema without visible fx requires CT evaluation
- Identify associated sacral stress/insufficiency fx

SELECTED REFERENCES

1. Bencardino JT et al: Imaging of hip disorders in athletes. Radiol Clin of N America 40(2):267-87, 2002
2. Spitz DJ et al: Imaging of stress fractures in athletes. Radiol Clin of N America 40(2):313-31, 2002
3. Mabrey JD et al: Periprosthetic fractures. Rockwood and green's fractures in adults. 5th ed. Philadelphia PA, Lippincott Wiliams & Wilkinson, 611-12, 2001
4. Hosono M et al: MR appearance of parasymphyseal insufficiency fractures of the os pubis. Skeletal Radiol 26(9):525-8, 1997
5. Otte MT et al: MR imaging of supra-acetabular insufficiency fractures. Skeletal Radiol 26(5):279-83, 1997
6. Schapira D et al: Insufficiency fractures of the pubic ramus. Semin Arthritis Rheum 25(6):373-82, 1996
7. Hill PF et al: Stress fracture of the pubic ramus in female recruits. J Bone Joint Surg Br 78(3):383-6, 1996
8. Peh WC et al: Imaging of pelvic insufficiency fractures. Radiographics 16(2):355-48, 1996
9. Pavlov H: Roentgen examination of groin and hip in the athlete. Clin in Sports Med 6(4):829-43, 1987
10. Noakes TD et al: Pelvic Stress fractures in long distance runners. Am J Sports Med 13:120, 1985
11. Pavlov H et al: Stress fractures of the pubic ramus. J Bone Joint Surg 64:1020, 1982
12. Koch R et al: Pubic symphysitis in runners. AM J Sports Med 9:62, 1981
13. Latshaw RF et al: A pelvic stress fracture in a female jogger. Am J Sports Med 9:54, 1981
14. McBryde Am Jr: Stress fractures in athletes. Am J Sports Med 3:212, 1976

PUBIC RAMI STRESS FRACTURES

IMAGE GALLERY

Variant

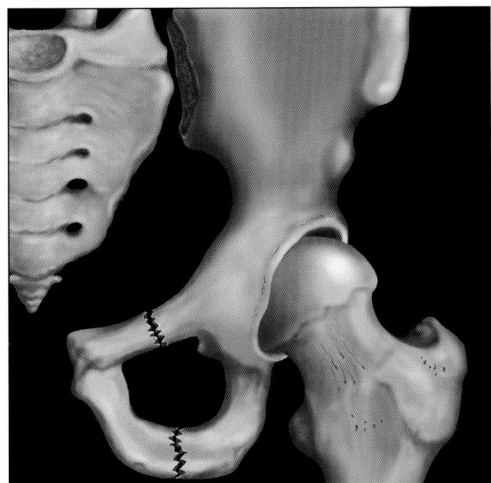

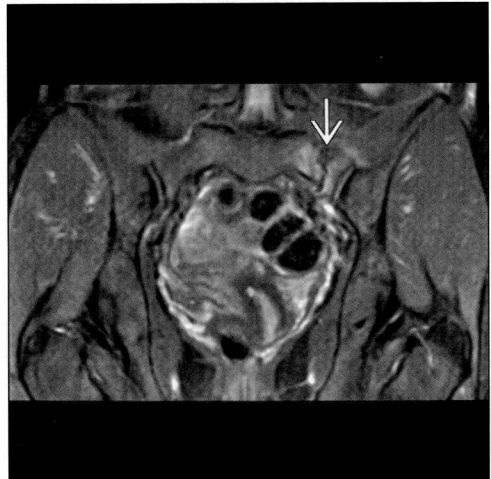

(Left) Coronal graphic shows Malgaigne fracture involving unilateral fracture of the ischiopubic rami and disruption of the ipsilateral sacroiliac joint. *(Right)* Coronal FS PD FSE MR shows unilateral sacroiliac disruption (arrow) associated with a left Malgaigne fracture.

Typical

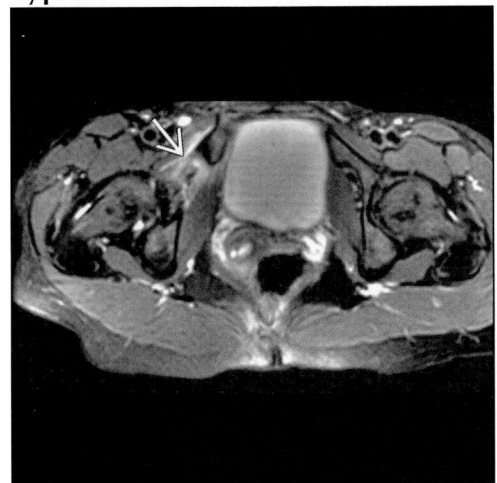

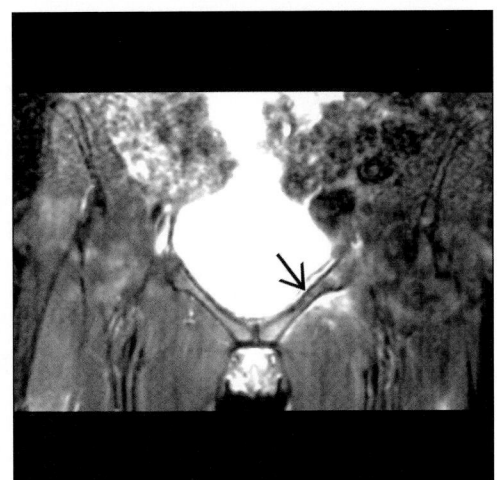

(Left) Axial FS PD FSE MR shows complete fracture (arrow) of the right superior pubic ramus with hyperintense soft tissue edema. *(Right)* Coronal FS PD FSE MR shows stress fracture of the left superior pubic ramus (arrow) with adjacent proximal adductor muscle edema.

Typical

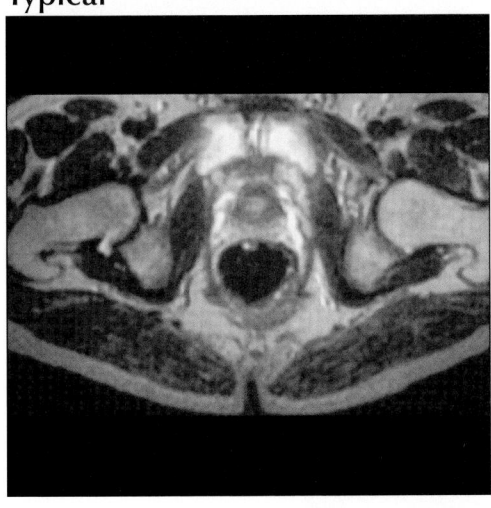

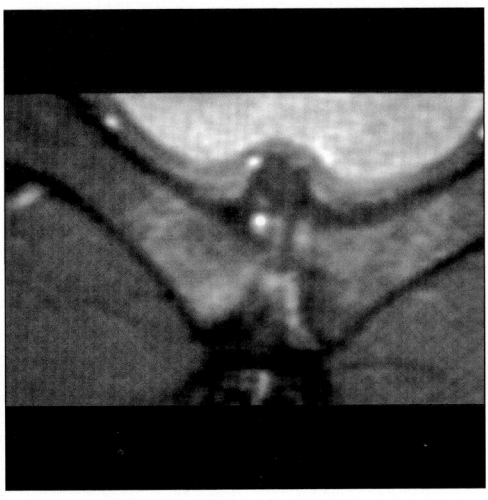

(Left) Axial T2WI MR shows hyperintense superior pubic rami adjacent to the symphysis from bilateral stress fractures in a marathon runner. *(Right)* Coronal FS PD FSE MR shows degenerative superior pubic rami without defined rami fractures.

SACRAL INSUFFICIENCY FRACTURES

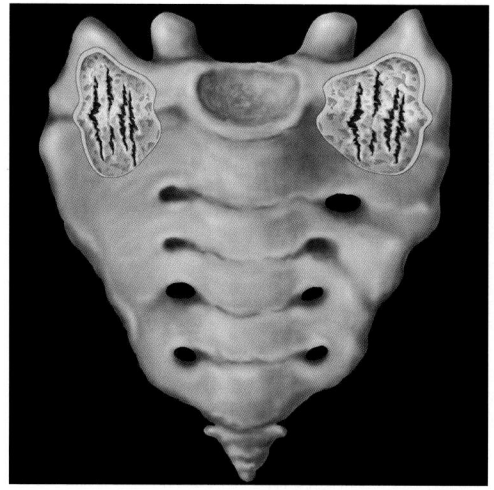

Coronal graphic shows bilateral sacral insufficiency fractures with vertical fracture orientation.

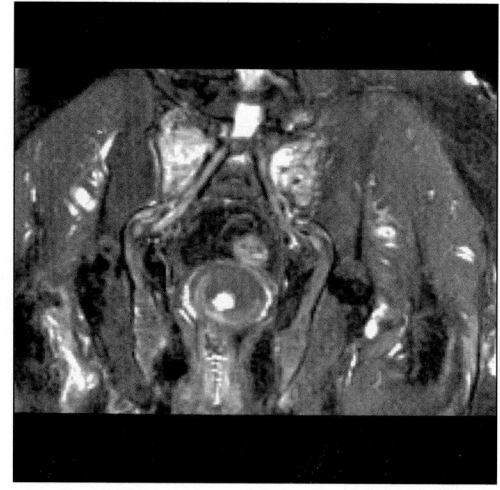

Coronal FS PD FSE MR shows diffuse hyperintense sacral alar marrow edema in bilateral sacral alar insufficiency fractures. The edema obscures fracture detail.

TERMINOLOGY

Abbreviations and Synonyms
- Insufficiency fracture (fx) sacrum, sacral alar fx

Definitions
- Stress fx of sacrum 2° to normal forces applied to weakened or abnormal bone

IMAGING FINDINGS

General Features
- Best diagnostic clue: Hyperintense sacral marrow on coronal oblique FS PD FSE or STIR images
- Location: Sacral ala
- Size
  - Unilateral or bilateral
  - Unilateral does not cross midline
- Morphology
  - Vertical fx with diffuse alar edema
  - "H" sign on MR for bilateral fx

Radiographic Findings
- Radiography
  - Insensitive
  - ± Osteopenia

CT Findings
- NECT
  - Indicated when MRI not available and bone scan inconclusive
  - Fx oriented vertically along sacral ala, parallel to sacroiliac (SI) joint
  - Linear fx with sclerosis
  - Fx unilateral or bilateral
  - Transverse fx component may not be visualized on axial images (fx in plane of scan)
  - Associated pubic arch fx 2° to altered biomechanics

MR Findings
- T1WI
  - Hypointense sacral ala
  - ± Visualized hypointense fx line
  - Fx lines parallel to SI joints
  - Transverse fx component in bilateral fx
- T2WI
  - Hyperintense sacral ala marrow edema
  - Hypointense fx line
  - "H" or "Honda" sign in bilateral fx connecting ala on T2WI
  - No trabecular destruction
  - ± Adjacent soft tissue edema (no mass)
  - ± Concomitant pubic arch stress fx
  - High resolution images may be required to identify fx

DDx: Sacral Insufficiency Fractures

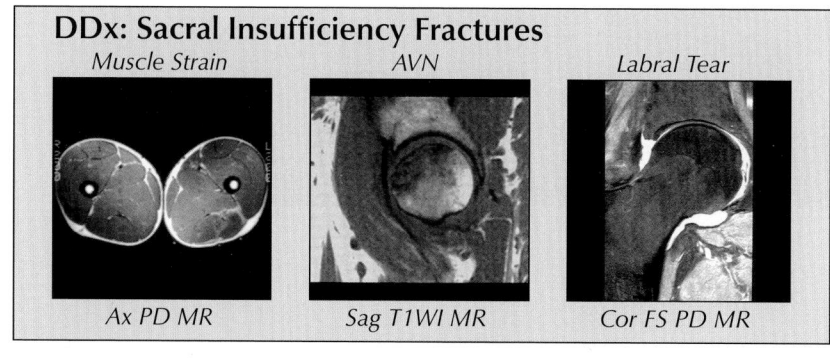

Muscle Strain	AVN	Labral Tear
Ax PD MR	Sag T1WI MR	Cor FS PD MR

SACRAL INSUFFICIENCY FRACTURES

Key Facts

Imaging Findings
- Best diagnostic clue: Hyperintense sacral marrow on coronal oblique FS PD FSE or STIR images
- Unilateral does not cross midline
- Vertical fx with diffuse alar edema
- "H" or "Honda" sign in bilateral fx connecting ala on T2WI

Top Differential Diagnoses
- Lumbar Radiculopathy
- Muscle Strain/Tear
- Bursitis (Trochanteric, Iliopsoas)
- Intrinsic Hip Pathology
- Femoral Neck Stress Fracture

Pathology
- Normal forces applied to abnormal bone (insufficiency) vs. abnormal forces to normal bone (stress)
- Runners susceptible
- Postmenopausal osteoporosis

Clinical Issues
- Most common signs/symptoms: Pain with weight-bearing or ambulation
- No history of trauma
- Symptoms > physical signs
- Gender: F > M

Diagnostic Checklist
- Coronal oblique + axial planes most useful

Nuclear Medicine Findings
- Bone Scan
  - Non-specific if atypical pattern of tracer uptake
  - Sensitive + moderate specificity if classic radiotracer distribution (bilateral involvement)
  - Classic "H" pattern or "Honda" sign with transverse component connecting 2 vertical fxs
  - Incomplete "H" or "Honda" sign in unilateral fx
  - Increased tracer uptake in sacrum + pubic bone = insufficiency fx

Imaging Recommendations
- Best imaging tool: MR identifies fx line, morphology, sacral alar edema + lack of osseous destruction
- Protocol advice: T1 (improved marrow fat contrast > PD) + FS PD FSE or STIR in coronal oblique + axial planes

DIFFERENTIAL DIAGNOSIS

Lumbar Radiculopathy
- Disk protrusion, extrusion, sequestration
- Foraminal or central stenosis
- Spondylolisthesis

Muscle Strain/Tear
- Overuse vs. indirect trauma
- Muscle + myotendinous tears
- Strains (grade I, II, III)
- Muscle hyperintensity secondary to hemorrhage on T2WI

Bursitis (Trochanteric, Iliopsoas)
- Lateral hip pain (trochanteric)
- Hyperintensity parallel to greater trochanter on FS PD FSE or STIR
- Iliopsoas bursal inflammation = groin pain + findings anterior to hip + lateral to neurovascular structures

Intrinsic Hip Pathology
- Hip dislocation
- Acetabular labral tears
- AVN of femoral head
- Osteoarthritis (OA)
- Femoroacetabular impingement (OA in younger patient without dysplastic hips)

Femoral Neck Stress Fracture
- Cyclic loading + microfracture
- Hypointense fx line + adjacent calcar hyperintensity (T2WI)
- Edema often more extensive than fx involvement

Pubic Stress Fracture
- Military recruits, long-distance runners
- Hypointense fx with parasymphyseal hyperintensity on FS PD FSE or STIR
- Vertical fx unilateral or bilateral

Metastatic Disease
- Interruption of cortex
- Destruction of cortex
- Marrow edema without defined fx
- May require CT documentation of loss of normal trabecular morphology

PATHOLOGY

General Features
- General path comments
  - Relevant anatomy
    - Pelvic ring = sacrum + 2 innominate bones
    - Innominate bone = fusion of 3 ossification centers (ilium, ischium, pubis)
    - SI joints = junction of innominate bones and sacrum posteriorly
    - Ligaments = posterior SI, sacrotuberous, sacrospinous, iliolumbar
    - Sciatic nerve (from roots of L4, L5, S1-3)
    - Lumbosacral trunk of lumbosacral plexus crosses anterior to sacral ala
- Etiology
  - Normal forces applied to abnormal bone (insufficiency) vs. abnormal forces to normal bone (stress)

SACRAL INSUFFICIENCY FRACTURES

- ○ Runners susceptible
- ○ Impact sport participants
- ○ Postmenopausal osteoporosis
- ○ Less common
  - ▪ Rheumatoid arthritis
  - ▪ Corticosteroid use
  - ▪ Pelvic irradiation
  - ▪ Tumor
- • Epidemiology
  - ○ 1% females > 55: Insufficiency fxs
  - ○ Stress fx of sacrum less common than pubis

Gross Pathologic & Surgical Features
- • Fx sacral ala
- • Vertical orientation of fx
- • Parallel to SI joints
- • ± Transverse fx component
- • Secondary pubic bone fx

Microscopic Features
- • Osteoclastic resorption > osteoblastic activity
- • Microfractures
- • Reduced bone mineral density

CLINICAL ISSUES

Presentation
- • Most common signs/symptoms: Pain with weight-bearing or ambulation
- • Clinical profile
  - ○ No history of trauma
  - ○ Minimal to low velocity trauma
  - ○ Hip, gluteal or groin pain
  - ○ May be non-ambulatory
  - ○ Point tenderness over sacrum
  - ○ Gait abnormality
  - ○ Limited range of motion
  - ○ Symptoms > physical signs

Demographics
- • Age: > 55 yrs
- • Gender: F > M

Natural History & Prognosis
- • Majority heal with conservative treatment
- • May progress to complete fx without treatment
- • Healing: Slow process (2-5 months)
- • Complications: Related to prolonged immobilization
  - ○ Deep venous thrombosis
  - ○ Pulmonary embolus
  - ○ Decubitus ulcers
  - ○ Falls (with use of crutches, walkers)

Treatment
- • Conservative
  - ○ Analgesics
  - ○ Bed rest
  - ○ Reduced weight bearing
  - ○ Physical therapy (range-of-motion, gait training, muscle strengthening/stretching)
- • Surgical = sacroplasty
  - ○ Interventional radiologic technique
  - ○ Similar to vertebroplasty
  - ○ Percutaneous injection polymethylmethacrylate

- ○ Nearly instantaneous relief of pain

DIAGNOSTIC CHECKLIST

Consider
- • Identify hypointense fx line, otherwise supplement with CT to assess trabecular bone destruction or microfracture
- • Associated pubic fx shown on T1, FS PD FSE or STIR
- • Coronal oblique + axial planes most useful
- • Sacral insufficiency fracture not to be confused with osteitis condensans ilii (mechanical stress induced osteosclerosis in the ilium involving inferior 1/3 of the SI joint)

SELECTED REFERENCES

1. Boissonnault WG et al: Differential diagnosis of a sacral stress fracture. J Orthop Sports Phys Ther 32(12):613-21, 2002
2. Shah MK et al: Sacral stress fractures: An unusual case of low back pain in an athlete. Spine 27(4):E104-8, 2002
3. Garant M: Sacroplasty: A new treatment for sacral insufficiency fracture. J of Vasc Interventional Radiol 12(12):1265-7, 2002
4. Springfield DS: Pathologic fractures. Rockwood and Green's fractures in adults. 5th ed. Philadelphia PA, Lippincott Williams and Wilkins, 578-9, 2001
5. Peh WC: Intrafracture fluid: A new diagnostic sign of insufficiency fractures of the sacrum and ilium. Br J Radiol 73(872):895-8, 2000
6. Major NM et al: Sacral stress fractures in long-distance runners. AJR 174(3):727-9, 2000
7. Oliver TB et al: Defects in the pelvic ring as a cause of sacral insufficiency fractures. Clin Radiol 12:852-4, 1999
8. Connolly JF: Fractures and dislocations: Closed management. 1st ed. Philadelphia PA, WB Saunders, 471-2, 1995
9. Weber M et al: Insufficiency fractures of the sacrum. Twenty cases and review of the literature. Spine 18(16):2507-12, 1993
10. Blomlie V et al: Radiation induced insufficiency fractures of the sacrum: Evaluation with MR imaging. Radiology 188:241-44, 1993
11. Daffner RH et al: Stress fractures: Current concepts. AJR 159:245-52, 1992
12. Peh WC et al: Tarlov Cysts; Another cause of sacral insufficiency fractures? Clin Radiol 46:329-30, 1992
13. Abe H et al: Radiation-induced insufficiency fractures of the pelvis: Evaluation with 99mTc-methylene diphosphonate scintigraphy. AJR 158:599-602, 1992
14. Brahme SK et al: Magnetic resonance appearance of sacral insufficiency fractures. Skeletal Radiol 19:489-493, 1990
15. Schneider R et al: Unsuspected sacral fractures: Detection by radionuclide bone scanning. AJR 144:337-41, 1985
16. Cooper KL et al: Supraacetabular insufficiency fractures. Radiology 157:15-17, 1985
17. DeSmet AA et al: Public and sacral insufficiency fractures: Clinical course and radiologic findings. AJR 145:601-6, 1985
18. Cooper KL et al: Insufficiency fractures of the sacrum. Radiology 156:15-20, 1985

SACRAL INSUFFICIENCY FRACTURES

IMAGE GALLERY

Typical

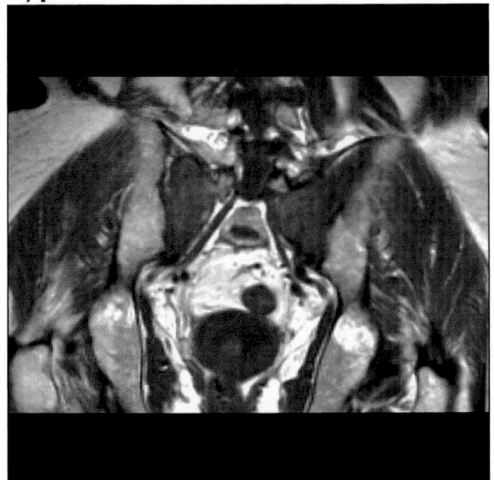

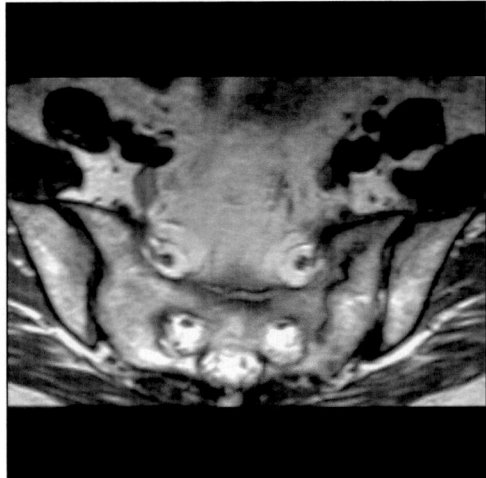

(Left) Coronal T1WI MR shows bilateral insufficiency fractures with diffuse hypointense marrow edema. *(Right)* Coronal T1WI MR shows left unilateral insufficiency fracture with a linear orientation.

Typical

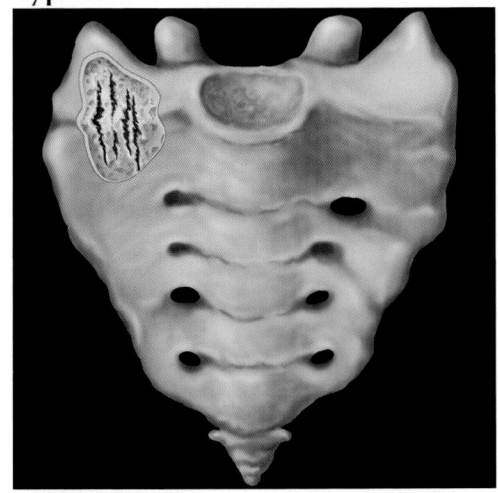

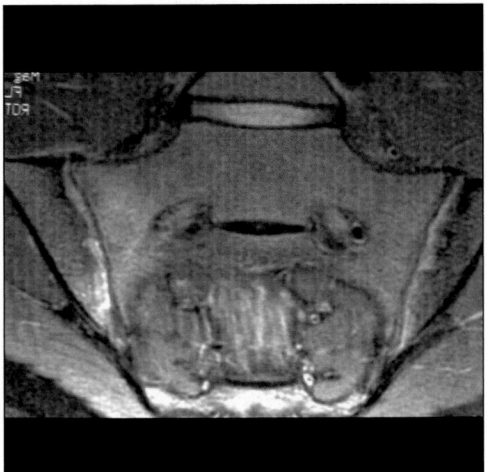

(Left) Coronal graphic shows unilateral sacral insufficiency fracture. *(Right)* Coronal FS PD FSE MR shows bilateral sacroiliitis with sacral erosions and marrow hyperintensity. The marrow edema may mimic an insufficiency fx.

Typical

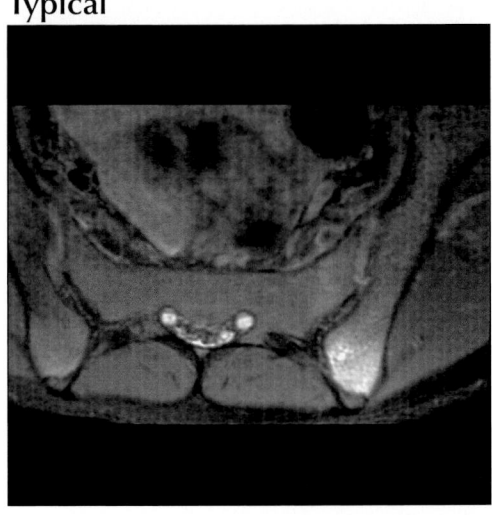

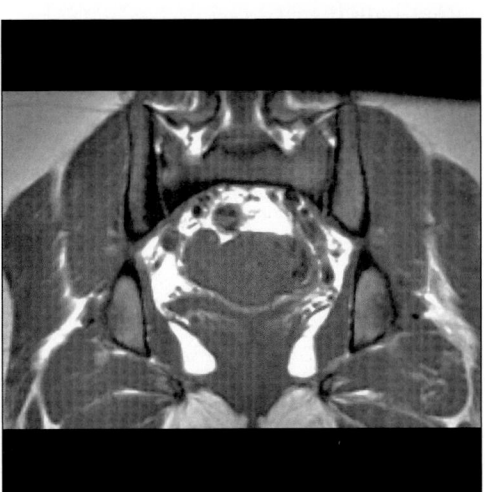

(Left) Coronal FS PD FSE MR shows subtle edema of left sacral ala in unilateral stress injury. *(Right)* Coronal T1WI MR shows hypointense sclerosis on the right in osteitis condensans ilii.

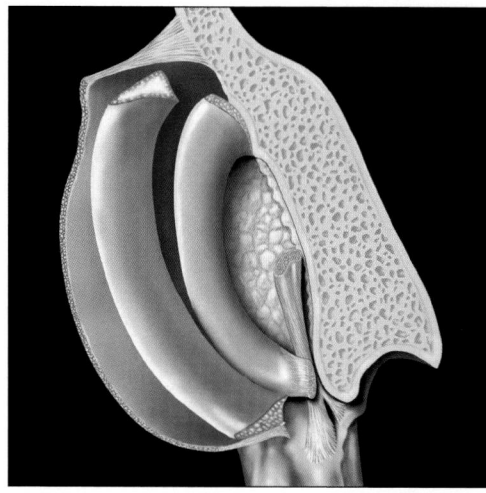

Coronal graphic shows labral detachment associated with labral degeneration and thickening (yellow).

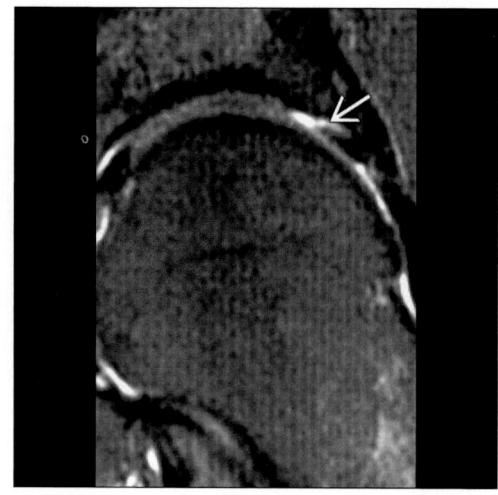

Coronal FS PD FSE MR shows hyperintense fluid signal within tear at the base of the acetabular labrum (arrow).

TERMINOLOGY

Abbreviations and Synonyms
- Acetabular labral tear, labral avulsion

Definitions
- Tear of acetabular labrum secondary to traumatic injury or degeneration of the labrum

IMAGING FINDINGS

General Features
- Best diagnostic clue: Linear hyperintensity within hypointense labrum on coronal FS PD FSE images
- Location: Anterosuperior + posterosuperior = common locations
- Size: Base of labrum or along long axis as a longitudinal tear
- Morphology: Linear tear to bucket-handle tear

Radiographic Findings
- Radiography
  - Usually negative in acute traumatic tears
  - ± Associated degenerative arthrosis
  - ± Developmental dysplasia of hip (DDH)

CT Findings
- NECT

- Subchondral cysts of the acetabulum
- Lateral acetabular rim/capsular avulsions
- Not sensitive for visualizing tear with or without contrast

MR Findings
- T1WI
  - Normal labrum
    - Hypointense
    - Covers hyaline articular cartilage at lateral peripheral margin of acetabulum
  - Intermediate linear signal vs. diffuse abnormal signal in labrum
  - Intralabral degeneration
  - Separation of the labrum at its base
  - Diastasis between acetabular articular cartilage + labral attachment
  - Assess for associated acetabular dysplasia on anterior coronal images
- T2WI
  - Linear hyperintensity contrasts hypointense labrum on FS PD FSE or STIR images
  - Radial images useful - perpendicular to tear plane
  - Hyperintense paralabral cyst on FS PD or T2 FSE or STIR images ± septations or lobulations
  - Surface irregularities associated with base of degenerated labrum

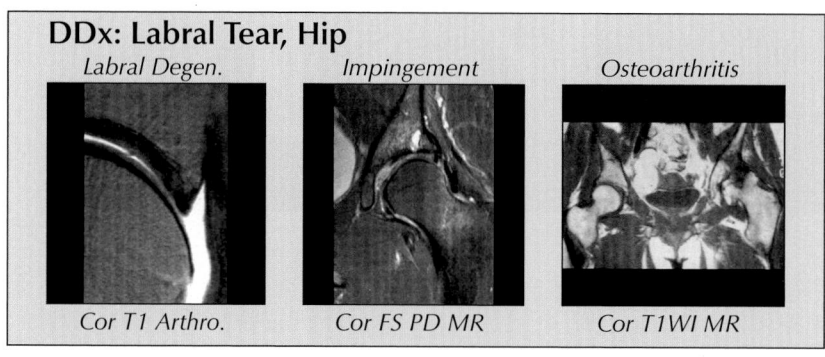

DDx: Labral Tear, Hip

Labral Degen.	Impingement	Osteoarthritis
Cor T1 Arthro.	Cor FS PD MR	Cor T1WI MR

LABRAL TEAR, HIP

Key Facts

Imaging Findings
- Best diagnostic clue: Linear hyperintensity within hypointense labrum on coronal FS PD FSE images
- Location: Anterosuperior + posterosuperior = common locations
- Morphology: Linear tear to bucket-handle tear

Top Differential Diagnoses
- Degenerative Labrum
- Normal Labral Attachment
- Femoroacetabular Impingement
- Osteoarthritis
- Developmental Dysplasia of Hip (DDH)

Pathology
- Acute, traumatic tears - common in sports requiring extreme hip rotation + flexion (soccer, hockey, golf, gymnastics, dancing, kickboxing)
- Degenerative tears - associated with degenerative disease of the hip
- Femoroacetabular impingement in younger population (< 50 years)

Clinical Issues
- Most common signs/symptoms: Hip pain
- Episodes of sharp pain associated with pivoting or twisting

Diagnostic Checklist
- Labral tear as part of femoroacetabular impingement syndrome

---

- ○ Femoroacetabular impingement: Associated labral tears + acetabular chondral erosions + subchondral acetabular hyperintensity
- ○ Hyperintense macerated to absent labrum in osteoarthritis
- ○ Labral displacement/bucket-handle tears
- ○ Loss of triangular morphology
- ○ Hyperintense joint effusion
- T1 C+
  - ○ Intraarticular contrast - fills tear
  - ○ Promotes uplifting or separation of torn labrum from acetabular articular cartilage
  - ○ Czerny classification: Based on MR arthrography (91% sensitive, 71% specific)

Imaging Recommendations
- Best imaging tool: MR for labral + chondral visualization
- Protocol advice
  - ○ T1 + FS PD FSE coronal, sagittal & axial planes
  - ○ Small FOV (16 to 18 cm) coronal ± intraarticular contrast

DIFFERENTIAL DIAGNOSIS

Degenerative Labrum
- Intralabral signal ± mild free edge blunting
- Normal margins
- No fluid across base of labrum

Normal Labral Attachment
- Normal intermediate signal intensity articular cartilage at labral base
- No contrast or fluid extension
- Normal fibrovascular bundles may mimic a tear

Femoroacetabular Impingement
- Osteoarthritis in younger patient population
- Acetabular sided pathology (chondral erosions)
- Femoral dysplasia - lateral femoral head/neck dysplastic bump
- Abnormal contact in flexion + internal rotation

Osteoarthritis
- Superior joint space narrowing
- Osteophytes
- Loss of femoral + acetabular articular cartilage

Developmental Dysplasia of Hip (DDH)
- Associated with labral pathology
- Predisposed to acetabular rim syndrome - similar to femoroacetabular impingement in nondysplastic hips
- Shallow acetabulum on anterior coronal images

Normal Iliopsoas Tendon
- Pitfall on axial and sagittal images
- Hypointense iliopsoas tendon anterior to anterior labrum ± associated fluid

Sublabral Foramen
- Inconsistent recess, sulcus or nonattachment without tear

PATHOLOGY

General Features
- General path comments
  - ○ Relevant anatomy = labrum
    - Fibrocartilaginous rim which deepens acetabulum
    - Attachment to osseous acetabular rim + transverse acetabular ligament
    - Not important in load transmission
- Etiology
  - ○ Acute, traumatic tears - common in sports requiring extreme hip rotation + flexion (soccer, hockey, golf, gymnastics, dancing, kickboxing)
  - ○ Trauma ranges from twisting injury to hip dislocation
  - ○ Degenerative tears - associated with degenerative disease of the hip
  - ○ Femoroacetabular impingement in younger population (< 50 years)
  - ○ DDH at increased risk
  - ○ Hip dislocations
- Epidemiology

LABRAL TEAR, HIP

- ○ 28% of asymptomatic individuals have labral abnormalities (includes labral degeneration)
- ○ 20% of symptomatic DDH - labral tears

Gross Pathologic & Surgical Features

- Reciprocal injury to femoral head chondral surface
- Anterosuperior labrum most frequent
- Posterosuperior more common in younger population
- Traumatic tears
  - ○ Radial flap = along inner free margin (most common)
  - ○ Longitudinal = ± unstable & displaced
- ± Associated paralabral cysts
- Subchondral acetabular cystic changes
- Gross labral detachment - less common
- Intraarticular displacement of labrum

Microscopic Features

- Degeneration
  - ○ Eosinophilic
  - ○ Mucoid
  - ○ Vascular
  - ○ Focal cavitation
  - ○ Cystic
  - ○ Separation from underlying bone interface
- Avascular regions preclude healing

Staging, Grading or Classification Criteria

- Czerny classification (MR arthrography)
  - ○ Stage IA: Hyperintense signal with no communication to articular surface + visualized perilabral sulcus
  - ○ Stage IB: No perilabral sulcus
  - ○ Stage IIA: Contrast extension into articular surface + visualized perilabral sulcus
  - ○ Stage IIB: No perilabral sulcus
  - ○ Stage IIIA: Labral detachment ± with triangular shape maintained + visualized perilabral sulcus
  - ○ Stage IIIB: Labral detachment + thickened labrum with labral hyperintensity + no perilabral sulcus
  - ○ Anterosuperior = common location for tears

CLINICAL ISSUES

Presentation

- Most common signs/symptoms: Hip pain
- Clinical profile
  - ○ Snapping
  - ○ Clicking
  - ○ Locking
  - ○ Episodes of sharp pain associated with pivoting or twisting
  - ○ Manipulation of hip from flexion, external rotation + abduction into extension + internal rotation + adduction = click for anterior labral tears
  - ○ Full flexion, adduction + internal rotation to extension + abduction + external rotation = symptoms of posterior labral tear
  - ○ Acetabular dysplasia associated
  - ○ Association with Legg-Calvé-Perthes and slipped capital femoral epiphysis
  - ○ End stage degenerative hip disease

Demographics

- Age
  - ○ 20 to 50 years = most common
  - ○ Spectrum ranges 18 to 75 years
  - ○ Young athletes = acute, traumatic
  - ○ Middle-aged associated with femoroacetabular impingement
  - ○ Older patients = degenerative tears
- Gender
  - ○ F slightly > M
    - ▪ Except increased male rate with high exposure to sports which increase the risk of femoroacetabular impingement

Natural History & Prognosis

- Progression of labral tear is typical
- Development of osteoarthritis especially as part of femoroacetabular impingement

Treatment

- Conservative
  - ○ Activity modification (limit flexion + internal rotation)
  - ○ Anti-inflammatory medication
  - ○ Intraarticular steroid injection during acute episodes of pain
- Surgical
  - ○ Debridement
  - ○ Modified Bankart

DIAGNOSTIC CHECKLIST

Consider

- Labral tear as part of femoroacetabular impingement syndrome
- Identify associated paralabral cysts
- Assess acetabular chondral surface for erosions

SELECTED REFERENCES

1. DeLee JC et al: Orthopaedic sports medicine. Principles and practice. vol 2. 2nd ed. Philadelphia PA, Saunders, 25(A):1443-63, 2003
2. McCarthy J et al: The role of hip arthroscopy in the elite athlete. Clin Orthop and Related Research 406:71-4, 2003
3. McCarthy J et al: Anatomy, pathologic features and treatment of acetabular labral tears. Clin Orthop and Related Research 406:38-47, 2003
4. Czerny C et al: Magnetic resonance imaging and magnetic resonance arthrography of the acetabular labrum: Comparison with surgical findings. Rofo Fortschr Geb Rontgenstr Neuen Bildgeb Verfahr 173(8):702-8, 2001
5. Aydingoz U et al: MR imaging of the acetabular labrum: A comparative study of both hips in 180 asymptomatic volunteers. Eur Radiol 11(4)567-74, 2001
6. Plotz GM et al: Magnetic resonance arthrography of the acetabular labrum. Macroscopic and histological correlation in 20 cadavers. J Bone Joint Surg Br 82(3)426-32, 2000
7. Abe I et al: Acetabular labrum: Abnormal findings at MR imaging in asymptomatic hips. Radiology 216(2)576-81, 2000

IMAGE GALLERY

Typical

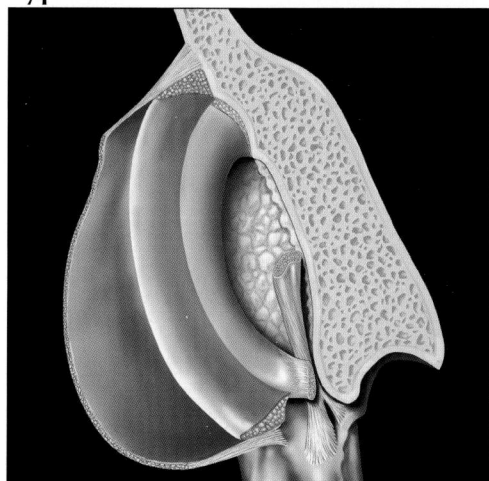
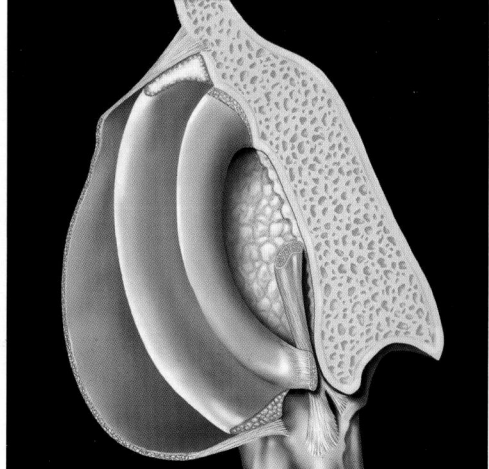

(Left) Coronal graphic shows normal acetabular labral anatomy. The normal labrum is triangular shaped with a well defined apex. *(Right)* Coronal graphic shows thickened labrum with fibrocartilaginous degeneration (yellow). No paralabral recess is identified.

Typical

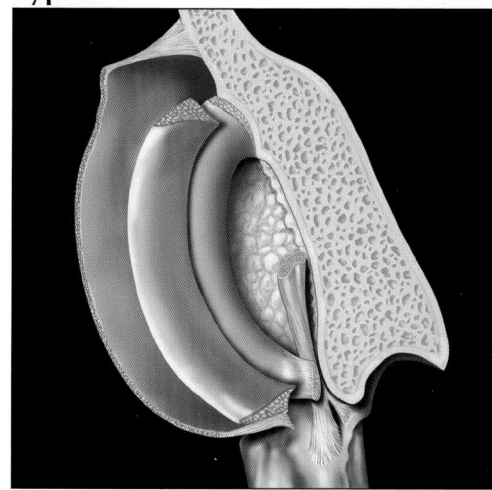
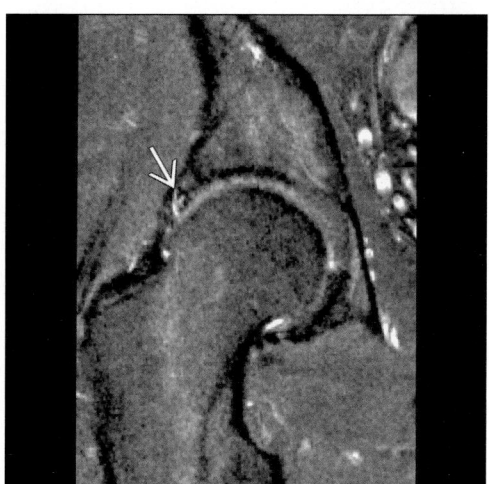

(Left) Coronal graphic shows normal undercutting of the labrum (gray) by articular cartilage (blue). *(Right)* Coronal FS PD FSE MR shows hyperintense longitudinal tear (arrow) of the labrum.

Variant

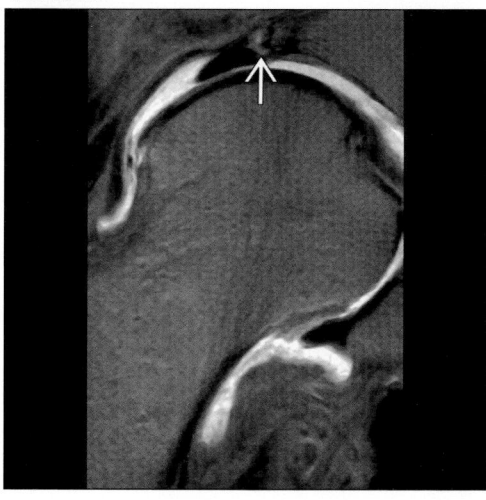
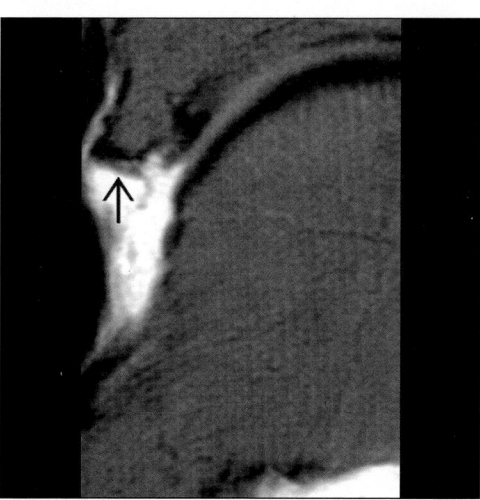

(Left) Coronal T1 C+ (MR arthrogram) shows hyperintense degeneration (arrow) at the base of an ossified labrum. *(Right)* Coronal T1 C+ (MR arthrogram) shows obliterated labrum (arrow) in osteoarthritis.

PARALABRAL CYSTS, HIP

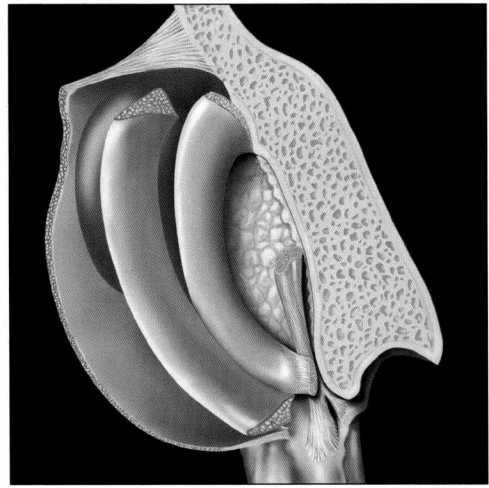

Coronal graphic shows paralabral cyst (blue) communicating with linear tear and detachment of the acetabular labrum.

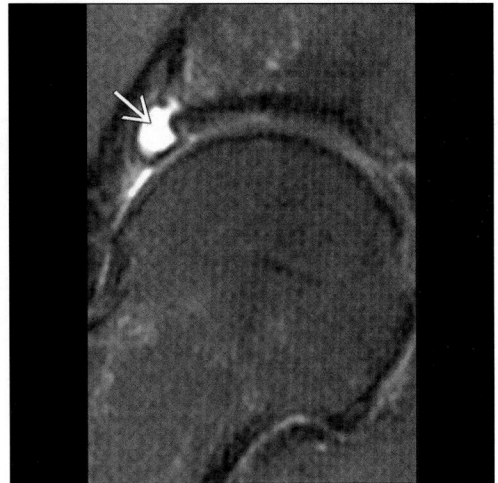

Coronal FS PD FSE MR shows hyperintense paralabral (intralabral) cyst (arrow) extending into the substance of acetabular labrum.

TERMINOLOGY

Abbreviations and Synonyms
- Ganglion cyst, synovial cyst of the hip, cystic degeneration of the labrum, acetabular ganglion cysts, para-acetabular soft tissue ganglion

Definitions
- Juxta-articular cyst formed secondary to a labral tear of the hip

IMAGING FINDINGS

General Features
- Best diagnostic clue: Hyperintense cyst adjacent to the labrum on coronal FS PD or T2 FSE images
- Location
  - Located lateral to anterosuperior or posterosuperior labrum
  - May communicate with any location of labral tear including anteroinferior or posteroinferior
- Size: Variable (1 mm to > 1 cm)
- Morphology: Septated & lobulated

Radiographic Findings
- Radiography
  - Usually normal
  - Acetabular dysplasia
  - Osteoarthritis
  - Not sensitive for femoroacetabular impingement

CT Findings
- NECT
  - Hypodense (fluid attenuation) juxta-articular mass
  - Labral tears cannot be reliably visualized, even with intraarticular contrast
  - Exclude intrinsic hip pathology

MR Findings
- T1WI
  - ± Septated + lobulated
  - Hypo to intermediate signal intensity
  - Well-defined margins without reactive soft tissue edema
  - Mucin contents may result in increased signal intensity
  - ± Associated hyperintense intraosseous ganglion cysts of acetabular roof or lateral rim
  - Associated intermediate signal in labral tear or separation of labrum at its base
- T2WI
  - Hyperintense juxta-articular mass
  - Longitudinal extension of cyst usually superior to inferior + anterior to posterior
  - Hypointense septations
  - Intermediate signal synovial thickening

DDx: Paralabral Cysts, Hip

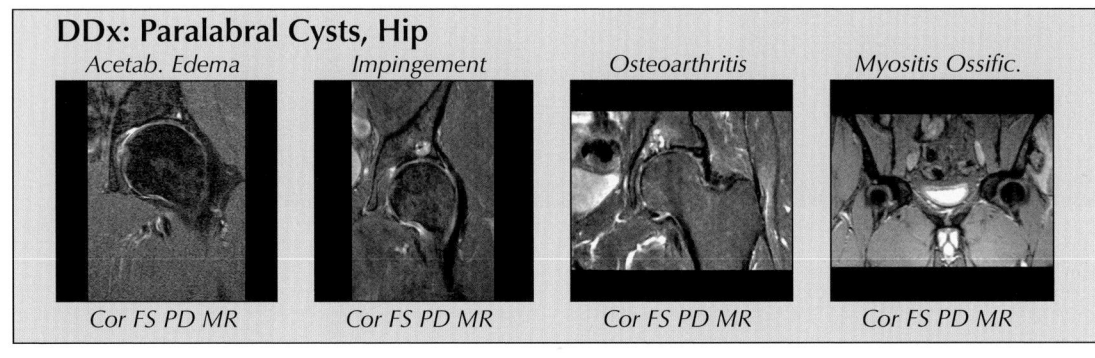

Acetab. Edema	Impingement	Osteoarthritis	Myositis Ossific.
Cor FS PD MR	Cor FS PD MR	Cor FS PD MR	Cor FS PD MR

PARALABRAL CYSTS, HIP

Key Facts

Imaging Findings
- Best diagnostic clue: Hyperintense cyst adjacent to the labrum on coronal FS PD or T2 FSE images
- Located lateral to anterosuperior or posterosuperior labrum
- May communicate with any location of labral tear including anteroinferior or posteroinferior
- Morphology: Septated & lobulated

Top Differential Diagnoses
- Femoroacetabular Impingement
- Osteoarthritis
- Developmental Dysplasia of the Hip (DDH)
- Soft Tissue Tumors

Pathology
- Increased/abnormal load on lateral aspect acetabular roof
- Increased intraarticular pressure forcing synovial fluid through a labral tear
- Anterosuperior > posterosuperior > inferior location

Clinical Issues
- Most common signs/symptoms: Hip pain
- Sudden sharp pain
- Clicking
- Locking of joint
- Deep anterior groin pain

Diagnostic Checklist
- Paralabral cysts may occur adjacent to any portion of the fibrocartilaginous labrum

   - ○ Linear hyperintense tear or detachment of adjacent labrum
   - ○ Femoroacetabular impingement
     - Hyperintense edema progressing to cyst formation in acetabular roof
     - Torn labrum
     - Acetabular roof chondral erosions
     - Dysplastic lateral femoral osseous bump lateral to physeal scar
   - ○ Hyperintense intraosseous ganglion + labral tear
   - ○ Associated acetabular dysplasia with shallow acetabulum on anterior coronal images
- T1 C+
   - ○ Intravenous contrast: Peripheral enhancement of cysts
   - ○ Intraarticular contrast: Variable demonstration of paralabral cyst (also requires FS PD FSE images to visualize cysts without joint communication)

Imaging Recommendations
- Best imaging tool: MR for labrum + cyst
- Protocol advice: T1 + FS PD FSE or STIR in coronal (+ small FOV), sagittal + axial planes

DIFFERENTIAL DIAGNOSIS

Femoroacetabular Impingement
- Osteoarthritis in younger patient population (< 50 years)
- Acetabular roof subchondral edema
- Labral tears associated in 50%
- Chondral erosions in acetabulum
- ± Femoral dysplastic osseous bump or lateral prominence

Osteoarthritis
- Superior joint space narrowing
- Chondral loss acetabulum + femoral head
- Joint effusion
- Osteophytes
- ± Subchondral marrow edema acetabulum + femoral head

Developmental Dysplasia of the Hip (DDH)
- Shallow acetabulum on anterior coronal images
- Associated with labral tears + cysts
- Subchondral sclerosis lateral acetabular rim
- Chondral fissures + erosions lateral acetabulum

Greater Trochanteric Bursitis
- Lateral hip pain
- Hyperintense fluid signal adjacent to and parallel with greater trochanter
- ± Associated with gluteus medius muscle-tendon pathology

Soft Tissue Tumors
- Lipoma
- Desmoid
- Malignant fibrous histiocytoma
- Liposarcoma
- Synovial cell sarcoma

Tumor-Like Soft Tissue Masses
- Abscess
- Hematoma
- Seroma
- Intramuscular cyst

Myositis Ossificans
- Calcified or ossified mass of granulation tissue
- History of blunt muscle trauma
- Inhomogeneity on T2WI ± surrounding edema

PATHOLOGY

General Features
- General path comments
   - ○ Relevant anatomy = labrum
     - Fibrocartilaginous rim - deepens acetabulum
     - Not important in load transmission
- Etiology
   - ○ Increased/abnormal load on lateral aspect acetabular roof
     - Femoroacetabular impingement

PARALABRAL CYSTS, HIP

- ■ Osteoarthritis
- ■ Developmental dysplasia
- ■ Femoral dysplasia (lateral aspect femoral head)
- ○ Intraosseous ganglion cyst becoming a soft tissue ganglion
- ○ Increased intraarticular pressure forcing synovial fluid through a labral tear
- ○ Post-traumatic
- • Epidemiology
  - ○ 28% of asymptomatic population have labral abnormalities (including labral degeneration)
  - ○ 20% of DDH with symptoms have a labral tear

Gross Pathologic & Surgical Features

- • Paralabral cysts adjacent to lateral acetabular labrum ± soft tissue dissection
- • Anterosuperior > posterosuperior > inferior location
- • Associated labral tears
  - ○ Traumatic
  - ○ Degenerative
- • ± Subchondral acetabular cystic changes + chondral erosions

Microscopic Features

- • Ganglion cyst
  - ○ Lined with connective tissue
  - ○ Contains mucinous material
  - ○ ± Communication with joint
- • Synovial cyst
  - ○ Lined with synovial cells
  - ○ Contains synovial fluid
  - ○ ± Communication with joint
- • Associated labral degeneration or tear
  - ○ Eosinophilic, mucoid, + vacuolar degeneration of labrum

CLINICAL ISSUES

Presentation

- • Most common signs/symptoms: Hip pain
- • Clinical profile
  - ○ Similar presentation as seen for labral tears
  - ○ Sudden sharp pain
  - ○ Clicking
  - ○ Popping & snapping
  - ○ Locking of joint
  - ○ Deep anterior groin pain
  - ○ Lateral hip ± gluteal radiation pain
  - ○ Symptoms correlate with underlying labral tear > than paralabral cyst
  - ○ A large paralabral cyst - symptoms of local mass effect

Demographics

- • Age
  - ○ 20 to 50 years most common for labral tears
  - ○ Age spectrum ranges from 18 to 75 years
  - ○ Common in sports requiring hip rotation + flexion: Golf, hockey, soccer, gymnastics, ballet
  - ○ Common in middle-aged adults secondary to degenerative labral tears in femoroacetabular impingement

- • Gender: Increased male rate as a function of sports related to risk of femoroacetabular impingement

Natural History & Prognosis

- • Will not spontaneously resolve
- • Conservative treatment for temporary pain relief
- • Labral tear or underlying labral abnormality (e.g., femoroacetabular impingement) must be addressed or cyst will recur

Treatment

- • Conservative
  - ○ Anti-inflammatories for pain relief
  - ○ Percutaneous aspiration: Temporary, as cyst will recur
  - ○ Intraarticular steroids
- • Surgical
  - ○ Repair/debridement/resection of labrum
  - ○ Debridement + microfracture of acetabular roof
  - ○ Femoral resurfacing in femoroacetabular impingement
  - ○ Acetabular osteotomy in femoroacetabular impingement
  - ○ Arthroscopic techniques available

DIAGNOSTIC CHECKLIST

Consider

- • Paralabral cysts are associated with acetabular labral tears
- • Paralabral cysts are seen in femoroacetabular impingement
- • Paralabral cysts may occur adjacent to any portion of the fibrocartilaginous labrum

SELECTED REFERENCES

1. McCarthy J et al: The role of hip arthroscopy in the elite athlete. Clin Orthop and Related Research 406:71-4, 2003
2. McCarthy J et al: Anatomy, pathologic features and treatment of acetabular labral tears. Clin Orthop and Related Research 406:38-47, 2003
3. Van Holsbeeck MT et al: Musculoskeletal ultrasound. 2nd ed. St. Louis MO, Mosby, 254-65, 2001
4. Mason JB: Acetabular labral tears in the athlete. Clin Sports Med 20(4):779-89, 2001
5. Aydingoz U et al: MR imaging of the acetabular labrum: A comparative study of both hips in 180 asymptomatic volunteers. Eur Radiol 11(4):567-74, 2001
6. Tan V et al: Contribution of acetabular labrum to articulating surface area and femoral head coverage in adult hip joints: An anatomic study in cadavera. Am J Orthop 30(11):809-12, 2001
7. Plotz GM et al: Magnetic resonance arthrography of the acetabular labrum. Macroscopic and histological correlation in 20 cadavers. J Bone Joint Surg Br 82(3):426-32, 2000
8. Abe I et al: Acetabular labrum: Abnormal findings at MR imaging in asymptomatic hips. Radiology 216(2):576-81, 2000
9. Lecouvet FE et al: MR imaging of the acetabular labrum: Variations in 200 asymptomatic hips. AJR 167(4):1025-8, 1996

PARALABRAL CYSTS, HIP

IMAGE GALLERY

Typical

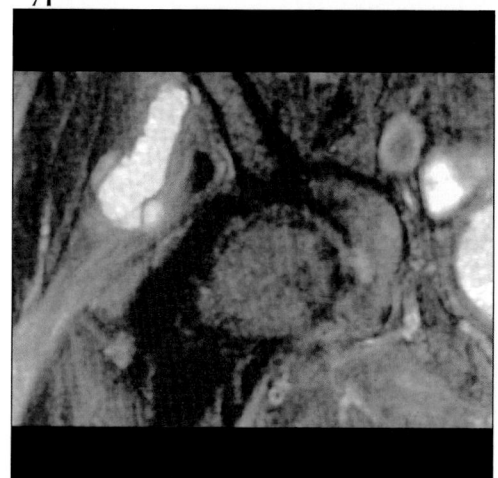 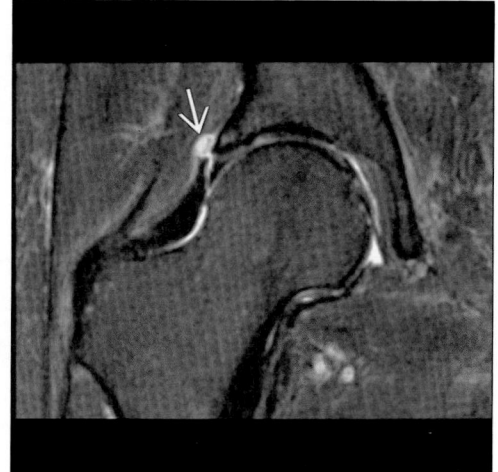

(Left) Coronal FS PD FSE MR shows lateral and superior dissection deep to the gluteus medius muscle. *(Right)* Coronal FS PD FSE MR shows focal paralabral cyst (arrow) undermining the superior acetabular labrum.

Typical

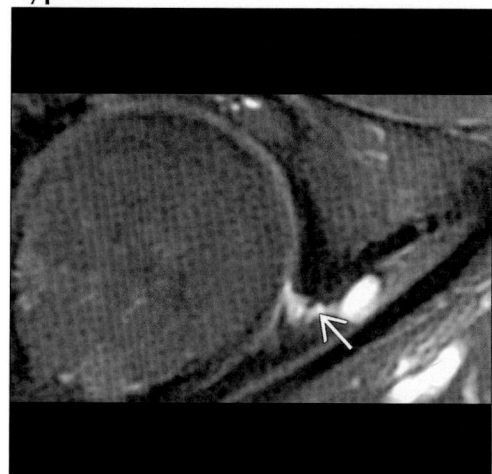 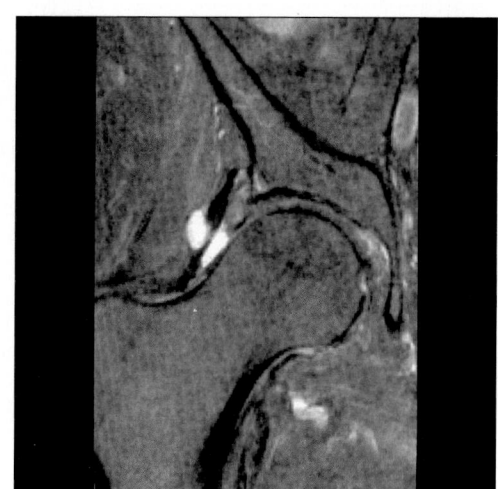

(Left) Axial FS PD FSE MR shows posterior paralabral cyst (arrow) in association with a posterosuperior labral tear. *(Right)* Coronal FS PD FSE MR shows extension of paralabral cyst lateral to the joint capsule (lateral to the iliofemoral ligament).

Typical

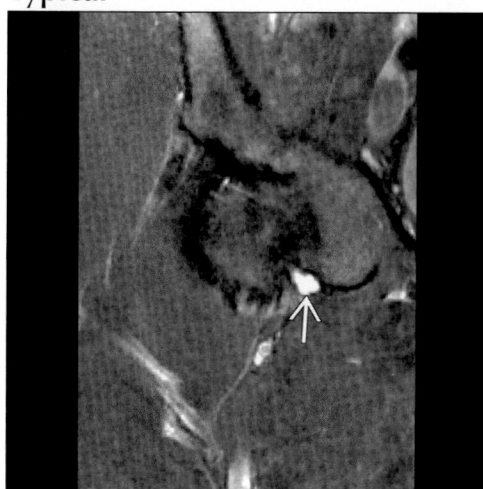 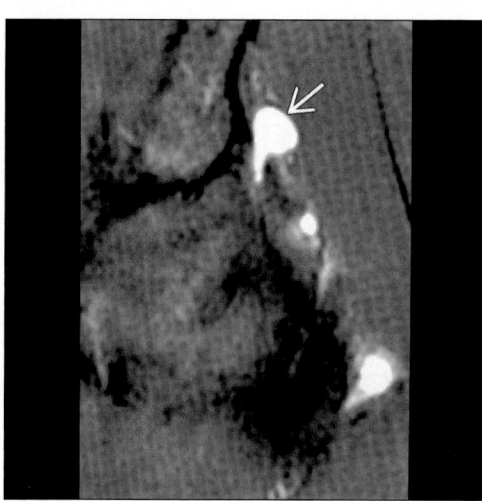

(Left) Anterior coronal FS PD FSE MR image shows paralabral cyst (arrow) presenting anteroinferiorly. *(Right)* Coronal FS PD FSE MR shows far anterior extension of an anterosuperior paralabral cyst (arrow).

FEMOROACETABULAR IMPINGEMENT

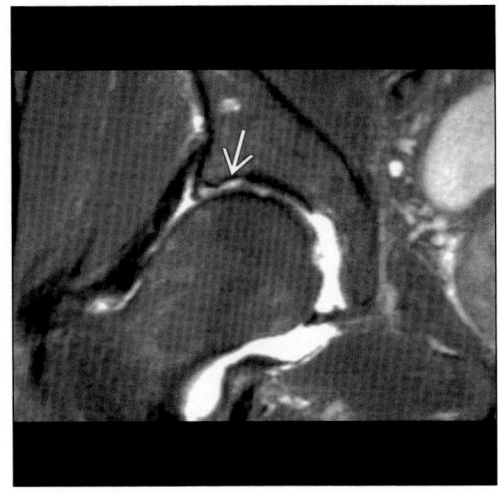

Coronal graphic shows femoroacetabular impingement with torn acetabular labrum, subchondral cystic change of lateral acetabular roof, dysplastic femoral "bump" and subchondral cyst.

Coronal FS PD FSE MR shows femoroacetabular impingement with articular cartilage erosion (arrow) of the lateral margin of the acetabular roof. The acetabular labrum is torn.

TERMINOLOGY

Abbreviations and Synonyms
- Cam-effect, acetabular rim syndrome

Definitions
- Repetitive microtrauma from impingement of femoral head against acetabulum
- Lateral acetabular rim syndrome is equivalent to femoroacetabular impingement in patients with hip dysplasia

IMAGING FINDINGS

General Features
- Best diagnostic clue: Abnormal signal of lateral femoral head + acetabular rim associated with labral tears & cartilage defects
- Location
  - Lateral femoral head
  - Acetabular rim
- Size
  - Variable acetabular subchondral cystic change, sclerosis + edema
  - Acetabular changes typically 5 mm to 2 cm in coronal plane
- Morphology

- Focal acetabular chondral erosions + focal underlying subchondral sclerosis, edema ± cyst
- ± Dysplastic lateral femoral bump adjacent to physeal scar

Radiographic Findings
- Radiography
  - Early stage: Normal
  - Advanced stage
    - Joint space narrowing
    - Subchondral sclerosis
    - Subchondral cysts
    - Osteophyte formation
  - Loss of anterior femoral offset (defined as anterior offset of head relative to anterior surface of femoral neck)

MR Findings
- T1WI
  - Hypointense edema + sclerosis lateral acetabular subchondral bone
  - Hypointense to intermediate signal intensity acetabular subchondral cysts
  - Abnormal contour (blunted) acetabular labrum
  - ± Dysplastic femoral "bump" lateral to physeal scar + loss of anterior femoral offset
- T2WI
  - Hyperintense subchondral marrow edema - laterally located

DDx: Femoroacetabular Impingement

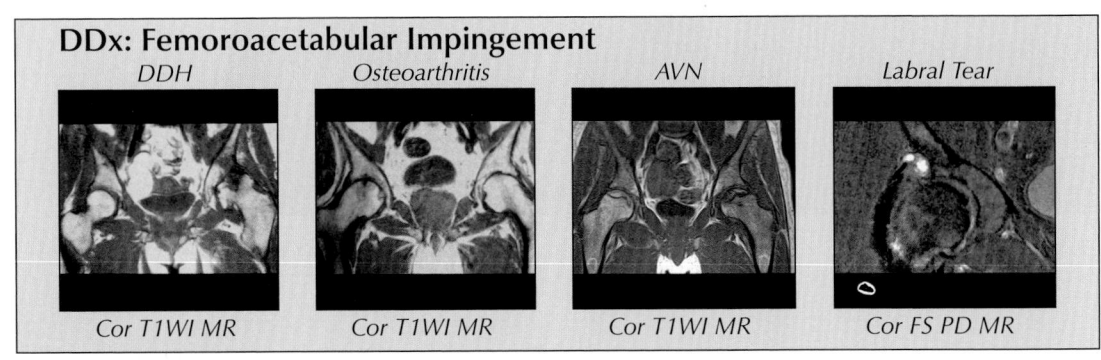

DDH	Osteoarthritis	AVN	Labral Tear
Cor T1WI MR	Cor T1WI MR	Cor T1WI MR	Cor FS PD MR

FEMOROACETABULAR IMPINGEMENT

Key Facts

Imaging Findings
- Best diagnostic clue: Abnormal signal of lateral femoral head + acetabular rim associated with labral tears & cartilage defects
- Focal acetabular chondral erosions + focal underlying subchondral sclerosis, edema ± cyst
- ± Dysplastic lateral femoral bump adjacent to physeal scar

Top Differential Diagnoses
- Developmental Dysplasia of the Hip (DDH)
- Osteoarthritis (OA)
- Avascular Necrosis (AVN) of the Hip
- Labral Tear

Pathology
- Labral damage occurs during impingement

- Occurs in non-dysplastic hips
- Femoral head is in contact with acetabular rim in flexion + internal rotation

Clinical Issues
- Most common signs/symptoms: Recurrent episodes of sharp hip, groin pain
- Pain with weight bearing
- Pain may also radiate laterally or posterolaterally
- Symptom increase with axial loading of hip - running
- Age: 20-50 years

Diagnostic Checklist
- Identify associated femoral dysplasia (anterior coronal images)

- ○ Intermediate signal labral degeneration
- ○ Hyperintense linear or diffuse signal in labral tear
- ○ Absent labral tissue
- ○ Inhomogeneous to hyperintense signal in acetabular subchondral cysts
- ○ Defect, attenuation or fissure in normally intermediate signal intensity articular cartilage
- ○ Dysplastic femoral "bump" - normal marrow fat signal or hyperintense + small hyperintense femoral head/neck cysts
- ○ Hypointense thickened hip capsule (iliofemoral ligament)
- T1 C+
  - ○ MR arthrography
    - Detects labral tears
    - Acetabular surface chondral erosions
    - Radial imaging useful
- Subchondral acetabular sclerosis hypointense on T1 + T2WI

Imaging Recommendations
- Best imaging tool: MR superior for early signs of acetabular chondral erosions + subchondral bone changes
- Protocol advice
  - ○ Coronal T1 for sclerosis + FS PD FSE (small FOV) to visualize extent of chondral fissures or erosions
  - ○ Radial imaging to improve sensitivity for labral tears
  - ○ Axial + sagittal planes also used

DIFFERENTIAL DIAGNOSIS

Developmental Dysplasia of the Hip (DDH)
- Shallow acetabulum
- Identified on anteroposterior (AP) radiograph or anterior slices of coronal MR

Osteoarthritis (OA)
- Joint space narrowing
- Osteophyte formation
- Cartilage thinning

Avascular Necrosis (AVN) of the Hip
- Wedge-shaped subchondral bone infarct
- Double line sign in 80%
- ± Femoral head + neck hyperintense edema
- Articular cartilage intact at presentation

Labral Tear
- ± Paralabral cyst
- Linear hyperintensity on T2WI
- Labral blunting
- Labral base degeneration
- Pain, clicking, locking

PATHOLOGY

General Features
- General path comments
  - ○ Intact labrum limits extent of cartilage deformation + stress through sealing mechanism
  - ○ Labral damage occurs during impingement
  - ○ Pain is result of stimulation of nociceptive and proprioceptive receptors in innervated labrum
  - ○ Femoroacetabular impingement represents a previously unrecognized cause of arthritis in young adults
- Etiology
  - ○ Occurs in non-dysplastic hips
  - ○ Repetitive microtrauma from impingement of femoral head against acetabulum
  - ○ Femoral head is in contact with acetabular rim in flexion + internal rotation
  - ○ Leads to degeneration of labrum + articular cartilage
  - ○ Might be due to anatomical variations of proximal femur
    - Reduction in mean femoral anteversion + mean head-neck offset relative to anterior aspect of neck
    - "Pistol-grip" or "post-slip" deformity
- Epidemiology
  - ○ Etiology of majority of "idiopathic" hip OA
  - ○ OA: 5%

FEMOROACETABULAR IMPINGEMENT

Gross Pathologic & Surgical Features
- Absent or thinned articular cartilage
- Polished subchondral bone if articular cartilage is absent
- Labral degeneration or tear
- Cystic changes: Cysts filled with loose fibromyxoid tissue
- Osteophytes

Microscopic Features
- Vertical clefting of articular cartilage
- Villous hyperplasia of synovium

CLINICAL ISSUES

Presentation
- Most common signs/symptoms: Recurrent episodes of sharp hip, groin pain
- Clinical profile
  - Pain out of proportion to radiographic findings
  - Positive impingement provocation test: Pain during flexion + internal rotation
  - Pain with weight bearing
  - Pain during hip flexion: Walking uphill, sitting, jumping
  - Pain may also radiate laterally or posterolaterally
  - Symptom increase with axial loading of hip - running

Demographics
- Age: 20-50 years
- Gender: M > F
- A function of hours of activity exposure with increasing age
- Flexion + internal rotation + axial loading activities at risk (e.g., kickboxing, squatting)

Natural History & Prognosis
- If unrecognized can lead to severe osteoarthritis requiring hip replacement
- Activity modification may stabilize symptoms with synovialization of subchondral cysts
- Full thickness chondral lesions of the acetabulum accelerate progression of joint space narrowing

Treatment
- Conservative
  - Non-weight bearing (short term)
  - Anti-inflammatory medication
  - Muscle strengthening to relieve hip joint stress
  - Non-loading activities (bicycle, elliptical) to cycle the hip joint while stimulating articular cartilage healing
- Surgical
  - Arthroscopic debridement of labral tears
  - Femoroacetabular debridement + femoral reshaping (resection of dysplastic "bump")
  - Periacetabular osteotomy
  - Hip replacement in advanced cases

DIAGNOSTIC CHECKLIST

Consider
- T1WI sensitive for acetabular roof subchondral sclerosis
- FS PD FSE coronal sensitive for subchondral edema, chondral fissures + labral tear
- Identify associated femoral dysplasia (anterior coronal images)

SELECTED REFERENCES

1. Siebenrock KA et al: Anterior femoro-acetabular impingement due to acetabular retroversion: Treatment with periacetabular osteotomy. J Bone Joint Surg Am 85-A(2):278-86, 2003
2. Schmidt MR et al: Cartilage lesions in the hip: Diagnostic effectiveness of MR arthrography. Radiol 226:382-6, 2002
3. Kloen P et al: Early lesions of the labrum and acetabular cartilage in osteonecrosis of the femoral head. J Bone Joint Surg Br 84(1):66-9, 2002
4. Notzli HP et al: The contour of the femoral head-neck junction as a predictor for the risk of anterior impingement. J Bone Joint Surg Br 84(4):556-60, 2002
5. Ito K et al: Femoroacetabular impingement and the cam-effect. A MRI-based quantitative anatomical study of the femoral head-neck offset. J Bone Joint Surg 83-B:171-6, 2001
6. Abe I et al: Acetabular labrum: Abnormal findings at MR imaging in asymptomatic hips. Radiol 216:576-81, 2000
7. Ferguson SJ et al: The influence of the acetabular labrum on hip cartilage consolidations: A poroelastic finite element model. J Biomechanics 33:953-60, 1999
8. Myers SR et al: Anterior femoroacetabular impingement after periacetabular osteotomy. Clin Orthop Rel Res 363:93-9, 1999
9. Toennis D et al: Acetabular and femoral anteversion: Relationship with osteoarthritis of the hip. J Bone Joint Surg 81-A:1747-70, 1999
10. McGibbon CA et al: Cartilage and subchondral bone thickness distribution with MR imaging. Acad Radiol 5(1):20-5, 1998
11. McGibbon CA et al: A general computing method for spatial cartilage thickness from co-planar MRI. Med Eng Phys 20(3):169-76, 1998
12. Leung M et al: Evaluation of the acetabular labrum by MR arthrography. J Bone Joint Surg 79-B:230-4, 1997
13. Varich L et al: Patterns of central acetabular osteophytosis in osteoarthritis of the hip. Invest Radiol 28(12):1120-7, 1993
14. Klaue K et al: The acetabular rim syndrome. A clincial presentation of dysplasia of the hip. J Bone Joint Surg 73-B:423-9, 1991
15. Kurrat HJ et al: The thickness of the cartilage in the hip joint. J Anat 126(1):145-55, 1978

FEMOROACETABULAR IMPINGEMENT

IMAGE GALLERY

Typical

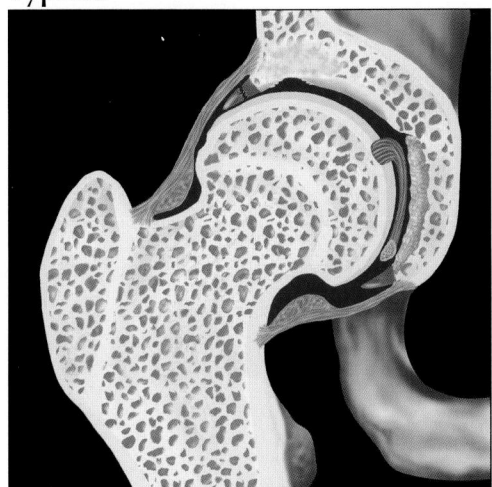
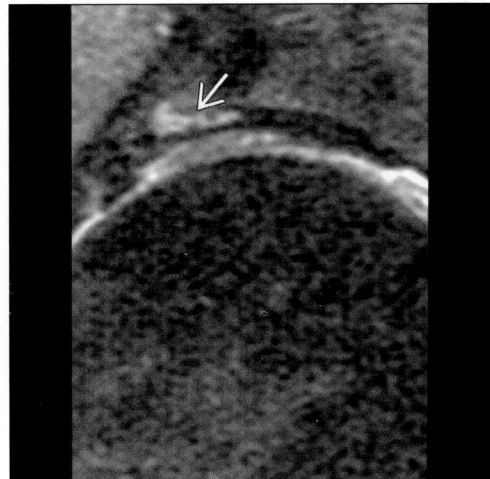

(Left) Coronal graphic shows femoroacetabular impingement with subchondral acetabular roof edema, focal chondral erosion, and labral tear. *(Right)* Coronal FS PD FSE MR shows early changes of femoroacetabular impingement with subchondral marrow edema *(arrow)* and articular cartilage fissures. The acetabular labrum is torn.

Typical

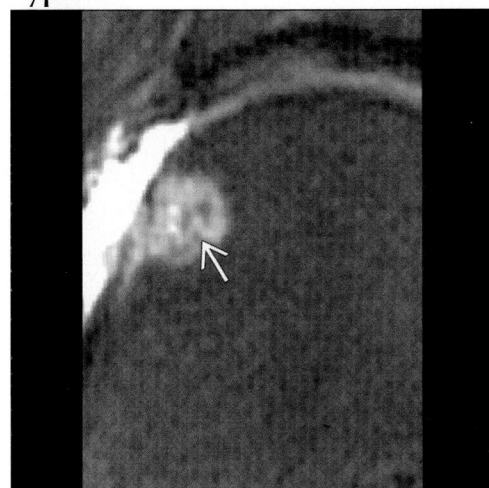
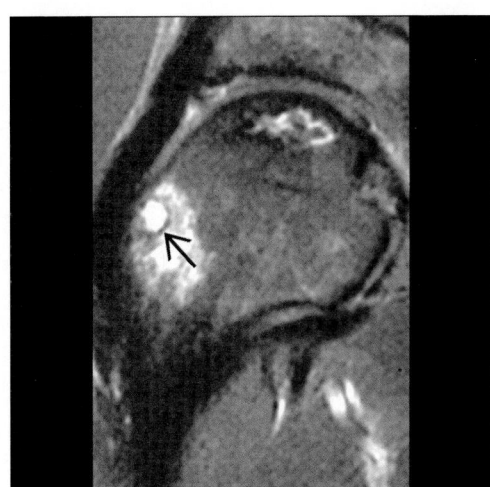

(Left) Coronal FS PD FSE MR shows hyperintense marrow edema *(arrow)* in an area of femoral dysplasia adjacent to the physeal scar. This is the contact point for impingement of the acetabular roof. *(Right)* Coronal FS PD FSE MR shows femoroacetabular impingement with dysplastic femoral "bump" and subchondral cyst *(arrow)*. Acetabular chondral erosions and labral tear are present. Incidental finding of AVN.

Typical

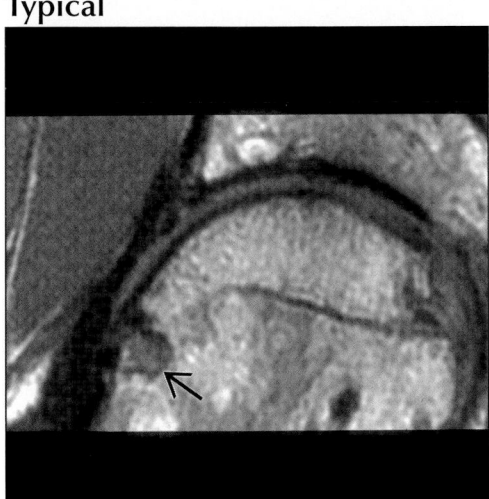
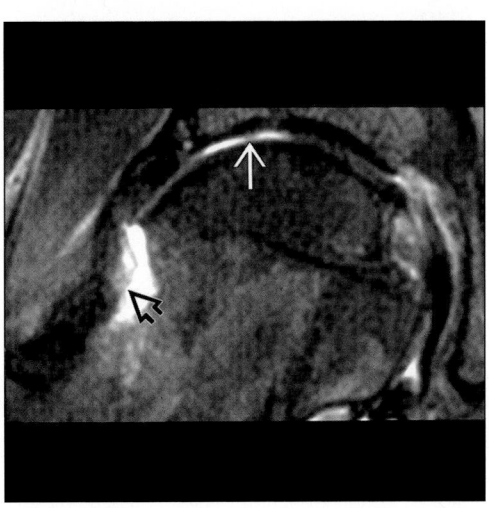

(Left) Coronal FS PD FSE MR shows lateral femoral subchondral cyst *(arrow)* characteristically located adjacent to the physeal scar. *(Right)* Coronal FS PD FSE MR shows postoperative removal of femoral cyst *(open arrow)* and debridement of acetabular *(arrow)* articular cartilage.

OSTEOARTHRITIS, HIP

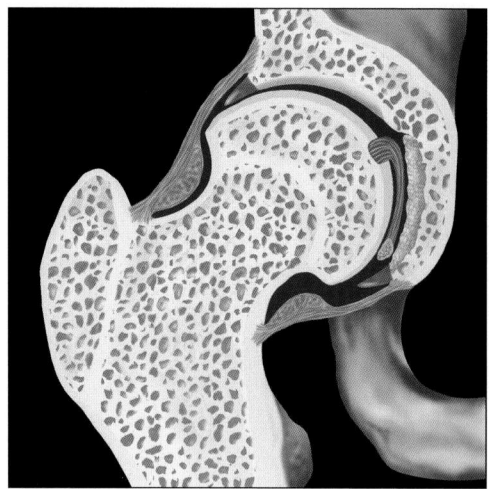

Coronal graphic shows superior joint space narrowing, acetabular and femoral subchondral cysts, chondral erosions, subcapital osteophytes. The acetabular labrum demonstrates degeneration.

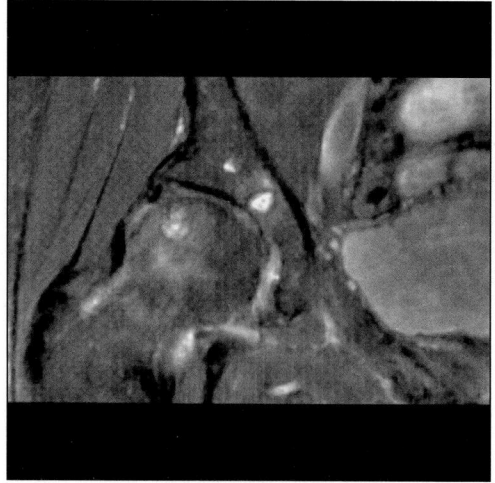

Coronal FS PD FSE MR shows hyperintense subchondral acetabular and femoral cysts and extended femoral head/neck marrow edema. Superior joint space narrowing and joint effusion are seen.

TERMINOLOGY

Abbreviations and Synonyms
- Degenerative joint disease (DJD), osteoarthritis (OA), femoroacetabular impingement

Definitions
- Articular cartilage degenerative change with hip joint space narrowing

IMAGING FINDINGS

General Features
- Best diagnostic clue: Superior joint space narrowing
- Location
  - OA changes
    - Acetabular roof
    - Chondral surfaces of acetabulum
    - Femoral head articular surface
- Size: Unilateral to bilateral involvement
- Morphology
  - Variable based on extent of cartilage loss
  - Active OA with extensive inflammatory reaction, osteophytes, subchondral cysts & sclerosis

Radiographic Findings
- Radiography
  - Narrowing of load-bearing joint space
  - Superior or superolateral migration femoral head (80%)
  - Medial migration plus protrusio acetabuli (20%)
  - Egger's subchondral acetabular cyst
  - Calcar buttressing
  - Ring of osteophytes (lateral acetabulum + medial subcapital)
  - Sclerosis of femoral head + acetabular roof

CT Findings
- NECT
  - Superior joint space narrowing
  - Sclerosis
  - Subchondral cysts
  - Osteophytes
  - Normal mineralization (no juxta-articular osteoporosis)

MR Findings
- T1WI
  - Attenuated or denuded chondral surface
  - Hypointense sclerosis acetabular roof + opposing surface femoral head
  - Hypointense effusion ± paralabral cysts
  - Marrow fat signal in osteophytes
  - Relative preservation of medial joint space relative to narrowed superior joint space
  - Single vs. multiple load-bearing zone subchondral cysts - hypointense to intermediate signal intensity

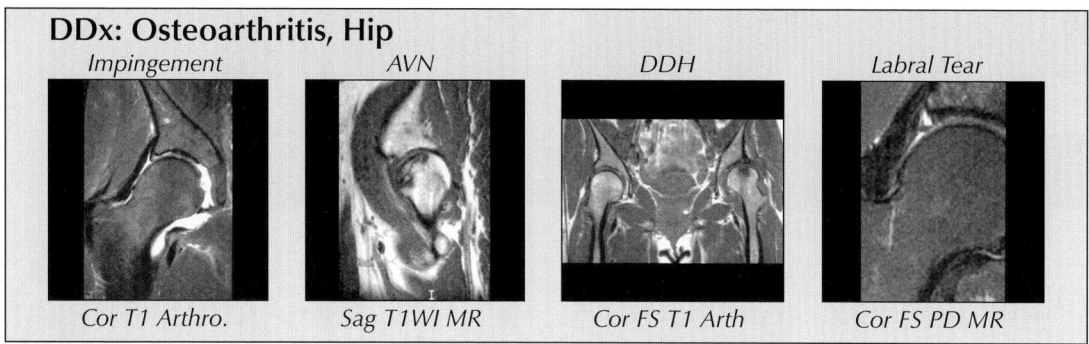

DDx: Osteoarthritis, Hip

Impingement	AVN	DDH	Labral Tear
Cor T1 Arthro.	Sag T1WI MR	Cor FS T1 Arth	Cor FS PD MR

OSTEOARTHRITIS, HIP

Key Facts

Imaging Findings

- Best diagnostic clue: Superior joint space narrowing
- Relative preservation of medial joint space relative to narrowed superior joint space
- Subchondral cysts hyperintense to intermediate signal + marginal hypointense sclerosis on T2WI

Top Differential Diagnoses

- Femoroacetabular Impingement
- Avascular Necrosis (AVN)
- Developmental Dysplasia of the Hip (DDH)
- Labral Tears
- Pigmented Villonodular Synovitis (PVNS)

Pathology

- Articular cartilage overload

- Primary (idiopathic) vs. secondary (pre-existing joint disorder)
- Fibrillation - fragmentation
- Joint space narrowing: Weight-bearing zones
- Subchondral cysts (detritic cysts)

Clinical Issues

- Most common signs/symptoms: Joint pain
- Insidious onset groin + thigh pain
- ± Gluteal pain radiation

Diagnostic Checklist

- Inflammatory OA with reactive subchondral edema involving both sides of joint
- Younger patient may present with femoroacetabular impingement as precursor to OA

- T2WI
  - Linear hyperintensity in chondral fissures
  - Subchondral hyperintensity lateral acetabular roof ± femoral head superior surface
  - Subchondral cysts hyperintense to intermediate signal + marginal hypointense sclerosis on T2WI
  - Subchondral cysts may be multiple + variable in size
  - Hyperintense paralabral cysts adjacent to acetabular labral tear
  - Hyperintense femoral head & neck edema in active OA
  - Hyperintense fluid + inhomogeneity of synovium in active inflammatory form of OA
- T1 C+: Intravenous contrast to enhance synovium
- Hypointense thickened stress trabeculae on T1 & T2WI

Imaging Recommendations

- Best imaging tool: MR indicated in early OA esp. younger population to identify femoroacetabular impingement, initial chondral degeneration, labral pathology + lateral acetabular roof edema
- Protocol advice
  - T1 (visualize sclerosis) + FS PD FSE in coronal, axial, sagittal planes
  - Non fat-suppressed PD imaging less sensitive to sclerosis & edema

DIFFERENTIAL DIAGNOSIS

Femoroacetabular Impingement

- Findings of OA in non-dysplastic hips in younger population
- Repetitive microtrauma 2° impingement of femoral head against acetabulum
- Hyperintense signal (T2WI) lateral femoral head + acetabular rim + labral tears & chondral defects

Avascular Necrosis (AVN)

- Wedge-shaped subchondral bone infarct
- Articular cartilage intact at presentation
- Double line sign on T2WI in 80%

Developmental Dysplasia of the Hip (DDH)

- Acetabular dysplasia - shallow acetabulum
- Lateral acetabular rim syndrome findings similar to femoroacetabular impingement in non-dysplastic hips
- Identified on anterior coronal images

Labral Tears

- Linear hyperintensity ± abnormal morphology on T2WI
- ± Paralabral cyst communicating with tear
- Associated with trauma, DDH or OA

Pigmented Villonodular Synovitis (PVNS)

- Proliferation of synovial lining
- Hemosiderin-containing
- Inhomogeneous signal on T2WI typically involving the medial capsule adjacent to femoral head/neck junction
- Hemosiderin - increased susceptibility on T2* GRE

Synovial Chondromatosis

- Multiple cartilaginous or osseous intraarticular loose bodies
- Related to synovial metaplasia
- Effusion + pain + restricted joint motion
- Loose bodies - round + hypointense to intermediate signal adjacent to hyperintense effusion on T2WI

Pyrophosphate Arthropathy

- CPPD (calcium pyrophosphate dihydrate crystal deposition disease)
- Calcified labrum
- Subchondral cysts
- Crystal deposition in chondral surfaces
- May cause or accelerate OA

Rheumatoid Diseases/Variants

- Hyperintense effusion on T2WI
- Intermediate signal synovial hypertrophy (T2WI)
- Bursal fluid distension
- Subchondral marrow edema on T2WI (FS PD FSE)
- Concentric joint space narrowing
- Synovial cysts

OSTEOARTHRITIS, HIP

PATHOLOGY

General Features
- General path comments
  - Relevant anatomy
    - Hyaline cartilage - resists mechanical stress (elastic)
    - Subchondral plate + calcified cartilage = less compressible than articular cartilage
    - Synovial fluid - produced by synoviocytes of synovial membrane (provides nutrients & viscosity + elasticity for shock absorption)
- Etiology
  - Articular cartilage overload
  - Primary (idiopathic) vs. secondary (pre-existing joint disorder)
  - Inflammation contributes to cartilage degeneration
  - Pathophysiologic changes also occur in synovial fluid, subchondral bone + capsular tissue
  - Cartilage may also be damaged by a metabolic process
- Epidemiology: 23% incidence at 55-74 years

Gross Pathologic & Surgical Features
- Articular cartilage
  - Fibrillation - fragmentation
- Pressure erosion
- Joint space narrowing: Weight-bearing zones
- Subchondral cysts
- Sclerosis, osteophytes & labral tear
- End-stage ankylosis

Microscopic Features
- Osteonecrosis of subchondral bone
- Hypervascularity
- Osteoblastic activity
- Trabecular thickening
- Subchondral cysts (detritic cysts)
  - Myxoid material
  - Proteoglycans
  - Articular cartilage fragments
  - Metaplastic cartilage
- Chondrocyte replication
- Decreased concentration of hyaluronic acid

Staging, Grading or Classification Criteria
- Grade I: Chondral inhomogeneity
- Grade II: Inhomogeneity + discontinuity of chondral surface & hypointensity of femoral head/neck on T1WI
- Grade III: Grade II + irregular cortical morphology of femoral head/acetabulum, cystic changes & indistinct zone between femoral head/acetabulum
- Grade IV: Addition of femoral head deformity

CLINICAL ISSUES

Presentation
- Most common signs/symptoms: Joint pain
- Clinical profile
  - Insidious onset groin + thigh pain
  - ± Gluteal pain radiation
  - Stiffness
  - Limited ability to sit, stand or walk
  - Symptoms worse in mornings & exacerbated by axial loading or weight-bearing activity
  - Pain & loss of internal rotation

Demographics
- Age: Usually > 55 years
- Gender: OA of hips > in males (OA knees > females)

Natural History & Prognosis
- Incidence of OA increases with age
- Clinical stabilization vs. progressive course
- Gait abnormalities
- Femoroacetabular impingement in the young patient may rapidly progress to advanced OA changes
- Unilateral involvement is common

Treatment
- Conservative
  - NSAIDs
  - Physical therapy
  - Intraarticular steroids in acute episodes
  - Intraarticular hyaluronate injections
- Surgical
  - Total hip arthroplasty

DIAGNOSTIC CHECKLIST

Consider
- Inflammatory OA with reactive subchondral edema involving both sides of joint
- Younger patient may present with femoroacetabular impingement as precursor to OA
- Primary process involves chondral degeneration as seen on FS PD FSE (small FOV) coronal images

SELECTED REFERENCES

1. DeLee JC et al: Orthopaedic sports medicine. Principles and practice. Hip and pelvis. vol 2. 2nd ed. Philadelphia PA, WB Saunders, (25):1443-62, 2003
2. Fitzgerald RH et al: Orthopaedics. Arthritis of the hip. St. Louis MO, Mosby, (6-8):869-76, 2002
3. Meyers S: Synovial fluid markers in osteoarthritis. Rheum Dis Clin North Am 25:433, 1999
4. Buckwalter J et al: Articular cartilage: Degeneration and osteoarthritis, repair, regeneration, and transplantation. Instr Course Lect. Rosemont IL, WB Saunders, 487, 1998
5. Vingard E et al: Sports and osteoarthritis of the hip. An epidemiological study. Am J Sports Med 21:195, 1993
6. Schumacher JR: Secondary osteoarthritis: Osteoarthritis: Diagnosis and management. Philadelphia PA, WB Saunders, 367-98, 1992
7. Haller J et al: Juxtaacetabular ganglionic (or synovial) cysts: CT and MR features. J Comput Assist Tomogr 13:976, 1989

OSTEOARTHRITIS, HIP

IMAGE GALLERY

Typical

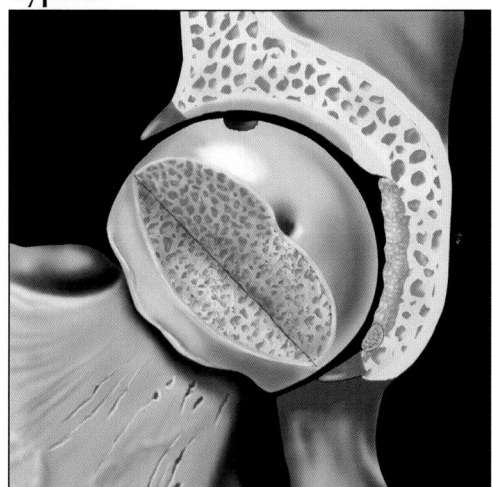

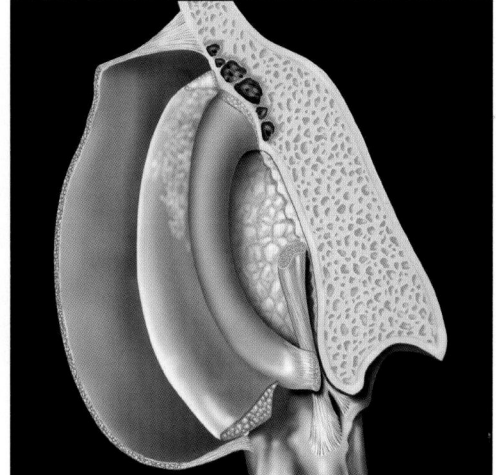

(Left) Coronal graphic shows focal femoral head chondral erosion. *(Right)* Coronal graphic shows degenerative acetabular labrum associated with subchondral acetabular cysts.

Typical

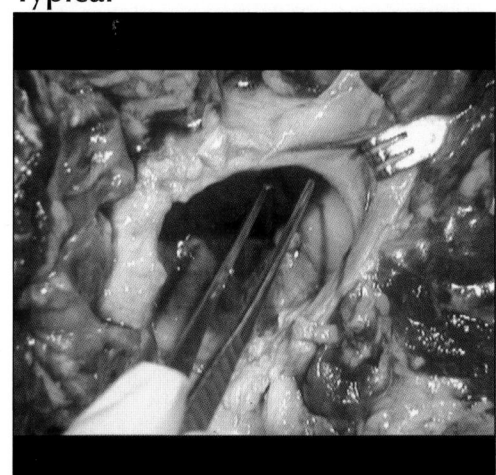

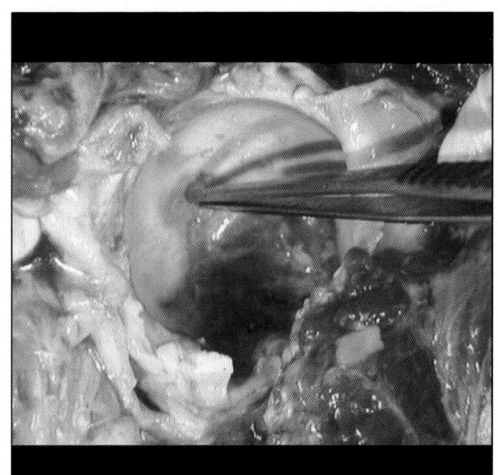

(Left) Surgical pathology shows intact labrum in a degenerative hip specimen. *(Right)* Surgical pathology shows chondral erosion of articular surface of acetabulum (lunate surface).

Typical

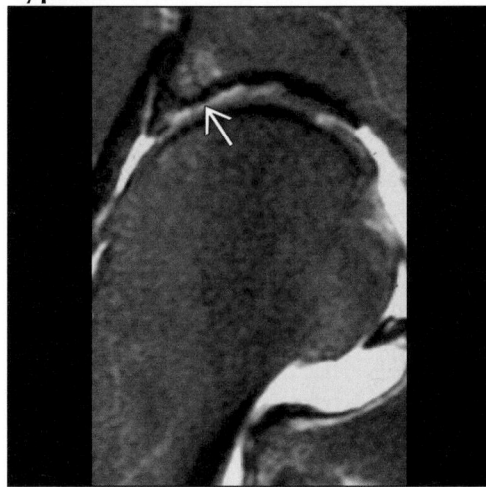

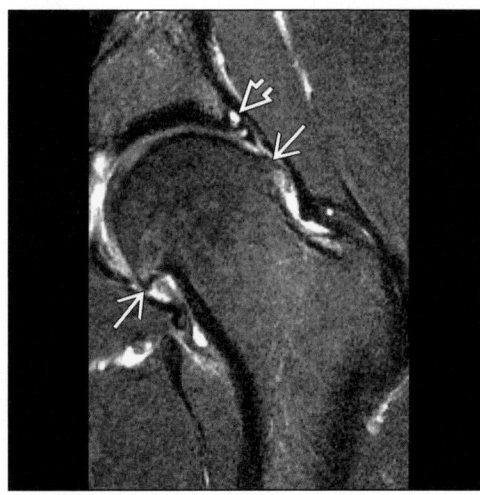

(Left) Coronal FS PD FSE MR shows superior joint space narrowing with full thickness acetabular chondral loss (arrow) and subchondral marrow edema. Osteophytes are present at the femoral head/neck junction. *(Right)* Coronal FS PD FSE MR shows narrowing of the superior joint space with loss of both femoral and acetabular articular cartilage. Subchondral cysts, (open arrow) labral tear, and osteophytes (arrows) are shown.

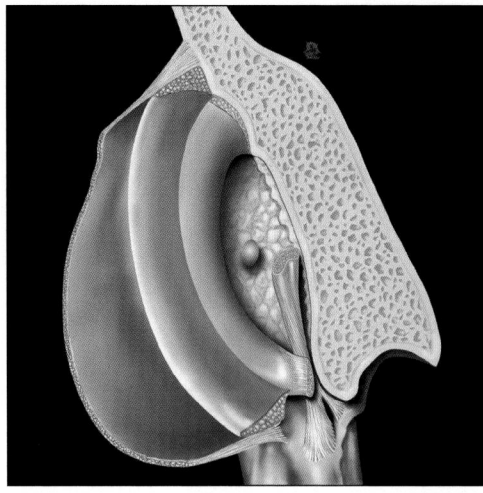

Coronal graphic shows loose body lodged within the acetabular fossa.

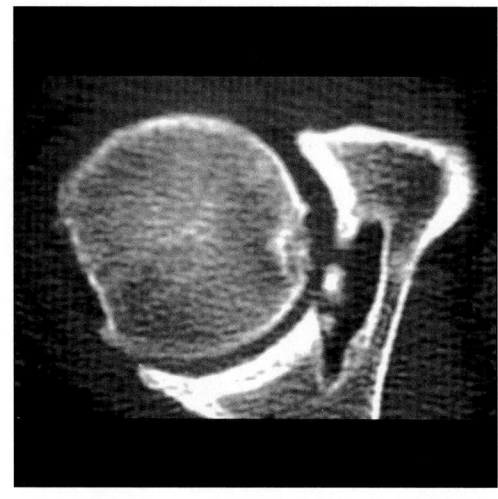

Axial NECT shows osseous loose bodies within the acetabular fossa.

TERMINOLOGY

Abbreviations and Synonyms
- Free fragments, joint mice, rice bodies

Definitions
- Free-floating or adherent intraarticular body

IMAGING FINDINGS

General Features
- Best diagnostic clue: Low to intermediate signal intensity focus within joint capsule on T1 & T2WI
- Location
  - Acetabular fossa common location
  - Other intracapsular locations including zona orbicularis
- Size: Variable from small chondral to larger osteochondral fragment
- Morphology: Round/oval to elongated

Radiographic Findings
- Radiography
  - Anteroposterior + frog-leg views
  - Usually insensitive, even for bony or calcified bodies
  - Chondral loose bodies (non-radiopaque) cannot be visualized
    - Particulate matter/debris typically cannot be visualized
    - Causative etiology or donor site can be identified
      - Fractures (acetabular, osteochondral, femoral head)
      - Osteoarthritis
      - Avascular necrosis (AVN) or Legg-Calvé-Perthes

CT Findings
- NECT
  - Excellent bony detail
  - Multi-planar capability
  - Chondral fragments cannot be visualized
  - Arthrography will increase sensitivity for non-ossified or non-calcified loose bodies
  - Associated fractures/dislocations
  - Causative etiology often identified
    - Fracture
    - Osteoarthritis (OA)
    - AVN
    - Osteochondral lesion

MR Findings
- T1WI
  - Hypointense to intermediate fragment
  - Less common - osteochondral fragment with marrow fat signal + hypointense sclerotic border
- T2WI
  - Hypointense to intermediate on T2WI

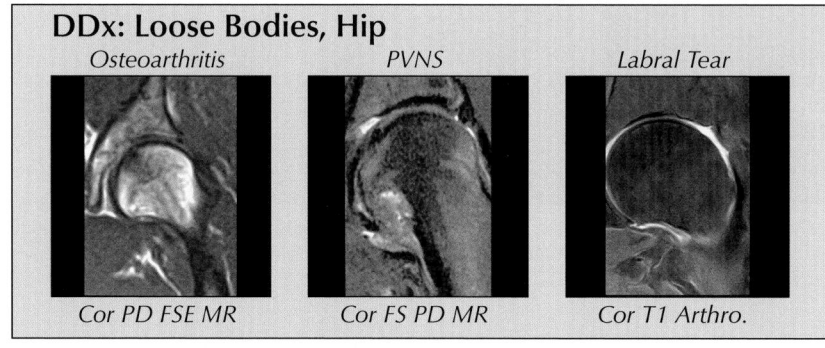

DDx: Loose Bodies, Hip

Osteoarthritis	PVNS	Labral Tear
Cor PD FSE MR	Cor FS PD MR	Cor T1 Arthro.

LOOSE BODIES, HIP

Key Facts

Imaging Findings
- Best diagnostic clue: Low to intermediate signal intensity focus within joint capsule on T1 & T2WI
- Acetabular fossa common location
- Hypointense to intermediate on T2WI
- Defect in chondral surface of femoral head or acetabulum

Top Differential Diagnoses
- Osteoarthritis
- Synovial Disorders
- Acetabular Labral Tears
- Artifacts

Pathology
- Trauma - commonly 2° to posterior dislocation + acetabular fracture

- Osteoarthritis
- PVNS
- Synovial chondromatosis/osteochondromatosis

Clinical Issues
- Pain secondary to retained material in acetabular fossa
- Clicking
- Snapping
- Popping
- Increased symptoms with activity

Diagnostic Checklist
- Match loose body with donor site if possible

- ○ Hyperintense adjacent synovial fluid
- ○ ± Adherent to synovium
- ○ Requires FS PD FSE or STIR
- ○ Donor site evaluation
  - ■ Defect in chondral surface of femoral head or acetabulum
- T1 C+
  - ○ MR arthrography
    - ■ Osseous, calcified, chondral, osteochondral bodies visualized
    - ■ Particulate matter/debris demonstrated
    - ■ Donor sites shown
    - ■ Less sensitive to subchondral changes or basal chondral degeneration

Ultrasonographic Findings
- Real Time
  - ○ Effusions help in searching for loose bodies
  - ○ Loose bodies = small hyperechoic foci in a hypo or anechoic background (effusion)
  - ○ Loose bodies in children with non-ossified epiphyses
  - ○ Particulate debris - tiny floating hyperechoic foci (inflammatory arthritis, infection)
  - ○ Chondral fragments: Hyperechoic, polygonal in shape
  - ○ Osseous or calcified loose bodies: Hyperechoic - may produce shadowing

Imaging Recommendations
- Best imaging tool: MR for spectrum of chondral to osteochondral fragments, donor site location + associated subchondral changes
- Protocol advice: T1 or PD + FS PD FSE or STIR in coronal, axial ± sagittal planes

DIFFERENTIAL DIAGNOSIS

Osteoarthritis
- Joint space narrowing
- Osteophytes
- Subchondral sclerosis
- Cystic changes

- Chondral degeneration anterosuperior femoral head or acetabulum

Synovial Disorders
- Rheumatoid - synovial proliferation
- Chondromatosis/osteochondromatosis - cartilaginous metaplasia
- Pigmented villonodular synovitis (PVNS) - periarticular erosions + synovial proliferation + hemosiderin
- Inflammatory osteoarthritis - synovitis ± reactive subchondral marrow edema

Acetabular Labral Tears
- Catching, locking, clicking and pain
- Associated with femoroacetabular impingement + osteoarthritis
- Bucket-handle labral tears

Artifacts
- Physiologic nitrogen
- Iatrogenically introduced air in MR arthrography
- Microscopic post-surgical metallic susceptibility artifact (MRI)

PATHOLOGY

General Features
- General path comments
  - ○ Relevant anatomy
    - ■ Inelastic fibrous capsule of hip - reinforced by iliofemoral, pubofemoral + ischiofemoral ligaments
    - ■ Zona orbicularis = deep circular fibers from ischiofemoral ligament (may be mistaken for labrum arthroscopically)
    - ■ Fovea capitis of femoral head = no articular cartilage surface
- Etiology
  - ○ Trauma - commonly 2° to posterior dislocation + acetabular fracture
  - ○ Osteoarthritis
  - ○ PVNS
  - ○ Synovial chondromatosis/osteochondromatosis

LOOSE BODIES, HIP

- ○ Crystal induced arthropathies
  - ▪ Gout
  - ▪ Calcium pyrophosphate dihydrate deposition (CPPD)
- ○ Rheumatoid arthritis
- ○ Infection/septic arthritis
- ○ AVN
- ○ Legg-Calvé-Perthes
- • Epidemiology
  - ○ Variable based on etiology
  - ○ Osteoarthritis - most common source of chondral debris

Gross Pathologic & Surgical Features

- • Osseous fracture fragment
- • Acetabular fractures
- • Osteochondral fractures
- • Chondral fractures
- • Traumatic labral tears + free-floating labral fragments
- • Chondral degeneration + sloughing
- • Synovial proliferations
- • Proteinaceous debris in setting of infection
- • Loose bodies may be identified in acetabular fossa, recesses around zona orbicularis

Microscopic Features

- • Proliferation of concentric layers of new cartilage + bone
- • Laminated appearance
- • Cartilaginous metaplasia in osteochondromatosis

CLINICAL ISSUES

Presentation

- • Most common signs/symptoms: Locking or catching
- • Clinical profile
  - ○ Pain secondary to retained material in acetabular fossa
  - ○ Clicking
  - ○ Snapping
  - ○ Popping
  - ○ Increased symptoms with activity

Demographics

- • Age: Older adults most commonly affected (due to association with OA)
- • Gender: M slightly > F

Natural History & Prognosis

- • Most loose bodies remain in joint unless surgically removed
- • May enlarge over time
- • Rarely resorb
- • Synovitis/debris
  - ○ Treated conservatively
  - ○ Improves when underlying pathology improves

Treatment

- • Conservative for bodies secondary to underlying joint disorder
  - ○ Synovitis
  - ○ ± Debris - particulate
  - ○ Infection - antibiotics to avoid joint destruction
- • Surgical

- ○ Most loose bodies arthroscopically removed
  - ▪ Osseous fracture fragments
  - ▪ Ossified or calcified loose bodies
  - ▪ Chondral/osteochondral fragments - reattach to donor site or remove
  - ▪ Chondromatosis/osteochondromatosis
  - ▪ PVNS
  - ▪ Free floating labral fragment

DIAGNOSTIC CHECKLIST

Consider

- • Match loose body with donor site if possible
- • FS PD FSE or STIR images to provide hyperintensity of joint fluid/effusion to facilitate loose body identification
- • Evaluate for underlying joint disorder with patient history of clicking, locking, trauma

SELECTED REFERENCES

1. Kramer J et al: MR arthrography of the lower extremity. Radiol Clin of N America 40(5):1211-32, 2002
2. Bencardino JT et al: Imaging of hip disorders in athletes. Radiol Clin of N America 40(2):267-87, 2002
3. Attarian DE et al: Observations on the growth of loose bodies in joints. Arthroscopy 18(8):930-4, 2002
4. Resnick D: Diagnosis of bone and joint disorders. Degenerative disease of extraspinal lesions. 4th ed. Philadelphia PA, WB Saunders, 1351-52, 2002
5. Van Holsbeeck MT et al: Musculoskeletal ultrasound. 2nd ed. St. Louis MO, Mosby, 265-8, 2001
6. McCarthy JC et al: The adult hip. Alternative to arthroplasty. vol 1. Iowa City IA, Lippincott-Raven, (43):721-36, 1998
7. Stoller DW: Magnetic resonance imaging in orthopaedics and sports medicine. 2nd ed. Philadelphia PA, WB Saunders, 802-12, 1997
8. McCarthy JC et al: The role of hip arthroscopy in the diagnosis and treatment of hip disease. Orthopaedics 18(8):753-6, 1995
9. Edwards DJ et al: Diagnosis of the painful hip by magnetic resonance imaging and arthroscopy. J Bone Joint Surg 77B(3):374-6, 1992
10. Berquist TH et al: Imaging of orthopaedic trauma. The pelvis and hips. 2nd ed. New York NY, Raven Press, 298-9, 1992
11. Hawkins RB: Arthroscopy of the hip. Clin Orthop 249:44-7, 1989
12. Harris WH: Etiology of osteoarthritis of the hip. Clin Orthop 213:20-33, 1986
13. Burman MS: Arthroscopy or the direct visulization of joints. J Bone Joint Surg 4:669-95, 1931

LOOSE BODIES, HIP

Typical

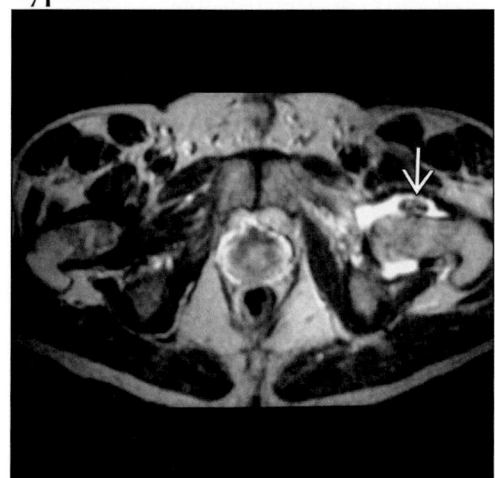

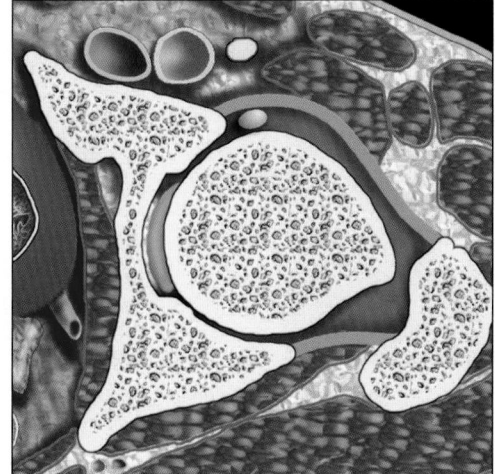

(Left) Axial T2WI MR shows cartilaginous loose body (arrow) in anterior left hip capsule. *(Right)* Axial graphic shows anterior capsule loose body.

Typical

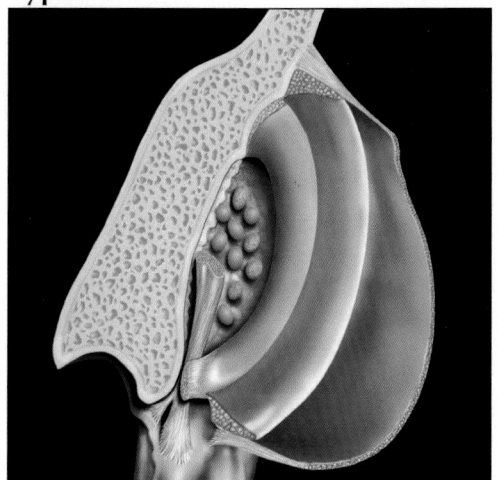

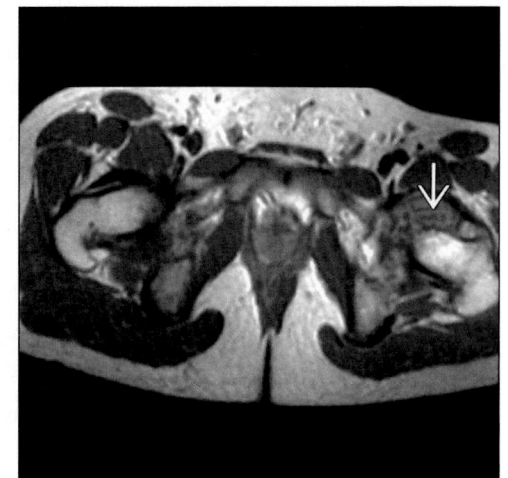

(Left) Coronal graphic shows synovial chondromatosis within the acetabular fossa. *(Right)* Axial PD/Intermediate MR shows synovial chondromatosis as hypointense defects (arrow) within the left hip joint effusion.

Typical

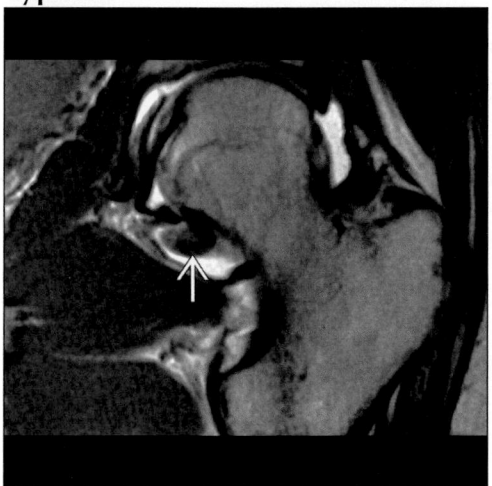

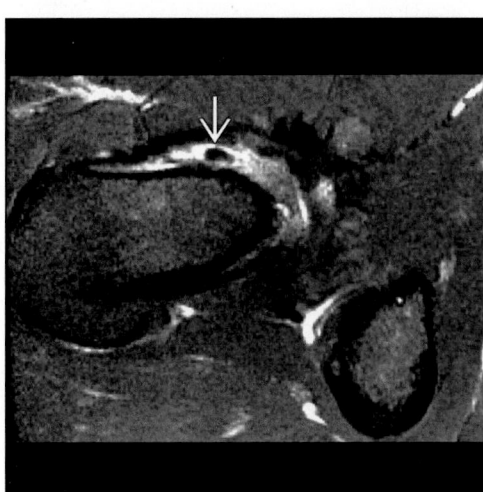

(Left) Coronal T1 C+ MR (MR arthrography) shows inferior capsule loose body (arrow) associated with adherent synovium. *(Right)* Axial FS PD FSE MR shows small corticated loose body (arrow) anterior to the femoral neck.

RHEUMATOID ARTHRITIS, HIP

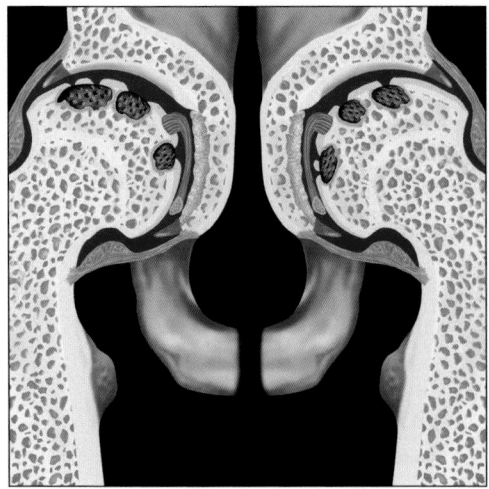

Coronal graphic shows multiple bilateral symmetric chondral and subchondral erosions in juvenile chronic arthritis.

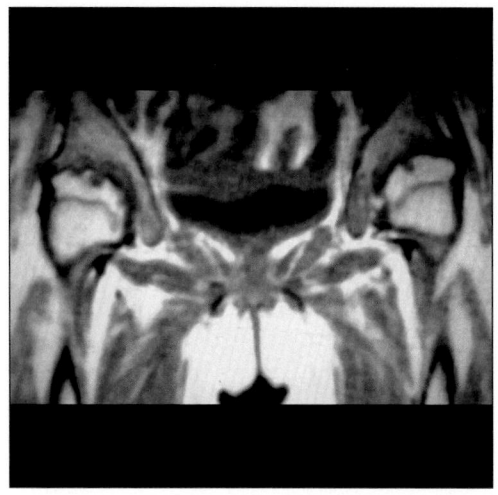

Coronal T1WI MR shows bilateral epiphyseal erosions in juvenile chronic arthritis.

TERMINOLOGY

Abbreviations and Synonyms
- RA, inflammatory arthritis, rheumatoid disease, juvenile chronic arthritis

Definitions
- Systemic autoimmune inflammatory disorder of unknown etiology primarily affecting synovial membranes + articular surfaces

IMAGING FINDINGS

General Features
- Best diagnostic clue: Effusion and synovial proliferation
- Location
  - Femoral head
  - Acetabulum
  - Joint capsule
- Size
  - Diffuse involvement of femoral head
  - Entire joint at risk
- Morphology
  - Concentric loss of joint space
  - Protrusio deformity (medial displacement of femoral head)

Radiographic Findings
- Radiography
  - Negative in early stages
  - Loss of joint space (chondral loss)
  - Progressive worsening of joint space loss
  - Juxta-articular osteoporosis
  - Soft tissue swelling
  - Loss of subchondral plate
  - Erosion - bare areas/capsular insertions
  - Subchondral cysts usually < 1 cm
  - Axial migration of femoral head
  - Protrusio acetabuli - medial femoral head cortex medial to ilioischial line

CT Findings
- NECT
  - Sensitive to subchondral erosions
  - Hypodense joint effusion
  - Joint space narrowing
  - ± Sclerosis, osteophytosis - superimposed osteoarthritic change

MR Findings
- T1WI
  - Hypointense joint effusion
  - Hypointense subchondral erosions
  - Hypointense mass - fluid in iliopsoas bursa
  - Hypointense acetabular + femoral head edema

DDx: Rheumatoid Arthritis, Hip

Impingement	AVN	DDH	Labral Tear	PVNS

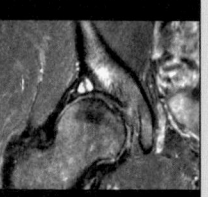

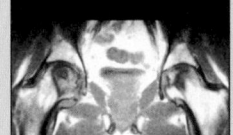

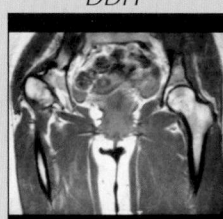

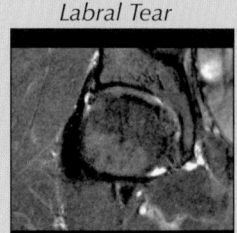

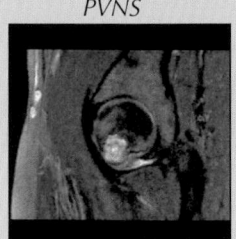

Cor FS PD MR	Cor T1WI MR	Cor T1WI MR	Cor FS PD MR	Sag FS PD MR

RHEUMATOID ARTHRITIS, HIP

Key Facts

Imaging Findings

- Best diagnostic clue: Effusion and synovial proliferation
- Concentric loss of joint space
- Protrusio deformity (medial displacement of femoral head)
- Inhomogeneity of effusions, synovium + debris relative to hyperintense fluid on T2WI

Top Differential Diagnoses

- Femoroacetabular Impingement
- Avascular Necrosis (AVN)
- Developmental Dysplasia of the Hip (DDH)
- Labral Tears
- Pigmented Villonodular Synovitis (PVNS)

Pathology

- Unknown etiology
- Bilateral, symmetrical joint involvement
- Hip joints involved later in disease process
- Inflammatory condition of synovial tissue
- Faulty immune response

Clinical Issues

- Most common signs/symptoms: Hip pain + stiffness
- Insidious onset
- Joint swelling, tenderness to palpation
- Pain with active/passive range of motion (ROM)

Diagnostic Checklist

- Intravenous contrast to enhance pannus

- T2WI
  - Hyperintense joint effusion
  - Capsular distension (joint capsule)
  - Demineralization (juxta-articular bone loss) with marrow hyperintensity on FS PD FSE or STIR
  - Attenuation/loss of subchondral plate (normally hypointense)
  - Intermediate to hyperintense subchondral cysts without sclerotic reactive interface
  - Femoral + acetabular erosions not confined to any specific quadrant (vs. osteoarthritis)
  - Hyperintense marrow edema
  - Inhomogeneity of effusions, synovium + debris relative to hyperintense fluid on T2WI
- T1 C+
  - Intravenous contrast to enhance pannus tissue
  - Map extent + distribution of synovial involvement

Imaging Recommendations

- Best imaging tool
  - MR
    - Detection of synovial pannus, erosions, cartilage loss, small subchondral cysts + marrow edema distribution
- Protocol advice: T1, FS PD FSE or STIR + FS T1 C+ in the coronal, axial, sagittal planes

DIFFERENTIAL DIAGNOSIS

Femoroacetabular Impingement

- Findings of osteoarthritis in non-dysplastic hips in younger patient population
- Repetitive microtrauma 2° impingement of femoral head against acetabulum
- Hyperintense signal (T2WI) of lateral femoral head + acetabular rim + labral tears & chondral defects

Avascular Necrosis (AVN)

- Wedge-shaped subchondral bone infarct
- Articular cartilage intact at presentation
- Double line sign on T2WI in 80%

Developmental Dysplasia of the Hip (DDH)

- Acetabular dysplasia - shallow acetabulum
- Lateral acetabular rim syndrome findings similar to femoroacetabular impingement in non-dysplastic hips
- Identified on anterior coronal images

Labral Tears

- Linear hyperintensity ± abnormal morphology on T2WI
- ± Paralabral cyst communication with tear

Pigmented Villonodular Synovitis (PVNS)

- Proliferation of synovial lining
- Hemosiderin-containing
- Inhomogeneous signal on T2WI typically involving the medial capsule adjacent to femoral head/neck junction
- Hemosiderin - increased susceptibility on T2* gradient echo

Synovial Chondromatosis

- Multiple cartilaginous or osseous intraarticular loose bodies
- Related to synovial metaplasia
- Effusion + pain + restricted joint motion

Pyrophosphate Arthropathy

- CPPD (calcium pyrophosphate dihydrate crystal deposition disease)
- Calcified labrum
- Subchondral cysts
- Crystal deposition in chondral surfaces
- May cause or accelerate osteoarthritis

Seronegative Arthritis

- Asymmetric
- Osteosclerosis
- Osseous proliferations
- Ankylosis

Inflammatory Systemic Connective Tissue Diseases

- Systemic lupus erythematosus

- Scleroderma
- Polymyositis & dermatomyositis

PATHOLOGY

General Features
- General path comments
  - Relevant anatomy
    - Subchondral plate - supports articular cartilage
    - Articular cartilage = hyaline
    - Joint capsule = fibrous + synovial lining
    - Synovial fluid - diffusion of nutrients to articular cartilage
- Genetics: Genetic predisposition - HLA-D antigen
- Etiology
  - Unknown etiology
  - Bilateral, symmetrical joint involvement
  - Hip joints involved later in disease process
  - Inflammatory condition of synovial tissue
  - Faulty immune response
  - Arthrotropic parvoviruses & lentiviruses - induce T4 helper cells + cytokine-medicated oligoclonal B cell response (IgG + IgM rheumatoid factors)
- Epidemiology: Prevalence of RA = 1% of population

Gross Pathologic & Surgical Features
- Synovial inflammation
- Pannus
- Tendon tears/ruptures
- Articular cartilage erosions
- Superior + medial protrusion of hip into pelvis
- Synovial cysts - subchondral

Microscopic Features
- Hyperplasia of synovial cells
  - Redundant synovial folds, villae + masses
- Lymphocytes + plasma cells infiltrate synovial membrane
- Fibrinous exudates

CLINICAL ISSUES

Presentation
- Most common signs/symptoms: Hip pain + stiffness
- Clinical profile
  - Insidious onset
  - 4 of 7 criteria for diagnosis
    - Morning stiffness > 1 hr., 3 or more joints, hand joints, symmetric, + Rh factor, nodules, radiographic changes
  - Malaise, weakness, weight loss, myalgias, fever
  - Joint swelling, tenderness to palpation
  - Pain with active/passive range of motion (ROM)
  - Rheumatoid factor
    - Serum IgM antibody - 70%
    - Directed against Fc fragment of IgG
    - 30% rheumatoid negative
  - Serum ANA (antinuclear antibodies) - 30%

Demographics
- Age
  - Adults - 25 to 60 years
  - Peak incidence 40-60 years

- Gender: F:M > 3:1

Natural History & Prognosis
- Slowly progressive disease with intermittent "flare-ups"
- ± Indolent course
- Joint destruction
- Complications
  - Joint effusions - capsular distention - pain
  - Large synovial cysts
  - Tendinous tears/disruptions
  - Cartilaginous destruction - joint obliteration
  - Osseous destruction
  - Fibrous/bony ankylosis
  - AVN (secondary to steroid use)

Treatment
- Conservative
  - Decrease inflammation, delay joint destruction + preserve function
  - Pharmacotherapy
    - Decrease inflammation
    - NSAIDs; immune mediating agents
  - Physical therapy
    - Heat, maintain ROM, strength, flexibility
- Surgical
  - Synovectomy (controversial)
  - Total hip arthroplasty - end stage disease

DIAGNOSTIC CHECKLIST

Consider
- Intravenous contrast to enhance pannus
- FS PD FSE or STIR for visualization of pannus + subchondral edema

SELECTED REFERENCES

1. Dablov G: Miscellaneous nontraumatic disorders: Cambell's operative orthopaedics. 10th ed. Philadelphia PA, Mosby, 905-13, 2003
2. Resnick D: Degenerative disease of extraspinal lesions: Diagnosis of bone and joint disorders. 4th ed. Philadelphia PA, WB Saunders, 891-939, 2002
3. Van Holsbeeck MT et al: Musculoskeletal ultrasound. 2nd ed. St. Louis MO, Mosby, 373-91, 2001
4. Mettler FA et al: Skeletal system: Essentials of nuclear medicine imaging. 4th ed. Philadelphia PA, WB Saunders, 326-9, 1998
5. Stoller DW: Magnetic resonance imaging in orthopaedics and sports medicine. 2nd Ed. Philadelphia PA, Lippincott Williams, 187-91, 1997
6. Anderson RJ: Rheumatoid arthritis: Primer on the rheumatic diseases. The arthritis foundation 90-5, 1993
7. Schumacher JR: Secondary osteoarthritis: Osteoarthritis-diagnosis and management. Philadelphia PA, WB Saunders, 367-98, 1992
8. Wallace CA et al: Juvenile rheumatoid arthritis: Outcome and treatment for the 1990's. Rheum Dis Clin North Am 17:891-906, 1991

IMAGE GALLERY

Typical

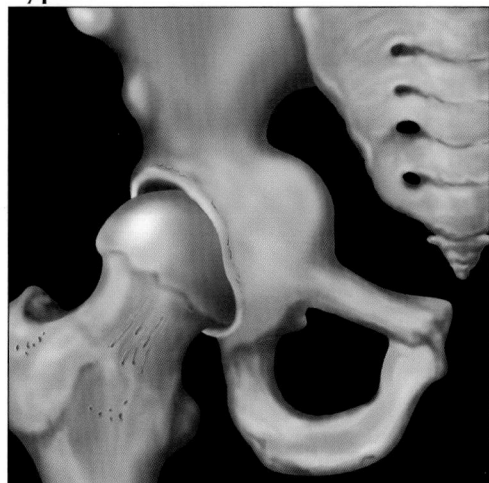

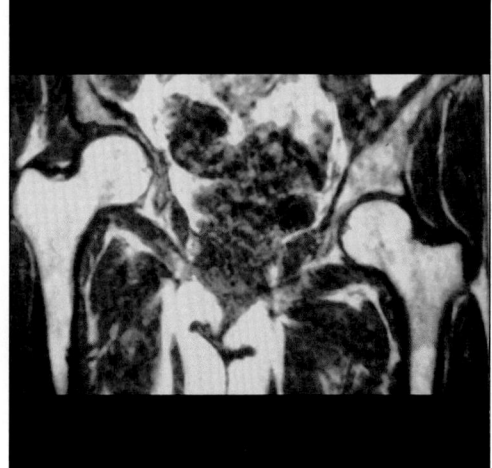

(Left) Coronal graphic shows protrusio acetabuli associated with rheumatoid arthritis. *(Right)* Coronal T1WI MR shows right protrusio acetabuli with medial femoral head located medial to the ilioischial line.

Typical

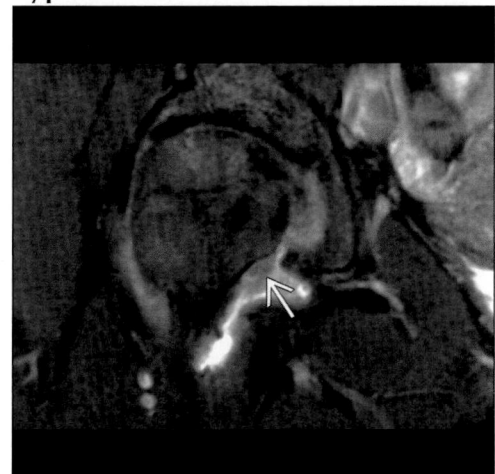

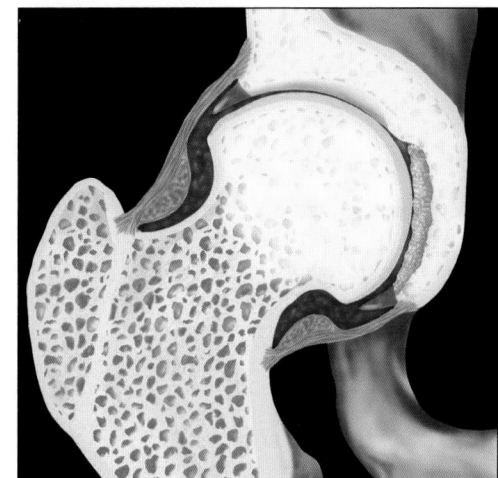

(Left) Coronal FS PD FSE MR shows hypertrophic synovium (arrow) associated with early rheumatoid arthritis. The synovium is intermediate in signal intensity. *(Right)* Coronal graphic shows hypertrophic synovium (red) with concentric joint space narrowing and reactive marrow edema on both sides of the joint.

Variant

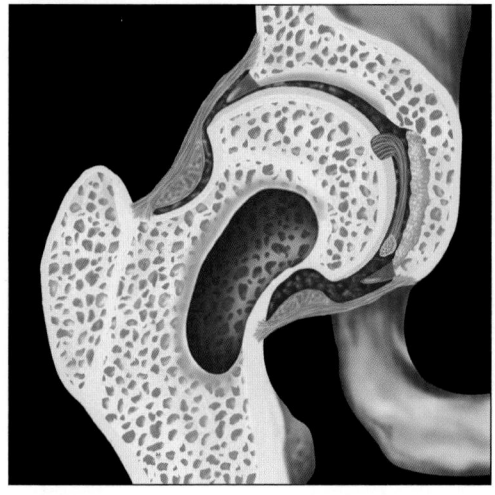

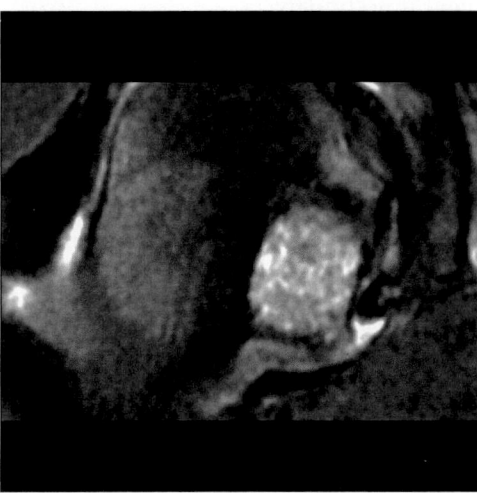

(Left) Coronal graphic shows subchondral cystic erosions of the medial femoral neck in PVNS. *(Right)* Coronal FS PD FSE MR shows characteristic location of PVNS erosion with intermediate signal of hypertrophic synovium. This erosion should not be mistaken for rheumatoid arthritis.

OSTEOMYELITIS, HIP

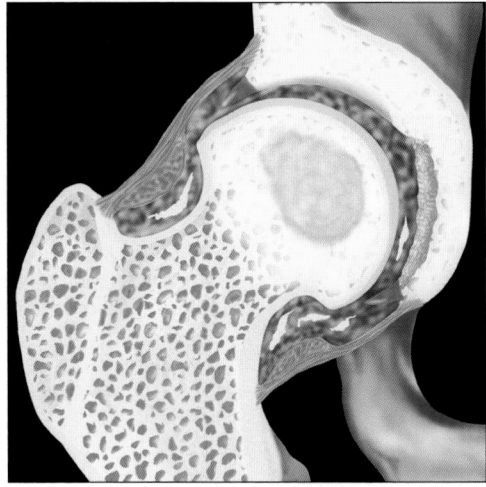

Coronal graphic shows synovitis and infectious nidus of the femoral head with reactive marrow edema involving both the acetabulum and femoral head.

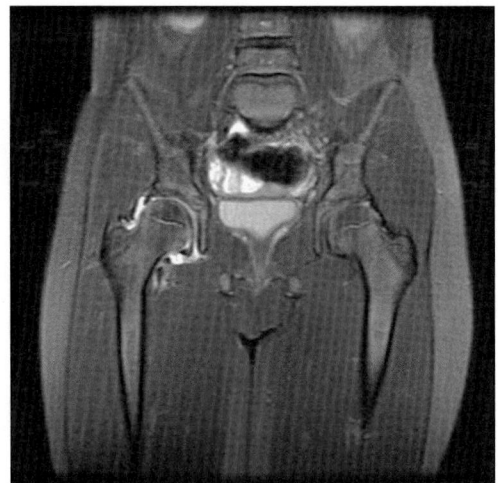

Coronal FS PD FSE MR shows septic right hip with hyperintense joint effusion and capsular distension.

TERMINOLOGY

Abbreviations and Synonyms
- Acute hematogenous osteomyelitis, chronic osteomyelitis

Definitions
- Acute hematogenous osteomyelitis in pediatric patient & chronic post-traumatic osteomyelitis in adult patient

IMAGING FINDINGS

General Features
- Best diagnostic clue: Bone marrow hyperintensity, erosion + sinus tract on T2WI
- Location
  - Bone marrow in hematogenous osteomyelitis
  - Osteitis ± marrow involvement in secondary (trauma or surgery) osteomyelitis
- Size: Variable from epiphyseal involvement to diaphyseal + soft tissue involvement
- Morphology: Focal, Brodie's abscess or larger area of medullary or cortical destruction

Radiographic Findings
- Radiography
  - Insensitive for early osteomyelitis
  - Changes delayed 10-14 days after onset of fever
  - Soft tissue edema/swelling
  - Focal lucency to frank destruction of bone
  - Periosteal elevation + underlying lucency (subperiosteal abscess)
  - Intramedullary abscess - focal lucency ± tract to cortical surface
  - Sequestration (necrotic fragments) + involucrum (periosteal bone) as parosteal ossification
  - Joint effusion - widening of affected hip joint

CT Findings
- NECT
  - Early bone destruction
  - Assessment of cortical + trabecular bone detail
  - Periosteal elevation, cortical destruction, intramedullary abscess + sinus tracts
  - Joint effusions = hypodense
- CECT
  - Infected regions enhance
  - Soft tissue complications: Abscesses enhance peripherally, sinus tracts enhance

MR Findings
- T1WI
  - Hypointense marrow edema + cortical destruction
  - Hypointense reactive joint effusion
  - Hypointense soft tissue abscess
  - Tract from skin to cortex

DDx: Osteomyelitis, Hip

TOH	AVN	Stress Fx	Amyloid	Myositis Ossific.
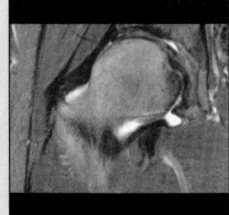	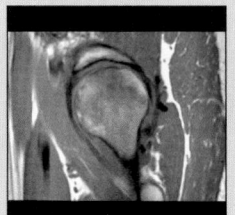	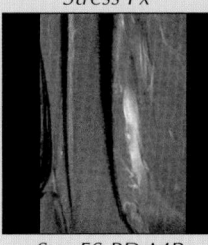	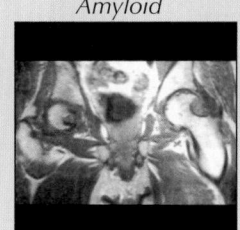	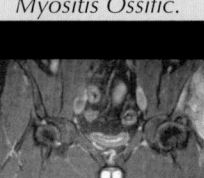
Cor PD FS MR	Sag T1WI MR	Sag FS PD MR	Cor T1WI MR	Cor FS PD MR

OSTEOMYELITIS, HIP

Key Facts

Imaging Findings
- Best diagnostic clue: Bone marrow hyperintensity, erosion + sinus tract on T2WI
- Sequestrum: Hypointense on T1 + T2WI
- Involucrum (periosteal reaction): Hypointense on T1 & T2WI

Top Differential Diagnoses
- Transient Osteoporosis of the Hip (TOH)
- Avascular Necrosis (AVN)
- Cellulitis
- Septic Arthritis
- Amyloid

Pathology
- Staph aureus = most common infecting organism in all age groups

Key Facts (right column)
- Chronic osteomyelitis = most common form of osteomyelitis in adult & 2° to trauma
- Hematogenous seeding
- Direct contamination
- Contiguous spread

Clinical Issues
- Most common signs/symptoms: Pain
- Fever

Diagnostic Checklist
- Identify marrow edema as well as associated extension through cortex + soft tissue tract
- Axial images to identify hypointense sequestrum

- ○ Hypointense to intermediate signal in metaphysis/diametaphysis in child
- T2WI
  - ○ Hyperintense marrow involvement
  - ○ Hyperintense intraosseous abscess
  - ○ Cortical destruction: Intermediate to hyperintense
  - ○ Cloaca (periosteal opening): Focal hyperintensity in hypointense periosteum
  - ○ Sinus tract: Intermediate to hyperintense
  - ○ Brodie's abscess (round abscess cavity representing a chronic pyogenic infection): Hyperintense + hypointense sclerotic rim
  - ○ Cellulitis: Reticulated subcutaneous hyperintensity
  - ○ Myositis: Hyperintense muscle + enlargement
- T1 C+
  - ○ Enhancement
    - ▪ Bone marrow - inflammation
    - ▪ Abscess - peripheral enhancement within medullary canal or soft tissue (thick wall)
    - ▪ Enhancement peripheral to sequestrum
    - ▪ Cortical erosion/destruction - ± enhancement
    - ▪ Sinus tract - peripheral enhancement
- Sequestrum: Hypointense on T1 + T2WI
- Involucrum (periosteal reaction): Hypointense on T1 & T2WI
  - ○ +/- Hyperintense adjacent soft tissue edema

Imaging Recommendations
- Best imaging tool: MR sensitive to marrow edema & soft tissue involvement
- Protocol advice: T1 + FS PD FSE or STIR in axial, coronal & sagittal planes

DIFFERENTIAL DIAGNOSIS

Transient Osteoporosis of the Hip (TOH)
- Middle-aged males
- Self-limited
- Hypointense on T1, hyperintense on T2WI

Avascular Necrosis (AVN)
- Trauma, steroid use, alcoholism
- Double-line sign on T2WI in 80%
- Fat signal in ischemic lesion in earlier stages
- ± Hyperintense marrow edema extending to femoral neck on T2WI

Fracture (Fx)
- Hyperintense fracture line on T2WI
- Adjacent hyperintensity of soft tissue without sinus tract or erosion

Cellulitis
- Subcutaneous fat involvement
- Hypointense on T1, hyperintense on T2WI
- Reticulated pattern on T1 & T2WI
- Underlying muscle or deep fascial planes intact

Septic Arthritis
- Large hyperintense (T2WI) joint effusion with capsular distension ± scalloping of capsule (synovitis)
- Diabetes, steroids, intravenous drug use = risk factors

Crystal-Induced Arthropathies
- Requires T2* gradient echo for visualization of susceptibility
- Effusion
- Degenerative findings including labral tears
- Chondral - hyaline cartilage degeneration

Tumor
- Ewing sarcoma
- Osteosarcoma
- Solid lesion = central enhancement & peritumoral edema

Amyloid
- Long-term hemodialysis
- Large cystic erosions
- B-microglobulin deposition

Legg-Calvé-Perthes
- Infarction of bony epiphysis of femoral head
- Age: 4-8 most common
- Hypointense capital epiphysis on T1 & T2WI

Eosinophilic Granuloma
- Proliferating histiocytes
- Punched-out calvarial lesions + button sequestrum
- Tubular bones - osteolytic destruction ± lamellar periosteal reaction

Osteoid Osteoma
- < 2 cm
- Painful lesion
- Requires FS PD or T2 or STIR to demonstrate hyperintensity of lesion + reactive edema

Myositis Ossificans
- Mass of calcified or ossified granulation tissue
- ± Reactive hyperintense soft tissue edema on T2WI adjacent to ossification

PATHOLOGY

General Features
- General path comments
  - Relevant anatomy for infection
    - Periosteum (periostitis)
    - Cortex (osteitis)
    - Marrow (osteomyelitis)
    - Metaphysis: > 1 year (physis acts as barrier to epiphyseal spread + metaphyseal capillary sinusoidal lakes and slow blood flow)
    - Metaphysis/epiphysis - hematogenous involvement in infants
    - Subcutaneous fat (cellulitis)
- Etiology
  - Staph aureus = most common infecting organism in all age groups
  - Other common organisms = streptococcus, pseudomonas, haemophilus, Enterobacter
- Epidemiology
  - Chronic osteomyelitis = most common form of osteomyelitis in adult & 2° to trauma
  - Staphylococcus aureus = 80-90% of cases

Gross Pathologic & Surgical Features
- Hematogenous seeding
  - Children
  - Vascular metaphyseal bone
- Direct contamination
  - Penetrating trauma
  - Post-surgical
- Contiguous spread
  - Soft tissue infection
  - Septic arthritis

Microscopic Features
- Leukocytic infiltration of marrow
- Vascular compression
- Necrosis, abscesses + sequestra

Staging, Grading or Classification Criteria
- Acute, subacute & chronic hematogenous forms
- Brodie's abscess
- Chronic recurrent multifocal osteomyelitis (CRMO)
- Post-traumatic osteomyelitis

CLINICAL ISSUES

Presentation
- Most common signs/symptoms: Pain
- Clinical profile
  - Fever
  - Restricted motion + point tenderness
  - Elevated sedimentation rate, C-reactive protein & WBC count
  - Soft tissue swelling + erythema + sinus tract

Demographics
- Age
  - Young children most commonly affected
  - Adults secondary to direct contamination (trauma, post-op)
- Gender: No bias

Natural History & Prognosis
- Osseous destruction will recur if untreated
- Prognosis good if treated early
- Progression to chronic infection
- Intramedullary, subperiosteal abscesses
- Soft tissue extension

Treatment
- Conservative
  - IV antibiotics
- Surgical
  - Debridement & antibiotic-impregnated beads

DIAGNOSTIC CHECKLIST

Consider
- Identify marrow edema as well as associated extension through cortex + soft tissue tract
- Axial images to identify hypointense sequestrum

SELECTED REFERENCES

1. Greenspan A: Orthopedic radiology: A practical approach. 3rd ed. Philadelphia PA, Lippencott Williams & Wilkins, 753-84, 2000
2. Mettler FA et al: Essentials of nuclear medicine imaging. 4th ed. Philadelphia PA, WB Saunders, 285-333, 1998
3. Resnick D: Internal derangements of joints: Emphasis on MR imaging. 1st ed. Philadelphia PA, WB Saunders, 473-554, 1997
4. Morrison WB et al: Diagnosis of osteomyelitis: Utility of fat-suppressed contrast-enhanced MR imaging. Radiology 189:251-7, 1993
5. Dangman BC et al: Osteomyelitis in children: Gadolinium-enhanced MR imaging. Radiology 182:743-7, 1992
6. Erdman WA et al: Osteomyelitis: Characteristics and pitfalls of diagnosis with MR imaging. Radiology 180:533-9, 1991
7. Gold RH et al: Bacterial osteomyelitis: Findings on plain radiography, CT, MR, and scintigraphy. AJR 157:365-70, 1991
8. Beltran J et al: Experimental infections of the musculoskeletal system: Evaluation with MR imaging and Tc-99m and Ga-67 scintigraphy. Radiology 167:167-72, 1988

OSTEOMYELITIS, HIP

IMAGE GALLERY

Typical

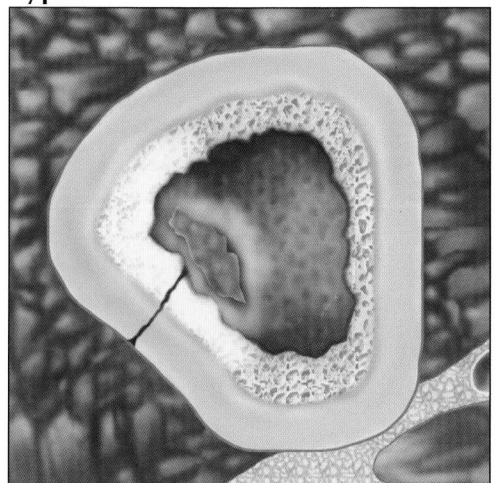
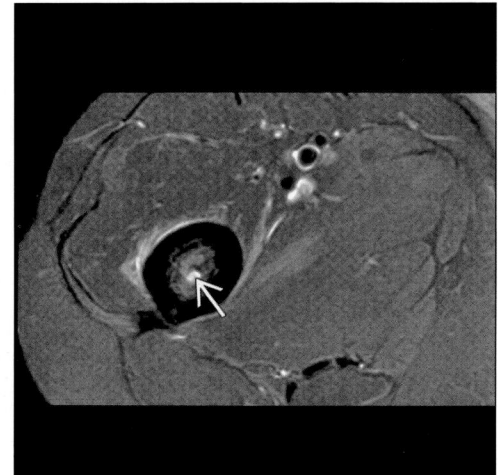

(Left) Axial graphic shows osteomyelitis with sequestrum and sinus tract. (Right) Axial FS PD FSE MR shows hyperintense signal in medullary cavity (arrow) of proximal femur from osteomyelitis. Periosteal hyperintense reaction identified as an early stage of the involucrum.

Variant

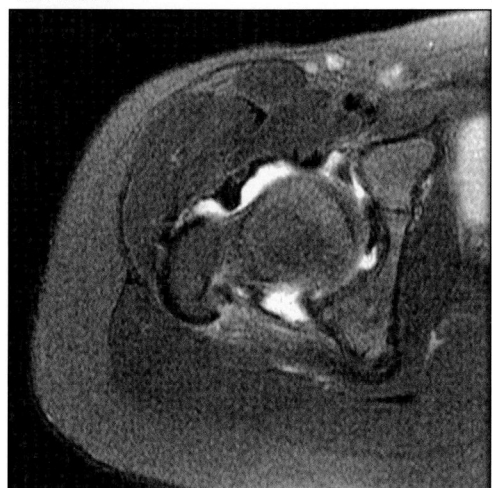
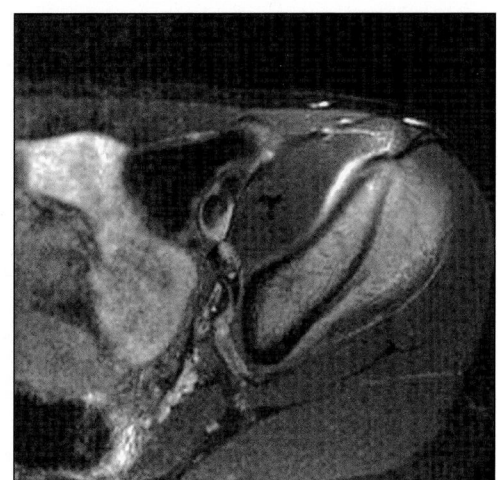

(Left) Axial FS PD FSE MR shows scalloping of capsular margins associated with infected joint fluid (septic hip). (Right) Axial FS PD FSE MR shows Ewing sarcoma mimicking soft tissue involvement and marrow edema as seen in osteomyelitis.

Variant

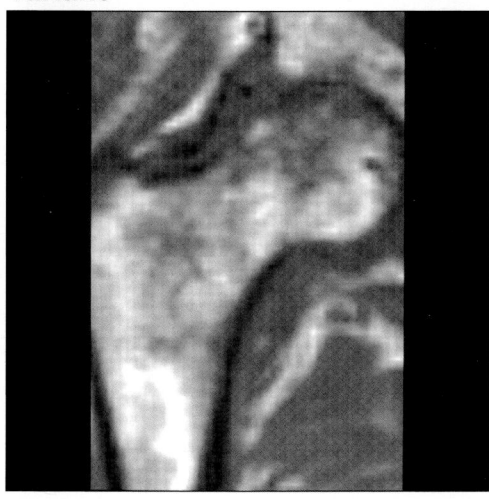
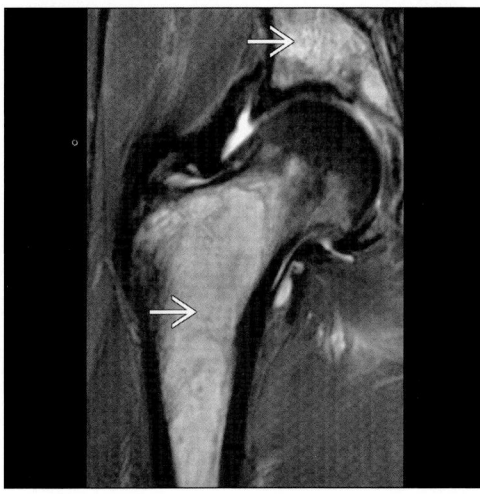

(Left) Coronal T1WI MR shows joint space collapse and subchondral marrow edema in active inflammatory osteoarthritis mimicking osteomyelitis. (Right) Coronal FS PD FSE MR shows diffuse involvement of multiple myeloma (arrows) in the acetabulum and femur mimicking osteomyelitis. Unlike osteomyelitis, there is relative sparing of marrow fat in the greater trochanter and femoral head.

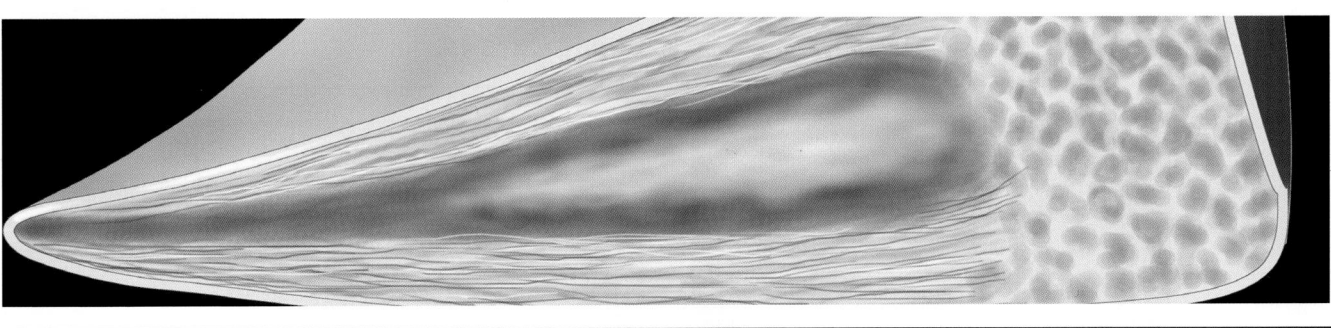

SECTION 5: Knee

DISCOID MENISCUS

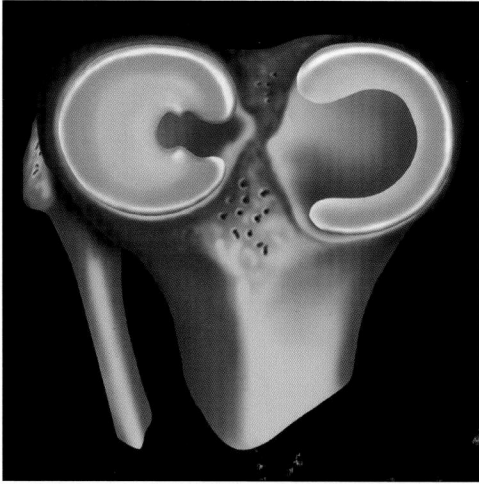

Axial graphic shows a discoid lateral meniscus with minimal resorption of the central portion of the meniscus.

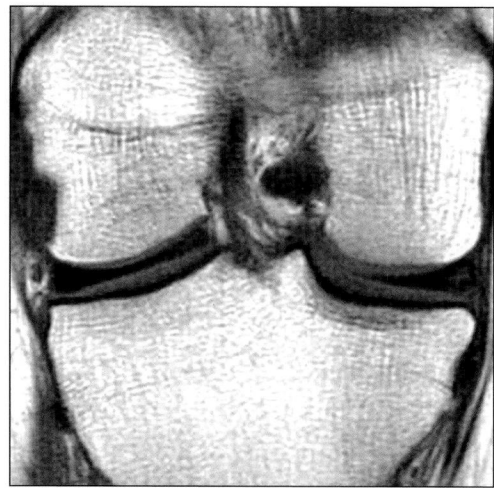

Coronal PD FSE MR shows a discoid lateral meniscus with meniscal tissue occupying the lateral compartment.

TERMINOLOGY

Abbreviations and Synonyms
- Discoid meniscus (DM)

Definitions
- Large, congenitally dysplastic meniscus with loss of normal semilunar shape
- Result of failure of resorption of central portion

IMAGING FINDINGS

General Features
- Best diagnostic clue: Large meniscus with loss of normal semilunar shape filling lateral or medial compartment (50% or greater coverage of lateral tibial plateau) on sagittal and coronal images
- Location
  - Lateral discoid meniscus is more common than medial discoid meniscus
  - Can be bilateral
- Size: > 13 mm
- Morphology
  - Pancake shaped meniscus with intact central portion
  - Large but incomplete disc commonly seen

Radiographic Findings
- Radiography

- Widening of joint space with hypoplastic femoral condyle and high fibular head in lateral discoid meniscus
- Cupping of lateral tibial plateau

MR Findings
- T1WI
  - Meniscal size > 13 mm in cross section
    - Normal hypointense meniscus is 5-13 mm from the capsular margin to the free edge on a central coronal image
  - Discoid meniscus exhibits continuous body segment appearance on ≥ 3 consecutive sagittal 4-5 mm thick images
- T2WI
  - Meniscus is hypointense
  - Intrameniscal mucoid degeneration or cyst may be intermediate to hyperintense on T2* GRE or FS PD FSE
- PD/Intermediate: Short TE sequence showing uniformly hypointense large meniscus
- T2* GRE
  - Mucinous degeneration and intrameniscal cystic cavities are hyperintense
  - Tear as hyperintense signal
  - Horizontal tear morphology common
  - Discoid meniscus is larger and disc shaped, filling a greater surface area of the central compartment
- Tear is seen as hyperintense signal (T1, PD, GRE T2*)

DDx: Discoid Meniscus

Displaced Bucket	Bucket-Handle	Flipped Meniscus
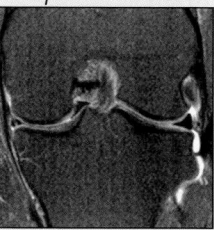	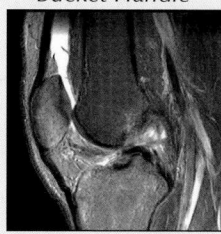	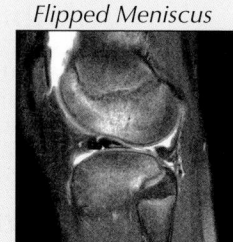
Cor FS PD FSE	Sag FS PD FSE	Sag FS PD FSE

DISCOID MENISCUS

Key Facts

Terminology
- Large, congenitally dysplastic meniscus with loss of normal semilunar shape

Imaging Findings
- Best diagnostic clue: Large meniscus with loss of normal semilunar shape filling lateral or medial compartment (50% or greater coverage of lateral tibial plateau) on sagittal and coronal images
- Lateral discoid meniscus is more common than medial discoid meniscus
- Can be bilateral
- Meniscal size > 13 mm in cross section
- Tear is seen as hyperintense signal (T1, PD, GRE T2*)

Top Differential Diagnoses
- Flipped Meniscus

- Bucket-Handle Tear

Pathology
- Etiology: Failure of resorption of the central portion of meniscus
- Microscopically normal meniscus

Clinical Issues
- Patients often present with pain, clicking and snapping
- Often asymptomatic in children

Diagnostic Checklist
- Identify the number of images with meniscus body segment visualized, if more than three consider DM
- Absent clear space at center of weightbearing surface of lateral compartment

---

- ○ Seen on all short TE sequences
- Complete discoid meniscus has "pancake" appearance
  - ○ Extending from intercondylar notch to the periphery of compartment
- MR arthrography
  - ○ Contrast extends into discoid meniscal tear
  - ○ Closed meniscal tears without contrast communication

Imaging Recommendations
- Best imaging tool: MRI
- Protocol advice
  - ○ Include short TE sequence to detect tears in discoid meniscus
    - ▪ FS PD FSE and T2* GRE
    - ▪ Direct axial images to show circumferential morphology

DIFFERENTIAL DIAGNOSIS

Vacuum Phenomenon
- Typically in hyperextended knee
- Decreased signal intensity on all pulse sequences in the joint between weightbearing surfaces
- Rarely homogeneous like discoid meniscus
- Exaggerated on T2* GRE MRI

Flipped Meniscus
- Meniscus is torn and often displaced anteriorly
- Portions of meniscus are missing - usually posterior horn "flipped" anteriorly
  - ○ Missing meniscus allows distinction from discoid meniscus
- +/- Extension block

Bucket-Handle Tear
- Displaced longitudinal tear
- Fragment usually migrates to notch of the knee
- Seen on coronal and sagittal images
- Donor site meniscal body usually smaller than normal
- Traumatic with identifiable antecedent event

Displaced Flap Meniscal Tear
- Meniscal donor site small
- Vertical signal in inner third of meniscus or blunted meniscal morphology
- Symptomatic adult
- Often reactive change in adjacent tibia
- = Oblique tear
- +/- Reactive tibial edema
- +/- MCL (medial collateral ligament) bursitis
- Hypointense mass on all pulse sequences = displaced fragment

PATHOLOGY

General Features
- General path comments: Pancake or large meniscus demonstrates intrameniscal degeneration or meniscal tear
- Genetics: Congenital deformities
- Etiology: Failure of resorption of the central portion of meniscus
- Epidemiology: 5% of population

Gross Pathologic & Surgical Features
- Pancake or large, otherwise normal-appearing meniscus in medial or lateral compartment
  - ○ Lateral compartment more common
- Wrisberg-ligament type discoid meniscus lacks posterior capsular (meniscotibial) attachment - unstable
  - ○ Horizontal tear in middle and posterior segments of meniscus

Microscopic Features
- Microscopically normal meniscus
  - ○ Meniscus may demonstrate mucinous intrasubstance degeneration +/- tearing
    - ▪ Tear - separating cleavage plane surrounded by regenerative chondrocytes
    - ▪ Degeneration - mucinous ground substance within the fibrocartilaginous meniscus +/- cystic areas or cavities

DISCOID MENISCUS

Staging, Grading or Classification Criteria

- Watanabe classification
  - Complete: Discoid meniscus extending into the intercondylar notch on coronal images
  - Incomplete: Partial discoid morphology +/- extension toward the intercondylar notch on coronal images
  - Wrisberg-ligament type: Lacks posterolateral meniscotibial attachment
- Classification by surface configuration - associated tear patterns (arthroscopic)
  - Vertical
    - Longitudinal tear (primary tear pattern is in vertical plane)
    - Flap tear (primary tear pattern is in vertical plane)
    - Radial tear
  - Horizontal
    - Horizontal cleavage tear
    - Longitudinal tear (primary tear pattern is in horizontal plane)
    - Flap tear (primary tear pattern is in horizontal plane)

CLINICAL ISSUES

Presentation

- Most common signs/symptoms
  - Patients often present with pain, clicking and snapping
  - Often asymptomatic in children
  - Locking is a common presentation in children
- Clinical profile
  - Symptoms may not develop until adolescence or young adulthood
  - Bilaterality: 20-90%
  - Click or clunk at the joint line during terminal 15-20 degrees of extension

Demographics

- Age
  - Children asymptomatic
  - Adults usually symptomatic
- Gender: No predilection

Natural History & Prognosis

- Extension loss
- Snapping (Wrisberg type)
- Giving way
- Palpable joint line mass
- Progression to a meniscal tear
- Painful intrameniscal cystic cavities of mucinous degeneration

Treatment

- Conservative initially
- Partial meniscectomy
- Saucerization/partial resection of the discoid portion to create a more normal shaped meniscus

DIAGNOSTIC CHECKLIST

Consider

- Displaced flap tear/bucket-handle tear as differential diagnosis

Image Interpretation Pearls

- Identify the number of images with meniscus body segment visualized, if more than three consider DM
- Absent clear space at center of weightbearing surface of lateral compartment
  - Less common involvement of medial compartment

SELECTED REFERENCES

1. Samoto N et al: Diagnosis of discoid lateral meniscus of the knee on MR imaging. Magn Reson Imaging 20(1):59-64, 2002
2. Choi NH et al: Medial and lateral discoid meniscus in the same knee. Arthroscopy 17(2):E9, 2001
3. Rao PS et al: Clinical, radiologic, and arthroscopic assessment of discoid lateral meniscus. Arthroscopy 17(3):275-7, 2001
4. Rohren EM et al: Discoid lateral meniscus and the frequency of meniscal tears. Skeletal Radiol 30(6):316-20, 2001
5. Arnold MP et al: Symptomatic ring-shaped lateral meniscus. Arthroscopy 16(8):852-4, 2000
6. Araki Y et al: MR imaging of meniscal tears with discoid lateral meniscus. Eur J Radiol 27(2):153-60, 1998
7. Raber DA et al: Discoid lateral meniscus in children. Long-term follow-up after total meniscectomy. Bone J Joint Surg 80(11):1579-86, 1998
8. Ryu KN et al: MR imaging of tears of discoid lateral menisci. AJR 171(4):963-7, 1998
9. Maffulli N et al: Knee arthroscopy in Chinese children and adolescents: An eight-year prospective study. Arthroscopy 13(1):18-23, 1997
10. Connolly B et al: Discoid meniscus in children: Magnetic resonance imaging characteristics. Canadian Association of Radiologists Journal 47(5):347-54, 1996
11. Washington ER et al: Discoid lateral meniscuc in children. Long-term follow-up after excision. Bone J Joint Surg 77(9):1357-61, 1995
12. Pellacci F et al: Lateral discoid meniscus: Treatment and results. Arthroscopy 8(4):526-30, 1992
13. Aichroth PM et al: Congenital discoid lateral meniscus in children. A follow-up study and evolution of management. Bone J Joint Surg 73(6):932-6, 1991
14. Fritschy D et al: Discoid lateral meniscus. International Orthopaedics 15(2):145-7, 1991
15. Sugawara O et al: Problems with repeated arthroscopic surgery in the discoid meniscus. Arthroscopy 7(1):68-71, 1991
16. Dimakopoulos P et al: Partial excision of discoid meniscus. Arthroscopic operation of 10 patients. Acta Orthopaedica Scandinavica 61(1):40-1, 1990
17. Bellier G et al: Lateral discoid menisci in children. Arthroscopy 5(1):52-6, 1989
18. Vandermeer RD et al: Arthroscopic treatment of the discoid meniscus: Results of long-term follow-up. Arthroscopy 5(2):101-9, 1989
19. Hayashi LK et al: Arthroscopic meniscectomy for discoid lateral meniscus in children. Bone J Joint Surg 70(10):1495-500, 1988
20. Dickhaut SD et al: The discoid lasteral-meniscus syndrome. J Bone Joint Surg 64:1068-73, 1982

DISCOID MENISCUS

IMAGE GALLERY

Typical

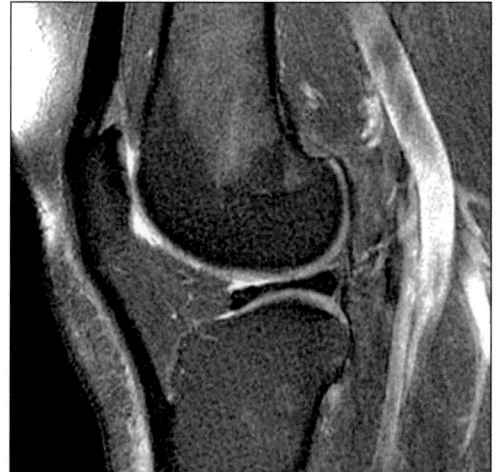

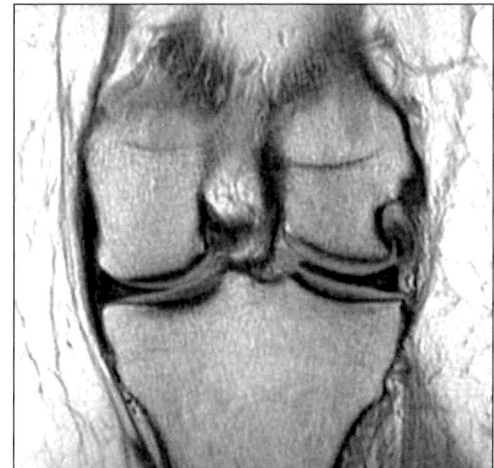

(Left) Sagittal FS PD FSE MR shows a discoid lateral meniscus. Meniscal tissue that is continuous with the anterior and posterior horn throughout multiple sagittal images is characteristic. *(Right)* Coronal PD FSE MR shows a discoid lateral meniscus.

Variant

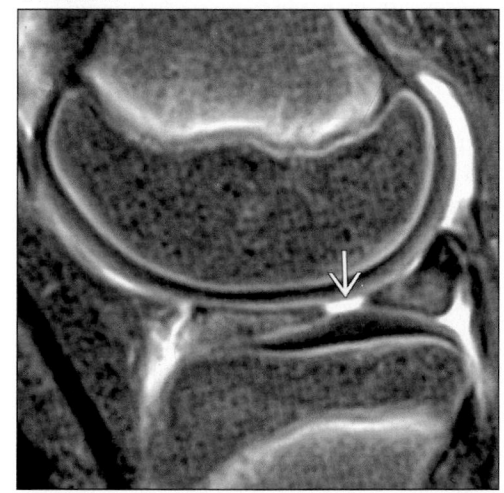

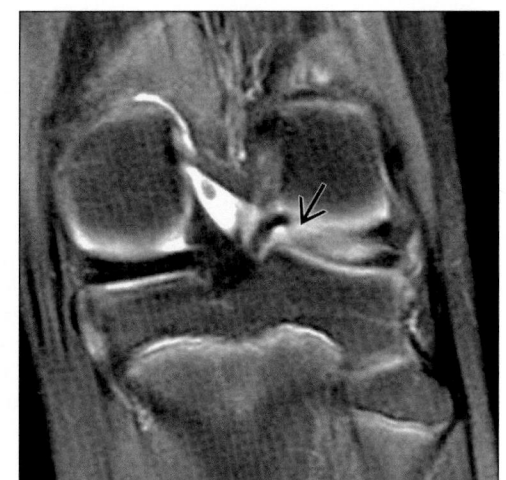

(Left) Sagittal FS PD FSE MR shows a torn and degenerated discoid lateral meniscus (arrow). *(Right)* Coronal FS PD FSE MR shows a torn and degenerated discoid lateral meniscus (arrow).

Variant

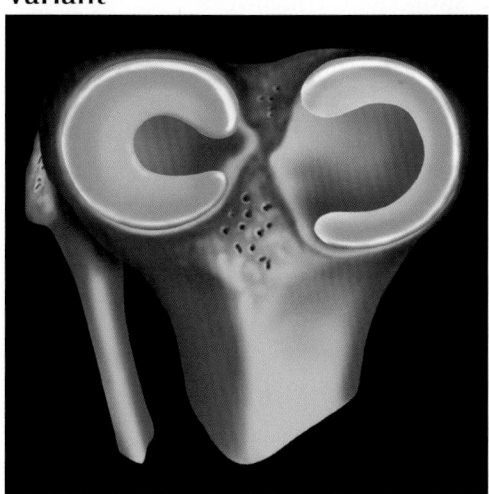

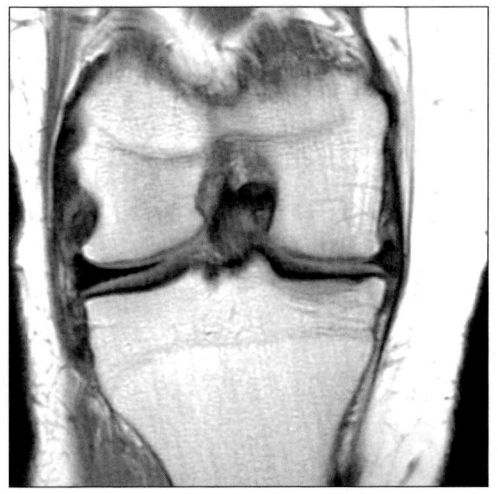

(Left) Axial oblique graphic shows a large lateral meniscus that is discoid-like. *(Right)* Coronal PD FSE MR shows a large, discoid-like lateral meniscus.

MENISCAL DEGENERATION

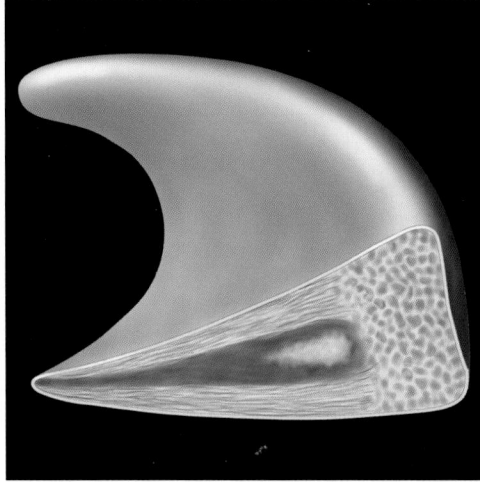

Sagittal graphic shows globular intrameniscal degeneration (yellow) within the central meniscal shear plane (dark blue).

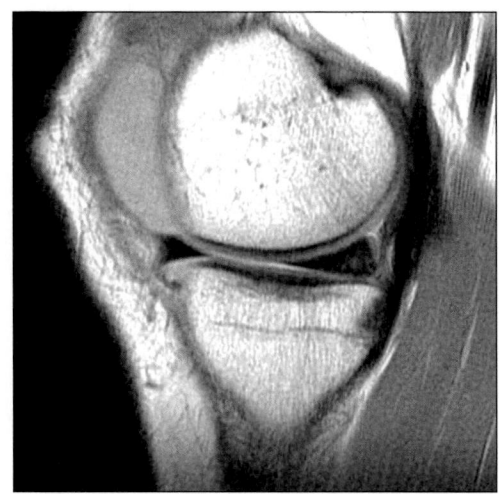

Sagittal PD FSE MR shows meniscal grade 1 signal intensity (degeneration) within the posterior horn of the medial meniscus. There is no extension (communication) with an articular surface.

TERMINOLOGY

Abbreviations and Synonyms
- Meniscal grade 1 and meniscal grade 2 signal intensity = meniscal degeneration, intrasubstance signal, intrasubstance degeneration

Definitions
- Internal degeneration of meniscal fibrocartilage resulting from chronic shear stresses + axial loading
- Caused by rotation, flexion & extension of knee during normal walking as well as cumulative effects of traumatic injuries of knee

IMAGING FINDINGS

General Features
- Best diagnostic clue: Increased signal intensity within meniscal substance on short TE MR images not extending to articular surface
- Location: Can occur in either meniscus but most common in posterior horn of medial meniscus
- Size: Variable from focal area to linear distribution - extending from capsular periphery
- Morphology
  - Nonarticular focal or globular intrasubstance increased signal intensity (grade 1 signal)
  - Horizontal linear intrasubstance increased signal intensity (grade 2 signal)

MR Findings
- T1WI
  - T1WI & short TE images are sensitive to meniscal degeneration
    - Short TE sequences: T1, PD, T2* GRE
- T2WI
  - Moderate to extensive lesions demonstrate mild increased signal intensity on T2WI
  - Intrameniscal degenerative cyst detection
    - Increased signal intensity (fluid) on T2WI
- Increased signal intensity
  - Globular
  - Linear
- Within the substance of the meniscus
- MR arthrography
  - Arthrography does not show communication with an articular surface of the meniscus

Imaging Recommendations
- Best imaging tool: MRI
- Protocol advice
  - Short TE images
    - T1, PD and/or gradient echo (T2* GRE) images

DDx: Meniscal Degeneration

Meniscus Vessels	Meniscus Vessels	Meniscal Ossicle	Magic Angle	Magic Angle

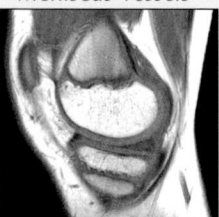 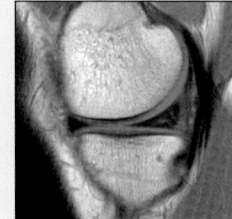 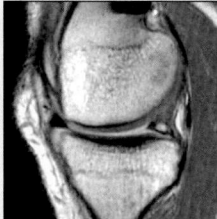 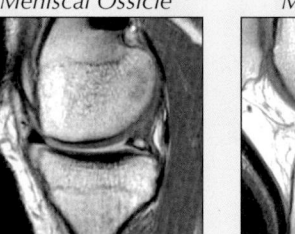 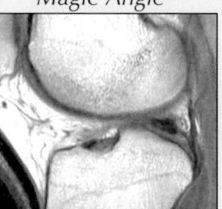 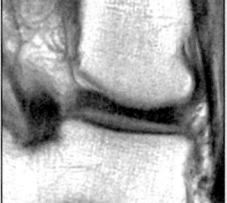

| *Sag PD FSE MR* | *Sag PD FSE MR* | *Sag PD FSE MR* | *Sag PD FSE MR* | *Cor PD FSE MR* |

MENISCAL DEGENERATION

Key Facts

Terminology
- Internal degeneration of meniscal fibrocartilage resulting from chronic shear stresses + axial loading
- Caused by rotation, flexion & extension of knee during normal walking as well as cumulative effects of traumatic injuries of knee

Imaging Findings
- Best diagnostic clue: Increased signal intensity within meniscal substance on short TE MR images not extending to articular surface
- Location: Can occur in either meniscus but most common in posterior horn of medial meniscus

Top Differential Diagnoses
- Prominent, Sometimes Linear Appearing Normal Vascularity Seen in Younger Patients

- Intrameniscal Tear not Communicating with an Articular Surface

Pathology
- Epidemiology: Common meniscal abnormality

Clinical Issues
- Typically asymptomatic
- Symptoms are suggestive of meniscal tear/intrameniscal closed tear
- Clinical profile: May present with pain without typical signs of clicking

Diagnostic Checklist
- Meniscal degeneration may be underestimated on FSE images secondary to blurring effect with increased echo spacing

---

DIFFERENTIAL DIAGNOSIS

Prominent, Sometimes Linear Appearing Normal Vascularity Seen in Younger Patients
- Typically less than 12 years of age
- Corresponds to mid perforating collagen bundle

Marrow Fat Containing Meniscal Ossicle
- Focally expansile without fluid intensity
- Corticated
- Posterior horn medial meniscus most common

Intrameniscal Tear not Communicating with an Articular Surface
- Prominent grade 2 signal
- Suggestive clinical signs and symptoms
- Grade 3 signal intensity which weakens as it approaches an articular surface = closed meniscal tear

Magic Angle Phenomenon in Upsloping Posterior Horn Lateral Meniscus
- Typical location
- Orientated 55 degrees to external magnetic field in 1.5T magnets
- Shift of position or longer TE values differentiates
- Common location for meniscal tear/injury in setting of anterior cruciate ligament (ACL) injury

Fat Planes within Meniscotibial Attachments
- Linear & vertical located at meniscal attachments only
- Anterior horn lateral meniscus
- Mimics meniscal tear

Meniscal Tear
- Signal abnormality extends to articular surface
- Communication with surface, maybe difficult to identify especially in peripheral body tears
- Suggestive clinical presentation
- +/- Displaced flap
- +/- Adjacent inflammatory change

PATHOLOGY

General Features
- General path comments: May be mimicked in young person by prominent, linear vascularity in plane of middle perforating collagen bundle
- Etiology
  - Internal degeneration of the meniscal substance resulting from chronic stresses (abnormal shear forces) caused by
    - Rotation, flexion and extension of knee during normal walking
    - Cumulative effects of traumatic injuries of the knee
- Epidemiology: Common meniscal abnormality

Gross Pathologic & Surgical Features
- Pale, often mucinous regions of discoloration in a variety of patterns within meniscal substance
- No tear identified

Microscopic Features
- Mucinous degeneration and chondrocyte deficient regions
  - Pale staining with hematoxylin and eosin (H&E)
- Increased production of mucopolysaccharide ground substance
  - Myxoid, mucinous or hyaline degeneration
- May have linear appearance (grade 2 degeneration)
  - Microscopic clefting and collagen fragmentation may be seen in hypocellular regions of the fibrocartilaginous matrix
- Central (middle) perforating bundle of the meniscus is a horizontal buffer zone between the different frictional forces
  - Between the femur and tibia is a preferential site for accumulation of mucinous ground substance (degeneration)
  - Common location for the development of grade 2 signal intensity

Staging, Grading or Classification Criteria
- Grading of meniscal signal

MENISCAL DEGENERATION

- ○ Grade 1: Nonarticular, focal or globular increased signal intensity within the meniscal substance on short TE sequences
- ○ Grade 2: Horizontal, linear increased signal intensity within the meniscal substance on short TE sequences
  - ▪ Extending from the capsular periphery of the meniscus but not extending to an articular surface
  - ▪ Histologically usually more extensive degeneration than that seen with MRI grade 1
- ○ Grade 3: Increased signal intensity that communicates or extends to at least one articular surface of the meniscus
  - ▪ Represents a meniscal tear with fibrocartilaginous separation
- • Classification based on location - vascular zones
  - ○ White zone (white/white zone)
    - ▪ Completely avascular central portion of the meniscus including inner one third
    - ▪ Menisci debrided
  - ○ Red-white junction (red/white zone)
    - ▪ Middle third between free edge and peripheral third
    - ▪ Incompletely vascularized area
    - ▪ Debridement vs. repair
    - ▪ Repair especially if vascular pedicle can be established
  - ○ Red zone (red/red zone)
    - ▪ Peripheral one third
    - ▪ Vascularized area
    - ▪ Primary repair usually possible if tear confined to red/red zone or peripheral portion of red/white zone

CLINICAL ISSUES

Presentation
- • Most common signs/symptoms
  - ○ Typically asymptomatic
  - ○ Symptoms are suggestive of meniscal tear/intrameniscal closed tear
- • Clinical profile: May present with pain without typical signs of clicking
- • If symptomatic with meniscal grade 2 signal, the findings may represent an intrameniscal closed tear
  - ○ A closed tear is associated with grade 3 signal intensity which weakens as it approaches an articular surface of the meniscus

Demographics
- • Age
  - ○ Typically older patient
  - ○ Also seen in younger, active patients
- • Gender: No predilection

Natural History & Prognosis
- • May progress to tear, especially horizontal cleavage tear when in the posterior horn of the medial meniscus
- • Does not necessarily indicate that a tear will occur
- • Mucinous degeneration does represent potential structural weakening within the meniscus

Treatment
- • Conservative
  - ○ Meniscal degeneration is treated conservatively
- • Surgical
  - ○ None for pure degeneration

DIAGNOSTIC CHECKLIST

Consider
- • Vascularity in a young person
- • Intrameniscal tear especially if fluid signal is present within the meniscus

Image Interpretation Pearls
- • Use short TE sequences
  - ○ T2* GRE images sensitive for intrasubstance degeneration
- • Meniscal degeneration may be underestimated on FSE images secondary to blurring effect with increased echo spacing
  - ○ Blurring seen with shorter effective TE, a longer echo train length & a lower acquisition matrix

SELECTED REFERENCES

1. Anderson MW: MR imaging of the meniscus. Radiol Clin North Am 40(5):1081-94, 2002
2. Fukuta SK et al: Prevalence of abnormal findings in magnetic resonance images of asymptomatic knees. J Orthop Sci 7(3):287-91, 2002
3. Greis PE et al: Meniscal injury: Management. J Am Acad Orthop Surg 10(3):177-87, 2002
4. Nawata K et al: Magnetic resonance imaging of meniscal degeneration in torn menisci: A comparison between anterior cruciate ligament deficient knees and stable knees. Knee Surg Sports Traumatol Arthrosc 7(5):274-7, 1999
5. Crues JV III: The impact of MRI on our understanding of the pathology of sports injuries. Sportverletz Sportschaden 8(4):156-9, 1994
6. Peterfy CG et al: "Magic-angle" phenomenon: A cause of increased signal in the normal lateral meniscus on short-TE MR images of the knee. AJR 163(1):149-54, 1994
7. Raunest J et al: Magnetic resonance imaging (MRI) and arthroscopy in the detection of meniscal degenerations: Correlation of arthroscopy and MRI with histology findings. Arthroscopy 10(6):634-40, 1994
8. Stoller DW et al: Meniscal tears: Pathologic correlation with MR imaging. Radiology 163(3):731-5, 1987

MENISCAL DEGENERATION

IMAGE GALLERY

Typical

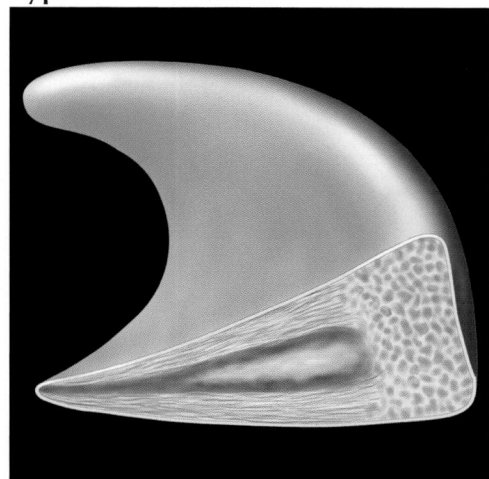
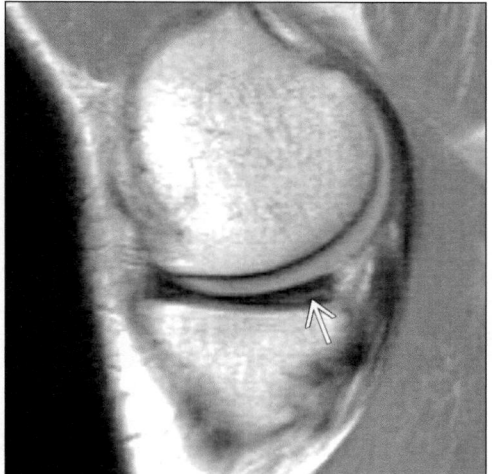

(Left) Sagittal graphic shows linear intrasubstance degeneration (grade 2 degeneration). *(Right)* Sagittal PD FSE MR shows linear grade 2 intrameniscal degeneration (arrow).

Variant

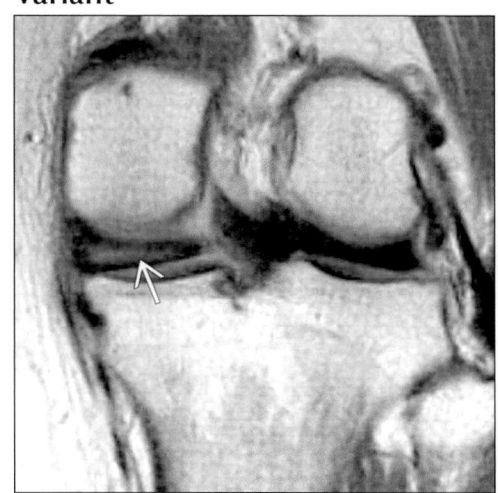
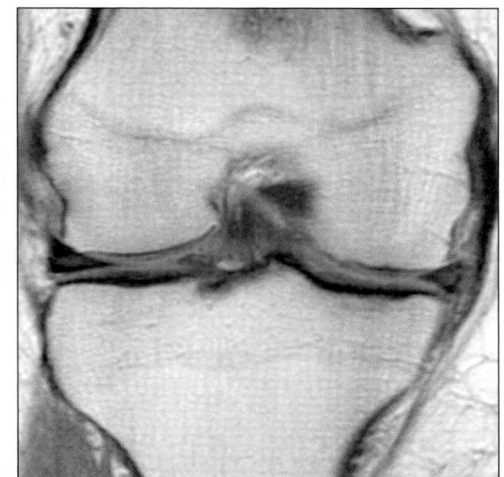

(Left) Coronal PD FSE MR shows diffuse intrameniscal degeneration (arrow) of the posterior horn of the medial meniscus adjacent to a radial tear of the posterior horn root attachment. There is slight enlargement of the degenerated posterior horn. *(Right)* Coronal PD FSE MR shows grade 2 intrameniscal degeneration of the lateral meniscus body and grade 1 intrameniscal degeneration of the medial meniscus body.

Typical

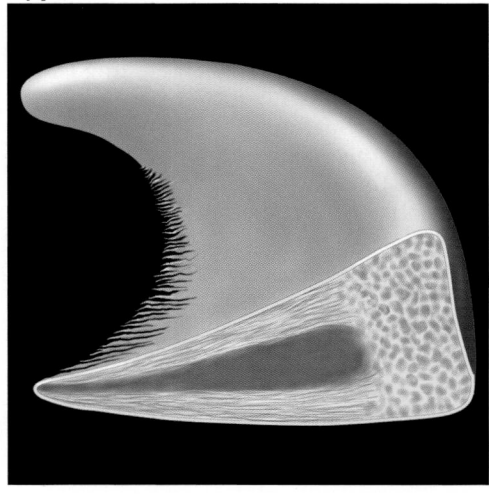
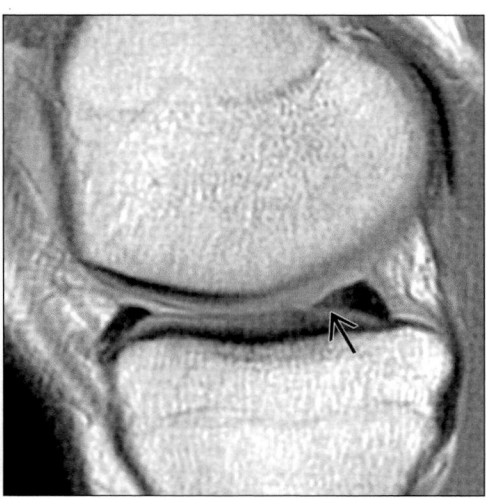

(Left) Sagittal graphic shows free edge fraying. *(Right)* Sagittal PD FSE MR shows increased signal (arrow) within the free edge of the medial meniscus confirmed at arthroscopy as free edge fraying.

MENISCAL HORIZONTAL TEAR

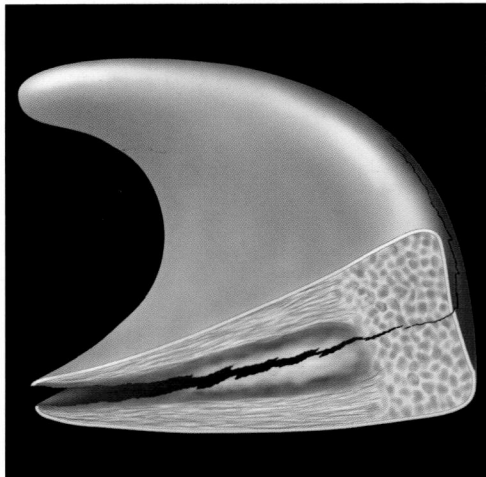

Sagittal graphic shows a horizontal tear extending from the free edge to an area of meniscal degeneration toward the more stable periphery of the meniscus.

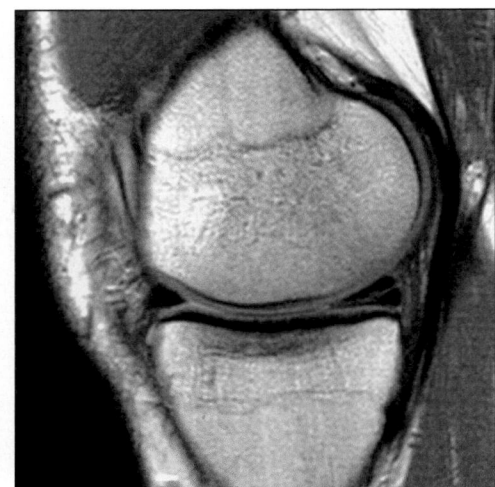

Sagittal PD FSE MR shows a horizontal medial meniscal tear with linear increased signal intensity reaching the surface at the free edge of the meniscus.

TERMINOLOGY

Abbreviations and Synonyms
- Horizontal tear (HT), cleavage tear, fishmouth tear

Definitions
- Meniscal tear that occurs in horizontal plane, dissecting through circumferential collagen fibers
- Tear most often extends from free edge inward along horizontally located central perforating bundle of meniscus, resulting in two separate shelves (leaves) of meniscal tissue

IMAGING FINDINGS

General Features
- Best diagnostic clue
  - Linear, horizontally-oriented, increased signal intensity on short TE sequences
    - Within meniscus extending from free edge inward
    - Short TE sequences: T1, PD, gradient echo
- Location
  - Most common within posterior horn of medial meniscus
  - Initially involves free edge then propagates transversely involving deeper substance then peripheral aspect

- Free edge: White zone
- Deeper substance: Red-white junction
- Peripheral aspect: Red zone
- Size: Varies from small tear involving free edge to completely bisecting meniscus
- Morphology
  - Horizontally-oriented (in superior to inferior plane)
  - Mesial to peripheral

CT Findings
- CT arthrography
  - Contrast extends into tear of meniscus body
- Sagittal, coronal reconstructions

MR Findings
- T1WI
  - Increased signal intensity extending to the articular surface in the plane of the middle perforating collagen fibers
    - Involves free edge
    - Horizontal orientation
- T2WI
  - Linear hyperintense signal on T2WI including FSE
    - Especially if fluid is present within tear and decompresses into a meniscal cyst
    - Posterior horn of the medial meniscus (PHMM) - hyperintense cystic mass
    - Communication with cyst often identified
- PD/Intermediate

DDx: Meniscal Horizontal Tear

Pediatric Vessels	Flap Tear	Normal Meniscus	Meniscal Degen	Meniscal Degen
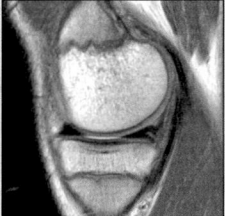	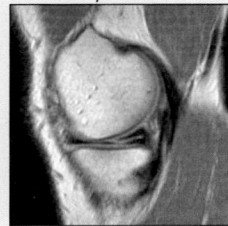	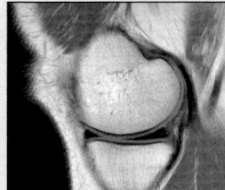	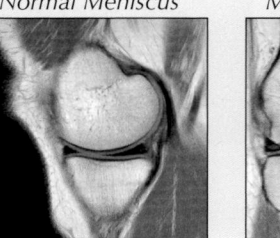	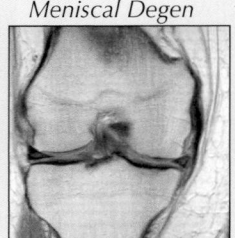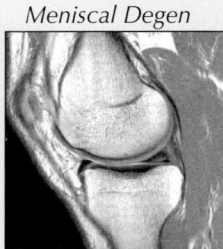
Sag PD FSE MR	Sag PD FSE MR	Sag PD FSE MR	Cor PD FSE MR	Sag PD FSE MR

MENISCAL HORIZONTAL TEAR

Key Facts

Terminology
- Meniscal tear that occurs in horizontal plane, dissecting through circumferential collagen fibers

Imaging Findings
- Linear, horizontally-oriented, increased signal intensity on short TE sequences
- Most common within posterior horn of medial meniscus
- Horizontally-oriented (in superior to inferior plane)

Top Differential Diagnoses
- Linear Intrameniscal Signal Abnormality
- Normal Vascularity Seen in Younger Patients
- Meniscal Flap Tear

Pathology
- Tear occurs in horizontal plane and dissects circumferential collagen fibers (splitting of fibers along their transverse axis)

Clinical Issues
- Tenderness typically at the joint line adjacent to the main portion of the tear if the tear reaches the peripheral, innervated, vascularized portion
- Asymptomatic if confined to the free edge and small in size

Diagnostic Checklist
- Signal intensity directed toward meniscal apex in horizontal plane (cleavage tear)

- o Linear hyperintensity extending to the articular surface = tear
  - o Parallels tibial articular surface orientation in cleavage tear
- MR arthrography
  - o Arthrogram - contrast extending into tear
  - o Arthrography typically not necessary
    - Useful in post operative setting
  - o May fill meniscal cyst if present
- +/- Separation of the two components of tear
- Coronal images - horizontal linear increased signal sequence intensity (short TE sequence) separating two resultant meniscal fragments
- Meniscal cyst formation

Imaging Recommendations
- Best imaging tool: Most accurately diagnosed on short TE MR images
- Protocol advice
  - o T1, PD and/or gradient echo (T2*) sequences
  - o FS PD FSE for detection of meniscal cyst

DIFFERENTIAL DIAGNOSIS

Linear Intrameniscal Signal Abnormality
- Linear degeneration
- Intrameniscal closed tear
- Visualized on short TE sequences

Normal Vascularity Seen in Younger Patients
- Typically less than 15 years of age
- Prominent, sometimes linear appearing
- Mimics meniscal tear/degeneration

Meniscal Flap Tear
- Complex tear of the meniscus with longitudinal and radial components
- Seen on short TE sequences
- +/- Displaced flap component
  - o Into meniscotibial or femoral attachment recesses

PATHOLOGY

General Features
- General path comments
  - o HT originates as a small free edge tear
    - After initial trauma in the setting of meniscal degeneration
  - o Tear occurs in horizontal plane and dissects circumferential collagen fibers (splitting of fibers along their transverse axis)
  - o Pure HT maintains a horizontal orientation toward meniscal apex
  - o Partial cleavage tear begins as horizontal tear
  - o Develop superior or inferior extension resulting in a mobile fragment of meniscus (flap of meniscus) known as flap tear
    - Flap tears may also result from a radial tear with secondary longitudinal component
  - o Most often occurs in a nontraumatic setting in an older person
- Etiology
  - o Shear forces resulting from difference in coefficient of friction between superior and inferior articular surfaces
    - Lead to horizontally-oriented degeneration
    - Eventually leading to tear after minor trauma
- Epidemiology: Common meniscal tear especially as a component of a flap tear

Gross Pathologic & Surgical Features
- Disruption of meniscal surface in a horizontal direction

Microscopic Features
- Mucinous ground substance within the fibrocartilaginous meniscus with a separating cleavage plane surrounded by regenerative chondrocytes along the free edge of the tear
- Variable degrees of synovial ingrowth
- Neovascularity in more chronic cases

MENISCAL HORIZONTAL TEAR

Staging, Grading or Classification Criteria
- Classification by surface configuration - tear patterns (arthroscopic)
  - Vertical
    - Longitudinal tear (primary tear pattern is in vertical plane)
    - Flap tear (primary tear pattern is in vertical plane)
    - Radial tear
  - Horizontal
    - Horizontal cleavage tear
    - Longitudinal tear (primary tear pattern is in horizontal plane)
    - Flap tear (primary tear pattern is in horizontal plane)
- Classification based on location-vascular zones
  - White zone (white/white zone)
    - Inner third of meniscus (free edge)
    - Debridement
  - Red-white junction (red/white zone)
    - Middle third between free edge and peripheral third
    - Debridement vs. repair
    - Repair especially if vascular pedicle can be established
  - Red zone (red/red zone)
    - Peripheral third
    - Vascularized
    - Primary repair usually possible if tear confined to red/red zone or peripheral portion of red/white zone

CLINICAL ISSUES

Presentation
- Most common signs/symptoms
  - Tenderness typically at the joint line adjacent to the main portion of the tear if the tear reaches the peripheral, innervated, vascularized portion
  - Tears involving only the free edge may be asymptomatic
  - Joint line tenderness and positive clinical meniscal testing
    - Positive McMurray's test, Steinmann's test, Apley's test
- Clinical profile
  - Middle aged or older patient, +/- physical activity
  - Patient often unaware when tear occurs

Demographics
- Age: Adult
- Gender: No predilection

Natural History & Prognosis
- Asymptomatic if confined to the free edge and small in size
- Progression to flap tear, fragment may displace peripherally into coronary recess or meniscofemoral attachment recess
- Reactive tibial edema common
- Small tears usually propagate peripherally
- Extension of debrided meniscus
  - Especially in traumatic setting
- Extensive resection may lead to osteoarthritis
- Clinical course depends in part on other structures damaged in traumatic cases
- Extensive injuries more likely to develop osteoarthritis

Treatment
- Conservative
  - If isolated to the peripheral third ("red zone") and small in size (uncommon)
- Surgical
  - Amenable to meniscal resection/debridement to stable intact or stable meniscus with residual grade 3 signal intensity (meniscal signal extending to an articular surface of either the superior or inferior leaf or apex)
- Complications
  - Immediate post operative complications include
    - Infection
    - Popliteal artery or venous thrombosis or laceration
    - Articular cartilage abrasions
    - Scuffing or defect formation
  - Development of osteoarthritis if the meniscus is resected
    - Altered load transfer
  - Malalignment secondary to meniscectomy

DIAGNOSTIC CHECKLIST

Consider
- In the absence of acute trauma
- A pseudolesion
  - Vascularity in a young patient
  - Grade 2 degeneration mistaken for grade 3 signal
    - Grade 2 degeneration: Linear intrasubstance meniscal signal
    - Grade 3 signal: Tear
- Could it be a flap tear with a secondary horizontal component vs. a classic horizontal cleavage tear which extends to the meniscal apex

Image Interpretation Pearls
- Utilize short TE images (T1, GRE, PD)
- Signal intensity directed toward meniscal apex in horizontal plane (cleavage tear)

SELECTED REFERENCES
1. Jee WH et al: Meniscal tear configurations: Categorization with MR imaging. AJR 180(1):93-7, 2003
2. Anderson MW: MR imaging of the meniscus. Radiol Clin North Am 40(5):1081-94, 2002
3. Greis PE et al: Meniscal injury: Management. J Am Acad Orthop Surg 10(3):177-87, 2002
4. Menetrey J et al: Medial meniscectomy in patients over the age of fifty: A six year follow-up study. Swiss Surg 8(3):113-9, 2002
5. Imhoff A et al: Comparison between magnetic resonance imaging and arthroscopy for the diagnosis of knee meniscal lesions. Rev Chir Orthop Reparatrice Appar Mot 83(3):229-36, 1997
6. Stoller DW et al: Meniscal tears: Pathologic correlation with MR imaging. Radiology 163(3):731-5, 1987

MENISCAL HORIZONTAL TEAR

IMAGE GALLERY

Variant

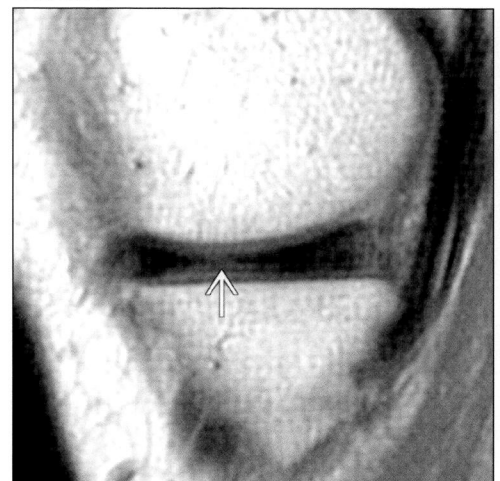 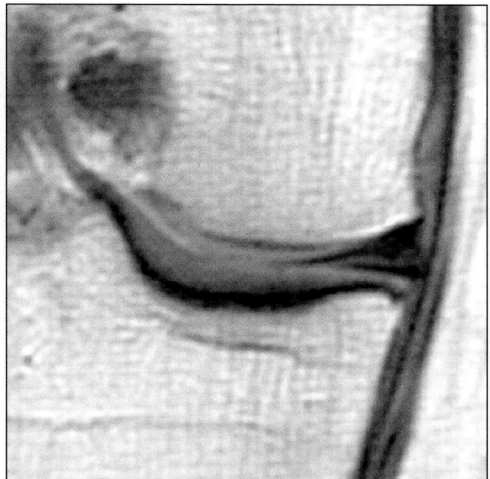

(Left) Sagittal PD FSE MR shows a subtle peripheral horizontal tear (arrow) of free edge of body of the medial meniscus. *(Right)* Coronal PD FSE MR shows the horizontal tear extending to the free edge of the body of the medial meniscus.

Typical

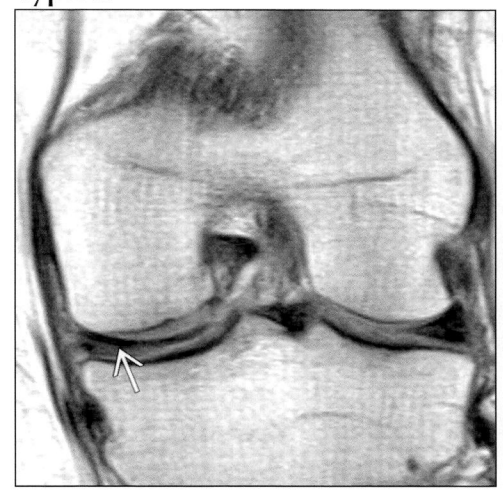 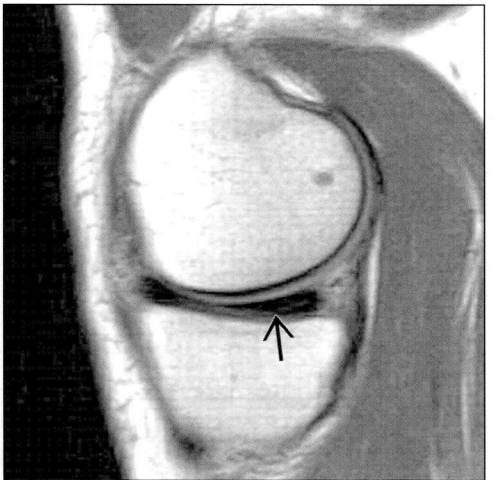

(Left) Coronal PD FSE MR shows a horizontal tear (arrow) of the body of the medial meniscus. *(Right)* Sagittal PD FSE MR (same case) shows where the tear (arrow) is difficult to identify due to involvement of the body of the meniscus. The findings include irregularity of the undersurface in this peripheral image.

Typical

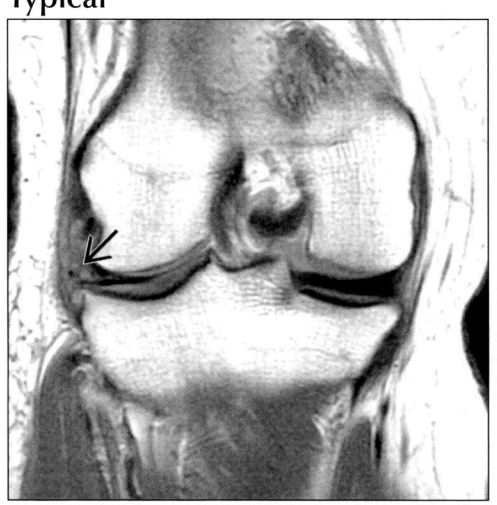 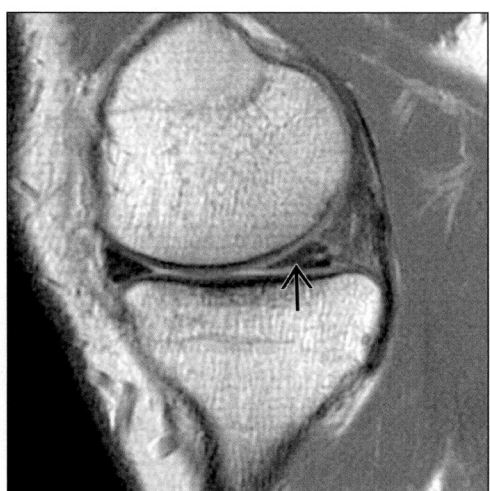

(Left) Coronal PD FSE MR shows an intrameniscal cyst (arrow) within the peripheral aspect of the body of the lateral meniscus adjacent to meniscal signal abnormality. *(Right)* Sagittal PD FSE MR shows inferior extension (arrow) of a horizontal tear. Note in this case the orientation of the tear is slightly oblique but would appear as a horizontal flap tear at arthroscopy.

MENISCAL CYST

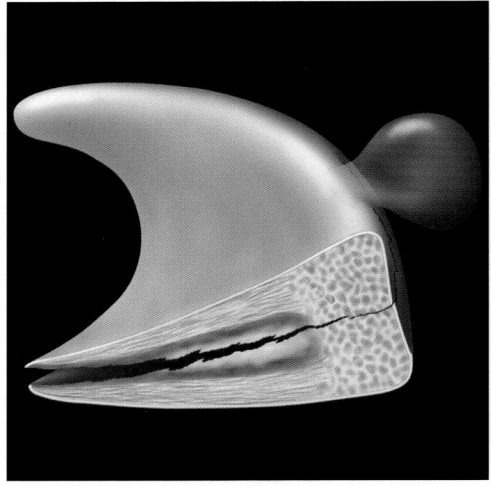

Sagittal graphic shows a horizontal tear of the body of the meniscus with associated meniscal cyst projecting peripherally.

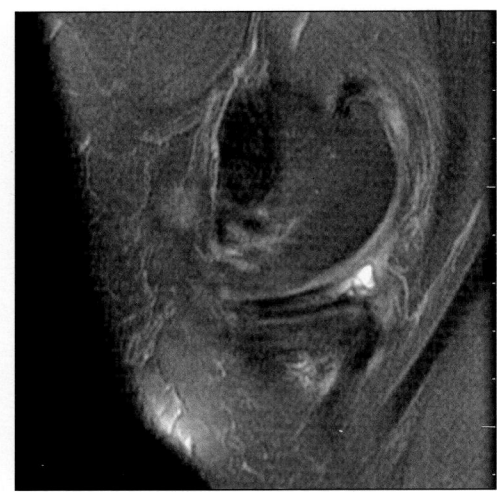

Sagittal FS PD FSE MR shows a horizontal tear of the peripheral aspect of the medial meniscus with a small posteriorly projecting meniscal cyst.

TERMINOLOGY

Abbreviations and Synonyms
- Parameniscal cyst, meniscal cyst (MC)

Definitions
- Cyst extending from meniscal tear
  - Horizontal tear most common

IMAGING FINDINGS

General Features
- Best diagnostic clue: Cystic mass extending from a meniscal tear
- Location
  - Most common locations
    - Anterior horn of the lateral meniscus (AHLM)
    - Posterior horn of the medial meniscus (PHMM)
- Size: Varies from a few mms to large dissecting cyst (> 1 cm)
- Morphology
  - Round +/- loculations
  - May be flattened
  - Dissection around medial collateral ligament (MCL) conforming to adjacent structures

- Cyst within (intrameniscal) or adjacent to (parameniscal) meniscus typically in continuity with meniscal tear
  - Meniscal tear horizontal cleavage or complex tear also known as a radial split tear with radial and horizontal component (lateral meniscus)
    - Posterior horn of medial meniscus
    - Anterior horn of lateral meniscus
    - Body of lateral meniscus
    - Lateral meniscal tear may be radial/complex

CT Findings
- CT arthrography
  - Contrast extends into tear
  - +/- Filling of cyst
    - Partial or complete filling

MR Findings
- T1WI
  - Intermediate to low signal intensity mass = cyst
  - If proteinaceous, the cyst may be of variable signal intensity
- T2WI
  - Rounded, homogenous increased signal intensity mass
  - If chronic, increased signal intensity hyperemia in adjacent tibia, femur = "reactive edema"
  - Increased signal intensity with soft tissue edema
- PD/Intermediate

DDx: Meniscal Cyst

SMTCL Bursitis	Pes Bursitis	Meniscal Ossicle	Pop Tendon Sheath
Sag FS PD FSE	Sag PD FSE	Cor PD FSE	Sag FS PD FSE

MENISCAL CYST

Key Facts

Imaging Findings
- Best diagnostic clue: Cystic mass extending from a meniscal tear
- Cyst within (intrameniscal) or adjacent to (parameniscal) meniscus typically in continuity with meniscal tear
- Rounded, homogenous increased signal intensity mass
- Protocol advice: T2WI show cyst as increased signal intensity mass (FS PD FSE is more sensitive)

Top Differential Diagnoses
- Synovial Cyst/Ganglion Cyst
- Bursitis
- Cystic Masses
- Meniscal Ossicle

Pathology
- Cyst develops from forcing of joint fluid into or through meniscal tear, typically horizontal tear

Clinical Issues
- Pain and palpable mass near joint line in cases of large cysts
- Palpable mass that disappears with flexion = Pisani's sign
- Cysts tend to be larger when lateral due to loose soft tissue constraints compared to the medial side

Diagnostic Checklist
- Bursitis, especially SMTCL bursitis if adjacent to PHMM and no tear seen
- Search for associated meniscal tear on short TE sequence

- ○ Intermediate signal intensity mass = cyst
- ○ PD intermediate = short TE sequence
- T2* GRE
  - ○ Intermediate to hyperintense mass = cyst
  - ○ GRE progressive T2* effect with increasing TE and decreased theta values
- T1 C+
  - ○ +/- Rim enhancement
  - ○ Greater enhancement if chronic cyst with thickened synovium
- Increased signal on short TE sequences extending to articular surface = tear
- Mass lobulated and septate especially if parameniscal location
- Cyst mass dissects around the knee into the paraarticular soft tissues
  - ○ When medial the cyst dissects around the MCL or between the deep and superficial components

Imaging Recommendations
- Best imaging tool: MRI
- Protocol advice: T2WI show cyst as increased signal intensity mass (FS PD FSE is more sensitive)

DIFFERENTIAL DIAGNOSIS

Synovial Cyst/Ganglion Cyst
- Does not originate from meniscal tear
- +/- Osteoarthritis (OA)
- Synovial cyst originates from joint
- Ganglion cyst - nonspecific origin
- May or may not contain synovial lining
- +/- History of trauma
- Often reflects past effusions (synovial cyst)

Bursitis
- Semimembranosus tibial collateral ligament (SMTCL) bursa mimics a medial parameniscal cyst (sagittal)
- Tibial collateral ligament bursa mimics a medial parameniscal cyst (coronal)
- Deep infrapatellar bursa can mimic anterior lateral parameniscal cyst with inferior extension

- Pes anserinus bursa mimics inferiorly dissecting medial cyst

Cystic Masses
- Neoplastic masses tend to be heterogeneous with visible cellular elements
  - ○ Hemangioma
  - ○ Varices
  - ○ Hematoma
  - ○ Neoplasm (rare)
- No demonstrable connection to meniscus
- MRI useful for differentiation

Meniscal Ossicle
- Hyperintense on T1/PD, not on conventional T2
  - ○ Due to marrow fat content
- Marrow fat ossicle may expand meniscus like intrameniscal cyst
- Posterior horn medial meniscus (PHMM) most common location
- Rare

Popliteus Tendon Sheath (Pop Tendon Sheath)
- Normal structure may be filled with fluid
- Mimics posterior horn lateral meniscus (PHLM) cyst
- In continuity with joint capsule
- Tendon within fluid-filled sheath

PATHOLOGY

General Features
- General path comments
  - ○ Results from "ball valve" mechanism
  - ○ Associated tear most commonly horizontal when associated with PHMM tear
  - ○ Associated tear most commonly complex when associated with AHLM tear
    - ■ Extends anteriorly from tear involving the body of the lateral meniscus

MENISCAL CYST

○ Associated tear most commonly complex when body segment of lateral meniscus is torn leading to cyst
  ▪ Prominent radial component
- Etiology
  ○ Cyst develops from forcing of joint fluid into or through meniscal tear, typically horizontal tear
  ○ Cyst arising from extrusion of joint fluid through meniscal tear often with a "ball valve" mechanism leading to build-up of pressure and cyst formation
- Epidemiology
  ○ Relatively common
  ○ 7% in surgically removed menisci
  ○ Seen in age groups in which meniscal tears are present

Gross Pathologic & Surgical Features
- Cyst filled with mucinous, proteinaceous fluid
  ○ Within or adjacent to meniscus
  ○ In continuity with horizontal cleavage meniscal tear or flap (oblique) tear with a predominately horizontal component
  ○ Associated with discoid menisci

Microscopic Features
- Cyst formed within meniscus lined by
  ○ Compressed meniscal collagen with areas of mucinous degeneration in adjacent meniscus
- Cyst outside the meniscus (parameniscal) formed by
  ○ Compressed, paraarticular loose areolar tissue with hemorrhage and inflammatory cells

CLINICAL ISSUES

Presentation
- Most common signs/symptoms
  ○ Pain and palpable mass near joint line in cases of large cysts
    ▪ Palpable mass that disappears with flexion = Pisani's sign
    ▪ Palpable cyst prominent at 15 to 30 degrees of flexion and disappears at full extension and flexion greater than 90 degrees
  ○ Cysts tend to be larger when lateral due to loose soft tissue constraints compared to the medial side
  ○ Vary in size depending on position of knee

Demographics
- Age: Adult patient
- Gender
  ○ More frequent in females
  ○ M:F = 1:1 to 1:10

Natural History & Prognosis
- Mass grows with time
- Will recur in cases of communicating meniscal tear
- If arthroscopy performed for meniscus, tear must be closed to prevent recurrence or growth of cyst

Treatment
- Arthroscopic resection of cyst and repair of tear

DIAGNOSTIC CHECKLIST

Consider
- Bursitis, especially SMTCL bursitis if adjacent to PHMM and no tear seen

Image Interpretation Pearls
- If communicating meniscal tear visualized or cyst is present at the joint line then assume the cyst is meniscal in origin
- Search for associated meniscal tear on short TE sequence
- Associated meniscal tear patterns include horizontal cleavage and radial split tears (horizontal and radial tear components)

SELECTED REFERENCES

1. Rath E et al: The menisci: Basic science and advances in treatment. Br J Sports Med 34(4):252-7, 2000
2. Stoller DW et al: Magnetic resonance imaging in orthopaedics and sports medicine. vol 1. 2nd ed. Philadelphia PA, J.B. Lippincott, 203-442, 1997
3. Rothstein CP et al: Semimembranosus-tibial collateral ligament bursitis: MR imaging findings. Am J Roentgenol 166(4):875-7, 1996
4. Steiner E et al: Ganglia and cysts around joints. Radiol Clin North Am 34(2):395-425, 1996
5. Janzen DL et al: Cystic lesions around the knee joint: MR imaging findings. Am J Roentgenol 163(1):155-61, 1994
6. Stoller DW et al: Meniscal tears: Pathologic correlation with MR imaging. Radiology 163(3):731-5, 1987
7. Fitzgerald R et al: Orthopaedics. Meniscal injury. 2nd ed. St Louis MO, Mosby, 663-77, 1984

MENISCAL CYST

Typical

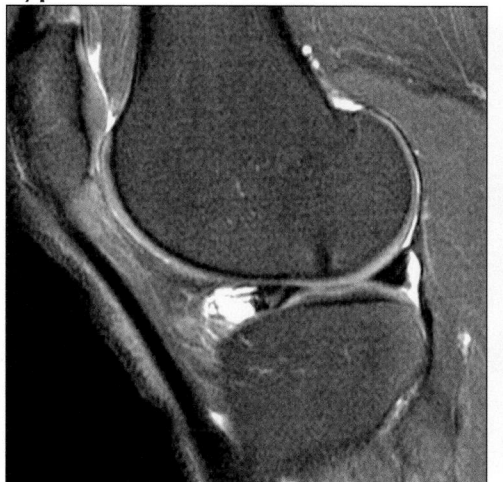 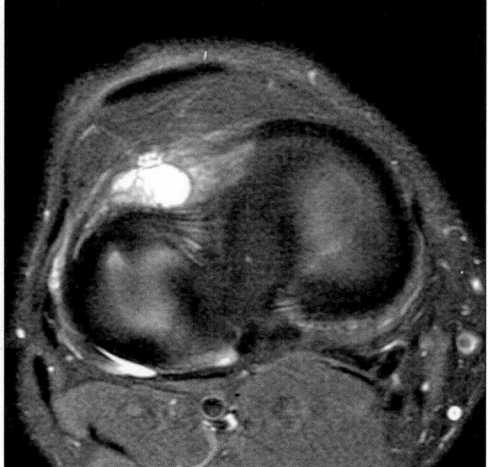

(Left) Sagittal FS PD FSE MR shows a hyperintense meniscal cyst arising from the anterior horn of the lateral meniscus - a common location. *(Right)* Axial FS PD FSE MR (same case) showing anterior soft tissue extension of the cyst .

Typical

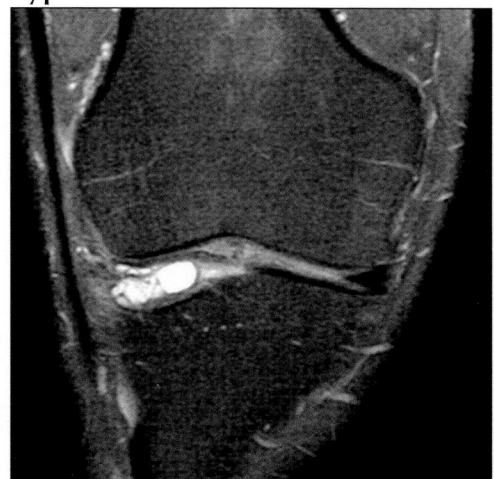 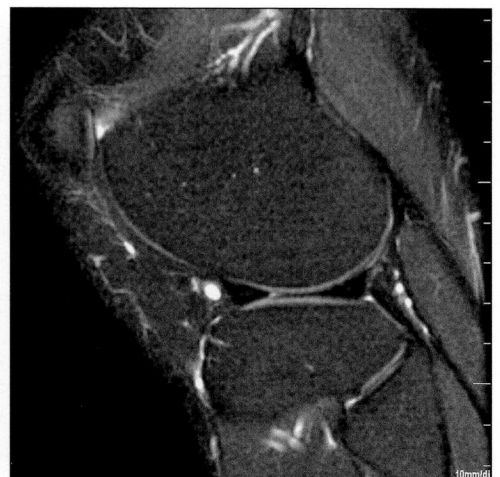

(Left) Coronal FS PD FSE MR shows a cyst anterior to the lateral meniscus, a common location for meniscal cysts. *(Right)* Sagittal FS PD FSE MR shows a small radial tear at the junction of the anterior horn and body of the lateral meniscus and an anteriorly projecting parameniscal cyst.

5

17

Typical

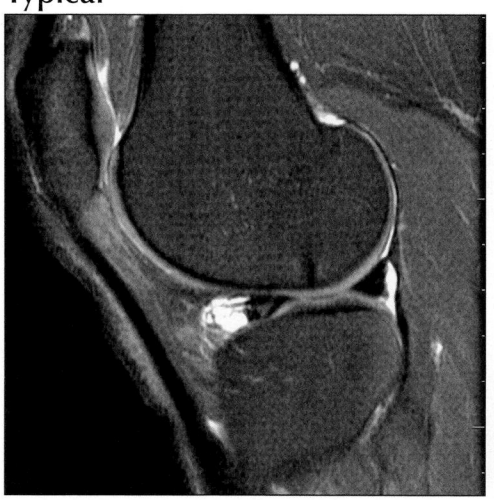 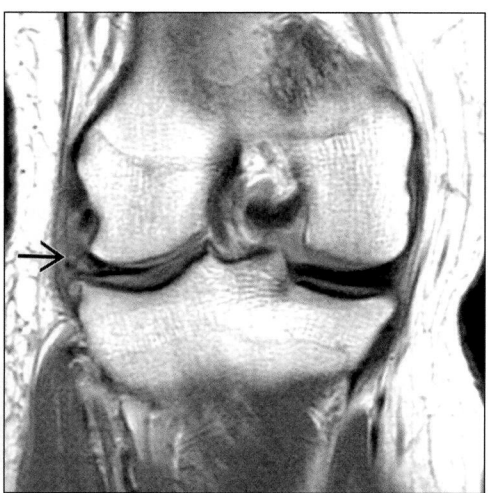

(Left) Sagittal FS PD FSE MR shows a moderate sized meniscal cyst projecting anteriorly from an anterior lateral meniscus tear. This is a common location for meniscal cyst. *(Right)* Coronal PD FSE MR shows a small meniscal cyst (arrow) adjacent to a lateral meniscal tear of the body segment.

MENISCAL LONGITUDINAL TEAR

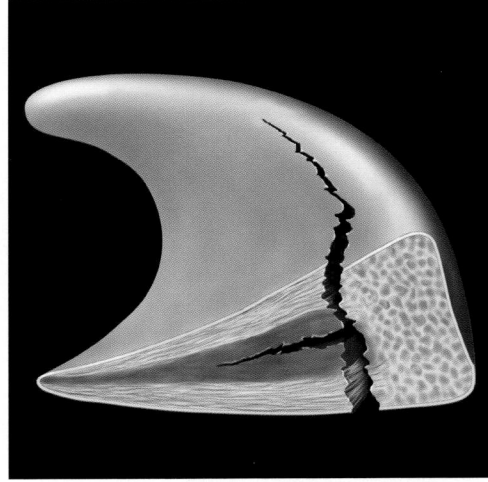

Sagittal graphic shows a longitudinal tear involving the peripheral aspect of the meniscus. A small horizontal intrameniscal component extends toward the free edge.

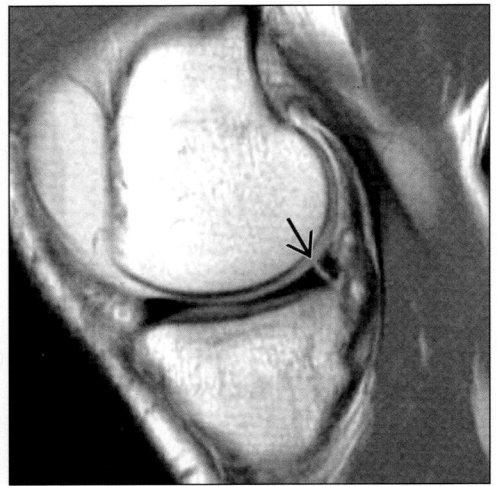

Sagittal PD FSE MR shows a longitudinal tear (arrow) within the posterior horn of the medial meniscus.

TERMINOLOGY

Abbreviations and Synonyms
- Vertical peripheral tear, longitudinal tear = LT

Definitions
- Tear along longitudinal axis of meniscus
- Begins in peripheral aspect of posterior horn and advances in direction of circumferential collagen fibers

IMAGING FINDINGS

General Features
- Best diagnostic clue
  - Linear, vertically oriented increased signal intensity on short TE sequences within the meniscus
  - Extends to superior articular surface, inferior articular surface or both
- Location
  - Typically within the outer third of the meniscus
    - Vascularized portion of the meniscus or "red zone"
  - Propagates longitudinally (circumferentially)
    - Posterior horn → body → anterior horn
    - Anterior horn rarely involved
- Size: Varies from small longitudinal tear to circumferential longitudinal tear
- Morphology

  - Vertically oriented tear in the superoinferior plane
  - Extends from posterior to anterior

Radiographic Findings
- Radiography
  - Associated fractures
  - Deepened sulcus terminalis of lateral femoral condyle
    - Associated with anterior cruciate ligament (ACL) tears

CT Findings
- NECT: +/- Fractures
- CT arthrography
  - Contrast extends into tear of meniscal body
  - Sagittal reconstructions

MR Findings
- T1WI
  - Increased signal intensity extending to the articular surface = tear
    - Typically peripheral; vertical orientation
- T2WI
  - Linear hyperintense signal if fluid is present within tear or when a T2* GRE sequence is used
    - T2* GRE is more sensitive (hyperintense) to meniscal degeneration and tears compared to conventional spin echo or fast spin echo

DDx: Meniscal Longitudinal Tear

Humphrey Lig	Humphrey Lig	Transverse Lig	Transverse Lig	Popliteus Tendon
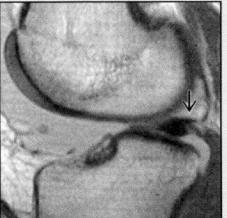	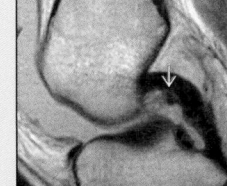	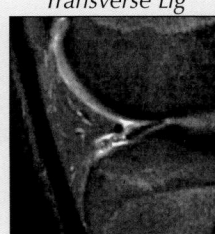	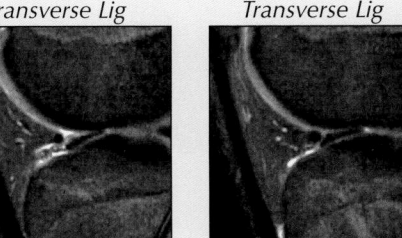	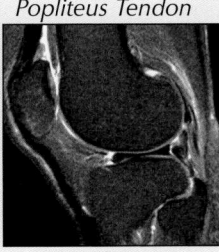
Sag PD FSE MR	Sag PD FSE MR	Sag FS PD FSE	Sag FS PD FSE	Sag FS PD FSE

MENISCAL LONGITUDINAL TEAR

Key Facts

Terminology
- Tear along longitudinal axis of meniscus
- Begins in peripheral aspect of posterior horn and advances in direction of circumferential collagen fibers

Imaging Findings
- Typically within the outer third of the meniscus
- Vascularized portion of the meniscus or "red zone"
- Size: Varies from small longitudinal tear to circumferential longitudinal tear

Top Differential Diagnoses
- Anterior Transverse Ligament Insertion
- Meniscofemoral Femoral Ligament Insertion
- Popliteus Tendon

Pathology
- Normal anatomic structures may mimic LT
- Insertion of anterior transverse intermeniscal ligament

Clinical Issues
- Conservative treatment most common

Diagnostic Checklist
- Identify vertical signal abnormality on sagittal and coronal images
- Signal intensity follows contour of meniscus on axial images in a longitudinal tear
- Meniscal tear pattern does not change direction on multiple sagittal images as seen in some flap tears

---

- PD/Intermediate: Increased signal on short TE sequences extending to the articular surface of the superior and/or inferior leaf of the meniscus: Vertical orientation common on meniscal cross section
- MR arthrography
  - Contrast extending into tear
  - MR arthrography not routinely used
    - Post operative setting for retear detection
- +/- Separation of two components of tear
  - Displacement (bucket-handle or flap tear)
- Often seen as a vertical tear within posterior horn
- Longitudinal tears also possible with horizontal component on meniscal cross section (sagittal plane)
- Coronal images identify body segment involvement
- Thin section axial images demonstrate linear signal intensity following the long axis of meniscus

Imaging Recommendations
- Best imaging tool: MRI
- Protocol advice
  - Accurately diagnosed on short TE MR images
    - T1 weighted, proton density weighted and/or T2* gradient echo images
  - PD FSE or T2* GRE

DIFFERENTIAL DIAGNOSIS

Anterior Transverse Ligament Insertion
- Ligament-meniscus interface (connects the anterior horns of the medial and lateral meniscus)
- Seen on successive sagittal images adjacent to anterior horn
- Isolated anterior meniscal tears are rare

Meniscofemoral Femoral Ligament Insertion
- Interface of the meniscofemoral ligament and posterior horn lateral meniscus (PHLM)
- Mesial third of posterior horn (near the posterior horn meniscotibial attachment)
- Ligament can be followed on successive contiguous images
- Ligament of Humphrey (anterior to PCL)

- Ligament of Wrisberg (posterior to PCL)

Popliteus Tendon
- Normal structure adjacent to posterior horn lateral meniscus
- Tendon sheath intracapsular at posterior aspect of joint
- Tendon may mimic posterior third of torn meniscus

PATHOLOGY

General Features
- General path comments
  - Normal anatomic structures may mimic LT
    - Insertion of anterior transverse intermeniscal ligament
    - Insertion of meniscofemoral (Humphrey's, Wrisberg's) ligament to PHLM
  - LT originates as a small longitudinal split
    - Disrupts posterior horn
    - Advances along the plane of circumferential collagen fibers
    - Splitting of the fibers along their long axis
  - Multiple tears can occur
  - Occurs in an acute traumatic setting
  - Accompanied by ACL and/or medial collateral ligament (MCL) tears
  - Inner fragment displaced resulting in a bucket-handle or flap fragment
- Etiology
  - Increased axial load (compressive force)
    - Resulting radial strain and subsequent splitting of meniscus longitudinally
- Epidemiology
  - Second most common tear pattern
  - Seen in ACL deficient knees

Gross Pathologic & Surgical Features
- Disruption of meniscal surface in longitudinal direction (parallel to the longitudinal axis)

MENISCAL LONGITUDINAL TEAR

Microscopic Features
- Mucinous ground substance within fibrocartilaginous meniscus with separating cleavage plane surrounded by regenerative chondrocytes and fibrosis
- Synovial ingrowth into the meniscal tear
- Neovascularity in chronic cases

Staging, Grading or Classification Criteria
- Classification by surface configuration - tear patterns (arthroscopic)
  - Vertical
    - Longitudinal tear (primary tear pattern is in vertical plane)
    - Flap tear (primary tear pattern is in vertical plane)
    - Radial tear
  - Horizontal
    - Horizontal cleavage tear
    - Longitudinal tear (primary tear pattern is in horizontal plane)
    - Flap tear (primary tear pattern is in horizontal plane)
  - Complex degenerative
- Classification based on location-vascular zones
  - White zone (white/white zone)
    - Menisci debrided in free edge (medial third)
  - Red-white junction (red/white zone)
    - Middle third between free edge and peripheral third
    - Debridement vs. repair
    - Repair if vascular pedicle can be established
  - Red zone (red/red zone)
    - Peripheral third
    - Vascularized
    - Primary repair usually possible if tear confined to red/red zone or peripheral portion of red/white zone

CLINICAL ISSUES

Presentation
- Most common signs/symptoms
  - Tenderness typically at the joint line adjacent to the apex of the tear
    - Due to greatest tension exerted on surrounding nerve fibers
  - Locking if inner fragment becomes displaced
    - Tension on the abnormally mobile fragment leads to pain and spasm
  - Posterior spring sign (clinically) which dissipates with general anesthesia
    - Spasmodic origin rather that true physical extension lock (displaced bucket-handle tear, flap tear or flipped meniscus)
  - Joint line tenderness and often positive clinical meniscal testing
    - Positive tests: McMurray's, Steinmann's & Apley's
- Clinical profile
  - Younger, physically active patient
  - Often posttraumatic and occurs after a single traumatic event
  - Common in a sports setting

Demographics
- Age: Younger patient
- Gender: M > F

Natural History & Prognosis
- May heal if isolated to the peripheral third ("red zone") and small in size
- Often propagates longitudinally
- Fragment may displace transiently giving a locked knee presentation (posterior spring sign)
- Small tear may heal
- Retear of repair in traumatic setting
- Extensive resection may lead to osteoarthritis
- Clinical course depends on associated injured structures
  - Extensive injuries have an increased chance of developing osteoarthritis

Treatment
- Conservative treatment most common
  - If isolated to the peripheral third ("red zone") and small in size
- Surgical
  - Amenable to meniscal repair if isolated to the peripheral third ("red zone")
  - Resection of the inner fragment if not amenable to repair
- Complications
  - Immediate post operative complications include infection, popliteal artery/venous thrombosis or laceration
  - Development of osteoarthritis if the meniscus is resected due to altered load transfer
  - Malalignment secondary to meniscectomy

DIAGNOSTIC CHECKLIST

Consider
- In the setting of trauma
- Signal hyperintensity could be pseudolesion: Meniscofemoral & anterior transverse ligament attachment
- Could the tear pattern identified on sagittal images represent a flap tear

Image Interpretation Pearls
- Identify vertical signal abnormality on sagittal and coronal images
- Signal intensity follows contour of meniscus on axial images in a longitudinal tear
- Meniscal tear pattern does not change direction on multiple sagittal images as seen in some flap tears

SELECTED REFERENCES
1. Jee WH et al: Meniscal tear configurations: Categorization with MR imaging. AJR 180(1):93-7, 2003
2. Greis PE et al: Meniscal injury: Management. J Am Acad Orthop Surg 10(3):177-87, 2002
3. Stoller DW et al: Meniscal tears: Pathologic correlation with MR imaging. Radiology 163(3):731-5, 1997

MENISCAL LONGITUDINAL TEAR

IMAGE GALLERY

Typical

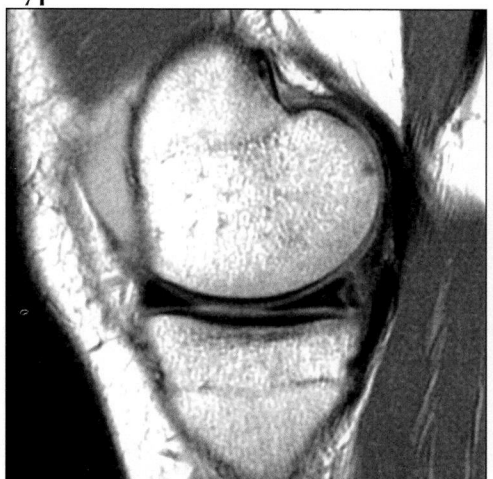
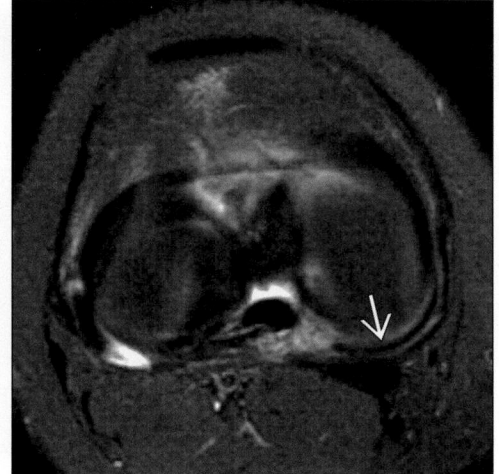

(Left) Sagittal PD FSE MR shows a typical nondisplaced longitudinal tear. *(Right)* Axial FS PD FSE MR shows longitudinal increased signal within the posterior horn of the medial meniscus (arrow) in the same case.

Typical

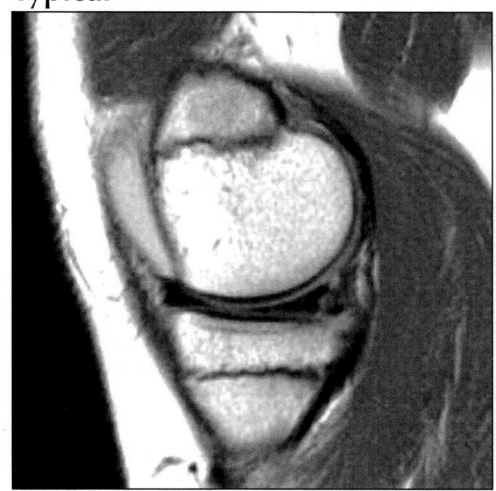
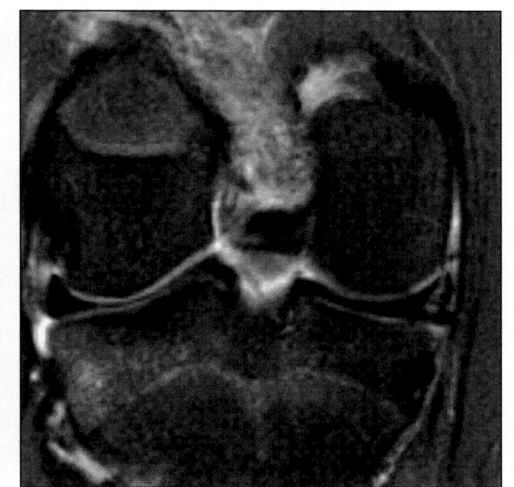

(Left) Sagittal PD FSE MR shows a vertical longitudinal tear through the posterior horn also referred to as a "corner fracture" seen in acute traumatic cases. *(Right)* Coronal FS PD FSE MR shows extension to and involvement of the peripheral aspect of the body of the meniscus.

Typical

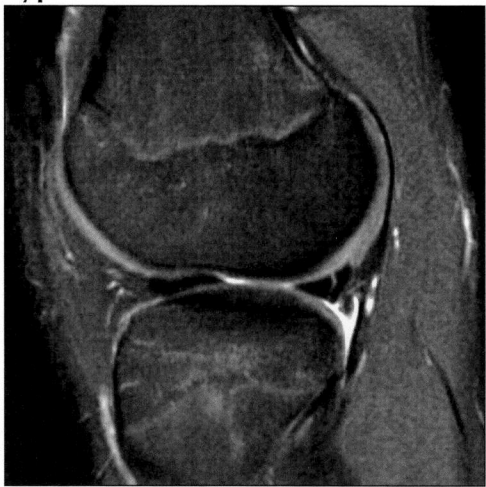
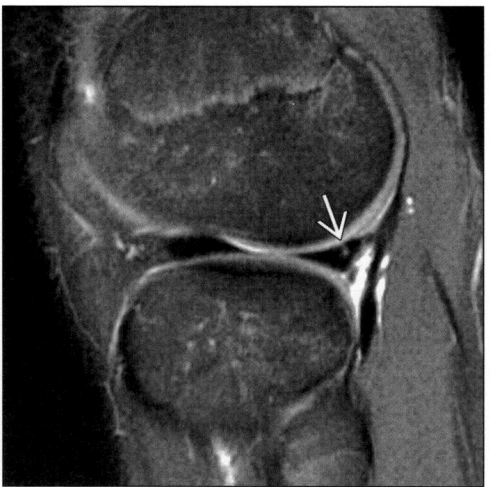

(Left) Sagittal FS PD FSE MR shows a longitudinal tear (lateral meniscus) at the insertion of the meniscofemoral ligament (Humphrey's or Wrisberg's ligament). This is seen with an ACL tear mechanism of injury. *(Right)* Sagittal FS PD FSE MR of the same case shows peripheral extension of the tear (arrow).

MENISCAL RADIAL TEAR

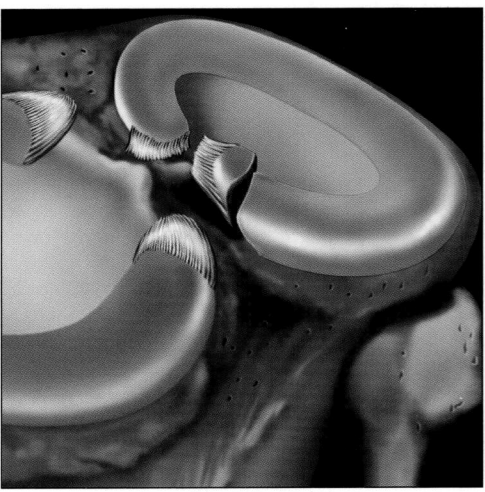

Axial oblique graphic shows a radial tear involving the posterior horn of the lateral meniscus at meniscotibial attachment.

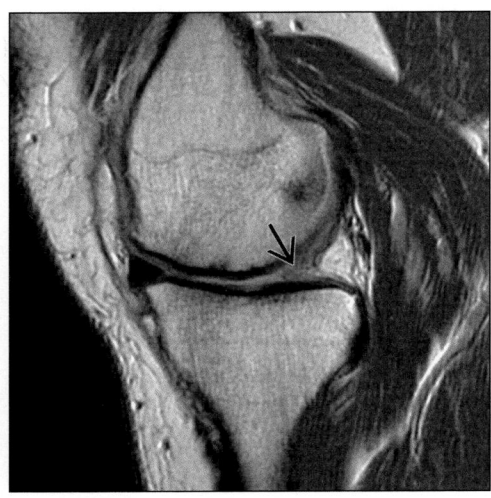

Sagittal PD FSE MR shows a radial tear (arrow) of posterior horn of the medial meniscus at the root attachment giving a "ghost meniscus" appearance.

TERMINOLOGY

Abbreviations and Synonyms
- Radial tear (RT)

Definitions
- Vertical tear oriented perpendicular to the free edge of meniscus
- Includes root tear at meniscotibial attachment

IMAGING FINDINGS

General Features
- Best diagnostic clue
  - Vertical tear perpendicular to the free edge of the meniscus
  - "Ghost meniscus" when in plane of acquisition in root tears
- Location
  - Most common at junction of the anterior horn and body of the lateral meniscus
  - Meniscotibial attachment posterior horn of the meniscus (root tear)
    - Common in posterior horn of medial meniscus as a degenerative tear
- Size: Small free edge tear, or tear through entire meniscus

- Morphology: Radially-oriented (perpendicular to long axis of meniscus)

Radiographic Findings
- Radiography
  - +/- Associated fractures in acute cases
  - Posterolateral tibia, anterolateral femur (sulcus terminalis) - with anterior cruciate ligament (ACL) tears

CT Findings
- NECT
  - +/- Associated fractures in acute cases
  - Posterolateral tibia, anterolateral femur (sulcus terminalis) - associated with ACL tears
- CT arthrography
  - Contrast extends into tear of meniscus body
  - Sagittal, coronal reconstructions

MR Findings
- T1WI
  - Increased signal intensity extending to articular surface = tear
    - Involves free edge extending variably to involve red-white junction, +/- red zone
    - Bisects meniscus in post traumatic cases
    - Radially-oriented (vertical on cross section)
- T2WI
  - Linear hyperintense signal on T2WI/(FSE PD FSE)

DDx: Meniscal Radial Tear

Degeneration	Meniscal Ossicle	Flap Tear	Post Operative	Post Operative
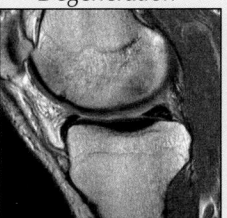	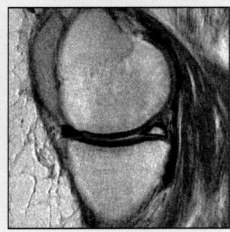	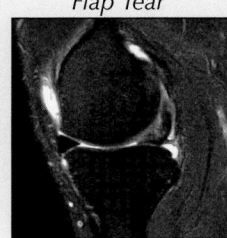	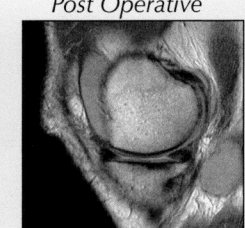	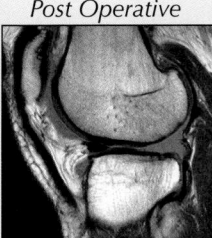
Sag PD FSE MR	Sag PD FSE MR	Sag FS PD FSE	Sag PD FSE MR	Sag PD FSE MR

MENISCAL RADIAL TEAR

Key Facts

Imaging Findings

- Vertical tear perpendicular to the free edge of the meniscus
- Morphology: Radially-oriented (perpendicular to long axis of meniscus)
- Diffuse, increased signal on one or two sagittal images seen in root attachment type of radial tears

Top Differential Diagnoses

- Meniscal Degeneration

Pathology

- Degenerative or acute (mostly a traumatic origin)
- Disruption of "hoop containment" results in subluxation of the body of the meniscus peripherally
- Posterior horn lateral meniscus radial tears associated with ACL tears

Clinical Issues

- Most common signs/symptoms: Pain after single traumatic event or insidious onset of pain
- Joint line tenderness anterior to lateral collateral ligament (LCL)
- Feeling of "giving way"
- Progresses to larger tear
- Asymptomatic if confined to the free edge & small in size
- Often propagates peripherally

Diagnostic Checklist

- Flap tear if not purely radial (radial + longitudinal)
- "Ghost meniscus" (root tear) if there is no history of surgery and posterior horn tissue is absent adjacent to the intercondylar notch

---

- ■ +/- Hyperintense bone edema = stress response/fx
  - ○ Associated with meniscal cyst - increased signal intensity mass on T2WI
    - ■ Body, anterior horn lateral meniscus
- PD/Intermediate
  - ○ Increased signal on short TE sequences extending to articular surface = tear
    - ■ Involves free edge extending variably to involve periphery
    - ■ Radially-oriented
- T2* GRE
  - ○ Radially-oriented increased signal extending to articular surface
    - ■ Involves free edge
- MR arthrography
  - ○ Arthrogram - contrast extending into tear
  - ○ Contrast may communicate with meniscal cyst if present
  - ○ Arthrography useful in post operative setting
- Diffuse, increased signal on one or two sagittal images seen in root attachment type of radial tears
  - ○ = "Ghost meniscus" in tear of root attachment
- Blunting of the free edge on coronal images

Imaging Recommendations

- Best imaging tool: MRI
- Protocol advice
  - ○ High resolution (ZIP512/interpolation) FSE
  - ○ Short TE sequences (T1, GRE, PD); PD FSE

DIFFERENTIAL DIAGNOSIS

Oblique Meniscal Tear/Flap Tear

- Contains longitudinal component in addition to radial component
- Associated with flap displacement
- No "ghost meniscus" sign
- Donor site may resemble radial tear

Meniscal Degeneration

- Leads to increased signal on short TE sequence without extending to surface

- May resemble "ghost meniscus" but surface integrity preserved
- Usually asymptomatic
- Free edge fraying

Meniscal Ossicle

- Rare
- Usually intrameniscal
- Leads to diffuse intrameniscal increased signal on T1WI and PD
- Ossicle low signal on fat suppressed images

Post Operative

- Meniscal resection mimics "ghost meniscus" sign
- Appropriate history for differentiation
- Variable amounts resected to stable fibrocartilage
- Increased signal on short TE sequences

PATHOLOGY

General Features

- General path comments
  - ○ Degenerative at junction of anterior horn/body lateral meniscus
  - ○ Involvement medially and laterally in acute setting
  - ○ Common posterior horn of lateral meniscus (PHLM) at meniscotibial attachment with ACL tear mechanism
- Etiology
  - ○ Degenerative or acute (mostly a traumatic origin)
  - ○ Usually develops insidiously in the lateral meniscus
    - ■ Rotational forces across meniscus at "fulcrum" of movement - junction of anterior horn and body
    - ■ Between the anterior and posterior horns: Susceptible to tear in the flexed and rotated (loaded) knee
    - ■ Screw home mechanism results in torque of the meniscal fibrocartilage
  - ○ Acutely with a sudden impact
- Epidemiology
  - ○ Up to 15% incidence

MENISCAL RADIAL TEAR

- ○ Recognized with greater frequency at posterior horn of medial meniscus (PHMM) root attachment
  - Degenerative tear
- Associated abnormalities
  - ○ Disruption of "hoop containment" results in subluxation of the body of the meniscus peripherally
  - ○ Loss of hoop containment leads to altered forces through joint: +/- Stress response, stress fx
  - ○ Posterior horn lateral meniscus radial tears associated with ACL tears
  - ○ Deepened sulcus terminalis with ACL tear mechanism

Gross Pathologic & Surgical Features
- Disruption of meniscal surface with a radial component (perpendicular to the longitudinal axis)
- May include displaced flap component

Microscopic Features
- Mucinous ground substance within the fibrocartilaginous meniscus with a separating cleavage plane surrounded by regenerative chondrocytes
- Variable degrees of synovial ingrowth
- Neovascularity in more chronic cases

Staging, Grading or Classification Criteria
- Classification by surface configuration - tear patterns (tear of meniscal root attachment also classified as a radial tear)
  - ○ Vertical
    - Longitudinal tear (primary tear pattern is in vertical plane)
    - Flap tear (primary tear pattern is in vertical plane)
    - Radial tear
  - ○ Horizontal
    - Horizontal cleavage tear
    - Longitudinal tear (primary tear pattern is in horizontal plane)
    - Flap tear (primary tear pattern is in horizontal plane)
- Classification based on location - vascular zones
  - ○ White zone (white/white zone)
    - Medial third of meniscus (free edge)
    - Debridement
  - ○ Red-white junction (red/white zone)
    - Middle third between free edge and peripheral third
    - Debridement vs. repair
    - Repair if vascular pedicle can be established
  - ○ Red zone (red/red zone)
    - Peripheral third
    - Vascularized
    - Primary repair possible if tear confined to red/red zone or peripheral portion of red/white zone
- MRI classification
  - ○ Parrot-beak
    - Poor terminology - not widely used
    - Radial tear + curved inner component
    - May in fact represent a flap tear (radial + longitudinal component)
  - ○ Four MR patterns based on location of the tear and imaging plane
    - Ghost (root tear)

- Cleft - free edge radial tear pattern
- Truncated triangle - free edge radial tear
- Marching cleft - free edge radial tear in different locations on consecutive sagittal images (this pattern may actually represent a developing flap tear)

CLINICAL ISSUES

Presentation
- Most common signs/symptoms: Pain after single traumatic event or insidious onset of pain
- Clinical profile
  - ○ Joint line tenderness anterior to lateral collateral ligament (LCL)
  - ○ Feeling of "giving way"
  - ○ Clicking
  - ○ Locking if fragment displaced
  - ○ "Pseudolocking" if hamstring spasm is present

Demographics
- Age: Adult
- Gender: No predilection

Natural History & Prognosis
- Progresses to larger tear
- Asymptomatic if confined to the free edge & small in size
- Often propagates peripherally
- Extension of debrided meniscus can occur
  - ○ Especially in traumatic setting
- Clinical course depends on associated structures damaged in traumatic cases

Treatment
- Debridement; repair in young individuals

DIAGNOSTIC CHECKLIST

Consider
- Flap tear if not purely radial (radial + longitudinal)
- Classic radial tear involves anterior horn body junction without root involvement
- "Ghost meniscus" (root tear) if there is no history of surgery and posterior horn tissue is absent adjacent to the intercondylar notch

Image Interpretation Pearls
- Consider radial tear if "ghost meniscus" (absent meniscus) appearance of posterior horn medial meniscus root attachment site on sagittal images

SELECTED REFERENCES
1. Anderson MW: MR imaging of the meniscus. Radiol Clin North Am 40(5):1081-94, 2002
2. Stoller DW et al: Magnetic resonance imaging in orthopaedics and sports medicine. vol 1. 2nd ed. Philadelphia PA, J.B. Lippincott, 203-442, 1997
3. Jones RS et al: Direct measurement of hoop strains in the intact and torn human medial meniscus. Clin Biomech 11(5):295-300, 1996

IMAGE GALLERY

Typical

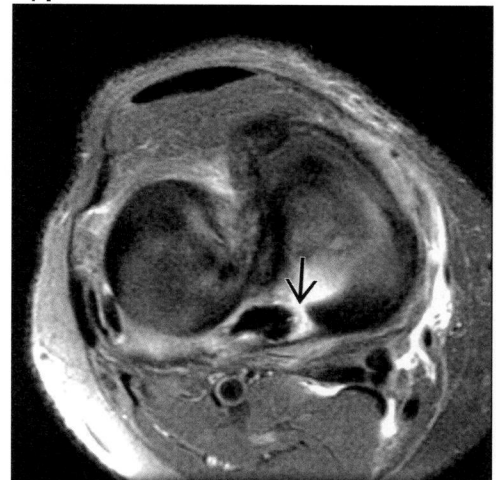 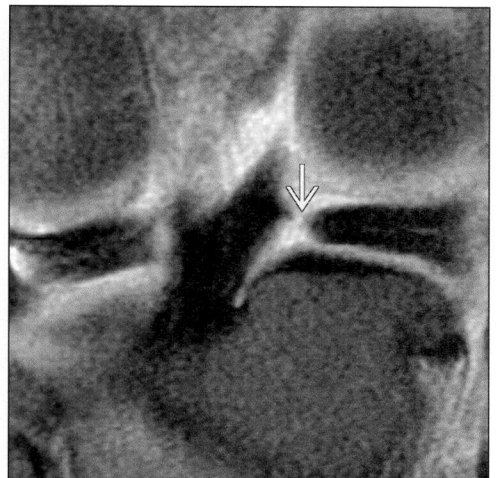

(Left) Axial FS PD FSE MR shows a radial tear of the posterior horn of the medial meniscus (arrow). The meniscus abruptly ends at the meniscotibial attachment. *(Right)* Coronal FS PD FSE MR shows the radial tear as increased signal through the meniscotibial attachment (arrow). This is associated with loss of "hoop containment" thereby leading to instability.

Typical

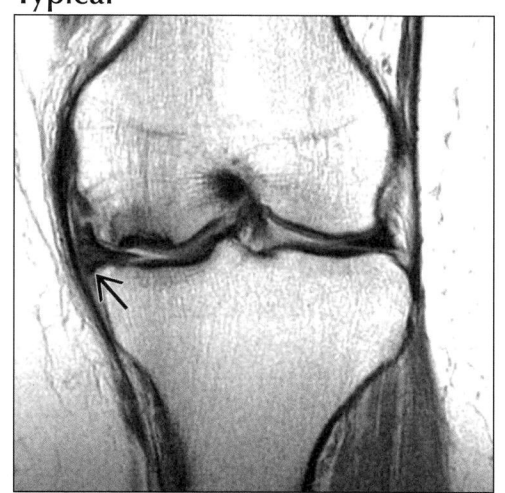 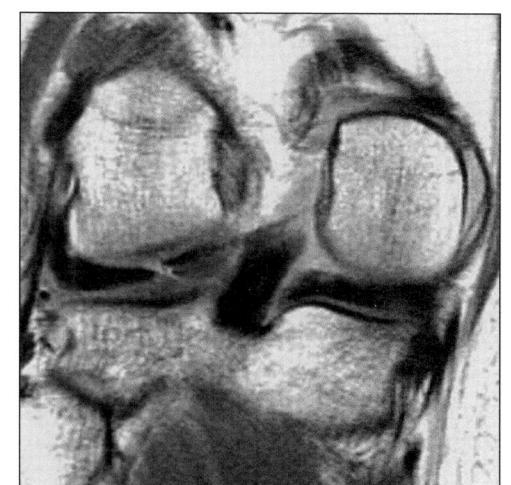

(Left) Coronal PD FSE MR shows subluxation (arrow) of body of meniscus as a result of meniscal instability and subchondral fracture. Instability leads to altered forces through joint and stress response, stress fractures, and/or osteoarthritis. *(Right)* Coronal PD FSE MR shows a obliquely oriented radial tear through posterior horn lateral meniscus associated with irregular tearing of the meniscotibial attachment. This type of tear is often associated with ACL tears.

5

25

Typical

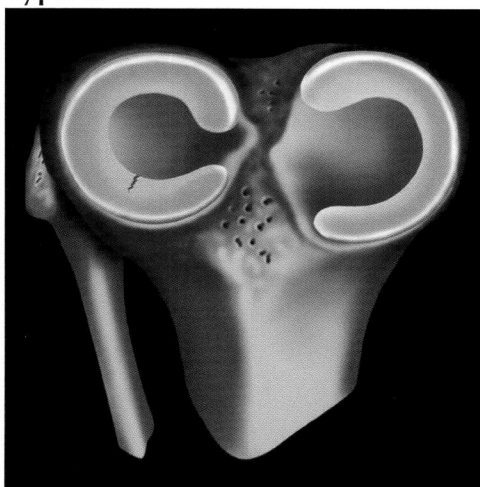 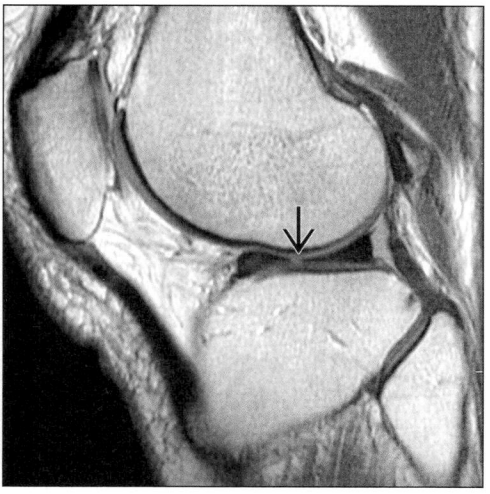

(Left) Axial oblique graphic shows a typical location for a degenerative radial tear at the junction of the anterior horn and body of the lateral meniscus which is the location of the fulcrum of movement of the meniscus with normal walking. *(Right)* Sagittal PD FSE MR shows a radial tear (arrow) at the junction of the anterior horn and body of the lateral meniscus as is depicted in the illustration.

MENISCAL FLAP TEAR

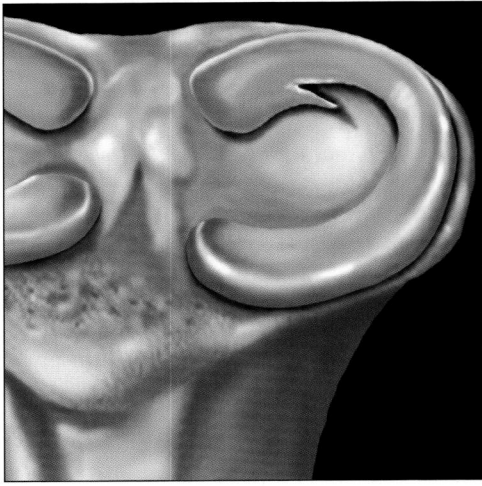

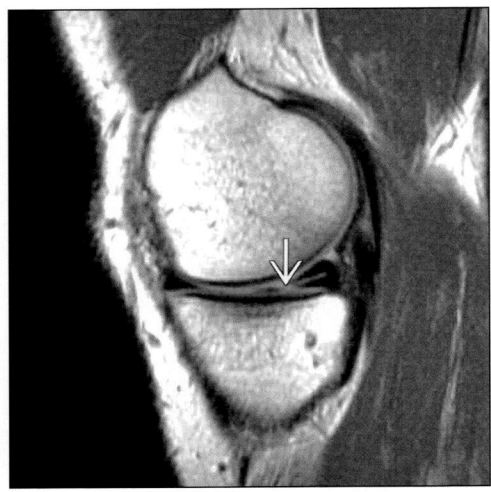

Axial oblique graphic shows a flap tear of the posterior horn of the medial meniscus.

Sagittal PD FSE MR shows displacement of a flap of the free edge (arrow) of the posterior horn of the medial meniscus in association with a large horizontal component.

TERMINOLOGY

Abbreviations and Synonyms
- Meniscus oblique tear, meniscus flap tear

Definitions
- Tear of the meniscus with both longitudinal and radial components forming a flap of meniscal tissue that may become displaced

IMAGING FINDINGS

General Features
- Best diagnostic clue
  - Obliquely oriented tear of the meniscus containing
    - Longitudinal (long axis of meniscus) component
    - Radial (perpendicular to long axis) component
- Location: Most commonly affects posterior horn and posterior aspect of body of medial meniscus
- Size: Varies from small (few mms) to large (cms)
- Morphology
  - Variable horizontal, radial components and connecting vertical/oblique components
  - Often begins as horizontal tear
    - Develops radial component resulting in flap at junction of horizontal tear and non-torn meniscus

Radiographic Findings
- Radiography
  - Subtle erosion due to chronic displaced flap
    - Involves tibia adjacent to coronary ligament insertion and meniscal body

CT Findings
- CT arthrography
  - Contrast extends into tear of meniscus body
    - +/- Displaced fragment surrounded by contrast
- Sagittal and coronal reconstructions helpful

MR Findings
- T1WI
  - Increased signal extending to the articular surface = tear
  - Horizontal tear + fragment
    - +/- Displacement
  - Fragment - decreased signal intensity of meniscal fragment with displacement peripherally
  - Increased signal of tear within donor meniscus +/- tearing of displaced fragment
- T2WI
  - +/- Fluid signal intensity in tear plane
    - Specific, not sensitive
  - Not sensitive for intrasubstance meniscal tear except when using T2* GRE sequence

---

DDx: Meniscal Flap Tear

Displaced Bucket	Loose Body	Chondral Shear	Meniscal Degen	Horizontal Tear

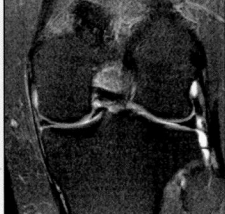
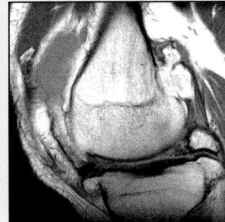
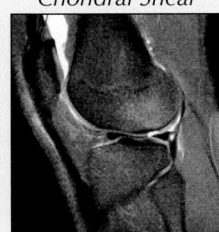
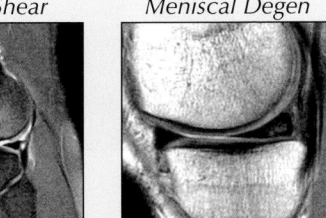
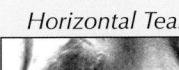
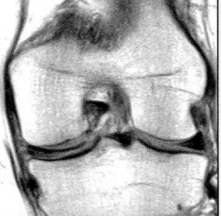

Cor FS PD FSE	Sag PD FSE MR	Sag FS PD FSE	Sag PD FSE MR	Cor PD FSE MR

MENISCAL FLAP TEAR

Key Facts

Terminology
- Meniscus oblique tear, meniscus flap tear

Imaging Findings
- Location: Most commonly affects posterior horn and posterior aspect of body of medial meniscus
- Variable horizontal, radial components and connecting vertical/oblique components
- Tear often horizontal on sagittal images originating along the inferior surface at the free edge

Top Differential Diagnoses
- Horizontal Cleavage Tear
- Bucket-Handle Tear with Displacement
- Chondral Lesions
- Loose Bodies
- Meniscal Degeneration (Meniscal Degen)

Pathology
- General path comments: Complex tear pattern
- Acutely with a sudden impact on the meniscus usually with a twisting component
- Insidiously as a result of chronic shear forces across the meniscus

Clinical Issues
- Most common signs/symptoms: Pain after single traumatic event or insidious onset of pain
- Joint line tenderness
- Feeling of "giving way"
- May progress to displaced flap

Diagnostic Checklist
- Use sagittal images to predict flap tear pattern

- If chronic, increased signal intensity hyperemia in adjacent tibia, femur = "reactive edema"
  - FS PD FSE shows hyperintense edema
- PD/Intermediate
  - Increased signal intensity extending to the articular surface is diagnostic of tear
    - Vertical peripheral tear giving rise to fragment and donor
  - Displaced fragment = decreased signal mass +/- displacement peripherally
    - Into coronary recess or between meniscofemoral ligament attachment and femur
  - Increased signal tear within donor meniscus body +/- tearing of displaced fragment
- T2* GRE
  - Increased signal, most often linear, extending to the articular surface = tear
  - +/- Displaced fragment
- MR arthrography
  - Contrast extending into tear
  - Arthrography typically not necessary
    - Useful in post operative setting
- Tear often horizontal on sagittal images originating along the inferior surface at the free edge
- Vertical tear also common involving inner third of meniscus on sagittal images
- Displaced fragment is decreased in signal intensity on all pulse sequences, located within
  - Recess formed by the coronary ligament
  - Meniscofemoral attachment
  - In case of displaced flap (sequestered fragment)

Imaging Recommendations
- Best imaging tool: MRI
- Protocol advice: Short TE MR images including T2* GRE (FS PD FSE for meniscal morphology)

DIFFERENTIAL DIAGNOSIS

Horizontal Cleavage Tear
- Lacks vertical component

- Degenerative tear extending from the free edge apex horizontally into the meniscus
- No displaced fragment

Bucket-Handle Tear with Displacement
- Originates from longitudinal vertical peripheral tear
- Inner fragment displaced
- Fragment displaced medially into notch (or towards notch)

Bone Trabecular Injuries
- Direct impact trauma vs. chronic repetitive microtrauma
- Diffuse increased signal intensity on T2WI
- FS PD FSE most sensitive
- Reactive and associated with meniscal tear

Chondral Lesions
- Hyaline chondral defect
- +/- Underlying bone marrow edema
- +/- Other findings of osteoarthritis (OA)
- Usually no displaced fragment in recesses

Loose Bodies
- May be displaced into recesses formed by meniscal attachments
- Often calcified
- +/- OA
- No donor meniscal site

Meniscal Degeneration (Meniscal Degen)
- Increased signal on short TE sequences without extension to surface
  - Short TE = T1, PD, T2* GRE
  - Globular or linear

PATHOLOGY

General Features
- General path comments: Complex tear pattern
- Etiology
  - Acutely with a sudden impact on the meniscus usually with a twisting component

MENISCAL FLAP TEAR

○ Insidiously as a result of chronic shear forces across the meniscus
• Epidemiology: Most common tear pattern

Gross Pathologic & Surgical Features
• Disruption of meniscal surface with variable longitudinal, radial and oblique (flap) components
• Displaced or coapted flap component

Microscopic Features
• Mucinous ground substance within fibrocartilaginous meniscus
• Separating cleavage plane surrounded by regenerative chondrocytes
• Variable synovial ingrowth
• Neovascularity in more chronic cases

Staging, Grading or Classification Criteria
• Classification by surface configuration - tear patterns (arthroscopic)
  ○ Vertical
    ▪ Longitudinal tear (primary tear pattern is in vertical plane)
    ▪ Radial tear
  ○ Flap tear (primary tear pattern is in vertical plane)
  ○ Horizontal
    ▪ Horizontal cleavage tear
    ▪ Longitudinal tear (primary tear pattern is in horizontal plane)
    ▪ Flap tear (primary tear pattern is in horizontal plane)
  ○ Flap tear also referred to as an oblique tear
• Classification based on location-vascular zones
  ○ White zone (white/white zone)
    ▪ Central third of meniscus (free edge)
    ▪ Debridement
  ○ Red-white junction (red/white zone)
    ▪ Middle third between free edge and peripheral third
    ▪ Debridement vs. repair
    ▪ Repair if vascular pedicle can be established
  ○ Red zone (red/red zone)
    ▪ Peripheral one third
    ▪ Vascularized
    ▪ Primary repair usually possible if tear confined to red/red zone or peripheral portion of red/white zone
• MRI classification of meniscal signal intensity
  ○ Grade 1: Globular increased signal intensity on short TE sequences within meniscus not extending to an articular surface
  ○ Grade 2: Linear increased signal intensity on short TE sequences not extending to an articular surface
  ○ Grade 3: Increased signal intensity on short TE sequences extending to an articular surface
  ○ Grade 1 and 2 are often referred to as meniscal degeneration, either globular or linear
  ○ Grade 3 signal represents a meniscal tear
• Criteria for prospective diagnosis (based on sagittal MR images) of flap tear morphology
  ○ Vertical tear inner one third of meniscus (coapted vs. noncoapted)
  ○ Blunted free edge of meniscus with displaced meniscal tissue inferior to periphery of meniscus
  ○ Relative deficiency of inner one third of inferior leaf with associated blunting
  ○ Changing slope of superior surface of meniscus as evaluated on a sagittal image

CLINICAL ISSUES

Presentation
• Most common signs/symptoms: Pain after single traumatic event or insidious onset of pain
• Clinical profile
  ○ Joint line tenderness
  ○ Feeling of "giving way"
  ○ Clicking
  ○ Locking with displaced fragment
  ○ "Pseudolocking" if hamstring spasm is present

Demographics
• Age: Adult (peak age: 31-40 years for men and 11-20 years for women)
• Gender: No predilection

Natural History & Prognosis
• May progress to displaced flap

Treatment
• Meniscal repair, debridement/partial meniscectomy
  ○ Partial meniscectomy for short flap tears
  ○ Repair for long tears to prevent loss of meniscal function

DIAGNOSTIC CHECKLIST

Consider
• Differentiate from horizontal cleavage tear
• Flap tear = oblique tear pattern

Image Interpretation Pearls
• Identify displaced flap especially within the coronary recess
• Use sagittal images to predict flap tear pattern

SELECTED REFERENCES

1. Boyd KT et al: Meniscus preservation: Rationale, repair techniques and results. 10(1):1-11, 2003
2. Jee WH et al: Meniscal tear configurations: Categorization with MR imaging. AJR 180(1):93-7, 2003
3. Greis PE et al: Meniscal injury: Management. J Am Acad Orthop Surg 10(3):177-87, 2002
4. Anderson MW: MR imaging of the meniscus. Radiol Clin North Am 40(5):1081-94, 2002
5. Matava MJ et al: Magnetic resonance imaging as a tool to predict meniscal reparability. Am J Sports Med. 27(4):436-43, 1999
6. Stoller DW et al: Magnetic resonance imaging in orthopaedics and sports medicine. vol 1. 2nd ed. Philadelphia PA, J.B. Lippincott, 203-442, 1997
7. Shino K et al: Arthroscopic repair for a flap tear of the posterior horn of the lateral meniscus adjacent to its tibial insertion. Arthroscopy 11(4):495-8, 1995
8. Belzer JP et al: Meniscus Tears: Treatment in the stable and unstable knee. J Am Acad Orthop Surg 1(1):41-7, 1993

MENISCAL FLAP TEAR

IMAGE GALLERY

Typical

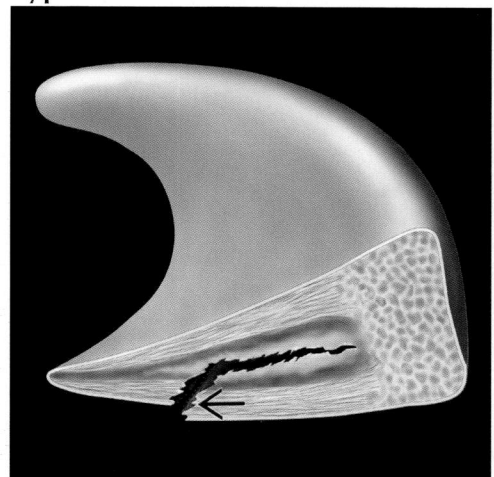

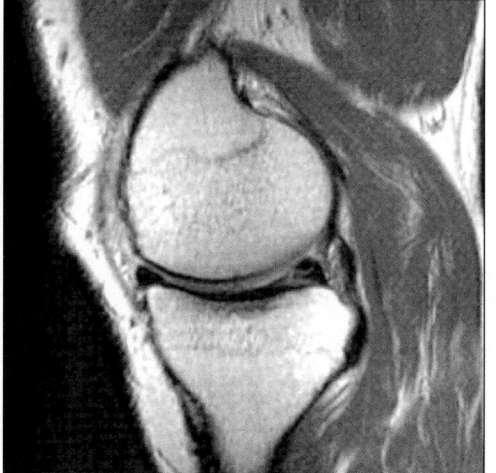

(Left) Sagittal graphic shows both a vertical and horizontal components to a flap tear. Note the blunting of the free edge of the inferior leaf (arrow). *(Right)* Sagittal PD FSE MR shows a slightly displaced flap tear of the medial meniscus with characteristic vertical signal intensity involving the inner third of the meniscal fibrocartilage.

Typical

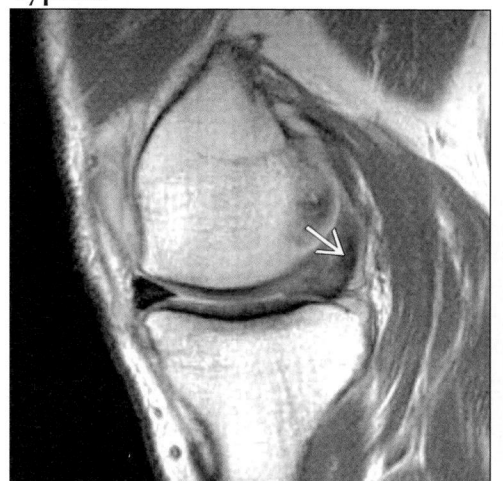

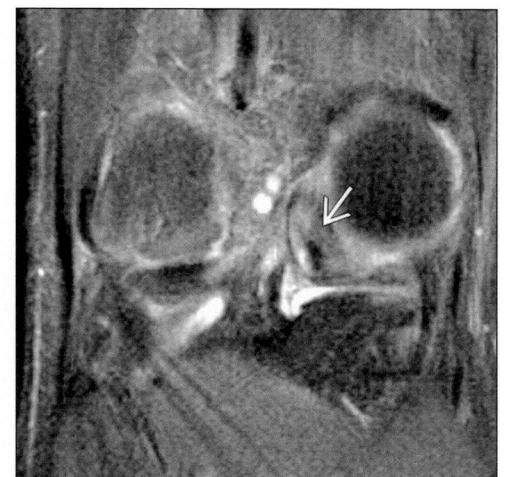

(Left) Sagittal PD FSE MR shows a large displaced meniscal flap (arrow) into a posterior superior recess adjacent to the posterior horn of the medial meniscus. *(Right)* Coronal FS PD FSE MR shows the large flap tear (arrow) extending into the notch of the knee.

Typical

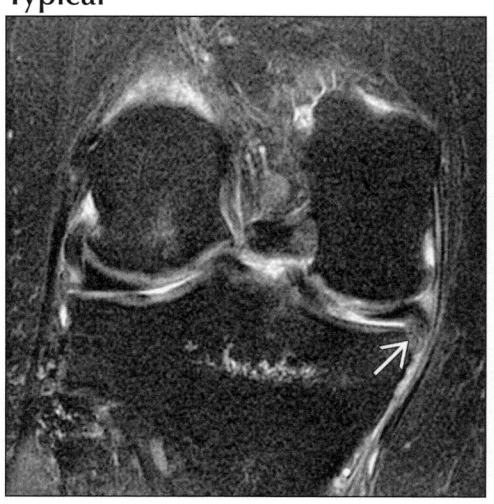

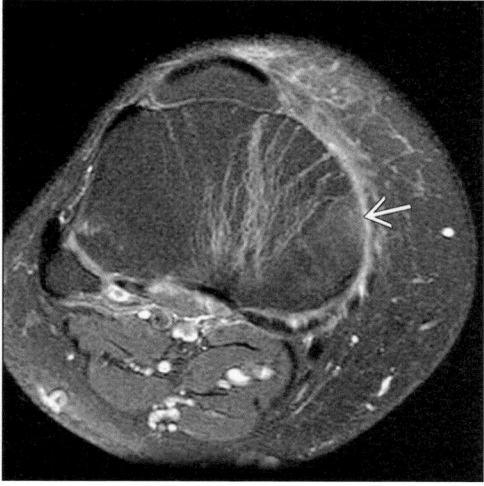

(Left) Coronal FS PD FSE MR shows a displaced flap (arrow) of inferior leaf into the recess formed by coronary ligament adjacent to body of medial meniscus with adjacent reactive hyperemia in the medial and proximal tibia. *(Right)* Axial FS PD FSE MR shows reactive hyperemia of medial tibia (arrow) as well as hyperemic vessel recruitment of the proximal medial tibia. Edema is likely a stress related response secondary to meniscal instability and load transference.

MENISCAL BUCKET-HANDLE TEAR

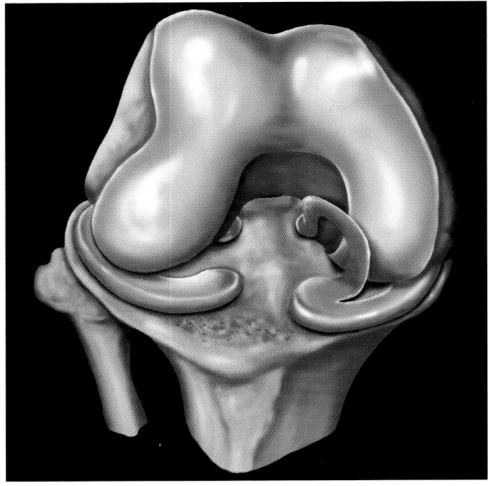

Axial oblique graphic shows a displaced bucket-handle tear of the medial meniscus.

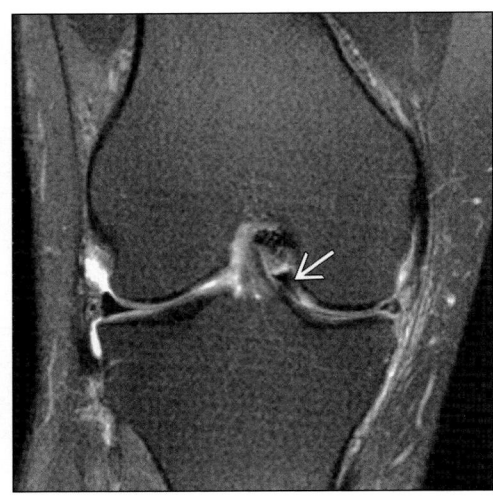

Coronal FS PD FSE MR shows a displaced bucket-handle fragment (arrow) of the medial meniscus into the intercondylar notch of the knee. The remnant of the body of the meniscus is small.

TERMINOLOGY

Abbreviations and Synonyms
- Bucket-handle tear (BHT)

Definitions
- Vertical peripheral tear with displaced mesial portion to the notch of knee

IMAGING FINDINGS

General Features
- Best diagnostic clue
  - Coronal images show small meniscus body and meniscal fragments at the notch resulting in 2 meniscal fragments
  - Double posterior cruciate ligament (PCL) sign on sagittal images
- Location: Medial > lateral meniscus
- Size: 2-5 mm displaced fragment (most common)
- Morphology
  - Displaced meniscus fragment resembles the handle of a bucket
    - Donor meniscus (residual body), remains in place - bucket
  - Displaced fragment partially displaced or displaced to the notch of knee
  - Displaced fragment attached to donor meniscus at both ends
    - Free at one end = displaced flap

CT Findings
- NECT
  - Displaced bucket-handle fragment - low density mass with variable displacement towards or into notch
  - Coronal and sagittal reconstructions helpful
- CT arthrography
  - Contrast extends into tear within donor meniscus body +/- tearing of displaced fragment

MR Findings
- T1WI
  - Increased signal on short TE sequences extending to the articular surface = tear
    - Vertical longitudinal tear giving rise to fragment and donor
  - Displaced bucket-handle fragment - decreased signal mass with variable displacement towards or into notch
  - Increased signal tear within donor meniscus body +/- tearing of displaced fragment
- T2WI
  - Not as sensitive for intrasubstance meniscal signal or tear unless T2* GRE sequence is used
  - Sensitive for morphology of meniscal fragments

DDx: Meniscal Bucket-Handle Tear

Chronic Torn ACL	Obl Intramen Lig	Obl Intramen Lig	Obl Intramen Lig	Flap Men Tear
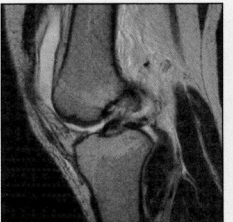	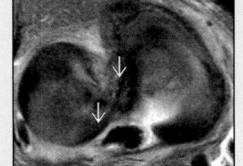	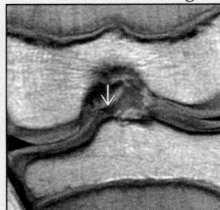	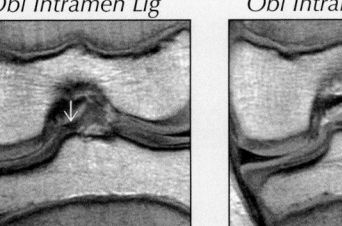	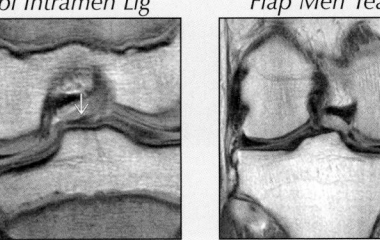
Sag T2 FSE MR	Ax FS PD FSE MR	Cor PD FSE MR	Cor PD FSE MR	Cor PD FSE MR

MENISCAL BUCKET-HANDLE TEAR

Key Facts

Terminology
- Vertical peripheral tear with displaced mesial portion to the notch of knee

Imaging Findings
- Coronal images show small meniscus body and meniscal fragments at the notch resulting in 2 meniscal fragments
- Location: Medial > lateral meniscus
- "Double PCL sign": Displaced fragment beneath the PCL at the notch of knee resembling two PCL ligaments
- "Double delta sign": Flipped inner meniscal fragment adjacent to anterior horn of the donor meniscus producing two triangle shaped structures adjacent to each other anteriorly

Top Differential Diagnoses
- Oblique Intermeniscal Ligament

Pathology
- General path comments: Typically an acute meniscal tear
- Displaced inner fragment of a vertical longitudinal tear of the meniscus

Clinical Issues
- Pain/locking after single traumatic event
- Locking, typically a block preventing full extension

Diagnostic Checklist
- Evaluate coronal and sagittal images for extra fragment within the intercondylar notch

---

- 3rd structure in notch (besides ACL & PCL)
  - Chronic, increased signal intensity hyperemia in adjacent tibia, femur = "reactive edema"
- PD/Intermediate
  - +/- Displaced bucket-handle fragment - hypointense meniscal fragment
  - Increased signal tear within donor meniscus body
    - +/- Tearing of displaced fragment
  - +/- Displaced anterior horn: Anterior to the bucket-handle fragment
- T2* GRE
  - 3D T2* GRE axial images provide direct visualization of bucket-handle tear pattern
  - Displaced bucket-handle fragment - best visualized on coronal and sagittal images
  - +/- Donor meniscus body tear
  - +/- Tearing of displaced fragment
- MR arthrography
  - Displaced bucket-handle fragment - surrounded by contrast
  - Contrast extends into tear within donor meniscus body +/- tearing of displaced fragment
- "Double PCL sign": Displaced fragment beneath the PCL at the notch of knee resembling two PCL ligaments
- "Double delta sign": Flipped inner meniscal fragment adjacent to anterior horn of the donor meniscus producing two triangle shaped structures adjacent to each other anteriorly
- Coronal and sagittal images demonstrate blunting of the meniscus donor with the remaining meniscus smaller than normal
- Axial images show fragment as deceased signal intensity linear/fusiform mass on all pulse sequences

Imaging Recommendations
- Best imaging tool: MRI
- Protocol advice
  - Sagittal and coronal images (T2* GRE, PD & FS PD FSE)
  - Axial FS PD FSE or 3D T2* GRE to show circumferential morphology of the bucket-handle tear

DIFFERENTIAL DIAGNOSIS

Oblique Intermeniscal Ligament
- Normal ligament extending between the menisci mimicking a displaced fragment
  - Anterior horn of the lateral meniscus to the posterior horn of the medial meniscus
  - Anterior horn of the medial meniscus to the posterior horn of the lateral meniscus
  - Both present rarely
  - Beneath synovium at arthroscopy
- The menisci are normal in size without a recognizable donor site

Scarred Chronic Disruption of the Anterior Cruciate Ligament (ACL)
- Normally two structures in the notch (ACL and PCL)
  - Bucket-handle = 3rd structure in notch
- History of trauma
- Associated typical bone injuries
- +/- Meniscal tear (non bucket handle)
- Torn ACL one of two structures in notch when bucket-handle tear not present

Meniscal Flap Tear
- A potential cause of locking of the knee joint
- Vertical peripheral tear, complex tear with horizontal, radial, +/- longitudinal components
- Anterior extension of the displaced flap is not seen

PATHOLOGY

General Features
- General path comments: Typically an acute meniscal tear
- Etiology: Acutely with sudden impact splitting the meniscus longitudinally
- Epidemiology: Relatively uncommon meniscal tear

Gross Pathologic & Surgical Features
- Displaced inner fragment of a vertical longitudinal tear of the meniscus

MENISCAL BUCKET-HANDLE TEAR

- Disruption of meniscal surface typically with a long longitudinal component involving the entire meniscus

Microscopic Features
- Mucinous ground substance within the fibrocartilaginous meniscus with a separating cleavage plane surrounded by regenerative chondrocytes
- Variable degrees of synovial ingrowth
- Neovascularity in more chronic cases

Staging, Grading or Classification Criteria
- Classification by surface morphology - tear patterns (bucket-handle = displaced longitudinal tear)
  ○ Vertical
    ▪ Longitudinal tear (primary tear pattern is in vertical plane)
    ▪ Flap tear (primary tear pattern is in vertical plane)
    ▪ Radial tear
  ○ Horizontal
    ▪ Horizontal cleavage tear
    ▪ Longitudinal tear (primary tear pattern is in horizontal plane)
    ▪ Flap tear (primary tear pattern is in horizontal plane)
- Classification of bucket-handle tears
  ○ Vertical longitudinal tears
    ▪ Single vertical longitudinal tears
    ▪ Displaced bucket-handle tears
    ▪ Broken bucket-handle tears
  ○ Horizontal (or cross section) longitudinal (circumferential) tears
    ▪ Also produces a nondisplaced or displaced bucket-handle tear
    ▪ Residual horizontal tear component seen in posterior horn
- Classification based on location-vascular zones
  ○ White zone (white/white zone)
    ▪ Free edge one third
    ▪ Debridement
  ○ Red-white junction (red/white zone)
    ▪ Middle third between free edge and peripheral third
    ▪ Debridement vs. repair
    ▪ Repair especially if vascular pedicle can be established
  ○ Red zone (red/red zone)
    ▪ Peripheral third
    ▪ Vascularized
    ▪ Primary repair usually possible if tear confined to red/red zone or peripheral portion of red/white zone

CLINICAL ISSUES

Presentation
- Most common signs/symptoms
  ○ Pain/locking after single traumatic event
  ○ Difficulty in ambulation secondary to extension block
    ▪ If displaced to central weightbearing surface or notch
- Clinical profile
  ○ Joint line tenderness

○ Feeling of "giving way"
○ Clicking
○ Locking, typically a block preventing full extension
  ▪ Results in difficulty in ambulation

Demographics
- Age: Usually younger patient, physically active
- Gender: M > F

Natural History & Prognosis
- Displacement leads to locked knee
  ○ Surgery necessary
  ○ Extension block

Treatment
- Repair if nondisplaced and affects the peripheral vascularized zone "red zone"
  ○ MR arthrography sometimes requested to check status of repaired meniscus
- Excision of fragment if tear extends through nonvascularized free edge or if fragment is separated from parent meniscus

DIAGNOSTIC CHECKLIST

Consider
- Oblique intermeniscal ligament
- Torn and chronically scarred ACL

Image Interpretation Pearls
- Evaluate coronal and sagittal images for extra fragment within the intercondylar notch

SELECTED REFERENCES

1. Elliott JM et al: MR appearances of the locked knee. Br J Radiol 73(874):1120-6, 2000
2. Sanders TG et al: Oblique meniscomeniscal ligament: Another potential pitfall for a meniscal tear--anatomic description and appearance at MR imaging in three cases. Radiology 213(1):213-6, 1999
3. Helms CA et al: The absent bow tie sign in bucket-handle tears of the menisci in the knee. AJR 170(1):57-61, 1998
4. Belzer JP et al: Meniscus tears: Treatment in the stable and unstable knee. J Am Acad Orthop Surg 1(1):41-7, 1993
5. Singson RD et al: MR imaging of displaced bucket-handle tear of the medial meniscus. Am J Roentgenol 156(1):121-4, 1991
6. Dandy DJ: The arthroscopic anatomy of symptomatic meniscal lesions. J Bone Joint Surg Br 72(4):628-33, 1990
7. Stoller DW et al: Meniscal tears: Pathologic correlation with MR imaging. Radiology 163(3):731-5, 1987
8. Northmore-Ball MD et al: Arthroscopic, open partial, and total meniscectomy. A comparative study. J Bone Joint Surg Br 65(4):400-4, 1983
9. Sprague NF III: The bucket handle meniscal tear. A technique using two incisions. Orthop Clin North Am 13(2):337-48, 1982

MENISCAL BUCKET-HANDLE TEAR

Variant

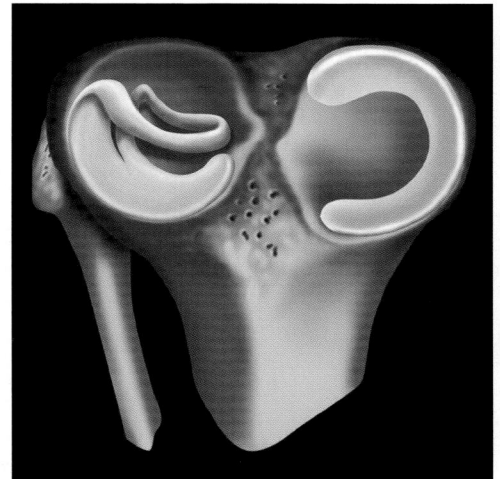
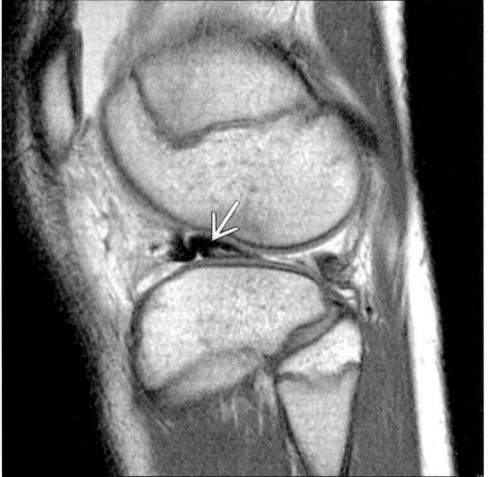

(Left) Axial oblique graphic shows a longitudinal tear of the lateral meniscus with a flipped anterior horn into the central portion of the lateral compartment. *(Right)* Sagittal PD FSE MR shows a "double delta" sign referring to a displaced posterior horn (arrow) compressing the free edge of the more anteriorly located anterior horn.

Typical

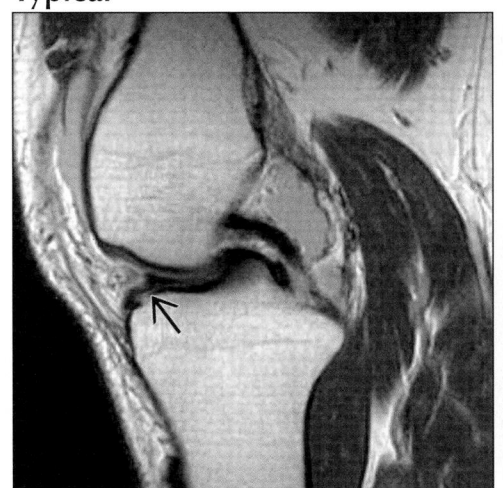
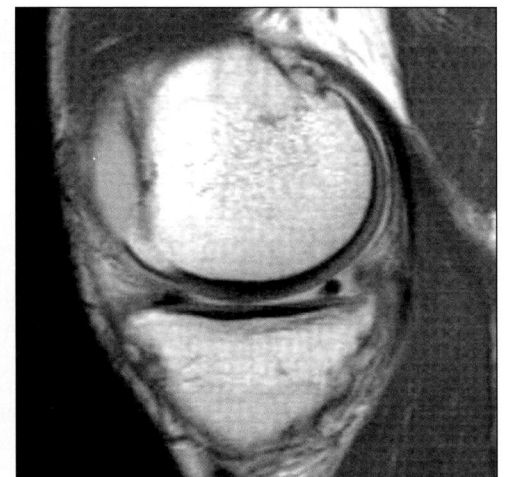

(Left) Sagittal PD FSE MR shows a bucket-handle fragment at the notch of knee producing a "double PCL" and a "double delta" (arrow) at the anterior aspect of the notch of knee indicating a displaced fragment. *(Right)* Sagittal PD FSE MR shows a small medial meniscus remnant indicating loss of meniscal tissue.

Typical

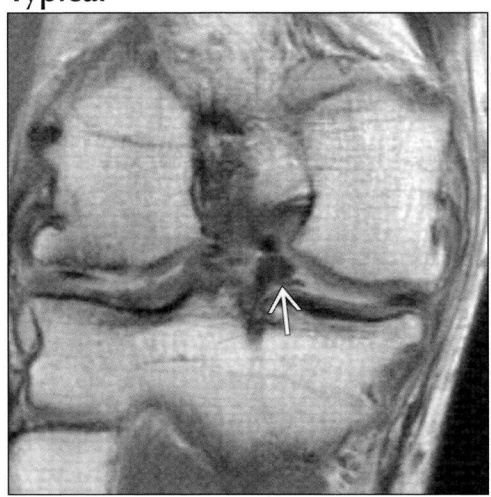
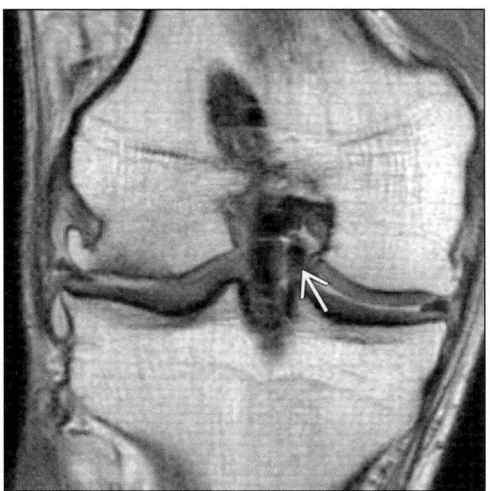

(Left) Coronal PD FSE MR shows a displaced medial meniscus bucket-handle fragment (arrow) at the notch of the knee producing an additional structure within the notch of the knee besides the ACL (graft) and PCL. *(Right)* Coronal PD FSE MR shows the 2 normal structures of the notch, the ACL and PCL, as well as a bucket-handle fragment (arrow).

MENISCOCAPSULAR SEPARATION

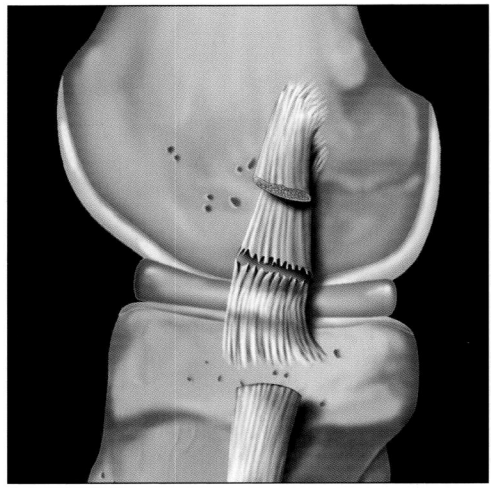

Sagittal graphic shows a tear of the meniscofemoral portion of the deep capsular attachment of the meniscus.

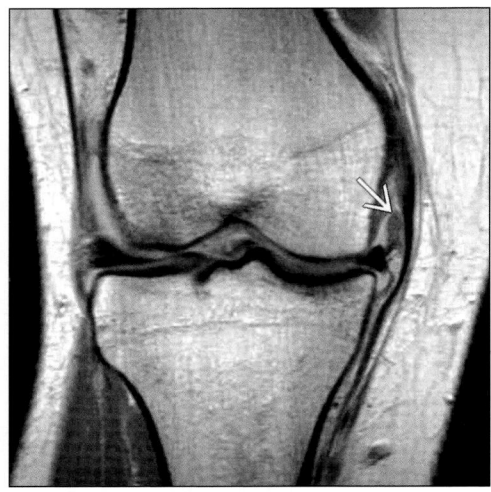

Coronal PD FSE MR shows a tear of the meniscofemoral attachment (arrow) from the femoral origin. There is medial meniscal subluxation.

TERMINOLOGY

Abbreviations and Synonyms
- Capsular sprain, fascicle tear, meniscocapsular separation (MCS)

Definitions
- Tear of the supporting meniscotibial (coronary) or meniscofemoral ligaments typically at attachment to meniscus

IMAGING FINDINGS

General Features
- Best diagnostic clue: Disruption of capsular attachment of meniscus, in trauma, with irregularity, and increased signal intensity within meniscofemoral or coronary ligament on T2WI
- Location: Most commonly adjacent to posterior horn/posterior aspect of body of medial meniscus
- Size: Varies from a few mms to more extensive tearing > 1 cm in size
- Morphology: Loss of normal linear ligamentous attachment

Radiographic Findings
- Radiography: +/- Associated fracture

CT Findings
- CT arthrography
  - Extravasation of contrast through defect

MR Findings
- T1WI
  - +/- Associated meniscal tear
    - Increased signal extending from meniscal substance to articular surface
  - Capsule thickened - decreased signal intensity
  - Associated fracture - decreased in signal intensity
    - +/- Surrounding hypointense edema
- T2WI
  - Irregularity + increased signal intensity within meniscofemoral or coronary ligament especially on T2WI
  - Hyperintense fluid interposed between peripheral portion of posterior horn of medial meniscus and joint capsule
    - Coronal & sagittal T2WI (FS PD FSE)
    - +/- Surrounding hyperintense edema
    - FS PD FSE more sensitive than PD FSE or T2* GRE
  - Osseous fx or contusion - increased in signal intensity
  - Medial collateral ligament (MCL) tear + meniscocapsular separation are associated injuries
- T2* GRE

DDx: Meniscocapsular Separation

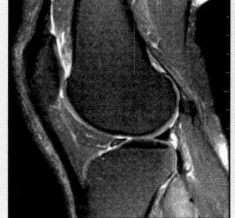 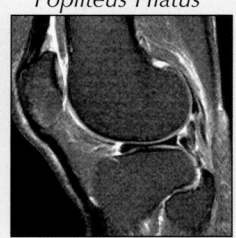 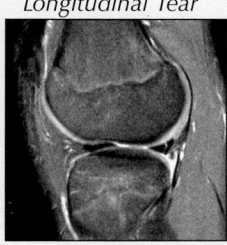 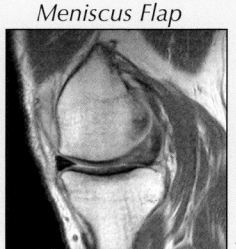

Popliteus Hiatus	Popliteus Hiatus	Longitudinal Tear	Meniscus Flap
Sag FS PD FSE	Sag FS PD FSE	Sag FS PD FSE	Sag PD FSE MR

MENISCOCAPSULAR SEPARATION

Key Facts

Terminology
- Tear of the supporting meniscotibial (coronary) or meniscofemoral ligaments typically at attachment to meniscus

Imaging Findings
- Best diagnostic clue: Disruption of capsular attachment of meniscus, in trauma, with irregularity, and increased signal intensity within meniscofemoral or coronary ligament on T2WI
- Meniscofemoral ligament tear frequently seen with medial collateral ligament disruption
- +/- Meniscal corner tear

Top Differential Diagnoses
- Popliteus Hiatus

- Fluid Distending the Normal Meniscal Attachment Recesses
- MCL Bursitis

Clinical Issues
- Tenderness and pain at site of the tear
- Less than 1 cm tear owing to a propensity to heal secondary to rich vascularity of peripheral aspect of meniscus
- Large tears are repaired

Diagnostic Checklist
- Bone injury of adjacent tibia is "signpost" often indicating injury to the meniscal attachments
- Always correlate meniscocapsular signal between sagittal and coronal images to increase diagnostic specificity

---

- o Increased signal intensity edema interposed between peripheral portion of posterior horn of medial meniscus and joint capsule (T2* GRE improves visualization of intrameniscal signal)
  - ▪ Coronal & sagittal images
  - o +/- Linear hyperintensity meniscal tear
    - ▪ Increased signal extending from meniscal substance to articular surface
- MR arthrography
  - o Interposition of contrast between the meniscus and the MCL
- Loss of the normal decreased signal intensity linear appearance of meniscal attachments (T1 & T2WI)
- Displacement of the posterior horn of the medial meniscus by ≥ 5 mm
  - o Measurement of this distance has been found to be unreliable
- Uncovering of the articular cartilage of the tibia
  - o Nonspecific
- Meniscofemoral ligament tear frequently seen with medial collateral ligament disruption
- A free floating meniscus or flipped meniscus, indicates a meniscocapsular disruption
- Adjacent bone injury (contusion) is common
  - o Edema visualized on fast spin echo images with fat saturation
- +/- Meniscal corner tear

Imaging Recommendations
- Best imaging tool: MR
- Protocol advice
  - o PD FSE or FS PD FSE
  - o Radial imaging to define meniscocapsular attachments

DIFFERENTIAL DIAGNOSIS

Popliteus Hiatus
- Normal hiatus laterally and posteriorly where the popliteus tendon pierces the capsule
- Posterolateral location
- Without history of trauma not likely to be tear

- Fascicles at this location can be torn in setting of trauma adjacent to the normal hiatus
  - o Discontinuity of fascicles
  - o Loss of the normal decreased signal intensity (all pulse sequences) linear ligamentous attachment
  - o Hemorrhage and surrounding edema
- A vertical longitudinal tear is frequently located parallel to the popliteus hiatus

Fluid Distending the Normal Meniscal Attachment Recesses
- Visualized laterally
- Rarely adjacent to the medial meniscus
  - o Large or chronic effusion

MCL Bursitis
- Fluid between deep and superficial components of MCL
- +/- Meniscal tear
- Post traumatic
  - o +/- Hemorrhage
- Increased signal on T2WI

Meniscal Tear and Cyst
- Meniscal tear usually visualized
- Extends between deep and superficial MCL
- Round or flattened cystic appearing mass
  - o Increased signal intensity on T2WI

MCL Superficial Tear, Joint Effusion
- Difficult to distinguish
- Valgus injury
- Hyperintense on T2WI

PATHOLOGY

General Features
- General path comments
  - o MCS originates as a tear of capsular attachment usually involving the posterior horn of the medial meniscus
  - o Multiple tears can occur and size varies
  - o Trauma

MENISCOCAPSULAR SEPARATION

- ▪ Twisting injury or impaction
- ○ Associated with an anterior cruciate ligament (ACL) and/or MCL tears
- ○ Associated with small "corner fracture tear" of the adjacent meniscus
- ○ The lateral capsule is more loosely attached to the lateral meniscus than is the medial attachments
  - ▪ The lateral attachments may balloon out when filled with fluid
  - ▪ + Effusion
  - ▪ Should not be misinterpreted as a tear
- • Etiology
  - ○ Injury/trauma: Twisting injury to knee
  - ○ MCL and deep medial capsular layer injured with valgus torque to the knee
  - ○ Direct blow to lateral knee with the foot planted
  - ○ Noncontact injuries
    - ▪ ACL injury mechanism
- • Epidemiology: Less common than superficial MCL tears

Gross Pathologic & Surgical Features

- • Disruption of the meniscotibial attachment, meniscofemoral attachment or both
- • Variable amounts of hemorrhage and swelling
- • Associated ACL tear usually present with tears of the meniscotibial, meniscofemoral ligament or intrasubstance tear of the meniscus

Microscopic Features

- • Disruption of collagenous, ligamentous structure(s)
- • Variable surrounding hemorrhage, edema and inflammatory cells

Staging, Grading or Classification Criteria

- • Tear less than 1 cm is often left alone because of propensity to heal due to rich vascularity of meniscal rim at the site of sprain
- • Tear greater than 1 cm may be surgically addressed (repaired) if discovered at arthroscopy

CLINICAL ISSUES

Presentation

- • Most common signs/symptoms
  - ○ Tenderness and pain at site of the tear
    - ▪ Nonspecific and may represent pain from other damaged structures
- • Clinical profile: Usually seen post trauma in young, active patients, especially athletes

Demographics

- • Age: Younger, physically active patient
- • Gender: M > F

Natural History & Prognosis

- • May heal especially if less than 1 cm in size
- • If large may lead to unstable meniscus
- • Excellent if the tear/separation is small
- • Meniscal instability if large and unrecognized

Treatment

- • Conservative

- ○ Less than 1 cm tear owing to a propensity to heal secondary to rich vascularity of peripheral aspect of meniscus
  - ▪ Fibrinogenic and other healing agents due to increased vascularity in this location (perimeniscal capillary plexus)
- • Surgical
  - ○ Large tears are repaired
- • Complications: Failure to diagnose or inadequate repair may lead to meniscal instability
  - ○ Subluxation
  - ○ Displacement
  - ○ Flipped meniscus

DIAGNOSTIC CHECKLIST

Consider

- • In the setting of trauma
- • Pseudolesions
  - ○ Popliteus hiatus
  - ○ Fluid distending the normal meniscal attachment recesses

Image Interpretation Pearls

- • Bone injury of adjacent tibia is "signpost" often indicating injury to the meniscal attachments
- • Meniscocapsular separation may be overestimated because knee is imaged in excessive external rotation
- • Always correlate meniscocapsular signal between sagittal and coronal images to increase diagnostic specificity

SELECTED REFERENCES

1. De Maeseneer M et al: Normal and abnormal medial meniscocapsular structures: MR imaging and sonography in cadavers. Am J Roentgenol 171(4):969-76, 1998
2. Stoller DW et al: Magnetic resonance imaging in orthopaedics and sports medicine. vol 1. 2nd ed. Philadelphia PA, J.B. Lippincott, 203-442, 1997
3. Applegate GR et al: MR diagnosis of recurrent tears in the knee: Value of intraarticular contrast material. Am J Roentgenol 161(4):821-5, 1993
4. Kimura M et al: Anatomy and pathophysiology of the popliteal tendon area in the lateral meniscus: Clinical investigation. Arthroscopy 8(4):424-7, 1992
5. Stoller DW et al: Meniscal tears: Pathologic correlation with MR imaging. Radiology 163(3):731-5, 1987
6. El-Khoury GY et al: Meniscotibial (coronary) ligament tears. Skeletal Radiol 11(3):191-6, 1984
7. Woods GW et al: Repairable posterior menisco-capsular disruption in anterior cruciate ligament injuries. Am J Sports Med 12(5):381-5, 1984

MENISCOCAPSULAR SEPARATION

IMAGE GALLERY

Typical

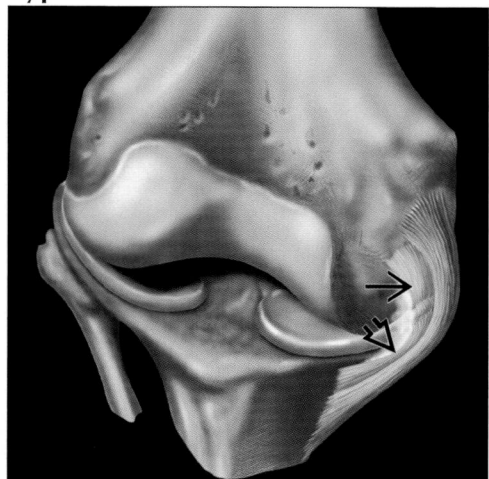

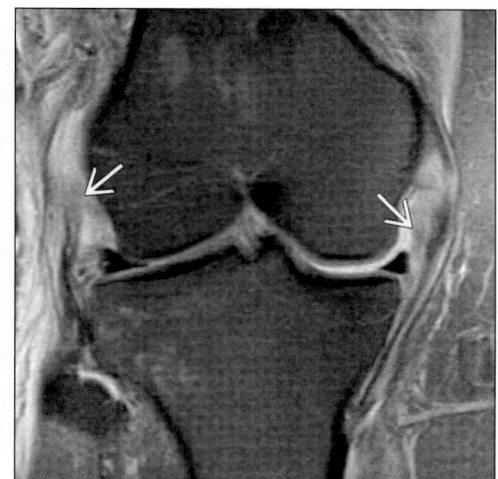

(Left) Coronal oblique graphic shows edema within the coronary (open arrow) and meniscofemoral (arrow) attachments of the medial meniscus associated with a grade I MCL sprain. *(Right)* Coronal FS PD FSE MR shows disruption of the lateral and medial meniscofemoral attachments (arrows) associated with lateral and medial collateral ligament injuries.

Typical

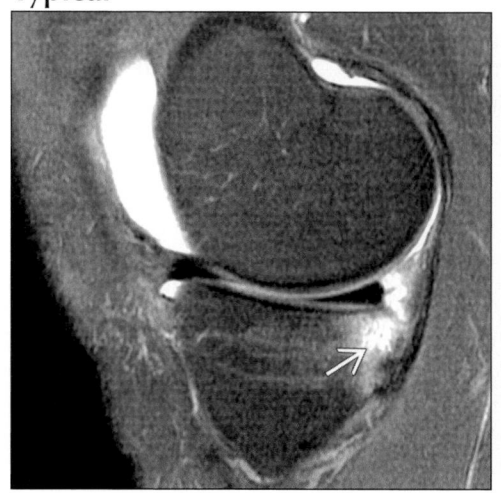

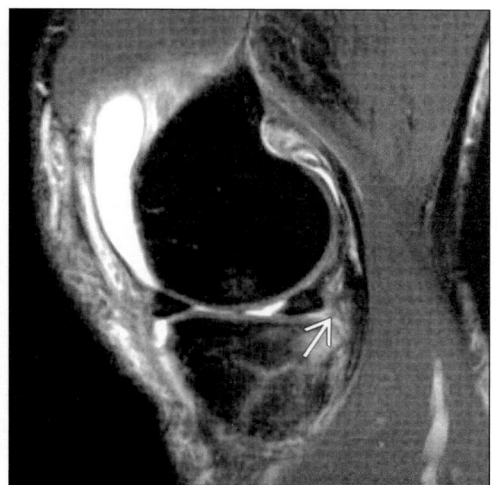

(Left) Sagittal FS PD FSE MR with a sprain of the coronary ligament attachment to the posterior horn of the medial meniscus. Trabecular injury of the posterior corner of the medial tibia is also noted (arrow) and commonly seen with ACL tears. *(Right)* Sagittal FS PD FSE MR shows a sprain of the coronary ligament (arrow) adjacent to a posteromedial tibial corner injury. There is a meniscal tear and small trabecular contusion of the femur associated.

Typical

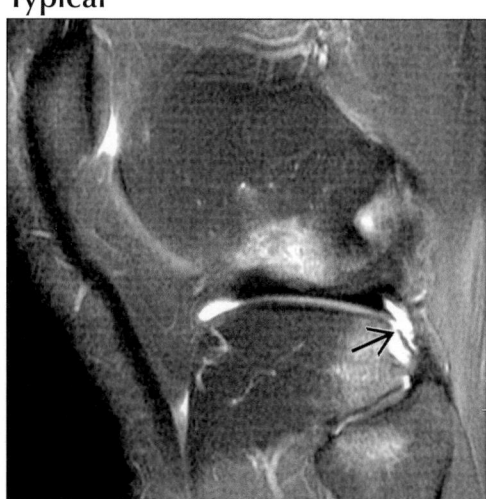

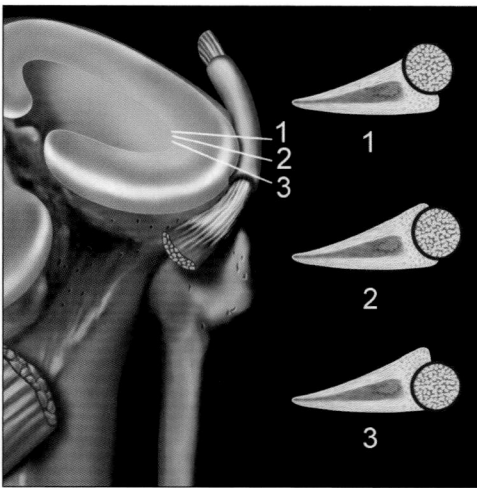

(Left) Sagittal FS PD FSE MR shows tear of coronary ligament (arrow) adjacent to attachment on the posterior horn of lateral meniscus. *(Right)* Sagittal graphic shows normal popliteus hiatus. Tendon pierces superior capsule lat. (#1) then travels through popliteus tendon sheath (#2) in communication with joint. Tendon pierces infer. meniscal attachment (coronary lig.) med. (#3).

POST-OPERATIVE MENISCUS CHANGE

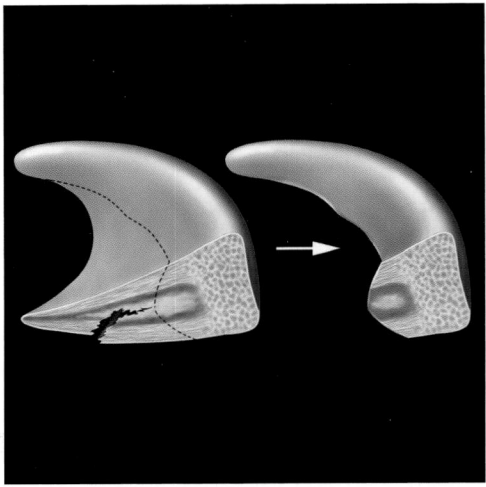

Sagittal graphic shows a meniscal tear trimmed back to intact meniscus. Note small amount of residual degeneration in post operative meniscus which may lead to increased signal.

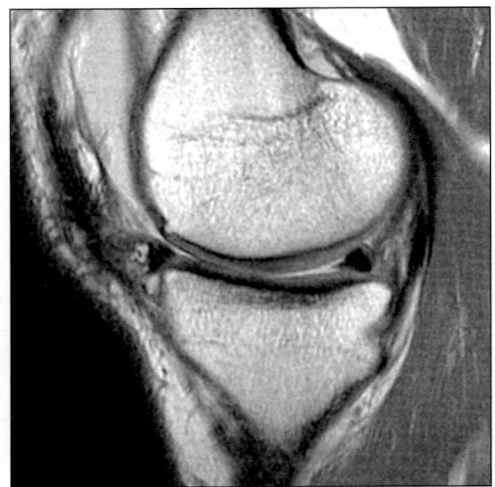

Sagittal PD FSE MR shows changes from a partial meniscectomy of the posterior horn medial meniscus with no residual degeneration.

TERMINOLOGY

Abbreviations and Synonyms
- Post op meniscus, post debridement meniscus
- Status post (S/p) surgery, post arthroscopy, S/p arthroscopy, S/p Sx (surgery), post meniscectomy, S/p meniscectomy

Definitions
- Meniscus that has been either repaired (primary repair) or partial/total meniscectomy has been performed

IMAGING FINDINGS

General Features
- Best diagnostic clue: Blunted appearance of meniscus, +/- micrometallic artifact
- Location: Medial, lateral meniscus, any location
- Size
  - Size of repair/resection area varies depending upon the amount of surgery performed
    - Depends on size of the original tear or amount debrided or resected
- Morphology
  - After primary repair the meniscus shape is preserved +/- surrounding metal artifact
  - After partial or complete (usually near complete) meniscectomy the meniscus is blunted
  - Regenerating meniscus is usually dark but smaller than normal meniscus

MR Findings
- T1WI
  - Small meniscus +/- blunting = partial meniscectomy/debridement
  - Free edge irregularity = fraying
  - Linear increased signal +/- surface extension residual tear vs. recurrent tear
    - +/- Arthrography to distinguish
    - Discrete linear signal on short TE sequence
    - Pre-existing meniscal signal changes mistaken for remnant tears
- T2WI
  - Fluid signal intensity extending into the meniscus on T2WI
    - 90% specific, 40-70% sensitive for retear
  - Grade 3 signal intensity in primary meniscal repair represents fibrovascular healing response without retear
- PD/Intermediate
  - Small meniscus +/- linear increased signal extending to surface
  - ~ 70% sensitive for retearing
  - +/- Susceptibility artifact in cases of meniscal repair of red zone tears

DDx: Post-Operative Meniscus Change

Radial Tear	Bucket Remnant	Bucket Tear	Frayed Remnant	OA Deg Men
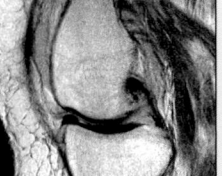	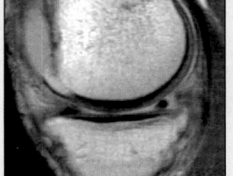	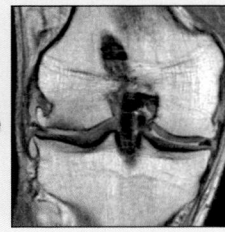	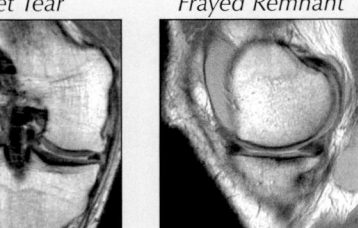	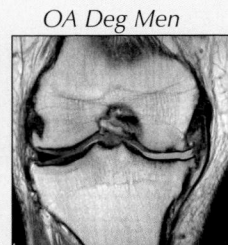
Sag PD FSE MR	Sag PD FSE MR	Cor PD FSE MR	Sag PD FSE	Cor PD FSE

POST-OPERATIVE MENISCUS CHANGE

Key Facts

Terminology
- Meniscus that has been either repaired (primary repair) or partial/total meniscectomy has been performed

Imaging Findings
- Best diagnostic clue: Blunted appearance of meniscus, +/- micrometallic artifact
- Fluid signal intensity extending into the meniscus on T2WI
- New area of high signal

Top Differential Diagnoses
- Displaced Flap Tear of Meniscus
- Chondrocyte "Healing" of the Tear or Area of Degeneration

Pathology
- Meniscal retear originates as a small split of meniscus at site of the old tear or in a new location
- Meniscal tear may undergo healing by fibrosis if the tear involves the vascularized "red zone"
- Healing tear may be blunted or irregular and still be intact

Clinical Issues
- Most common signs/symptoms: Post operative pain
- Arthritis
- Loose body – causes grinding, locking, pain

Diagnostic Checklist
- Recurrent symptoms after meniscal surgery
- Consider MR arthrography in post-op setting

- Usually longitudinal tears
  - ○ Residual grade 3 signal without imbibed fluid may exist in meniscal remnant
  - ○ Evaluate collagen meniscus implants (CMI) and meniscal transplants
- T2* GRE: Susceptibility may obscure recurrent tear in case of meniscal repair
- MR arthrography
  - ○ Dilute gadolinium into meniscus at site of retear or new tear in previously normal area of the meniscus
  - ○ Dilute gadolinium - increased signal intensity on T1 and proton density weighted images
  - ○ 88-95% sensitivity
- New area of high signal
  - ○ Previous study to directly compare
- Displaced meniscal fragment (decreased signal intensity structure) on all pulse sequences
- Regenerating meniscus (at the vascularized rim – "red zone")
  - ○ Fibrous in composition
  - ○ Generally decreased or intermediate in signal intensity on all pulse sequences
- Primary meniscal repairs +/ - diffuse or linear high signal (residual degeneration), on short TE sequence
- Short TE sequences ~ 70% sensitive in the setting of discrete signal abnormality
- MRI 66% accuracy overall in the post operative meniscus setting without arthrography

Imaging Recommendations
- Best imaging tool: In the setting of prior partial or complete meniscectomy, MRI arthrography or FS PD FSE recommended
- Protocol advice
  - ○ Most accurately diagnosed on short TE MR images
    - T1, PD, FS PD FSE or GRE sequences

DIFFERENTIAL DIAGNOSIS

Displaced Flap Tear of Meniscus
- Blunted appearance of the meniscal free edge

- With or without surgical changes elsewhere in the knee

Chondrocyte "Healing" of the Tear or Area of Degeneration
- Leading to recurrent or persistent intermediate signal at the former tear site (T1& T2WI)
- MR arthrography to identify free influx of contrast

Bucket-Handle Tear in Post Operative Setting Where a Meniscal Repair was not Performed
- Leaves a small meniscal remnant mimicking a partial meniscectomy
- Radial tear
- Partial remnant visualized as a foreshortened meniscus

Osteoarthritis (OA)
- +/- New degeneration, osteophytes

PATHOLOGY

General Features
- General path comments
  - ○ Meniscal retear originates as a small split of meniscus at site of the old tear or in a new location
  - ○ Simple/or complex pattern retear
  - ○ Meniscal tear may undergo healing by fibrosis if the tear involves the vascularized "red zone"
    - Peripheral one third
  - ○ Tear may heal with increased regenerative chondrocyte activity
    - Decreased signal intensity relative to original tear
- Etiology: Post operative state
- Epidemiology
  - ○ Meniscal tears - 50% of knee injuries that require surgery
  - ○ Healing rate 90% for lesions in 3 mm peripheral location
  - ○ Healing rate 50-60% for treated lesions 5 mm or greater from periphery

POST-OPERATIVE MENISCUS CHANGE

Gross Pathologic & Surgical Features
- Meniscal retear - disruption of meniscal substance
- Healing tear may be blunted or irregular and still be intact

Microscopic Features
- Meniscal retear
- Mucinous ground substance within the fibrocartilaginous meniscus
- With a separating cleavage plane surrounded by regenerative chondrocytes and fibrosis
- Peripheral synovial ingrowth
- Regenerating meniscus (at the vascularized rim – red zone)
  - Composed of fibrous tissue
  - Typically smaller than adjacent meniscus

Staging, Grading or Classification Criteria
- Meniscal shape and post operative arthritis (Smith and colleagues)
  - Group I menisci – near normal length, no osteoarthritis
  - Group II menisci – significantly shortened menisci, no osteoarthritis
  - Group III menisci – any length but with superimposed osteoarthritis

CLINICAL ISSUES

Presentation
- Most common signs/symptoms: Post operative pain
- Clinical profile: Patients of any age who have had meniscal surgery
- Retear of meniscus
  - Tenderness at joint line adjacent to apex of the tear
    - Due to the greatest tension being exerted on the surrounding nerve fibers
  - Joint line tenderness and often positive clinical meniscal testing
    - Positive McMurray's test, Steinmann's test and Apley's test
- Displaced meniscal fragment - locking if the inner fragment becomes displaced
- Arthritis
  - Grinding, pain locking
  - Patients with preexisting arthritic change may have a greater propensity to progression of arthritis after meniscectomy than individuals without preexisting disease
- Loose body - causes grinding, locking, pain
- Malalignment
  - Preexisting or the result of meniscectomy

Demographics
- Age: No predilection
- Gender: No predilection

Natural History & Prognosis
- Patients status post meniscal surgery may show resolution of symptoms or recurrent symptoms
  - Abnormal intermediate to hyperintense signal may persist up to 27 months postoperatively
- Causes of recurrent symptoms include

- Meniscal retear
- Development or progression of arthritis
- Malalignment develops
- Osteonecrosis (possible stress or insufficiency fracture)
- Arthrofibrosis (adhesions)
- Fragment from retear may displace transiently giving a locked knee presentation (posterior spring sign)
- Meniscectomy outcome generally favorable but these results may deteriorate over time
- Variations in outcome attributed to a poor prognosis
  - Amount of meniscus resected; greater amount resected
  - Degree of preexisting arthritic change
    - Greater the degree of preexisting arthritis
  - Limb alignment
    - Greater the degree of preexisting malalignment
  - Location of meniscal tear
    - Lateral meniscus surgery (increased incidence of lateral compartment arthrosis)
  - Ligamentous instability
    - Greater the degree of preexisting ligamentous instability
  - Age: Increased age at time of operation

Treatment
- Conservative
  - If retear is isolated to the peripheral one third ("red zone"), small in size (uncommon)
- Surgical
  - Reoperation of those tears that are amenable to meniscal resection/debridement back to stable meniscus
- Complications following surgery
  - 13% incidence
  - Osteonecrosis
    - Esp. in older patients, post meniscal surgery
    - May represent insufficiency fractures of weightbearing surface in osteoporotic especially immobile patients
  - Arthrofibrosis (adhesions)
  - Deep venous thrombosis

DIAGNOSTIC CHECKLIST

Consider
- Recurrent symptoms after meniscal surgery

Image Interpretation Pearls
- Consider MR arthrography in post-op setting
- FS PD FSE demonstrates post operative meniscal morphology

SELECTED REFERENCES

1. Rangger C et al: Osteoarthritis after arthroscopic partial meniscectomy. Am J Sports Med 23:240, 1995
2. Applegate GR et al: MR diagnosis of recurrent tears in the knee. Value of intraarticular contrast material. AJR 161(4):821-5, 1993
3. Ihn JC et al: In vitro study of contact area and pressure distribution in the human knee after partial and total meniscectomy. Int Orthop 17(4):214-8, 1993

POST-OPERATIVE MENISCUS CHANGE

IMAGE GALLERY

Variant

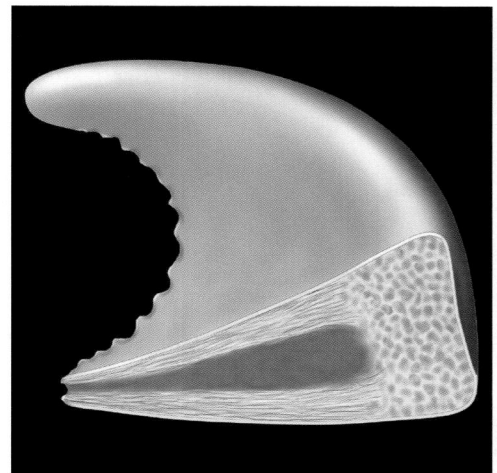 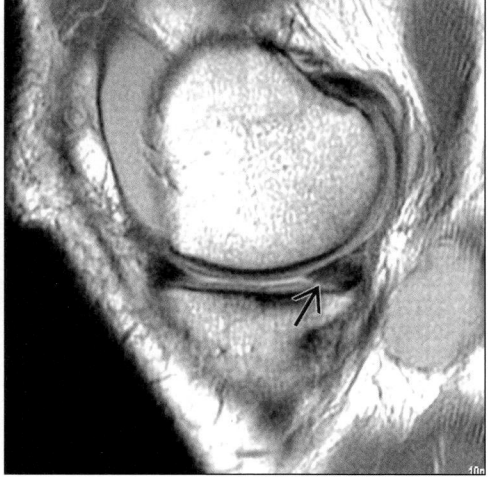

(Left) Sagittal graphic shows an irregular free edge of the meniscus after debridement. This will mimic free edge fraying at MRI evaluation. *(Right)* Sagittal PD FSE MR shows degeneration of the meniscus remnant with fraying (arrow) of the free edge and inferior surface.

Typical

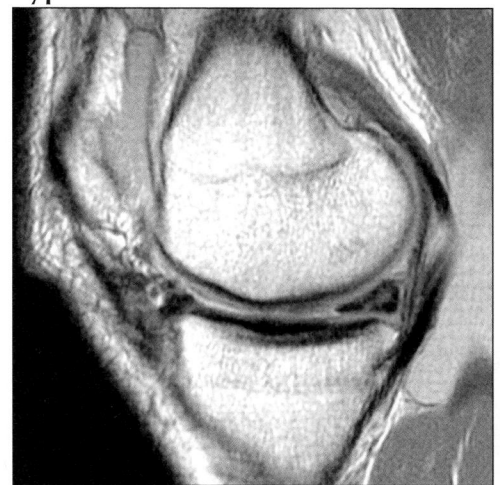 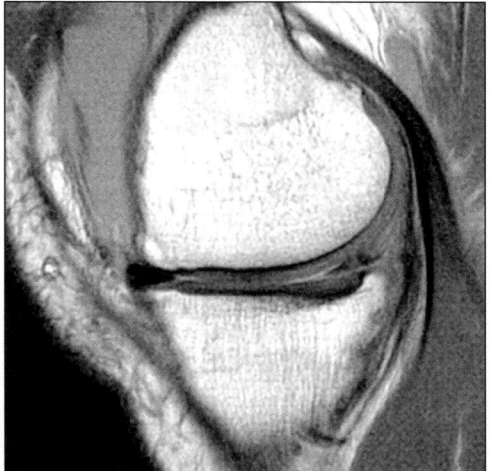

(Left) Sagittal PD FSE MR shows linear increased signal intensity within posterior horn meniscal remnant. This appearance is associated with a 70% sensitivity for retear at second look arthroscopy. *(Right)* Sagittal PD FSE MR shows a healing cleft within the posterior horn of the medial meniscus remnant. There was no retear at arthroscopy and in this case MR arthrography would be of benefit to exclude a retear.

Typical

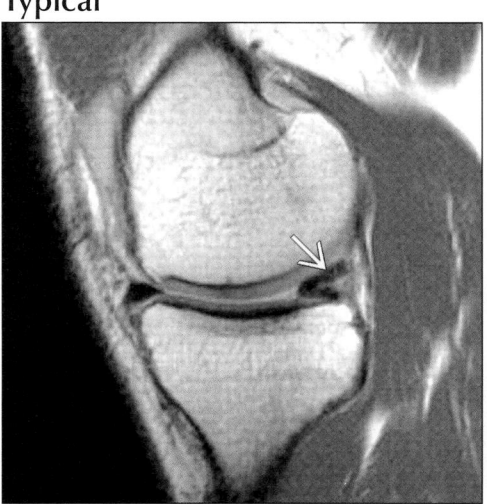 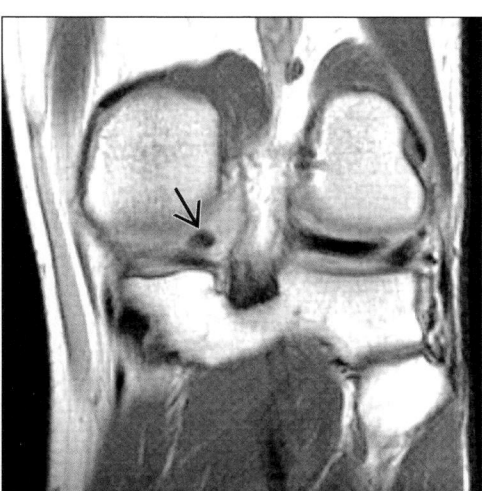

(Left) Sagittal PD FSE MR shows a failed repair of the posterior horn of the medial meniscus with a displaced fragment (arrow) flipped superior to the posterior horn. *(Right)* Coronal PD FSE MR shows the displaced meniscal fragment (arrow) from a failed repair adjacent to the posterior horn at the meniscotibial attachment.

ANTERIOR CRUCIATE LIGAMENT (ACL) TEAR

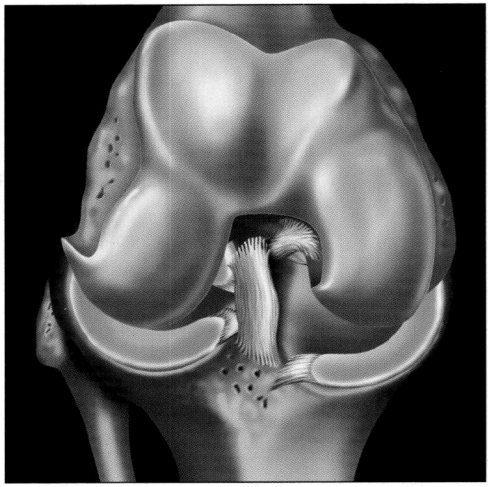

Coronal graphic shows a grade III tear of the proximal aspect of the anterior cruciate ligament.

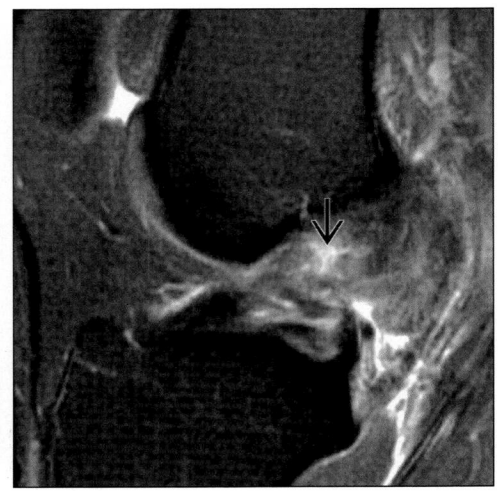

Sagittal FS PD FSE MR shows a grade III tear (arrow) of the anterior cruciate ligament resulting in a "blowout" appearance. This is often seen in contact sports and downhill snow skiing.

TERMINOLOGY

Abbreviations and Synonyms
- ACL tear, ACL rupture

Definitions
- Disruption of ACL

IMAGING FINDINGS

General Features
- Best diagnostic clue: Disruption of normal continuous low signal intensity ACL with irregularity and increased signal on T2WI
- Location: ACL in the intercondylar notch of knee
- Size: Tear may be small discrete or complete "blowout"
- Morphology
  - Disruption of linear ligament appearance
  - Torn ligament no longer parallel to Blumensaat's line (intercondylar notch roof angle)

Radiographic Findings
- Radiography
  - Deepening of the lateral femoral condylar notch "lateral notch sign" of the condylopatellar sulcus terminalis
    - Depression > 1.5 mm in depth at sulcus terminalis
  - Segond fracture (associated with ACL tear)

- Avulsion of meniscotibial portion of the middle third of lateral capsular ligament from the lateral tibial plateau

CT Findings
- NECT
  - Associated fractures
    - Posterolateral and posteromedial tibia
    - Sulcus terminalis of lateral femoral condyle
- CT arthrography
  - Chondral defects seen as contrast collection/ulceration of articular surface

MR Findings
- T1WI
  - Intermediate signal intensity of disrupted pattern of ACL fascicles
  - Bone injuries appear as hypointense edematous contusions
    - +/- Fracture (nondisplaced)
- T2WI
  - Increased signal intensity with disorganized and thickened fibers + discontinuity
  - Increased signal intensity with or without fracture lines or subchondral contusions involving
    - The posterolateral corner of tibia
    - Lateral femoral condyle
    - +/- Posteromedial tibial plateau

Tear leg mucosa

DDx: Anterior Cruciate Ligament (ACL) Tear

Partial PL Bundle	PL Bundle Tear	Mucoid Degen	Radial Tear Lt Mn	B-H Meniscal Tear
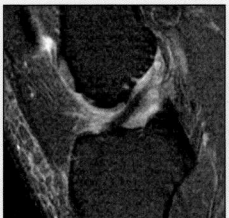	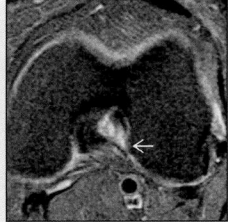	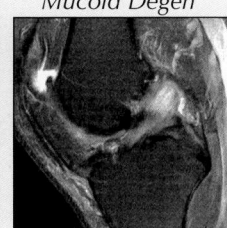	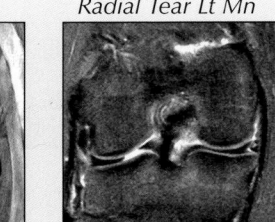	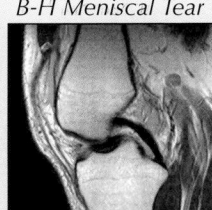
Sag FS PD FSE	Sag FS PD FSE	Sag FS PD FSE	Cor FS PD FSE	Sag PD FSE MR

ANTERIOR CRUCIATE LIGAMENT (ACL) TEAR

Key Facts

Terminology
- Disruption of ACL

Imaging Findings
- Best diagnostic clue: Disruption of normal continuous low signal intensity ACL with irregularity and increased signal on T2WI
- Size: Tear may be small discrete or complete "blowout"
- Segond fracture (associated with ACL tear)
- Avulsion fracture of anterior tibial spine (especially in children)

Top Differential Diagnoses
- Partial Tear
- Bucket-Handle Meniscal Tear
- Mucoid Degeneration of ACL (Mucoid Degen)

Pathology
- Tears are most commonly caused by forward translation of the tibia, external rotation of the femur with respect to the tibia, valgus stress and axial loading

Clinical Issues
- Anterior drawer sign (forward translation of tibia)
- Lachman's test (drawer test performed with 15 to 30 degrees knee flexion)
- ACL reconstruction in active patients

Diagnostic Checklist
- Coronal images can increase sensitivity and specificity for the detection of partial (grade I and II) ACL tears

---

- Axial images - thickening and increased signal intensity adjacent to the lateral intercondylar notch wall
  - Normal ligament - flat, decreased in signal intensity adjacent to lateral wall of intercondylar notch
- Coronal images show increased signal intensity replacing normal hypointense ligament
- Increased signal intensity hemorrhagic effusion common
- FS PD FSE sensitive for hyperintense edema associated with ACL tear
- T2* GRE
  - Associated fractures as increased signal line
    - Not sensitive for bone edema
- Disruption of normal linear low signal intensity ligament within the notch of knee on all sequences
- Avulsion fracture of anterior tibial spine (especially in children)
- Buckling of posterior cruciate ligament (PCL) on sagittal images due to anterior translation of tibia
- Difficult to identify ACL fiber morphology secondary to increased sensitivity to ligamentous edema on T2* GRE or STIR

Imaging Recommendations
- Best imaging tool: MRI
- Protocol advice
  - Sagittal axial and coronal FS PD FSE and T1/PD FSE for detection of tear
  - Coronal images very sensitive to partial ACL tears on T1 or PD FSE images (intermediate signal within normally hypointense ligament)

DIFFERENTIAL DIAGNOSIS

Partial Tear
- May be difficult to diagnose on MRI
  - Grade I vs. grade II partial tears
- Thickening, disruption or abnormal orientation of some fibers

- Anteromedial bundle (AM) disruption more common than posterolateral (PL) bundle disruption

Bucket-Handle Meniscal Tear
- Bucket-handle fragment mimics chronically torn, fibrotic ACL
- Horizontally oriented fragment seen as "extra structure" in the notch in addition to ACL and PCL
- Difficult to identify on clinical exam in setting of an ACL tear

Mucoid Degeneration of ACL (Mucoid Degen)
- Expands ligament
- Increased signal within ligament on T2WI (FS PD FSE)
- "Celery stalk" appearance of fluid + ACL fascicles

Radial Tear Lateral Meniscus (Radial Tear Lt Mn)
- Associated with ACL tear
- Posterolateral pain

PATHOLOGY

General Features
- General path comments
  - Most commonly disrupted ligament in the knee
  - Partial tear may affect posterolateral bundle or anteromedial bundle
    - Bundles not histologically distinct
    - Posterolateral bundle tightened in extension, larger and bulkier than anteromedial bundle
    - Anteromedial band = primary restraint against anterior translation of tibia on the femur when anterior drawer test performed in usual manner (the knee flexed)
- Etiology
  - Three common mechanisms of injury (force that stresses the ligament and exceeds its capacity to maintain integrity)

ANTERIOR CRUCIATE LIGAMENT (ACL) TEAR

○ Tears are most commonly caused by forward translation of the tibia, external rotation of the femur with respect to the tibia, valgus stress and axial loading
  ▪ Associated with posterolateral corner injury and lateral femoral condylar injury
  ▪ Seen with foot plant and external rotation of the thigh
○ Varus stress (associated with Segond fracture)
○ Hyperextension (uncommon)
• Epidemiology
  ○ Common injury especially in sports where foot plant is a risk
    ▪ Football, soccer, rugby, snow skiing and tennis
  ○ Incidence in general population is 1 in 3000
• Associated abnormalities
  ○ Bone trabecular injuries or impaction fractures of the posterolateral tibia and weight-bearing surface of lateral femoral condyle (sulcus)
  ○ Meniscal tears (lateral greater than medial)
  ○ Posterolateral corner injuries
    ▪ Lateral collateral ligament
    ▪ Arcuate ligament
    ▪ Popliteus tendon
    ▪ Posterolateral capsule
    ▪ Popliteofibular ligament

Gross Pathologic & Surgical Features
• Disruption of ligament within its midsubstance, origin, or at its attachment associated with hemorrhage and synovitis
• Avulsion of anterior tibial spine seen in younger patients
• Empty lateral wall sign (absent attachment to lateral femoral condyle)
• Fallen ACL (loss of normal tension & tear)
• ± Stenotic notch

Microscopic Features
• Disruption of normal collagen bundles accompanied by hemorrhage of fibrosis, and inflammatory infiltration
• Normal ACL cells resemble fibrocartilage
• Femoral and tibial attachment sites consist of four morphologic zones from flexible tissue to rigid bone (for dissipation of shearing forces)
  ○ Zone 1 - ligament proper
  ○ Zone 2 - fibrocartilage
  ○ Zone 3 - tidemark and mineralized fibrocartilage
  ○ Zone 4 - bone
• ACL matrix - primarily type I collagen

Staging, Grading or Classification Criteria
• Grade I: Intraligamentous injury
• Grade II: Intraligamentous injury + increase in ligament length
• Grade III: Complete ligament disruption

CLINICAL ISSUES

Presentation
• Most common signs/symptoms
  ○ Physical examination findings

▪ Joint effusion in the acute case
▪ Anterior drawer sign (forward translation of tibia)
▪ Lachman's test (drawer test performed with 15 to 30 degrees knee flexion)
▪ Pivot shift test - applied valgus force during flexion and extension to accentuate subluxation or reduction of the tibia
▪ KT-1000 arthrometry for partial tears vs. complete tears
• Clinical profile
  ○ Athletically active individuals
  ○ Common injury in sports activities characterized by rapid stopping, starting and pivoting
    ▪ Snow skiing, soccer, football, basketball, tennis

Demographics
• Age: Younger active patients
• Gender
  ○ F > M
  ○ Increased rate of ACL injuries in women collegiate athletes
  ○ Risk factor 4-8 times greater in women (basketball/soccer)

Natural History & Prognosis
• Partial tears (difficult to assess)
  ○ Less than 25% fiber disruption associated with more favorable prognosis
  ○ > 50% leads to insufficiency
  ○ Excellent results in 80 to 90% of ACL reconstructions

Treatment
• Conservative treatment may be effective
  ○ Osteoarthritis is a possibility in active patient without reconstruction
• ACL reconstruction in active patients
  ○ Bone-patellar tendon-bone graft
    ▪ Associated with patellar fractures if activity is resumed too quickly
  ○ Hamstring graft
    ▪ Quadruped hamstring (semitendinosus ± gracilis)

DIAGNOSTIC CHECKLIST

Consider
• Bucket-handle tear of meniscus as a differential for chronically torn, fibrotic ACL on MRI

Image Interpretation Pearls
• Coronal images can increase sensitivity and specificity for the detection of partial (grade I and II) ACL tears

SELECTED REFERENCES
1. Fithian DC et al: Fate of the anterior cruciate ligament-injured knee. Orthop Clin North Am 33(4):621-36, 2002
2. Fujimoto E et al: Spontaneous healing of acute anterior cruciate ligament (ACL) injuries - conservative treatment using an extension block soft brace without anterior stabilization. Arch Orthop Trauma Surg 122(4):212-6, 2002

IMAGE GALLERY

Typical

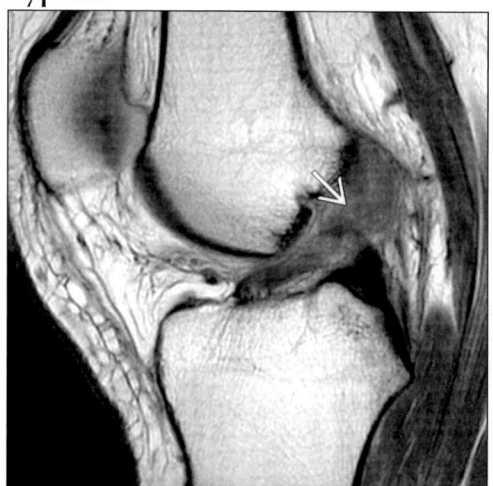 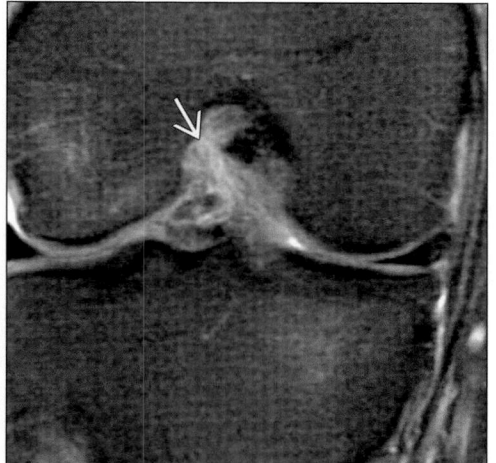

(Left) Sagittal PD FSE MR shows the typical appearance of a proximal ACL tear (arrow). *(Right)* Coronal FS PD FSE MR shows an "empty lateral intercondylar notch wall" representing a grade III ACL tear (arrow).

Typical

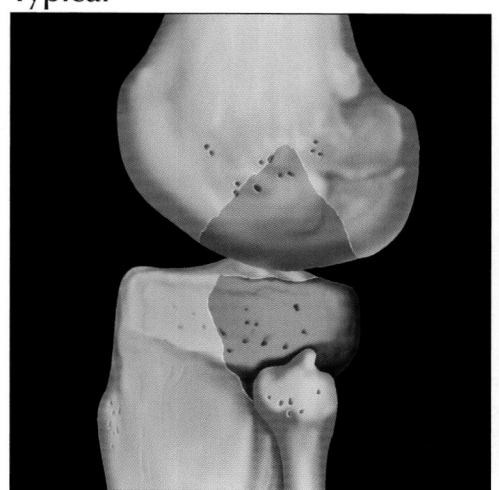 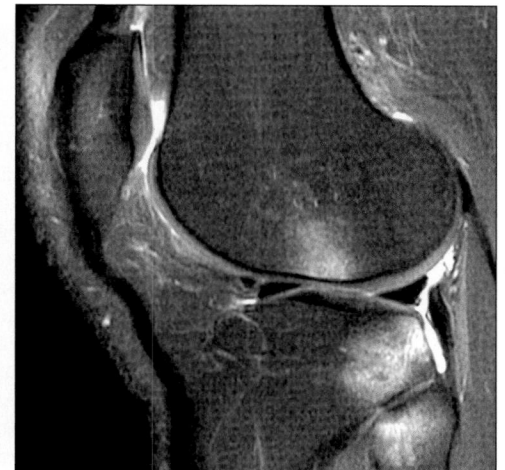

(Left) Sagittal graphic shows the associated bone contusions after an internal rotation valgus mechanism of injury involving the lateral femoral condyle (sulcus terminalis) and the posterolateral tibia. *(Right)* Sagittal FS PD FSE MR shows the lateral bone injuries associated with an ACL tear including the posterolateral tibia and sulcus terminalis of the lateral femoral condyle. The proximal fibula is also injured (osseous contusion).

Variant

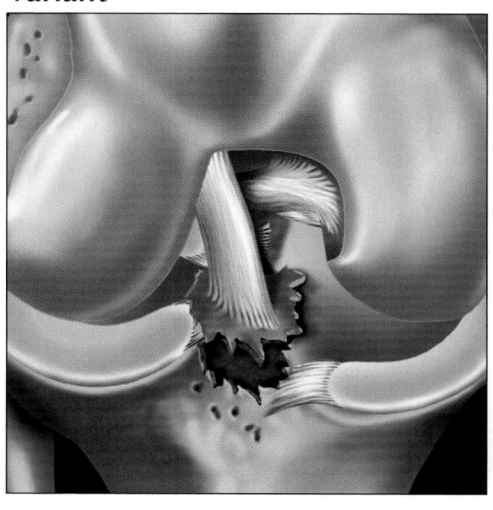 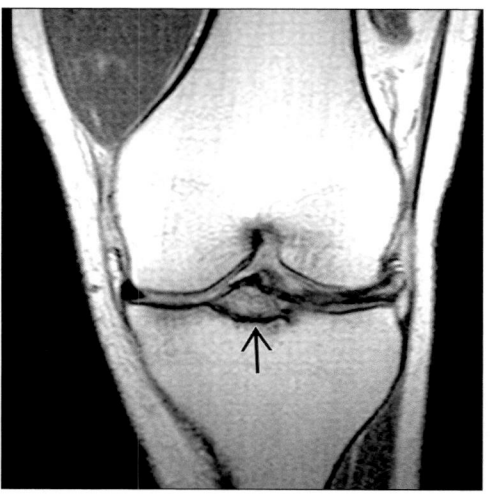

(Left) Coronal oblique graphic shows avulsion fracture of the tibial spine at the insertion of the ACL. This injury is often seen in younger patients. *(Right)* Coronal PD FSE MR shows a nondisplaced tibial spine fracture (arrow).

5

45

ACL RECONSTRUCTION

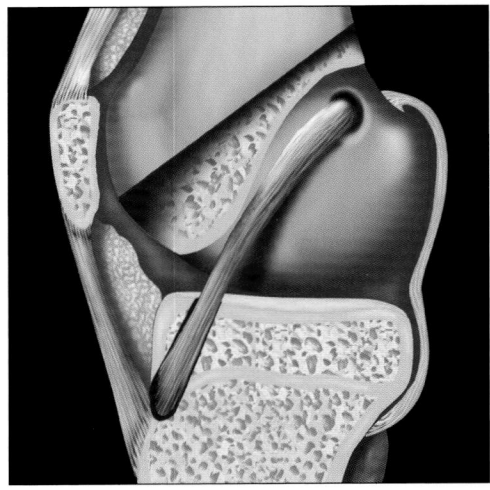

Sagittal graphic shows fraying of the anterior aspect of the graft from chronic roof impingement by the adjacent intercondylar notch roof.

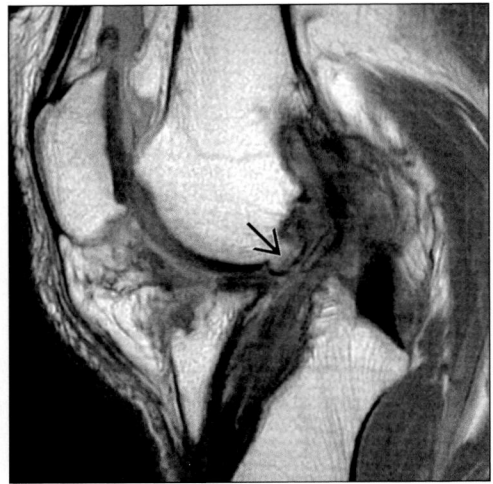

Sagittal PD FSE MR shows a degenerated partially torn graft secondary to impingement by an osteophyte (arrow) of the adjacent intercondylar notch roof.

TERMINOLOGY

Abbreviations and Synonyms
- Anterior cruciate ligament (ACL), ACL reconstruction

Definitions
- Operative (open or arthroscopic) replacement of ACL
- Graft disruption after trauma
- Graft disruption secondary to chronic frictional trauma = roof impingement

IMAGING FINDINGS

General Features
- Best diagnostic clue
  - Normal bone-patellar tendon-bone graft = continuous linear structure coursing through the notch
  - Normal hamstring graft seen as two linear hypointense structures on all pulse sequences
  - Other grafts (including synthetic) seen as linear hypointense structures on all pulse sequences
  - Disruption of graft as discontinuous fibers within the notch + associated hemorrhage and generalized increased signal intensity of grafts on T2WI

- Location: Tibial tunnel superior through anterior medial aspect of tibia at notch (spine) to posterolateral intercondylar notch wall to femoral tunnel
- Size
  - Complete replacement of the ACL by graft approximating normal ACL size
  - Tears may be small partial or large complete disruptions
- Morphology
  - Bone-patellar tendon-bone graft - linear graft
  - Hamstring graft - 2 linear grafts adjacent to each other (quadrupled hamstring)
    - Semitendinosus +/- gracilis tendon
    - Increased signal intensity between grafts on all sequences (fluid and/or synovium)
  - Allograft (patellar tendon/Achilles)
- Normal graft
  - Linear hypointense signal intensity (T1 and T2WI) structure parallel to the roof of intercondylar notch (Blumensaat's line)
  - Tibial tunnel
    - Posterior to the midpoint of the tibial ACL footprint
    - Posterior and parallel to Blumensaat's line tibial intersection in knee extension
  - Femoral tunnel
    - Intersection of posterior femoral cortex and the physeal scar

DDx: ACL Reconstruction

Pseudo Impinge.	Fractured Screw	Pat. Tendonitis	Tunnel Cyst	Patellar Fx

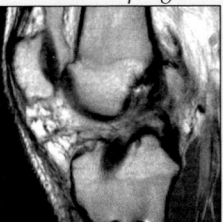 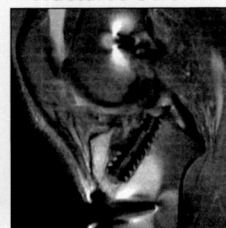 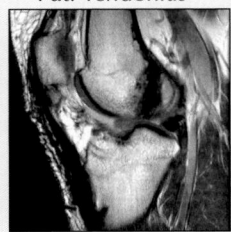 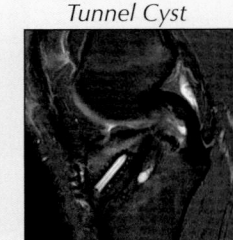 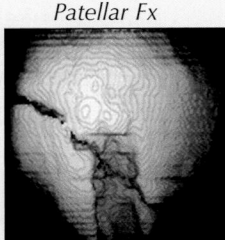

Sag PD FSE MR	Sag FS PD FSE	Sag PD FSE MR	Sag FS PD FSE	Cor NECT

ACL RECONSTRUCTION

Key Facts

Terminology
- Operative (open or arthroscopic) replacement of ACL
- Graft disruption after trauma
- Graft disruption secondary to chronic frictional trauma = roof impingement

Imaging Findings
- Normal bone-patellar tendon-bone graft = continuous linear structure coursing through the notch
- Cyclops lesion - rounded decreased SI mass (fibrotic) on all sequences anterior to the graft

Top Differential Diagnoses
- Apparent Anterior Placement of Tibial Tunnel Mimicking Roof Impingement (Pseudo Impinge)
- Revascularization
- Fractured Hardware

Pathology
- General path comments: Bone-patellar tendon-bone and hamstring grafts most common

Clinical Issues
- Most common signs/symptoms: Pain, instability after operation and usually after repeat trauma if failed reconstruction
- Maintenance of ligament isometric tension to keep distance between tibial & femoral attachment points from changing > 2-3 mm through 0 to 90° flexion

Diagnostic Checklist
- Roof impingement if osteophyte develops at the notch in a symptomatic patient

---

- Intermediate SI on short TE sequence from 1 to 6 months after grafting due to ligamentization and development of a synovial envelope

MR Findings
- T1WI
  - Intermediate to increased signal intensity 6 weeks to 8 months after grafting (revascularization)
  - Torn graft intermediate to increased signal with disorganized graft fibers
    - Typical bone injuries appear as hypointense edematous regions
    - +/- Fracture
- T2WI
  - Normal bone-patellar tendon-bone graft is hypointense
  - Hamstring graft +/- small amounts of increased signal intensity between two components within tibial or femoral tunnel
  - Intermediate to increased signal intensity 6 to 8 months after grafting (revascularization)
  - Graft rupture
    - Increased signal intensity with discontinuity +/- thickening and laxity of graft
    - Axial images - thickening and increased signal intensity adjacent to the lateral intercondylar notch wall
    - Increased signal intensity with nondisplaced fractures or subchondral impaction involving the lateral compartment similar to native ACL tear
    - Reinjury, improper graft placement and failure bone plug/interference screw fixation
- T1 C+
  - Synovial envelope will enhance after I.V. gadolinium administration
    - Confirms intact graft
- Graft impingement
  - Forward placement of tibial tunnel with impingement of intercondylar notch roof on graft (roof impingement)
  - Sidewall impingement (less common) secondary to incomplete notchplasty

- Increased signal on all sequences and variable disruption of fibers
- Graft disruption - associated findings
  - Discontinuous fibers, associated with meniscal tears, bony injuries & collateral ligament tears
    - As with native ACL tears
- Cyclops lesion - rounded decreased SI mass (fibrotic) on all sequences anterior to the graft
  - Extension block and pain

Imaging Recommendations
- Best imaging tool: MRI
- Protocol advice
  - FS PD and FS PD FSE in all planes
    - Consider T1 C+ in difficult cases to enhance synovial reflection

DIFFERENTIAL DIAGNOSIS

Apparent Anterior Placement of Tibial Tunnel Mimicking Roof Impingement (Pseudo Impinge)
- Forward translation of tibia may result from graft/disruption & tibial translation and 2° instability
- Not due to improper surgical placement

Revascularization
- Graft may exhibit intermediate signal on short TE sequence normally from 6 weeks to 8 months after repair
- Important to have accurate history of surgery, and presence of pain

Fractured Hardware
- Pain and graft dysfunction
- Visualized on MR, radiographs

Meniscal Tear with Resultant Locking
- Mimics cyclops lesion clinically
- Increased signal on short TE sequence extending to surface of meniscus
  - Usually associated with displaced fragment

ACL RECONSTRUCTION

○ Bucket-handle tear

Osteochondral Injury
- Posttraumatic pain, +/- locking, +/- graft tear
- Acute on chronic injury with acute development of hyperintense (T2WI) bone contusions

Donor Site Abnormalities
- Patellar tendonitis
  ○ Thickened increased signal intensity of tendon on T2WI, +/- tear
  ○ Normal post surgical (persist up to 18 months post harvest)
- Post graft patellar insufficiency fracture
  ○ Decreased surface area and secondary weakening of bone
  ○ Premature resumption of sport activities

Tunnel Cyst
- +/- Mass effect, pain
- Hamstring grafts
- Tibial tunnel
- Hyperintense on T2WI

PATHOLOGY

General Features
- General path comments: Bone-patellar tendon-bone and hamstring grafts most common
- Etiology
  ○ Most ACL reconstructions (intraarticular): Either hamstring or bone-patellar tendon-bone grafts
  ○ Abnormal placement of tibial tunnel (usually anterior) can result in graft impingement
- Epidemiology: Common procedure of ACL tear in active patients to prevent development of arthritis

Gross Pathologic & Surgical Features
- Disrupted graft: Discontinuous tendon fibers within notch of knee with variable degrees of hemorrhage and synovitis

Microscopic Features
- Tendon grafts progress through 4 stages of "ligamentization"
  ○ Avascular necrosis
  ○ Revascularization
  ○ Cellular proliferation
  ○ Remodeling, resulting in histology closely resembling native ACL
- Fibroblast healing occurs through synovial membrane
- Revascularization occurs from the synovial membrane and endosteal vessels

CLINICAL ISSUES

Presentation
- Most common signs/symptoms: Pain, instability after operation and usually after repeat trauma if failed reconstruction
- Reconstruction goal

○ Maintenance of ligament isometric tension to keep distance between tibial & femoral attachment points from changing > 2-3 mm through 0 to 90° flexion
- Graft placement depends upon activity level of patients
  ○ Active patients are encouraged to undergo reconstruction to prevent development of osteoarthritis
- Roof impingement leads to pain and may eventually lead to graft disruption
  ○ Associated findings of impingement
    ▪ Joint effusion, decreased extension, pain, and recurrent instability
- Cyclops lesion may lead to pain and extension block
- Patellar tendinitis can occur at donor site
  ○ Middle third of patellar tendon

Demographics
- Age: Typically younger active patient
- Gender: F > M

Natural History & Prognosis
- Post operative patient does well with no new trauma
  ○ Helps prevent arthritis (seen with unstable patient)

Treatment
- Graft impingement treated with resection of osteophytes and replacement of graft if torn
- Cyclops lesion resected if symptomatic

DIAGNOSTIC CHECKLIST

Consider
- Roof impingement if osteophyte develops at the notch in a symptomatic patient

Image Interpretation Pearls
- Intact graft as continuous fibers
- Evaluate the posterolateral tibial plateau articular cartilage for erosions secondary to osteochondral injury associated with the initial ACL tear

SELECTED REFERENCES
1. Boni DM et al: Hamstring tendon graft for anterior cruciate ligament reconstruction. Aorn J 76(4):610-5, 617-9, 621-4; quiz 625-8, 2002
2. Jansson KA et al: MRI of anterior cruciate ligament repair with patellar and hamstring tendon autografts. Skeletal Radiol 30(1):8-14, 2001
3. Jarvela TP et al: Anterior cruciate ligament reconstruction in patients with or without accompanying injuries. A re-examination of subjects 5 to 9 years after reconstruction. Arthroscopy 17(8):818-25, 2001
4. Veselko MA et al: Cyclops syndrome occurring after partial rupture of the anterior cruciate ligament not treated by surgical reconstruction. Arthroscopy 16(3):328-31, 2000

IMAGE GALLERY

Variant

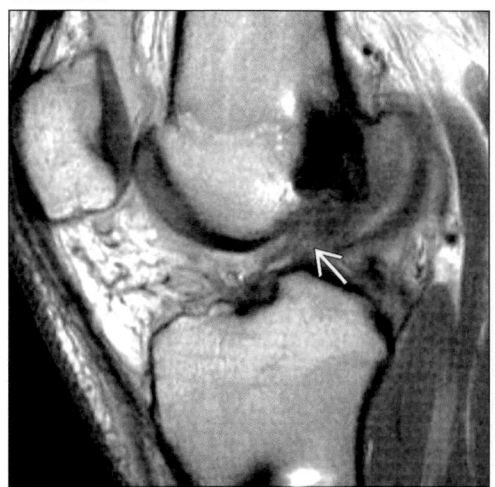

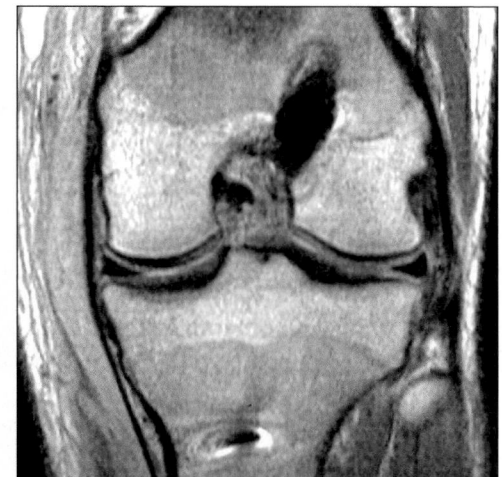

(Left) Sagittal PD FSE MR shows a torn ACL graft. Note the discontinuous and lax fibers (arrow) and anterior displacement of the tibia as a result of the instability. *(Right)* Coronal PD FSE MR shows the torn graft in the notch of the knee. The fibers are discontinuous and distorted. Note the soft tissue edema adjacent to the MCL indicating recent injury.

Variant

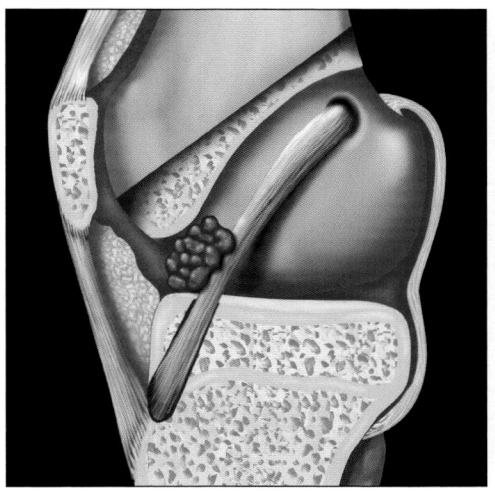

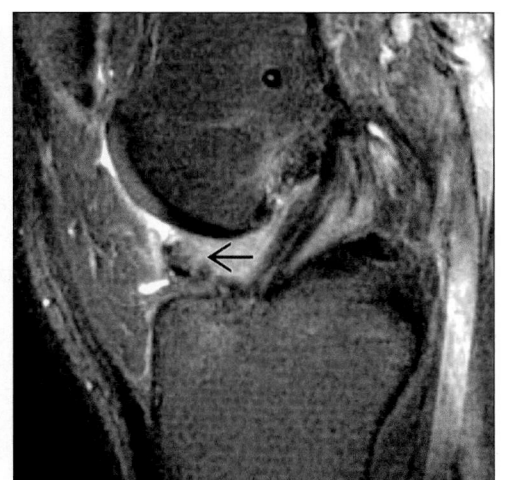

(Left) Sagittal graphic shows arthrofibrosis of the anterior intercondylar notch adjacent to the ACL graft (mass like = cyclops lesion). This may result in terminal extension block. *(Right)* Sagittal FS PD FSE MR shows an intact ACL graft with a rounded decreased signal intensity mass in the anterior notch consistent with a cyclops lesion (arrow). There is surrounding synovial proliferation.

5

49

Typical

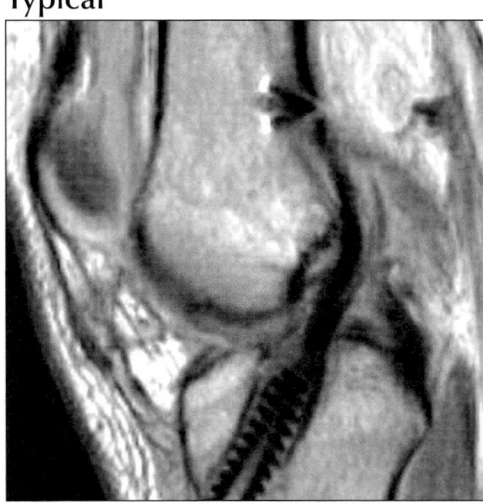

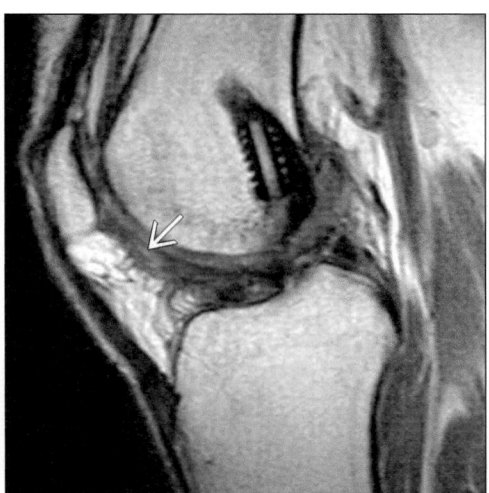

(Left) Sagittal PD FSE MR shows an intact ACL graft with decreased signal intensity. *(Right)* Sagittal PD FSE MR shows fixation of ACL graft within femoral tunnel. There is scarring of Hoffa's fat pad (arrow). A cyclops lesion is usually more round and well-defined.

POSTERIOR CRUCIATE LIGAMENT TEAR

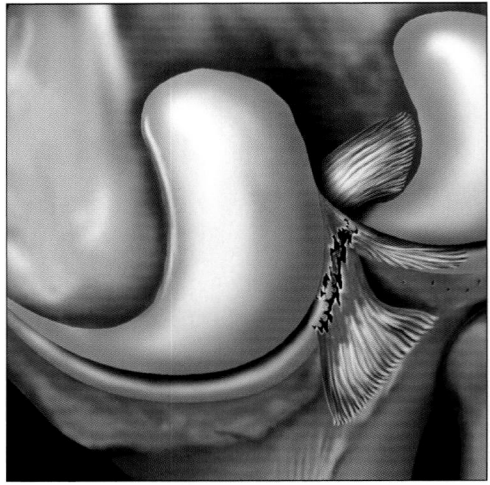

Coronal oblique graphic shows a torn PCL.

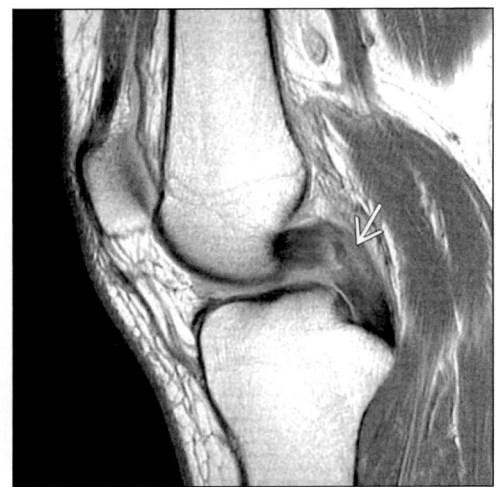

Sagittal PD FSE MR shows a high grade partial tear (arrow) in the middle third of the PCL.

TERMINOLOGY

Abbreviations and Synonyms
- Posterior cruciate ligament (PCL) tear

Definitions
- Disruption of the PCL usually after forced posterior displacement of the tibia

IMAGING FINDINGS

General Features
- Best diagnostic clue: Discontinuous and/or thickened PCL fibers of increased signal intensity on all pulse sequences
- Location: Posterior tibia insertion site avulsion fracture common
- Size: Small discrete tear to complex tear
- Morphology: Discrete to complete disorganized tear

Radiographic Findings
- Radiography
  ○ Avulsion fractures of the posterior tibia
  ○ Subtle anterior impaction fractures
  ○ Reverse Segond fracture rare
    ▪ Avulsion at tibial insertion site at deep portion of MCL associated with PCL & peripheral medial meniscus tear

CT Findings
- NECT
  ○ Associated fractures
    ▪ Anterior hyperextension fractures
- CT arthrography
  ○ Torn ligament seen in contrast pool
  ○ Chondral defects seen as contrast collection/ulceration of chondral surface if fractured

MR Findings
- T1WI
  ○ Complete rupture - decreased signal intensity and discontinuous fibers
    ▪ +/- Thickening of attached ligament portions
  ○ Partial tear (grade I and II sprains) - variable thickening, decreased signal intensity continuous fibers partially intact
  ○ Avulsion fractures of the posterior mid-tibia hypointense line
    ▪ Hypointense fx surrounded by hypointense edema
- T2WI
  ○ Interstitial tear: Diffuse thickening, increased signal intensity
  ○ Complete rupture: Increased signal intensity and discontinuous fibers
  ○ Partial tear (grade I and II sprains) - variable thickening, increased signal intensity, continuous fibers generally intact

DDx: Posterior Cruciate Ligament Tear

Fx Normal PCL	PCL Graft Intact	Post Lat Cor Sx	PCL Cyst	Mucoid Degen

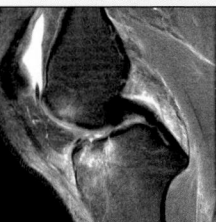 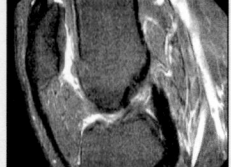 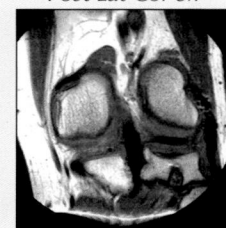 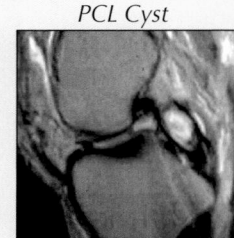 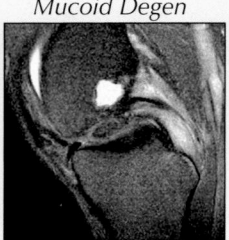

Sag FS PD FSE	Sag STIR MR	Cor PD FSE MR	Sag T2 FSE MR	Sag FS PD FSE

POSTERIOR CRUCIATE LIGAMENT TEAR

Key Facts

Terminology
- Disruption of the PCL usually after forced posterior displacement of the tibia

Imaging Findings
- Best diagnostic clue: Discontinuous and/or thickened PCL fibers of increased signal intensity on all pulse sequences
- Normal ligament appears as decreased signal intensity on all pulse sequences "hockey stick" in the notch of the knee (sagittal images)
- Protocol advice: FS PD FSE in sagittal and coronal planes

Top Differential Diagnoses
- Mucoid Degeneration
- Osteochondral Injuries

- PCL Graft Surgery
- Posterolateral Corner (PLC) Injury/Surgery (Post Lat Cor Sx)

Pathology
- Most commonly occurs by direct trauma impacting the anterior knee in a posterior direction (dashboard injury with the knee in flexion)

Clinical Issues
- Most common signs/symptoms: Positive posterior drawer sign (excessive mobility of the tibia posteriorly)

Diagnostic Checklist
- In setting of anterior tibial trabecular injury

- o Coronal images - thickening and increased intensity within the medial intercondylar notch
  - Partial or complete tear
  - Replacing normal "hockey puck" appearance
- o Avulsion fractures of the posterior mid tibia - hypointense fracture line
  - Surrounded by hyperintense edema
- o Anterior tibial trabecular injury or fracture + posterior femur injury (hyperintense contusion)
  - Forced posterior displacement of tibia in a flexed knee
  - Dashboard injury
- o Increased signal intensity anterior tibia and anterior femur "kissing fractures" = hyperextension injury
- o FS increases conspicuity of edema
- PD/Intermediate
  - o Interstitial tear may appear as diffuse thickening and increased signal intensity
  - o Complete rupture seen as increased signal intensity and discontinuous fibers
- STIR
  - o Hyperintensity similar to FS PD FSE
  - o Fat saturation increases edema conspicuity
- T2* GRE
  - o Complete rupture: Increased signal intensity and discontinuous fibers
  - o Interstitial tear: Diffuse thickening and increased signal intensity
- Increased signal intensity on all pulse sequences is abnormal
  - o Tear vs. degeneration maybe difficult to differentiate
- Normal ligament appears as decreased signal intensity on all pulse sequences "hockey stick" in the notch of the knee (sagittal images)

Imaging Recommendations
- Best imaging tool: MRI
- Protocol advice: FS PD FSE in sagittal and coronal planes

DIFFERENTIAL DIAGNOSIS

Mucoid Degeneration
- Normal aging of ligament
- Increased signal intensity of PCL and slight thickening on T2WI
- +/- Intraligamentous cyst

Osteochondral Injuries
- "Kissing fractures" of hyperextension in absence of PCL tear
- Hypointense fx line on all pulse sequences
- Hyperintense edema on T2WI

PCL Graft Surgery
- Graft normally decreased in signal
- Retear
- Enters posterior tibia at notch

Posterolateral Corner (PLC) Injury/Surgery (Post Lat Cor Sx)
- Posterolateral corner injury associated with PCL tears
- PLC injury + PCL arthritis/instability
- Hyperintense ligaments/tendons
  - o Including popliteus, arcuate complex, posterolateral capsule

PATHOLOGY

General Features
- General path comments
  - o PCL is twice as strong as anterior cruciate ligament (ACL)
  - o Posteromedial bundle of PCL is taut in extension and lax in flexion
  - o Anterolateral bundle is tight in flexion and lax in extension
  - o PCL fibers attach in an anterior-to-posterior direction on the femur and medial-to-lateral direction on the tibia
  - o Medial intercondylar notch wall origin (in the form of a semicircle)

POSTERIOR CRUCIATE LIGAMENT TEAR

○ PCL insertion = central fovea on the posterior tibia 1.5 cm inferior to the joint line
○ Humphry's (anterior) and Wrisberg's (posterior) meniscofemoral ligaments extend from posterior horn lateral meniscus to insert anteriorly & posteriorly relative to the PCL on the medial femoral condyle
○ Main vascular supply of the cruciate ligaments = middle geniculate artery
• Etiology
○ Most commonly occurs by direct trauma impacting the anterior knee in a posterior direction (dashboard injury with the knee in flexion)
○ Also occurs in hyperextension, dislocation and rotational injuries
○ Flexed knee decelerates quickly - fall on flexed knee
• Epidemiology
○ Accounts for only 5 to 20% of all knee ligament injuries (38% incidence reported in regional trauma centers)
○ Less common than other ligament tears of the knee
• Associated abnormalities
○ Posterolateral corner injury
  ▪ Early arthritis/instability if unrecognized
○ Hyperextension "kissing fractures"
  ▪ Anterior tibia
  ▪ Anterior femur
  ▪ Increased signal T2WI
  ▪ +/- Hypointense (all pulse sequences) fracture line

Gross Pathologic & Surgical Features
• Disruption of the ligament within midsubstance, at origin, or at attachment
• +/- Hemorrhage and synovitis (in chronic cases)

Microscopic Features
• Disruption of normal collagen bundles
○ Hemorrhage
○ Fibrosis
○ Inflammatory infiltration

Staging, Grading or Classification Criteria
• Grade I sprain: Minimal tear without joint laxity
○ Intraligamentous injury
• Grade II sprain: Moderate tear with joint laxity
• Grade III sprain: High grade sprain to complete tear with no firm endpoint
○ > 10 mm of tibial translation

CLINICAL ISSUES

Presentation
• Most common signs/symptoms: Positive posterior drawer sign (excessive mobility of the tibia posteriorly)
• Clinical profile
○ Posterior drawer test
  ▪ Accurate test for PCL integrity
  ▪ Patient supine, knee flexed 90° + posterior directed force on tibia
○ Posterior sag test in complete tears (Godfrey's test)
  ▪ Tibia sags into a posterior subluxation relative to femur with patient supine and knee flexed to 90 degrees

○ Quadriceps active test results in translation of tibia anteriorly during quadriceps contraction
○ External rotation of the tibia (Dial test)
  ▪ To evaluate posterolateral structures (PLS)
  ▪ Patient prone + external rotation force to feet (knee in 30° and 90° of flexion)
  ▪ 10° difference with contralateral side is abnormal
○ Reverse pivot shift test
  ▪ Passive extension of knee from 90° of flexion with foot externally rotated + valgus force applied to the tibia
  ▪ Positive result = reduction of tibial plateau at 20-30° of flexion

Demographics
• Age: Children or adults
• Gender
○ No predilection
○ 2% of National Football League players have PCL instability

Natural History & Prognosis
• Patient may do without intervention for isolated PCL injuries
• Increased articular cartilage wear as tibiofemoral contact shifts anteriorly

Treatment
• Usually conservative
• Repair if multiple abnormalities associated with ligament tear

DIAGNOSTIC CHECKLIST

Consider
• In setting of anterior tibial trabecular injury

Image Interpretation Pearls
• FS PD FSE in sagittal and coronal planes show lesion as loss of "hockey stick" appearance (sagittal) or hockey puck (coronal)

SELECTED REFERENCES

1. DeLee J et al: Orthopaedics sports medicine. vol 1. 2nd ed. Philadelphia PA, Saunders, 1577-2154, 2003
2. Freeman RT et al: Combined chronic posterior cruciate and posterolateral corner ligamentous injuries. vol 9. Philadelphia PA, Elsevier (4):309-12, 2002
3. Bergfeld JA et al: The effects of tibial rotation on posterior translation in knees in which the posterior cruciate ligament has been cut. J Bone Joint Surg Am 83-A(9):1339-43, 2001
4. Covey DC: Injuries of the posterolateral corner of the knee. J Bone Joint Surg Am 83-A(1):106-18, 2001
5. Feltham GT et al: The diagnosis of PCL injury: Literature review and introduction of two novel tests. Iowa Orthop J 21:36-42, 2001
6. Fanelli GC: Treatment of combined anterior cruciate ligament-posterior cruciate ligament-lateral side injuries of the knee. Clin Sports Med. 19(3):493-502, 2000

IMAGE GALLERY

Typical

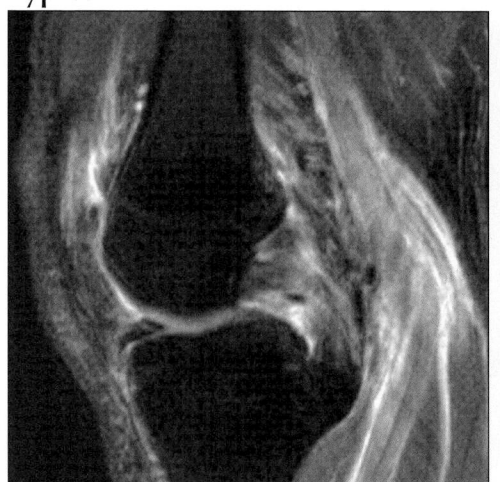 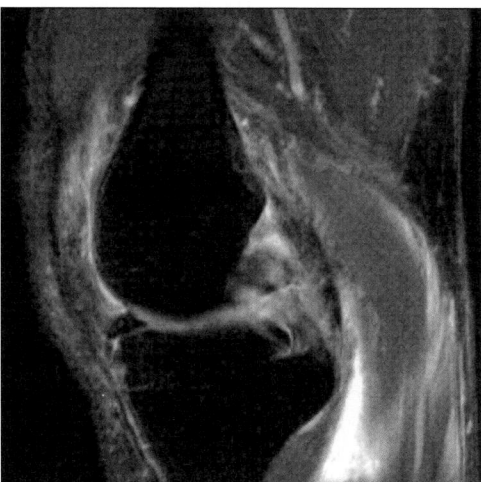

(Left) Sagittal FS PD FSE MR shows a complete tear of the PCL. *(Right)* Sagittal FS PD FSE MR shows a complete tear of the PCL mid portion.

Typical

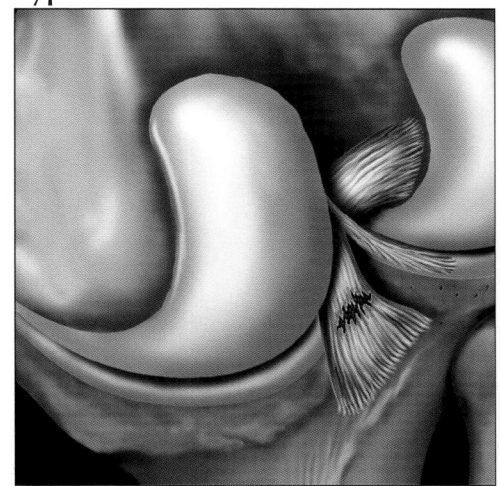 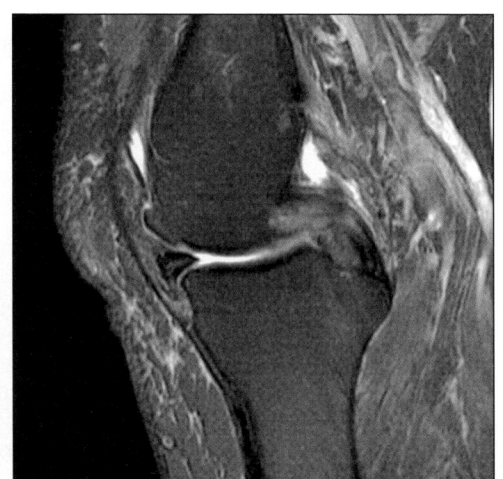

(Left) Coronal oblique graphic shows a partial tear of the PCL. *(Right)* Sagittal FS PD FSE MR shows a partial PCL tear of the proximal and mid portion.

Typical

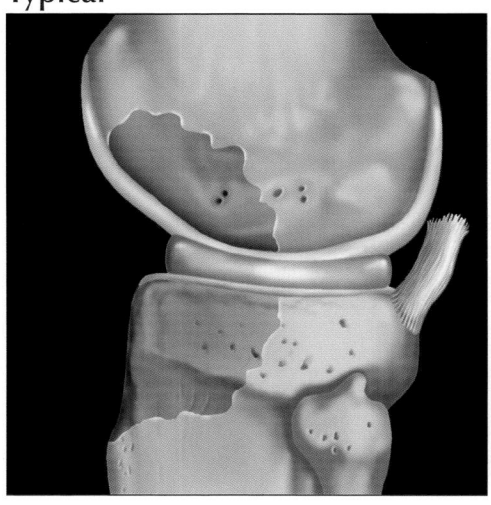 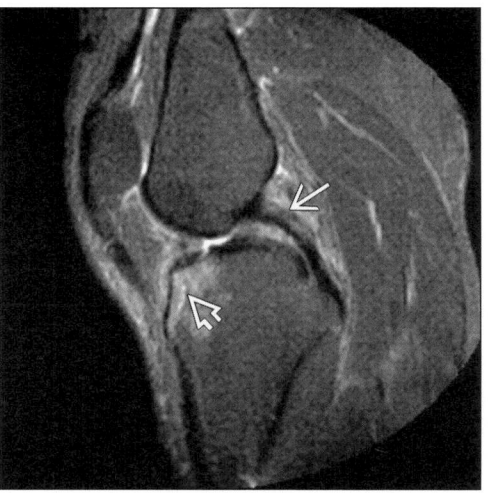

(Left) Sagittal graphic shows the typical anterior bone contusion pattern of hyperextension often seen with PCL tears. *(Right)* Sagittal STIR MR shows a partial PCL tear (arrow) and an anterior subchondral contusion of the tibia (open arrow) in a patient who suffered a dashboard injury.

5

53

MEDIAL COLLATERAL LIGAMENT TEAR

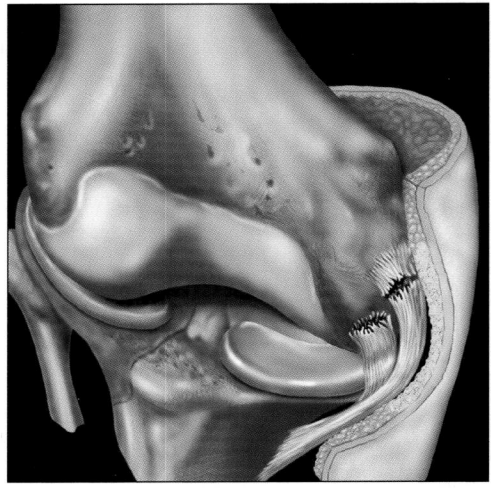

Coronal oblique graphic shows a grade III tear of the proximal aspect of the medial collateral ligament. Both the superficial and deep layers are torn. Note the soft tissue edema.

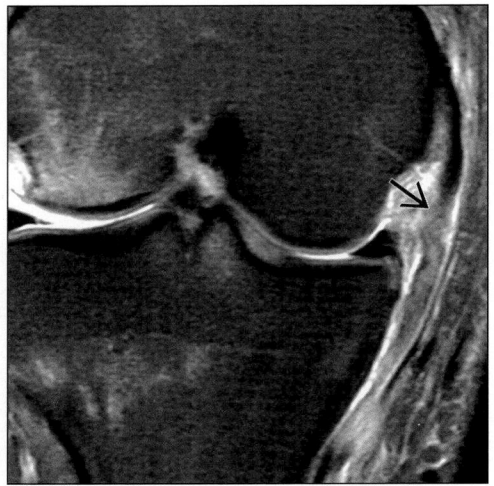

Coronal FS PD FSE shows a grade III MCL tear (arrow) after valgus injury.

TERMINOLOGY

Abbreviations and Synonyms
- Medial collateral ligament (MCL) tear, tibial collateral ligament tear

Definitions
- Disruption of MCL fibers after trauma
- Secondary to valgus stress

IMAGING FINDINGS

General Features
- Best diagnostic clue: Discontinuous MCL with thickening and increased signal intensity on all sequences within ligament remnant
- Location
  - Superficial and deep (medial capsular ligament) layers can be disrupted completely or partially
    - Superficial component: Medial (tibial) collateral ligament proper
    - Deep layer: Meniscofemoral and meniscotibial attachments
- Size: Tears vary from small discrete partial disruption to complete grade III "blowout"
- Morphology
  - Varies from discrete tear to massive disruption
  - Disruption of normal continuous linear ligament appearance

CT Findings
- NECT
  - Nonspecific soft tissue edema
  - Heterotopic ossification if Pellegrini-Stieda lesion
  - +/- Fracture

MR Findings
- T1WI
  - Intermediate signal intensity of disorganized appearing ligament
  - +/- Bone trabecular injury
    - Medial femoral condyle - direct impact
    - Lateral femoral condyle - clipping injury
  - Heterotopic ossification (Pellegrini-Stieda disease)
    - Increased signal (fat in bone marrow) corticated structure
    - = Chronic tear
- T2WI
  - Increased signal intensity disorganization and often thickening within the normally hypointense ligament
  - Increased signal intensity with or without visible fracture lines or subchondral impaction involving
    - Medial femoral condyle
    - Posterolateral femoral condyle
    - Lateral tibial plateau

DDx: Medial Collateral Ligament Tear

Tear Hyperemia	SM Tendinosis	TCL Bursitis	Hyperemia (Infla)	Plateau Fx
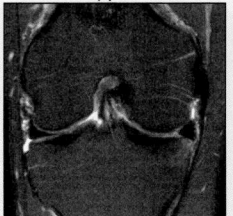	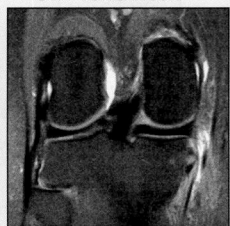	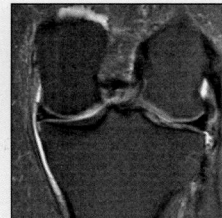	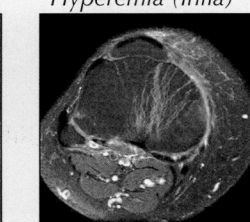	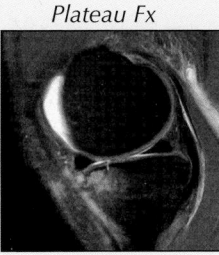
Cor FS PD FSE	Cor FS PD FSE	Cor FS PD FSE	Ax FS PD FSE MR	Sag FS PD FSE

MEDIAL COLLATERAL LIGAMENT TEAR

Key Facts

Imaging Findings
- Best diagnostic clue: Discontinuous MCL with thickening and increased signal intensity on all sequences within ligament remnant
- Superficial and deep (medial capsular ligament) layers can be disrupted completely or partially
- Coronal and axial FS PD FSE, for diagnosis and characterization

Top Differential Diagnoses
- Tibial Collateral Ligament Bursitis (TCL Bursitis)
- Semimembranosus Tibial Collateral Ligament Bursitis
- Semimembranosus Tendinosis

Pathology
- Ligament disrupted by valgus stress on the knee which "opens up" the medial joint

- Anterior cruciate ligament (ACL) tear in injury to peripheral aspect of the medial meniscus or meniscal attachments

Clinical Issues
- Child or adult after valgus injury
- Usually heals, even grade III disruptions with no associated "collateral" damage to other structures in the joint
- Isolated MCL sprains are treated with functional rehabilitation

Diagnostic Checklist
- Damage to other ligaments or menisci may necessitate surgery
- Coronal and axial images show either proximal or distal tears

---

- Hyperintense hemorrhagic effusion common
- Coronal images show increased signal intensity with disorganized tissue replacing normal hypointense ligament
- FS PD FSE sensitive for edema associated with MCL tear
- PD/Intermediate
  - Heterotopic ossification (Pellegrini-Stieda disease): Increased signal (fat in bone marrow), corticated structure
  - Loss of normal decreased signal intensity ligament in tear
- STIR
  - Increased signal within the ligament
  - Disorganization of fibers and thickening within the normally decreased signal intensity ligament
- Discontinuity of ligament fibers
- Bone contusions involving the lateral femur and lateral tibia indicating valgus stress
- Partial tear: Some fibers are still continuous and intact

Imaging Recommendations
- Best imaging tool: MRI
- Protocol advice
  - Coronal and axial FS PD FSE, for diagnosis and characterization
    - T2* GRE for Pellegrini-Stieda

DIFFERENTIAL DIAGNOSIS

Osseous Injury
- Medial bone trabecular or osteochondral injuries
- History of trauma common
- Affects chondral surface and subchondral bone
- Increased signal on T2WI

Tibial Collateral Ligament Bursitis (TCL Bursitis)
- Fluid signal intensity between layers of MCL
  - Increased signal on T2WI
- +/- Trauma
- Hemorrhagic with trauma

- +/- Intact ligament
- Inflammatory condition
- +/- Hyperemia (reactive) in tibia and/or femur in inflammation
  - Edema in association with meniscal tear

Semimembranosus Tibial Collateral Ligament Bursitis
- Fluid signal intensity posterior to semimembranosus (SM)
  - Increased signal on T2WI
- +/- Trauma
- +/- SM tendinosis
- Inflammatory condition

Semimembranosus Tendinosis
- Overuse syndrome
- Increased (relative) signal intensity on all pulse sequences within SM attachment
- Associated with tibial collateral ligament semimembranosus bursitis

Medial Meniscus Tear
- Linear increased signal intensity on short TE sequences extending to the articular margin of the meniscus
- Positive clinical signs of meniscal tear - i.e., McMurray test
- +/- Associated edema within the medial tibia and femur (tear hyperemia)

PATHOLOGY

General Features
- Etiology
  - Ligament disrupted by valgus stress on the knee which "opens up" the medial joint
  - Acute with valgus stress injury
  - Acute episode superimposed on chronic repetitive valgus stress
- Epidemiology: Common in sports injuries (5-10% of college football players)
- Associated abnormalities

MEDIAL COLLATERAL LIGAMENT TEAR

- o Anterior cruciate ligament (ACL) tear in injury to peripheral aspect of the medial meniscus or meniscal attachments
- o Pellegrini-Stieda disease is a chronic ligament sprain
  - Calcification or ossification of proximal ligament adjacent to the medial femoral epicondyle

Gross Pathologic & Surgical Features
- Thickened, partially or completely torn ligament
- Disruption of ligament within its midsubstance, at its origin, or at its attachment accompanied by surrounding hemorrhage

Microscopic Features
- Degeneration, partial or complete rupture
- Variable amounts of hemorrhage and inflammatory cells
- MCL heals with scar formation
  - o Scar contracts (3-14 weeks) then stretches
  - o Scar is biomechanically inferior to normal ligament
  - o Increased cellularity, decreased total collagen and increased type III (immature) collagen

Staging, Grading or Classification Criteria
- MR (grades)
  - o Grade I: Hyperintensity in soft tissues medial to MCL
  - o Grade II: Hyperintensity in soft tissues medial to MCL + hyperintensity within a portion of the MCL itself
  - o Grade III: Complete disruption of MCL fibers + interposed fluid or fibrosis (chronic)
- Clinical (grades)
  - o Grade 1 sprain: Interstitial tear with no joint laxity
    - No increased medial opening to valgus stress
  - o Grade 2 sprain: Partial tear
    - 1+ or 2+ mm opening
    - No pathologic laxity
  - o Grade 3 sprain: Complete tear with no firm endpoint to abduction stress
    - 3+ mm opening (pathologic laxity)
- Pathologic laxity grades (amount of joint opening with displacing forces)
  - o 0 = normal
  - o I = 1 to 4 mm
  - o II = 5 to 9 mm
  - o III = 10 to 15 mm

CLINICAL ISSUES

Presentation
- Most common signs/symptoms
  - o Child or adult after valgus injury
  - o Pain (grade I sprain)
  - o Pain and instability (grade II and grade III sprains)

Demographics
- Age: Child or adult
- Gender: M > F

Natural History & Prognosis
- Usually heals, even grade III disruptions with no associated "collateral" damage to other structures in the joint

- Stage 1: Inflammation
  - o Within 3 days of injury
  - o Fibroblasts produce type III collagen
- Stage 2: Repair and regeneration
  - o 6 weeks after injury
  - o Type I collagen replaces type III collagen
- Stage 3: Remodeling
  - o Continues for up to and > 1 year after injury
  - o 50-70% of elasticity and strength by 1 year
- Injury characteristics that slow healing
  - o Grade III sprains heal < grades I and II

Treatment
- Isolated MCL sprains are treated with functional rehabilitation
- MCL sprains associated with ACL injuries are treated by repair of the ACL tear
  - o +/- MCL repair

DIAGNOSTIC CHECKLIST

Consider
- Damage to other ligaments or menisci may necessitate surgery

Image Interpretation Pearls
- Coronal and axial images show either proximal or distal tears

SELECTED REFERENCES

1. Twaddle BC et al: Knee dislocations: Where are the lesions? A prospective evaluation of surgical findings in 63 cases. J Orthop Trauma 17(3):198-202, 2003
2. Borden PS et al: Medial collateral ligament reconstruction with allograft using a double-bundle technique. Arthroscopy 18(4):E19, 2002
3. Bergin D et al: A traumatic medial collateral ligament edema in medial compartment knee osteoarthritis. Skeletal Radiol 31(1):14-8, 2002
4. Koehle MS et al: Alpine ski injuries and their prevention. Sports Med 32(12):785-93, 2002
5. Gardiner JC et al: Strain in the human medial collateral ligament during valgus loading of the knee. Clin Orthop (391):266-74, 2001
6. Woo SL et al: Injury and repair of ligaments and tendons. Annu Rev Biomed Eng 2:83-118, 2000
7. Woo SL et al: Healing and repair of ligament injuries in the knee. J Am Acad Orthop Surg 8(6):364-72, 2000
8. Elliott JM et al: MR appearances of the locked knee. Br J Radiol 73(874):1120-6, 2000
9. Lundberg M et al: Ten-year prognosis of isolated and combined medial collateral ligament ruptures. A matched comparison in 40 patients using clinical and radiographic evaluations. Am J SPorts Med 25(1):2-6, 1997
10. Stoller DW et al: Magnetic resonance imaging in orthopaedics and sports medicine. vol 1. 2nd ed. Philadelphia PA, Lippincott Williams & Wilkins, 203-442, 1997
11. Reider B et al: Medial collateral ligament injuries in athletes. Sports Med 21(2):147-56, 1996
12. Albright JP et al: Medial collateral ligament knee sprains in college football. Effectiveness of preventive braces. Am J Sports Med 22(1):12-8, 1994

IMAGE GALLERY

Variant

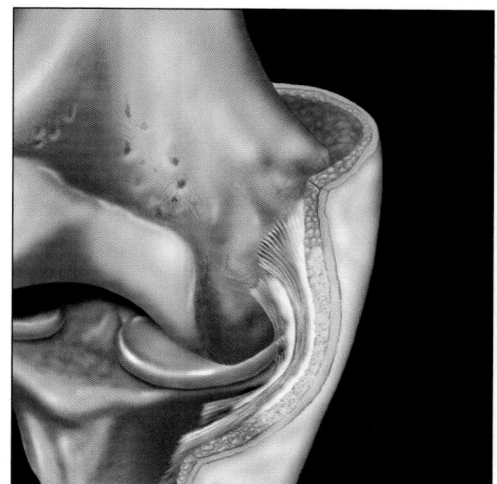 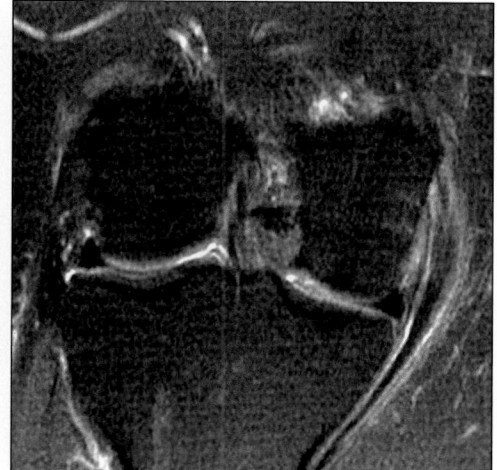

(Left) Coronal oblique graphic shows a grade I sprain of the MCL with adjacent edema. (Right) Coronal FS PD FSE MR shows a grade II sprain of the MCL. Note the intraligamentous hyperintensity.

Variant

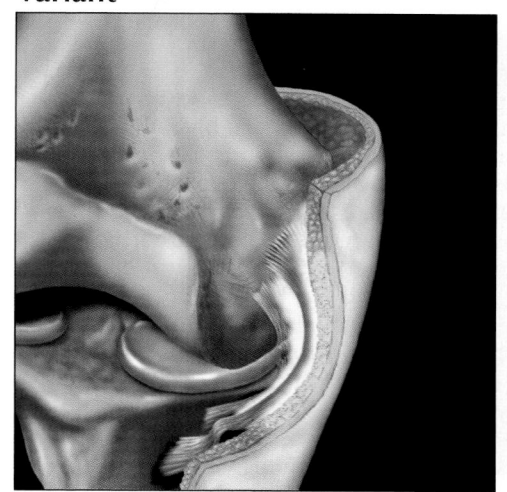 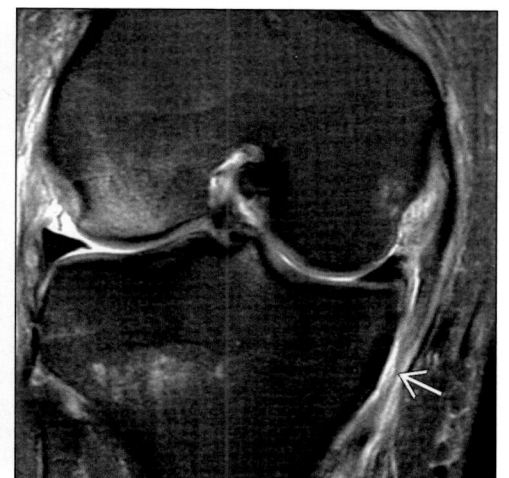

(Left) Coronal graphic shows a grade III sprain of the distal MCL. Note laxity of distal fibers. (Right) Coronal FS PD FSE MR shows a grade III sprain of the distal MCL (arrow). Laxity of distal fibers are demonstrated.

Variant

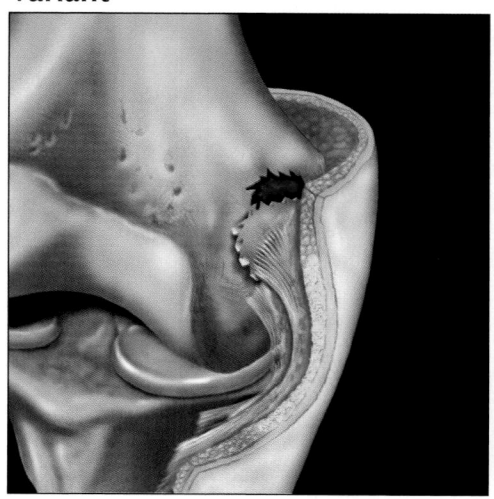 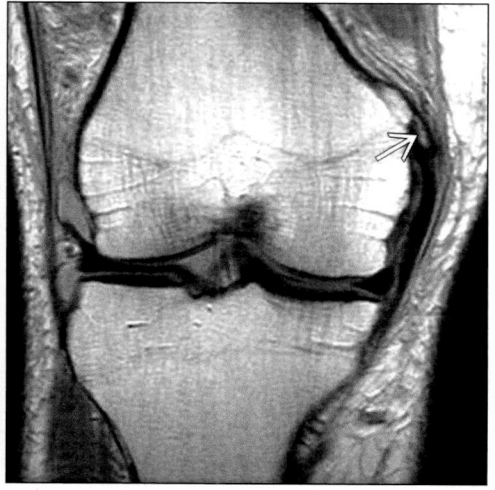

(Left) Coronal graphic shows an avulsion fracture (Stieda fracture) at the origin of the MCL with adjacent hemorrhage in surrounding soft tissues. (Right) Coronal PD FSE MR shows osseous marrow signal (arrow) of the proximal aspect of the MCL consistent with Pellegrini-Stieda disease. This represents the ossification of a chronic tear.

5

57

MEDIAL BURSITIS, KNEE

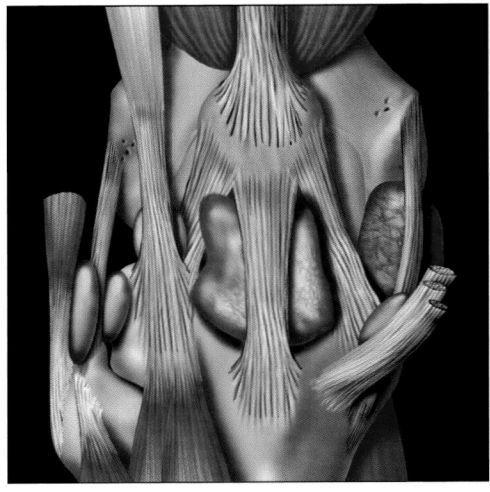

Coronal graphic shows the tibial collateral ligament bursa deep to the superficial component of the ligament. The pes anserinus bursa is beneath the insertion of the pes anserine tendons.

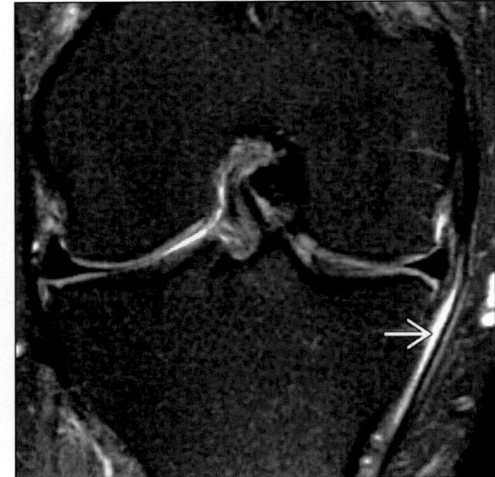

Coronal FS PD FSE MR shows hyperintense fluid signal intensity (arrow) within the TCL bursa consistent with bursitis.

TERMINOLOGY

Abbreviations and Synonyms
- Pes anserinus (PA) bursitis
- Medial collateral ligament (MCL) bursitis
- Tibial collateral ligament (TCL) bursitis
- Semimembranosus-tibial collateral ligament (SMTCL) bursitis

Definitions
- Synovial lining: Inflammation of the medial bursae of the knee
  - Including TCL bursa (bursa of Voshell between superficial and deep layers of MCL)
  - Pes bursa overlies tendinous attachments of sartorius, gracilis and semitendinosus tendons distal to Voshell's bursa

IMAGING FINDINGS

General Features
- Best diagnostic clue: Fluid containing mass (fluid signal intensity) in location of a medial bursae
- Location
  - MCL bursa
    - Between deep and superficial components of medial collateral ligament

- Five locations described including between the meniscofemoral attachment and superficial MCL, coronary ligament and superficial MCL, and an anterior to posterior distribution/location
  - Semimembranosus tibial collateral ligament bursa
    - Posteromedial to semimembranosus tendon extending anteriorly for variable distance
  - Pes anserinus bursa
    - Interposed between tendons of pes anserine (sartorius, gracilis, semitendinosus) and medial tibia
    - Approximately 1-2 cm below joint line
- Size: Varies from a few mms to several cms depending on amount of fluid contained
- Morphology
  - Flattened synovial sacs not usually visualized on MRI unless distended with fluid
  - Moderate amount of fluid - distended bursa with oval shaped morphology
  - Large amount of fluid distends bursa proximally toward knee joint
  - Semimembranosus tibial collateral ligament bursa - inverted "U" shape (drapes over semimembranosus tendon)

Radiographic Findings
- Radiography
  - Nonspecific soft tissue swelling of medial knee
  - +/- Well-defined medial mass

DDx: Medial Bursitis, Knee

Fluid In Recess	SM Tendinosis	Hemangioma	Meniscal Cyst	Meniscal Cyst

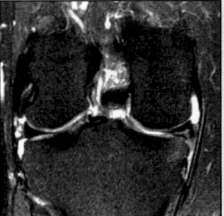 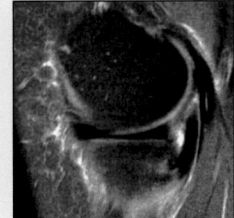 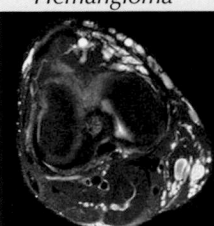 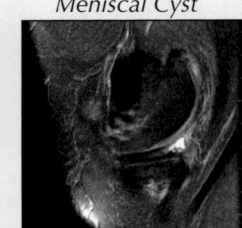 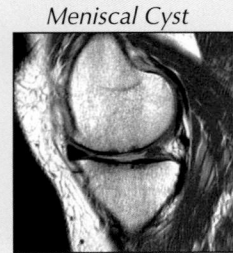

Cor FS PD FSE	Sag FS PD FSE	Ax FS PD FSE	Sag FS PD FSE	Sag PD FSE MR

MEDIAL BURSITIS, KNEE

Key Facts

Terminology
- Synovial lining: Inflammation of the medial bursae of the knee

Imaging Findings
- Best diagnostic clue: Fluid containing mass (fluid signal intensity) in location of a medial bursae
- Flattened synovial sacs not usually visualized on MRI unless distended with fluid

Top Differential Diagnoses
- Meniscal Cyst
- Fluid Distending Normal Meniscal Attachment Recesses
- Hemorrhage between Deep & Superficial Components of MCL in Trauma
- Soft Tissue Cystic Appearing Mass adjacent to Bursa

- MCL Sprain or Stress Response
- Semimembranosus (SM) Tendinosis

Pathology
- Epidemiology: Common; accompanies meniscal tears

Clinical Issues
- Medial to anterior knee pain and well-localized tenderness
- Conservative: Local injection of corticosteroids - good relief and confirmation of diagnosis

Diagnostic Checklist
- FS PD FSE most sensitive to fluid collections and synovial thickening

MR Findings
- T1WI
  - Homogeneous decreased signal intensity mass in characteristic location
  - Associated tendinosis of semimembranosus with SMTCL bursitis
    - Thickening and increased signal intensity of insertion
  - Decreased signal in adjacent bone if reactive edema
  - +/- Meniscal tear
    - Increased signal in substance of meniscus extending to surface
    - Bursitis associated as "reactive" phenomenon
- T2WI
  - Hyperintense fluid distending bursa
  - Hyperintense flattened, oval, or round shaped cystic masses in characteristic locations
  - Hypointense structures if calcified
  - Intermediate signal debris during inflammatory, hemorrhagic or exudative process
  - +/- Rice bodies in patients with rheumatoid arthritis
    - Intermediate to decreased signal "rice" shaped fibrinous bodies
  - +/- Associated tendinosis of semimembranosus
    - Thickening and variable increased signal intensity of insertion
    - +/- Associated bursitis
  - Decreased signal in adjacent bone if reactive edema
- T2* GRE
  - Fluid intensity masses
  - Decreased signal intensity rim if hemorrhagic
- T1 C+
  - +/- Rim enhancement
  - Greater enhancement if longstanding with thickened synovium

Ultrasonographic Findings
- Typically hypo or anechoic mass with through transmission

Imaging Recommendations
- Best imaging tool: MRI

- Protocol advice: T2WI, especially FS PD FSE demonstrates fluid-filled bursa

DIFFERENTIAL DIAGNOSIS

Meniscal Cyst
- +/- Meniscal tear
- SMTCL bursitis commonly mistaken for meniscal cyst (sagittal)
- TCL bursa mimics meniscal cyst (coronal)
- Usually deep to capsule
- Immediately adjacent to meniscus

Fluid Distending Normal Meniscal Attachment Recesses
- Deep to the coronary ligament
- Deep to meniscofemoral attachment
- Lateral meniscus more common, larger recess

Hemorrhage between Deep & Superficial Components of MCL in Trauma
- Appropriate history
- +/- MCL tear
- Frequently indistinguishable

Synovial/Ganglion Cyst
- Ganglion cyst - nonspecific origin
- Synovial cyst - from joint
- +/- Synovial lining
- Variable location
- +/- History of trauma
- Often reflects past effusions (synovial cyst)

Soft Tissue Cystic Appearing Mass adjacent to Bursa
- No demonstrable connection to bursa
- Different anatomic location
- MRI useful for differentiation
- Varices may mimic distended bursa

Meniscal Tear
- Associated bursitis common

MEDIAL BURSITIS, KNEE

- See reactive edema "hyperemia" in tibia and femur commonly
- Increased signal on short TE sequences within meniscus extending to surface

MCL Sprain or Stress Response
- Edema within, around ligament
- +/- Osteoarthritis (OA)
- Acute traumatic event
- Chronic repetitive microtrauma

Semimembranosus (SM) Tendinosis
- Thickening and variable increased signal intensity of insertion on all pulse sequences
- +/- Bursitis (common)
- Chronic repetitive microtrauma

PATHOLOGY

General Features
- General path comments: Fluid distending normal meniscal attachment recesses mimic bursitis, especially TCL bursitis
- Etiology: Chronic frictional trauma or overuse centered upon bursal glide plane results in inflammation of bursa
- Epidemiology: Common; accompanies meniscal tears

Gross Pathologic & Surgical Features
- Synovial lined bursal sac
- Variable degrees of thickening of the lining
- Variable amounts of fluid

Microscopic Features
- Thickened synovial lining with variable degree of inflammatory infiltration
- Rice bodies especially in bursitis associated with rheumatoid arthritis
- Variable degrees of hemorrhagic byproducts
- Exudate in case of infectious bursitis

Staging, Grading or Classification Criteria
- No grading criteria described for imaging

CLINICAL ISSUES

Presentation
- Most common signs/symptoms
  - Medial to anterior knee pain and well-localized tenderness
  - Fullness, ranging from joint line to extend approx. 5 cm distally (medial portion of knee to anterior tibia)
- Clinical profile
  - Overweight, middle-aged or elderly women
  - Medial to anterior knee pain
  - Localized tenderness
  - OA of knee common and may mask presentation of bursitis
  - Athletes - overuse phenomenon

Demographics
- Age: Middle age or elderly

Natural History & Prognosis
- Presents insidiously or after athletic activity
- +/- Resolution with cessation of activities that led to condition
- Conservative treatment usually successful

Treatment
- Conservative: Local injection of corticosteroids - good relief and confirmation of diagnosis
- Surgical extirpation for
  - Recalcitrant cases
  - Infectious bursitis
- Complications
  - Tendon weakening, +/- tear, if corticosteroid injected into bursa and onto tendon

DIAGNOSTIC CHECKLIST

Consider
- In overuse
  - Consider mimickers such as
    - Meniscal cyst
    - Fluid in normal joint recesses
    - Hematoma

Image Interpretation Pearls
- FS PD FSE most sensitive to fluid collections and synovial thickening

SELECTED REFERENCES

1. Koh WL et al: Clinics in diagnostic imaging (77). Pes anserine bursitis. Singapore Med J 43(9):485-91, 2002
2. Uson J et al: Pes anserinus tendino-bursitis: What are we talking about? Scand J Rheumatol 29(3):184-6, 2000
3. Kerlan RK et al: Tibial collateral ligament bursitis. Am J Sports Med 16(4):344-6, 1998
4. Handy JR et al: Anserine bursitis: A brief review. South Med J 90(4):376-7, 1997
5. Rothstein CP et al: Semimembranosus-tibial collateral ligament bursitis: MR imaging findings. AJR 166(4):875-7, 1996
6. Cohen SE et al: Anserine bursitis and non-insuln dependent diabetes mellitus. J Rheumatol 24(11): 2162-5, 1995
7. Forbes JR et al: Acute pes anserine bursitis: MR imaging. Radiology 194(2):525-7, 1995
8. Zeiss J et al: Chronic bursitis presenting as a mass in the pes anserine bursa: MR diagnosis. J Comput Assist Tomogr 17(1):137-40, 1993

MEDIAL BURSITIS, KNEE

Typical

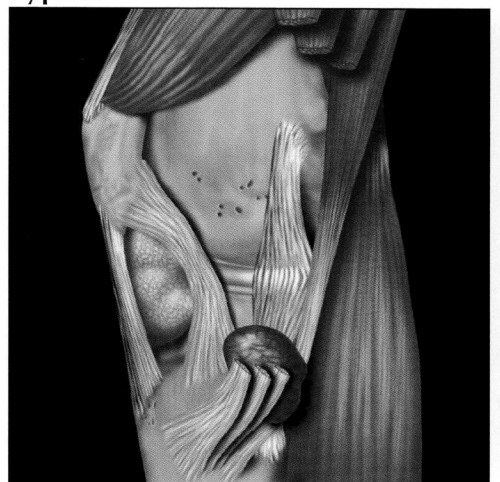
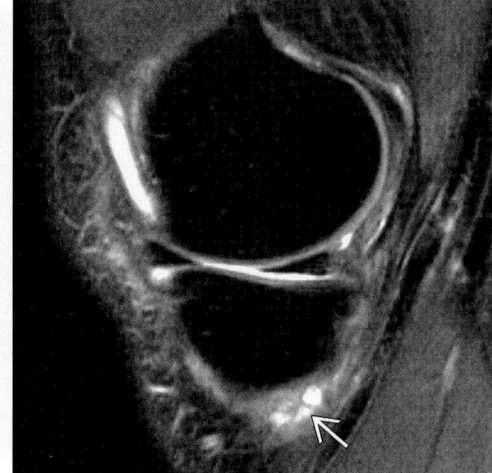

(Left) Sagittal graphic demonstrates distention of the pes anserinus bursa indicating inflammation. *(Right)* Sagittal FS PD FSE MR shows a small amount of fluid within the pes anserinus bursa in a patient with pain approximately 2 cm below joint line (arrow).

Typical

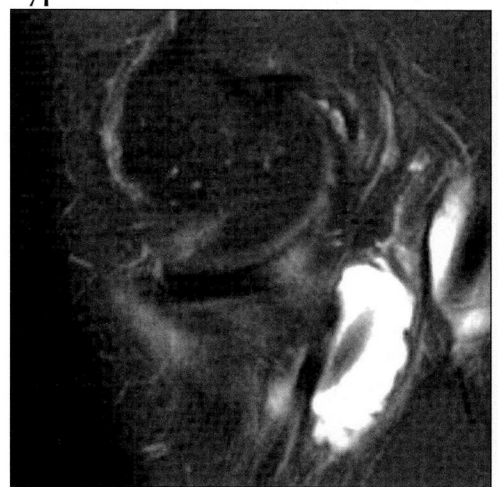
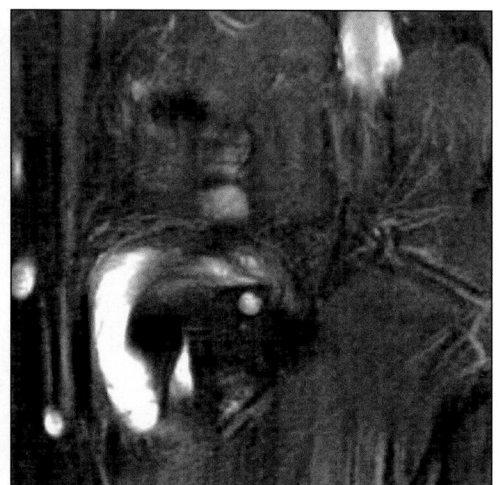

(Left) Sagittal FS PD FSE MR shows the typical appearance of semimembranosus tibial collateral ligament bursitis. The bursa has been described as "U" or "7" shaped in the sagittal plane. There is a small amount of fluid within a popliteal cyst. *(Right)* Coronal FS PD FSE MR at the posterior aspect of the joint shows the distended bursa.

Typical

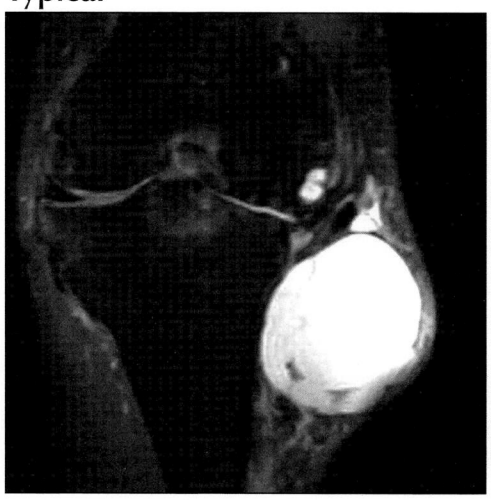
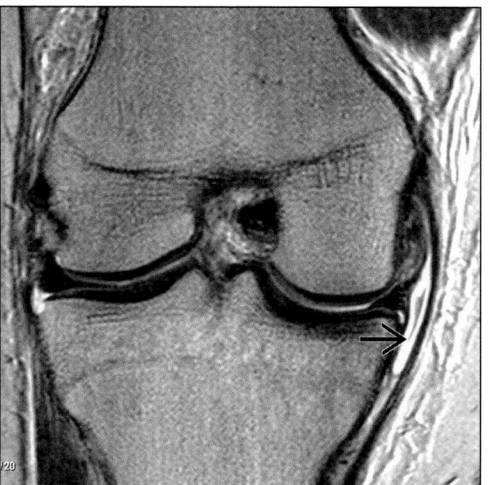

(Left) Coronal FS PD FSE MR shows a large distended pes anserinus bursa in a severe case of bursitis. A mass was palpable. *(Right)* Coronal T2 FSE MR shows TCL bursitis with thickened synovial tissue (arrow).

LATERAL COLLATERAL LIGAMENT (LCL) TEAR

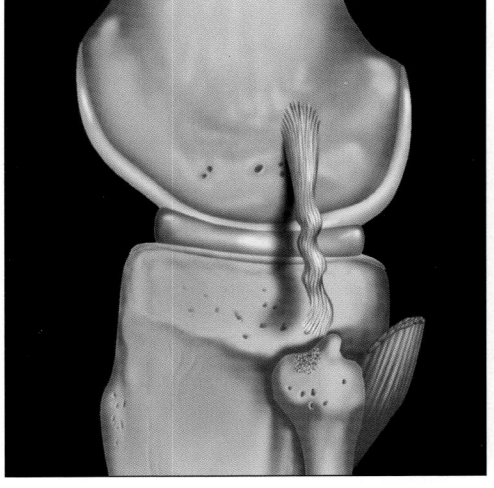

Sagittal graphic shows a tear of the distal aspect of the lateral collateral ligament with mild retraction of the ligament proximally.

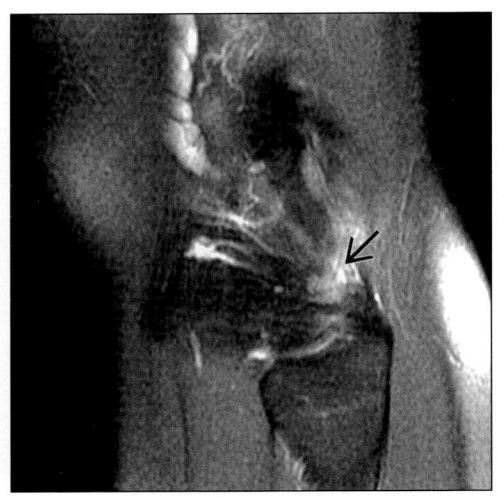

Sagittal FS PD FSE MR shows a tear of the lateral collateral ligament (arrow).

TERMINOLOGY

Abbreviations and Synonyms
- Lateral collateral ligament (LCL) tear, fibular collateral ligament (FCL) tear, FCL = LCL

Definitions
- Tear of the lateral collateral ligament after varus +/- external rotation stress

IMAGING FINDINGS

General Features
- Best diagnostic clue: Discontinuous LCL fibers +/- thickening, hyperintense on FS PD FSE or T2WI
- Location
  - Extends from lateral femoral condyle to insertion with the biceps femoris on the fibular head
    - Injury usually occurs at the proximal origin
- Size: Normal size 5-7 cm
- Morphology
  - Alteration in the linear shape of normal ligament
  - Relevant anatomy
    - Normal ligament is extracapsular and free from meniscal attachment

Radiographic Findings
- Radiography

  - +/- Associated fracture of femur or tibia
  - +/- Effusion

CT Findings
- NECT
  - Associated fractures seen and characterized
    - Fibular head, adjacent tibia, medial or lateral femur
    - +/- Effusion

MR Findings
- T1WI
  - Intermediate signal intensity with disorganized appearing ligament
  - Typical bone injuries appear as hypointense edematous regions
    - +/- Fracture (fx)
  - Effusions - hypointense
- T2WI
  - Discontinuous fibers +/- thickening and increased signal intensity on FS PD FSE
  - Increased signal intensity bone injury
    - Impaction bone trabecular injuries of medial femur and tibia indicating varus injury
    - +/- Decreased signal intensity fx line
  - Injury to other posterolateral ligamentous and capsular supporting structures

---

DDx: Lateral Collateral Ligament (LCL) Tear

Arcuate and LCL	PCL Popliteus	Lat Tib Plt Fx	Lat Men Tear	Osteochondral Inj

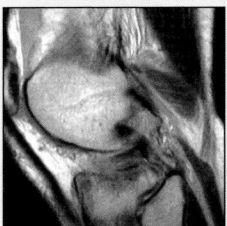 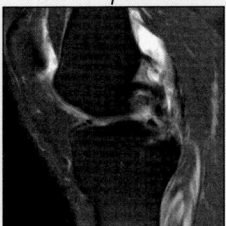 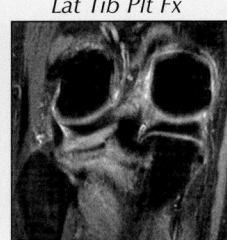 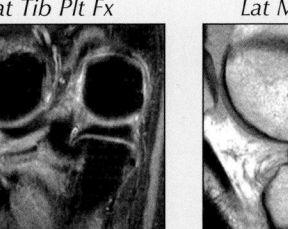 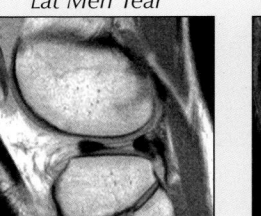 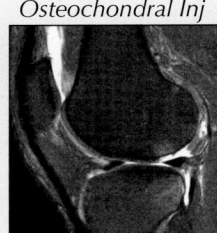

Sag PD FSE MR	Sag FS PD FSE	Cor FS PD FSE	Sag PD FSE MR	Sag FS PD FSE

LATERAL COLLATERAL LIGAMENT (LCL) TEAR

Key Facts

Terminology
- Tear of the lateral collateral ligament after varus +/- external rotation stress

Imaging Findings
- Best diagnostic clue: Discontinuous LCL fibers +/- thickening, hyperintense on FS PD FSE or T2WI
- Protocol advice: Best seen on FS PD FSE or T2WI

Top Differential Diagnoses
- Lateral Bone Trabecular/Capsular Injuries
- Isolated cases of LCL injury are rare
- Lateral Gastrocnemius Insertional Tear/Tendinosis
- Popliteus Insertional Tendinosis/Tear

Pathology
- Rarely torn in isolation

- Associated with tear of other posterolateral corner structures
- Ligament disrupted by varus stress on the knee (a blow to the medial aspect of the knee)

Clinical Issues
- Posterolateral pain
- Posterolateral rotatory instability if combined with injury to other posterolateral supporting structures
- Effusion indicates associated intraarticular pathology
- Healing ligament scars and stability gradually restored unless major posterolateral corner disruption

Diagnostic Checklist
- Damage to other posterolateral corner ligaments as isolated LCL tears are unusual

---

- Arcuate complex, biceps femoris tendon, popliteus tendon, popliteofibular & fabellofibular ligaments, and posterolateral capsule
  - Discontinuous fibers +/- thickening
  - Increase in signal intensity
  - Visualized on FS PD FSE to T2WIs
  - Hemorrhage = diffuse increased signal intensity
  - Associated tears of the iliotibial band and popliteus tendon (posterolateral corner)
    - Discontinuous fibers +/- hyperintense
- T2* GRE
  - Associated fractures seen as increased signal line in acute stage
    - Not sensitive for the identification of bone edema
    - Sensitive for fracture morphology

Imaging Recommendations
- Best imaging tool: MRI
- Protocol advice: Best seen on FS PD FSE or T2WI

DIFFERENTIAL DIAGNOSIS

Lateral Bone Trabecular/Capsular Injuries
- Isolated cases of LCL injury are rare
- +/- Posterolateral tendon ligament tears
  - Popliteus strain/tear
  - Arcuate complex sprain/tear

Lateral Gastrocnemius Insertional Tear/Tendinosis
- Chronic repetitive microtrauma
- Pain at insertion site
- Thickening +/- increased signal intensity on all pulse sequences
- FS PD FSE images in sagittal plane

Popliteus Insertional Tendinosis/Tear
- Acute trauma
- Chronic repetitive microtrauma
- Thickening +/- increased signal intensity on all pulse sequences
- Visualized on FS PD FSE

Lateral Meniscal Tear
- Pain with twisting movements
- Visualized on MRI as increased signal intensity linear region on short TE sequences
- Tear at posterior peripheral aspect may mimic LCL sprain
- Acutely after trauma
- +/- Meniscal cyst

Posterior Cruciate Ligament (PCL) Tear
- Associated with posterolateral corner injury
- Failure of recognition of associated injury may lead to osteoarthritis (OA), dysfunction
- Seen as discontinuous fibers or thickening with an increase in signal intensity on all pulse sequence
- Visualized on FS PD FSE sagittal images

Lateral Tibial Plateau Fracture (Lat Tib Plt Fx)
- Depressed vs. nondepressed
- Bumper Fx
- Associated with lateral meniscus tear, +/- capsular injury
- +/- LCL sprain
- Osteochondral injury

PATHOLOGY

General Features
- General path comments
  - Rarely torn in isolation
  - Associated with tear of other posterolateral corner structures
  - Lateral collateral ligament - primary restraint to varus angulation
  - Primary restraint to external rotation in the posterolateral complex
  - LCL resists internal rotation forces
  - Transecting LCL with either ACL or PCL results in large increase in varus instability
- Etiology
  - Ligament disrupted by varus stress on the knee (a blow to the medial aspect of the knee)

LATERAL COLLATERAL LIGAMENT (LCL) TEAR

○ Varus force + full knee extension is associated with LCL and PCL involvement and straight lateral instability
- Straight lateral instability = disruption of all lateral ligaments, the PCL +/- the ACL
- Epidemiology
  ○ Isolated LCL injuries - 2% or knee ligament injuries
  ○ Associated LCL injury - 4% or knee ligament injuries
- Associated abnormalities
  ○ Injury to other posterolateral corner structures
  ○ Fracture of proximal fibula

Gross Pathologic & Surgical Features
- Thickened, partially torn or completely torn ligament

Microscopic Features
- Degeneration, partial or complete rupture
- Variable amounts of hemorrhage and inflammatory cells

Staging, Grading or Classification Criteria
- General MRI grading of ligamentous disruptions
  ○ Grade I: Mild sprain (stretching of ligament)
  ○ Grade II: Intermediate grade
  ○ Grade III: High grade to complete disruption (instability with > 10 mm of medial joint opening)

CLINICAL ISSUES

Presentation
- Most common signs/symptoms
  ○ Posterolateral pain
  ○ Buckling into hyperextension with weightbearing
  ○ Varus instability
  ○ Posterolateral rotatory instability if combined with injury to other posterolateral supporting structures
  ○ +/- Cruciate and lateral meniscus tears
    - Pain with clinical meniscal testing
- Clinical profile
  ○ Seen in sports activities: Football, soccer, tennis
  ○ Motor vehicle accident, motorcycle accident
  ○ Adduction or varus stress test with knee in 30 degrees of flexion (no resistance from secondary restraints)
  ○ Effusion indicates associated intraarticular pathology
  ○ Varus alignment
  ○ Medial thrust on weightbearing
  ○ +/- Injury to peroneal nerve

Demographics
- Age: Typically young active patient
- Gender: No predilection

Natural History & Prognosis
- Healing ligament scars and stability gradually restored unless major posterolateral corner disruption
- Stage 1: Inflammation
  ○ 3 days of injury
  ○ Fibroblasts-type III collagen
- Stage 2: Repair and regeneration
  ○ 6 weeks after injury
  ○ Type I collagen replaces type III collagen
- Stage 3: Remodeling
  ○ Continues for up to and > 1 year after injury

- Injury characteristics that slow healing
  ○ Grade III sprains heal < grades I and II
  ○ LCL tears heal more slowly than MCL tears

Treatment
- Conservative
  ○ Isolated tears of the LCL are treated conservatively (closed)
    - Similar to treatment of most MCL tears
  ○ Splint in full extension for two weeks
  ○ Motion and weightbearing as tolerated afterward
- Surgical
  ○ Open fixation
    - Cases where cruciate abnormalities or extensive posterolateral corner injuries are additionally involved

DIAGNOSTIC CHECKLIST

Consider
- Damage to other posterolateral corner ligaments as isolated LCL tears are unusual

Image Interpretation Pearls
- FS PD FSE sensitive for detecting tears

SELECTED REFERENCES

1. Twaddle BC et al: Knee dislocations: Where are the lesions? A prospective evaluation of surgical findings in 63 cases. J Orthop Trauma 17(3):198-202, 2003
2. Huang GS et al: Avulsion fracture of the head of the fibula (the "arcuate" sign): MR imaging findings predictive of injuries to the posterolateral ligaments and posterior cruciate ligament. AJR 180(2):381-7, 2003
3. Munshi M et al: MR Imaging, MR arthrography, and specimen correlation of the posterolateral corner of the knee: An anatomic study. AJR 180(4):1095-101, 2003
4. Krudwig WK et al: Posterolateral aspect and stability of the knee joint. Posterolateral instability and effect of isolated and combined posterolateral reconstruction on knee stability: A biomechanical study. Knee Surg Sports Traumatol Arthrosc 10(2):91-5, 2002
5. Fitzgerald R et al: Knee ligaments injuries: Epidemiology, mechanism, diagnosis and natural history. Orthopaedics. St. Louis, MO, Mosby, 564-76, 2002
6. Chen CH et al: Lateral collateral ligament reconstruction using quadriceps tendon-patellar bone autograft with bioscrew fixation. Arthroscopy 17(5):551-4, 2001
7. Meister BR et al: Anatomy and kinematics of the lateral collateral ligament of the knee. Am J Sports Med 28(6):869-78, 2000
8. Harfe DT et al: Elongation patterns of the collateral ligaments of the human knee. Clin Biomech (Bristol, Avon) 13(3):163-75, 1998

LATERAL COLLATERAL LIGAMENT (LCL) TEAR

IMAGE GALLERY

Typical

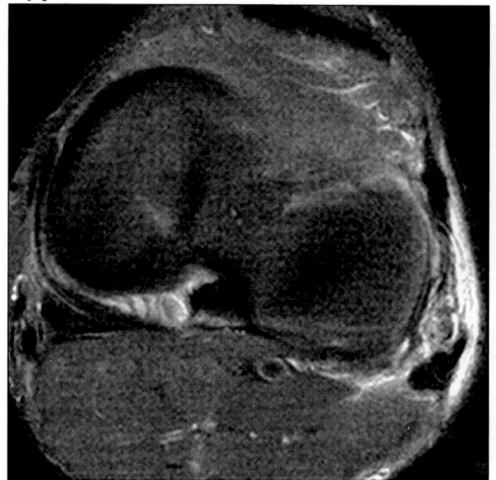 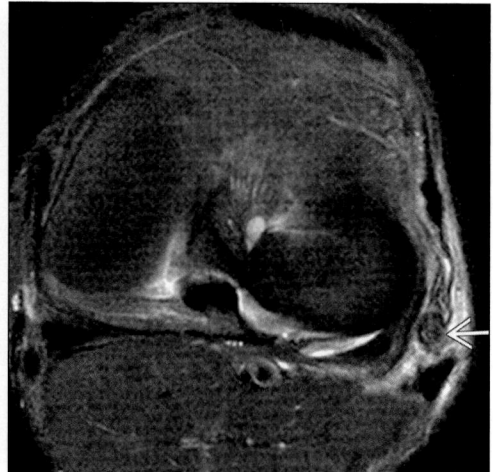

(Left) Axial FS PD FSE MR shows the torn LCL deep to the conjoined tendon. *(Right)* Axial FS PD FSE MR adjacent image shows the thickened edematous LCL *(arrow)*.

Typical

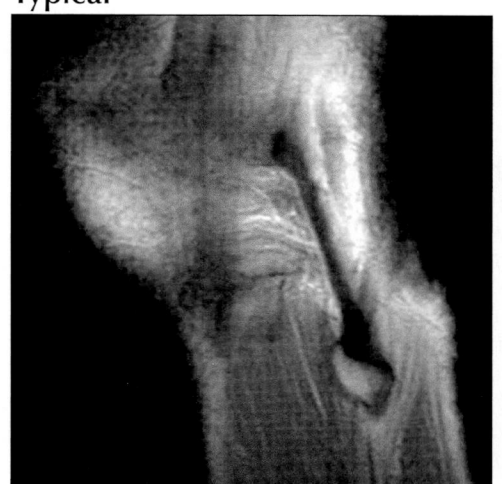 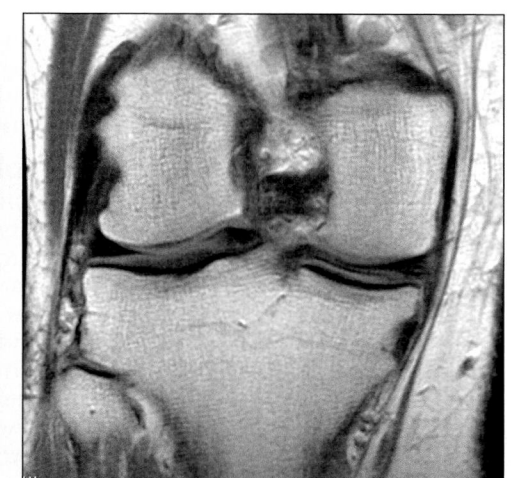

(Left) Sagittal PD FSE MR shows a normal LCL. *(Right)* Coronal PD FSE MR shows a normal LCL.

Typical

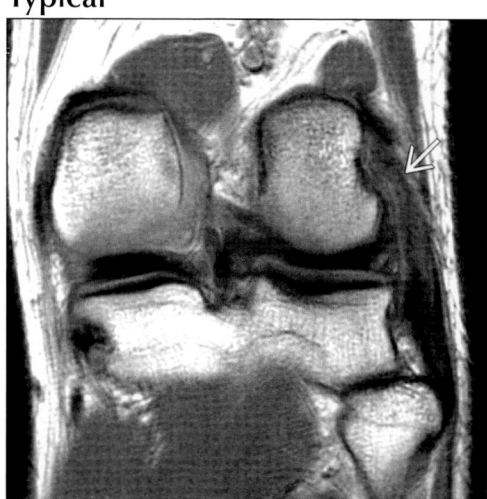 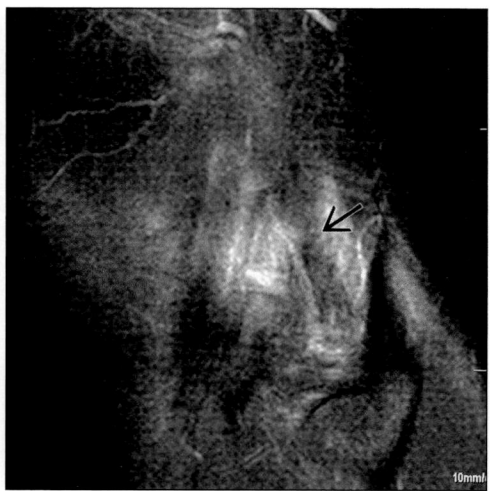

(Left) Coronal PD FSE MR shows a grade III sprain *(arrow)* of the proximal aspect of the LCL. *(Right)* Sagittal FS PD FSE MR shows a mid and distal aspect LCL tear *(arrow)*.

POSTEROLATERAL COMPLEX INJURIES

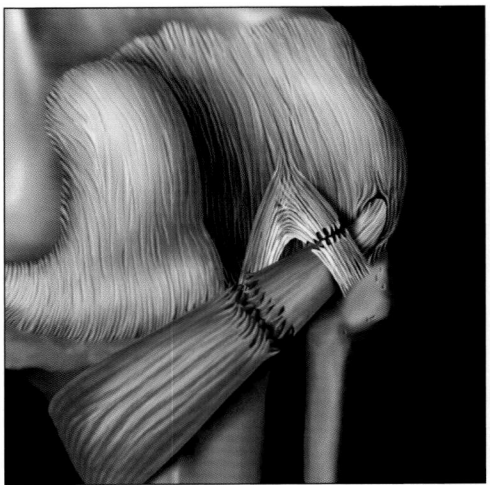

Coronal oblique graphic shows a tear of the lateral aspect of the arcuate ligament and tear of the popliteus muscle.

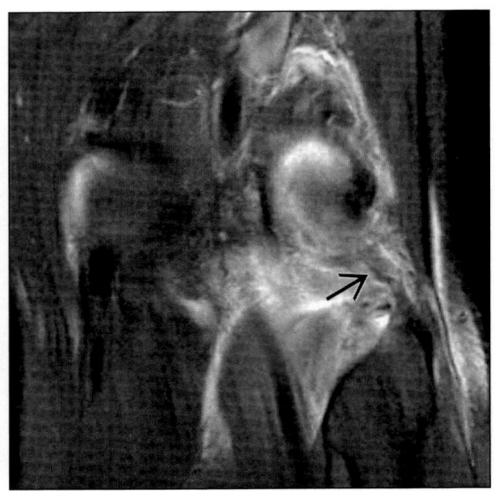

Coronal FS PD FSE MR shows a sprain of the popliteofibular ligament/arcuate complex (arrow) and surrounding edema.

TERMINOLOGY

Abbreviations and Synonyms

- Posterolateral corner injuries (PLCI), posterolateral complex (PLC) injuries, posterolateral instability (PLI), arcuate complex injuries

Definitions

- Sprain/strain of the supporting structures of the posterolateral corner of the knee
  - Arcuate ligament, medial & lateral limbs
  - Popliteal tendon
  - Lateral (fibular) collateral ligament
  - Fabellofibular ligament
  - Popliteofibular ligament
  - Posterolateral joint capsule; many of the ligaments represent thickenings of the posterolateral capsule

IMAGING FINDINGS

General Features

- Best diagnostic clue
  - Discontinuous ligament +/- tendon fibers + edema in the posterolateral aspect of the knee
    - Posttraumatic, best seen on FS PD FSE
- Location: Adjacent to tibiofibular joint

- Size: Tear of structures varies from grade I sprain/strain to grade III "blowout"
- Morphology: Disrupted fibers ranging from discrete tear to markedly irregular ligamentous thickened fibers
- Varus overload with variable degrees of rotation

Radiographic Findings

- Radiography
  - +/- Fractures
    - Posterolateral tibia
    - Fibular styloid
    - Sulcus terminalis - lateral femoral condyle
    - Segond fracture - lateral tibia avulsion fx
    - Posterior tibia at notch at posterior cruciate ligament insertion
    - Reverse Segond medial tibia avulsion fx (rare with posterolateral corner (PLC) injury)
    - = Fractures seen with anterior cruciate ligament (ACL), and posterior cruciate ligament (PCL) tears
  - Effusion
  - Posterolateral soft tissue swelling

CT Findings

- NECT
  - Associated fractures assessed and characterized
  - Reconstructions used in comminuted fracture cases

MR Findings

- T1WI

DDx: Posterolateral Complex Injuries

ITB Friction	Popliteus Hiatus	Fibular Fracture	Fibular Fracture	Popliteus Strain

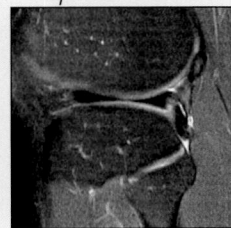 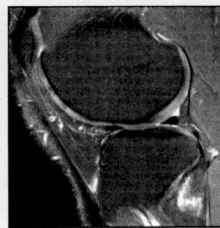 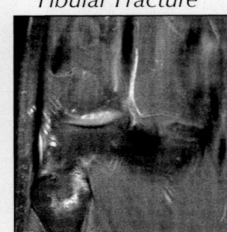 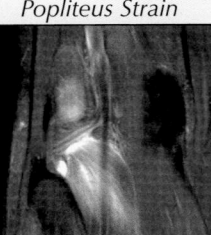

Cor FS PD FSE	Sag FS PD FSE	Sag FS PD FSE	Cor FS PD FSE	Cor FS PD FSE

POSTEROLATERAL COMPLEX INJURIES

Key Facts

Terminology
- Sprain/strain of the supporting structures of the posterolateral corner of the knee

Imaging Findings
- Discontinuous ligament +/- tendon fibers + edema in the posterolateral aspect of the knee
- Fibular head avulsion fracture diagnostic of posterolateral complex injuries

Top Differential Diagnoses
- Lateral Meniscus Tear
- Iliotibial Band Friction Syndrome
- Popliteus Hiatus
- Fracture without PLC Ligament/Tendon Involvement
- Popliteus/Biceps Strain

Pathology
- Leg internal rotation valgus stress: Typical ACL mechanism
- Direct blow to the tibia with the knee flexed or extended
- Associated abnormalities: Associated with cruciate ligament tears: ACL > PCL

Clinical Issues
- Posterolateral pain
- Buckling in hyper-extension with weight bearing and variable instability
- Combined PCL and posterolateral complex injuries are often missed at initial clinical presentation

Diagnostic Checklist
- Use FS PD FSE in all three planes (sagittal = key plane)

- o Complete rupture - decreased signal intensity and discontinuous fibers
  - +/- Thickening of attached ligament portions
- o Partial tear (grade I and II sprains) - variable thickening, decreased signal intensity some continuous fibers intact
- o Fractures - hypointense linear signal abnormality
  - Surrounded by hypointense edema
- T2WI
  - o Increased signal intensity within the structures of the arcuate complex
    - +/- Thickening of attached ligament portions
    - Hyperintense fluid posterior to popliteus tendon sheath
  - o Complete rupture - increased signal intensity and discontinuous fibers
    - +/- Thickening of attached ligament portions
  - o Partial tear (grade I and II sprains) - variable thickening, increased signal intensity some continuous fibers intact
  - o Fractures: Decreased signal intensity fracture lines surrounded by hyperintense edema
    - Assessed on FS PD FSE/STIR
    - Involve posterolateral tibia, sulcus terminalis, Segond and reverse Segond, lateral tibial plateau fracture
    - Other knee fractures possible
  - o Soft tissue edema best assessed at level of and surrounding fibular head
  - o ACL/PCL sprain
    - Variable thickening, increased signal intensity +/- continuous fibers
    - Traumatic history, appropriate mechanism of injury
- STIR
  - o Increased signal intensity of the posterolateral corner structures
  - o Fractures: Decreased signal intensity fracture lines surrounded by hyperintense edema
  - o Sensitive for edema but less signal than FS PD FSE
- Fibular head avulsion fracture diagnostic of posterolateral complex injuries

Imaging Recommendations
- Best imaging tool: MRI
- Protocol advice: FS PD FSE or STIR images; FS PD FSE - increased signal, optimized spatial resolution

DIFFERENTIAL DIAGNOSIS

Lateral Meniscus Tear
- No injury to capsule, ligaments or tendons
- Suggestive clinical testing
- Increased signal intensity on short TE sequence extending to articular surface
- +/- Cyst

Iliotibial Band Friction Syndrome
- Chronic frictional trauma iliotibial band and lateral femoral condyle
  - o Increased signal intensity between the two structures
  - o FS PD weighted images most sensitive
  - o +/- Thickening and increased signal intensity within iliotibial band (ITB)
- Suggestive history
- Anterolateral pain

Popliteus Hiatus
- Normal anatomy
- Popliteus tendon sheath pierces inferior capsule medial aspect/superior capsule lateral aspect
  - o Behind lateral meniscus
  - o Contiguous with joint
  - o +/- Fluid
- May be mistaken for meniscal tear/ligament tear

Fracture without PLC Ligament/Tendon Involvement
- Posterior lateral corner
- Unusual, typically associated with ligamentous/capsular/tendon injuries
- Decreased signal intensity line surrounded by hyperintense edema on T2WI

POSTEROLATERAL COMPLEX INJURIES

Popliteus/Biceps Strain
- Antagonist force on contracted muscle
- Thickened, increased signal tendon and/or muscle belly on T2WI
- FS PD FSE used to identify edema

PATHOLOGY

General Features
- General path comments
  - Posterolateral complex includes
    - LCL
    - Popliteal tendon
    - Arcuate ligament
    - Popliteofibular ligament
    - Fabellofibular ligament
    - Posterolateral capsule
    - Lateral head of the gastrocnemius muscle (also part of the arcuate ligament complex as defined by Baker)
    - The biceps femoris tendon + ITB although not usually listed as components of complex contribute to stability of lateral and posterolateral knee
  - The arcuate complex stabilizes posterolateral aspect of knee against varus stress + external rotation
  - Isolated lateral collateral ligament injury is less common than medial collateral ligament injury
  - Lateral collateral ligament joins tendon of the biceps femoris - conjoined tendon
    - Rarely injured alone without injury to the remainder of the PLC
- Etiology
  - Leg internal rotation valgus stress: Typical ACL mechanism
  - Direct blow to the tibia with the knee flexed or extended
  - Rotational injury +/- cruciate ligament disruption and/or posterolateral instability
  - Varus stress
  - Noncontact hyperextension is the mechanism for isolated posterolateral rotatory instability
  - Blow to anteromedial tibia in knee extension results in arcuate ligament disruption and PLI
- Epidemiology
  - Overall common injury in athletics
    - Especially snow skiing, soccer, football, tennis
- Associated abnormalities: Associated with cruciate ligament tears: ACL > PCL

Gross Pathologic & Surgical Features
- Tear of the structures of the PLC with variable amounts of hemorrhage

Microscopic Features
- Microscopic and macroscopic tearing of the posterolateral corner structures
- Variable amounts: Hemorrhage + inflammatory cells

Staging, Grading or Classification Criteria
- Ligament injury
  - Grade I: Pain without instability, minimal tear
  - Grade II: Partial tear with some instability (50% or greater)
  - Grade III: Complete disruption
- PLI types
  - A = increased external rotation without varus instability (injury to popliteofibular ligament and popliteus tendon)
  - B = increased external rotation + moderate varus laxity (injury to popliteofibular ligament, popliteus tendon and LCL)
  - C = increased external rotation plus complete varus laxity (injury to popliteofibular ligament, popliteus tendon, LCL, lateral capsule and cruciate ligaments)

CLINICAL ISSUES

Presentation
- Most common signs/symptoms
  - Posterolateral pain
  - Buckling in hyper-extension with weight bearing and variable instability
  - +/- Cruciate ligament instability
- Clinical profile
  - Posttraumatic abnormality secondary to rotational mechanisms of injury described above
  - Combined PCL and posterolateral complex injuries are often missed at initial clinical presentation

Demographics
- Age: Children & adults, active adolescents & adults more common
- Gender: M > F

Natural History & Prognosis
- Grade III - posterolateral rotatory instability can develop

Treatment
- Ligament & tendon disruptions treated with repair
- Cruciate ligament disruption associated with PCL injury - cruciate is repaired to prevent instability

DIAGNOSTIC CHECKLIST

Consider
- This injury is in association with cruciate ligament tears

Image Interpretation Pearls
- Use FS PD FSE in all three planes (sagittal = key plane)

SELECTED REFERENCES

1. Fitzgerald R et al: Orthopaedics. Knee ligament injuries: Epidemiology, mechanism, diagnosis, and natural history. St. Louis MO, Saunders, 619-35, 2003
2. Huang GS et al: Avulsion fracture of the head of the fibula (the "arcuate" sign): MR imaging findings predictive of injuries to the posterolateral ligaments and posterior cruciate ligament. AJR 180(2):381-7, 2003
3. Munshi M et al: MR Imaging, MR Arthrography, and specimen correlation of the posterolateral corner of the knee: An Anatomic Study. AJR 180(4):1095-1101, 2003

POSTEROLATERAL COMPLEX INJURIES

IMAGE GALLERY

Variant

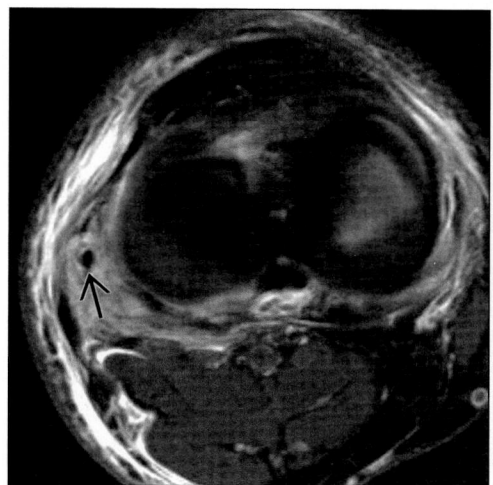
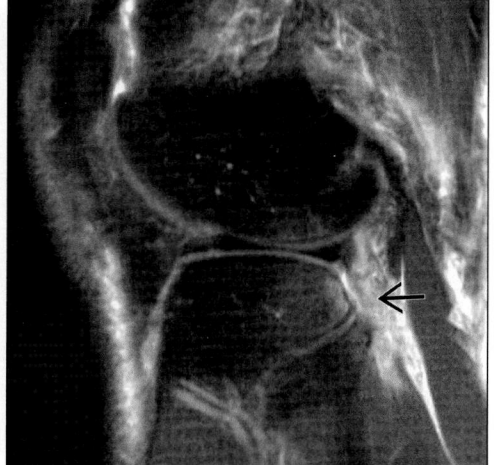

(Left) Axial FS PD FSE MR shows a sprain of the posterolateral corner structures after a fall while snow skiing. Note the intact (at this axial level) fibular collateral ligament (arrow). *(Right)* Sagittal FS PD FSE MR shows the sprain of the posterolateral corner structures including a grade III sprain of the arcuate complex (arrow).

Typical

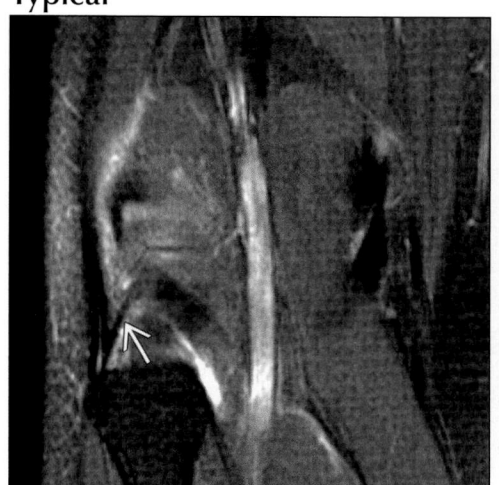
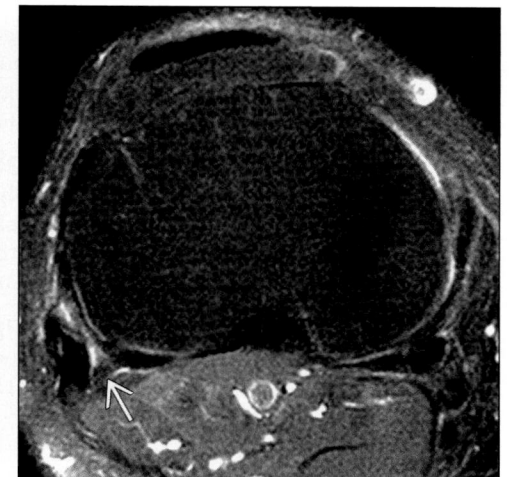

(Left) Coronal FS PD FSE MR shows a normal popliteofibular ligament extending from the fibular styloid to the popliteus tendon (arrow). *(Right)* Axial FS PD FSE MR shows the normal anatomy of the posterolateral corner. Note the lack of edema and observe the popliteofibular ligament (arrow) extending obliquely from the conjoined tendon medially to the popliteus tendon.

Typical

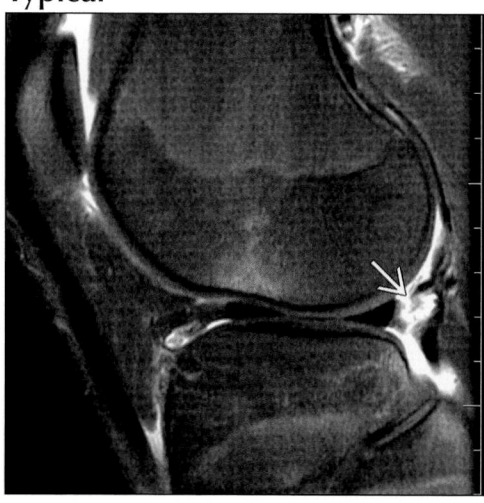
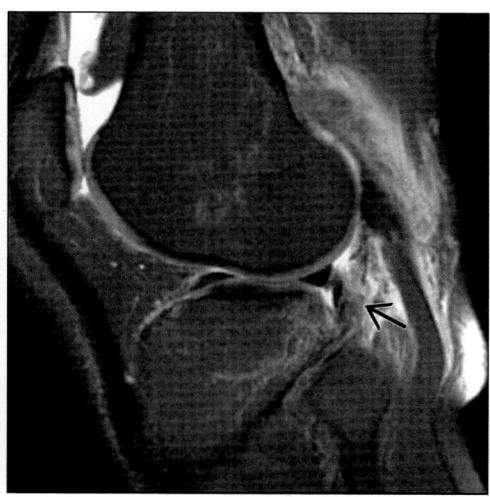

(Left) Sagittal FS PD FSE MR shows a torn superior fascicle of the posterior horn of the lateral meniscus (arrow). *(Right)* Sagittal FS PD FSE MR shows a lateral head of the gastrocnemius strain and sprain of the posterolateral corner ligaments (arrow).

ILIOTIBIAL BAND SYNDROME

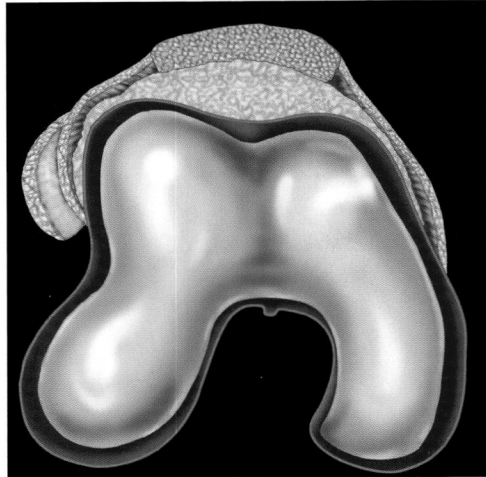

Axial graphic shows edema interposed between the iliotibial band and lateral femoral condyle. Associated thickening of the iliotibial band may be present.

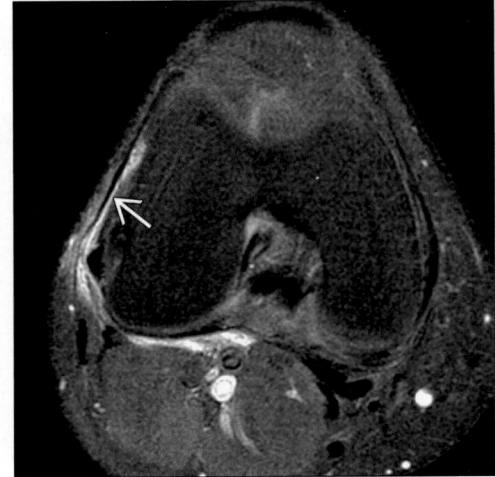

Axial FS PD FSE MR shows hyperintense edema (arrow) between iliotibial band and lateral femoral condyle in a runner with lateral pain and suspected lateral meniscal tear.

TERMINOLOGY

Abbreviations and Synonyms
- Iliotibial friction syndrome, iliotibial band (ITB) syndrome, ITB friction

Definitions
- Inflammatory overuse disorder affecting soft tissues caused by chronic frictional trauma
  - Interposed between iliotibial band and lateral femoral condyle (LFC)

IMAGING FINDINGS

General Features
- Best diagnostic clue
  - Increased signal intensity within soft tissues interposed between iliotibial band and lateral femoral condyle on T2WI
    - Coronal and axial plane
    - History of running activity helpful
- Location
  - Lateral aspect of knee joint
  - Soft tissues interposed between
    - ITB and lateral femoral condyle, ITB itself, lateral condyle and lateral synovial recess
- Size

- Subjective thickening of the ITB
  - No specific size criteria established
- Thickening typically adjacent to insertion on tibia
- Morphology: Normal to thickened ITB, +/- fraying and longitudinal partial tearing

Radiographic Findings
- Radiography
  - Nonspecific soft tissue swelling interposed between ITB and LFC
  - Usually negative

MR Findings
- T1WI: Hypointense edema in soft tissues interposed between ITB and LFC
- T2WI
  - Increased signal intensity within soft tissues interposed between iliotibial band and lateral femoral condyle
    - = Edema
    - On T2WIs and FS PD FSE sequence
    - Best seen in coronal and axial plane
- STIR: Sensitive to underlying subchondral edema of lateral femoral condyle
- T2* GRE
  - Hyperintense soft tissues interposed between the iliotibial band and lateral femoral condyle
    - Coronal and axial plane
- +/- Thickened ITB

DDx: Iliotibial Band Syndrome

Infrapat Bursitis	LTPl Fx	Meniscal Cyst	Segond Fx	Ex Lat Pressure
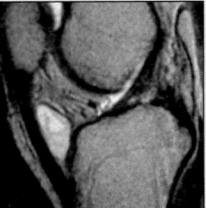	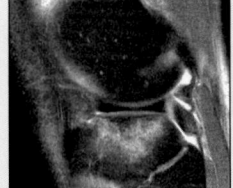	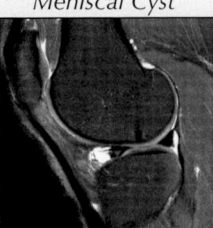	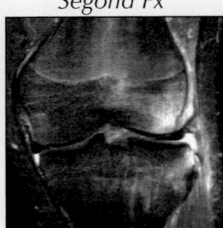	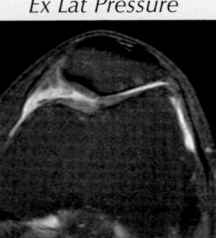
Sag T2WI MR	Sag FS PD FSE	Sag FS PD FSE	Cor FS PD FSE	Ax FS PD FSE

ILIOTIBIAL BAND SYNDROME

Key Facts

Terminology
- Inflammatory overuse disorder affecting soft tissues caused by chronic frictional trauma

Imaging Findings
- Increased signal intensity within soft tissues interposed between iliotibial band and lateral femoral condyle on T2WI
- Protocol advice: FS PD FSE in coronal and axial planes

Top Differential Diagnoses
- Large Joint Effusion Distending Lateral Synovial Recess
- Lateral Meniscus Tear/Cyst
- Lateral Collateral Ligament (LCL) Injuries
- Excessive Lateral Pressure Syndrome (Ex Lat Pressure)

Pathology
- Lateral synovial recess of the knee can be visualized arthroscopically
- Typically not inflamed or distended with fluid unless ITB friction syndrome is present
- Chronic frictional trauma when ITB rubs on outer aspect of the lateral femoral condyle

Clinical Issues
- Most common signs/symptoms: Patients present with anterolateral knee pain at the level of ITB
- Responds to conservative therapy

Diagnostic Checklist
- Consider when history suggests lateral meniscal tear in athlete

---

- Lateral synovial recess of knee may contain fluid and findings of synovitis

Imaging Recommendations
- Best imaging tool: MRI
- Protocol advice: FS PD FSE in coronal and axial planes

DIFFERENTIAL DIAGNOSIS

Large Joint Effusion Distending Lateral Synovial Recess
- Associated with synovitis
- May be posttraumatic
- +/- Hemorrhage
- +/- Osteoarthritis
- Hyperintense on T2WI

Lateral Meniscus Tear/Cyst
- Suggestive clinical examination symptoms
- Antecedent trauma
- MRI diagnostic
- Tear often filled with fluid
  - Hyperintense on T2WI
- Anterior horn/body

Lateral Collateral Ligament (LCL) Injuries
- Posttraumatic
- Pain with stress on injured structures
- Varus stress injury or complex twisting injury
- Hyperintense on T2WI

Popliteus Tendinosis
- Pain during external rotation
- May be posttraumatic or often due to chronic microtrauma
- +/- Fluid in tendon sheath

Lateral Hamstring (Biceps Femoris) Strains
- Painful to direct palpation
- More posterior to ITB
- Posttraumatic or due to chronic microtrauma
- Hyperintense on T2WI
- Isolated injury is rare

- +/- Injury to anterior oblique band

Excessive Lateral Pressure Syndrome (Ex Lat Pressure)
- Chondromalacia of lateral patella
- Edema in superolateral Hoffa's fat pad
- Abnormal tracking of patella
- Chronic microtrauma
- Hyperintense on T2WI

Infrapatellar Bursitis (Infrapat Bursitis)
- Fluid inferior and anterior to ITB on MRI
  - Hyperintense fluid on T2WI
- More anterior than lateral pain
- Seen with occupational stresses
  - Carpet layers, housemaids

Lateral Bone Injuries Including Lateral Tibial Plateau (LTPl Fx)
- Posttraumatic
- Associated with ACL tears
- Segond fx (avulsion fx of lateral tibial plateau)
- Posterior lateral tibia fx
- Sulcus terminalis impaction fx

PATHOLOGY

General Features
- General path comments
  - Lateral synovial recess of the knee can be visualized arthroscopically
    - Typically not inflamed or distended with fluid unless ITB friction syndrome is present
  - Contact of the ITB against the condyle greatest between 20° and 30°
  - Adventitial bursal extension from the synovial capsule deep to ITB and superficial to LFC
    - = Lateral synovial recess (LSR)
    - +/- Inflammation
- Etiology
  - Chronic frictional trauma when ITB rubs on outer aspect of the lateral femoral condyle

ILIOTIBIAL BAND SYNDROME

○ Overuse injury especially in runners
○ Nonrunning knee flexion activities are also at risk
- Cyclists
- Football
- Soccer
- Tennis players
- Skiers
- Weightlifters
- Epidemiology
  ○ 1.6-52% depending on the population studied
  ○ Most common cause of lateral knee pain in long-distance runners

Gross Pathologic & Surgical Features
- Nonspecific soft tissue edema
- Thickened iliotibial band in some cases
- Inflamed lateral synovial recess of the knee

Microscopic Features
- Nonspecific soft tissue edema and inflammatory infiltration within soft tissues
- Thickened synovium with variable amount of inflammation within the lateral synovial recess

Staging, Grading or Classification Criteria
- Extrinsic - training technique
- Intrinsic - patient's anatomic alignment

CLINICAL ISSUES

Presentation
- Most common signs/symptoms: Patients present with anterolateral knee pain at the level of ITB
- Clinical profile
  ○ Typically seen in runners (especially long distance), cyclists and in some contact sport athletes
  ○ Point tenderness - 3 cm proximal to lateral joint line (superficial to lateral epicondyle)
  ○ Full extension
    - Iliotibial band anterior to femoral epicondyle
  ○ With flexion - iliotibial band rides over lateral epicondyle
  ○ Symptoms progressive usually after 2 to 3 miles of running
  ○ Asymptomatic at rest
- Clinical tests
  ○ Ober's test to assess iliotibial band tightness
    - Affected knee is flexed to 90 degrees with ipsilateral hip abduction and hyperextension
    - Positive Ober's test: Tight iliotibial band prevents leg from dropping inferior to a horizontal plane (patient is on their side with examined extremity on top)
  ○ Positive Noble's test
    - Patient lying supine with kneed flexed 90 degrees
    - Pain at 30 to 40 degrees of flexion with applied pressure to iliotibial band during knee extension

Demographics
- Age: Young active patient
- Gender: No predilection

Natural History & Prognosis
- Responds to conservative therapy
- Resolution of symptoms excellent with cessation of inciting activity

Treatment
- Conservative
  ○ Steroid injection into painful site
  ○ Orthotics designed to alleviate frictional trauma

DIAGNOSTIC CHECKLIST

Consider
- Synovitis or other cause of effusion distending the lateral aspect of the joint

Image Interpretation Pearls
- FS PD FSE most sensitive
- Consider when history suggests lateral meniscal tear in athlete

SELECTED REFERENCES

1. DeLee J et al: Orthopaedic sports medicine: Principles and practice. vol 1. 2nd ed. Philadelphia PA, Saunders 28:1577-2154, 2003
2. Farrell KC et al: Force and repetition in cycling: Possible implications for iliotibial band friction syndrome. Philadelphia PA, Elsevier Science 10(1):103-9, 2003
3. Kirk KL et al: Iliotibial band friction syndrome. Orthopedics. 23(11):1209-14; discussion 1214-5; quiz 1216-7, 2000
4. Muhle C et al: Iliotibial band friction syndrome: MR imaging findings in 16 patients and MR arthrographic study of six cadaveric knees. Radiology 212(1):103-10, 1999
5. Krivickas LS: Anatomical factors associated with overuse sports injuries. Sports Med 24(2):132-46, 1997
6. Nemeth WC et al: The lateral synovial recess of the knee: Anatomy and role in chronic Iliotibial band friction syndrome. Arthroscopy 12(5): 574-80, 1996
7. Orchard JW et al: Biomechanics of iliotibial band friction syndrome in runners. Am J Sports Med 24(3): 375-9, 1996
8. Messier SP et al: Etiology of iliotibial band friction syndrome in distance runners. Med Sci Sports Exerc 27(7):951-60, 1995
9. DeLee JC: Orthopaedic sports medicine: Principles and practice. vol 2. Philadelphia PA, WB Saunders, 1251-2, 1994
10. Ekman EF et al: Magnetic resonance imaging of iliotibial band syndrome. Am J Sports Med 22(6):851-4, 1994
11. Holmes JC et al: Iliotibial band syndrome in cyclists. Am J Sports Med 419-24, 1993
12. Firer P et al: Results of surgical management for iliotibial band friction syndrome. Clin J Sport Med 2:247-50, 1992
13. Linenger JM et al: Is iliotibial band syndrome overlooked? Phys Sports Med 20:98-108, 1992
14. Murphy BJ et al: Iliotibial band friction syndrome: MR imaging findings. Radiology 185(2):569-71, 1992
15. Lebsack D et al: Iliotibial band friction syndrome. JNATA 356-61,1990
16. Noble CA: Iliotibial band friction syndrome in runners. Am J Sports Med 8(4):232-4, 1980

ILIOTIBIAL BAND SYNDROME

IMAGE GALLERY

Typical

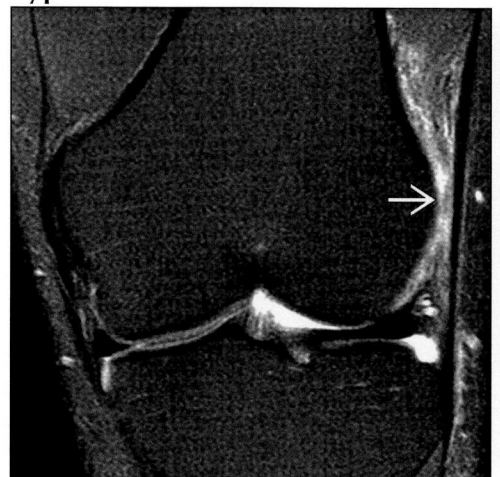

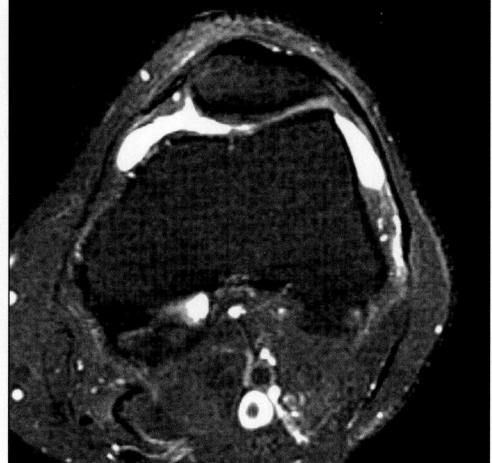

(Left) Coronal FS PD FSE MR shows edema (arrow) interposed between the iliotibial band and the lateral femoral condyle in a cyclist complaining of anterolateral knee pain. (Right) Axial FS PD FSE MR demonstrates edema/hyperemia posterior to the lateral suprapatellar joint recess.

Typical

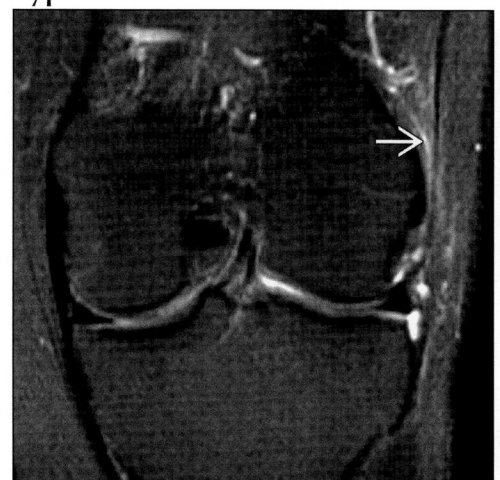

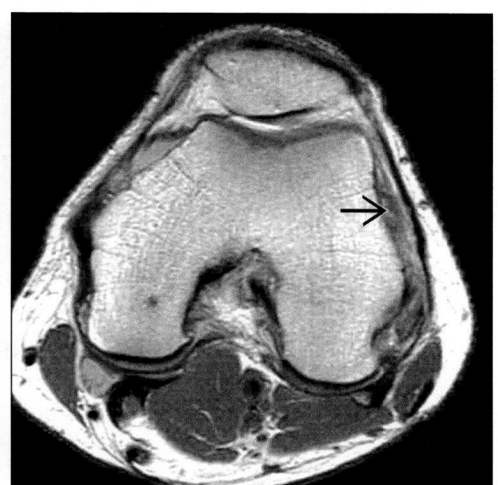

(Left) Coronal FS PD FSE MR shows the typical findings of ITB friction with edema (arrow) interposed between the ITB and the lateral femoral condyle in a runner with lateral knee pain. (Right) Axial PD FSE MR shows thickened indurated soft tissue (arrow) between the ITB and LFC.

Variant

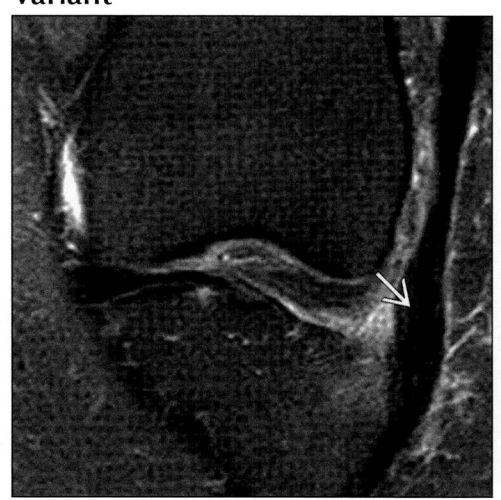

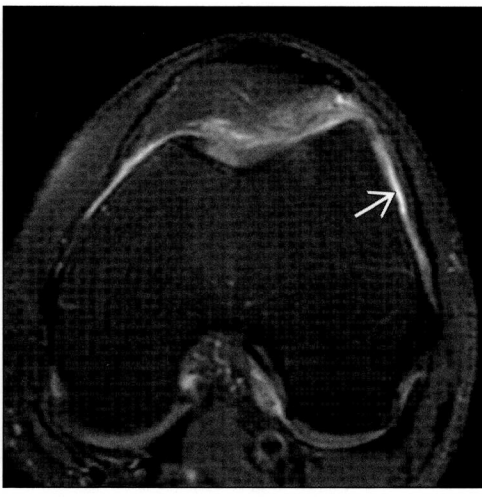

(Left) Coronal FS PD FSE MR shows a thickened ITB (arrow) with surrounding edema in a patient with chronic symptoms of ITB friction. (Right) Axial FS PD FSE MR shows edema and fluid in the superolateral aspect of Hoffa's fat pad as well as deep to the ITB (arrow) in association with femoral trochlear chondromalacia. Chronic frictional syndromes may coexist.

OSTEOCHONDRAL INJURIES, KNEE

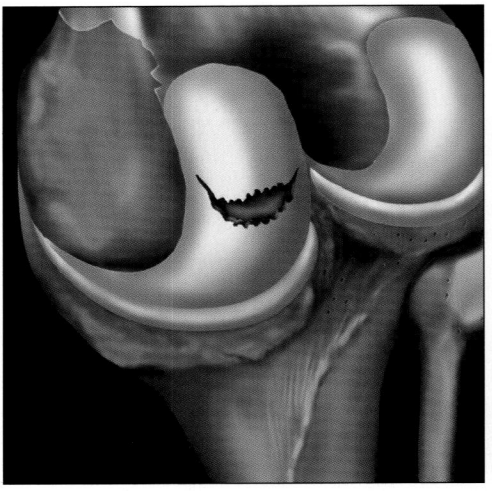

Coronal oblique graphic shows a grade IV chondral defect of the posterior medial femoral condyle. Note the underlying edema of the medial femoral condyle.

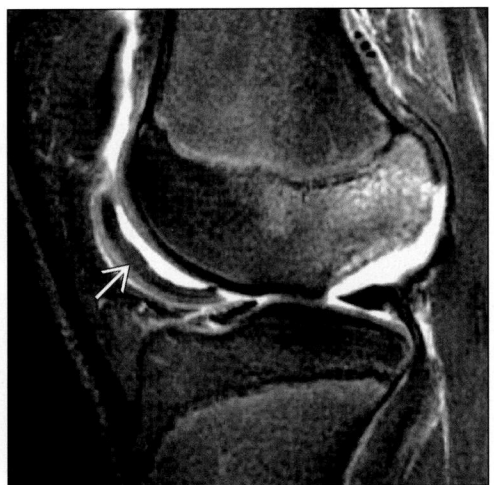

Sagittal FS PD FSE MR shows a large osteochondral defect of the posterior lateral femoral condyle with a displaced fragment (arrow) into the anterior aspect of the joint.

TERMINOLOGY

Abbreviations and Synonyms
- Osteochondral injury (OCI)

Definitions
- Injury to articular cartilage, +/- underlying bone fracture, bone trabecular injury or associated reactive stress response

IMAGING FINDINGS

General Features
- Best diagnostic clue: Alteration in contour and/or signal of hyaline articular cartilage with underlying bone changes
- Location
  - Weight bearing hyaline cartilaginous surfaces of the knee
    - Medial compartment four times more common than lateral compartment
- Size: From small chondral defect (mm) to large area of cartilage injury including denudation
- Morphology: Varies from well-defined to irregular chondral defect, associated with underlying bone changes

Radiographic Findings
- Radiography
  - +/- Fracture
  - +/- Subchondral sclerosis in chronic cases

CT Findings
- NECT
  - +/- Visible fracture
  - +/- Subchondral sclerosis in chronic cases
- CT arthrography
  - Chondral defect filled with contrast

MR Findings
- T1WI
  - Hypointense subchondral edema
  - +/- Hypointense fracture
- T2WI
  - Focal hyaline articular cartilage defect
  - Well-defined chondral defect or defect with irregular borders, +/- filled with hyperintense fluid
  - +/- Underlying bone marrow edema (hyperintense)
  - +/- Hypointensity - trabecular compaction
  - FS PD FSE - increased signal intensity in hyaline articular cartilage defects
    - Bone marrow edema (hyperintense) associated with presence of chondral injury
    - Chondral defect visualized with hyperintense tissue, flap or full thickness gap

DDx: Osteochondral Injuries, Knee

Physeal Closure	Physeal Closure	OCD	Bucket-Handle	Healing NOF
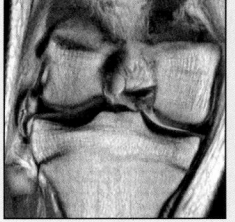	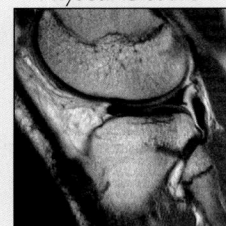	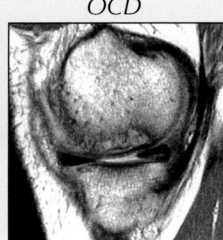	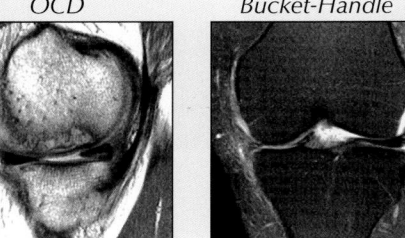	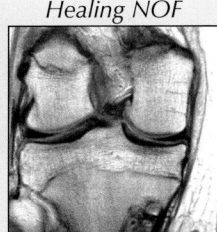
Cor PD FSE MR	*Sag PD FSE MR*	*Sag PD FSE MR*	*Cor FS PD FSE*	*Cor PD FSE MR*

OSTEOCHONDRAL INJURIES, KNEE

Key Facts

Terminology
- Injury to articular cartilage, +/- underlying bone fracture, bone trabecular injury or associated reactive stress response

Imaging Findings
- Best diagnostic clue: Alteration in contour and/or signal of hyaline articular cartilage with underlying bone changes
- Focal hyaline articular cartilage defect
- FS PD FSE - increased signal intensity in hyaline articular cartilage defects
- Protocol advice: FS PD FSE in at least 2 planes

Pathology
- Etiology: Rotational forces and direct trauma most common, may secondarily involve subchondral bone

- Meniscal tears, ligamentous sprains, soft tissue injuries, hematomas
- Loose bodies

Clinical Issues
- Most common signs/symptoms: Intermittent locking, recurrent effusions, crepitus, and persistent pain
- Chondral repair or isolated defect with secondary arthritic change

Diagnostic Checklist
- Underlying bone marrow edema associated with presence of chondral injury
- Check for increased signal intensity or fluid in hyaline cartilage

---

- Chondral fragments are intermediate in signal intensity +/- displacement
  - T2 FSE similar to FS PD FSE except marrow edema is not well shown
- PD/Intermediate
  - Increased signal intensity in hyaline articular cartilage defect
  - Suboptimal visualization of subchondral marrow edema or sclerosis
- STIR
  - Hyperintense as in FS PD FSE but with less spatial resolution
  - Increased signal intensity in hyaline articular cartilage +/- underlying bone
  - Chondral defect +/- filled with hyperintense fluid more difficult to appreciate than on T2WI at high field strength
- T2* GRE
  - Bone marrow edema can be obscured by susceptibility artifact
  - T2* WI shows joint fluid isointense to cartilage
    - Defects difficult to visualize
    - Useful for free fragment (hypointense) visualization within joint capsule

Nuclear Medicine Findings
- Bone Scan: Increased uptake of radiotracer in case of bone involvement

Imaging Recommendations
- Best imaging tool: MRI
- Protocol advice: FS PD FSE in at least 2 planes

DIFFERENTIAL DIAGNOSIS

Osteochondritis Dissecans (OCD)
- Affects specific areas in adolescent patients
  - Lateral aspect of medial femoral condyle
  - +/- Synovitis
  - Single focal area
  - Variant of osteochondral defect

Osteoarthritis (OA)
- Initial osteochondral injury/defect
- Gradual, insidious onset
- Subchondral cysts
- Subchondral edema
- Subchondral sclerosis
- Older patient and/or post traumatic patient

Magic Angle Artifact
- Mild high signal especially with shorter TE sequence
- In areas oriented at 55 degrees to the external magnetic field
  - Upsloping areas of hyaline articular cartilage adjacent to the notch

Bucket-Handle Tear
- Displaced hypointense meniscus into intercondylar notch
- Foreshortened posterior horn of meniscus
- Locked knee in flexion

Healing Nonossifying Fibroma (NOF)
- Not subchondral
- Well-defined sclerotic border
- Eccentric

Physeal Closure
- Normal development
- Mimics subchondral fracture
- Mistaken for avascular necrosis (AVN) sclerotic interface

PATHOLOGY

General Features
- General path comments
  - Tidemark zone is the weakest part of hyaline articular cartilage and is most often disrupted
    - Between the overlying cartilage and subchondral bone
  - Shearing injuries often produce chondral rather than osteochondral injury

- o Mild lesion as increased signal intensity on FS PD FSE in hyaline articular cartilage
- o Fibrillation, fissuring, flap lesion, defect or osteochondral fracture in severe case
- Etiology: Rotational forces and direct trauma most common, may secondarily involve subchondral bone
- Epidemiology: Occurs in young active patients
- Associated abnormalities
  - o Meniscal tears, ligamentous sprains, soft tissue injuries, hematomas
  - o Loose bodies

Gross Pathologic & Surgical Features

- Mild lesion on MRI may show minimal abnormality at gross inspection
- Progresses to mild fibrillation (discoloration with soft cartilage)
- Fissures to chondral flaps followed by partial and full thickness chondral defects
- Bone injuries ranging from bone trabecular injury to displaced fracture

Microscopic Features

- Chondrocyte disruption followed by swelling
- If underlying bone is involved, blood vessels are ruptured & hematoma is formed
- Bone cells without blood flow die, while perfused bone cells undergo healing process

Staging, Grading or Classification Criteria

- Outerbridge classification for chondromalacia
  - o Grade 0: Normal cartilage
  - o Grade I: Chondral softening and swelling
    - MRI: Increased signal intensity
  - o Grade II: Partial thickness defect with fissuring surface that does not extend to subchondral bone or defect which does not exceed 1.5 cm in diameter
    - MRI: Surface irregularity
  - o Grade III: Fissuring to the level of subchondral bone in an area with a diameter more than 1.5 cm
    - MRI: Partial to small full thickness defect
  - o Grade IV: Exposed bone
    - MRI: Subchondral involvement

CLINICAL ISSUES

Presentation

- Most common signs/symptoms: Intermittent locking, recurrent effusions, crepitus, and persistent pain

Demographics

- Age: Younger active patient, usually < 40 years
- Gender: M > F

Natural History & Prognosis

- Chondral repair or isolated defect with secondary arthritic change

Treatment

- Conservative
  - o Rest followed by physical therapy
  - o NSAIDs
  - o Glucosamine/Chondroitin
    - Not monitored by FDA
    - Improve mobility, decrease pain
    - No long term benefits reported
- Surgical
  - o Abrasion chondroplasty vs. debridement
    - Debridement alone - 66% good results at 5 years
  - o Chondral resurfacing techniques
    - Chondral defects without malalignment and intact meniscus
  - o Microfracture-marrow stimulating procedure causing development of fibrocartilage/hyaline cartilage
    - 97% compliance, improvement at follow up - Steadman technique
  - o Osteochondral autografts = OATS
    - Resurfacing grade IV defects with small plugs
    - OATS small plugs (mosaicplasty) - multiple small plugs, 4 mm
    - OATS large plugs – 6-10 mm plugs, greater stability
    - Favorable results – 80-94% improvement
  - o Osteochondral allograft – larger defects, tumor, OCD
    - Increased complications compared to autografts - infection
  - o Autologous chondrocyte implantation (ACI)
    - Large defects (> 15 mm) – femur, patella, trochlea
    - Unipolar lesion in normally aligned knee, intact meniscus, no inflammatory disease
    - Expensive
    - Biopsies have shown more fibrocartilage in ACI vs. hyaline cartilage in OATS

DIAGNOSTIC CHECKLIST

Consider

- In posttraumatic setting
- Underlying bone marrow edema associated with presence of chondral injury

Image Interpretation Pearls

- Check for increased signal intensity or fluid in hyaline cartilage

SELECTED REFERENCES

1. McCauley TR: MR imaging of chondral and osteochondral injuries of the knee. Radiol Clin North Am 40(5):1095-107, 2002
2. Morelli M et al: Management of chondral injuries of the knee by osteochondral autogenous transfer (mosaicplasty). J Knee Surg 15(3):185-90, 2002
3. Hjelle K et al: Articular cartilage defects in 1,000 knee arthroscopies. Arthroscopy 18(7):730-4, 2002
4. Wang CJ: Treatment of focal articular cartilage lesions of the knee with autogenous osteochondral grafts A2 - to 4-year follow-up study. Arch Orthop Trauma Surg 122(3):169-72, 2002
5. Sanders TG et al: Autogenous osteochondral "plug" transfer for the treatment of focal chondral defects: Postoperative MR appearance with clinical correlation. Skeletal Radiol 30(10):570-8, 2001
6. Sledge SL: Microfracture techniques in the treatment of osteochondral injuries. Clin Sports Med 20(2):365-77, 2001

IMAGE GALLERY

Variant

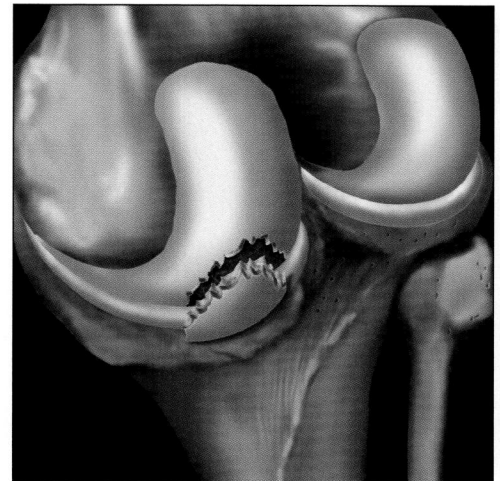 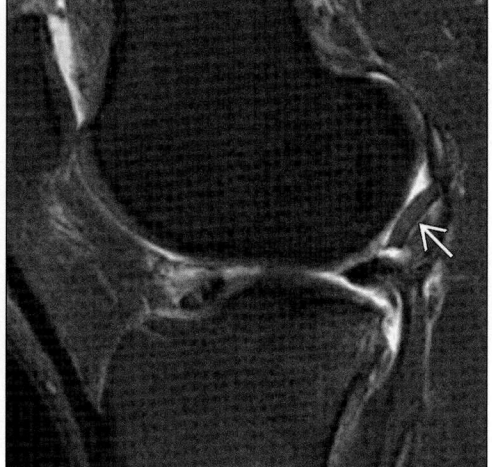

(Left) Sagittal oblique graphic shows an osteochondral defect with slight displacement of the weightbearing surface of the medial femoral condyle. *(Right)* Sagittal FS PD FSE MR shows a hyaline chondral fracture with the flipped cartilaginous fragment (arrow) located adjacent to the donor site of lateral femoral condyle.

Typical

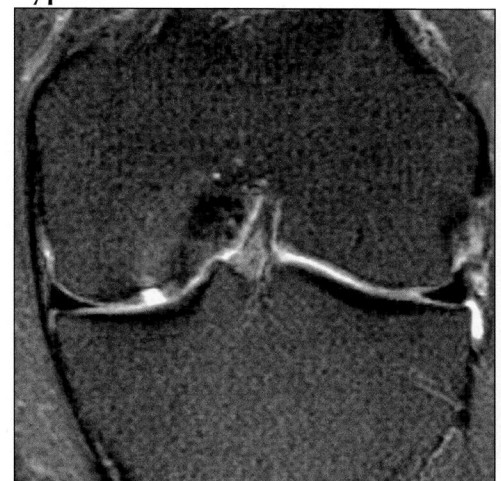 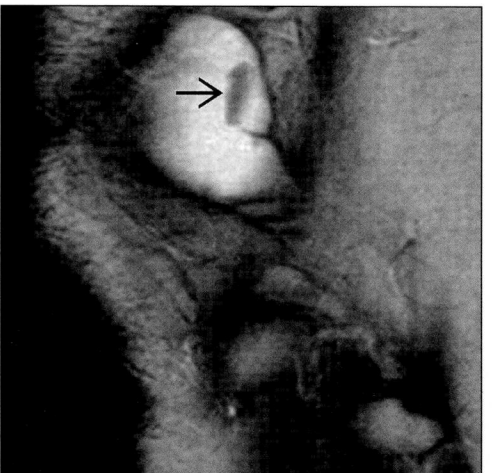

(Left) Coronal FS PD FSE MR shows a grade IV chondral defect of the weightbearing surface of the lateral femoral condyle with underlying edema. *(Right)* Sagittal T2 FSE MR shows a displaced hyaline chondral fragment (arrow) within the suprapatellar recess laterally.

Variant

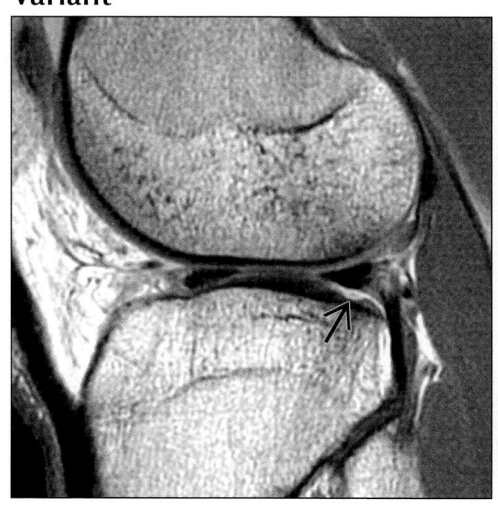 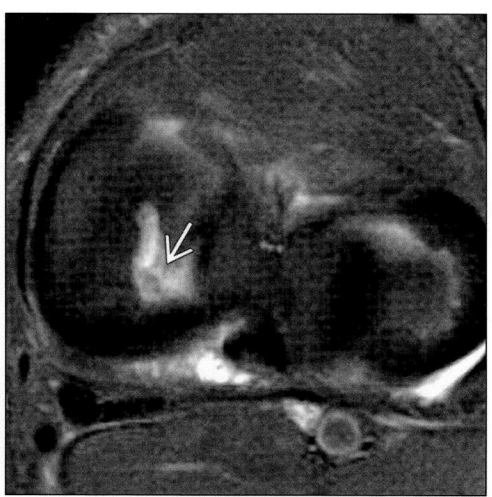

(Left) Sagittal PD FSE MR shows a grade II-III hyaline chondral defect (arrow) of the posterolateral tibial plateau. *(Right)* Axial FS PD FSE MR shows a chondral defect (arrow) of the medial femoral condyle. On axial images the fluid filled defect appears as a puddle giving rise to the "puddle sign."

OSTEOCHONDRITIS DISSECANS, KNEE

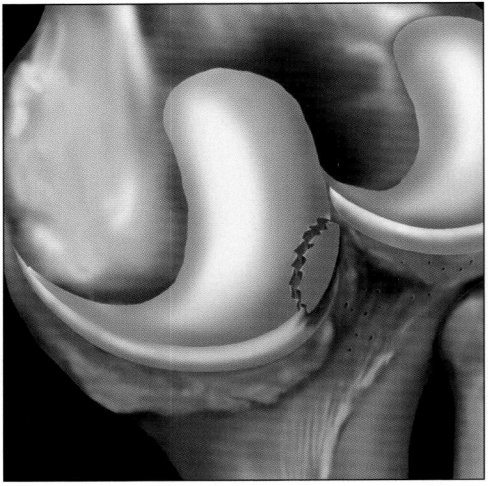

Coronal oblique graphic shows an osteochondral defect of the lateral aspect of the weightbearing surface of the medial femoral condyle. This findings is characteristic of OCD.

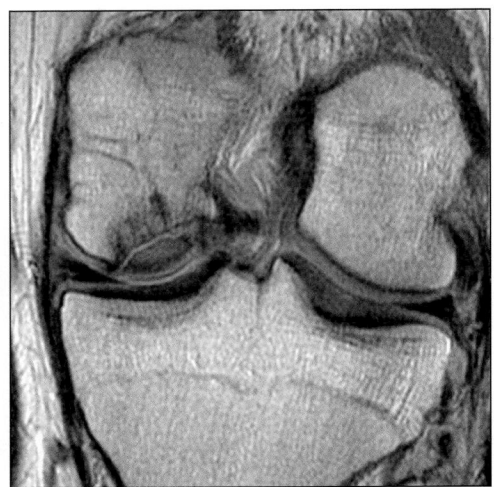

Coronal PD FSE MR shows osteochondritis dissecans of the lateral aspect of the medial femoral condyle. This is a classic location for this lesion.

TERMINOLOGY

Abbreviations and Synonyms
- Osteochondritis dissecans (OCD)

Definitions
- Osteochondrosis/osteonecrosis followed by reossification and healing

IMAGING FINDINGS

General Features
- Best diagnostic clue: Osteochondral segment with +/- stable or unstable osteochondral fragment in typical location in young males
- Location: Lateral aspect of medial femoral condyle subarticular surface, can also affect weight bearing surface of the lateral femoral condyle, tibia or patella
- Size: Osteochondral fragment of variable size either contiguous with the donor site or detached from it
- Morphology: Hyaline cartilage with underlying bone forming a crescentic/oval bone/cartilage fragment
- Predictors of instability of bone/cartilage fragment include
  - Large size (greater than 1 cm)
  - Fluid interface between the fragment and donor site
  - Cystic areas within the donor site
  - Enhancement of granulation tissue on post MR contrast enhanced images between donor site and fragment

Radiographic Findings
- Radiography
  - Area of sclerosis
    - Affecting the lateral aspect of the medial femoral condyle with or without loose fragment

CT Findings
- NECT
  - Osteochondral fragment
  - Helpful in identifying and characterizing fragments
- CT arthrography
  - Contrast beneath fragment - indicator for instability
  - Loose fragments identified within contrast pool

MR Findings
- T1WI
  - Osteochondritis dissecans site
    - Hypointense intensity with variable amounts of edema
    - +/- Adjacent donor site
  - Hypointense subchondral edema
  - Slightly hyperintense thickened synovium = synovitis
- T2WI
  - Osteochondritis dissecans site

DDx: Osteochondritis Dissecans, Knee

Insufficiency Fx	Normal Ossificat.	Chon Defect LFC	Volume Averaging	Osteochondral Inj
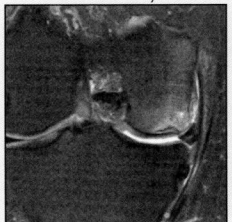	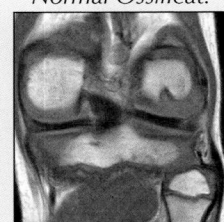	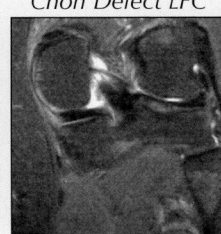	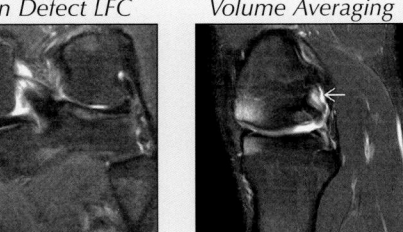 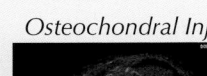	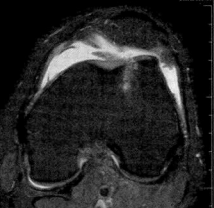
Cor FS PD FSE	Cor PD FSE MR	Cor FS PD FSE	Sag FS PD FSE	Ax FS PD FSE MR

OSTEOCHONDRITIS DISSECANS, KNEE

Key Facts

Terminology
- Osteochondrosis/osteonecrosis followed by reossification and healing

Imaging Findings
- Best diagnostic clue: Osteochondral segment with +/- stable or unstable osteochondral fragment in typical location in young males
- Location: Lateral aspect of medial femoral condyle subarticular surface, can also affect weight bearing surface of the lateral femoral condyle, tibia or patella

Top Differential Diagnoses
- Osteochondral Fracture
- Normal Pediatric Fusing Apophysis

Pathology
- Unstable lesions
- Loose fragment

Clinical Issues
- Insidious onset with gradual increase in pain followed by healing
- Predisposing trauma history found in approximately 50% of patients
- Spontaneously heal unless unstable fragment forms

Diagnostic Checklist
- Measure size of fragment and evaluate underlying bone for stability

- Hyperintense signal intensity with variable amounts of edema
  - FS PD FSE demonstrates direct extension of subchondral fluid indicating instability
  - +/- Hyperintense subchondral edema
  - +/- Hyperintense subchondral cysts
- PD/Intermediate
  - Focus of osteochondritis dissecans
    - Hyperintense with variable amounts of edema
    - Edema may be relatively isointense to marrow
  - Hyperintense thickened synovium = synovitis
- MR arthrography
  - Contrast beneath fragment - indicator for instability
  - Loose fragments
- All pulse sequences may demonstrate loose osteochondral fragments

Nuclear Medicine Findings
- Bone Scan: Increased uptake with bone reactive change +/- instability

Imaging Recommendations
- Best imaging tool: MRI, MR arthrography
- Protocol advice
  - Overlying defects in articular cartilage best appreciated on FS PD FSE and STIR
  - Chondral fragments are best seen on FS PD FSE
  - MR arthrography: Improves visualization of fluid across the articular cartilage surface thus helping determine whether the lesion is stable or unstable

DIFFERENTIAL DIAGNOSIS

Insufficiency Fracture
- Typically older osteoporotic patient
- Spontaneous osteonecrosis (SONK)
- Postoperative patient with disuse osteoporosis

Stress Fracture
- Usually in sports setting
- Hyperintense subchondral edema (T2)
- Stress response without fracture line

Osteochondral Fracture
- Post traumatic
- Not in typical OCD location

Normal Pediatric Fusing Apophysis
- Posterior lateral femoral condyle
- Can be medial
- Usually asymptomatic

Volume Averaging
- May mimic OCD in region of intercondylar notch
- Not typical location of OCD

PATHOLOGY

General Features
- General path comments
  - Unstable lesions
    - Large size (typically > 1 cm)
    - Cyst-like lesion beneath osteochondrotic lesion
    - Contains loose granulation tissue
  - Loose fragment
    - Fluid insinuating beneath the fragment at arthrography
    - Loose body formation and residual deformity often present
- Etiology
  - Idiopathic
    - Trauma implicated in up to 50%
    - Cyclic, cumulative stress to subchondral bone
- Epidemiology
  - Common disorder in young adults
  - Peak prevalence in preteen age group
- Distribution
  - Bilaterality in 20-25%
    - Bilateral lesions - asymmetric

Gross Pathologic & Surgical Features
- Lateral posterior aspect of medial femoral condyle in 70-80% of cases
- Necrotic desiccated bone fragment in unstable lesions

- Extended classic lesion also involves medial femoral trochlea

Microscopic Features
- Osteonecrosis with variable amounts of healing
- Fracture, inflammation and vascular compromise
- Subchondral avascularity
- Alteration of articular cartilage basilar growth
- Creeping substitution in revascularization
- Inadequate repair - avascular centrum + articular cartilage disruption
- Modulus mismatch between lesion and surrounding articular surface + subchondral zones
  - Subchondral fracture
- Synovial fluid intrusion at junction of subchondral centrum
  - Limits healing

Staging, Grading or Classification Criteria
- Based on arthroscopic findings
  - Stage 1: Lesion measures 1 to 3 cm with intact articular cartilage
  - Stage 2: Articular cartilage defect without loose body
  - Stage 3: Partially detached osteochondral fragments with or without fibrous tissue interposition
  - Stage 4: Loose body formation
- Cahill classification into five stages based on radiographic and bone scan findings
  - Stage 0: Normal
  - Stage I: Radiographs abnormal and normal bone scan
  - Stage II: Increased uptake on bone scan
  - Stage III: Increased bone scan uptake in lesion and femoral condyle
  - Stage IV: Increased uptake in adjacent tibial plateau

CLINICAL ISSUES

Presentation
- Most common signs/symptoms
  - Insidious onset with gradual increase in pain followed by healing
    - Locking/pain if unstable fragment forms
- Clinical profile
  - Predisposing trauma history found in approximately 50% of patients
  - Young athletes
  - Activity-related pain
  - +/- Clicking and catching
  - Localized tenderness over the lesion
  - Antalgic gait

Demographics
- Age: Primarily affects patients 10 to 20 years
- Gender: M > F (M:F = 5:3)

Natural History & Prognosis
- Spontaneously heal unless unstable fragment forms

Treatment
- Conservative
  - Rest followed by physical therapy
  - NSAIDs
  - Glucosamine/chondroitin

- Not monitored by FDA
- Might lead to improved mobility, decreased pain
- No long term benefits reported
- Chondral resurfacing technique
  - Chondral defects without malalignment and with intact meniscus
- Microfracture - marrow stimulating procedure
  - Leads to development of fibrocartilage/hyaline cartilage
  - 97% compliance, improvement at follow up - Steadman technique
- Osteochondral autografts = OATS
  - Resurfacing of full thickness defects with small plugs
  - OATS small plugs (mosaicplasty) - multiple small plugs, 4 mm
  - OATS large plugs - 6-10 mm plugs, greater stability
    - Favorable results - 80-94% improvement
    - Donor site morbidity
- Osteochondral allograft - gross, larger defects, tumor, OCD
  - Increased complications compared to autografts - infection
- Chondrocyte implantation
  - Large defects (> 15 mm) - femur, patella, trochlea
  - Unipolar lesion in normally aligned knee, intact meniscus, no inflammatory disease
  - Expensive
  - Good results

DIAGNOSTIC CHECKLIST

Consider
- If osseous fragment is in lateral aspect of medial femoral condyle

Image Interpretation Pearls
- Measure size of fragment and evaluate underlying bone for stability

SELECTED REFERENCES

1. DeLee J et al: Orthopaedics. vol 1. 2nd ed. Philadelphia PA, Saunders, 1577-2154, 2003
2. Yoshizumi Y et al: Cylindrical osteochondral graft for osteochondritis dessecans of the knee: A report of three cases. Am J Sports Med 30(3):441-5, 2002
3. Fitzgerald R Jr et al: Orthopaedics. Pediatric orthopaedics. St. Louis MO, Mosby, 1489-95, 2002
4. Gaweda K et al: Repair of focal chondral lesions of femoral condyles treated with osteochondral autograft. Ruchu Ortop Pol 67(3):247-53, 2002
5. Farmer JM et al: Chondral and osteochondral injuries. Diagnosis and management. Clin Sports Med 20(2):299-320, 2001
6. Sales de Gauzy JC et al: Natural course of osteochondritis dissecans in children. J Pediatr Orthop B 8(1):26-8, 1999
7. Long G et al: Magnetic resonance imaging of injuries in the child athlete. Clin Radiol 54(12):781-91, 1999
8. Lafforgue P et al: Insufficiency fractures of the medial femoral condyle. Rev Rhum Engl Ed 63(4):262-9, 1996
9. Cahill BR: Osteochondritis dissecans of the knee: Treatment of juvenile and adult forms. J Am Acad Orthop Surg 3(4)237-47, 1995

OSTEOCHONDRITIS DISSECANS, KNEE

IMAGE GALLERY

Typical

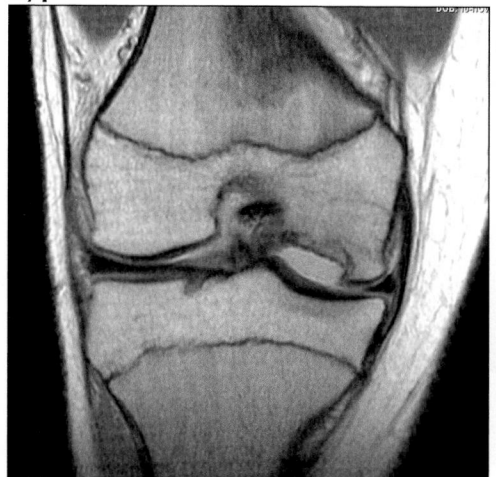 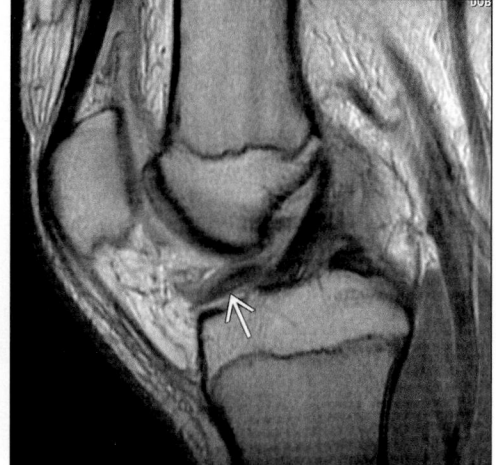

(Left) Coronal PD FSE MR shows a large defect indicating a displaced fragment. *(Right)* Sagittal PD FSE MR shows the inverted fragment (arrow) in the anterior aspect of the notch of the knee, anterior to the ACL.

Typical

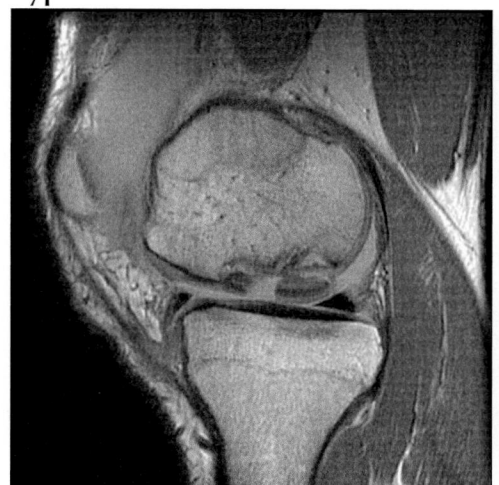 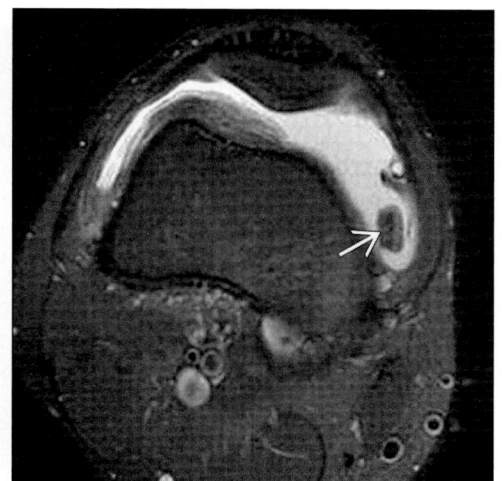

(Left) Sagittal PD FSE MR shows a fragmented OCD lesion with a grade IV defect (full thickness) of the anterior aspect. This finding should prompt a search for a loose fragment in other joint recesses. *(Right)* Axial FS PD FSE MR shows the free osteochondral fragment (arrow) within the suprapatellar pouch.

Typical

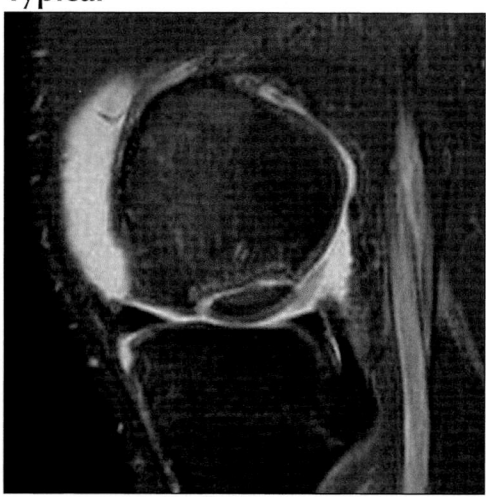 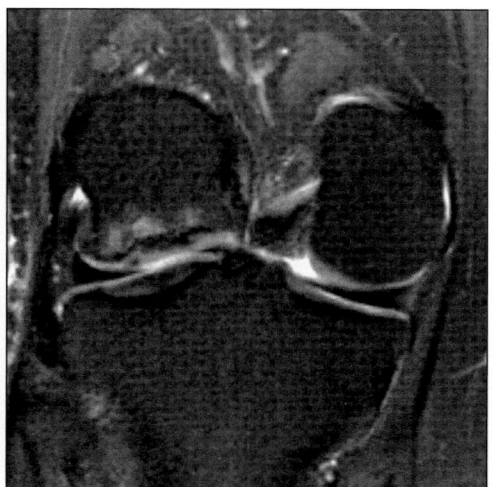

(Left) Sagittal FS PD FSE MR shows an osteochondritis lesion greater than 1 cm with fluid signal intensity between the fragment and the donor site. These are signs of instability even if the fragment is "in situ". *(Right)* Coronal FS PD FSE MR shows high signal at the base of the osteochondrotic lesion. Note the congruous hyaline cartilage surface. This lesion has remained stable.

BONE INFARCT, KNEE

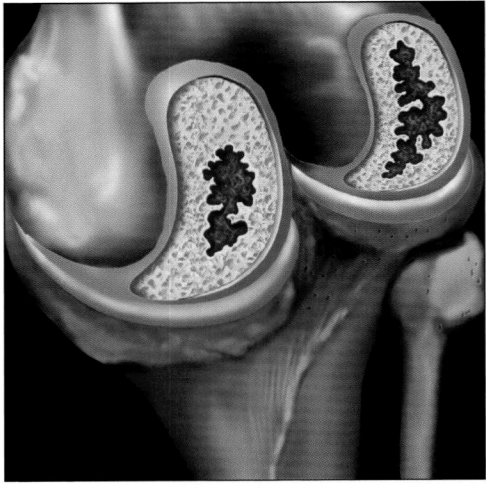

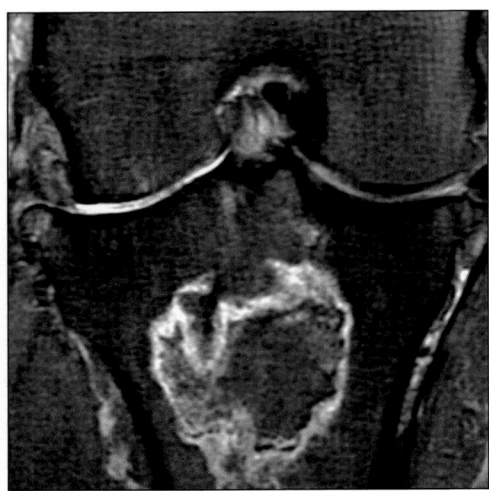

Coronal graphic shows medullary infarcts involving the posterior aspect of the femoral condyles. Note the geographic appearance of the infarcts.

Coronal FS PD FSE MR shows the double line sign of a medullary infarct in the proximal tibia.

TERMINOLOGY

Abbreviations and Synonyms
- Bone infarct (BI), avascular necrosis (AVN), osteonecrosis, aseptic necrosis, ischemic necrosis, ischemic bone death, bone necrosis, bone death

Definitions
- Ischemic death of cellular elements of bone and marrow

IMAGING FINDINGS

General Features
- Best diagnostic clue
  ○ Serpiginous border or outline in subchondral cancellous marrow
  ○ "Double line sign" of decreased signal intensity periphery with adjacent increased signal intensity inner border on T2WI
- Location
  ○ Subchondral cancellous bone, can extend to subchondral plate
  ○ Metaphyseal more common than epiphyseal or diaphyseal
- Size: Varies from small to large areas of affected bone
- Morphology

○ Irregular serpiginous linear structures described as "chinese figures"
○ Serpiginous hypointense peripheral sclerosis and central marrow fat signal intensity

Radiographic Findings
- Radiography
  ○ Epiphysis: Arc-like, subchondral, lucent lesion +/- areas of patchy bone loss mixed with sclerotic areas (subchondral fracture may occur)
  ○ In diametaphyseal region, sheetlike lucency surrounded by shell-like sclerosis and/or calcification and periostitis
  ○ Findings delayed from initial event

CT Findings
- NECT
  ○ Serpiginous outline
  ○ Increased density

MR Findings
- T1WI
  ○ Serpiginous lines of decreased signal intensity
  ○ Edema: Moderate decrease in signal intensity
- T2WI
  ○ Double line sign of decreased signal intensity periphery with adjacent hyperintense inner border

DDx: Bone Infarct, Knee

Healing NOF	Healing NOF	OCD	OCD	Normal Marrow
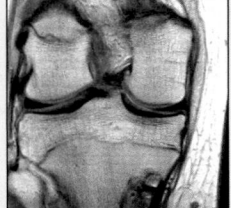	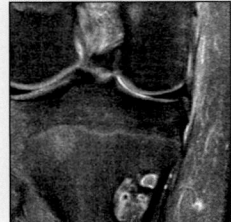	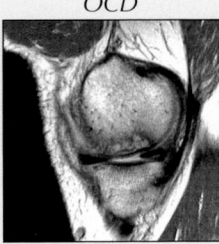	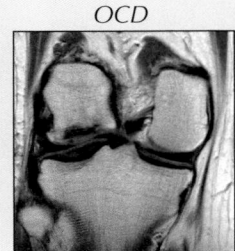	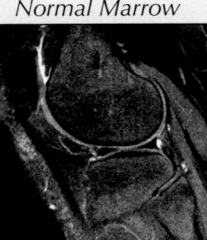
Cor PD FSE MR	Cor FS PD FSE	Sag PD FSE MR	Cor PD FSE MR	Sag FS PD FSE

BONE INFARCT, KNEE

Key Facts

Terminology
- Ischemic death of cellular elements of bone and marrow

Imaging Findings
- "Double line sign" of decreased signal intensity periphery with adjacent increased signal intensity inner border on T2WI
- Protocol advice: T1, FS PD FSE or T2WI and STIR sensitive

Top Differential Diagnoses
- Osteoarthritis (OA)
- Enchondroma (MRI and Radiography)
- Osteochondral Injury

Pathology
- General path comments: Patient with predisposing factor - steroid use or underlying disease such as sickle cell anemia
- Compromises of blood supply to the bone
- Steroid-induced osteonecrosis: 2% to > 25%

Clinical Issues
- Clinical features of bone infarct depend on stage of disease, often asymptomatic

Diagnostic Checklist
- Underlying abnormality that led to infarct
- In contrast to spontaneous osteonecrosis infarcts are usually metaphyseal

---

- o Double lines may form pseudomass in chronic cases and internal marrow fat is preserved distinguishing infarct from tumor
- o Variable degrees of collapse of articular surface in advanced cases
- o Acute infarct as a less well-defined area of edema within cancellous bone
- o Well-marginated cyst in cystic degeneration
- PD/Intermediate
  - o Generally same as T2 but less sensitive for edema
  - o PD FSE less sensitive for sclerosis compared to T1WI
  - o FS PD FSE contrast with increased sensitivity for edema compared to PD or T2 FSE
  - o To evaluate overlying chondral surfaces in subarticular infarcts
- STIR: More hyperintense periphery but with less spatial resolution than FS PD FSE
- T2* GRE
  - o Double line sign
  - o Edema may be obscured because of susceptibility
- T1 C+: Peripheral rim of reactive tissue may enhance

Nuclear Medicine Findings
- Bone Scan
  - o "Cold spot" (no uptake) in region of disrupted blood supply
  - o Uptake in acute cases where revascularization has occurred (nonspecific and somewhat diffuse)

Imaging Recommendations
- Best imaging tool: MRI - T1 and T2 are diagnostic
- Protocol advice: T1, FS PD FSE or T2WI and STIR sensitive

DIFFERENTIAL DIAGNOSIS

Osteoarthritis (OA)
- Subchondral changes
  - o Chronic symptoms and typical radiographic and MRI findings
  - o Chondromalacia
  - o Subchondral cysts, edema, sclerosis

Stress Fracture
- Lacks double line sign morphology
- Abnormal stresses of activity (usually athletic) on normal bone
- Suggestive history

Enchondroma (MRI and Radiography)
- Marrow involved in center of lesion on MRI
- Chondroid matrix

Infection
- Vague areas of radiolucencies in infarct may mimic infection

Marrow Tumor
- Areas of radiolucencies in infarct may mimic neoplastic processes
- Medullary marrow replaced in neoplasm
- Lack of cortical disruption in infarct
- Well-marginated cyst differentiates cystic degeneration of infarct from malignant degeneration

Non Ossifying Fibroma (NOF)
- Children and adolescents
- Healing NOF may mimic infarct
  - o Seen in younger patients without predisposing disease

Osteochondral Injury
- History of trauma
- Affects chondral surface and subchondral bone
- Osteochondritis dissecans (OCD) +/- history of trauma
  - o Young patient

Normal Marrow
- Red marrow inhomogeneity in metaphyseal region will not extend distal to physeal scar

BONE INFARCT, KNEE

PATHOLOGY

General Features
- General path comments: Patient with predisposing factor - steroid use or underlying disease such as sickle cell anemia
- Etiology
  - Compromises of blood supply to the bone
  - Intrinsic or extrinsic abnormality in blood vessel supplying part of the bone may lead to infarct
  - Predisposing factor or disease
    - Trauma
    - Renal transplant
    - Steroids (endogenous and exogenous including Cushing's syndrome)
    - Collagen vascular disease (e.g., systemic lupus erythematosus - SLE)
    - Pancreatitis
    - Alcoholism
    - Gaucher's disease, Fabry's disease, sickle cell anemia, gout
    - Arteritis (radiation and other causes)
- Epidemiology
  - Steroid-induced osteonecrosis: 2% to > 25%
  - SLE: 5-40%
  - Alcohol: Up to 60%
- Associated abnormalities: Secondary osteoarthritis may occur with associated complications

Gross Pathologic & Surgical Features
- Pale bone marrow with variable degrees of necrosis depending on age of infarct and duration of ischemia
- Secondary osteoarthritis develops after structural failure and collapse of articular surface cartilage
- Cystic degeneration in areas of bone infarction in diaphysis of femur and tibia

Microscopic Features
- Medullary necrosis appears yellowish with occasional flecks of calcium
- Serpiginous capsule of grayish glistening collagen may surround the area of necrosis
- Variability in depth of the yellow necrotic marrow in subchondral necrosis
- Vascular granulation tissue or grayish glistening collagen separates dead tissue from underlying viable bone
- At border zone between dead and living bone
  - Dead bone trabeculae may be broadened by formation of new bone on surface
    - Leads to decreased and increased signal intensity of double line sign

Staging, Grading or Classification Criteria
- Stage 0: Asymptomatic, normal radiograph, abnormal histology
- Stage 1: +/- Symptoms, normal radiograph, abnormal signal on MRI, abnormal histology
- Stage 2: Symptomatic, radiograph shows osteopenia, sclerosis, MRI characteristic (serpiginous line/double line sign)
- Stage 3: Symptomatic, subchondral lucency, subchondral collapse, joint space preserved
- Stage 4: Articular surface collapse + superimposed osteoarthritic changes

CLINICAL ISSUES

Presentation
- Most common signs/symptoms
  - Clinical features of bone infarct depend on stage of disease, often asymptomatic
  - +/- Generalized pain

Demographics
- Age
  - Varies and depends on underlying disease
    - Patients with sickle cell anemia may present with bone infarcts in the first few decades of life
- Gender
  - Posttraumatic infarcts are more common in young males
  - Spontaneous infarcts around knee in adults, F > M
  - Malignant transformation occurs more frequently in men
- Ethnicity
  - Infarcts associated with sickle cell anemia are seen in patients of African descent
  - Bone infarcts associated with Gaucher's disease are seen in the Ashkenazi population

Natural History & Prognosis
- Occurs suddenly and often heals without residue unless progression of underlying disease
- Malignant transformation rare

Treatment
- Idiopathic lesions treated conservatively

DIAGNOSTIC CHECKLIST

Consider
- Underlying abnormality that led to infarct

Image Interpretation Pearls
- Infarct in case of serpiginous line/double line findings
- In contrast to spontaneous osteonecrosis infarcts are usually metaphyseal
- Epiphyseal and diaphyseal locations also occur for bone infarcts

SELECTED REFERENCES

1. Lau WF et al: Extensive bone infarct in myeloid leukemia correlation of bone scan and magnetic resonance imaging. Clin Nucl Med 26(2):165-6, 2001
2. Skaggs DL et al: Differentiation between bone infarction and acute osteomyelitis in children with sickle-cell disease with use of sequential radionuclide bone-marrow and bone scans. J Bone Joint Surg Am 83(12):1810-3, 2001
3. Cerilli LA et al: Angiosarcoma arising in a bone infarct. Ann Diagn Pathol 3(6):370-3, 1999
4. Ahn BC et al: Intramedullary fat necrosis of multiple bones associated with pancreatitis. J Nucl Med 39(8):1401-4, 1998.

5

84

BONE INFARCT, KNEE

IMAGE GALLERY

Typical

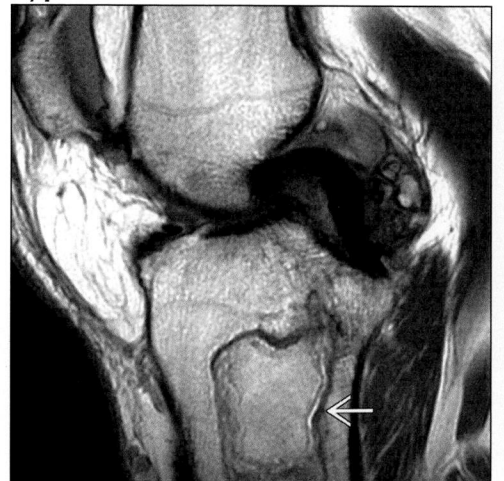

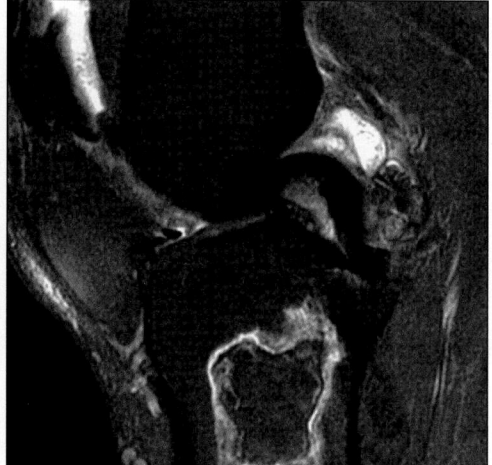

(Left) Sagittal PD FSE MR shows an extensive infarct of the proximal tibia with a characteristic double line sign (arrow). *(Right)* Sagittal FS PD FSE MR shows the T2-like appearance of the chronic infarct.

Typical

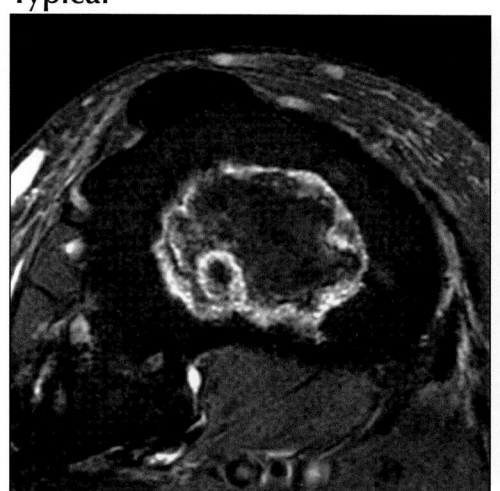

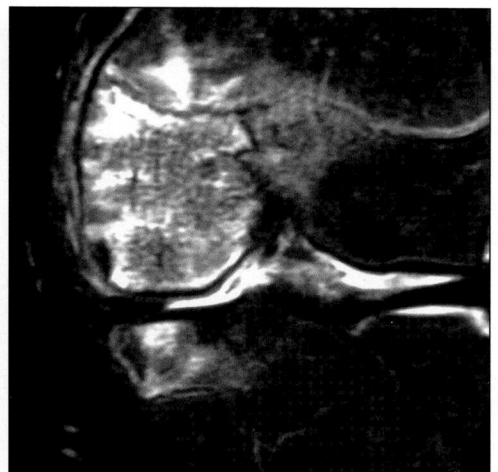

(Left) Axial FS PD FSE MR shows a chronic medullary infarct with lack of internal edema. The patient is asymptomatic. *(Right)* Coronal FS PD FSE MR shows an acute hyperintense infarct of the medial femoral condyle & tibial plateau.

Typical

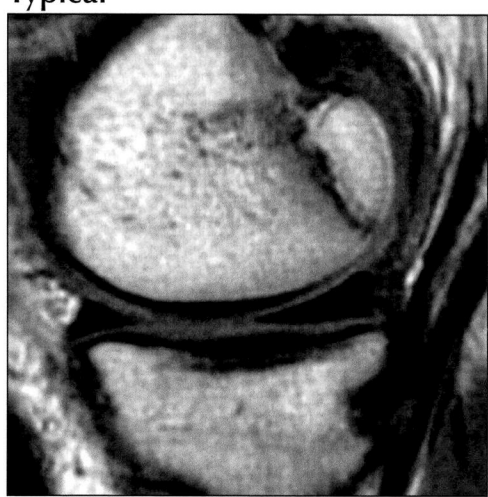

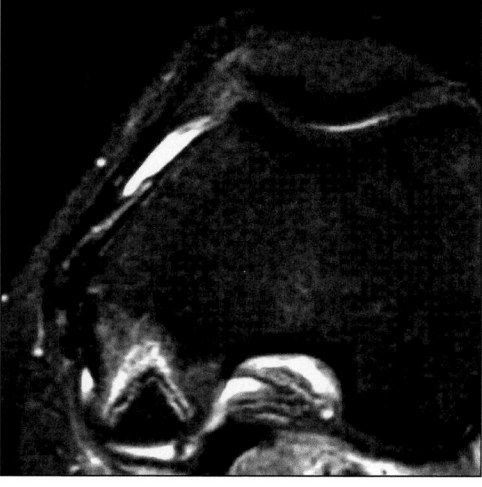

(Left) Sagittal PD FSE MR shows a chronic infarct within the posterior aspect of the medial femoral condyle. Note the preservation of bone marrow within the borders of the lesion differentiating this from a neoplasm. *(Right)* Axial FS PD FSE MR shows a chronic infarct of the posterior aspect of the medial femoral condyle with acute edematous changes at the anterior margin = extending infarct.

SPONTANEOUS OSTEONECROSIS, KNEE

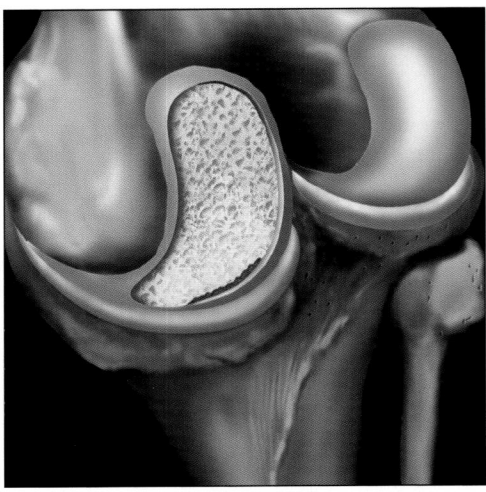

Oblique coronal graphic shows a focus of subchondral devitalized bone involving the weightbearing surface of the medial femoral condyle.

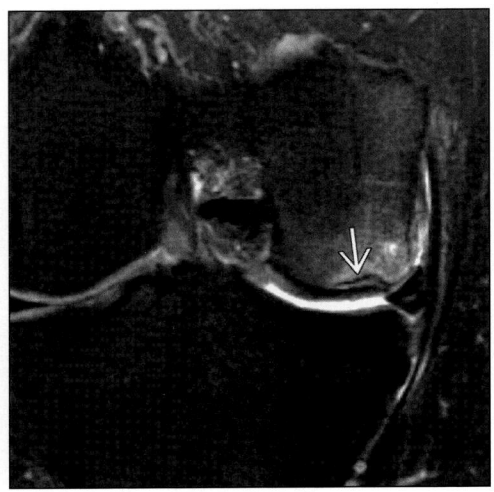

Coronal FS PD FSE MR shows SONK of the medial femoral condyle as a nondisplaced fx (arrow), in an elderly osteoporotic female with pain after climbing stairs with a heavy sack of groceries.

TERMINOLOGY

Abbreviations and Synonyms
- Spontaneous osteonecrosis (SONK), spontaneous idiopathic osteonecrosis, Ahlbäck disease

Definitions
- Necrosis of the weight-bearing portion of the femur or tibia with associated subchondral fracture and collapse
  - Affects weight-bearing portion of the medial femoral condyle
  - May affect lateral femoral condyle

IMAGING FINDINGS

General Features
- Best diagnostic clue
  - Diffuse increased signal intensity on FS PD FSE within subchondral bone
  - Crescentic linear subchondral fracture line common
  - Elderly patient, usually female
- Location
  - Weight-bearing portion of the medial femoral condyle
  - +/- Weight-bearing portion of the lateral femoral condyle or either tibial plateau
- Size

  - Focus of edema varies from small to large area of the condyle
  - Fracture line (if present) varies from few millimeters to centimeters
- Morphology: Diffuse increased signal intensity (edema) within the subchondral bone +/- crescentic linear fracture line in subchondral location

Radiographic Findings
- Radiography
  - +/- Subchondral sclerosis
  - +/- Articular surface collapse
  - Effusion

MR Findings
- T1WI
  - Necrosis: Discrete area of subchondral decreased signal intensity
  - Lesion surrounded by area of intermediate signal intensity
    - Mixture of edema and normal fatty marrow
- T2WI
  - Focus of low signal intensity ischemia or fracture surrounded by diffuse increased signal intensity edema
  - +/- Linear often serpiginous low signal abnormality adjacent to the edema
    - Probable fracture
  - +/- Articular surface collapse

DDx: Spontaneous Osteonecrosis, Knee

Geode	Stress Respone	Fracture	Hyperemia/Stress	Osteoarthritis
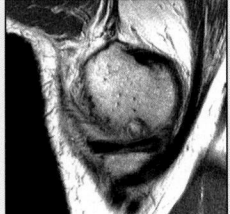	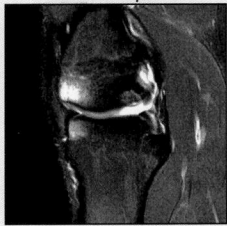	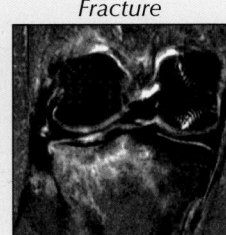	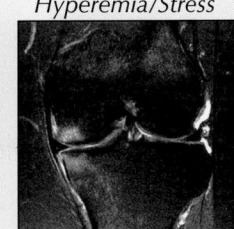	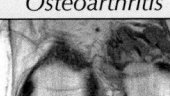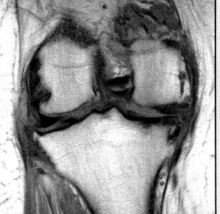
Sag PD FSE MR	Sag FS PD FSE	Cor FS PD FSE	Cor FS PD FSE	Cor PD FSE MR

SPONTANEOUS OSTEONECROSIS, KNEE

Key Facts

Terminology
- Necrosis of the weight-bearing portion of the femur or tibia with associated subchondral fracture and collapse
- Affects weight-bearing portion of the medial femoral condyle

Imaging Findings
- Morphology: Diffuse increased signal intensity (edema) within the subchondral bone +/- crescentic linear fracture line in subchondral location
- Focus of low signal intensity ischemia or fracture surrounded by diffuse increased signal intensity edema
- +/- Linear often serpiginous low signal abnormality adjacent to the edema

- +/- Articular surface collapse

Top Differential Diagnoses
- Subchondral Fracture
- Osteoarthritis
- Osteochondritis Dissecans (OCD)
- Meniscal Tears

Clinical Issues
- Intense pain often after trivial trauma, typically in elderly female

Diagnostic Checklist
- Elderly patients, especially female who experiences sudden onset of pain after trivial trauma
- Identify subchondral fracture line in patient with typical clinical profile

---

- ○ Overlying hyaline articular cartilage may remain intact or may become detached
  - ■ Hypointense, hyperintense or normal signal
- ○ Advanced cases may be accompanied by secondary degenerative changes in the adjacent or opposing bone
  - ■ Osteophyte formation
  - ■ Subchondral sclerosis
  - ■ Subchondral cyst formation
- ○ Hyperintense effusion
- ○ +/- Synovial thickening
- ○ Subchondral marrow edema shows the greatest hyperintensity on FS PD FSE or STIR images

Nuclear Medicine Findings
- Bone Scan: Positive after 72 hours

Imaging Recommendations
- Best imaging tool: MRI
- Protocol advice: FS PD FSE coronal & sagittal

DIFFERENTIAL DIAGNOSIS

Subchondral Fracture
- Younger active patient
- May be indistinguishable
- Stress fx, insufficiency fx (typically older or post-op) or posttraumatic fx

Osteoarthritis
- Diffuse edema in the early stages before cyst formation (hyperemia)
- Hyperintense T2WI
- +/- Overlying chondromalacia
- +/- Subchondral cyst (geode)
- +/- Subchondral sclerosis

Osteochondritis Dissecans (OCD)
- Lateral aspect of the medial femoral condyle (most common)
  - ○ Non-weight bearing portion
- Teenage males
- Usually insidious onset of pain

- ○ 50% association with trauma as opposed to sudden onset with SONK
- Bone typically not necrotic unless completely detached in OCD

Meniscal Tears
- Grade 3 meniscal signal (hyperintensity extending to meniscal articular surface or apex)
- Increased signal on short TE sequence
- Normal femoral condyle
- SONK associated with meniscal tears

Medial Bursitis
- Fluid deep to superficial medial collateral ligament
- Fluid-filled mass at insertion of pes anserine bursa (hyperintense T2WI)
- Pain inferior to joint line

Stress Response/Fracture (Hyperemia/Stress)
- Hyperintense edema on T2WI
- Reactive edema to adjacent inflammation vs. response to increased mechanical stress
- +/- Meniscal tear
- +/- Fracture line

PATHOLOGY

General Features
- General path comments: Subchondral osteonecrosis often following trauma in elderly osteoporotic patient
- Etiology
  - ○ Controversial
    - ■ Traumatic theory - osteoporotic patient suffers insufficiency fracture following trivial trauma, bone subsequently becomes necrotic
    - ■ Vascular theory – thrombotic venous occlusion leading to venous hypertension and hypoxic death - recently less accepted in the knee
- Epidemiology: Middle-aged and elderly patients
- Distribution
  - ○ Weight bearing portion of medial femoral condyle

SPONTANEOUS OSTEONECROSIS, KNEE

Gross Pathologic & Surgical Features
- Early stage: Area of slight flattening or discoloration in the articular cartilage over an area of the condyle of variable size, similar to the indentation of a golf ball
  - Irregular line of demarcation at the edge of the lesion on the surface with a ridge of blemished chondral surface
- Later stages: Demarcation line becomes more pronounced and flap develops
- Advanced stages: Fragmentation and degenerative changes

Microscopic Features
- Early stages: Fibrillation/erosions appear in the layer of the tidemark
  - Marrow cell lysis, fat cell necrosis, trabecular area demonstrates osteolytic areas
- Advanced cases: Advanced necrosis with dusky appearance to marrow
  - Necrotic trabeculae fibrovascular granulation and histiocytic and osteoclastic resorption of necrotic tissue
  - New bone formation surrounding crater

Staging, Grading or Classification Criteria
- Based on radiography (femoral condyle)
  - Stage I: Normal, lesion may resolve, may be diagnosed at MRI with diffuse edema, serpiginous fracture line
  - Stage II: Subtle flattening of condyle
  - Stage III: Lucent subchondral area with sclerotic halo
  - Stage IV: Sclerotic halo enlarges, collapse ensues
  - Stage V: Stage IV and degenerative changes

CLINICAL ISSUES

Presentation
- Most common signs/symptoms
  - Intense pain often after trivial trauma, typically in elderly female
  - Osteoporotic
- Clinical profile: Elderly female

Demographics
- Age: Elderly, most patients > 60 years
- Gender: F > M

Natural History & Prognosis
- Resolve spontaneously
- Advance with development of secondary degenerative change requiring knee replacement
- Satisfactory result: Decrease in symptoms after 6 weeks with persistent mild pain for up to 15 months
  - Radiographically normal or small lesion
- Poor result: Lesions with greater than 50% of femoral condylar width on radiography/MRI and persistent symptoms proceeding to destruction

Treatment
- Conservative
  - Small lesions
  - Protective weightbearing and analgesia

- Surgical
  - Core decompression
    - Stage I and II lesions
  - Osteochondral allograft
    - Variable results
  - Proximal tibial osteotomy
    - Younger active patients with varus deformity due to collapse of femoral condyle
    - Often performed with arthroscopy for inspection and loose body removal
  - Knee replacement
    - Advanced cases
- Complications
  - Immediate post-operative complications including infection, popliteal artery or venous thrombosis or laceration, articular cartilage abrasions, scuffing or defect formation
  - Development of progressive osteoarthritis
  - Malalignment (varus or valgus)

DIAGNOSTIC CHECKLIST

Consider
- Elderly patients, especially female who experiences sudden onset of pain after trivial trauma

Image Interpretation Pearls
- Identify subchondral fracture line in patient with typical clinical profile

SELECTED REFERENCES

1. Pape D et al: Prevalence of spontaneous osteonecrosis of the medial femoral condyle in elderly patients. Knee Surg SportsTraumatol Arthrosc 10(4):233-40, 2002
2. Yamamoto T et al: Spontaneous osteonecrosis of the knee: The result of subchondral insufficiency fracture. J Bone Joint Surg Am 82(6):858-66, 2002
3. Ecker ML: Spontaneous osteonecrosis of the distal femur. Instr Course Lect 50:495-8, 2001
4. Patel DV et al: Osteonecrosis of the knee: Current clinical concepts. Knee Surg Sports Traumatol Arthrosc 6(1):2-11, 1998
5. Stoller DW et al: Magnetic resonance imaging in orthopaedics and sports medicine, vol 1. 2nd ed. Philadelphia PA, J.B. Lippincott, 203-442, 1997
6. Perez Carro L et al: Core decompression and arthroscopic bone grafting for avascular necrosis of the knee. Arthroscopy 12(3):323-6, 1996
7. Ecker ML et al: Spontaneous osteonecrosis of the knee. J Am Acad Orthop Surg 2(3):173-178, 1994

SPONTANEOUS OSTEONECROSIS, KNEE

IMAGE GALLERY

Typical

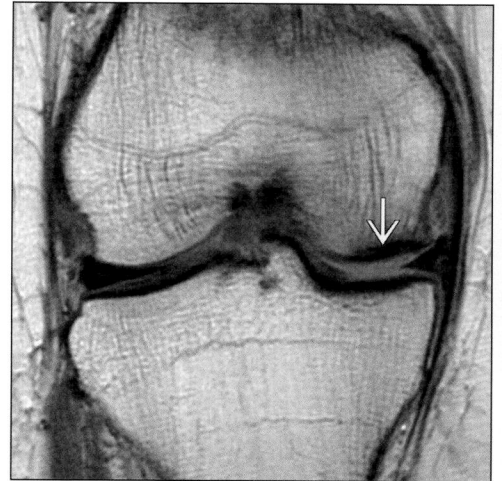
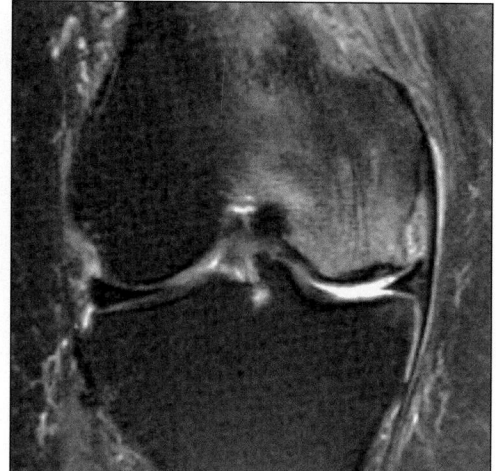

(Left) Coronal PD FSE MR shows changes of SONK including a subchondral fracture (arrow) in the MFC in an elderly female who complained of sudden excruciating pain after stepping off of a curb. *(Right)* Coronal STIR MR shows the edema in the medial femoral condyle.

Typical

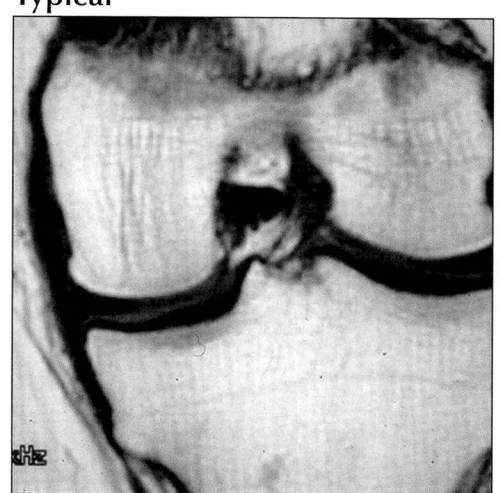
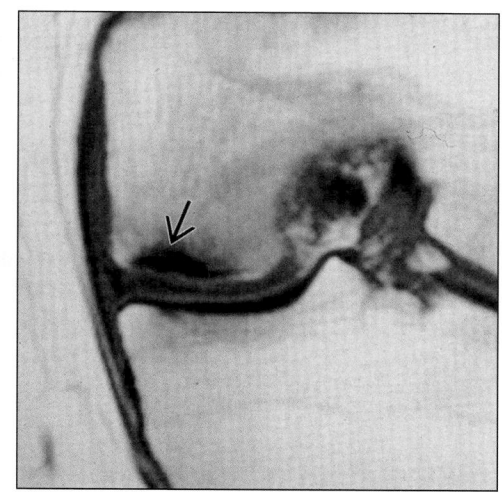

(Left) Coronal T1WI MR of a preoperative patient with osteopenia of the medial femoral condyle without SONK. *(Right)* Coronal T1WI MR of the same patient post operatively after sudden onset of pain shows subchondral hypointense sclerosis (arrow). Spontaneous osteonecrosis may represent an insufficiency fracture.

Typical

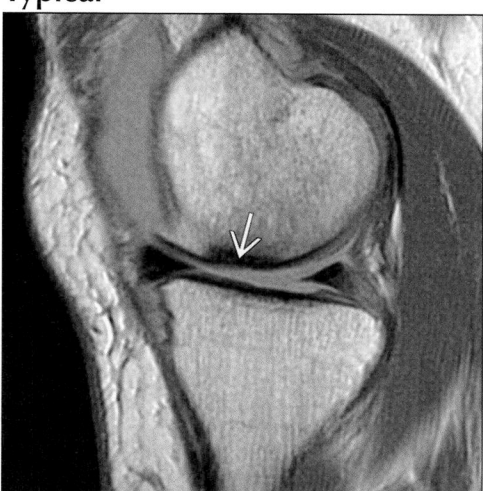
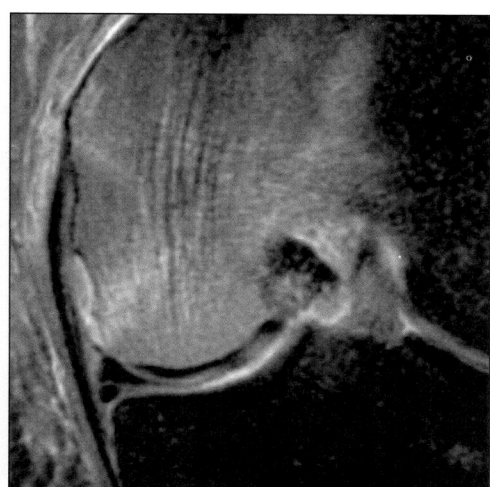

(Left) Sagittal PD FSE MR Shows a SONK lesion (arrow) with underlying edema but no evidence of subchondral collapse. *(Right)* Coronal FS PD FSE MR shows the SONK lesion of the medial femoral condyle. There is diffuse hyperintense edema within the medial condyle.

PATELLAR FRACTURE

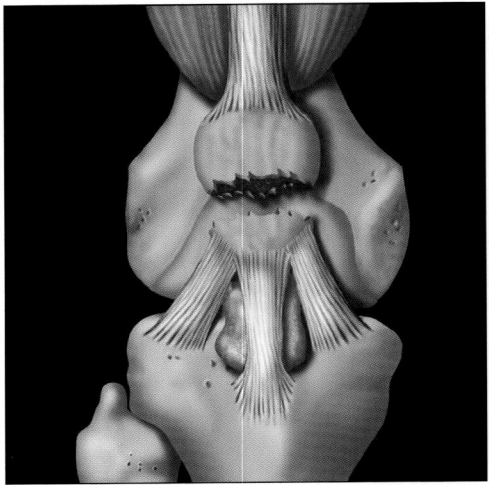

Coronal graphic shows a transverse fracture through the inferior half of the patella.

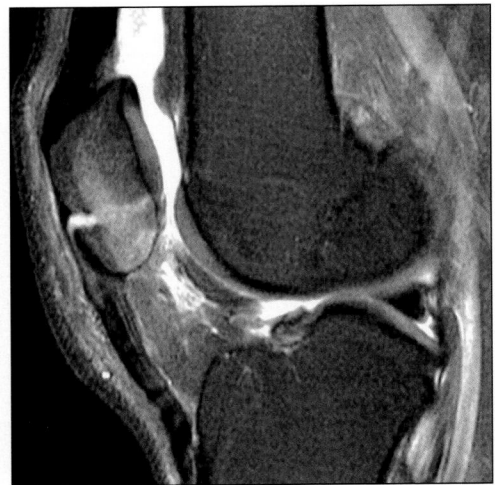

Sagittal FS PD FSE MR shows a transverse fracture of the lower third of patella with hyperintense bone marrow edema.

TERMINOLOGY

Abbreviations and Synonyms
- Kneecap fracture, fractured kneecap, fractured patella

Definitions
- Fracture of the patella either transverse, vertical, marginal, or osteochondral

IMAGING FINDINGS

General Features
- Best diagnostic clue
  - Linear decreased signal intensity on all pulse sequence within the patella
  - Variable displacement of fragments
- Location: Within patella
- Size: Fracture sizes vary from small nondisplaced to large and completely displaced
- Morphology: Transverse, vertical, marginal, or osteochondral

Radiographic Findings
- Radiography
  - Linear lucency representing fracture line with variable degrees of comminution and/or displacement
  - Include anteroposterior (AP), lateral, tangential, or Merchant views
  - Cross-table lateral radiographs demonstrate lipohemarthrosis
  - Occult on plain films (bone trabecular injury)
  - Fracture line or comminuted fragment

CT Findings
- NECT
  - Linear lucency representing fracture line with variable comminution and/or displacement of fragments
  - Localization of the fragments in case of reconstruction
  - Confirm anatomic relationship of fracture fragments with complex fractures

MR Findings
- T1WI
  - Variable comminution (multifragmentary) and displacement of fracture fragments
  - High-energy fractures - highly comminuted (stellate)
  - Decreased signal intensity in single fracture line
  - Decreased signal intensity marrow edema
- T2WI
  - Linear decreased signal intensity within the patella, increased signal bone marrow and surrounding soft tissue edema
    - Variable displacement of fragments, comminution

DDx: Patellar Fracture

Bipartite Stress	Sinding-L-J	Bipartite	Failure Fat Sat	Chondromalacia
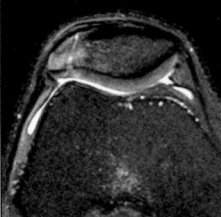	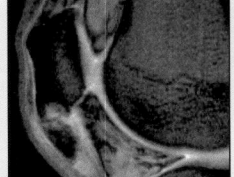	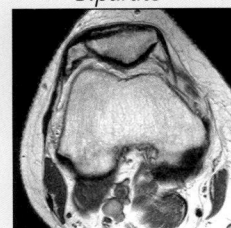	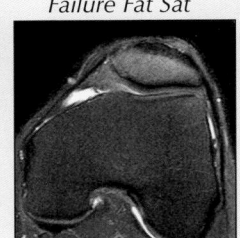	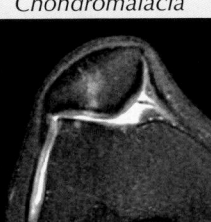
Ax FS PD FSE	*Sag T2* GRE MR*	*Ax PD FSE*	*Ax FS PD FSE*	*Ax FS PD FSE*

PATELLAR FRACTURE

Key Facts

Terminology
- Fracture of the patella either transverse, vertical, marginal, or osteochondral

Imaging Findings
- Morphology: Transverse, vertical, marginal, or osteochondral
- Linear decreased signal intensity within the patella, increased signal bone marrow and surrounding soft tissue edema

Top Differential Diagnoses
- Dorsal Defect of the Patella
- Extensor Tendonitis/Tear
- Sinding-Larsen-Johansson Syndrome (SLJ or Sinding-L-J)
- Bipartite Patella

- Failure of Fat Saturation (Failure Fat Sat)
- Chondromalacia Patella

Pathology
- Direct and indirect mechanisms
- Direct, e.g., fall, usually greater comminution, less displacement, more articular cartilage damage

Clinical Issues
- Persistent patellar tenderness and pain and/or joint effusion with history of direct or indirect injury

Diagnostic Checklist
- Patella alta on sagittal images associated with patellar fracture or patellar tendon rupture
- Evaluate for displacement, loose chondral fragments
- FS PD FSE or T2WI sensitive for edema

- Variable displacement of fragments, comminution
  - +/- Ligament, tendon tears
    - Increased signal within thickened ligament/tendon
    - Discontinuous fibers
  - Hemorrhagic effusion: Increased (fluid) signal intensity, +/- fluid-fluid level and debris/synovitis
  - Non-hemorrhagic effusion = hyperintense fluid in joint without fluid-fluid layering of hemorrhagic components
- STIR: Hypointense fracture line + surrounding hyperintense edema
- T2* GRE
  - Fracture line emphasized secondary to loss of trabeculae
  - Identify longitudinal displacement
  - Step-off between fragments at the articular surface
  - Detection for associated injuries including other bone, or soft tissue injury (retinaculum), and loose bone fragments

Nuclear Medicine Findings
- Bone Scan: Increased uptake typically after 24-72 hours indicating fracture

Imaging Recommendations
- Best imaging tool: MRI, CT
- Protocol advice: FS PD FSE or T2 or STIR to show fracture and edema

DIFFERENTIAL DIAGNOSIS

Dorsal Defect of the Patella
- Benign defect of the posterior patella covered by articular cartilage
- Developmental variation, +/- symptomatic
- Mimics osteochondral defect

Extensor Tendonitis/Tear
- Jumping sports activities
- Increased signal within thickened tendon on all pulse sequences
- +/- Tear (hyperintense on T2WI)

Sinding-Larsen-Johansson Syndrome (SLJ or Sinding-L-J)
- Osteochondrosis of the distal pole of the patella at the tendinous insertion
- Related to chronic traction injury
- Hypertrophic bone +/- stress edema

Bipartite Patella
- Secondary ossification center in superolateral pole (type III in the Saupe's classification of accessory ossification centers) is most common location
- Usually asymptomatic
- May include stress response
- Male to female ratio of 9:1

Failure of Fat Saturation (Failure Fat Sat)
- Susceptibility artifact
  - Due to curved surface "bump" of patella, disrupting cylinder of remainder of knee
- Hyperintense fat signal without edema

Chondromalacia Patella
- Increased signal with surface irregularity on FS PD FSE
- Anterior pain, especially with stair climbing

PATHOLOGY

General Features
- General path comments
  - Direct and indirect mechanisms
    - Direct, e.g., fall, usually greater comminution, less displacement, more articular cartilage damage
    - Indirect, e.g., forced flexion on tight quadriceps - jumping, less comminution, increased displacement, less articular cartilage damage
  - Transverse fractures primarily indirect mechanism
    - Displaced or nondisplaced
    - Central or distal third
    - +/- Comminution
  - Vertical fractures rare
  - Marginal fractures - edge of the patella, no extension across the bone

PATELLAR FRACTURE

- Not associated with disruption of extensor mechanism
  - o Osteochondral defect or injury usually medial or inferior, result of dislocation of the patella
    - Associated with lateral femoral condyle (LFC) and retinacular injury
    - Medial patellofemoral ligament (MPFL)
    - Vastus medialis obliquus (VMO)
  - o Sleeve fracture
    - Avulsion of portion of the articular surface (typically involves periphery)
    - Forced extension on flexed knee - lower pole
    - Small inferior fragment with articular cartilage and large superiorly migrated superior fragment
  - o Lateral stress avulsion may occur at vastus lateralis insertion
  - o Pathologic fractures can occur
- Etiology
  - o Direct trauma or indirect mechanism
    - Rapid or forced flexion on extended knee or extension on a flexed knee
  - o Secondary to anterior cruciate ligament (ACL) reconstruction with an autologous patellar tendon at site of bone plug removal
- Epidemiology
  - o 1% of all skeletal injuries in both adults and children
  - o 5% of all acute dislocations of the patella in children
- Associated abnormalities
  - o Quadriceps tears
  - o Patellar tendon tears
  - o Retinacular injury
  - o LFC injury
  - o Loose bodies

Gross Pathologic & Surgical Features
- Fracture of patella with variable degrees of comminution, displacement

Microscopic Features
- Disruption of cortex and trabecula with hemorrhage, osteoblasts, osteoclasts and inflammatory cells depending on the age of fracture

Staging, Grading or Classification Criteria
- Transverse, vertical, marginal, or osteochondral
- Comminuted
- Pediatric sleeve fracture with large chondral component

CLINICAL ISSUES

Presentation
- Most common signs/symptoms
  - o Persistent patellar tenderness and pain and/or joint effusion with history of direct or indirect injury
  - o Swelling, tenderness and hemarthrosis
  - o Proximal displacement of the patella, difficulty weight bearing and extending knee
- Clinical profile
  - o Child or adolescent after injury, often indirect trauma
  - o Child or adult after fall onto patella

Demographics
- Age: Children or adolescents > adults
- Gender: M = F

Natural History & Prognosis
- If displaced, considered relative surgical emergency to prevent fibrosis with resulting inability to reduce

Treatment
- Conservative
  - o Nondisplaced vertical, peripheral, comminuted, and transverse fractures with step-off of ≤ 2 mm
    - Immobilization cylinders or above-the-knee cast with the knee in extension for 4-6 weeks
- Surgical
  - o Surgical treatment, displaced fractures - step-off of > 2 mm or separation > 3 mm
  - o Patellar fracture fixation
    - Modified tension band wiring (circular configuration)
    - Modified tension band wiring (figure-eight)
    - Lag screw
    - Lag screw + tension band wiring
  - o Patellectomy

DIAGNOSTIC CHECKLIST

Consider
- In setting of acute trauma with patellar pain
- Rule out bipartite patella

Image Interpretation Pearls
- Patella alta on sagittal images associated with patellar fracture or patellar tendon rupture
- Evaluate for displacement, loose chondral fragments
- FS PD FSE or T2WI sensitive for edema

SELECTED REFERENCES

1. DeLee J et al: Orthopaedic sports medicine. Knee. vol 1. 2nd ed. Philadelphia PA, Saunders, 1577-2154, 2003
2. Fortis AP et al: Experimental investigation of the tension band in fractures of the patella. Injury 33(6):489-93, 2002
3. DuMontier TA et al: Patella fracture after anterior cruciate ligament reconstruction with the patellar tendon: A comparison between different shaped bone block excisions. Am J Knee Surg 14(1):9-15, 2001
4. Atkinson PJ et al: Injuries produced by blunt trauma to the human patellofemoral joint vary with flexion angle of the knee. J Orthop Res 19(5):827-33, 2001
5. Dai LY et al: Fractures of the patella in children. Knee Surg Sports Traumatol Arthrosc 7(4):243-5, 1999
6. Kaeding CC et al: Musculoskeletal injuries in adolescents. Prim Care 25(1):211-23, 1998
7. Stoller DW: Patellofemoral joint and the extensor mechanism. Magnetic resonance imaging in orthopaedics and sports medicine. vol 1. 2nd ed. Philadelphia PA, Lippincott-Raven, 361-85, 1997
8. Brownstein B: Patella fractures associated with accelerated ACL rehabilitation in patients with autogenous patella tendon reconstructions. J Orthop Sports Phys Ther 26(3):168-72, 1997

IMAGE GALLERY

Typical

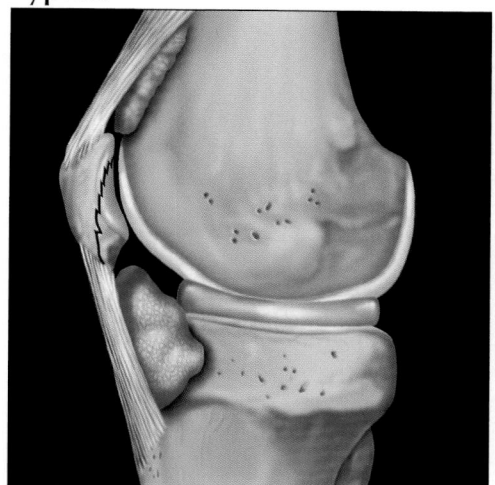
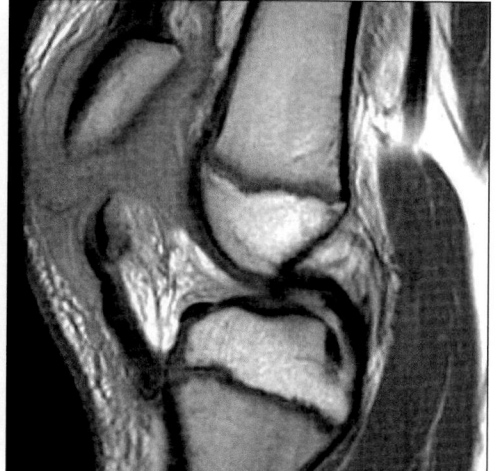

(Left) Sagittal graphic shows a patellar sleeve avulsion (oblique fracture of the patella with segment of articular cartilage making up a large part of one of the fragments). (Right) Sagittal PD FSE MR shows a complete fracture through the inferior aspect of the patella with retraction. This is considered an indication for an urgent surgical repair to prevent fibrosis.

Typical

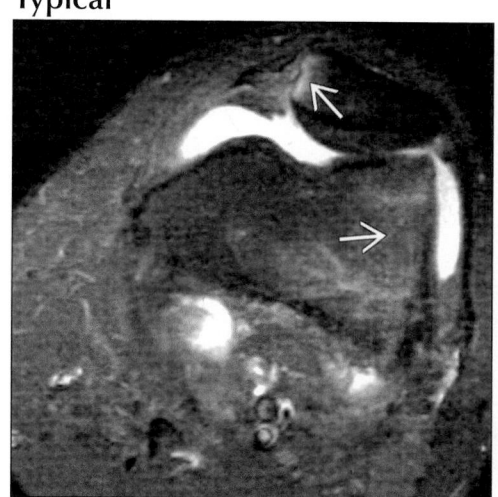
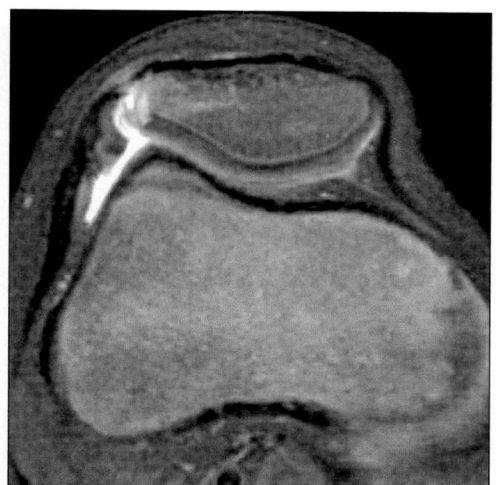

(Left) Axial FS PD FSE MR shows findings of patellar dislocation including bone injury (arrows) of lateral femoral condyle and medial patella. There is mild sprain of medial retinaculum and its patellar interface. (Right) Axial FS PD FSE MR shows a vertical fracture through the lateral aspect of the patella with slight distraction of the fracture fragments. This fracture was probably through a preexisting bipartite patella.

Typical

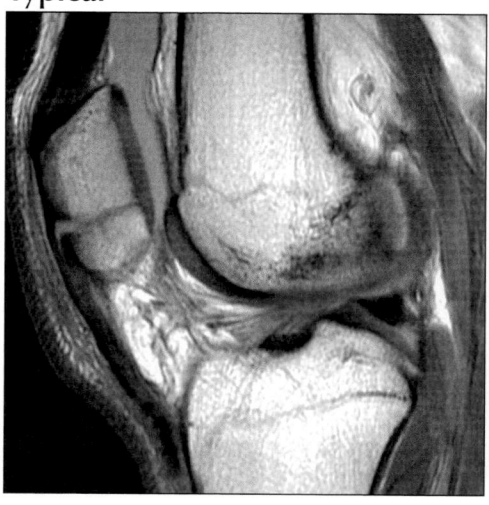
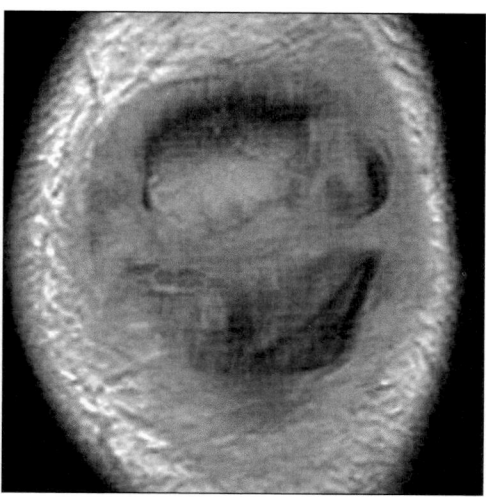

(Left) Sagittal PD FSE MR shows a transverse fracture of the patella with minimal distraction of the fracture fragments. (Right) Coronal PD FSE MR shows a transverse fracture through the central portion of the patella.

LATERAL TIBIAL PLATEAU FRACTURE

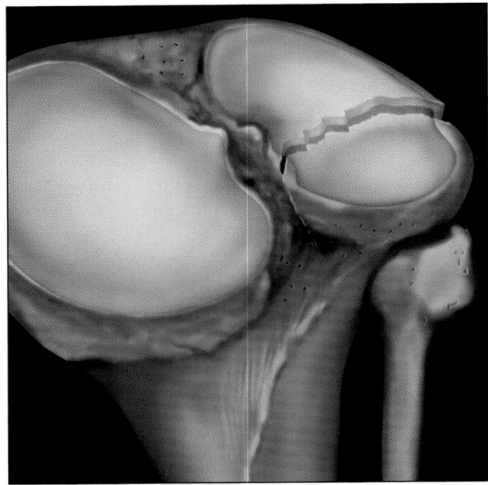

Axial oblique graphic shows a coronally oriented nondepressed tibial plateau fracture.

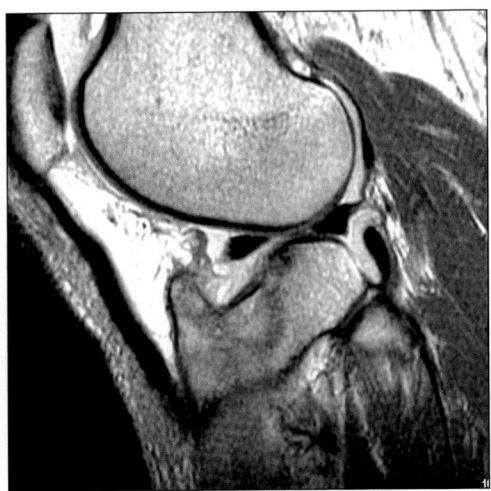

Sagittal PD FSE MR shows a depressed lateral tibial plateau fracture.

TERMINOLOGY

Abbreviations and Synonyms
- Lateral tibial plateau (LTP) fracture, bumper or fender fracture

Definitions
- Fracture of LTP as a result of axial loading, +/- rotational injury, +/- valgus angulation

IMAGING FINDINGS

General Features
- Best diagnostic clue: Oblique or vertical linear decreased signal intensity fracture line (all pulse sequences)
- Location: LTP with variable extension medially to involve intercondylar eminence +/- medial plateau
- Size: Varies from trabecular injury to small nondisplaced fracture to comminuted depressed fracture
- Morphology
  - Vertical splitting fracture: Younger patients
  - Depressed fractures: More common in older osteoporotic patients
  - Depressed split fractures - lateral articular surface
  - Depressed LTP, with no splitting through the articular surface
  - Medial tibial plateau (+/- associated with lateral plateau fx in type V and VI tibial plateau fx)
    - +/- Split fractures
    - +/- Depression
  - Split fractures of medial + lateral tibial plateaus
  - Severe fx + dissociation of tibial plateau from diaphysis

Radiographic Findings
- Radiography
  - Most depressed fractures of tibial plateau can be diagnosed by conventional radiography
  - Oblique views helpful
  - Cross-table lateral radiographs - lipohemarthrosis
  - +/- Occult on conventional radiography
  - Fracture line or comminuted fragment

CT Findings
- NECT
  - Confirm anatomic relationship of fracture fragments - more complex and nondisplaced fractures
  - Precise localization of surgical landmarks and fracture fragments
  - Surgical planning for Schatzker type IV, V, and VI fractures

DDx: Lateral Tibial Plateau Fracture

Med Plateau Fx	Medial Condyle Fx	Segond Fx	Tibial Osteotomy	PL Corner Injury
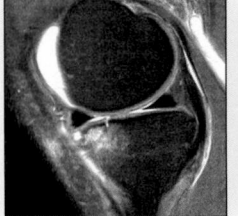	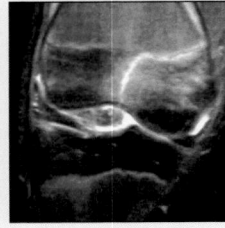	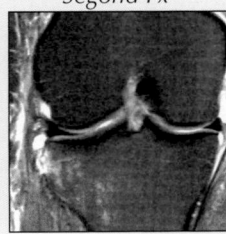	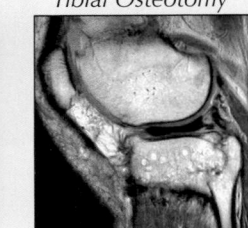	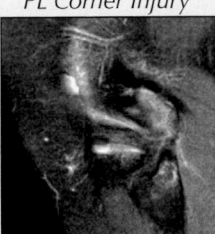
Sag FS PD FSE	*Cor FS PD FSE*	*Cor FS PD FSE*	*Sag PD FSE MR*	*Sag FS PD FSE*

LATERAL TIBIAL PLATEAU FRACTURE

Key Facts

Imaging Findings
- Best diagnostic clue: Oblique or vertical linear decreased signal intensity fracture line (all pulse sequences)
- Location: LTP with variable extension medially to involve intercondylar eminence +/- medial plateau
- Size: Varies from trabecular injury to small nondisplaced fracture to comminuted depressed fracture
- Vertical splitting fracture: Younger patients
- Depressed fractures: More common in older osteoporotic patients

Top Differential Diagnoses
- Medial Condyle Fracture (Med Condyle Fx)
- Segond Fracture

- Posterolateral Corner Injury (PL Corner Injury)

Pathology
- LTP fxs - more common than medial
- Trauma with axial load +/- blending force

Clinical Issues
- Most common signs/symptoms: Knee effusion, pain, and joint stiffness after trauma
- Typically older person, female, after fall or twisting injury

Diagnostic Checklist
- Posterolateral tibial corner injury typically associated with ACL tears
- Measure degree of depression

MR Findings
- T1WI
  - Decreased signal intensity fracture line
    - Fracture may propagate inferiorly, vertically, horizontally, medially
  - Decreased signal intensity (hypointense) edema
  - Depression of fragments seen and measured
  - +/- Meniscal tear
    - Increased signal intensity within meniscus extending to surface on short TE sequences
- T2WI
  - Decreased signal intensity fracture line with surrounding increased signal intensity edema
  - +/- Ligament tendon tears
    - Thickened increased signal within ligament/tendon
    - Discontinuous fibers
  - Hemorrhagic effusion as increased (fluid) signal intensity effusion, +/- fluid-fluid level
- STIR: Decreased signal intensity fracture line with surrounding increased signal intensity edema
- T2* GRE: Fracture line visualized secondary to loss of normal trabeculae

Imaging Recommendations
- Best imaging tool: CT with 3D reconstruction, MRI (direct visualization of fracture components in 3 planes)
- Protocol advice
  - CT 3D with sagittal and coronal reconstruction
  - MRI
    - FS PD FSE for diagnosis and hyaline cartilage involvement, and associated injury to soft tissue structures
    - Short TE sequence for menisci (T1, PD or T2* GRE)

DIFFERENTIAL DIAGNOSIS

Medial Condyle Fracture (Med Condyle Fx)
- Uncommon

- Decreased signal intensity fracture line on all pulse sequences
- Surrounding increased signal intensity edema on T2WI
- ± Associated medial tibial plateau fracture

Segond Fracture
- Associated with anterior cruciate ligament (ACL) tears
- Small avulsion of lateral tibial plateau margin
- +/- Meniscal tear

Tibial Osteotomy
- Correct varus deformity usually
- Treatment for osteoarthritis, malalignment
- Healed changes mimic chronic LTP Fx

Posterolateral Corner Injury (PL Corner Injury)
- Posterior lateral bone bruise associated with ACL tears
- LTP fx variant
- Injury to arcuate ligament, lateral collateral ligament (LCL), popliteofibular & fabellofibular ligaments, + popliteus & lateral head of gastrocnemius strains

PATHOLOGY

General Features
- General path comments
  - LTP fxs - more common than medial
    - Medial plateau of tibia is stronger than lateral
    - Varus stresses less common than valgus stresses due to carrying angle of knee and protection by other extremity
  - Forces producing LTP fxs (75-80% of fractures) directed medially
  - +/- Tear of ACL, medial collateral ligament (MCL)
  - Forces producing MTP fxs (5-10% of fractures) directed laterally are much more violent
  - Tear posterior cruciate ligament (PCL), popliteal artery, or lateral ligaments
- Etiology
  - Trauma with axial load +/- blending force

LATERAL TIBIAL PLATEAU FRACTURE

○ Fall, +/- with twisting and valgus force, leading to LTP fxs
○ Motor vehicle accident
- Epidemiology: 1% of all fractures (approximately)
- Associated abnormalities
  ○ Soft tissue abnormalities including menisci and ligaments
  ○ Posttraumatic osteoarthritis

Gross Pathologic & Surgical Features
- Fractured tibial plateau with varying degrees of depression/displacement
- Surrounding hemorrhage and soft tissue injury

Microscopic Features
- Disruption of bone cortex and trabeculae with surrounding hemorrhage in acute cases

Staging, Grading or Classification Criteria
- Schatzker classification is the most widely accepted (tibial plateau fractures)
  ○ Type I - split fractures LTP, usually younger patients, no depression
  ○ Type II - depressed split fractures lateral articular surface, usually older patients + osteoporosis
  ○ Type III - depressed LTP, no splitting through the articular surface
  ○ Type IV - medial tibial plateau and may be split fractures with or without depression
  ○ Type V - split fractures of both medial and lateral tibial plateaus
  ○ Type VI - severe stress resulting in dissociation of the tibial plateau from the underlying diaphysis
    ▪ Fracture component separates metaphysis from diaphysis

CLINICAL ISSUES

Presentation
- Most common signs/symptoms: Knee effusion, pain, and joint stiffness after trauma
- Clinical profile
  ○ Typically older person, female, after fall or twisting injury
  ○ Called bumper fracture because of auto bumpers (25%) as etiology
  ○ Compartment syndrome of the leg must be ruled out
  ○ Open wounds need to be identified
  ○ Varus & valgus stress test to the knee in full extension
    ▪ Laxity > 10 degrees = articular depression/ligamentous injury

Demographics
- Age: Incidence in older persons > general population secondary to osteoporosis
- Gender
  ○ Older patients: F > M, because of greater incidence of osteoporosis in women
  ○ Younger patients: M > F, because of involvement in high-energy contact sports

Natural History & Prognosis
- Nondepressed fractures may heal with conservative management
- Posttraumatic osteoarthritis from associated ligamentous injuries/instability

Treatment
- Conservative for nondepressed (under 4-5 mm) lesions
- Surgical treatment for those with 4-5 mm of articular depression and 3-4 mm of diastasis
  ○ Goal of therapy is to reduce the fracture and begin early mobilization
  ○ If patient immobilized for > 3 weeks, joint often will not return to full range of motion
  ○ Inadequately corrected depression results in a varus or valgus deformity and accelerated osteoarthritis

DIAGNOSTIC CHECKLIST

Consider
- Posterolateral tibial corner injury typically associated with ACL tears

Image Interpretation Pearls
- FS PD FSE identifies subchondral marrow edema and associated ligament pathology
- T1WI provides accurate visualization of fracture morphology
- Measure degree of depression

SELECTED REFERENCES

1. Patel RV et al: Diagnosis and immediate care of fractures of the knee. Hosp Med 63(4):238-9, 2002
2. Bai B et al: Effect of articular step-off and meniscectomy on joint alignment and contact pressures for fractures of the lateral tibial plateau. J Orthop Trauma 15(2):101-6, 2001
3. Wicky S et al: Comparison between standard radiography and spiral CT with 3D reconstruction in the evaluation, classification and management of tibial plateau fractures. Eur Radiol 10(8):1227-32, 2000
4. Schwartsman R et al: Patient self-assessment of tibial plateau fractures in 40 older adults. Am J Orthop 27(7):512-9, 1998
5. Dirschl DR et al: Current treatment of tibial plateau fractures. J South Orthop Assoc 6(1):54-61, 1997
6. Bernfeld BM et al: Arthroscopic assistance for unselected tibial plateau fractures. Arthroscopy 12(5):598-602, 1996
7. Cameron HU: Lateral tibial plateau fractures. Can J Surg 39(4):339, 1996
8. Colletti P et al: MR findings in patients with acute tibial plateau fractures. Comput Med Imaging Graph 20(5):389-94, 1996
9. Barrow BA et al: Tibial plateau fractures: Evaluation with MR imaging. Radiographics 14(3):553-9, 1994
10. Watson JT et al: High-energy fractures of the tibial plateau. Orthop Clin North Am 25(4):723-52, 1994
11. Kode L et al: Evaluation of tibial plateau fractures: Efficacy of MR imaging compared with CT. AJR 163(1):141-7, 1994
12. Benirschke SK et al: Open reduction internal fixation of complex proximal tibial plateau fractures. J Orthop Trauma 5:236, 1991
13. Anglen Jo et al: Tibial plateau fractures. Orthopedics 11(11):1527-34, 1988

LATERAL TIBIAL PLATEAU FRACTURE

Typical

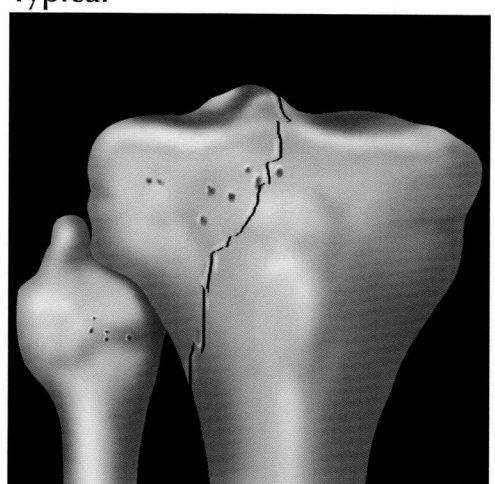

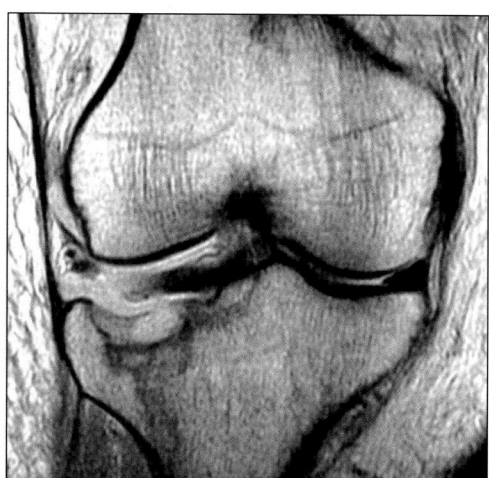

(Left) Coronal graphic shows a type I lateral tibial plateau fracture. (Right) Coronal PD FSE MR shows depressed (type II) lateral tibial plateau fracture.

Typical

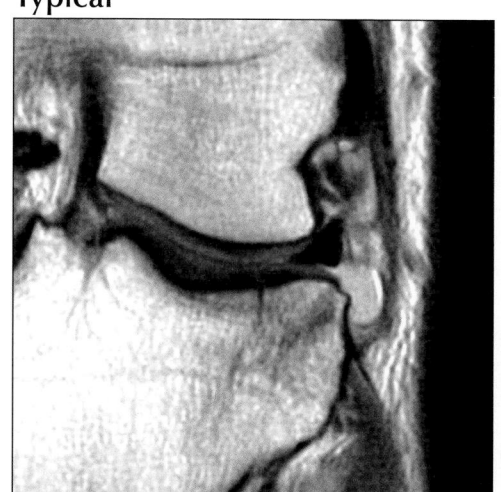

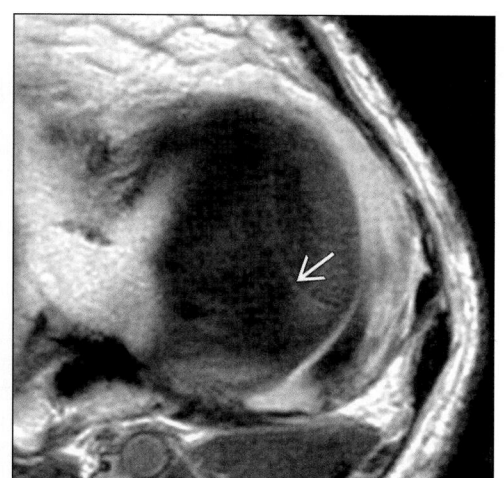

(Left) Coronal PD FSE MR shows a nondisplaced lateral tibial plateau fracture including a fracture line through the hyaline articular cartilage. (Right) Axial PD FSE MR shows a fracture line (arrow) through the hyaline cartilage of the lateral tibial plateau.

Variant

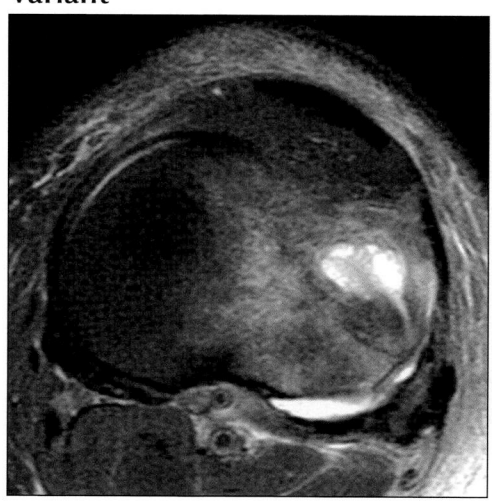

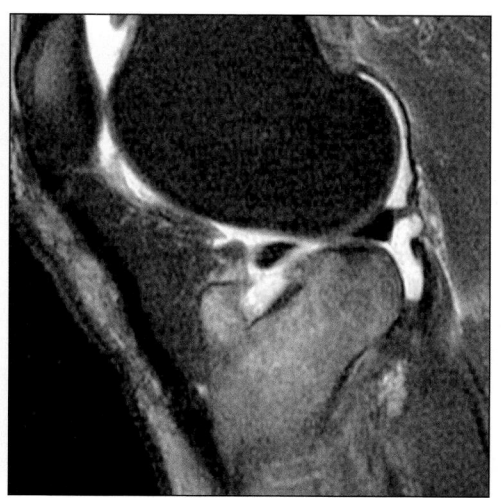

(Left) Axial FS PD FSE MR shows a fracture through the lateral tibial plateau with a depressed (hyperintense) central component. (Right) Sagittal FS PD FSE MR shows the depressed lateral tibial plateau fracture involving the hyaline articular cartilage and subchondral plate. Tibial edema is hyperintense.

PATELLAR TENDINITIS

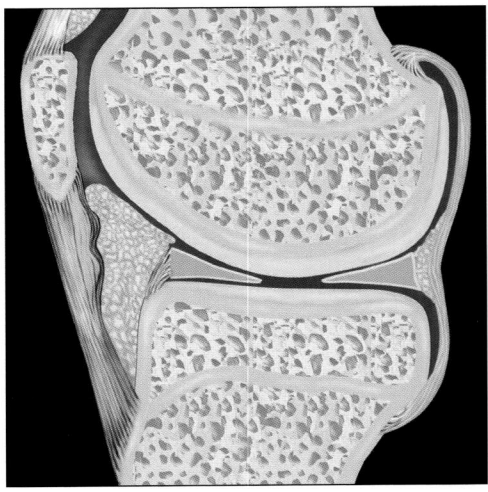

Sagittal graphic shows degeneration (tendinosis) of the proximal patellar tendon.

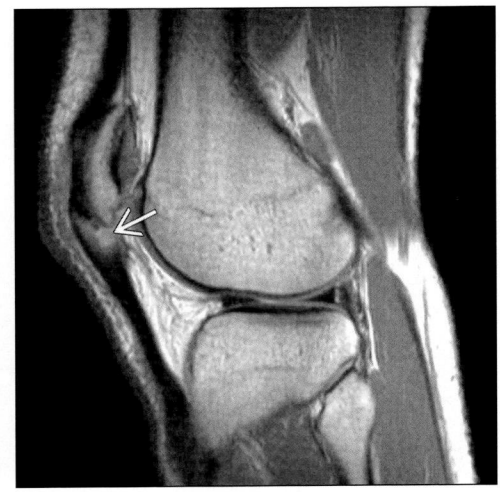

Sagittal PD FSE MR shows patellar tendinitis (tendinosis) involving proximal posterior fibers with tendon thickening and hyperintensity (arrow).

TERMINOLOGY

Abbreviations and Synonyms
- Jumper's knee, chronic patellar tendinitis, patellar tendinosis, patellar tendinopathy

Definitions
- Inflammation (tendinosis) of patellar tendon secondary to repetitive trauma (jumping sports)

IMAGING FINDINGS

General Features
- Best diagnostic clue: MRI demonstrates patellar tendon thickening, +/- partial or complete tearing and edema
- Location: Most commonly affects the proximal third of the patellar tendon (proximal posterior fibers)
- Size: Affected tendon (medial to central tendon involvement) usually thickened/expanded
- Morphology
  - Increased signal intensity of thickened tendon on short TE sequence
  - Increased anterior to posterior dimension with convex posterior margin

Radiographic Findings
- Radiography
  - Thickening of the patellar tendon

- +/- Tibial tubercle hypertrophy/fragmentation = Osgood-Schlatter disease

CT Findings
- NECT
  - Thickening of the patellar tendon with edematous changes within Hoffa's fat pad
  - Sagittal reconstruction to show tendon in long axis + fat pad
  - Axial or coronal images to identify medial or central involvement

MR Findings
- T1WI
  - Hypointense edema in the peritenon without visible change in the tendon itself (early)
  - Chronic tendinosis
    - Thickening and areas of intermediate signal intensity (collagen degeneration)
    - Decreased (normal) signal intensity indicates fibrosis in chronic tendinosis
  - Hypointense fluid signal intensity within the substance of the tendon = partial tear
  - Hypointense reactive edema within the lower pole of the patella (reactive osteitis)
  - Hypointense edema of adjacent proximal Hoffa's fat pad
- T2WI

DDx: Patellar Tendinitis

Bursitis	Enthesophytes/OA	Prepat Hematoma	Magic Angle	Prepatellar Edema
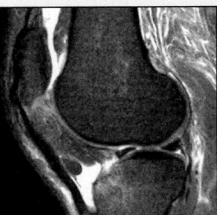	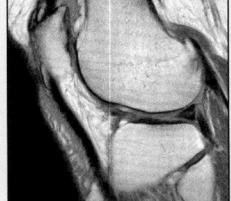	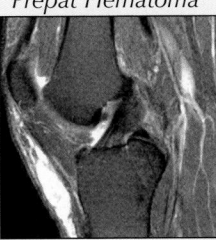	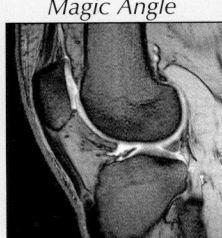	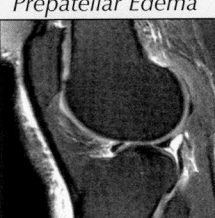
Sag FS PD FSE	*Sag PD FSE MR*	*Sag FS PD FSE*	*Sag T2* GRE MR*	*Sag FS PD FSE*

PATELLAR TENDINITIS

Key Facts

Imaging Findings

- Best diagnostic clue: MRI demonstrates patellar tendon thickening, +/- partial or complete tearing and edema
- Location: Most commonly affects the proximal third of the patellar tendon (proximal posterior fibers)
- Hyperintense edema in the peritenon without visible change in the tendon itself (early) on T2WI
- Chronic tendinitis - thickening and areas of intermediate to hyperintense signal intensity (collagen degeneration)
- Protocol advice: Sagittal FS PD FSE or T2* GRE

Top Differential Diagnoses

- Prepatellar Bursitis (Housemaid's Knee)
- Stress Response/Fracture of the Patella

- Osgood-Schlatter Disease
- Sinding-Larsen-Johansson Disease
- Magic Angle Artifact

Pathology

- Chronic overuse tendinitis often due to sports containing jumping activities (jumper's knee)
- Usually thickened, indurated tendon

Clinical Issues

- Will heal/subside with cessation of jumping sports
- May progress to tear

Diagnostic Checklist

- Identify fluid signal intensity in tendon on T2WI
- T2* GRE sagittal images are most sensitive & specific sequence for identifying tendon degeneration

---

- o Hyperintense edema in the peritenon without visible change in the tendon itself (early) on T2WI
- o Chronic tendinitis - thickening and areas of intermediate to hyperintense signal intensity (collagen degeneration)
- o Affected tendon may maintain hypointensity on T2WI unless T2* GRE or STIR sequence used
- o Hyperintense fluid signal intensity within the substance of the tendon = partial tear
- o Hyperintense reactive edema within the lower pole of the patella (reactive osteitis) and adjacent fat pad
- T2* GRE
  - o Chronic tendinitis - thickening and areas of hyperintense signal intensity
  - o Involvement typical in proximal posterior fibers
  - o T2* shows greater sensitivity for tendon hyperintensity
  - o T2* is often positive for tendon degeneration when FS PD FSE is normal
  - o T2* not as sensitive to edema of Hoffa's fat pad or pre/infrapatellar bursa compared to FS PD FSE

Ultrasonographic Findings

- Thickened hypoechoic tendon

Imaging Recommendations

- Best imaging tool: MRI
- Protocol advice: Sagittal FS PD FSE or T2* GRE

DIFFERENTIAL DIAGNOSIS

Prepatellar Bursitis (Housemaid's Knee)

- Localized fluid and inflammatory debris in the prepatellar bursa
- Occupational
- Cystic appearing mass
  - o Hyperintense on T2WI

Stress Response/Fracture of the Patella

- Increased signal intensity with or without fracture lines in the presence of a normal patellar tendon on T2WI
- +/- Trauma

- +/- Repetitive microtrauma
- +/- Chondromalacia patella

Osgood-Schlatter Disease

- Osteochondrosis with variable hypertrophy of the tibial tuberosity
- +/- Deep and/or superficial infrapatellar bursitis
- Childhood/adolescence presentation
- Adults (usually chronic)

Sinding-Larsen-Johansson Disease

- Osteochondrosis of the distal pole of the patella
- +/- Irregularity/fragmentation
- Inferior patellar pain
- Adolescent/adult

Magic Angle Artifact

- At 55 degrees to external magnetic field
- Proximal mid and distal patellar tendon
- Short TE sequences
  - o T1WI
  - o PD/Intermediate WI
  - o T2*GRE WI
- Tendon not thickened
- Asymptomatic

Prepatellar Edema

- Nonspecific anterior edema
- Hyperintense on T2WI (FS PD FSE)
- +/- Trauma
- Common finding

Prepatellar Hematoma (Prepat Hematoma)

- Trauma history
- Hyperintense prepatellar fluid collection on T2WI
- +/- Hyperintensity on T1WI related to hemorrhage
- Hemosiderin as hypointense rim on T2* GRE WI
- Mimics prepatellar bursitis

Osteoarthritis (OA)

- Degenerative arthritis
- +/- Osteophytes/enthesophytes
  - o Enthesophytes at patellar tendon origin or quadriceps tendon insertion

PATELLAR TENDINITIS

○ Marrow fat in osteophyte/enthesophyte hyperintense (fat signal) on T1WI, saturates with FS PD FSE
- +/- Hyperintense cysts on T2WI
- +/- Hyperintense marrow edema on T2WI
- +/- Chondromalacia

PATHOLOGY

General Features
- General path comments
  ○ Degeneration, thickening and edema with collagen breakdown
  ○ Short TE sequences sensitive to early changes > long TE (T2WI)
    - Short TE = T1WI, GRE, PD/Intermediate
    - Increased signal intensity as a result of degeneration
    - Magic angle mimics tendinosis
  ○ Earliest changes manifest as edema in peritenon + normal tendon
- Etiology
  ○ Chronic overuse tendinitis often due to sports containing jumping activities (jumper's knee)
  ○ In collagen vascular diseases along with tendinosis of other tendons
  ○ May occur acutely but usually in the setting of preexisting tendinosis
  ○ Malalignment of the extensor mechanism
- Epidemiology
  ○ Common in athletes participating in jumping sports
    - Basketball, tennis

Gross Pathologic & Surgical Features
- Usually thickened, indurated tendon
- Loss of integrity of tendon fibers in partially or completely torn tendons
- Partial tear may be proximal or distal

Microscopic Features
- Collagen degeneration without influx of inflammatory cells: "Tendinosis" is more accurate term than tendinitis
- Tenocyte hyperplasia
- Angiogenesis with endothelial hypoplasia
- Loss of collagen architecture
- Microtears with collagen fiber separation
- Bursal, articular or interstitial partial tears vs. through-and-through torn tendon fibers
- Fatty infiltration of muscle tissue in chronically torn tendons
- Affected tendon tissue with increased levels of cyclooxygenase-2 (COX-2)
  ○ COX-2 - enzyme which controls production of proinflammatory prostaglandins (PGE2)

Staging, Grading or Classification Criteria
- Phase I: Pain after activity
- Phase II: Pain/discomfort during activity, without interfering with participation
- Phase III: Pain during & after participation, which interferes with activity
- Phase IV: Complete tendon disruption

CLINICAL ISSUES

Presentation
- Most common signs/symptoms: Pain, excessive foot pronation, and tenderness over the patellar tendon +/- inferior pole of patella, especially with resisted extension

Demographics
- Age
  ○ Usually occurs in adults
  ○ Athletic adolescents
- Gender: No predilection

Natural History & Prognosis
- Will heal/subside with cessation of jumping sports
- May progress to tear
  ○ Acute direct trauma, laceration risk for full thickness tear

Treatment
- Conservative at first
  ○ Rest
  ○ Ice
  ○ Non steroidal anti-inflammatory agents
  ○ Steroids - may lead to increase risk of rupture
- Surgical
  ○ Maquet's procedure - anterior tibial tubercle elevation
    - Decrease in the forces that lead to overuse

DIAGNOSTIC CHECKLIST

Consider
- Diagnosis with anterior knee pain and increased signal in proximal tendon especially on short TE sequences
- Magic angle artifact may mimic tendon degeneration

Image Interpretation Pearls
- Identify fluid signal intensity in tendon on T2WI
- T2* GRE sagittal images are most sensitive & specific sequence for identifying tendon degeneration

SELECTED REFERENCES

1. McGrory JE: Disruption of the extensor mechanism of the knee. J Emerg Med 24(2):163-8, 2003
2. Panni AS et al: Overuse injuries of the extensor mechanism in athletes. Clin Sports Med 21(3):483-98, 2002
3. Kasten P et al: Rupture of the patellar tendon: A review of 68 cases and a retrospective study of 29 ruptures comparing two methods of augmentation. Arch Orthop Trauma Surg 121(10):578-82, 2001
4. Duri ZA et al: Patellar tendonitis and anterior knee pain. Am J Knee Surg 12(2):99-108, 1999
5. Verheyden FG et al: Jumper's knee: Results of surgical treatment. Acta Orthop Belg 63(2):102-5, 1997
6. Stoller DW: Magnetic resonance imaging in orthopaedics and sports medicine. vol 1. 2nd ed. Philadelphia PA, J.B. Lippincott, 203-442, 1997

PATELLAR TENDINITIS

IMAGE GALLERY

Typical

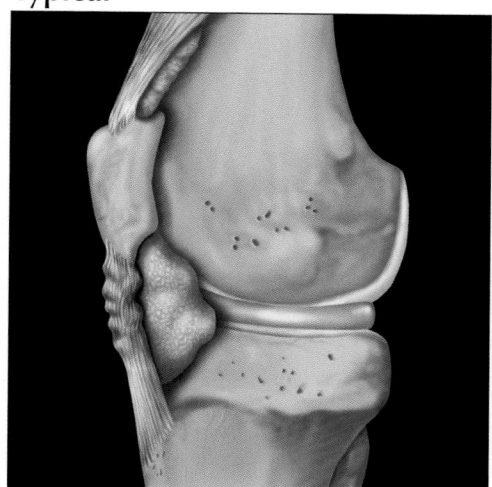
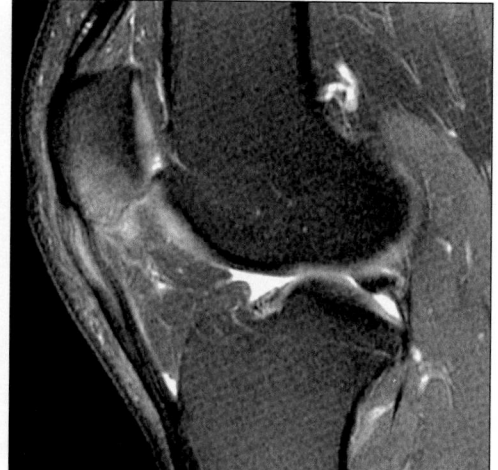

(Left) Sagittal graphic shows severe patellar tendinosis of the proximal aspect of the tendon. *(Right)* Sagittal FS PD FSE MR shows severe proximal patellar tendinosis with slight expansion of the tendon and surrounding edema.

Typical

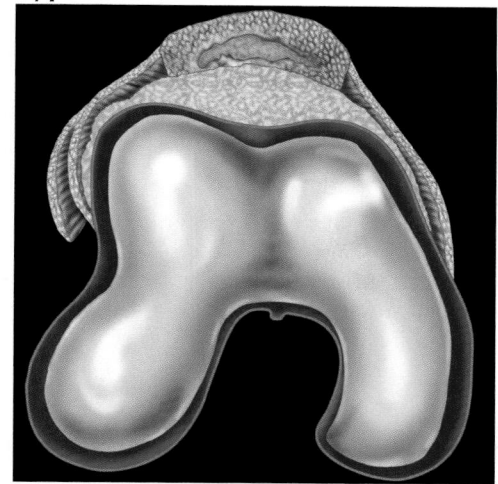
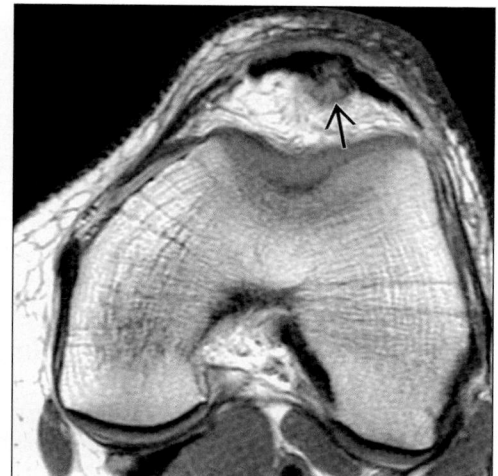

(Left) Axial graphic shows severe tendinosis of the proximal aspect of the tendon. There is an interstitial partial tear present. *(Right)* Axial PD FSE MR shows a focus of increased signal intensity within the tendon consistent with a focus of tendinosis (arrow). Note greater involvement of posterior fibers.

Typical

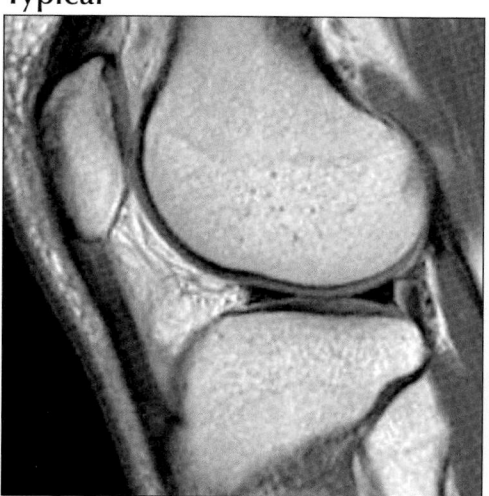
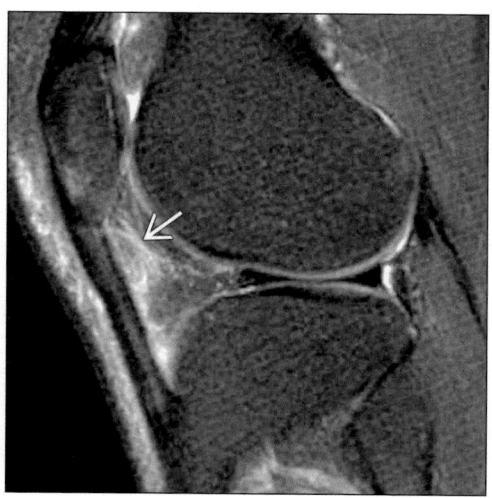

(Left) Sagittal PD FSE MR shows a thickened indurated tendon with surrounding edema consistent with tendinosis. *(Right)* Sagittal FS PD FSE MR shows the surrounding edema. Note the reactive edema within the infrapatellar soft tissues and Hoffa's fat pad (arrow).

OSGOOD-SCHLATTER DISEASE

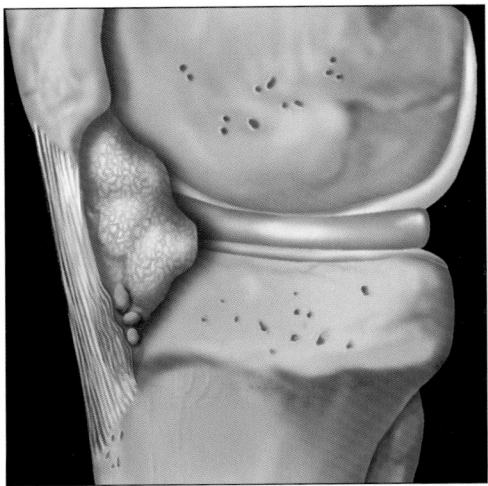

Sagittal graphic shows distal patellar tendinosis with adjacent deep infrapatellar bursal inflammation. Tibial tubercle hypertrophy and fragmentation with adjacent edema may also be seen.

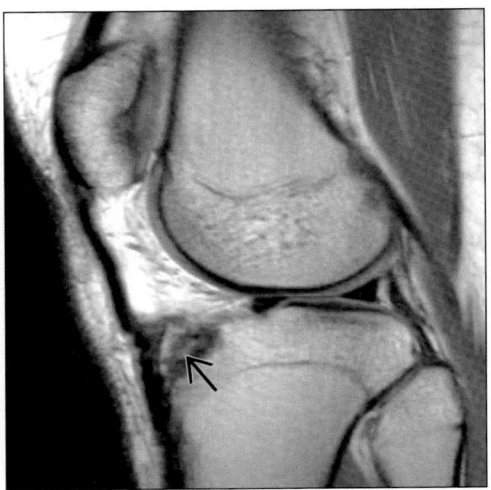

Sagittal PD FSE MR shows fragmentation (arrow) of the tibial tuberosity in a patient with pain over this region consistent with Osgood-Schlatter disease. The patient is an athlete.

TERMINOLOGY

Abbreviations and Synonyms
- Osgood-Schlatter disease (OSD), tibial osteochondrosis

Definitions
- Traction apophysitis of the patellar ligament insertion on the tibial tubercle

IMAGING FINDINGS

General Features
- Best diagnostic clue
  - Acute: Increased signal intensity on FS PD images
    - Within and around the distal patellar tendon at its insertion on tibial tubercle
    - Variable amounts of fluid within the surrounding infrapatellar bursae
  - Deep infrapatellar bursa can normally contain a small amount of fluid and should not be confused with OSD
- Location: Tibial tubercle apophysis and distal patellar ligament
- Size: Tibial tubercle and patellar tendon of normal size or enlarged
- Morphology
  - +/- Hypertrophy of the tibial tubercle

  - +/- Distension of deep and/or superficial infrapatellar bursae
  - +/- Thickening of the distal patellar ligament (tendon)
  - +/- Fragmentation of the tibial tubercle

Radiographic Findings
- Radiography
  - Hypertrophy of the tibial tubercle on lateral view
  - +/- Fragmentation
  - Greater than 4 mm soft tissue swelling over the anterior proximal surface of tibia

CT Findings
- NECT
  - Hypertrophic change of the tibial tubercle
  - +/- Fragmentation of the ossific nucleus, on sagittal reconstruction views
  - Sagittal and 3D reconstruction helpful

MR Findings
- T1WI
  - Hypertrophy and/or fragmentation of the tibial tubercle
  - Fragmentation of the ossific nucleus with a discrete ossicle
  - Heterotopic ossification within the distal patellar tendon
- T2WI

DDx: Osgood-Schlatter Disease

SLJ	SLJ	S Infra Bursitis	S Infra Bursitis	Normal Tubercle
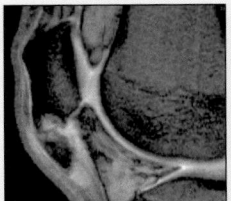	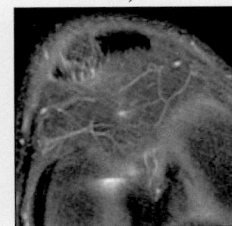	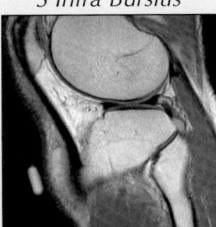	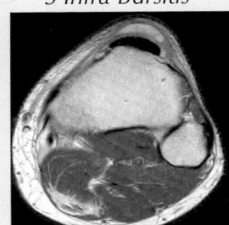	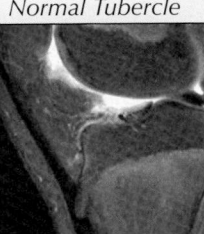
Sag T2* GRE MR	Ax FS PD FSE	Sag PD FSE MR	Ax PD FSE MR	Sag FS PD FSE

OSGOOD-SCHLATTER DISEASE

Key Facts

Terminology

- Osgood-Schlatter disease (OSD), tibial osteochondrosis
- Traction apophysitis of the patellar ligament insertion on the tibial tubercle

Imaging Findings

- Acute: Increased signal intensity on FS PD images
- Location: Tibial tubercle apophysis and distal patellar ligament
- +/- Hypertrophy of the tibial tubercle
- +/- Distension of deep and/or superficial infrapatellar bursae
- +/- Thickening of the distal patellar ligament (tendon)

Top Differential Diagnoses

- Isolated Deep or Superficial Infrapatellar Bursitis (S Infra Bursitis)
- Patellar Tendonitis

Pathology

- General path comments: Traction apophysitis
- Repetitive microtraction trauma

Clinical Issues

- Most common signs/symptoms: Insidious onset of low-grade ache associated with activity localized to tibial tubercle

Diagnostic Checklist

- Hypertrophied, edematous tibial tubercle on FS PD FSE key for diagnosis

---

- ○ Distension of the deep and/or superficial infrapatellar bursae indicating reactive bursitis
- ○ Non-specific edema can be seen in the surrounding soft tissues including Hoffa's fat pad on FS PD images
- ○ FS PD FSE and T2* GRE are the most sensitive sequences
  - ▪ Signal increase is variable: From intermediate to hyperintense (subchondral edema of tibial tubercle)
  - ▪ Thickening of the distal patellar ligament (tendon) with increase in signal intensity

Nuclear Medicine Findings

- Bone Scan: Positive in cases of tubercle apophysitis

Imaging Recommendations

- Best imaging tool: MRI
- Protocol advice
  - ○ Edema and tendon tears are identified on FS PD FSE, T2* GRE or STIR images
  - ○ Bony hypertrophy is visualized on T1 or PD FSE images
  - ○ FS PD FSE in sagittal and axial plane

DIFFERENTIAL DIAGNOSIS

Isolated Deep or Superficial Infrapatellar Bursitis (S Infra Bursitis)

- Patients with kneeling occupations
- Different age group compared to OSD
- Fluid signal intensity on T2WI

Patellar Tendonitis

- Jumper's knee
- Same age group and similar circumstances as OSD
- May be differentiated by MRI in many cases

Sinding-Larsen-Johansson Disease (SLJ Disease)

- Traction apophysitis of inferior pole of patella

- Irregular and sometimes fragmented appearance of inferior patella
  - ○ Bony avulsion
  - ○ Soft tissue calcification
  - ○ Elongation of inferior pole of patella
- Pain superiorly located compared to OSD

PATHOLOGY

General Features

- General path comments: Traction apophysitis
- Etiology
  - ○ Repetitive microtraction trauma
    - ▪ Anterior tibial tubercle
    - ▪ During formation of the secondary ossification center
  - ○ Multiple submaximal avulsion fractures of patellar tendon insertion caused by traction microtrauma
    - ▪ Occurs particularly during eccentric contractions of strong extensor mechanism
    - ▪ Common in jumping sports: Basketball and volleyball – boys; gymnastics, soccer, other jumping sports - girls
- Associated abnormalities: Patellar tendon tears (partial tears) in some cases
- Distribution: Young active patients

Gross Pathologic & Surgical Features

- Thickened, indurated patellar tendon
- Multiple ossific bodies may be present within the tendon or about the tubercle

Microscopic Features

- Focal tendon collagen degeneration
- Tendon microtears
- Influx of inflammatory cells in surrounding soft tissues
- Bursal synovial hypertrophy and inflammatory infiltrate
- Heterotopic bone formation and/or fragmentation
- Three normal histologic zones within immature tibial tubercle

OSGOOD-SCHLATTER DISEASE

- ○ Proximal - columnar cartilage
- ○ Midzone - fibrocartilage
- ○ Distal - fibrous tissue blending with tibial perichondrium
- Physiologic epiphysiodesis of the tubercle starts proximally and extends centrifugally and distally

CLINICAL ISSUES

Presentation

- Most common signs/symptoms: Insidious onset of low-grade ache associated with activity localized to tibial tubercle
- Clinical profile
  - ○ Young active patient with anterior knee pain
  - ○ Symptoms occur during rapid growth period as tibial tubercle is maturing
  - ○ Aggravated by acceleration/deceleration, direct blows
  - ○ Bilateral 20-30%
  - ○ Tubercle prominence often bilateral although symptoms are usually unilateral
- Ossicle at tibial tubercle in 30-50% of cases
- +/- Tenderness also around patella and patellar tendon
- Quadriceps atrophy
- Extensor lag
- Tightness
  - ○ Quadriceps
  - ○ Hamstrings
  - ○ Gastrocnemius
  - ○ Iliotibial band
- Resisted knee extension = pain

Demographics

- Age
  - ○ Typically occurs at the onset of the adolescent growth spurt, ranging from 10-15 years of age
    - ▪ 10-15 years of age boys
    - ▪ 8-13 years of age girls
  - ○ Increasing in girls usually at age 10-11 years (range 8-13 years)
    - ▪ Skeletal maturity equivalent to boys at age 13-14
- Gender: M > F

Natural History & Prognosis

- Usually self-limited
- Patellar tendinitis and bursitis are common sources of pain independent of fracture healing
- Residual hypertrophy of the tibial tubercle or fragmentation
- Ossification within the patellar tendon
- Prognosis excellent
- Post surgical prognosis improved in older child near skeletal maturity

Treatment

- Conservative
  - ○ Exercises to restore strength and flexibility of the extensor mechanism
- Surgical
  - ○ For recalcitrant cases
  - ○ For those patients with ossification around the tibial tubercle or within the patellar tendon

- ○ Tuberosity drilling: Less common
- ○ Bone plug placement: Less common
- ○ Tuberosity debulking
- ○ Linear osteotomy with excision of the tuberosity
- Complications: Excision before skeletal maturity can result in
  - ○ Residual prominence of the tubercle
  - ○ Decreased range of motion
  - ○ Recurvatum deformity

DIAGNOSTIC CHECKLIST

Consider

- Uncomplicated patellar tendonitis in the absence of tuberosity changes

Image Interpretation Pearls

- Hypertrophied, edematous tibial tubercle on FS PD FSE key for diagnosis

SELECTED REFERENCES

1. Adirim TA et al: Overview of injuries in the young athlete. Sports Med 33(1):75-81, 2003
2. Delee J et al: Orthopaedic Sports Medicine. Hip and Pelvis. vol 1. 2nd ed. Philadelphia PA, Saunders, 25:1443-80, 2003
3. Olivieri I et al: Enthesitis of spondylarthritis can masquerade as Osgood-Schlatter disease by radiographic findings. Arthritis Rheum 49(1):147-8, 2003
4. Duri ZA et al: The immature athlete. Clin Sports Med 21(3):461-82, 2002
5. Hirano A et al: Magnetic resonance imaging of Osgood-Schlatter disease. The course of the disease. Skeletal Radiol 31(6):334-42, 2002
6. Orava S et al: Results of surgical treatment of unresolved Osgood-Schlatter lesion. Ann Chir Gynaecol 89(4):298-302, 2000
7. Nowinski RJ et al: Hyphenated history: Osgood-Schlatter disease. Am J Orthop 27(8):584-5, 1998
8. de Inocencio J: Musculoskeletal pain in primary pediatric care: Analysis of 1000 consecutive general pediatric clinic visits. Pediatrics 102(6):E63, 1998
9. Aparicio G et al: Radiologic study of patellar height in Osgood-Schlatter disease. J Pediatr Orthop 17(1):63-6, 1997
10. McCarroll JR et al: Anterior cruciate ligament reconstruction in athletes with an ossicle associated with Osgood-Schlatter's disease. Arthroscopy 12(5):556-60, 1996

OSGOOD-SCHLATTER DISEASE

IMAGE GALLERY

Typical

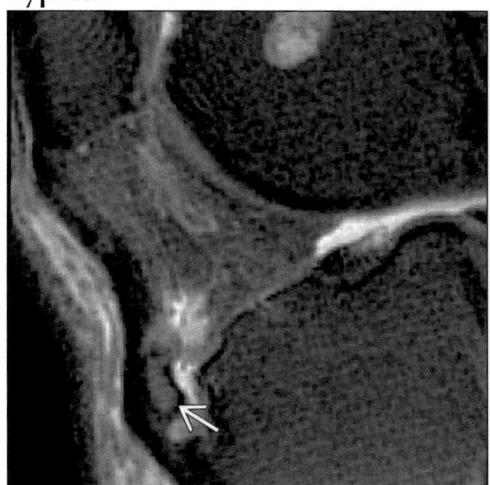
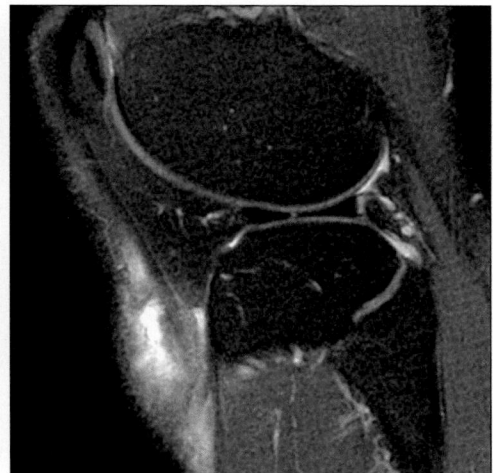

(Left) Sagittal FS PD FSE MR shows findings of Osgood-Schlatter disease including edema within the nonfused tibial tubercle apophysis *(arrow)* and surrounding edema. *(Right)* Sagittal FS PD FSE MR shows hyperintense inflammation at the patellar tendon insertion site in a patient with Osgood-Schlatter disease.

Typical

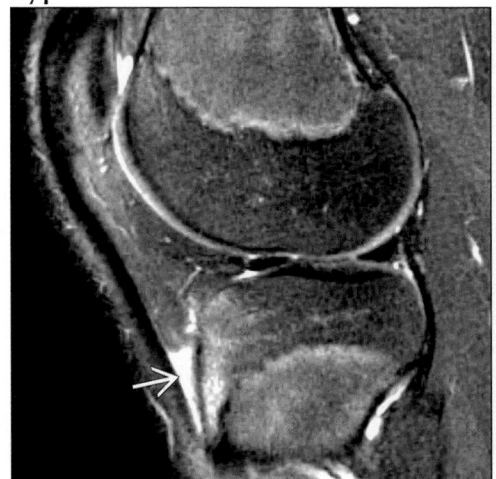
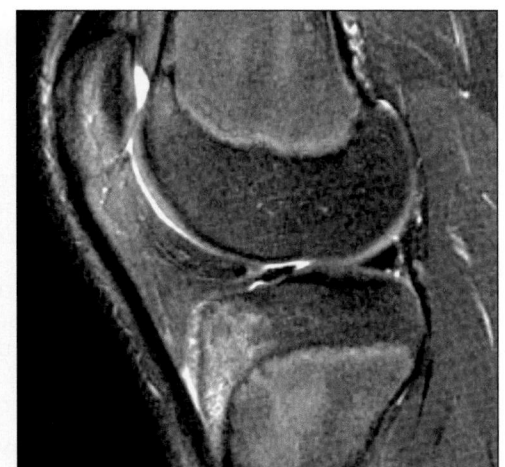

(Left) Sagittal FS PD FSE MR shows inflammation within the deep infrapatellar bursa *(arrow)* and reactive edema within the anterior proximal tibia in a patient with clinical presentation of acute Osgood-Schlatter disease. *(Right)* Sagittal FS PD FSE MR of the same patient shows the associated edema within the anterior tibia.

Typical

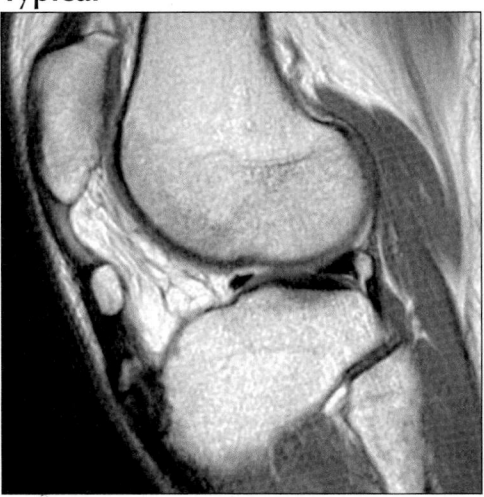
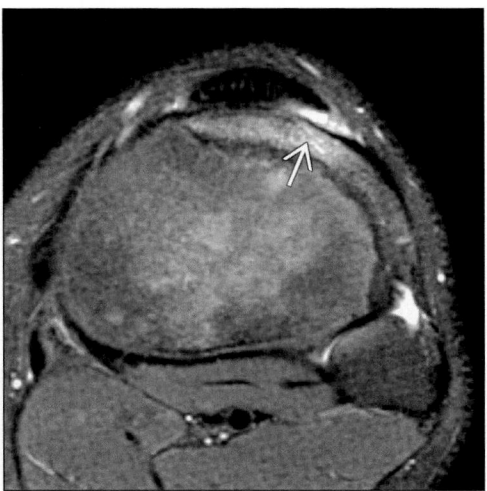

(Left) Sagittal PD FSE MR shows heterotopic ossification within the patellar tendon and at the tibial tubercle as well as patellar tendinosis in a patient with chronic Osgood-Schlatter disease. *(Right)* Axial FS PD FSE MR shows minimal amount of fluid in deep infrapatellar bursa, tendinosis of the distal patellar tendon and edema in the adjacent tibia *(arrow)* in patient with acute changes superimposed upon chronic Osgood-Schlatter disease.

PATELLAR (ANTERIOR) BURSITIS

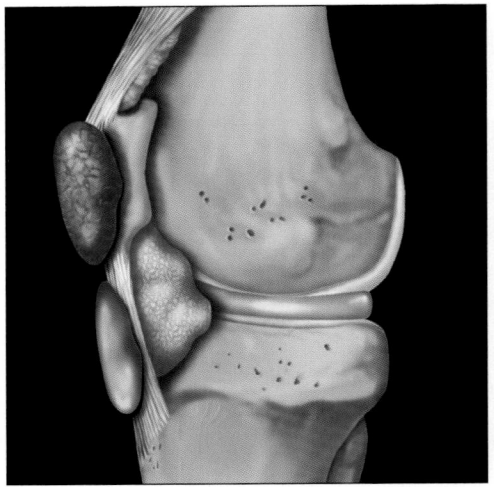

Sagittal graphic shows an inflamed fluid-filled prepatellar bursa (purple).

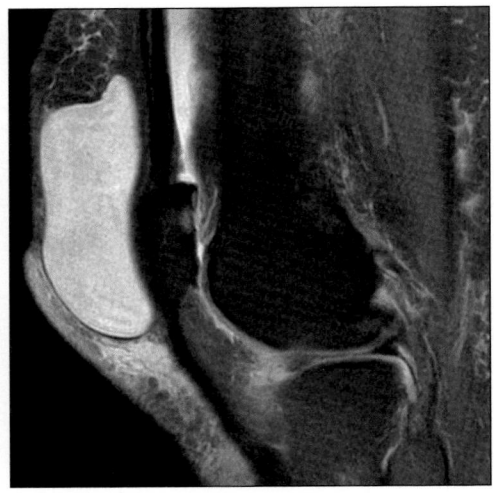

Sagittal FS PD FSE MR shows large amount of hyperintense fluid within the prepatellar bursa in prepatellar bursitis.

TERMINOLOGY

Abbreviations and Synonyms
- Prepatellar bursitis, deep infrapatellar bursitis, superficial infrapatellar bursitis, housemaid's knee (prepatellar), preachers's or clergyman's knee (superficial infrapatellar)

Definitions
- Inflammation of synovial lining of bursae
  - Prepatellar bursitis - anterior to inferior pole of the patella and proximal patellar tendon
  - Deep infrapatellar bursitis - between the patellar tendon and anterior aspect of the proximal tibia
  - Superficial infrapatellar bursitis - anterior and superficial to distal aspect of patellar tendon

IMAGING FINDINGS

General Features
- Best diagnostic clue
  - Fluid containing mass (fluid signal intensity) in one of the anterior bursae of knee
  - History of occupation or activities including large amounts of kneeling
- Location
  - Prepatellar bursa

- Superficial infrapatellar bursa
- Deep infrapatellar bursa
  - Small amount of fluid may be found normally in the deep infrapatellar bursa
- Size: Few mms to several cms depending on the distension of involved bursae
- Morphology
  - Bursae present as flattened synovial sacs are usually not visualized on MRI unless distended with fluid
  - If filled with mild amount of fluid, bursa may remain flattened or collapsed
  - If distended with moderate amount of fluid, bursa may be oval shaped
  - If distended with extensive amount of fluid, bursa may be rounded (convex margins)

Radiographic Findings
- Radiography
  - Soft tissue swelling in anterior soft tissues of the patellofemoral joint
  - +/- Anterior mass

MR Findings
- T1WI
  - Homogeneous decreased signal intensity mass
  - Associated tendinosis of patellar tendon common
    - Thickening and increased signal intensity of tendon origin

DDx: Patellar (Anterior) Bursitis

Hematoma	Hematoma	Anterior Edema	Bursal Hemorrhage	Varicies
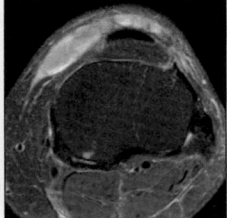	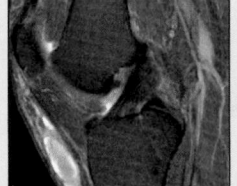	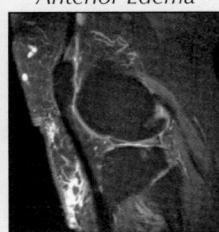	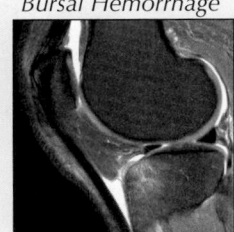	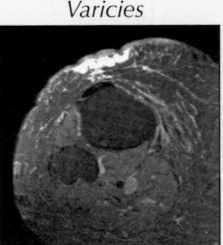
Ax FS PD FSE	*Sag FS PD FSE*	*Sag FS PD FSE*	*Sag FS PD FSE*	*Ax FS PD FSE*

PATELLAR (ANTERIOR) BURSITIS

Key Facts

Terminology
- Inflammation of synovial lining of bursae

Imaging Findings
- Fluid containing mass (fluid signal intensity) in one of the anterior bursae of knee
- Prepatellar bursa
- Superficial infrapatellar bursa
- Deep infrapatellar bursa
- Small amount of fluid may be found normally in the deep infrapatellar bursa

Top Differential Diagnoses
- Meniscal Cyst
- Hemorrhage
- Ganglion Cyst
- Cystic Appearing Mass in or near Bursa

Pathology
- Found in occupations requiring kneeling
- Housemaids, clergy, carpet layers
- Bursal sac with variable thickening of the synovial-like lining

Clinical Issues
- Most common signs/symptoms: Anterior knee pain, +/- mass
- Local injection of corticosteroids with pain relief helps for confirmation of diagnosis

Diagnostic Checklist
- Hyperintense fluid in collection anterior, anteroinferior or inferior and deep to the patellar on FS PD FSE

- ○ Decreased signal in adjacent patella if reactive edema
- T2WI
  - ○ Fluid signal intensity of flattened, oval, or round cystic mass in characteristic location
  - ○ Follows fluid signal intensity on all pulse sequences unless containing inflammatory debris or calcification
    - ▪ Decreased signal structures if calcified
    - ▪ Intermediate signal if contains inflammatory, hemorrhagic or exudative debris
  - ○ Rice bodies especially in patients with rheumatoid arthritis (fibrin filled synovium and thickened synovial membrane forming villous projections that become detached)
    - ▪ Intermediate to decreased signal "rice" shaped fibrinous bodies
  - ○ +/- Associated tendinosis of patellar/quadriceps tendon(s)
    - ▪ Thickening and variable increased signal intensity of tendon insertion with associated bursitis
- T2* GRE
  - ○ Hyperintense fluid intensity structures
  - ○ Decreased signal intensity bursal rim if hemorrhagic
- T1 C+
  - ○ +/- Rim enhancement
  - ○ Greater enhancement if longstanding with thickened synovium

Imaging Recommendations
- Best imaging tool: MRI
- Protocol advice: T2WI, + fat saturation (FS PD FSE) demonstrates fluid-filled bursa

DIFFERENTIAL DIAGNOSIS

Meniscal Cyst
- Visible meniscal tear (most commonly)
- May be mistaken for deep infrapatellar bursitis
- + Meniscal test (clinically)
- +/- Dissection into Hoffa's fat pad

Hemorrhage
- Appropriate history
  - ○ Posttraumatic
- Often accompanied by patellar bone trabecular injury
- Prepatellar soft tissues
- Within bursa proper
  - ○ Hemorrhagic bursitis

Ganglion Cyst
- Nonspecific origin
- +/- Synovial lining
- Hoffa's fat pad near the deep infrapatellar bursa
- Uncommon

Cystic Appearing Mass in or near Bursa
- Rare
- Neoplasm
- Varices
- Hemangioma

Patellar Chondromalacia
- Increased signal with surface irregularity on FS PD FSE
- +/- Surface defect
- +/- Decreased signal abnormalities (desiccation)
- Anterior pain, especially with stair climbing

Patellar Tendinitis
- Jumping sports activities
- Increased signal within thickened proximal posterior tendon fibers on all pulse sequences
  - ○ Hypointense fibrosis + thickening = chronic tendinosis
- +/- Tear (hyperintense on T2WI)

PATHOLOGY

General Features
- General path comments: Inflammation of bursa with effusion
- Etiology

PATELLAR (ANTERIOR) BURSITIS

o Chronic frictional trauma or overuse centered upon the bursal glide plane resulting in inflammation of the bursa
o Infected in case of penetrating trauma
o Crystalline deposit (gout)
• Epidemiology
o Found in occupations requiring kneeling
   ▪ Housemaids, clergy, carpet layers
   ▪ 9% incidence in wrestlers

Gross Pathologic & Surgical Features
• Bursal sac with variable thickening of the synovial-like lining
• Contains variable amounts of fluid
• Three potential bursal spaces anterior to patella
o Prepatellar bursa
   ▪ Most superficial bursa
   ▪ Between skin and arciform fascia (transverse fibers from iliotibial tract extending over patellar tendon)
o Bursa between the arciform layer and the intermediate oblique layer (intermediate layer between arciform layer and deeper longitudinal fibers of the rectus femoris)
o Bursa between intermediate oblique layer and deep fibers of the rectus femoris
• Deep infrapatellar bursa
o Integral to the extensor mechanism
o Scarring or adherence to patellar tendon associated with trochlear groove chondral abnormalities
o Infrapatellar bursa, Hoffa's fat pad and tibial tuberosity prevent impingement between the patellar tendon and bone in full knee flexion

Microscopic Features
• Thickened synovial lining with variable degree of inflammatory infiltration
• Rice bodies can be seen, especially in bursitis associated with rheumatoid arthritis
• Hemorrhagic by-products
• Exudate in infectious bursitis
• Polymorphonuclear cell percentage greater than 75% in fluid
• Infection related to Staphylococcus aureus or Streptococcus

CLINICAL ISSUES

Presentation
• Most common signs/symptoms: Anterior knee pain, +/- mass
• Clinical profile
o Typically middle aged or older patients with anterior knee pain and localized tenderness
o Sometimes with puffiness, ranging from level of the patella to about 5 cm below knee joint to anterior tibia
• Extensor mechanism abnormalities of knee are often present and may distract from clinical consideration of bursitis
• In athletes as overuse phenomenon
• Prepatellar bursal hematoma can be present after direct trauma

Demographics
• Age: Usually adult
• Gender
o Prepatellar bursitis - F > M
o Superficial infrapatellar bursitis - M > F

Natural History & Prognosis
• Insidiously or after athletic/work activity
• Found in patients with predisposing activities
o Repetitive kneeling
• May resolve with cessation of activities that led to condition
• Conservative treatment leads to resolution

Treatment
• Conservative
o Local injection of corticosteroids with pain relief helps for confirmation of diagnosis
o Antibiotics used if infectious
• Surgical
o Extirpation for recalcitrant cases
o Extirpation for infectious bursitis and in some cases calcific bursitis
o Extirpation for selected cases with rice bodies
• Complications
o Tendon weakening and/or tearing if corticosteroid injected into bursa and surrounding tendon

DIAGNOSTIC CHECKLIST

Consider
• In the setting of overuse or if typical patient profile is met
o Anterior trauma (wrestling)
o Work-related kneeling
• Consider mimics such as
o Hematoma
o Small amount of fluid in normal deep infrapatellar bursa

Image Interpretation Pearls
• Hyperintense fluid in collection anterior, anteroinferior or inferior and deep to the patellar on FS PD FSE

SELECTED REFERENCES

1. DeLee J et al: Orthopaedic sports medicine. vol 2. Philadelphia Pennsylvania, Saunders, 1577-2135, 2003
2. Stell IM: Management of acute bursitis: Outcome study of a structured approach. J R Soc Med 92(10):516-21, 1999
3. Gomez-Rodriguez N et al: Infectious bursitis: Study of 40 cases in the pre-patellar and olecranon regions. Enferm Infecc Microbiol Clin 15(5):237-42, 1997
4. Dawn B et al: Prepatellar bursitis: A unique presentation of tophaceous gout in an normouricemic patient. J Rheumatol 24(5):976-8, 1997
5. Butcher JD et al: Lower extremity bursitis. Am Fam Physician 53(7):2317-24, 1996
6. Davis JM et al: Prepatellar bursitis caused by Brucella abortus. Med J Aust 165(8):460, 1996
7. Myllymaki T et al: Carpet-layer's knee. An ultrasonographic study. Acta Radiol 34(5):496-9, 1993

IMAGE GALLERY

Typical

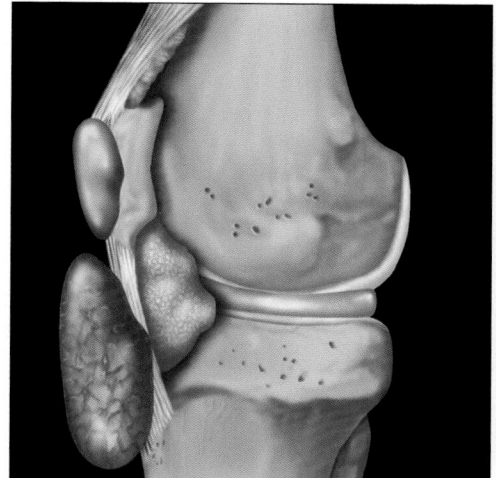
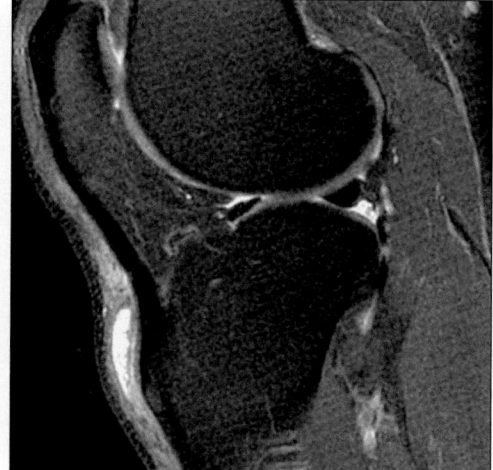

(Left) Sagittal graphic shows an inflamed superficial infrapatellar bursa. Deep infrapatellar bursitis (along the deep surface of the distal tendon) often accompanies Osgood-Schlatter disease or may be isolated. (Right) Sagittal FS PD FSE MR shows fluid within the superficial infrapatellar bursa in a patient with bursitis and clinical "preacher's knee".

Typical

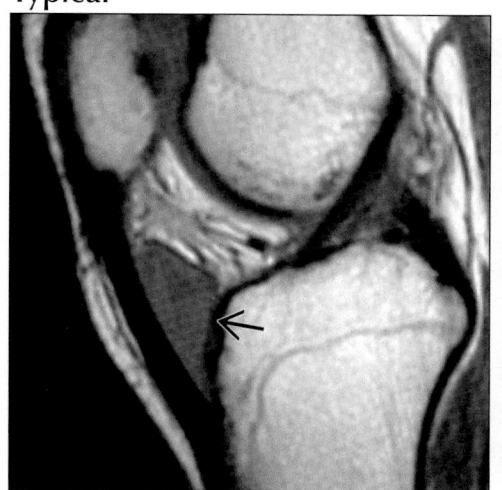
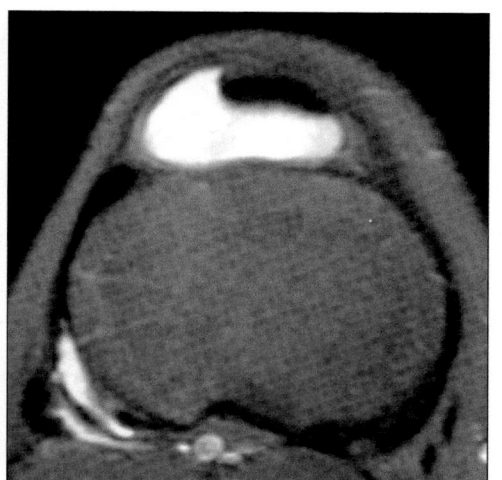

(Left) Sagittal PD FSE MR shows deep infrapatellar bursitis (arrow). (Right) Axial FS PD FSE MR of the same patient shows a large amount of fluid within the deep infrapatellar bursa.

5

109

Typical

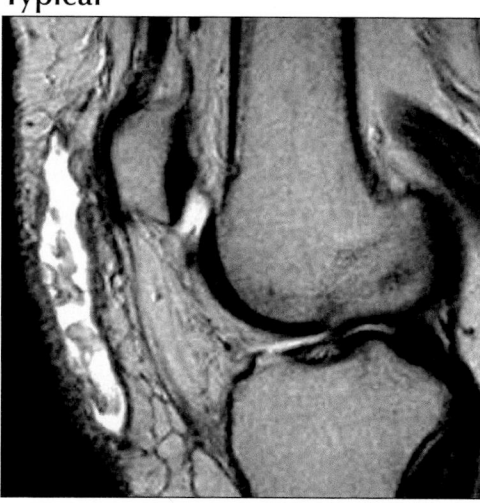
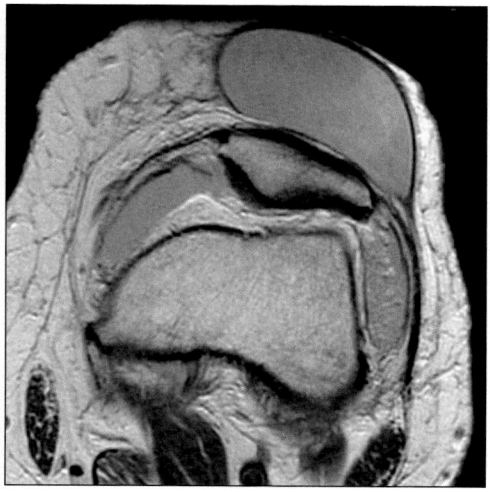

(Left) Sagittal T2 FSE MR shows prepatellar bursitis with the bursal fluid collection containing a large amount of debris. (Right) Axial PD FSE MR shows a large prepatellar bursal fluid collection.

SYNOVITIS, KNEE

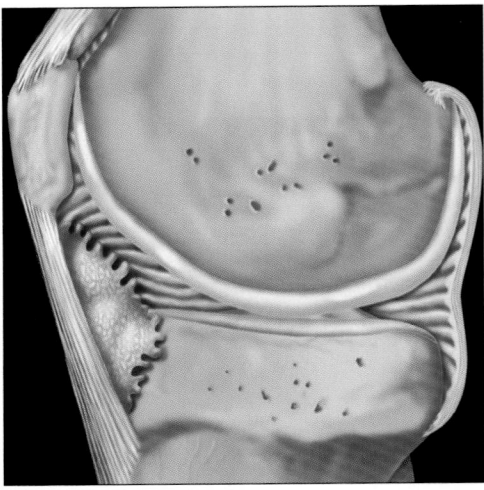

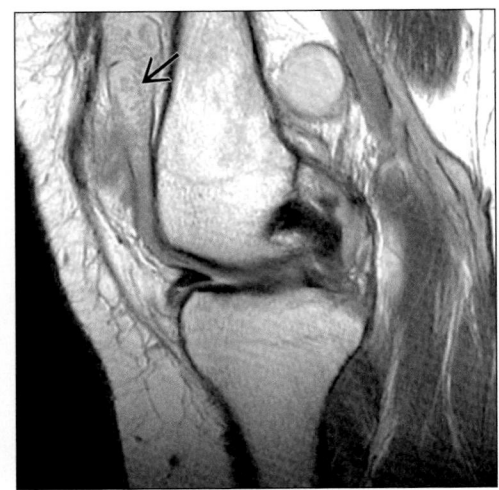

Sagittal graphic shows an inflamed thickened synovium in this patient with Lyme arthritis. Note the irregular free edge of Hoffa's fat pad.

Sagittal PD FSE MR shows extensive synovial thickening (arrow) consistent with synovitis. Hypertrophied synovium is seen adjacent to suprapatellar joint fluid.

TERMINOLOGY

Abbreviations and Synonyms
- Synovitis, Hoffa's disease, irregular fat pad sign

Definitions
- Inflammation of the synovial lining of the knee from various causes including trauma (hemorrhagic effusions), inflammatory arthritis, PVNS, Lyme arthritis, crystal deposition, metal deposition, infection, and neoplasm
- Hoffa's disease = inflammation and enlargement of the synovium of Hoffa's fat pad with variable enlargement of the fat pad itself on either side of the patellar tendon with pain or aching in the anterior compartment

IMAGING FINDINGS

General Features
- Best diagnostic clue
  - Thickened intermediate signal intensity of synovium between periarticular fat and joint fluid on proton density images (PD or FS PD FSE)
    - + Effusion
- Location: Synovial lining of the joint adjacent to Hoffa's fat pad and in the suprapatellar pouch

- Size: Thickened synovium in the case of synovitis varies from a few millimeters to greater than 1 cm with hypertrophic villous fronds
- Morphology
  - Normal synovium is not seen on MRI as a distinct structure
  - Thickening indicates synovitis
  - Relevant anatomy
    - Prefemoral fat and Hoffa's fat pad may have variable morphology - pliability of adipose tissue with respect to joint capsule
    - Should not be confused with synovitis

Radiographic Findings
- Radiography: Effusion

CT Findings
- NECT: Effusion
- CECT
  - Inflamed synovium enhances markedly
  - +/- Villous fronds

MR Findings
- T1WI
  - Low to intermediate in signal intensity in suprapatellar bursa and posterior to free edge of Hoffa's fat pad
    - Irregular fat pad sign (irregular free edge contour of Hoffa's fat pad)

DDx: Synovitis, Knee

Ex Lateral Press	Hemorrhagic Eff.	JCA	RA	PVNS
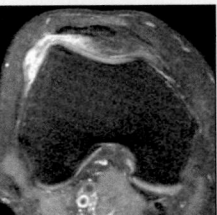	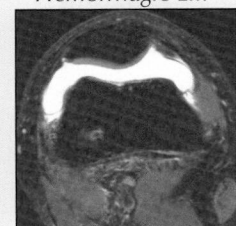	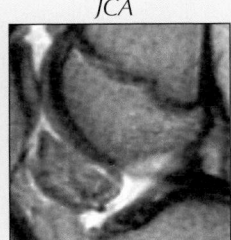	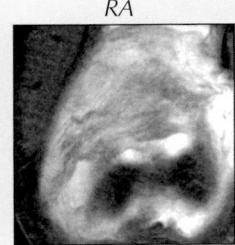	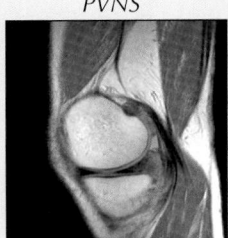
Ax FS PD FSE	Ax FS PD FSE	Sag T2 FSE MR	Cor FS PD FSE	Sag PD FSE MR

SYNOVITIS, KNEE

Key Facts

Terminology
- Inflammation of the synovial lining of the knee from various causes including trauma (hemorrhagic effusions), inflammatory arthritis, PVNS, Lyme arthritis, crystal deposition, metal deposition, infection, and neoplasm

Imaging Findings
- Thickened intermediate signal intensity of synovium between periarticular fat and joint fluid on proton density images (PD or FS PD FSE)
- Location: Synovial lining of the joint adjacent to Hoffa's fat pad and in the suprapatellar pouch
- Thickening indicates synovitis

Top Differential Diagnoses
- Post Traumatic Synovitis
- Indolent Infection
- Inflammatory Arthritis
- Degenerative Arthritis
- Neoplasm/Pseudoneoplasm

Pathology
- Synovial inflammation

Clinical Issues
- Most common signs/symptoms: Synovitis is a cause of knee pain and should be considered as an etiology
- Commonly seen as reaction to underlying internal derangement of a joint

Diagnostic Checklist
- Irregular contour to free edge of Hoffa's fat pad

- T2WI
  - Hyperintense effusion
  - FS PD FSE low to intermediate in signal intensity
- PD/Intermediate
  - Thickened intermediate signal intensity interposed between periarticular fat and joint fluid
    - Effusion relatively hypointense
  - Synovial signal intensity varies depending on the cause of synovitis
  - Hemorrhagic areas of decreased signal intensity within the thickened synovium - hemosiderin deposition
    - Due to trauma, pigmented villonodular synovitis, hemophilia or any cause of hemorrhage
- T2* GRE
  - Low to intermediate signal intensity in hemorrhage related synovitis
  - Blooming can be seen in the synovium in cases of iron deposition, hemosiderin along synovial reflection
- T1 C+
  - Inflamed synovium enhances markedly
  - Visualization of irregular contour of Hoffa's fat pad
- Fibrinous villous hypertrophy can lead to the formation of rice bodies
- Micrometallic artifact on all pulse sequences can be seen in the synovium in cases of metallic deposition
- Decreased signal intensity foci on all pulse sequences indicate calcification
- Ossified bodies in synovial osteochondromatosis

Imaging Recommendations
- Best imaging tool: MRI
- Protocol advice
  - PD and FS PD FSE images to define irregular free edge of Hoffa's fat pad and synovial thickening within joint capsule
  - T1 C+ (intravenous contrast) + FS is sensitive and specific for synovitis

DIFFERENTIAL DIAGNOSIS

Post Traumatic Synovitis
- +/- Hemorrhagic effusion
- Appropriate history
- Sports trauma
- Mildly thickened synovium
- +/- Periarticular inflammatory change
- Chronic frictional trauma
  - Iliotibial band (ITB) syndrome
  - Excessive lateral pressure syndrome (Ex Lat Press)

Indolent Infection
- Tuberculosis
- Lyme arthritis
  - Consider the above in cases of marked effusion and synovitis without trauma or internal derangement

Inflammatory Arthritis
- Rheumatoid arthritis (RA)
- Juvenile chronic arthritis (JCA)
- Other collagen vascular disease
  - Scleroderma, systemic lupus erythematosus

Degenerative Arthritis
- Degenerative arthritis - +/- synovitis in inflammatory osteoarthritis
  - Chondromalacia and underlying bone reactive changes
- Crystal induced arthropathies may demonstrate decreased signal intensity foci on all pulse sequence
- Intra- or periarticular

Neoplasm/Pseudoneoplasm
- Pigmented villonodular synovitis (PVNS)
  - Decreased signal intensity on all pulse sequences synovial thickening
  - Hemosiderin deposition in macrophages
  - Focal nodular or diffuse
  - Hemophilic arthropathy has a similar MR appearance with respect to synovial involvement
- Synovioma
  - Nonspecific focal synovial mass
  - Diffuse enhancement characteristic

SYNOVITIS, KNEE

- Osteochondromatosis
  - Synovial masses of various sizes of intermediate to decreased signal intensity on all pulse sequences depending on composition
  - +/- Calcification
- Synovial hemangioma
  - Increased signal intensity mass (T2WI) with septated, tubular structures
  - FS PD FSE useful
- Rice bodies
  - Fibrin filled villous structures typically found in rheumatoid arthritis
  - Typically fragments from the synovium to fill the joint or a nearby bursa with masses that resemble rice

PATHOLOGY

General Features
- General path comments
  - Synovial inflammation
  - Inflammation + enlargement of the synovium of Hoffa's fat pad with variable enlargement of the fat pad itself + pain or aching in the anterior compartment
- Genetics: ± Genetic predisposition in cases of inflammatory arthritis
- Etiology: Varied depending on cause, may be seen in posttraumatic setting, osteoarthritis and rheumatoid arthritis
- Epidemiology
  - Commonly observed after variety of insults to knee
  - 75 to 85% of older individuals with arthritis and synovitis

Gross Pathologic & Surgical Features
- Thick dull opaque synovium develops as a result of synovitis
  - Normally transparent, smooth and thin
- Turns red with hemorrhagic synovitis and turns reddish-brown with chronic hemarthrosis due to hemosiderin
  - May turn purple in chronic, severe cases
- Darkening maybe result of metallic deposition
- Ochronosis can result in grey appearance
- White foci may indicate crystal deposition or calcification

Microscopic Features
- Degenerative joint disease - mild villous hypertrophy without pannus formation
- Rheumatoid arthritis – nodular lymphocyte and plasma cell infiltration + villous hypertrophy & proliferation of synoviocytes
- Septic arthritis - leukocytic infiltration
- Traumatic synovitis - fibrinous change
- Neuropathic joint – bone and cartilage detritus

Staging, Grading or Classification Criteria
- Staging criteria have been proposed based on individual arthritides
  - Conventional radiographs insensitive to mild effusions and irregular Hoffa's fat pad sign

CLINICAL ISSUES

Presentation
- Most common signs/symptoms: Synovitis is a cause of knee pain and should be considered as an etiology
- Clinical profile
  - Depending on the underlying disease
  - Commonly seen as reaction to underlying internal derangement of a joint

Demographics
- Age: Varies (greater than 45 years for arthritis population)
- Gender: Depends on specific disease state

Natural History & Prognosis
- Resolves in uncomplicated posttraumatic synovitis

Treatment
- Conservative - minor trauma
- Surgical - neoplasm, pseudoneoplasm, severe cases (synovectomy)

DIAGNOSTIC CHECKLIST

Image Interpretation Pearls
- Thickened synovium with intermediate to increased signal intensity: Posttraumatic, degenerative arthritis, inflammatory arthritis, neoplasm, crystal deposition, infection
- Thickened synovium with decreased signal intensity: PVNS, synovial osteochondromatosis (ossified bodies), any cause of hemorrhagic synovitis, crystal deposition disease in some cases, metallic deposition (lead synovitis)
- Irregular contour to free edge of Hoffa's fat pad
- Synovitis will enhance with intravenous contrast

SELECTED REFERENCES

1. Saito I et al: Increased cellular infiltrate in inflammatory synovia of osteoarthritic knees. Osteoarthritis Cartilage 10(2):156-62, 2002
2. Abdelwahab F et al: True bursal pigmented villonodular synovitis. Skeletal Radiol 31(6):354-8, 2002
3. Dabby D et al: Synovial knee pain arising from chronic inflammatory disorders of the knee. J Knee Surg 15(1):53-6, 2002
4. Gibbons CE et al: Long-term results of arthroscopic synovectomy for seropositive rheumatoid arthritis: 6-16 year review. Int Orthop, 26(2):98-100, 2002
5. Hoffman EB et al: Tuberculosis of the knee. Clin Orthop (398):100-6, 2002
6. Jackson RW: Arthroscopic synovectomy. J Rheumatol 28(7):1474-5, 2001
7. Jaswal TS et al: Synovial hemangioma--a case report. Indian J Pathol Microbiol 44(3):353-4, 2001
8. Hill CL et al: Knee effusions, popliteal cysts, and synovial thickening: Association with knee pain in osteoarthritis. J Rheumatol 28(6):1330-7, 2001
9. Bredella MA et al: Reactive synovitis of the knee joint: MR imaging appearance with arthroscopic correlation. Skeletal Radiol 29(10):577-82, 2000

SYNOVITIS, KNEE

IMAGE GALLERY

Typical

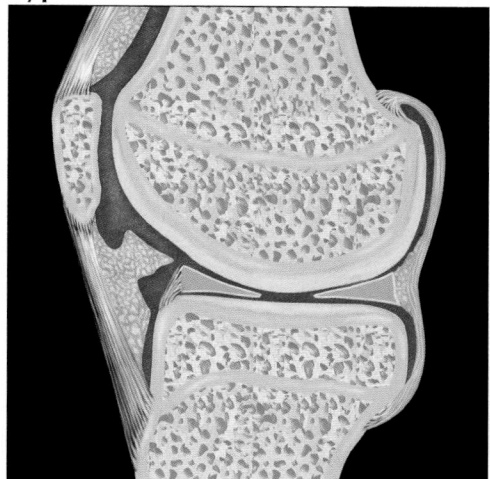
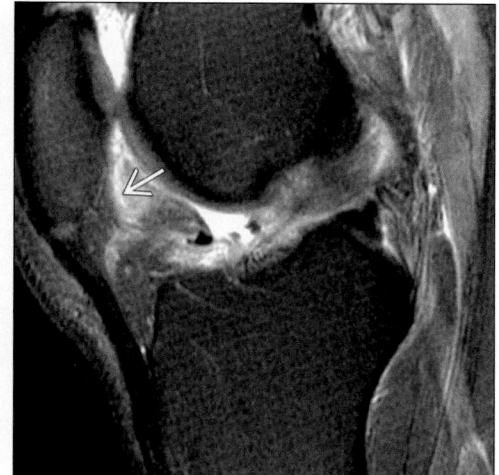

(Left) Sagittal graphic shows Hoffa's irregular fat pad sign. An irregular posterior surface indicates synovitis in this location. *(Right)* Sagittal FS PD FSE MR shows synovitis (arrow) along the posterior margin of Hoffa's fat pad.

Typical

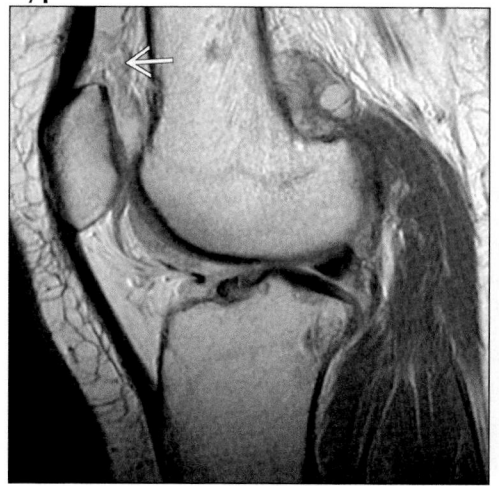
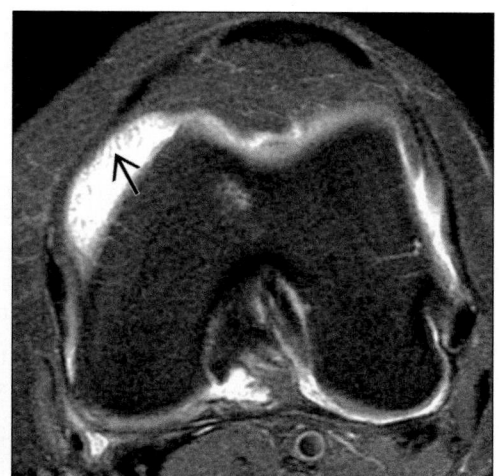

(Left) Sagittal PD FSE MR shows synovitis (arrow) in the suprapatellar pouch and an irregular fat pad sign. *(Right)* Axial FS PD FSE MR shows thickened synovium as frond-like projections (arrow) into the suprapatellar portion of the joint. This synovitis has the arthroscopic appearance of "hair".

5

113

Typical

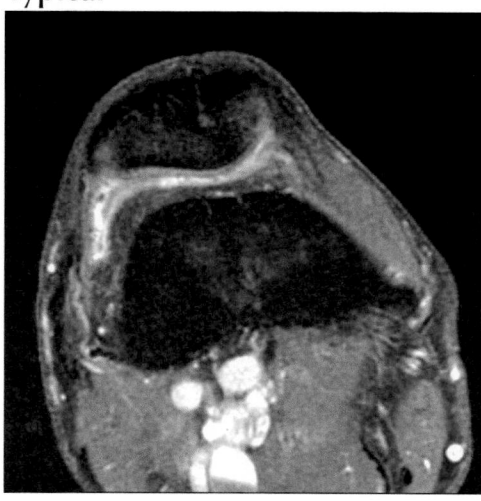
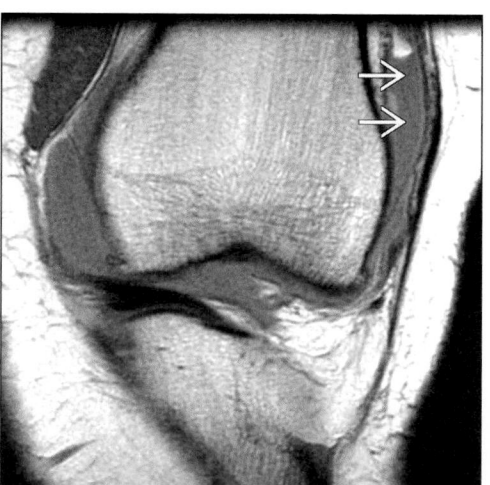

(Left) Axial T1 C+ MR shows synovial enhancement consistent with synovitis. Normal synovium does not enhance. *(Right)* Coronal PD FSE MR shows subtle synovitis as thickened, intermediate signal intensity synovium (arrows) compared to slightly decreased signal intensity joint fluid best seen laterally.

PATELLAR TENDON TEARS

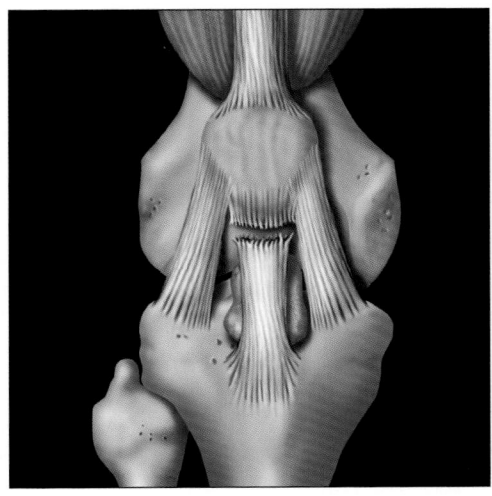

Coronal graphic shows a tear of the proximal patellar tendon (ligament). This is often considered an orthopedic emergency and is treated quickly to prevent fibrosis after retraction.

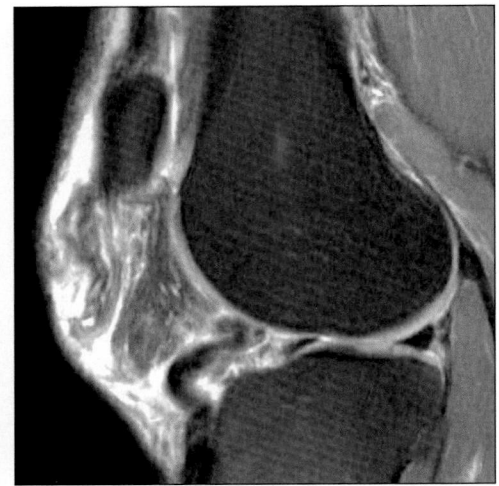

Sagittal FS PD FSE shows rupture of patellar tendon with preexisting patellar tendinitis in a patient who had multiple steroid injections. Patient was performing a "lay-up" basketball move.

TERMINOLOGY

Abbreviations and Synonyms
- Patellar tendon rupture

Definitions
- Disruption of the patellar tendon

IMAGING FINDINGS

General Features
- Best diagnostic clue: Tear or gap in patellar tendon, +/- hemorrhage & granulation tissue
- Location
  - Proximal third of the patellar tendon (most common)
  - Inferior pole of patellar
- Size: Range from mm to several cms
- Morphology: Irregular thickened tendon edges, retracted

Radiographic Findings
- Radiography: Lateral radiograph - small avulsion at inferior patellar pole, patella alta

MR Findings
- T2WI: Fluid signal intensity filling a gap in the tendon, +/- surrounding reactive edema

Imaging Recommendations
- Best imaging tool: MRI to document partial vs. complete retraction
- Protocol advice: FS PD FSE & T2* GRE

DIFFERENTIAL DIAGNOSIS

Patellar Tendinitis/Tendinosis without Tear
- Jumper's knee, injured by steroid use
- +/- Deep infrapatellar bursal fluid

Hematoma
- Increased signal mass on T2WI

Sinding-Larsen-Johansson Disease
- Traction apophysitis at inferior pole of patella

Bipartite Patella
- Failure of superolateral ossification fusion, +/- stress response/fracture

PATHOLOGY

General Features
- General path comments
  - Degeneration & deterioration as a predisposing factor to tendon rupture

---

DDx: Patellar Tendon Tears

Deep Bursitis	Stress Bipartite	Hematoma	Tendinitis
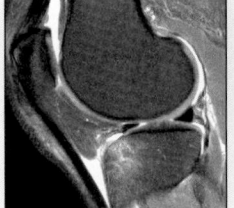	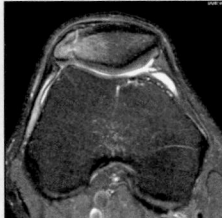	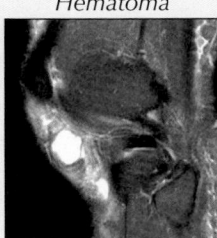	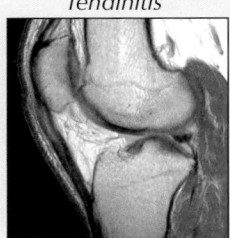
Sag FS PD FSE	Ax FS PD FSE	Sag FS PD FSE	Sag PD FSE MR

PATELLAR TENDON TEARS

Key Facts

Terminology
- Patellar tendon rupture

Imaging Findings
- Best diagnostic clue: Tear or gap in patellar tendon, +/- hemorrhage & granulation tissue
- Proximal third of the patellar tendon (most common)
- Radiography: Lateral radiograph - small avulsion at inferior patellar pole, patella alta
- T2WI: Fluid signal intensity filling a gap in the tendon, +/- surrounding reactive edema

Top Differential Diagnoses
- Patellar Tendinitis/Tendinosis without Tear
- Hematoma
- Sinding-Larsen-Johansson Disease
- Bipartite Patella

Pathology
- Degeneration & deterioration as a predisposing factor to tendon rupture
- Etiology: Jumping sports (dynamic loading), steroid injections, previous surgery (ACL reconstruction)

Clinical Issues
- Complete tear results in inability to extend knee
- Partial tear: Incomplete knee extension without full range of motion

Diagnostic Checklist
- Partial tear in the setting of peripatellar pain
- FS PD FSE sagittal images demonstrate tendon tear morphology

---

- Tensile & viscoelastic properties of the patellar tendon, however remain relatively stable between younger and older age groups
- Etiology: Jumping sports (dynamic loading), steroid injections, previous surgery (ACL reconstruction)
- Epidemiology
  - Acute tear in patient < 40 yrs of age, +/- preexisting disease (e.g., rheumatoid arthritis, diabetes)
  - Less common than quadriceps tendon rupture

Gross Pathologic & Surgical Features
- Thickened, indurated tendon edges with discontinuity

Microscopic Features
- Preexisting collagen degeneration without significant influx of inflammatory cells

Staging, Grading or Classification Criteria
- Grade I - mild strain with minimal functional impairment, grade II - intermediate tear, grade III - complete disruption

CLINICAL ISSUES

Presentation
- Most common signs/symptoms: Pain, physical examination reveals palpable defect in patellar ligament with complete tear
- Clinical profile
  - Complete tear results in inability to extend knee
  - Partial tear: Incomplete knee extension without full range of motion

Demographics
- Age: Physically active patients < 40 years
- Gender: Male > female

Natural History & Prognosis
- Complete tear requires surgical repair and is often considered an orthopedic emergency

Treatment
- Conservative: Partial tear can be treated with immobilization for 3-6 weeks

- Surgical: Repair using end-to-end sutures, +/- delayed or late repair

DIAGNOSTIC CHECKLIST

Consider
- Partial tear in the setting of peripatellar pain

Image Interpretation Pearls
- FS PD FSE sagittal images demonstrate tendon tear morphology

SELECTED REFERENCES
1. McGrory JE: Disruption of the extensor mechanism of the knee. J Emerg Med 24(2):163-8, 2003
2. Enad JG et al: Primary patellar tendon repair and early mobilization: Results in an active-duty population. J South Orthop Assoc 10(1):17-23, 2001
3. Kasten P et al: Rupture of the patellar tendon: A review of 68 cases and a retrospective study of 29 ruptures comparing two methods of augmentation. Arch Orthop Trauma Surg 121(10):578-82, 2001
4. Casey MR et al: Neglected ruptures of the patellar tendon. A case series of four patients. Am J Sports Med 29(4):457-60, 2001

IMAGE GALLERY

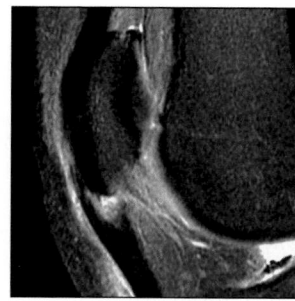 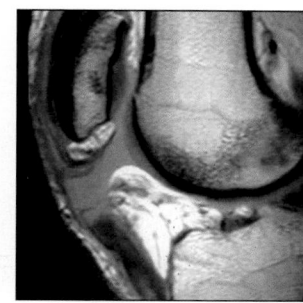

(Left) Sagittal FS PD FSE MR shows a partial patellar tendon tear. *(Right)* Sagittal PD FSE MR shows a complete rupture of the patellar tendon.

CHONDROMALACIA PATELLA

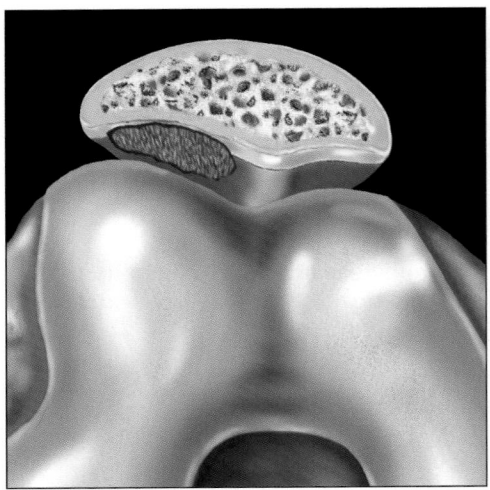

Axial graphic shows thinning and irregularity of the hyaline cartilage of the lateral patellar facet consistent with chondromalacia.

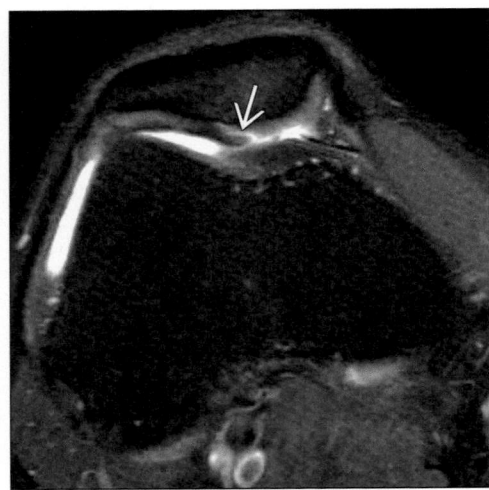

Axial FS PD FSE MR shows chondromalacia of the patella with a developing chondral flap (arrow) and underlying bone marrow edema at the lateral aspect of the median ridge.

TERMINOLOGY

Abbreviations and Synonyms
- Chondromalacia patella (CMP)

Definitions
- Degradation and eventually ulceration of hyaline cartilage of the patella usually with underlying bone reactive changes

IMAGING FINDINGS

General Features
- Best diagnostic clue: Signal alteration of patella hyaline cartilage with variable degrees of ulceration and underlying bone reactive change
- Location: Patellar hyaline cartilage
- Size: Varies from small area to entire chondral surface
- Morphology: Varies from small well-defined defect to larger irregular region

Radiographic Findings
- Radiography
  - Osteoarthritic changes are late findings and include
    - Osteophyte formation
    - Subchondral cyst formation
    - Bone attrition and remodeling
    - Subchondral sclerosis

MR Findings
- T1WI
  - Area of hypointensity within hyaline articular cartilage
  - Subchondral reactive change includes bone marrow edema, cyst formation and sclerosis - hypointense
  - Surface irregularity not well seen on T1WI
- T2WI
  - FS PD & PD FSE MR sequences sensitive to the changes of chondromalacia
  - Increased or less commonly decreased signal intensity on fat saturated fast spin echo images
    - Due to alterations in water content
  - Focal areas of hyperintensity on FS PD FSE within normal contour - early stages (softening)
    - Blister-like swelling with focal cartilage convexity and signal change
  - Fraying of hyaline articular cartilage surface (crab meat morphology by arthroscopy and MRI) - intermediate stage
  - Partial thickness chondral defect - more advanced stage
  - Full thickness chondral loss & subchondral erosion - end stage
  - Fissures or chondral defects often are seen as hyperintensity in contrast to the adjacent intermediate signal cartilage
  - Bone marrow and edema within the adjacent patella

DDx: Chondromalacia Patella

Normal Arthrogram	Trochlea Chondro	Pat Tendinitis	Prepat Edema

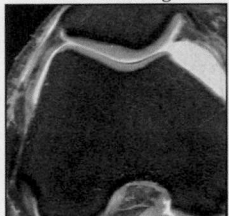 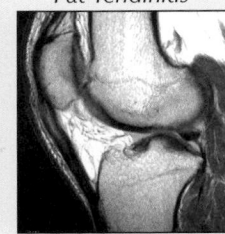 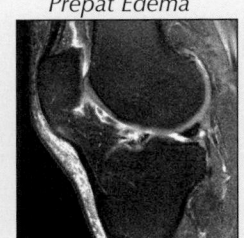

Ax FS PD FSE	Sag FS PD FSE	Sag PD FSE MR	Sag FS PD FSE

CHONDROMALACIA PATELLA

Key Facts

Terminology
- Degradation and eventually ulceration of hyaline cartilage of the patella usually with underlying bone reactive changes

Imaging Findings
- Best diagnostic clue: Signal alteration of patella hyaline cartilage with variable degrees of ulceration and underlying bone reactive change
- FS PD & PD FSE MR sequences sensitive to the changes of chondromalacia
- Fraying of hyaline articular cartilage surface (crab meat morphology by arthroscopy and MRI) - intermediate stage
- Full thickness chondral loss & subchondral erosion - end stage

Top Differential Diagnoses
- Osteochondral Injuries of Femoral Trochlea
- Patellar Tendinitis
- Dorsal Defect of Patella

Pathology
- Degenerative in nature (50%) but can be acute and posttraumatic (15%)

Clinical Issues
- Anterior knee pain

Diagnostic Checklist
- Chondral edema as an early marker of articular cartilage softening

---

- Acute changes (acute inflammatory chondromalacia)
  - Stress vs. a bone trabecular injury in cases of direct trauma
  - Subchondral cysts are seen in more chronic cases and are hyperintense
    - Identified with full thickness chondral loss
- T2* GRE
  - T2* weighted GRE demonstrates larger defects as hyperintense
    - Normal cartilage may be isointense to joint fluid and therefore surface defects may be inconspicuous
    - T2 * GRE not a recommended cartilage imaging sequence (not sensitive to fibrillation & fissures)

Imaging Recommendations
- Best imaging tool
  - MRI
    - Detects early & late stages of chondromalacia
- Protocol advice: PD or FS PD FSE in axial plane for patellar facets and sagittal plane for trochlear groove

DIFFERENTIAL DIAGNOSIS

Osteochondral Injuries of Femoral Trochlea
- Hyaline articular cartilage abnormalities of femoral trochlea
- +/- Underlying bone changes
- +/- Normal patella
- Traumatic - direct impact
- Chronic microtrauma and associated with CMP
- Associated with thickened infrapatellar plica

Patellar Tendinitis
- Increased signal intensity and/or thickening within the patellar tendon
- Associated with jumping sports activity
- Pain at proximal tendon inferior to patella

Dorsal Defect of Patella
- Located along the superolateral aspect of the articular surface of patella

- Radiolucency with sclerotic margins and intact overlying articular cartilage

Anterior Meniscal Tears
- Uncommon as isolated abnormality
- ± Horizontal tear and meniscal cyst
- Diagnostic MRI finding of increased signal on short TE sequence extending to surface

Inflammation of Hoffa's Fat Pad (Hoffitis)
- Associated with generalized synovitis
- Irregular posterior margin
  - Irregular fat pad sign

Prepatellar Edema (Prepat Edema)
- Superficial subcutaneous edema
- ± Associated trauma
- Nonspecific

PATHOLOGY

General Features
- General path comments: Softening of articular cartilage with associated degenerative changes includes fissuring, ulceration, chondral defects and underlying bone changes
- Etiology
  - Degenerative in nature (50%) but can be acute and posttraumatic (15%)
  - 20% secondary to tracking abnormalities - lateral patellar compression syndrome
  - 15% secondary to chronic dislocations
  - Causes of acute chondromalacia include instability, direct trauma, and fracture
  - Causes of chronic chondromalacia include
    - Patellar subluxation, increased quadriceps angle (Q-angle), quadriceps imbalance, posttraumatic malalignment, excessive lateral pressure syndrome and posterior cruciate ligament (PCL) injuries
  - Painful chondromalacia
    - Excessive mechanical overload
    - Increased intraosseous pressure of the patella

- ■ Transient venous outflow obstruction (pain with prolonged knee flexion)
- ■ Excessive load transference to innervated subchondral and cancellous bone
- ■ Malalignment - shifting and transference of load with excessive mechanical forces
- ■ Chronic triggering of pain producing cytokines
- Epidemiology: Young women
- Associated abnormalities: Patella alta, increased valgus angle, and femoral condyle hypoplasia

Gross Pathologic & Surgical Features
- Softening, discoloration, fissuring and/or ulceration and desiccation

Microscopic Features
- Histologic changes of articular cartilage softening occur in transitional zone deep to superficial zone
  - ○ Reorientation and disorganization of collagen and fibers into collapsed segments associated with decrease in matrix proteoglycans

Staging, Grading or Classification Criteria
- MRI adaptation of Outerbridge arthroscopic grading system
  - ○ Grade 1
    - ■ FS PD FSE display focal areas of hyperintensity within normal contour
    - ■ ± Focal basal degeneration
    - ■ Softening by arthroscopy
  - ○ Grade 2
    - ■ FS PD FSE demonstrates blister-like swelling of articular cartilage extending to surface
    - ■ Fissuring and fibrillation within soft areas of articular cartilage and extending to a depth of 1 to 2 mm within an area of 1.3 cm or less in diameter arthroscopically
  - ○ Grade 3
    - ■ FS PD FSE demonstrates focal ulcerations and "crab meat" lesions
    - ■ Partial thickness cartilage loss (> 2 mm depth in area and > 1.3 cm in diameter) arthroscopically
  - ○ Grade 4
    - ■ FS PD FSE demonstrate full thickness cartilage loss with underlying bone reactive changes
    - ■ Ulceration with exposed subchondral bone (end-stage) arthroscopically

CLINICAL ISSUES

Presentation
- Most common signs/symptoms
  - ○ Anterior knee pain
  - ○ Patellofemoral joint pain
    - ■ Especially during flexion as can occur in ascending or descending stairs: Associated crepitus

Demographics
- Age: Most often affects adolescents and young adults
- Gender: F > M

Natural History & Prognosis
- Insidious onset or acute onset subsequent to patellar trauma

Treatment
- Initial treatment is conservative and consists of rest and rehabilitation
- If instability is present surgical correction may be needed
- Direct surgical treatment of chondromalacia includes chondroplasty microfracturing and chondral implantation

DIAGNOSTIC CHECKLIST

Image Interpretation Pearls
- Utilize FS PD FSE and PD FSE axial images to optimize visualization of cartilage fibrillation, blister, fissure, ulceration and fragmentation
- Chondral edema as an early marker of articular cartilage softening

SELECTED REFERENCES

1. Peterson L et al: Treatment of osteochondritis dissecans of the knee with autologous chondrocyte transplantation: Results at two to ten years. J Bone Joint Surg Am 85-A Suppl 2:17-24, 2003
2. Fitzgerald R Jr et al: Orthopaedics. Pediatric Orthopaedics. St. Louis, MO, Mosby, 1489-95, 2002
3. Kerrigan DC et al: Women's shoes and knee osteoarthritis. Lancet 357(9262):1097-8, 2001
4. Outerbridge RE: The etiology of chondromalacia patellae. Clin Orthop (389):5-8, 2001
5. Bosch JJ: Chondromalacia patella. J Pediatr Health Care 13(3:1):144; quiz 155-6, 1999
6. Kim BS et al: Selective patellar nonresurfacing in total knee arthroplasty. 10 year results. Clin Orthop (367):81-8, 1999
7. Kannus P et al: An outcome study of chronic patellofemoral pain syndrome. Seven-year follow-up of patients in a randomized, controlled trial. J Bone Joint Surg Am 81(3):355-63, 1999
8. Holmes SW Jr et al: Clinical classification of patellofemoral pain and dysfunction. J Orthop Sports Phys Ther 28(5):299-306, 1998
9. Johnson LL et al: Clinical assessment of asymptomatic knees: Comparison of men and women. Arthroscopy 14(4):347-59, 1998
10. Barrack RL et al: Resurfacing of the patella in total knee arthroplasty. A prospective, randomized, double-blind study. J Bone Joint Surg Am 79(8):1121-31, 1997
11. Minas T et al: Current concepts in the treatment of articular carilage defects. Orthopaedics 20:525-38, 1997
12. Van Leersum M et al: Chondromalacia patellae: An in vitro study. Comparison of MR criteria with histologic and macroscopic findings. Skeletal Radiol 25(8):727-32, 1996
13. Joshi AB et al: Total knee arthroplasty after patellectomy. J Bone Joint Surg 76(6):926-9,1994
14. Kelly MA et al: Historical perspectives of chondromalacia patellae. Orthop Clin North Am 23(4):517-21, 1992
15. Kolettis GT et al: Patellar resurfacing for patellofemoral arthritis. Orthop Clin North Am 23(4):665-73, 1992

CHONDROMALACIA PATELLA

Typical

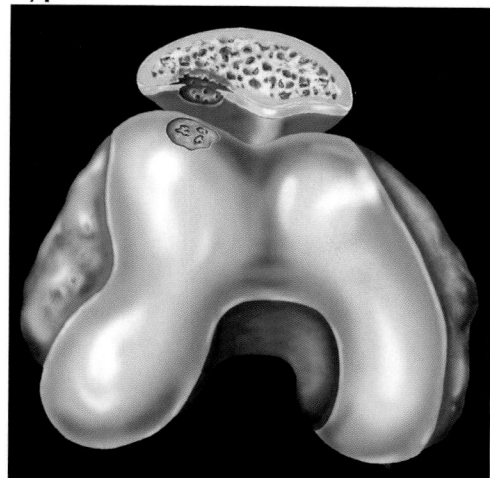

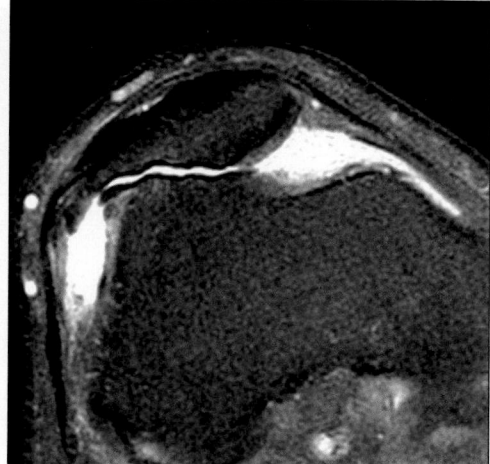

(Left) Axial graphic demonstrates chondromalacia of the lateral patella and femoral trochlea with underlying cystic resorptive changes of the subchondral bone. This constellation of findings is associated with excessive lateral pressure syndrome. *(Right)* Axial FS PD FSE MR shows patellofemoral arthrosis with full thickness chondral loss and subchondral irregularity of the lateral facet.

Typical

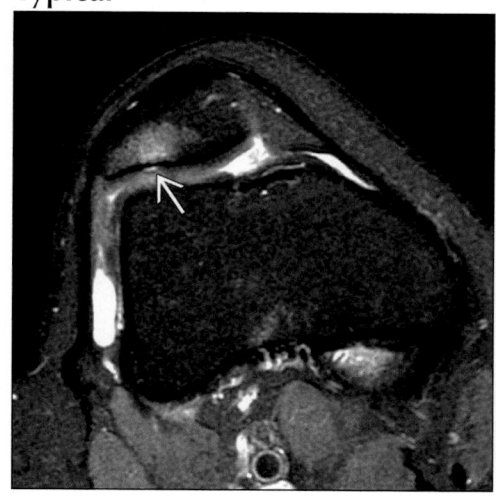

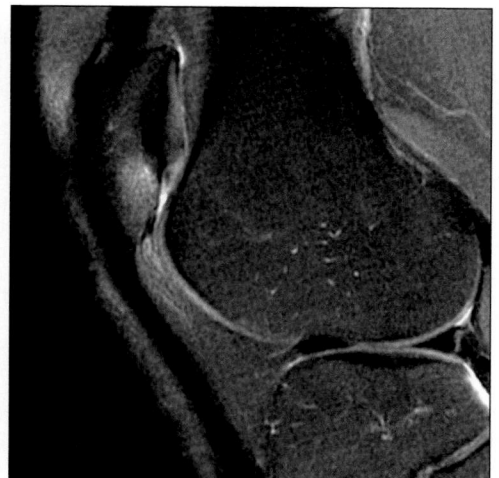

(Left) Axial FS PD FSE MR shows a "subchondral bubble" area (arrow) of chondral dehiscence with adjacent bone marrow edema, also referred to as "acute inflammatory chondromalacia". *(Right)* Sagittal FS PD FSE MR of the same patient demonstrates hyperintense inferior pole edema.

5

119

Typical

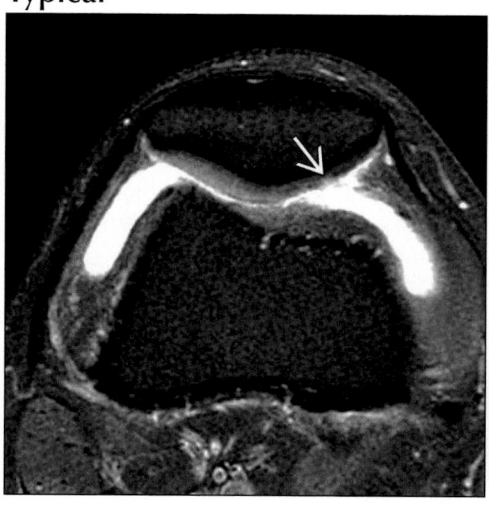

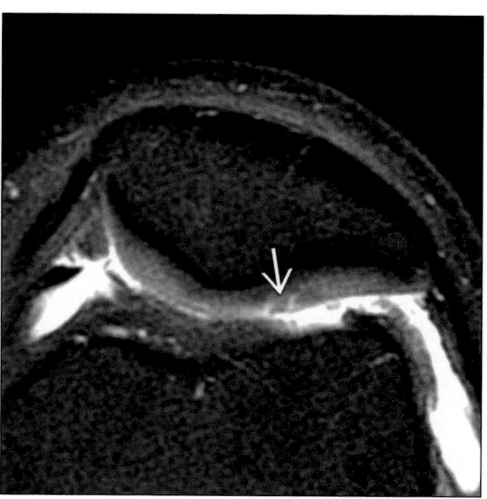

(Left) Axial FS PD FSE MR shows mild surface irregularity (arrow) in early chondromalacia (arrow). *(Right)* Axial FS PD FSE MR shows lateral patellar facet chondral fissuring (arrow) and a thick medial plica with a normal medial facet.

QUADRICEPS TENDON TEAR

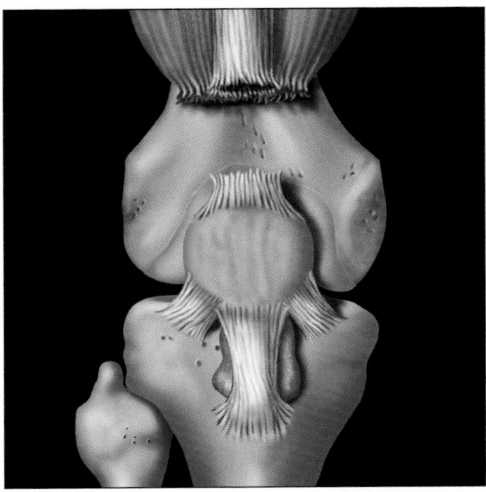

Coronal graphic shows a complete tear of the quadriceps tendon adjacent to the patellar insertion site.

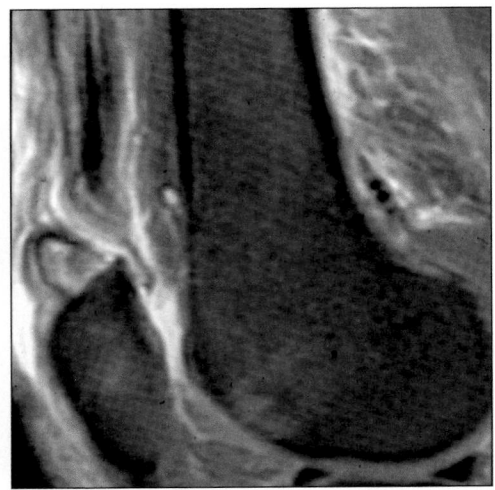

Sagittal FS PD FSE MR shows a complete tear of the distal quadriceps tendon. Associated patella baja is demonstrated.

TERMINOLOGY

Abbreviations and Synonyms
- Quadriceps tendon rupture (quad rupture)

Definitions
- Rupture of the quadriceps tendon at the patellar insertion site

IMAGING FINDINGS

General Features
- Best diagnostic clue
  - Discontinuous hypointense signal (T1 & T2WI) fibers of the quadriceps tendon
    - Interposed with surrounding edema/hemorrhage
- Location
  - Commonly occurs above level of the patellar insertion site of the tendon (expansion)
  - Usually initiated centrally and progresses peripherally
  - Rupture often extends through the vastus intermedius tendon
    - Proximal to a rupture involving the rectus femoris tendon
- Size: Varies from small interstitial or partial surface tear to large tear with gap

- Morphology
  - From small interstitial or surface partial gap in the tendon to large tear with irregular borders
    - Variable retraction

Radiographic Findings
- Radiography
  - Patella may migrate inferiorly with full thickness tear (patella baja)
    - +/- Soft tissue swelling

MR Findings
- T1WI
  - Normal quadriceps tendon has a laminated appearance
  - Discontinuous hypointense fibers of the tendon
  - Interposed with surrounding decreased signal intensity edema/hemorrhage
  - +/- Patella baja
  - +/- Patella with decreased signal intensity edema
- T2WI
  - Hyperintense fluid/hemorrhage in tear site, +/- tendon retraction (FS PD FSE)
  - Tendon diastasis
  - Complete ruptures seen as increased signal intensity and discontinuous fibers
  - Partial tear (grade I and II strain) - variable thickening, increased signal intensity, continuity of fibers remain intact

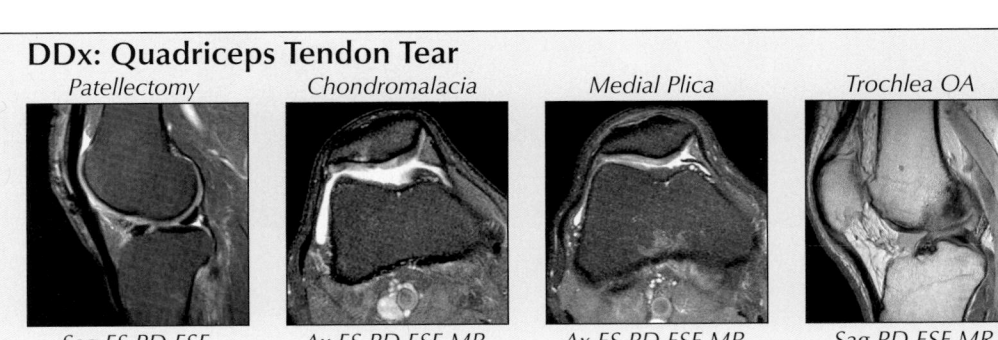

DDx: Quadriceps Tendon Tear

Patellectomy	Chondromalacia	Medial Plica	Trochlea OA
Sag FS PD FSE	Ax FS PD FSE MR	Ax FS PD FSE MR	Sag PD FSE MR

QUADRICEPS TENDON TEAR

Key Facts

Terminology
- Rupture of the quadriceps tendon at the patellar insertion site

Imaging Findings
- Discontinuous hypointense signal (T1 & T2WI) fibers of the quadriceps tendon
- Commonly occurs above level of the patellar insertion site of the tendon (expansion)

Top Differential Diagnoses
- Patellar Chondromalacia
- Patellar Tendinosis
- Medial Plica
- Osteoarthritis/Chondromalacia Patella
- Surgery

Pathology
- Begins centrally and progresses peripherally

Clinical Issues
- Large hemarthrosis with freely mobile patella
- Age: 5th and 6th decade
- Full thickness tears need to be repaired within 48 hours if possible

Diagnostic Checklist
- Expanding FOV to completely evaluate tendon rupture
- Identify discontinuous fibers on FS PD FSE in the sagittal plane
- Evaluate superior aspect of the sagittal images to detect tendinosis or tear

---

- ○ T2 FSE is less sensitive for the depiction of edema compared to FS PD FSE
- ○ +/- Inferior migration of patella
- ○ Surrounding soft tissue hyperintensity edema
- PD/Intermediate: Less sensitive for the depiction of edema compared to FS PD FSE or STIR
- STIR
  - ○ Hyperintense fluid as FS PD FSE except with less resolution of tendon
  - ○ Superior soft tissue contrast including degenerative area within tendon
  - ○ Altered tendon structure (incomplete ruptures with focal discontinuities of individual layers)
  - ○ Tendon laxity secondary to loss of extensor mechanism tension
  - ○ +/- Patellar hyperintense edema
- T2* GRE
  - ○ Discontinuous fibers of the tendon with intermediate to hyperintense signal in tendon edges
  - ○ Magic angle may cause increased signal intensity at tendon patella junction

Imaging Recommendations
- Best imaging tool: MRI
- Protocol advice: FS PD FSE images preferably in the sagittal and axial planes

DIFFERENTIAL DIAGNOSIS

Patellar Chondromalacia
- Increased signal with surface irregularity on FS PD FSE
- +/- Surface defect
- +/- Decreased signal (FS PD FSE) abnormalities (desiccation)
- Anterior knee pain, especially with stair climbing
- Trochlear osteoarthritis (OA)

Patellar Tendinosis
- Jumping sports
- Increased signal on short TE sequence
- +/- Partial tear/tear

Magic Angle Artifact
- At 55° to external magnetic field
- Upper patellar tendon
- Short TE sequences
  - ○ T1WI
  - ○ PD/intermediate
  - ○ T2* GRE
- Tendon not thickened
- Asymptomatic
- Quad patella interface
- Unusual cause of increased signal
  - ○ Less common than in patellar tendon

Stress Response/Fracture of the Patella
- Increased signal intensity on T2WI with or without fracture lines in the presence of a normal quadriceps tendon
- +/- Trauma
- +/- Repetitive microtrauma
- +/- Chondromalacia patella

Medial Plica
- Failure of resorption of embryologic remnant
- +/- Thickening of plica (hypointense on T1 and T2WI)
- Adolescent/young adult usually
- Medial anterior pain and sometimes suprapatellar pain

Osteoarthritis/Chondromalacia Patella
- Subchondral cysts
- Subchondral edema
- Subchondral sclerosis
- Anterior pain, especially with stair climbing

Surgery
- Post operative healing - thickening/fibrosis
- Patellectomy
- Appropriate history

PATHOLOGY

General Features
- General path comments

- ○ Begins centrally and progresses peripherally
- ○ Superficial and deep tears rarely involve the trilaminar tendon at the same level
- Etiology
  - ○ Decreased vascularity, predisposing conditions
    - ■ Cortisone injections
    - ■ Diabetes
    - ■ Chronic renal failure
    - ■ Hyperthyroidism
    - ■ Gout
  - ○ Acute flexion of extended knee
    - ■ Usually in setting of preexisting tendinosis
    - ■ Chronic repetitive microtrauma - tendinosis
    - ■ Eccentric contraction leads to tendon failure
- Epidemiology: Uncommon < 1%
- Associated abnormalities: Inferior migration of patella in complete tears

Gross Pathologic & Surgical Features

- Discontinuous tendon fibers with surrounding edema/hemorrhage in complete tears

Microscopic Features

- Discontinuous tendon fibers with surrounding edema/hemorrhage
- Tendinosis associated with neovascularization
  - ○ Attempt at healing
- Tendinosis with angioblastic hyperplasia
- Absence of inflammatory cells in tendon microtears/partial rupture

Staging, Grading or Classification Criteria

- Tendon strain
  - ○ Grade I (mild)
    - ■ Tear of only few tendon fibers
    - ■ + Mild swelling, pain, disability
    - ■ Functional, painful, muscle contractions
  - ○ Grade II (moderate)
    - ■ Moderate disruption of a number tendon fibers
    - ■ Muscle-tendon unit still intact
    - ■ Moderate swelling, pain and disability
    - ■ Weak and painful, muscle contractions
  - ○ Grade III (high grade)
    - ■ Near complete to complete disruption of tendon unit
    - ■ Extremely weak but painless attempts at muscle contraction

CLINICAL ISSUES

Presentation

- Most common signs/symptoms
  - ○ Large hemarthrosis with freely mobile patella
  - ○ Loss of extensor function with full thickness tears
  - ○ Palpable defect with full thickness tears
  - ○ Partial tears present with extensor lag
- Clinical profile
  - ○ A "pop" felt or heard in acute rupture
  - ○ Inability to walk with full thickness tears
  - ○ More commonly associated with pain than Achilles tears

Demographics

- Age: 5th and 6th decade

- Gender: No predilection

Natural History & Prognosis

- Full thickness tears need to be repaired within 48 hours if possible

Treatment

- Conservative: Partial tears with immobilization and early range of motion exercises
- Surgical: Within 48 hours as early intervention allows end-to-end repair of the tendon

DIAGNOSTIC CHECKLIST

Consider

- Expanding FOV to completely evaluate tendon rupture
  - ○ If history of injury is absent or technologist unaware of diagnosis, rupture may be incompletely imaged

Image Interpretation Pearls

- Identify discontinuous fibers on FS PD FSE in the sagittal plane
- Evaluate superior aspect of the sagittal images to detect tendinosis or tear

SELECTED REFERENCES

1. McGrory JE: Disruption of the extensor mechanism of the knee. J Emerg Med 24(2):163-8, 2003
2. Shah MK: Simultaneous bilateral rupture of quadriceps tendons: Analysis of risk factors and associations. South Med J 95(8):860-6, 2002
3. Richards DP et al: Repair of quadriceps tendon ruptures using suture anchors. Arthroscopy 18(5):556-9, 2003
4. Panni AS et al: Overuse injuries of the extensor mechanism in athletes. Clin Sports Med 21(3):483-98, 2002
5. De Baere T et al: Functional results after surgical repair of quadriceps tendon rupture. Acta Orthop Belg 68(2):146-9, 2002
6. Bikkina RS et al: Magnetic resonance imaging of simultaneous bilateral quadriceps tendon rupture in a weightlifter: Case report. J Trauma 52(3):582-4, 2002
7. O'Shea K et al: Outcomes following quadriceps tendon ruptures. Injury 33(3):257-60, 2002
8. Omololu B et al: Quadriceps tendon rupture in an adolescent. West Afr J Med 20(3):272-3, 1998
9. Konrath GA et al: Outcomes following repair of quadriceps tendon ruptures. J. Orthop Trauma. vol 12. (4)273-279, 1998

QUADRICEPS TENDON TEAR

IMAGE GALLERY

Typical

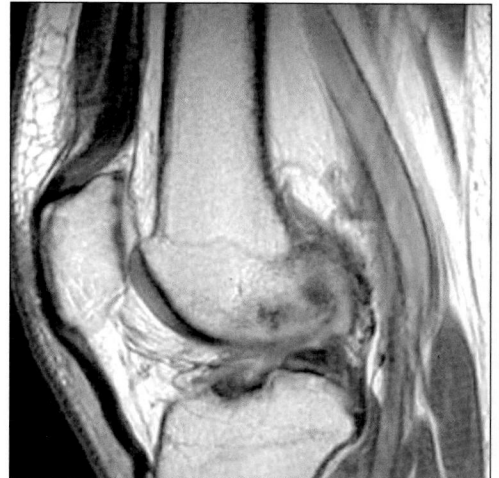
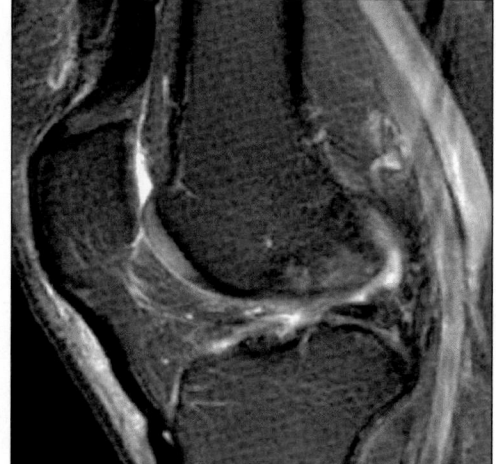

(Left) Sagittal PD FSE MR shows marked thickening of the quadriceps tendon consistent with tendinosis. *(Right)* Sagittal FS PD FSE MR shows the tendinosis in the anterior aspect of the quadriceps tendon.

Typical

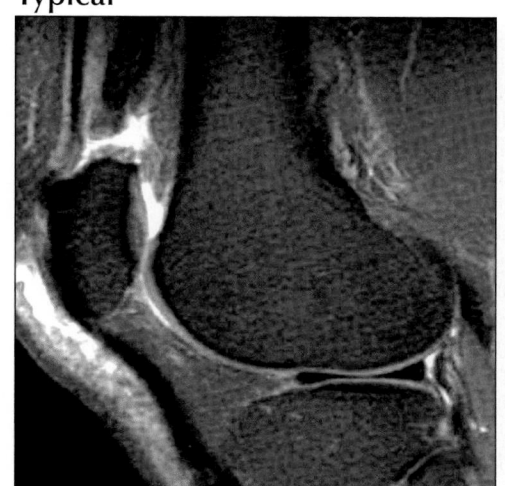
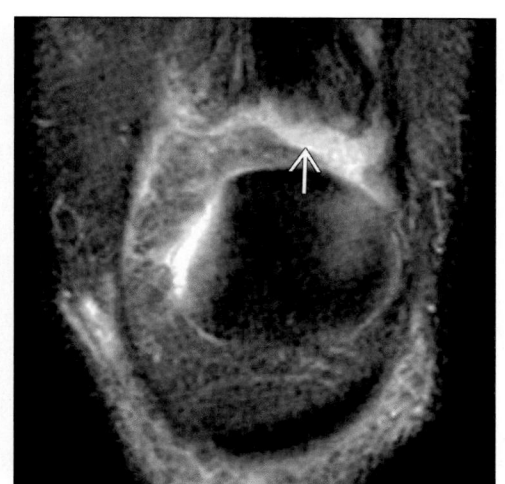

(Left) Sagittal FS PD FSE MR shows an extensive partial tear through the posterior two-thirds of the quadriceps tendon. *(Right)* Coronal FS PD FSE MR shows the high grade partial tear (arrow) with retraction.

Typical

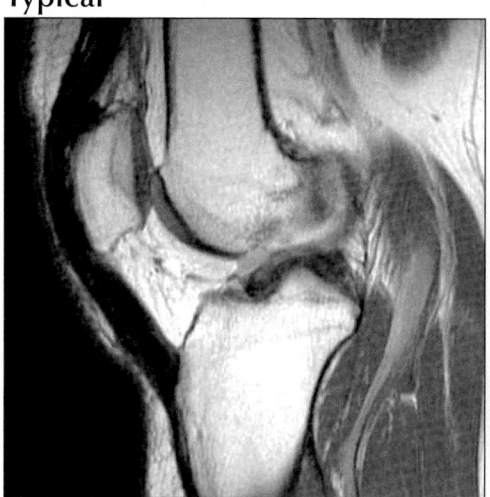
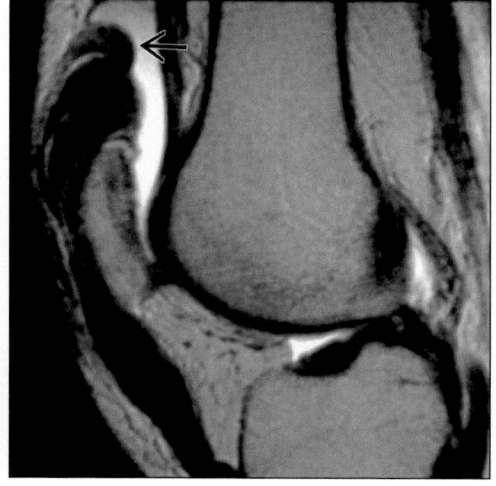

(Left) Sagittal PD FSE MR shows thickening of the quadriceps and patellar tendons consistent with tendinosis. *(Right)* Sagittal T2 FSE MR shows a full thickness quadriceps tendon tear (arrow) at the top of the field of view. These complete tears may be overlooked at the edge of the FOV especially if appropriate history is not available.

TRANSIENT PATELLAR DISLOCATION

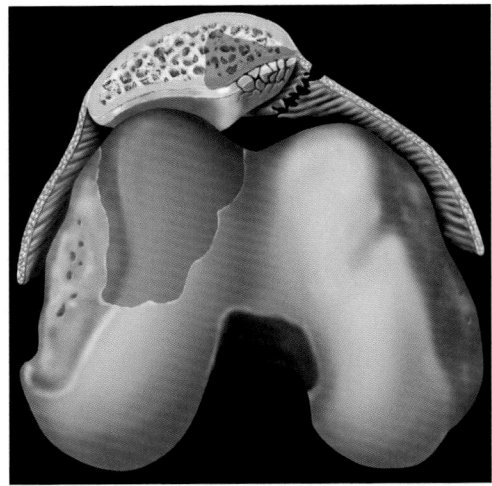

Axial graphic shows the hallmarks of a transient patellar dislocation: Osteochondral injury of medial patella, lateral femoral condyle contusion and medial retinacular tear.

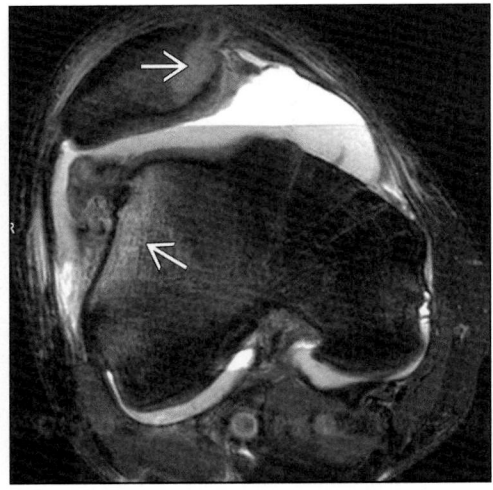

Axial FS PD FSE shows osseous contusions (arrows) of the medial facet and lateral aspect of the lateral femoral condyle. Medial retinacular tear and hemorrhagic fluid level are present.

TERMINOLOGY

Abbreviations and Synonyms
- Patellar dislocation, patellar subluxation

Definitions
- Dislocation of the patella laterally as the result of twisting injury with valgus stress or as the result of direct trauma

IMAGING FINDINGS

General Features
- Best diagnostic clue
  - Bone contusions of the anterior lateral femoral condyle and medial patella are diagnostic
    - Includes osteochondral fracture
- Location: Patellofemoral joint
- Size: Osteochondral defects small and nondisplaced to large +/- displaced
- Morphology: Intact posttraumatic structures to edematous, torn and/or fractured

Radiographic Findings
- Radiography: Fracture of the patella or anterior lateral femoral condyle may be seen

MR Findings
- T1WI
  - Bone contusion (hypointense edema) of medial patella + lateral aspect of lateral femoral condyle characteristic
  - Decreased signal intensity edema
  - + Hypointense effusion
  - +/- Hypointense fracture of medial patella (osteochondral fracture)
  - +/- Fracture of anterior lateral femur (osteochondral fracture) - hypointense
  - +/- Hypointense chondral fracture anterior femur
  - +/- Discontinuous medial patellofemoral ligament at femoral origin or attachment to medial facet
- T2WI
  - Bone contusion (hyperintense edema) of medial patella + anterior lateral femur (lateral aspect of lateral femoral condyle)
  - Disruption of the origin of the medial patellofemoral ligament - increased signal intensity at femoral origin or from medial patellar facet
    - Disruption of this ligament is often surgically treated
    - Partial or complete retinacular tear identified on axial FS PD FSE
  - Hemarthrosis - fluid signal intensity on T2WI (hyperintense)
    - Decreased signal intensity, debris

DDx: Transient Patellar Dislocation

Valgus Injury	Bipartite Patella	Post Lat Tib Fx	Chondromalacia	Vastus Hemangioma
Cor FS PD FSE	Ax PD FSE MR	Sag FS PD FSE	Ax FS PD FSE	Ax FS PD FSE

TRANSIENT PATELLAR DISLOCATION

Key Facts

Terminology
- Dislocation of the patella laterally as the result of twisting injury with valgus stress or as the result of direct trauma

Imaging Findings
- Bone contusions of the anterior lateral femoral condyle and medial patella are diagnostic
- +/- Hyperintense fracture of anterior lateral femur (osteochondral fracture)

Top Differential Diagnoses
- Patellar Osteochondral Injury
- Lateral Femoral Bone Injury

Pathology
- Secondary to a shallow trochlear groove, ligamentous laxity or both
- Intrinsic muscle abnormalities and soft tissue damage predispose to dislocation

Clinical Issues
- Patella often spontaneously reduces into trochlear groove with extension following the injury

Diagnostic Checklist
- Direct impact injury
- Consider patellar dislocation in case of injury to lateral aspect of lateral femoral condyle
- Axial images show typical pattern of bone contusions/fractures, retinacular tear and chondral injuries

---

- +/- Fluid-fluid level
- Chondral or osteochondral fragments often free floating within an effusion
  - Important to identify intermediate signal chondral fragments or hypointense osteochondral fragments
- + Hyperintense effusion
- +/- Hyperintense fracture of medial patella (osteochondral fracture)
- +/- Hyperintense fracture of anterior lateral femur (osteochondral fracture)
- +/- Hyperintense chondral fracture anterior femur
- Edema in muscle stain of vastus medialis obliquus (VMO) muscle
  - Stripping of the VMO away from the adductor magnus tendon

Imaging Recommendations
- Best imaging tool: MRI
- Protocol advice
  - FS PD FSE in the axial and coronal planes
  - Axial images to define medial retinacular tear at medial patellar facet vs. adductor tubercle

DIFFERENTIAL DIAGNOSIS

Anterior Cruciate Ligament (ACL) Tear with Hemarthrosis
- May mimic transient patellar dislocation clinically
- +/- Valgus injury
- Posterolateral tibia plateau contusion
- Lateral femoral condyle (sulcus) contusion

Patellar Osteochondral Injury
- Direct trauma
- Sleeve avulsion
- Sudden quadriceps contraction
- +/- Chondral displacement

Lateral Femoral Bone Injury
- Valgus stress
- Direct trauma

- +/- ACL tear

Bipartite Patella
- Normal variant
- Failure of fusion of secondary ossification center
- Superolateral pole patella (not medial)

High Signal T2 Mass
- Hemangioma medially may mimic retinacular damage
- Rare
- FS PD FSE most sensitive
  - Increased venous vascularity

Chondromalacia Patella
- FS PD FSE sequence for chondral evaluation
- Axial images to identify patellar facets and sagittal images for the trochlear groove
- +/- Hyperintense collagen matrix on FS PD FSE
- +/- Underlying patellar bone edema
  - Hyperintense T2WI
- +/- Subchondral cysts
  - Hyperintense on T2WI
- +/- Trochlea osteoarthritis
- +/- Medial plica

PATHOLOGY

General Features
- General path comments
  - Traumatic patellar dislocation occurs laterally
  - Usually iatrogenic
  - Secondary to realignment procedures, +/- previous surgery
- Etiology
  - Two common mechanisms
    - Noncontact, indirect injury
    - Direct mechanism secondary to a blow to knee
  - Knee in internal rotation and valgus vs. forced external rotation of the tibia (less common)
  - Secondary to a shallow trochlear groove, ligamentous laxity or both
  - Abnormal iliotibial band and vastus lateralis attachment produce a lateral patellar pull

TRANSIENT PATELLAR DISLOCATION

- ○ Intrinsic muscle abnormalities and soft tissue damage predispose to dislocation
- ○ Variation of patellar shapes (Wiberg types) may predispose to dislocations including type 3 (small and convex medial patellar facet) and type 5 (Jagerhut or hunter's cap) patella
  - ▪ Patella alta with subsequent loss of containment by the lateral femoral condyle predisposes to dislocations
- • Epidemiology: Uncommon injury, 1% of general population
- • Associated abnormalities
  - ○ Osteochondral injuries of the patella and lateral femoral condyle
  - ○ +/- Tear of the medial retinaculum
  - ○ +/- Strain of the vastus medialis obliquus
  - ○ +/- Disruption of the medial patellofemoral ligament

Gross Pathologic & Surgical Features
- • Injury/hemorrhage/edema of medial patella, lateral femoral condyle, medial patellofemoral ligament, VMO
- • Osteochondral fracture
  - ○ Medial patellar facet
  - ○ Lateral lip of trochlear
  - ○ Lateral trochlear fractures result in patellofemoral instability
- • Rupture of vastus medialis obliquus muscle is usually interstitial (insertional rupture when present can be sutured surgically)

Microscopic Features
- • Fracture, ligamentous disruption, chondral injury

Staging, Grading or Classification Criteria
- • Classification (Fulkerson)
  - ○ I: Subluxation
  - ○ II: Subluxation and tilt
  - ○ III: Tilt
  - ○ IV: No malalignment
- • Associated with each class
  - ○ A: Absence of articular lesion
  - ○ B: Presence of minimal chondromalacia
  - ○ C: Presence of osteoarthritis
- • Wiberg classification for patella shape; no predisposition for dislocation
  - ○ Type 1: Concave facets, symmetrical and equal in size (10%)
  - ○ Type 2: Medial facet is smaller; lateral facet is concave (65%)
  - ○ Type 3: Medial facet is distinctly smaller with marked lateral predominance (25%)

CLINICAL ISSUES

Presentation
- • Most common signs/symptoms
  - ○ Anterior and anterolateral knee pain after twisting injury
  - ○ ACL tear often suspected clinically
- • Clinical profile
  - ○ Children with congenitally shallow trochlear groove

- ○ Occurs throughout adulthood secondary to twisting injury, valgus stress or direct blow

Demographics
- • Age: Younger patient to adult
- • Gender: No predilection

Natural History & Prognosis
- • Patella often spontaneously reduces into trochlear groove with extension following the injury
- • Torn medial patellofemoral ligament (especially from medial femoral epicondylar insertion) predisposes patella to recurrent dislocations
- • Torn medial patellofemoral ligament (MPFL) usually repaired

Treatment
- • Non operative treatment includes
  - ○ Cast immobilization and rehabilitation with early return of range of motion and strength
- • Arthroscopy is used in
  - ○ Diagnosis and treatment of osteochondral fragments and associated intraarticular pathology
  - ○ Selective lateral retinacular release
    - ▪ Lateral retinacular release relieves the retinacular pull
- • +/- Medial patellofemoral ligament repair to medial femoral epicondyle and use of adductor magnus tendon for reinforcement

DIAGNOSTIC CHECKLIST

Consider
- • Direct impact injury
- • Consider patellar dislocation in case of injury to lateral aspect of lateral femoral condyle

Image Interpretation Pearls
- • Axial images show typical pattern of bone contusions/fractures, retinacular tear and chondral injuries
- • Distinguish between medial retinacular tear to medial facet vs. disruption to adductor tubercle attachment (insertion to the medial femoral epicondyle)

SELECTED REFERENCES

1. Arendt EA et al: Current concepts of lateral patella dislocation. Clin Sports Med 21(3):499-519, 2002
2. Bharam S et al: Knee fractures in the athlete. Orthop Clin North Am 33(3):565-74, 2002
3. Elias DA et al: Acute lateral patellar dislocation at MR imaging: Injury patterns of medial patellar soft tissue restraints and osteochondral injuries of the inferomedial patella. Radiology 225(3):736-43, 2002
4. Drez D et al: Results of medial patellofemoral ligament reconstruction in the treatment of patellar dislocation. Arthroscopy 17(3):298-306, 2001
5. Sanders TG et al: Medial patellofemoral ligament injury following acute transient dislocation of the patella: MR findings with surgical correlation in 14 patients. J Comput Assist Tomogr 25(6):957-62, 2001
6. Pope TL Jr: MR imaging of patellar dislocation and relocation. Semin Ultrasound CT MR 22(4):371-82, 2001

TRANSIENT PATELLAR DISLOCATION

IMAGE GALLERY

Typical

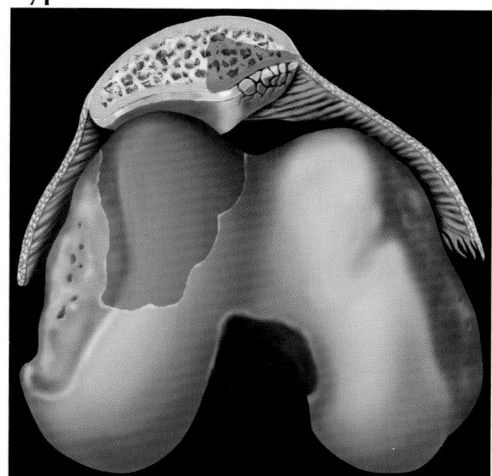
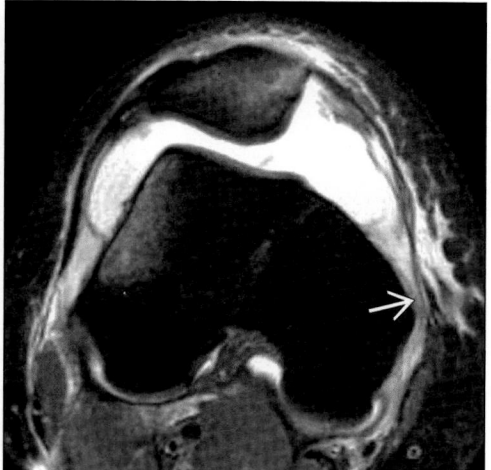

(Left) Axial graphic shows an intact patellar attachment of the medial retinaculum after dislocation. The medial patellofemoral ligament is torn at the medial femoral epicondyle. Fragmentation of medial patellar chondral surface is shown. *(Right)* Axial FS PD FSE MR shows a dislocation osseous injury pattern associated with a disruption of the origin of the medial patellofemoral ligament from the medial femoral epicondyle (arrow).

Typical

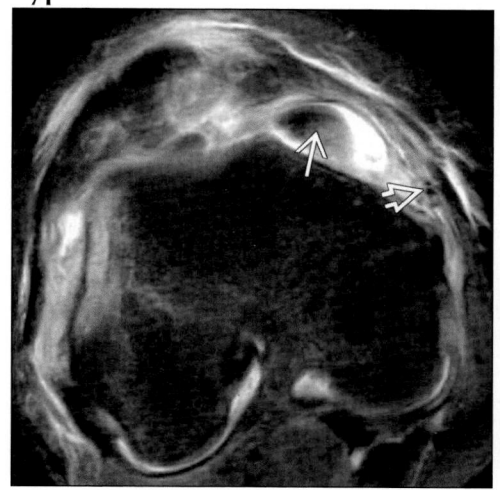
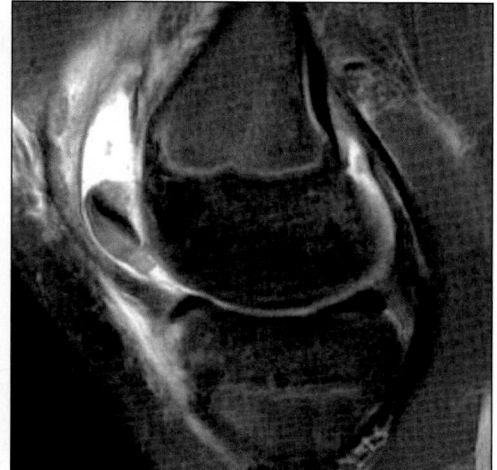

(Left) Axial FS PD FSE MR shows an impaction fracture of anterior aspect of lateral femoral condyle and a loose osteochondral fragment (arrow) within the medial joint recess. Origin of the medial patellofemoral ligament is disrupted (open arrow). *(Right)* Sagittal FS PD FSE MR of the same patient shows the large displaced osteochondral fragment within the medial suprapatellar joint recess.

Typical

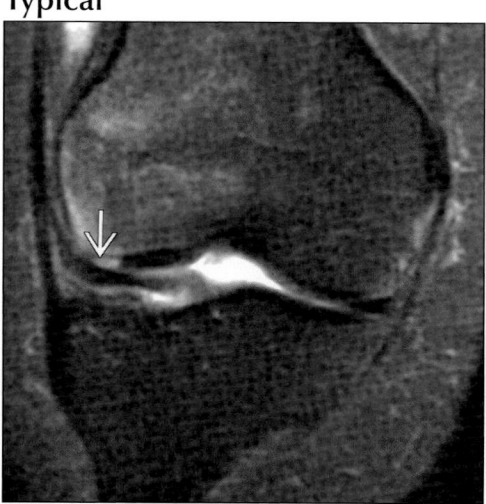
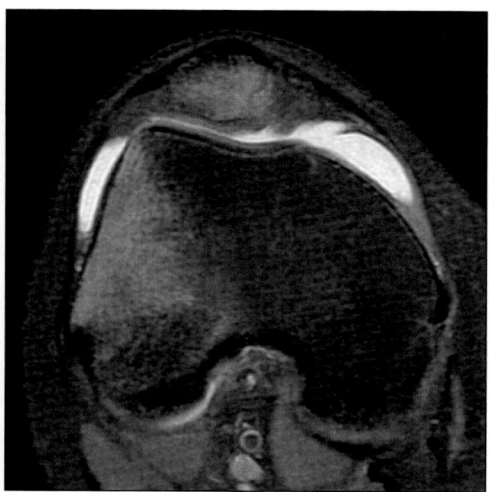

(Left) Coronal FS PD FSE MR shows an osteochondral injury, including a chondral defect (arrow), of the anterior lateral femoral condyle. *(Right)* Axial FS PD FSE MR shows the typical bone injury pattern (edema of lateral femoral condyle and medial patellar facet) of a recent patellar dislocation. The medial patellofemoral ligament origin, however is intact.

MEDIAL PLICA SYNDROME

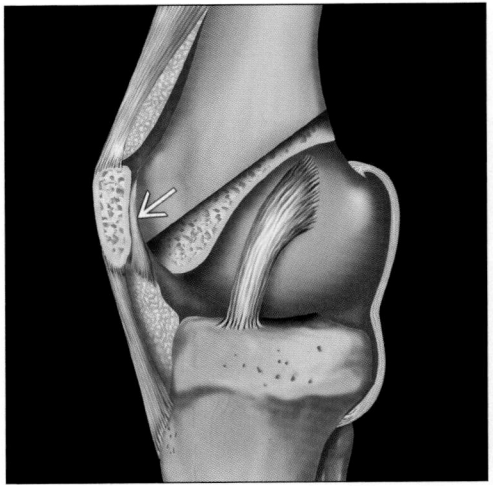

Sagittal graphic shows a thickened medial plica (arrow) interposed between the patella and medial femoral condyle.

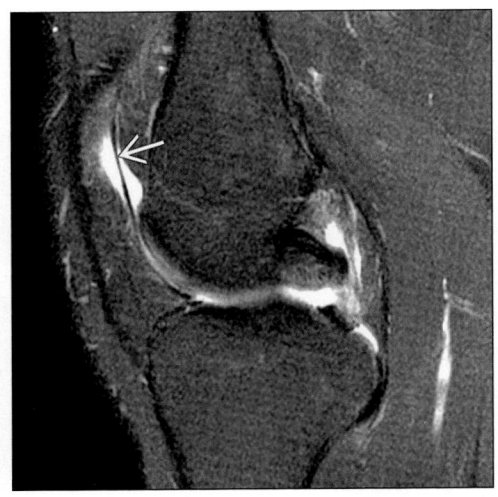

Sagittal FS PD FSE MR shows a slightly thickened hypointense medial plica (arrow) in medial aspect of the suprapatellar bursa.

TERMINOLOGY

Abbreviations and Synonyms
- Medial plica syndrome (MPS), medial shelf, mediopatellaris, Iino's band

Definitions
- Inflamed synovial plica leading to pain, crepitus and/or pseudolocking

IMAGING FINDINGS

General Features
- Best diagnostic clue: Low signal intensity linear structure (usually thickened if symptomatic) on all sequences at expected location in a patient with dull aching medial knee pain
- Location
  ○ Originates on medial side of knee joint adjacent to medial patella
  ○ Oblique, course from superior/midpatellar medial capsule towards synovium covering medial aspect of fat pad
- Size: Varies from 1 to several mm in thickness
- Morphology
  ○ Thin in case of normal variant
  ○ Thickens and fibrotic when symptomatic
  ○ Elongated and thin or thickened

MR Findings
- T1WI
  ○ Abnormal plica as thickened band of low signal intensity
  ○ Subchondral cystic changes of medial patella well-defined, with low signal intensity
  ○ Focal synovitis - increased in signal intensity relative to adjacent fluid
  ○ Subchondral reactive decreased signal intensity changes in the medial anterior femur (trochlea) (rare)
- T2WI
  ○ Thickened band of low signal intensity
  ○ Chondromalacia of medial patellar facet
    ▪ Increased signal intensity within hyaline articular cartilage
    ▪ Surface ulceration
    ▪ FS PD FSE (hyperintense erosions)
  ○ Increased signal intensity synovitis
    ▪ Intermediate signal relative to joint fluid
- PD/Intermediate
  ○ Intermediate signal intensity synovitis adjacent to patella in medial joint
  ○ Joint fluid is slightly decreased in signal compared to inflamed synovium
- T2* GRE
  ○ Plica thicker if hemorrhagic

DDx: Medial Plica Syndrome

Pat Tendonitis	Chondro Patella	Trochlea Chondro	Pat Bone Inj
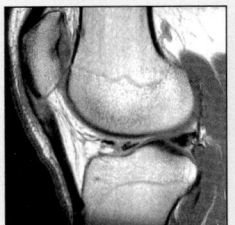	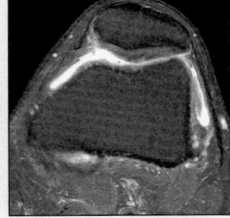	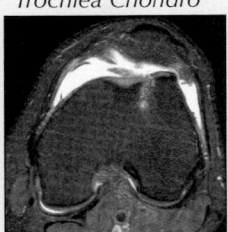	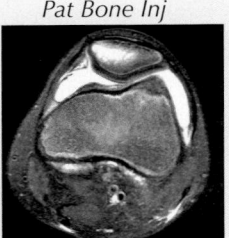
Sag PD FSE MR	Ax FS PD FSE MR	Ax FS PD FSE MR	Ax FS PD FSE MR

MEDIAL PLICA SYNDROME

Key Facts

Terminology
- Inflamed synovial plica leading to pain, crepitus and/or pseudolocking

Imaging Findings
- Best diagnostic clue: Low signal intensity linear structure (usually thickened if symptomatic) on all sequences at expected location in a patient with dull aching medial knee pain
- Originates on medial side of knee joint adjacent to medial patella
- Thin in case of normal variant

Top Differential Diagnoses
- Patellar Chondromalacia (Chondro Patella)
- Femoral Trochlear Osteoarthritic Change (Trochlea Chondro)

- Suprapatellar Plica

Pathology
- Incomplete/partial resorption of synovial membrane that divides medial knee during embryologic development = medial plica
- Thickened, indurated and inflamed often fibrotic synovial membrane

Clinical Issues
- Most common signs/symptoms: Dull aching medial knee pain sometimes worsened by activity or prolonged sitting
- Age: Adolescent and athletic population

Diagnostic Checklist
- Thickened elongated plica especially on axial images

- ■ Due to blooming/susceptibility
  - ○ Sensitivity similar to FS PD FSE for identification of plica
- No measurements have been described to define plical thickening
  - ○ Thickening is a subjective determination in a symptomatic patient
- Sagittal images show elongated plica as linear hypointense structure anterior to the anterior horn of the medial meniscus

Imaging Recommendations
- Best imaging tool: MRI
- Protocol advice
  - ○ Axial & sagittal FS PD FSE for demonstrating thickened plica
    - ■ FS PD FSE demonstrate associated chondromalacia in medial patella facet

DIFFERENTIAL DIAGNOSIS

Medial Meniscal Tear
- Positive clinical signs (e.g., Lachman's test)
- Increased signal abnormality on short TE sequences extending to articular surface
  - ○ T1, PD/Intermediate, T2* GRE
- +/- Reactive edema in medial tibia
- +/- Medial bursitis

Patellar Chondromalacia (Chondro Patella)
- Tenderness along medial patellar facet
- Imaging helpful to define chondral erosions
- Common abnormality often without symptomatic plica
- +/- Medial plica
  - ○ Thin plica may be incidental
- Typically older patient population

Hoffa's Impingement (Excessive Lateral Pressure Syndrome)
- More often lateral/superior when due to chronic frictional trauma

- ○ Excessive lateral pressure syndrome when lateral and superior

Femoral Trochlear Osteoarthritic Change (Trochlea Chondro)
- Includes chondromalacia, subchondral reactive edema +/- cystic change, sclerosis and/or osteophyte formation
- +/- Associated thickened infrapatellar plica
- Posttraumatic associated with impact of patella on trochlea

Suprapatellar Plica
- May form complete shelf (suprapatellar septum) and result in fluid build up in suprapatellar pouch
  - ○ Mimics mass
  - ○ Child to adolescent
- Rarely become inflamed and symptomatic
- One-way valve theory
  - ○ Trapping of fluid in bursa
  - ○ Small perforation or porta in plica allows passage of fluid & results in sequestration of loose bodies

Infrapatellar Plica
- Extends into intercondylar notch to anterior cruciate ligament (ACL)
- Associated with trochlear chondromalacia

Patellar Tendinitis (Pat Tendinitis)
- Jumper's knee
- Anterior infrapatellar pain
- Hyperintensity of proximal posterior fibrosis on FS PD FSE or T2* GRE

Patellar Bone Injury (Pat Bone Inj)
- Direct impact vs. avulsive stress
- Increased signal on T2WI (esp. FS PD FSE)
- Stress related (chronic frictional)

PATHOLOGY

General Features
- Etiology

MEDIAL PLICA SYNDROME

- o Incomplete/partial resorption of synovial membrane that divides medial knee during embryologic development = medial plica
- o Asymptomatic plica may become symptomatic after injury
  - Effusion and synovitis cause plica to become edematous causing fibrotic reaction
  - Leads to tightening, bowstringing and impingement against medial femoral condyle and/or medial patellar facet
  - Vicious cycle of further thickening and contraction
- o Intraarticular pathology contributes to symptomatic plica secondary to inflammation and hemorrhage
  - Osteochondritis dissecans
  - Loose bodies
  - Meniscal pathology
- Epidemiology
  - o Four types of plica
    - Suprapatellar (89% incidence)
    - Medial (18-30% incidence)
    - Infrapatellar (common)
    - Lateral (rare)
- Associated abnormalities
  - o In association with or in continuity with a suprapatellar plica
  - o Chondromalacia of the medial patellar facet

Gross Pathologic & Surgical Features
- Thickened, indurated and inflamed often fibrotic synovial membrane
- Loss of elastic properties

Microscopic Features
- Bland fibrous synovial membrane
- Fibrous tissue
- Hyalinization
- Calcification

Staging, Grading or Classification Criteria
- Arthroscopic
  - o Type A: Cord-like elevation of the medial wall
  - o Type B: Shelf-like appearance that does not cover anterior surface of medial condyle
  - o Type C: Shelf-like appearance that covers the anterior surface of medial condyle
  - o Type D: Double insertions onto the medial wall (separation between the shelf and synovial wall, creating a bucket-handle component)

CLINICAL ISSUES

Presentation
- Most common signs/symptoms: Dull aching medial knee pain sometimes worsened by activity or prolonged sitting
- Clinical profile
  - o Often adolescent
    - Mechanical symptoms such as crepitus
  - o Pressure erosions of articular cartilage of medial femoral condyle and patella
  - o Exacerbated discomfort/pain with repetitive flexion-extension motions

- Rowing
- Swimming
- Cycling
- o Snap and roll of medial plica with applied pressure to medial femoral condyle
- o Pop between 60 and 45 degrees of knee flexion (with applied pressure to patella medially)

Demographics
- Age: Adolescent and athletic population
- Gender: No predilection

Natural History & Prognosis
- Symptoms may resolve but are often progressive with fibrosis, especially if repeated injuries occur
- Best results with treatment in teenagers because of less damage to articular cartilage

Treatment
- Conservative
  - o Activity reduction, NSAIDs, physical therapy
- Surgical
  - o Arthroscopic resection for recalcitrant cases
  - o 66-90% success reported

DIAGNOSTIC CHECKLIST

Consider
- In correct clinical setting
- Evaluate for different cause of anterior knee pain
  - o Differentiate medial plica from patellofemoral syndrome and meniscal tear

Image Interpretation Pearls
- Thickened elongated plica especially on axial images
- Medial sagittal images through suprapatellar bursa helpful

SELECTED REFERENCES

1. DeLee J et al: Orthopaedics sports medicine. Knee. vol 1. 2nd ed. Philadelphia PA, Saunders, 1577-2135, 2003
2. Calpur OU et al: United unresorbed medial and lateral plicae as anterior mesenchymal synovial septal remnant. Knee Surg Sports Traumatol Arthrosc 10(6):378-80, 2002
3. Calpur OU et al: Arthroscopic mediopatellar plicectomy and lateral retinacular release in mechanical patellofemoral disorders. Knee Surg Sports Traumatol Arthrosc 10(3):177-83, 2002
4. Duri ZA et al:The immature athlete. Clin Sports Med 21(3):461-82, 2002
5. Kim SJ et al: Pathologic infrapatellar plica. Arthroscopy 18(5):E25, 2002
6. Garcia-Valtuille R et al: Anatomy and MR imaging appearances of synovial plicae of the knee. Radiographics 22(4):775-84, 2002
7. Rang M et al: The Story of Orthopaedics. Philadelphia PA, WB Saunders, 493-7, 2000
8. Thomee RJ et al: Patellofemoral pain syndrome: A review of current issues. Sports Med 28(4):245-62, 1999
9. Bae DK et al: The clinical significance of the complete type of suprapatellar membrane. Arthroscopy 14(8):830-5, 1998

130

MEDIAL PLICA SYNDROME

IMAGE GALLERY

Variant

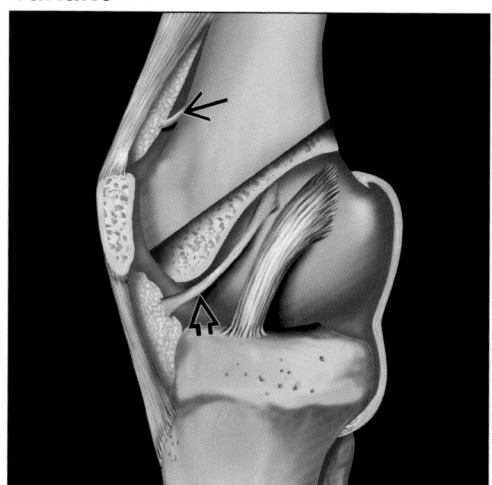 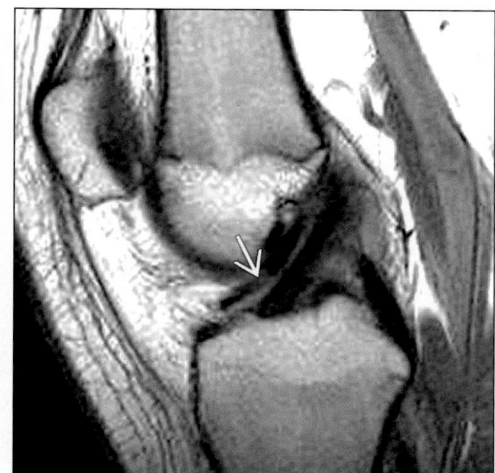

(Left) Sagittal graphic shows a suprapatellar plica (arrow) in the superior aspect of the suprapatellar pouch and an infrapatellar plica (open arrow) anterior to the anterior cruciate ligament. *(Right)* Sagittal PD FSE MR shows a thick infrapatellar plica (arrow). This plica has been implicated as a cause of femoral trochlear chondromalacia.

Typical

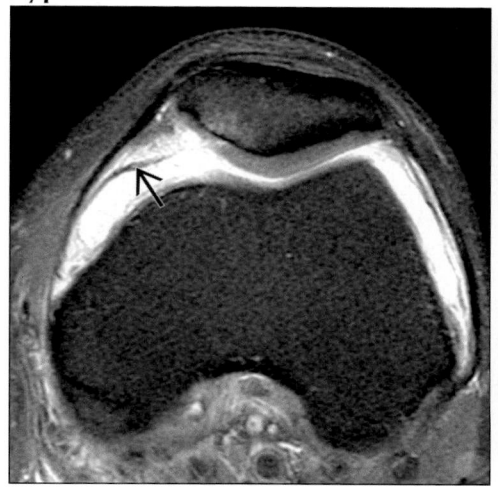 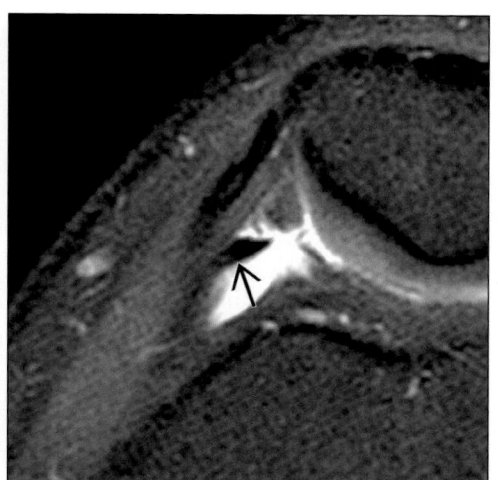

(Left) Axial FS PD FSE MR shows an irregular, elongated medial plica (arrow) with adjacent chondromalacia of the patella and reactive marrow edema within the patella. *(Right)* Axial FS PD FSE MR shows a thick medial plica (arrow) without associated medial patellar chondromalacia.

Typical

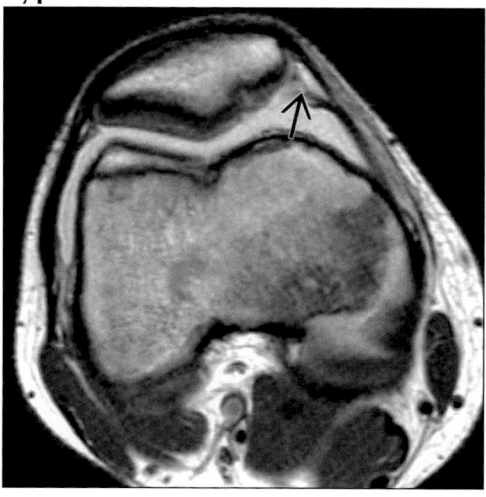 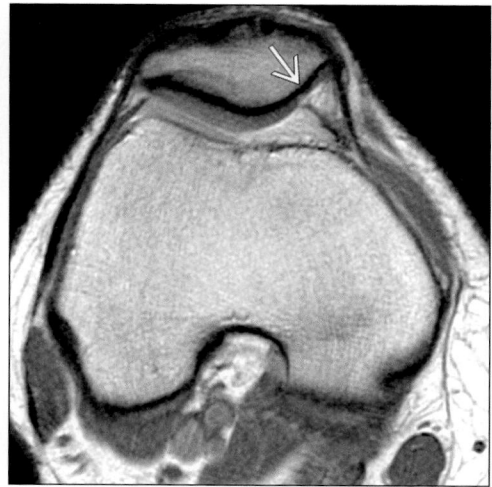

(Left) Axial PD FSE MR shows a thickened and frayed medial plica (arrow) and adjacent patellar chondromalacia. *(Right)* Axial PD FSE MR shows a mildly thickened medial plica with adjacent patellar chondromalacia (arrow).

OSTEOARTHRITIS, KNEE

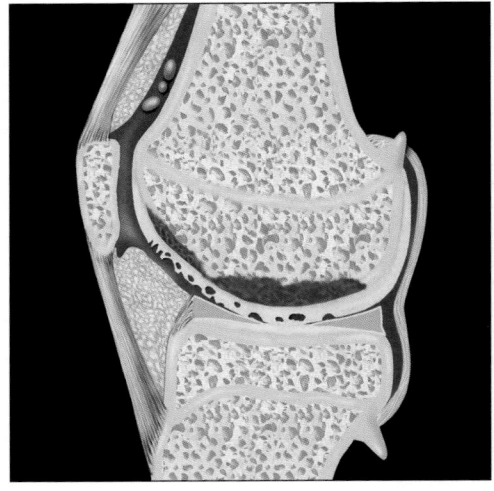

Sagittal graphic shows findings of osteoarthritis including chondral erosions, subchondral sclerosis (eburnation) and fibrinous rice bodies as a result of synovitis.

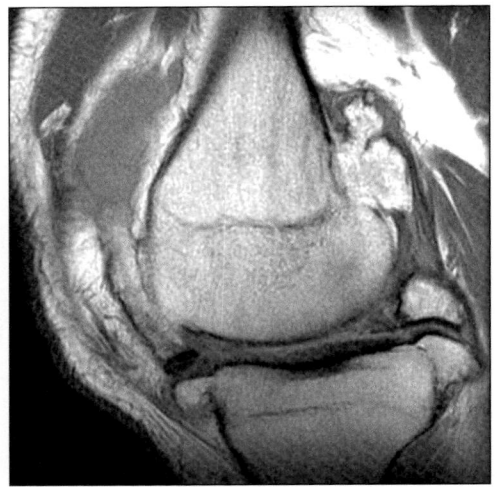

Sagittal PD FSE MR shows large osteophytes, cartilage loss, meniscal tear, and synovitis consistent with osteoarthritis.

TERMINOLOGY

Abbreviations and Synonyms
- Osteoarthritis (OA), degenerative joint disease (DJD)

Definitions
- Primary - gradual process of destruction & regeneration as result of chronic microtrauma
- Secondary - non-inflammatory degenerative joint disease resulting from predisposing events such as previous trauma, congenital deformity, infection or metabolic disorder

IMAGING FINDINGS

General Features
- Best diagnostic clue: Chondromalacia often accompanied by subchondral sclerosis, subchondral cysts, osteophytes and/or edema
- Location: Hyaline chondral surfaces of the knee
- Size: Can affect small localized area (typically post trauma), compartment, or whole knee
- Morphology: Progressive loss of articular cartilage with associated new bone formation and capsular fibrosis

Radiographic Findings
- Radiography: Joint space narrowing, subchondral sclerosis/eburnation, subchondral cysts, and osteophyte formation

MR Findings
- T1WI
  - Decreased signal intensity - subchondral cysts, marrow fat signal can be seen extending into osteophytes
    - Subchondral decreased signal indicating sclerosis and/or edema
- T2WI
  - Variable degree of high signal in hyaline cartilage, subchondral bone marrow edema (bright signal)
    - Decreased signal indicating sclerosis in subchondral bone
    - General thinning of articular (hyaline) cartilage with occasional focal defects
  - FS PD FSE - increased signal in hyaline cartilage erosions and subchondral bone marrow edema
    - Thinning of hyaline cartilage +/- focal defects and underlying bone change
    - Edema (hyperintense) demonstrated with fat saturation
    - Subchondral decreased signal indicating sclerosis
    - Associated findings including subchondral cysts (bright signal), and osteophytes

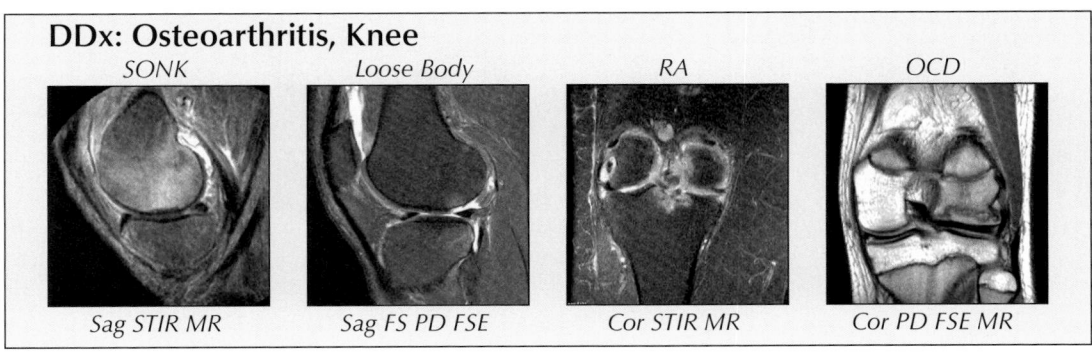

DDx: Osteoarthritis, Knee

SONK	Loose Body	RA	OCD
Sag STIR MR	Sag FS PD FSE	Cor STIR MR	Cor PD FSE MR

5

132

OSTEOARTHRITIS, KNEE

Key Facts

Terminology
- Primary - gradual process of destruction & regeneration as result of chronic microtrauma
- Secondary - non-inflammatory degenerative joint disease resulting from predisposing events such as previous trauma, congenital deformity, infection or metabolic disorder

Imaging Findings
- Best diagnostic clue: Chondromalacia often accompanied by subchondral sclerosis, subchondral cysts, osteophytes and/or edema
- Radiography: Joint space narrowing, subchondral sclerosis/eburnation, subchondral cysts, and osteophyte formation
- Variable degree of high signal in hyaline cartilage, subchondral bone marrow edema (bright signal)

Pathology
- Epidemiology: Affects 90% of patients older than 40 years
- Degraded cartilage with fissured and/or ulcerated cartilage surface, loss of surface sheen

Clinical Issues
- Pain with utilization of joint and variable joint capsular swelling (effusion)

Diagnostic Checklist
- Secondary OA in cases of focal findings
- Utilize FS PD FSE to visualize chondral erosions and subchondral edema

---

- o T2 FSE
  - Edema not as hyperintense compared to FS PD FSE because of the high signal intensity of fat on non fat suppressed FSE images
- PD/Intermediate
  - o PD FSE - cartilage not as well seen unless resolution is increased
    - Synovial thickening seen well
    - Sclerosis is difficult to appreciate without T1 contrast
    - Edema difficult to appreciate without fat suppression
- T2* GRE
  - o With fat suppression, cartilage abnormalities are visualized as decreased signal areas on T1 weighted GRE images
  - o T2* demonstrates loose bodies as hypointense structures within joint capsule
- T1 C+
  - o Synovium enhances in cases of synovitis
    - Irregular free edge of Hoffa's fat pad in inflammatory OA

Nuclear Medicine Findings
- Bone Scan: Increased tracer uptake with subchondral fractures, cysts, or general sclerosis

Imaging Recommendations
- Best imaging tool: MRI for cartilage visualization
- Protocol advice
  - o FS PD FSE
  - o GRE imaging to demonstrate loose bodies

DIFFERENTIAL DIAGNOSIS

Inflammatory Arthritis
- Polyarticular systemic disease
- Serum indicators
- Synovitis +/- erosions

Crystal Deposition Disease
- Polyarticular with crystals in joint aspirates
- Calcium pyrophosphate dihydrate (CPPD), gout

- Crystals identified at microscopy
- +/- Erosions

Osteochondral Abnormalities
- History of trauma
- Underlying edema common
- Osteoarthritis (OA) as a complication
- Osteochondritis dissecans (OCD) may mimic or lead to OA
- Spontaneous osteonecrosis (SONK) may lead to OA

PATHOLOGY

General Features
- General path comments
  - o Begins as fatigue fracture of the collagen meshwork followed by increased hydration of the articular cartilage (as opposed to desiccated cartilage seen with aging)
    - Fibrillation of the cartilage followed by deep clefts and regeneration/proliferation of chondrocytes
    - Proliferative changes occur at the joint margins with formation of osteophytes
    - Articular cartilage thins and is fissured in areas of maximum mechanical stress, underlying bone becomes sclerotic and subchondral cysts form
    - Compression of weakened bone with variable degrees of collapse
    - Loose bodies are followed by fragmentation of osteochondral surfaces
    - Synovial hypertrophy - joint pain by nerve stimulation
    - Synovial fluid - increased intraarticular pressure "stretching the joint lining," causing pain
    - Increased levels of degrading enzymes including matrix metalloproteinases (MMPs), collagenase, gelatinase, and stromelysin
    - Loss of proteoglycans from the matrix into the synovial fluid
  - o Molecular changes in osteoarthritic cartilage include
    - Increased water
    - Weakening of type II collagen network

OSTEOARTHRITIS, KNEE

- Shorter collagen chains
- Alteration of proteoglycans
- Etiology
  - Multiple theories - chronic microtrauma (primary) leading to disruption of the articular surface, fibrillation, eburnation, subchondral cysts, and osteophytes
    - Secondary OA results from healing of major trauma or other predisposing events
    - Joint instabilities may be predisposing
  - Associated injuries with OA
    - Meniscal tears (and partial meniscectomy)
    - Cruciate ligament damage
- Epidemiology: Affects 90% of patients older than 40 years
- Associated abnormalities
  - Deformities
  - Subluxations
  - Ankylosis
  - Loose bodies with catching and locking

Gross Pathologic & Surgical Features
- Degraded cartilage with fissured and/or ulcerated cartilage surface, loss of surface sheen
  - Subchondral geodes (cysts) containing variable amounts of debris
  - Buttressing osteophytes to increase surface area
  - Articular surface collapse

Microscopic Features
- Diminution of chondrocytes in superficial zones with chondrocyte swelling
- Cartilage matrix loses its ability to stain for proteoglycans with Alcian blue or safranin-O
- Matrix chondrocytes demonstrate proliferation in clusters (brood capsules)
- Neovascularity penetrates layer of calcified cartilage and new chondrocytes extend up from deeper layers
- Hypertrophied synovium becomes folded into villous folds with variable infiltration of plasma cells, and lymphocytes

Staging, Grading or Classification Criteria
- Primary osteoarthritis
  - Hip, knee, first metacarpophalangeal and interphalangeal articulations
- Secondary (following a preexisting joint disorder)
  - Shoulder, elbow, foot and ankle
- Articular cartilage damage (stages)
  - I: Edema
  - II: Articular fissuring
  - III: "Crabmeat" changes
  - IV: Full thickness defect + subchondral erosions

CLINICAL ISSUES

Presentation
- Most common signs/symptoms
  - Pain with utilization of joint and variable joint capsular swelling (effusion)
    - Often with antecedent traumatic history
- Clinical profile: Catching, locking or grinding in older patient

Demographics
- Age: Typically older patients (over 50) unless history of trauma
- Gender: M > F for knee joint

Natural History & Prognosis
- Progressively debilitating disease without medical intervention

Treatment
- Conservative
  - Protection of knee from overloading including weight loss
  - Exercise of supporting muscles around joints to increase stability and avoid wasting
  - Pain management by analgesics or NSAIDs
  - Hyaluronic acid injections, glucosamine & chondroitin supplements
- Surgical
  - Indicated for patients with persistent symptoms and pain
  - Arthroscopy (debridement)
  - Arthroplasty
  - Realignment osteotomies may be performed in younger patients to redistribute weight bearing load to prevent progression
  - Newer treatments include
    - Soft tissue periosteal and perichondral grafts
    - Chondrocyte transplantation, mosaicplasty
    - Artificial matrix - carbon fiber, collagen, polylactic acid, fresh osteochondral grafts, doxycycline therapy, and transforming growth factor beta (TGF beta)

DIAGNOSTIC CHECKLIST

Consider
- Secondary OA in cases of focal findings

Image Interpretation Pearls
- Utilize FS PD FSE to visualize chondral erosions and subchondral edema
- Irregular fat pad sign in OA + synovitis on sagittal images

SELECTED REFERENCES

1. Saito I et al: Increased cellular infiltrate in inflammatory synovia of osteoarthritic knees. Osteoarthritis Cartilage 10(2):156-62, 2002
2. Hill CL et al: Knee effusions, popliteal cysts, and synovial thickening: Association with knee pain in osteoarthritis. J Rheumatol 28(6):1330-7, 2001

OSTEOARTHRITIS, KNEE

IMAGE GALLERY

Typical

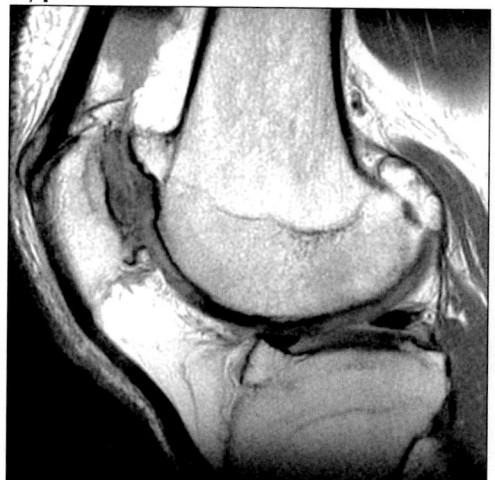

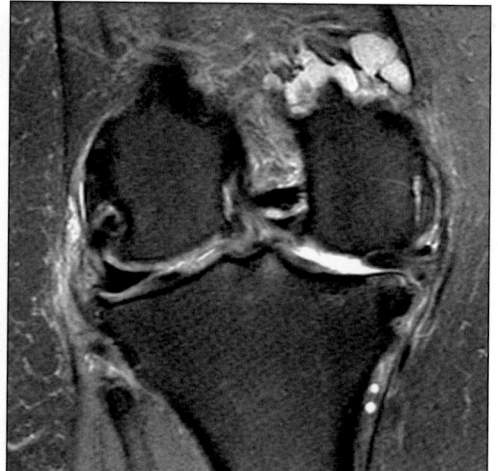

(Left) Sagittal PD FSE MR shows the typical findings of OA including chondromalacia, osteophytes, and synovitis. *(Right)* Coronal FS PD FSE MR shows OA of the medial compartment greater than the lateral compartment. Note the synovial cyst extending superiorly from the posterosuperior medial joint as a result of chronic increased joint pressure.

Typical

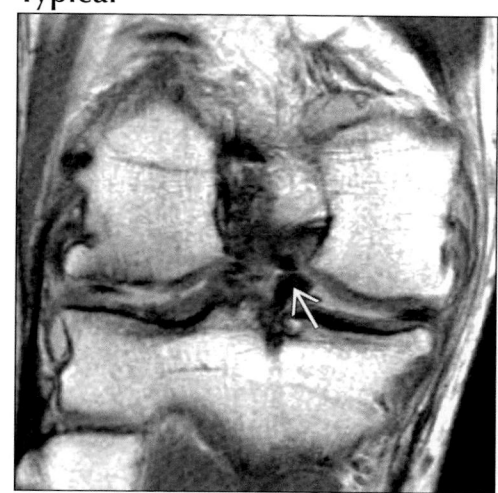

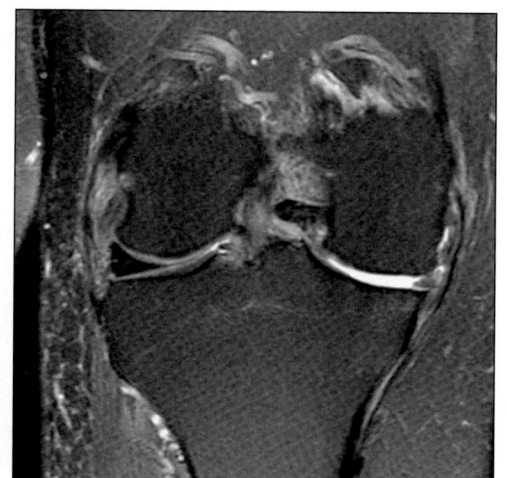

(Left) Coronal PD FSE MR shows OA in a post operative setting. Note the displaced bucket-handle tear (arrow) of the medial meniscus. *(Right)* Coronal FS PD FSE MR demonstrates medial compartment OA after partial meniscectomy.

Typical

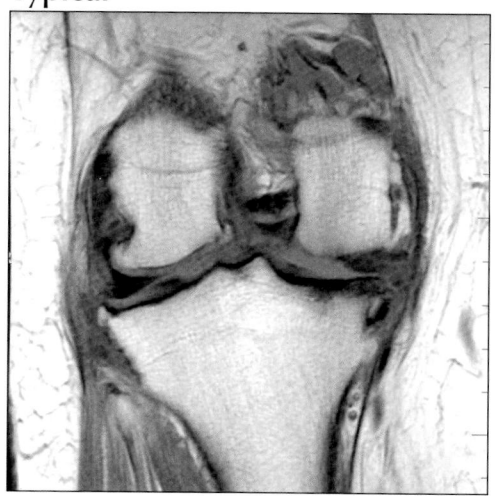

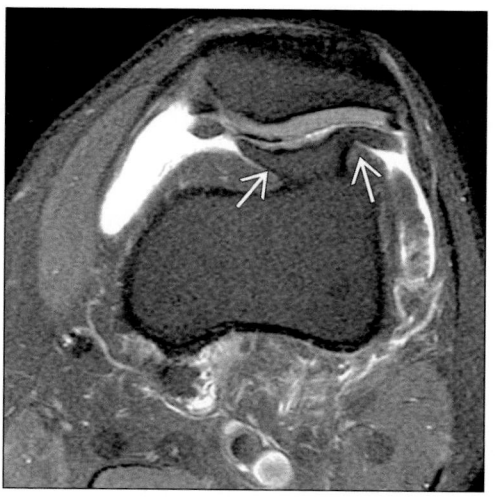

(Left) Coronal PD FSE MR shows medial compartment OA including a meniscal tear. *(Right)* Axial FS PD FSE MR shows very large femoral osteophytes in effect creating a new femoral trochlea (arrows).

RHEUMATOID ARTHRITIS, KNEE

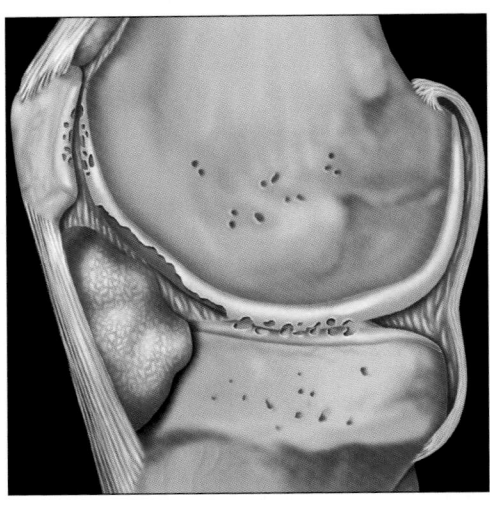

Sagittal graphic shows MRI findings of rheumatoid arthritis including synovitis and cartilage degradation. Periarticular erosions and cysts are characteristic findings as well.

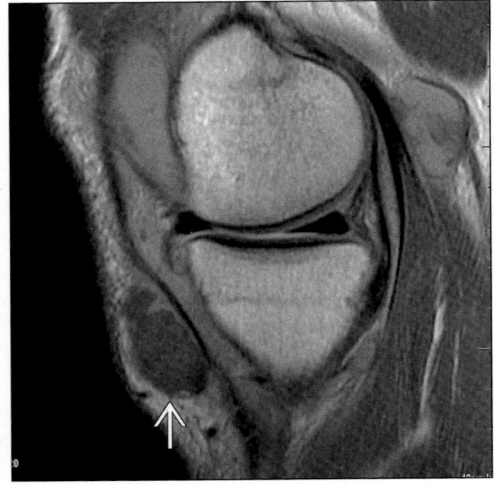

Sagittal PD FSE MR shows synovitis and a hypointense rheumatoid nodule (arrow) within the superficial infrapatellar bursa in a patient with rheumatoid arthritis.

TERMINOLOGY

Abbreviations and Synonyms
- Rheumatoid arthritis (RA)

Definitions
- Systemic inflammatory arthritic condition requiring the presence of 4 out of the following 7 criteria for > 6 weeks
- Classification criteria for rheumatoid arthritis
  - Morning stiffness
  - Oligo or polyarthritis in three or more joints or several joint groups
  - Arthritis of either wrist, metacarpophalangeal joint or proximal interphalangeal joint
  - Symmetric arthritis
  - Rheumatoid nodules over bony prominences, extensor surfaces or juxta-articular
  - Abnormal amounts of serum rheumatoid factor
  - Radiographic changes including erosions and juxta-articular demineralization

IMAGING FINDINGS

General Features
- Best diagnostic clue

  - Thickened edematous knee synovium in association with effusion in patient with suggestive clinical symptomatology
  - Erosions common
- Location
  - Affects synovium first, then cartilage and bone with destructive changes leading to deformity
  - +/- Nodules
    - 20% of RA patients
    - Mixed signal intensity masses in the skin, synovium, tendons, sclera, viscera
- Size: Variable involvement of synovium or tenosynovium
- Morphology
  - Thickened irregular synovium usually in the presence of a joint effusion
    - Synovitis followed by erosive/destructive changes

Radiographic Findings
- Radiography
  - Osteopenia
  - Periarticular erosions
  - Joint space narrowing (symmetric)
  - Effusion and soft tissue swelling
  - +/- Cyst formation (cystic rheumatoid)
  - Destruction (late)

DDx: Rheumatoid Arthritis, Knee

Traumatic Effus	PVNS	Synovial Cysts	Trauma	JCA
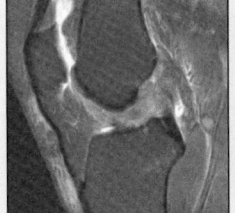	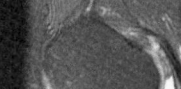	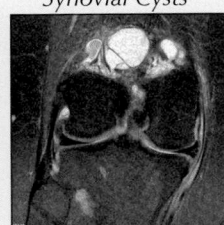	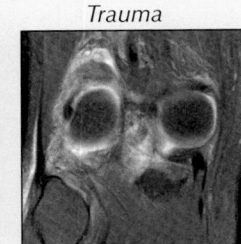	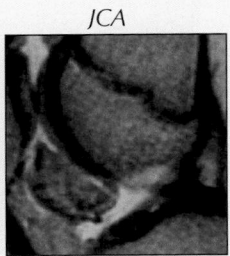
Sag FS PD FSE	Sag FS PD FSE	Cor FS PD FSE	Cor FS PD FSE	Sag T2 MR

RHEUMATOID ARTHRITIS, KNEE

Key Facts

Terminology
- Systemic inflammatory arthritic condition requiring the presence of 4 out of the following 7 criteria for > 6 weeks

Imaging Findings
- Thickened edematous knee synovium in association with effusion in patient with suggestive clinical symptomatology
- Diffuse hyaline articular cartilage loss
- Erosions: Increased signal intensity defects in the subchondral bone at the joint edges
- FS PD FSE demonstrates synovium as intermediate signal and hyperintense joint fluid

Top Differential Diagnoses
- Synovitis

Pathology
- Combination of genetic and environmental factors
- Felty's syndrome characterized by splenomegaly and leukopenia
- Juvenile chronic arthritis (JCA)
- Still's disease characterized by fever, rash and splenomegaly

Clinical Issues
- 10% improve after first attack of synovitis and up to 60% can have remissions

Diagnostic Checklist
- Causes of synovitis: What is the clinical picture, is presentation monoarticular or polyarticular

CT Findings
- NECT: Joint space narrowing, effusion, occasional cyst formation (cystic rheumatoid) followed by destruction

MR Findings
- T1WI
  - Erosions - decreased in signal intensity
  - Hypointense subchondral edema and effusion
  - Lateral compartment involvement frequent
    - Valgus deformity
- T2WI
  - Joint effusion: Increased signal intensity
    - Popliteal cyst
  - Diffuse hyaline articular cartilage loss
  - Erosions: Increased signal intensity defects in the subchondral bone at the joint edges
  - Hyperintense subchondral edema
- PD/Intermediate
  - Inflamed synovium = increased signal intensity in thickened joint lining
  - PD FSE shows hypointense to intermediate signal in synovium
  - FS PD FSE demonstrates synovium as intermediate signal and hyperintense joint fluid
  - Poor contrast visualization of subchondral marrow edema unless fat suppression or STIR sequence used
- STIR
  - Generally less effective because of poor signal to noise and blurring
  - Useful at low and mid field - edema is of increased signal intensity
- T2* GRE: Shows subchondral erosions although masks subchondral edema
- T1 C+
  - Marked synovium enhancement especially with fat saturation
  - FS T1 (+ contrast) - enhancement of thickened edematous synovium and subchondral edema

Nuclear Medicine Findings
- Bone Scan: Bone reactive change will demonstrate increased uptake

Imaging Recommendations
- Best imaging tool: MR to show thickened synovium, cartilage loss, subchondral edema and early erosions
- Protocol advice: FS PD FSE

DIFFERENTIAL DIAGNOSIS

Systemic Lupus Erythematosus
- Characteristic rash and other symptoms/signs (especially bone involvement) different from RA
- Erosions uncommon
- +/- Subluxation

Psoriatic Arthritis
- Primarily involves wrist/hands, feet, sacroiliac joint and spine
- Asymmetric destructive erosive articular process
- Sausage digits

Synovitis
- Thickened increased signal synovium best seen on PDWI
- Multiple causes, including RA
- + Enhancement with gadolinium

Trauma
- Effusion, +/- thickened synovium
- Soft tissue edema
- +/- Fracture
- Asymmetrical

Pigmented Villonodular Synovitis (PVNS)
- Monoarticular
- Hemosiderin laden macrophages
- Decreased signal synovium on all pulse sequences

Synovial Cyst
- Atypical location
- May extend from popliteus tendon sheath/tibiofibular joint
- +/- Synovial lining

RHEUMATOID ARTHRITIS, KNEE

PATHOLOGY

General Features
- General path comments
  - IgM: Rheumatoid factor (RF)
  - Affects synovium first, then cartilage and bone leading to deformity
  - Lab tests (RF) alone do not confirm diagnosis of RA
    - RF can be present (usually low titers) in normal individuals and other diseases
- Genetics: HLA-D allele DR4 is associated with RA patients
- Etiology
  - Combination of genetic and environmental factors
  - Interaction of antigen presenting macrophages with T cells (helper/inducer) - likely inciting event
  - Complexes of IgM & IgG rheumatoid factor can deposit in blood vessels and lead to vasculitis
  - Hepatitis B vaccine may be causative in a small number of patients
- Epidemiology: 1-2% of general population
- Associated abnormalities
  - Felty's syndrome characterized by splenomegaly and leukopenia
  - Juvenile chronic arthritis (JCA)
  - Still's disease characterized by fever, rash and splenomegaly
  - Sjögren syndrome: Decreased salivary and lacrimal gland secretion and lymphoid proliferation
  - Extraarticular manifestations
    - Nodules, lymphadenopathy, splenomegaly, vasculitis, myopathy, sensory changes from neuropathy or direct compression from synovitis
    - Visceral changes including pericarditis, pulmonary fibrosis, nodules, and pleuritic pain

Gross Pathologic & Surgical Features
- Pannus (exuberant inflammatory synovium) tissue erodes cartilage & bone
  - Direct extension of pannus occurs at the margins of the joint
  - Tendon sheaths also involved with pannus (tendinomuscular involvement)
- Synovial cysts (popliteal fossa)
- Sinus tracts

Microscopic Features
- Thickening of the synovial membrane
- Edematous, villous projections
- Multilayering of synoviocytes over thickened villous membrane
- Infiltration of synovia
  - Macrophages, lymphocytes, plasma cells
- ± Fibrin deposition and necrosis within synovia
- RA cells (neutrophils)
  - Granular intracytoplasmic inclusions of phagocytized immune complexes
- Rheumatoid nodules
  - Central fibrinoid necrosis
  - Inflammatory infiltrate of palisaded epithelioid cells and surrounding lymphocytes, macrophages, and plasma cells

Staging, Grading or Classification Criteria
- Fundamental imaging signs
  - Soft tissue swelling and direct visualization of pannus tissue
  - Juxta-articular osteoporosis (marrow inhomogeneity)
  - Loss of subchondral plate
  - Erosion
  - Subchondral cysts
  - Joint space narrowing

CLINICAL ISSUES

Presentation
- Most common signs/symptoms
  - See 7 inclusion criteria (described in definition)
  - Knee stiffness, pain, swelling

Demographics
- Age: Adult (22 to 55 years) for classical RA, variants (juvenile - JCA) affect younger patients
- Gender: F:M = 3:1

Natural History & Prognosis
- 10% improve after first attack of synovitis and up to 60% can have remissions
- Up to 10% can become disabled
- Poor prognostic indicators include
  - Elevation of RF, periarticular erosions, rheumatoid nodules, muscle wasting, joint contractures

Treatment
- Conservative
  - Rest, physical therapy
  - Pyramid pharmaceutical approach including NSAIDs, antimalarials, disease modifying agents (MTX, sulphasalazine, gold, penicillamine), steroids and cytotoxic drugs
- Surgical
  - Synovectomy
  - Arthroplasty, arthrodesis, osteotomy

DIAGNOSTIC CHECKLIST

Consider
- Causes of synovitis: What is the clinical picture, is presentation monoarticular or polyarticular

Image Interpretation Pearls
- Evaluate PD & FS PD images for synovial thickening, effusions and erosions
  - FS PD FSE to detect hyperintense subchondral edema

SELECTED REFERENCES
1. Usatine RP et al: A swollen knee. J Fam Pract 52(1):53-5, 2003
2. Dabby D et al: Synovial knee pain arising from chronic inflammatory disorders of the knee. J Knee Surg 15(1):53-6, 2002

IMAGE GALLERY

Typical

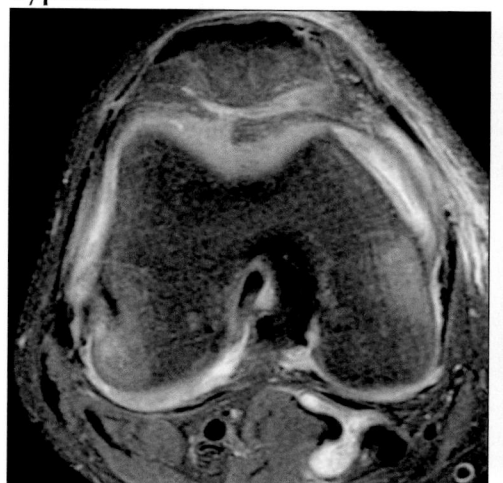

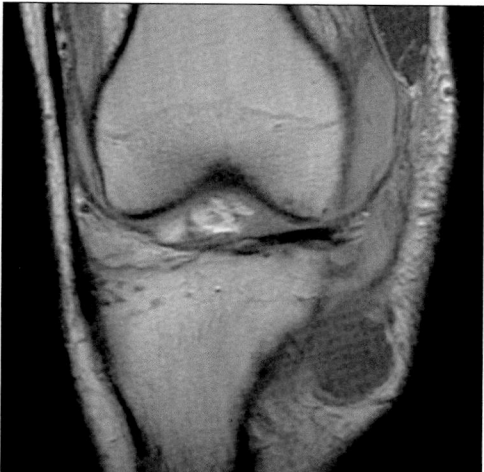

(Left) Axial FS PD FSE MR shows erosions, synovitis and reactive edema in a patient with RA. *(Right)* Coronal PD FSE MR shows an anterior rheumatoid nodule and synovitis in a patient with RA.

Typical

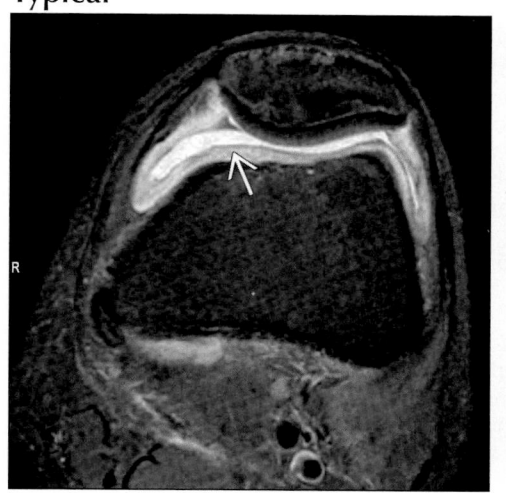

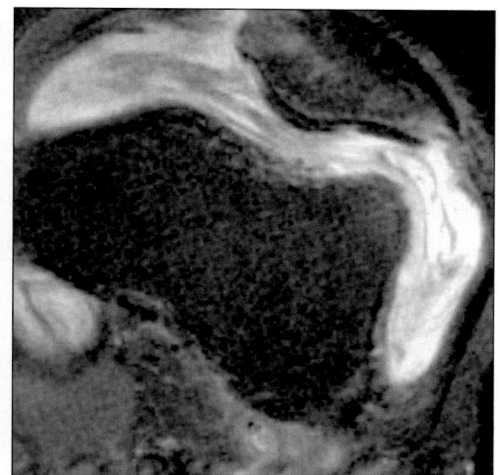

(Left) Axial FS PD FSE MR demonstrating a thick rind (arrow) of synovial hypertrophy lining the suprapatellar bursa. *(Right)* Axial FS PD FSE MR shows hypertrophic synovium (intermediate signal) involving the suprapatellar bursa.

Typical

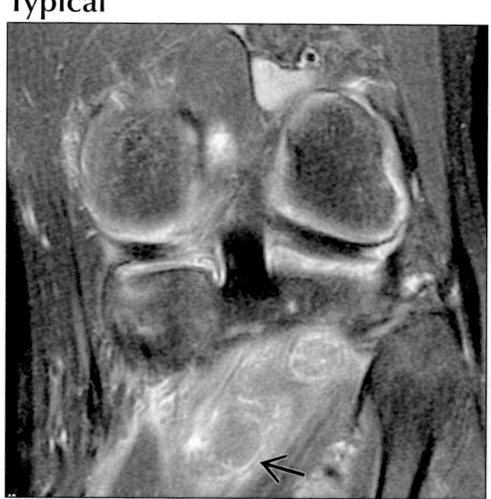

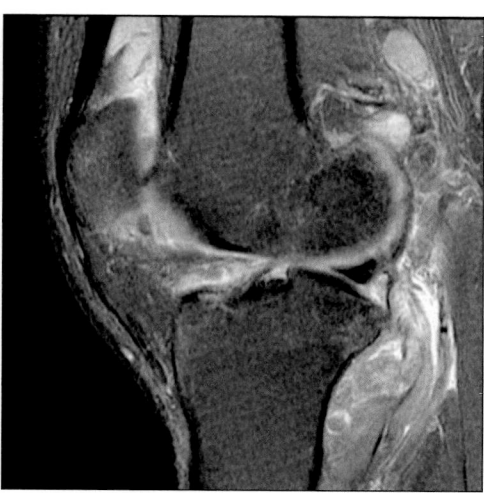

(Left) Coronal FS PD FSE MR shows edematous synovium/pannus (arrow) extending into the popliteus tendon sheath in a patient with RA. *(Right)* Sagittal STIR MR shows synovitis, erosions, edema and adenopathy in a patient with RA.

5

139

PIGMENTED VILLONODULAR SYNOVITIS, KNEE

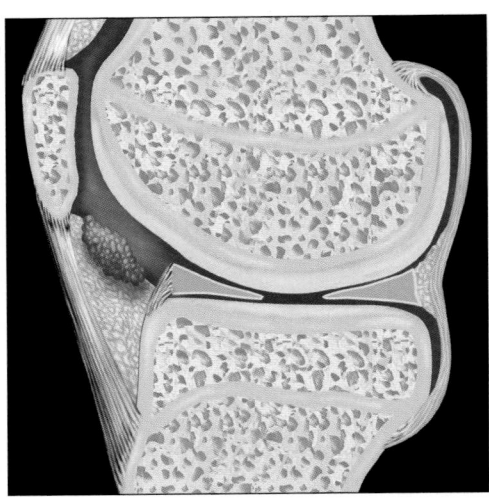

Sagittal graphic shows a focal nodular synovitis lesion in a typical location immediately adjacent to the posterior aspect of Hoffa's fat pad.

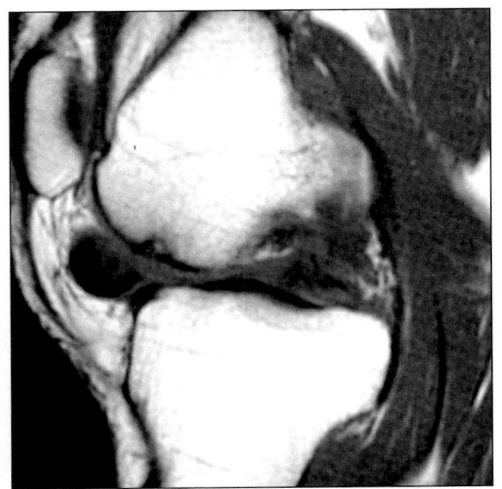

Sagittal PD/Intermediate MR shows hypointense focal nodular PVNS deforming the posterior margin of Hoffa's fat pad.

TERMINOLOGY

Abbreviations and Synonyms

- Pigmented villonodular synovitis (PVNS)

Definitions

- Monoarticular synovial proliferative disorder characterized by hemosiderin laden macrophages within hypertrophic synovial masses often associated with sclerotic rimmed bone erosions

IMAGING FINDINGS

General Features

- Best diagnostic clue: Hypertrophic synovium which is of variable intermediate to decreased signal intensity on T1 and T2WI
- Location: Focal nodular form found posterior to Hoffa's fat pad
- Size: Thickened synovium masses ranging from a few mms to cms in size
- Morphology
  - Diffusely thickened synovium which is of intermediate to decreased signal intensity on all pulse sequences
  - May be focal especially adjacent to Hoffa's fat pad = focal nodular PVNS (localized PVNS)

Radiographic Findings

- Radiography
  - +/- Effusion
  - +/- Variable-sized erosions with sclerotic margins
    - Where adjacent synovium is located
  - Absence of calcification within hyperplastic synovium

CT Findings

- NECT
  - No calcification is demonstrated in synovial mass
  - +/- Effusion
  - +/- Chronic erosive changes
  - Involvement of any synovial tissue
- CT arthrography
  - Irregular and thickened synovium +/- erosions
  - Nodular filling defects

MR Findings

- T1WI
  - Intermediate to decreased signal intensity masses
  - +/- Hypointense erosions
    - +/- Surrounding hypointense edema
  - Erosions well-defined with thin margin
  - Hypointense effusion
- T2WI
  - Hypointense to intermediate signal secondary to paramagnetic effect of iron

---

DDx: Pigmented Villonodular Synovitis, Knee

Synovial Cyst	Hemophilia	RA	Hem Synovitis	Synovial Scar
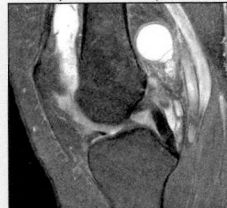	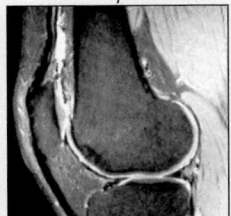	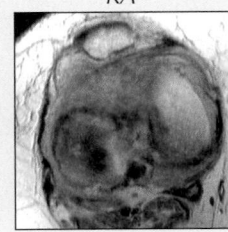	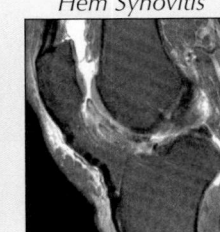	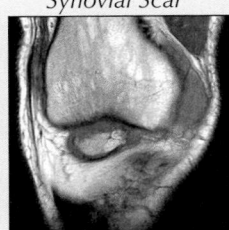
Sag FS PD FSE	Sag T2* GRE MR	Ax PD FSE MR	Sag FS PD FSE	Cor PD FSE MR

PIGMENTED VILLONODULAR SYNOVITIS, KNEE

Key Facts

Terminology
- Monoarticular synovial proliferative disorder characterized by hemosiderin laden macrophages within hypertrophic synovial masses often associated with sclerotic rimmed bone erosions

Imaging Findings
- Best diagnostic clue: Hypertrophic synovium which is of variable intermediate to decreased signal intensity on T1 and T2WI
- May be focal especially adjacent to Hoffa's fat pad = focal nodular PVNS (localized PVNS)

Top Differential Diagnoses
- Hemophilic Arthropathy
- Hemorrhagic Synovitis

Pathology
- Found in any recess in communication with joint
- Diffuse form and focal nodular form

Clinical Issues
- Monoarticular synovial disorder
- Nonpainful soft tissue mass

Diagnostic Checklist
- Monoarticular arthritis characterized by decreased signal intensity synovial thickening is diagnostic
- Hypointense (intermediate to hypointense) synovial mass posterior to free edge of Hoffa's fat pad
- T2* GRE identifies hemosiderin components (hypointense)

- +/- Intermediate signal erosions
  - +/- Surrounding hyperintense edema
  - FS PD FSE less sensitive to hemosiderin in pannus tissue and synovium than T2* GRE
- Hyperintense effusion
- PD/Intermediate
  - Decreased signal intensity masses
  - Hemosiderin deposits in synovium - decreased signal
- T2* GRE
  - Decreased signal intensity masses
  - Condylar erosions associated with synovial mass and fibrous tissue
  - Foci of hypointensity due to hemosiderin deposits in synovium
    - GRE sensitive to hemosiderin
    - Involved synovium found in all potential joint recesses in diffuse form
- T1 C+
  - Inflamed synovium enhances
  - Hemosiderin - infiltrated synovial masses show only minimal enhancement
- Diffuse form: Diffusely thickened synovium with variable degrees of decreased signal intensity on all pulse sequences
- Focal nodular form
  - Adjacent to the patella and Hoffa's fat pad
    - Variable but generally decreased signal intensity on all pulse sequences
    - Hemosiderin laden macrophages in synovium

Imaging Recommendations
- Best imaging tool: MRI
- Protocol advice: GRE images demonstrate hemosiderin component due to susceptibility of hemosiderin

DIFFERENTIAL DIAGNOSIS

Hemophilic Arthropathy
- Clinical history
- Diffuse form most common
- Familial (X-linked)
- Decreased signal masses on all pulse sequences

- T2* GRE sensitive

Hemorrhagic Synovitis
- Posttraumatic
  - Traumatic history
- Hypointense synovium on all pulse sequences

Hypertrophic Synovitis
- Thickened synovium
- Absence of decreased signal masses unless hemorrhagic
- Focal or nodular presentation unusual
  - Inflammatory, posttraumatic, infectious

Rheumatoid Arthritis (RA)
- Systemic inflammatory disorder
- Polyarticular
- + RA factor usually
- Thick synovium (cause of synovitis)

Synovial Cyst
- Usually reflects repeated effusions
- Can extrude from joint at many locations
- Hyperintense on T2WI
- Often exits the joint posteriorly

Scar/Adhesions
- Posttraumatic
- Post surgical
- Hypointense cicatricial change on all pulse sequence

PATHOLOGY

General Features
- General path comments
  - Monoarticular synovial proliferative disorder
  - Found in any recess in communication with joint
    - Popliteus tendon sheath
    - Coronary recess
    - Meniscofemoral recess
    - Suprapatellar pouch
    - Popliteal cyst
    - Intercondylar notch

PIGMENTED VILLONODULAR SYNOVITIS, KNEE

- Etiology
  - Idiopathic monoarticular disorder
  - Hemosiderin laden macrophages
- Epidemiology: > 1% general population

Gross Pathologic & Surgical Features
- Localized/nodular type
  - Well-circumscribed
  - Lobular
  - Usually < 4 cm in diameter
  - Cut surface with white, yellow, gray and brown areas (fat and hemosiderin)
  - Soft and elastic vs. fibrous scarring in later stages
- Diffuse type
  - Multiple, soft, spongy lesions
  - Brown, yellow, or rust-like (based on hemosiderin content)
  - No well defined collagenous capsule

Microscopic Features
- Localized/nodular type
  - Dense, collagenous capsule
  - Fibrous scarring
  - Multinucleated giant cells
  - Mononuclear cells
  - Xanthoma cells
  - Histiofibroblastic hyperplasia
  - Small cystic spaces
  - Hemosiderin (less than diffuse type of PVNS)
- Diffuse type
  - Hemosiderin within histiocytes
  - Villous hyperplasia of synovial membrane & capillary hyperplasia
  - Sheets of polymorphic/rounded cells
  - Cystic clefts
  - Decreased number of multinucleated giant cells relative to localized type
  - Collagen in stroma ± hyalinized appearance

Staging, Grading or Classification Criteria
- Diffuse form and focal nodular form
  - Diffuse form: Throughout joint
  - Focal nodular form: Adjacent to patellofemoral joint (adherent to posterior surface of Hoffa's fat pad)

CLINICAL ISSUES

Presentation
- Most common signs/symptoms
  - Monoarticular synovial disorder
  - Nonpainful soft tissue mass

Demographics
- Age: Typically found in adults (common age range between 20 & 50 years)
- Gender: Predilection for females

Natural History & Prognosis
- Progressive synovitis with pain and effusions

Treatment
- Synovectomy

DIAGNOSTIC CHECKLIST

Consider
- Hemophilia or any cause of hemorrhagic synovitis

Image Interpretation Pearls
- Monoarticular arthritis characterized by decreased signal intensity synovial thickening is diagnostic
- Hypointense (intermediate to hypointense) synovial mass posterior to free edge of Hoffa's fat pad
- T2* GRE identifies hemosiderin components (hypointense)

SELECTED REFERENCES

1. Calmet J et al: Localized pigmented villonodular synovitis in an unusual location in the knee. Arthroscopy 19(2):144-9, 2003
2. Adem C et al: Recurrent and non-recurrent pigmented villonodular synovitis. Ann Pathol 22(6):448-52, 2002
3. Abdelwahab Fet al: True bursal pigmented villonodular synovitis. Skeletal Radiol 31(6):354-8, 2002
4. Fitzgerald RH et al: Orthopaedics. St Louis MO, Mosby, 2002
5. Durr HR et al: Pigmented villonodular synovitis. Review of 20 cases. J Rheumatol 28(7):1620-30, 2001
6. DiCaprio MR: Pigmented villonodular synovitis of the elbow: A case report and literature review. J Hand Surg Am 24(2): 386-91, 1999
7. Lin J et al: Pigmented villonodular synovitis and related lesions: The spectrum of imaging findings. Am J Roentgenol 172:191-7, 1999
8. Lindenbaum BL et al: An unusual presentation of pigmented villonodular synovitis. Clin Orthop 122:263-7, 1999
9. Lee B et al: Localized pigmented villonodular synovitis of the knee: Arthroscopic treatment. Arthroscopy 14(7):764-8, 1998
10. Mancini GB et al: Localized pigmented villonodular synovitis of the knee. Arthroscopy. 14(5):532-6, 1998
11. Aigner TS et al: Iron deposits, cell populations and proliferative activity in pigmented villonodular synovitis of the knee joint. Verh Dtsch Ges Pathol 82:327-31, 1998
12. Bertoni F et al: Malignant giant cell tumor of the tendon sheaths and joints (malignant pigmented villonodular synovitis). Am J Surg Pathol 21(2):153-63, 1997
13. Stoller DW et al: Magnetic resonance imaging in orthopaedics and sports medicine. vol 1. 2nd ed. Philadelphia PA, J.B. Lippincott, 203-442, 1997
14. Aboulafia AJ et al: Neuropathy secondary to pigmented villonodular synovitis of the hip. Clin Orthop 174-80, 1996
15. Bravo SM et al: Pigmented villonodular synovitis. Radiol Clin North Am 34(2):311-26, 1996
16. Gezen F et al: Spinal pigmented villonodular synovitis: A case report. 21(5):642-5, 1996
17. Giannini C et al: Pigmented villonodular synovitis of the spine: A clinical, radiological, and morphological study of 12 cases. J Neurosurg 84(4):592-7, 1996
18. Budny PG et al: Localized nodular synovitis: A rare cause of ulnar nerve compression in Guyon's canal. J Hand Surg Am 17(4):663-4, 1992
19. Schwartz HS et al: Pigmented villonodular synovitis. A retrospective review of affected large joints. Clin Orthop 247:243-55, 1989

IMAGE GALLERY

Typical

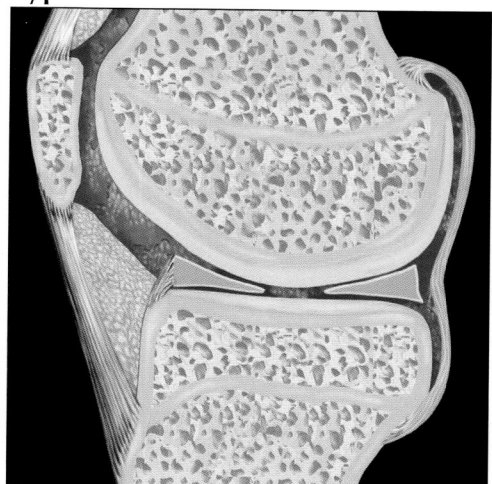 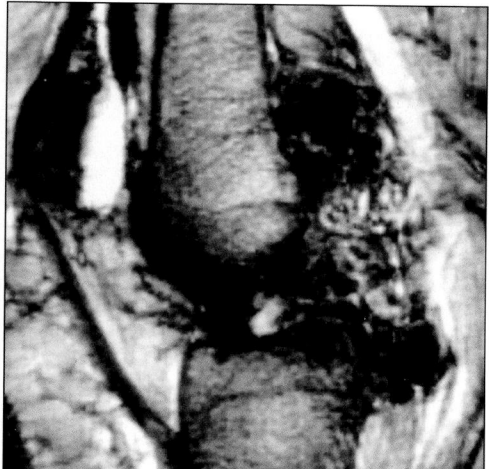

(Left) Sagittal graphic shows the diffuse form of PVNS. *(Right)* Sagittal T2* GRE MR shows diffuse PVNS predominately in the posterior aspect of the joint.

Variant

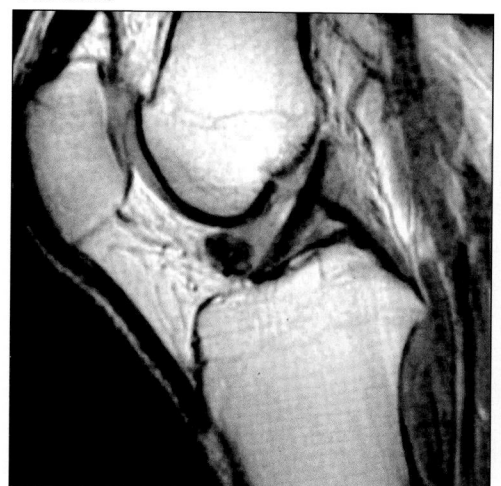 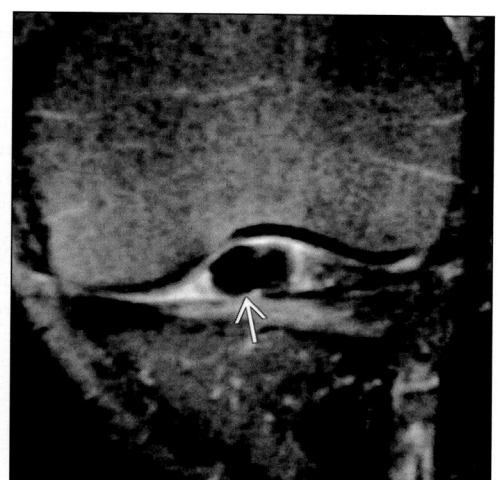

(Left) Sagittal PD MR shows focal nodular PVNS adjacent to Hoffa's fat pad. *(Right)* Coronal FS PD FSE MR shows the focus of focal nodular PVNS at the anterior aspect of the joint (arrow). The patient had an extension block and was suspected of having a bucket-handle meniscus tear.

5

143

Typical

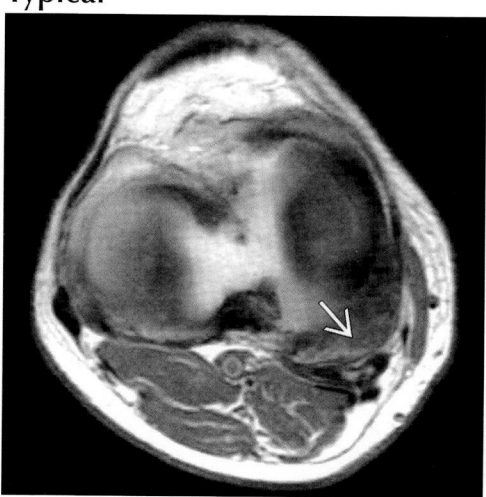 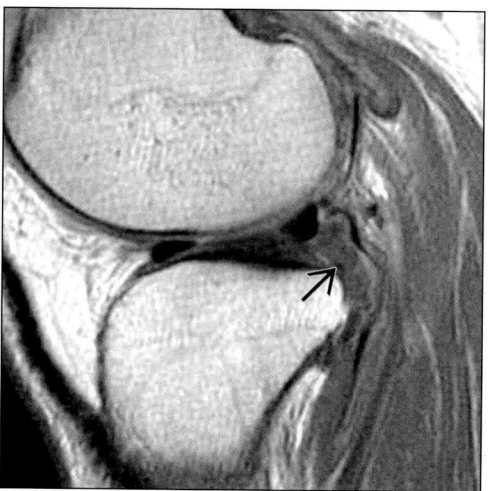

(Left) Axial PD FSE MR shows PVNS (arrow) in the popliteus tendon sheath. *(Right)* Sagittal PD FSE MR shows intermediate signal intensity PVNS (arrow) in the popliteus tendon sheath.

LIPOMA ARBORESCENS, KNEE

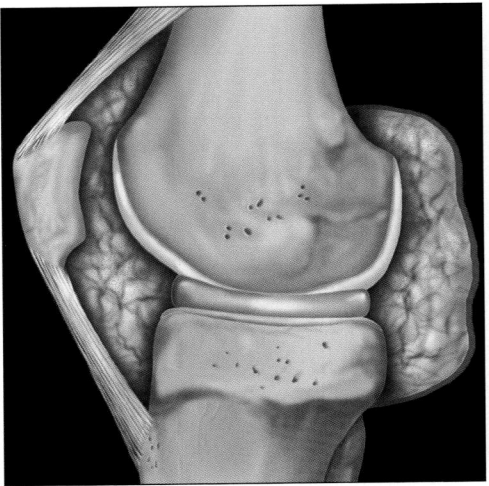

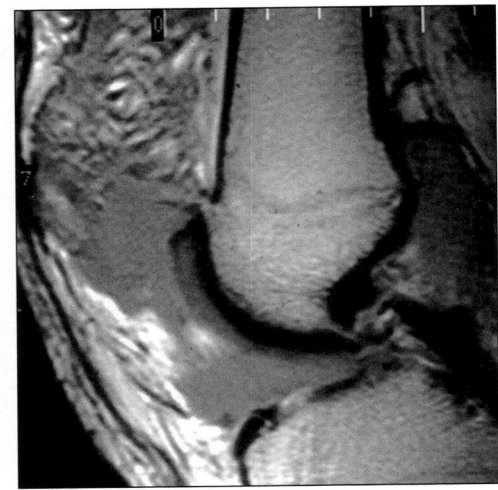

Sagittal graphic shows fatty infiltration of the synovium resulting in distention of the joint capsule.

Sagittal PD FSE MR shows intraarticular lipoma arborescens occupying the suprapatellar pouch.

TERMINOLOGY

Abbreviations and Synonyms
- Lipoma arborescens (LA)

Definitions
- Fatty synovial/subsynovial infiltration

IMAGING FINDINGS

General Features
- Best diagnostic clue: Increased (fat) signal thickening of the synovium on T1WI, PD FSE & FS PD FSE MR
- Location: Within capsule of knee joint, most common in suprapatellar pouch (bursa)
- Size: Small fronds of affected synovium to large infiltrated fronds filling the joint
- Morphology: Usually frond-like until large then globular and rounded masses

Radiographic Findings
- Radiography: Increased lucency in joint (fat density)

CT Findings
- NECT: Decreased density synovial masses

MR Findings
- T1WI: Increased signal intensity synovial masses (fat signal intensity)
- T2WI: Signal intensity decreases as with subcutaneous fat or saturates with FS PD FSE
- STIR: Fat within synovial masses saturates (hypointense)

Imaging Recommendations
- Best imaging tool: MRI, NECT
- Protocol advice: T1 and FS PD FSE

DIFFERENTIAL DIAGNOSIS

Synovial Lipoma
- Found in/on Hoffa's fat pad, single mass

Synovial Osteochondromatosis
- Calcific masses

Synovitis
- Visualized as thickened synovium but without saturation with fat saturation techniques
- +/- Synovial fronds

Loose Bodies
- Decreased signal structures most often calcified
- +/- Cortical rim

DDx: Lipoma Arborescens, Knee

Volume Averaging	Synovitis	Normal Prefem Fat
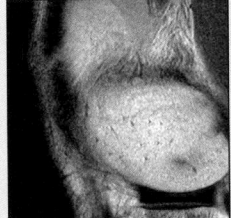	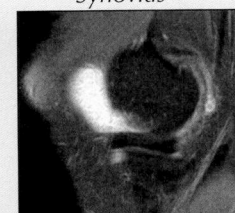	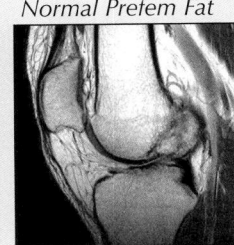
Sag PD FSE MR	*Sag FS PD FSE*	*Sag PD FSE MR*

LIPOMA ARBORESCENS, KNEE

Key Facts

Terminology
- Fatty synovial/subsynovial infiltration

Imaging Findings
- Best diagnostic clue: Increased (fat) signal thickening of the synovium on T1WI, PD FSE & FS PD FSE MR
- Size: Small fronds of affected synovium to large infiltrated fronds filling the joint
- Morphology: Usually frond-like until large then globular and rounded masses
- NECT: Decreased density synovial masses

Top Differential Diagnoses
- Synovial Lipoma
- Synovitis
- Normal Fat around the Joint

Pathology
- General path comments: Infiltration of fat tissue at synovium and subsynovial tissue forming frond-like masses
- Etiology: Idiopathic, unusual response to chronic synovial irritation, +/- underlying degenerative joint disease
- Epidemiology: Rare

Clinical Issues
- Most common signs/symptoms: Swelling, usually painless

Diagnostic Checklist
- Saturation of synovial masses (esp. frond-like) on FS PD FSE is diagnostic

---

- +/- Marrow fat vs. sclerotic hypointense signal

Normal Fat around the Joint
- Volume averaged mimicking LA, e.g., normal prefemoral fat (Normal Prefem Fat)

PATHOLOGY

General Features
- General path comments: Infiltration of fat tissue at synovium and subsynovial tissue forming frond-like masses
- Etiology: Idiopathic, unusual response to chronic synovial irritation, +/- underlying degenerative joint disease
- Epidemiology: Rare
- Associated abnormalities: Joint effusion

Gross Pathologic & Surgical Features
- Fatty enlargement of the synovium with frond-like architecture
- Fatty appearing globules and villous projections seen at arthroscopy

Microscopic Features
- Mature adipocytes within subsynovium and enlarged synovial fronds

CLINICAL ISSUES

Presentation
- Most common signs/symptoms: Swelling, usually painless
- Clinical profile: Painless effusion

Demographics
- Age: Reported in adolescents - adults
- Gender: No predilection

Natural History & Prognosis
- Painless swelling usually without complete regression

Treatment
- Synovectomy

DIAGNOSTIC CHECKLIST

Consider
- Other causes of synovial proliferation

Image Interpretation Pearls
- Saturation of synovial masses (esp. frond-like) on FS PD FSE is diagnostic

SELECTED REFERENCES

1. Al-Ismail K et al: Bilateral lipoma arborescens associated with early osteoarthritis. Eur Radiol 12(11):2799-802, 2002
2. Ikushima K et al: Lipoma arborescens of the knee as a possible cause of osteoarthrosis. Orthopedics 24(6):603-5, 2001
3. Kloen P et al: Lipoma arborescens of the knee. J Bone Joint Surg Br 80(2):298-301, 1998
4. Feller JF et al: Lipoma arborescens of the knee: MR demonstration. AJR 163(1):162-4, 1994

IMAGE GALLERY

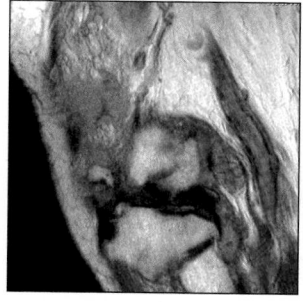
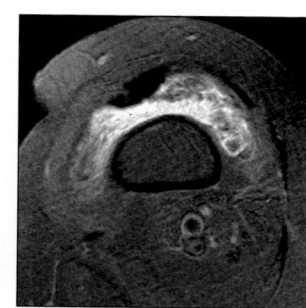

(Left) Sagittal PD FSE MR shows lipoma arborescens within the suprapatellar pouch at the lateral aspect of the joint in this arthritic knee. *(Right)* Axial FS PD FSE MR shows fat saturation of the lipomatous masses.

REFLEX SYMPATHETIC DYSTROPHY, KNEE

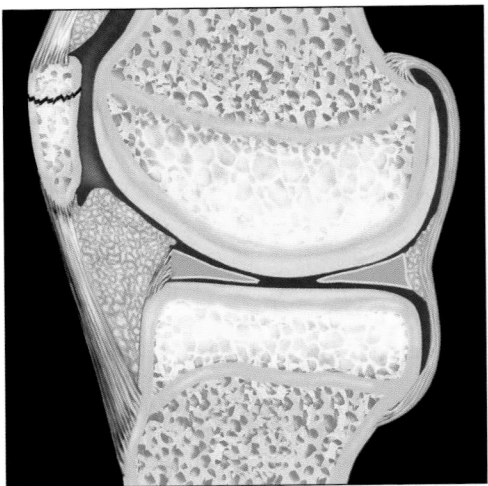

Sagittal graphic shows patchy edema within the femur, tibia and patella. There is an associated fracture of the patella. Chronic intractable disproportionate pain characterizes RSD.

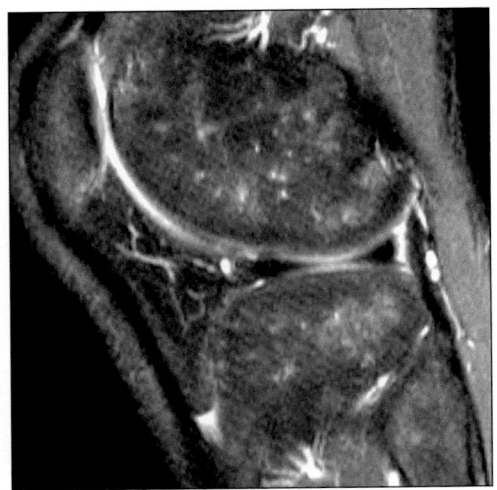

Sagittal FS PD FSE MR shows patchy bone marrow edema in a patient three months post trauma with a pain syndrome clinically characteristic of reflex sympathetic dystrophy.

TERMINOLOGY

Abbreviations and Synonyms
- Reflex sympathetic dystrophy (RSD), complex regional pain syndrome (CRPS)

Definitions
- Chronic pain disorder of the sympathetic nervous system, usually result of trauma or complication of surgery, infection, casting or splitting
  - Normal system of pain perception "misfires" leading to abnormal cycle of intractable pain
  - With progression, effect on other areas of the body can result in varying degrees of disability as recruitment of other systems occurs
- Complex regional pain syndrome - type I (RSD) = initiating noxious event, or a cause of immobilization
  - Pain, allodynia, or hyperalgesia with which the pain is disproportionate to inciting event
  - Edema, changes in skin blood flow (skin color changes, skin temperature changes more than 1.1°C difference from the homologous body part), or abnormal pseudomotor activity in region of the pain
  - Nerve injury cannot be immediately identified
- Complex regional pain syndrome - type II (causalgia)
  - Type I + continuing pain, allodynia, or hyperalgesia after nerve injury, not necessarily limited to distribution of the injured nerve
  - Distinct "major" nerve injury
- CRPS = injury to a nerve or soft tissue (e.g., osseous fracture) that does not follow the normal healing path

IMAGING FINDINGS

General Features
- Best diagnostic clue
  - Clinical: Prolonged, intractable pain more severe than expected with original injury
  - Patchy areas of bone marrow edema on FS PD FSE
- Location: Bones of the knee (subarticular in patella, femur, tibia, and fibula)
- Size: Patchy areas of edema vary in size
- Morphology: Patchy or smaller diffuse punctate pattern bone changes (edema)

Radiographic Findings
- Radiography: Osteopenia - not sensitive

CT Findings
- NECT: Osteopenia and focal lucencies

MR Findings
- T1WI
  - Foci of hypointense bone marrow edema
    - Proper clinical setting

DDx: Reflex Sympathetic Dystrophy, Knee

Normal Marrow	Normal Marrow	Metastasis	Infarct	Tibial Fracture

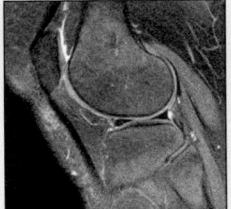 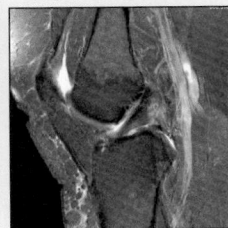 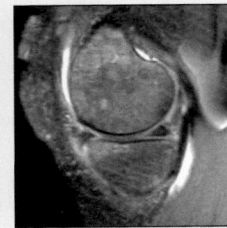 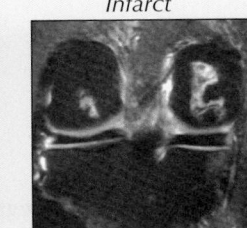 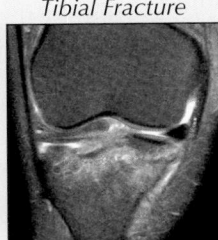

| Sag FS PD FSE | Sag FS PD FSE | Sag FS PD FSE | Cor FS PD FSE | Cor FS PD FSE |

REFLEX SYMPATHETIC DYSTROPHY, KNEE

Key Facts

Terminology

- Chronic pain disorder of the sympathetic nervous system, usually result of trauma or complication of surgery, infection, casting or splitting

Imaging Findings

- Clinical: Prolonged, intractable pain more severe than expected with original injury
- Patchy areas of bone marrow edema on FS PD FSE

Top Differential Diagnoses

- Normal Marrow
- Metastasis
- Bone Infarct
- Fracture/Bone Trabecular Injury

Pathology

- Fatty atrophy in later stages

Clinical Issues

- Most common signs/symptoms: Severe chronic pain out of proportion to trauma
- Patient with severe pain out of proportion to frequent trivial trauma, skin changes (swelling and redness in the affected area)

Diagnostic Checklist

- Interpret images in setting of proper clinical history for RSD diagnosis
- Use T1 and FS PD FSE images to identify changes in subarticular marrow signal intensity

---

- ○ +/- Healing/healed fracture (if posttraumatic) (hypointense)
- ○ +/- Healing/healed ligamentous changes (if posttraumatic)
  - ▪ +/- Thickening/fibrosis hypointensity
- T2WI
  - ○ FS PD FSE
    - ▪ Skin thickening, soft tissue edema = stage I
    - ▪ Skin thickening/thinning without edema = stage II
    - ▪ Muscle atrophy = stage III
  - ○ Patchy bone marrow edema - hyperintensity
    - ▪ Proper clinical setting
  - ○ +/- Healing/healed fracture (if posttraumatic)
    - ▪ +/- Hyperintensity
    - ▪ Proper clinical setting
  - ○ +/- Healing/healed ligamentous changes (if posttraumatic)
    - ▪ Proper clinical setting
- PD/Intermediate
  - ○ Intermediate "sponge painted" bone marrow appearance
    - ▪ PD FSE usually insensitive to marrow signal changes relative to T1WI or FS PD FSE and STIR
- STIR
  - ○ Patchy bone marrow edema - hyperintensity
  - ○ +/- Healing/healed fracture (if posttraumatic) (+/- hyperintensity)
  - ○ +/- Healing/healed ligamentous changes if posttraumatic (typically hypointense)

Nuclear Medicine Findings

- Bone Scan: +/- Increased uptake

Imaging Recommendations

- Best imaging tool: MRI
- Protocol advice: FS PD FSE, STIR, T1

DIFFERENTIAL DIAGNOSIS

Normal Marrow

- Red marrow mimicking bone marrow edema
- Brighter than normal skeletal muscle on T1WI

- Younger patients
- Patients on hormonal therapy
- Seen in proliferative states
  - ○ Anemia
  - ○ Perimenopausal hormone therapy
  - ○ Obesity (occasionally)

Metastasis

- Older age group
- Positive history
- Often multifocal

Bone Infarct

- Serpiginous region of signal abnormality
- Result of vascular compromise
- Predisposing condition
  - ○ Steroids
  - ○ Caisson's disease
  - ○ Pancreatitis
- Double line sign
- Location not restricted to metaphyseal areas

Fracture/Bone Trabecular Injury

- +/- Decreased signal intensity fracture line
- Trabecular injury with increased signal intensity on T2WI
- Focal involvement

PATHOLOGY

General Features

- General path comments: Sympathetic nervous system dysfunction
- Etiology
  - ○ Result of minor trauma, inflammation following surgery, infection, lacerations, degenerative joint disease, burns and compression such as casting or swelling due to injury that may cause prolonged pressure on peripheral nerves
  - ○ Sympathetic nervous system dysfunction
    - ▪ Nociceptors transmit pain syndrome to spinal cord

REFLEX SYMPATHETIC DYSTROPHY, KNEE

- Atypical sympathetic reflex results in tissue edema, capillary collapse, and ischemia
- Wide dynamic range neurons stimulated increasing sympathetic activity from the spinal cord to the periphery
- Release of norepinephrine in the periphery has effect on the blood vessels causing vasoconstriction and pain
- Recruitment of receptors = allodynia = pain from light touch
- Vasoconstriction = increased pain + sympathetic nervous system stimulation = Substance P and prostaglandin increase in nociceptor stimulation
- Other theories for abnormal pain include unregulated sensitivity of α-adrenoreceptors for catecholamines or an exaggeration of the peripheral neural inflammatory response
- Epidemiology: May follow 5% of all injuries
- Associated abnormalities: Muscle atrophy, chronic pain

Gross Pathologic & Surgical Features
- Skin edema, swelling progress to skin thinning, and muscle atrophy

Microscopic Features
- Fatty atrophy in later stages

Staging, Grading or Classification Criteria
- RSD stages
  - Stage I (traumatic): Up to 3 months after injury, swelling and redness of affected area
  - Stage II (dystrophic): 3-9 months after injury, affected area becomes blue and cold + increased pain, stiffness, +/- osteoporosis
    - Skin temperature decreases, mottled skin tone, pseudomotor dysfunction, +/- osteoporosis
    - Most difficult stage to treat
  - Stage III (atrophic): 9-18 months after injury, wasting of affected muscles, contraction of tendons, atrophy

CLINICAL ISSUES

Presentation
- Most common signs/symptoms: Severe chronic pain out of proportion to trauma
- Clinical profile
  - Patient with severe pain out of proportion to frequent trivial trauma, skin changes (swelling and redness in the affected area)
  - Types I and II CRPS have similar clinical symptoms and progression of disease
    - No known nerve injury in type I
  - If regional sympathetic block provides immediate relief, diagnosis can be sympathetically maintained pain (RSD)
    - If symptoms remit only after a complete nerve block then diagnosis may be nerve entrapment
  - Acetone drop test can be done to demonstrate allodynia

- Alcohol applied on affected limb then blow on the area - evaporation will stimulate cold hyperalgesia in RSD patient

Demographics
- Age: Children and adults
- Gender
  - Females predominate
    - Lower extremity

Natural History & Prognosis
- Often improves but may progress to atrophy and chronic dysfunction

Treatment
- Drug therapy, nerve blocks, physical therapy, transcutaneous electrical stimulator
- Implantable devices: Spinal cord stimulator, drug delivery infusion pump
- Sympathectomy

DIAGNOSTIC CHECKLIST

Consider
- Any etiology of bone marrow edema
- Complex regional pain syndrome (CRPS) is divided into two types
  - Type I replaces the term reflex sympathetic dystrophy
  - Type II replaces the term causalgia

Image Interpretation Pearls
- Interpret images in setting of proper clinical history for RSD diagnosis
- Use T1 and FS PD FSE images to identify changes in subarticular marrow signal intensity

SELECTED REFERENCES

1. Cuckler J.M: The stiff knee: Evaluation and management. Orthopedics 25(9):969-70, 2002
2. Papadopoulos GS et al: The treatment of reflex sympathetic dystrophy in a 9 year-old boy with long standing symptoms. Minerva Anestesiol 67(9):659-63, 2001
3. Leitha T: Reflex sympathetic dystrophy after arthroscopy. Clin Nucl Med 25(12):1028-9, 2000
4. Poncelet C et al: Reflex sympathetic dystrophy in pregnancy: Nine cases and a review of the literature. Eur J Obstet Gynecol Reprod Biol 86(1):55-63, 1999
5. Braverman DL et al: Recurrent spontaneous hemarthrosis associated with reflex sympathetic dystrophy. Arch Phys Med Rehabil 79(3):339-42, 1998
6. Stanton-Hicks M et al: Reflex sympathetic dystrophy: Changing the concepts and taxonomy. Pain 63:127-133, 1995
7. Merskey H et al: Classification of chronic pain: Descriptions of chronic pain syndromes and definitions of pain terms. 2nd ed. Seattle WA, IASP Press, 1994
8. Michell SW et al: Gunshot wounds and injuries of nerves. New York NY, JB Lippincott, 1989

IMAGE GALLERY

Typical

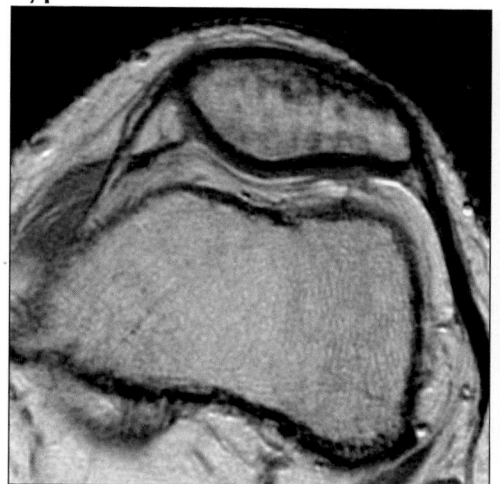 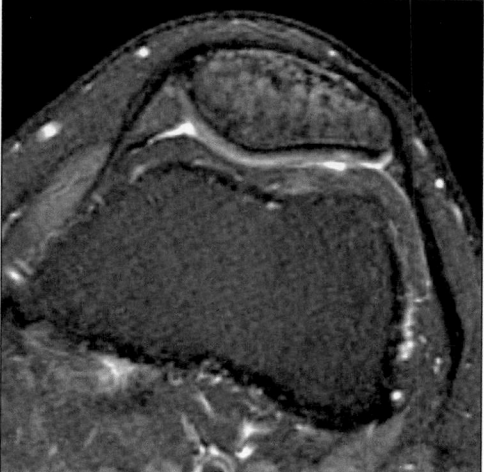

(Left) Axial PD FSE MR shows RSD changes of the patella in a patient s/p trauma. (Right) Axial FS PD FSE MR shows the patchy high signal intensity edema within the patella. This patient had a clinical presentation of RSD.

Typical

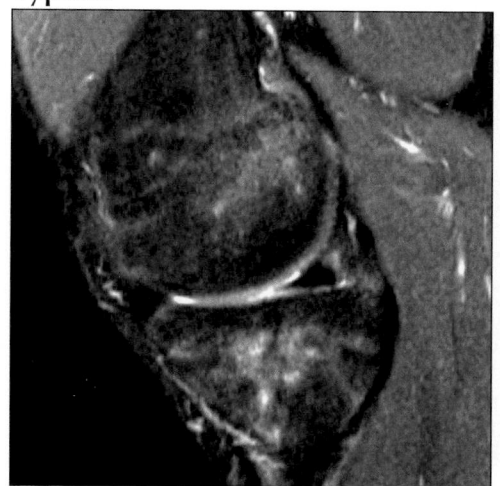 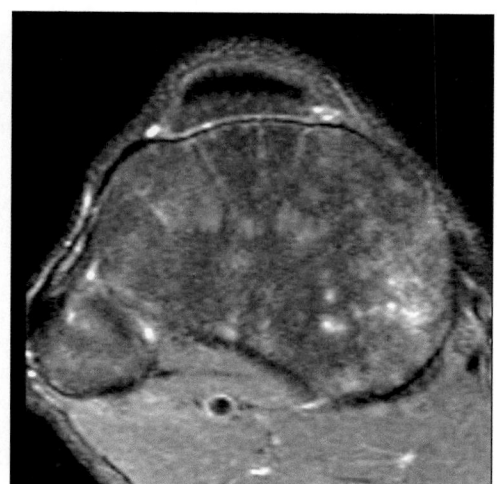

(Left) Sagittal FS PD FSE MR shows RSD hyperintense RSD changes in the femur and tibia in a patient without history of a nerve injury. (Right) Axial FS PD FSE MR image of the same patient shows the hyperintense inhomogeneity of the tibia and fibula.

5

149

Typical

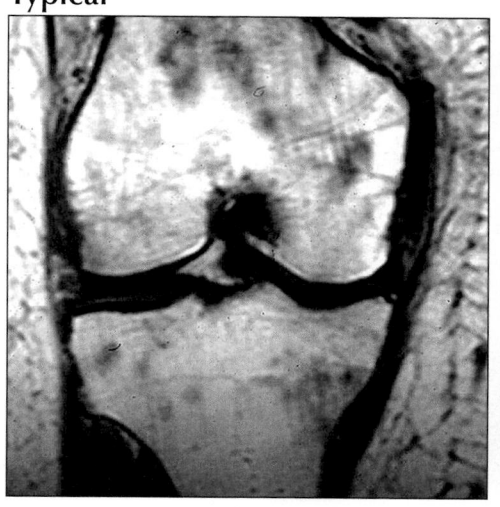 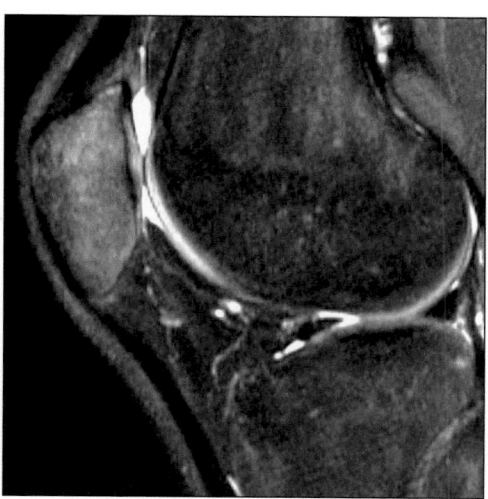

(Left) Coronal T1WI MR shows hypointense areas of marrow involvement with RSD. (Right) Sagittal FS PD FSE MR shows isolated involvement of the patella (hyperintense edema) in this patient with RSD and no history of patellar trauma.

CHONDROCALCINOSIS, KNEE

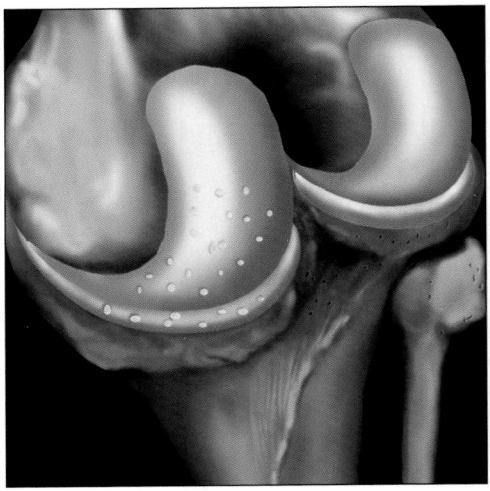

Coronal oblique graphic shows the typical appearance of chondrocalcinosis at gross pathologic inspection with white calcium deposits within the hyaline and fibrocartilage.

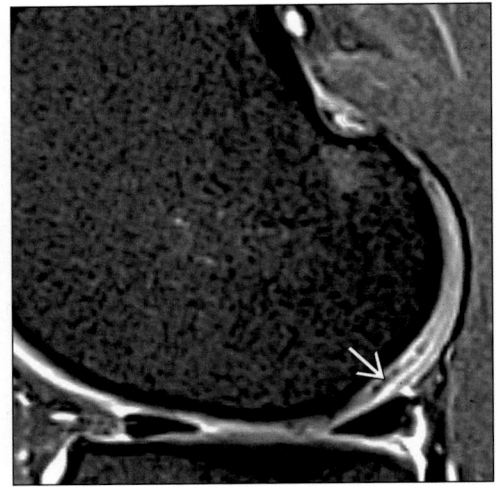

Sagittal T2 GRE MR shows hypointense chondrocalcinosis (arrow) within the hyaline articular cartilage of the posterior lateral femoral condyle.*

TERMINOLOGY

Abbreviations and Synonyms
- Calcium pyrophosphate dihydrate deposition (CPPD) disease (CPPDD), pseudogout, tophaceous pseudogout

Definitions
- Chondrocalcinosis = visible calcification within tissues on imaging study
- CPPD represents deposition of calcium pyrophosphate crystals in hyaline cartilage, synovial tissue, capsule, meniscus
  ○ Chondrocalcinosis not synonymous with CPPD
- CPPD represents chemical manifestation of separate, yet related diseases
  ○ Pseudogout
    ▪ Acute presentation appears very similar to gout
    ▪ + Crystals (no urate as in gout)
  ○ Tophaceous pseudogout
    ▪ Produces pseudotumor
    ▪ Rare in knee
  ○ Familial calcium pyrophosphate dihydrate deposition
    ▪ Appears at earlier age (as early as third decade of life)
    ▪ More aggressive & poor long-term prognosis
  ○ Osteoarthritis (OA)
    ▪ Pyrophosphate arthropathy

    ▪ Symptoms are identical to those of patients with OA + calcium pyrophosphate crystals
    ▪ Common in orthopedic practices
  ○ Chondrocalcinosis
    ▪ Asymptomatic

IMAGING FINDINGS

General Features
- Best diagnostic clue
  ○ Radiography valuable for showing chondrocalcinosis (pathognomonic)
  ○ Decreased signal intensity calcium deposition in soft tissues on all sequences
- Location: Knee - most often affected joint in the body
- Size: Small to large areas of calcific depositions
- Morphology: Small to large irregular depositions of calcium crystals

Radiographic Findings
- Radiography
  ○ Foci of increased density (calcification = chondrocalcinosis)
  ○ Chondrocalcinosis in hyaline cartilage, menisci, synovium

CT Findings
- NECT

DDx: Chondrocalcinosis, Knee

Trochlear Chondro	OCD	Chondromalacia	Chondromalacia
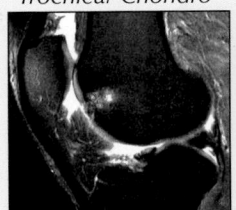	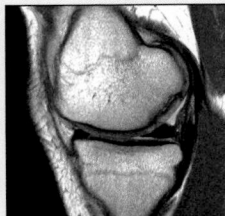	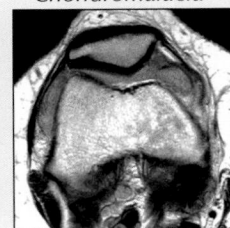	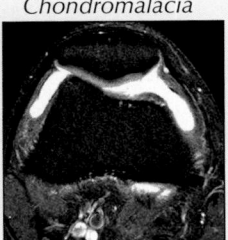
Sag FS PD FSE	Sag PD FSE MR	Ax PD FSE MR	Ax FS PD FSE

CHONDROCALCINOSIS, KNEE

Key Facts

Terminology
- Calcium pyrophosphate dihydrate deposition (CPPD) disease (CPPDD), pseudogout, tophaceous pseudogout
- Chondrocalcinosis = visible calcification within tissues on imaging study

Imaging Findings
- Chondrocalcinosis within hyaline articular cartilage as decreased signal intensity foci (GRE most sensitive technique)

Top Differential Diagnoses
- Gout
- Osteoarthritis without CPPD

Pathology
- Pyrophosphate arthropathy resembles osteoarthritis ± intermittent attacks of pseudogout

Clinical Issues
- Pseudogout - begins in galloping fashion, peak within hours, + pain, swelling, heat, and redness
- 50% of patients have fever
- Associated with OA in older patient
- Spontaneous resolution over several days to weeks

Diagnostic Checklist
- Evaluate hyaline articular cartilage on MR images
- T2* GRE is the most sensitive sequence for the detection of CPPD crystal deposition

---

- ○ Chondrocalcinosis in hyaline cartilage, menisci, synovium
- ○ Changes of OA (in pyrophosphate arthropathy)
  - Subchondral sclerosis, cysts, osteophytes
- CECT: Enhancing synovium in case of synovitis

MR Findings
- T1WI
  - ○ Chondrocalcinosis: Decreased signal intensity foci within hyaline articular cartilage
  - ○ Menisci demonstrate punctate irregularities within degenerated foci
  - ○ T1WI not sensitive to calcium pyrophosphate dihydrate crystals
  - ○ Synovitis - thickened intermediate signal intensity joint lining compared to hypointense fluid
  - ○ Association with osteoarthritis
    - Osteophytes, joint space narrowing, subchondral sclerosis, chondral erosions
- T2WI
  - ○ Intermediate sensitivity compared to GRE
  - ○ Difficult to visualize articular cartilage or meniscal crystal deposition even when using FS PD FSE or STIR
- PD/Intermediate
  - ○ Synovitis - relatively increased signal intensity thickened joint lining compared to hypointense fluid
    - Sensitive for synovitis
  - ○ Decreased signal intensity foci within hyaline articular cartilage
  - ○ Difficult to visualize on either PD or FS PD FSE
- T2* GRE
  - ○ Chondrocalcinosis within hyaline articular cartilage as decreased signal intensity foci (GRE most sensitive technique)
  - ○ Menisci may demonstrate punctate irregularities within degeneration foci
  - ○ 3-dimensional fat saturated gradient echo technique superior to radiography for the detection of crystals in articular cartilage
- Calcium deposition (decreased signal intensity) in soft tissues is characteristic on all sequences

- ○ Inflamed synovium will enhance

Imaging Recommendations
- Best imaging tool: Radiography, MRI
- Protocol advice
  - ○ Include GRE if index of suspicion is high, otherwise calcium deposition is poorly visualized on other sequences
    - Findings are often subtle (hypointense deposits within hypointense menisci on T1 and T2WI)

DIFFERENTIAL DIAGNOSIS

Gout
- Monosodium urate monohydrate crystals
- Needle shaped negatively birefringent crystals
  - ○ Pseudogout in comparison = rhomboid shaped crystals with weak positive birefringence as seen with calcium pyrophosphate dihydrate crystals
- Hyaline cartilage calcification not characteristic

Tumoral Calcinosis
- Mimics tophaceous pseudogout

Osteoarthritis without CPPD
- Absence of CPPD crystals on T2* GRE confirms diagnosis
- Typical changes of subchondral reaction
  - ○ +/- Cysts, edema, sclerosis, osteophytes

Chondromalacia (Chondro)
- Desiccation of hyaline cartilage may be associated with decreased signal intensity (FS PD FSE)
  - ○ Usually early stage before defined defect
- +/- Associated subchondral bone reactive changes
  - ○ Subchondral cysts
  - ○ Edema
  - ○ Sclerosis
- Posttraumatic
- Early OA

Osteochondral Injuries
- Chondromalacia + underlying bone edema +/- fracture

CHONDROCALCINOSIS, KNEE

- Posttraumatic
- Osteochondritis dissecans (OCD) +/- history of trauma
- Well defined chondral defect rather than foci of chondrocalcinosis

PATHOLOGY

General Features
- General path comments
  - CPPD crystal
  - Pyrophosphate arthropathy resembles osteoarthritis ± intermittent attacks of pseudogout
  - Crystals are identified in synovial fluid
- Genetics
  - Autosomal dominant mode of inheritance in familial form of CPPD
    - Chromosome 8q
- Etiology
  - Deposition of calcium pyrophosphate crystals into soft tissue
  - Chondrocyte and surrounding matrix
    - Noxious event incites cascade - hypertrophy and degeneration of chondrocytes
    - Separation of calcium-binding effect of the matrix
    - Crystals grow adjacent to hypertrophic chondrocytes within affected matrix
    - Collagen cells - probable source of inorganic pyrophosphate
- Epidemiology
  - 4 to ≥ 25% of the population by age 80 years
    - Half as common as gout in typical practice
- Associated abnormalities: Hyperparathyroidism, hemochromatosis, hemosiderosis, hypomagnesemia, hypophosphatemia

Gross Pathologic & Surgical Features
- White crystal precipitation in various joints
- +/- OA

Microscopic Features
- Crystal deposition with adjacent chondroid metaplasia
- +/- Synovial hyperplasia with inflammatory changes
  - Mononuclear cells
- Tophaceous pseudogout +/- giant cells
- CPPD crystals identified from joint fluid by polarized light microscopy

Staging, Grading or Classification Criteria
- Clinical syndromes of calcium pyrophosphate dihydrate crystal deposition disease
  - Chondrocalcinosis (asymptomatic)
  - Pseudogout (acute crystal synovitis)
  - Pyrophosphate arthropathy
    - Osteoarthritis-like
    - Neuropathic-like

CLINICAL ISSUES

Presentation
- Most common signs/symptoms
  - Pseudogout - begins in galloping fashion, peak within hours, + pain, swelling, heat, and redness
    - 50% of patients have fever

- Clinical profile
  - Associated with OA in older patient
  - After injury or surgery to affected area
  - Pseudogout identified following parathyroid adenoma excision

Demographics
- Age: Elderly, increases with age
- Gender: M:F = 1.4:1

Natural History & Prognosis
- Spontaneous resolution over several days to weeks
- Treatment accelerates recovery

Treatment
- Conservative: Depends on degree of involvement
  - Treat as OA in most common presentation
  - Modified activity, physical therapy, NSAIDs
- Surgical treatment: Recalcitrant cases
  - Arthrocentesis + intraarticular steroid = prompt relief
  - Arthroscopic debridement: +/- Helpful
  - Patients with OA form
    - Surgical debridement
    - Microfracture chondroplasty
    - Radiofrequency chondroplasty
    - Osteochondral transfers
    - Osteotomy
    - Partial or total joint replacement

DIAGNOSTIC CHECKLIST

Consider
- In setting of acute arthritis (esp. with findings of OA and radiographic findings of calcium deposition)

Image Interpretation Pearls
- Evaluate hyaline articular cartilage on MR images
- T2* GRE is the most sensitive sequence for the detection of CPPD crystal deposition

SELECTED REFERENCES

1. Al-Arfaj AS: The relationship between chondrocalcinosis and osteoarthritis in Saudi Arabia. Clin Rheumatol 21(6):493-6, 2002
2. Canhao H et al: Cross-sectional study of 50 patients with calcium pyrophosphate dihydrate crystal arthropathy. Clin Rheumatol 20(2):119-22, 2001
3. Sagarin MJ: Pseudogout. J Emerg Med 18(3):373-4, 2000
4. Oni OO: Crystal deposition in normal and diseased articular cartilage. An extended report. Afr J Med Med Sci 28(3-4):181, 1999
5. Concoff AL et al: What is the relation between crystals and osteoarthritis? Curr Opin Rheumatol 11(5):436-40, 1999
6. Gunther KP et al: Reliability of radiographic assessment in hip and knee osteoarthritis. Osteoarthritis Cartilage 7(2):239-46, 1999
7. Beltran J et al: Chondrocalcinosis of the hyaline cartilage of the knee: MRI manifestations. Skeletal Radiol 27(7):369-74, 1998
8. Baldwin CT et al: Linkage of early-onset osteoarthritis and chondrocalcinosis to human chromosome 8q. Am J Hum Genet 56(3):692-7, 1995

CHONDROCALCINOSIS, KNEE

IMAGE GALLERY

Typical

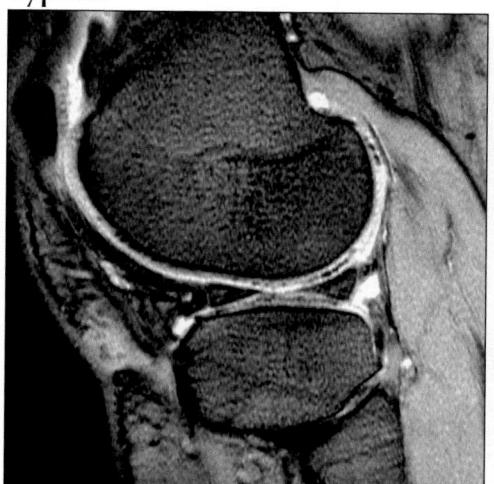 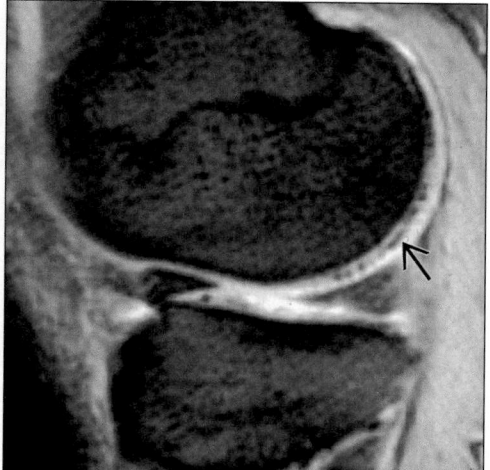

(Left) Sagittal T2* GRE MR shows chondrocalcinosis within the hyaline cartilage of the lateral compartment in a patient with CPPD. *(Right)* Sagittal T2* GRE MR shows the hypointense punctate foci of chondrocalcinosis (arrow) in a patient with CPPD. Gradient echo images often show these calcifications secondary to increased magnetic susceptibility.

Typical

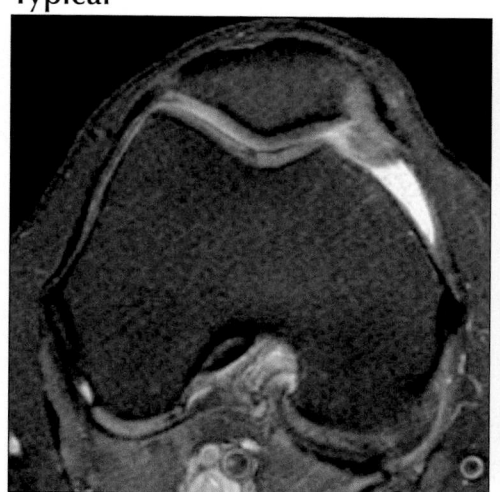 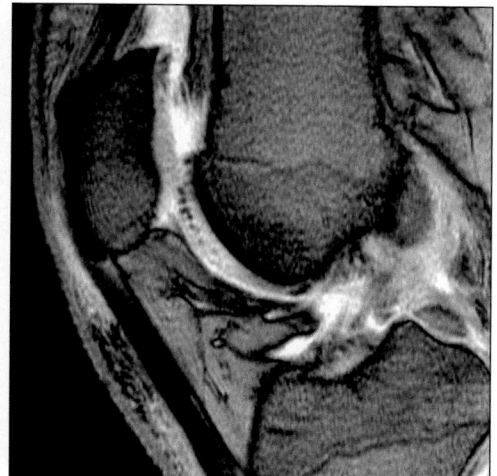

(Left) Axial FS PD FSE MR shows subtle chondrocalcinosis within the trochlear hyaline cartilage. *(Right)* Sagittal T2* GRE (more sensitive technique) MR shows chondrocalcinosis within the patellofemoral hyaline articular cartilage.

Typical

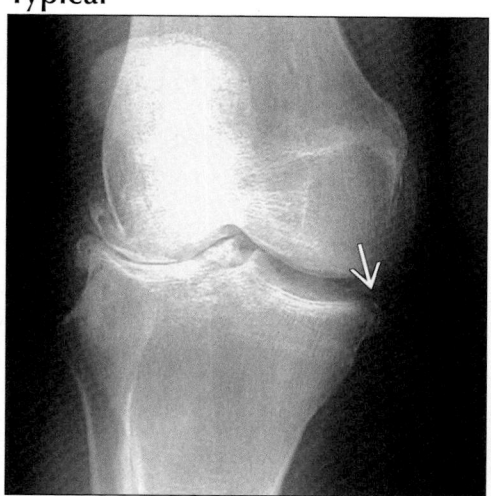 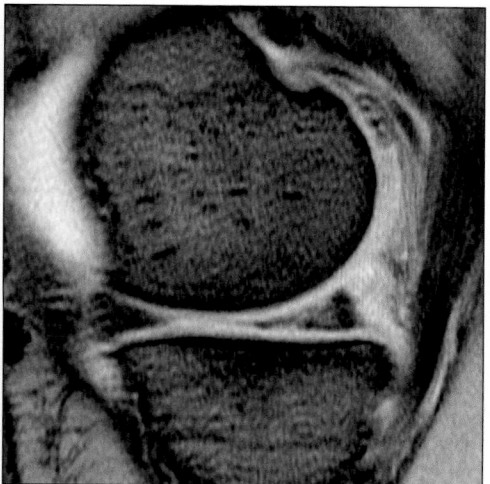

(Left) Anteroposterior radiography shows calcification (arrow) within the medial meniscus. *(Right)* Sagittal T2* GRE MR shows chondrocalcinosis within the meniscus as irregular hypointense heterogeneous signal in addition to meniscal degenerative tearing.

INTERCONDYLAR NOTCH CYST

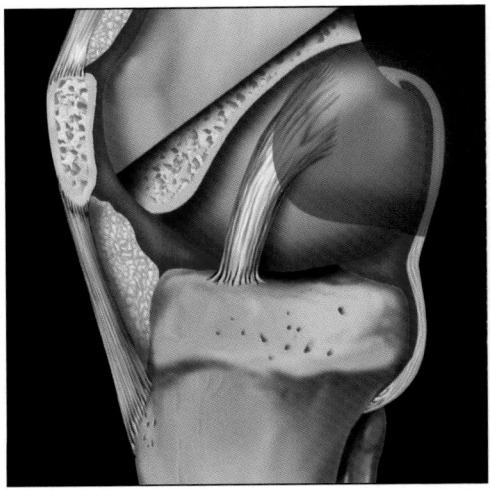 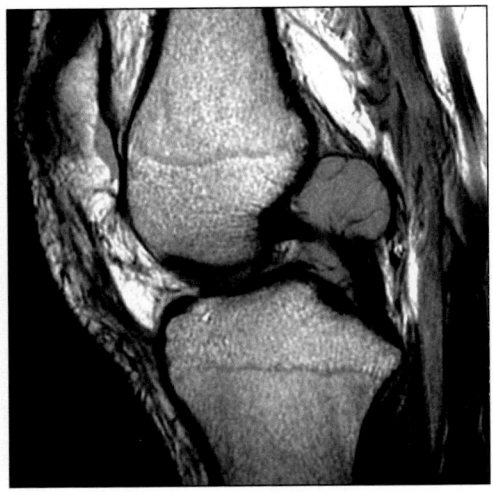

Sagittal graphic shows an intercondylar notch cyst associated with proximal fibers of the ACL.

Sagittal PD FSE MR shows the classical appearance of an intercondylar notch cyst posterior to the proximal PCL.

TERMINOLOGY

Abbreviations and Synonyms
- Cruciate cyst

Definitions
- Cyst within or extending from the intercondylar notch
- Cyst containing thick, sticky, clear, colorless, jellylike material (cruciate ganglion)
- Mucoid degeneration of a cruciate ligament
  - Contains mucinous material from degeneration of a cruciate ligament
    - Fatty material occasionally expressed at arthroscopy
  - Often associated with adjacent edema, +/- degenerative cysts at origin (femur) or insertion (tibia) of ligament

IMAGING FINDINGS

General Features
- Best diagnostic clue
  - Increased signal intensity (T2WI) mass expanding and/or extending from a cruciate ligament
    - Hyperintense on T2WI (FS PD FSE), T2* GRE, and STIR

- Location
  - Intercondylar notch of knee
  - +/- Within cruciate ligament
  - More common in anterior cruciate ligament
- Size: Mild expansion of cruciate ligament to cyst, several centimeters in size
- Morphology
  - Simple cyst
    - Oval expansion of ligament to round or multiloculated cyst
  - Mucoid degeneration
    - "Celery stalk" appearance
    - Fusiform enlargement with preservation of some fibers

Radiographic Findings
- Radiography: Enlarged notch with large cyst (rare)

CT Findings
- NECT
  - Homogeneous decreased attenuation (0-20 HU) mass
    - Degenerative cruciate or small cyst may not be visualized as separate structures
- CECT: +/- Rim enhancement if inflamed

MR Findings
- T1WI

DDx: Intercondylar Notch Cyst

Meniscal Cyst	Meniscal Cyst	Meniscal Cyst	Popliteal Cyst	Popliteal Cyst

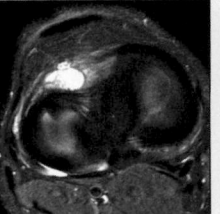 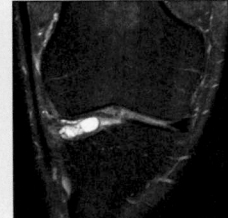 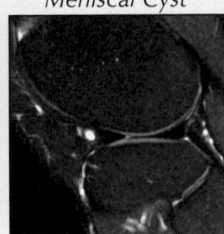 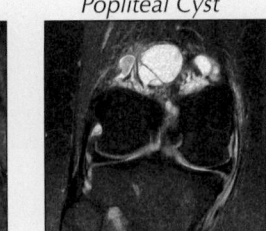 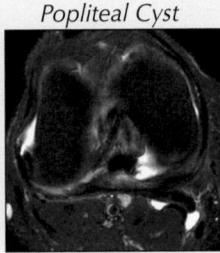

Ax FS PD FSE MR	*Cor FS PD FSE*	*Sag FS PD FSE*	*Cor FS PD FSE*	*Ax FS PD FSE MR*

INTERCONDYLAR NOTCH CYST

Key Facts

Terminology
- Cyst within or extending from the intercondylar notch
- Cyst containing thick, sticky, clear, colorless, jellylike material (cruciate ganglion)

Imaging Findings
- Increased signal intensity (T2WI) mass expanding and/or extending from a cruciate ligament
- Size: Mild expansion of cruciate ligament to cyst, several centimeters in size
- Protocol advice: FS PD FSE

Top Differential Diagnoses
- Meniscal Cyst
- Popliteal Cyst

Pathology
- Asymptomatic or variable presentation of pain
- Related to trauma followed by tissue breakdown of cruciate ligament or adjacent tissue
- Epidemiology: 1% of MR knee studies

Clinical Issues
- Usually asymptomatic but may present as dull non-focal pain
- Pain if associated with erosions

Diagnostic Checklist
- Visible cyst extending from cruciate ligament on MRI
- Pitfall - mistaking an ACL cyst for an intraarticular tumor

---

- Homogeneous decreased signal intensity mass within or extending from intercondylar notch
- Mucoid degeneration: Fusiform enlargement of intermediate to hypointense cruciate ligament
- Subchondral sclerosis/cysts in adjacent lateral femur or in tibia - hypointense
  - Sclerosis/cysts seen as reactive phenomenon especially with mucoid degeneration
- T2WI
  - Homogeneous increased signal intensity mass within or extending from the intercondylar notch - simple cyst
  - FS PD FSE shows hyperintense fluid due to saturation of surrounding fat increasing cyst contrast
  - Mucoid degeneration appears as fusiform enlargement of intermediate to hyperintense cruciate
    - "Celery stalk" appearance
  - Subchondral cysts in adjacent lateral femur or in tibia - hyperintense
  - Surrounding reactive edema - hyperintense
- STIR
  - Increased signal intensity cyst within or extending from intercondylar notch
  - Mucoid degeneration fusiform enlargement of intermediate to hyperintense cruciate
  - Hyperintense subchondral cysts in adjacent lateral femur or tibia
  - Surrounding reactive edema - hyperintense
  - Superior contrast with decreased spatial resolution
- T1 C+
  - +/- Rim enhancement if inflamed
  - Enhancing synovitis

Ultrasonographic Findings
- Visualize cystic mass from posterior approach
- Through transmission (simple cysts)
- Mucoid degeneration may not be seen

Imaging Recommendations
- Best imaging tool: MRI
- Protocol advice: FS PD FSE

DIFFERENTIAL DIAGNOSIS

Meniscal Cyst
- May extend into notch
- Associated with meniscal tear
- Posterior horn medial meniscus
- Anterior horn lateral meniscus

Cyst within Tibial Tunnel after ACL Surgery
- ± Extension into notch
- Mass effect causing knee extension difficulty or limitation

Partial Tear of Cruciate
- Associated with intracruciate hemorrhage
- Expansion of cruciate may occur with attempted healing

Joint Fluid
- Loculated in or near notch
- Associated with synovitis
- Hemorrhage
  - Inhomogeneous on T2WI

Popliteal Cyst
- In association with joint fluid
- Seen with joint synovitis
- ± Hemorrhagic
- Often reflects intraarticular pathology
- Typical (medial) or atypical (lateral) location

PATHOLOGY

General Features
- General path comments
  - One large cyst or several smaller cysts
    - Common stalk connects multiple small cysts
    - Multiloculation common
  - Asymptomatic or variable presentation of pain
  - Mucoid degeneration +/- history of trauma
    - Chronic partial tear or in asymptomatic patient with no instability
    - Cyst may develop without history of trauma

INTERCONDYLAR NOTCH CYST

- Etiology
  - Related to trauma followed by tissue breakdown of cruciate ligament or adjacent tissue
  - Defect or weakness of synovial lining of cruciate ligament
- Epidemiology: 1% of MR knee studies
- Associated abnormalities
  - If cyst is large, results in pressure erosion of adjacent bone
  - +/- Reactive edema
  - +/- Sclerosis
  - +/- Subchondral cysts

Gross Pathologic & Surgical Features

- Cyst contains thick, sticky, clear, colorless, jellylike material seen as bulge or synovial covered mass

Microscopic Features

- Inflammatory cells contained in cyst
- Mucoid degeneration contains fatty material

CLINICAL ISSUES

Presentation

- Most common signs/symptoms
  - Usually asymptomatic but may present as dull non-focal pain
    - Pain if associated with erosions
    - Chronic in case of trauma with associated pathology/instability
- Clinical profile: Usually incidental finding

Demographics

- Age: Adults
- Gender: M >/= F

Natural History & Prognosis

- May regress, remain unchanged, or enlarge causing mass effect

Treatment

- Conservative
  - Anti-inflammatory drugs for dull general pain
- Surgical
  - Arthroscopic aspiration/resection if
    - Large and seen at arthroscopy
    - Associated with erosions
    - Symptomatic at physical exam

DIAGNOSTIC CHECKLIST

Consider

- Meniscal tear with associated cyst or partial tear of cruciate with associated hemorrhage

Image Interpretation Pearls

- Visible cyst extending from cruciate ligament on MRI
- Pitfall - mistaking an ACL cyst for an intraarticular tumor

SELECTED REFERENCES

1. Sanders TG et al: Fluid collections in the osseous tunnel during the first year after anterior cruciate ligament repair using an autologous hamstring graft: natural history and clinical correlation. J Comput Assist Tomogr 26(4):617-21. 2002
2. Fealy S et al: Mucoid degeneration of the anterior cruciate ligament. Arthroscopy 17(9):E37, 2001
3. Kim MG et al: Intra-articular ganglion cysts of the knee: Clinical and MR imaging features. Eur Radiol 11(5):834-40, 2001
4. McIntyre JS et al: Mucoid degeneration of the anterior cruciate ligament mistaken for ligamentous tears. Skeletal Radiol 30(6):312-5, 2001
5. Sung MS et al: Myxoid liposarcoma: Appearance at MR imaging with histologic correlation. Radiographics 20(4):1007-19, 2000
6. Bui-Mansfield LT et al: Intraarticular ganglia of the knee: prevalence, presentation, etiology, and management. AJR 168(1):123-7, 1997
7. Lepore L et al: Bilateral baker's cyst in a patient with psoriatic arthritis of pediatric onset. Clin Exp Rheumatol 14(1):109-10, 1996
8. Takano Y et al: Is Baker's cyst a risk factor for pulmonary embolism? Intern Med 35(11):886-9, 1996
9. Szer IS et al: Ultrasonography in the study of prevalence and clinical evolution of popliteal cysts in children with knee effusions. J Rheumatol 19(3):458-62, 1992
10. Toolanen G et al: Sonography of popliteal masses. Acta Orthop Scand 59(3):294-6, 1988
11. Kattapuram SV et al: Case report 181: Calcified popliteal cyst (Baker cyst). Skeletal Radiol 7(4):279-81, 1982
12. Goldberg RP et al: Calcified bodies in popliteal cysts: A characteristic radiographic appearance. AJR 131(5):857-9, 1978
13. Houston CS: Pitfalls to avoid. When is fabella not a fabella not a fabella? J Can Assoc Radiol 29(3):193, 1978

INTERCONDYLAR NOTCH CYST

IMAGE GALLERY

Typical

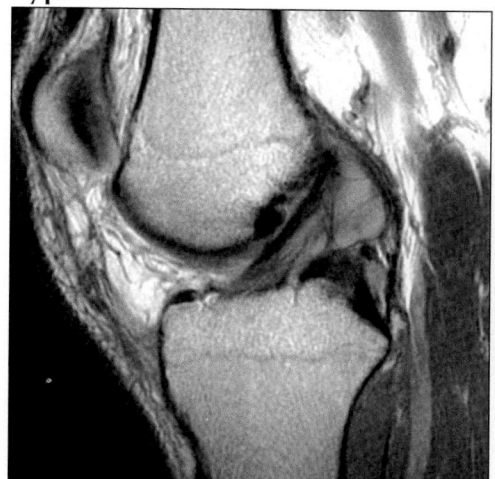
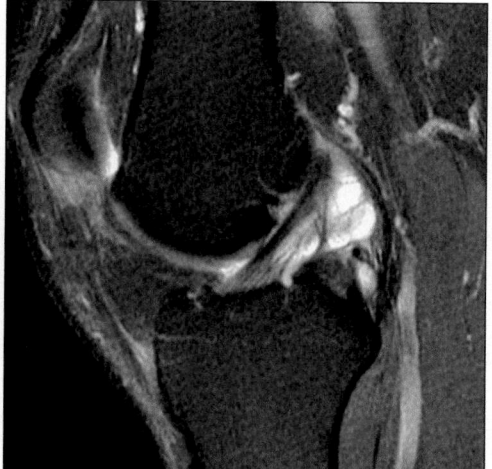

(Left) Sagittal PD FSE MR shows an intercondylar notch cyst communicating with the proximal ACL. *(Right)* Sagittal FS PD FSE MR shows the hyperintense cyst with septations.

Typical

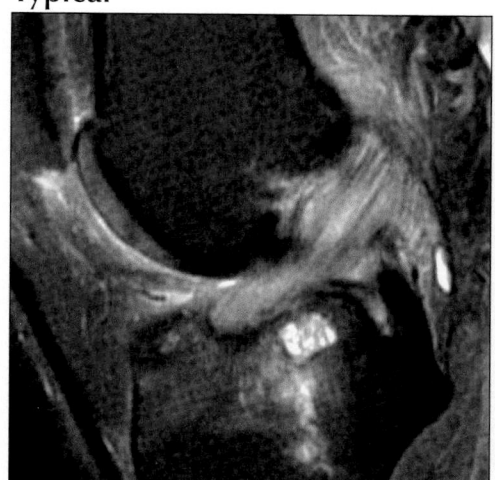
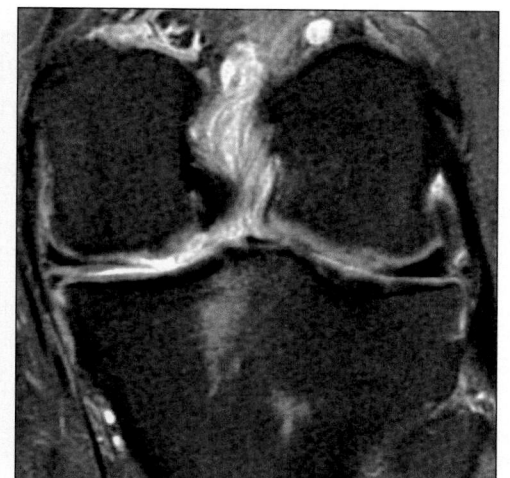

(Left) Sagittal FS PD FSE MR shows expansion of the ACL and a "celery stalk" appearance secondary to mucoid degeneration. There is reactive cystic intraosseous change in the tibia - a common association. *(Right)* Coronal FS PD FSE MR shows the "celery stalk" appearance of mucoid degeneration of the ACL.

Typical

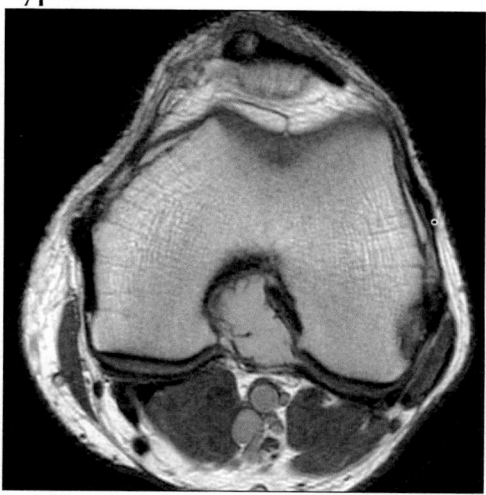
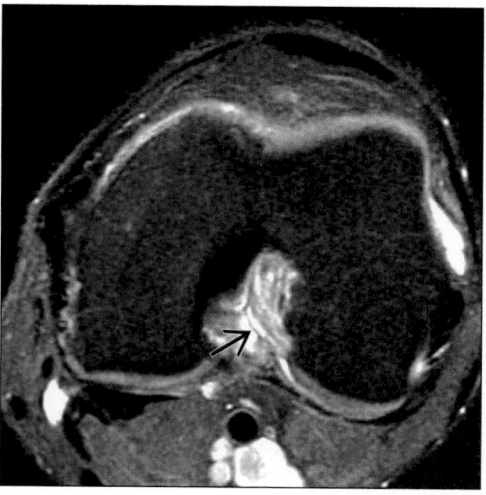

(Left) Axial PD FSE MR shows an intercondylar notch cyst. There is also proximal patellar tendinosis. *(Right)* Axial FS PD FSE MR shows the expanded appearance of mucoid degeneration of the ACL (arrow).

POPLITEAL CYST

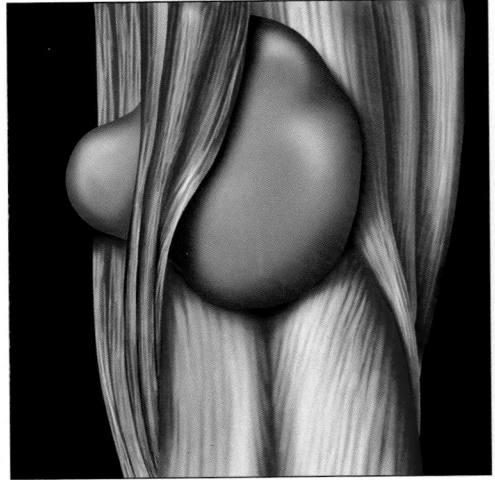

Coronal graphic shows a large popliteal cyst originating from gastrocnemius semimembranosus bursa.

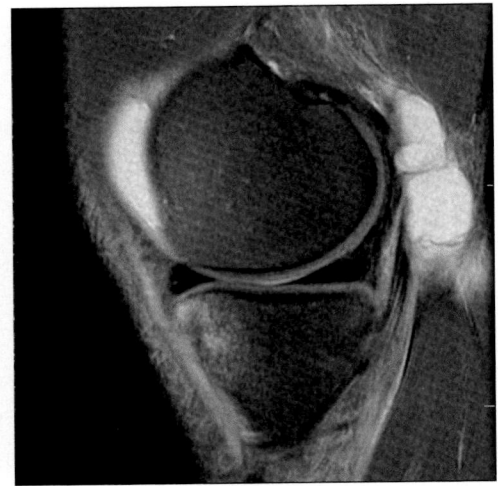

Sagittal FS PD FSE MR shows a medial popliteal cyst in a patient post trauma.

TERMINOLOGY

Abbreviations and Synonyms
- Pop cyst = popliteal cyst, Baker's cyst, gastrocnemius/semimembranosus bursa

Definitions
- Fluid distension of gastrocnemius/semimembranosus bursa which is usually in communication with the knee joint

IMAGING FINDINGS

General Features
- Best diagnostic clue: Fluid signal intensity mass in typical location (gastrocnemius/semimembranosus bursa)
- Location: Posterior to the medial femoral condyle between tendons of medial head gastrocnemius and semimembranosus
- Size
  ○ Range from 1-30+ cm³ (median 3cm³)
  ○ When large may dissect into calf
- Morphology: Flattened sac to oval shaped cystic mass depending on the amount of fluid

Radiographic Findings
- Radiography
  ○ Soft tissue swelling in posteromedial knee
    ▪ +/- Displacement of popliteal artery
    ▪ +/- Calcified debris

MR Findings
- T1WI
  ○ Decreased signal intensity mass
  ○ +/- Adjacent hypointense edema
  ○ Variable size
  ○ Gastrocnemius/semimembranosus bursa distension
  ○ Extends in multiple different directions (multiple appearances)
  ○ Subacute hemorrhage in cyst seen with areas of hyperintensity
- T2WI
  ○ Increased signal intensity mass: Gastrocnemius/semimembranosus bursa
    ▪ +/- Debris
    ▪ +/- Hemorrhage (fluid level/hypointensity foci - hemosiderin)
    ▪ Calcification/loose bodies (hypointense)
    ▪ Thick synovial rind
  ○ +/- Hyperintense surrounding edema
    ▪ = Leakage/rupture
- PD/Intermediate: Intermediate signal intensity mass within gastrocnemius/semimembranosus bursa
- STIR: Increased signal intensity fluid within gastrocnemius/semimembranosus bursa
- T2* GRE

DDx: Popliteal Cyst

Pop A Aneurysm	Pop A Aneurysm	Synovial Cyst	Synovial Cyst	DVT
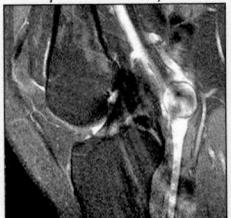	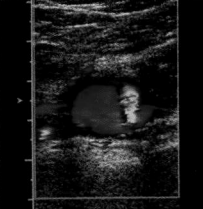	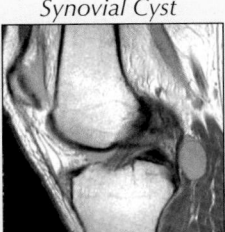	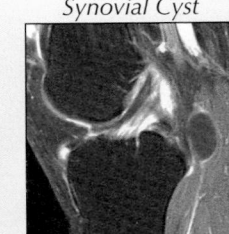	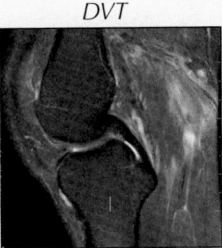
Sag FS PD FSE	Sag Doppler US	Sag PD FSE MR	Sag T1 C+ MR	Sag FS PD FSE

POPLITEAL CYST

Key Facts

Terminology
- Fluid distension of gastrocnemius/semimembranosus bursa which is usually in communication with the knee joint

Imaging Findings
- Best diagnostic clue: Fluid signal intensity mass in typical location (gastrocnemius/semimembranosus bursa)
- Morphology: Flattened sac to oval shaped cystic mass depending on the amount of fluid
- Typical findings of fluid-filled mass on ultrasound
- Best imaging tool: MRI

Top Differential Diagnoses
- Meniscal Cyst
- Cystic Adventitial Degeneration of a Popliteal Artery

- Popliteal Artery Aneurysm

Pathology
- Baker's cyst usually communicates with the joint at posteromedial knee
- Fluid from joint effusion extending into cyst

Clinical Issues
- Popliteal mass, swelling, dull ache, knee effusion
- Cyst may regress or enlarge

Diagnostic Checklist
- Evaluate underlying disorder as a popliteal cyst is common and is frequently associated with intraarticular pathology
- Follow the course of the popliteal cyst proximally for confirmation of orgin and joint communication

---

- ○ Increased signal intensity mass in typical location: Gastrocnemius/semimembranosus bursa
  - ▪ Sensitive to hypointense foci of hemosiderin
- T1 C+
  - ○ Rim enhancement
    - ▪ Inflamed synovial lining
  - ○ Recommended to evaluate atypical cyst locations, morphology or matrix

Ultrasonographic Findings
- Typical findings of fluid-filled mass on ultrasound
- Pure cystic structure or complex cyst
- Anechoic mass with posterior acoustic enhancement
  - ○ +/- Identifiable communication with knee joint

Imaging Recommendations
- Best imaging tool: MRI
- Protocol advice: FS PD FSE shows cystic mass intermediate to hyperintense located medial to medial head of the gastrocnemius muscle

DIFFERENTIAL DIAGNOSIS

Meniscal Cyst
- Associated with meniscal tear
- Increased signal extending to articular surface on short TE sequences
- Posterior horn of medial meniscus (PHMM)

Cystic Adventitial Degeneration of a Popliteal Artery
- Cystic degeneration of arterial adventitia
- Color Doppler helpful in differentiating popliteal cyst
- Rare

Popliteal Artery Aneurysm
- Color Doppler imaging can confirm the absence of vascular flow within the mass
- Continuous with artery
- Pulsatile
- +/- History of sharp trauma

Ganglion/Synovial Cyst
- Atypical location compared to popliteal cyst
- Variable location around knee joint
  - ○ Tibiofibular joint
  - ○ Bursa between lateral head gastrocnemius muscle and biceps femoris
- May extend from popliteus tendon sheath/tibiofibular joint
- +/- Synovial lining

Deep Venous Thrombosis (DVT)
- Mimics rupture or leak of popliteal cyst
- Irritating nature of synovial fluid on the interstitial soft tissues
- Hyperintense on T2WI in soft tissues
- Venous collaterals developing in medial head of gastrocnemius

Semimembranosus Tibial Collateral Ligament Bursitis
- Bursal fluid distention
- Hyperintense on T2WI
- Inverted "U" shape
- +/- Semimembranosus tendinosis

PATHOLOGY

General Features
- General path comments
  - ○ Baker's cyst usually communicates with the joint at posteromedial knee
  - ○ Cyst represents pressure relief valve for joint effusions
  - ○ Often acts as ball valve with fibrin in the joint preventing fluid return
  - ○ Cyst has projections away from tendons that may preferentially become filled with fluid leading to slight change in location
    - ▪ Can be followed to bursa
- Etiology
  - ○ Fluid from joint effusion extending into cyst

POPLITEAL CYST

- Fluid may communicate freely or be restricted to the cyst via a ball valve mechanism
- Epidemiology
  - 5-58% of general population
  - Most common with effusion producing disorder such as rheumatoid arthritis (RA), osteoarthritis (OA) or trauma
- Associated abnormalities
  - Underlying knee disorders
    - Arthritis (inflammatory or degenerative), trauma, infection, other synovial processes

Gross Pathologic & Surgical Features
- Fluid-filled bursal sac in popliteal space
- Lining may be indurated
- Sac may contain debris
- Arise in bursa deep to medial head gastrocnemius
- Some cysts arise laterally
- Alternative site of orgin = herniation through posterior joint capsule

Microscopic Features
- Lined by synovium - extension of the knee joint
- Four histopathologic types of popliteal cyst
  - Fibrous
  - Synovial
  - Inflammatory
  - Transitional

Staging, Grading or Classification Criteria
- Primary/idiopathic cyst - valvular connection with joint
- Secondary/symptomatic cyst communicates freely with joint with normal synovial fluid
  - + Underlying articular disorder

CLINICAL ISSUES

Presentation
- Most common signs/symptoms
  - Popliteal mass, swelling, dull ache, knee effusion
  - Symptoms from underlying derangement such as meniscal tear, etc.
- Clinical profile: Adult patient with recurrent knee effusions

Demographics
- Age
  - 6.3% of children's knee MRI studies
  - Popliteal cysts in children may be isolated bursal sac formations without associated intraarticular pathology
  - Associated with intraarticular pathology in adult population
- Gender: More common in males

Natural History & Prognosis
- Cyst may regress or enlarge
- Good prognosis

Treatment
- Conservative
  - Treatment of underlying cause

- Nonsteroidal anti-inflammatory agents, ice, assisted weight bearing
- Surgical
  - Radioactive synoviorthosis - radionuclide agents instilled at arthrography
    - After documentation of cyst integrity
    - Leakage is contraindication
  - Cyst excision when other treatment fails

DIAGNOSTIC CHECKLIST

Consider
- Evaluate underlying disorder as a popliteal cyst is common and is frequently associated with intraarticular pathology

Image Interpretation Pearls
- Follow the course of the popliteal cyst proximally for confirmation of orgin and joint communication

SELECTED REFERENCES

1. Zandman-Goddard G et al: Coexisting chondrocalcinosis, osteoarthritis and popliteal cyst. Isr Med Assoc J 5(1):74-5, 2003
2. Torreggiani WC et al: The imaging spectrum of Baker's (Popliteal) cysts. Clin Radiol 57(8):681-91, 2002
3. Hsu WH et al: Dissecting popliteal cyst resulting from a fragmented, dislodged metal part of the patellar component after total knee arthroplasty. J Arthroplasty 17(6):792-7, 2001
4. Garcia-Porrua C et al: Atypical Baker's cyst as a presenting sign of osteomyelitis superimposed on avascular necrosis of the knee. Clin Exp Rheumatol 20(1):118, 2001
5. Rupp S et al: Long-term results after excision of a popliteal cyst. Unfallchirurg 104(9):847-51, 2001
6. Hill CL et al: Knee effusions, popliteal cysts, and synovial thickening: Association with knee pain in osteoarthritis. J Rheumatol 28(6):1330-7, 2001
7. Handy JR: Popliteal cysts in adults: A review. Semin Arthritis Rheum 31(2):108-18, 2001
8. De Maeseneer M et al: Popliteal cysts in children: Prevalence, appearance and associated findings at MR imaging. Pediatr Radiol 29(8):605-9, 1999
9. Dunlop D et al: Ruptured baker's cyst causing posterior compartment syndrome. Injury 28(8):561-2, 1997
10. Krome J et al: Acute compartment syndrome in ruptured Baker's cyst. J South Orthop Assoc 6(2):110-4, 1997
11. Langsfeld M et al: Baker's cysts mimicking the symptoms of deep vein thrombosis: Diagnosis with venous duplex scanning. J Vasc Surg 25(4):658-62, 1997
12. Baker WM: On the formation of synovial cysts in the leg in connection with disease of the knee joint. 1887. Clin Orthop (299):2-10, 1994
13. Fielding JR et al: Popliteal cysts: A reassessment using magnetic resonance imaging. Skeletal Radiol 20(6):433-5, 1991
14. Fergusson C et al: An unusual loose body in the knee. Clin Orthop (206):233-5, 1986
15. Fam AG et al: Ultrasound evaluation of popliteal cysts on osteoarthritis of the knee. J Rheumatol 9(3):428-34, 1982
16. Onetti CM et al: Synoviorthesis with 32P-colloidal chromic phosphate in rheumatoid arthritis--clinical, histopathologic and arthrographic changes. J Rheumatol 9(2):229-38, 1982

POPLITEAL CYST

IMAGE GALLERY

Typical

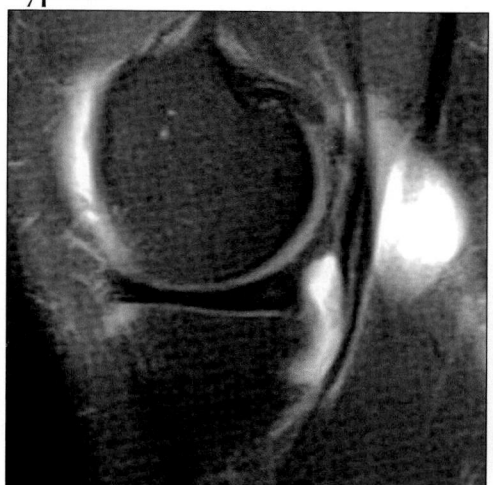
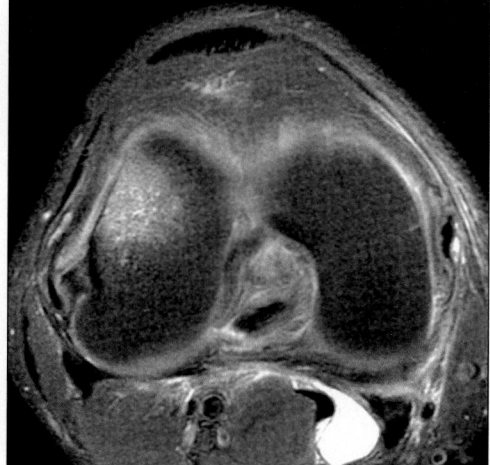

(Left) Sagittal FS PD FSE MR shows a popliteal cyst and tibial collateral ligament semimembranosus bursitis. *(Right)* Axial FS PD FSE MR shows a popliteal cyst - expansion of the gastrocnemius - semimembranosus bursa. There is a bone trabecular contusion of the lateral femoral condyle.

Typical

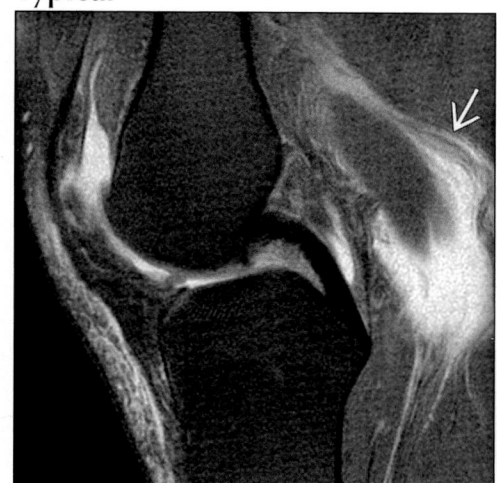
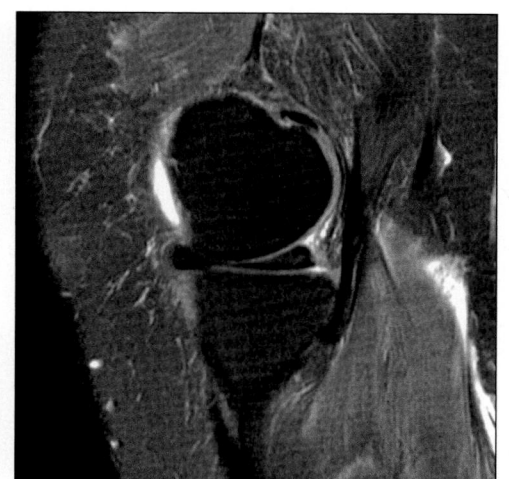

(Left) Sagittal FS PD FSE MR shows a leaking popliteal cyst with surrounding inflammation (arrow). *(Right)* Sagittal FS PD FSE MR shows recently ruptured popliteal cyst.

Typical

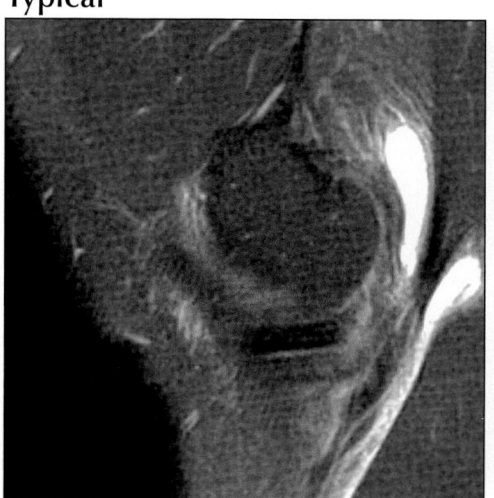
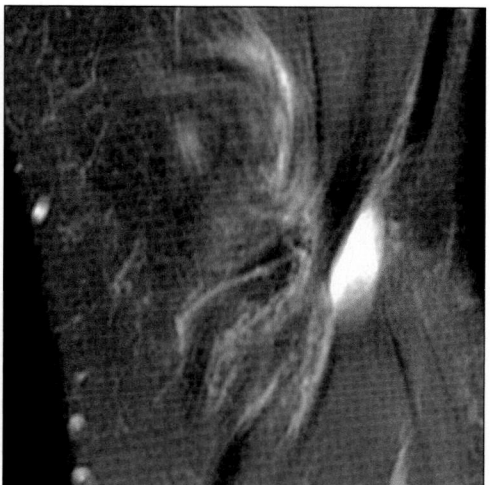

(Left) Sagittal FS PD FSE MR shows a popliteal cyst adjacent to the semimembranosus tendon. *(Right)* Sagittal FS PD FSE MR shows the medial soft tissue extension of a popliteal cyst.

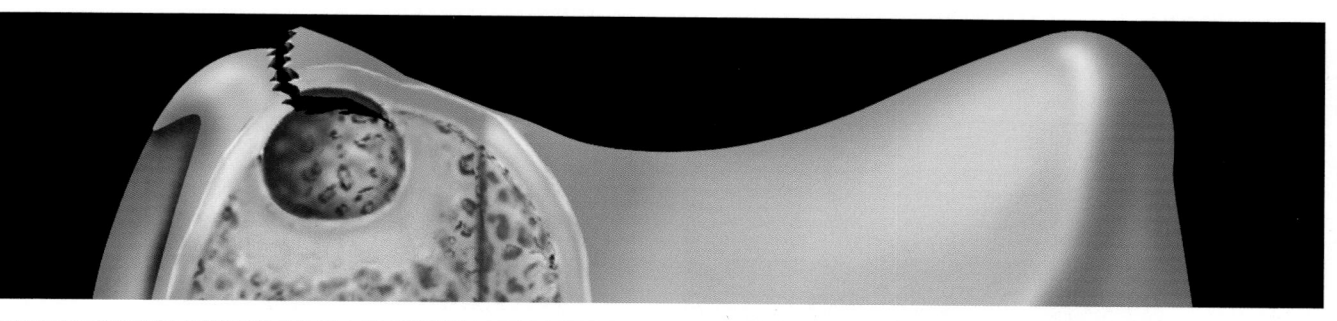

SECTION 6: Ankle and Foot

Tendons

Ligaments

Osseous Fractures

Overuse Syndromes and Soft Tissue Injury

ACHILLES TENDINITIS

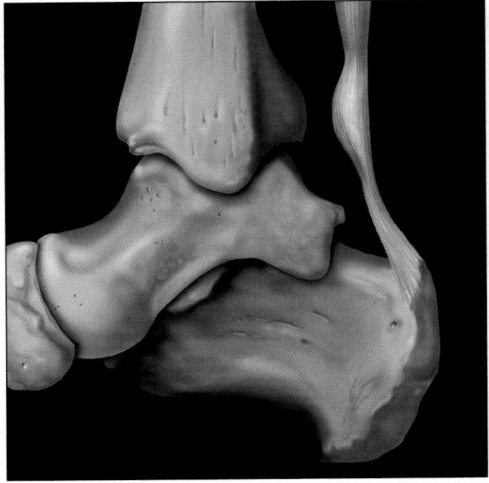

Sagittal graphic shows non-insertional Achilles tendinosis with anterior tendon convexity proximal to the os calcis. Mucoid degeneration shown in yellow.

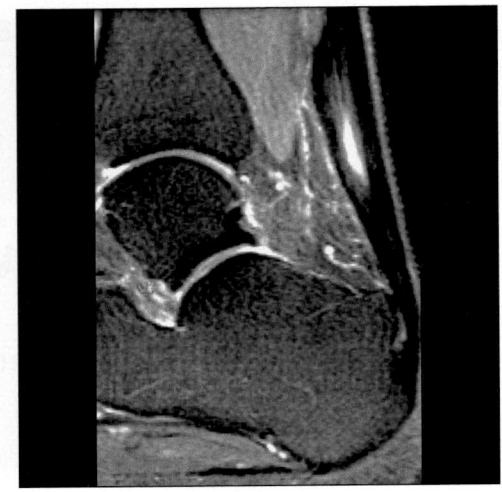

Sagittal FS PD FSE MR shows non-insertional Achilles tendinosis with hyperintense mucoid degeneration and anterior tendon convexity.

TERMINOLOGY

Abbreviations and Synonyms
- Tendo Achilles tendinitis; Achilles tendinopathy

Definitions
- Tendinosis or tendinopathy represents intrasubstance tendon degeneration
- Paratenon-connective tissue envelope surrounding tendon (also referred to as peritenon)
- Paratendinitis as generalized inflammation of tissues surrounding the Achilles tendon
- Paratendinitis with tendinosis as inflammation of surrounding tissues with tendon degeneration
- Paratenonitis as inflammation of connective tissue envelope
- Tendinitis as clinical symptoms develop in association with degenerative process of tendinosis

IMAGING FINDINGS

General Features
- Best diagnostic clue: Focal thickening or diffusely enlarged tendon
- Location
  - Non-insertional

- Hypovascular area 2-6 cm proximal to Achilles insertion
  - Insertional
    - Distal calcaneal tendon insertion
- Size: Variable in longitudinal extent + anteroposterior thickening within watershed region of decreased vascular perfusion
- Morphology
  - Anterior tendon convexity
  - Nodular thickening

Radiographic Findings
- Radiography
  - Enlarged Achilles tendon
  - Blurring between anterior tendon margin and pre-Achilles fat on lateral radiograph

MR Findings
- T1WI
  - Increased cross sectional diameter on axial images
  - Increased anteroposterior dimensions
  - Prominent anterior convexity with focal or diffuse thickening in sagittal plane
  - Thickening + intermediate signal of peritendinous tissue dorsal, medial, & lateral to Achilles tendon
  - Assess lesion size, extent of tendinopathy and severity of degeneration
  - Intermediate signal intensity effacement of peritendinous tissue anterior to Achilles tendon

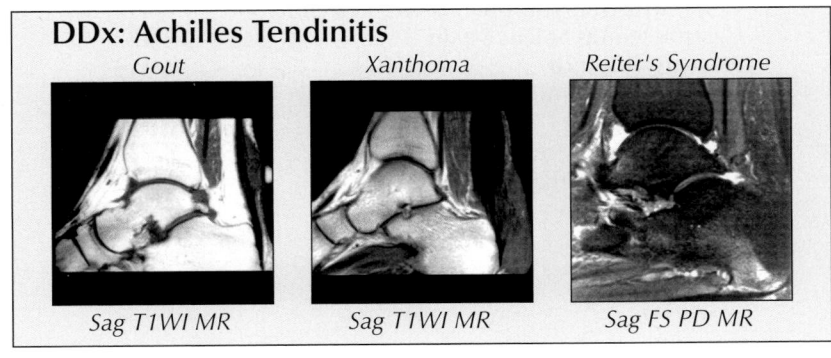

DDx: Achilles Tendinitis

Gout	Xanthoma	Reiter's Syndrome
Sag T1WI MR	Sag T1WI MR	Sag FS PD MR

6

2

ACHILLES TENDINITIS

Key Facts

Imaging Findings
- Best diagnostic clue: Focal thickening or diffusely enlarged tendon
- Non-insertional
- Insertional
- Anterior tendon convexity

Top Differential Diagnoses
- Gout
- Spondyloarthropathies
- Xanthoma
- Rheumatoid Arthritis

Pathology
- Hypovascular watershed zone 2-6 cm proximal to calcaneal insertion
- Eccentric loading of a fatigued muscle-tendon unit

- Hyperpronation

Clinical Issues
- Most common signs/symptoms: Pain with weight bearing
- Symptoms proximal to retrocalcaneal bursa
- Tenderness with deep palpation
- Tenderness at os calcis tendon insertion in Haglund's deformity
- Partial tears associated with regions of tendinosis

Diagnostic Checklist
- MR to identify coexistent partial tears of Achilles tendon on sagittal FS PD FSE images

---

- T2WI
  - Hypointense to intermediate signal within enlarged tendon
  - Hyperintense inflammatory fluid anterior to tendon
  - Tendinous mucoid degeneration may show increased signal on FS PD FSE or STIR images
  - Associated partial tears hyperintense on FS PD FSE or STIR images
  - Haglund's deformity - insertional tendinitis with reactive calcaneal marrow edema, and constellation of thickened tendon, retrocalcaneal/Tendo Achilles bursitis, and calcaneal bony prominence
  - Effacement + edema of pre-Achilles fat body may exist with normal tendon morphology/signal
- T1 C+: Soft tissue inflammatory fluid enhancement in paratendinitis

Ultrasonographic Findings
- Operator dependent
- Increased fibril thickness
- Disruption fibrillar bundles
- Fragmentation
- Decreased echogenicity associated with extent of disease
- Nodularity with small hypoechoic focal lesions

Imaging Recommendations
- Best imaging tool: MR for superior soft tissue contrast
- Protocol advice: Requires both T1 (or PDWI) and FS PD FSE sagittal & axial images

DIFFERENTIAL DIAGNOSIS

Gout
- Intermediate signal intensity urate tophi

Spondyloarthropathies
- Band of reactive marrow edema in calcaneus
- Inflammatory enthesopathy with insertional tendinitis

Xanthoma
- Infiltrating mass with large soft tissue component

Rheumatoid Arthritis
- Identify intermediate signal rheumatoid nodules ± synovitis, reactive osseous marrow edema

PATHOLOGY

General Features
- General path comments
  - Relevant anatomy
    - Achilles tendon has no synovial sheath
    - Retrocalcaneal bursae between Achilles insertion and calcaneus
    - Tendo Achilles bursa located posterior to Achilles tendon
- Etiology
  - Direct trauma to Achilles tendon
    - Hematoma
    - Inflammation
    - Fibrosis with restricted tendon sliding
  - Hypovascular watershed zone 2-6 cm proximal to calcaneal insertion
  - Eccentric loading of a fatigued muscle-tendon unit
    - Overtraining
    - Runners susceptible in both acceleration (sprinting) and deceleration (eccentric contraction)
  - Hyperpronation
    - Leg and foot generate opposing forces of rotation
    - Subtalar joint pronates
    - Calcaneus everts
    - Knee extends
  - Forefoot varus
  - Cavus foot
  - Equinus deformity
    - Triceps surae contracture
  - Insertional changes
    - Calcaneus bony prominence
  - Hypertrophic spur or enthesophyte
  - Systemic arthropathy
    - HLA-B27 antigen
    - Rheumatoid arthritis

ACHILLES TENDINITIS

- Epidemiology
  - 11% incidence in runners
  - 9% in dancers

Gross Pathologic & Surgical Features
- Inadequate healing
- Adhesions
- Fibrotic changes of peritenon
- Loss of normal tendon luster
- Nodular thickening
- Calcification
- Inflamed peritenon

Microscopic Features
- Chronic paratendinitis
  - Hypertrophic connective tissue
  - Increased capillary infiltration
  - Regional blood vessel degeneration
  - Fibrinogen deposition and fibrinoid necrosis
  - Round cell infiltrate
  - Increase in glycosaminoglycans (chondroitin sulfate) and mucoid degeneration
  - Leakage plasma proteins secondary to disruption of local blood flow
  - Absence of tendon inflammatory response (separate from inflammatory disease of peritendinous tissues and peritenon)

CLINICAL ISSUES

Presentation
- Most common signs/symptoms: Pain with weight bearing
- Clinical profile
  - Non-insertional
    - Acute pain with altered biomechanics
    - Symptoms proximal to retrocalcaneal bursa
    - Tenderness with deep palpation
    - Palpable tendon nodularity
    - Occurs in higher level athlete
  - Insertional tendinitis
    - Tenderness at os calcis tendon insertion in Haglund's deformity
    - Older, less athletic or sedentary population

Demographics
- Age
  - Adult ages 30-40 most at risk
  - Also young athletes, sedentary individuals and older population
- Gender: Pronounced lesions associated with male gender
- Activity
  - 6.5-18% incidence of non-insertional Achilles tendinitis in runners

Natural History & Prognosis
- Chronic tendinopathy
  - Perfusion insufficiency with vascular proliferation
  - Abnormal tendon fiber morphology
  - Hypercellularity
  - 90% symptomatic
  - Partial tears associated with regions of tendinosis

- Tendinosis may be precursor lesion to final stage of partial or complete tendon tear

Treatment
- Conservative - to decrease symptoms of tendinopathy
  - Therapeutic rest
  - Stretching exercises
  - Cross training or alternative exercise
  - Antiinflammatory medications
  - Immobilization
  - Orthoses to correct hyperpronation
  - Brisement to lift adherent paratenon
- Surgical
  - Release ± excision paratenon in paratenonitis (improved success relative to cases of intrinsic tendon degeneration)
  - Excision of calcaneal prominence in insertional tendinopathy
  - Partial tears repaired
  - Mucoid degeneration treated with debridement

DIAGNOSTIC CHECKLIST

Consider
- Evaluate paratenon connective tissue envelope and paratendinous tissue for inflammatory change separate from tendon degeneration
- MR to identify coexistent partial tears of Achilles tendon on sagittal FS PD FSE images

SELECTED REFERENCES

1. Paavola M et al: Achilles tendinopathy. J Bone Joint Surg Am 84-A(11):2062-76, 2002
2. Shalabi A et al: Dynamic contrast-enhanced MR imaging and histopathology in chronic Achilles tendinosis. A longitudinal MR study of 15 patients. Acta Radiol 43(2):198-206, 2002
3. Banks A et al: McGlamry's comprehensive textbook of foot and ankle surgery. vol 1. Philadelphia PA, Lippincott Williams & Wilkins, (35):1091- 152, 2001
4. Myerson M: Foot and ankle disorders. vol 2. Philadelphia PA, Lippincott Raven, (55):1367-98, 2000
5. Stoller D: Magnetic resonance Imaging in orthopaedics & sports medicine. 2nd ed. Philadelphia PA, Lippincott Williams & Wilkins, (8):443-595, 1997
6. Resnick D et al: Internal derangement of joints: Emphasis on MR imaging. Philadelphia PA, Saunders WB, (17):787-925, 1997
7. Astrom M et al: Chronic Achilles tendinopathy. A survey of surgical & histopathologic findings. Clin Orthop 316:151-64, 1995
8. Clement DR et al: Achilles tendonitis and peritendonitis: Etiology and treatment. AMJ Sports Med 12(3):197-84, 1984
9. Neuhold A et al: Degenerative Achilles tendon disease: Assessment by magnetic resonance and ultrasonography. Eur J Radiol 4(4):145-50, 1976

IMAGE GALLERY

Typical

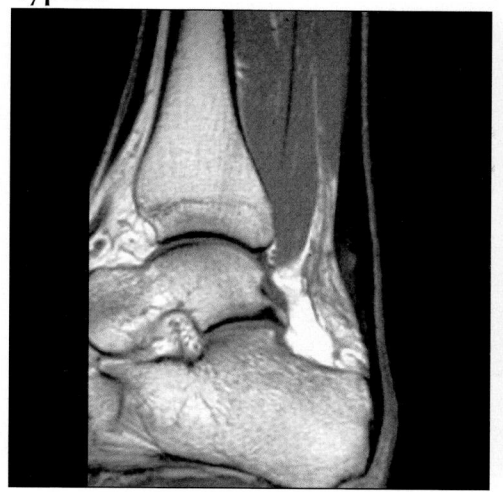
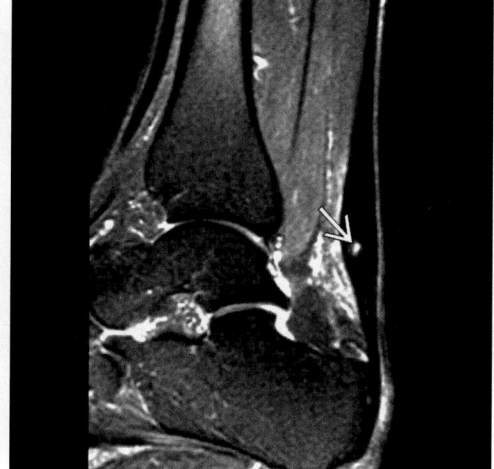

(Left) Sagittal T1WI MR shows non insertional Achilles tendinosis with focal degeneration and paratendinitis. *(Right)* Sagittal FS PD FSE MR shows hyperintense mucoid degeneration (arrow) and paratendinitis.

Typical

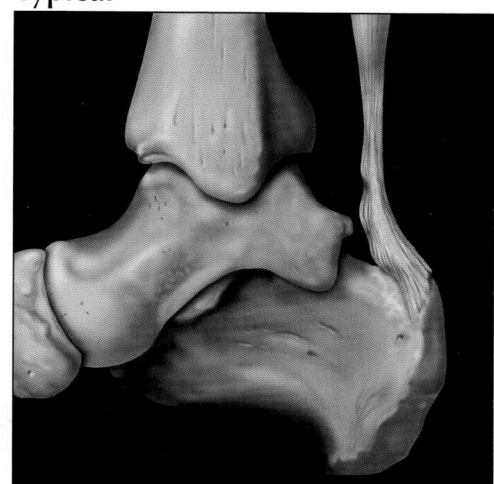
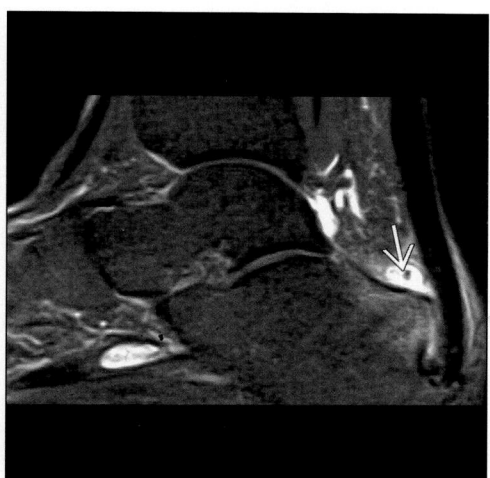

(Left) Sagittal graphic of insertional Achilles tendinitis. *(Right)* Sagittal FS PD FSE MR shows Haglund's deformity with insertional tendinitis and calcaneal marrow edema plus hyperintense retrocalcaneal (arrow) and retro-Achilles bursa.

Variant

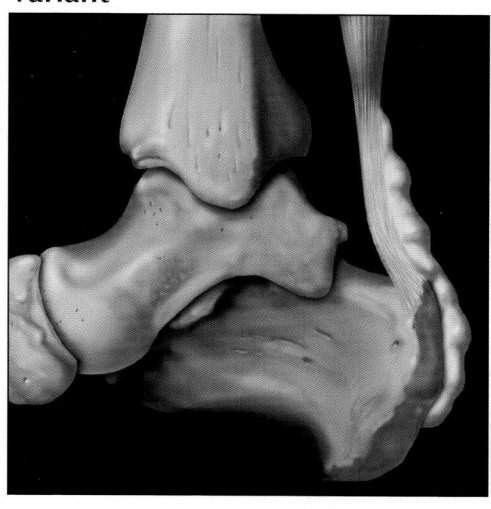
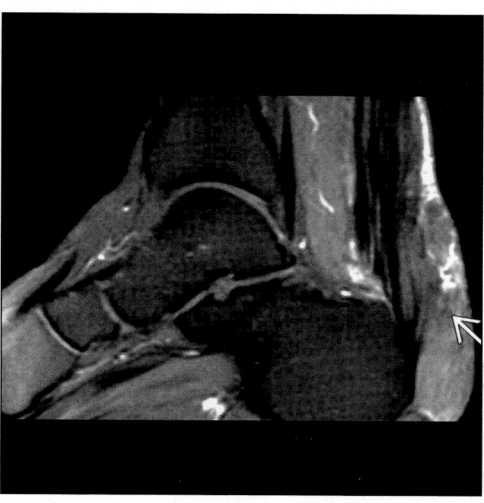

(Left) Sagittal graphic shows xanthoma with infiltrating soft tissue mass in yellow. *(Right)* Sagittal FS PD FSE MR shows posterior infiltrating intermediate signal xanthomatous soft tissue mass (arrow).

6

5

ACHILLES TENDON TEAR

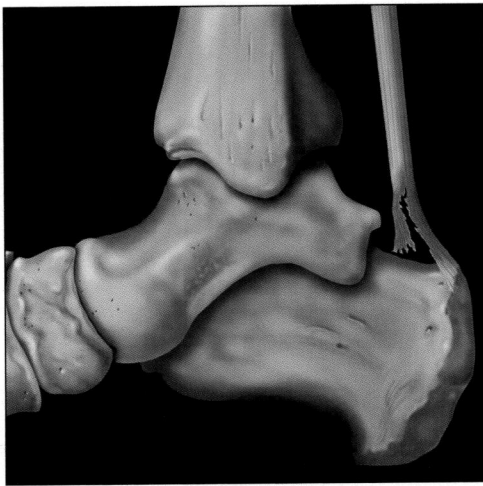
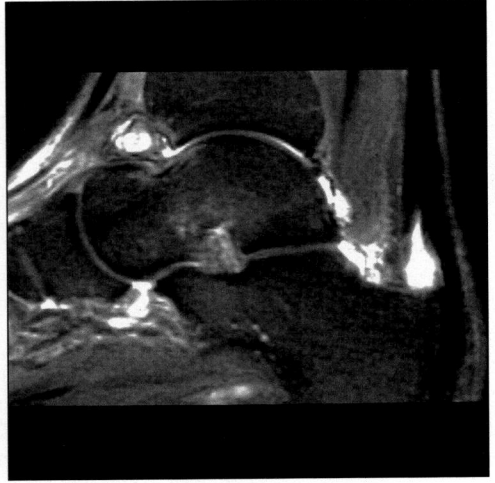

Sagittal graphic shows high grade partial tear of the distal Achilles tendon.

Sagittal FS PD FSE MR shows hyperintense signal in partial tear of the distal Achilles tendon (insertional tear).

TERMINOLOGY

Abbreviations and Synonyms
- Achilles tendon rupture

Definitions
- Partial or complete discontinuity ± tendinous gap in Achilles

IMAGING FINDINGS

General Features
- Best diagnostic clue: Hyperintense fluid-filled tendinous gap
- Location: Rupture 2-6 cm superior to the os calcis
- Size: Variable based on tendon retraction
- Morphology: Diffuse convexity anterior margin and enlarged tendon ends at tear site

MR Findings
- T1WI
  - Effacement of Kager's triangle
  - Intratendinous degeneration as intermediate signal intensity
  - Assess morphology of tendon edges
  - Assess tendon enlargement + retraction
- T2WI
  - Hemorrhage or edema in intratendinous or peritendinous soft tissue: Hyperintense (FS PD FSE)
  - Normal Achilles tendon is of uniform hypointensity
  - Rupture/tear = disruption with discontinuity ± wavy retracted tendon
  - Hyperintense fluid-filled gap ± interposed fat
  - Proximal tendon retraction associated with fraying or corkscrewing of tendon edges
  - Intratendinous fluid: May be seen up to six months post surgical treatment or conservative management (a widened tendon up to 12 months)
  - Enlarged proximal and distal ends may be associated with an attenuated union bridging the tear site
  - Surgical repair healing response: Increased size of tendon associated with decreased tendinous signal intensity secondary to scar tissue
  - Associated edema in peritendon and preachilles fat pad is a common finding
- T1 C+: FS T1 C+ to enhance tear site and define margins

Imaging Recommendations
- Best imaging tool
  - MR superior to ultrasound and CT for partial and complete tears especially intratendinous lesions
  - MR imaging identifies tendinous gap - important for conservative management (retracted tendons are less likely to heal with large diastasis)
- Protocol advice

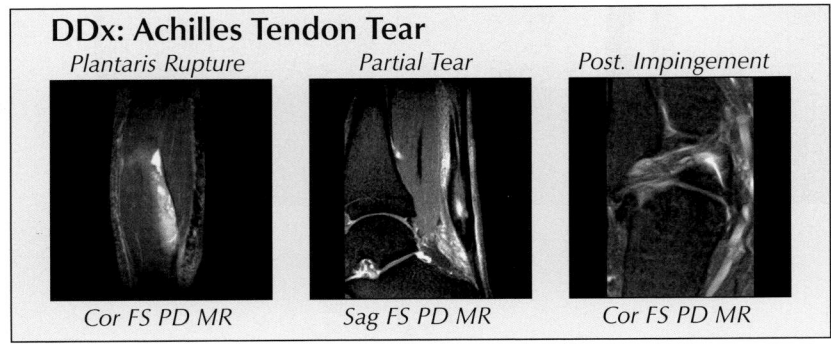

DDx: Achilles Tendon Tear

Plantaris Rupture	Partial Tear	Post. Impingement
Cor FS PD MR	Sag FS PD MR	Cor FS PD MR

ACHILLES TENDON TEAR

Key Facts

Imaging Findings
- Best diagnostic clue: Hyperintense fluid-filled tendinous gap
- Location: Rupture 2-6 cm superior to the os calcis
- Assess tendon enlargement + retraction
- Hemorrhage or edema in intratendinous or peritendinous soft tissue: Hyperintense (FS PD FSE)

Top Differential Diagnoses
- Partial Tear of the Achilles Tendon
- Plantaris Tendon Tear
- Posterior Impingement

Pathology
- Indirect trauma common
- Repetitive microtrauma

- Forced dorsiflexion of foot against contracting force (triceps surae group) or eccentric loading in a sudden stretch
- Direct trauma: Rupture at the myotendinous junction
- Posterior fibers rupture first (partial tearing may exist in anterior fibers which are under less tension)

Clinical Issues
- Pain and soft tissue swelling (hemorrhage)
- Athletic activity in middle-aged males
- Musculotendinous junction in younger population
- Surgical repair usually required

Diagnostic Checklist
- Identify proximal and distal tendon ends on sagittal images

---

- ○ MR
  - ■ T1 and FS PD FSE or STIR sagittal and axial images required

DIFFERENTIAL DIAGNOSIS

Partial Tear of the Achilles Tendon
- Without tendinous gap

Plantaris Tendon Tear
- A torn plantaris tendon may mimic an Achilles tendon tear on medial sagittal images (an intact plantaris tendon may also be seen in the presence of an Achilles tendon rupture)
- Fluid between plantaris and Achilles may mimic a tear

Posterior Impingement
- Hyperintensity of posterior ligaments or interposed ganglion ± synovitis

PATHOLOGY

General Features
- General path comments
  - ○ No true synovial sheath
  - ○ Mesotendon provides blood supply through anterior mesentery
  - ○ Kager's triangle = triangular fat pad anterior to Achilles tendon
- Etiology
  - ○ Indirect trauma common
  - ○ Repetitive microtrauma
  - ○ Over pronation of foot or heel stress leads to micro tears
  - ○ Forced dorsiflexion of foot against contracting force (triceps surae group) or eccentric loading in a sudden stretch
  - ○ Direct trauma: Rupture at the myotendinous junction
  - ○ Atrophy of soleus muscle
  - ○ Rheumatoid arthritis, systemic lupus, diabetes mellitus and gout

- ○ Acute rupture: Predisposing factors include chronic tendonitis and partial tears
- ○ Use of fluoroquinolone antibiotics
- Epidemiology: Third most frequent tendon rupture

Gross Pathologic & Surgical Features
- Tear 2-3 cm proximal to calcaneal insertion
- Reduced anterior mesenteric blood supply with increasing age
- Posterior fibers rupture first (partial tearing may exist in anterior fibers which are under less tension)
- Plantaris usually intact secondary to a more anterior calcaneal insertion

Microscopic Features
- Degeneration with decreased collagen cross-linking
  - ○ Increased stiffness
  - ○ Loss of viscoelasticity

Staging, Grading or Classification Criteria
- Type 1
  - ○ Partial ruptures of 50% or less
- Type 2
  - ○ Complete rupture with tendinous gap 3 cm or less
- Type 3
  - ○ Complete rupture with tendinous gap 3 cm to 6 cm
- Type 4
  - ○ Complete rupture with defect of greater than 6 cm
  - ○ Associated with neglected ruptures

CLINICAL ISSUES

Presentation
- Most common signs/symptoms
  - ○ Pain and soft tissue swelling (hemorrhage)
  - ○ Clinical assessment can be incorrect up to 25%
- Clinical profile
  - ○ Athletic activity in middle-aged males
  - ○ Hyperdorsiflexion sign
  - ○ O'Brien's needle test to detect proximal tendon motion as a sign of tendon continuity in acute ruptures
  - ○ Palpable tendon defect

ACHILLES TENDON TEAR

- o Thompson test positive if squeezing calf does not produce plantar flexion response

Demographics
- Age
  - o After age 30 (30 to 50 years most common)
  - o Musculotendinous junction in younger population
- Gender
  - o M:F = 5:1 to 6:1 for complete rupture secondary to indirect trauma
  - o Concentric loading
    - Basketball
    - Tennis
    - Racquetball

Natural History & Prognosis
- Non-surgical rate of rerupture 20.8%
- Surgical rate of rerupture 1.7%
- Recurrent rupture
  - o 10 to 30% with conservative treatment
  - o 5% with a surgical reinforcement

Treatment
- Non-operative
  - o Cast immobilization
    - Above knee cast with equinus for 4 weeks
    - Below knee cast with decreased equinus
  - o Often indicated for acute ruptures < 48 hours
    - Steroid induced ruptures
- Surgical repair usually required
  - o Type 1 and 2 ruptures repaired with an end-to-end anastomosis
  - o Type 3 rupture requires autogenous tendon graft flap
  - o Type 4 requires a free tendon graft or synthetic graft
- Suture techniques
  - o Bunnell
  - o Kessler
  - o Krackow (locking loop) with four sutures across repair site
  - o Percutaneous repair
  - o Synthetic graft materials
- Alternative function bracing
- Plantaris reinforcement

DIAGNOSTIC CHECKLIST

Consider
- Identify proximal and distal tendon ends on sagittal images
- Use axial FS PD FSE images to confirm complete rupture (an intact plantaris may simulate an intact tendon in sagittal plane)
- Identify surface contour irregularity to differentiate partial tears vs. nonretracted complete ruptures

SELECTED REFERENCES

1. Dwornik L et al: Radiologic case study. Acute Achilles tendon rupture. Orthopedics 25(11):1239, 1318-20, 2002
2. Marshall H et al: Contrast enhanced magic-angle MR imaging of the Achilles tendon. AJR 179(1): 187-92, 2002
3. Schepsis AA et al: Achilles tendon disorders in athletes. Am J Sports Med 30(2): 287-305, 2002
4. Banks A et al: McGlamry's comprehensive textbook of foot and ankle surgery. vol 1. 3rd ed. Philadelphia, Lippincott Williams & Wilkins, 1706-23, 2001
5. Myerson M et al: Foot and ankle disorders. vol 1. Philadelphia, W.B. Saunders, 1367-98, 2000
6. Saltzman C et al: Achilles tendon injuries. J Am Acad Orthop Surg 6(5):316-23, 1998
7. Stoller D et al: Magnetic resonance imaging in orthopaedics & sports medicine. 2nd ed. Philadelphia, Lippincott Williams & Wilkins, 443-595, 1997
8. Resnick D et al: Internal Derangements of Joints: Emphasis on MR imaging. 1st ed. Philadelphia, W.B. Saunders, 787-925, 1997
9. Karjalainen PT et al: Magnetic resonance imaging during healing of surgically repaired Achilles tendon ruptures. Am J Sports Med 25:164-71, 1997
10. Astrom M et al: Imaging in chronic Achilles tendinopathy: A comparison of ultrasonography, magnetic resonance imaging and surgical findings in 27 histologically verified cases. Skeletal Radiol 25:615-20, 1996
11. Cetti R et al: Operative versus nonoperative treatment of Achilles tendon rupture. A prospective randomized study and review of the literature. Am J Sports Med 21(6):791-9, 1993
12. Schweitzer ME: Magnetic resonance imaging of the foot and ankle. Magn Reson Q 9(4):214-34, 1993
13. Kier R et al: MR imaging of the normal ligaments and tendons of the ankle. J Comput Assist Tomogr 15(3):477-82, 1991
14. Mink JH et al: Tendon injuries of the lower extremity: Magnetic resonance assessment. Top Magn Reson Imaging 3(4):23-38, 1991
15. Keene JS et al: Magnetic resonance imaging of Achilles tendon ruptures. Am J Sports Med 17:333-7, 1989
16. Hamilton WG: Foot and ankle injuries in dancers. Clin Sports Med 7(1):143-73, 1988
17. Quinn SF et al: Achilles tendon: MR imaging at 1.5 T. Radiology 164:767-70, 1987
18. Reinig JW et al: MR imaging of a ruptured Achilles tendon: Case report. J Comput Assist Tomogr 9:1131-4, 1985
19. Clement P et al: Achilles tendinitis and peritendinitis: Etiology and treatment. Am J Sports Med 12:179-84, 1984
20. James S et al: Injuries to runners. Am J Sports Med 6:40-50, 1978

IMAGE GALLERY

Typical

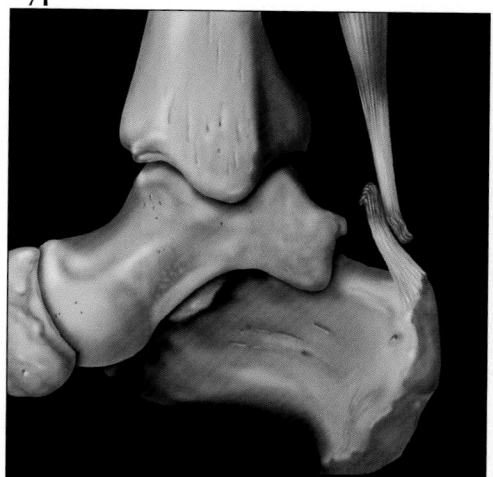

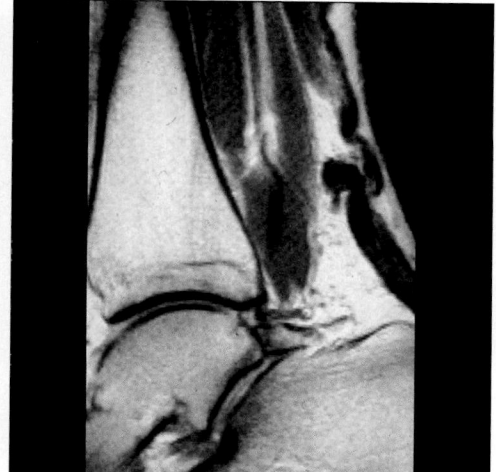

(Left) Sagittal graphic shows Achilles tendon rupture with overlapping proximal and distal tendon segments. (Right) Sagittal T1WI MR shows complete rupture of Achilles tendon with approximation of proximal and distal tendon fibers.

Typical

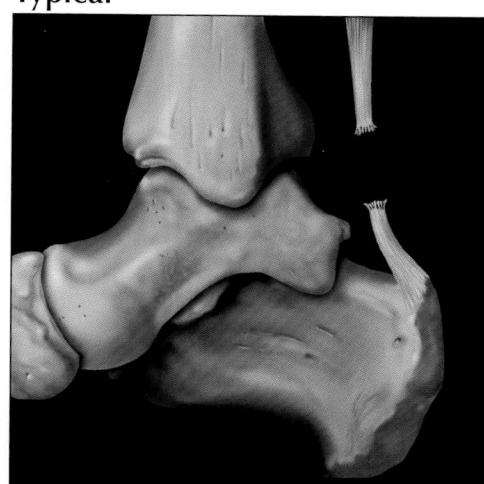

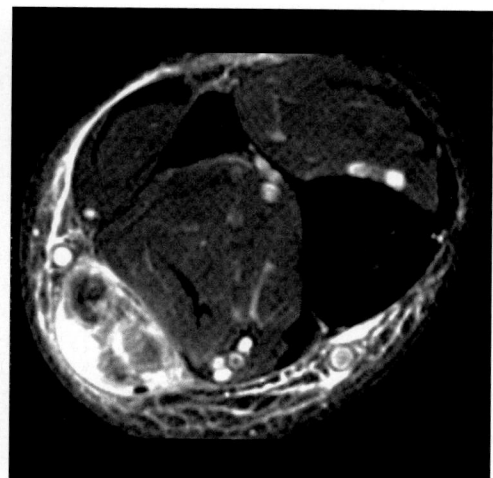

(Left) Sagittal graphic shows Achilles tendon tear with tendinous gap and retraction. (Right) Axial FS PD FSE MR shows hyperintensity at hemorrhagic tear site in a complete tendon rupture.

Typical

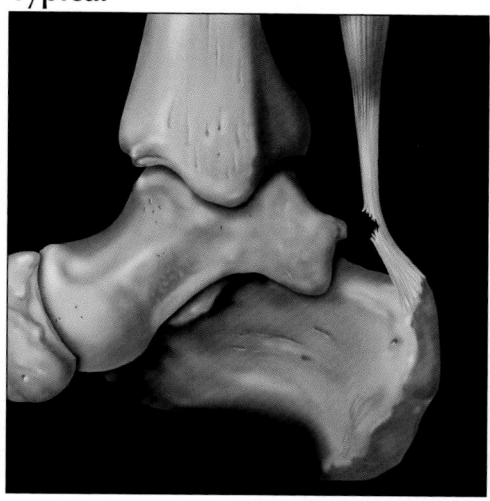

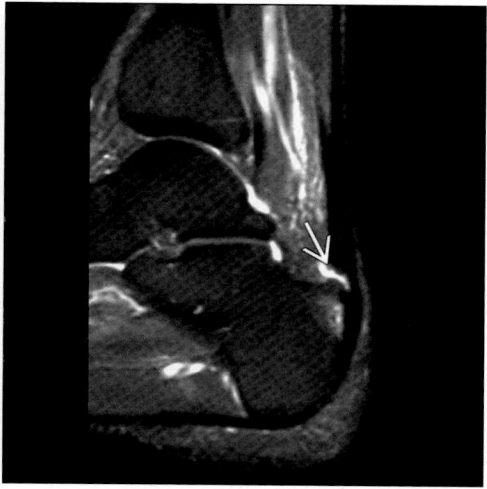

(Left) Sagittal graphic shows anterior tendon deformity with partial Achilles tear. (Right) Sagittal FS PD FSE MR shows hyperintense linear signal in an insertional Achilles partial tear (arrow) with reactive calcaneal marrow edema.

6

9

TIBIALIS POSTERIOR TENDON TEAR

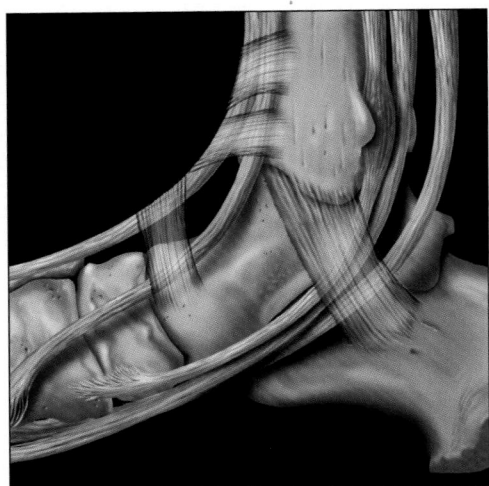

Sagittal graphic shows tibialis posterior tendon tear type 1 with medial malleolar spur opposite area of interstitial longitudinal split. Abnormal segment of tendon shown in red.

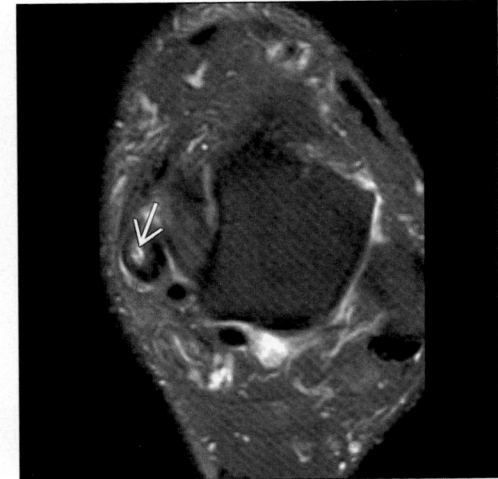

Axial FS PD FSE MR shows type 1 tibialis posterior tendon tear with hyperintense signal (arrow) within an enlarged tendon. Involved tendon is shown posterior to the deltoid ligament.

TERMINOLOGY

Abbreviations and Synonyms
- Tibialis posterior tendon dysfunction; tibialis posterior tendon insufficiency, tibialis posterior tendon rupture

Definitions
- Tendinopathy and progressive tendon tear resulting in collapsed pes valgus deformity

IMAGING FINDINGS

General Features
- Best diagnostic clue: A change in tendon size, morphology and/or signal intensity
- Location
  - Mid portion of tendon involved at level of and immediately distal to medial malleolus
  - Corresponds to relative zone of tendon hypovascularity
- Size
  - Normal tibialis posterior 2x size of flexor digitorum longus
  - Tibialis posterior tendon tear presents as spectrum of tendon hypertrophy, attenuation or disruption
- Morphology
  - Bulbous cross sectional enlargement
  - Attenuation in a curvilinear orientation
  - Complete tendinous gap

MR Findings
- T1WI
  - Type 1 tear
    - Intrasubstance vertical split
    - Enlarged tendon diameter ± intrasubstance intermediate signal
  - Type 2 tear
    - Thin or attenuated tendon with variable intratendinous signal change
  - Type 3 tear
    - Complete tendinous discontinuity with low to intermediate signal intensity fluid-filled gap
    - Presence of sub-tendons in partial tears
    - Associated findings: Hypertrophy medial tubercle of navicular, abnormal talonavicular alignment, accessory navicular, loss of longitudinal arch on sagittal images
    - Normal variant of increased signal intensity + girth at distal tendon insertion to navicular (intrasubstance striations)
    - Osseous spur ± fatty marrow signal posteromedial aspect medial malleolus
    - Uncommon to see tendon dislocation, associated with disruption of flexor retinaculum
- T2WI

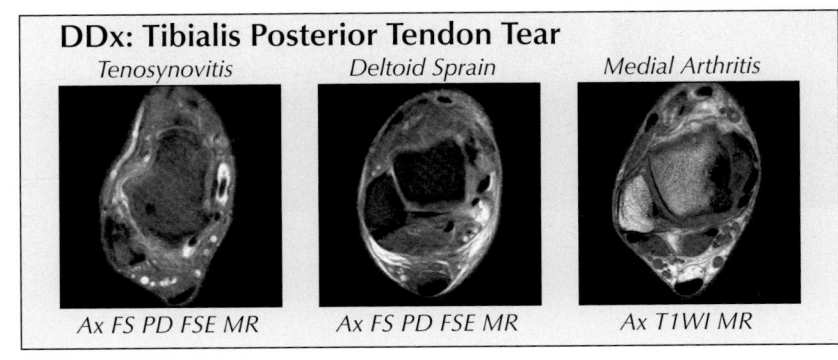

DDx: Tibialis Posterior Tendon Tear

Tenosynovitis	Deltoid Sprain	Medial Arthritis
Ax FS PD FSE MR	Ax FS PD FSE MR	Ax T1WI MR

TIBIALIS POSTERIOR TENDON TEAR

Key Facts

Imaging Findings
- Best diagnostic clue: A change in tendon size, morphology and/or signal intensity
- Mid portion of tendon involved at level of and immediately distal to medial malleolus
- Presence of sub-tendons in partial tears

Top Differential Diagnoses
- Tenosynovitis
- Tibialis Posterior Tendon Insertion
- Deltoid Sprain
- Medial Tibiotalar Arthritis

Pathology
- Acute trauma less common than degenerative
- Degenerative is most frequent etiology of tibialis posterior dysfunction

- Type 1 tear: Tendon hypertrophy with vertical split
- Type 2 tear: Attenuated section of tendon at level of medial malleolus with sub-tendons
- Type 3 tear: Complete with tendinous gap

Clinical Issues
- Most common signs/symptoms: Pain, swelling, tenderness and flattening of medial longitudinal arch
- Age: Fifth and sixth decades
- Gender: Two-thirds cases female population
- Plantar fasciitis
- Severe pes planus

Diagnostic Checklist
- Assess tendon morphology otherwise may overlook type 2 tears

---

- ○ Tendon hypertrophy with heterogenous signal intensity (FS PD FSE) in type 1 vertical split
- ○ Thickening flexor retinaculum
- ○ Tenosynovitis
  - ▪ Hyperintense fluid seen associated with degeneration and tendon tears
- ○ Hyperintense fluid-filled gap or diastasis at tendon rupture site
- ○ Chronic dysfunction: Spring ligament laxity or rupture
  - ▪ Superomedial calcaneal navicular component usually injured
- STIR
  - ○ Tenosynovitis: Seen in tears and degeneration as hyperintense fluid
  - ○ Subchondral marrow edema

Imaging Recommendations
- Best imaging tool: MR superior to CT for tendon morphology, vertical splits, tenosynovitis and edema
- Protocol advice
  - ○ T1 or PD FSE and FS PD FSE axial, sagittal and coronal planes
  - ○ Axial plane key in evaluating changes of tendon morphology
  - ○ Coronal and sagittal planes used for secondary confirmation of tendon pathology

DIFFERENTIAL DIAGNOSIS

Tenosynovitis
- Tendon morphology is maintained without intrinsic tendinopathy

Tibialis Posterior Tendon Insertion
- Normal broadening of tendon restricted to navicular insertion

Deltoid Sprain
- Superficial or deep layer hyperintensity on T2WI

Medial Tibiotalar Arthritis
- Sclerosis (hypointense) between medial malleolus + talus

Magic Angle Effect
- Increased signal where tendon alignment is approximately 55° relative to main magnetic field (e.g., at medial malleolus)
- Lengthening of T2 relaxation
- Seen on short echo sequences (typically TE is less than 40 ms)
- Not present on long TE sequences

PATHOLOGY

General Features
- General path comments
  - ○ Relevant anatomy
    - ▪ Tibialis posterior superficial to superomedial calcaneal navicular component of spring ligament
    - ▪ Synergistic relationship of tibialis posterior tendon with spring ligament
  - ○ Insertion
    - ▪ Proximal on navicular tuberosity
    - ▪ Extensive plantar insertions
  - ○ Relevant function
    - ▪ Supports medial arch
    - ▪ Stabilizes foot
    - ▪ High inversion moment arm
    - ▪ Supination of foot
    - ▪ Pulley action with medial malleolus
- Etiology
  - ○ Traumatic
    - ▪ Acute trauma less common than degenerative
    - ▪ Minor trauma
    - ▪ Lacerations and puncture
    - ▪ Rupture usually associated with indirect trauma (sprains and/or fractures)
  - ○ Chronic
    - ▪ Degenerative is most frequent etiology of tibialis posterior dysfunction

- o Systemic inflammatory disease
  - Rheumatoid arthritis
- o Seronegative spondyloarthropathies
  - Psoriasis
  - Ankylosing spondylitis
  - Reiter's
  - Enteropathic arthritis
  - Associated with sites of enthesopathy
- o Infections
  - Gonococcal
  - Tubercular
- o Tendon hypovascularity
  - Zone of hypovascularity in mid portion of tendon, at and distal to medial malleolus
  - At risk for rupture
  - Diminished arterial perfusion (age-related) leading to tendon ischemia
  - Acute angulation of tendon posterior to medial malleolus compounds hypovascularity
  - Pronation of hindfoot causes tendon compression
- o Biomechanical
  - Overuse
  - Pes valgus
  - Equinus
  - Increased stress on tibialis posterior with decreased medial longitudinal arch support
- o Abnormal insertion
  - Accessory navicular
  - Prominent medial navicular tubercle
  - Associated with tendon degeneration secondary to change in leverage
- o Iatrogenic tendon dysfunction
  - Medial ankle/tarsal tunnel surgery
  - Steroid use
- Epidemiology: Patients > 50 years: 60% associated with hypertension, diabetes + obesity

Gross Pathologic & Surgical Features
- Longitudinal split
- Tendon laxity and elongation
- Irregular surface
- Adhesions with sheath and flexor retinaculum
- Elongated and fibrotic tendon
- Bone proliferation
- Atrophic sheath
- Tendon rupture
- Scarred and frayed proximal and distal tendon ends

Microscopic Features
- Intrasubstance degeneration

Staging, Grading or Classification Criteria
- MR criteria
  - o Type 1 tear: Tendon hypertrophy with vertical split
  - o Type 2 tear: Attenuated section of tendon at level of medial malleolus with sub-tendons
  - o Type 3 tear: Complete with tendinous gap

CLINICAL ISSUES

Presentation
- Most common signs/symptoms: Pain, swelling, tenderness and flattening of medial longitudinal arch

- Clinical profile
  - o Weakness of inversion
  - o Severe pes planus deformity
  - o Heel valgus, talar plantar flexion and forefoot abduction

Demographics
- Age: Fifth and sixth decades
- Gender: Two-thirds cases female population
- Distribution
  - o Unilateral (90%) and left sided predominance

Natural History & Prognosis
- Change in foot shape
- Decreased exercise tolerance
- Plantar fasciitis
- Tarsal tunnel associated with tenosynovitis and tendon hypertrophy
- Severe pes planus
- Tenderness sinus tarsi and lateral ankle pain in advanced deformity

Treatment
- Conservative
  - o Tendon must be intact without significant degeneration
  - o Orthotics, medial heel wedge (support medial longitudinal arch)
  - o Non-steroidal antiinflammatory drugs
  - o Physical therapy
- Surgical
  - o Primary repair
  - o Excision of segmental defects with reanastomosis or grafting
  - o Reinforcement with flexor digitorum longus or tibialis anterior
  - o Osteotomies + limited fusions

DIAGNOSTIC CHECKLIST

Consider
- Assess tendon morphology otherwise may overlook type 2 tears
- Identify associated sub-tendons
- Confirm tendon anatomy on coronal and sagittal images

SELECTED REFERENCES

1. Banks AS et al: McGlamry's comprehensive textbook of foot and ankle surgery. vol 1. 3rd ed. Philadelphia PA, Lippincott Williams & Wilkins, 862-99, 2001
2. Myerson M: Foot and ankle disorders. vol 2. Philadelphia PA, Lippincott Raven:1017-39, 2000
3. Karasick D et al: Tear of the posterior tibial tendon causing asymmetric flatfoot: Radiologic findings. AJR 161:1237, 1993

IMAGE GALLERY

Typical

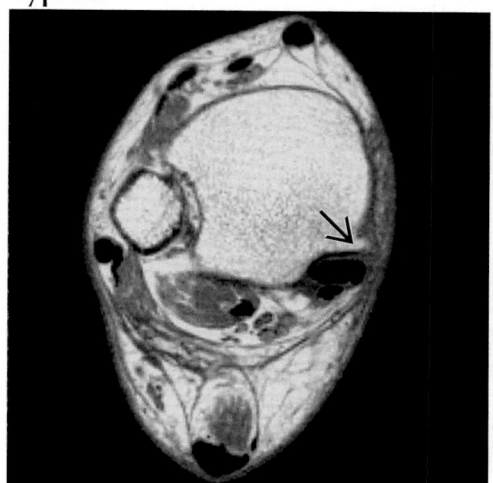 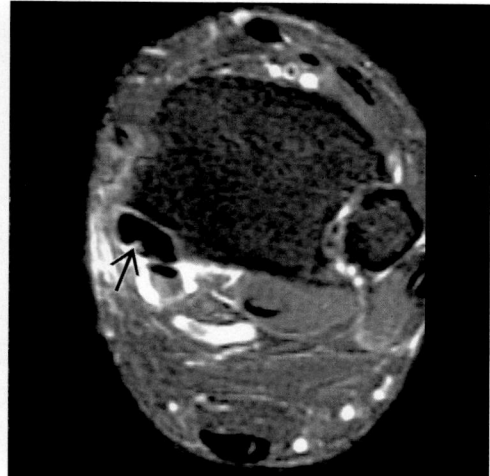

(Left) Axial T1WI MR shows enlarged tibialis posterior tendon in type 1 tear with posterior medial malleolus spur. The medial spur *(arrow)* is marrow containing. *(Right)* Axial FS PD FSE MR shows hyperintense signal *(arrow)* in partial tear *(type 1)* of the posterior aspect of the tibialis posterior tendon. Adjacent soft tissue edema is hyperintense.

Typical

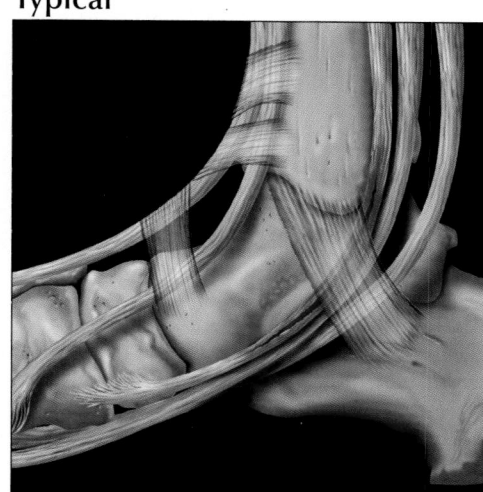 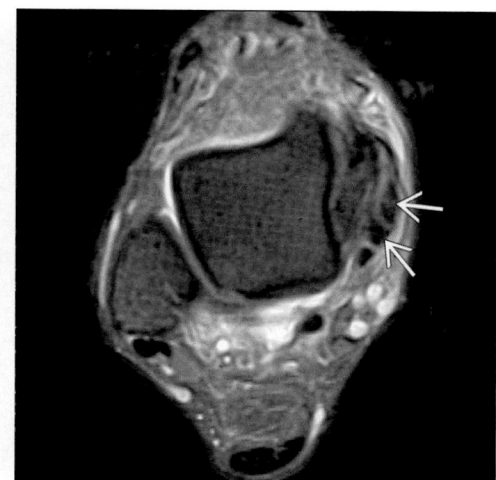

(Left) Sagittal graphic shows longitudinal split of the tibialis posterior tendon into two subtendons. Subtendons and abnormal tendon section shown in red. *(Right)* Axial FS PD FSE MR shows the anterior and posterior subtendons of a type 2 tibialis posterior tendon tear. Subtendons *(arrows)* are posterior to the deltoid ligament and anterior to the flexor digitorum longus tendon.

Typical

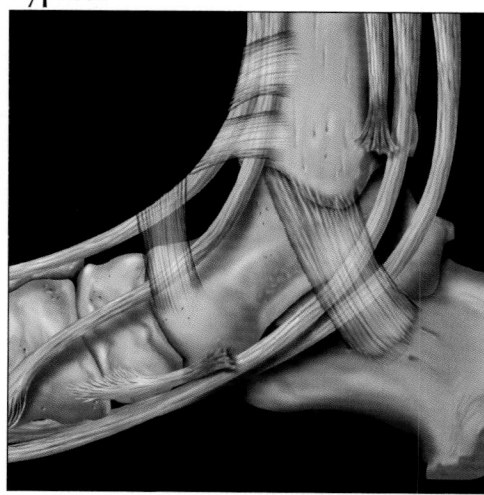 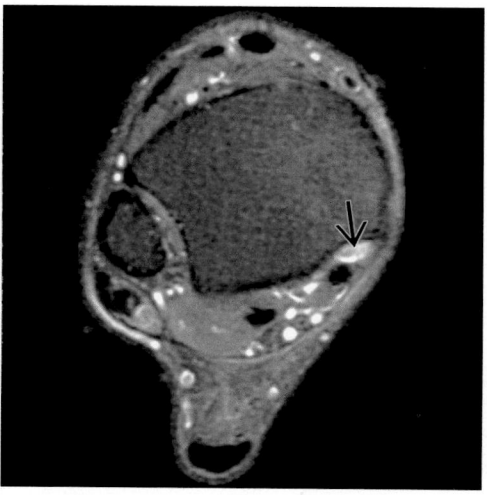

(Left) Sagittal graphic shows complete rupture of the tibialis posterior tendon with retracted tendon stumps. *(Right)* Axial FS PD FSE MR shows hyperintense fluid *(arrow)* occupying area of absent tibialis posterior tendon in a type 3 tendon tear. Fluid is anterior to the flexor digitorum longus tendon.

6

13

FLEXOR HALLUCIS LONGUS ABNORMALITIES

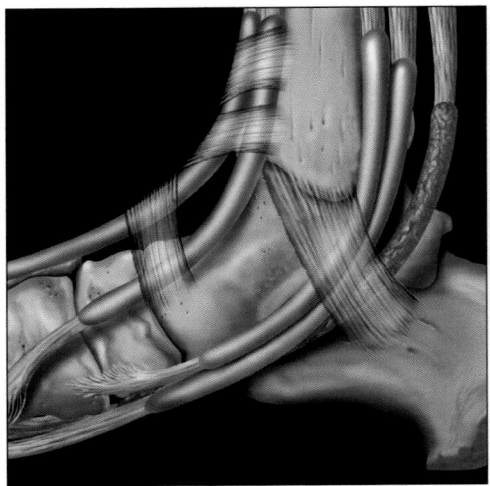

Sagittal graphic shows flexor hallucis longus tenosynovitis in red.

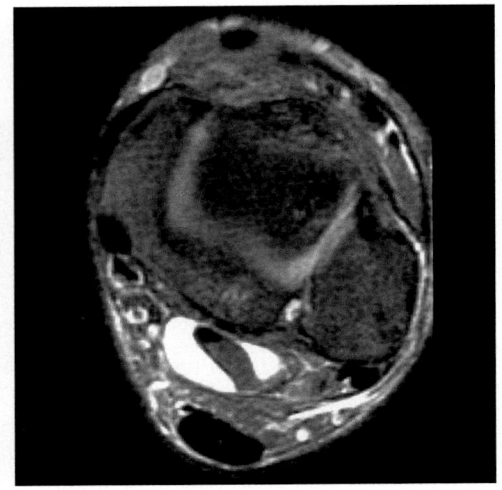

Axial FS PD FSE MR shows hemorrhagic tenosynovitis with layering of fluid in the flexor hallucis longus tendon sheath.

TERMINOLOGY

Abbreviations and Synonyms
- Tendinosis; tenosynovitis; muscle-tendon unit (MTU) strain; tethering; tear

Definitions
- Susceptible to tendinosis + rupture through tarsal tunnel

IMAGING FINDINGS

General Features
- Best diagnostic clue: Hyperintense fluid (FS PD FSE) in synovial sheath disproportionate to quantity of tibiotalar joint fluid
- Location
  - Runs posterior to medial malleolus, through tarsal tunnel, to Henry's knot
    - Plantar to base of first metatarsal
- Size
  - Muscle - focal or involving entire cross sectional diameter
  - Tendon sheath - variable
- Morphology
  - Restricted to muscle or tendon sheath
  - Muscle tendon unit injuries with diffuse edema ± focal muscle hemorrhage
  - Tenosynovitis with hyperintense fluid on FS PD/T2 images (circular to elongated fluid collection)

MR Findings
- T1WI: Hypointense to intermediate signal intensity fluid
- T2WI
  - Hyperintense fluid in tendon sheath on FS PD or T2 FSE images
    - Commonly identified between tibial plafond + calcaneus
    - Fluid generally uniform hyperintensity ± septation
    - Disproportionate fluid in flexor hallucis longus (FHL) tendon sheath relative to tibiotalar joint
  - Muscle strain: Hyperintense edema or hemorrhage radiating from trauma epicenter
    - Foci of hemosiderin within muscle
  - Ruptured retracted FHL tendon enlarged in cross sectional area

Imaging Recommendations
- Best imaging tool
  - MR to identify
    - Tendon sheath fluid
    - Muscle signal changes
    - Tendon morphology
- Protocol advice

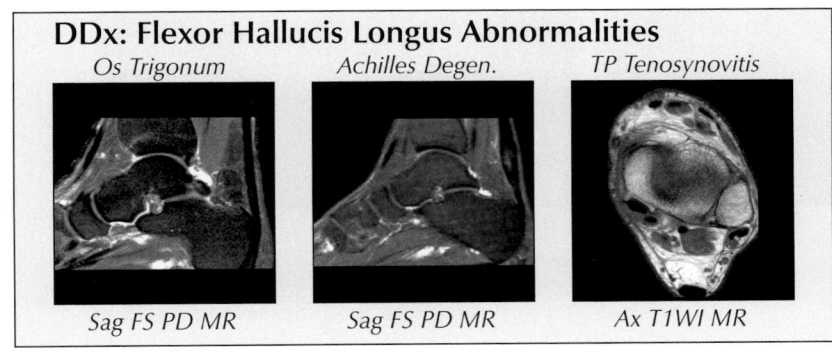

DDx: Flexor Hallucis Longus Abnormalities

Os Trigonum	Achilles Degen.	TP Tenosynovitis
Sag FS PD MR	Sag FS PD MR	Ax T1WI MR

FLEXOR HALLUCIS LONGUS ABNORMALITIES

Key Facts

Imaging Findings

- Best diagnostic clue: Hyperintense fluid (FS PD FSE) in synovial sheath disproportionate to quantity of tibiotalar joint fluid
- Muscle tendon unit injuries with diffuse edema ± focal muscle hemorrhage
- Tenosynovitis with hyperintense fluid on FS PD/T2 images (circular to elongated fluid collection)
- Ruptured retracted FHL tendon enlarged in cross sectional area

Top Differential Diagnoses

- Os Trigonum Syndrome
- Fluid in Tendon Sheath 2° to Ankle Effusion
- Achilles Tendonitis
- Tibialis Posterior (TP) Tenosynovitis

Pathology

- Repetitive plantar flexion and dorsiflexion lead to tenosynovitis
- Twisting injury ankle
- Paratendinitis (tenosynovitis) most common abnormality

Clinical Issues

- Most common signs/symptoms: Pain, swelling and tenderness posterior ankle
- Repetitive stress may result in chronic muscle strain ± hemorrhage
- Release constricting FHL tendon sheath

Diagnostic Checklist

- Tendon sheath fluid may be a normal finding and should be correlated with ankle joint fluid volume

---

- ○ Routine ankle using FS PD FSE in axial, sagittal, and coronal planes
  - ▪ Coronal images through the foot for distal rupture

DIFFERENTIAL DIAGNOSIS

Os Trigonum Syndrome

- Hypertrophy of the os trigonum

Fluid in Tendon Sheath 2° to Ankle Effusion

- Fluid may be present in association with tibiotalar effusion (pseudo-tenosynovitis)
- Communication with ankle joint in 70%

Achilles Tendonitis

- Thickening Achilles tendon

Tibialis Posterior (TP) Tenosynovitis

- Fluid in tendon sheath
- ± Associated tendinopathy of tibialis posterior

PATHOLOGY

General Features

- General path comments
  - ○ Relevant anatomy
    - ▪ Fibroosseous tunnel deep to flexor retinaculum (between medial + lateral tubercles of posterior talar process)
    - ▪ Passes underneath sustentaculum tali
    - ▪ Sheaths of FHL and flexor digitorum longus cross at master knot of Henry
    - ▪ Plantar insertion base distal phalanx great toe
    - ▪ Os trigonum - ununited lateral tubercle of posterior talar process
- Etiology
  - ○ Repetitive plantar flexion and dorsiflexion lead to tenosynovitis
  - ○ Low-lying FHL muscle creating impingement
  - ○ Partial tearing or thickening with nodule development and hallux triggering (hallux sultans)

- ○ Fixed or locked FHL within sheath associated with severe tenosynovitis
- Epidemiology
  - ○ Twisting injury ankle
  - ○ Calcaneal fracture with involvement of sustentaculum tali
  - ○ Ballet dancing
    - ▪ FHL termed the Achilles tendon of the foot or "dancer's Achilles heel"
  - ○ Paratendinitis (tenosynovitis) most common abnormality

Gross Pathologic & Surgical Features

- Tendon thickening with tendinosis and partial tear
- Fluid proximal to talar fibroosseous tunnel in stenosing tenosynovitis
- Complete tendon rupture in talar fibroosseous tunnel uncommon
- Midfoot rupture more frequent at distal insertion
- Paratenonitis in three anatomic sites
  - ○ Fibroosseous tunnel between medial and lateral tubercles of posterior talar process
  - ○ Deep to flexor retinaculum
  - ○ Level of sesamoids within distal hallux tunnel

Microscopic Features

- Inflammatory reaction surrounding FHL

CLINICAL ISSUES

Presentation

- Most common signs/symptoms: Pain, swelling and tenderness posterior ankle
- Clinical profile
  - ○ Demipointe to pointe in ballet (balled foot to toe position)
  - ○ Condition exacerbated by hyper plantar flexion

Demographics

- Age: Young athletes and dancers
- Gender: More common in female than male dancers

FLEXOR HALLUCIS LONGUS ABNORMALITIES

Natural History & Prognosis
- Repetitive stress may result in chronic muscle strain ± hemorrhage
- Stenosing tenosynovitis
- Partial or complete tendon tear

Treatment
- Conservative
  - Antiinflammatory agents
  - Rest
  - Modification of dance or related causative activities
  - Immobilization
- Surgical
  - Release constricting FHL tendon sheath
  - Excision of an associated symptomatic os trigonum

DIAGNOSTIC CHECKLIST

Consider
- Chronic muscle changes in dancers at muscle tendon junction
- Follow distal course of FHL to exclude distal rupture
- Tendon sheath fluid may be a normal finding and should be correlated with ankle joint fluid volume

SELECTED REFERENCES

1. Sitler DF et al: Posterior ankle arthroscopy: An anatomic study. J Bone Joint Surg AM 84A(5):763-9, 2002
2. Banks A et al: McGlamry's comprehensive textbook of foot and ankle surgery. vol 1. Philadelphia PA, Lippincott Williams & Wilkins, (35):1091-152, 2001
3. Myerson M: Foot and ankle disorders. vol 2. Philadelphia PA, Lippincott Raven, (39):942-71, 2000
4. Bureau NJ et al: Posterior ankle impingement syndrome: MR imaging findings in seven patients. Radiology 215(2): 497-503, 2000
5. Cooper ME et al: Os trigonum syndrome with flexor hallucis longus tenosynovitis in a professional football referee. Med Sci Sports Exerc 31:S493-96, 1999
6. Sammarco GJ et al: Flexor hallucis longus tendon injury in dancers and nondancers. Foot Ankle Int 19(6):356-62, 1998
7. Sammarco GJ et al: Flexor hallucis longus tendon injury in dancers and nondancers. Foot Ankle Int 19:356-63, 1998
8. Inokuchi S et al: Closed complete rupture of the flexor hallucis longus tendon at the groove of the talus. Foot Ankle Int 18:47-9, 1997
9. Kolettis GJ et al: Release of the flexor hallucis longus tendon in ballet dancers. J Bone Joint Surg Am 78A:1386-90, 1996
10. Hamilton WG et al: Pain in the posterior aspect of the ankle in dancers. Differential diagnosis and operative treatment. J Bone Joint Surg Am 78:1491-1500, 1996
11. Chandnani VP et al: Achilles tendon and miscellaneous tendon lesions. Magn Reson Imaging Clin N Am 2(1):89-96, 1994
12. Schweitzer ME et al: Fluid in normal and abnormal ankle joints: Amount and distribution as seen on MR images. AJR 162(1):111-4, 1994
13. Coghlan BA et al: Traumatic rupture of the flexor hallucis longus tendon in a marathon runner. AM J Sports Med Assoc 21:617-18, 1993
14. Mink JH et al: Tendon injuries of the lower extremity: Magnetic resonance assessment. Top Magn Reson Imaging 3(4):23-38, 1991
15. Floyd DW et al: Tendon lacerations in the foot. Foot Ankle 4:8-14, 1983
16. Cowell HR et al: Bilateral tendonitis of the flexor hallucis longus in a ballet dancer. J Pediatr Orthop 2:582-86, 1982
17. Garth WP Jr: Flexor hallucis tendinitis in a ballet dancer. A case report. J Bone Joint Surg Am 63:1489, 1981
18. Krackow KA: Acute, traumatic rupture of a flexor hallucis longus tendon: A case report. Clin Orthop 150:261-2, 1980
19. Frenette JP et al: Lacerations of the flexor hallucis longus in the young athlete. J Bone Joint Surg Am 59:673-76, 1977
20. Hamilton WG: Tendonitis about the ankle joint in classical ballet dancers. Am J Sports Med 5:84-8, 1977

IMAGE GALLERY

Typical

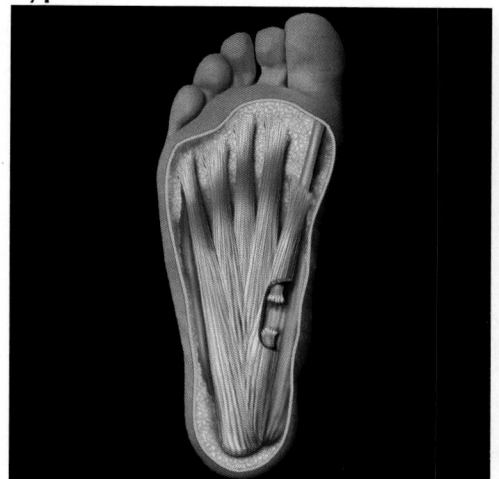 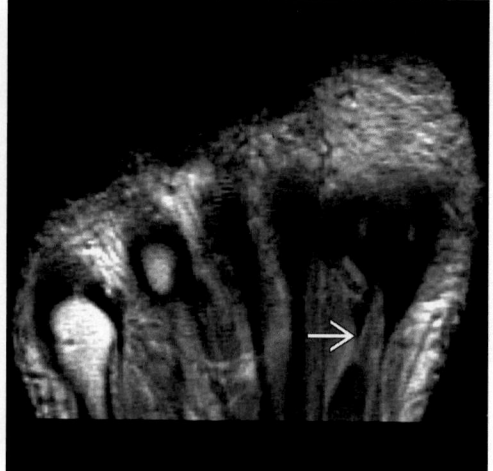

(Left) Axial graphic of plantar rupture of flexor hallucis longus tendon. *(Right)* Axial FS PD FSE MR of distal rupture (arrow) with retraction of flexor hallucis longus tendon. Retracted tendon shows enlarged distal contour.

Typical

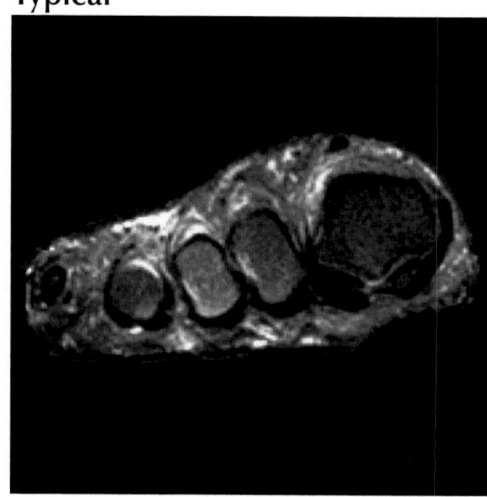 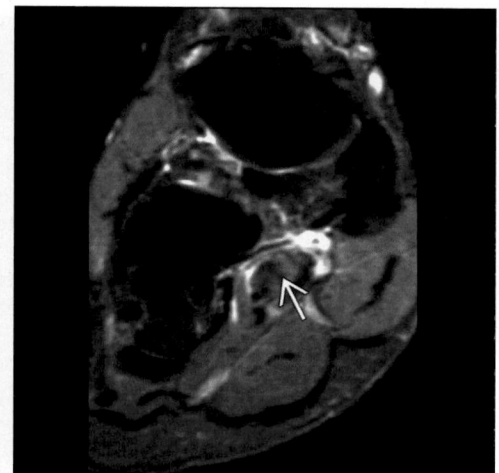

(Left) Coronal FS PD FSE MR showing absence of distal flexor hallucis longus tendon between the sesamoids of the first metatarsal. *(Right)* Coronal FS PD FSE MR of retracted flexor hallucis longus tendon surrounded by hyperintense fluid at the level of the master knot of Henry (arrow).

6

17

Typical

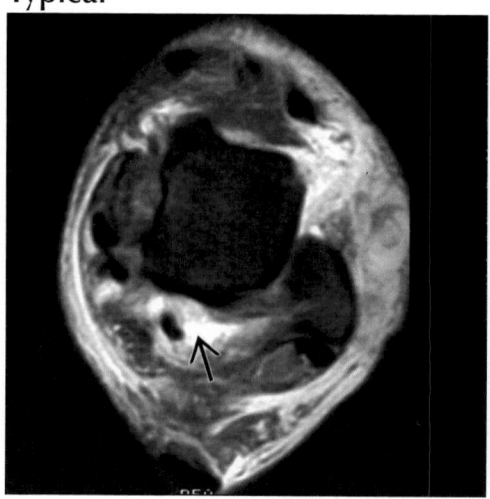 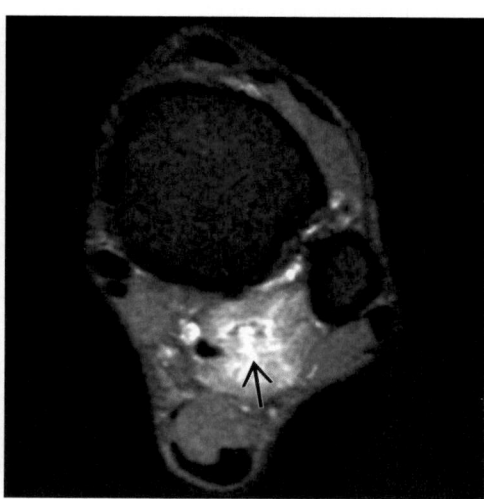

(Left) Axial FS PD FSE MR shows hyperintense traumatic tenosynovitis distending the flexor hallucis longus tendon sheath (arrow). *(Right)* Axial FS PD FSE MR shows chronic flexor hallucis longus muscle tendon unit injury. Hyperintense edema (arrow) and chronic hypointense hemorrhage are present within the belly of the flexor hallucis longus muscle.

TIBIALIS ANTERIOR TENDON TEAR

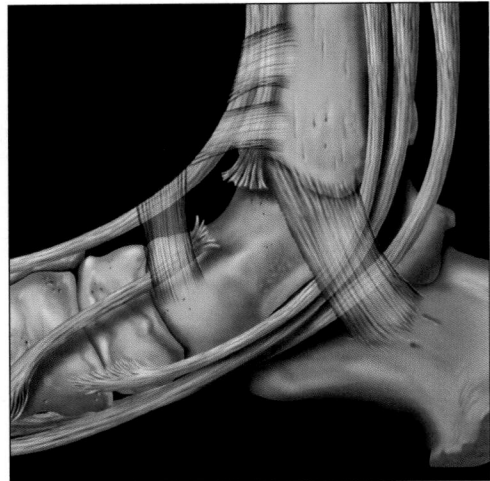

Sagittal graphic shows rupture of tibialis anterior with tendinous gap. Frayed tendon ends are shown in red. Tear site is located between slips of the inferior extensor retinaculum.

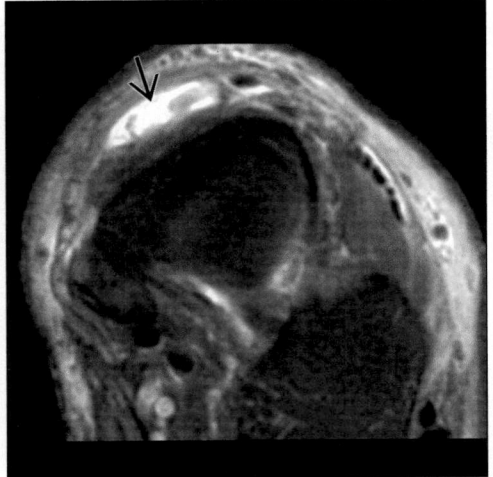

Coronal FS PD FSE MR shows complete tear (arrow) of the tibialis anterior tendon on image acquired perpendicular to the long axis of the tendon. Hyperintense fluid occupies tear site.

TERMINOLOGY

Abbreviations and Synonyms
- Tibialis anterior tendon rupture

Definitions
- Rupture between extensor retinaculum and insertion onto medial first cuneiform and adjacent base first metatarsal

IMAGING FINDINGS

General Features
- Best diagnostic clue: Tendinous gap
- Location
  - Between superior and inferior extensor retinaculum
  - 1.5-3 cm proximal to insertion site
- Size
  - Variable based on retraction of torn tendon deep to superior slip of inferior extensor retinaculum
  - Retraction limited to level of ankle joint secondary to inferior extensor retinaculum
- Morphology
  - High grade partial to complete tear (normal width 1 cm)
  - Mass secondary to protrusion of proximal tendon above inferior retinaculum

MR Findings
- T1WI
  - Enlarged tendon and sheath
  - Intermediate signal intensity in tendinous gap
  - Variable increased signal intensity (intermediate) in frayed tendon ends
  - Partial tendon continuity with preserved hypointense tendon fibers in high grade partial tear
  - Absence of tendon at tear site
  - Associated dorsal osteophyte in ruptures at medial tarsometatarsal joint
- T2WI
  - Partial tear: Focal enlargement with high grade discontinuity, hyperintense on FS PD or T2 FSE
  - Complete rupture: Hyperintense fluid filled gap with proximal tendon retraction
  - Hyperintense fluid within tendon sheath
  - Absent tendon at tear site (empty sheath)
  - Inhomogeneity of associated hemorrhage
- T1 C+
  - Enhancement of tendon ends
  - Enhancement of inflamed sheath

Imaging Recommendations
- Best imaging tool: MR imaging provides greater soft tissue resolution and contrast relative to CT
- Protocol advice
  - FS PD FSE in axial and sagittal planes required

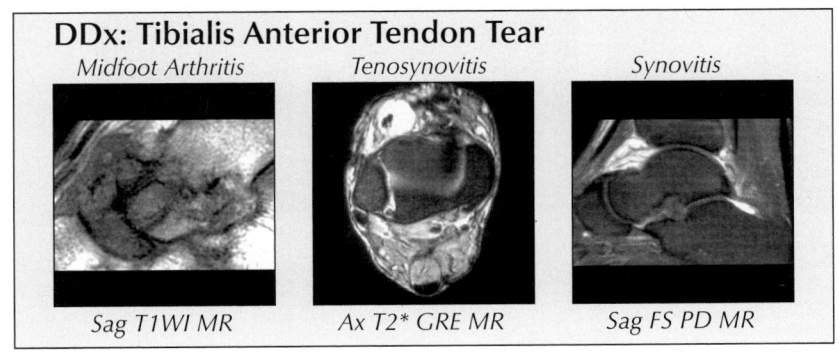

DDx: Tibialis Anterior Tendon Tear

Midfoot Arthritis	Tenosynovitis	Synovitis
Sag T1WI MR	Ax T2* GRE MR	Sag FS PD MR

6

18

TIBIALIS ANTERIOR TENDON TEAR

Key Facts

Imaging Findings
- Best diagnostic clue: Tendinous gap
- Between superior and inferior extensor retinaculum
- Absent tendon at tear site (empty sheath)
- Supplement with oblique axial images perpendicular to tendon at level of medial malleolus

Top Differential Diagnoses
- Partial Tear Versus Complete Tear
- Peroneal Nerve Palsy
- Midfoot Arthritis
- Tenosynovitis
- Tibiotalar Synovitis

Pathology
- Spontaneous rupture is rare
- Forceful contraction against forced plantar flexed foot

- Inferior edge of extensor retinaculum as abrading surface
- Spontaneous rupture associated with diabetes, gout and rheumatoid arthritis
- Dorsal exostosis

Clinical Issues
- Most common signs/symptoms: Weakness with attempted dorsiflexion
- Local tenderness and foot drop
- Palpable mass and/or defect
- Age: Spontaneous rupture - over 45 yrs. (usually > 60)
- Mechanical irritation

Diagnostic Checklist
- Differentiate partial vs. complete rupture using axial and coronal oblique images

---

- ○ Supplement with oblique axial images perpendicular to tendon at level of medial malleolus
- ○ Oblique coronal images parallel to long axis

DIFFERENTIAL DIAGNOSIS

Partial Tear Versus Complete Tear
- Axial oblique and coronal oblique images required

Peroneal Nerve Palsy
- Extensor hallucis longus + extensor digitorum longus innervated by deep peroneal nerve
- Peroneus longus + brevis innervated by superficial peroneal nerve

Midfoot Arthritis
- Sclerosis
- Erosions
- Osteophytes

Tenosynovitis
- Hyperintense fluid surrounding tendon

Tibiotalar Synovitis
- Intermediate to hyperintense inhomogeneity in anterior joint capsule

PATHOLOGY

General Features
- General path comments
  - ○ Tendon inserts onto medial cuneiform
  - ○ Dorsiflexor of the ankle
  - ○ Invertor of subtalar + metatarsal joint
  - ○ Blood supply exclusively from anterior tibial artery - at risk for ischemia
  - ○ Musculotendinous junction at level of mid to distal third of tibia (tendinosis rare finding at surgery)
- Etiology
  - ○ Spontaneous rupture is rare
  - ○ Plantar flexion places eccentric stress on tibialis anterior

- ○ Repetitive dorsiflexion and plantar flexion
- ○ Forceful contraction against forced plantar flexed foot
- ○ Rupture proximal to insertion however no zone of hypovascularity documented
- ○ Inferior edge of extensor retinaculum as abrading surface
- ○ Steroid injections predispose to rupture
- ○ Spontaneous rupture associated with diabetes, gout and rheumatoid arthritis
- Epidemiology: 1% of muscle + tendon injuries

Gross Pathologic & Surgical Features
- Tendon retraction
- Mass effect produced secondary to tendon protrusion relative to inferior extensor retinaculum
- Secondary inflammation of adjacent tendon sheaths
- Hemorrhage
- Empty tendon sheath
- Dorsal exostosis

Microscopic Features
- Peritenonitis inflammatory changes
- Lack of intrinsic tendon degeneration

CLINICAL ISSUES

Presentation
- Most common signs/symptoms: Weakness with attempted dorsiflexion
- Clinical profile
  - ○ Local tenderness and foot drop
  - ○ Palpable mass and/or defect
  - ○ Initial symptoms may be minimal

Demographics
- Age: Spontaneous rupture - over 45 yrs. (usually > 60)
- Gender: Male athletes: Runners, soccer players, hikers
- Activity
  - ○ Related to eccentric contraction during midfoot and forefoot forced plantar flexion
  - ○ Mechanical irritation
    - ▪ Ski boots and hockey skates

TIBIALIS ANTERIOR TENDON TEAR

Natural History & Prognosis
- Diagnosis frequently delayed
- Critical history may be related to minor injury
- Association with chronic rupture tibialis posterior tendon
- History of steroid injections
- Avulsion fracture medial cuneiform
- Initially patients adapt gait to compensate
- Foot slapping
- Dragging toes
- Inability to heel walk
- Eversion of foot with active dorsiflexion
  - Engaged extensor hallucis longus and extensor digitorum longus
- Complications
  - Progressive flat foot deformity in older patients
  - Equinocavus deformity and Achilles tendon contracture in children

Treatment
- Conservative
  - Displacement of tendons < 5 mm ± osseous fragments
  - Less active or older population treated with below knee non-weight bearing cast
- Surgical
  - Young and active population within 3 to 4 months of injury
  - End-to-end repair
  - Sliding tendon graft + extension hallucis transfer
  - Tendon grafts if increased tendon gap (use of extensor digitorum longus, free peroneus brevis for tendon lengthening)

DIAGNOSTIC CHECKLIST

Consider
- Differentiate partial vs. complete rupture using axial and coronal oblique images

SELECTED REFERENCES
1. Aydingoz U et al: Spontaneous rupture of the tibialis anterior tendon in a patient with psoriasis. Clin Imaging 26(3):209-11, 2002
2. Lohman M et al: MRI abnormalities of foot and ankle in asymptomatic, physically active individuals. Skeletal Radiol 30(2):61-6, 2001
3. Banks AS et al: McGlamry's comprehensive textbook of foot and ankle surgery. vol 1. 3rd ed. Philadelphia, Lippincott Williams & Wilkins, 1683-705, 2001
4. Maganaris CN: In vivo measurement-based estimations of the moment arm in the human tibialis anterior muscle-tendon unit. J Biomech 33(3):375-9, 2000
5. Myerson M: Foot and ankle disorders. vol 2. Philadelphia, W.B. Saunders Company, 942-71, 2000
6. Jacobson JA: Musculoskeletal sonography and MR imaging. A role for both imaging methods. Radiol Clin North Am 37(4):712-35, 1999
7. Khoury NJ et al: Rupture of the anterior tibial tendon: Diagnosis by MR imaging. AJR 167:351, 1996
8. Aerts P et al: Abnormalities of the foot and ankle: MR imaging findings. Am J Roentgenol (165):119-24, 1995
9. Brandser EA et al: Tendon injuries: Application of magnetic resonance imaging. Can Assoc Radiol J 46:9-18, 1995
10. Ouzounian TJ et al: Anterior tibial tendon rupture. Foot Ankle 16:406, 1995
11. Bernstein RM: Spontaneous rupture of the tibialis anterior tendon. Am J Orthop 24(4):354-6, 1995
12. Barnett T et al: Anterior tibial tendon rupture. Contemp Orthop 23(4):365-7, 1991
13. Mensor MC et al: Traumatic subcutaneous rupture of the tibialis anterior tendon. J Bone Joint Surg Am 35(30):675-80, 1953
14. Moberg E: Subcutaneous rupture of the tendon of the tibialis anterior muscle. Acta Chir Scand 95:455-60, 1947
15. Lapidus PW: Indirect subcutaneous rupture of the anterior tibial tendon. Bull Hosp Joint Dis Orthop Inst 2:119-27, 1941
16. Burman MS: Subcutaneous rupture of the tendon of the tibialis anticus. Ann Surg 100:368-72, 1934

IMAGE GALLERY

Typical

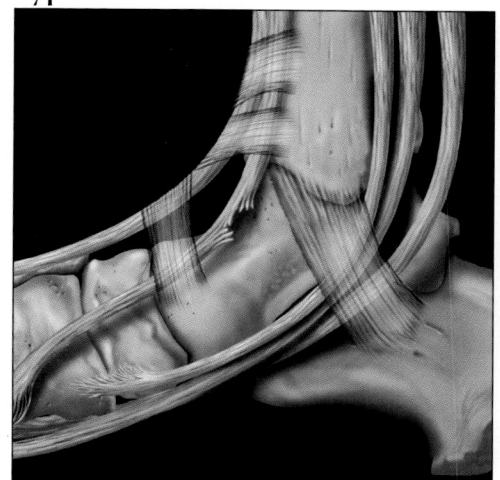
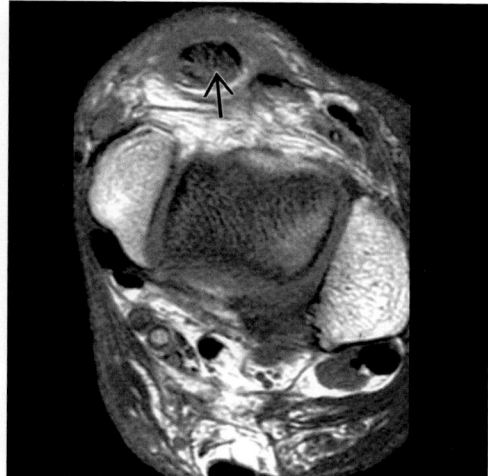

(Left) Sagittal graphic shows partial tear of the tibialis anterior tendon (posterior surface). *(Right)* Axial FS PD FSE MR shows partial tear (arrow) of tibialis anterior tendon with enlargement of cross sectional diameter.

Variant

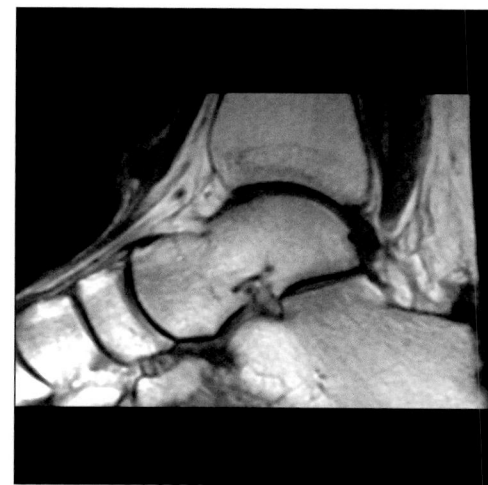
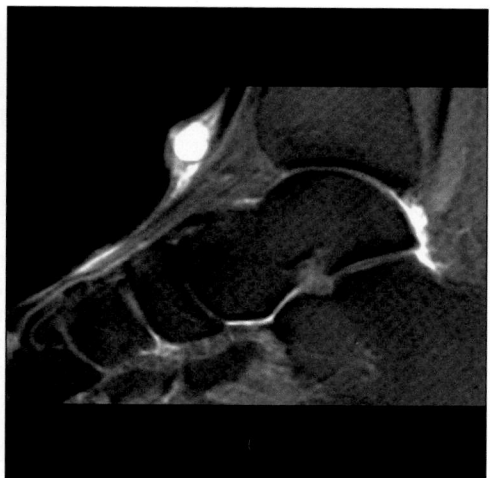

(Left) Sagittal T1WI MR shows hypointense ganglion associated with tibialis anterior tendon sheath. *(Right)* Sagittal FS PD FSE MR shows hyperintense ganglion anterior to tibialis anterior tendon in the absence of tendon fiber disruption.

Variant

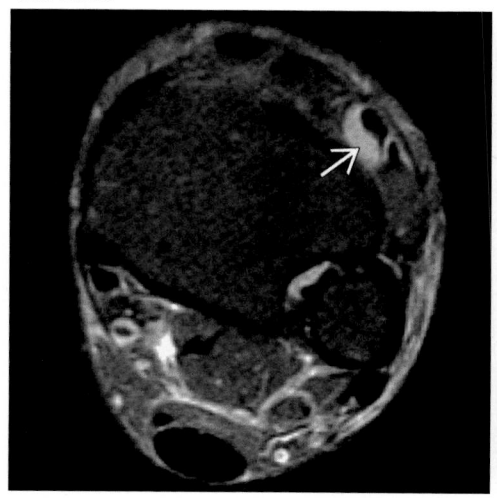
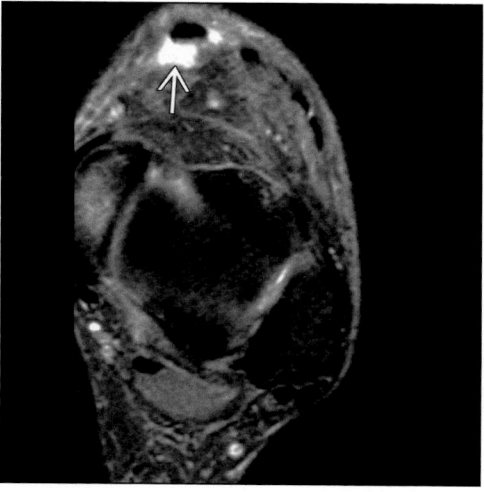

(Left) Axial FS PD FSE MR shows hyperintense tenosynovitis of the more laterally located extensor digitorum longus tendon (arrow). This could be mistaken for clinical symptoms of tibialis anterior dysfunction. *(Right)* Axial FS PD FSE MR shows tenosynovitis (arrow) of the tibialis anterior as hyperintense signal secondary to a traumatic eccentric overload stress.

PERONEUS BREVIS TENDON TEAR

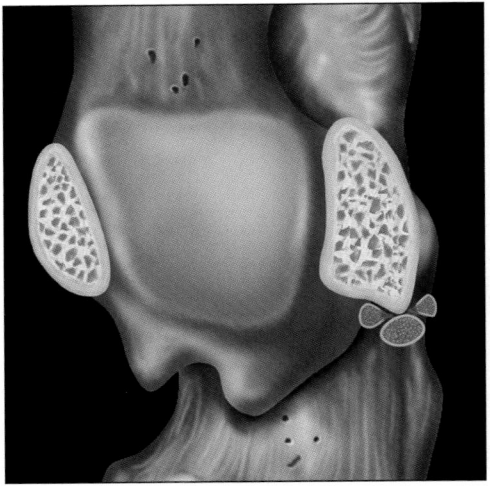

Axial graphic shows split peroneus brevis tendon posterior to the lateral malleolus.

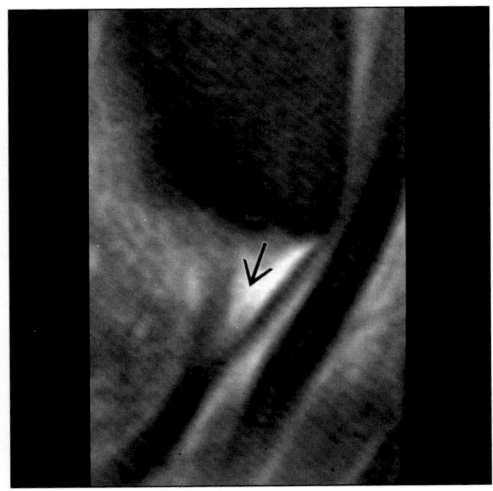

Sagittal FS PD FSE MR shows anterolateral subluxation of split (arrow) peroneus brevis tendon immediately distal to the lateral malleolus.

TERMINOLOGY

Abbreviations and Synonyms
- Peroneus brevis split tear; peroneus brevis split syndrome

Definitions
- Longitudinal split tear within tendon substance
- Division of tendon into two subtendons

IMAGING FINDINGS

General Features
- Best diagnostic clue: Split of peroneus brevis tendon into two subtendons
- Location
  - Centered at retrofibular groove near distal tip lateral malleolus
  - Tear extends distally or proximally or both directions
- Size: Longitudinal tears 2.5 to 5 cm in length
- Morphology: C-shaped split configuration relative to peroneus longus

MR Findings
- T1WI
  - Hypointense subtendons
  - Irregular contour
  - Decrease in cross sectional diameter
  - Anteroposterior separation of split components of tendon
  - Peroneus longus tendon may interpose between two subtendons of brevis
  - Intermediate signal in degenerative tendon
- T2WI
  - Fluid hyperintense in association with tenosynovitis
  - Associated sprain with discontinuity or laxity of superior peroneal retinaculum and/or lateral ligamentous complex
  - Hyperintense fluid between split subtendons
  - Clefts within tendon
  - Split brevis tendon wraps around longus tendon
  - Attenuated tendons without subtendons in partial tears

Imaging Recommendations
- Best imaging tool: MR preferred over ultrasound
- Protocol advice: FS PD FSE and T1 or PD axial and sagittal images to detect longitudinal splits (secondary visualization on coronal images)

DIFFERENTIAL DIAGNOSIS

Peroneal Tenosynovitis
- Hyperintense fluid with tendon cleft (T2WI)
- May be associated with tendon degeneration

DDx: Peroneous Brevis Tendon Tear

Tenosynovitis	PVNS	Calcaneal Fx	Retinaculum Tear	Os Peroneum Abn.

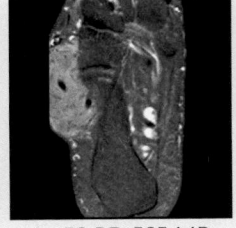
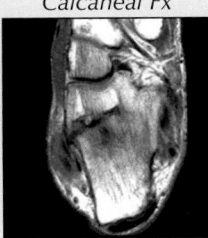
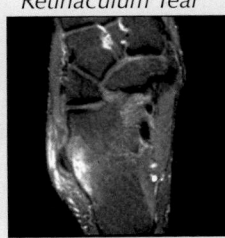
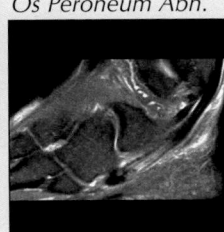

Sag FS PD MR	Ax FS PD FSE MR	Ax T1WI MR	Ax FS PD FSE MR	Sag FS PD MR

PERONEUS BREVIS TENDON TEAR

Key Facts

Imaging Findings
- Best diagnostic clue: Split of peroneus brevis tendon into two subtendons
- Centered at retrofibular groove near distal tip lateral malleolus
- Morphology: C-shaped split configuration relative to peroneus longus
- Peroneus longus tendon may interpose between two subtendons of brevis

Top Differential Diagnoses
- Peroneal Tenosynovitis
- Synovitis
- Anterolateral Ankle Instability
- Fractures
- Painful Os Peroneum Syndrome

Clinical Issues
- Most common signs/symptoms: Chronic ankle pain
- Edema within peroneal sheath
- Popping and clicking with active foot eversion
- Pain with peroneal compression test (compression of longus against brevis)
- Peroneal tendon instability with disruption of superior peroneal retinaculum

Diagnostic Checklist
- Split tendon syndrome may be part of lateral ligamentous injury complex
- Identify any disruption or laxity of superior peroneal retinaculum and associated tendon instability

---

Synovitis
- Hyperintense fluid and intermediate signal intensity synovium (T2WI)
- Pigmented villonodular synovitis (PVNS)

Anterolateral Ankle Instability
- Anterior talofibular ± calcaneofibular ligament tear

Fractures
- Distal fibula
- Lateral process talus
- Anterior process calcaneus
- Fifth metatarsal base
- Lateral calcaneal fracture

Retinacular Tear
- Complete brevis rupture may be associated with reactive calcaneal marrow edema at lateral attachment of inferior peroneal retinaculum (peroneal tubercle)
- Associated subluxation or dislocation of peroneal tendons with brevis displaced anterolaterally
  - Stripping of periosteum with superior peroneal retinaculum

Painful Os Peroneum Syndrome
- Displacement or fracture of os peroneum may be associated with peroneus longus dysfunction
- Associated peroneus longus tear

PATHOLOGY

General Features
- General path comments
  - Relevant anatomy and function
    - Peroneal tendons are lateral stabilizers of the ankle joint
    - Brevis contributes to eversion
    - Brevis and longus share a common synovial sheath posterior to lateral malleolus
    - Brevis located anterior to longus in retrofibular groove

- Superior peroneal retinaculum (restrains tendon subluxation or dislocation) inserts into medial and lateral ridges of the tendon sulcus
- Distal to lateral malleolus, brevis tendon is above calcaneal peroneal tubercle in osseoaponeurotic canal formed by inferior peroneal retinaculum
- Close relationship of calcaneofibular ligament (CFL) + common peroneal tendon sheath
- Etiology
  - Overuse syndrome with repetitive trauma
  - Chronic injury
  - Mechanical friction and shearing injury induces degeneration
  - Degenerative changes precede longitudinal splits
  - Dynamic injury associated with CFL sprain
  - Shallow fibular groove
  - Superior peroneal retinacular laxity
  - Lateral ligament tears and laxity of superior peroneal retinaculum leads to split and tendon subluxation
  - Anatomic factors
    - Hypertrophic fibular ridge
    - Peroneus quartus
    - Accessory or anomalous peroneal tendon
  - Calcaneal friction associated with entrapment or tear
- Epidemiology
  - Spontaneous ruptures less common than traumatic
  - Partial tears more common than complete

Gross Pathologic & Surgical Features
- Synovial proliferation
- Degenerative tendon
- Longitudinal split
- Frayed tendon

Microscopic Features
- Disruption of fibrillar arrangement
- Inflammation tendon sheath
- Mucoid tendon degeneration
- Increased vascular and fibroblastic growth

Staging, Grading or Classification Criteria
- Grade I: < 50% cross sectional tendon area
- Grade II: > 50% cross sectional tendon area

PERONEUS BREVIS TENDON TEAR

CLINICAL ISSUES

Presentation
- Most common signs/symptoms: Chronic ankle pain
- Clinical profile
  - Insidious onset
  - Edema within peroneal sheath
  - Popping and clicking with active foot eversion
  - Subclinical subluxation
  - Crepitus
  - Pain with peroneal compression test (compression of longus against brevis)

Demographics
- Age: Young adults for spontaneous rupture and athletic trauma; older adults for degenerative tendon splits
- Gender: Soccer players with indirect and direct trauma without sex bias

Natural History & Prognosis
- Peroneal tendon instability with disruption of superior peroneal retinaculum
- Progression of tendon fissuring
- Frank tendon rupture
- Concomitant involvement of peroneus longus
- Stenosing tenosynovitis

Treatment
- Conservative
  - Limited immobilization
  - Antiinflammatory medications
  - Physical therapy
  - Orthotics
- Surgical
  - Primary anastomosis
  - Tendon debridement
  - Excision tenosynovial inflammation

DIAGNOSTIC CHECKLIST

Consider
- Split tendon syndrome may be part of lateral ligamentous injury complex
- Identify any disruption or laxity of superior peroneal retinaculum and associated tendon instability

SELECTED REFERENCES

1. Fitzgerald RA et al: Orthopaedics. St Louis MO, Mosby, (39):942-71, 2002
2. Banks AS et al: McGlamry's comprehensive textbook of foot and ankle surgery. vol 1. 3rd ed. Philadelphia PA, Lippincott Williams and Wilkins, (33):1091-152, 2001
3. Myerson MS: Foot and ankle disorders. vol 2. Philadelphia PA, WB Saunders, (39):942-71, 2000
4. DIGiovanni BF et al: Associated injuries found in chronic lateral ankle instability. Foot Ankle Int 21(10):809-15, 2000
5. Major NM et al: The MR imaging appearance of longitudinal split tears of the peroneus brevis tendon. Foot Ankle Int 21(6): 514-9, 2000
6. Rademaker J et al: Tear of the peroneus longus tendon: MR imaging features in nine patients. Radiology 214(3):700-4, 2000
7. Rosenberg ZS et al: MR features of longitudinal tears of the peroneus brevis tendon. AJR 168:141-7, 1997
8. Schweitzer ME et al: Using MR imaging to differentiate peroneal splits from other peroneal disorders. AJR 168:129-33, 1997
9. Tjin A et al: MR imaging of peroneal tendon disorders. AJR 168:134-40, 1997
10. Khoury NJ et al: Peroneus longus and brevis tendon tears: MR imaging evaluation. Radiol 200:833, 1996
11. Geppert MJ et al: Lateral ankle instability as a cause of superior peroneal retinacular laxity: An anatomic and biomechanical study of cadaveric feet. Foot Ankle 14:330, 1993
12. Mink JH et al: MRI of the foot and ankle. New York, Raven Press 160-171, 1993
13. Link SC et al: MR imaging of the ankle and foot: Normal structures and anatomic variants that simulate disease. AJR 607-12, 1993
14. Munk RL et al: Longitudinal rupture of the peroneus brevis tendon. J Trauma 803-6, 1976
15. Eckert WR et al: Acute rupture of the peroneal retinaculum. J Bone Joint Surg 670-3, 1976

PERONEUS BREVIS TENDON TEAR

Typical

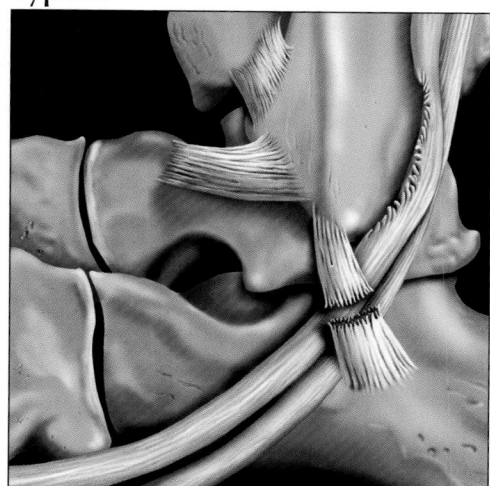
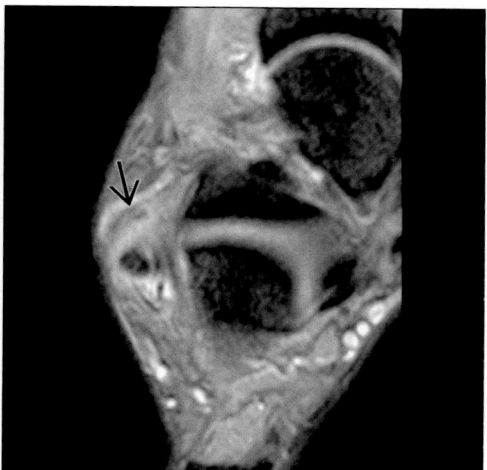

(Left) Sagittal graphic shows peroneus brevis tendon tear with frayed tendon posterior to the lateral malleolus. Associated lateral subluxation of peroneus brevis is identified. *(Right)* Axial FS PD FSE MR shows split peroneus brevis tendon (arrow) anterior to normal hypointense peroneus longus tendon. Fluid signal is hyperintense.

Typical

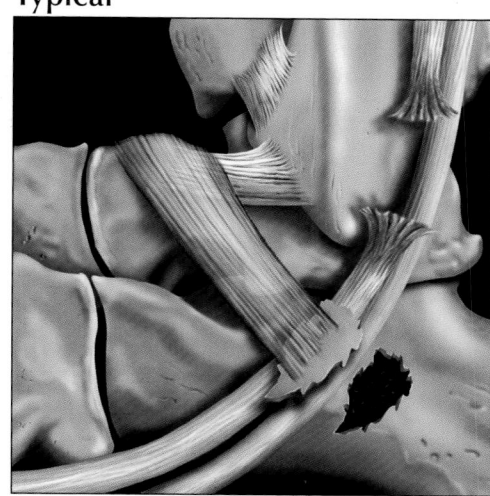
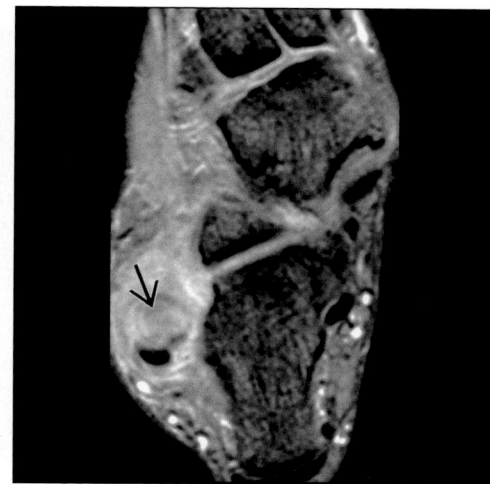

(Left) Sagittal graphic shows complete rupture of peroneus brevis tendon with avulsion of the inferior peroneal retinaculum. Osseous avulsion of calcaneal fragment from the inferior peroneal tubercle is shown attached to the inferior retinaculum. *(Right)* Axial FS PD FSE MR shows complete rupture (arrow) of the peroneus brevis tendon.

Variant

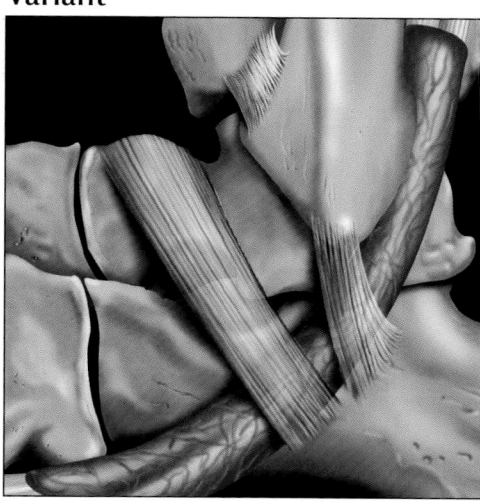
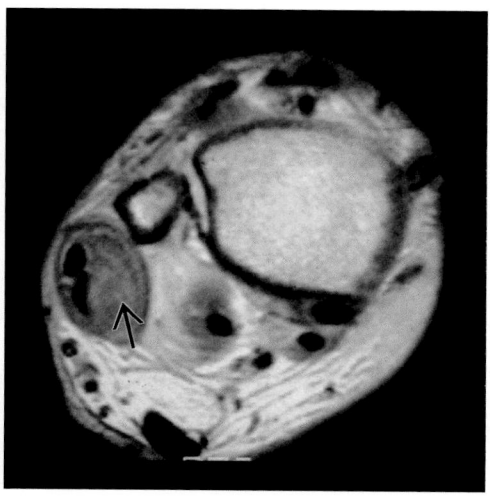

(Left) Sagittal graphic shows chronic stenosing tenosynovitis of the peroneal tendons. Thickened and chronically inflamed tendon sheath in red. *(Right)* Axial PD MR shows chronic stenosing tenosynovitis with intermediate signal granulation tissue encasing (arrow) the peroneus brevis and longus tendons.

ANTERIOR TALOFIBULAR LIGAMENT TEAR

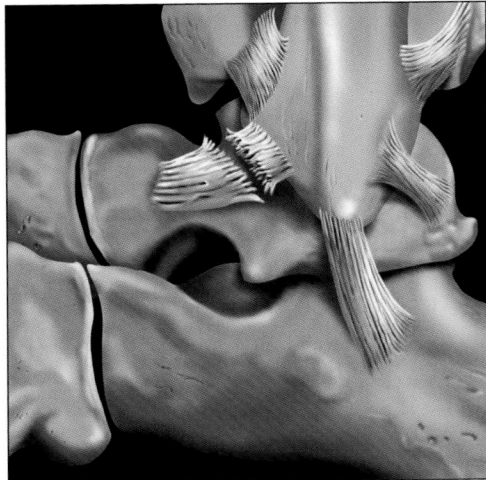

Sagittal graphic shows tear of the ATFL.

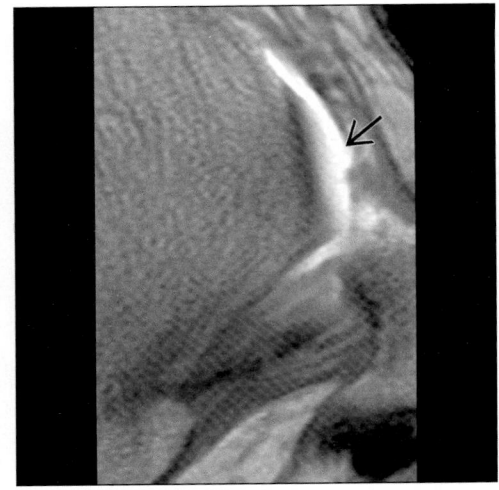

Axial T1 C+ MR (intraarticular contrast) shows complete tear (arrow) and absence of the ATFL.

TERMINOLOGY

Abbreviations and Synonyms
- Anterior talofibular ligament (ATFL) tear; anterior talofibular ligament sprain or injury

Definitions
- Partial to complete disruption of anterior talofibular ligament fibers

IMAGING FINDINGS

General Features
- Best diagnostic clue: Loss of normal ligament morphology and/or continuity
- Location
  - Along course of ligament from anterior border lateral malleolus to its talar insertion anterior to lateral articular facet
  - Midsubstance rupture or a talar avulsion
- Size
  - Interstitial involvement, avulsion to complete ligamentous disruption of both larger upper and smaller lower band
  - ATFL: 5 mm width + 12 mm length
- Morphology
  - Partial or complete ligament interruption
  - Ligament laxity
  - Thickening (acute + chronic) or attenuation (chronic) of ligament fibers
  - Irregularity of ligament contours

Radiographic Findings
- Radiography
  - Avulsion fracture distal fibula
  - Stress radiographs
    - Anterior drawer test: Test for ATFL rupture with > 4 mm anterior displacement of talus relative to tibia
    - Stress inversion test: Test for combined ATFL and calcaneofibular ligament injury using talar tilt comparison
    - Stress applied to plantar flexed talus to evaluate ATFL function

MR Findings
- T1WI
  - Change from hypointense to intermediate signal intensity
  - Interruption of a segment or entire ligament
  - Blurring of anterior + posterior ligament margins on T1WI
  - Acute injuries with thickening of ligament or absence of ligament on T1WI

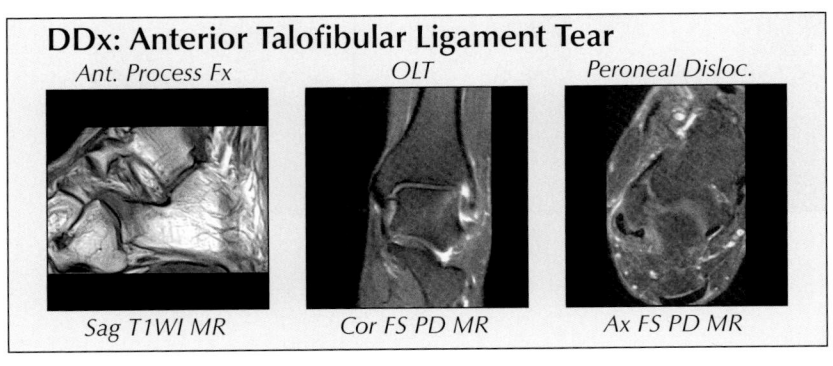

DDx: Anterior Talofibular Ligament Tear

Ant. Process Fx	OLT	Peroneal Disloc.
Sag T1WI MR	Cor FS PD MR	Ax FS PD MR

ANTERIOR TALOFIBULAR LIGAMENT TEAR

Key Facts

Imaging Findings

- Best diagnostic clue: Loss of normal ligament morphology and/or continuity
- Interstitial involvement, avulsion to complete ligamentous disruption of both larger upper and smaller lower band
- Blurring of anterior + posterior ligament margins on T1WI
- Acute injuries with thickening of ligament or absence of ligament on T1WI

Top Differential Diagnoses

- Stress Fracture
- Anterior Process Fracture Calcaneus
- Osteochondral Lesion of the Talus (OLT)
- Peroneal Tendon Dysfunction

Pathology

- Inversion + internal rotation & plantar flexion
- Grade I: ATFL stretching
- Grade II: ATFL partial tear with stretching of CFL
- Grade III: Complete tear ATFL and CFL

Clinical Issues

- Most common signs/symptoms: Pain + swelling lateral ankle
- ATFL tenderness
- Pop followed by pain + swelling in acute grade III

Diagnostic Checklist

- Use T1WI or PDWI to increase sensitivity for grade I + II ankle sprains

---

- o Chronic instability associated with attenuated or hypoplastic ligament with sharper, more defined ligament margins
- o Reinjury with continued stress may produce ligament hyperplasia
- o Avulsed ligament ± distal fibula avulsion fracture
- T2WI
  - o Hyperintensity of ATFL along its course in a 45° angle from lateral malleolus to talus
  - o Associated capsular rupture
  - o Extension of hyperintense fluid anterolaterally into soft tissues
  - o Acute tears associated with partial to complete absence of ligament
  - o Subacute to chronic tears may be hyperintense with only mild residual thickening
  - o Intermediate to hyperintense inflamed synovium
  - o Inhomogeneity + hypointense hemosiderin associated with hemorrhage
  - o Hyperintense soft tissue edema adjacent to anterolateral gutter
  - o Bone marrow edema distal fibular or talar insertion
  - o Hyperintense fluid in tibiotalar effusion and adjacent tendon sheaths (peroneal tendons)

Imaging Recommendations

- Best imaging tool: MRI superior for extent of injury, chronicity + acute ligamentous defects
- Protocol advice
  - o Requires axial T1 or PD and FS PD FSE images
  - o Secondary ligament visualization in lateral sagittal images + coronal images

DIFFERENTIAL DIAGNOSIS

Stress Fracture

- Navicular
- Metatarsal
- Mimics grade I injuries clinically

Anterior Process Fracture Calcaneus

- Identified on lateral sagittal images adjacent to calcaneocuboid joint

Lateral Process Fracture Talus

- Visualized on coronal images
- Symptoms similar to grade II or III lateral sprain
- Snowboarders fracture

Osteochondral Lesion of the Talus (OLT)

- Lesion medial or lateral talar dome
- Associated with ankle instability

Peroneal Tendon Dysfunction

- Differential for grade II and III sprain
- Displacement peroneus brevis (split) and longus over posterior lateral distal fibula

Fibula Fracture

- May have associated deltoid ligament injury

Calcaneus and Talar Neck Fractures

- Differential for grade III sprain
- Tenderness over medial and lateral calcaneal tuberosity
- Talar neck fracture anterior to tibiotalar joint

PATHOLOGY

General Features

- General path comments
  - o Relevant anatomy
    - ATFL separated into two distinct bands
    - Taut in plantar flexion
    - Lateral collateral ligament complex also includes calcaneofibular ligament (CFL) + posterior talofibular ligament
- Etiology
  - o Inversion + internal rotation & plantar flexion
  - o Loading ball of foot with landing from a jump or fall
  - o Talus moves anteriorly and is unlocked from mortise in ankle plantar flexion

ANTERIOR TALOFIBULAR LIGAMENT TEAR

- ○ ATFL tight in plantar flexion + susceptible to injury vs. CFL which is taut in neutral position
- ○ ATFL weakest of lateral collateral ligaments
- Epidemiology
  - ○ 85% of ankle sprains occur laterally
  - ○ Represents 12% of emergency room trauma
  - ○ 25-50% of lateral sprains occur in running + jumping sports

Gross Pathologic & Surgical Features

- Ligament fiber disruption + hemorrhage
- Anterior displacement talus
- Combined ligament injury with CFL = widening of lateral joint space + medial tilt of talus

Microscopic Features

- Acute injuries with hyperplastic synovial reaction + hemosiderin
- Chronic injury either fibrous ingrowth with hyperplastic ligament vs. hypoplastic ligament

Staging, Grading or Classification Criteria

- Lateral ankle sprains
  - ○ Grade I: ATFL stretching
  - ○ Grade II: ATFL partial tear with stretching of CFL
  - ○ Grade III: Complete tear ATFL and CFL

CLINICAL ISSUES

Presentation

- Most common signs/symptoms: Pain + swelling lateral ankle
- Clinical profile
  - ○ Most common among athletes
  - ○ ATFL tenderness
  - ○ Pop followed by pain + swelling in acute grade III
  - ○ Difficult to bear weight on affected ankle in acute grade II and III
  - ○ Sense of giving way = functional instability
  - ○ Joint instability

Demographics

- Age: 15 to 35 years most common
- Gender
  - ○ Males predominate in 15 to 35 year group
  - ○ Females with higher incidence after 40 years

Natural History & Prognosis

- Scarred ligament with return of biomechanics
- Anterolateral impingement
- Chronic lateral ankle instability

Treatment

- Conservative
  - ○ Early functional rehabilitation for acute injuries beginning with immobilization + range-of-motion exercises
  - ○ Functional CAM walker (controlled ankle motion) for stability + protected weight bearing
- Surgical
  - ○ Acute grade III sprain + chronic lateral ankle instability
  - ○ Primary repair

- ○ Arthroscopy to address impingement + osteochondral lesions
- ○ Evans procedure: Transposition of entire peroneus brevis through distal fibula
- ○ Watson-Jones procedure: Tenodesis of peroneus brevis for single ligament replacement to replace the ATFL
- ○ Bronstrom procedure: Suturing with end-to-end ligament repair
- ○ Modified Bronstrom: Capsular shift
- ○ Bronstrom/Evans: Tenodesis peroneus brevis with fibular tunnel
- ○ Christman-Snook procedure (modification of Elmslie repair, with split peroneus brevis tendon instead of fascia lata): Tenodesis of peroneus brevis for a double ligament replacement of ATFL and CFL

DIAGNOSTIC CHECKLIST

Consider

- Use T1WI or PDWI to increase sensitivity for grade I + II ankle sprains
- Evaluate for associated impingement, osteochondral lesion and other ligament injuries

SELECTED REFERENCES

1. Uys HD et al: Clinical association of acute lateral ankle sprain with syndesmotic involvement: A stress radiography and magnetic resonance imaging study. Am J Sports Med 30(6):816-22, 2002
2. Banks A et al: McGlamry's comprehensive textbook of foot and ankle surgery: Chronic ankle conditions. vol 1. 3rd ed. Philadelphia, Lippincott Williams & Wilkins, 1091-152, 2001
3. Myerson M: Foot and ankle disorders: Injuries about the ankle: Instability of the ankle and subtalar joint. vol 1. Philadelphia, W.B. Saunders, 1399-419, 2000
4. Jordan LK 3rd et al: Magnetic resonance imaging findings in anterolateral impingement of the ankle. Skeletal Radiol 29(1):34-9, 2000
5. Tochigi Y et al: Acute inversion injury of the ankle: Magnetic resonance imaging and clinical outcomes. Foot Ankle Int 19(11):730-4, 1998
6. Colville MR: Reconstruction of the lateral ankle ligaments. J Bone Joint Surg (AM) 76A:1092, 1994
7. Rijke AM et al: MRI of lateral ankle ligaments injuries. AM J Sports Med 21:527, 1994
8. Erickson SJ et al: MR imaging of the lateral collateral ligament of the ankle. AJR 156:131, 1991
9. Kier R et al: MR imaging of the normal ligaments and tendons of the ankle. J Comput Assist Tomogr 15:477-82, 1991
10. Kannus P et al: Treatment for acute tears of the lateral ligaments of the ankle. J Bone Joint Surg 73A:305-12, 1991
11. Beltran J et al: Ligaments of the lateral aspect of the ankle and sinus tarsi: An MR imaging study. Radiology 177:455-8, 1990
12. Kneeland JB et al: MR imaging of the normal ankle: Correlation with anatomic sections. AJR 151:117-23, 1988
13. Hamilton WG: Foot and ankle injuries in dancers. Clin Sports Med 7(1):143-73, 1988
14. Perlman M et al: Inversion lateral ankle trauma: Differential diagnosis, review of the literature, and prospective study. J Foot Surg 26(2):95-133, 1987

ANTERIOR TALOFIBULAR LIGAMENT TEAR

IMAGE GALLERY

Typical

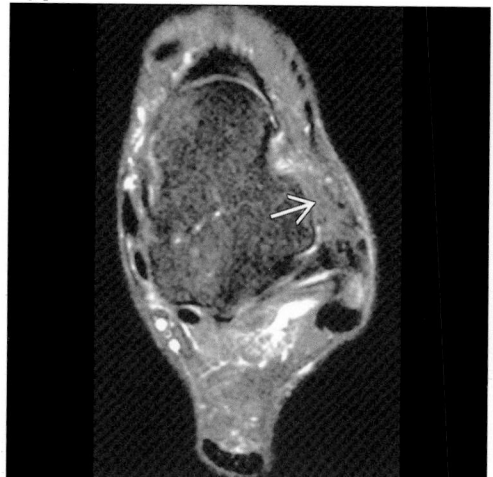
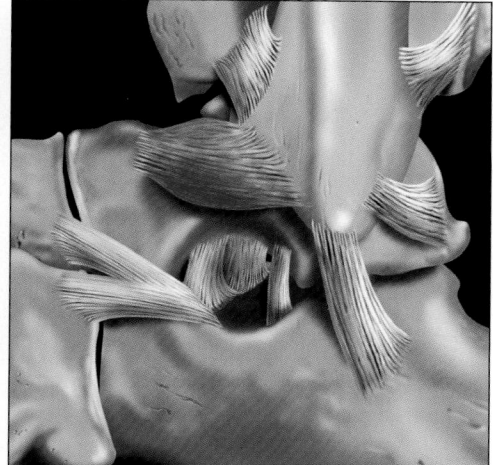

(Left) Axial FS PD FSE MR shows grade II tear (arrow) of the ATFL with ligament thickening and hyperintensity. *(Right)* Sagittal graphic shows chronically thickened ATFL secondary to grade II sprain.

Typical

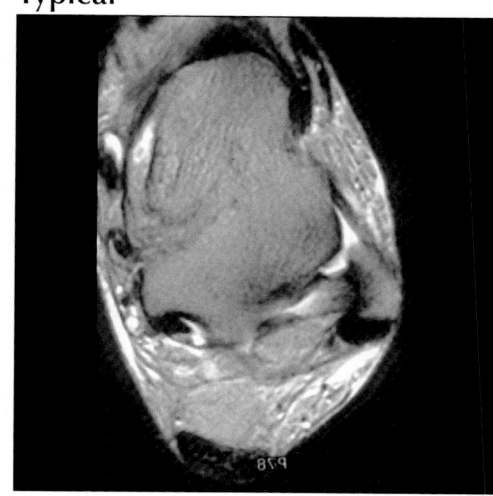
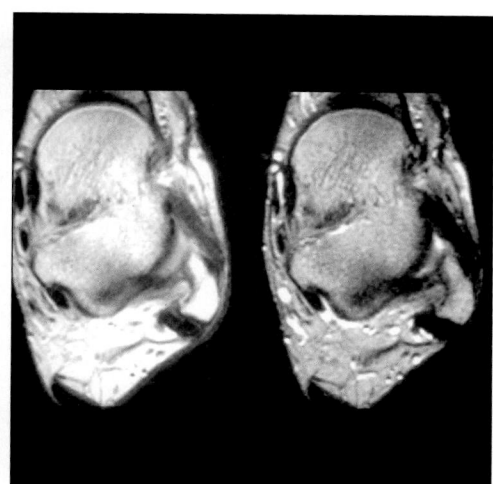

(Left) Axial FS PD FSE MR shows normal morphology of the ATFL with hyperintense fluid in the lateral gutter. *(Right)* Axial T2WI MR showing intermediate signal intensity with increased sensitivity on the first echo (left image) of a dual echo sequence in a chronic grade II ankle sprain. Ligament is hypointense on second echo image (right).

Typical

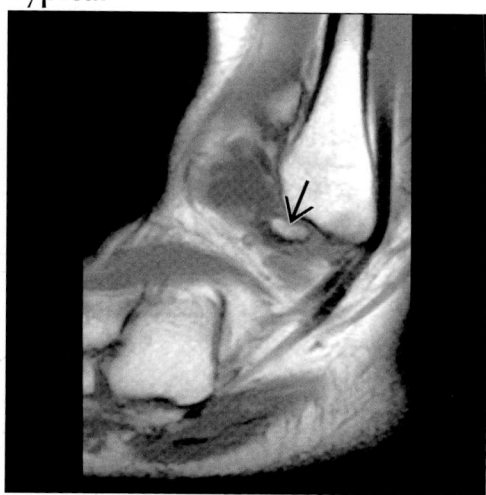
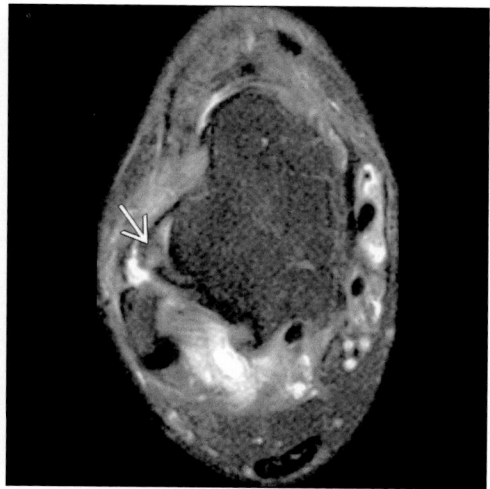

(Left) Sagittal T1WI MR shows edema without normal morphology of the ATFL. Associated marrow containing avulsion fragment (arrow) is present anterior to the lateral malleolus. *(Right)* Axial FS PD FSE MR shows osseous avulsion injury (arrow) with the ATFL attached to the displaced osseous fragment.

CALCANEOFIBULAR LIGAMENT SPRAIN

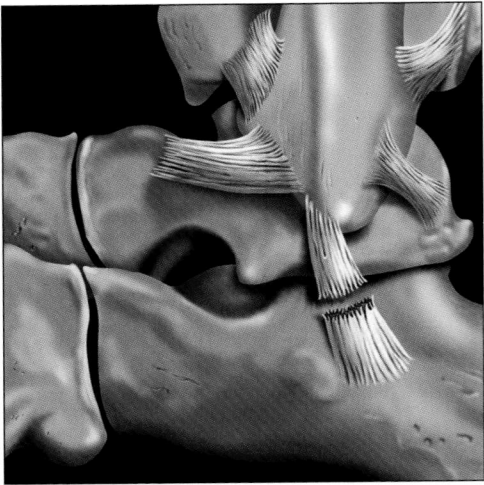

Sagittal graphic shows mid substance tear of the CF ligament.

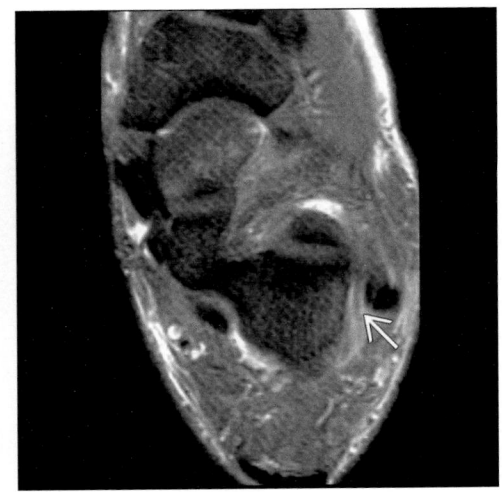

Axial FS PD FSE MR shows attenuated CFL (arrow) with associated hyperintense edema in a grade II ligament sprain.

TERMINOLOGY

Abbreviations and Synonyms
- CFL sprain; calcaneofibular ligament injury

Definitions
- Stretching, partial to complete tear of calcaneofibular ligament (CFL)

IMAGING FINDINGS

General Features
- Best diagnostic clue: Loss of normal ligament morphology associated with hyperintense fluid signal intensity on T2WI
- Location
  - Along course of ligament from distal lateral malleolus to lateral surface of calcaneus
  - Midsubstance rupture complex of both anterior talofibular ligament (ATFL) + CFL + intervening capsule
- Size
  - Cordlike structure
  - 2 cm length/4 to 6 mm diameter
- Morphology
  - Partial or complete ligament interruption
  - Ligament laxity

- Irregular ligament contour
- Attenuated ligament fibers
- Edematous soft tissue mass

Radiographic Findings
- Radiography
  - Stress radiography/talar tilt test
    - Varus stress applied with neutral dorsiflexion of talus to isolate CFL function
    - Talar tilt > 18 degrees associated with rupture of ATFL and CFL
  - Arthrography
    - Leakage of contrast into peroneal tendon sheath up to one week post CFL tear

MR Findings
- T1WI
  - Hypointense to intermediate signal intensity ligament
  - Segmental interruption of ligament
  - Blurring of medial and lateral margins of ligament
  - Absence of ligament
- T2WI
  - Tenosynovitis
  - Hyperintense edema surrounding ligament between calcaneus and peroneal tendons
  - Associated tear of peroneal tendon sheath
  - Attenuated ligament + adjacent edema or hemorrhage

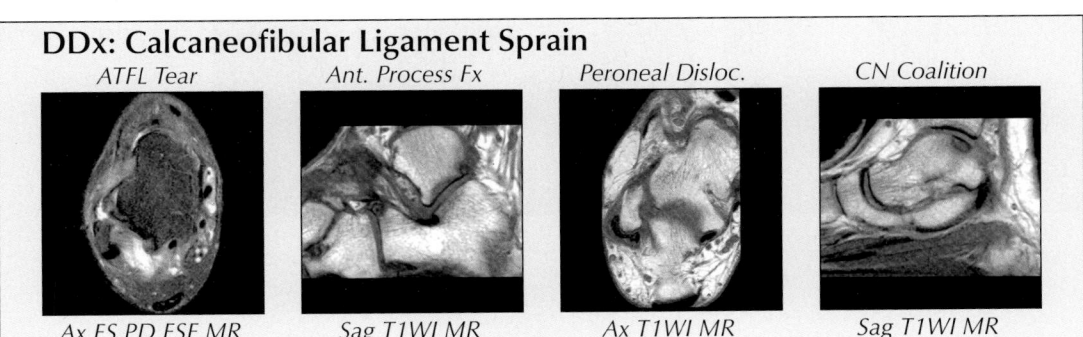

DDx: Calcaneofibular Ligament Sprain

ATFL Tear	Ant. Process Fx	Peroneal Disloc.	CN Coalition
Ax FS PD FSE MR	Sag T1WI MR	Ax T1WI MR	Sag T1WI MR

CALCANEOFIBULAR LIGAMENT SPRAIN

Key Facts

Imaging Findings
- Best diagnostic clue: Loss of normal ligament morphology associated with hyperintense fluid signal intensity on T2WI
- Midsubstance rupture complex of both anterior talofibular ligament (ATFL) + CFL + intervening capsule
- Blurring of medial and lateral margins of ligament

Top Differential Diagnoses
- ATFL Sprain
- Anterior Process Fracture Calcaneus
- Lateral Process Fracture Talus
- Peroneal Tendon Subluxation/Dislocation
- Osteochondral Lesion of Talar Dome

Pathology
- CFL partial or complete tear in combination with complete tear ATFL
- Peroneal retinacular thickening
- Edematous mass or synovial reaction + influx of fluid associated with hemorrhage

Clinical Issues
- Most common signs/symptoms: Pain + swelling lateral ankle
- Tenderness at both ATFL and CFL
- Increased varus tilt of talar dome

Diagnostic Checklist
- CFL sprain as an associated injury with ATFL tear

- ○ Loss of linear or cordlike morphology
- ○ Peroneal retinacular thickening
- ○ Associated peroneal tendon subluxation

Imaging Recommendations
- Best imaging tool
  - ○ MR for acute, subacute and chronic injuries
  - ○ Associated lesions of talar dome, peroneal tendons and subtalar sinus tarsi ligaments visualized on MRI
- Protocol advice: Axial FS PD FSE to visualize ligament deep to peroneal tendons

DIFFERENTIAL DIAGNOSIS

ATFL Sprain
- Pain and tenderness anterior to CFL

Anterior Process Fracture Calcaneus
- Pain isolated to anterior process inferior and distal to sinus tarsi

Lateral Process Fracture Talus
- Snowboarder's fracture
- Tender distal to tip of fibula

Peroneal Tendon Subluxation/Dislocation
- Pain posterior border fibula

Osteochondral Lesion of Talar Dome
- Tibiotalar pain referred medial or laterally + osteochondral fracture

Lisfranc Sprain
- Midfoot dorsal tenderness base of first and second metatarsals

Fracture Base of Fifth Metatarsal
- Pain, swelling and tenderness distal and inferior to ATFL and CFL

Subtalar Coalition
- Direct visualization with MRI for talocalcaneal or calcaneonavicular coalition (CN coalition)

Bifurcate Ligament Sprain
- Associated with plantar flexion-inversion mechanism
- ± Anterior process fracture calcaneus

Fibular Fracture
- Tenderness at osseous fracture site (not over CF ligament)

PATHOLOGY

General Features
- General path comments
  - ○ Relevant anatomy and function
    - CFL crossed superficially by peroneal tendons and their sheaths
    - CFL is extracapsular and stabilizes both tibiotalar and subtalar joints
    - Normal CFL/ATFL angle between 70 and 140 degrees
- Etiology
  - ○ Twisting injuries
  - ○ Dorsiflexion and internal rotation
  - ○ CFL alignment parallel to tibia in neutral dorsiflexion placing CFL at risk for sprain
- Epidemiology
  - ○ CFL second most frequently injured ankle ligament
  - ○ CFL partial or complete tear in combination with complete tear ATFL

Gross Pathologic & Surgical Features
- Ligament fiber disruption and hemorrhage
- Combined ligament injury of ATFL and CFL = widening of lateral joint space + varus tilt of talus
- Peroneal retinacular thickening
- Peroneal tenosynovitis

Microscopic Features
- Edematous mass or synovial reaction + influx of fluid associated with hemorrhage
- Chronic scarring with hypoplastic ligament

CALCANEOFIBULAR LIGAMENT SPRAIN

Staging, Grading or Classification Criteria
- Lateral ankle sprains
  - Grade I = ATFL stretching
  - Grade II = ATFL tear with stretching CFL
  - Grade III = complete tear ATFL and CFL

CLINICAL ISSUES

Presentation
- Most common signs/symptoms: Pain + swelling lateral ankle
- Clinical profile
  - Tenderness at both ATFL and CFL
  - Increased varus tilt of talar dome
  - Unstable ankle in acute grade III injury
  - Grade III sprain associated with pop followed by severe pain + swelling
  - Inability to continue physical activity in severe lateral ankle sprains
  - Ecchymosis

Demographics
- Age: 15 to 35 years most common
- Gender: Males predominate in 15 to 35 year group

Natural History & Prognosis
- Scarred ligament
- Chronic instability with persistent laxity
- History of frequent ankle sprains: Subtalar injury with associated sinus tarsi ligament injury
- Associated injuries include osteochondral lesion + peroneal tendon instability

Treatment
- Conservative
  - Rest, ice, compression, elevation (RICE)
  - Range of motion
  - Protected weight bearing
  - Functional Cam walker for stability
  - Cast immobilization
  - Early mobilization with improved stability
- Surgical
  - Acute grade III sprains or chronic instability
  - Primary repair - acute/subacute disruption
  - Ligament reconstruction - chronic instability: Evans, Watson-Jones, Elmslie, Chrisman and Snook
    - Evans: Transposition of entire peroneus brevis through distal fibula
    - Watson-Jones procedure: Reconstruction with peroneus brevis tenodesis to replace ATFL without anatomic replacement of CFL
    - Modified Watson-Jones: Use of split peroneus longus tendon, split peroneus brevis, plantaris tenodesis (or graft) and split Achilles tenodesis
    - Elmslie-fascia lata graft to replace or augment ATFL and CFL (more anatomic than modified Watson-Jones)
    - Chrisman and Snook-modification of Elmslie repair with split peroneus brevis tendon instead of fascia lata to replace the ATFL and CFL (more anatomic than modified Watson-Jones)
    - Modified Broström repair - primary tendon repair + augmentation using extensor retinaculum

DIAGNOSTIC CHECKLIST

Consider
- CFL sprain as an associated injury with ATFL tear
- Axial T2WI using FS PD or T2 FSE best to visualize status of ligament morphology and adjacent hyperintense edema

SELECTED REFERENCES

1. DeLee JC et al: Orthopaedic sports medicine. Principles and practice. Ligament injuries of the foot and ankle in the athlete. vol 2. 2nd Ed. Philadelphia PA, Saunders, (E):2323-71, 2003
2. Fitzgerald RH et al: Orthopaedics. Ligament injuries of the foot and ankle. St. Louis, Missouri, Mosby Inc, 1607-21, 2002
3. Uys HD et al: Clinical association of acute lateral ankle sprain with syndesmotic involvement: A stress radiography and magnetic resonance imaging study. Am J Sports Med 30(6):816-22, 2002
4. Banks A et al: McGlamry's comprehensive textbook of foot and ankle surgery. Chronic ankle conditions. vol 1. Philadelphia PA, Lippincott Williams & Wilkins (35):1091-152, 2001
5. Kreitner KF et al: Injuries of the lateral collateral ligaments of the ankle: Assessment with MR imaging. Eur Radiol 9(3):519-24, 1999
6. Tochigi Y et al: Acute inversion injury of the ankle: Magnetic resonance imaging and clinical outcomes. Foot Ankle Int 19(11):730-4, 1998
7. Zanetti M et al: Magnetic resonance imaging of injuries to the ankle joint: Can it predict clinical outcome? Skeletal Radiol 26(2):82-8, 1997
8. Nishimura G: Trabecular trauma of the talus and medial malleolus concurrent with lateral collateral ligamentous injuries of the ankle: Evaluation with MR imaging. Skeletal Radiol 25(1):49-54, 1996
9. Chandnani VP et al: Chronic ankle instability: Evaluation with MR arthrography, MR imaging, and stress radiography. Radiology 192(1):189-94, 1994
10. Mink JH et al: MRI of the foot and ankle. Ligaments of the ankle. New York, Raven Press, 173-8, 1992
11. Schneck CD et al: MR imaging of the most commonly injured ankle ligaments. Part I. Normal anatomy. Radiology 499-506, 1992
12. Schneck CD et al: MR imaging of the most commonly injured ankle ligaments. Part II. Ligament injuries. Radiology 507-12, 1992
13. Kannus et al: Treatment for acute tears of the lateral ligaments of the ankle. J Bone Joint Surg 305-12, 1991
14. Erickson SJ et al: MR imaging of the lateral collateral ligament of the ankle. AJR 131-6,1991
15. Kier R et al: MR imaging of the normal ligaments and tendons of the ankle. J Comput Assist Tomogr 477-82, 1991
16. Beltran J et al: Ligaments of the lateral aspect of the ankle and sinus tarsi: An MR imaging study. Radiology 455-8, 1990

CALCANEOFIBULAR LIGAMENT SPRAIN

IMAGE GALLERY

Typical

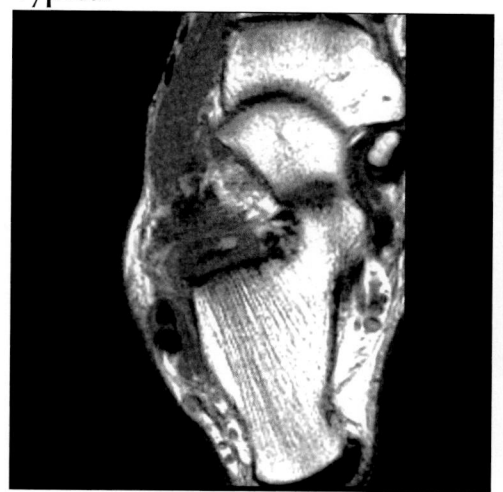 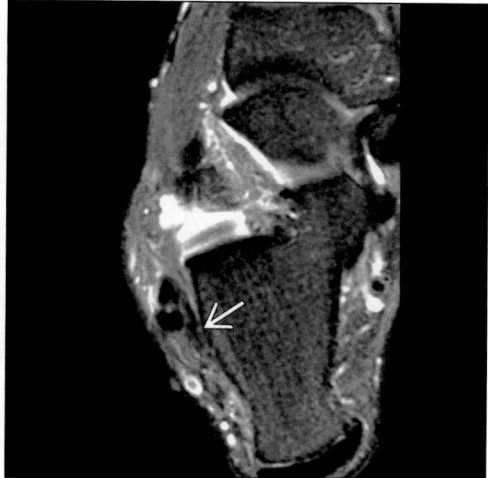

(Left) Axial T1WI MR shows edema associated with CFL sprain deep to the peroneal tendons. (Right) Axial FS PD FSE MR shows intact CFL (arrow) fibers status post grade I sprain.

Typical

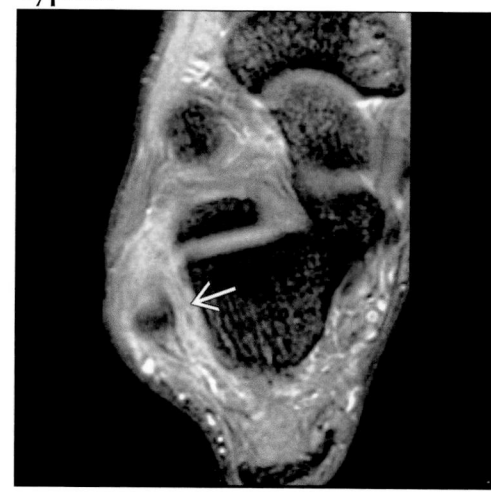 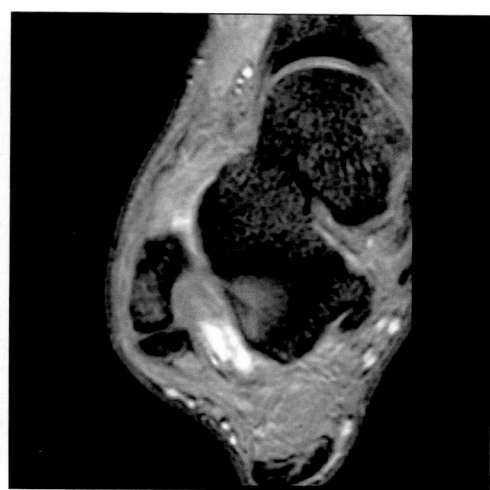

(Left) Axial T2* GRE MR shows absent CFL (arrow) in a severe lateral ligamentous sprain. (Right) Axial T2* GRE MR shows associated lateral ligamentous complex injury with torn ATFL.

Typical

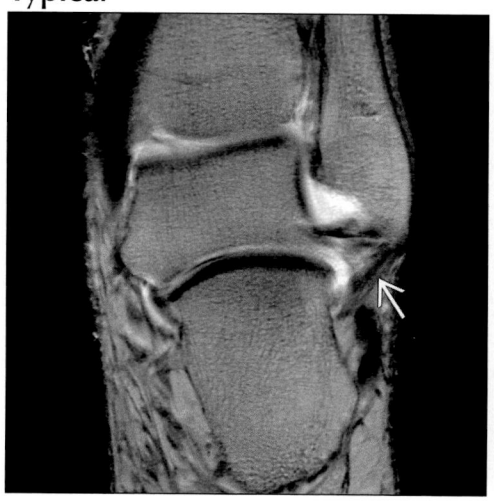 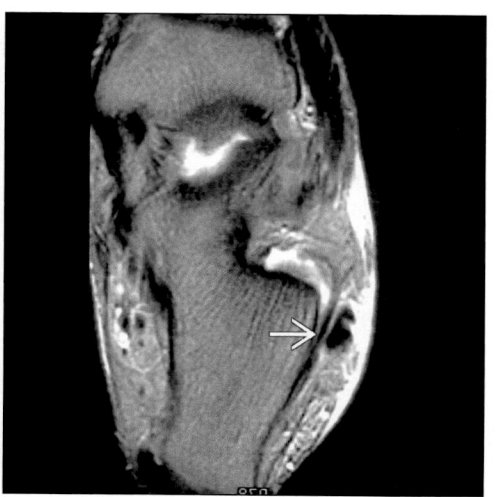

(Left) Coronal T1 C+ MR (intraarticular contrast) shows normal oblique orientation of the CFL (arrow) in the coronal plane. (Right) Axial T1 C+ MR (intraarticular contrast) shows normal linear morphology of CFL (arrow) deep to the peroneus brevis and longus tendons.

DELTOID LIGAMENT SPRAIN

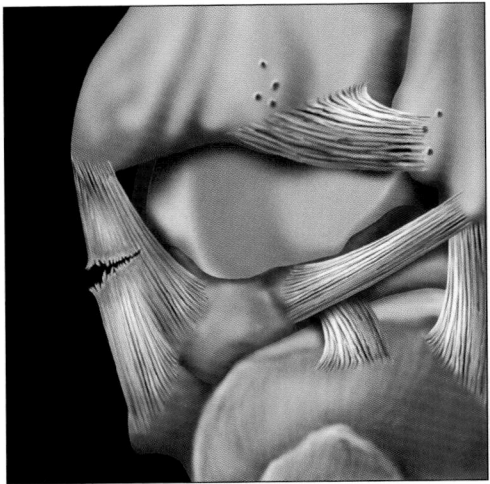

Coronal graphic shows partial tear of the superficial and deep layers of the deltoid ligament.

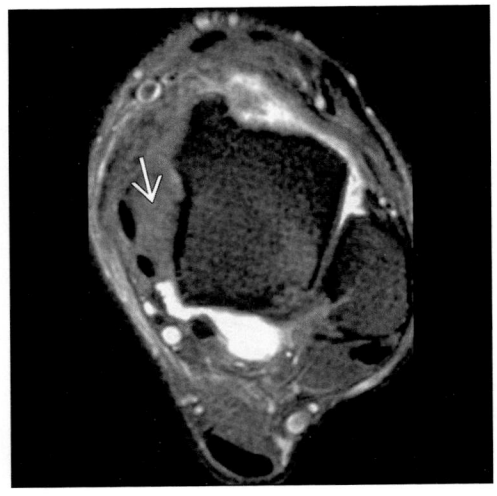

Axial FS PD FSE MR shows hyperintensity and inhomogeneity (arrow) of the deltoid ligament fibers.

TERMINOLOGY

Abbreviations and Synonyms
- Deltoid ligament tear; medial ankle sprain

Definitions
- Partial or complete disruption of deltoid ligaments fibers

IMAGING FINDINGS

General Features
- Best diagnostic clue: Interstitial hyperintensity on T2WI
- Location: Midsubstance close to medial malleolus
- Size
  - Superficial component longer than deep with tibiocalcaneal ligament 2 cm length and 1 cm wide at insertion
  - Deep component shorter with small anterior component + strong posterior talotibial ligament
    - 1.5 cm length, 1.5 cm width and 1.0 cm thickness at origin
- Morphology
  - Superficial layer: Wide triangular ligaments
  - Deep layer: Conical posterior talotibial ligaments

- Complete disruption of fiber morphology with absent ligament less common

Radiographic Findings
- Radiography
  - Weight bearing
  - Associated malleolar fracture
  - Osteochondral lesion
  - Avulsion fracture
  - Deltoid ossification
  - Increased medial clear space
  - Stress radiograph
    - Valgus stress test with anteroposterior radiograph
    - Valgus tilt greater than 2 degrees with deltoid ligament injury
  - Arthrography - not commonly used
    - Leakage at level of medial malleolus in partial deltoid rupture

MR Findings
- T1WI
  - Interstitial intermediate signal intensity
  - Loss of fiber striation
  - Medial malleolus fracture
  - Hypointense medial malleolus subchondral edema
  - Marrow containing ligament ossification
  - Talar displacement laterally or posterolaterally
  - Coronal images to separate superficial from deep layer sprains

DDx: Deltoid Ligament Sprain

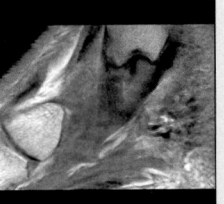
Intact Deltoid

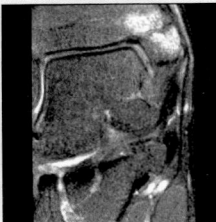
Medial Mall. Fx

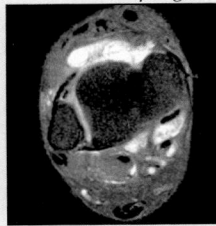
Medial Imping.

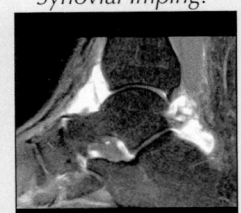
Synovial Imping.

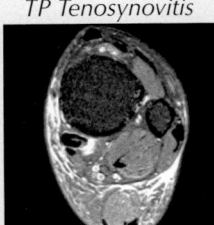
TP Tenosynovitis

Sag T1WI MR   Cor FS PD FSE   Ax FS PD FSE   Sag FS PD MR   Ax FS PD FSE MR

6

34

DELTOID LIGAMENT SPRAIN

Key Facts

Imaging Findings
- Best diagnostic clue: Interstitial hyperintensity on T2WI
- Loss of fiber striation
- Diffuse amorphous hyperintensity on FS PD and T2 FSE
- Mass-like morphology in disruption with associated edema, hemorrhage and granulation tissue

Top Differential Diagnoses
- Normal Deltoid Ligament
- Fracture
- Impingement
- Tibialis Posterior (TP) Tendon Dysfunction

Pathology
- Increased load: Deep deltoid ligament last to fail

- End stage of supination external rotation injury
- Partial tear more common than complete ligamentous disruption

Clinical Issues
- Most common signs/symptoms: Swelling and tenderness over deltoid ligaments + surrounding soft tissue
- Anteromedial or medial pain
- Medial sprains more painful than lateral sprains
- Associated lateral ligamentous injury, fibular fracture and/or syndesmosis injuries

Diagnostic Checklist
- Correlate axial and coronal images to define extent of injury in superficial and deep layers of deltoid

---

- o Loss of detail in individual ligamentous components on medial sagittal image through superficial layer
- o Absence of ligamentous fibers
- o Osseous degenerative change medial malleolar talar articulation
- T2WI
  - o Diffuse amorphous hyperintensity on FS PD and T2 FSE
  - o Indistinct margins and loss of fiber striation especially talotibial (tibiotalar) fibers of deep layer
  - o Axial + coronal images to separate superficial from deep layer sprains
  - o Mass-like morphology in disruption with associated edema, hemorrhage and granulation tissue
  - o Axial FS PD FSE to assess associated tendon and neurovascular structures
  - o Fluid-filled gap in complete disruption
- T1 C+: Useful in peripherally enhancing partial tears, synovi and inflammatory fluid collections

Imaging Recommendations
- Best imaging tool: MR superior to CT and ultrasound
- Protocol advice
  - o Axial T1 or PD and FS PD FSE and coronal FS PD FSE image for partial or complete ligament tears
  - o Superficial layer of deltoid seen on coronal images or on a single medial sagittal image with T1, PD or FS PD FSE sequence

DIFFERENTIAL DIAGNOSIS

Normal Deltoid Ligament
- Interposed fatty tissue
- Partial volume of periligamentous fatty or fibrocartilaginous tissue

Fracture
- Medial malleolus fracture may be isolated or associated with deltoid ligament injury
- Edema and fracture line on coronal and sagittal images

Impingement
- Anterior or medial soft tissue impingement

- Synovial thickening and fluid on FS PD FSE axial images

Tibialis Posterior (TP) Tendon Dysfunction
- Tenosynovitis, degeneration and tear on axial images

Accessory Ossification Center
- Accessory navicular medially
- Hyperintense edema across synchondrosis
- Degenerative changes across synchondrosis

PATHOLOGY

General Features
- General path comments
  - o Superficial layer
    - Superficial anterior tibiotalar
    - Tibionavicular
    - Tibioligamentous (tibiospring)
    - Tibiocalcaneal
    - Superficial posterior tibiotalar
  - o Deep layer
    - Small anterior component: Anterior talotibial (tibiotalar)
    - Strong posterior talotibial (tibiotalar)
- Etiology
  - o Increased load: Deep deltoid ligament last to fail
  - o Associated with ankle fractures
  - o Abduction (deep deltoid injury)
  - o External rotation (anterior deltoid injury)
  - o Eversion
  - o End stage of supination external rotation injury
  - o Significant ankle trauma
- Epidemiology
  - o 10 to 15% of all ankle sprains
  - o Less frequent than lateral injury
  - o 10% have associated syndesmosis injury
  - o Isolated injury rare

Gross Pathologic & Surgical Features
- Weakest to strongest components
  - o Tibiocalcaneal, tibionavicular, tibiospring and posterior tibiotalar

DELTOID LIGAMENT SPRAIN

- Disruption of tibiocalcaneal fibers of superficial layer results in talocrural increase contact pressure and decrease contact area
- Medial malleolus fracture with posterior deep tibiotalar (talotibial) ligament tear
- Partial tear more common than complete ligamentous disruption
- Hemorrhage
- Increased valgus talar tilt

Microscopic Features
- Acute injuries with hyperplastic synovial reaction and hemosiderin
- Chronic injury with fibrous ingrowth or scar

Staging, Grading or Classification Criteria
- Grade I - stretch injury
- Grade II - partial tear
- Grade III - complete ligamentous disruption

CLINICAL ISSUES

Presentation
- Most common signs/symptoms: Swelling and tenderness over deltoid ligaments + surrounding soft tissue
- Clinical profile
  o Anteromedial or medial pain
  o Blister formation
  o Gross deformity
  o Ecchymosis
  o Medial sprains more painful than lateral sprains
  o Tender over deltoid + distal tip medial malleolus
  o Mechanical instability

Demographics
- Age: 15 to 35 years most common
- Gender
  o Males predominates in 15 to 35 year group
  o Females with higher incidence after 40 years

Natural History & Prognosis
- Associated lateral ligamentous injury, fibular fracture and/or syndesmosis injuries
- Fullness in region of retromalleolar tendons secondary to chronic irritation and inflammation
- Widened ankle mortise more common with deltoid injuries with preexisting lateral complex injuries
- Alignment and translation deformity
- Chronic medial ankle pain + instability
- Heals in lengthened position
- Deltoid ossification

Treatment
- Conservative
  o Rest, ice, compression and elevation (RICE)
  o Range of motion
  o Protected weight bearing
  o Grade III requires complete immobilization with short leg cast
- Surgical
  o Infrequently used
  o Debride symptomatic anterior deltoid ossicle
  o Imbrication

  o Delayed primary repair
  o Ligament reconstruction with tendon transfer or graft

DIAGNOSTIC CHECKLIST

Consider
- Associated injury to lateral ligamentous complex
- Assess medial malleolus
- Correlate axial and coronal images to define extent of injury in superficial and deep layers of deltoid

SELECTED REFERENCES

1. DeLee JC et al: Orthopaedic sports medicine. Principles and practice: Ligament injuries of the foot and ankle in the athlete. vol 1. 2nd ed. Philadelphia, Elsevier Science, 2323-91, 2003
2. Fitzgerald RH et al: Orthopaedics: Ligament injuries of the foot and ankle. 2nd ed. Philadelphia, J.B. Lippincott Company, 1607-21, 2002
3. Banks A et al: McGlamry's comprehensive textbook of foot and ankle surgery: Chronic ankle conditions. vol 1. 3rd ed. Philadelphia Lippincott, Williams & Wilkins,1091-152, 2001
4. Tochigi Y et al: Acute inversion injury of the ankle: Magnetic resonance imaging and clinical outcomes. Foot Ankle Int 19(11):730-4, 1998
5. Egol KA et al: Impingement syndrome of the ankle caused by a medial meniscoid lesion. Arthroscopy 13(4):522-5, 1997
6. Klein MA: MR imaging of the ankle: Normal and abnormal findings in the medial collateral ligament. AJR 162(2):377-83, 1994
7. Deutsch AL et al: MRI of the foot and ankle: Ligaments of the ankle. New York, Raven Press, 173-8, 1992
8. Schneck CD et al: MR imaging of the most commonly injured ankle ligaments. Part I. Normal anatomy. Radiology 184:499-506, 1992
9. Schneck CD et al: MR imaging of the most commonly injured ankle ligaments. Part II. Ligament injuries. Radiology 184:507-512, 1992
10. Kier R et al: MR imaging of the normal ligaments and tendons of the ankle. J Comput Assist Tomogr 15:477-482, 1991
11. Kneeland JB et al: MR imaging of the normal ankle: Correlation with anatomic sections. AJR 151:117-123, 1988
12. Siegler S et al: The mechanical characteristics of the collateral ligaments of the human ankle joint. Foot Ankle 8:234-42, 1988
13. Perlman M et al: Inversion lateral ankle trauma: Differential diagnosis, review of the literature, and prospective study. J Foot Surg 26(2):95-133, 1987

DELTOID LIGAMENT SPRAIN

IMAGE GALLERY

Typical

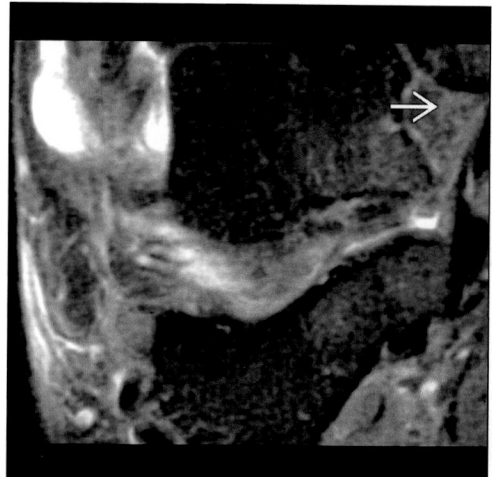
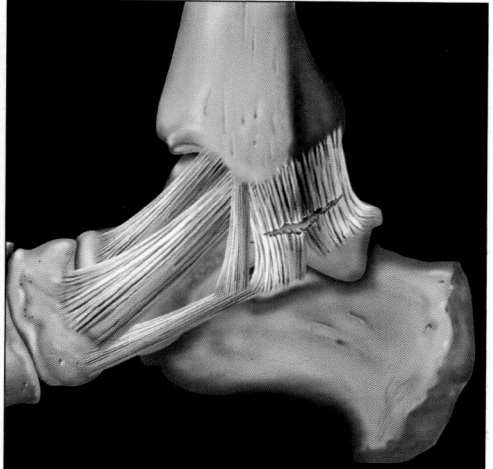

(Left) Coronal FS PD FSE MR shows partial tear (arrow) of deep fibers of the deltoid. (Right) Sagittal graphic with partial tearing of the tibiocalcaneal and superficial posterior tibiotalar components of the superficial deltoid.

Typical

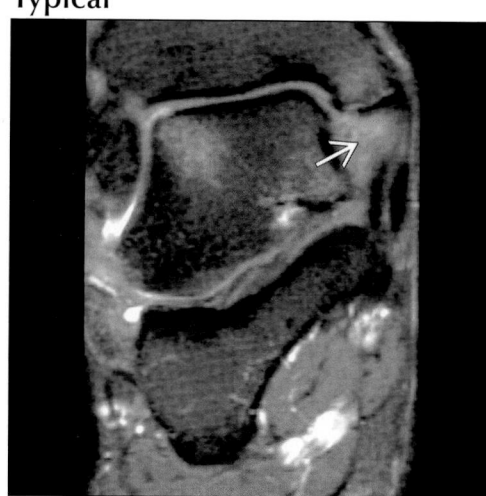
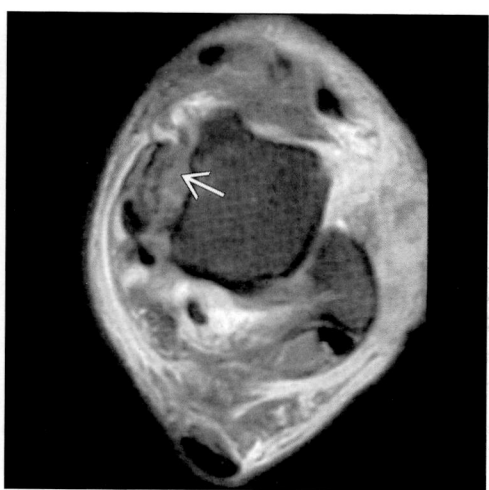

(Left) Coronal FS PD FSE MR shows osteochondral lesion of the lateral talus in association with a grade II deltoid sprain (arrow). Medial malleolar and talar edema is hyperintense. (Right) Axial FS PD FSE MR shows complete disruption of both the medial (arrow) and lateral ligamentous complexes.

Typical

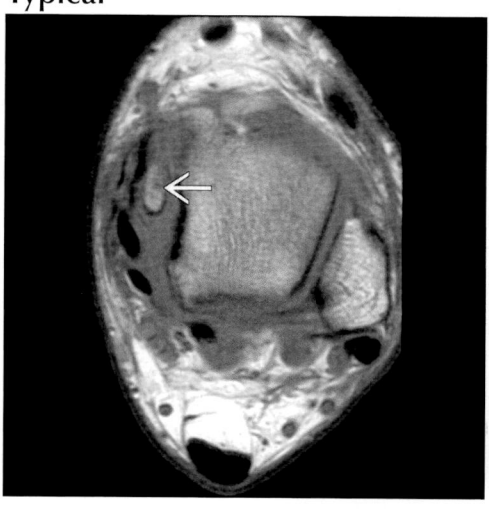
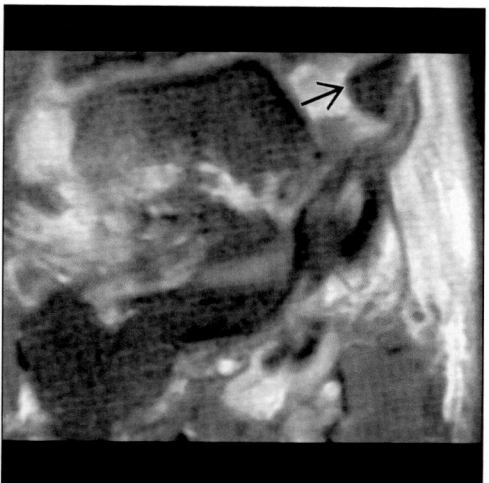

(Left) Axial T1WI MR shows chronic deltoid tear with absent ligament and marrow containing osseous avulsion (arrow). Note lack of deltoid ligament striations deep to the tibialis posterior tendon. (Right) Coronal FS PD FSE MR shows avulsed fracture (arrow) of the medial malleolus with osseous displacement. Superficial component of the deltoid ligament is attached to the displaced medial malleolus.

SYNDESMOSIS SPRAIN

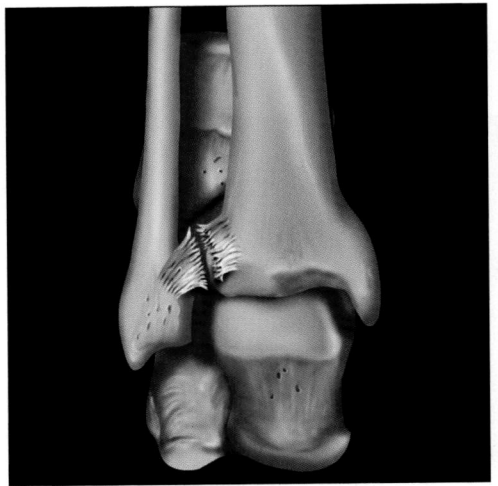

Coronal graphic shows anterior syndesmotic (anterior inferior tibiofibular) ligament tear.

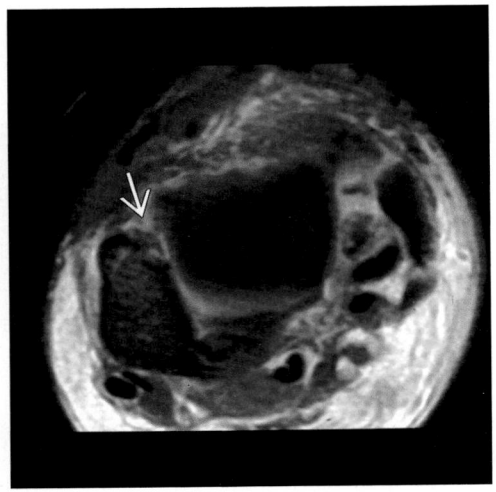

Axial FS PD FSE MR shows syndesmotic ligament disruption (arrow) associated with disruption of medial ankle ligaments.

TERMINOLOGY

Abbreviations and Synonyms
- Syndesmotic injury; tibiofibular diastasis, high ankle sprain

Definitions
- Stretching, partial tear or tear of distal tibiofibular syndesmotic ligaments

IMAGING FINDINGS

General Features
- Best diagnostic clue: Associated fluid and ligamentous edema of syndesmotic ligaments
- Location
  - Anterior inferior tibiofibular (AITF) ligament
  - Posterior inferior tibiofibular (PITF) ligament
  - Transverse tibiofibular ligament
  - Interosseous membrane
- Size: Diastasis of 2.3 mm to 7.3 mm
- Morphology
  - AITF
    - Flat band
    - Two or three bands
    - Multifascicular
    - 20% intraarticular
  - PITF
    - Thick band
    - Quadrilateral shape
    - Transverse tibiofibular ligament (deep and inferior component)
    - True posterior labrum
    - Interosseous membrane
    - Short fibrous bands

Radiographic Findings
- Radiography
  - Weight-bearing views
  - Medial clear space on mortise view (normal < 4 mm)
  - Syndesmotic clear space on anteroposterior (AP) and mortise (normal < 6 mm)
  - Tibiofibular overlap on AP or mortise (normal > 6 mm)
  - Stress testing for dysfunction and instability
  - External rotation stress test = widening of mortise

CT Findings
- NECT: More sensitive for 1 to 3 mm diastasis compared to radiographs

MR Findings
- T1WI
  - Intermediate signal intensity and blurring syndesmotic ligaments
  - Lateral fibular subluxation

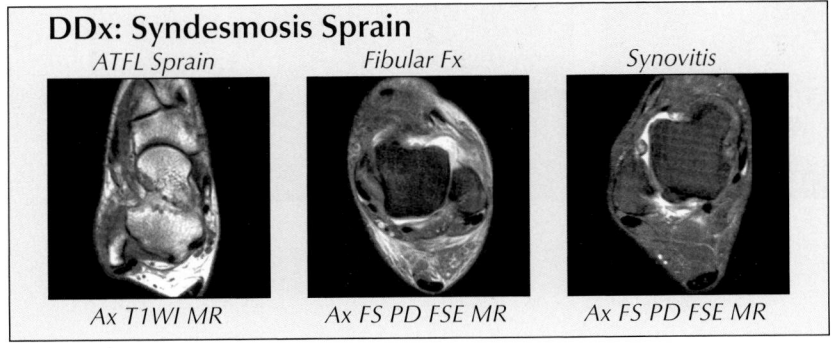

DDx: Syndesmosis Sprain

ATFL Sprain	Fibular Fx	Synovitis
Ax T1WI MR	Ax FS PD FSE MR	Ax FS PD FSE MR

SYNDESMOSIS SPRAIN

Key Facts

Imaging Findings

- Best diagnostic clue: Associated fluid and ligamentous edema of syndesmotic ligaments
- Size: Diastasis of 2.3 mm to 7.3 mm
- Contour irregularity of syndesmotic ligaments (AITF or PITF)
- Fluid hyperintensity and diastasis of AITF and PITF on T2WI

Top Differential Diagnoses

- Lateral Ankle Instability
- Fibular Fracture
- Compartment Syndrome
- Posterior Impingement

Pathology

- Abduction, external rotation and dorsiflexion of ankle/lower leg
- Substantial tearing AITF, PITF and interosseous membrane

Clinical Issues

- Most common signs/symptoms: Severe pain with external rotation
- Pain anterolateral leg
- Palpable tenderness over syndesmosis
- Age: Young persons/high-contact athletic injuries

Diagnostic Checklist

- Evaluate congruity and diastasis of syndesmosis on axial images

---

- ○ Calcification interosseous membrane
- ○ Fibular shortening
- ○ Tibiofibular diastasis
- T2WI
  - ○ Ligament thickening: Increased anteroposterior (AP) dimension of anterior or posterior syndesmotic ligament
  - ○ Intraligamentous hyperintensity
  - ○ Contour irregularity of syndesmotic ligaments (AITF or PITF)
  - ○ Frank discontinuity of ligaments
  - ○ Fluid hyperintensity and diastasis of AITF and PITF on T2WI
  - ○ Interosseous membrane linear hyperintensity
  - ○ Interosseous membrane hemosiderin, fibrosis or calcification

Imaging Recommendations

- Best imaging tool: MR to identify anterior and posterior syndesmotic ligaments
- Protocol advice: Axial FS PD FSE

DIFFERENTIAL DIAGNOSIS

Lateral Ankle Instability

- Positive anterior drawer and talar tilt
- Tear of ATFL and calcaneofibular ligament (CFL)
- Synovitis
- MR documents intact syndesmotic ligaments

Fibular Fracture

- Point tenderness over lateral malleolus

Compartment Syndrome

- Pain out of proportion to injury

Posterior Impingement

- Synovitis of posterior ankle ligaments

PATHOLOGY

General Features

- Etiology
  - ○ Abduction, external rotation and dorsiflexion of ankle/lower leg
  - ○ Relevant causative factors
    - Football
    - Soccer
    - Basketball
  - ○ Complication of fractures
- Epidemiology
  - ○ Syndesmotic injuries: 10% to 20% of ankle sprains
  - ○ Second most common ankle injury after lateral ligament injury
- AITF
  - ○ Oblique from anterior inferior lateral malleolus to anterolateral tubercle tibia
  - ○ Contacts lateral ridge talar trochlear surface in plantarflexion
- PITF
  - ○ Posterior lateral malleolus to posterolateral tibial tubercle
  - ○ Transverse tibiofibular ligament: Deep and inferior to PITF
    - From fibular tubercle + digital fossa to posterior tibial articular surface/medial border medial malleolus
    - True posterior labrum: Projects below posterior tibial margin
  - ○ Tibial slip: Posterior talofibular ligament to posterior tibia + transverse tibiofibular ligament
  - ○ Interosseous membrane
    - Medial distal fibular shaft to lateral distal tibia
    - Vault over tibiofibular synovial recess

Gross Pathologic & Surgical Features

- Substantial tearing AITF, PITF and interosseous membrane
- Hemorrhage
- Associated bi- and tri-malleolar fractures
- Fibular subluxation
- Plastic deformation fibula

- Posterior rotation and subluxation fibula
- Talus dislocated superiorly

Microscopic Features
- Hemorrhagic cellular elements
- Soft tissue hyperplasia
- Heterotopic calcification

Staging, Grading or Classification Criteria
- Clinical
  - Grade I: Stretch
  - Grade II: Partial tear
  - Grade III: Complete rupture
- Frank diastasis: Identified on unstressed radiographs
- Latent diastasis: Identified on stress radiographs
- Radiologic types of frank injuries
  - Type I: Straight lateral fibular subluxation and increased medial clear space
  - Type II: Straight lateral fibular subluxation and plastic/angular deformation fibula
  - Type III: Posterior rotation and subluxation distal fibula
  - Type IV: Talus dislocated superiorly and increased intermalleolar distance

CLINICAL ISSUES

Presentation
- Most common signs/symptoms: Severe pain with external rotation
- Clinical profile
  - Pain anterolateral leg
  - Palpable tenderness over syndesmosis
  - Pain on squeeze test of fibula and tibia
  - Swollen leg
  - Mild pain over ATFL and CFL
  - Instability
  - Unable to bear weight
  - Muscular splinting/reflex spasm

Demographics
- Age: Young persons/high-contact athletic injuries
- Gender: Male predominance

Natural History & Prognosis
- Chronic instability of distal tibiofibular syndesmosis
- Reduction of syndesmosis necessary to minimize dysfunction and arthritis
- Tibiofibular joint snapping
- Syndesmotic impingement: Inflamed synovium, AITF scarring, talar chondromalacia and osteophytes

Treatment
- Open reduction/internal fixation
- Repair AITF using plantaris or peroneal tendons
- Arthrodesis for severe pain & degenerative changes

DIAGNOSTIC CHECKLIST

Consider
- In more severe ankle sprains
- MRI to document disruption of AITF, PITF or interosseous membrane

- Evaluate congruity and diastasis of syndesmosis on axial images

SELECTED REFERENCES

1. DeLee JC et al: Orthopaedic sports medicine. Principles and practice: Ligament injuries of the foot and ankle in the athlete. vol 2. 2nd ed. Philadelphia, Saunders, 2323-75, 2003
2. Uys HD et al: Clinical association of acute lateral ankle sprain with syndesmotic involvement: A stress radiography and magnetic resonance imaging study. Am J Sports Med 30(6):816-22, 2002
3. Banks A et al: McGlamry's comprehensive textbook of foot and ankle surgery. vol 1. Philadelphia, Lippincott Williams & Wilkins, 1091-152, 2001
4. Ogilvie-Harris DJ et al: Disruption of the ankle syndesmosis: Diagnosis and treatment by arthroscopic surgery. Arthroscopy 10:561, 1994
5. Schneck CD et al: MR imaging of the most commonly injured ankle ligaments. Part I. Normal anatomy. Radiology 184:499, 1992
6. Mink JH: MRI of the foot and ankle: Ligaments of the ankle. New York, Raven Press, 185-9, 1992
7. Schneck CD et al: MR imaging of the most commonly injured ankle ligaments. Part II. Ligament injuries. Radiology 184:499-506, 1992
8. Erickson SJ et al: MR imaging of the lateral collateral ligament of the ankle. AJR 156:131-6, 1991
9. Noto A et al: MR imaging of the ankle: Normal variants. Radiology 170:121-4, 1989
10. Fritschy D: An unusual ankle injury in top skiers. Am J Sports Med 17(2):282, 1989
11. Sclafini S: Ligamentous injury of the lower tibiofibular syndesmosis: Radiographic evidence. Radiology 56:21-7, 1985
12. Monk C: Injuries to the tibo-fibular ligaments. J Bone Joint Surg 51B:330-7, 1969

SYNDESMOSIS SPRAIN

IMAGE GALLERY

Typical

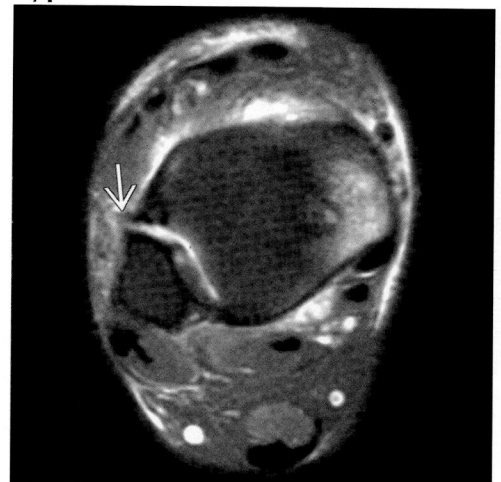
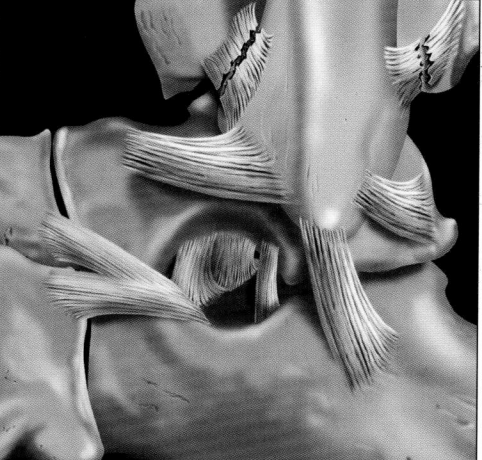

(Left) Axial FS PD FSE MR shows discontinuity (arrow) of anterior syndesmotic ligament (anterior inferior tibiofibular ligament) with associated hyperintense contusion of the medial malleolus. *(Right)* Sagittal graphic shows disruption of both the anterior and posterior syndesmotic ligaments.

Typical

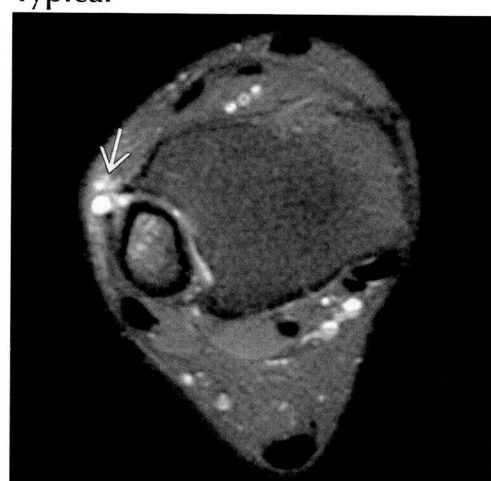
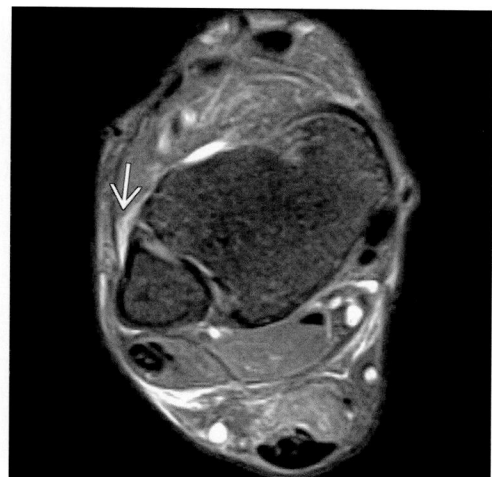

(Left) Axial FS PD FSE MR shows posttraumatic ganglion cyst (arrow) formation adjacent to anterior syndesmotic ligament tear. *(Right)* Axial FS PD FSE MR shows linear fluid collection (arrow) anterior to partial tear of the anterior syndesmotic ligament.

Typical

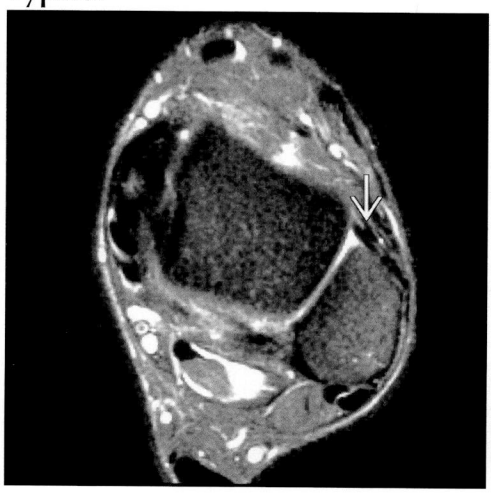
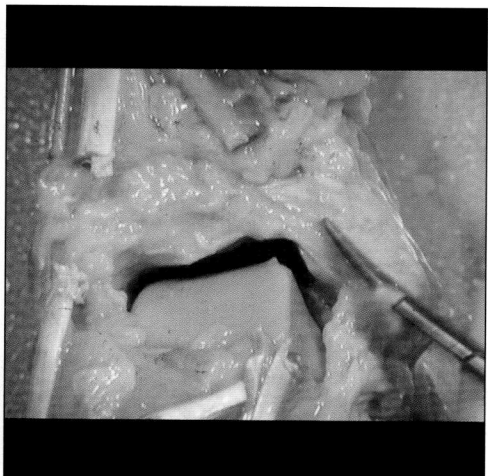

(Left) Axial FS PD FSE MR shows normal hypointense anterior inferior tibiofibular ligament (arrow). This ligament may be divided into two or three bands or may be multifascicular. *(Right)* Surgical pathology shows location of the oblique course of the anterior syndesmotic ligament (anterior inferior tibiofibular ligament at tip of probe).

ANTEROLATERAL IMPINGEMENT

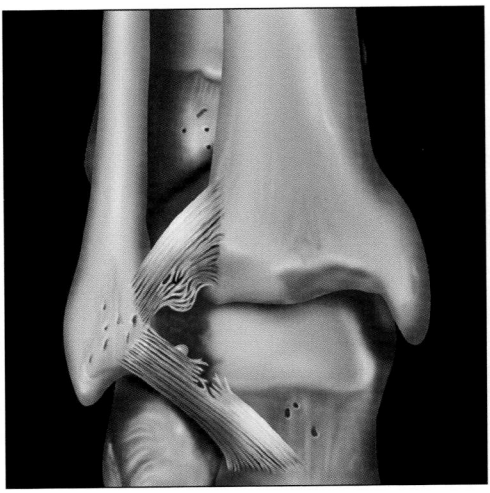

Coronal graphic shows anterolateral soft tissue impingement with synovitis (red), fibrosis, and chondromalacia in the anterolateral gutter. Small ossicle is located deep to the ATFL.

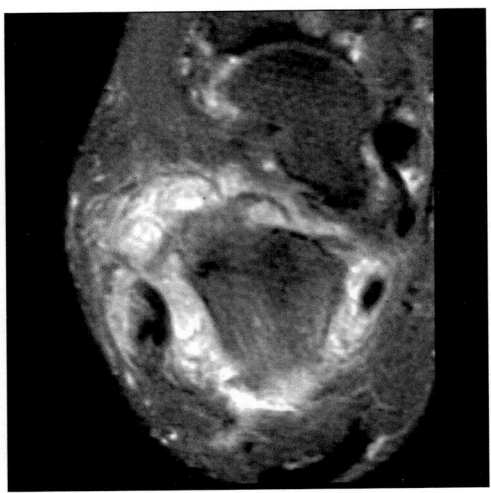

Axial FS PD FSE MR shows hypertrophic synovial tissue anterior to and within the lateral gutter.

TERMINOLOGY

Abbreviations and Synonyms
- Anterolateral impingement syndrome; anterolateral soft tissue impingement

Definitions
- Synovitis and fibrosis of anterior inferior tibiofibular ligament (AITF), anterior talofibular ligament (ATFL) and lateral gutter

IMAGING FINDINGS

General Features
- Best diagnostic clue: Soft tissue thickening anterior aspect lateral gutter
- Location
  - AITF
  - Lateral gutter
  - ATFL
- Size: Variable synovitis, fibrosis, chondromalacia - relative to lateral gutter
- Morphology
  - Thickened adhesive bands and synovium
  - Osteophytes
  - Loose bodies
  - Meniscoid-shaped lesion

MR Findings
- T1WI
  - Hypointense to intermediate signal intensity in anterolateral gutter
  - Effacement of fat signal anterior to AITF
  - Hypointense fluid to intermediate signal synovium deep to AITF
  - Hypointense ossicle/loose body in soft tissues at tip of fibula
- T2WI
  - Intermediate signal intensity hyalinized mass
  - Associated injury to AITF and ATFL
  - Hyperintense fluid and intermediate signal synovium anterolateral gutter
  - Hypointense fibrosis/scar band
  - Talar chondromalacia - denuded intermediate signal chondral surface
  - Hypointense loose body surrounded by hyperintense fluid
- T1 C+: Enhanced synovium

Imaging Recommendations
- Best imaging tool
  - MR superior
  - Radiographs, bone scan, CT often negative
- Protocol advice: Axial FS PD FSE and FS T1 C+

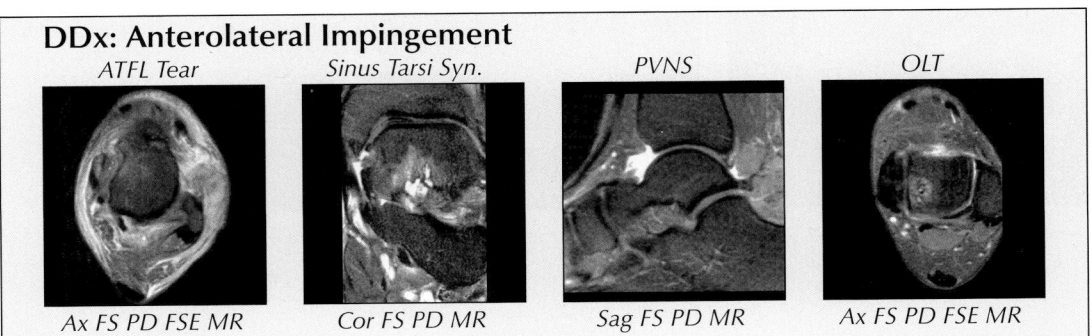

DDx: Anterolateral Impingement

ATFL Tear	Sinus Tarsi Syn.	PVNS	OLT
Ax FS PD FSE MR	Cor FS PD MR	Sag FS PD MR	Ax FS PD FSE MR

ANTEROLATERAL IMPINGEMENT

Key Facts

Imaging Findings

- Best diagnostic clue: Soft tissue thickening anterior aspect lateral gutter
- Size: Variable synovitis, fibrosis, chondromalacia - relative to lateral gutter
- Thickened adhesive bands and synovium
- Associated injury to AITF and ATFL

Top Differential Diagnoses

- Retracted ATFL Tear
- Sinus Tarsi Syndrome
- Pigmented Villonodular Synovitis (PVNS)
- Idiopathic Synovial (Osteo) Chondromatosis
- Ganglion Cysts
- Osteochondral Lesion of Talus (OLT)

Pathology

- Posttraumatic with plantar flexion inversion most common
- Partial/complete tear AITF or ATFL
- Synovial hyperplasia and compression

Clinical Issues

- Most common signs/symptoms: Vague pain anterolateral ankle
- Tenderness along syndesmosis + anterior gutter
- Inflammatory tissue lateral gutter + syndesmosis between tibia/fibula

Diagnostic Checklist

- Contrast to enhance scar/fibrosis

DIFFERENTIAL DIAGNOSIS

Retracted ATFL Tear

- Without synovitis/fibrosis

Sinus Tarsi Syndrome

- Pathology of sinus tarsi ligaments
- Synovitis/ligament tearing

Pigmented Villonodular Synovitis (PVNS)

- Hemosiderin/intermediate signal tissue: Diffuse or nodular

Idiopathic Synovial (Osteo) Chondromatosis

- Multiple loose bodies not restricted to anterolateral gutter

Ganglion Cysts

- T2WI - focal hyperintense cyst

Osteochondral Lesion of Talus (OLT)

- MR sensitive and specific for talar subchondral sclerosis, edema and cystic change

PATHOLOGY

General Features

- General path comments
  - Relevant anatomy
    - AITF
    - ATFL
    - Syndesmosis
    - Lateral gutter
- Etiology
  - Posttraumatic with plantar flexion inversion most common
  - Synovial and capsular irritation
  - Infection
  - Rheumatologic
  - Degenerative
- Epidemiology
  - Subset of inversion injury population
  - True meniscoid lesion less common
    - 20-40% occur post ankle sprain = chronic ankle pain

Gross Pathologic & Surgical Features

- Partial/complete tear AITF or ATFL
- Intraarticular hemorrhage
- Synovial hyperplasia and compression
- Entrapment synovial membrane
- Hyalinized scar/meniscoid lesions
  - Hyalinized tissue post lateral sprain
  - Synovial impingement lesion
  - Attached to anteroinferior talofibular joint capsule
  - Extension into lateral gutter
  - Fibrocartilaginous consistency
  - 5 mm width
  - Anterior to fibula
  - Between lateral talus + distal medial fibula
  - Associated with synovitis, chondromalacia + osteophytes
  - Morphology similar to hypertrophic synovitis
- Chondral erosion lateral talar dome

Microscopic Features

- Synovial hyperplasia
- Subsynovial capillary proliferation
- Hyaline cartilage degenerative change/fibrosis
- Chronic inflammatory process
- Absence of ligamentous tissue on histology

CLINICAL ISSUES

Presentation

- Most common signs/symptoms: Vague pain anterolateral ankle
- Clinical profile
  - Pain absent at rest
  - Pain with activity/cutting + pivoting movement
  - Tenderness along syndesmosis + anterior gutter
  - +/- Tenderness posterior subtalar joint + sinus tarsi

Demographics

- Age: Younger population post inversion injury to lateral ligament

- Gender: Male predominance in athletic population

Natural History & Prognosis
- Heterotropic bone interosseous space
- Ossicles at tip of fibula and talar dome
- Chronic lateral ankle pain
- Inflammatory tissue lateral gutter + syndesmosis between tibia/fibula

Treatment
- Conservative
  - Physical therapy
  - NSAIDs
- Surgical
  - Arthroscopic with shavers, burrs, graspers and baskets
  - Debridement: Removing inflamed synovium, thickened adhesive bands, osteophytes and loose bodies
  - Involved tissue excised down to underlying cartilage
  - Removal synovium and inflamed capsular and ligamentous tissue
  - ATFL remnant not excised
- Post surgical splint
- CAM walker

DIAGNOSTIC CHECKLIST

Image Interpretation Pearls
- Axial images to identify synovitis anterior + posterior to ATFL/AITF
- Contrast to enhance scar/fibrosis
- Identify associated talar chondral erosions

SELECTED REFERENCES

1. Robinson P et al: Soft-tissue and osseous impingement syndromes of the ankle: Role of imaging in diagnosis and management. Radiographics 6:1457-69, 2002
2. Banks A et al: McGlamry's comprehensive textbook of foot and ankle surgery. Philadelphia PA, Lippincott Williams & Wilkins, 1091-152, 2001
3. Robinson P et al: Anterolateral ankle impingement: MR arthrographic assessment of the anterolateral recess. Radiology 221(1):186-90, 2001
4. Trnka HJ et al: Arthrography of the foot and ankle. Ankle and subtalar joint. Foot Ankle Clin 5(1):49-62, 2000
5. DIGiovanni BF et al: Associated injuries found in chronic lateral ankle instability. Foot Ankle Int 21(10):809-15, 2000
6. Rosenberg ZS et al: From the RSNA refresher courses, Radiological Society of North America. MR imaging of the ankle and foot. Radiographics 20 (Spec No:S153-79): Review, 2000
7. Jordan LK 3rd et al: Magnetic resonance imaging findings in anterolateral impingement of the ankle. Skeletal Radiol 29(1):34-9, 2000
8. Akseki D et al: The distal fascicle of the anterior inferior tibio-fibular ligament as a cause of anterolateral ankle impingement: Results of arthroscopic resection. Acta Orthop Scand 70(5):478-82, 1999
9. Farooki S et al: Anterolateral impingement of the ankle: Effectiveness of MR imaging. Radiology 207(2):357-60, 1998
10. Skib RA: Anterolateral soft tissue impingement of the ankle. Radiology 209(3):855, 1998
11. Resnick D et al: Internal Derangement of Joints. Emphasis on MR Imaging. Philidelphia PA, WB Saunders. Chap 17, 1997
12. Rubin DA et al: Anterolateral soft-tissue impingement in the ankle: Diagnosis using MR imaging. AJR 169(3):829-35, 1997
13. Mink JH: MRI of the foot and ankle. Ligaments of the ankle. New York, Raven Press, 178-185, 1992
14. Bassett F et al: Talar impingement by the anteroinferior tibiofibular ligament. J Bone Joint Surg 72A:55-59, 1990
15. Martin D et al: Operative ankle arthroscopy. Long term follow-up. Am J Sports Med 17(1):16-23, 1989
16. Martin D et al: Arthroscopic treatment of chronic synovitis of the ankle. Arthroscopy 5(2):110-14,1989
17. Ferkel R et al: Progress in ankle arthroscopy. Clin Orthop Rel Res 210-20, 1988
18. McCarrol J et al: Meniscoid lesions of the ankle in soccer players. Am J sports Med 15:255-7, 1987

ANTEROLATERAL IMPINGEMENT

Typical

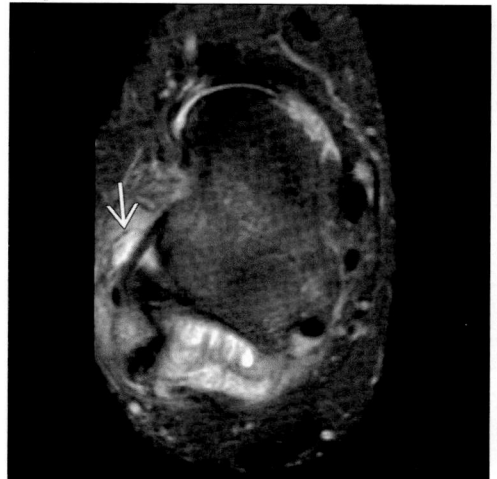 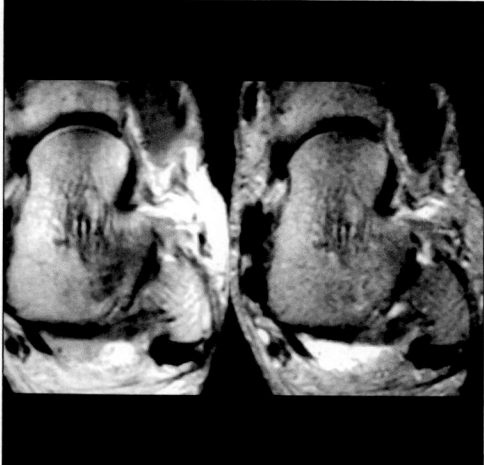

(Left) Axial FS PD FSE MR shows hyperintense synovitis anterior (arrow) and posterior to the ATFL. *(Right)* Axial T2WI MR shows synovitis in area of previous ATFL disruption.

Typical

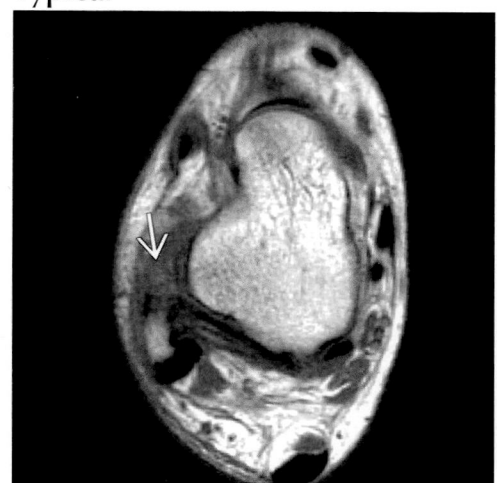 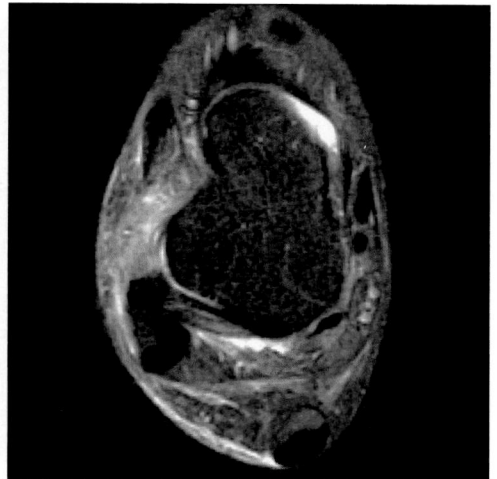

(Left) Axial T1WI MR shows soft tissue thickening (arrow) and scar tissue corresponding to ATFL sprain. *(Right)* Axial PD FSE MR shows hyperintense edema and thickening in area of previous ATFL sprain.

Typical

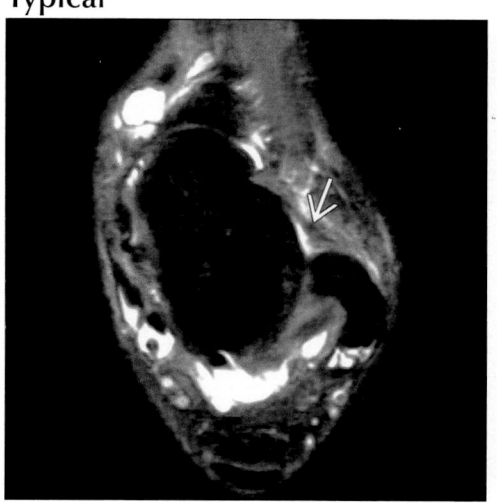 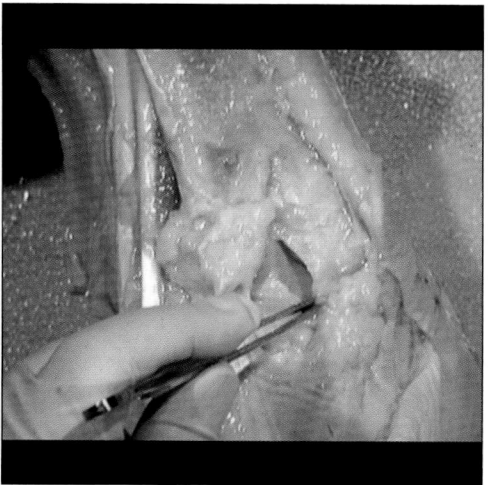

(Left) Axial FS PD FSE MR shows scarred ATFL (arrow) with fluid and synovitis anterior and posterior to its fibers. *(Right)* Coronal surgical pathology shows location for anterolateral impingement at the level of the anterior aspect of the lateral gutter. Absent ATFL is indicated.

6

45

ANTERIOR IMPINGEMENT

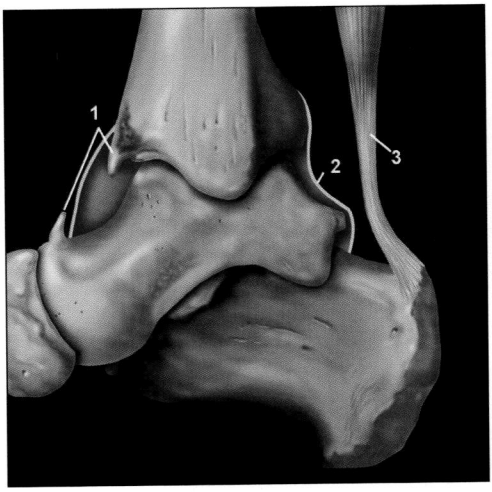

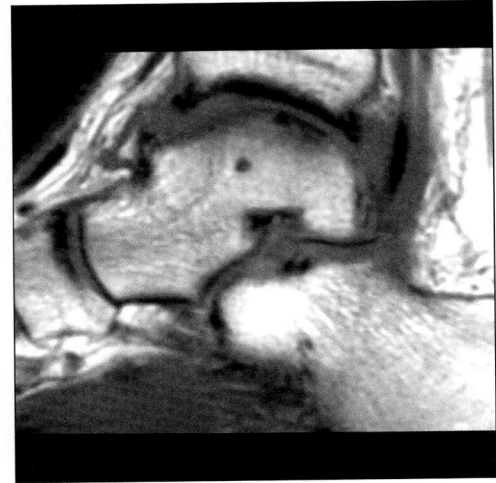

Sagittal graphic shows anterior spur formation of the anterior tibial plafond and dorsal surface talar neck. (1) capsular contraction (2) and Achilles tendon shortening (3) are associated.

Sagittal T1WI MR shows hypointense sclerotic anterior osteophytes of the tibia and talus contributing to anterior tibiotalar impingement.

TERMINOLOGY

Abbreviations and Synonyms
- Anterior impingement syndrome; athlete's or football player's ankle

Definitions
- Spur formation anterior inferior tibial plafond + talar neck

IMAGING FINDINGS

General Features
- Best diagnostic clue: Distal anterior tibial osteophyte
- Location: Between anterior surface tibia and superior aspect neck of talus
- Size: Osteophyte greater than 1 cm in grade 3 and 4 lesions
- Morphology: Triangular shaped osteophyte - tibia side spur with narrower base than talar spur

Radiographic Findings
- Radiography: Anterior tibial exostosis on lateral radiograph

CT Findings
- NECT
  - Tibial and talar osteophyte on sagittal reformations
  - Less sensitive for associated effusion, chondral surfaces and marrow changes

MR Findings
- T1WI
  - Low signal intensity osteophytes
  - Fat signal intensity osteophytes
  - Intermediate signal fluid + synovium between tibial osteophyte and talus at capsular attachment
  - Hypointense subchondral sclerosis
- T2WI
  - Low to intermediate signal osteophytes
  - Hyperintense tibiotalar effusion
  - Intermediate to hyperintense fluid + synovium adjacent to anterior talar neck
  - Hyperintense talar + anterior distal tibial subchondral edema
  - Discrete cartilaginous defects/trough of talus = tram track lesion
  - Hypointense fibrous overgrowth
- T1 C+: Variable enhancement of inflamed synovium + fibrous tissue

Imaging Recommendations
- Best imaging tool: MR superior for talar longitudinal chondral defects
- Protocol advice: Sagittal T1/PD + FS PD FSE

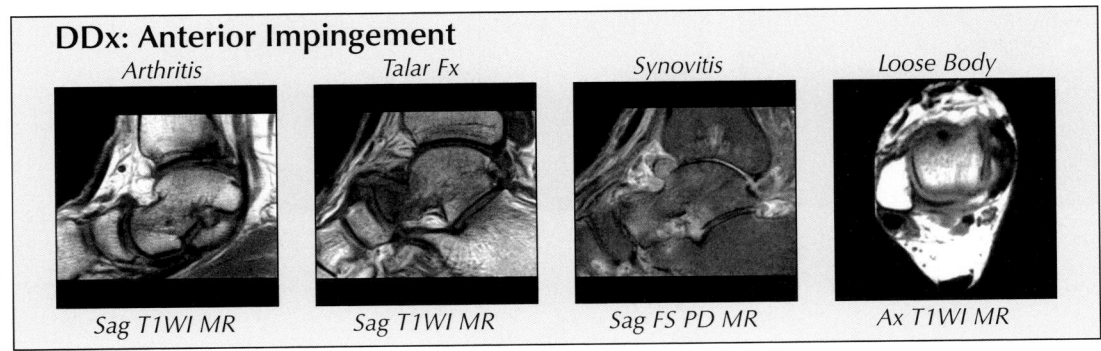

DDx: Anterior Impingement

Arthritis	Talar Fx	Synovitis	Loose Body
Sag T1WI MR	Sag T1WI MR	Sag FS PD MR	Ax T1WI MR

ANTERIOR IMPINGEMENT

Key Facts

Imaging Findings

- Best diagnostic clue: Distal anterior tibial osteophyte
- Location: Between anterior surface tibia and superior aspect neck of talus
- Morphology: Triangular shaped osteophyte - tibia side spur with narrower base than talar spur

Top Differential Diagnoses

- Generalized Tibiotalar Arthritis
- Talar Fracture (Fx)
- Synovitis - Tibiotalar Joint
- Loose Body

Pathology

- Osteophytes on distal tibio + talar neck decrease tibio-talar angle to < 60 degrees
- Direct tibial talar repetitive + forceful microtrauma

- Not secondary to single episode of acute trauma
- Full thickness talar chondral defects
- Synovial hyperplasia

Clinical Issues

- Most common signs/symptoms: Generalized anterior ankle pain
- Pain augmented by dorsiflexion
- Pain at end-range of motion
- Restricted dorsiflexion capacity
- Arthroscopy: Decompression + resection hypertrophic synovitis

Diagnostic Checklist

- Sagittal MR images to differentiate anterior impingement from generalized tibiotalar arthritis

DIFFERENTIAL DIAGNOSIS

Generalized Tibiotalar Arthritis

- Narrowing of entire articulation
- Osteochondral defects
- Subchondral sclerosis anterior tibial plafond

Talar Fracture (Fx)

- Edema talar head/neck + linear trabecular fracture segments

Synovitis - Tibiotalar Joint

- Tibiotalar effusion
- Anterior capsular distention with intermediate signal intensity hyperplastic synovium (on T2WI)

Loose Body

- Chondral or osteochondral fragment in anterior joint capsule

PATHOLOGY

General Features

- General path comments
  - Relevant anatomy
    - Talar sulcus normally seen superior aspect talar neck
    - Normal tibial-dorsal talar neck angle = 60 degrees
    - Osteophytes on distal tibio + talar neck decrease tibio-talar angle to < 60 degrees
- Etiology
  - Hyperdorsiflexion
  - Direct tibial talar repetitive + forceful microtrauma
  - Spur formation anterior inferior tibial plafond + neck of talus (capsular attachment site)
    - Synovial impingement + tibial spur
    - Osteochondral reaction - exostosis formation
    - Exostosis ± fragmentation + secondary dorsal talar spur ± fragmentation of secondary osteophytes
    - Pantalocrural arthritic destruction (degenerative)
  - Not secondary to single episode of acute trauma
  - Lateral ankle ligament laxity

  - Equinus foot
- Epidemiology
  - Subset chronic ankle pain population
  - Activity at risk: Hyperdorsiflexion
    - Runners
    - High jumpers
    - Rock climbers
    - Gymnasts

Gross Pathologic & Surgical Features

- Superior dorsally projecting talar + anteriorly projecting tibial osteophytes
- Exuberant bone: Focal or bridging
- "Door jam" effect between osteophytes
- Fracture/fragmentation of osteophytes
- Full thickness talar chondral defects

Microscopic Features

- Inflammatory cellular response
- Synovial hyperplasia
- Fibrous ingrowth

Staging, Grading or Classification Criteria

- Grade 1: Abnormal osseous contour, anteroinferior tibia
- Grade 2: Sharp interface of hypertrophic bone
- Grade 3: Tibial exostosis 3/8 to 1/2 inch (1-1.3 cm) with sharply defined margins
- Grade 4: Tibial exostosis > 1/2 inch (> 1.3 cm), poorly defined apex/base ± fragmentation

CLINICAL ISSUES

Presentation

- Most common signs/symptoms: Generalized anterior ankle pain
- Clinical profile
  - Pain augmented by dorsiflexion
  - Pain at end-range of motion
  - Restricted dorsiflexion capacity
  - Divot in anterior talar neck in soccer players secondary to tibial spur abutment

o "Tram track" lesions in soccer players - contact by prominent tibial osteophyte with talar dome articular cartilage

Demographics

- Age: Younger age/athletes (< 40 years)
- Gender
  - Present in male and female sport activities
    - Football, dancing, soccer

Natural History & Prognosis

- Pronounced ankle restriction
- Progressive hypertrophic bone
- Inflammation
- Spur fragmentation
- Synovitis

Treatment

- Conservative
  - Activity modification
  - Immobilization
  - Antiinflammatory agents
  - Steroid compounds
- Surgical
  - Arthroscopy: Decompression + resection hypertrophic synovitis
  - Open surgical: Resection of large exostosis

DIAGNOSTIC CHECKLIST

Consider

- Sagittal MR images to differentiate anterior impingement from generalized tibiotalar arthritis
- T2WI to identify effusion, marrow edema, acute fragmentation of osteophytes + associated chondral lesions

6

48

SELECTED REFERENCES

1. DeLee JC et al: Orthopaedic sports medicine. Principles and practice. Ligament Injuries of the foot and ankle in the athlete. Osteochondroses and related problems of the foot and ankle. vol 2. 2nd ed. Philadelphia PA, Saunders, 2587-623, 2003
2. Robinson P et al: Soft-tissue and osseous impingement syndromes of the ankle: Role of imaging in diagnosis and management. Radiographics 22(6):1457-69, 2002
3. Tuite MJ: MR imaging of the tendons of the foot and ankle. Semin Musculoskelet Radiol 6(2):119-31, 2002
4. Robinson P et al: Anteromedial impingement of the ankle: Using MR arthrography to assess the anteromedial recess. AJR 178(3):601-4, 2002
5. Banks A et al: McGlamry's comprehensive textbook of foot and ankle surgery. Philadelphia PA, Lippincott Williams & Wilkins, 1091-152, 2001
6. Haverstock BD: Anterior ankle abutment. Clin Podiart Med Surg 18(3):457-65, 2001
7. Jordon LK 3rd et al: Magnetic resonance imaging findings in anterolateral impingement of the ankle. Skeletal Radiol 29(1):34-9, 2000
8. Farooki S et al: Anterolateral impingement of the ankle: Effectiveness of MR imaging. Radiology 207(2):357-60, 1998
9. Rubin DA et al: Anterolateral soft-tissue impingement in the ankle: Diagnosis using MR imaging. AJR 169(3):829-35, 1997
10. Khan K et al: Overuse injuries in classical ballet. Sports 19:341, 1995
11. Cutsuries AM et al: Arthroscopic arthroplasty of the ankle joint. Clin Podiatr Med Surg 11(3):449-67, 1994
12. Vogler HW et al: Anterior ankle impingement arthropathy. The role of anterolateral arthrotomy and arthroscopy. Clin Podiatr Med Surg 11(3):425-47, 1994
13. Ogilvie-Harris DJ et al: Anterior impingement of the ankle treated by arthroscopic removal of bony spurs. J Bone Joint Surg 75:437, 1993
14. Ferkel RD et al: Arthroscopy of the ankle and foot. J Bone Joint Surg 75:1233, 1993
15. Hardaker WT Jr et al: Foot and ankle injuries in theatrical dancers. Foot Ankle 6:59, 1985
16. King JW et al: Lesions of the feet in athletes. South Med J 64:45, 1971
17. Brodelius A et al: Osteoarthritis of the talar joints in footballers and ballet dancers. Acta Orthop Scand 30:309, 1960
18. O'Donoghue DH et al: Impingement exostoses of the talus and tibia. J Bone Joint Surg 39:835, 1957
19. McMurray TP et al: Footballer's ankle. J Bone Joint Surg 32:68, 1950
20. Morris LH et al: Athlete's ankle. J Bone Joint Surg 25:220, 1943

IMAGE GALLERY

Typical

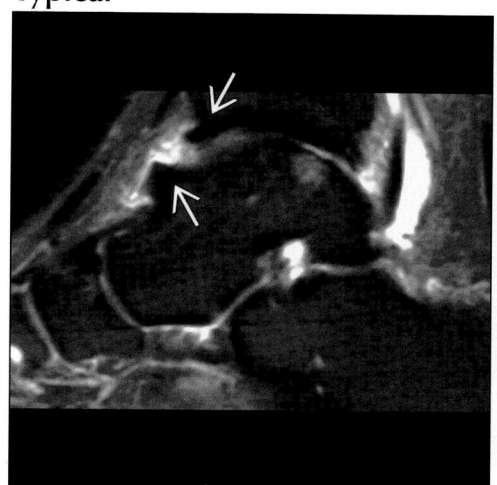

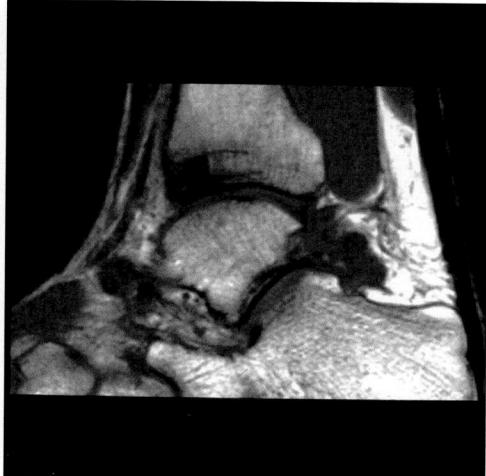

(Left) Sagittal FS PD FSE MR shows anterior osteophytes (arrows) with tibiotalar joint effusion. *(Right)* Sagittal T1WI MR shows anterior tibial plafond sclerosis.

Typical

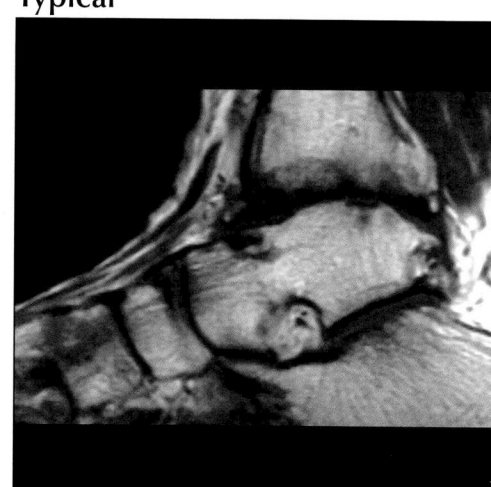

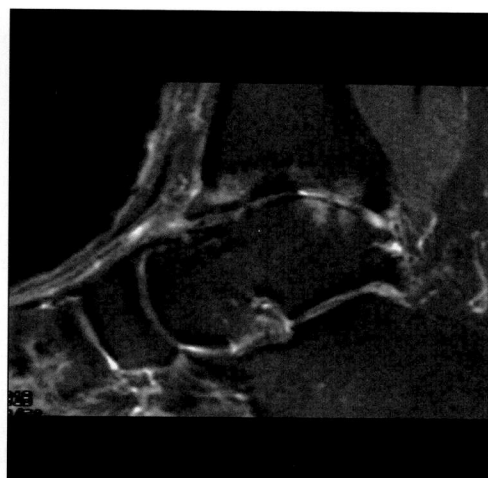

(Left) Sagittal T1WI MR shows prominent anterior osteophytes associated with tibiotalar arthritis. *(Right)* Sagittal FS PD FSE MR shows hyperintense degenerative edema in anterior tibial plafond osteophyte.

Typical

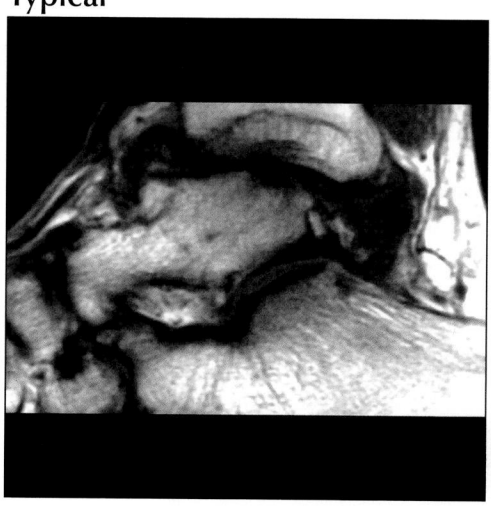

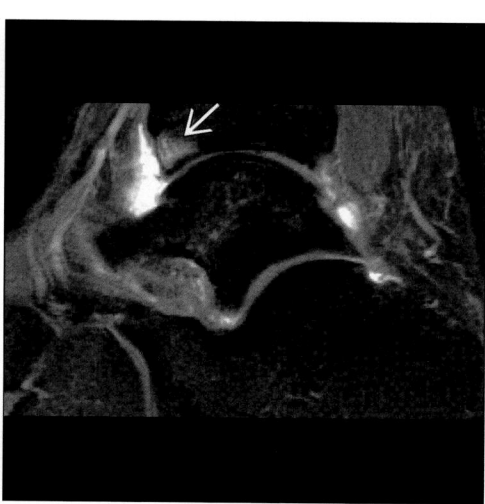

(Left) Sagittal T1WI MR shows secondary synovial inflammatory reaction in the tibiotalar joint associated with hypertrophic bone. *(Right)* Sagittal FS PD FSE MR shows early hyperintense stress (arrow) reaction in the anterior inferior distal tibia.

SYNDESMOTIC IMPINGEMENT

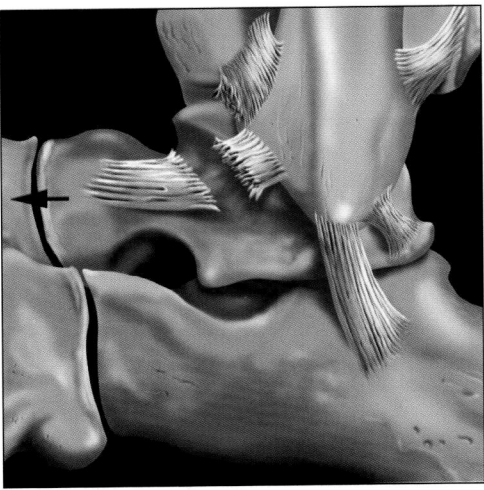

Sagittal graphic shows tear of the ATFL associated with lateral ankle laxity and anterior extrusion of the talar dome. There is impingement of the distal AITF against the talus.

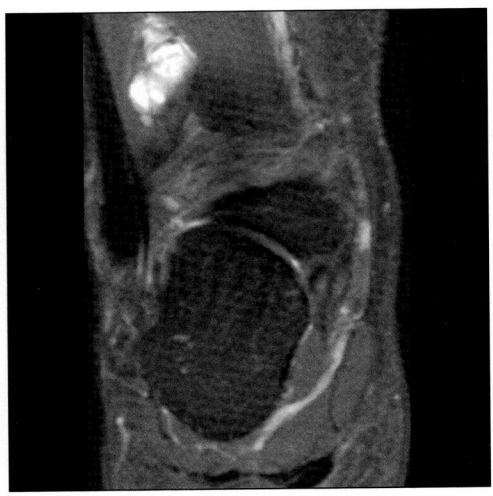

Coronal FS PD FSE MR shows ganglion at the level of the posterior syndesmotic ligament.

TERMINOLOGY

Abbreviations and Synonyms
- Syndesmotic impingement syndrome

Definitions
- Synovitis and scar post injury to syndesmotic ligaments

IMAGING FINDINGS

General Features
- Best diagnostic clue: Tissue thickening in syndesmotic space on axial images between tibia and fibula
- Location
  - Anterior inferior tibiofibular ligament (AITF)
  - Interosseous membrane
  - Posterior inferior tibiofibular ligament (PITF)
  - Abnormal fascicle AITF which rubs over talar dome = Bassett's ligament
- Size: Varies with involvement of anterior, central or posterior syndesmosis
- Morphology
  - Inflamed synovium envelops AITF
  - Synovial nodules

MR Findings
- T1WI
  - Intermediate signal inflamed synovium
  - Hypointense to intermediate signal synovial nodules
  - ± Tear AITF
  - Hypointense loose bodies
  - Hypointense osteophytes
- T2WI
  - Hyperintense fluid in syndesmosis
  - Chondromalacia of talar dome with focal hyperintense fissures
  - Hypointense filling defects in fluid
  - Hypointense/intermediate signal AITF ligament
  - Intermediate signal distal fascicle AITF
- T1 C+: Enhanced synovium

Imaging Recommendations
- Best imaging tool: MR
- Protocol advice
  - Axial FS PD FSE
  - ± T1 C+

DIFFERENTIAL DIAGNOSIS

Osteochondral Lesion (OLT)
- Focal edema ± interruption chondral surface talus

Peroneal Tendon Dysfunction
- Subluxation/dislocation peroneal tendons

DDx: Syndesmotic Impingement

OLT	P. Brevis Tear	Achilles Tear	Ant. Impingement
Cor T1WI MR	Ax FS PD MR	Sag FS PD MR	Sag FS PD MR

6

50

SYNDESMOTIC IMPINGEMENT

Key Facts

Imaging Findings
- Best diagnostic clue: Tissue thickening in syndesmotic space on axial images between tibia and fibula
- Abnormal fascicle AITF which rubs over talar dome = Bassett's ligament
- Inflamed synovium envelops AITF
- Synovial nodules

Top Differential Diagnoses
- Osteochondral Lesion (OLT)
- Peroneal Tendon Dysfunction
- Fracture Base 5th Metatarsal
- Achilles Tendon Injury
- Anterior Impingement
- Posterior Impingement

Pathology
- Mechanism = external rotation or hyperdorsiflexion
- Syndesmotic sprains - 10% of ankle injuries

Clinical Issues
- Most common signs/symptoms: Tenderness along syndesmosis + interosseous membrane
- Anterior popping sensation
- Age: Young high-performance athletes
- Talar dome extrudes anteriorly with dorsiflexion

Diagnostic Checklist
- Evaluate the entire anteroposterior extent of syndesmosis on axial cross-sectional images

Fracture Base 5th Metatarsal
- Edema and hypointense fracture line

Achilles Tendon Injury
- Tendinosis or partial tear on axial/sagittal images

Anterior Impingement
- Anterior osteophytes tibiotalar joint

Posterior Impingement
- Posterior talofibular, posterior syndesmotic + tibial slip

PATHOLOGY

General Features
- General path comments
  - Relevant anatomy
    - AITF
    - PITF
    - Inferior transverse tibiofibular ligament (just inferior to PITF)
    - Interosseous membrane
    - 20% AITF is intraarticular
- Etiology
  - With sprains + fractures
  - Collision sports: Hockey, football, soccer
  - Mechanism = external rotation or hyperdorsiflexion
  - Tibiofibular joint mechanics
    - Width trochlear surface of talus smaller posteriorly/lateral malleolus pulled superiorly with fibula medial rotation
- Epidemiology
  - Syndesmotic sprains - 10% of ankle injuries
  - Impingement - 3% of ankle injuries
  - Syndesmosis injuries underestimated clinically

Gross Pathologic & Surgical Features
- Inflamed synovium
- AITF involvement
- Inferior articulation tibia/fibula
- Synovial nodules
- Frayed AITF
- Chondromalacia of talus
- Osteophytes involving syndesmosis

Microscopic Features
- Synovial hyperplasia
- Capillary proliferation
- Chondral degeneration

CLINICAL ISSUES

Presentation
- Most common signs/symptoms: Tenderness along syndesmosis + interosseous membrane
- Clinical profile
  - Syndesmosis palpation elicits symptoms
  - Squeeze test: Compressing fibula against tibia proximal to mid calf
  - External rotation test: Pain with external rotation foot
    - Knee 90 degrees flexion
  - Passive dorsiflexion test
  - Anterior popping sensation

Demographics
- Age: Young high-performance athletes
- Gender: Male predominance: Military cadets, football players

Natural History & Prognosis
- Laxity lateral ankle
- Talar dome extrudes anteriorly with dorsiflexion
- Tibiofibular synostosis
- Pain with push-off
- Restricted dorsiflexion
- Ossification between distal tibia and fibula
- Talar surface degeneration

Treatment
- Conservative
  - Physical therapy
  - NSAIDs
- Surgery
  - Arthroscopy

- o Debridement AITF + hypertrophic synovium
- o Partial ligament excision
- o Removal synovial nodules in tibiofibular interspace

DIAGNOSTIC CHECKLIST

Consider
- Evaluate the entire anteroposterior extent of syndesmosis on axial cross-sectional images
- Visualize distal fascicle AITF and talar chondral surface

SELECTED REFERENCES

1. DeLee JC et al: Orthopaedic sports medicine. Principles and practice: Ligament injuries of the foot and ankle in the athlete. vol 2. 2nd ed. Philadelphia, Saunders, 2323-75, 2003
2. Uys HD et al: Clinical association of acute lateral ankle sprain with syndesmotic involvement: A stress radiography and magnetic resonance imaging study. Am J Sports Med 30(6):816-22, 2002
3. Banks A et al: McGlamry's comprehensive textbook of foot and ankle surgery. vol 1. 3rd ed. Philadelphia, Lippincott Williams & Wilkins, 1091-152, 2001
4. Tourne Y et al: Surgical treatment of bi- and trimalleolar ankle fractures: Should the medial collateral ligament be sutured or not? J Foot Ankle Surg 38(1):24-9, 1999
5. Ogilvie-Harris DJ et al: Chronic pain following ankle sprain in athletes: The role of arthroscopic surgery. Arthroscopy 13(5):564-74, 1997
6. Rubin A et al: Evaluation and diagnosis of ankle injuries. Am Fam Physician 54(5):1609-18, 1996
7. Ogilvie-Harris DJ et al: Disruption of the ankle syndesmosis: Diagnosis and treatment by arthroscopic surgery. Arthroscopy 10:561, 1994
8. Schneck CD et al: MR imaging of the most commonly injured ankle ligaments. Part I. Normal anatomy. Radiology 184:499, 1992
9. Mink JH: MRI of the foot and ankle: Ligaments of the ankle. New York, Raven Press, 185-9, 1992
10. Schneck CD et al: MR imaging of the most commonly injured ankle ligaments. Part II. Ligament injuries. Radiology 184:507-12, 1992
11. Erickson SJ et al: MR imaging of the lateral collateral ligament of the ankle. AJR 156:131-6, 1991
12. Fritschy D: An unusual ankle injury in top skiers. Am J Sports Med 17(2):282, 1989
13. Noto A et al: MR imaging of the ankle: Normal variants. Radiology 170:121-4, 1989
14. Sclafini S: Ligamentous injury of the lower tibiofibular syndesmosis: Radiographic evidence. Radiology 56:21-7, 1985
15. Monk C: Injuries to the tibio-fibular ligaments. J Bone Joint Surg 51B:330-7, 1969

SYNDESMOTIC IMPINGEMENT

IMAGE GALLERY

Typical

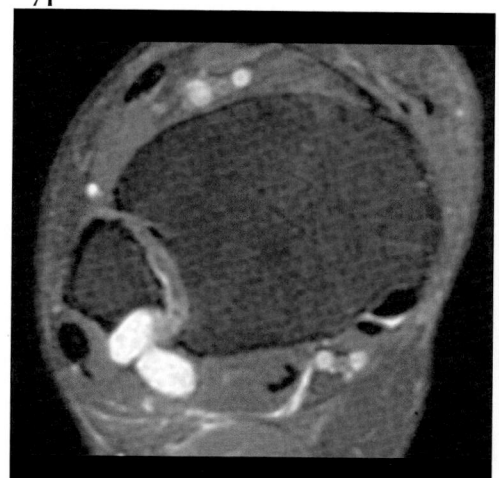

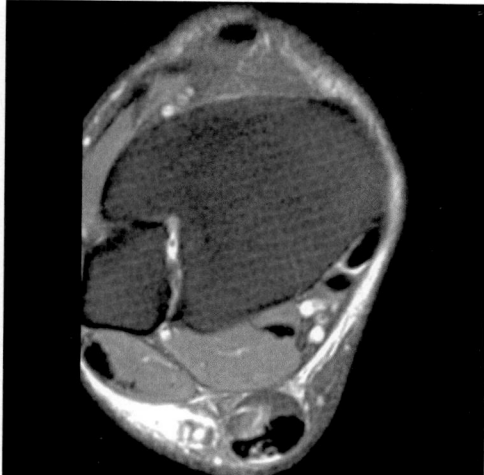

(Left) Axial FS PD FSE MR shows multilobulated posterior syndesmotic ganglion. *(Right)* Axial FS PD FSE MR shows abnormal osseous syndesmosis.

Typical

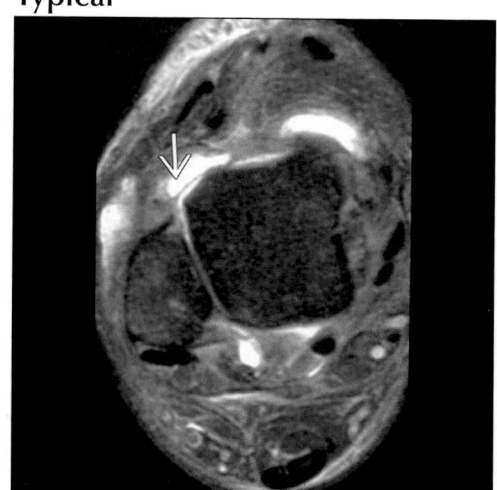

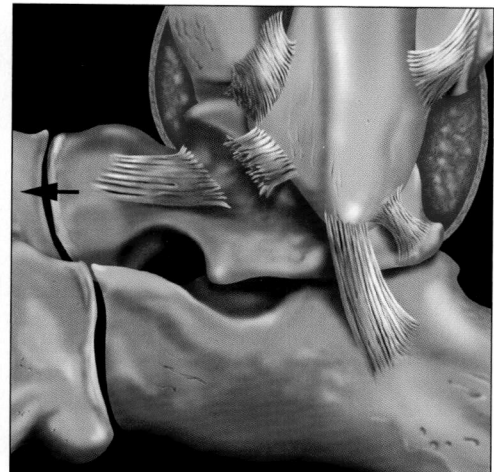

(Left) Axial FS PD FSE MR shows anterior syndesmotic synovitis (arrow). *(Right)* Sagittal graphic shows inflamed synovium enveloping frayed anterior inferior tibiofibular ligament and joint capsule. There is ligamentous impingement against the talus in dorsiflexion.

Typical

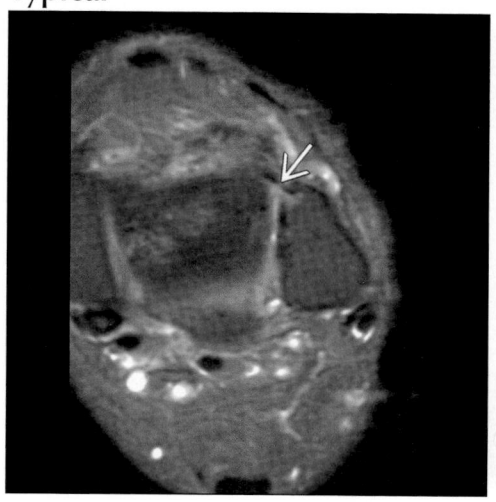

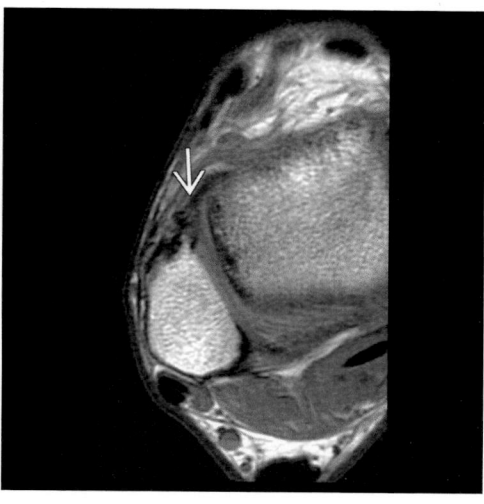

(Left) Axial FS PD FSE MR shows attenuated anterior syndesmotic ligament (arrow). *(Right)* Axial T1WI MR shows chronic thickening (arrow) with scar formation of anterior inferior tibiofibular ligament.

6

53

POSTERIOR IMPINGEMENT

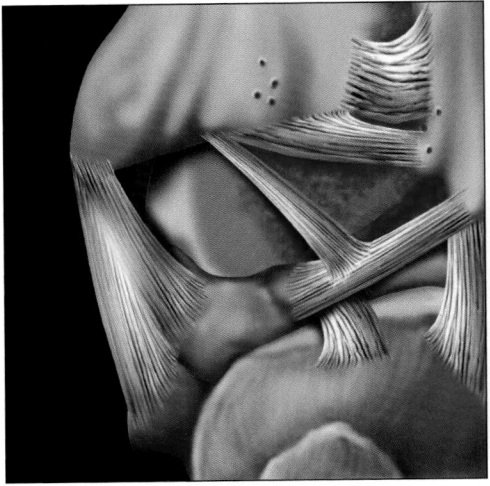

Coronal graphic shows synovitis, fibrosis, and capsulitis involving the posterior ligaments (posterior syndesmotic, transverse, posterior talofibular ligaments, tibial slip).

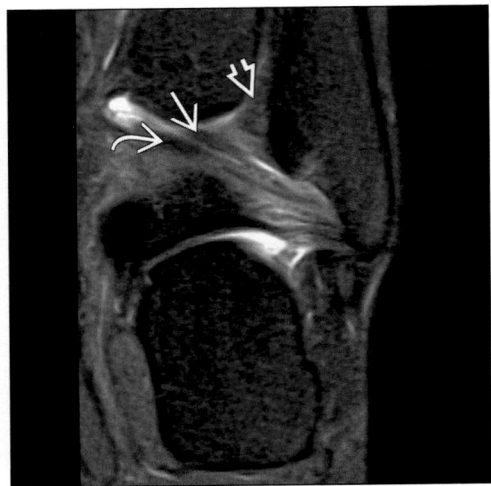

Coronal FS PD FSE MR shows hyperintense synovitis at level of posterior syndesmotic (open arrow), transverse (arrow), posterior talofibular ligaments as well as tibial slip (curved arrow).

TERMINOLOGY

Abbreviations and Synonyms
- Posterior soft tissue impingement; posterolateral soft tissue impingement

Definitions
- Soft tissue impingement posterolateral ankle

IMAGING FINDINGS

General Features
- Best diagnostic clue: Edema and fluid associated with posterior talofibular ligament (PTFL), transverse tibiofibular ligament, or tibial slip
- Location: Lateral side posterior ankle from posterior syndesmosis proximally to PTFL distally
- Size: Variable relative to synovitis, ganglion formation + combination of ligaments involved
- Morphology
  - Hypertrophy/tear of posterior ligaments
  - Posterior labrum enlargement (transverse ligament)
  - Bucket-handle tear tibial slip

MR Findings
- T1WI
  - Hypointense to intermediate signal fluid and synovium encasing posterior ligaments
  - Intermediate signal capsular thickening
  - Hypointense fibrosis
  - Enlarged labrum (transverse ligament)
    - Hypointense to intermediate signal
  - Periostitis
- T2WI
  - Inhomogeneous fluid/synovium combination surrounding posterior ligaments
  - Hyperintense ganglion cysts protruding between posterior ligaments
  - Interstitial hyperintensity posterior ligaments
  - Gross enlargement of tibial slip or labrum (transverse ligament)
  - Synovial nodule intermediate signal
- T1 C+: Enhanced synovium

Imaging Recommendations
- Best imaging tool: MR
- Protocol advice
  - FS PD FSE posterior coronal and sagittal images to identify individual components of posterior ligament complex
  - T1 C+ selective enhancement of thickened synovium or synovial nodule

---

DDx: Posterior Impingement

Os Trigonum	OLT	PTFL Sprain	Peroneal Sublux.	Subtalar DJD

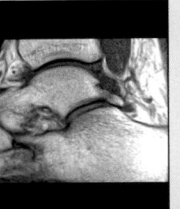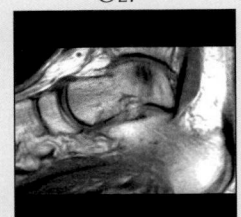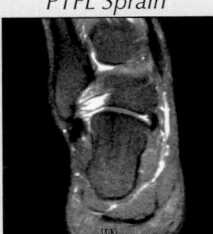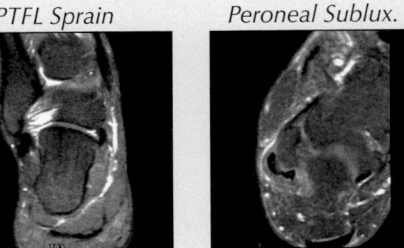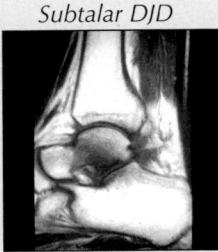

Sag T1WI MR	Sag T1WI MR	Cor FS PD MR	Ax FS PD MR	Sag T1WI MR

POSTERIOR IMPINGEMENT

Key Facts

Imaging Findings
- Best diagnostic clue: Edema and fluid associated with posterior talofibular ligament (PTFL), transverse tibiofibular ligament, or tibial slip
- Intermediate signal capsular thickening
- Hypointense fibrosis
- Enlarged labrum (transverse ligament)

Top Differential Diagnoses
- Os Trigonum Syndrome
- Osteochondral Lesion Talus (OLT)
- Posterior Talofibular Ligament Sprain

Pathology
- Isolated or in combination with anterolateral + syndesmosis impingement

- Plantar flexion mechanism with trauma/repetitive stress
- Predisposed with prominent posterior labrum or tibial slip
- Fibrosis

Clinical Issues
- Most common signs/symptoms: Pain/tenderness posterior ankle
- Posterior soft tissue fullness
- Chronic plantar flexion associated with fibrosis thickened synovium + ganglion

Diagnostic Checklist
- Identify posterior ligaments as potential sites of impingement on direct posterior coronal and sagittal images

DIFFERENTIAL DIAGNOSIS

Os Trigonum Syndrome
- Compression flexor hallucis longus tendon against medial edge ununited lateral tubercle of posterior talar process
- Osseous form of posterior ankle impingement

Osteochondral Lesion Talus (OLT)
- Compressed or avulsed talar dome fracture

Posterior Talofibular Ligament Sprain
- Associated with severe lateral ankle sprain
- Severe acute trauma + fracture

Peroneal Subluxation
- Sprain superior peroneal retinaculum/lateral ligament complex

Subtalar Arthrosis
- Subchondral sclerosis ± cystic change posterior facet subtalar joint

Tarsal Coalition
- Lateral cuneonavicular osseous, fibrocartilaginous or fibrous coalition with restricted motion

PATHOLOGY

General Features
- General path comments
  - Relevant anatomy
    - Posterior inferior tibiofibular ligament (PITF): From posterior lateral malleolus upward medially to posterolateral tibial tubercle
    - Transverse tibiofibular ligament: Deep/inferior to PITF (deep component of PITF)
    - Tibial slip: Superior border PTFL to posterior tibial margin + transverse tibiofibular ligament (insertion to posterior surface medial malleolus) = posterior intermalleolar ligament

    - PTFL: From medial/posterior lateral malleolus to insertion tubercle posterior talus lateral to flexor hallucis longus (FHL) groove
- Etiology
  - Isolated or in combination with anterolateral + syndesmosis impingement
  - Plantar flexion mechanism with trauma/repetitive stress
  - Athletes: Plantar flexion/inversion
  - Predisposed with prominent posterior labrum or tibial slip
  - Pseudomeniscus lesion on tibial slip ± displacement into joint
  - Ballet predisposes: Forced turn out and foot plant
- Epidemiology: Subset of ballet dancing, gymnastics, football players with plantarflexion activity

Gross Pathologic & Surgical Features
- Fibrosis
- Capsulitis
- Synovial swelling
- Hypertrophy transverse tibiofibular ligament or tibial slip
- Pseudomeniscus/tibial slip
- Synovial nodule

Microscopic Features
- Synovial hyperplasia
- Subsynovial capillary proliferation
- Chronic inflammatory process
- Fibrous ingrowth

CLINICAL ISSUES

Presentation
- Most common signs/symptoms: Pain/tenderness posterior ankle
- Clinical profile
  - Pain reproduced with passive plantar flexion ankle
  - Posterior soft tissue fullness

6

55

POSTERIOR IMPINGEMENT

Demographics
- Age: Younger population participating in plantar flexion sports
- Gender
  - Female predominance in ballet and gymnastics
  - Male involvement in football

Natural History & Prognosis
- Improvement with rest
- Chronic plantar flexion associated with fibrosis thickened synovium + ganglion
- Chronic ankle pain

Treatment
- Conservative
  - NSAIDs
  - Alteration of foot plantar flexion mechanics
  - Corticosteroid injection (lateral approach)
- Surgical
  - Arthroscopic
    - Debridement: Synovium + fibrosis

DIAGNOSTIC CHECKLIST

Consider
- Identify posterior ligaments as potential sites of impingement on direct posterior coronal and sagittal images
- Use T2WI (FS PD FSE) to identify hyperintense ganglion between posterior ligaments
- Normal variations exist in size of tibial slip and transverse ligament, evaluate gross hypertrophy of these structures

SELECTED REFERENCES

1. Robinson P et al: Soft tissue and osseous impingement syndromes of the ankle: Role of imaging in diagnosis and management. Radiographics 1457-69, 2002
2. Bureau NJ et al: Posterior ankle impingement syndrome: MR imaging findings in seven patients. Radiology 497-503, 2000
3. Fiorella D et al: The MR imaging features of the posterior intermalleolar ligament in patients with posterior impingement syndrome of the ankle. Skeletal Radiol 573-6, 1999
4. Steinbach LS: Painful syndromes around the ankle and foot: Magnetic resonance imaging evaluation. Top Magn Reson Imaging 311-26, 1998
5. Masciocchi C et al: Ankle impingement syndromes. Eur J Radiol Suppl 1:S70-3,1998
6. Masciocchi C et al: Overload syndromes of the peritalar region. Eur J Radiol 46-53,1997
7. Rosenberg ZS et al: Posterior intermalleolar ligament of the ankle: Normal anatomy and MR imaging features. AJR Am J Roentgenol 387-90, 1995
8. Hedrick MR et al: Posterior ankle impingement. Foot Ankle 15:2-8, 1994
9. Schweitzer ME et al: Magnetic resonance imaging of the foot and ankle. Magn Reson Q 214-34, 1993
10. Gibson JN et al: Arthroscopic lavage and debridement for osteoarthritis of the knee. J Bone Joint Surg Br 74:534-7, 1992
11. Marotta JJ et al: Os trigonum impingement in dancers. Am J Sports Med 20:533-6, 1992
12. Glick J et al: Ankle arthroscopy: Instructional course. Presented at the annual meeting of the American academy of orthopaedics surgeons, New Orleans, February 1990
13. Holt K et al: Isolated ruptures of the flexor hallucis longus tendon: A case report. Am J Sports Med 18:645, 1990
14. Martin DF et al: Operative ankle arthroscopy copy. Am J Sports Med 17:16-23, 1989
15. Hamilton WG: Foot and ankle injuries in dancers. Clin Sports Med 7:160-6, 1988
16. Kleiger B et al: The posterior tibiotalar impingement syndrome in dancers. Bull Hosp Jt Dis Orthop Inst 47:203-10, 1987
17. Brodsky EAE et al: Talar compression syndrome. Am J Sports Med 472-6, 1986
18. Glick JM et al: Ankle and foot fractures in athletics. The lower extremity and spine in sports medicine. St Louis, Mosby, 526-40, 1986
19. Andrews JR et al: Arthroscopy of the ankle: Technique and normal anatomy. Foot Ankle 6:29-33, 1985
20. Paulos LE et al: Posterior compartment fractures of the ankle: A commonly missed athletic injury. Am J Sports Med 11:439-43, 1983
21. Hamilton WG et al: Stenosing tenosynovitis of the flexor hallucis longus tendon and posterior impingement upon the os trigonum in ballet dancers. Foot Ankle 3:74-80, 1982
22. Howse AJG et al: Posterior block of the ankle joint in dancers. Foot Ankle 3:81-4, 1982

IMAGE GALLERY

Typical

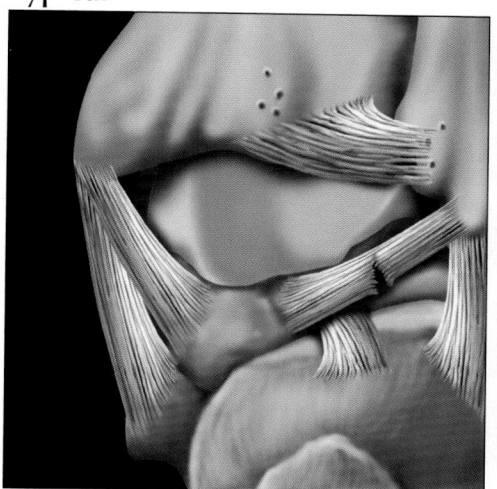
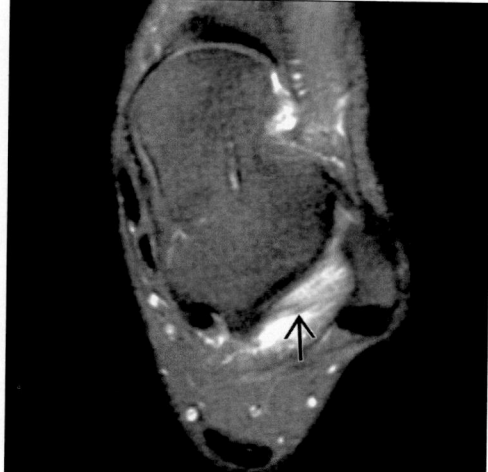

(Left) Coronal graphic shows partial tear of the posterior talofibular ligament. Frayed ligament fibers are shown in red. Enlargement of the posterior talofibular ligament may represent a potential site for posterior impingement. *(Right)* Axial FS PD FSE MR shows hyperintense edema (arrow) and synovitis associated with sprain of the posterior talofibular ligament.

Typical

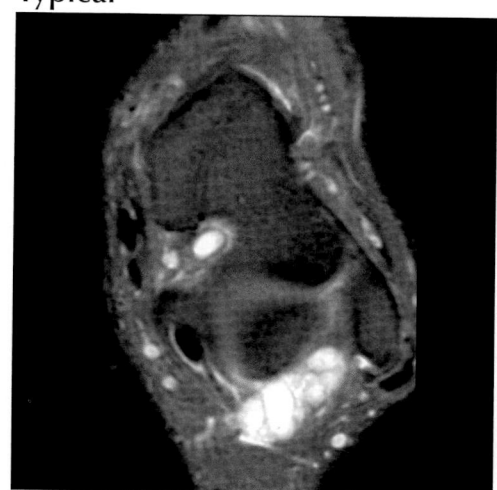
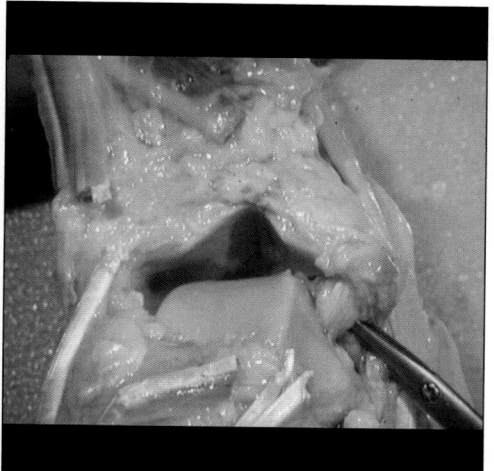

(Left) Axial FS PD FSE MR shows posterior impingement with multilobulated and septated ganglion associated with the posterior talofibular ligament. *(Right)* Coronal surgical pathology shows normal morphology of the posterior talofibular ligament which courses horizontally to insert on the posterior surface of the talus lateral to the groove for the FHL tendon.

Typical

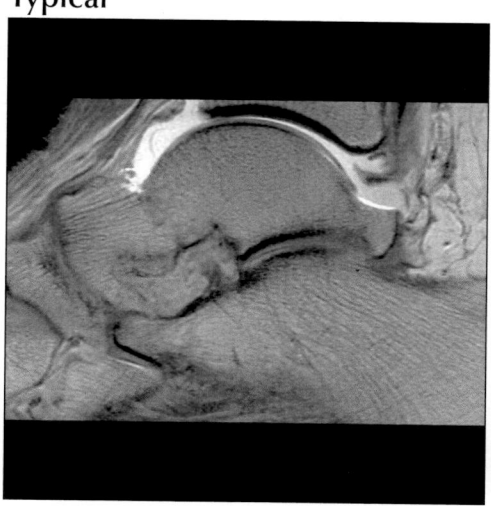
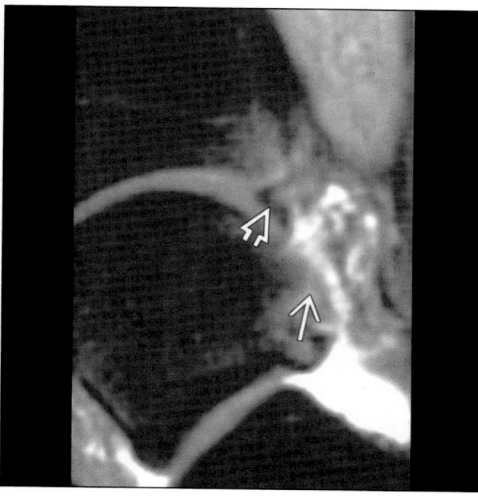

(Left) Sagittal T1 C+ (MR arthrogram) shows posterior inferior tibiofibular ligament and transverse tibiofibular ligament which projects inferior to posterior margin of distal tibia, anterior to posterior capsule. *(Right)* Sagittal FS PD FSE shows posterior impingement with hyperintense edema, synovitis, fluid involving posterior syndesmotic, transverse, (open arrow) posterior talofibular (arrow) ligaments. Hyperintense tibial bone marrow edema is also noted.

SINUS TARSI SYNDROME

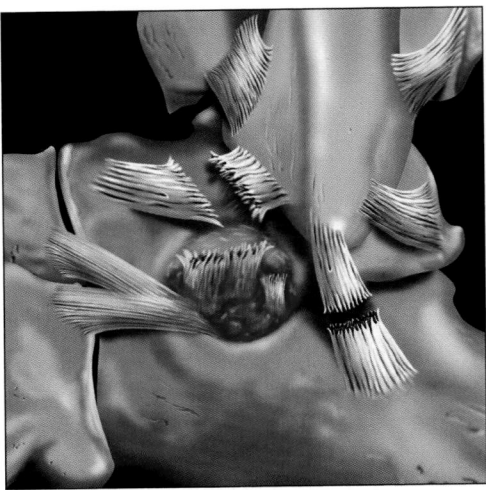

Sagittal graphic shows sinus tarsi syndrome with synovitis (in red) and tearing of the sinus tarsi ligaments. There is an associated tear of the ATFL.

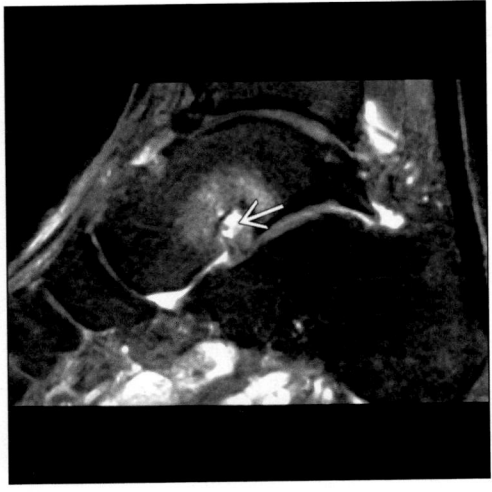

Sagittal FS PD FSE MR shows hyperintense bone marrow edema of the roof of the sinus tarsi with partial tearing (arrow) of the normally hypointense interosseous talocalcaneal ligament.

TERMINOLOGY

Abbreviations and Synonyms
- Sinus tarsi pathology

Definitions
- Sinus tarsi + lateral hindfoot pain and instability with injury to the contents of the tarsal canal and sinus

IMAGING FINDINGS

General Features
- Best diagnostic clue: Synovitis and poorly defined sinus tarsi ligaments
- Location
  - Anterior to posterior facet subtalar joint
  - Between inferior surface talus and superior surface calcaneus
  - Posterior to talocalcaneonavicular joint
  - Sinus tarsi continuous medially with narrower tarsal canal
- Size
  - Sinus tarsi + tarsal canal separates subtalar joint into anterior and posterior articulations
  - Larger lateral opening of tarsal canal = sinus tarsi
  - Tarsal canal
    - 10 to 15 mm high
    - 3 to 5 mm wide
    - 15 to 20 mm long
- Morphology
  - Sinus tarsi = funnel-shaped channel
  - 45 degree angle between long axis sinus tarsi & lateral aspect calcaneus

Radiographic Findings
- Radiography
  - Negative for degenerative findings
  - Normal stress radiography
  - Arthrography - decreased microrecesses/loss of sinus tarsi filling

MR Findings
- T1WI
  - Effacement sinus tarsi fat with intermediate signal fluid, synovitis ± fibrosis on T1WI
  - Poorly defined margins of interosseous and cervical ligaments
  - Secondary sclerosis and subchondral cystic change roof of sinus tarsi
  - Osseous flattening subchondral hypointense sclerosis posterior facet subtalar joint
  - Subchondral erosions within critical angle of Gissane
- T2WI
  - Hypointense/intermediate synovial fibrosis
  - Inhomogeneous synovitis

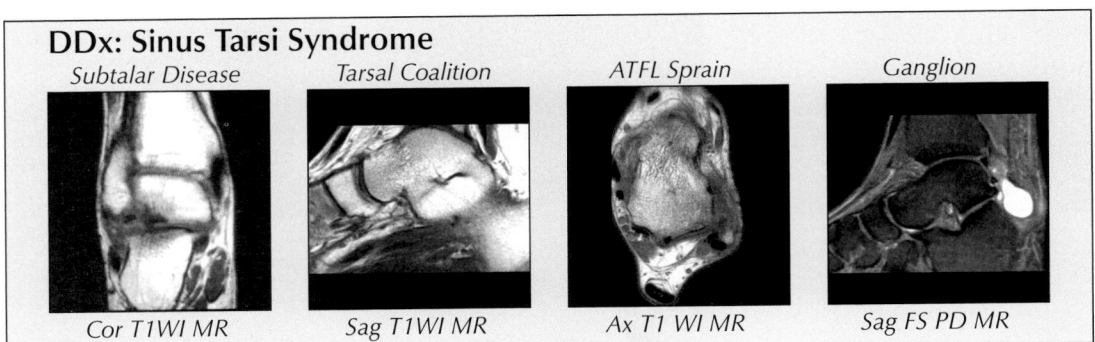

DDx: Sinus Tarsi Syndrome

Subtalar Disease	Tarsal Coalition	ATFL Sprain	Ganglion
Cor T1WI MR	Sag T1WI MR	Ax T1 WI MR	Sag FS PD MR

6

58

SINUS TARSI SYNDROME

Key Facts

Imaging Findings

- Best diagnostic clue: Synovitis and poorly defined sinus tarsi ligaments
- Larger lateral opening of tarsal canal = sinus tarsi
- Effacement sinus tarsi fat with intermediate signal fluid, synovitis ± fibrosis on T1WI
- Poorly defined margins of interosseous and cervical ligaments
- Secondary sclerosis and subchondral cystic change roof of sinus tarsi

Top Differential Diagnoses

- Subtalar Arthrosis
- Tarsal Coalition
- Lateral Ankle Ligament Sprain
- Ganglion

Pathology

- Initial traumatic event: Decreased venous outflow
- Fibrosis with vascular engorgement or nerve irritation
- Interosseous ligament tears

Clinical Issues

- Most common signs/symptoms: Pain lateral aspect sinus tarsi
- Previous ankle sprain in 70%
- Tibialis posterior tendon disruption
- Association of subtalar ± lateral ankle instability

Diagnostic Checklist

- Document condition of interosseous talocalcaneal and cervical ligaments in sagittal plane

---

- ○ Tears ± absence normally hypointense interosseous talocalcaneal and cervical ligaments
- ○ Increased signal intermediate and medial roots inferior extensor retinaculum
- ○ Synovitis anterior capsule of posterior talocalcaneal joint
- ○ Talar + calcaneal subchondral cystic degeneration
- ○ Lateral ankle ligament sprain
  - Anterior talofibular
  - Calcaneofibular
- ○ Complete rupture interosseous talocalcaneal + cervical ligaments = subtalar joint dislocation
- ○ Associated tibialis posterior tendon dysfunction
- T1 C+
  - ○ Enhancement of chronic synovitis inflammation
  - ○ Peripheral enhancement synovial cysts

Imaging Recommendations

- Best imaging tool: MRI indicated for nonlocalized symptoms, persistent pain, failed conservative treatment or associated injuries
- Protocol advice
  - ○ Sagittal T1/PD and FS PD FSE
  - ○ FS T1 C+ for selective enhancement hypertrophic synovium

DIFFERENTIAL DIAGNOSIS

Subtalar Arthrosis

- Subchondral sclerosis and degeneration isolated to posterior facet > middle facet without sinus tarsi involvement

Tarsal Coalition

- Osseous or fibrous talocalcaneal or calcaneonavicular

Lateral Ankle Ligament Sprain

- Localized to anterior talofibular (ATFL) or calcaneofibular ligaments and not sinus tarsi ligaments

Bifurcate Ligament Sprain

- Localized to anterior subtalar and calcaneocuboid articulation (bifurcate ligament connects anterior process calcaneus to navicular and cuboid)

Ganglion

- Extension through sinus tarsi without sprain of sinus ligaments
- Hyperintense on T2WI

Lipomas

- Mass effect secondary to extrinsic compression on sinus tarsi contents
- Fat signal suppresses on FS PD FSE or STIR

Inflammatory Arthritis

- Seropositive (reactive synovial hyperplasia)
- Seronegative
- Calcium pyrophosphate dihydrate deposition (CPPD)

PATHOLOGY

General Features

- General path comments
  - ○ Relevant anatomy
    - Fat pad
    - Arterial anastomosis (branches of posterior tibial and peroneal arteries)
    - Proprioceptive nerves
    - Bursal projection
    - Ligaments: Medial and intermediate roots inferior extensor retinaculum; cervical ligaments; talocalcaneal interosseous ligament of tarsal canal
- Etiology
  - ○ Initial traumatic event: Decreased venous outflow
  - ○ Fibrosis with vascular engorgement or nerve irritation
  - ○ Inversion injury ankle or hindfoot
  - ○ Ligament injury sequence
    - Calcaneofibular ligament
    - Lateral talocalcaneal ligament
    - Interosseous ligament

SINUS TARSI SYNDROME

- Subtalar joint sprain
- Epidemiology: Posttraumatic = 70% of cases

Gross Pathologic & Surgical Features
- Interosseous ligament tears
- Osteoarthrosis
- Arthrofibrosis
- Partial tears calcaneofibular ligament
- Synovial hypertrophy

Microscopic Features
- Scarring
- Synovial hyperplasia
- Chronic synovitis
- Hemosiderin

Staging, Grading or Classification Criteria
- Clinical signs
  - Tenderness with palpation
  - Instability on uneven terrain
  - Pain relief with local anesthetic block
  - Failure to reproduce instability clinically or radiographically

CLINICAL ISSUES

Presentation
- Most common signs/symptoms: Pain lateral aspect sinus tarsi
- Clinical profile
  - Previous ankle sprain in 70%
  - Deep aching
  - Throbbing
  - Subtalar instability
  - Symptoms exacerbated with weight bearing
  - Swelling/edema in acute setting
  - Relief of pain with local anesthetic injection
  - Tibialis posterior tendon disruption

Demographics
- Age: 20 to 40 years
- Gender: Slight male predominance as a function of chronic ankle sprain history

Natural History & Prognosis
- Association of subtalar ± lateral ankle instability
- > 50% respond to conservative treatment

Treatment
- Conservative
  - Physical therapy
  - NSAID's
  - Steroid injections into sinus tarsi
  - Orthotics
  - Casting/aircast splints
- Surgery
  - Sinus tarsi evacuation
  - Subtalar arthroscopy/debridement of posterior subtalar joint and sinus tarsi
  - Removal hypertrophic synovium and scarred ligamentous tissue
  - Arthrodesis for posterior facet arthrosis subtalar joint

DIAGNOSTIC CHECKLIST

Consider
- Document condition of interosseous talocalcaneal and cervical ligaments in sagittal plane
- Evaluate arthrosis of posterior facet of subtalar joint on sagittal images
- Use of T1 C+ if severe synovial hypertrophy present

SELECTED REFERENCES

1. Banks A et al: McGlamry's comprehensive textbook of foot and ankle surgery. vol 1. Philadelphia PA, Lippincott Williams & Wilkins, 1091-152, 2001
2. Lektrakul N et al: Tarsal sinus: Arthrographic, MR imaging MR arthrographic, and pathologic findings in cadavers and retrospective study data in patients with sinus tarsi syndrome. Radiology 19(3):802-10, 2001
3. Myerson M: Foot and ankle disorders. vol 2. Philadelphia PA, Lippincott Raven, 1399-419, 2000
4. Rosenberg ZS et al: From RSNA refresher courses. Radiologic Society of North America. MR imaging of the ankle and foot. Radiographics 20 S153-79, 2000
5. Steinbach LS: Painful syndromes around the ankle and foot: Magnetic resonance imaging evaluation. Top Magn Reson Imaging 9(5):311-26, 1998
6. Beltran J: Sinus tarsi syndrome. Magn Reson Imaging Clin N Am 2(1):59-65, 1994
7. Klein MA et al: MR imaging of the tarsal sinus and canal: Normal anatomy, pathologic findings, and features of the sinus tarsi syndrome. Radiology 186(1):233-40, 1993
8. Keeland JB et al: Magnetic resonance imaging of the foot and ankle. Magn Reson Q 8(2):97-115 review, 1992
9. Regnauld B: The foot: Pathology, etiology, semiology, clinical investigation, and therapy. Sinus tarsi syndrome. New York NY. Springer-Ver-lag, 298, 1986
10. Taillard W et al: The sinus tarsi syndrome. Int Orthop 5:117, 1981
11. Meyer JM et al: Post-traumatic sinus tarsi syndrome: An anatomical and radiological study. Acta Orthop Scand 48:121, 1977
12. Cahill DR et al: The anatomy and function of the contents of the human tarsal sinus and canal. Anat Rec 153:1, 1965
13. O'Connor D et al: Sinus tarsi syndrome - a clinical entity. J Bone Joint Surg 40A:720, 1958

SINUS TARSI SYNDROME

IMAGE GALLERY

Typical

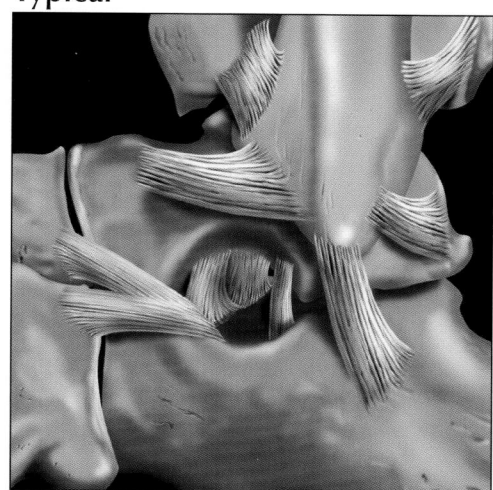
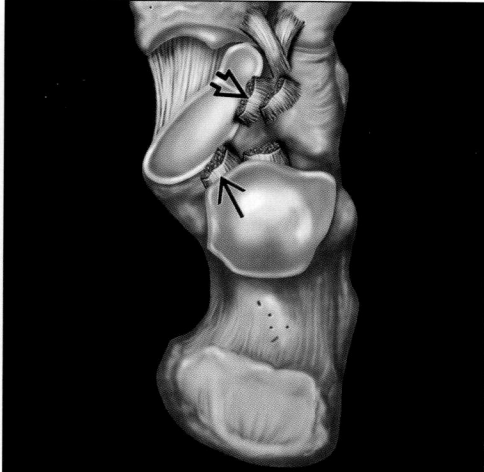

(Left) Sagittal graphic shows intact cervical and interosseous talocalcaneal ligaments of the sinus tarsi. The sinus tarsi and tarsal canal separate the anterior and posterior articulations of the subtalar joints. *(Right)* Axial graphic shows normal 45 degree angle of the long axis of the sinus tarsi relative to the lateral aspect of the calcaneus. The cervical ligament (open arrow) is anterolateral to the interosseous talocalcaneal ligament (arrow).

Typical

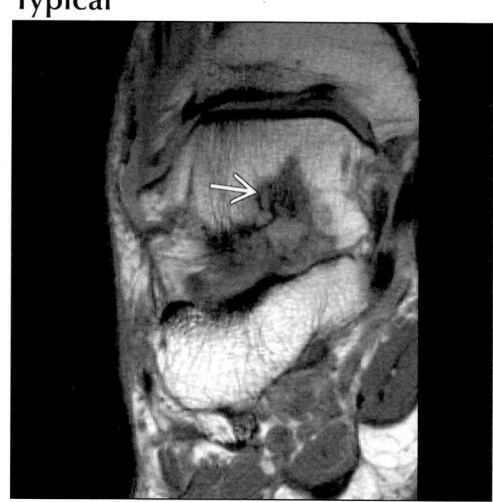
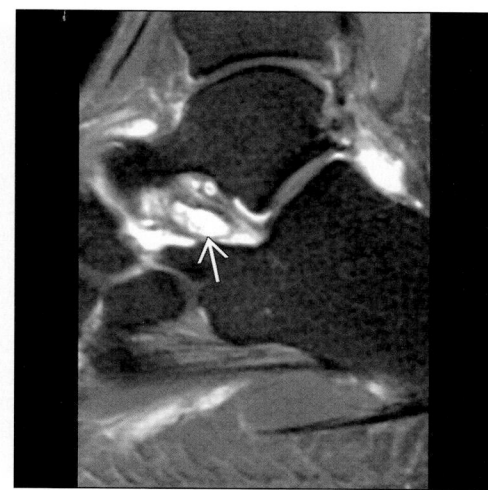

(Left) Coronal T1WI MR shows subchondral sclerosis (arrow) and cystic change of the roof of sinus tarsi with poorly defined margins of the sinus tarsi ligaments. *(Right)* Sagittal FS PD FSE MR shows hyperintense cystic changes (arrow) and synovitis within the sinus tarsi ligaments.

Variant

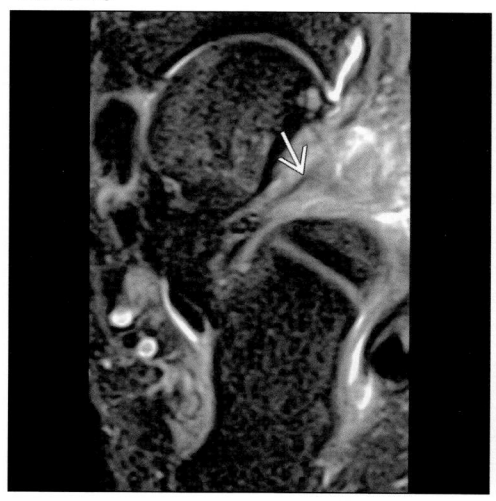
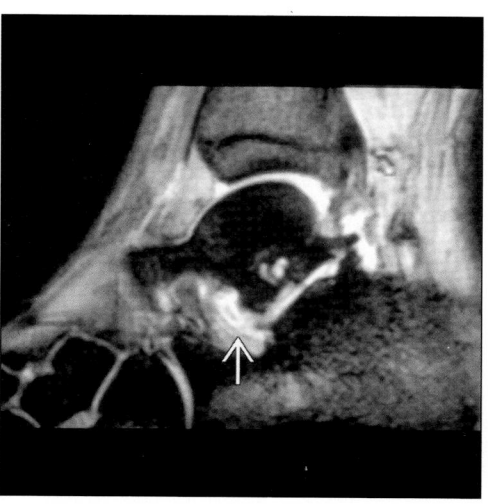

(Left) Axial FS PD FSE MR shows synovitis with hypertrophic synovium (arrow) encasing the sinus tarsi and tarsal canal. *(Right)* Sagittal FS PD FSE MR shows subtalar arthrosis with anteriorly projecting synovium (arrow) mimicking posterior sinus tarsi pathology.

ANKLE FRACTURES

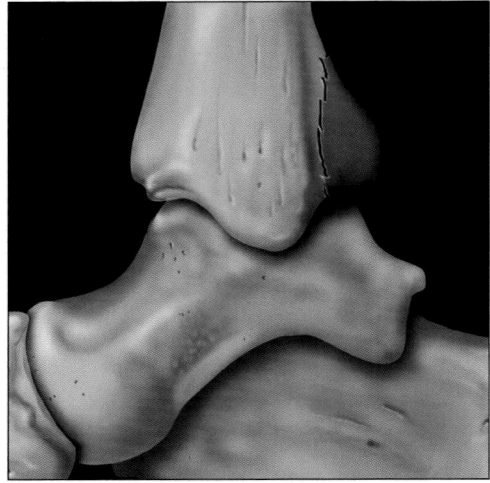

Sagittal graphic shows non-displaced posterior malleolar fracture.

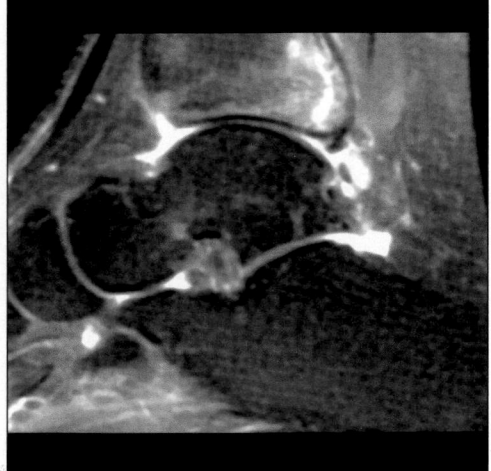

Sagittal FS PD FSE MR shows hyperintense edema involving the posterior tubercle of the distal tibia (fracture of the posterior or third malleolus).

TERMINOLOGY

Abbreviations and Synonyms
- Malleolar; distal tibia or pilon; Tillaux (lateral margin tibia); triplanar or Marmor-Lynn (lateral distal tibia epiphysis); distal third fibular or Pott fracture; Dupuytren or fibular (proximal to distal tibiofibular syndesmosis); Maisonneuve (proximal half fibula)

Definitions
- Fracture of malleoli, distal tibia and fibula

IMAGING FINDINGS

General Features
- Best diagnostic clue: Complete cortical fracture malleoli, distal tibia or fibula
- Location
  - Medial, lateral and posterior malleoli
  - Pilon = distal tibia with + intraarticular extension
  - Tillaux = lateral margin distal tibia to distal articular surface
  - Juvenile Tillaux = Salter-Harris (S-H) type III distal tibial growth plate
  - Triplanar = S-H type IV, lateral distal tibial epiphysis with sagittal, axial and coronal plane components
  - Pott = distal third fibula

- Dupuytren = fibula 2 to 7 cm proximal to distal tibiofibular syndesmosis
- Maisonneuve = proximal fibula at proximal/middle thirds diaphysis
- Size: Variable based on location (malleoli vs. tibia vs. fibular) and pathomechanics
- Morphology
  - Malleoli - transverse to oblique to vertical (posterior malleolus)
  - Pilon - comminution distal tibia + extension through tibial plafond
  - Tillaux - horizontal physeal component + vertical extension to distal tibia articular surface
  - Triplane = vertical in sagittal plane + horizontal in axial plane + oblique in coronal plane
  - Fibular fractures - horizontal to oblique

Radiographic Findings
- Radiography
  - Routine anteroposterior (AP), lateral & oblique internal rotation (mortise)
  - ± Full-length views for proximal tibia/fibula
  - ± Stress views

CT Findings
- NECT
  - Extent & position articular fragments
  - Degree of comminution
  - Associated osteochondral lesions talus

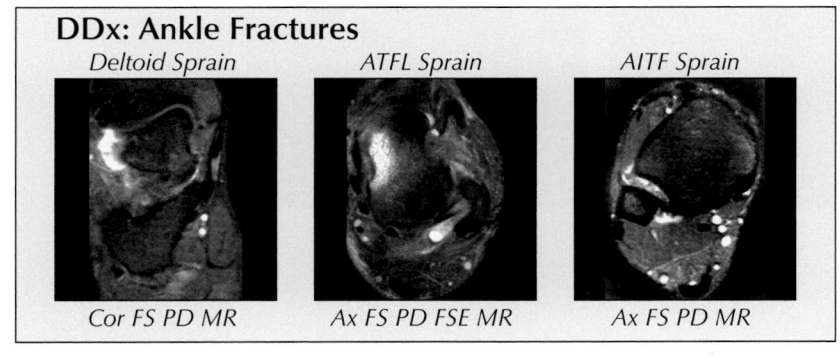

DDx: Ankle Fractures

Deltoid Sprain	ATFL Sprain	AITF Sprain
Cor FS PD MR	Ax FS PD FSE MR	Ax FS PD MR

ANKLE FRACTURES

Key Facts

Imaging Findings
- Best diagnostic clue: Complete cortical fracture malleoli, distal tibia or fibula
- Pilon = distal tibia with + intraarticular extension
- Tillaux = lateral margin distal tibia to distal articular surface
- Triplanar = S-H type IV, lateral distal tibial epiphysis with sagittal, axial and coronal plane components

Top Differential Diagnoses
- Medial Ankle Sprain
- Lateral Ankle Sprain
- Syndesmotic Sprain

Pathology
- Position of foot and direction of force at time of loading = injury type

- Eccentric vertical loading = asymmetric compression
- Torsional loading = helical fracture patterns
- Combined loading most common = medial, lateral, torsional, axial
- Epidemiology: Supination - external rotation - most common mechanism = 40 to 75% all malleolar fractures

Clinical Issues
- Most common signs/symptoms: Localized pain & tenderness over malleoli, distal tibia, fibula
- Degenerative changes in 85% if not anatomically reduced

Diagnostic Checklist
- Associated ligamentous injuries - medial, lateral or syndesmotic ligaments

MR Findings
- T1WI
  - Malleoli: Hypointense fracture line ± hypointense marrow edema
  - Pilon
    - Separate comminuted distal tibial fragment
    - Hypointense fracture extension to tibial plafond
    - ± Displacement
  - Tillaux: Vertical hypointense fracture line perpendicular to epiphysis + thick hypointense lateral physis with lateral fracture extension
  - Triplanar: Separate hypointense fractures oriented anteroposterior in axial plane, proximal to distal in coronal plane, oblique in sagittal plane
  - Fibular: Hypointense transverse to oblique
- T2WI
  - Malleoli: Diffuse marrow edema to localized edema adjacent to fracture site
  - Distal tibia
    - Localized edema adjacent to fracture site vs. more diffuse pattern of edema
    - Variable proximal extension of hyperintense signal
    - Interruption of distal chondral surface with hyperintense fluid signal

Imaging Recommendations
- Best imaging tool: MR, except CT for complex pilon fractures with displacement of weight-bearing segments
- Protocol advice
  - Coronal, sagittal and axial T1 (note PD - poor marrow contrast)
  - Coronal, sagittal and axial FS PD FSE or STIR

DIFFERENTIAL DIAGNOSIS

Medial Ankle Sprain
- Sprained deltoid > complete tear
- Associated osseous avulsions
- ± Fibular fracture

- Widened mortise in preexisting lateral complex injuries

Lateral Ankle Sprain
- Pain & tenderness & swelling anterior to fibular ligament distribution
- ± Calcaneofibular ligament involvement
- ± Anterior displacement talus
- ± Widened mortise

Syndesmotic Sprain
- Pain over anterior inferior tibiofibular ligament (AITF) most common
- Diastasis syndesmosis at level of tibial plafond
- Hemorrhage ± fibrosis in syndesmosis ± interosseous membrane involvement

PATHOLOGY

General Features
- General path comments
  - Relevant anatomy
    - Load-bearing surface = pilon = lower tibial metaphyseal expansion
- Etiology
  - Eversion fractures
    - Pott
    - Maisonneuve
    - Dupuytren
    - Tillaux
  - Position of foot and direction of force at time of loading = injury type
  - Eccentric vertical loading = asymmetric compression
  - Torsional loading = helical fracture patterns
  - Combined loading most common = medial, lateral, torsional, axial
  - Pilon: Pronation/dorsiflexion
- Epidemiology: Supination - external rotation - most common mechanism = 40 to 75% all malleolar fractures

Gross Pathologic & Surgical Features
- Supination - adduction (Lauge-Hansen)

- Stage I = lateral ligamentous failure + lateral malleolus avulsion (transverse fracture at level of plafond)
  - Stage II = vertical, medially displaced fracture medial malleolus
- Supination - external rotation
  - Stage I = tear anterior talofibular ligament (ATFL)
  - Stage II = spiral oblique fracture lateral malleolus from plafond extending proximally
  - Stage III = tear posterior inferior tibiofibular ligament/fracture posterior malleolus
  - Stage IV = medial malleolus fracture ± rupture deep deltoid ligament
- Pronation - abduction
  - Stage I = transverse avulsion fracture medial malleolus or deltoid ligament rupture
  - Stage II = rupture anterior and posterior inferior tibiofibular syndesmotic ligaments
  - Stage III = horizontal, oblique fibular fracture above the joint (plafond)
- Pronation - external rotation
  - Stage I = rupture deltoid ligament or medial malleolus transverse fracture
  - Stage II = tear anterior inferior tibiofibular ligament
  - Stage III = oblique/spiral fibular fracture above plafond
  - Stage IV = tear posterior inferior tibiofibular ligament or posterior malleolus fracture
- Pilon
  - Type I = fissure fracture undisplaced
  - Type II = displaced + articular incongruity
  - Type III = compression fracture + displacement weight-bearing segments (crushing subchondral cancellous bone)
- Tillaux: Fracture line from distal tibial articular surface proximally + toward lateral cortex
- Triplane: Fracture - vertical, horizontal & oblique
- Maisonneuve: Spiral fracture proximal fibula + unstable ankle injury

Microscopic Features
- Fracture site
  - Hematoma
  - Revascularization
  - Primary heading vs. callus
  - Collagen separation of ligamentous structures

Staging, Grading or Classification Criteria
- Danis - Weber type A = Lauge - Hansen supination - adduction
- Danis - Weber type B = Lauge - Hansen supination external rotation or pronation - abduction
- Danis - Weber type C = Lauge - Hansen pronation - external rotation

CLINICAL ISSUES

Presentation
- Most common signs/symptoms: Localized pain & tenderness over malleoli, distal tibia, fibula
- Clinical profile
  - Deformity = dislocation
  - Swelling

- Ecchymosis
- Fibular compression test

Demographics
- Age
  - Variable
  - Tillaux as juvenile Tillaux pattern in children
  - Pediatric ankle fracture = most common is Salter I physis injury
- Gender: Non-specific for gender
- Related activity
  - High energy (e.g., motorcycle)
  - Low energy - seen as mechanism for medial malleolar injuries

Natural History & Prognosis
- Arthritis - based on severity
- Degenerative changes in 85% if not anatomically reduced

Treatment
- Conservative: Closed reduction
- Surgical: Open reduction with internal fixation (ORIF)

DIAGNOSTIC CHECKLIST

Consider
- Associated ligamentous injuries - medial, lateral or syndesmotic ligaments
- CT may be useful for displaced distal tibial pilon fractures
- Evaluate for osteochondral lesions of the talus (OLT)

SELECTED REFERENCES

1. Vander Griend et al: Fractures of the ankle and distal parts of the tibia. Inst Course Lect 46:311-21, 1997
2. Petit P et al: Acute fracture of the distal tibial physis: Role of gradient-echo MR imaging versus plain film examination. AJR 166(5):1203-6, 1996
3. Michelson JD: Fractures about the ankle. J Bone Joint Surg Am 77:142-52, 1995
4. Karas EH et al: Displaced pilon fractures: An update. Orthop Clin North Am 25:651, 1994
5. Schils JP et al: Medial malleolar stress fractures in seven patients: Review of the clinical and imaging features. Radiology 185:219, 1992
6. Michelson JD et al: Examination of the pathologic anatomy of ankle fractures. J Trauma 32:65, 1992
7. Harper MC et al: Posterior malleolar fractures of the ankle associated with external rotation-abduction injuries: Results with and with-out internal fixation. J Bone Joint Surg Am 70:1348, 1988
8. Bauer M et al: Supination-eversion fractures of the ankle joint: Changes in incidence over 30 years. Foot Ankle 8:26-28, 1987
9. Lindsjo U: Classification of ankle fractures: The Lauge-Hansen or AO system? Clin Orthop 199:12, 1985

ANKLE FRACTURES

IMAGE GALLERY

Typical

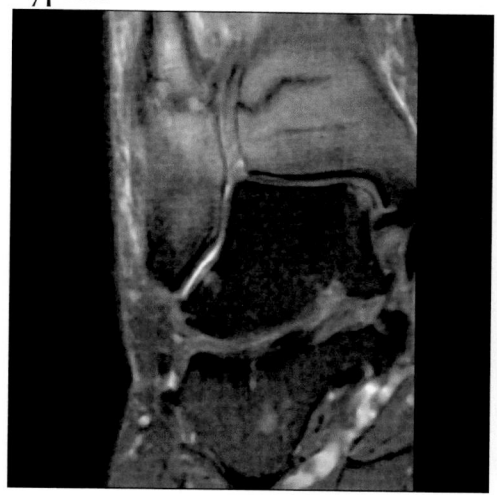
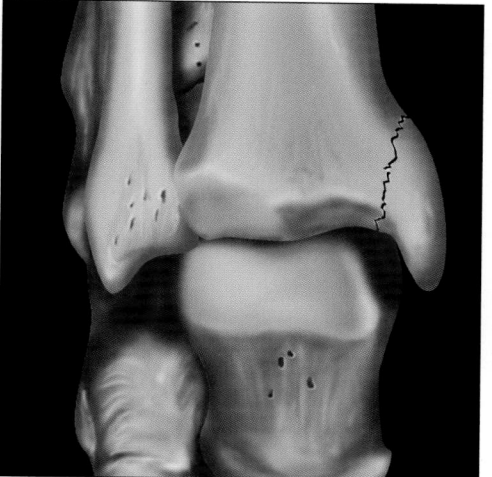

(Left) Coronal FS PD FSE MR shows transverse fractures of the distal tibia and fibula with hyperintense edema. Tibiotalar joint instability and medial OLT are present. *(Right)* Coronal graphic shows medial malleolar fracture.

Typical

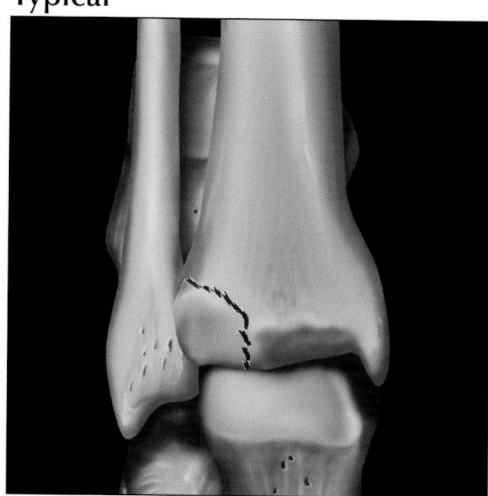
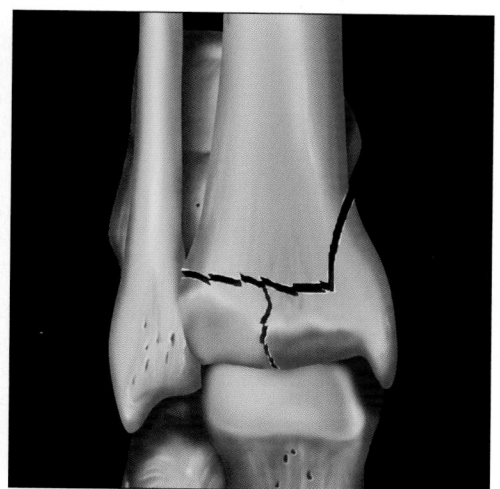

(Left) Coronal graphic shows Tillaux fracture with avulsion of the lateral margin of the distal tibia. *(Right)* Coronal graphic shows triplane injury with fracture involving the sagittal, axial, and coronal planes.

Typical

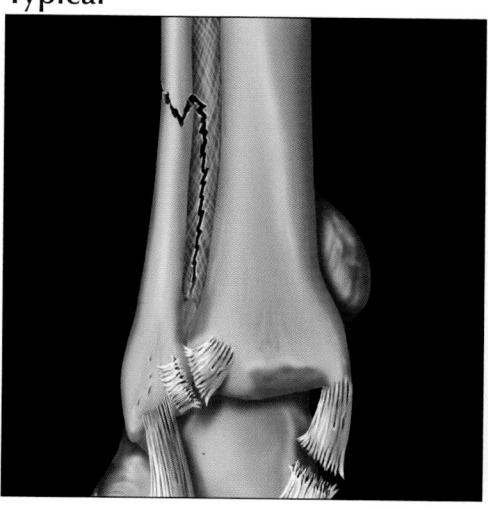
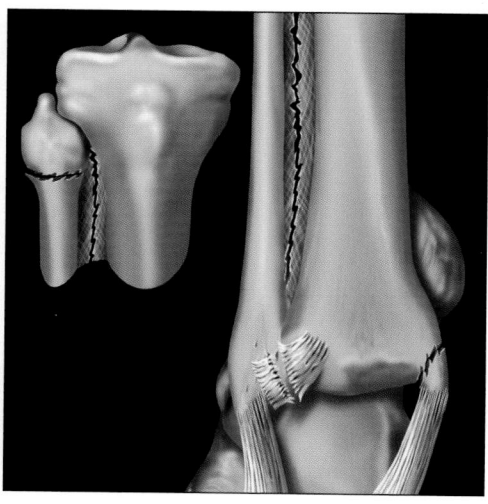

(Left) Coronal graphic shows Dupuytren fracture of the fibular diaphysis with deltoid ligament, interosseous membrane, and syndesmosis disruption. This also represents a Weber type C fracture. *(Right)* Coronal graphic shows Maisonneuve fracture involving the proximal fibula with disruption of the interosseous membrane and syndesmotic ligament.

TALUS FRACTURES

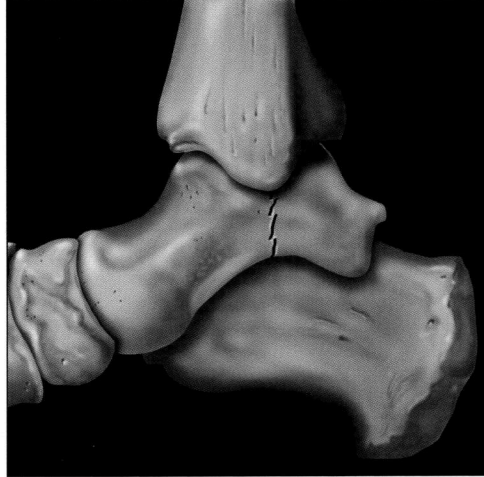

Sagittal graphic shows fracture of the talar body.

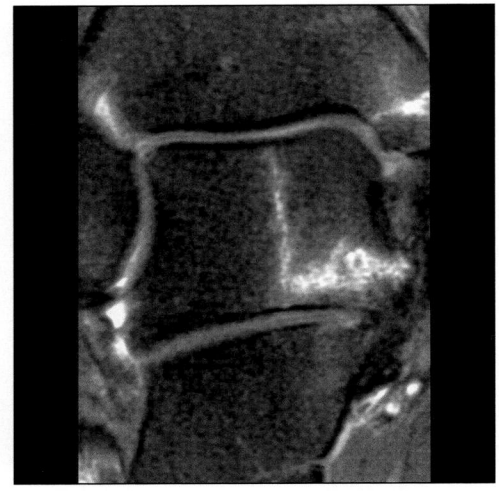

Coronal FS PD FSE MR shows vertical non-displaced fracture of the talar body. Hyperintense edema of the fracture is oriented in the sagittal plane.

TERMINOLOGY

Abbreviations and Synonyms
- Fractures of the talus

Definitions
- Fracture of talar head, neck, body, lateral or posterior process

IMAGING FINDINGS

General Features
- Best diagnostic clue: Linear, usually vertical fracture segments
- Location
  - Talar head, neck + body
  - Lateral + posterior process
- Size
  - Variable
    - Nondisplaced
    - Displaced
    - Open fractures
- Morphology
  - Head of talus
    - Avulsion
    - Peripheral
    - Compression
  - Lateral process
    - Comminuted
    - Large fragment (noncomminuted)
  - Posterior process
    - Os trigonum - vertical fracture at synchondrosis
  - Talar neck: Vertical
  - Body
    - Coronal
    - Sagittal
    - Horizontal

Radiographic Findings
- Radiography
  - Head of talus
    - Lateral view: Fracture pattern
    - Sagittal view: Displacement
    - Oblique views: Extent of fracture
  - Lateral process
    - AP or mortise
  - Posterior process
    - Lateral view
  - Talar neck
    - Lateral view: ± Subluxation/dislocation
  - Talar body
    - Lateral view

CT Findings
- NECT
  - Direct coronal + axial, sagittal reformations

DDx: Talar Fractures

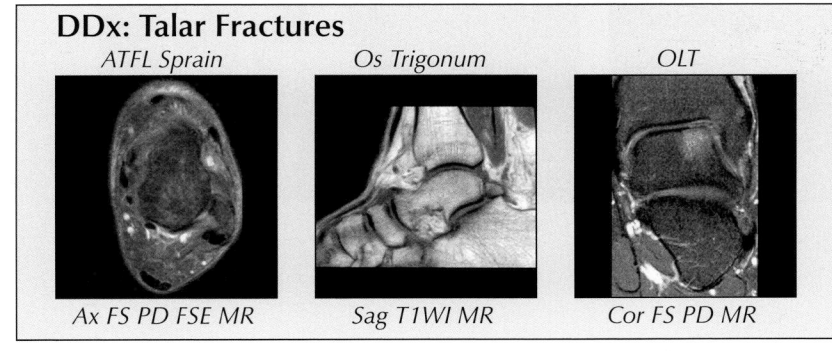

ATFL Sprain	Os Trigonum	OLT
Ax FS PD FSE MR	Sag T1WI MR	Cor FS PD MR

6

66

TALUS FRACTURES

Key Facts

Imaging Findings
- Best diagnostic clue: Linear, usually vertical fracture segments
- Talar head, neck + body
- Lateral + posterior process
- Best imaging tool: MR - to appreciate marrow edema, chondral involvement + AVN

Top Differential Diagnoses
- Ankle Sprains
- Os Trigonum
- Osteochondral Lesions (OLT)

Pathology
- Articular cartilage = 60% talar surface
- High-energy trauma: Falls + motor vehicle accidents (MVA)

- 0.5% of all fractures
- Talar neck = 50% of talar injuries (most common talar fracture) + associated with calcaneus + spine + medial malleolus fractures
- Talar neck = Hawkins classification

Clinical Issues
- Most common signs/symptoms: Ankle/foot pain
- 15% talar fractures = open
- Associated injuries = calcaneus + medial malleolus
- Arthritis: 40-90%

Diagnostic Checklist
- Evaluate for AVN with talar neck fractures

○ Used in comminuted fractures

MR Findings
- T1WI
  - Head of talus
    - Avulsion usually medially
    - Intraarticular displacement/dislocation talonavicular joint
    - Single vs. multiple hypointense fracture lines
    - Associated diffuse hypointensity
  - Lateral process
    - Hypointense edema in comminuted fracture
    - Oblique/vertical single fracture (hypointense) + intraarticular displacement
  - Posterior process
    - Fracture vs. painful os trigonum difficult on T1WI
    - Irregular separation on sagittal = talus + fragment
  - Talar neck
    - Posterior to transverse sulcus
    - Vertical hypointense nondisplaced segment (type I)
    - Subluxation/dislocation talus in subtalar joint (type II)
    - Displacement of talar body (type III)
  - Talar body
    - Comminuted
    - Primary fracture in any of three orthogonal planes
    - Hypointense fracture line
- T2WI
  - Head of talus
    - Hyperintense talar head
    - Edema ± obscures fracture line
    - Chondral extension to talonavicular joint
  - Lateral process
    - Hyperintense edema on coronal/sagittal images
    - Increased hyperintense subtalar fluid + chondral interruption
  - Posterior process
    - Complete hyperintense vertical fluid gap between talus/posterior process
    - Adjacent marrow edema
    - Hyperintense soft tissue fluid + edema

- Hyperintense fluid flexor hallucis longus tendon sheath
  - Talar neck
    - Hyperintense fluid + inhomogeneity of hemorrhage with separation between head and neck/body
    - Adjacent fragment hyperintense marrow
    - Sagittal plane to document extrusion of talus from subtalar joint (Hawkins type III injury)
  - Talar body
    - Hyperintense edema across fracture plane (coronal, sagittal or axial)
    - Soft tissue hyperintense edema/hemorrhage
- T2* GRE
  - Head of talus
    - T2* gradient reduce edema, define fracture pattern

Imaging Recommendations
- Best imaging tool: MR - to appreciate marrow edema, chondral involvement + AVN
- Protocol advice: Coronal, sagittal and axial T1, PD FSE + FS PD FSE

DIFFERENTIAL DIAGNOSIS

Ankle Sprains
- Fracture of lateral and posterior process mistaken for ligament injury
- Anterior drawer sign with ligament tear

Os Trigonum
- Vs. fracture posterior process
- Os trigonum - smooth cortical border

Osteochondral Lesions (OLT)
- Subchondral fracture medial/lateral talar dome

PATHOLOGY

General Features
- General path comments
  - Relevant anatomy

- ■ Articular cartilage = 60% talar surface
- Etiology
  - ○ High-energy trauma: Falls + motor vehicle accidents (MVA)
  - ○ Head of talus
    - ■ Plantarflexed foot is forcefully dorsiflexed
    - ■ Axial load = shearing force
  - ○ Lateral process
    - ■ Inversion + dorsiflexion + compressive force
    - ■ Snowboarder's fracture: Flexible boots + increased subtalar motion
    - ■ MVA
  - ○ Posterior process
    - ■ Forced plantarflexion + compression
  - ○ Talar neck
    - ■ Forced dorsiflexion - contact between anterior lip tibia + dorsal talar neck sulcus
  - ○ Talar body
    - ■ Axial compression + plantarflexed talus
- Epidemiology
  - ○ 0.5% of all fractures
  - ○ Talar neck = 50% of talar injuries (most common talar fracture) + associated with calcaneus + spine + medial malleolus fractures

Gross Pathologic & Surgical Features

- Head of talus
  - ○ Periphery of head (medially)
  - ○ Subtalar dislocation
  - ○ Comminution vs compression
- Lateral process
  - ○ Comminuted fracture, minimal displacement
  - ○ Larger fragment ± displacement
- Posterior process
  - ○ Irregular separation from talus
- Talar neck
  - ○ Head + neck separated from talar body
  - ○ ± Failure interosseous talocalcaneal ligament
  - ○ ± Disruption vascular supply
  - ○ ± Talar dislocation from mortise
- Talar body
  - ○ Comminuted fractures without dislocations
  - ○ Less comminuted fractures associated with dislocations ankle + subtalar joint
  - ○ Simple fracture

Microscopic Features

- Fracture site
  - ○ Hematoma
  - ○ Revascularization
  - ○ Haversian canal formation in primary healing
  - ○ Callus formation
  - ○ Lamellar bone - remodeling

Staging, Grading or Classification Criteria

- Talar neck = Hawkins classification
  - ○ Type I (11 - 21%): No talar displacement
  - ○ Type II (40 - 42%): Subluxation/dislocation talus with respect to subtalar joint (dislocation posterior facet)
  - ○ Type III (23 - 47%): Displacement talar body (ankle and subtalar dislocation)
  - ○ Type IV (rare): Additional dislocation talonavicular joint

CLINICAL ISSUES

Presentation

- Most common signs/symptoms: Ankle/foot pain
- Clinical profile
  - ○ Swelling
  - ○ Ecchymosis
  - ○ 15% talar fractures = open
  - ○ Associated injuries = calcaneus + medial malleolus

Demographics

- Age: Talar neck = 30-38 years
- Gender: Talar neck: M:F = 3:1

Natural History & Prognosis

- Outcomes related to fracture type
- Malunion in comminuted fractures
- Arthritis: 40-90%
- Complications: AVN

Treatment

- Conservative: Short cast
- Surgical: Open reduction with internal fixation (ORIF)
  - ○ Body fracture, displaced
  - ○ Lateral process, displaced
  - ○ Talar neck, type III

DIAGNOSTIC CHECKLIST

Consider

- Evaluate for AVN with talar neck fractures
- Coronal, sagittal and axial planes to characterize fracture pattern
- Associated injuries visualized include medial malleolus and calcaneus

SELECTED REFERENCES

1. Banks A et al: McGlamry's comprehensive textbook of foot and ankle surgery. Talar fractures. vol 1. 3rd ed. Philadelphia PA, Lippincott Williams & Wilkins, 1865-96, 2001
2. Sijbrandij EJ et al: Posttraumatic subchondral bone contusions and fractures of the talotibial joint: Occurrence of "kissing" lesions. AJR 175(6):1707-10, 2000
3. Adellar RS: Complex fractures of the talus. Instr Course Lect. Review (46):323-38, 1997
4. Thordarson DB et al: Magnetic resonance imaging to detect avascular necrosis after open reduction and internal fixation of talar neck fractures. Foot Ankle Int 17(12):742-7, 1996
5. Nishimura G et al: Trabecular trauma of the talus and medial malleolus concurrent with lateral collateral ligamentous injuries of the ankle: Evaluation with MR imaging. Skeletal Radiol 25(1):49-54, 1996

TALUS FRACTURES

IMAGE GALLERY

Typical

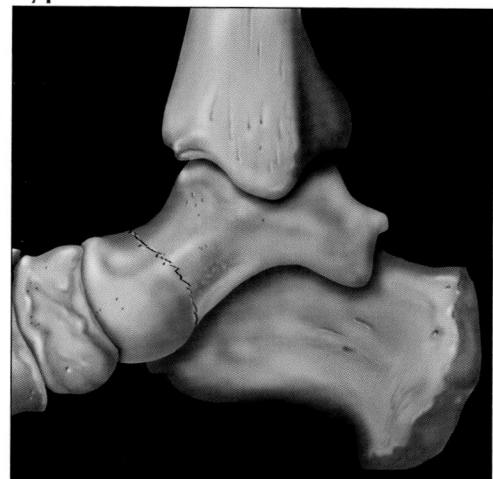
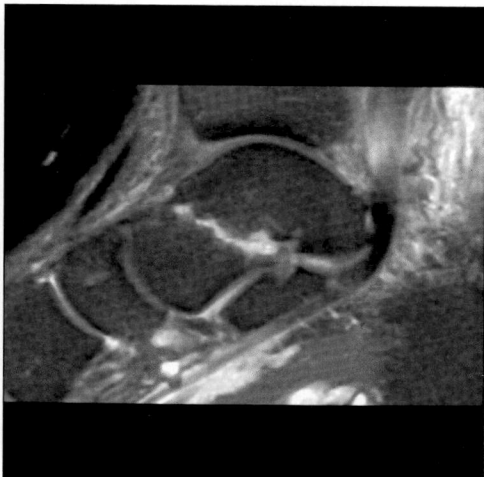

(Left) Sagittal graphic shows talar neck fracture. *(Right)* Sagittal FS PD FSE MR shows hyperintense non-displaced fracture of the talar neck.

Typical

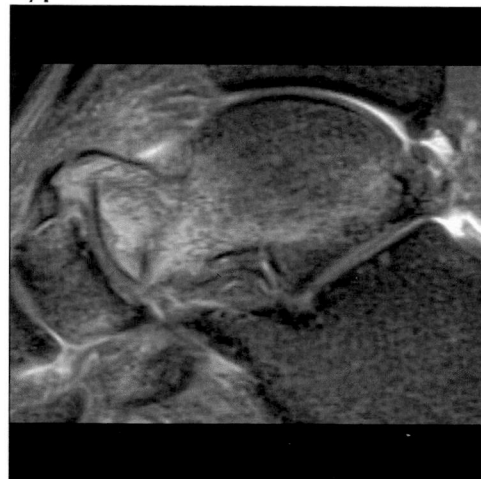
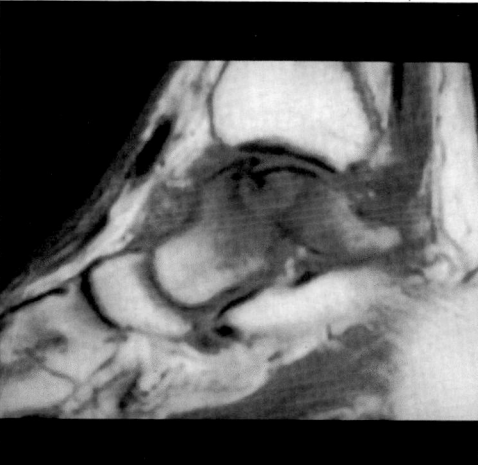

(Left) Sagittal FS PD FSE MR shows hyperintense marrow edema in talar head fracture. Intraarticular extension to the talonavicular joint is present in the plantar aspect of the fracture. *(Right)* Sagittal T1WI MR shows comminuted talar body fracture.

Typical

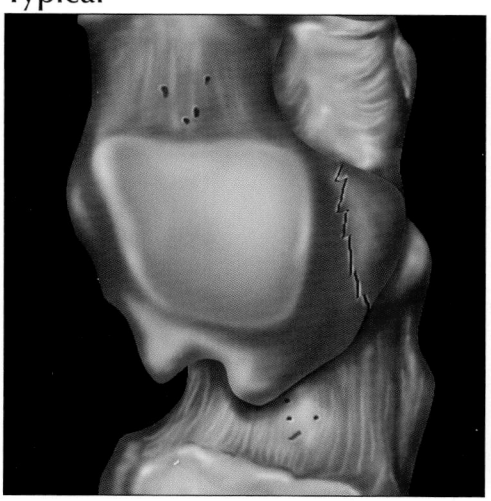
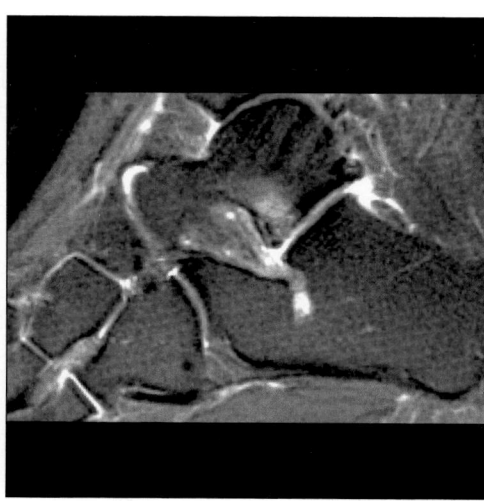

(Left) Axial graphic shows lateral process fracture of the talus. *(Right)* Sagittal FS PD FSE MR shows hyperintense edema in lateral process fracture.

CALCANEAL FRACTURES

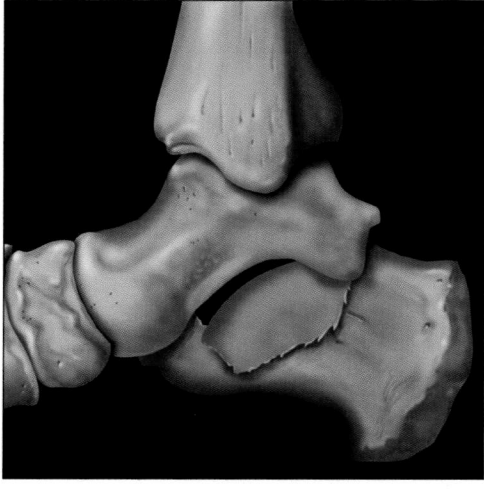

Sagittal graphic shows Essex Lopresti type B intraarticular joint depression fracture of the calcaneus.

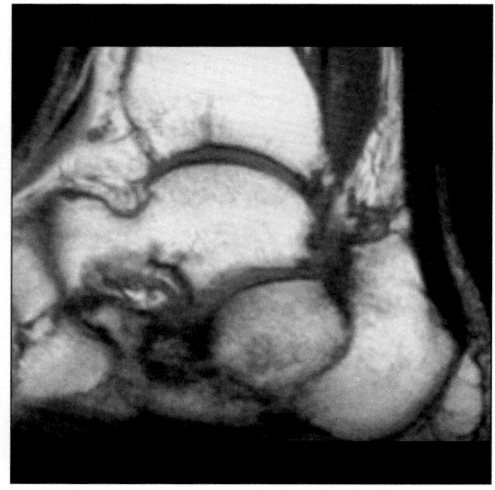

Sagittal T1WI MR shows central joint depression pattern with posterior extension to the posterior facet of the subtalar joint.

TERMINOLOGY

Abbreviations and Synonyms
- Fracture of the calcaneus

Definitions
- Extraarticular or intraarticular fracture of the calcaneus

IMAGING FINDINGS

General Features
- Best diagnostic clue: Fracture line ± extension into subtalar joint
- Location
  - Extraarticular
  - Intraarticular
    - Essex Lopresti type A: Tongue-type
    - Essex Lopresti type B: Joint depression
    - Fracture line vertical from Gissane's crucial angle (anterior lateral aspect tarsal canal) to calcaneal plantar surface
    - Secondary fracture line: Tongue type extends posterior to posterior facets + dorsal calcaneal tuberosity; depression type extends to fractured articular surface posterior facet
- Size: Varies from localized tuberosity, sustentaculum, process, avulsion, depression to comminution

- Morphology
  - Sanders classification = number of fragments in posterior facet on coronal CT
  - Intraarticular fracture
    - Y-shaped on lateral perspective
    - Secondary fracture: Tongue-type = horizontal extension to posterior tuberosity; joint depression = vertical to thalamic fragment (lateral articular posterior facet)

Radiographic Findings
- Radiography
  - Lateral foot, axial heel (Harris view)
  - AP + oblique foot - fracture calcaneocuboid joint and lateral wall displacement
  - Foot dorsiflexed and internal rotation to visualize posterior facet
  - Normal Bohler's angle = 20 to 40 degrees
  - Normal Gissane's critical angle = 120 to 145 degrees

CT Findings
- NECT
  - Coronal and axial images, sagittal reformations, ± three dimensional reconstruction
  - Sanders classification: Number of posterior facet fragments on coronal CT

MR Findings
- T1WI

DDx: Calcaneal Fractures

ATFL Sprain	Sinus Tarsi Synd.	Achilles Tear	PB Split	Tarsal Tunnel

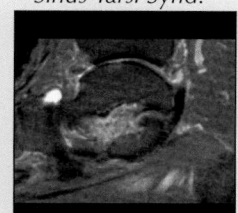 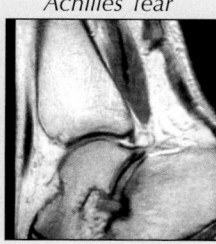 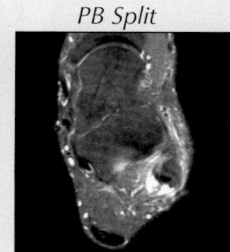 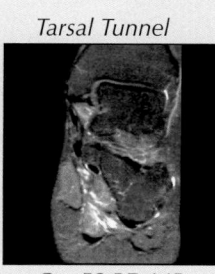

Sag T1WI MR	Sag FS PD MR	Sag T1WI MR	Ax FS PD FSE MR	Cor FS PD MR

CALCANEAL FRACTURES

Key Facts

Imaging Findings
- Best diagnostic clue: Fracture line ± extension into subtalar joint
- Extraarticular
- Intraarticular

Top Differential Diagnoses
- Lateral Ankle Ligament Sprain
- Sinus Tarsi Syndrome
- Achilles Tendon Tear
- Peroneal Tendon (PB, PL) Dysfunction
- Deltoid Ligament

Pathology
- Axial loading of hindfoot + downward talar force
- Primary fracture line - shears calcaneus obliquely (anteromedial + posterolateral portions)

- Secondary fracture line - divides calcaneus transversely
- 75% intraarticular in adults (25% in children)

Clinical Issues
- Most common signs/symptoms: Ankle pain
- Inability to ambulate
- Ecchymosis (heel + arch)
- Limited ankle motion (flattened calcaneus + talar dorsiflexion)
- Surgical for displaced intraarticular
- Complications: Compartment syndrome

Diagnostic Checklist
- Determine presence of subtalar joint extension

- Anterior process fracture (Rowe type I)
  - Avulsion at origin bifurcate ligament: Hypointense to intermediate edema vs. chronic hypointense sclerosis
  - Compression fracture - hypointense fracture extension to calcaneocuboid joint
- Sustentaculum tali (Rowe type I)
  - ± Medial displacement
- Beak and avulsion fxs (Rowe type II)
  - Hypointense edema in beak or avulsed tuberosity
  - Attached Achilles tendon to superior tuberosity
- Calcaneal body (Rowe type III)
  - No subtalar joint communication
  - Sagittal images to exclude posterior facet involvement
- Intraarticular
  - Coronal images for widening of calcaneus
  - Sagittal images to separate central depression from tongue-like fracture
- Stress fractures
  - Hypointense linear lines posterior calcaneus perpendicular to long axis vs. more diffuse posterior calcaneus trabecular microfracture edema
- T2WI
  - Anterior process fracture (Rowe type I)
    - Hyperintense edema lateral sagittal images
    - ± Bifurcate ligament edema
    - Increase signal extensor digitorum brevis muscle and calcaneocuboid ligament
    - Compression fracture ± avulsion navicular tuberosity with hyperintense edema; ± calcaneocuboid joint
  - Sustentaculum tali (Rowe type I)
    - Hyperintense edema, fluid or hemorrhage - axial/coronal
  - Beak and avulsion fxs (Rowe type II)
    - Beak - smaller
    - Avulsion - larger 2° sudden contraction Achilles tendon
    - Hyperintense fracture line posterior-superior calcaneus
  - Calcaneal body (Rowe type III)

  - Single hyperintense fracture line posterior to posterior facet vs. comminution
- Intraarticular
  - Hyperintense edema - in joint - depression vs. tongue-type fracture
  - Chondral extension
  - Free fragments - hypointense bodies outlined by hyperintense fluid
- Stress fracture
  - Posterior calcaneal hyperintensity in linear pattern parallel to posterior tuberosity vs. diffuse hyperintense edema

Imaging Recommendations
- Best imaging tool
  - MR for extraarticular and noncomminuted intraarticular
  - CT superior for multifragment involvement, fracture displacement, loose bodies
- Protocol advice: T1/PD + FS PD FSE in all 3 orthogonal planes

DIFFERENTIAL DIAGNOSIS

Lateral Ankle Ligament Sprain
- Not tender over anterior process
- Tear of anterior talofibular (ATFL) or calcaneofibular ligament

Sinus Tarsi Syndrome
- Abnormal sinus tarsi edema + sinus tarsi ligament pathology
- Sinus tarsi pain in anterior process fracture

Achilles Tendon Tear
- Severe tendinosis and tear with no associated posterior superior calcaneal avulsion

Peroneal Tendon (PB, PL) Dysfunction
- Tenosynovitis, tendinosis or splint without fracture of calcaneal body
- Lateral wall blow-out fracture - impingement of peroneal tendons

CALCANEAL FRACTURES

- Medial ankle ligament sprain

Deltoid Ligament
- Stretch or tear without fractured sustentaculum

PATHOLOGY

General Features
- General path comments
  - Relevant anatomy
    - Middle third calcaneus supports posterior facet
    - Posterior facet separated from anterior + middle facets by tarsal canal + sinus tarsi
    - Anterior = calcaneocuboid joint
    - Thalamic bone = cortical bone supporting posterior facet
    - Angle of Gissane - thick cortex of anterior lateral tarsal canal
- Etiology
  - Axial loading of hindfoot + downward talar force
  - Primary fracture line - shears calcaneus obliquely (anteromedial + posterolateral portions)
  - Secondary fracture line - divides calcaneus transversely
  - Posterior facet - impacted into body + rotated anteriorly
  - Lateral wall = blown out
  - Direct trauma
  - Stress/overuse in athletes
- Epidemiology
  - 2% of all fractures
  - 60% of tarsal bone injuries
  - 5-9% = bilateral
  - 75% = fall from height
  - 10% associated with thoracic/lumbar (T12-L2) compression injuries
  - 25 to 70% associated with lower extremity injuries
  - 15 to 25% = extraarticular fractures
  - 75% intraarticular in adults (25% in children)

Gross Pathologic & Surgical Features
- Rowe classification
  - Type I (21%): Fracture of tuberosity, sustentaculum tali, anterior process
  - Type II (3.8%): Beak + avulsion fractures/Achilles tendon insertion
  - Type III (19.5%): Oblique fractures (no subtalar involvement)
  - Type IV (24.7%): Fracture involving subtalar joint
  - Type V (31%): Central depression ± comminution

Microscopic Features
- Fracture site
  - Vascular disruption (hematoma)
  - Revascularization
  - Haversian canal - formation in primary healing
  - Callus formation response to micromotion at fracture (fibrous tissue, cartilage + woven bone)
  - Lamellar bone - remodeling

Staging, Grading or Classification Criteria
- Sanders classification: Coronal CT based, number of fragments involving post facet (sustentaculum, medial, central + lateral columns)

- Rowe classification

CLINICAL ISSUES

Presentation
- Most common signs/symptoms: Ankle pain
- Clinical profile
  - Inability to ambulate
  - Swelling, tenderness
  - Ecchymosis (heel + arch)

Demographics
- Age: Working age population (30-50 years)/fall from height (3-50 feet)
- Gender: M:F = 5:1

Natural History & Prognosis
- Sequelae include widened heel (blown out lateral wall); shortened heel (anterior process split)
- Limited ankle motion (flattened calcaneus + talar dorsiflexion)

Treatment
- Conservative for nondisplaced/minimally displaced intraarticular
  - Early range of motion without reduction
  - Closed reduction ± fixation
- Surgical for displaced intraarticular
  - Open reduction + internal fixation
  - Arthrodesis - comminuted
- Complications: Compartment syndrome

DIAGNOSTIC CHECKLIST

Consider
- MR or CT with coronal + sagittal planes to identify fracture type
- Determine presence of subtalar joint extension
- CT superior for severe comminuted + displaced fragments

SELECTED REFERENCES

1. Banks A et al: McGlamry's comprehensive textbook of foot and ankle surgery. Calcaneal fractures. vol 1. Philadelphia PA, Lippincott Williams & Wilkins, (57):1819-64, 2001
2. Karr JC: Magnetic resonance imaging evaluation of heel pain. J Am Podiatr Med Assoc 89(7):364-7, 1999
3. Robbins MI et al: MR imaging of anterosuperior calcaneal process fractures. AJR 172(2):475-9, 1999
4. Born CT et al: Imaging of calcaneal fractures. Clin Podiatr Med Surg 14(2):337-56, 1997
5. Berger PE et al: MRI demonstration of radiographically occult fractures: What have we been missing? Radiographics 9:407, 1989
6. Lee YK et al: Stress fractures: MR imaging. Radiology 169:217, 1989

IMAGE GALLERY

Typical

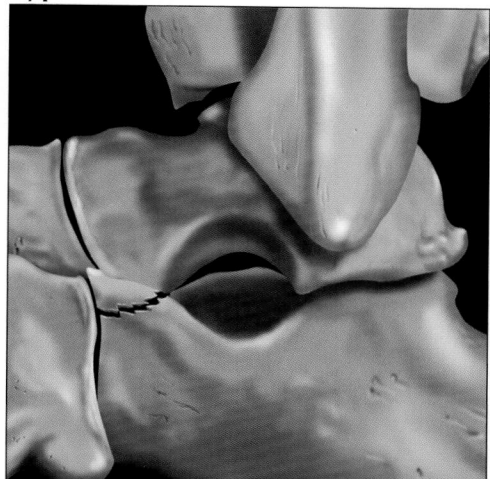
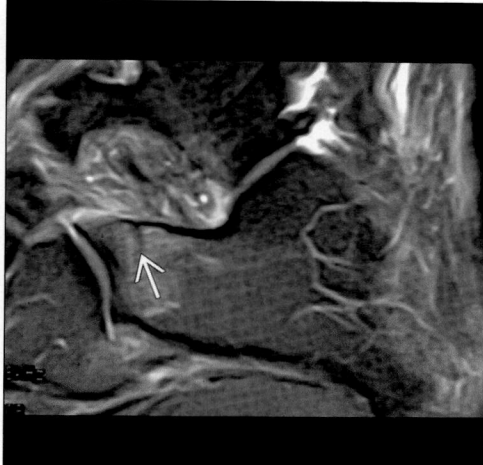

(Left) Sagittal graphic shows anterior process fracture adjacent to the calcaneocuboid joint. *(Right)* Sagittal FS PD FSE MR shows anterior process fracture (arrow) with hyperintense marrow edema adjacent to the origin of the bifurcate ligament.

Typical

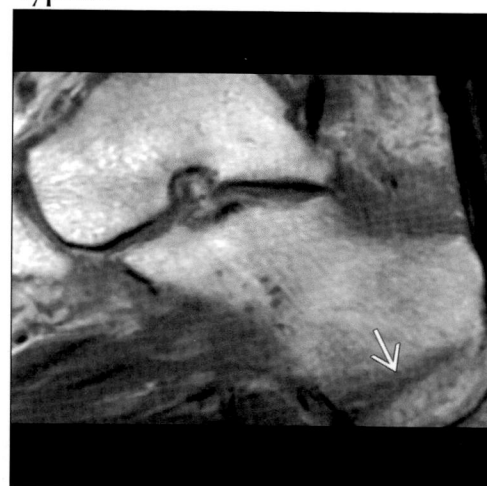
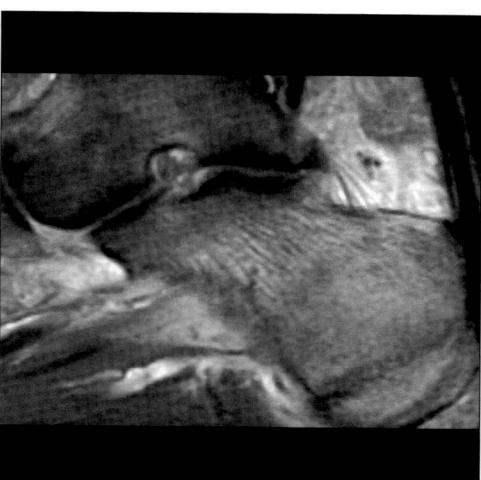

(Left) Sagittal T1WI MR shows calcaneal stress fracture with hypointense fracture line (arrow) perpendicular to the long axis of the calcaneus. *(Right)* Sagittal FS PD FSE MR shows calcaneal stress fracture with extensive hyperintense marrow edema.

Typical

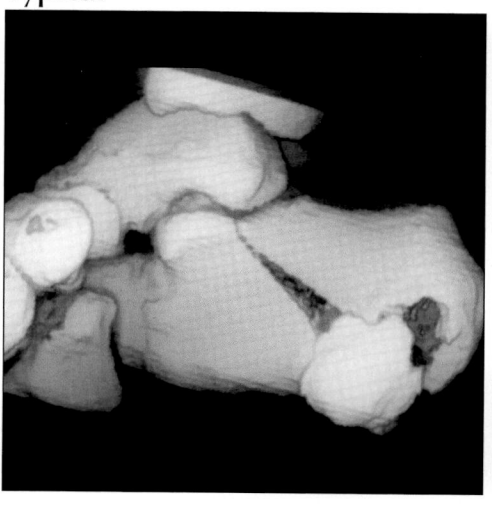
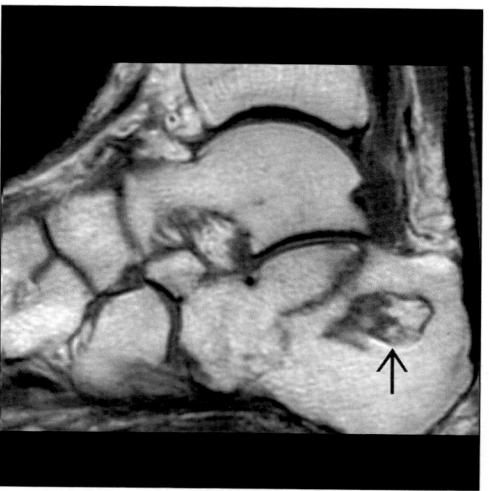

(Left) Sagittal NECT (3 D rendering) shows Essex Lopresti type A joint tongue-type intraarticular calcaneal fracture. *(Right)* Sagittal T1WI MR shows calcaneal body fracture and anterior process fracture complicated by infarction (arrow) of the posterior calcaneus.

NAVICULAR FRACTURES

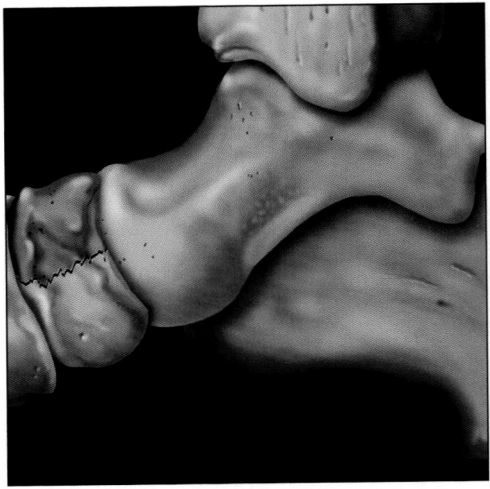

Sagittal graphic shows non-displaced stress fracture of the navicular. The dorsal fragment is sclerotic.

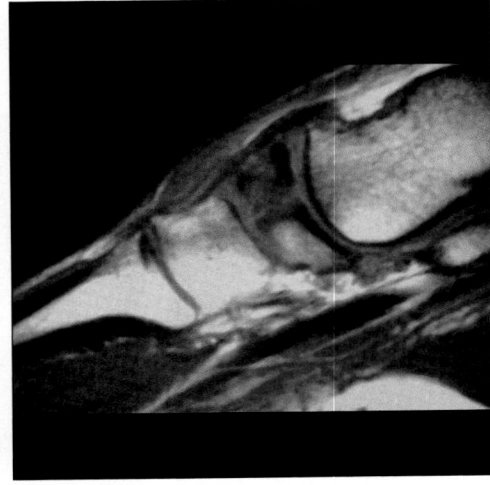

Sagittal T1WI MR shows navicular stress fracture with involvement of the proximal and distal cortices in a world-class sprinter. The dorsal fragment shows hypointense sclerosis.

TERMINOLOGY

Abbreviations and Synonyms
- Fractures of the navicular

Definitions
- Fractures of the navicular: Tuberosity, body, avulsion or stress

IMAGING FINDINGS

General Features
- Best diagnostic clue: Linear fracture line usually perpendicular to long axis of navicular
- Location
  ○ Avulsion
    ■ Dorsal lip
    ■ At insertion of dorsal tibionavicular ligament (tibialis posterior insertion)
  ○ Navicular tuberosity fx
  ○ Body fx
  ○ Stress fx
    ■ Middle third
- Size
  ○ Avulsion
    ■ Cortical avulsion: Part of dorsal cortex
  ○ Tuberosity

- Variable with size of tuberosity
- Minimally displaced
  ○ Body
    ■ Nondisplaced most common
  ○ Stress
    ■ Anteroposterior/short axis length of navicular
    ■ In sagittal plane/central third navicular
    ■ 96% are partial fxs
- Morphology
  ○ Avulsion
    ■ Elongated cortical fragment
  ○ Tuberosity
    ■ Fracture sharp/jagged edges
  ○ Body
    ■ Horizontal
    ■ Crush
    ■ Displaced
  ○ Stress
    ■ Complete
    ■ Incomplete

Radiographic Findings
- Radiography: Conventional radiographs - often negative for stress fractures

CT Findings
- NECT
  ○ Stress (most useful indication)
    ■ Direct coronal

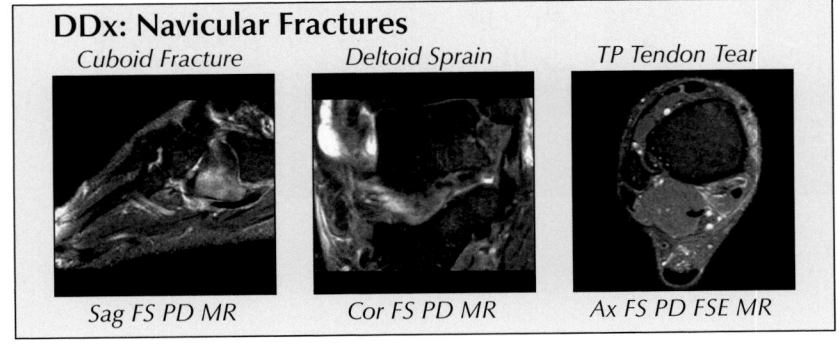

DDx: Navicular Fractures

Cuboid Fracture	Deltoid Sprain	TP Tendon Tear
Sag FS PD MR	Cor FS PD MR	Ax FS PD FSE MR

NAVICULAR FRACTURES

Imaging Findings

- Best diagnostic clue: Linear fracture line usually perpendicular to long axis of navicular
- Avulsion
- Navicular tuberosity fx
- Body fx
- Stress fx

Top Differential Diagnoses

- Cuboid Fracture
- Deltoid Ligament Sprain
- Tibialis Posterior (TP) Tendon Tear

Pathology

- Central third navicular avascular (at risk for stress fracture + nonunion)
- Dorsal avulsion = 47% of navicular fractures

Key Facts

- Tuberosity = 24% of navicular fractures
- Body = 29% of navicular fractures

Clinical Issues

- Most common signs/symptoms: Midfoot pain
- Avulsion = tenderness + edema at fracture site
- Tuberosity = tenderness medial navicular
- Body = pain mid medial arch & local tenderness & swelling
- Stress = poorly localized dorsum pain + medial longitudinal arch/minimal swelling

Diagnostic Checklist

- Correlate navicular edema with axial or coronal images to confirm a stress fracture

---

  - Direct axial
  - Confirm diagnosis: CT visualizes central third navicular

MR Findings

- T1WI
  - Avulsion
    - Elongated hypointense dorsal cortical fragment
    - Adjacent dorsal soft tissue hypointense edema
    - ± Hypointensity dorsal tibionavicular component deltoid
  - Tuberosity
    - Hypointense subchondral edema across tuberosity fracture
    - Irregular edges at fracture site
  - Body
    - Hypointense vertical or horizontal fracture line + edema
    - Hypointense subchondral edema
  - Stress
    - Hypointense fracture line on direct coronal or axial images
    - Hypointense marrow edema ± visualized fracture on sagittal
- T2WI
  - Avulsion
    - Fragment remains hypointense (cortically based)
    - Adjacent edema/hyperintensity (soft tissue + navicular)
  - Tuberosity
    - Variable hyperintensity across fracture site
    - Hyperintense fluid/hemorrhage at fracture site
    - Hyperintense fluid involving tibialis posterior tendon
  - Body
    - Hyperintensity epicentered in coronal plane, from dorsolateral to plantar medial within navicular or comminution in sagittal plane
  - Stress
    - Hyperintensity ± diffuse marrow edema in acute injuries

Imaging Recommendations

- Best imaging tool
  - MR with improved multiplanar display especially in stress fractures
  - MR useful for tuberosity fractures vs accessory navicular
- Protocol advice: Coronal, sagittal + axial T1 or PD FSE + FS PD FSE

DIFFERENTIAL DIAGNOSIS

Cuboid Fracture

- Edema + fracture line in cuboid
- Associated with navicular tuberosity fracture
- ± Associated cuneiform fracture

Deltoid Ligament Sprain

- Vs. dorsal avulsion fracture of navicular
- Normal dorsal margin navicular on sagittal

Tibialis Posterior (TP) Tendon Tear

- Intrinsic hypertrophy, attenuated or complete tear
- Mimics avulsion fracture navicular tuberosity

Bipartite Tarsal Navicular

- Vs. true fracture of body
- Bipartite = smooth interface

PATHOLOGY

General Features

- General path comments
  - Relevant anatomy
    - Central third navicular avascular (at risk for stress fracture + nonunion)
- Etiology
  - Avulsion
    - Plantar displacement foot + inversion or eversion
    - Dorsal tibionavicular ligament taut = dorsal cortex avulsion at insertion
  - Tuberosity

NAVICULAR FRACTURES

- Avulsion - tibialis posterior
- Forceful eversion - contraction tibialis posterior
- Body
  - Direct or indirect mechanism
  - Fall + foot plantarflexion
  - Plantarflexion + abduction metatarsal joint
- Stress
  - Excessive pronation
  - Running
- Epidemiology
  - 62% of midfoot fractures
  - 37% of all foot fractures
  - Dorsal avulsion = 47% of navicular fractures
  - Tuberosity = 24% of navicular fractures
  - Body = 29% of navicular fractures

Gross Pathologic & Surgical Features
- Avulsion
  - Fragment may contain segment of articular cartilage
- Tuberosity
  - Nondisplaced most common
  - Associated injury calcaneocuboid joint
- Body
  - Nondisplaced most common
  - ± Navicular compressed between talar head & cuneiform
- Stress
  - 96% incomplete
  - Complete fracture ± dislocation

Microscopic Features
- Fracture site
  - Hemorrhage
  - Revascularization
  - Primary healing with haversian canal
  - Callus formation
  - Remodeling with lamellar bone

Staging, Grading or Classification Criteria
- Body fractures
  - Type 1: Transverse + dorsal fragment (< 50% body)
  - Type 2: Transverse from dorsolateral to plantar medial across body (major fragment = dorsomedial; smaller comminuted fracture = plantar lateral)
  - Type 3: Central or lateral comminution (major fragment = medial)

CLINICAL ISSUES

Presentation
- Most common signs/symptoms: Midfoot pain
- Clinical profile
  - Avulsion = tenderness + edema at fracture site
  - Tuberosity = tenderness medial navicular
  - Body = pain mid medial arch & local tenderness & swelling
  - Stress = poorly localized dorsum pain + medial longitudinal arch/minimal swelling

Demographics
- Age
  - Stress fractures in athletes + recreational age
  - Ages 20 to 50 years
- Gender: Stress fracture in male & female population

- Related causes
  - Stress fractures in sprints, hurdles and jumps
  - Body fractures - fall from great height or motor vehicle accident

Natural History & Prognosis
- Avulsion
  - If displaced - closed reduction usually unstable
- Tuberosity
  - 50% calcaneocuboid joint injury = persistent pain
  - Edema decreases after 72 hours
- Body
  - Remain nondisplaced
  - Heal without sequelae
- Stress
  - Under-diagnosed
  - Symptoms increased with activity
  - Failure to treat = delayed or nonunion

Treatment
- Conservative
  - Short leg cast
- Surgical
  - Avulsion: Open reduction with internal fixation (ORIF) if > 20% articular cartilage
  - Tuberosity: Reattachment for displacement; resection
  - Body: Displacement requires ORIF vs. closed reduction vs. K-wires
  - Stress: Displaced, nonunions, comminuted or cyst formation requires graft vs. excision vs. ORIF
- Complications
  - Degenerative arthritis
  - Nonunion

DIAGNOSTIC CHECKLIST

Consider
- Stress fractures associated with running & jumping athletic activity
- High axial compression related to acute navicular fractures
- Correlate navicular edema with axial or coronal images to confirm a stress fracture

SELECTED REFERENCES

1. Coris EE et al: Tarsal navicular stress fractures. Am Fam Physician. 67(1)85-90, 2003
2. Choi CH et al: Occult osteochondral fractures of the subtalar joint: A review of 10 patients. J Foot Ankle Surg 40-3, 2002
3. Ostlie DK et al: Tarsal navicular stress fracture in a young athlete: Case report with clinical, radiologic, and pathophysiologic correlations. J Am Board Fam Pract 381-5, 2001
4. Banks A et al: McGlamry's comprehensive textbook of foot and ankle surgery. Midfoot fractures. vol 1. Philadelphia PA, Lippincott Williams & Wilkins (35):1791-818, 2001
5. Myerson M: Foot and ankle disorders. Fractures of the midfoot and forefoot. vol 2. Philadelphia PA, Lippincott Raven (52):1265-96, 2000

NAVICULAR FRACTURES

IMAGE GALLERY

Typical

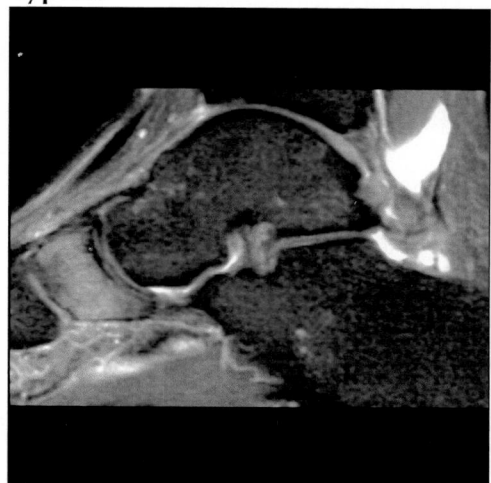

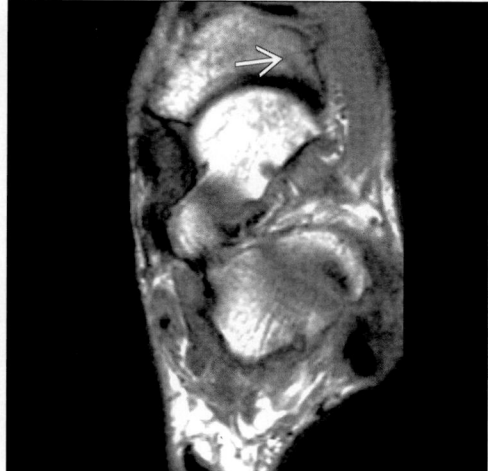

(Left) Sagittal FS PD FSE MR shows diffuse hyperintense marrow edema in the plane of the navicular fracture. *(Right)* Axial T1WI MR shows fracture (arrow) of the proximal medial navicular (tuberosity fracture).

Typical

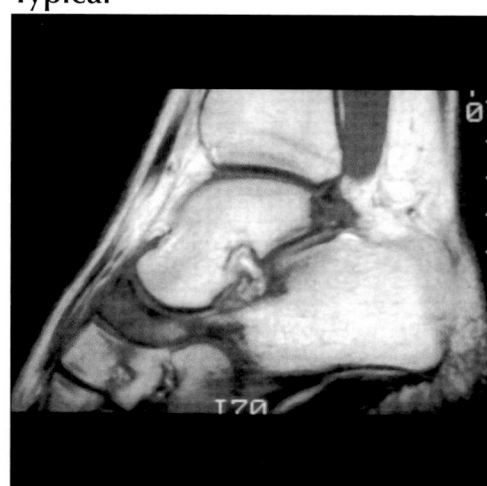

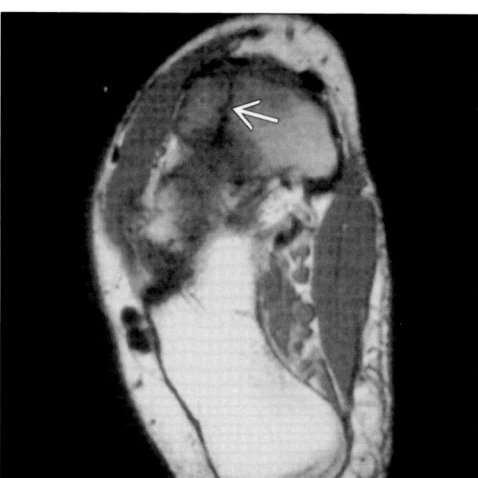

(Left) Sagittal T1WI MR shows diffuse hypointensity without direct visualization of the fracture. *(Right)* Axial T1WI MR shows stress fracture (arrow) perpendicular to the long axis of the navicular.

Typical

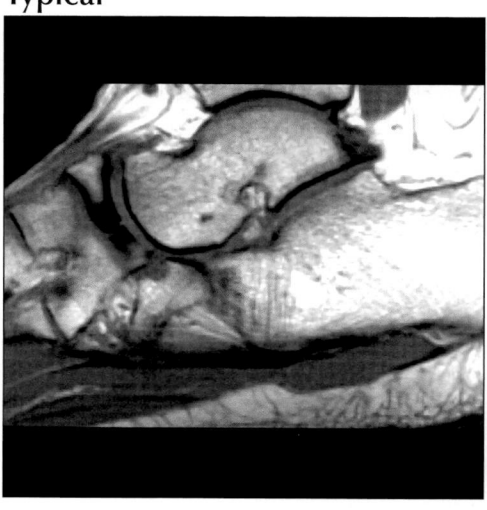

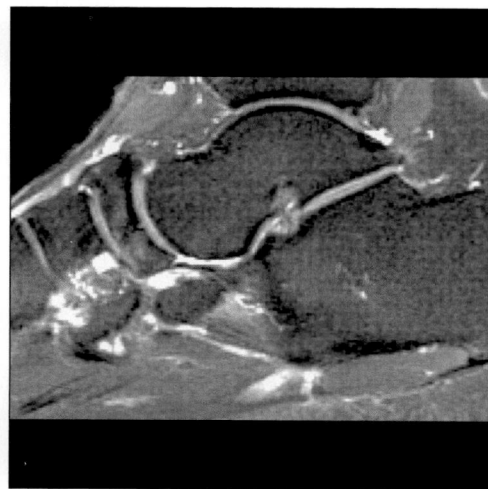

(Left) Sagittal T1WI MR shows chronic changes of navicular fracture with sclerosis and foreshortening. *(Right)* Sagittal FS PD FSE MR shows complication of navicular fracture with dorsal subluxation deformity.

METATARSAL FRACTURES

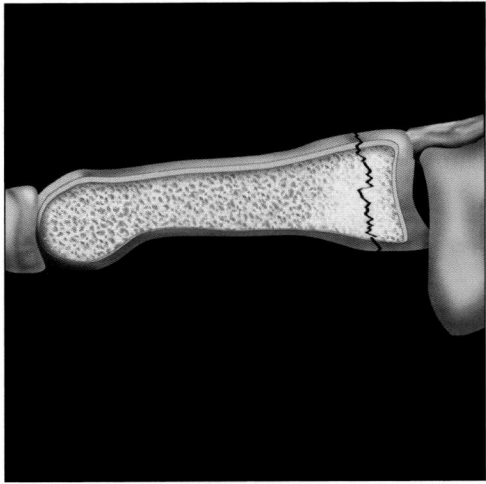

Sagittal graphic shows stress fracture of the proximal metatarsal with associated bone marrow edema.

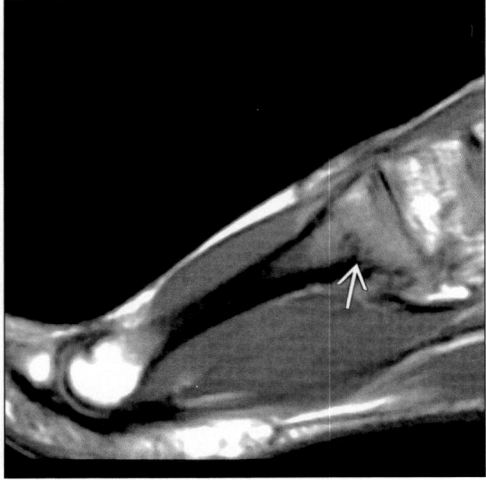

Sagittal T1WI MR shows second metatarsal stress fracture (arrow) in a ballet dancer.

TERMINOLOGY

Abbreviations and Synonyms
- Fractures of the metatarsals

Definitions
- Metatarsal fracture: Stress, head, neck, mid shaft, base, first, central (2nd, 3rd, 4th), or 5th fracture

IMAGING FINDINGS

General Features
- Best diagnostic clue: Bone marrow edema + fracture line
- Location
  - Stress - proximal third, common in dancers
  - Head, neck, shaft, base, central
- Size
  - Variable
    - Stress - perpendicular to long axis
    - Head - ± shortening in impaction injuries
    - Neck - ± displacement & ± multisegment involvement
    - Mid shaft - size related to oblique, transverse, spiral & comminuted patterns
    - Base - usually minimal displacement & good alignment
    - First - direct ± comminution, indirect ± avulsion
    - Central - displacement in same direction
    - Fifth - avulsion or transverse Jones fracture
- Morphology
  - Stress - transverse ± angulation ± periosteal reaction/exuberant callus
  - Head - ± angulation or rotation
  - Neck - ± plantar + lateral displacement
  - Mid shaft - oblique, transverse, spiral or comminuted
  - Base - associated with Lisfranc's fracture-dislocation (alignment usually maintained)
  - First - direct with comminution vs. indirect with avulsion
  - Central - usually transverse + parallel relationship of fractured segments
  - Fifth - transverse pattern in Jones fracture

Radiographic Findings
- Radiography
  - Confirms fracture location
  - Three views recommended
  - ± Comparison study uninvolved extremity
  - Healing = new bone formation

CT Findings
- NECT
  - For fracture displacement & dislocation of metatarsals

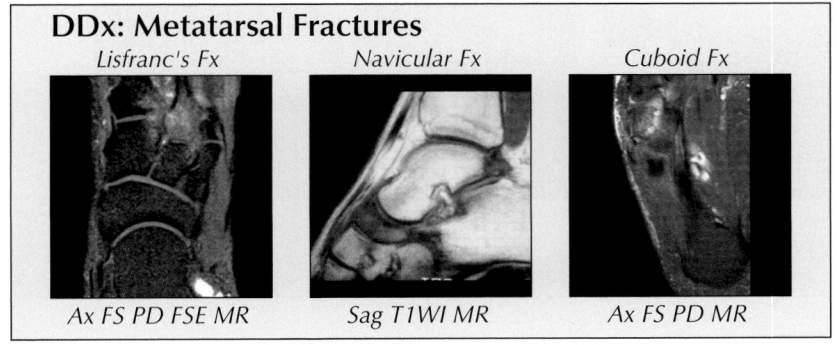

DDx: Metatarsal Fractures

Lisfranc's Fx	Navicular Fx	Cuboid Fx
Ax FS PD FSE MR	Sag T1WI MR	Ax FS PD MR

METATARSAL FRACTURES

Key Facts

Imaging Findings
- Best diagnostic clue: Bone marrow edema + fracture line
- Stress - proximal third, common in dancers
- Head, neck, shaft, base, central
- Best imaging tool: MR to identify marrow edema in nondisplaced fractures

Top Differential Diagnoses
- Lisfranc's Fracture
- Navicular Fracture
- Cuboid & Cuneiform Fracture

Pathology
- Direct - crushing, blunt trauma or penetrating injuries
- Indirect - axial loading

- Overuse: Running or dancing
- Fifth metatarsal > 3rd > 2nd > 1st > 4th for gross involvement
- Stewart classification of fifth metatarsal base fractures

Clinical Issues
- Most common signs/symptoms: Pain at fracture site
- Stress - focal tenderness + pain with activity (diaphysis or neck most common)
- First metatarsal - altered gait
- Age: Stress fractures: Young runners, dancers, marchers

Diagnostic Checklist
- Metatarsal marrow edema often indicative of a stress fracture

---

  - Documents cortical thickening in stress fractures

MR Findings
- T1WI
  - Stress
    - Subchondral hypointensity
    - Asymmetric thickening of hypointense cortex
    - Hypointense fracture line (single or multiple)
    - Usually perpendicular to metatarsal long axis
  - Head
    - Displacement
    - Hypointense edema metatarsal head
    - ± Dislocation
  - Neck
    - Hypointense oblique or transverse fracture & edema
    - ± Plantar displacement
  - Mid shaft
    - Oblique or transverse + hypointense marrow edema
    - ± Shortening, angulation, displacement
  - Base
    - Hypointense marrow edema
    - Identify multiple metatarsal involvement
  - First
    - ± Extensive soft tissue effacement with hypointense edema/hemorrhage
    - Comminution in direct injuries
    - Avulsion fragment
  - Central: Displacement as unit
  - Fifth: Hypointensity of base ± extension into proximal diaphysis
- T2WI
  - Stress
    - Hyperintense medullary edema
    - ± Soft tissue hyperintensity
    - Edema without fracture line visualization in acute stage
  - Head
    - Angulation or rotation of articular surface on sagittal images
    - Chondral fracture with interruption of intermediate signal intensity articular cartilage

  - Neck
    - Hyperintense marrow ± soft tissue edema
    - Tendinous interposition
    - Muscle hyperintensity
  - Mid shaft: Variable proximal/distal diaphysis edema
  - Base
    - Hyperintense base ± visualized fracture fragment in Lisfranc injuries
    - Chip fractures - variable marrow hyperintensity
  - First
    - ± Association with Lisfranc injuries
    - Marrow hyperintensity
  - Central
    - Multiple metatarsal involvement (second, third + fourth)
    - Displacement with extensive soft tissue + muscular hyperintense edema
  - Fifth
    - Increased fracture gap in nonunion
    - Marrow hyperintensity vs. hypointensity of fibrous tissue or sclerosis

Imaging Recommendations
- Best imaging tool: MR to identify marrow edema in nondisplaced fractures
- Protocol advice
  - T1/PD FSE + FS PD FSE
    - Direct axial for Lisfranc joint
    - Coronal for displacement & dislocation
    - Sagittal for shortening and angulation

DIFFERENTIAL DIAGNOSIS

Lisfranc's Fracture
- Tarsometatarsal involvement
- Homolateral vs. divergent displacement
- Axial plane to diagnose

Navicular Fracture
- Dorsal avulsion
- Tuberosity
- Body

METATARSAL FRACTURES

Cuboid & Cuneiform Fracture
- Cuneiform associated with tarsometatarsal dislocations
- Cuboid associated with fractures of calcaneus, fifth metatarsal or navicular

PATHOLOGY

General Features
- General path comments
  - Relevant anatomy
    - Metatarsal structure = base, diaphysis, neck & head
    - Base - broad & cancellous with strong plantar ligaments
    - Diaphysis - origin of intrinsic foot muscles
    - Neck - strong intermetatarsal ligaments
    - Metatarsal heads - weightbearing
- Etiology
  - Direct vs. indirect force
    - Direct - crushing, blunt trauma or penetrating injuries
    - Indirect - axial loading
  - Stress
    - Overuse: Running or dancing
    - Decrease bone density: Amenorrhea
  - Head: Direct trauma
  - Neck: Shearing force vs. direct trauma
  - Mid shaft: Direct, blunt vs. torsional
  - Base: Direct trauma = motor vehicle accident or fall from a height
  - First metatarsal: Crush vs. twisting
  - Central metatarsals: Direct impact or crushing
  - Fifth metatarsal: Plantarflexion + inversion vs. direct impact
- Epidemiology: 35% of foot fractures

Gross Pathologic & Surgical Features
- Fifth metatarsal > 3rd > 2nd > 1st > 4th for gross involvement
- Stress mechanism to complex trauma
- Malalignment post fracture = displacement, shortening, or angulation

Microscopic Features
- Fracture site
  - Hematoma
  - Revascularization
  - Primary healing vs. callus

Staging, Grading or Classification Criteria
- Stewart classification of fifth metatarsal base fractures
  - Type I: Jones fracture
  - Type II: Intraarticular
  - Type III: Avulsion
  - Type IV: Comminuted intraarticular
  - Type V: Apophysis

CLINICAL ISSUES

Presentation
- Most common signs/symptoms: Pain at fracture site

- Clinical profile
  - Stress - focal tenderness + pain with activity (diaphysis or neck most common)
  - First metatarsal - altered gait

Demographics
- Age: Stress fractures: Young runners, dancers, marchers
- Gender
  - Females more susceptible in military context (thinner cortices)
  - Level of fitness most important determinant (stress fractures)

Natural History & Prognosis
- Bridging callus - good prognosis
- Complications: Non-union, malunion, unresolving pain

Treatment
- Conservative
  - Stress fracture - decreased/altered activity to immobilization
  - Head - closed treatment if intact nondisplaced articular surface
  - Neck, base, central, fifth = immobilization/cast for nondisplaced fractures
- Surgical: Head, neck, mid shaft, base, 1st, central, 5th for displacement
  - Open reduction with internal fixation (ORIF)

DIAGNOSTIC CHECKLIST

Consider
- Metatarsal marrow edema often indicative of a stress fracture
- Axial plane to visualize Lisfranc tarsometatarsal articulations

SELECTED REFERENCES

1. Banks A et al: McGlamry's comprehensive textbook of foot and ankle surgery. Metatarsal fractures. vol 1. 3rd ed. Philadelphia PA, Lippincott Williams & Wilkins, (55):1775-90, 2001
2. Ashman CJ et al: Forefoot pain involving the metatarsal region: Differential diagnosis with MR imaging. Radiographics 21(6):1425-40, 2001
3. Harmath C et al: Stress fracture of the fifth metatarsal. Orthopedics 24(2):111, 204-8 Review, 2001
4. Chowchuen P et al: Stress fractures of the metatarsal heads. Skeletal Radiol 27(1):22-5, 1998
5. Harrington T et al: Overuse ballet injury of the base of the second metatarsal. A diagnostic problem. Am J Sports Med 21(4):591-8, 1993

METATARSAL FRACTURES

Typical

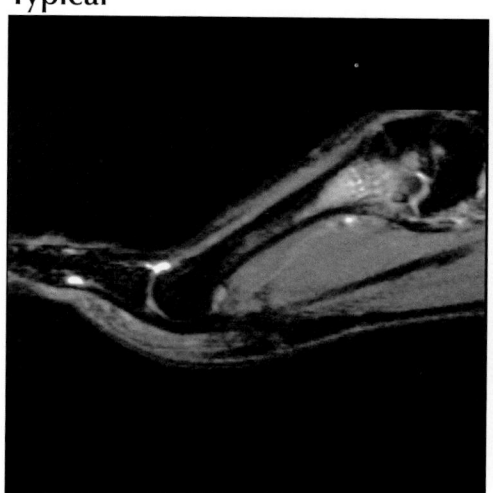
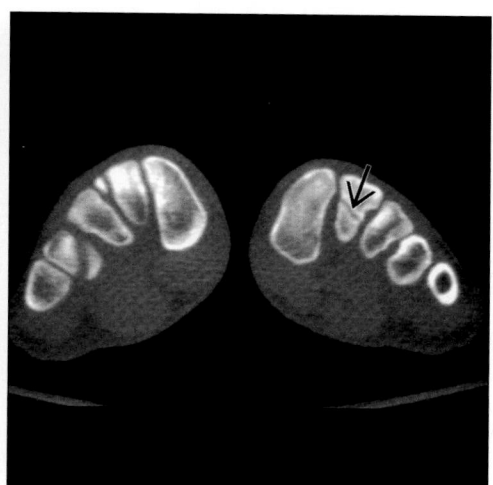

(Left) Sagittal FS PD FSE MR shows hyperintense bone marrow edema in second metatarsal stress fracture. (Right) Coronal NECT shows fracture (arrow) of the second metatarsal base.

Typical

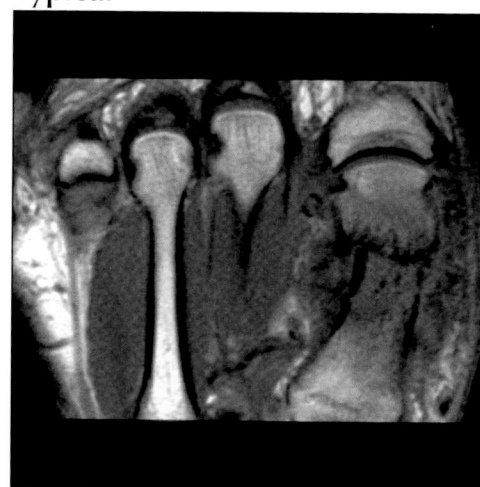
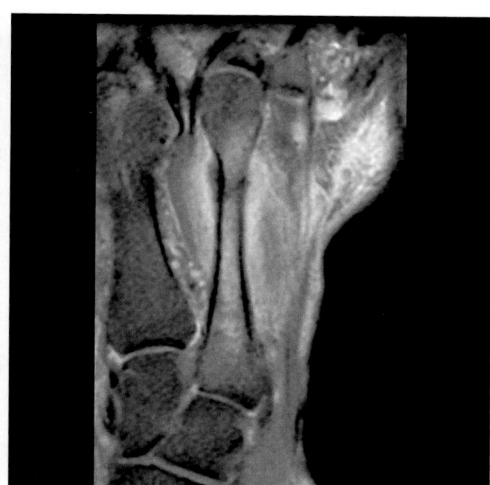

(Left) Axial T1WI MR shows first distal transverse metatarsal fracture. (Right) Axial FS PD FSE MR shows diaphyseal fracture with hyperintense marrow edema and soft tissue reaction. Asymmetric periosteal reaction is noted.

Typical

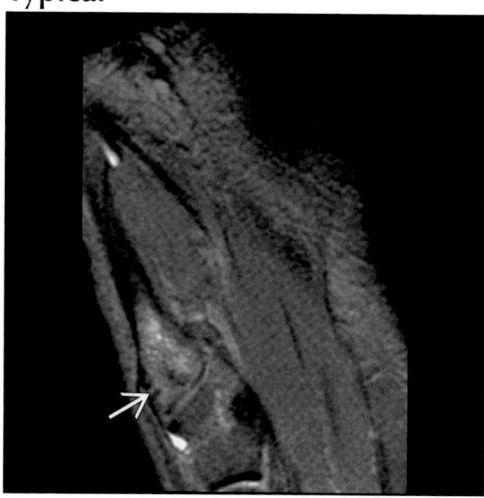
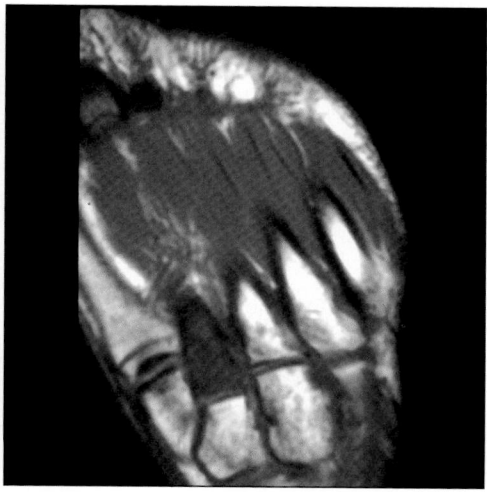

(Left) Axial FS PD FSE MR shows hyperintense marrow edema (arrow) in a fracture of the base of the fifth metatarsal (Jones fracture). (Right) Axial T1WI MR shows diffuse hypointense edema and sclerosis of a proximal second metatarsal fracture.

LISFRANC FRACTURE-DISLOCATION

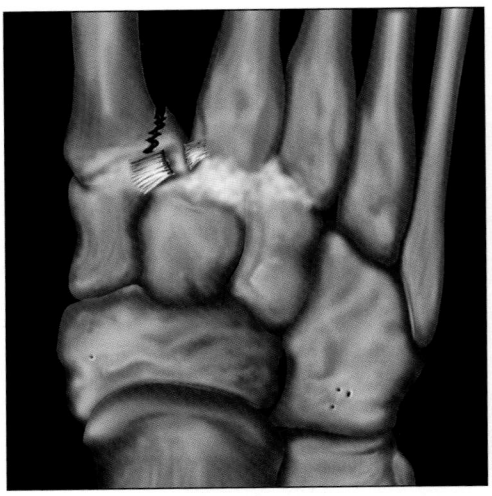

Axial graphic shows fracture of the base of the 1st metatarsal with disruption of Lisfranc's ligament. Homolateral displacement of the metatarsals is shown.

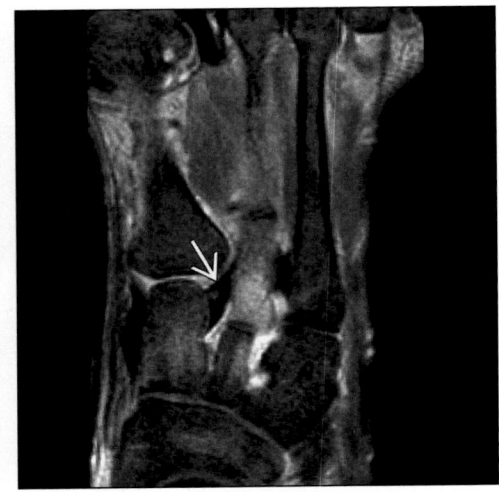

Axial FS PD FSE MR shows fracture with hyperintense edema at the base of 2nd metatarsal and trabecular injury of 1st and intermediate cuneiforms. The Lisfranc ligament (arrow) is intact.

TERMINOLOGY

Abbreviations and Synonyms
- Tarsometatarsal fracture-dislocation; tarsometatarsal dislocation

Definitions
- Dorsal dislocation as homolateral or divergent + associated fractures at tarsometatarsal joints

IMAGING FINDINGS

General Features
- Best diagnostic clue: Lateral offset lateral aspect 1st metatarsal relative to medial cuneiform + medial aspect 2nd metatarsal relative to medial aspect intermediate cuneiform
- Location
  - Fractures at bases 2nd and 3rd metatarsals
  - Dislocation metatarsocuneiform joint
  - Lateral shift 2nd - 5th metatarsals
  - Homolateral - 1st to 5th metatarsals dislocated laterally
  - Divergent - 1st metatarsal medially dislocated
- Size: Variable based on associated ligament disruption, fractures and static vs. dynamic displacement of metatarsals

- Morphology
  - Homolateral
  - Divergent
  - Fracture base 2nd metatarsal
  - Pathognomonic flock fracture proximal medial 2nd metatarsal

Radiographic Findings
- Radiography
  - Lateral view: Uneven osseous dorsal contour
  - AP view: Metatarsal cuneiform offset
  - Stress radiographs

CT Findings
- NECT
  - Direct axial
  - Superior to standard radiography: Tarsometatarsal joints without overlap
  - Dislocation detection as subtle as 1 mm
  - Confirms chip fractures

MR Findings
- T1WI
  - Axial: Lateral displacement 1st to 5th homolaterally; 1st metatarsal medially dislocated + lateral dislocation metatarsals 2 through 5 in divergent form

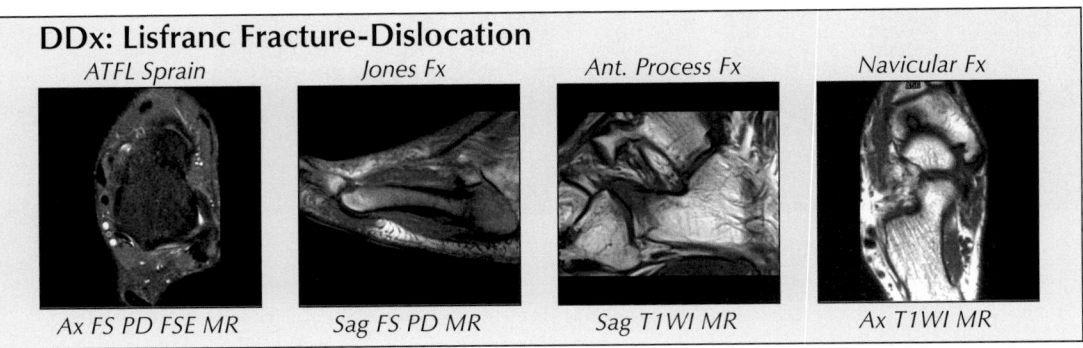

DDx: Lisfranc Fracture-Dislocation

ATFL Sprain	Jones Fx	Ant. Process Fx	Navicular Fx
Ax FS PD FSE MR	Sag FS PD MR	Sag T1WI MR	Ax T1WI MR

LISFRANC FRACTURE-DISLOCATION

Key Facts

Imaging Findings

- Best diagnostic clue: Lateral offset lateral aspect 1st metatarsal relative to medial cuneiform + medial aspect 2nd metatarsal relative to medial aspect intermediate cuneiform
- Homolateral - 1st to 5th metatarsals dislocated laterally
- Divergent - 1st metatarsal medially dislocated

Top Differential Diagnoses

- Lateral Ligamentous Sprain
- Jones Fracture
- Navicular Fracture
- Subtalar Sprain

Pathology

- Forced plantar flexion of forefoot on rearfoot (e.g., stepping off curb)
- Direct: Blow/crush (e.g., foot run over by motor vehicle)
- Osseous avulsion (Lisfranc ligament)

Clinical Issues

- Most common signs/symptoms: Pain tarsometatarsal joint and midfoot
- Pain with weightbearing

Diagnostic Checklist

- Identify Lisfranc ligament between medial cuneiform & proximal 2nd metatarsal

---

- Fractures hypointense at base 2nd or 3rd metatarsals, medial/intermediate cuneiform or navicular
- Impaction injury cuboid + abduction deformity forefoot = lateral column shortening
- Disruption dorsal arch on direct coronal (2nd metatarsal normally at apex of arch)
- Intermediate signal or discontinuity Lisfranc ligament medial cuneiform to medial proximal 2nd metatarsal
- Hypointense edema at Lisfranc's ligament avulsion fracture, proximal medial aspect 2nd metatarsal
- T2WI
  - Hyperintense subchondral marrow edema tarsometatarsal joints = chip or trabecular fractures
  - Oblique (Lisfranc) ligament frayed or torn ± synovitis and hyperintensity
  - Intramedullary hyperintensity in displaced metatarsals seen in cross section on direct coronal plane
  - Arterial injury on coronal images
  - Charcot arthropathy with superimposed neuropathic hyperintensity throughout midfoot + Lisfranc fracture-dislocation
  - Cuboid marrow hyperintensity with trabecular impaction injury
  - Widening 1st/2nd metatarsal interspace-axial plane

Imaging Recommendations

- Best imaging tool
  - MR sensitive to nondisplaced fractures with presence of marrow edema
  - CT delineates cortical detail of chip fractures after initial workup with MR
- Protocol advice: T1 and FS PD FSE axial images with entire midfoot tarsometatarsal articulation in plane

DIFFERENTIAL DIAGNOSIS

Lateral Ligamentous Sprain

- Partial or complete tear localized to anterior talofibular ligament (ATFL) or calcaneofibular ligament (CFL)

- Thickened or attenuated scarred ligaments
- Inversion of plantar flexed ankle

Jones Fracture

- Fifth metatarsal base fracture
- Avulsion force + supination of foot

Navicular Fracture

- May involve naviculocuneiform & calcaneocuboid joints
- Repetitive stress - running + jumping
- Body fractures 2° to axial compression
- Avulsion fracture of tuberosity - pull of tibialis posterior
- Dorsal avulsion - talonavicular or deltoid + forced plantar flexion

Subtalar Sprain

- Mild to complete subtalar + talonavicular dislocation
- Associated with lateral ankle sprain
  - Superficial layer (lateral root inferior extensor retinaculum, lateral talocalcaneal, calcaneofibular, posterior talocalcaneal + medial talocalcaneal)
  - Intermediate layer (intermediate root inferior extensor retinaculum + cervical ligament)
  - Deep layer (medial root inferior extensor retinaculum + interosseous talocalcaneal ligament)

Bifurcate Sprain

- Ligament spans from anterior process calcaneus to navicular and cuboid
- Midfoot remains stable with this injury
- Anterior process fracture

PATHOLOGY

General Features

- General path comments
  - Relevant anatomy
    - Recessed second metatarsal base
    - Metatarsals bound by transverse dorsal + stronger plantar ligaments

- No ligament directly attaching 1st metatarsal base to base of lesser (2nd-5th) metatarsals
- Dorsal medial ligament (medial cuneiform - 1st metatarsal)
- Lisfranc ligament medial cuneiform to 2nd metatarsal base (medial aspect 2nd metatarsal base)
- Etiology
  - Forced plantar flexion of forefoot on rearfoot (e.g., stepping off curb)
  - Plantarflexed foot + longitudinal force (e.g., equestrian injury - foot caught in stirrup)
  - Direct: Blow/crush (e.g., foot run over by motor vehicle)
  - Motor vehicle + industrial injuries = majority
- Epidemiology
  - 1 in 55,000 people per year
  - 0.2% of all fractures
  - 67% motor vehicle related; motorcade + crush = high energy injuries
  - < 1% dislocations

Gross Pathologic & Surgical Features
- Osseous avulsion (Lisfranc ligament)
- Lisfranc ligament disruption
- Homolateral displacement all rays laterally
- Divergent displacement - 1st ray medial, 2nd-5th rays laterally
- Widened intermetatarsal space (between 1st + 2nd)
- Malalignment metatarsals and cuneiforms
- Associated fractures

Microscopic Features
- Hemorrhagic elements; soft tissue edema
- Fracture cortical, subchondral + trabecular
- Ligamentous microtears to complete collagen fiber disruption
- Chondrolysis
- Arterial spasm (at risk - branch between dorsalis pedis/plantar arterial arch)

Staging, Grading or Classification Criteria
- Type A
  - Total incongruity
  - Displacement metatarsals 1st-5th lateral or dorsoplantar
- Type B
  - Partial incongruity
  - Medial dislocation 1st metatarsal
  - Lateral dislocation tarsometatarsal joints (metatarsals 2-5)
- Type C
  - Divergent; partial or total displacement
  - 1st metatarsal medially + lesser metatarsals laterally

CLINICAL ISSUES

Presentation
- Most common signs/symptoms: Pain tarsometatarsal joint and midfoot
- Clinical profile
  - Pop or snap
  - Edema midfoot

- Shortening foot
- Forefoot abducted/adducted
- Palpation dorsal or plantar displacement 2nd metatarsal
- Plantar ecchymosis sign
- Pain with weightbearing
- Excessive range of motion (hypermobility)

Demographics
- Age
  - High energy trauma not age specific
  - Athletic injury in younger population (collegiate age): Basketball, running, gymnastics, football
  - Charcot arthropathy in older diabetic population
- Gender: Increase male predominance in athletic activities and motorcycle accidents

Natural History & Prognosis
- Initial evaluation - 20% missed diagnosis
- Delayed treatment - chronic instability
- Complication - compartment syndrome
- Long term morbidity high
- Osteoarthritis - posttraumatic arthritis
- Fracture-dislocation/instability requires surgical treatment

Treatment
- Conservative
  - Rest, ice, compression, elevation (RICE)
  - Non-weight bearing
  - Stretch/partial tear capsule + ligament use cast boot
  - Physical therapy + orthotic
- Surgical
  - Nondisplaced unstable - percutaneous wire fixation
  - Displaced or angled - open reduction with internal fixation (ORIF) with cannulated screws
  - Anatomic reduction improves outcome

DIAGNOSTIC CHECKLIST

Consider
- Align metatarsal bases with respective cuneiforms on direct axial images to show tarsometatarsal joints in same plane of section
- Identify Lisfranc ligament between medial cuneiform & proximal 2nd metatarsal
- Use direct coronal images to appreciate dorsal/plantar displacement

SELECTED REFERENCES

1. Peicha G et al: The anatomy of the joint as a risk factor for Lisfranc dislocation and fracture-dislocation. An anatomical and radiological case control study. J Bone Joint Surg Br 84(7):981-5, 2002
2. Banks A et al: McGlamry's comprehensive textbook of foot and ankle surgery. Talar fractures. vol 1. 3rd ed. Philadelphia PA, Lippincott Williams & Wilkins, 1091-152, 2001
3. Preidler KW et al: Conventional radiography, CT, and MR imaging in patients with hyperflexion injuries of the foot: Diagnostic accuracy in the detection of bony and ligamentous changes. AJR 173(5):1673-7, 1999

LISFRANC FRACTURE-DISLOCATION

Typical

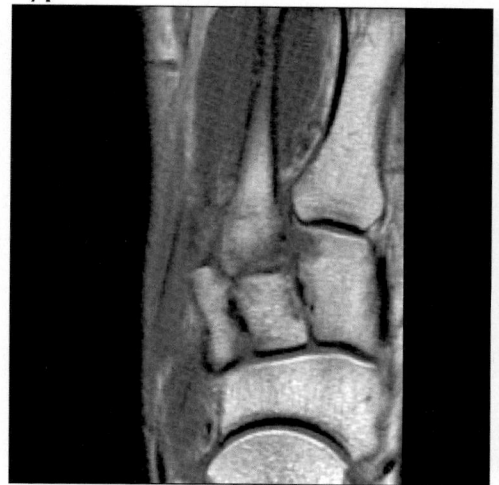 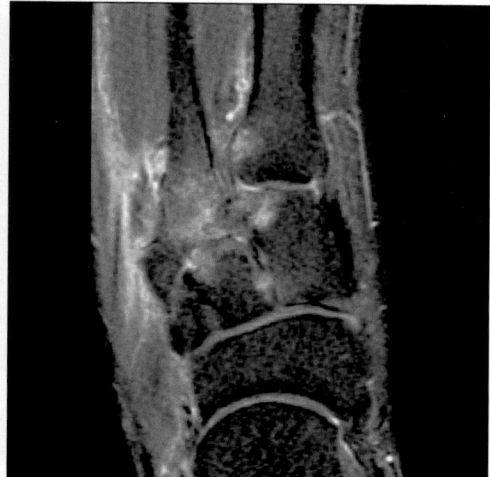

(Left) Axial T1WI MR shows Lisfranc fracture with lateral displacement of the 1st and 2nd metatarsals relative to the medial and intermediate cuneiforms. *(Right)* Axial FS PD FSE MR shows extensive trabecular marrow edema pattern in metatarsal bases and distal cuneiforms associated with partial tearing of Lisfranc's ligament.

Typical

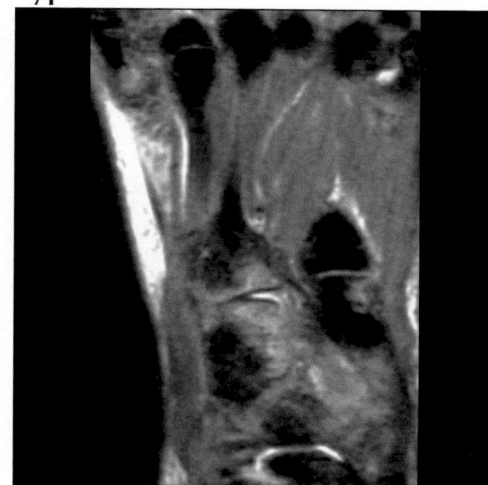 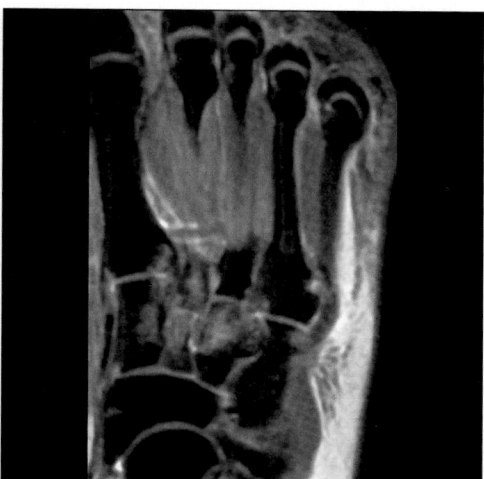

(Left) Axial FS PD FSE MR shows more extensive pattern of cuneiform fracture involving the medial, intermediate, and lateral cuneiforms. *(Right)* Axial FS PD FSE MR shows avulsion fracture with attached Lisfranc ligament. Hyperintense midfoot edema is present.

6

85

Typical

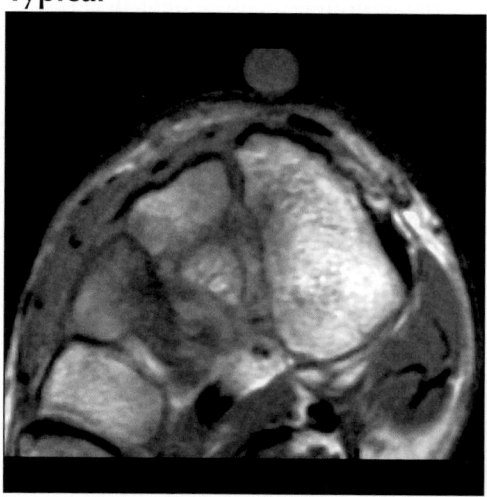 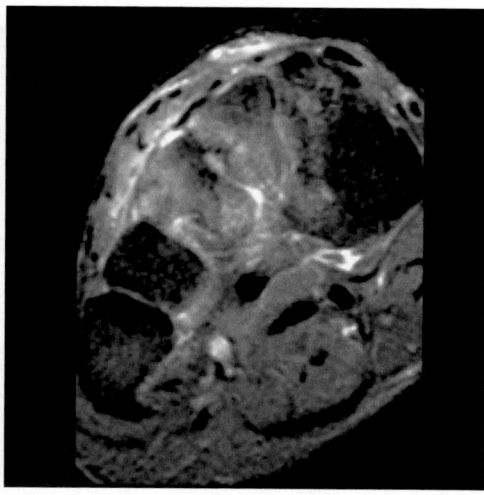

(Left) Coronal T1WI MR shows fracture at the level of the cuneiforms. *(Right)* Coronal FS PD FSE MR shows hyperintense edema and fractures of the intermediate and lateral cuneiforms.

OSTEOCHONDRAL LESION OF THE TALUS

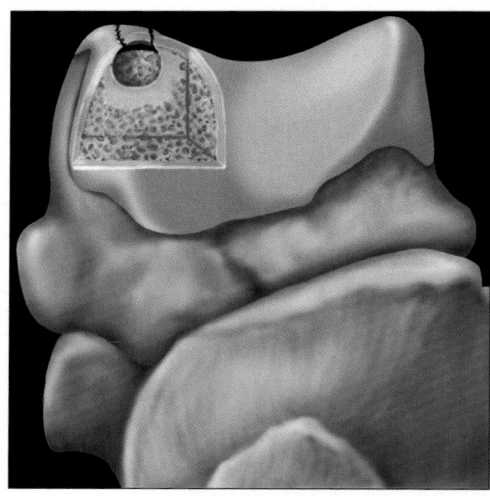

Coronal graphic shows stage III OLT with unattached and nondisplaced chondral fragment. Associated subchondral bone marrow edema in yellow.

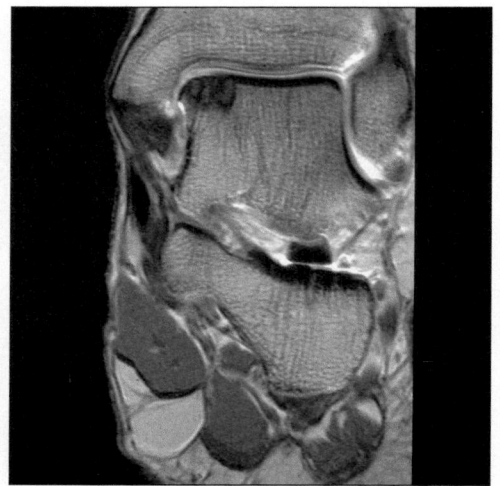

Coronal T1 C+ MR (intraarticular contrast) shows medial talar dome OLT with attenuated overlying articular cartilage.

TERMINOLOGY

Abbreviations and Synonyms
- OLT, transchondral fracture, osteochondral fracture, osteochondritis dissecans, talar dome fracture, flake fracture

Definitions
- Chronic phase of compressed or avulsed talar dome fracture

IMAGING FINDINGS

General Features
- Best diagnostic clue: Focal talar dome subchondral hypointensity on T1, hyperintensity on T2WI
- Location
  - Medial: Middle/posterior third
  - Lateral: Middle or anterior
  - Exceptions
    - Anteromedial corner
    - Posterolateral corner
    - Central lesions
    - Multiple sites
- Size
  - Variable size from 1 mm to > 1 cm
  - Perilesional edema larger than osteochondral focus

- Morphology
  - Lateral: Shell/wafer shaped ± displaced
  - Medial
    - Deeper/cup-shaped
    - Usually not displaced

Radiographic Findings
- Radiography
  - Conventional radiographs insensitive to occult OLT (stage I)
  - Unable to assess integrity of hyaline articular cartilage
  - Difficult to differentiate grades I, II, III
  - Berndt and Harty's original classification
    - Stage I: Subchondral compression
    - Stage II: Partially detached osteochondral fragment
    - Stage III: Completely detached fragment without displacement from crater
    - Stage IV: Osteochondral fragment detached + displaced from crater

CT Findings
- NECT
  - Stage I
    - Cystic lesion + intact roof
  - Stage IIA
    - Cystic lesion + communication with talar dome
  - Stage IIB

DDx: Osteochondral Lesion of Talus

OL Tibia	Tibial Infarct	Talar Fx	Arthritis
Sag FS PD MR	Sag T1WI MR	Ax FS PD FSE MR	Sag T1WI MR

OSTEOCHONDRAL LESION OF THE TALUS

Key Facts

Imaging Findings
- Best diagnostic clue: Focal talar dome subchondral hypointensity on T1, hyperintensity on T2WI
- Variable size from 1 mm to > 1 cm
- Perilesional edema larger than osteochondral focus
- Conventional radiographs insensitive to occult OLT (stage I)

Top Differential Diagnoses
- Osteochondral Lesion Tibia
- Osteonecrosis
- Fracture
- Arthritis

Pathology
- Direct trauma
- Repetitive microtrauma

- Compressed/avulsed talar dome fracture
- Increased joint pressures forces synovial fluid into fracture site - prevents healing

Clinical Issues
- Most common signs/symptoms: Persistent ankle pain post inversion injury
- Swelling
- Catching
- Giving way
- Reduced motion

Diagnostic Checklist
- Coronal FS PD FSE coronal images to define morphology of overlying chondral surface

---

- Open articular surface lesion + nondisplaced fragment
  - Stage III
    - Nondisplaced lesion + lucency
  - Stage IV
    - Displaced fragment

MR Findings
- T1WI
  - Detached cortical fragment: Hypointense
  - Attenuated or irregular subchondral plate
  - Subchondral lesion: Hypointense to intermediate (function of fluid and fibrous tissue)
  - Subchondral edema: Hypointense
- T2WI
  - Fluid: Hyperintense
  - Hypointense reactive bone sclerosis
  - Adjacent subchondral talar marrow edema
    - Extends beyond focus of necrosis
    - Hyperintense on FS PD FSE/STIR
  - Chondral thinning, bowing, nodularity and disruption (fissures and flap lesions)
  - Unattached fragment: Complete ring of hyperintense fluid
- T1 C+
  - Intravenous contrast
    - Congruity of chondral surface
    - Enhance subchondral edema
    - Enhance synovial tissue
  - Intraarticular
    - Unstable fragment - free fragment/loose body
    - Communication with subchondral cyst
- MR classification (T1 + T2WI)
  - Stage I: Subchondral trabecular compression and marrow edema
  - Stage IIA: Subchondral cyst
  - Stage II: Incomplete separation fragment
  - Stage III: Unattached, nondisplaced fragment + synovial fluid surrounding fragment
  - Stage IV: Displaced fragment

Imaging Recommendations
- Best imaging tool: MR: Superior for articular cartilage + marrow edema
- Protocol advice
  - FS PD FSE all orthogonal planes
  - 10 cm FOV coronal FS PD FSE to define talar chondral surface
  - T1WI to correlate lesion subchondral sclerosis

DIFFERENTIAL DIAGNOSIS

Osteochondral Lesion Tibia
- Similar subchondral ± chondral lesion tibia

Osteonecrosis
- Sclerosis subchondral bone with infarct like morphology

Fracture
- Sclerosis or edema in body fractures; discrete linear fracture line identified
- Talar neck fracture ± complicated by avascular necrosis (AVN)

Arthritis
- Usually posttraumatic
- Joint space narrowing

Transient Osteoporosis
- Edema without subchondral lesion
- Resolution on follow up MR

PATHOLOGY

General Features
- General path comments
  - Relevant anatomy
    - Wider anterior talus
    - Narrower posterior talus
    - Ankle mortise = medial + lateral malleolus
- Etiology

OSTEOCHONDRAL LESION OF THE TALUS

- o Direct trauma
- o Repetitive microtrauma
- o Compressed/avulsed talar dome fracture
- o Trauma + predisposition to talar dome ischemia
- o Increased joint pressures forces synovial fluid into fracture site - prevents healing
- o Subchondral fracture susceptible to AVN
- o Torsional impaction
- o Lateral lesions
  - ▪ Strong inversion force + dorsiflexed foot + internal rotation tibia
  - ▪ Lateral talar margin impacted/compressed against medial fibula = shear end compression
- o Medial lesions
  - ▪ Strong inversion force + plantarflexed foot + lateral rotation tibia on talus (external rotation)
  - ▪ Posteromedial edge talar dome impacted against posteromedial tibia + shear stress
- o Shear stress > bone = subchondral fracture + intact articular cartilage
- o Shear stress > bone + cartilage = complete displaced osteochondral lesion
- • Epidemiology
  - o 0.09% of all fractures
  - o 1% of talar fractures
  - o 4% of cases of osteochondritis
  - o 6.5% of sprained ankles
  - o Lateral lesions (44%): Trauma (94%)
  - o Medial lesions: Trauma (62%)
  - o Bilateral (10 to 30%)

Gross Pathologic & Surgical Features
- • Cartilage
  - o Soft, frayed
- • Subchondral plate defect/cyst
- • Loose bodies
- • Effusion
- • Stable vs. unstable fragment in crater

Microscopic Features
- • Cartilage
  - o Chondrocytes viable
  - o Fibrillation
  - o Fissures
  - o Fracture
- • Fibrous granulation tissue
- • Poor capillary ingrowth
- • Trabecular compression and necrosis subchondral bone
- • Synovial hyperplasia

Staging, Grading or Classification Criteria
- • Surgical grade - articular cartilage
  - o Grade A: Smooth, intact + soft
  - o Grade B: Rough surface
  - o Grade C: Fibrillations/fissures
  - o Grade D: Flap/exposed bone
  - o Grade E: Loose, undisplaced fragment
  - o Grade F: Displaced fragment

CLINICAL ISSUES

Presentation
- • Most common signs/symptoms: Persistent ankle pain post inversion injury
- • Clinical profile
  - o Chronic ankle pain/sprain
  - o Stiffness
  - o Swelling
  - o Ecchymosis
  - o Catching
  - o Clicking
  - o Locking
  - o Giving way
  - o Reduced motion

Demographics
- • Age
  - o Average age = 25 years
  - o Also occurs fifth/sixth decades
  - o Children - not common
- • Gender: Male = 67%; female = 33%

Natural History & Prognosis
- • Joint stiffness
- • Ankle instability
- • Stable fragment = healing
- • Healing + motion = fibrous tissue at fracture + sequestration
- • Degenerative arthritis

Treatment
- • Conservative
  - o Stage I and II, medial stage III lesions
  - o Reduced activity, limited ankle motion - stage I
  - o Casting - acute stage II
- • Surgical = stage III + IV lesions
  - o Free fragment excision
  - o Curettage
  - o Drilling
  - o Abrasion arthroplasty
- • Complications
  - o Continued pain
  - o Degenerative joint arthrosis

DIAGNOSTIC CHECKLIST

Consider
- • T1WI most accurate to assess sclerosis
- • Do not overestimate size of lesion by including adjacent marrow edema in lesion dimensions
- • Coronal FS PD FSE coronal images to define morphology of overlying chondral surface

SELECTED REFERENCES
1. Banks A et al: McGlamry's comprehensive textbook of foot and ankle surgery. vol 1. Philadelphia PA, Lippincott Williams & Wilkins, (35):1091-152, 2001
2. Loredo R et al: Imaging of osteochondral injuries. Clin Sports Med 20(2):249-78, 2001

IMAGE GALLERY

Typical

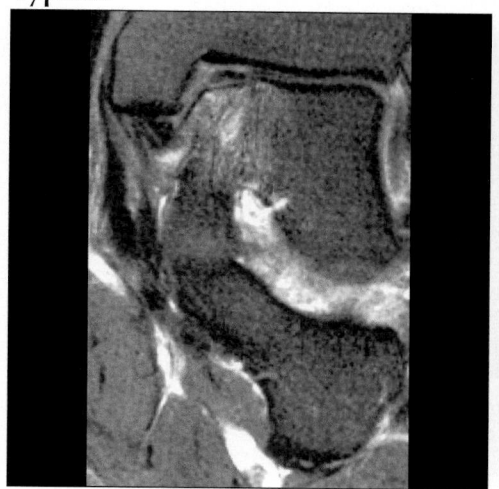

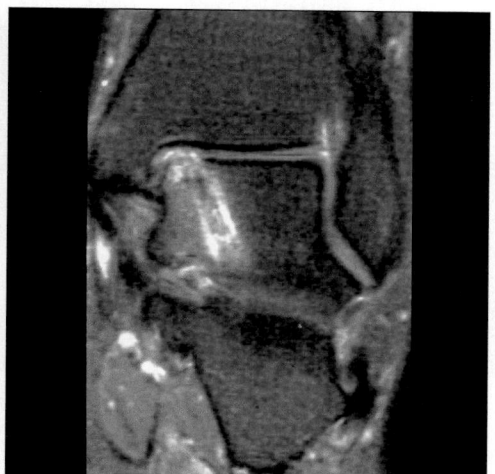

(Left) Coronal FS PD FSE MR shows stage III OLT with joint fluid undermining the osteochondral fracture. There is interruption of the subchondral plate with associated bone marrow edema. *(Right)* Coronal FS PD FSE MR shows hyperintense surgical drilling tract for the treatment of a stage III OLT.

Typical

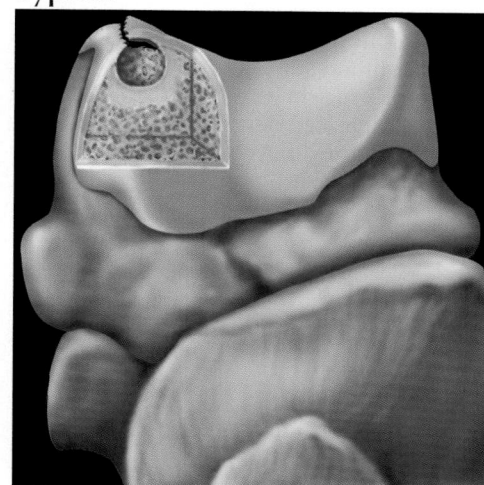

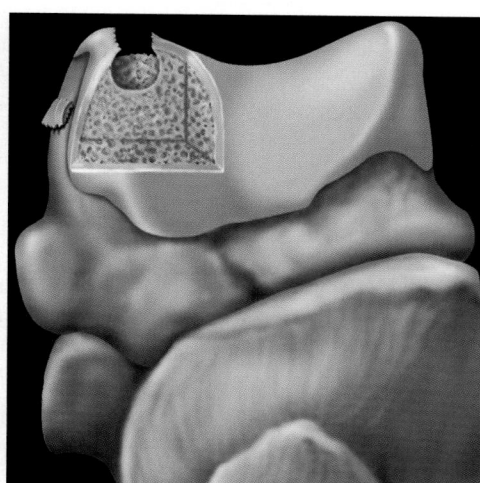

(Left) Coronal graphic shows stage II OLT with partial osteochondral fracture. Bone marrow edema in yellow. *(Right)* Coronal graphic shows stage IV OLT with loss of articular cartilage, interruption of the subchondral plate, and displaced medial fragment. There is a lack of bone marrow edema in this chronic lesion.

Typical

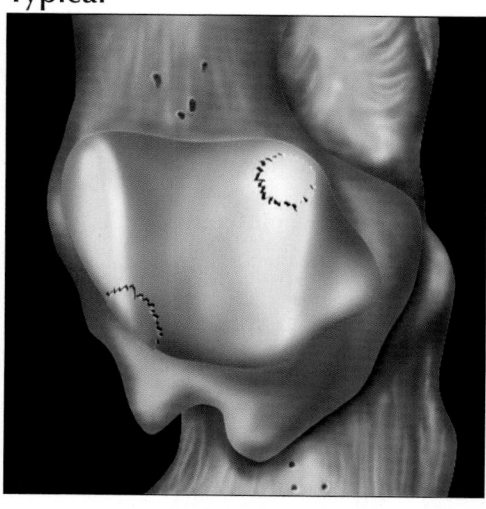

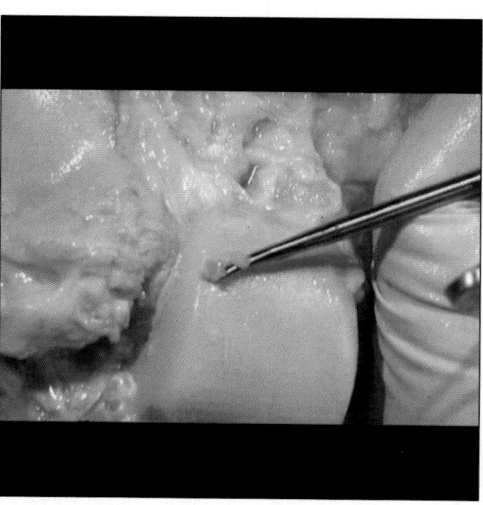

(Left) Axial graphic shows the posteromedial (cup-shaped) and anterolateral (wafer-shaped) appearance of OLT. *(Right)* Surgical pathology showing the posteromedial OLT location in the talar dome.

AVASCULAR NECROSIS (AVN) OF THE TALUS

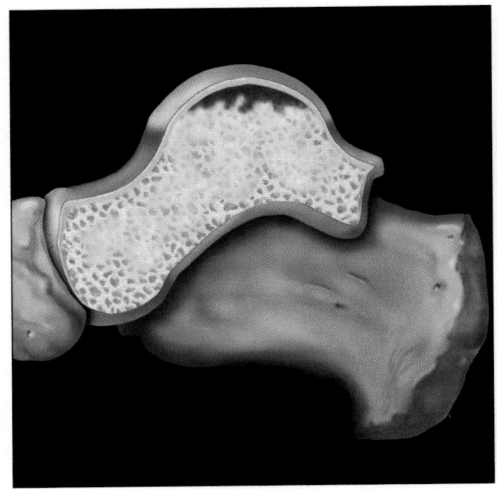

Sagittal graphic shows subchondral ischemic focus (dark) of the talus with associated diffuse bone marrow edema pattern.

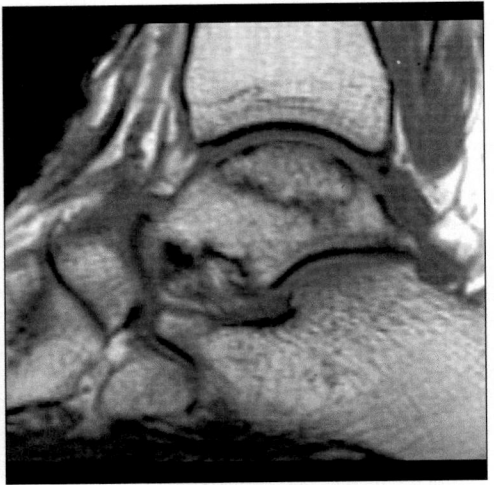

Sagittal T1WI MR shows central marrow containing ischemic region outlined by sclerotic periphery.

TERMINOLOGY

Abbreviations and Synonyms

- Avascular necrosis of the talus (AVN); osteonecrosis of the talus

Definitions

- Ischemic injury to the talar bone

IMAGING FINDINGS

General Features

- Best diagnostic clue: Localized subchondral ischemic focus + bone marrow edema
- Location
  - Central subchondral talus (talar dome)
  - Diffuse infarction pattern entire body of talus
- Size: Variable from small focus to entire talar volume
- Morphology
  - Well-demarcated linear subchondral lesion
  - Long axis directed from anterior to posterior
  - Ovoid ischemic area with sharply defined serpiginous perimeter
  - Diffuse bone infarct pattern with serpiginous sclerotic border

Radiographic Findings

- Radiography

  - Dome of talus
  - Localized subchondral rarefaction = Hawkins sign, indicative of intact blood supply
  - Subchondral sclerotic region = AVN
  - Body of talus with increased density relative to adjacent osseous structures = AVN (osteolysis with well-marginated sclerotic rim)

CT Findings

- NECT
  - Subchondral fracture
  - Collapse of articular surface
  - Mixed sclerotic pattern
  - Assess percentage of affected talus

MR Findings

- T1WI
  - Small hypointense necrotic focus superior talar dome
  - Hypointense sclerotic line directly adjacent to subchondral plate
  - Hypointense sclerotic line marginating central marrow fat signal
  - Diffuse osteonecrosis: Serpiginous bone infarct pattern
  - Association with talar neck fractures
- T2WI
  - Ischemic focus remains hypointense

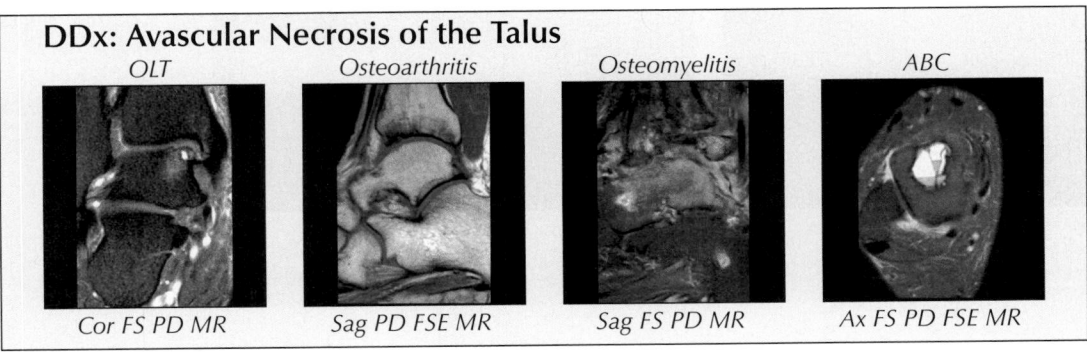

DDx: Avascular Necrosis of the Talus

OLT	Osteoarthritis	Osteomyelitis	ABC
Cor FS PD MR	Sag PD FSE MR	Sag FS PD MR	Ax FS PD FSE MR

AVASCULAR NECROSIS (AVN) OF THE TALUS

Key Facts

Imaging Findings
- Best diagnostic clue: Localized subchondral ischemic focus + bone marrow edema
- Central subchondral talus (talar dome)
- Diffuse infarction pattern entire body of talus
- Marrow edema most hyperintense adjacent to ischemic focus (with ischemia, edema commonly seen with focus of AVN) on T2WI

Top Differential Diagnoses
- Osteochondral Lesion of the Talus (OLT)
- Osteoarthritis
- Bone Marrow Edema Syndrome
- Osteomyelitis

Pathology
- Post-traumatic

- Atraumatic
- Bilateral involvement: 30 to 70%
- Talar neck fracture
- Subtalar/talar dislocation

Clinical Issues
- Most common signs/symptoms: Pain with weight bearing
- Limited range of motion
- Effusion
- Bilateral with asynchrony
- Delayed onset AVN: 3 months or greater post trauma

Diagnostic Checklist
- Repeat with serial MR to document resolution of edema to help define AVN focus

---

- ○ Disproportionate hyperintense diffuse marrow edema
- ○ Signal-void secondary to necrosis centrally with hyperintense rim (fat suppressed sequences)
- ○ Marrow edema most hyperintense adjacent to ischemic focus (with ischemia, edema commonly seen with focus of AVN) on T2WI
- ○ Chronic
  - ■ Resolution of bone marrow edema
  - ■ Persistent well demarcated focus osteonecrosis
- ○ Double line sign
  - ■ Hypointense outer line (sclerosis + fibrosis)
  - ■ Hyperintense inner line (granulation tissue)
- T1 C+: Enhancement - periphery of necrosis

Imaging Recommendations
- Best imaging tool: MRI - to diagnose and determine extent of talar involvement
- Protocol advice
  - ○ Coronal and axial T1WI and FS PD FSE MR
  - ○ High resolution coronal or sagittal T1WI to identify subtle subchondral fracture
  - ○ T1 C+/fat suppression to assess reparative process

DIFFERENTIAL DIAGNOSIS

Osteochondral Lesion of the Talus (OLT)
- Chronic phase of compressed/avulsed talar dome fracture
- Cup-shaped/deep medial lesions
- Wafer-shaped/thin lateral lesions
- Less extensive pattern of talar edema

Osteoarthritis
- Joint space narrowing
- Osteophytes
- Sclerosis both sides tibiotalar joint
- No discrete ischemic focus

Bone Marrow Edema Syndrome
- Transient + self-limiting
- No associated subchondral ischemic focus

- Edema may be centered in distal 1/2 of talus (talar head and neck)

Osteomyelitis
- Erosions
- Soft tissue involvement including sinus tracts
- Adjacent joint involvement

Tumors
- Trabecular destruction
- Cortical breakthrough
- Space-occupying
- Matrix often appreciated

PATHOLOGY

General Features
- General path comments
  - ○ Relevant anatomy
    - ■ Neck of talus - susceptible to fracture
    - ■ Subtalar region - dislocation
    - ■ Posterolateral corner talus = poorest blood supply
- Etiology
  - ○ Post-traumatic
    - ■ Talar neck fracture
    - ■ Talar dislocation
  - ○ Atraumatic
    - ■ Vasculitis or fat/arterial embolism
    - ■ Diabetes mellitus
    - ■ Systemic lupus erythematosus/vasculitis
    - ■ Sickle cell anemia
    - ■ Corticosteroids
- Epidemiology
  - ○ Incidence: Less frequent relative to AVN of femoral head, Kienböck's, scaphoid fracture necrosis and Freiberg's
  - ○ 40% AVN: Talar neck fracture + subtalar dislocation
  - ○ 90% AVN: Complete talar dislocation + subtalar dislocation
  - ○ 100% AVN: Comminuted fracture body of talus
  - ○ Bilateral involvement: 30 to 70%

AVASCULAR NECROSIS (AVN) OF THE TALUS

Gross Pathologic & Surgical Features
- Talar neck fracture
- Subtalar/talar dislocation
- Disruption tarsal canal artery - a posterior tibial artery branch
- Subchondral collapse + necrotic focus
- Focal vs. entire body of talus

Microscopic Features
- Arterial/venous insufficiency
- Intraluminal capillary obstruction and compression
- Ischemic marrow edema
- Increased intraosseous pressure
- Necrosis (vascular insufficiency)
- Trabecular insufficiency and subchondral plate fracture

Staging, Grading or Classification Criteria
- 0: Ischemia
- I: Necrotic focus + edema
- II: Large defined necrotic area
- III: Subchondral fracture (analogous to Ficat III in hip)
- IV: Subchondral collapse + secondary osteoarthrosis

CLINICAL ISSUES

Presentation
- Most common signs/symptoms: Pain with weight bearing
- Clinical profile
  - Inability to walk
  - Limited range of motion
  - Effusion
  - Compensatory weight shift
  - Bilateral with asynchrony

Demographics
- Age: Peak = fourth decade
- Gender: Not specific

Natural History & Prognosis
- Delayed onset AVN: 3 months or greater post trauma
- Revascularization of avascular fragment: Up to 24 months
- Risk of osseous collapse: Dependent on vertical load
- Collapse and repair = change in talar morphology
- Osteoarthritis: Degenerative process
  - Joint space narrowing
  - Ankylosis

Treatment
- Conservative
  - Protection from weight bearing during revascularization phase
  - Bracing
  - Nonsteroidal antiinflammatory agents
  - Orthotic support
- Surgical
  - Anatomic reduction of talar fracture: Screw fixation
  - Decompression (core) of necrosis
  - Debridement and autogenous grafting
  - External fixation
  - Ankle and subtalar arthrodesis

DIAGNOSTIC CHECKLIST

Consider
- Bone marrow edema syndrome without focal necrotic focus
- Repeat with serial MR to document resolution of edema to help define AVN focus
- Exclude bilateral involvement if atraumatic etiology

SELECTED REFERENCES

1. Fitzgerald RH et al: Orthopaedics. Trauma. 2nd ed. St. Louis Missouri, Mosby Inc 250-6, 2002
2. Banks A et al: McGlamry's comprehensive textbook of foot and ankle surgery. Talar fractures. vol 1. Philadelphia PA, Lippincott Williams & Wilkins 1865-96, 2001
3. Myerson M: Foot and ankle disorders. Fractures of the Hindfoot. vol 2. Philadelphia PA, Lippincott Raven 1297-340, 2000
4. Agnew PS: Avascular necrosis of the talus in a toddler. J Foot Ankle Surg 34(2):132-4, 1995
5. Mitchell MJ: The foot and ankle. Top Magn Reson Imaging 1:57-73, 1989
6. DeLee JC et al: Subtalar dislocation of the foot. J Bone Joint Surg 433-7, 1982
7. Dunn A: Peritalar dislocation. Orthop Clin North Am 7-18, 1974
8. Hawkins LG: Fractures of the neck of the talus. J Bone Joint Surg Am 52A:991-1002, 1970
9. Detenbeck LC et al: Total dislocation of talus. J Bone Joint Surg 283-8, 1969

AVASCULAR NECROSIS (AVN) OF THE TALUS

IMAGE GALLERY

Typical

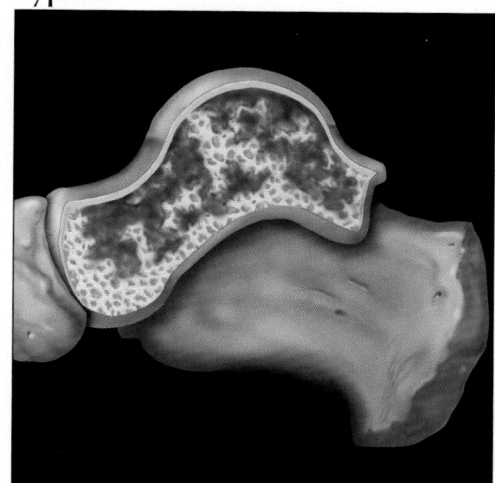 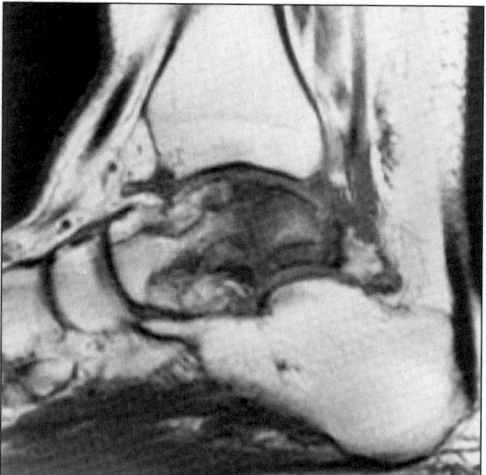

(Left) Sagittal graphic shows diffuse pattern of talar osteonecrosis. (Right) Sagittal T1WI MR shows diffuse infarct pattern involving the entire talus.

Typical

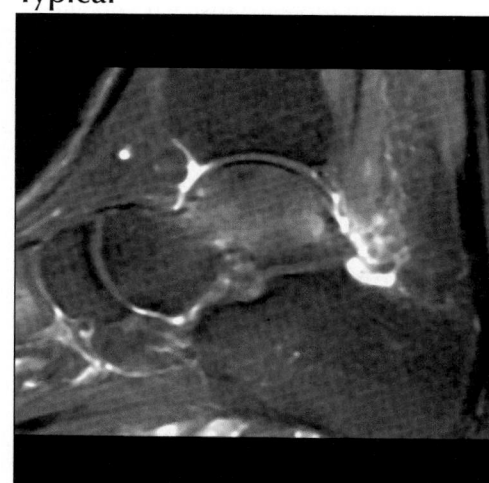 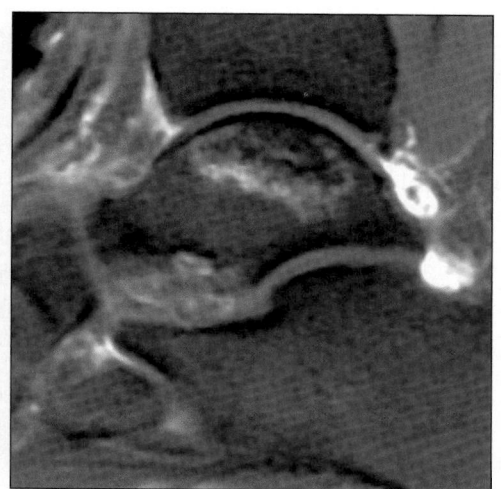

(Left) Sagittal FS PD FSE MR shows hyperintense marrow edema of the talar body associated with a subtle ischemic focus. (Right) Sagittal FS PD FSE MR shows hyperintense periphery in localized ischemia of the talus.

Variant

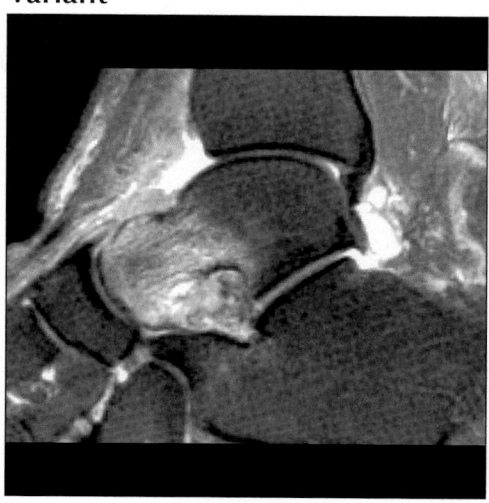 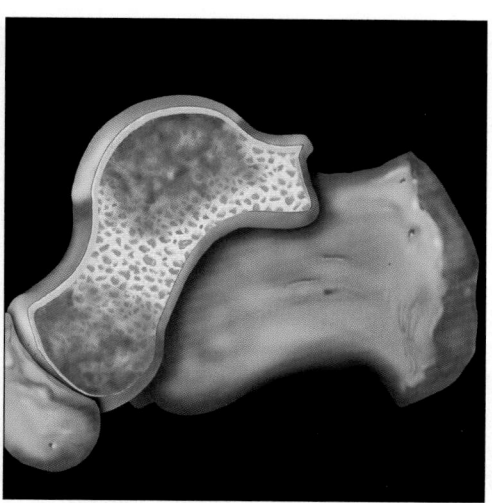

(Left) Sagittal FS PD FSE MR shows regional migratory osteoporosis with hyperintense signal involving the talar head and neck. No fracture or ischemic focus is identified. (Right) Sagittal graphic shows osteomyelitis involving the metaphyseal equivalent locations of the talus (not to be mistaken for AVN).

FREIBERG'S INFRACTION

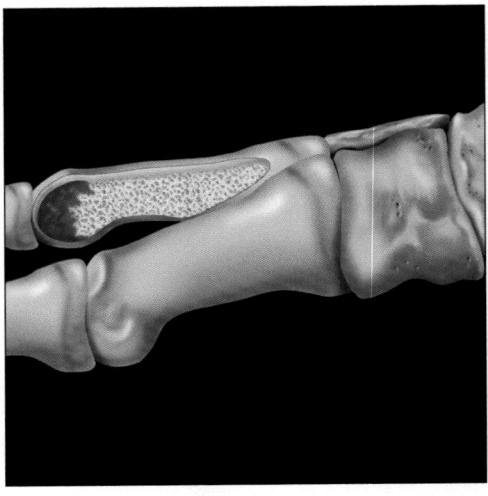

Sagittal graphic shows Freiberg's infraction with osteonecrosis of the 2nd metatarsal head.

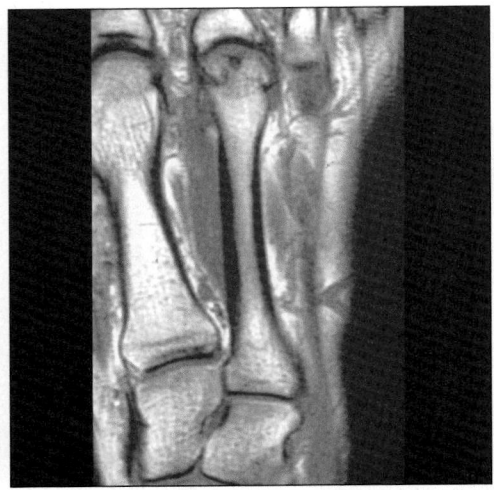

Axial T1WI MR shows sclerosis and flattening of the distal subchondral plate with mild hypertrophy of the metatarsal head.

TERMINOLOGY

Abbreviations and Synonyms
- Freiberg disease; Köhler-Freiberg disease

Definitions
- Articular osteochondrosis metatarsal head

IMAGING FINDINGS

General Features
- Best diagnostic clue: Sclerosis and flattening of second metatarsal head
- Location
  - Most frequently involves second metatarsal head
  - Less common involvement of third + fourth metatarsal heads
  - Rarely first metatarsal heads
  - Unilateral characteristic
  - Bilateral involvement and changes in two or more metatarsal heads possible
- Size
  - Initially restricted to distal dorsocentral subchondral bone
  - Focal hypointense sclerosis

- Advanced changes with more extensive involvement of distal metatarsal associated with central collapse and articular cartilage separation
- Morphology
  - Flattening metatarsal head
  - Periostitis
  - Cortical thickening adjacent metaphysis + diaphysis
  - Cystic lesion metatarsal head
  - Enlargement metatarsal head

Radiographic Findings
- Radiography
  - Initial radiographs normal
  - Subtle flattening distal subchondral plate
  - Increased sclerosis
  - Cystic lucency
  - Metatarsophalangeal (MTP) joint widening to joint space collapse
  - Osteochondral fragment
  - Periostitis
  - Metatarsal metaphysis + distal diaphysis cortical thickening
  - Premature physeal closure
  - MTP joint osseous fragments
  - Endstage with marked metatarsal head flattening + hypertrophy

CT Findings
- NECT

DDx: Freiberg's Infraction

Midfoot Arthritis	MTP Arthritis	Lisfranc Fx	Neuropathic Fx
Ax T1WI MR	Sag T1WI MR	Ax T1WI MR	Sag T1WI MR

FREIBERG'S INFRACTION

Key Facts

Imaging Findings
- Best diagnostic clue: Sclerosis and flattening of second metatarsal head
- Most frequently involves second metatarsal head
- Initially restricted to distal dorsocentral subchondral bone
- Variable degenerative subchondral marrow change with hyperintense edema

Top Differential Diagnoses
- Osteoarthritis
- Trauma
- Rheumatoid Arthritis

Pathology
- Long 2nd metatarsal susceptible to increased stresses
- Trauma is primary event

- Single event or repeated microtrauma
- Vascular damage/compression
- Long involved second metatarsal: 85%

Clinical Issues
- Most common signs/symptoms: Localized pain (metatarsalgia)
- Focal tenderness
- Swelling
- Decreased range of motion at MTP joint
- Peak = 11 to 17 years
- Gender: M:F = 1:3 up to 1:11

Diagnostic Checklist
- Confirm contour abnormality of metatarsal head

- ○ Metatarsal head deformity on sagittal reformations
- ○ Sclerosis + osteophytes using bone window algorithm

MR Findings
- T1WI
  - ○ Hypointense sclerosis
  - ○ Subchondral plate flattening metatarsal head on sagittal images
  - ○ Fragmentation subchondral plate
- T2WI
  - ○ Variable degenerative subchondral marrow change with hyperintense edema
  - ○ Hyperintense joint effusion MTP joint
  - ○ Intermediate to hypointense loose bodies
  - ○ Fragmentation of chondral surface metatarsal head on FS PD FSE images

Imaging Recommendations
- Best imaging tool: MRI subsequent to conventional radiography
- Protocol advice
  - ○ T1 axial and sagittal images to assess sclerosis
  - ○ FS PD FSE axial and sagittal images for chondral surface evaluation
  - ○ Direct coronal FS PD FSE for MTP joint capsule visualization in cross section

DIFFERENTIAL DIAGNOSIS

Midfoot Arthritis
- Degenerative sclerosis

Metatarsal Phalangeal Joint Arthritis
- Joint space narrowing + sclerosis 1st or 2nd digits

Lisfranc Fracture
- Tarsometatarsal articulation

Neuropathic Joint
- Erosion, sclerosis, + marrow changes

Osteoarthritis
- Degenerative changes in malpositioned toes

- Hallux valgus
  - ○ Hyperostosis + cystoid osseous transformation
  - ○ Bursitis

Trauma
- Stress fractures + osseous contusions
  - ○ Subchondral marrow edema without metatarsal head flattening

Rheumatoid Arthritis
- Metatarsal heads commonly involved
  - ○ Involvement from lateral to medial
- Forefoot deformities
  - ○ Hallux valgus
  - ○ Hammer toe
  - ○ MTP joint lateral subluxation
  - ○ Dorsiflexion + lateral deviation of toes
  - ○ Interphalangeal + intertarsal erosions later in disease

Calcium Pyrophosphate Dihydrate Crystal Deposition
- Productive + erosive process
- T2* images to identify crystal deposition

Diabetes Mellitus
- Neuropathic arthropathy
  - ○ Destructive arthropathy with erosive + productive changes

Gout
- First MTP joint
  - ○ Gouty tophus
  - ○ Normal bone density
  - ○ Sharply marginated erosions

PATHOLOGY

General Features
- General path comments
  - ○ Relevant anatomy
    - ▪ Long 2nd metatarsal susceptible to increased stresses

FREIBERG'S INFRACTION

- Second metatarsal head epiphysis unique vascular pattern of penetrating radial arteries to periosteal shaft network
- Etiology
  - Trauma is primary event
    - Single event or repeated microtrauma
  - Vascular damage/compression
  - Long involved second metatarsal: 85%
  - Biomechanical stress (e.g., high heel shoes)
- Distribution
  - Unilateral involvement predominates

Gross Pathologic & Surgical Features
- Vascular occlusion
- Subchondral trabecular fracture
- Secondary compression of chondral surface
- Cortical thickening

Microscopic Features
- Necrosis trabecular marrow
- Revascularization
  - Vascular invasion from periosteum and metaphyseal regions
- Necrotic trabeculae resorption
- Subperiosteal osseous apposition

Staging, Grading or Classification Criteria
- Bragard classification
  - Stage I subchondral decreased density plus metatarsal head flattening
  - Stage II with sclerotic and radiolucent areas leading to fragmentation, metatarsal head deformity + enlargement, cortical thickening + physeal fusion
  - Stage III with degenerative osteoarthritis

CLINICAL ISSUES

Presentation
- Most common signs/symptoms: Localized pain (metatarsalgia)
- Clinical profile
  - Focal tenderness
  - Swelling
  - Decreased range of motion at MTP joint
  - Vague forefoot pain which increases with weight bearing and/or activity
  - Pain with extreme range of motion

Demographics
- Age
  - Peak = 11 to 17 years
  - Degenerative arthrosis in adulthood
- Gender: M:F = 1:3 up to 1:11

Natural History & Prognosis
- Asymptomatic to symptomatic
- Associated
  - Periarticular edema
  - Soft tissue thickening
  - Localized warmth
  - Synovitis
- Antalgic gait to compensate for metatarsalgia
- Later findings
  - Enlarged metatarsal head

- Dorsal osteophyte
- Loose body
- Proliferative changes proximal aspect adjacent proximal phalanx
- Complications
  - Related to fragmentation of cartilage + subchondral bone
- Prognosis
  - Decreased symptoms with protecting metatarsal head during remodeling

Treatment
- Nonoperative
  - Cast immobilization
  - Non weight bearing
  - Corticosteroids
- Surgical
  - Second metatarsal head debridement + synovectomy
  - Metatarsal head excision or reshaping
  - Cheilectomy of osteophytes
  - Dorsiflexion osteotomy
  - Joint replacement

DIAGNOSTIC CHECKLIST

Consider
- Confirm contour abnormality of metatarsal head
- Metatarsal symptoms may be related to a stress fracture
- Exclude an associated systemic disorder (e.g., rheumatoid arthritis)

SELECTED REFERENCES

1. Banks A et al: McGlamry's comprehensive textbook of foot and ankle surgery. Osteochondroses of the foot and ankle. vol 1. Philadelphia PA, Lippincott Williams & Wilkins, (66):2075-96, 2001
2. Myerson M: Foot and ankle disorders. Osteochondroses of the foot. vol 2. Philadelphia PA, Lippincott Raven, (31):785-99, 2000
3. Chao KH et al: Surgery for symptomatic Freiberg's disease: Extraarticular dorsal closing-wedge osteotomy in 13 patients followed for 2-4 years. Acta Orthop Scand 70(5):483-6, 1999
4. Maresca G et al: Arthroscopic treatment of bilateral Freiberg's infraction. Arthroscopy 12(1):103-8, 1996
5. Kinnard P et al: Freiberg's disease and dorsiflexion osteotomy. J Bone Joint Surg Br. 864-5, 1991
6. Walsh HPJ et al: Etiology of Freiberg's disease: Trauma. J Foot Surg 27:243-4, 1988
7. Wiley JJ et al: Freiberg's disease. J Bone Joint Surg Br 63:459, 1981

FREIBERG'S INFRACTION

IMAGE GALLERY

Typical

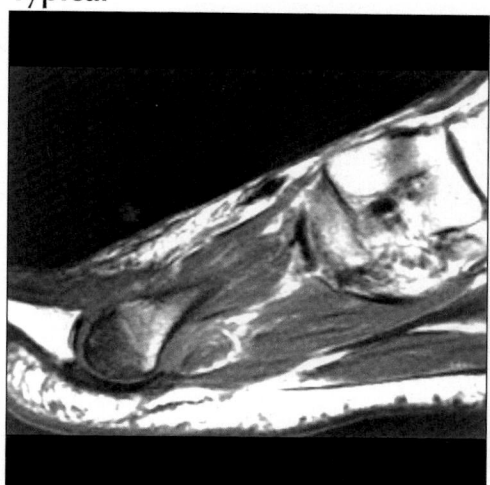 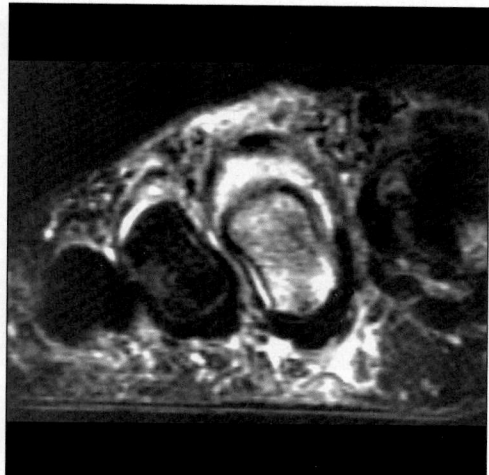

(Left) Sagittal T1WI MR shows early flattening of the metatarsal head in Freiberg's infraction. Osteonecrosis is hypointense. *(Right)* Coronal STIR MR shows hyperintense edema in the necrotic focus in the distal metatarsal head.

Typical

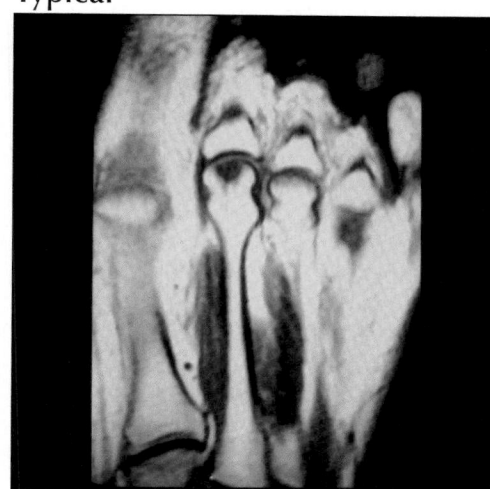 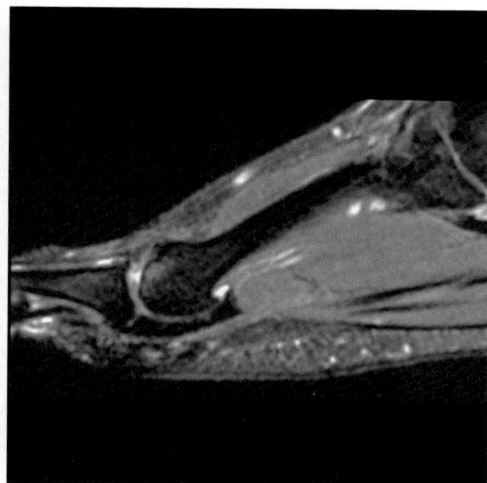

(Left) Axial T1WI MR shows focal well marginated sclerosis of 2nd metatarsal head. There is no fragmentation of the subchondral plate. *(Right)* Sagittal FS PD FSE MR shows dorsocentral flattening of the metatarsal head with adjacent subchondral bone marrow edema.

Typical

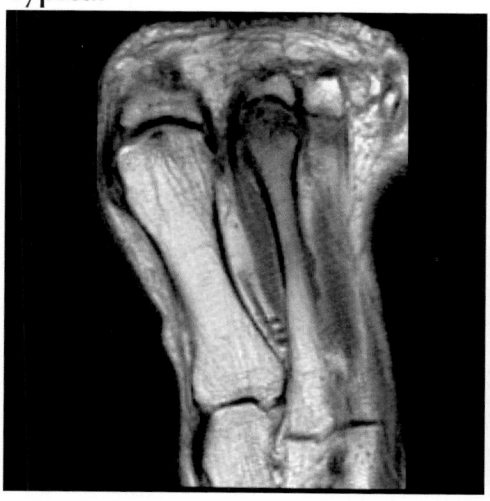 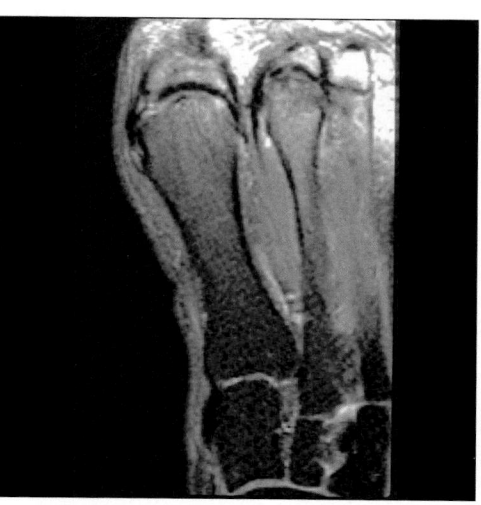

(Left) Axial T1WI MR shows advanced changes of Freiberg's infraction with flattening and fragmentation of the 2nd metatarsal head. *(Right)* Axial FS PD FSE MR shows subchondral cystic changes adjacent to fragmentation of subchondral plate.

6

97

MEDIAL TIBIAL STRESS SYNDROME

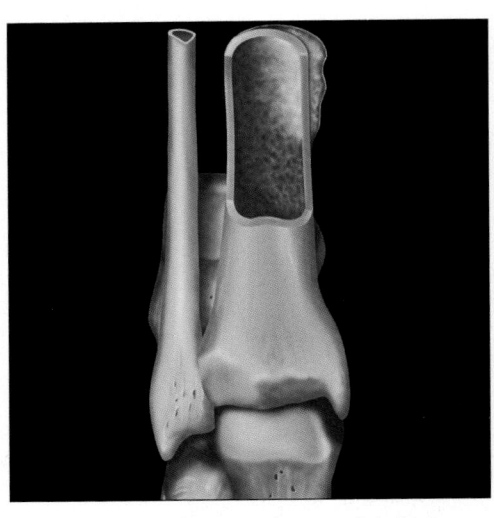

Coronal graphic shows grade II medial tibial stress syndrome with bone marrow and periosteal edema.

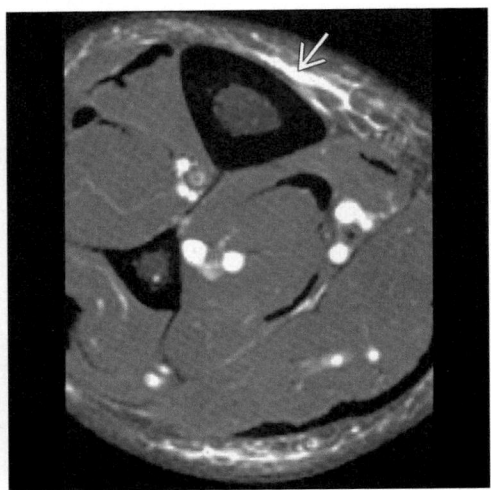

Axial FS PD FSE MR shows hyperintense anteromedial periosteal edema (arrow) in grade I medial tibial stress syndrome.

TERMINOLOGY

Abbreviations and Synonyms
- Medial tibial stress; shin splint syndrome; shin splints

Definitions
- Leg pain + discomfort secondary to repetitive overuse in running + hiking

IMAGING FINDINGS

General Features
- Best diagnostic clue: Hyperintense edema/fluid signal (T2WI) medial tibial border
- Location
  - Posteromedial to anteromedial tibia
  - Medial periosteum
  - Intracortical
  - Medullary cavity
- Size
  - Middle + distal third of leg
  - 4 cm proximal to medial malleolus ± proximal extension up to 12 cm
- Morphology
  - Linear edema/fluid applied to medial periosteum
  - Linear to globular intracortical increased signal

- Eccentric curvilinear to more diffuse marrow signal change

Radiographic Findings
- Radiography
  - Usually negative
  - ± Posteromedial tibial cortex - hypertrophy (remodeling)

MR Findings
- T1WI
  - Intermediate signal within deep subcutaneous tissue overlying medial tibial cortex
  - Intermediate signal within normally hypointense cortex
  - Eccentric hypointense marrow in medullary bone of diaphysis
- T2WI
  - Linear hyperintense periosteal edema/fluid in direct contact with medial tibial cortex
  - Anteromedial to posteromedial extension
  - Hyperintense edema/fluid extends to orgin of soleus posteromedially (soleus bridge)
  - Marrow hyperintensity (common anterior or posteromedially)
  - Intermediate/hyperintense focus or linearity anterior tibial cortex
- T1 C+
  - May enhance medial periosteal interface

DDx: Medial Tibial Stress Syndrome

Tibial Stress Fx	DVT	Gastroc Strain	Cellulitis	Fascia Herniation
Sag T1WI MR	Ax FS PD FSE MR	Ax FS PD FSE MR	Ax FS PD FSE MR	Ax T1WI MR

MEDIAL TIBIAL STRESS SYNDROME

Key Facts

Imaging Findings

- Best diagnostic clue: Hyperintense edema/fluid signal (T2WI) medial tibial border
- Linear hyperintense periosteal edema/fluid in direct contact with medial tibial cortex
- Anteromedial to posteromedial extension
- Hyperintense edema/fluid extends to orgin of soleus posteromedially (soleus bridge)

Top Differential Diagnoses

- Stress Fracture of the Tibia
- Deep Venous Thrombosis (DVT)
- Gastrocnemius - Soleus Strain
- Cellulitis

Pathology

- Periosteal avulsion + periostitis = medial soleus insertional stress
- Velocity of pronation = stress/strain of supporting musculature + soleus bridge

Clinical Issues

- Most common signs/symptoms: Tenderness posteromedial tibial border - mid to distal third
- Pain on exertion

Diagnostic Checklist

- FS PD FSE or STIR to identify subtle periosteal edema requires axial plane of section

---

- ○ Variable marrow enhancement

Nuclear Medicine Findings

- Bone Scan
  - ○ Radionuclide activity posteromedial border tibia- delayed images - involves 1/3 length of tibia
  - ○ Perfusion and blood pool phases = normal in medial tibial stress
  - ○ Uptake - soleus muscle origin (posteromedially)

Imaging Recommendations

- Best imaging tool: MR more specific for staging and morphology of medial tibial stress
- Protocol advice
  - ○ Axial FS PD FSE or STIR images required
  - ○ Sagittal/coronal plane to visualize longitudinal extent of tibial involvement in a single image

DIFFERENTIAL DIAGNOSIS

Stress Fracture of the Tibia

- Transverse fracture
- Posteromedially (compression side of tibia)
- Continuum from medial tibial stress syndrome to frank fracture
- Interruption of cortex

Deep Venous Thrombosis (DVT)

- Perivascular hyperintensity - neurovascular bundle at or distal to popliteal fossa
- Enlargement and thrombus popliteal vein
- Muscle infarct
- Venous Doppler confirmation

Gastrocnemius - Soleus Strain

- Medial head gastrocnemius strain
- Hyperintense edema or hemorrhage medial head gastrocnemius

Cellulitis

- Subcutaneous edema extension beyond anterior/posteromedial tibia

Popliteal Artery Entrapment Syndrome

- Exercise - induced claudication
- Anomalies or anatomic variation of popliteal artery - fibrous bands, third head of gastrocnemius

Chronic Exertional Compartment Syndrome

- Increased compartmental pressure in leg with exercise
- Compartment tightness to palpation

Accessory Soleus

- ± Overuse symptoms with exercise
- Fullness or bulge medial ankle + lower 1/3 leg
- Sensory nerve findings
- ± Calcaneal nerve involvement
- Less commonly plantar nerve involvement

Fascial Herniation

- Localized asymmetric bulge or prominence of muscle group contour without muscle strain

PATHOLOGY

General Features

- General path comments
  - ○ Relevant anatomy
    - Soleus bridge = medial origin of investing fascia posteromedially
    - Deep posterior compartment = anterior to soleus muscle
- Etiology
  - ○ Periosteal avulsion + periostitis = medial soleus insertional stress
  - ○ Velocity of pronation = stress/strain of supporting musculature + soleus bridge
  - ○ Hyperpronation foot - increase stress medial soleus
  - ○ Not related to tibialis posterior overload
  - ○ Varus hindfoot
  - ○ Genu valgum
  - ○ Excessive femoral anteversion
  - ○ External tibial torsion
  - ○ Decreased heel cord flexibility
  - ○ Change in activity or intensity of training

MEDIAL TIBIAL STRESS SYNDROME

- Epidemiology
  - 13% of injuries in runners
  - 4.07% in Naval Academy cadets

Gross Pathologic & Surgical Features
- Hypertrophy posteromedial tibial cortex
- Surface scalloping anterior or medial tibia
- Avulsion periosteum
- Periostitis + inflammatory response

Microscopic Features
- Increased erythrocytes - vascular congestion + thrombosis within bone
- Osteoclastic resorption
- Periosteal reaction - increase in osteoblasts
- Osseous remodeling
- Periosteal callus - cortical hypertrophy
- Increased mineralization with repetitive stress

Staging, Grading or Classification Criteria
- Grade I: Periosteal edema (T2WI)
- Grade II: Periosteal and marrow edema (T2WI)
- Grade III: Marrow edema (T1 and T2WI)
- Grade IV: Fracture line

CLINICAL ISSUES

Presentation
- Most common signs/symptoms: Tenderness posteromedial tibial border - mid to distal third
- Clinical profile
  - Pain with active resistance plantar flexion and toe raises
  - Pain on exertion
  - Dull ache
  - Soreness
  - Mild swelling
  - Tenderness more diffuse relative to complete stress fracture

Demographics
- Age: Uncommon < 15 years
- Gender
  - Females at increased risk: Smaller bone size + amenorrhea in competitive runners
  - Female runners up to 12x risk stress fracture vs. male counterparts

Natural History & Prognosis
- 7-10 days - return to low impact activity
- Recurrent pain (premature return to training)
- Development complete fracture line = tibial stress fracture (end stage of medial tibial stress syndrome)

Treatment
- Conservative
  - Rest - relative
  - Antiinflammatory medication
  - Heel cord stretching
  - Casting
  - Evaluate gait mechanics + lower limb alignment
  - Heel cup for hindfoot valgus
  - Orthotic for excessive foot pronation
  - Cushion insoles to decrease velocity of foot pronation on heel strike (decreases eccentric muscle stress)
- Surgical
  - Resistant medial tibial stress syndrome
  - Release soleus investing fascia
  - Cauterization posteromedial tibial periosteum

DIAGNOSTIC CHECKLIST

Consider
- Advanced grade medial tibial stress syndrome = tibial stress fracture
- FS PD FSE or STIR to identify subtle periosteal edema requires axial plane of section

SELECTED REFERENCES

1. DeLee JC et al: Orthopaedic sports medicine. Principles and practice. The Leg. vol 2. 2nd ed, Philadelphia PA, Saunders, (29):2155-82, 2003
2. Spitz DJ et al: Imaging of stress fractures in the athlete. Radiol Clin North Am 40(2):313-31, 2002
3. Magnusson HI et al: Abnormally decreased regional bone density in athletes with medial tibial stress syndrome. Am J Sports Med 29(6):712-5, 2001
4. Bennett JE et al: Factors contributing to the development of medical tibial stress syndrome in high school runners. J Orthop Sports Phys Ther 31(9):504-10, 2001
5. Gibbon WW: Shin splits. Radiology 207(3):826-7, 1998
6. Beck BR: Tibial stress injuries. An etiological review for the purposes of guiding management. Sports Med 26(4):265-79, 1998
7. Anderson MW et al: Shin splints: MR appearance in a preliminary study. Radiology 204(1):177-80, 1997
8. Deutsch A et al: Imaging of stress injuries to bone. Clin Sports Med 16:275-90, 1997
9. Beck BR: Medial tibial stress syndrome. The location of muscles in the leg in relation to symptoms. J Bone Joint Surg Am 76(7):1057-61, 1994
10. Clanton T et al: Chronic leg pain in the athlete. Clin Sports Med 13:743-59, 1994
11. Detmer DE: Chronic shin splints. Classification and management of medial tibial stress syndrome. Sports Med 3:436-46, 1986
12. Stafford S et al; MRI in stress fracture. AJR 147:553-6, 1986
13. Michael RH et al: The soleus syndrome. A cause of medial tibial stress (shin splints). Am J Sports Med 13:87-94, 1985
14. Milgrom C et al: The long term follow-up of soldiers with stress fractures. Am J Sports Med 13:398-400, 1985
15. Mubarak SJ et al: The medial tibial stress syndrome. A cause of shin splints. Am J Sports med 10:201-05, 1982
16. James SL et al: Injuries to runners. Am J Sports Med 6:40-50, 1978
17. Stanitski C et al: On the nature of stress fractures. Am J Sports Med 6:391-6,1978
18. Andrish JT et al: A prospective study on the management of shin splints. J Bone Joint Surg Am 56:1697-700, 1974
19. Darling R et al: Intermittent claudication in young athletes: Popliteal artery entrapment syndrome. J Trauma 14:543-52, 1974

MEDIAL TIBIAL STRESS SYNDROME

IMAGE GALLERY

Typical

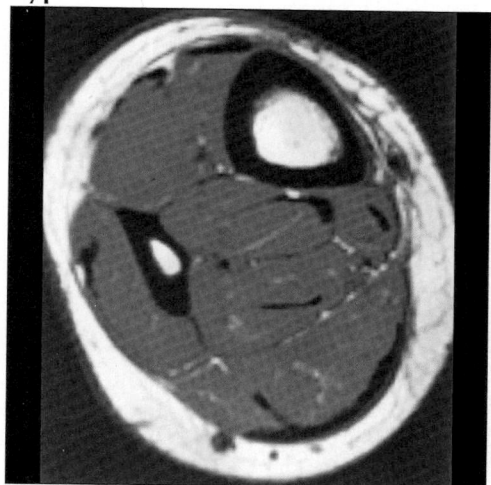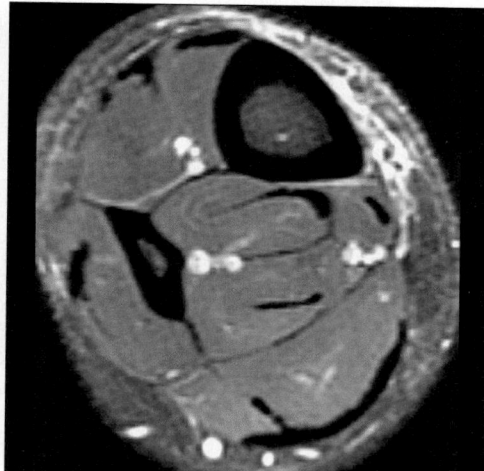

(Left) Axial T1WI MR shows hypointense anteromedial periosteal edema with normal bone marrow signal. *(Right)* Axial FS PD FSE MR shows hyperintense periosteal edema involving the anteromedial and posteromedial tibial periosteum in a grade I medial tibial stress syndrome.

Typical

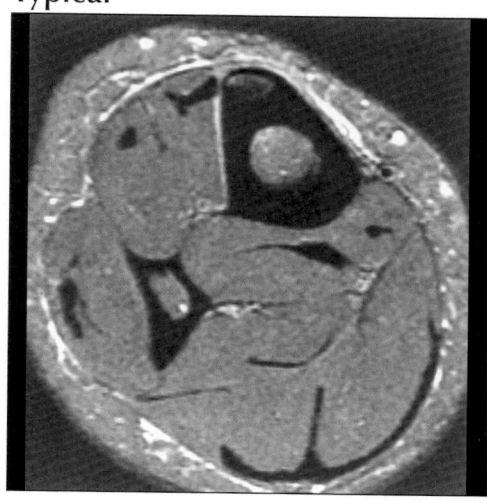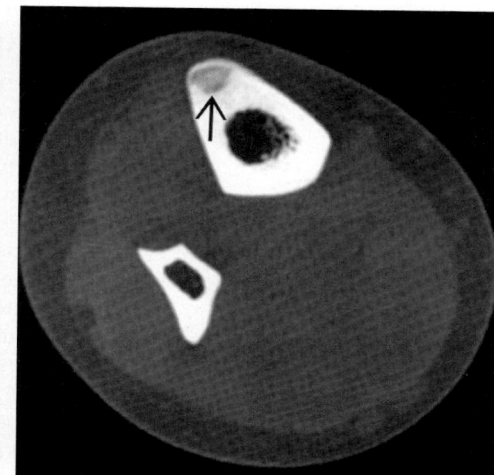

(Left) Axial FS PD FSE MR shows hyperintense signal within the anterior medullary cavity, intracortical cystic change, and medial periosteal edema. This represents medial tibial stress syndrome in a sprinter. *(Right)* Axial NECT shows intracortical cystic reaction (arrow) with remodeling of repeated cortical stress fractures.

Typical

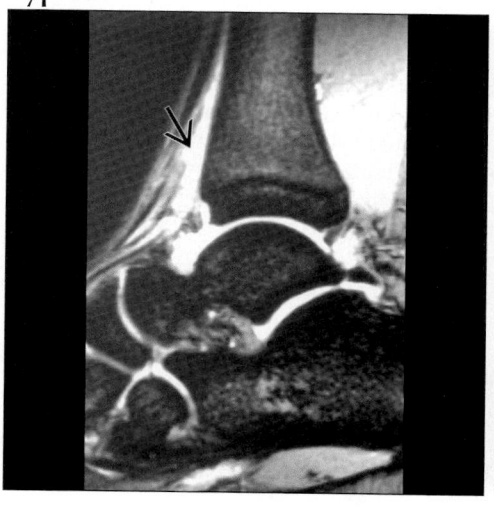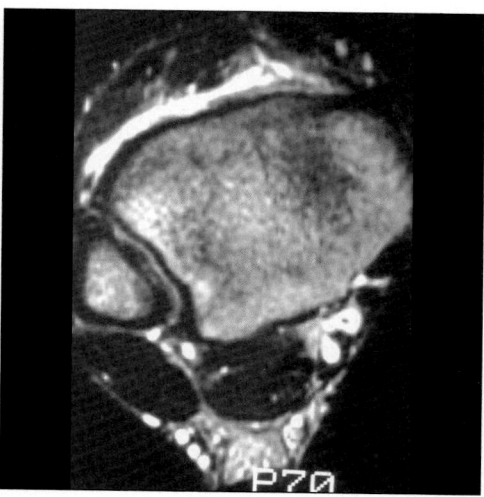

(Left) Sagittal T2* GRE MR shows edema applied to the periosteum (arrow) of the anterior tibial cortex. *(Right)* Axial T2WI MR shows hyperintense edema extending from the medial to the lateral aspect of the distal tibia.

TARSAL COALITION

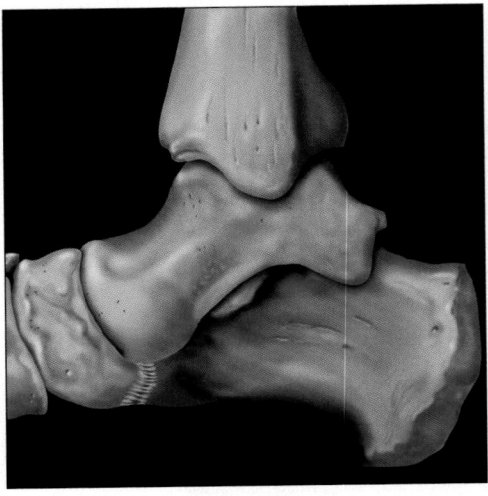

Sagittal graphic shows calcaneonavicular fibrocartilaginous coalition.

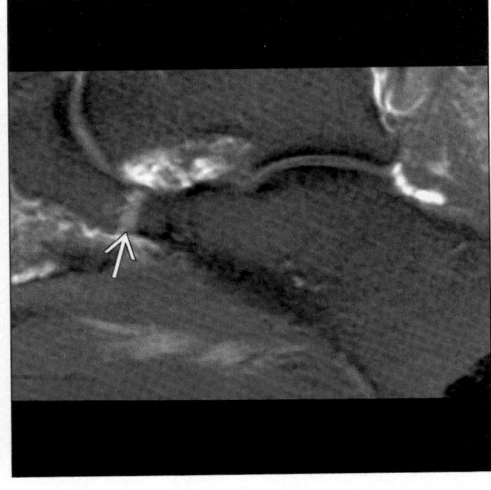

Sagittal FS PD FSE MR shows intermediate signal with mild reactive osseous changes in calcaneonavicular fibrous coalition (arrow).

TERMINOLOGY

Abbreviations and Synonyms
- Coalitions

Definitions
- Osseous, cartilaginous or fibrous union of two or more bones involving hindfoot or midfoot

IMAGING FINDINGS

General Features
- Best diagnostic clue: Approximation or incorporation of talus + calcaneus through middle facet vs. calcaneus to navicular through anterior facet
- Location
  ○ Talocalcaneal
  ○ Calcaneonavicular
  ○ Talonavicular (less common)
  ○ Cubonavicular (less common)
- Size: Variable based on location + synostosis vs. synchondrosis vs. syndesmosis or combination
- Morphology
  ○ Synostosis = complete coalition
  ○ Synchondrosis = cartilaginous
  ○ Syndesmosis = fibrous
  ○ Extraarticular = bars (e.g., calcaneonavicular)
  ○ Intraarticular = bridges (e.g., talocalcaneal)

Radiographic Findings
- Radiography
  ○ Calcaneonavicular coalition
    ■ 45° internal oblique view
    ■ Comma sign = protrusion of calcaneus toward navicular on oblique view
    ■ Anterior nose sign = anterior extension of calcaneus on lateral view
    ■ Connecting bar between anterolateral process calcaneus + dorsal lateral margin navicular = osseous, cartilaginous, fibrous or mixed
    ■ Sclerosis + osseous marrow irregularity at interface in cartilaginous + fibrous coalitions
    ■ ± Hypoplasia talar head
    ■ Flattening navicular adjacent to calcaneus
  ○ Talocalcaneal coalition
    ■ Lateral radiograph + axial views (Harris-Beath) for visualization posterior and middle facets
    ■ Joint space absent/diminished
    ■ Middle facet involvement (less frequently anterior + posterior facets)
    ■ Narrowing posterior facet subtalar joint
    ■ Talar beak (limited subtalar joint motion + dorsal subluxation navicular)
    ■ C sign - prominence inferior border sustentaculum tali + medial outline talar dome on lateral view

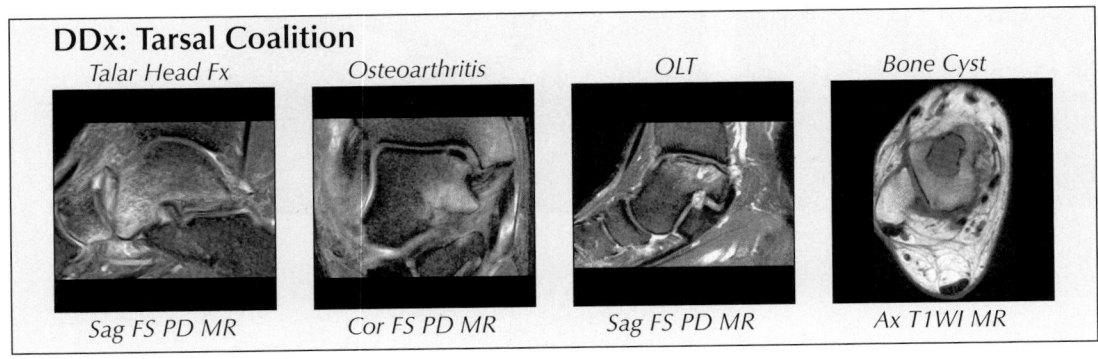

DDx: Tarsal Coalition

Talar Head Fx	Osteoarthritis	OLT	Bone Cyst
Sag FS PD MR	Cor FS PD MR	Sag FS PD MR	Ax T1WI MR

TARSAL COLITION

Key Facts

Imaging Findings
- Best diagnostic clue: Approximation or incorporation of talus + calcaneus through middle facet vs. calcaneus to navicular through anterior facet
- Synostosis = complete coalition
- Synchondrosis = cartilaginous
- Syndesmosis = fibrous

Top Differential Diagnoses
- Subtalar Fractures
- Osteoarthritis
- Osteochondral Lesion of the Talus (OLT)

Pathology
- Congenital = failure of differentiation + segmentation of primitive mesenchyme
- Acquired = arthritis, infection, trauma + neoplasm

- 90% coalition = talocalcaneal + calcaneonavicular

Clinical Issues
- Most common signs/symptoms: Limitation of subtalar joint motion; pain
- Talocalcaneal coalition = rearfoot pain with localization to sustentaculum medially + sinus tarsi laterally
- Limitation of subtalar + mid tarsal joint motion including peroneal muscle spasm
- Tarsal coalition = most common cause of peroneal spastic flatfoot

Diagnostic Checklist
- Talocalcaneal coalitions require coronal images

- ± Ball-and-socket ankle joint - decreased subtalar motion with concavity proximal talar surface + concavity distal tibial surface

CT Findings
- NECT
  - Requires direct axial + coronal images
  - Requires sagittal reformations
  - Section thickness = 1.5 cm or less
  - Calcaneonavicular coalition
    - Narrowing + sclerosis between calcaneus + navicular on sagittal reformations
    - Medial broadening anterior + dorsal aspects calcaneus at navicular
  - Talocalcaneal
    - Direct coronal CT to visualize connection between talus + calcaneus through middle facet
    - Solid osseous continuity
    - Fibrous/fibrocartilaginous coalition with sclerosis + irregular articular interface ± cystic subchondral changes
    - Change in sustentaculum tali slope from upward medially to downward or laterally
    - ± Sustentaculum hypoplasia

MR Findings
- T1WI
  - Calcaneonavicular coalition
    - Sagittal plane to visualize osseous vs. cartilaginous vs. fibrous
    - ± Hypointense subchondral sclerosis at synchondrosis or syndesmosis
    - Narrowing calcaneal navicular interface
  - Talocalcaneal
    - Coronal plane
    - Osseous connection with fat signal bone marrow continuity between talus and calcaneus
    - Narrowing with irregular articular interface ± sclerosis across middle facet in cartilaginous, fibrous or fibrocartilaginous unions
    - ± Hypoplastic sustentaculum tali
    - Talar beaking + degenerative dorsal changes calcaneocuboid joint on lateral sagittal images

- Talar neck concavity on sagittal views
- T2WI
  - Calcaneonavicular
    - ± Linear hyperintense calcaneonavicular interface in non-osseous coalition
    - Irregular interface contour
    - ± Hyperintense reactive subchondral marrow edema
    - Solid continuous marrow continuity between calcaneus and navicular on lateral sagittal images
  - Talocalcaneal
    - Continuity of marrow across middle facet on coronal images
    - Variable increased subchondral signal + degenerative changes in fibrous, cartilaginous or fibrocartilaginous coalitions
    - Intermediate signal on fibrocartilaginous interface
    - Low to intermediate signal in fibrous tissue syndesmosis

Imaging Recommendations
- Best imaging tool: MR with direct three plane visualization + identification of subchondral marrow edema and non-osseous cartilaginous + fibrous unions
- Protocol advice
  - Coronal T1/PD + FS PD FSE for talocalcaneal coalition
  - Sagittal T1/PD + FS PD FSE for calcaneonavicular coalition
  - Sagittal plane for secondary osseous changes including talar beaking

DIFFERENTIAL DIAGNOSIS

Subtalar Fractures
- Head of talus, lateral process, posterior process, talar neck + body
- Calcaneal extra + intraarticular fractures

Osteoarthritis
- Subtalar arthrosis middle or posterior facet with sclerosis + subchondral cystic change

TARSAL COALITION

- Calcaneocuboid sclerosis

Osteochondral Lesion of the Talus (OLT)
- Antecedent trauma (e.g. torsional impaction)
- Chronic phase of compressed or avulsed talar dome fracture

Tumor
- Bone cyst
- Secondary osseous invasion (e.g., synovial sarcoma)

Rheumatoid Arthritis
- Retrocalcaneal bursitis
- Posterior calcaneal erosion
- Pannus formation/hypertrophied synovium

Recurrent Ankle Sprains
- Injured lateral ligament complex with inversion + internal rotation + plantar flexion
- Complication = anterolateral impingement

Sinus Tarsi
- Lateral foot pain + tenderness
- Tears of sinus tarsi ligaments
- Subtalar microinstability

PATHOLOGY

General Features
- General path comments
  - Relevant anatomy
    - Subtalar articulation through anterior, middle + posterior facet
    - Transverse tarsal joint: Calcaneocuboid + talonavicular joints
    - Normal subtalar motion + rotation + gliding
- Genetics: Genetic mutation autosomal gene, autosomal dominant
- Etiology
  - Congenital = failure of differentiation + segmentation of primitive mesenchyme
  - Acquired = arthritis, infection, trauma + neoplasm
- Epidemiology
  - 1% incidence of talocalcaneal coalitions
  - 90% coalition = talocalcaneal + calcaneonavicular
  - Talocalcaneal slightly more common than calcaneonavicular
  - Talonavicular = 3rd most common
  - 22 - 60% bilateral rate - talocalcaneal
  - 40 - 68% bilateral rate - calcaneonavicular

Gross Pathologic & Surgical Features
- Osseous
- Cartilaginous
- Fibrous

Microscopic Features
- Nonosseous coalitions - no neural elements
- Microfracture = pain generator
- Osseous remodeling = pain generator
- Vascular proliferation
- Osteoblastic + osteoclastic activity
- Fibrous connective tissue, cellular components

CLINICAL ISSUES

Presentation
- Most common signs/symptoms: Limitation of subtalar joint motion; pain
- Clinical profile
  - Asymptomatic to symptomatic
  - Talocalcaneal coalition = rearfoot pain with localization to sustentaculum medially + sinus tarsi laterally
  - Limitation of subtalar + mid tarsal joint motion including peroneal muscle spasm
  - Tarsal coalition = most common cause of peroneal spastic flatfoot

Demographics
- Age: Second decade
- Gender: Slight male predominance

Natural History & Prognosis
- Coalitions are initially cartilaginous and progress to ossification
- Decreased rearfoot motion results in increased laxity ankle ligaments (susceptible to sprain)
- Decreased subtalar & midtarsal joint motion

Treatment
- Conservative
  - Shoe modification, orthotics ± casting
- Surgical
  - Resection of coalition
  - Fusion of involved joint

DIAGNOSTIC CHECKLIST

Consider
- Talocalcaneal coalitions require coronal images
- Calcaneonavicular coalitions require sagittal images

SELECTED REFERENCES

1. Sijbrandij ES et al: Bone marrow ill-defined hyperintensities with tarsal coalition: MR imaging findings. Eur J Radiol 43(1):61-5, 2002
2. Lee MF et al: Tarsal tunnel syndrome caused by talocalcaneal coalition. Clin Imaging 26(2):140-3, 2002
3. Banks A et al: McGlamry's comprehensive textbook of foot and ankle surgery. Tarsal coalition. vol 1. Philadelphia PA, Lippincott Williams & Wilkins (31):99-1032, 2001
4. Newman JS et al: Congenital tarsal coalition: Multimodality evaluation with emphasis on CT and MR imaging. Radiographics 20(2):321-32, 2000
5. Skellariou A et al: Tarsal coalition. Orthopedics 22(11):1066-73, discussion 1073-4 Review, 1999
6. Emery KH et al: Tarsal coalition: A blinded comparison of MRI and CT. Pediatr Radiol 28(8):612-6, 1998

TARSAL COALITION

IMAGE GALLERY

Typical

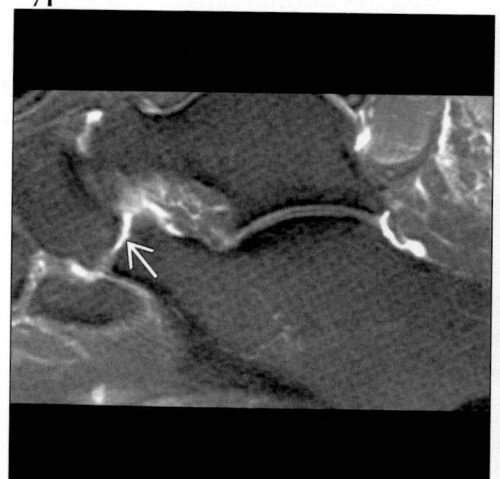

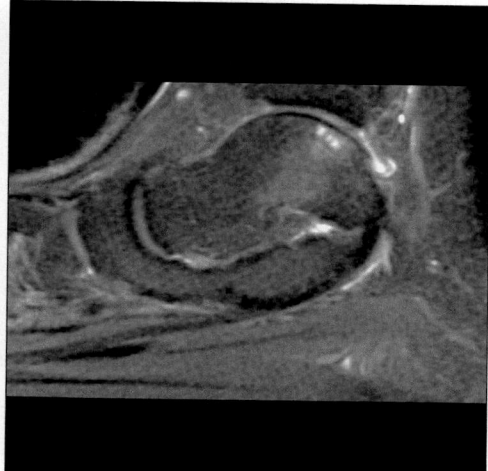

(Left) Sagittal FS PD FSE MR shows hyperintensity (arrow) in calcaneonavicular fibrocartilaginous coalition. *(Right)* Sagittal FS PD FSE MR shows solid extraarticular synostosis representing a calcaneonavicular bar.

Typical

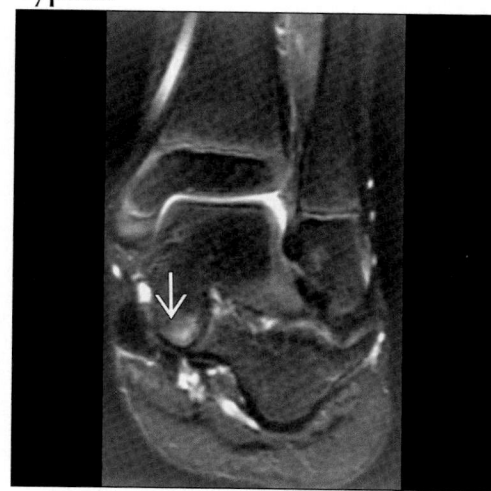

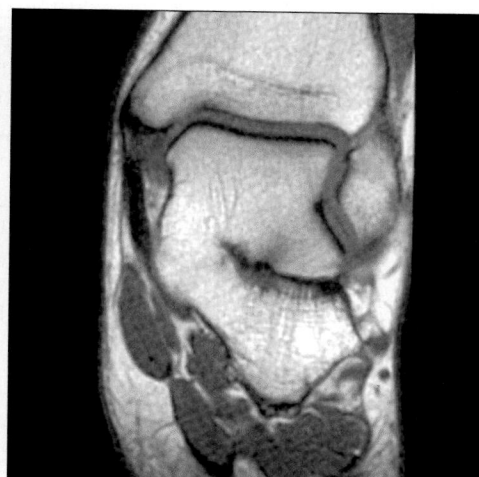

(Left) Coronal FS PD FSE MR shows symptomatic fibrocartilaginous talocalcaneal coalition with hyperintense subchondral bone marrow edema (arrow) on the talar side of the middle facet. *(Right)* Coronal T1WI MR shows complete intraarticular bridge representing a talocalcaneal synostosis. There is complete continuity of bone marrow across the sustentaculum tali.

Typical

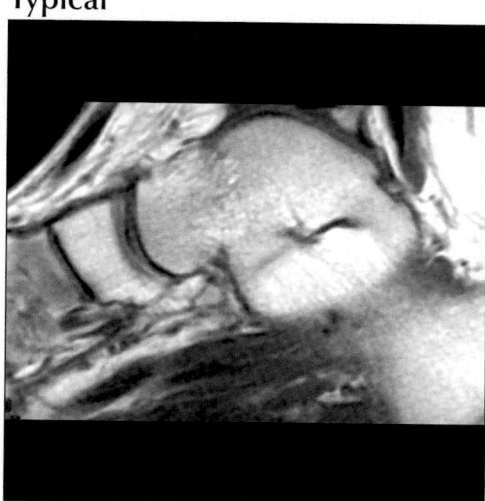

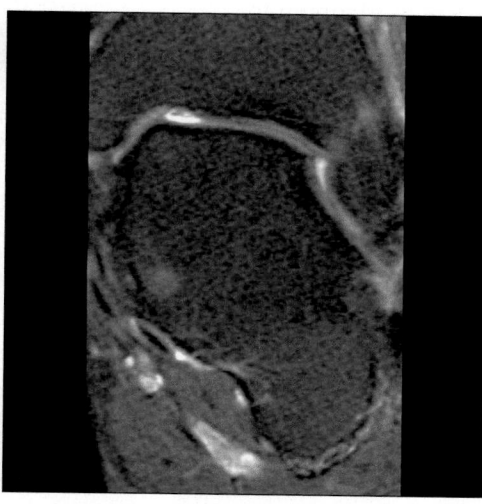

(Left) Sagittal T1WI MR shows solid talocalcaneal coalition involving both the middle and posterior facets of the subtalar joints with obliteration of the sinus tarsi. *(Right)* Coronal FS PD FSE MR shows complete synostosis of the talus and calcaneus in talocalcaneal coalition.

OS TRIGONUM SYNDROME

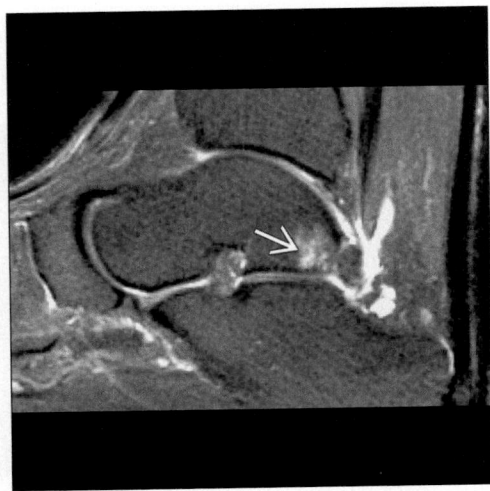

Sagittal graphic shows triangular shaped os trigonum at the level of the lateral tubercle of the posterior talar process. Surrounding edema is highlighted in yellow.

Sagittal FS PD FSE MR shows hyperintensity of the posterior talus (arrow) with fluid signal and synovitis surrounding the os trigonum.

TERMINOLOGY

Abbreviations and Synonyms
- Talar compression syndrome; posterior ankle impingement syndrome; posterior impingement syndrome

Definitions
- Pain with disruption of cartilaginous synchondrosis between os trigonum + lateral tubercle of posterior talar process

IMAGING FINDINGS

General Features
- Best diagnostic clue: Hyperintensity across synchondrosis on T2WI
- Location: Lateral tubercle of posterior talar process
- Size: Variable size from absence of os trigonum to grossly enlarged
- Morphology
  - Round
  - Oval
  - Triangular

Radiographic Findings
- Radiography
  - Smooth edges + dense cortical bone

  - Well-rounded osseous body
  - Prominent os trigonum or trigonal process
  - Irregular gap between talus and os trigonum on lateral view

MR Findings
- T1WI
  - Enlarged fat marrow containing os trigonum
  - Hypointense degenerative sclerosis/cystic change between os trigonum & talus
  - Hypointense sclerosis, edema in a trigonal process
  - Hypointense fluid, effacement of surrounding soft tissues
- T2WI
  - Os trigonum or trigonal process hyperintensity on PD T2 FSE or STIR
  - Hyperintensity in synchondrosis or posterior talus
  - Hyperintense edema/synovitis posterior to talus + superior to os trigonum
  - Hyperintense edema/synovitis posterior to os trigonum on sagittal images
  - Isolated hyperintense tenosynovitis flexor hallucis longus (FHL) tendon sheath (partial tethering FHL tendon)
  - Hyperintense degenerative cystic changes between os trigonum and talus
  - ± Intraarticular loose bodies

DDx: Os Trigonum Sydrome

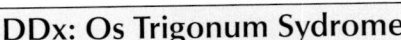

Shepherd's Fx	Impingement	FHL Tenosynovitis	Tibial Fx

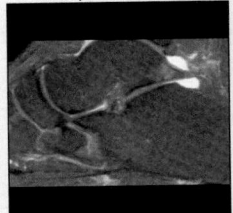 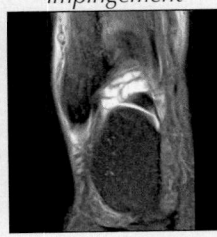 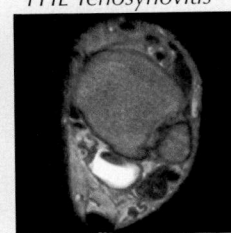 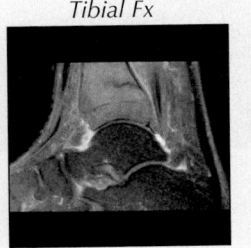

Sag FS PD MR	Cor FS PD MR	Ax T2WI MR	Sag FS PD MR

OS TRIGONUM SYNDROME

Key Facts

Imaging Findings

- Best diagnostic clue: Hyperintensity across synchondrosis on T2WI
- Location: Lateral tubercle of posterior talar process
- Size: Variable size from absence of os trigonum to grossly enlarged
- Os trigonum or trigonal process hyperintensity on PD T2 FSE or STIR

Top Differential Diagnoses

- Fracture of Lateral Tubercle (Shepherd's Fracture)
- Posterior Soft Tissue Impingement
- Flexor Hallucis Longus (FHL) Tenosynovitis

Pathology

- Repetitive microtrauma
- Forceful repetitive ankle joint plantar flexion

- Extreme ankle dorsiflexion = compression of ossicle between FHL + posterior talofibular ligament (PTFL)
- End-range plantar flexion = compression ossicle between calcaneus + tibia
- Enlarged os trigonum - not required

Clinical Issues

- Most common signs/symptoms: Posterior ankle pain
- Tenderness posterior ankle
- Soft tissue swelling posterior ankle
- Pain exaggerated by plantarflexion + weight-bearing activities
- Decreased subtalar range of motion

Diagnostic Checklist

- Identify signal changes across synchondrosis + os trigonum

Imaging Recommendations

- Best imaging tool: MR: Identifies marrow edema, synchondrosis and soft tissue changes
- Protocol advice
  - T1 sagittal, coronal + axial to evaluate marrow signal changes (sclerosis vs. edema)
  - FS PD FSE sagittal, coronal + axial for edema, fluid + synovitis
  - Sagittal plane required for accurate diagnosis

DIFFERENTIAL DIAGNOSIS

Fracture of Lateral Tubercle (Shepherd's Fracture)

- Irregular jagged separation between talar body and fragment
- Progressive widening/diastasis of fracture site

Posterior Soft Tissue Impingement

- Posterolateral side of ankle joint
- Posterior tibiofibular ligament
- Transverse tibiofibular ligament
- Tibial slip
- Impingement = fibrosis + capsulitis + synovial swelling

Flexor Hallucis Longus (FHL) Tenosynovitis

- Fluid in FHL tendon sheath
- Scar + fibrosis in chronic overuse injury

Dancer's Foot

- Subchondral sclerosis posterior facet + calcaneocuboid joint
- Secondary to vertical loading stress
- Pain posterior subtalar area or laterally

Flexor Hallucis Longus Checkrein Deformity

- Fixed tethering FHL at or proximal to flexor retinaculum
- Flexion contracture interphalangeal joint of hallux + claw hallux
- Posttraumatic adhesions with healing of distal tibial fracture

PATHOLOGY

General Features

- General path comments
  - Relevant anatomy = os trigonum
    - Triangular ossicle posterior to lateral tubercle of posterior talar process
    - Articulates with posterolateral process talus + superior aspect calcaneus
    - Ossicle united to posterior process by cartilaginous, fibrous or fibrocartilaginous tissue
    - Stieda's process = posterior extension lateral tubercle talus
- Etiology
  - Repetitive microtrauma
  - Forceful repetitive ankle joint plantar flexion
  - Ballet associated
  - Extreme ankle dorsiflexion = compression of ossicle between FHL + posterior talofibular ligament (PTFL)
  - End-range plantar flexion = compression ossicle between calcaneus + tibia
  - High-arched or supinated foot = traction force on posterolateral talar process by PTFL
  - Pronated foot = traction force on posterolateral talar process by posterior talocalcaneal ligament
  - Calcaneal eversion = impingement between superior surface calcaneus/ossicle + tibia
  - Plantarflexion + dorsiflexion = irritation of FHL at level of posterior talar process
- Epidemiology
  - 0.2% incidence of syndrome in ankle sprain population
  - Os trigonum common bilaterally (50%)
  - Bipartite morphology is rare
  - Os trigonum bone present in 10% of population

Gross Pathologic & Surgical Features

- FHL tendon sheath thickening
- Accessory bone = os trigonum
- Synchondrosis fissuring
- Arthritic process between talar projection + calcaneus
- Degenerative changes across synchondrosis
- Enlarged os trigonum - not required

OS TRIGONUM SYNDROME

Microscopic Features
- Chronic inflammation
- Synovial hyperplasia
- Tendinosis FHL
- Periostitis of FHL sulcus

Staging, Grading or Classification Criteria
- Anatomic variations posterolateral talus
  - Type I = normal tubercle
  - Type II = Steida's process/enlarged tubercle
  - Type III = accessory bone or os trigonum
  - Type IV = fused os trigonum via synchondrosis or syndesmosis with talus

CLINICAL ISSUES

Presentation
- Most common signs/symptoms: Posterior ankle pain
- Clinical profile
  - Tenderness posterior ankle
  - Soft tissue swelling posterior ankle
  - Pain exaggerated by plantarflexion + weight-bearing activities
  - Pain = deep and aching
  - Decreased subtalar range of motion
  - Peroneal spasm
  - ± Impingement FHL tendon
  - Ballet dancers: Seen with demipointe, full pointe, tendu, frappé, relevé, jump (weight bearing in plantar flexion)
  - Onset associated with chronic ankle sprain

Demographics
- Age
  - Fusion of os trigonum: 8 to 11 years
  - Ossification os trigonum: Second decade
  - Pain syndrome: 20 to 35 years
- Gender: > Female involvement in dancers

Natural History & Prognosis
- Symptoms frequently relieved with rest
- Recalcitrant pain
- Fracture
- FHL stenosing tenosynovitis

Treatment
- Conservative
  - Splinting
  - Antiinflammatory agents
  - Steroid injection
  - Non-weight bearing vs. weight bearing cast
- Surgical - for recalcitrant pain or fracture
  - Resection of os trigonum
  - Recontouring of prominences in superior calcaneus + posterolateral talus
  - Resection of hypertrophic or fibrotic tissue
  - Resection of hypertrophic or scarred FHL sheath
  - Arthroscopic technique available
- Complications
  - Arthritis
  - Impingement of soft tissue

DIAGNOSTIC CHECKLIST

Consider
- Identify signal changes across synchondrosis + os trigonum
- Evaluate fluid and morphology of adjacent FHL tendon + sheath
- Anatomic variations exist in lateral tubercle

SELECTED REFERENCES

1. Banks A et al: McGlamry's comprehensive textbook of foot and ankle surgery. Chronic ankle conditions. vol 1. Philadelphia PA, Lippincott Williams & Wilkins (35):1091-152, 2001
2. Bureau NJ et al: Posterior ankle impingement syndrome: MR imaging findings in seven patients. Radiology 215(2):497-503, 2000
3. Masciocchi C et al: Ankle impingement syndromes. Eur J Radiol 27 Suppl 1:S70-3, 1998
4. Wakeley CJ et al: The value of MR imaging in the diagnosis of the os trigonum syndrome. Skeletal Radiol 25(2):133-6, 1996
5. Karasick D et al: The os trigonum syndrome: Imaging features. AJR 166:125-9, 1996

OS TRIGONUM SYNDROME

IMAGE GALLERY

Typical

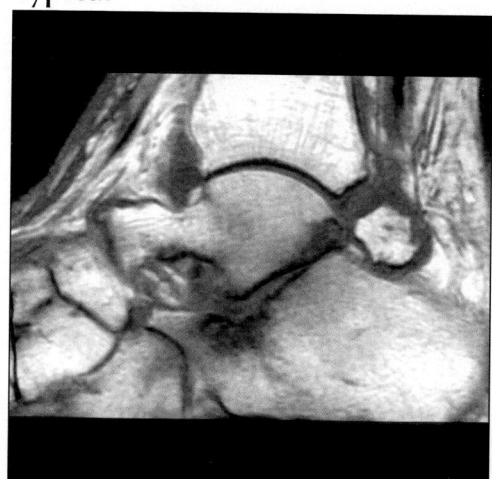
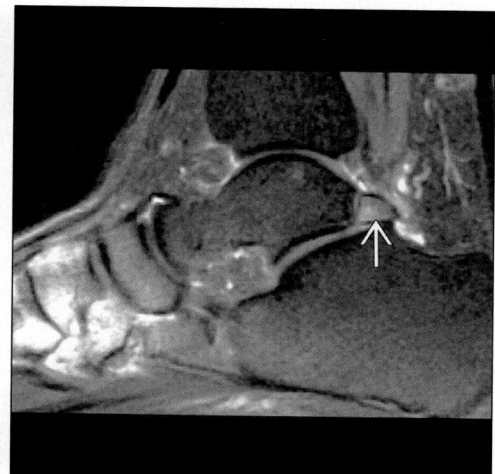

(Left) Sagittal T1WI MR shows enlarged os trigonum surrounded by hypointense fluid. *(Right)* Sagittal FS PD FSE MR shows os trigonum hyperintensity (arrow) with normal talar marrow signal.

Typical

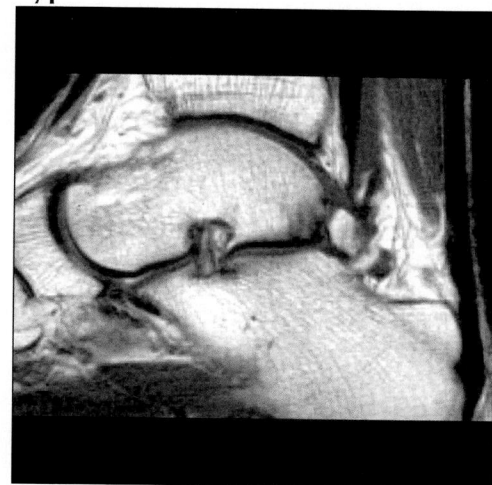
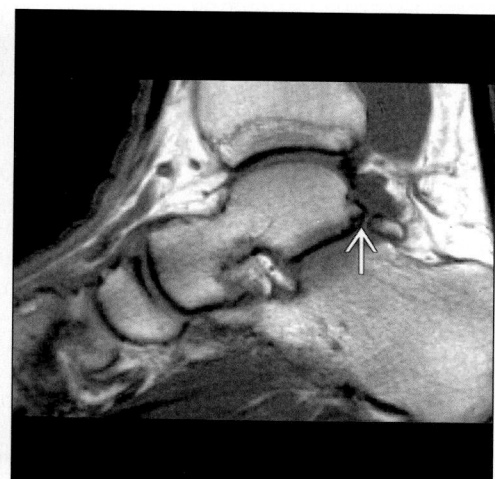

(Left) Sagittal T1WI MR shows os trigonum with hypointense degenerative changes on the talar side of the synchondrosis. *(Right)* Sagittal T1WI MR shows gross separation (arrow) of the os trigonum at the level of the synchondrosis.

Variant

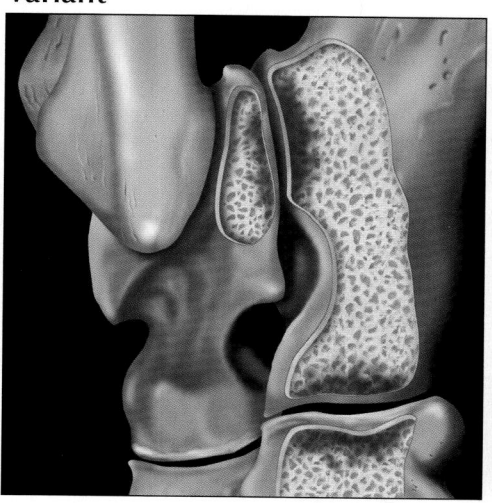
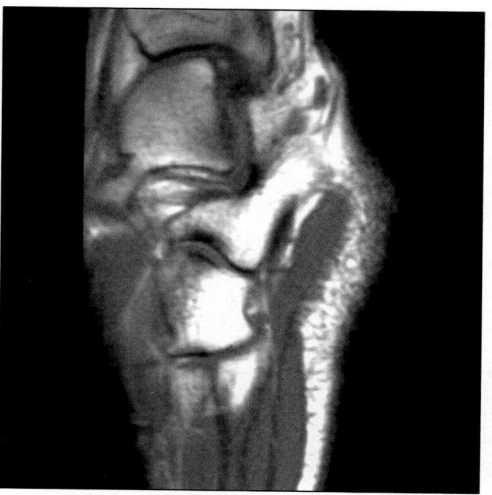

(Left) Sagittal graphic shows subchondral sclerosis across the posterior facet of the subtalar joint and calcaneocuboid articulation in the en-point position of a dancer. These changes may mimic os trigonum syndrome. *(Right)* Sagittal T1WI MR shows posterior subtalar and calcaneocuboid sclerosis in the weight bearing en-point position. Extreme plantar flexion can produce compression of the os trigonum between the calcaneus and the tibia.

ACCESSORY NAVICULAR

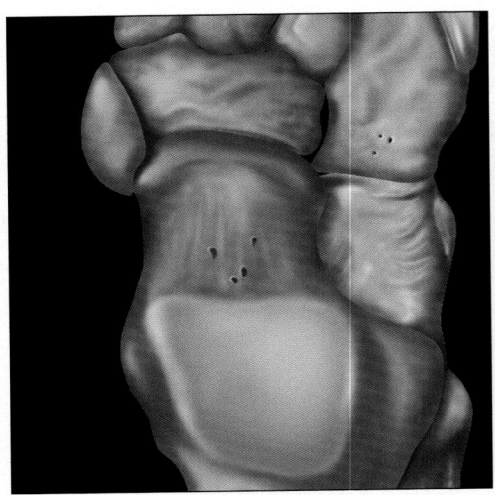

Axial graphic shows type II accessory navicular.

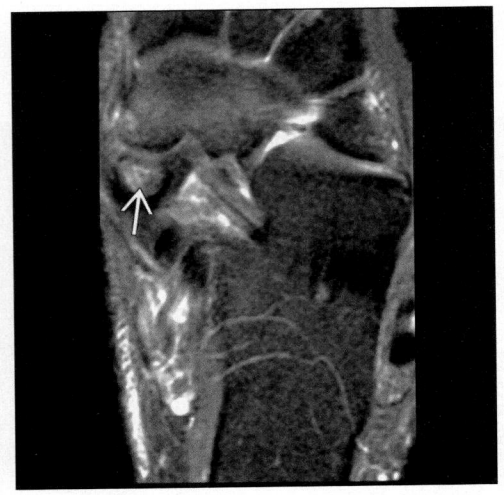

Axial FS PD FSE MR shows symptomatic accessory (arrow) tarsal navicular with bone marrow edema of the accessory navicular and tuberosity.

TERMINOLOGY

Abbreviations and Synonyms

- Os tibiale externum; navicular secundum; pre hallux; bifurcate navicular; accessory tarsal scaphoid; extrascaphoid + divided navicular

Definitions

- Congenital development of navicular tuberosity from a secondary center of ossification with synchondrosis to the navicular body

IMAGING FINDINGS

General Features

- Best diagnostic clue: Unattached accessory bone or synchondrosis within medial navicular
- Location
  - Medial navicular
  - Accessory bone/sesamoid of tibialis posterior (TP) tendon in plantar portion at level of inferior calcaneonavicular ligament
  - Tuberosity separated from medial part of navicular body
- Size
  - Type I accessory navicular = 4 to 6 mm ossicle
  - Type II with non-ossified zone of 1 to 3 mm

  - Type III cornuate or enlarged navicular tuberosity
- Morphology
  - Type I - true sesamoid within TP tendon
  - Type II - triangular or heart shaped
  - Type III - enlarged medial extension of navicular

Radiographic Findings

- Radiography
  - Type I = small ossicle proximal to navicular tuberosity on anteroposterior and lateral radiographs
  - Type II = extension of navicular radiographically + connection by a radiolucent zone, produces double density on lateral radiograph with proximal extension of navicular overlapping digital calcaneus
  - Type III = navicular extends medially proximal to talar head

MR Findings

- T1WI
  - Type I
    - Small (4 to 6 mm) usually marrow fat containing ossicle proximal to navicular tuberosity
    - Within hypointense to intermediate signal intensity distal tibialis posterior tendon
    - 5 to 7 mm separation from navicular
  - Type II

DDx: Accessory Navicular

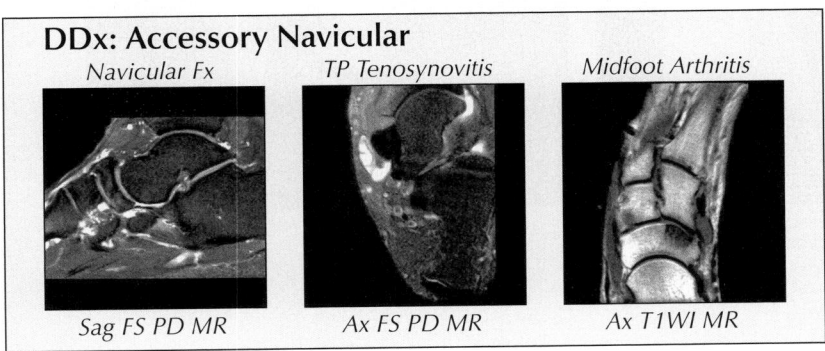

Navicular Fx	*TP Tenosynovitis*	*Midfoot Arthritis*
Sag FS PD MR	*Ax FS PD MR*	*Ax T1WI MR*

ACCESSORY NAVICULAR

Key Facts

Imaging Findings

- Best diagnostic clue: Unattached accessory bone or synchondrosis within medial navicular
- Accessory bone/sesamoid of tibialis posterior (TP) tendon in plantar portion at level of inferior calcaneonavicular ligament
- Marrow fat containing triangular or heart-shaped ossicle with direct connection to medial navicular through a synchondrosis
- Symptomatic = usually ± hyperintense marrow edema + degenerative hyperemia subchondral bone

Top Differential Diagnoses

- Navicular Tuberosity Fracture
- Tibialis Posterior (TP) Tendon Tear

Pathology

- Type I = small ossicle
- Type II = synchondrosis
- Type III = cornuate or enlarged medial tuberosity

Clinical Issues

- Most common signs/symptoms: Medial navicular pain
- Type I = symptoms of tibialis posterior tendinosis ± associated pes valgo planus
- Type II = navicular pain, shoe irritation
- Type III = complaint of shoe irritation + superficial pain

Diagnostic Checklist

- Evaluate status of tibialis posterior tendon

- Marrow fat containing triangular or heart-shaped ossicle with direct connection to medial navicular through a synchondrosis
- Non-ossified synchondrosis low to intermediate signal intensity
- Associated degenerative sclerosis ± subchondral cystic degeneration = hypointensity across synchondrosis
- Medial hypointense to intermediate signal intensity bursitis
- Distal thickening in tibialis posterior tendinosis
- Intermediate signal intensity in partial tear of tibialis posterior
  - Type III
    - Enlarged or cornuate marrow fat signal intensity extension of medial navicular proximally
    - No hypointense synchondrosis present
- T2WI
  - Type I
    - Suppressed fat signal in ossicle
    - Ossicle may be difficult to differentiate from surrounding hypointense tibialis posterior
  - Type II
    - Asymptomatic = normal fat suppressed marrow signal intensity
    - Symptomatic = usually ± hyperintense marrow edema + degenerative hyperemia subchondral bone
    - Hyperintense overlying bursitis
    - Hyperintense tibialis posterior tenosynovitis ± partial to complete tibialis posterior tendon tear
    - Hyperintensity may involve synchondrosis directly
    - Osseous edema may involve accessory navicular, accessory + navicular tuberosity or tuberosity alone
  - Type III
    - Normal marrow fat characteristics on T2 or fat suppressed PD or T2 or STIR
    - No synchondrosis present

Imaging Recommendations

- Best imaging tool: MR to visualize the signal intensity of marrow, bursitis and integrity of the synchondrosis
- Protocol advice: T1 and FS PD FSE or STIR direct axial images required

DIFFERENTIAL DIAGNOSIS

Navicular Tuberosity Fracture

- Navicular tuberosity = 24% of navicular fractures
- Avulsion injuries
- Usually non-displaced
- If abduction force involved ± osseous trauma to calcaneocuboid joint

Tibialis Posterior (TP) Tendon Tear

- Site of rupture within 6 cm of navicular insertion
- Spectrum of degeneration and longitudinal splitting
- Collapse of medial longitudinal arch

Midfoot Arthritis

- Sclerosis ± joint space narrowing between navicular + medial cuneiform

Köhler's Disease

- Fragmented ossification in skeletally immature patient
- Tarsal navicular fragmentation in previously documented normal navicular
- Pain at site of fragmentation

PATHOLOGY

General Features

- General path comments
  - Relevant anatomy = medial osseous prominences
    - Head of talus
    - Tuberosity of navicular
    - Accessory ossicles
    - Combination of above
- Etiology

ACCESSORY NAVICULAR

- Congenital navicular variations from a secondary center of ossification
- Type I
  - ± Tibialis posterior tendinosis
- Type II
  - Chronic stress
- Type III
  - Irritation of navicular prominence
- Epidemiology
  - 2 to 20% incidence of accessory ossicle
  - Os tibiale externum = 2nd most common accessory bone of foot (1st = os peroneum)
  - Type I = 30% of accessory naviculars
  - Type II & III = 70%

Gross Pathologic & Surgical Features

- Synchondrosis
  - Fibrous
  - Cartilaginous
  - Fibrocartilaginous
  - Partially osseous

Microscopic Features

- Inflammatory chondro-osseous changes
- Microfracture
- Cellular proliferation/repair

Staging, Grading or Classification Criteria

- Type I = small ossicle
- Type II = synchondrosis
- Type IIa = more superior placement of accessory bone (at risk for avulsion + tension force)
- Type IIb = more inferior placement of accessory bone (at risk for shearing forces)
- Type III = cornuate or enlarged medial tuberosity
- Combination prominence

CLINICAL ISSUES

Presentation

- Most common signs/symptoms: Medial navicular pain
- Clinical profile
  - Type I = symptoms of tibialis posterior tendinosis ± associated pes valgo planus
  - Type II = navicular pain, shoe irritation
  - Type III = complaint of shoe irritation + superficial pain

Demographics

- Age
  - Os tibiale externum ossifies age 9 to 11 years
  - Symptoms after 5 years of age
  - Symptoms most common during adolescence
- Gender: More frequent in females

Natural History & Prognosis

- Symptoms may occur or exacerbate post local trauma to foot and ankle
- Chronic irritation + bursa development over bony protuberance
- Degenerative change - progressive at synchondrosis
- ± Height loss medial longitudinal arch
- Intact range of motion of ankle, subtalar & transverse tarsal joints

Treatment

- Conservative
  - Type I, II & III = orthotic, shielding, shoe modifications
- Surgical
  - Kidner operation - to remove accessory navicular prominence & reinsertion of tibialis posterior
  - Type I - removal of ossicle from tibialis posterior tendon in symptomatic tibialis posterior tendinosis
  - Type II - resection entire non-ossified synchondrosis or bone graft + arthrodesis
  - Type III
    - Surgical remodeling
    - Reconstructive procedures for pes valgo planus
- Complications
  - Weakness tibialis posterior muscle post excision Type I, II or III navicular prominences

DIAGNOSTIC CHECKLIST

Consider

- Evaluate status of tibialis posterior tendon
- Need adequate fat suppression - T2WI in axial plane to appreciate hyperintense edema
- Identify associated bursa of soft tissue inflammatory changes

SELECTED REFERENCES

1. Banks A et al: McGlamry's comprehensive textbook of foot and ankle surgery. Common Pedal Prominences. vol 1. Philadelphia PA, Lippincott Williams & Wilkins, (11):419-40, 2001
2. Demeyere N et al: Quiz case. Symptomatic type II accessory navicular. Eur J Radiol 37(1):60-3, 2001
3. Kiter E et al: Tibialis posterior tendon abnormalities in feet with accessory navicular bone and flatfoot. Acta Orthop Scand 70(6):618-21, 1999
4. Steinbach LS: Painful syndromes around the ankle and foot: Magnetic resonance imaging evaluation. Top Magn Reson Imaging 9(5):311-26, 1998
5. Bencardino J et al: Os sustentaculi: Depiction on MR images. Skeletal Radiol 26(8):505-6, 1997
6. Miller TT: The symptomatic accessory tarsal navicular bone: Assessment with MR imaging. Radiology 195(3):949-53, 1995

ACCESSORY NAVICULAR

IMAGE GALLERY

Typical

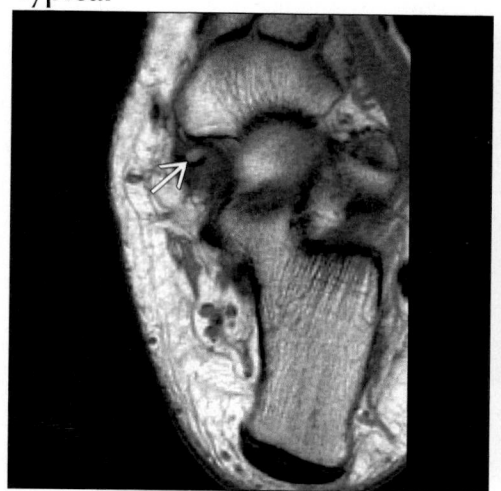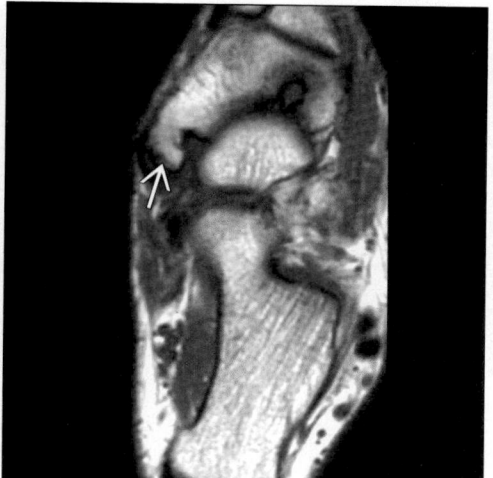

(Left) Axial T1WI MR shows type I (arrow) accessory navicular as a true sesamoid. *(Right)* Axial T1WI MR shows type III accessory navicular with enlarged medial extension (arrow) of the tuberosity (cornuate navicular).

Typical

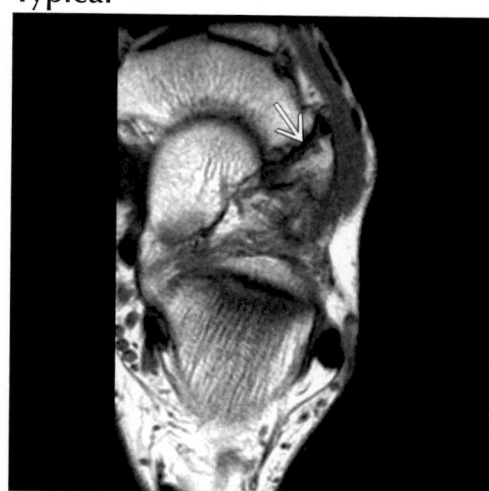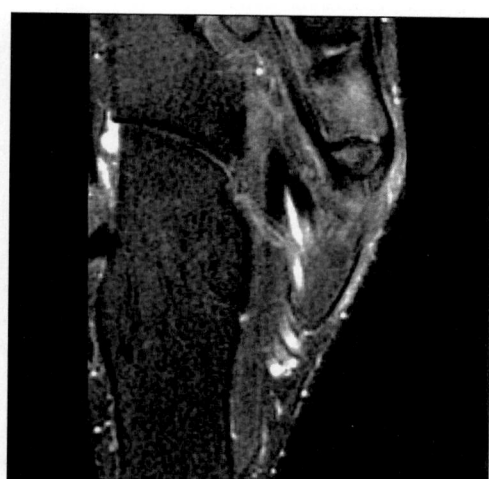

(Left) Axial T1WI MR shows degenerative changes (arrow) with sclerosis and erosions with the type II triangular navicular. The non ossified zone is 1-3 mm in thickness. *(Right)* Axial FS PD FSE MR shows hyperintense bone marrow edema of a type II accessory navicular on both sides of the non ossified synchondrosis.

Typical

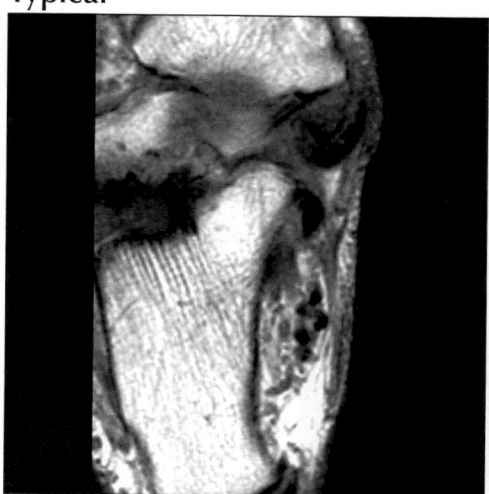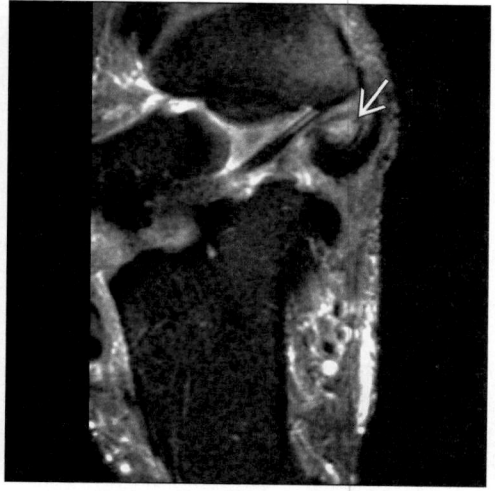

(Left) Axial T1WI MR shows sclerotic hypointense marrow in a type II accessory navicular. *(Right)* Axial FS PD FSE MR shows intermediate to hyperintense signal in the synchondrosis of the type II accessory navicular (arrow). Bone marrow edema is present in both the navicular and accessory navicular.

6

113

SESAMOID DYSFUNCTION

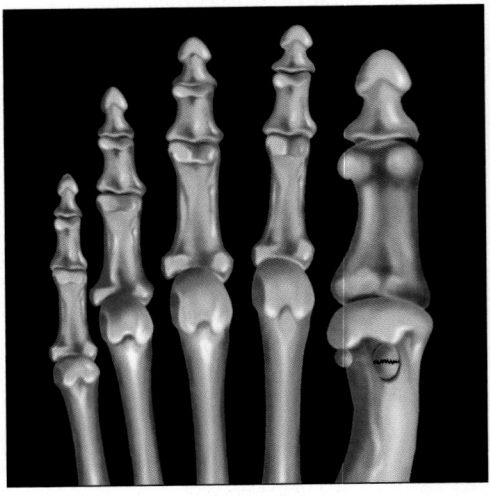

Axial graphic shows medial tibial sesamoid fracture.

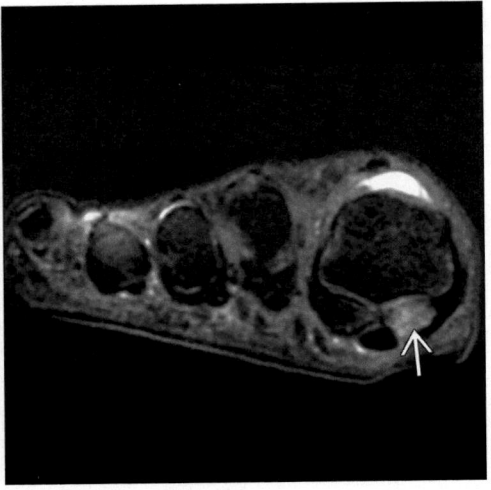

Coronal FS PD FSE MR shows hyperintense medial tibial sesamoid edema (arrow) secondary to fracture.

TERMINOLOGY

Abbreviations and Synonyms
- Sesamoid disorders

Definitions
- Bipartite sesamoids; fractures, turf toe, osteochondritis + avascular necrosis; sesamoiditis, arthritis

IMAGING FINDINGS

General Features
- Best diagnostic clue: Altered signal intensity or morphology of sesamoids
- Location: Within double tendon of flexor hallucis brevis, the two plantar sesamoids articulate with the 1st metatarsal head
- Size: Medial sesamoid slightly > lateral sesamoid
- Morphology: Ovoid morphology separated by intersesamoidal ridge or crista to articulate with concave facets of first metatarsal head

Radiographic Findings
- Radiography
  - Anteroposterior to show limited (obscured by metatarsal head) view of medial (tibial) and lateral (fibular) sesamoids
  - Lateral view - overlap of sesamoids

- Oblique view for fibular sesamoid
- Axial view for both sesamoids

MR Findings
- T1WI
  - Bipartite sesamoids
    - More frequent involvement of medial sesamoid
    - Identical vs. asymmetric division with marrow fat signal intensity
    - Lateral sesamoid rarely separated into > than 2 fragments
    - Smooth margins (rounded edges)
  - Fracture
    - Sharp or discrete linear hypointense line
    - Replacement of marrow fat with hypointense edema
    - Hypointense adjacent capsular/soft tissue edema
  - Turf toe
    - Disruption plantar joint capsule = discontinuity
    - Disruption plantar plate = hypointense to intermediate signal of fluid in sesamoid attachment to base of proximal phalanx
  - Osteochondritis and avascular necrosis
    - Fragmentation of involved sesamoid
    - Hypointense signal
    - Greater involvement of lateral sesamoid
  - Sesamoiditis
    - Hypointense effusion 1st metatarsophalangeal (MTP) joint

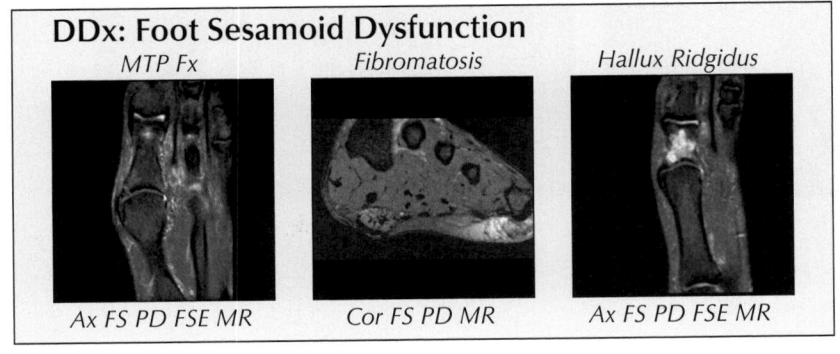

DDx: Foot Sesamoid Dysfunction

MTP Fx	Fibromatosis	Hallux Ridgidus
Ax FS PD FSE MR	*Cor FS PD MR*	*Ax FS PD FSE MR*

SESAMOID DYSFUNCTION

Key Facts

Terminology
- Sesamoid disorders

Imaging Findings
- Best diagnostic clue: Altered signal intensity or morphology of sesamoids
- Morphology: Ovoid morphology separated by intersesamoidal ridge or crista to articulate with concave facets of first metatarsal head

Top Differential Diagnoses
- Stress Fracture
- Synovitis

Pathology
- Irregular ossification in medial bipartite sesamoid
- Sudden loading or repetitive stress

Clinical Issues
- Most common signs/symptoms: Pain over plantar aspect sesamoids
- Fracture = nonspecific swelling first MTP joint + discomfort on passive range of motion
- Osteochondritis = tenderness on palpation
- Turf toe = pain with dorsiflexion + weight bearing
- Sesamoiditis = pain weight bearing + athletic activity (e.g. running) + localized tenderness + MTP swelling
- Osteoarthritis - in association with hallux valgus + rigidus

Diagnostic Checklist
- Distinguish between fracture line vs. normal bipartite morphology

---

- Mild subchondral sclerosis (hypointense) between 1st metatarsal facets + dorsal articular surface sesamoids
  - Arthritis
    - Marrow fat signal maintained
    - Subchondral hypointense sclerosis at articulation with 1st metatarsal head
    - Osteophytic spurring
    - MTP joint hypointense joint fluid
- T2WI
  - Bipartite sesamoids
    - No increase in signal intensity on T2 or fat suppressed T2WI
    - Normal surrounding soft tissue + capsular structures
  - Fracture
    - Hyperintense linear transverse fracture ± displacement of fragment
    - Serrated + irregular edges
    - Variable subchondral hyperintense edema in one or both fragments
  - Turf toe
    - ± Plantar subchondral hyperintense edema 1st metatarsal head
    - Hyperintense edema/fluid associated with capsular + plantar plate injury
    - ± Discontinuity in intersesamoid ligament associated with sesamoid displacement/dislocation
  - Osteochondritis and avascular necrosis
    - Chronic phase with hypointensity
    - Acute/subacute with variable increased signal intensity
  - Sesamoiditis
    - Hyperintense effusion + synovitis 1st MTP joint
    - Dorsal sesamoid chondral degeneration with narrowing relative to metatarsal concave articular facets
  - Arthritis
    - Osteophytes maintain marrow fat signal intensity
    - ± Hyperintense 1st metatarsophalangeal joint effusion
    - Sclerosis hypointense

Imaging Recommendations
- Best imaging tool: MR for detection of sesamoid marrow edema + identification of capsular structures
- Protocol advice
  - Coronal, axial & sagittal T1 + FS PD FSE or STIR
  - Coronal plane to visualize both sesamoids + flexor hallucis longus in one image

DIFFERENTIAL DIAGNOSIS

Stress Fracture
- Distal third metatarsal except dancers (proximal third)
- Bone callus
- Subchondral marrow edema

Synovitis
- Hyperintense fluid (T2WI)
- Intermediate signal synovium (T2WI)
- Capsular distention

Metatarsal Fracture
- Proximal fracture base 1st metatarsal

Plantar Fibromatosis
- Inhomogeneous mass medial plantar fascia

Morton's Neuroma
- Localized enlargement interdigital nerve
- Between third + fourth metatarsal heads
- Lateral branch medial plantar nerve to third interspace

Hallux Limitus & Hallus Rigidus
- Painful, acquired, arthritis first MTP joint
- Inadequate sagittal mobility
- Limitus = precursor to rigidus
- Rigidus = ankylosis of sesamoids to plantar surface 1st metatarsal

PATHOLOGY

General Features
- General path comments

SESAMOID DYSFUNCTION

- ○ Relevant anatomy
    - Sesamoid + collateral ligaments = stabilize 1st MTP joint
    - Dorsal surface of sesamoids = cartilaginous to articulate with first metatarsal head
- Etiology
    - ○ Bipartite sesamoids
        - Irregular ossification in medial bipartite sesamoid
    - ○ Fracture
        - Sudden loading or repetitive stress
        - Increase weight bearing function medial
        - Dorsiflexion or hyperflexion
    - ○ Turf toe
        - Extreme dorsiflexion + valgus/varus strain MTP joint in turf toe injuries
        - Associated with artificial sports surfaces
    - ○ Sesamoiditis
        - Associated with trauma
        - Sesamoid chondromalacia is sesamoiditis
    - ○ Arthritis: ± Progression sesamoiditis, chondromalacia or trauma
- Distribution
    - ○ 90% bipartite sesamoids = bilateral
    - ○ Up to 90% bipartite sesamoids = tibial or medial
    - ○ Tibial sesamoid divided into two or three fragments

Gross Pathologic & Surgical Features
- Bipartite sesamoids
    - ○ Asymmetrical division bipartite sesamoid
    - ○ Medial sesamoid
    - ○ Metatarsophalangeal joint swelling
- Fracture
    - ○ Transverse cleft ± displacement
    - ○ Irregular fracture interface
- Turf toe
    - ○ Ruptured sesamoid complex
    - ○ ± Proximal vs. distal migration
    - ○ ± Sesamoid fracture
- Osteochondritis and avascular necrosis
    - ○ Fragmentation
    - ○ Stress fracture
- Sesamoiditis
    - ○ MTP joint swelling
    - ○ Inflammation plantar sesamoid complex
- Arthritis
    - ○ Erosion articular cartilage
    - ○ Osteophytes

Microscopic Features
- Bipartite sesamoids = articular cartilage between fragments
- Osteochondritis - stress fracture + healing = fragmentation

CLINICAL ISSUES

Presentation
- Most common signs/symptoms: Pain over plantar aspect sesamoids
- Clinical profile
    - ○ Fracture = nonspecific swelling first MTP joint + discomfort on passive range of motion
    - ○ Osteochondritis = tenderness on palpation

- ○ Turf toe = pain with dorsiflexion + weight bearing
- ○ Sesamoiditis = pain weight bearing + athletic activity (e.g. running) + localized tenderness + MTP swelling
- ○ Arthritis = warmth + swelling + restricted range of motion + pain to palpation
- ○ Osteoarthritis - in association with hallux valgus + rigidus

Demographics
- Age
    - ○ Ossification hallucal sesamoids - 7 to 10 years
    - ○ Sesamoiditis - young athletes
- Gender: Ossification sesamoids in females earlier

Natural History & Prognosis
- Fracture = bony consolidation vs fibrous union
- Osteochondritis = fragmentation
- Sesamoiditis = reduce weight bearing
- Turf toe = improved recurrent with sprains vs. continued pain with rupture of sesamoid complex

Treatment
- Conservative
    - ○ Fracture: Below knee walking cast
    - ○ Osteochondritis = avascular necrosis: Shoe insert/pad + nonsteroidal anti-inflammatory medication
    - ○ Turf toe: Below knee cast
    - ○ Sesamoiditis: Activity modification + reduced weight bearing
    - ○ Arthritis: Orthotic, stiff insole + padding + nonsteroidal anti-inflammatory medications
- Surgical: Excision - for failed conservative treatment + chronically painful sesamoid

DIAGNOSTIC CHECKLIST

Consider
- Identify sesamoid edema on FS PD FSE or STIR
- Distinguish between fracture line vs. normal bipartite morphology

SELECTED REFERENCES

1. DeLee JC et al: Orthopaedic sports medicine. Principles and practice. Ligament injuries of the foot and ankle in the athlete. Foot and ankle, conditions of the forefoot. Sesamoid dysfunction. vol 2. 2nd ed. Philadelphia PA, Saunders 2510-20, 2003
2. Ashman CJ et al: Forefoot pain involving the metatarsal region: Differential diagnosis with MR imaging. Radiographics 21(6):1425-40, Review, 2001
3. Karasick D et al: Disorders of the hallux sesamoid complex: MR features. Skeletal Radiol 27:411-8, 1998

SESAMOID DYSFUNCTION

IMAGE GALLERY

Typical

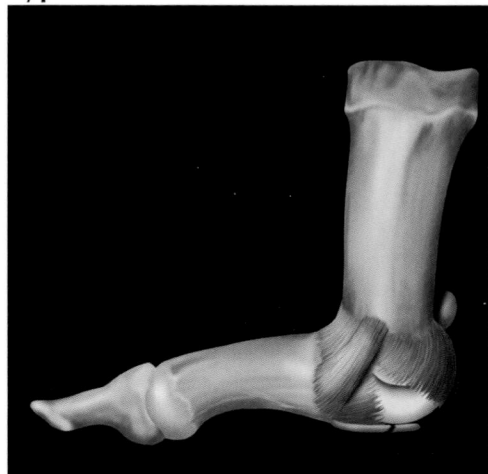
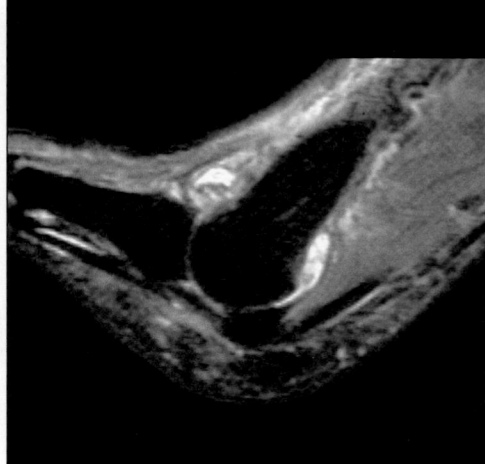

(Left) Sagittal graphic shows disruption of the MTP joint capsule. *(Right)* Sagittal FS PD FSE MR shows hyperintense joint effusion associated with capsular sprain in turf toe.

Typical

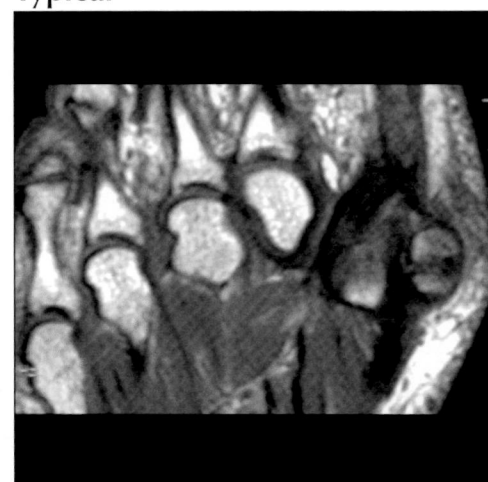
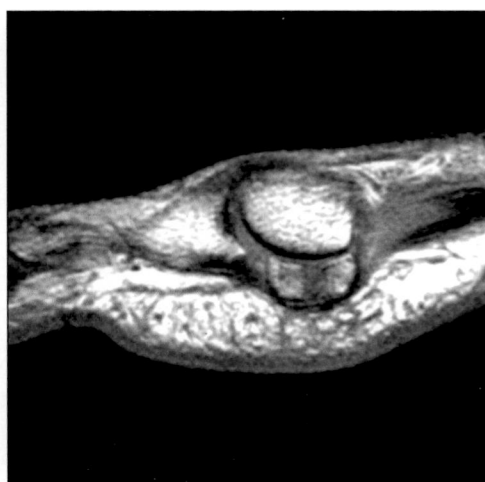

(Left) Axial T1WI MR shows bipartite medial tibial sesamoid. The normal medial sesamoid is larger than the lateral sesamoid. *(Right)* Sagittal T1WI MR shows normal marrow fat signal in a bipartite medial tibial sesamoid.

Typical

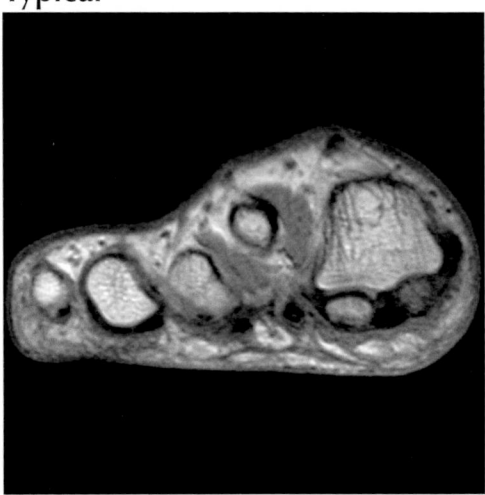
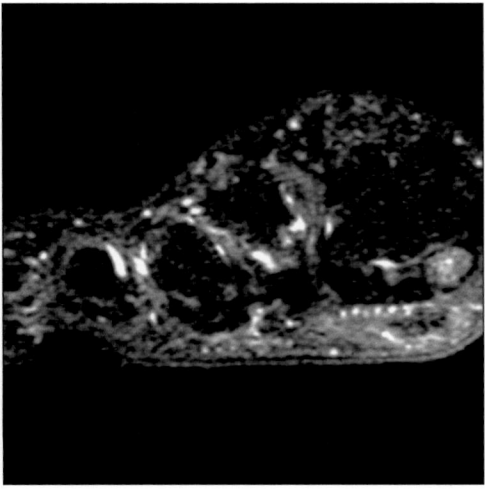

(Left) Coronal T1WI MR shows hypointense marrow edema in the acute phase of osteochondritis of the medial tibial sesamoid. *(Right)* Coronal FS PD FSE MR shows bone marrow edema in osteochondritis of the sesamoid.

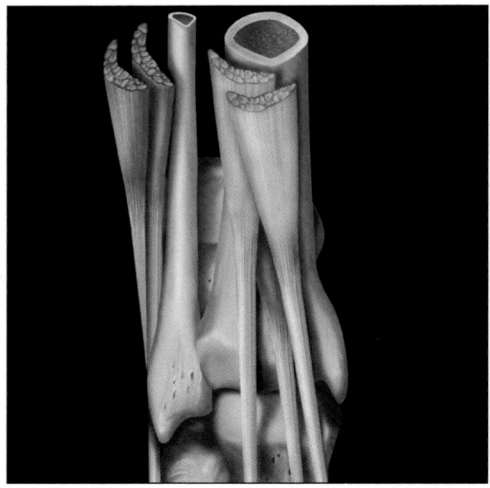

Coronal graphic shows anterior compartment muscle edema.

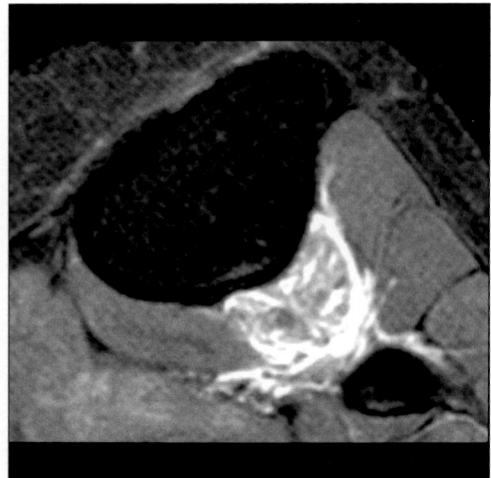

Axial FS PD FSE MR shows edema of the tibialis posterior muscle in deep posterior compartment syndrome.

TERMINOLOGY

Abbreviations and Synonyms
- Acute compartment syndrome; chronic (exertional) compartment syndrome

Definitions
- Circulation + function of tissue within anatomically confined space/fibro-osseous compartment are damaged by elevated pressure

IMAGING FINDINGS

General Features
- Best diagnostic clue: Diffuse hyperintensity on T2WI (FS PD FSE or STIR) within affected compartment muscle or muscles
- Location
  - Anterior, lateral, superficial + deep posterior compartments of the leg (tibialis posterior may be classified as its own compartment)
  - Medial, central, lateral + interosseous + calcaneal compartments of the foot
- Size
  - Variable as a function of affected muscle group or groups within a compartment
  - Combined foot + leg compartment syndromes may occur
- Morphology: Diffuse along affected muscle group/compartment of leg and/or foot

MR Findings
- T1WI
  - Intermediate signal intensity within edematous muscle
  - Loss of normal muscle striations
  - ± Increased signal in subacute hemorrhage
  - Hypointense hemosiderin foci
  - Enlargement of affected muscle group ± peripheral convex bowing
  - Hypointense calcification in chronic compartment syndrome
  - Hyperintense fat in muscle atrophy/chronic compartment syndrome
  - Chronic fibrous replacement = hypointensity
  - Calcific myonecrosis - intermediate signal liquefied necrotic muscle & hypointense calcific shell
  - T1 ± normal in exertional compartment syndrome
- T2WI
  - Hyperintense diffusely within cross sectional anatomic boundaries of affected muscle + proximal/distal extension on T2WI
  - Hyperintense fluid/hemorrhage/edema also between muscles in fascial planes

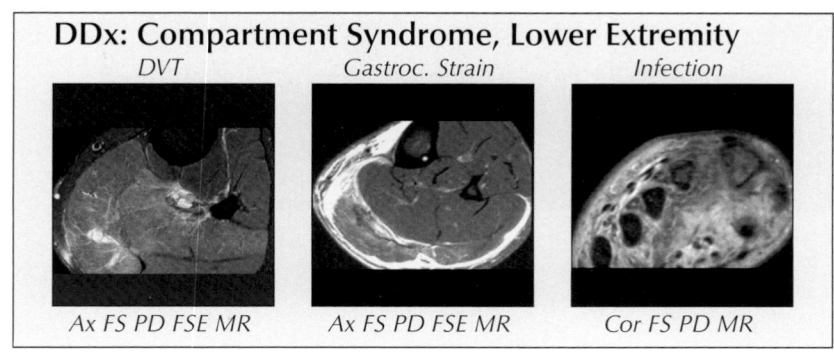

DDx: Compartment Syndrome, Lower Extremity
DVT	Gastroc. Strain	Infection
Ax FS PD FSE MR	Ax FS PD FSE MR	Cor FS PD MR

6

118

COMPARTMENT SYNDROME, LOWER EXTREMITY

Key Facts

Imaging Findings
- Best diagnostic clue: Diffuse hyperintensity on T2WI (FS PD FSE or STIR) within affected compartment muscle or muscles
- Hyperintense diffusely within cross sectional anatomic boundaries of affected muscle + proximal/distal extension on T2WI

Top Differential Diagnoses
- Deep Vein Thrombosis (DVT)
- Gastrocnemius - Soleus Muscle Strain
- Cellulitis
- Tumors

Pathology
- Arteriovenous gradient theory
- Ischemia - reperfusion theory

- Muscle hernias in 40% of chronic compartment syndrome
- Acute compartment syndrome in leg usually related to tibial fractures

Clinical Issues
- Most common signs/symptoms: Disproportionate pain relative to injury
- Palpable swelling (± tense skin), pain, pallor, paralysis + paresthesias
- Acute = fasciotomy/open procedure

Diagnostic Checklist
- Use axial images to identify diffuse muscle edema + compartmental bulging

---

- ○ Hyperintensity associated with both edema + rhabdomyolysis
- ○ Atrophied muscle suppresses without associated hyperintensity
- ○ ± Subcutaneous tissue hyperintense edema
- ○ Intermediate to increased signal of muscle in exertional compartment syndrome (FS PD FSE or STIR)
- ○ Calcification + fibrosis remain hypointense
- • ± Associated muscle herniation on T1WI + T2WI

Imaging Recommendations
- Best imaging tool
  - ○ MR superior to bone scan, radiography and CT
  - ○ Edema, fibrosis + fatty infiltration contrast best visualized on MR
  - ○ Conventional radiography and CT limited to ruling out associated injuries
- Protocol advice
  - ○ T1 + FS PD FSE or STIR axial, coronal, + sagittal images
  - ○ Axial plane required for cross-sectional muscle compartment + neurovascular relationship

DIFFERENTIAL DIAGNOSIS

Deep Vein Thrombosis (DVT)
- Neurovascular bundle perivascular edema
- Edema in watershed distribution ± medial head gastrocnemius + soleus
- ± Enlarged popliteal vein with thrombus occlusion ± collateral venous structures

Gastrocnemius - Soleus Muscle Strain
- Grade 1 to 2 muscle/muscle tendon unit partial tear
- Feathery/diffuse edema hyperintense on FS PD FSE or STIR
- Partial intermuscular septum disruption
- ± Plantaris muscle myotendinous rupture between medial head gastrocnemius + soleus

Cellulitis
- Reticular to circumscribed subcutaneous (superficial + deep) edema
- No muscle compartment involvement or fascial extension

Tumors
- Intramuscular lipoma or hemangioma

Myositis Ossificans
- Localized soft tissue ossifications (circumscripta)
- Damage to interstitium not muscle directly
- Proximal involvement > distal
- Soft tissue mass + periosteal reaction to peripheral calcification to circumscribed pattern of bone
- ± Periosteal enhancement or edema

PATHOLOGY

General Features
- General path comments
  - ○ Relevant anatomy
    - Anterior compartment (leg) muscles = tibialis anterior, extensor hallucis longus, extensor digitorum longus + peroneus tertius
    - Anterior compartment neurovascular bundle = deep peroneal nerve + anterior tibial artery
    - Posterior compartment divided by deep transverse fascia into superficial and deep sections
    - Superficial posterior compartment muscles = gastrocnemius, plantaris + soleus
    - Deep posterior compartment muscles = popliteus, flexor digitorum longus, flexor hallucis longus + tibialis posterior
    - Neurovascular supply posterior compartment = tibial nerve + posterior tibial artery
    - Anterolateral compartment muscles = peroneus longus + peroneus brevis
    - Neurovascular supply anterolateral compartment = superficial peroneal nerve + branches peroneal artery
- Etiology

COMPARTMENT SYNDROME, LOWER EXTREMITY

- ○ Arteriovenous gradient theory
  - Compromised blood flow - arterial, capillary or venous
  - Reduced blood flow: Hypotension, increased vascular resistance (shock or arterial spasm), increased tissue pressure (extravasated blood)
- ○ Ischemia - reperfusion theory
  - Compromised blood flow
  - Ischemia
  - Impaired cellular metabolism
  - Interstitial edema
  - Increased compartmental pressure
- ○ Reperfusion: Restore cellular activity vs. worsen preexisting cellular damage
- ○ Fractures leading to compartment syndrome
  - Proximal + middle thirds tibia
  - Open tibial fractures
- ○ Acute compartment pressure elevation
  - Fractures (tibia)
  - Muscle rupture
  - Crush injuries
  - Burns
- ○ Chronic: Exercise induced chronic compartment syndrome
- ○ Foot compartment syndrome: Calcaneal fractures
- Epidemiology
  - ○ Open tibial fractures = 20% complicated by compartment syndrome
  - ○ Muscle hernias in 40% of chronic compartment syndrome
  - ○ 5% calcaneal fractures develop compartment syndrome of the foot
  - ○ Acute compartment syndrome in leg usually related to tibial fractures
  - ○ Bivalving a cast = 85% reduction in intracompartmental pressure

Gross Pathologic & Surgical Features
- Fracture ± open
- Hemorrhage
- Inflammation
- Decreased compartment size (pressure dressings)
- Venous obstruction

Microscopic Features
- Tissue - cellular damage (muscle + nerve ischemia)
- Neutrophils + leukocytes with reestablished flow
- Interstitial edema
- Local vasodilation

Staging, Grading or Classification Criteria
- Acute
  - ○ Resting intracompartment pressures > 30 mm Hg (Wick catheter measurement)
- Chronic
  - ○ Resting intramuscular pressure > 10 mm Hg
  - ○ Elevated tissue pressure of 15 mm Hg at 15 minutes post exercise

CLINICAL ISSUES

Presentation
- Most common signs/symptoms: Disproportionate pain relative to injury
- Clinical profile
  - ○ Palpable swelling (± tense skin), pain, pallor, paralysis + paresthesias
  - ○ Distal pedal pulses usually intact
  - ○ Crush injuries to the foot: Massive swelling + fractures or dislocations
  - ○ Chronic - exercise related, anterior or deep posterior compartment
  - ○ Acute compartment syndrome uncommon in athletic population
  - ○ Chronic compartment syndrome - in runners

Demographics
- Age: Nonspecific
- Gender: No gender bias

Natural History & Prognosis
- Nerve + muscle ischemia > 12 hours = permanent injury
- Muscle necrosis
- Volkmann's contracture (fibrous contracture + neurologic damage)
- Complication: Reperfusion injury

Treatment
- Conservative: Not an option
- Surgical
  - ○ Acute = fasciotomy/open procedure
  - ○ Chronic = surgical decompression - fasciotomy
  - ○ Techniques for fasciotomies: Fibulectomy, perifibular fasciotomy or double-incision fasciotomy

DIAGNOSTIC CHECKLIST

Consider
- Use axial images to identify diffuse muscle edema + compartmental bulging
- T2WI (FS PD FSE or STIR) visualizes fluid in fascial boundaries
- T1 + T2WI to identify loss of normal muscle striations
- T1WI characterizes the associated atrophy and fibrosis in chronic compartment syndrome

SELECTED REFERENCES

1. DeLee JC et al: Orthopaedic sports medicine. Principles and practice. Ligament injuries of the foot and ankle in the athlete. The Leg. vol 2. 2nd ed. Philadelphia PA, Saunders, (29):2155-82, 2003
2. Lauder TD et al: Exertional compartment syndrome and the role of magnetic resonance imaging. Am J Phys Med Rehabil 81(4):315-9, 2002
3. Brown RR et al: MR imaging of exercise-induced lower leg pain. Magn Reson Imaging Clin N Am 9(3):533-52, 2001
4. Matsen F et al: Diagnosis and management of compartment syndromes. J Bone Joint Surg Am 62:286-291, 1980

COMPARTMENT SYNDROME, LOWER EXTREMITY

IMAGE GALLERY

Typical

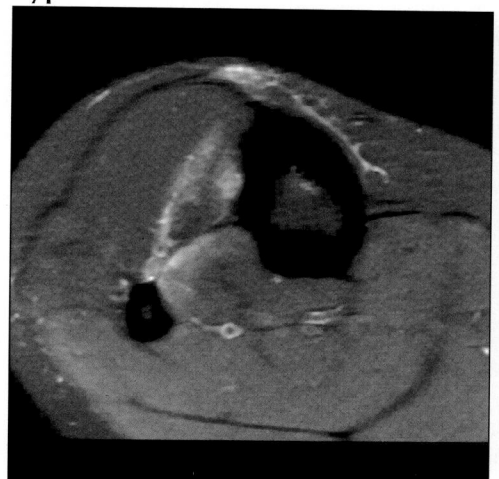

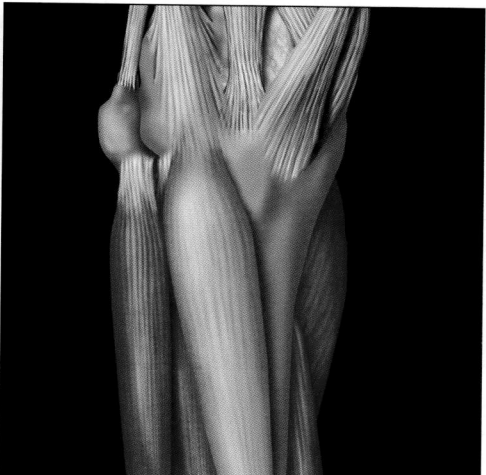

(Left) Axial FS PD FSE MR shows hyperintense edema of the posterior fibers of the tibialis anterior muscle. *(Right)* Coronal graphic shows edema of the tibialis anterior in the anterior compartment.

Typical

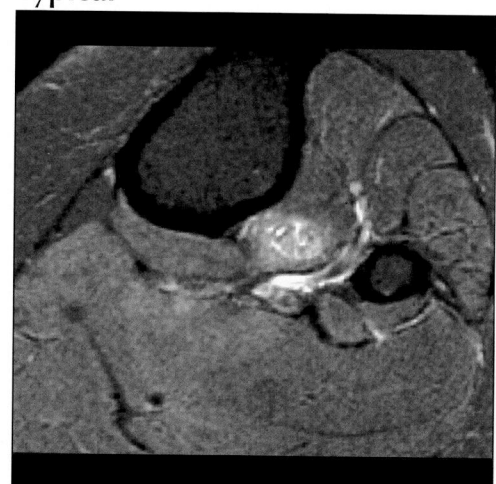

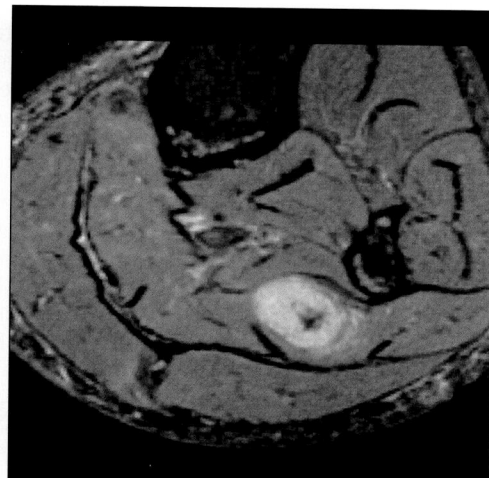

(Left) Axial FS PD FSE MR shows compartment syndrome with hyperintense edema of the tibialis posterior muscle. *(Right)* Axial FS PD FSE MR shows intramuscular hemangioma with central hemosiderin focus and reactive muscle edema of the soleus.

Typical

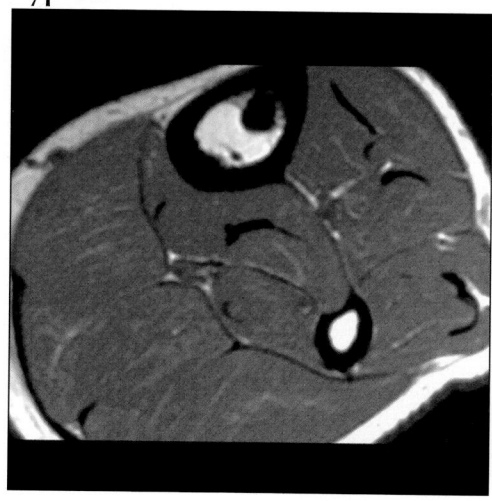

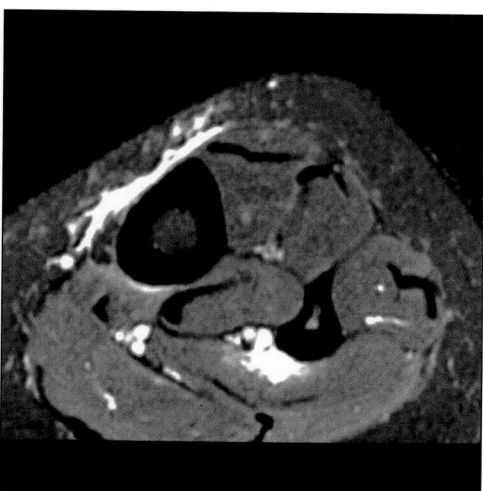

(Left) Axial T1WI MR shows lateral herniation of the crural fascia with associated peroneus brevis and longus muscles. *(Right)* Axial FS PD FSE MR shows hyperintense hemangioma between the posterior fibula and soleus muscle group in a runner presenting with compartment syndrome. Anteromedial periosteal edema in medial tibial stress syndrome is also shown.

GASTROCNEMIUS SOLEUS STRAIN

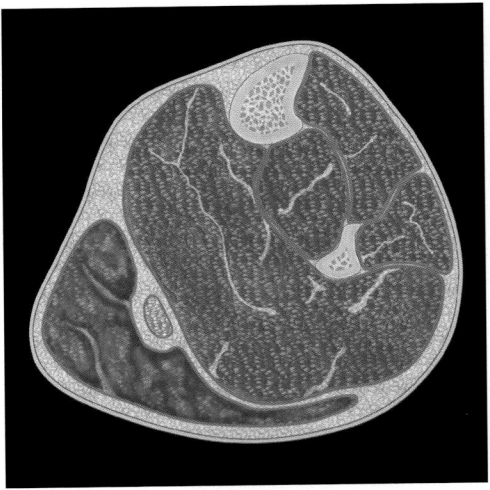 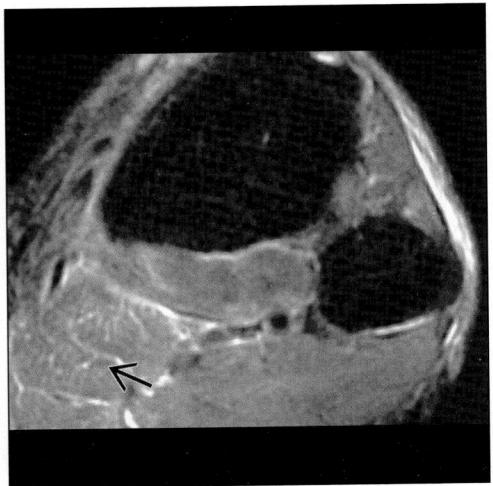

Axial graphic shows subtle edema of the medial head of the gastrocnemius in a grade 1 strain.

Axial FS PD FSE MR shows feathery distribution (arrow) of muscle edema in the medial head of the gastrocnemius in a grade 1 injury.

TERMINOLOGY

Abbreviations and Synonyms
- Gastrocnemius-soleus complex injury; tennis leg (has been used for either injury to medial head gastrocnemius or plantaris tendon rupture)

Definitions
- Partial to complete tear medial head of gastrocnemius muscle

IMAGING FINDINGS

General Features
- Best diagnostic clue: Diffuse hyperintensity within medial head gastrocnemius ± soleus muscle
- Location: Medial head gastrocnemius at muscle-tendon junction ± associated soleus muscle
- Size: Variable from a portion to entire cross sectional areas of medial gastrocnemius
- Morphology
  - Feathery or diffuse edema pattern
  - Irregularity of intermuscular fascia
  - ± Localized muscle hemorrhage in grade 2 tears
  - Muscle discontinuity in grade 3 disruption

MR Findings
- T1WI
  - Intermediate signal edema medial head
  - Subacute hemorrhage as hyperintensity
  - Laxity intermuscular septum between gastrocnemius and soleus
  - Intermediate signal fluid deep to subcutaneous tissue
- T2WI
  - Hyperintensity in edematous muscle fibers
  - Fascial discontinuity
  - Fluid between gastrocnemius & soleus
  - Fluid filled gap (hyperintense) in myofascial separation
- T2* GRE: Hypointense signal in hemosiderin foci especially on T2* gradient echo

Imaging Recommendations
- Best imaging tool: MR - demonstrates cross sectional muscle morphology and distribution of edema/hemorrhage
- Protocol advice
  - Axial T1 and FSE or STIR
  - Secondary - coronal and sagittal FS PD FSE or STIR

DIFFERENTIAL DIAGNOSIS

Plantaris Tendon Rupture
- Intermuscular hematoma - between medial head gastrocnemius & soleus

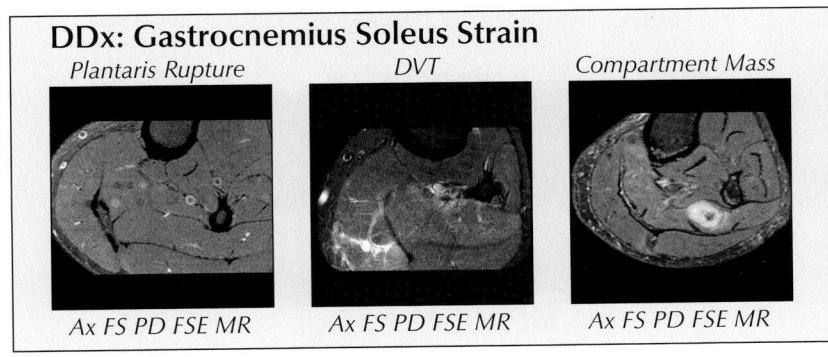

DDx: Gastrocnemius Soleus Strain

Plantaris Rupture	DVT	Compartment Mass
Ax FS PD FSE MR	*Ax FS PD FSE MR*	*Ax FS PD FSE MR*

GASTROCNEMIUS SOLEUS STRAIN

Key Facts

Terminology
- Gastrocnemius-soleus complex injury; tennis leg (has been used for either injury to medial head gastrocnemius or plantaris tendon rupture)

Imaging Findings
- Location: Medial head gastrocnemius at muscle-tendon junction ± associated soleus muscle
- ± Localized muscle hemorrhage in grade 2 tears
- Fascial discontinuity

Top Differential Diagnoses
- Plantaris Tendon Rupture
- Deep Venous Thrombosis (DVT)
- Posterior Compartment Syndrome

Pathology
- Overstretching - forced dorsiflexion & extended knee
- Tear medial head gastrocnemius at muscle-tendon junction
- Hemorrhage between medial head & soleus without plantaris tear

Clinical Issues
- Most common signs/symptoms: Acute onset calf pain
- Calf swelling (pain & swelling develop 1st 24 hours)
- Gastrocnemius pain with localized tenderness to medial head gastrocnemius ± soleus

Diagnostic Checklist
- Axial images to identify fascial disruption

- Retracted plantaris tendon & mass effect

Deep Venous Thrombosis (DVT)
- Calf swelling, tenderness & pain with dorsiflexion
- Duplex ultrasound vs. venography
- MR: Peri-neurovascular edema with watershed edema medial head gastrocnemius
- Prominent venous collaterals extending into gastrocnemius

Posterior Compartment Syndrome
- Progressive pain, exceeding degree of injury
- Paresthesias
- Weakness
- Requires direct measurement of compartment pressure

PATHOLOGY

General Features
- General path comments
  - Relevant anatomy
    - Medial larger than lateral head gastrocnemius
    - Gastrocnemius crosses two joints (knee & ankle)
    - Gastrocnemius = fast twitch fibers
    - Soleus muscle = slow twitch fibers
    - Medial head origin = medial condyle & adjacent femur & capsule of knee joint
    - Medial head insertion = Achilles tendon into calcaneus
- Etiology
  - Overstretching - forced dorsiflexion & extended knee
  - Eccentric action - increased force during muscle fiber lengthening
  - Jump injury (plyometric muscle activity)
  - Running
- Epidemiology
  - Muscle strains = 30% sports injuries
  - Gastrocnemius, rectus femoris, hamstring & adductor longus - most susceptible
  - Passive stretch - causative if too aggressive
  - Gastroc-soleus activated during stretch

- Eccentric action - muscle forces high during fiber lengthening

Gross Pathologic & Surgical Features
- Tear medial head gastrocnemius at muscle-tendon junction
- Hemorrhage between medial head & soleus without plantaris tear
- Partial tear of fascia between medial head gastrocnemius & soleus
- Partial tear transverse intermuscular septum at border of superficial posterior & deep posterior compartment

Microscopic Features
- Muscle strain in fast-twitch type II fibers of medial head gastrocnemius
- Muscle-tendon unit (MTU) = weak link
- Inflammatory cell infiltrate
- Separation of muscle fibers from tendon or fascia

Staging, Grading or Classification Criteria
- Grade 1 strain
  - No myofascial disruption
  - Edema
  - Swelling
- Grade 2 strain
  - Weakness
  - Variable separation muscle from tendon or fascia
- Grade 3 strain
  - Myofascial separation complete
  - Lack of muscle function

CLINICAL ISSUES

Presentation
- Most common signs/symptoms: Acute onset calf pain
- Clinical profile
  - Young - middle-aged recreational athlete
  - History running & sudden stop or change in direction
  - Calf swelling (pain & swelling develop 1st 24 hours)
  - Gastrocnemius pain with localized tenderness to medial head gastrocnemius ± soleus

○ Difficulty in walking (activity results in stress in preexisting MTU injury)

Demographics
- Age: Middle-aged
- Gender: Based on eccentric muscle activation - non gender specific

Natural History & Prognosis
- Improvement with non weight-bearing & rest
- 1st 24 hours = greatest pain & swelling
- Reinjury common if premature return to activity

Treatment
- Conservative
  ○ Supportive wraps
  ○ Ice
  ○ Anti-inflammatory medications
  ○ Cam walker - ambulation without crutches (no activation of injured MTU)
  ○ Early ankle motion
  ○ Stretching exercises as pain decreases
  ○ Strengthening to follow stretching
  ○ Criteria for return to activity - pain free motion & 90% return of gastrocnemius muscle strength
- Surgical
  ○ Compartment syndrome requires fasciotomy
- Complication
  ○ Acute posterior compartment syndrome (deep or superficial)
  ○ Anterior compartment syndrome
  ○ Lateral compartment syndrome

DIAGNOSTIC CHECKLIST

Consider
- Evaluate soleus muscle in association with medial head gastrocnemius strain
- DVT if perivascular hyperintensity, watershed distribution of muscle edema or prominent venous collaterals
- Axial images to identify fascial disruption

SELECTED REFERENCES

1. DeLee JC et al: Orthopaedic sports medicine. Principles and practice: Ligament injuries of the foot and ankle in the athlete. vol 2. 2nd ed. Philadelphia PA, Saunders, 2323-71, 2003
2. Clarkson PM et al: Exercise-induced muscle damage in humans. Am J Phys Med Rehabil 81(11 Suppl):S52-69, 2002
3. Boutin RD et al: Imaging of sports-related muscle injuries. Radiol Clin North Am 40(2):333-62, Review, 2002
4. Delgado GJ et al: Tennis leg: Clinical US study of 141 patients and anatomic investigation of four cadavers with MR imaging and US. Radiology 224(1):112-9, 2002
5. Bencardino JT et al: Traumatic musculotendinous injuries of the knee: Diagnosis with MR imaging. Radiographics 20 Spec No:S103-20, 2000
6. Nguyen B et al: Pains, strains and fasciculations: Lower extremity muscle disorders. Magn Reson Imaging Clin N Am 8(2):391-408, 2000
7. Leekham R et al: Using sonography to diagnose injury of plantaris muscles and tendons. AJR 172:185-9, 1999
8. Bianchi S et al: Sonographic evaluation of tears of the gastrocnemius medial head ("tennis leg"). J Ultrasound Med 17:157-62, 1998
9. Pomphrey MM Jr: More comments on tennis calf or tennis leg. Orthopedics 19(8):643, 1996
10. Menz MJ et al: Magnetic resonance imaging of a rupture of the medial head of the gastrocnemius muscle. A case report. J Bone Joint Surg 73(8):1260-2, 1991
11. Gecha S et al: Knee injuries in tennis. Clin Sports Med 7:435-52, 1988
12. Leach R: Leg and foot injuries in racquet sports. Clin Sports Med 7:359-70, 1988
13. Anouchi Y et al: Posterior compartment syndrome of the calf resulting from misdiagnosis of a rupture of the medial head of the gastrocnemius. J Trauma 27:678-80, 1987
14. Straehley D et al: Acute compartment syndrome (anterior lateral, and superficial posterior) following tear of the medial head of the gastrocnemius muscle. Am J Sports Med 14:96-9, 1986
15. Sutro C et al: The medial head of the gastrocnemius: A review of the basis for partial rupture and for intermittent claudication. Bull Hosp Jt Dis 45:150-7, 1985
16. Daffner RH: Anterior tibial striations. AJR 143:651-3, 1984
17. Severance H et al: Rupture of the plantaris - does it exist? J Bone Joint Surg Am 64:1387-8, 1982
18. Miller W: Rupture of the musculotendinous juncture of the medial head of the gastrocnemius muscle. Am J Sports Med 5:191-3, 1977
19. Froimson A: Tennis leg. JAMA 209:415-6, 1969

GASTROCNEMIUS SOLEUS STRAIN

Typical

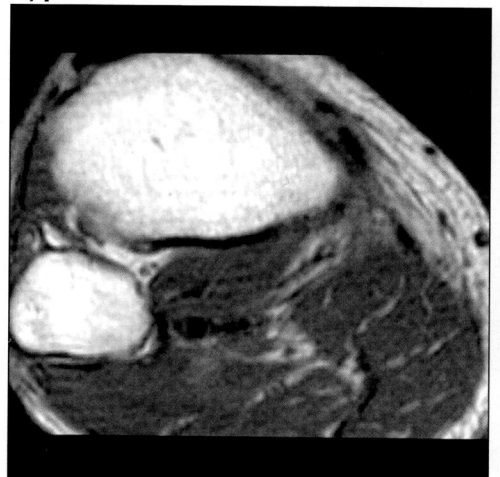 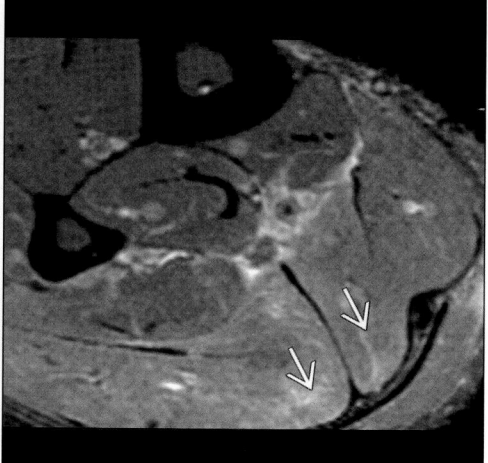

(Left) Axial T1WI MR shows isointense changes in a grade 1 medial head strain indistinguishable from normal muscle. *(Right)* Axial FS PD FSE MR shows soleus muscle edema (arrows) involving both medial and lateral aspects.

Typical

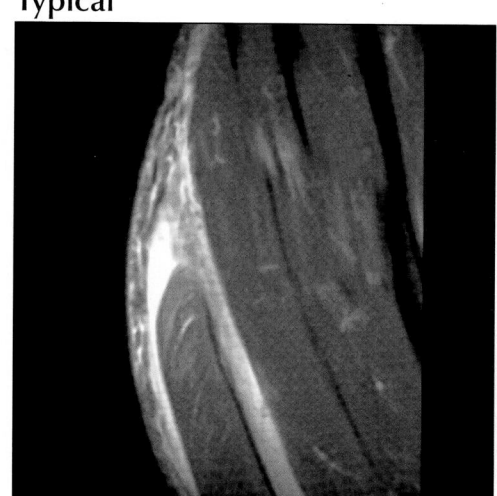 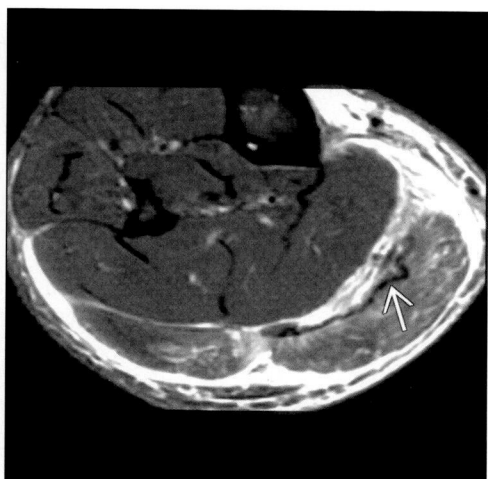

(Left) Coronal T2 FSE MR shows retracted medial head of the gastrocnemius muscle. *(Right)* Axial FS PD FSE MR shows gastrocnemius muscle-tendon-unit (MTU) injury with laxity (arrow) of fascia, edema of the gastrocnemius muscle, and intermuscular fluid.

Typical

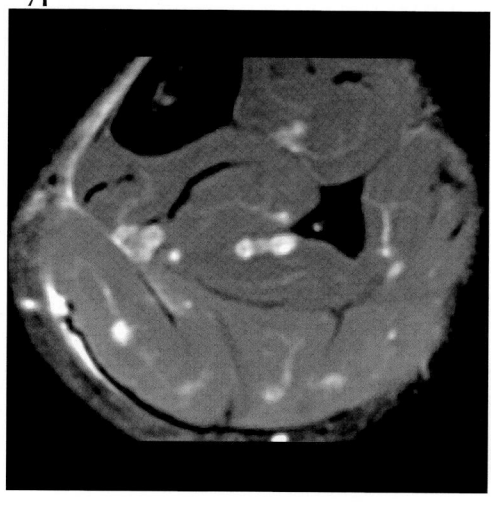 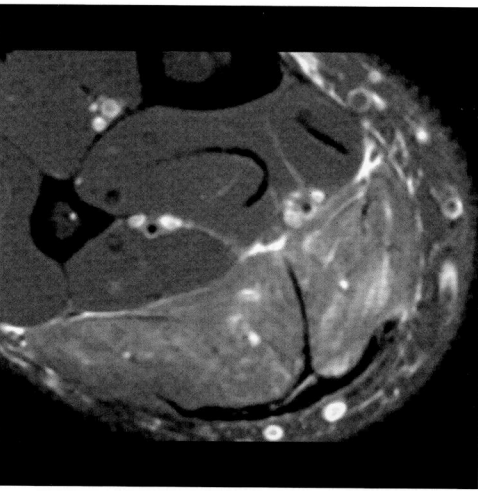

(Left) Axial FS PD FSE MR shows subtle MTU injury involving the medial aspect of the soleus muscle. *(Right)* Axial FS PD FSE MR shows diffuse hyperintense edema involving the medial and lateral aspects of the soleus muscle. The intramuscular soleus tendon is perpendicular to the tendo calcaneus tendon posteriorly.

PLANTARIS RUPTURE

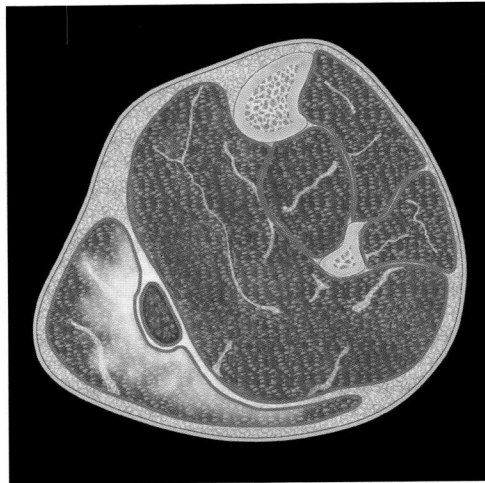

Axial graphic shows enlarged retracted plantaris tendon with associated edema of adjacent muscle fibers of the medial head of the gastrocnemius muscle.

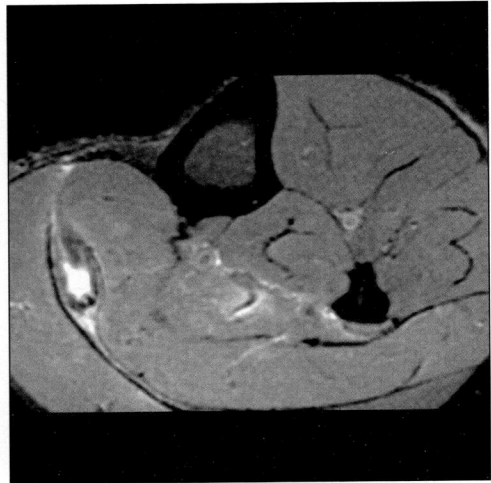

Axial FS PD FSE MR shows rupture of plantaris tendon with intermuscular hemorrhage between the soleus and medial head of the gastrocnemius muscle groups. Hemosiderin ring is hypointense.

TERMINOLOGY

Abbreviations and Synonyms
- Plantaris tendon tear
- Tennis leg (has been used for both injury to medial head gastrocnemius and plantaris tendon rupture)

Definitions
- Myotendinous junction rupture

IMAGING FINDINGS

General Features
- Best diagnostic clue: Hemorrhage & mass effect
- Location: Between medial head gastrocnemius and soleus muscles
- Size: Variable: Tendon & hemorrhage may extend up to 50% anteroposterior length of fascial division between soleus and medial head
- Morphology
  - Tubular hemorrhagic fluid collection
  - Tendon mass & hemorrhage with convex medial/lateral margins

MR Findings
- T1WI
  - Intermediate signal mass ± hypointense hemosiderin between medial head gastrocnemius & soleus
  - Hyperintense subacute hemorrhage
  - Variable intermediate signal within adjacent medial head gastrocnemius ± soleus
  - Distal tears with absence of distal course of plantaris less common
  - Proximal tears associated with anterior cruciate ligament (ACL) injuries (± anterior translation of tibial relative to femur)
- T2WI
  - Hyperintense hemorrhage ± hypointense hemosiderin ring & inhomogeneity in restricted tendon
  - Hyperintense edema within a portion or complete cross sectional area at a specified level
  - ± Hyperintense edema soleus and less commonly lateral head gastrocnemius
  - Hyperintense hemorrhagic fluid tracks medially deep to subcutaneous tissue
  - Hyperintense fluid ± anterolateral & posteromedial extension between subcutaneous tissue and medial head/soleus plane
  - Fluid ± extension anteromedial to tibia
  - Disruption of fascia separating medial head gastrocnemius and soleus
  - Less commonly associated with strain tibialis posterior

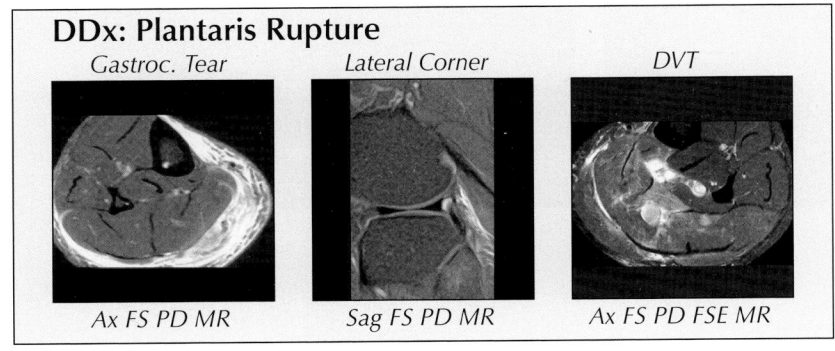

DDx: Plantaris Rupture

Gastroc. Tear	Lateral Corner	DVT
Ax FS PD MR	Sag FS PD MR	Ax FS PD FSE MR

PLANTARIS RUPTURE

Key Facts

Imaging Findings
- Best diagnostic clue: Hemorrhage & mass effect
- Location: Between medial head gastrocnemius and soleus muscles
- Tubular hemorrhagic fluid collection
- Tendon mass & hemorrhage with convex medial/lateral margins

Top Differential Diagnoses
- Gastrocnemius - Soleus Muscle Strain
- Posterolateral Corner Sprain
- Deep Venous Thrombosis (DVT)

Pathology
- Forceful muscle contraction
- Overstretching - forced dorsiflexion & extended knee
- Eccentric loading

- Less common incidence relative to gastrocnemius muscle strain

Clinical Issues
- Most common signs/symptoms: Acute onset calf pain
- Sudden pop followed by calf swelling & tenderness
- Difficulty in walking
- Impaired weight bearing
- Symptoms localized more proximally in association with myotendinous and posterolateral complex injuries
- Improvement with non weight-bearing & rest

Diagnostic Checklist
- Hemorrhage within the gastrocnemius - soleus plane may present without plantaris rupture

---

- o Proximal injuries at muscle-tendon junction ± ACL tears or hyperintense fluid in posterolateral corner sprains
- o Hyperintense curvilinear "comet sign" of fluid extending along distal course of plantaris adjacent to Achilles tendon
- o Absent plantaris muscle in proximal tears in sagittal plane through knee joint

Imaging Recommendations
- Best imaging tool: MR - demonstrates retracted tendon/hemorrhage mass in axial plane & localizes proximal vs. distal injury
- Protocol advice
  - o T1, FS PD FSE or STIR axial images (T2* gradient echo optional for hemosiderin detection)
  - o Additional sagittal images for posterolateral corner complex injury with proximal tears
  - o Coronal images to define lateral to medial course of hemorrhage

DIFFERENTIAL DIAGNOSIS

Gastrocnemius - Soleus Muscle Strain
- Partial to complete tear medial head gastrocnemius
- Absence of retracted plantaris tendon

Posterolateral Corner Sprain
- Fluid posterior to popliteus tendon & disruption arcuate ligament
- Strain to partial tear popliteus muscle & muscle tendon junction

Deep Venous Thrombosis (DVT)
- Calf swelling, tenderness & pain with dorsiflexion
- Duplex ultrasound vs. venography
- MR findings: Perivascular edema & watershed muscle edema & venous collaterals & popliteal venous obstruction

Posterior Compartment Syndrome
- Progressive pain, exceeding degree of injury
- Paresthesias

- Weakness
- Requires direct measurement of compartment pressure

PATHOLOGY

General Features
- General path comments
  - o Relevant anatomy
    - Plantaris anterior to lateral head gastrocnemius at level of knee joint
    - Extends obliquely from lateral to medial
    - Medial to Achilles tendon in distal course
    - Origin = distal lateral supracondylar line femur
    - Myotendinous junction = level of soleus origin from tibia
    - Plantaris plane = between medial head gastrocnemius & soleus
- Etiology
  - o Forceful muscle contraction
  - o Overstretching - forced dorsiflexion & extended knee
  - o Eccentric loading
  - o Plyometric muscle action - jumping
  - o Running - uneven terrain
- Epidemiology
  - o Plantaris normally absent 7-10% population
  - o Less common incidence relative to gastrocnemius muscle strain

Gross Pathologic & Surgical Features
- Myotendinous junction tear vs. distal tendon avulsion (less common)
- Myotendinous proximal tear associated with distal retraction

Microscopic Features
- Muscle-tendon unit (MTU) failure
- Inflammatory cell infiltrate
- Hemorrhagic cellular elements

Staging, Grading or Classification Criteria
- First degree strain
  - o No myofascial disruption

PLANTARIS RUPTURE

○ Edema
○ Swelling
- Second degree strain
  ○ Weakness
  ○ Variable separation of muscle from tendon or fascia
- Third degree strain
  ○ Myofascial separation complete
  ○ Lack of muscle function

CLINICAL ISSUES

Presentation
- Most common signs/symptoms: Acute onset calf pain
- Clinical profile
  ○ Sudden pop followed by calf swelling & tenderness
  ○ Difficulty in walking
  ○ Impaired weight bearing
  ○ Symptoms localized more proximally in association with myotendinous and posterolateral complex injuries
  ○ Tenderness medial to Achilles in cases of distal rupture

Demographics
- Age: Young - middle aged recreational athlete
- Gender: Non gender specific

Natural History & Prognosis
- Improvement with non weight-bearing & rest
- 1st 24 hours = greatest pain & swelling
- Recovery also based on associated injuries
  ○ Posterolateral corner
  ○ Anterior cruciate ligament
  ○ Popliteus muscle sprain
  ○ Lateral head gastrocnemius sprain

Treatment
- Conservative
  ○ Supportive wraps
  ○ Ice
  ○ Antiinflammatory medications
  ○ Cam walker
  ○ Stretching and strengthening of gastrocnemius - soleus complex after acute phase
- Surgical
  ○ Not required for plantaris tendon
  ○ Compartment syndrome not common unless severe hemorrhage with compartment constriction

DIAGNOSTIC CHECKLIST

Consider
- Evaluate plantaris proximally on sagittal and axial images and distally to the calcaneus on axial images
- Cases of suspected plantaris rupture are usually medial head gastrocnemius partial tears
- Hemorrhage within the gastrocnemius - soleus plane may present without plantaris rupture

SELECTED REFERENCES

1. Delgado GJ et al: Tennis leg: Clinical US study of 141 patients and anatomic investigation of four cadavers with MR imaging and US. Radiology 244(1):112-9, 2002
2. Pomphrey MM Jr: More comments on tennis calf or tennis leg. Orthopedics 19(8):643, 1996
3. Brown TR et al: Diagnoses of popliteus injuries with MR imaging. Skel Radiol 24:511-4, 1995
4. Menz MJ et al: Magnetic resonance imaging of a rupture of the medial head of the gastrocnemius muscle. A case report. J Bone Joint Surg AM 73(8):1260-2, 1991
5. Leach R: Leg and foot injuries in racquet sports. Clin Sports Med 7:359-70, 1988
6. Gecha S et al: Knee injuries in tennis. Clin Sports Med 7:435-52, 1988
7. Sutro C et al: The medial head of the gastrocnemius: A review for the basis for partial rupture and for intermittent claudication. Bull Hosp Jt Dis 45:150-7, 1985
8. Daffner RH: Anterior tibial striations. AJR 143:651-3, 1984
9. Severance H et al: Rupture of the plantaris - does it exist? J Bone Joint Surg Am 64:1387-8, 1982

PLANTARIS RUPTURE

IMAGE GALLERY

Typical

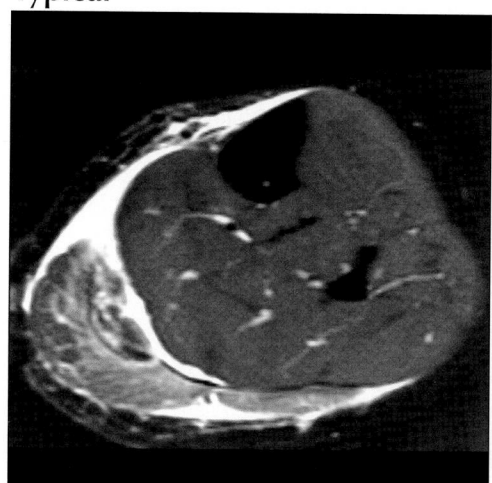 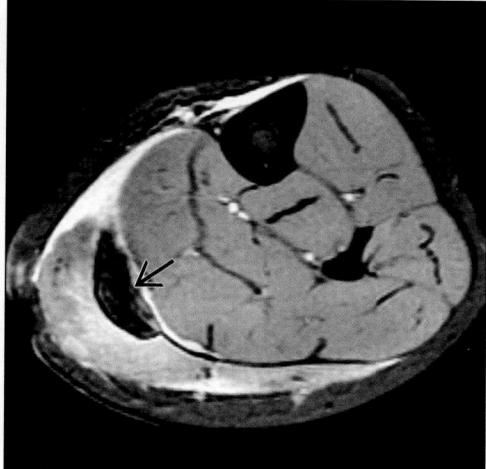

(Left) Axial FS PD FSE MR shows plantaris rupture with intramuscular hemorrhage with associated edema of the medial head of the gastrocnemius muscle. *(Right)* Axial T2* GRE MR shows magnetic susceptibility (arrow) effect of hemorrhage within plane of injury.

Typical

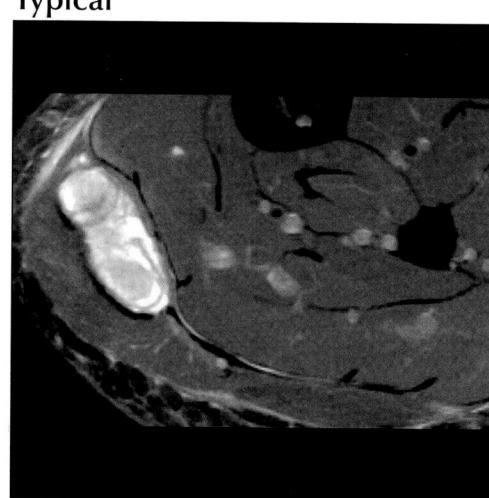 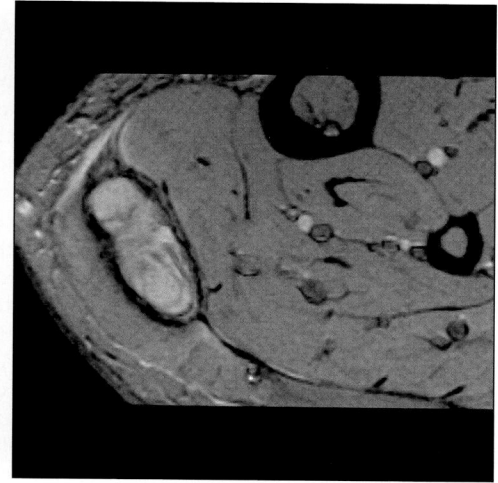

(Left) Axial FS PD FSE MR shows hemorrhagic mass associated with a plantaris tendon rupture. Plantaris tendon tissue is not visualized. *(Right)* Axial T2* GRE MR shows well circumscribed hemosiderin ring surrounding hemorrhagic fluid collection associated with an absent plantaris tendon.

Typical

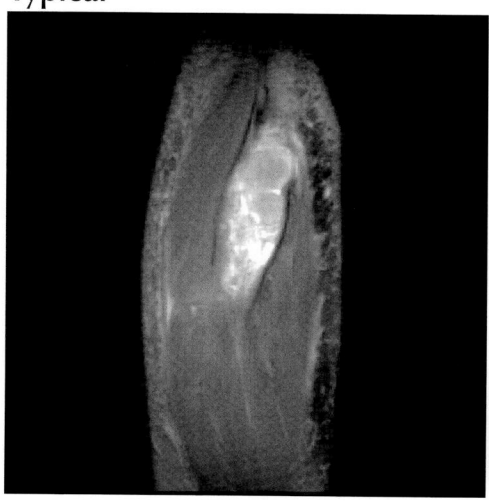 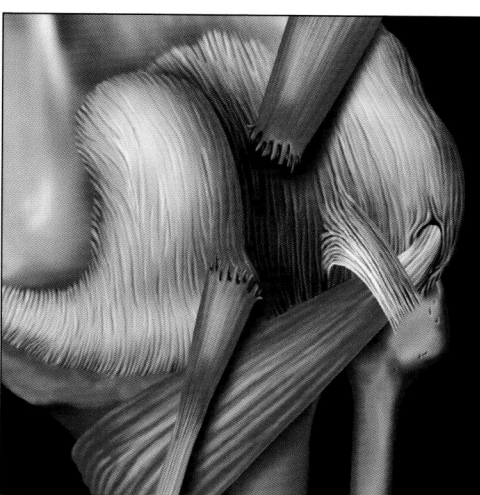

(Left) Coronal FS PD FSE MR shows longitudinal distribution of hemorrhage corresponding to the course of the retracted plantaris tendon. *(Right)* Coronal graphic shows rupture of the plantaris tendon at the muscle-tendon junction. Tendon retraction is illustrated.

TARSAL TUNNEL SYNDROME

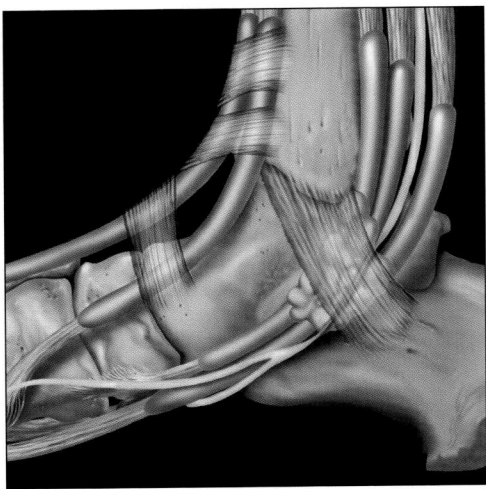

Sagittal graphic shows compression neuropathy of the posterior tibial nerve secondary to a space occupying ganglion deep to the flexor retinaculum.

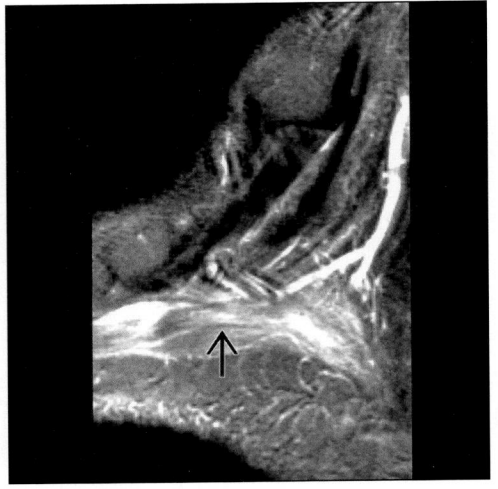

Sagittal FS PD FSE MR shows hyperintensity (muscle denervation) of the abductor hallucis (arrow) from tarsal tunnel syndrome secondary to varicose veins.

TERMINOLOGY

Abbreviations and Synonyms
- Tibial neuropathy

Definitions
- Entrapment or compression neuropathy of posterior tibial nerve

IMAGING FINDINGS

General Features
- Best diagnostic clue: Space occupying lesion ± muscle denervation supplied by posterior tibial nerve or one of its branches
- Location: Fibroosseous tunnel deep to flexor retinaculum posterior/inferior to medial malleolus
- Size: Variable based on involvement of posterior tibial nerve or one of its branches + etiology (e.g., trauma vs. space-occupying lesions)
- Morphology
  - Morphology based on causative factor (e.g., fracture vs. varicosities, ganglion, lipomas, neurilemomas, thickened flexor retinaculum, accessory muscles)
  - Distribution of associated muscle denervation supplied by medial or lateral plantar nerves

MR Findings
- T1WI
  - Fractures
    - Sustentaculum tali
    - Medial tubercle posterior process talus
  - Serpiginous venous signal (intermediate) - varicosities
  - Hypointense ganglia
  - Hyperintense lipomas
  - Intermediate signal neurilemomas
  - Hypointense thickened flexor retinaculum (lacinate ligament)
  - Muscle signal in presence of accessory muscle
  - Intermediate signal proliferative synovitis
  - Fat marrow signal in bony vs. low to intermediate signal fibrous coalition
  - Fat marrow signal in talar exostosis
- T2WI
  - Hyperintense edema associated with fractures of talus/calcaneus
  - Hyperintense tangle of venous varicosities
  - Hypointense lipomas (FS PD FSE or STIR)
  - Hyperintense neurilemomas
  - Intermediate to hyperintense synovitis
  - Diffuse hyperintense muscle edema in muscle groups supplied by posterior tibial nerve + its branches (abductor hallucis/medial plantar nerve + abductor digiti quinti/lateral plantar nerve)

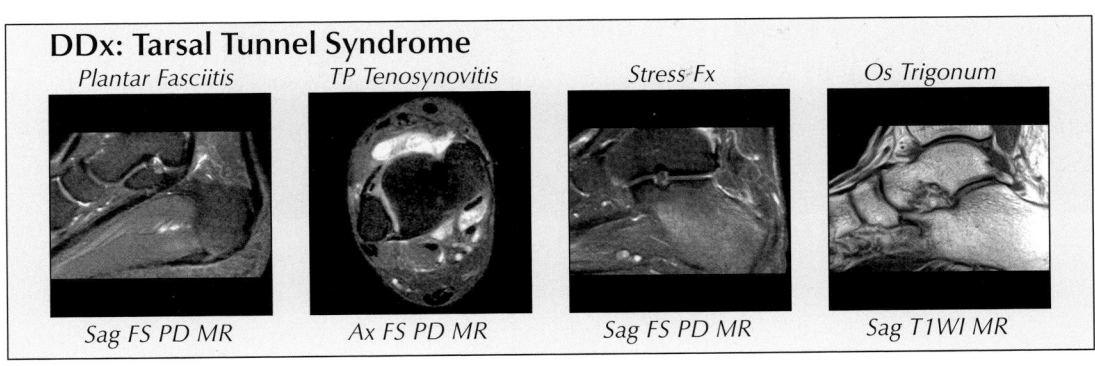

DDx: Tarsal Tunnel Syndrome

Plantar Fasciitis	TP Tenosynovitis	Stress Fx	Os Trigonum
Sag FS PD MR	Ax FS PD MR	Sag FS PD MR	Sag T1WI MR

TARSAL TUNNEL SYNDROME

Key Facts

Imaging Findings
- Best diagnostic clue: Space occupying lesion ± muscle denervation supplied by posterior tibial nerve or one of its branches
- Morphology based on causative factor (e.g., fracture vs. varicosities, ganglion, lipomas, neurilemomas, thickened flexor retinaculum, accessory muscles)
- Distribution of associated muscle denervation supplied by medial or lateral plantar nerves

Top Differential Diagnoses
- Interdigital Neuroma
- Plantar Fasciitis
- Tibialis Posterior (TP) Tenosynovitis
- Tarsal Coalition

Pathology
- Idiopathic - up to 50%
- Varicosities 13%
- 34.4% association with systemic disease
- Inflammation posterior tibial nerve

Clinical Issues
- Most common signs/symptoms: Pain plantar aspect foot
- Burning
- Numbness
- Positive Tinel's sign (percussion of tibial nerve over tarsal tunnel) + sensory impediment

Diagnostic Checklist
- Associated denervation muscle hyperintensity (e.g., abductor hallucis) with space-occupying lesions

---

- ○ Tenosynovitis - hyperintense fluid flexor hallucis sheath
- T1 C+: To differentiate enhancing neurilemomas vs. nonenhancing synovial cysts

Imaging Recommendations
- Best imaging tool: MR to identify space-occupying soft tissue lesions + denervation hyperintensity
- Protocol advice: Axial, coronal and sagittal T1 or PD + FS PD FSE

DIFFERENTIAL DIAGNOSIS

Interdigital Neuroma
- Morton's neuroma
- Metatarsalgia + localized enlargement interdigital nerve
- Between third + fourth metatarsal heads
- Lateral branch medial plantar nerve to third interspace

Plantar Fasciitis
- Inflammation plantar aponeurosis
- Associated calcaneal spur, inflammatory changes ± thickening fascia
- Hyperintense plantar aponeurosis os calcis attachment

Tibialis Posterior (TP) Tenosynovitis
- Fluid signal hyperintensity in tendon sheath
- Spectrum of degeneration + longitudinal splitting + tearing

Radiculopathy
- Disc protrusion lower lumbar discs on sagittal and axial images
- L5 or S1 radiculopathy

Tarsal Coalition
- Talocalcaneal coalition between sustentaculum tali + middle facet of subtalar joint
- Visualized on T1 coronal image

Diabetic Neuropathy
- Osseous hyperemia
- Associated chronic stenosing tenosynovitis

Calcaneal Stress Fracture
- Posterior calcaneal subchondral edema
- Discrete linear calcaneal fracture lines perpendicular to long axis

Os Trigonum Syndrome
- Pain + disruption cartilaginous synchondrosis between os trigonum and lateral tubercle of posterior process talus

PATHOLOGY

General Features
- General path comments
  - ○ Relevant anatomy: Tarsal tunnel
    - Distal deep posterior compartment leg forms tarsal tunnel
    - Posterior to medial malleolus
    - Fibroosseous space
    - Formed by medial talar wall, sustentaculum tali + medial calcaneal wall
    - Flexor retinaculum = lacinate ligament = roof of tarsal tunnel
    - Contents: Tibialis posterior, flexor digitorum longus + flexor hallucis longus tendons; neurovascular (N/V) bundle
    - Posterior tibial nerve terminal branches = medial + lateral plantar nerves
    - Posterior tibial nerve usually bifurcates within tarsal tunnel
    - Third branch of posterior tibial nerve = medial calcaneal nerve (may arise from lateral plantar nerve)
- Etiology
  - ○ Idiopathic - up to 50%
  - ○ Trauma: Fractured sustentaculum tali or medial tubercle posterior talar process
  - ○ Varicosities
  - ○ Ganglia
  - ○ Lipomas
  - ○ Neurilemomas

TARSAL TUNNEL SYNDROME

- o Thickened flexor retinaculum
- o Accessory muscle
- o Synovitis (inflammatory arthropathies)
- o Tarsal coalition
- o Diabetes
- o Valgus heel + pronated forefoot
- Epidemiology
  - o Trauma incidence 17%
  - o Varicosities 13%
  - o Fibrosis 9%
  - o Heel valgus 8%
  - o 34.4% association with systemic disease

Gross Pathologic & Surgical Features
- Accessory flexor digitorum longus muscle
- Proliferative synovitis
- Ganglia
- Varicosities
- Lipomas
- Neurilemomas

Microscopic Features
- Inflammation posterior tibial nerve
- Axonal compression
- Vascular changes
- Atrophy innervated muscles

CLINICAL ISSUES

Presentation
- Most common signs/symptoms: Pain plantar aspect foot
- Clinical profile
  - o Burning
  - o Tingling
  - o Numbness
  - o Pain localized to posterior tibial nerve or one of its three terminal branches
  - o Pain aggravated with activity + prolonged standing
  - o Nocturnal paresthesias
  - o Valleix's phenomenon = radiation of paresthesias proximally to calf + leg
  - o Positive Tinel's sign (percussion of tibial nerve over tarsal tunnel) + sensory impediment
  - o Tenderness to palpation
  - o Motor symptoms = less common
  - o Perthes' tourniquet test for varicosities = test deep venous system/posterior tibial venae comitantes by occluding superficial venous system

Demographics
- Age: Average = 47 years
- Gender: Female = 56% predilection

Natural History & Prognosis
- Varies with etiology
- Synovitis responds to rest + antiinflammatory medications (NSAIDs)
- Space-occupying lesions usually require surgical decompression

Treatment
- Conservative

- o NSAIDs to decrease posterior tibial nerve inflammation
- o Corticosteroid injections
- o Orthotics
- o Physical therapy
- o Compressive stockings
- o Immobilization
- Surgical
  - o Surgical decompression
  - o Excision of space-occupying lesion
  - o Release flexor retinaculum, abductor fascia + decompress posterior tibial nerve/branches
- Complications
  - o Recurrent tarsal tunnel syndrome
  - o Space-occupying lesions + coalitions = better post surgical result vs. trauma or idiopathic

DIAGNOSTIC CHECKLIST

Consider
- Associated denervation muscle hyperintensity (e.g., abductor hallucis) with space-occupying lesions
- Use of T1 C+ to distinguish between cysts and neural tumors
- T1/PD coronal images to exclude tarsal coalition

SELECTED REFERENCES

1. Kinoshita M et al: Tarsal tunnel syndrome associated with an accessory muscle. Foot Ankle Int 24(2):132-6, 2003
2. Lee MF et al: Tarsal tunnel syndrome caused by talocalcaneal coalition. Clin Imaging 26(2):140-3, 2002
3. Banks A et al: McGlamry's comprehensive textbook of foot and ankle surgery. vol 1. Philadelphia PA, Lippincott Williams & Wilkins, 1266-78, 2001
4. Still GP: Neurilemoma of the medial plantar nerve: A case report. J Foot Ankle Surg 40(4):236-9, 2001
5. Garchar DJ et al: Hypertrophic sustentaculum tali causing a tarsal tunnel syndrome: A case report. J Foot Ankle Surg 40(2):110-2, 2001
6. Rosenberg ZS et al: From the RSNA refresher courses. Radiological Society of North America. MR imaging of the ankle and foot. Radiographics 20 Spec No:s153-79 Review, 2000
7. Narvaez JA et al: Painful heel: MR imaging findings. Radiographics 20(2):333-52, 2000
8. Steinbach LS: Painful syndromes around the ankle and foot: Magnetic resonance imaging evaluation. Top Magn Reson Imaging 9(5):311-26, 1998
9. Turan I et al: Tarsal tunnel syndrome. Outcome of surgery in longstanding cases. Clin Orthop 343:151-6, 1997
10. Kerr R et al: MR imaging in tarsal tunnel syndrome. J Comput Assist Tomogr 15:280-6, 1991
11. Zeiss J et al: Normal magnetic resonance anatomy of the tarsal tunnel. Foot Ankle 10:214-18, 1990
12. Havel PE et al: Tibial nerve branching in the tarsal tunnel. Foot Ankle 10:214-18, 1990
13. Dellon AL et al: Tibial nerve branching in the tarsal tunnel. Arch Neurol 41:645-46, 1984

TARSAL TUNNEL SYNDROME

IMAGE GALLERY

Typical

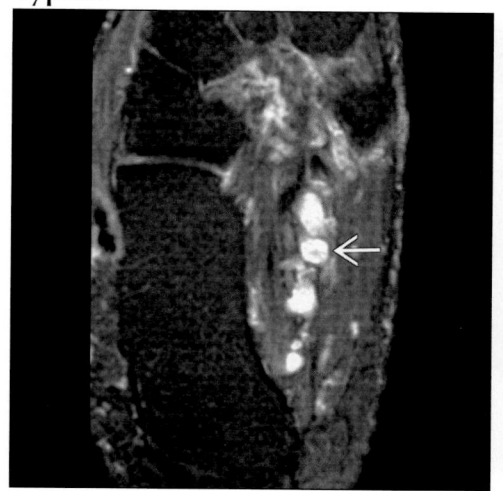
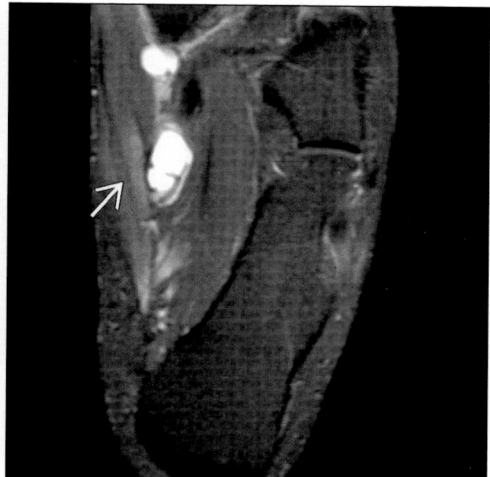

(Left) Axial FS PD FSE MR shows hyperintense varicosities (arrow) within the tarsal tunnel. *(Right)* Axial FS PD FSE MR shows enlarged varicose veins with associated muscle denervation (arrow) of the abductor hallucis muscle (medial to the veins).

Typical

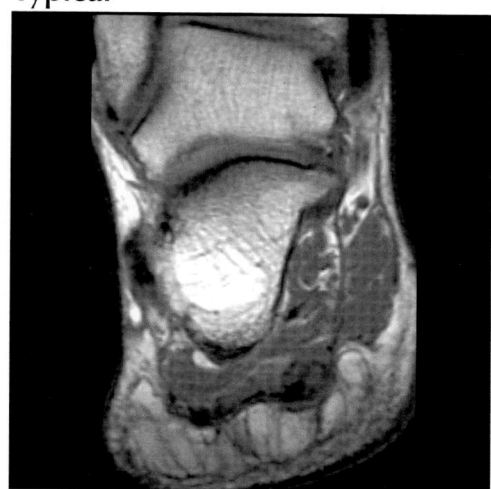
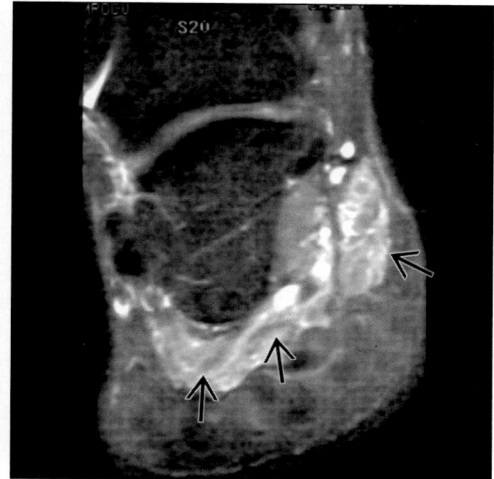

(Left) Coronal T1WI MR shows muscle denervation isointense to adjacent muscle in the acute phase. *(Right)* Coronal FS PD FSE MR shows hyperintense muscle denervation (arrows) involving the abductor hallucis, flexor digitorum brevis, and abductor digiti minimi. Both the medial and lateral (abductor digiti minimi) plantar nerves are involved.

Typical

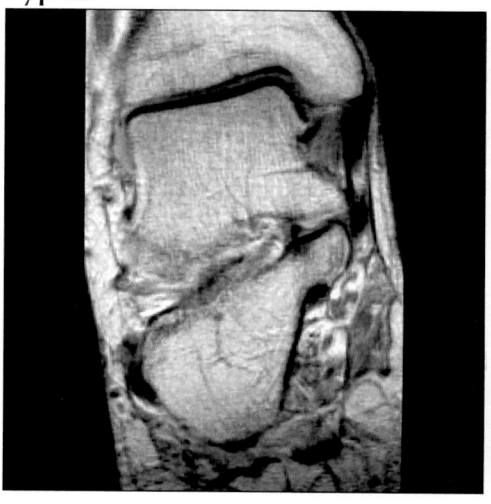
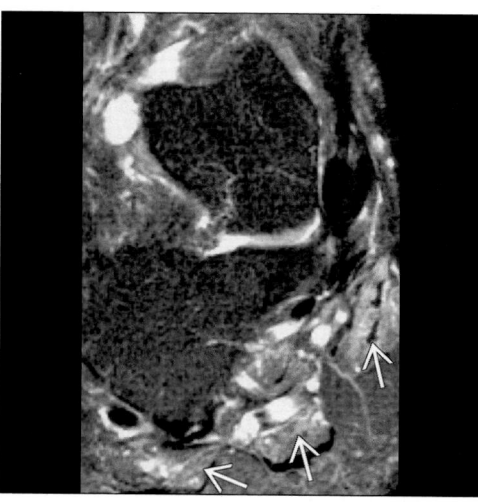

(Left) Coronal T1WI MR shows chronic changes of compression neuropathy with fatty atrophy developing in the abductor hallucis, flexor digitorum brevis, and abductor digiti minimi. *(Right)* Coronal FS PD FSE MR shows prominent varicose veins with muscle hyperintensity (arrows) of the abductor hallucis, flexor digitorum brevis, and abductor digiti minimi.

PLANTAR FASCIITIS

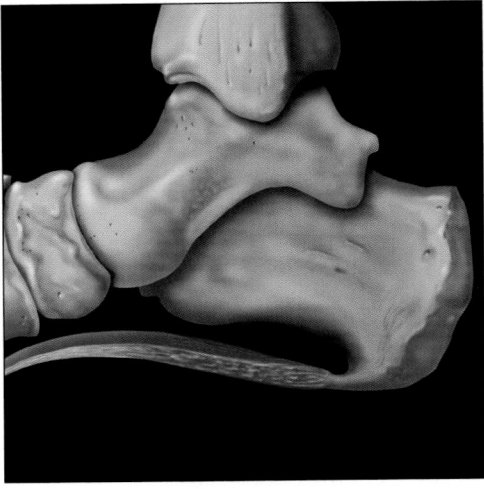

Sagittal graphic shows inflamed and thickened plantar fascia (in red). Adjacent plantar calcaneal enthesophyte is attached to the plantar fascia.

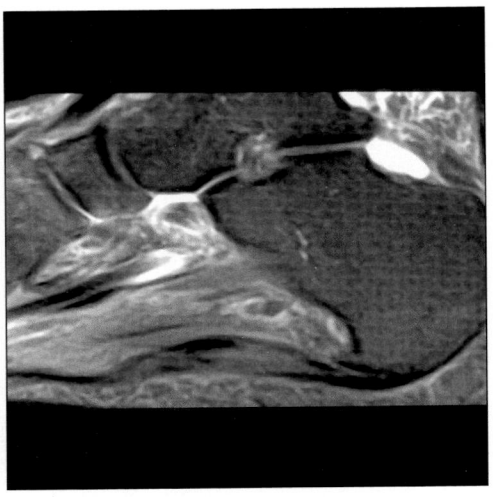

Sagittal FS PD FSE MR shows long segment of proximal plantar fascia with hyperintensity and convex dorsal thickening of the aponeurosis.

TERMINOLOGY

Abbreviations and Synonyms
- Proximal plantar fasciitis, heel pain syndrome, subcalcaneal pain syndrome

Definitions
- Inflammation of plantar aponeurosis

IMAGING FINDINGS

General Features
- Best diagnostic clue: Hyperintensity (T2WI) of plantar aponeurosis adjacent to os calcis attachment
- Location
  - Medial/lateral cords or central attachment of plantar fascia to os calcis
  - Most common site = origin of plantar fascia from medial calcaneal tuberosity
- Size
  - Variable in proximal/distal extent (usually posterior third or 1-2 cm plantar fascia)
  - Increased plantar fascia thickness to 7 or 8 mm (normal thickness 3 or 4 mm)
- Morphology: Superior to inferior thickening directed along long axis

MR Findings
- T1WI
  - Initial prefascial thickening = hypointense to intermediate effacement of subcutaneous tissue superficial (plantar) to os calcis attachment
  - Hypointense thickening of plantar fascia
  - ± Enthesophyte
  - Enthesophyte ± marrow containing fat signal
  - Partial detachment of medial or lateral cord
  - ± Adjacent calcaneal erosions (tuberosity of calcaneus)
- T2WI
  - Intermediate to hyperintense thickening proximal plantar fascia on T2WI
  - Hyperintense subcutaneous tissue edema
  - Hyperintense reactive calcaneal marrow edema
  - Subcutaneous tissue hyperintensity + edema deep to plantar fascia
  - Rupture both mid portion and at proximal segment
  - Hyperintense fluid-filled gap in fascial rupture

Imaging Recommendations
- Best imaging tool: MR superior for edema in subcutaneous tissue + fascia
- Protocol advice
  - T1WI sagittal for enthesophyte and subcutaneous tissue effacement

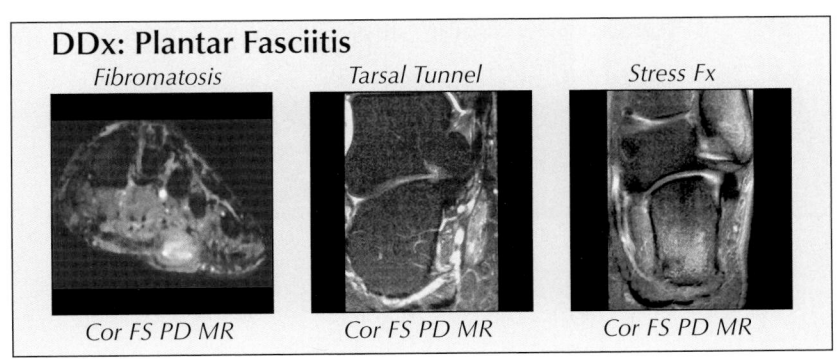

DDx: Plantar Fasciitis

Fibromatosis	Tarsal Tunnel	Stress Fx
Cor FS PD MR	Cor FS PD MR	Cor FS PD MR

PLANTAR FASCIITIS

Key Facts

Imaging Findings
- Best diagnostic clue: Hyperintensity (T2WI) of plantar aponeurosis adjacent to os calcis attachment
- Increased plantar fascia thickness to 7 or 8 mm (normal thickness 3 or 4 mm)
- Intermediate to hyperintense thickening proximal plantar fascia on T2WI

Top Differential Diagnoses
- Plantar Fibromatosis
- Tarsal Tunnel Syndrome
- Calcaneal Stress Fracture
- Entrapment of 1st Branch of Lateral Plantar Nerve

Pathology
- Microtrauma of plantar fascia

- ± Nerve entrapment or irritation of medial calcaneal N. or lateral plantar N. to abductor digiti quinti
- Repetitive tensile overload affecting central band
- Reparative inflammatory response to traumatic overload
- Calcaneal spur - within flexor brevis origin

Clinical Issues
- Most common signs/symptoms: Pain medial tuberosity calcaneus
- Affects medial aspect foot & heel
- Severe inflammation - unable to weight bear on heel
- Medial tuberosity enthesophyte

Diagnostic Checklist
- Locate involvement in medial, lateral or central portions

- ○ FS PD FSE coronal + sagittal for identifying cords of involvement (medial, lateral or central)

DIFFERENTIAL DIAGNOSIS

Plantar Fibromatosis
- Fibrous proliferation + replacement of plantar aponeurosis
- Nodules
- Solitary or multiple

Tarsal Tunnel Syndrome
- Entrapment or compression neuropathy
- Affecting posterior tibial nerve in fibroosseous tunnel deep to flexor retinaculum
- Pain + sensory deficit sole + foot
- Intrinsic muscle weakness

Calcaneal Stress Fracture
- Trabecular fractures perpendicular to long axis of calcaneus
- Posterior subchondral bone calcaneus (not plantar)
- Extensive posterior calcaneal marrow edema

Entrapment of 1st Branch of Lateral Plantar Nerve
- At level of medial plantar aspect heel
- Between fascia of abductor hallucis + medial head quadratus plantae

Sarcoidosis
- Bilateral heel pain occurring with or prior to onset of sarcoid arthritis

PATHOLOGY

General Features
- General path comments
  - ○ Relevant anatomy = plantar aponeurosis
    - Origin = os calcis
    - Plantar fascia = multilayered fibrous aponeurosis
    - Three segments or cords + distal superficial tracts

- Central segment = largest + extends from plantar posteromedial calcaneal tuberosity to proximal phalanges + skin, ball of foot
- Lateral cord = from lateral process os calcis tuberosity to base of fifth metatarsal
- Medial cord = thin + covers plantar aspect abductor hallucis
- Medial calcaneal nerve (N.) in subcutaneous tissue between plantar fascia + skin
- Nerve to abductor digiti quinti (from lateral plantar nerve) passes between long plantar ligament & calcaneal plantar enthesophyte
- Etiology
  - ○ Microtrauma of plantar fascia
  - ○ ± Nerve entrapment or irritation of medial calcaneal N. or lateral plantar N. to abductor digiti quinti
  - ○ Repetitive tensile overload affecting central band
  - ○ Reparative inflammatory response to traumatic overload
  - ○ Heel cord contracture
  - ○ Pes planus association
  - ○ Pes cavus association
  - ○ Calcaneal spur - within flexor brevis origin
- Epidemiology
  - ○ 50% of adult plantar heel pain patients
    - Calcaneal enthesophyte (enthesophyte actually located in short toe flexor origins and not aponeurosis)

Gross Pathologic & Surgical Features
- Inflamed proximal plantar fascia
- Thickened fascia from normal thickness of 3 mm to mean thickness of 7.4 mm
- Calcaneal enthesophyte
- Fatigue fractures/periosteitis medial calcaneal tuberosity

Microscopic Features
- Angiofibroblastic hyperplasia
- Collagen degenerative/necrosis
- Chondroid metaplasia
- Matrix calcification

PLANTAR FASCIITIS

Staging, Grading or Classification Criteria
- Acute plantar fascia rupture - less common, with palpable defect distal to medial calcaneal tuberosity
- Chronic proximal plantar fasciitis

CLINICAL ISSUES

Presentation
- Most common signs/symptoms: Pain medial tuberosity calcaneus
- Clinical profile
  - Slow gradual onset pain
  - Pain with dorsiflexion toes
  - Pain ± associated with twisting injury to foot
  - Affects medial aspect foot & heel
  - Pain worse in AM
  - Severe inflammation - unable to weight bear on heel
  - Medial tuberosity enthesophyte
  - ± Seronegative spondyloarthritis (HLA-B27 antigen positive)
  - ± History increased stress on foot either standing or activity related

Demographics
- Age: Average = 45 years
- Gender: 2 times more common in women

Natural History & Prognosis
- Pain partially resolves during day
- Exacerbated by prolonged standing or athletic activity
- 90% patients improve with conservative treatment

Treatment
- Conservative
  - Nonsteroidal antiinflammatory medications
  - Rest
  - Orthotics
  - Physical therapy with stretching
  - Immobilization with cast
  - Steroid injection - controversial
- Surgical
  - Plantar fasciotomy
  - Excision calcaneal spur
  - Release of nerve to abductor digiti quinti
  - Endoscopic plantar fascia release
- Complications
  - Steroid injections associated with rupture of plantar fascia & fat pad atrophy
  - Endoscopic release: Stress fractures, pseudoaneurysm, recurrence of pain

DIAGNOSTIC CHECKLIST

Consider
- Identify associated plantar fascial tearing
- Locate involvement in medial, lateral or central portions
- Early diagnosis by visualizing subcutaneous fat effacement by edema on T1WI in sagittal plane

SELECTED REFERENCES

1. McGonagle D et al: The rule of biomechanical factors and HLA-B27 in magnetic resonance imaging-determined bone changes in plantar fascia enthesopathy. Arthritis Rheum 46(2):489-93, 2002
2. Recht MP et al: Magnetic resonance imaging of the foot and ankle. J Am Acad Orthop Surg 9(3):187-99, 2001
3. Balen PF et al: Association of posterior tibial tendon injury with spring ligament injury, sinus tarsi abnormality, and plantar fasciitis on MR imaging. AJR 176(5):1137-43, 2001
4. Theodorou DJ et al: Disorders of the plantar aponeurosis: A spectrum of MR imaging findings. AJR 176(1):97-104, 2001
5. Theodorou DJ et al: Plantar fasciitis and fascial rupture: MR imaging findings in 26 patients supplemented with anatomic data in cadavers. Radiographics 20 Spec No:S181-97, 2000
6. Narvaez JA et al: Painful heel: MR imaging findings. Radiographics 20(2):333-52, 2000
7. Yu JS et al: Foot pain after a plantar fasciotomy: An MR analysis to determine potential causes. J Comput Assist Tomogr 23(5):707-12, 1999
8. Yu JS et al: The plantar fasciotomy: MR imaging findings in asymptomatic volunteers. Skeletal Radiol 28(8):447-52, 1999
9. Grasel RP et al: MR imaging of plantar fasciitis: Edema, tears, and occult marrow abnormalities correlated with outcome. AJR 173(3):699-701, 1999
10. Schepsis AA et al: Plantar fasciitis. Etiology, treatment, surgical results, and review of the literature. Clin Orthop Rel Res 266:185-196, 1991
11. Berkowitz JF et al: Plantar fasciitis: MR imaging. Radiology 179:665-7, 1991
12. Amis J et al: Painful heel syndrome: Radiographic assessment. Foot Ankle 9:91-5, 1988
13. Kwong PK et al: Plantar fasciitis: Mechanics and pathomechanics of treatment. Clin Sports Med 7:119-26, 1988
14. Williams RL et al: Imaging study of the painful heel syndrome. Foot Ankle 7:345-9, 1987
15. Baxter DE et al: Heel pain operative results. Foot Ankle 5:16-25, 1984
16. Clancy WG Jr. et al: Tendinitis and plantar fasciitis in runners. Orthopedics 6:217-33, 1983
17. Graham CE: Painful heel syndrome: Rational of diagnosis and treatment. Foot Ankle 3:261-7, 1983
18. Snider MP et al: Plantar fascia release for chronic plantar fasciitis in runners. Am J Sports Med 11:215-9, 1983

IMAGE GALLERY

Typical

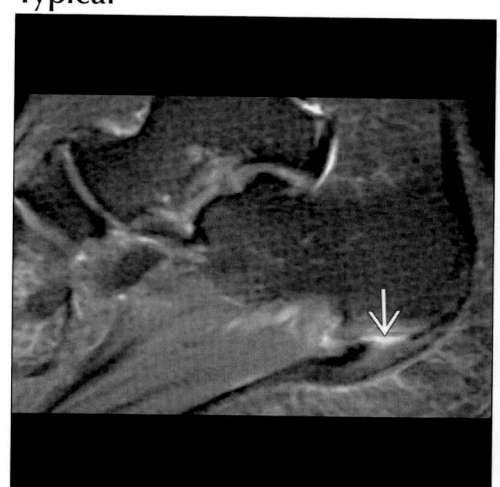
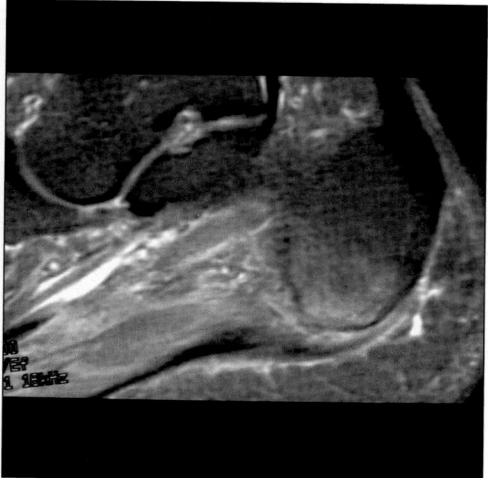

(Left) Sagittal FS PD FSE MR shows partial detachment (arrow) of plantar fascia adjacent to plantar enthesophyte and os calcis attachment. Partial retraction of the plantar fascia contributes to the thickening of the proximal aponeurosis. *(Right)* Sagittal FS PD FSE MR shows high grade tear of the plantar fascia with adjacent inflammatory change, calcaneal subchondral marrow edema, and hyperintensity of the flexor digitorum brevis.

Typical

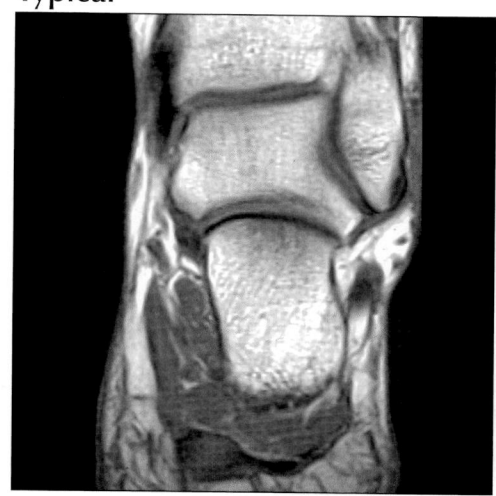
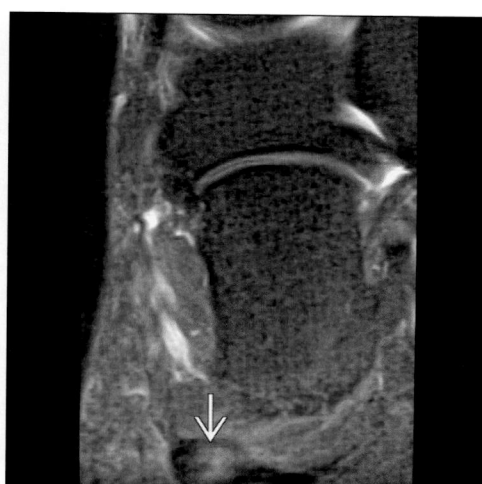

(Left) Coronal T1WI MR shows preferential involvement of the medial cord (band) of the plantar fascia with convex dorsal and plantar margins and central intermediate signal. *(Right)* Coronal FS PD FSE MR shows hyperintense inflammatory change of the medial cord (arrow) of the plantar fascia.

6

137

Typical

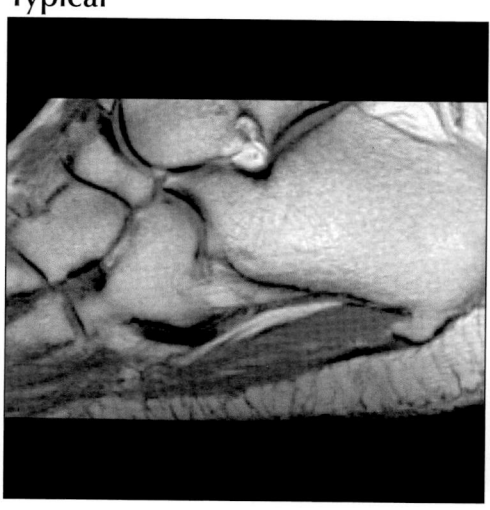
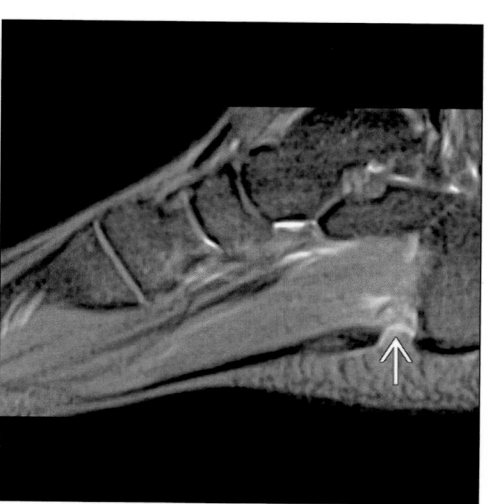

(Left) Sagittal T1WI MR shows large calcaneal enthesophyte adjacent to plantar fascia. Plantar enthesophyte is usually located in the toe flexor origins and not the aponeurosis. *(Right)* Sagittal FS PD FSE MR shows surgical release (arrow) of the plantar fascia origin.

PLANTAR FIBROMATOSIS

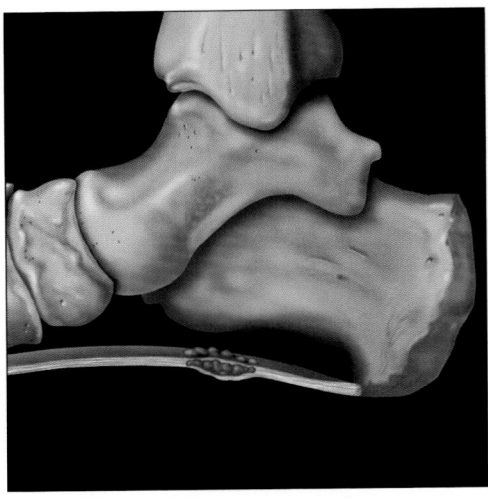

Sagittal graphic shows localized plantar fibromatosis with nodular thickening.

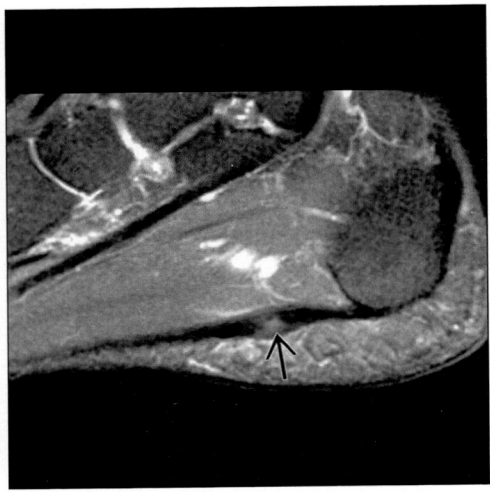

Sagittal FS PD FSE MR shows central hyperintense signal (arrow) in early lesion consisting of proliferating fibroblasts.

TERMINOLOGY

Abbreviations and Synonyms
- Collagenous fibromatosis, plantar fibromas

Definitions
- Fibrous and collagenous nodular development in plantar aponeurosis

IMAGING FINDINGS

General Features
- Best diagnostic clue: Nodular thickening in plantar aponeurosis
- Location: Plantar fascia + subcutaneous tissue usually medial
- Size: Usually less than 1 cm diameter
- Morphology: Nodular single or multiple lesions

MR Findings
- T1WI
  - Hypointense nodule
  - Central region of low to intermediate signal intensity
  - ± Low signal intensity effacement of plantar subcutaneous tissue
  - Long axis of nodule along long axis of plantar fascia
  - Normal thickness of adjacent plantar fascia
- T2WI
  - Mild hyperintensity plantar subcutaneous tissue
  - Convex dorsal (deep) and plantar (superficial) margins
  - ± Intermediate signal in adjacent unaffected plantar fascia
  - ± Infiltrative upper margins
  - ± Lesions deep to plantar aponeurosis
- T1 C+
  - ± Enhancement
  - Plantar margin more defined vs. infiltrative upper margin
  - ± Identification of multiple lesions
- Intermediate central signal intensity on FS PD FSE, STIR or T2* gradient echo imaging

Imaging Recommendations
- Best imaging tool: MR to identify location, morphology and extension relative to plantar aponeurosis
- Protocol advice: FS PD or T2 FSE or STIR sagittal images

DIFFERENTIAL DIAGNOSIS

Plantar Fasciitis
- Hyperintensity in thickened plantar fascial attachment to os calcis

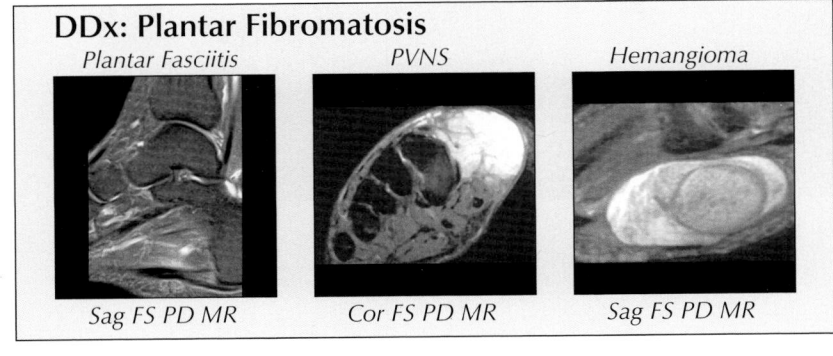

DDx: Plantar Fibromatosis

Plantar Fasciitis	PVNS	Hemangioma
Sag FS PD MR	Cor FS PD MR	Sag FS PD MR

PLANTAR FIBROMATOSIS

Key Facts

Imaging Findings
- Best diagnostic clue: Nodular thickening in plantar aponeurosis
- Morphology: Nodular single or multiple lesions
- Convex dorsal (deep) and plantar (superficial) margins
- Intermediate central signal intensity on FS PD FSE, STIR or T2* gradient echo imaging

Top Differential Diagnoses
- Plantar Fasciitis
- Lipoma
- Ganglion Cyst
- Pigmented Villonodular Synovitis (PVNS)

Pathology
- Superficial collagenous fibromatoses group

- Nodular or poorly defined aggregates of fibroblasts + dense collagen
- Infiltration of surrounding structures without malignant transformation

Clinical Issues
- Most common signs/symptoms: Mild plantar pain
- Asymptomatic vs. pain + discomfort with walking or prolonged standing
- ± Dupuytren's contracture (palmar)
- Nodules = firm and fixed to plantar aponeurosis

Diagnostic Checklist
- Use FS PD FSE, STIR or contrast to appreciate increased signal

---

- No discrete nodular thickening
- Partial detachment medial or lateral cord

Lipoma
- Subcutaneous tissue location
- Fat signal with suppression on STIR or FS PD or T2
- Heterotopic lipomas = intramuscular, intermuscular, lipoma of tendon sheath

Ganglion Cyst
- Common on dorsum of foot
- Round morphology
- Hypointense on T1WI
- Hyperintense on T2WI

Pigmented Villonodular Synovitis (PVNS)
- Inhomogeneous hyperintensity with hypointense hemosiderin (T2WI)

Hemangioma
- Dilated, serpiginous vessels
- Hypointense on T1WI
- Hyperintense on FS PD FSE, STIR or T2* gradient echo
- Extension to skin + subcutaneous tissue

Schwannoma
- Benign peripheral nerve sheath tumor
- Grows eccentrically from nerve
- Painless mass relative to major nerve
- ± Cystic degeneration

Neurofibromas
- Develop within a peripheral nerve
- Painless mass
- Minority of patients develop multiple neurofibromas (syndrome of neurofibromatosis)
- Target lesions with hypointense center + hyperintense periphery

Synovial Sarcoma
- Hypointense mass on T1WI
- Hyperintense mass on T2WI (FS or STIR)
- ± Adjacent osseous invasion
- Tracking along adjacent tendons

- Biphasic histology of epithelioid cells + fibroblastic spindle cells
- Occur in close proximity to joints

PATHOLOGY

General Features
- General path comments
  - Relevant anatomy = plantar fascia
    - From calcaneus to metatarsal heads and distally
    - Central, lateral + medial parts or cords
    - Central section ± contributions from plantaris + Achilles tendon
    - Lateral plantar aponeurosis = plantar to abductor digiti minimi muscle
    - Medial plantar aponeurosis = plantar to abductor hallucis muscle
- Genetics: Proposed genetic link based on occurrence of plantar + palmar fibromatosis together in some individuals
- Etiology
  - Superficial collagenous fibromatoses group
  - Association with Peyronie's disease + Dupuytren's contracture hand
- Associated abnormalities: Association with other collagenous fibromatoses (palmar + penile)
- Distribution
  - Solitary, multiple, unilateral or bilateral
  - Less common than palmar fibromatosis

Gross Pathologic & Surgical Features
- Similar to palmar fibromatosis - except without flexion contractures
- Single or multiple lesions
- Firm
- Thin poorly defined capsule
- Cut surface gray-white or gray-yellow

Microscopic Features
- Nodular or poorly defined aggregates of fibroblasts + dense collagen
- Myofibroblasts

PLANTAR FIBROMATOSIS

- Infiltration of surrounding structures without malignant transformation
- Mitotic figures uncommon

Staging, Grading or Classification Criteria
- Proliferative phase = fibroblastic activity & cellular proliferation
- Involutional phase = active phase with nodule formation
- Residual phase = reduced fibroblastic activity + collagen maturation

CLINICAL ISSUES

Presentation
- Most common signs/symptoms: Mild plantar pain
- Clinical profile
  - Asymptomatic vs. pain + discomfort with walking or prolonged standing
  - ± Dupuytren's contracture (palmar)
  - Nodules = firm and fixed to plantar aponeurosis

Demographics
- Age: Fibromatosis usually in ages 65 and older (especially palmar fibromatosis)
- Gender: Slight predilection for men

Natural History & Prognosis
- ± Gradual enlargement
- More extensive distribution
- Increasing number of nodules
- No contractures of toes

Treatment
- Conservative
  - Orthotics
  - ± Anti-inflammatory agents
- Surgical
  - Excision
- Complications
  - Local recurrence

DIAGNOSTIC CHECKLIST

Consider
- Occurs in more distal location compared to plantar fasciitis
- Use FS PD FSE, STIR or contrast to appreciate increased signal
- Upper or dorsal margins frequently infiltrative

SELECTED REFERENCES

1. Recht MP et al: Magnetic resonance imaging of the foot and ankle. J Am Acad Orthop Surg 9(3):187-99, 2001
2. Ng A et al: Atypical presentation of plantar fasciitis secondary to soft-tissue mass infiltration. J Am Podiatr Med Assoc 91(2):89-92, 2001
3. Theodorou DJ et al: Disorders of the plantar aponeurosis: A spectrum of MR imaging findings. AJR 176(1):97-104, 2001
4. Timins ME: MR imaging of the foot and ankle. Foot Ankle Clin 5(1):83-101, Review, 2000
5. Yu JS: Pathologic and post-operative conditions of the plantar fascia: Review of MR imaging appearances. Skeletal Radiol 29(9):491-501, Review, 2000
6. Llauger J et al: MR imaging of benign soft-tissue masses of the foot and ankle. Radiographics 18(6):1481-98, Review, 1998
7. Ericson SJ et al: MR imaging of the ankle and foot. Radiol Clin North Am 35(1):163-92, Review, 1997
8. Morrison WB et al: Plantar fibromatosis: A benign aggressive neoplasm with a characteristic appearance on MR images. Radiology 193(3):841-5, 1994
9. Pasternack WA et al: Plantar fibromatosis: Staging by magnetic resonance imaging. J Foot Ankle Surg 32(4):390-6, 1993
10. Berquist TH et al: Value of MR imaging in differentiating benign from malignant soft tissue masses. AJR 1251-55, 1990
11. Kirby EJ et al: Soft tissue tumors and tumor-like lesions of the foot. An analysis of eighty-three cases. J Bone Joint Surg Am 621-26,1989
12. Kransdorf MJ et al: Soft tissue masses: Diagnosis using MR imaging. AJR Am J Roentgenol 541-7, 1989
13. Chang AE et al: Magnetic resonance imaging versus computed tomography in the evaluation of soft tissue tumors of the extremities. Ann Surg 340-8,1987
14. Simon MA et al: Diagnostic strategy for bone and soft tissue tumors. Instr Course Lect 527-36, 1987
15. Totty WG et al: Soft tissue tumors: MR imaging. Radiology 135-41, 1986

IMAGE GALLERY

Typical

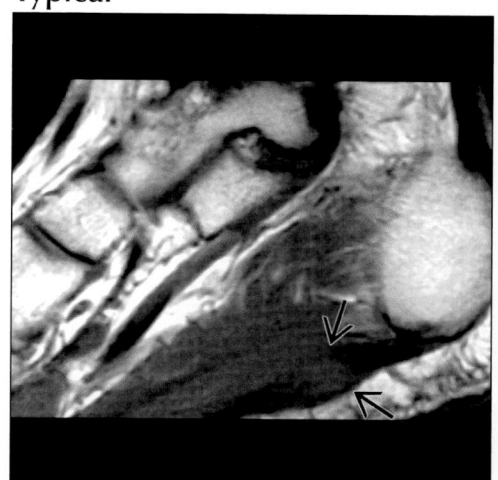
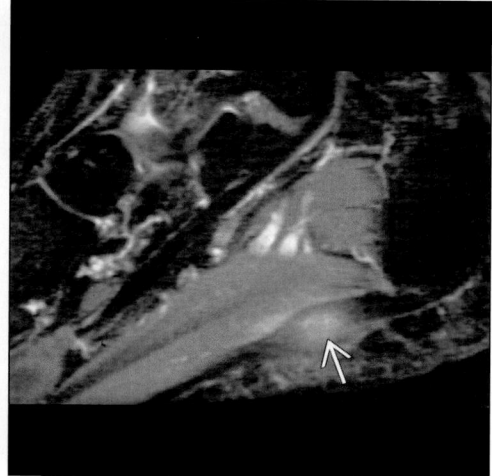

(Left) Sagittal T1WI MR shows convex margins (arrows) of plantar fibromatosis oriented along the long axis of the plantar fascia. *(Right)* Sagittal FS PD FSE MR shows convex deep and superficial margins with central hyperintensity (arrow).

Typical

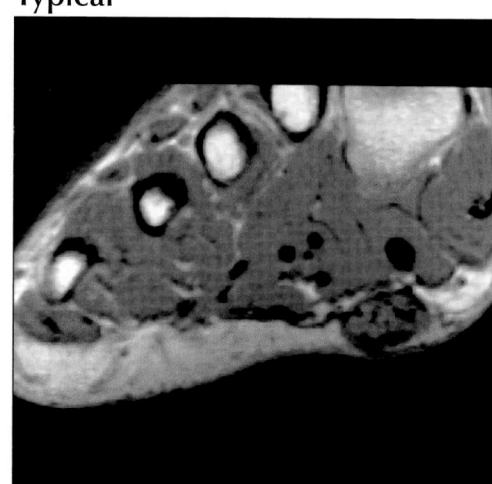
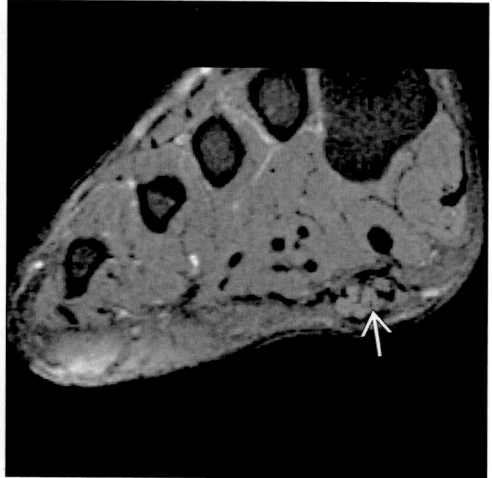

(Left) Coronal T1WI MR shows preferential involvement of the medial plantar fascia with large single nodular lesion. *(Right)* Coronal T2* GRE MR shows intermediate central SI with inhomogeneity of medial plantar fibromatosis (arrow).

6

141

Typical

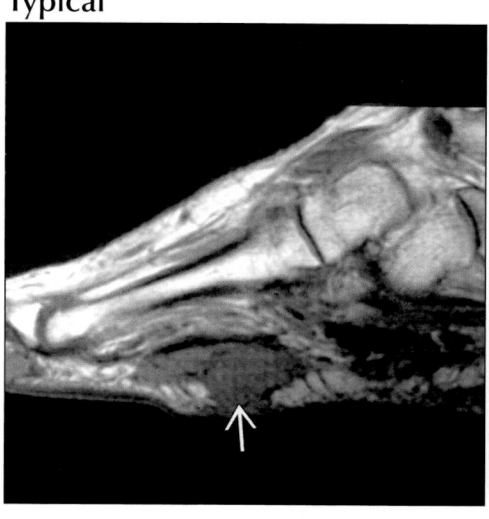
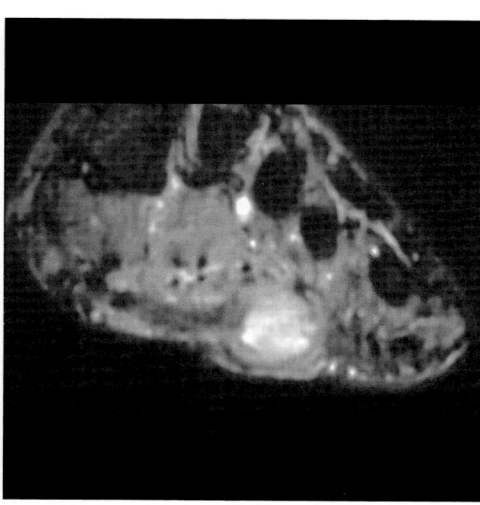

(Left) Sagittal T1WI MR shows plantar subcutaneus tissue extension (arrow) of the plantar fibroma. *(Right)* Coronal FS PD FSE MR shows well defined plantar margin and more infiltrative upper margins characteristic of plantar fibromatosis.

MORTON'S NEUROMA

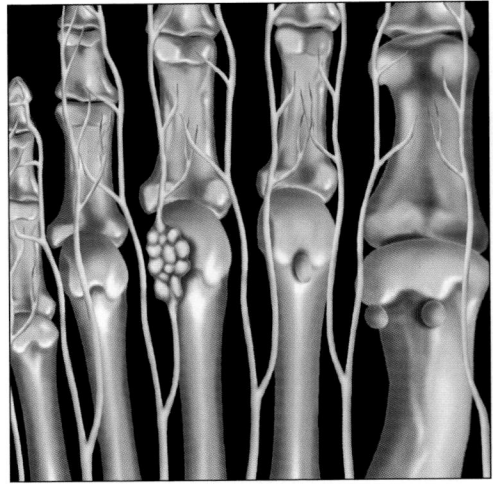

Axial graphic shows Morton's neuroma with localized enlargement of the interdigital nerve branch between the 3rd and 4th metatarsal heads.

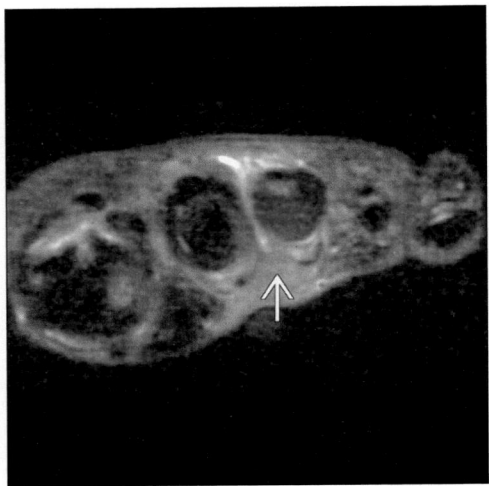

Coronal FS PD FSE MR shows hyperintense mass (arrow) plantar to the metatarsal heads in the 2nd interspace.

TERMINOLOGY

Abbreviations and Synonyms
- Metatarsalgia, interdigital neuralgia

Definitions
- Metatarsalgia + localized enlargement of the interdigital nerve between 3rd + 4th metatarsal heads

IMAGING FINDINGS

General Features
- Best diagnostic clue: Soft tissue mass between ± distal to 3rd + 4th metatarsal heads
- Location: 3rd common digital branch of medial plantar nerve, plantar to deep transverse intermetatarsal ligament
- Size: 5 mm or greater in diameter (normal interdigital nerve diameter = 2 mm)
- Morphology: Fusiform teardrop-shaped enlargement with bulbous plantar extension

Radiographic Findings
- Radiography
  - Increased intermetatarsal angle of affected interspace
  - Neuroma not visible

MR Findings
- T1WI
  - Hypointense to intermediate on coronal T1WI
  - Teardrop-shaped mass
  - Plantar to metatarsal heads in third interspace
  - Fat signal plantar subcutaneous tissue visualized superficial to mass
  - ± Hypointensity extending dorsal to transverse metatarsal ligament in a thickened/inflamed intermetatarsal bursa
- T2WI
  - Intermediate to hyperintense on FS PD FSE + STIR images
  - Intermediate without areas of hyperintensity on conventional or non-fat suppressed sequences
  - Effacement of plantar subcutaneous fat by convex border of teardrop-shaped mass
  - Inhomogeneity modified by degree of fibrosis
  - Hyperintense intermetatarsal bursal fluid
- T2* GRE: Intermediate to hyperintense
- T1 C+
  - Diffuse hyperintense enhancement
  - Enhanced lining of inflamed intermetatarsal bursa
- Epineurium fibrosis intermediate signal on T1+ T2WI

Imaging Recommendations
- Best imaging tool: MR for direct coronal cross sectional images in initial diagnosis and recurrence

---

DDx: Morton's Neuroma

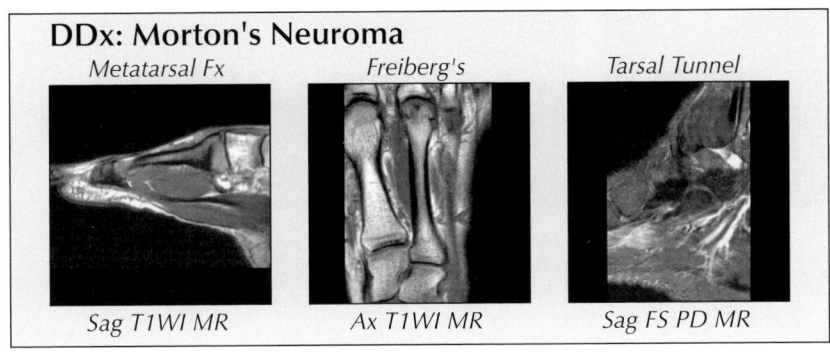

Metatarsal Fx	Freiberg's	Tarsal Tunnel
Sag T1WI MR	Ax T1WI MR	Sag FS PD MR

MORTON'S NEUROMA

Key Facts

Imaging Findings
- Best diagnostic clue: Soft tissue mass between ± distal to 3rd + 4th metatarsal heads
- Location: 3rd common digital branch of medial plantar nerve, plantar to deep transverse intermetatarsal ligament
- Intermediate to hyperintense on FS PD FSE + STIR images
- Effacement of plantar subcutaneous fat by convex border of teardrop-shaped mass

Top Differential Diagnoses
- Metatarsal Stress Fracture
- Osteochondrosis (Freiberg's Infraction)
- Tarsal Tunnel Syndrome
- Neurofibroma

- Intermetatarsal Bursitis

Pathology
- Entrapment neuropathy secondary to compressive forces against deep transverse intermetatarsal ligament
- Fibrotic response: Not true tumor
- Inflammation intermetatarsal bursa
- Dense fibrosis of axons and sheath (Schwann cells)

Clinical Issues
- Most common signs/symptoms: Plantar foot pain
- Paroxysmal burning sensation
- Neurologic pain in toe ± interdigital space

Diagnostic Checklist
- T1C+ useful especially in post operative recurrence

- Protocol advice: FS PD FSE or STIR or T1C+ direct coronal images

DIFFERENTIAL DIAGNOSIS

Metatarsal Stress Fracture
- Discrete fracture line/metatarsal edema
- Cortical thickening

Osteochondrosis (Freiberg's Infraction)
- Flattening second metatarsal head
- Subchondral fracture
- Sclerosis

Tarsal Tunnel Syndrome
- Medial tarsal tunnel mass
- Denervation hyperintensity

Neurofibroma
- Hyperintense on conventional, non-fat suppressed T2 as well as FS PD FSE images
- Morton's neuroma requires STIR or FS PD FSE or T1C+

Intermetatarsal Bursitis
- Hyperintense fluid between metatarsals (on T2WI)
- No focal soft tissue mass superficial to transverse metatarsal ligament

Rheumatoid Arthritis
- Inflammation intermetatarsal bursa
- Rheumatoid nodules
- Chronic joint involvement = synovitis = pannus
- Involvement begins at fifth ray metatarsal head + progresses medially

PATHOLOGY

General Features
- General path comments
  - Relevant anatomy
    - Third common digital branch of medial plantar nerve
    - Communicating branch lateral plantar nerve may contribute to 3rd common digital nerve (also supplies 3rd interspace)
    - Plantar nerve superficial to deep transverse intermetatarsal ligament
    - Third plantar metatarsal artery and veins also superficial (plantar) to transverse metatarsal ligament
    - Tendon of third lumbrical muscle - also superficial to transverse metatarsal ligament
    - Pacinian corpuscles in subcutaneous tissue
    - Fat pad of subcutaneous tissue superficial to plantar nerve
- Etiology
  - Entrapment neuropathy secondary to compressive forces against deep transverse intermetatarsal ligament
  - Localized enlargement third common digital branch medial plantar nerve
  - Fibrotic response: Not true tumor
  - Tethering 3rd common digital branch medial plantar nerve by anastomotic or communicating branch between medial + lateral plantar nerves
  - Traction on 3rd interspace nerve by hindfoot valgus, intermetatarsal bursitis or extreme dorsiflexion of toes (high-heeled shoes)
- Distribution
  - 93% of patients with foot pain
  - 64% to 91% third intermetatarsal space
  - Bilateral lesions in 0 to 12%
  - < 4% involvement in two intermetatarsal spaces

Gross Pathologic & Surgical Features
- Benign fusiform enlargement third common digital nerve
- Perineural fibroma
- Shiny + glistening white to yellowish surface
- Bifurcating digital branches + fusiform enlargement in resected neuroma
- Nodule ± attached to intermetatarsal bursa
- Inflammation intermetatarsal bursa

MORTON'S NEUROMA

Microscopic Features
- Neural proliferation
- Dense fibrosis of axons and sheath (Schwann cells)
- Degeneration
- Endoneural + neural edema (early)
- Perineural + epineural fibrosis + hypertrophy (late stages)
- Endoneural blood vessel wall hyalinization
- Perivascular fibrosis
- Vascular occlusion
- Endoneural + perineural mucinous change
- Demyelination + axonal loss
- Renaut's bodies (hyaline granules) in endoneural tissue in response to compressive nerve trauma
- Wallerian or fatty degeneration
- Axon regeneration

Staging, Grading or Classification Criteria
- Early stage = endoneural + neural edema
- Late stage = perineural, epineural & endoneural fibrosis

CLINICAL ISSUES

Presentation
- Most common signs/symptoms: Plantar foot pain
- Clinical profile
  - Pain = sharp, dull or throbbing
  - Paroxysmal burning sensation
  - Neurologic pain in toe ± interdigital space
  - Tingling toe or forefoot
  - Increased pain with walking also ± night pain
  - ± Numbness third + fourth toes
  - Exacerbation with wearing shoes + activity
  - Relief by rest
  - Positive Mulder's sign with palpation plantar interspace distal to metatarsal heads

Demographics
- Age
  - 40 to 60 years of age
  - Less common in teenagers
- Gender: Increased incidence in women

Natural History & Prognosis
- Tenderness with applied pressure to metatarsophalangeal joints
- Palpable mass dorsal or plantar
- Associated inflammation intermetatarsal bursa
- < 60% success for conservative treatment

Treatment
- Conservative
  - Avoid high-heeled shoes
  - Wider shoes + arch support
  - Metatarsal of pads
  - Injection of corticosteroids
- Surgical
  - Excision involved interdigital nerve
  - Epineural neurolysis or decompression
  - Endoscopic instrumentation
  - Percutaneous electrocoagulation
  - Carbon dioxide laser techniques

- Complications
  - Hematoma
  - Vascular ischemia
  - Hammer toes related to division of deep transverse intermetatarsal ligament
  - Painful stump neuroma
  - Continued pain
  - Subcutaneous fat pad atrophy with steroid injections

DIAGNOSTIC CHECKLIST

Consider
- Use FS PD FSE or STIR in the direct coronal plane to identify Morton's neuroma
- T2* gradient echo techniques can be used if there is inhomogeneity on fat-suppressed images
- T1C+ useful especially in post operative recurrence

SELECTED REFERENCES

1. Weishaupt D et al: Morton neuroma: MR imaging in prone, supine, and upright weight-bearing body positions. Radiology 266(3):849-56, 2003
2. Gentili A et al: MR imaging of soft tissue masses of the foot. Semin Musculoskelet Radiol 6(2):141-52, 2002
3. Banks A et al: McGlamry's comprehensive textbook of foot and ankle surgery. Morton's Neuroma. vol 1. Philadelphia PA, Lippincott Williams & Wilkins, (8):231-52, 2001
4. Still GP: Neurilemoma of the medial plantar nerve: A case report. J Foot Ankle Surg 40(4):236-9, 2001
5. Ashman CJ et al: Forefoot pain involving the metatarsal region: Differential diagnosis with MR imaging. Radiographics 21(6):1425-40, 2001
6. Bencardino J et al: Morton's neuroma: Is it always symptomatic? AJR 175(3):649-53, 2000
7. Morscher E et al: Morton's intermetatarsal neuroma: Morphology and histological substrate. Foot Ankle Ing 21(7):558-62, 2000
8. Zanetti M et al: Morton neuroma: Effect of MR imaging findings on diagnostic thinking and therapeutic decisions. Radiology 213(2):583-8, 1999
9. Llauger J et al: MR imaging of benign soft-tissue masses of the foot and ankle. Radiographics 18(6):1481-98, 1998
10. Zanetti M et al: Efficacy of MR imaging in patient suspected of having Morton's neuroma. AJR 529-32, 1997
11. Terk MR et al: Morton neuroma: Evaluation with MR imaging performed with contrast enhancement and fat suppression. Radiology 516-20, 1997
12. Williams JW et al: MRI in the investigation of Morton's neuroma: Evaluation with MR imaging performed with contrast enhancement and fat suppression. Radiology 239-41,1989
13. Sartoris DJ et al: Magnetic resource images: Interdigital or Morton's neuroma. J Foot Surg 78-82, 1989

MORTON'S NEUROMA

IMAGE GALLERY

Typical

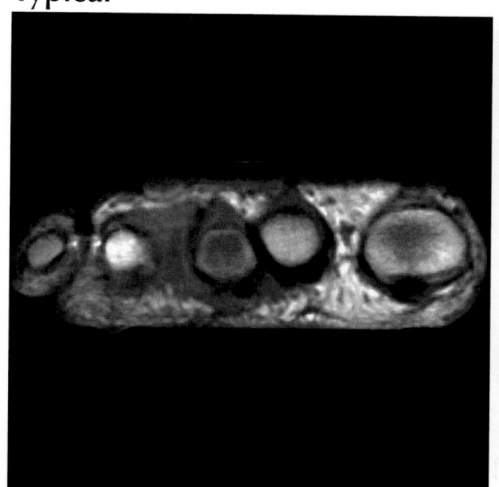
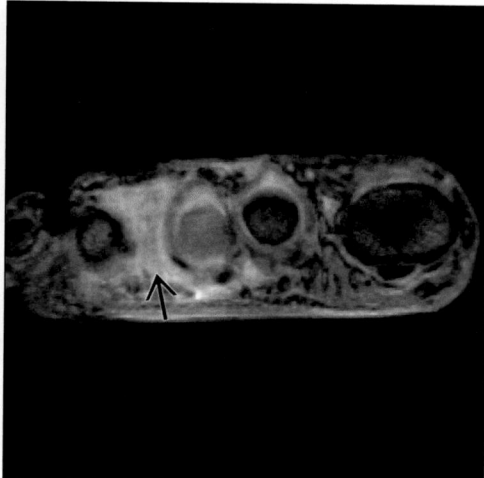

(Left) Coronal T1WI MR shows hypointense intermetatarsal bursal fluid associated with epineurium fibrosis. *(Right)* Coronal FS PD FSE MR shows hyperintense intermetatarsal fluid and inhomogeneity of Morton's neuroma (arrow) modified by the presence of fibrosis.

Typical

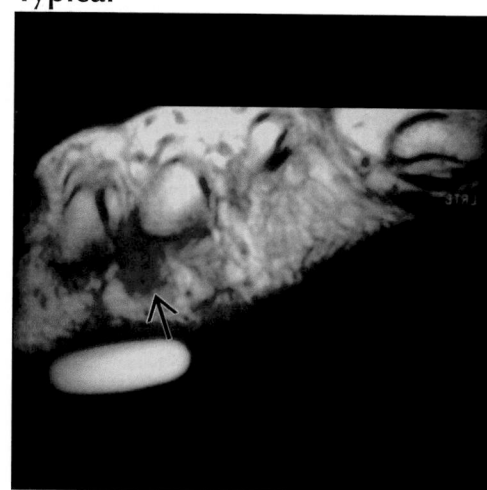
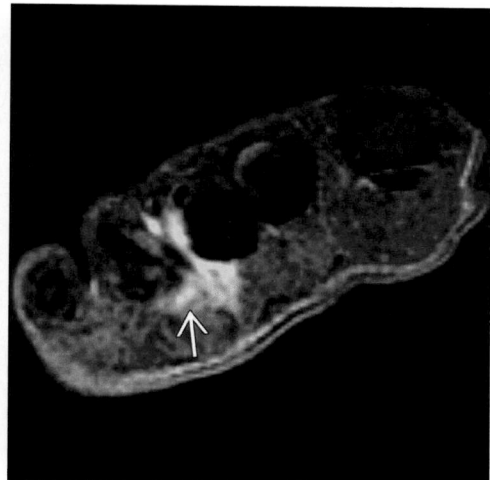

(Left) Coronal T1WI MR shows hypointense teardrop-shaped mass (arrow) projecting plantar to the metatarsal heads of the 3rd interspace. *(Right)* Coronal T1 C+ MR shows recurrence of a Morton's neuroma on a gadolinium-enhanced fat suppressed image. Intermetatarsal bursal enhancement medially is greater than the recurrent neuroma laterally (arrow).

Typical

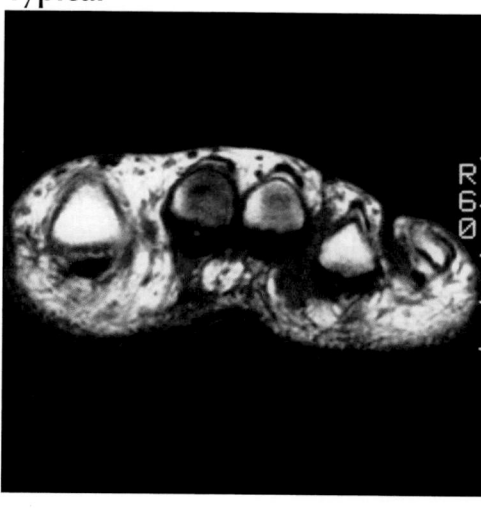
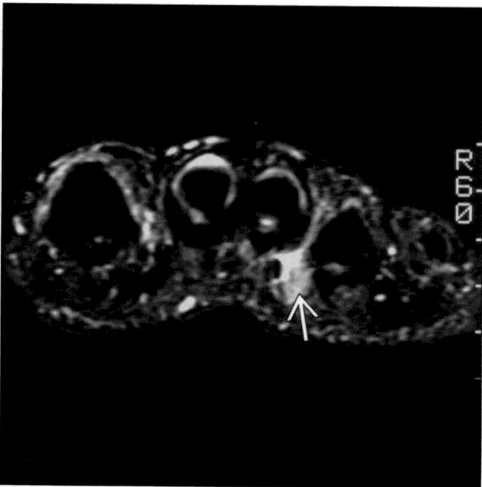

(Left) Coronal T1WI MR shows isointense Morton's neuroma with adjacent inflammation. *(Right)* Coronal STIR MR shows contrast differentiation between hyperintense inflammation medially and intermediate to hyperintense reactive connective tissue proliferation and nerve degeneration laterally (arrow).

DIABETIC FOOT

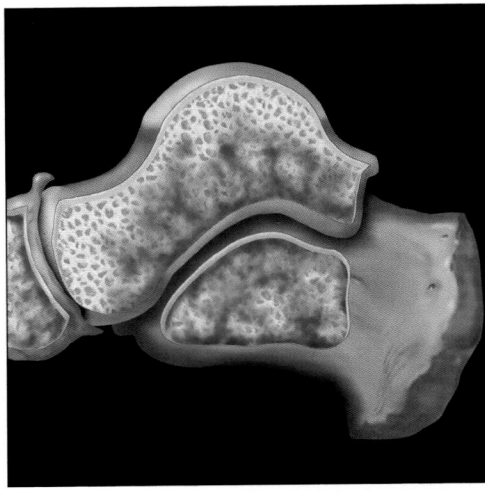

Sagittal graphic shows neuropathic edema (in red) involving the subarticular portions of the talus and adjacent calcaneus.

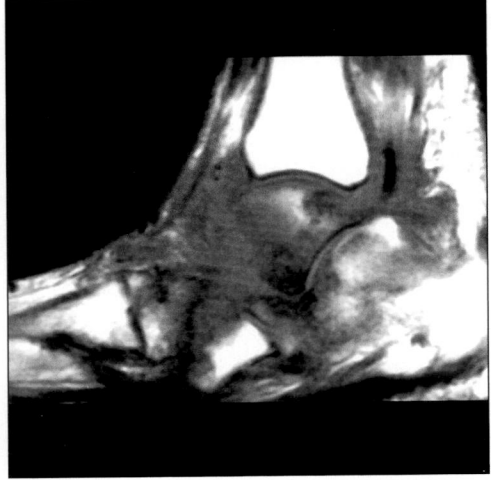

Sagittal T1WI MR shows neuropathic hyperemic marrow with hypointense signal changes involving the talus and calcaneus.

TERMINOLOGY

Abbreviations and Synonyms
- Diabetic foot ulcers and infection; neuropathic arthropathy

Definitions
- Soft tissue infection, osteomyelitis
- Neuropathic changes

IMAGING FINDINGS

General Features
- Best diagnostic clue
  - Osteomyelitis associated with pressure point ulcers + hyperintense osseous signal on T2WI
  - Neuropathic arthropathy - involves midfoot joints with intermediate to hyperintense signal on T2WI without overlying ulcer or pressure point
- Location
  - Pressure lesions in foot/infection sites
    - Plantar relative to 1st + 5th metatarsal heads
    - Calcaneal tuberosity
    - Malleoli
    - Medial to 1st metatarsal head
  - Neuropathic: Midfoot or multiple joints without overlying ulcers

- Size: Variable, with neuropathic joint involvement over several tarsal bones
- Morphology
  - Ulcers - curve of 1st + 5th metatarsal heads
  - Neuropathic ulcer - under metatarsal head + thick hyperkeratosis
  - Ischemic ulcer - fibrotic base without hyperkeratosis
  - Charcot foot - foot collapse, arch flattens + osseous destruction + bone formation and subluxation/dislocation
  - Osteomyelitis - soft tissue infection ± skin tract from ulcer to bone

Radiographic Findings
- Radiography
  - Limited for acute osteomyelitis
  - Infection associated with periosteal reaction, lytic lesions or sclerotic sequestra
  - ± Osteolysis distal forefoot to mid-metatarsal level + neuropathic process
  - Charcot process - osteopenia + fracture/dislocation or fragmentation

MR Findings
- T1WI
  - Hypointense to intermediate signal in ulcer
  - Ulcer ± cystic component
  - Pressure lesion/ulcer with hypointense effacement of subcutaneous fat or fat plane

---

DDx: Diabetic Foot

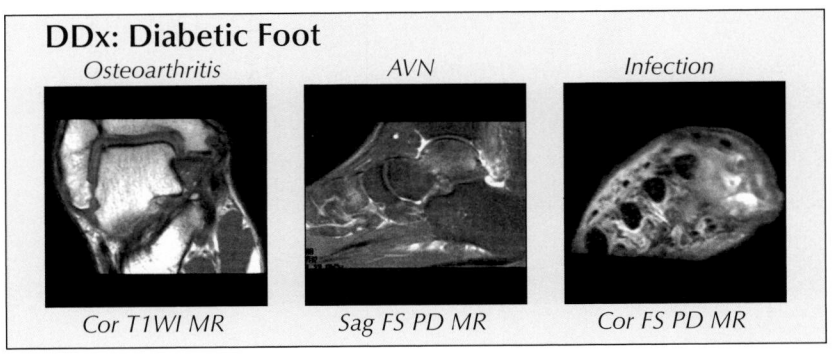

Osteoarthritis	AVN	Infection
Cor T1WI MR	Sag FS PD MR	Cor FS PD MR

DIABETIC FOOT

Key Facts

Terminology
- Neuropathic changes

Imaging Findings
- Osteomyelitis associated with pressure point ulcers + hyperintense osseous signal on T2WI
- Neuropathic changes common: Metatarsophalangeal, tarsometatarsal, intertarsal joints
- Neuropathic + osteomyelitis change hyperintense on FS PD FSE or STIR
- Primary findings in osteomyelitis = hyperintense soft tissue tract from skin ulcer to bone + osseous erosion and marrow edema on T2WI

Top Differential Diagnoses
- Osteoarthritis
- Osteonecrosis

- Infection

Pathology
- Neuropathy - sensory type responsible for diabetic foot complications
- Charcot's neuroarthropathy = motor + autonomic
- Plantar surface forefoot ulcers in diabetic feet

Clinical Issues
- Diabetic foot ulcer = non-healed plantar ulcer
- Charcot's joint = painless swelling + erythema of foot + ankle
- Charcot's joints = fragmentation or dislocation

Diagnostic Checklist
- STIR or FS PD or T2 FSE = hyperintense for both osteomyelitis & neuropathic joints

---

- Neuropathic arthropathy hypointense replacement of fat marrow
- Neuropathic changes common: Metatarsophalangeal, tarsometatarsal, intertarsal joints
- Periosteal reaction + cortical destruction in osteomyelitis or neuropathic
- Muscle atrophy with fat signal intensity in neuropathic foot
- T2WI
  - Pressure lesions/ulcer intermediate signal intensity
  - Necrotic cystic center of ulcer = hyperintense
  - Cellulitis = hyperintense soft tissue
  - Abscesses - thick wall = central hyperintense necrosis
  - Neuropathic + osteomyelitis change hyperintense on FS PD FSE or STIR
  - Focal area of greatest hyperintensity = osteomyelitis superimposed over neuropathic change
  - Primary findings in osteomyelitis = hyperintense soft tissue tract from skin ulcer to bone + osseous erosion and marrow edema on T2WI
  - Neuropathic changes associated with joint based abnormalities including fragmentation + resorption
  - Reactive marrow edema in area adjacent to soft tissue inflammation visualized on STIR & FS PD FSE
- T2* GRE: Osteomyelitis frequently hyperintense on T2* gradient echo vs. neuropathic marrow which is not hyperintense
- T1 C+
  - Abscess enhances along peripheral wall
  - Enhancement may be present in both neuropathic + osteomyelitis
  - Cellulitis = larger area of diffuse enhancement

Imaging Recommendations
- Best imaging tool: MR to identify ulcer, cellulitis, soft tissue tract, osteomyelitis vs. neuropathic marrow signal
- Protocol advice
  - T1 - to assess marrow fat replacement and subcutaneous tissue effacement
  - FS PD FSE or STIR - for marrow edema

- T2* gradient echo to help differentiate osteomyelitis from neuropathic change

DIFFERENTIAL DIAGNOSIS

Osteoarthritis
- Cartilage destruction; lack of erosions
- Osteophytes; subchondral sclerosis + cysts

Osteonecrosis
- Avascular necrosis (AVN) - body of talus
- Localized ischemia produces diffuse marrow edema vs. diffuse infarction pattern

Infection
- Sinus tracts, multiple abscesses
- Loss of subcutaneous tissue planes

Calcium Pyrophosphate Dihydrate Crystal Deposition Disease
- Mixed erosive + productive process
- Subchondral cysts
- Intraarticular + paraarticular crystal deposition
- Uniform cartilage destruction

PATHOLOGY

General Features
- General path comments
  - Relevant anatomy - at risk
    - Metatarsal heads, calcaneal tuberosity
    - Tendo Achilles bursa
    - Soft tissue medial to 1st metatarsal head
    - Malleoli, distal toes
    - Tarsometatarsal joints
- Etiology
  - Neuropathy - sensory type responsible for diabetic foot complications
  - Neuropathy theories - sorbitol accumulation, glycosylation of proteins
  - Motor neuropathy - intrinsic muscle atrophy, weakness + foot deformity

DIABETIC FOOT

- ○ Charcot's neuroarthropathy = motor + autonomic
- ○ Arteriosclerotic disease - lower extremity ischemia
- ○ Biomechanics - decrease range of motion + tightness gastrocnemius/soleus complex
- ○ Posterior heel ulcers = heel pressure; ulcers sides + dorsum related to footwear
- • Epidemiology
  - ○ Diabetes mellitus = 5.9% population
  - ○ Foot problems = 20 to 25% of admissions for diabetic population
  - ○ Diabetic foot ulcers divided into 1/3 neuropathic; 1/3 ischemic + 1/3 mixed
  - ○ 2-4% diabetic patients = diabetic foot ulcers or deep infections

Gross Pathologic & Surgical Features
- • Diabetic foot ulcers
  - ○ Plantar surface forefoot ulcers in diabetic feet
  - ○ Associated claw toes and Charcot's midfoot
- • Charcot's joints
  - ○ Fracture
  - ○ Subluxation, dislocation
  - ○ Resorption + new bone formation

Microscopic Features
- • Diabetic foot ulcers
  - ○ Platelets, cytokines, neutrophils
  - ○ Chemotactic fractures
  - ○ Granulocytes + lymphocytes
  - ○ ± Fibroblastic + endothelial cell migration
  - ○ Failure of wound remodeling
- • Charcot's neuroarthropathy
  - ○ Osseous resorption + new bone formation in neuropathic joints
  - ○ Detritic synovitis with cartilaginous + osseous debris

Staging, Grading or Classification Criteria
- • Diabetic foot ulcers: Based on depth + ischemia
- • Charcot's joints
  - ○ Stage I = acute inflammatory process
  - ○ Stage II = reparative process
  - ○ Stage III = consolidation stage of healing

CLINICAL ISSUES

Presentation
- • Most common signs/symptoms
  - ○ Diabetic foot ulcer = non-healed plantar ulcer
  - ○ Charcot's joint = painless swelling + erythema of foot + ankle
- • Clinical profile
  - ○ Ulcer = tracks, abscess, bone or joint involvement
  - ○ Charcot's joints = fragmentation or dislocation

Demographics
- • Age
  - ○ Diabetic elderly population at risk
  - ○ Charcot's joint diagnosed in patients with diabetes for 10 years
- • Gender
  - ○ Neuropathic arthropathy - no sex predilection
  - ○ Neuroarthropathy associated with connective tissue disorders - more common in females

- ○ Neuroarthropathy associated with alcoholism + trauma - more frequent in males

Natural History & Prognosis
- • Diabetic foot ulcers
  - ○ At risk for infection = spontaneous drainage, erythema, cellulitis, ± lymphadenitis, osteomyelitis
- • Charcot's neuroarthropathy: Fixed deformity
- • Complications: Infection = polymicrobial

Treatment
- • Conservative
  - ○ Diabetic foot ulcers = bedrest, orthotics, casting, cast boots, crutches, walker or wheelchair
  - ○ Charcot's neuroarthropathy = non-weight bearing, cast, orthotic walker (total contact cast)
- • Surgical
  - ○ Diabetic foot ulcers = debridement + off-loading
  - ○ Charcot's neuroarthropathy = exostosectomy, arthrodesis, open reduction + internal fixation, reconstruction, + fusion
- • Complications
  - ○ Surgery in Charcot's joints associated with prolonged healing times
  - ○ ± Amputations for infections

DIAGNOSTIC CHECKLIST

Consider
- • Osteomyelitis associated with soft tissue ulcers at pressure points
- • Neuropathic joints - usually independent of soft tissue ulcers + typically involve joints
- • Hyperintensity on T2* gradient echo when present seen in osteomyelitis and not neuropathic marrow
- • STIR or FS PD or T2 FSE = hyperintense for both osteomyelitis & neuropathic joints

SELECTED REFERENCES

1. Fitzgerald RH et al: Orthopaedics. Sec 11 foot and ankle. The diabetic foot. 2nd ed. St Louis Missouri, Mosby Inc (11-5):1665-80, 2002
2. Morrison WB et al: Work-up of the diabetic foot. Radiol Clin North Am 40(5):1171-92, 2002
3. Ledermann HP et al: Tendon involvement in pedal infection: MR analysis of frequency, distribution, and spread of infection. AJR 179(4):939-47, 2002
4. Ledermann HP et al: Pedal abscesses in patients suspected of having pedal osteomyelitis: Analysis with MR imaging. Radiology 224(3):649-55, 2002
5. Ledermann HP et al: MR image analysis of pedal osteomyelitis: Distribution, patterns of spread, and frequency of associated ulceration and septic arthritis. Radiology 223(3):747-55, 2002

DIABETIC FOOT

IMAGE GALLERY

Typical

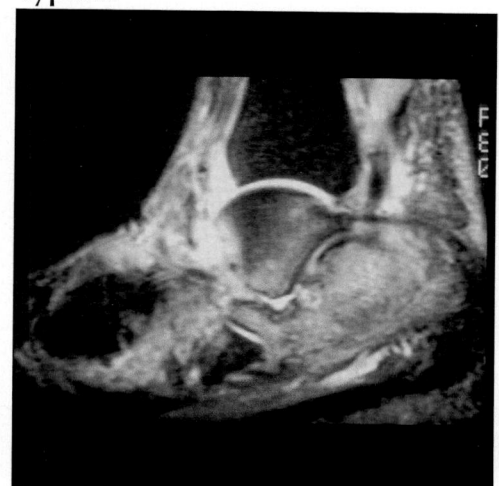 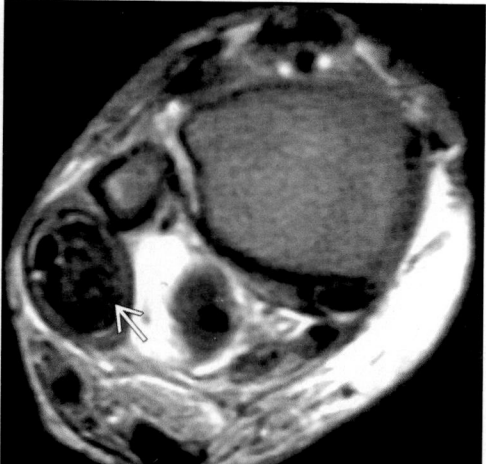

(Left) Sagittal STIR MR shows hyperintense neuropathic changes of the hindfoot associated with soft tissue inflammation. The differentiation between neuropathy and osteomyelitis may be more difficult with STIR imaging. *(Right)* Axial T2WI MR shows hypointense encasement (arrow) of the peroneal tendons with granulation tissue in a diabetic patient.

Typical

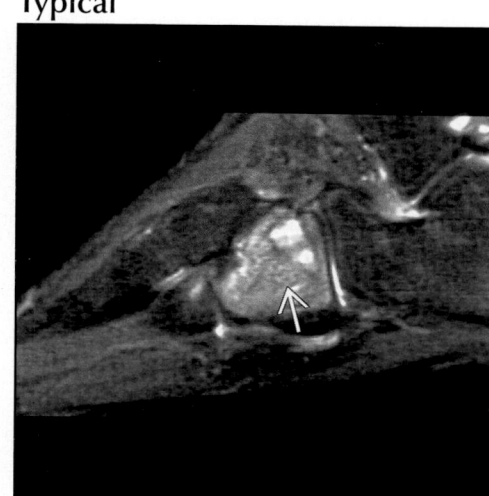 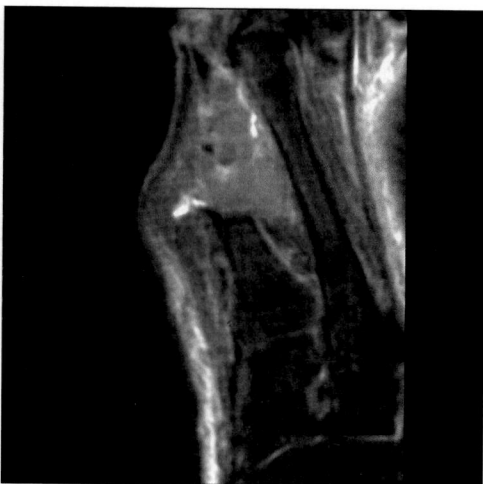

(Left) Sagittal FS PD FSE MR shows selective involvement of the cuboid (arrow) with osteomyelitis in a diabetic patient. Erosions are present in the proximal dorsal aspect of the cuboid. *(Right)* Axial FS PD FSE MR post amputation shows residual chronic soft tissue inflammation without osteomyelitis of the proximal metatarsal stump.

Typical

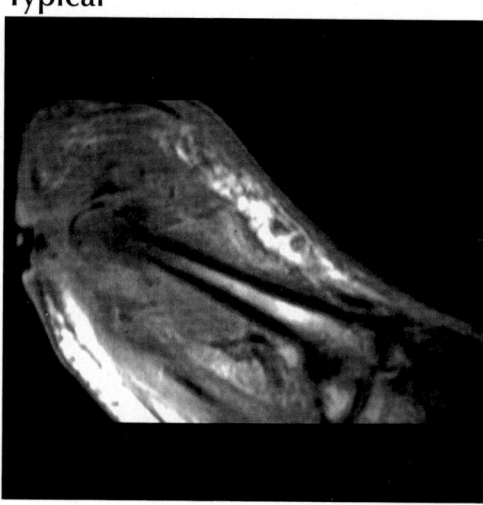 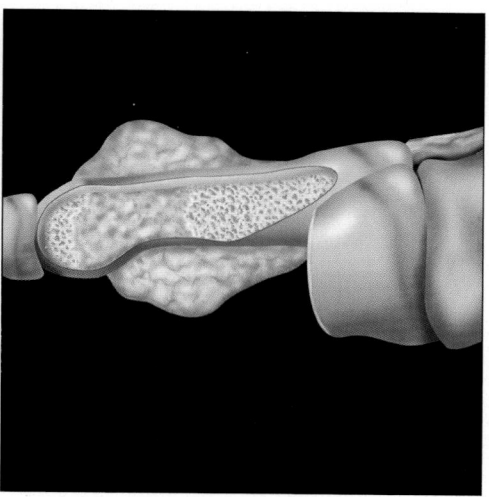

(Left) Sagittal T1WI MR shows osteomyelitis of the distal metatarsal in a diabetic patient. Marrow involvement and loss of distal cortices are best visualized on T1 WI MR. *(Right)* Sagittal graphic shows metatarsal osteomyelitis with medullary and soft tissue extension.

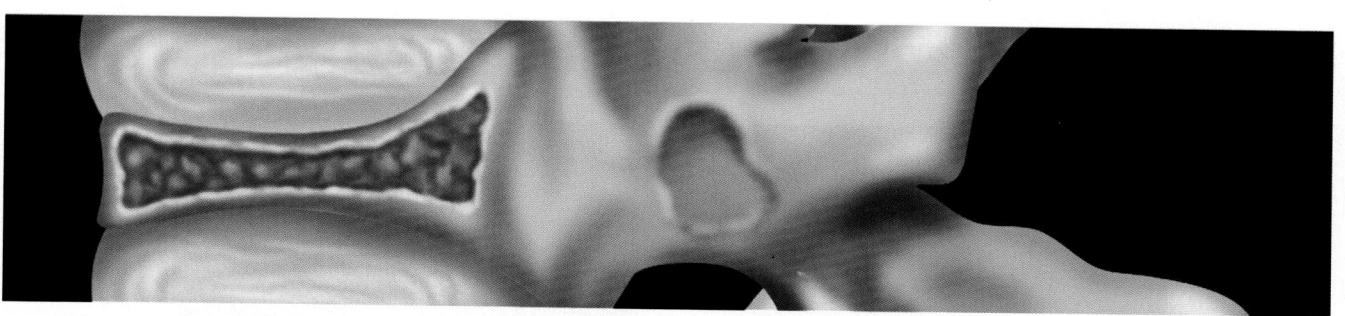

SECTION 7: Bone Marrow

1

LANGERHANS CELL HISTIOCYTOSIS

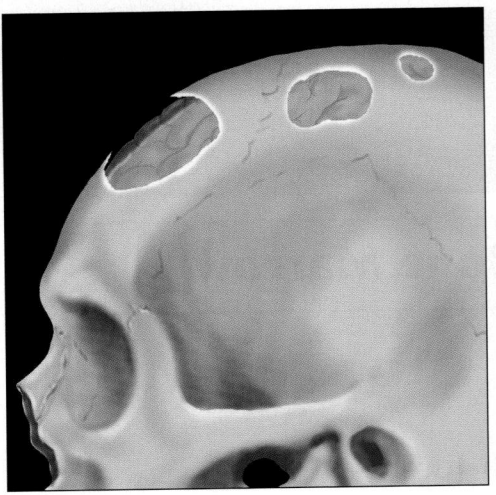

Sagittal graphic shows multiple lytic "punched-out" lesions of the skull. Note the well-defined beveled margins.

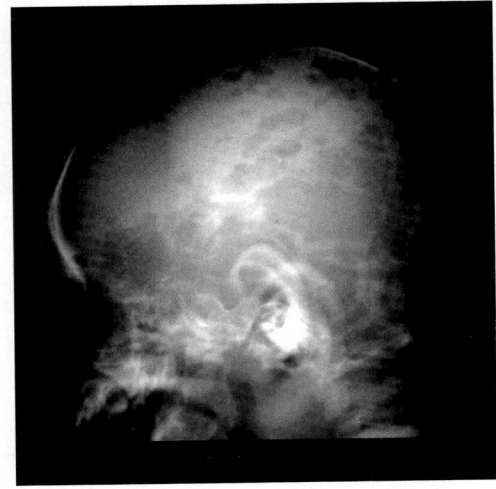

Lateral radiography in a child with disseminated Langerhans cell histiocytosis shows multiple well-defined lytic lesions involving the calvarium.

TERMINOLOGY

Abbreviations and Synonyms
- Histiocytosis X, eosinophilic granuloma (EG), Hand-Schüller-Christian disease, Letterer-Siwe disease

Definitions
- Group of disorders characterized by proliferation of Langerhans cells

IMAGING FINDINGS

General Features
- Best diagnostic clue: Well-defined lytic lesion without sclerotic rim
- Location
  - Flat bones: 70%
    - Calvarium
    - Mandible
    - Pelvis
  - Long bones: 30%
    - Metadiaphysis
  - Spine: 9%
  - Monostotic involvement: 50-75%
  - Multifocal involvement: 10-20%
    - Osseous lesions appear simultaneously or within 1-2 years

- If new lesions occur four years after initial diagnosis it should be interpreted as localized form
- Size: 1-15 cm, mean: 4-6 cm
- Morphology: Lytic and sharply demarcated "punched-out" lesions

Radiographic Findings
- Radiography
  - Skull
    - Well-defined lytic lesion without sclerotic rim
    - Sclerotic rim during healing phase
    - Occasional cortical destruction
    - Coalescence of lesions, geographic skull
    - Hole-within-a-hole appearance
    - Outer table of skull more destroyed than inner table; button sequestrum
    - Beveled edges
    - Soft tissue mass overlying lytic lesion
    - Floating tooth: Lesion in alveolar portion of mandible
  - Appendicular skeleton
    - Expansile lytic lesion with ill-defined, sclerotic edges
    - Endosteal scalloping, widening of medullary cavity
    - Lesions respect joint space/growth plate
    - Intramedullary in majority, can be intracortical
  - Ribs

DDx: Langerhans Cell Histiocytosis

Osteomyelitis	Ewing Sarcoma	Hemangioma	Leukemia	Metastases

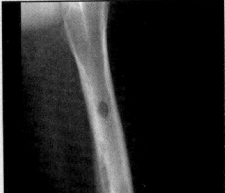
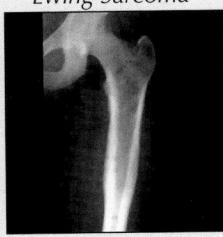
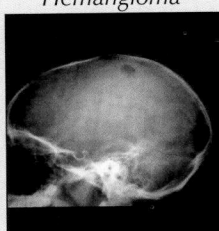
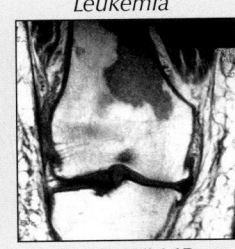
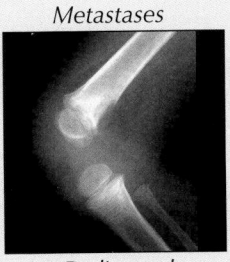

AP Radiography	AP Radiography	Lat Radiography	Cor T1WI MR	Lat Radiography

LANGERHANS CELL HISTIOCYTOSIS

Key Facts

Imaging Findings
- Best diagnostic clue: Well-defined lytic lesion without sclerotic rim

Top Differential Diagnoses
- Osteomyelitis
- Ewing Sarcoma
- Hemangioma
- Lymphoma
- Metastases

Pathology
- 1% of biopsied primary bone tumors

Clinical Issues
- Most common signs/symptoms: Local pain, tenderness, swelling

- Fever, elevated sedimentation rate, leukocytosis, peripheral eosinophilia
- Eosinophilic granuloma: Lung and lymph node involvement common
- Chronic disseminated form: Christian's triad (lytic skull lesion, exophthalmus, diabetes insipidus)
- Acute disseminated form: Acute onset of hepatosplenomegaly, rash, lymphadenopathy
- Benign course with healing of lesions after curettage
- Eosinophilic granuloma has best prognosis
- Spontaneous remission of bone lesions within 3 months to 2 years
- Acute disseminated form often fatal
- Observation
- Curettage with bone grafting of large lesions at risk of pathologic fracture

---

- Lytic expansile lesion
- Can have permeative appearance
  - Spine
    - Vertebra plana: Complete collapse of vertebral body
  - Pelvis
    - Involved in young children

CT Findings
- NECT
  - Helpful to assess extent of disease
  - Can show periosteal reaction, reactive sclerosis, beveled edges

MR Findings
- T1WI: Low signal intensity
- T2WI: High signal intensity
- T1 C+: Marked enhancement
- Destructive lesion with surrounding edema
- Can show early bone marrow involvement in absence of radiographic findings

Nuclear Medicine Findings
- Bone Scan
  - Increased uptake of radiotracer in majority of cases
  - Decreased uptake with surrounding halo of increased uptake
  - Normal uptake in 35%

Imaging Recommendations
- Best imaging tool: Radiographs, MRI
- Protocol advice
  - Radiographs diagnostic
  - Bone scan or skeletal survey to look for additional lesions
  - T1, FS T2 or STIR, T1 C+ MR to evaluate extent of lesion
  - Chest CT to evaluate for pulmonary involvement

DIFFERENTIAL DIAGNOSIS

Osteomyelitis
- Moth eaten appearance

- Periosteal reaction

Ewing Sarcoma
- Permeative bone destruction
- Lamellated periosteal reaction
- Progression of tumor
  - Langerhans cell histiocytosis: "Tempo phenomenon" rapid progression and disappearance of lesion

Hemangioma
- Calvarium: Radiating thickened trabeculae
- Greater expansion of outer than inner table

Lymphoma
- Older patients
- Permeative bone destruction

Metastases
- Metastatic neuroblastoma, rhabdomyosarcoma
- Permeative bone destruction
- Multifocal

PATHOLOGY

General Features
- General path comments
  - Letterer-Siwe (acute disseminated form): 10%
  - Hand-Schüller-Christian (chronic disseminated form): 20%
  - Eosinophilic granuloma (only bone involvement): 70%
- Etiology
  - Group of disorders involving abnormal proliferation of histiocytes in organs of reticuloendothelial system
  - Disorder of immune regulation rather than neoplastic process
- Epidemiology
  - 1% of biopsied primary bone tumors
  - Incidence: 0.05-0.5 per 100,000 children per year in the US

LANGERHANS CELL HISTIOCYTOSIS

Gross Pathologic & Surgical Features
- Sharply demarcated yellow, gray, or brown tumor mass with hemorrhagic areas
- Cortical disruption common
- Large areas of soft yellow tissue (representing lipid filled histiocytes) in lesions that undergo spontaneous involution

Microscopic Features
- Proliferation of Langerhans cells: Mononuclear histiocyte-like cells
  - Produce prostaglandin, causes bone resorption
  - Prominent indentation of nuclear membrane (nuclear groove), coffee bean nuclei
  - Low phagocytic activity, Birbeck granules (racquet shaped cytoplasmatic organelles)
  - Immunohistochemistry: Positive for S-100 protein and CD1a
- Infiltrate of histiocytes, eosinophils, lymphocytes, neutrophils, plasma cells
- Eosinophils may aggregate with necrosis (eosinophilic abscess)

CLINICAL ISSUES

Presentation
- Most common signs/symptoms: Local pain, tenderness, swelling
- Clinical profile
  - Soft tissue mass
  - Fever, elevated sedimentation rate, leukocytosis, peripheral eosinophilia
  - Fulminant forms can be associated with lymphoma
  - Eosinophilic granuloma: Lung and lymph node involvement common
    - Can be isolated to bone or lung
  - Chronic disseminated form: Christian's triad (lytic skull lesion, exophthalmus, diabetes insipidus)
    - Massive lymph node involvement, hepatosplenomegaly, pulmonary fibrosis, seborrhea
  - Acute disseminated form: Acute onset of hepatosplenomegaly, rash, lymphadenopathy
    - Skeletal involvement can be absent
  - Multiple lesions more frequently associated with involvement of parenchymal organs and skin
  - Mandibular involvement: Floating teeth, fractures
  - Pathologic fractures
  - Back pain from compression fractures (vertebra plana)

Demographics
- Age
  - 0-30 years, mean age: 5-10 years
  - 80% < 30 years, 50% < 10 years
  - Disseminated form can occur during first two years of life
- Gender: M:F = 2:1
- Ethnicity: More common in Caucasians

Natural History & Prognosis
- Benign course with healing of lesions after curettage
- Eosinophilic granuloma has best prognosis
  - Spontaneous remission of bone lesions within 3 months to 2 years
- Acute disseminated form often fatal

Treatment
- Observation
- Curettage with bone grafting of large lesions at risk of pathologic fracture
  - Usually no local recurrence
- Steroid injections
- Radiation therapy for inaccessible lesion
- Neurologic impairment from spinal involvement: Decompression, spinal fusion

DIAGNOSTIC CHECKLIST

Consider
- Important to differentiate localized from disseminated disease (different prognosis)

Image Interpretation Pearls
- Langerhans histiocytosis is "great imitator" of various benign and malignant bone lesions

SELECTED REFERENCES

1. Kilborn TN et al: Paediatric manifestations of Langerhans cell histiocytosis: A review of the clinical and radiological findings. Clin Radiol 58:269-78, 2003
2. Arico M et al: Clinical aspects of Langerhans cell histiocytosis. Hematol Oncol Clin North Am 12:247-58, 1998
3. Broadbent V et al: Current therapy for Langerhans cell histiocytosis. Hematol Oncol Clin North Am 12:327-38, 1998
4. Greenspan A et al: Differential diagnosis of tumors and tumor-like lesions of bones and joints. 1st ed. Philadelphia PA, Lippincott-Raven, 247-55, 1998
5. Lieberman PH et al: Langerhans cell (eosinophilic) granulomatosis. A clinicopathologic study encompassing 50 years. Am J Surg Pathol 20:519-52, 1996
6. Fisher AJ et al: Quantitative analysis of the plain radiographic appearance of eosinophilic granuloma. Invest Radiol 30:466-73, 1995
7. Kilpatrick SE et al: Langerhans cell histiocytosis (histiocytosis X) of bone. A clinicopathologic analysis of 263 pediatric and adult cases. Cancer 76:2471-84, 1995
8. Beltran J et al: Eosinophilic granuloma: MRI manifestations. Skeletal Radiol 22:157-61, 1993
9. David R et al: Radiologic features of eosinophilic granuloma of bone. Am J Roentgenol 153:1021-6, 1989

LANGERHANS CELL HISTIOCYTOSIS

Typical

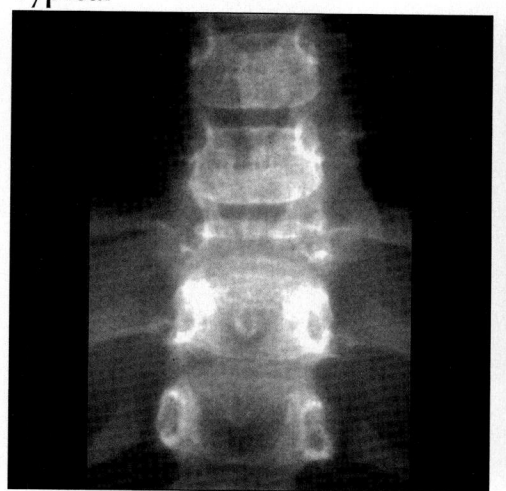
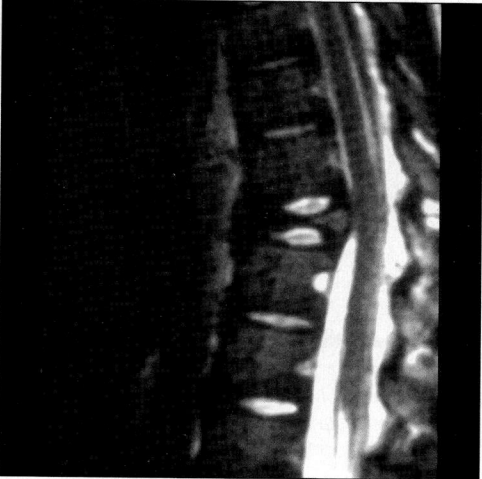

(Left) Anteroposterior radiography shows collapse of the T10 vertebral body, consistent with vertebra plana. *(Right)* Sagittal FS T2 FSE MR shows vertebra plana in the thoracic spine. Note preservation of intervertebral disk spaces.

Typical

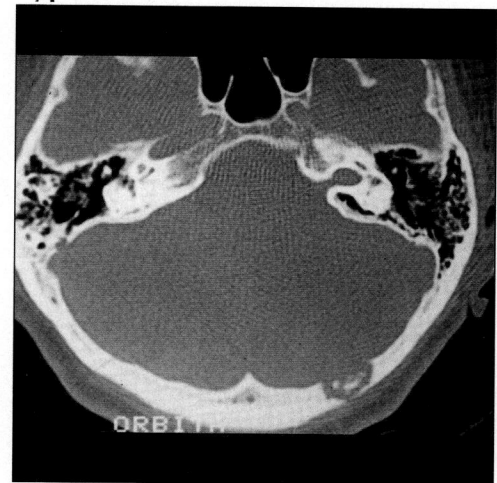
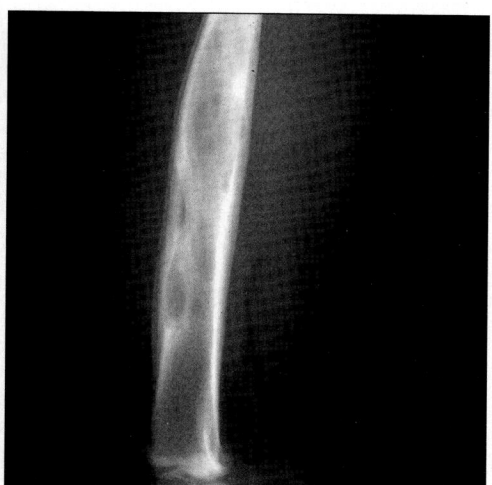

(Left) Axial NECT shows lytic lesion in the posterior left calvarium. Sclerotic central focus is consistent with a button sequestrum. *(Right)* Lateral radiography shows lytic lesions in the femoral diaphysis with sclerotic areas and periosteal reaction. These changes are seen in the healing phase of the disease. In this stage the lesion can be mistaken for osteomyelitis.

Typical

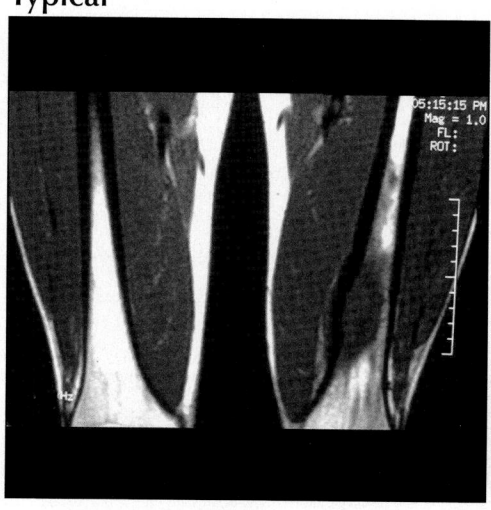
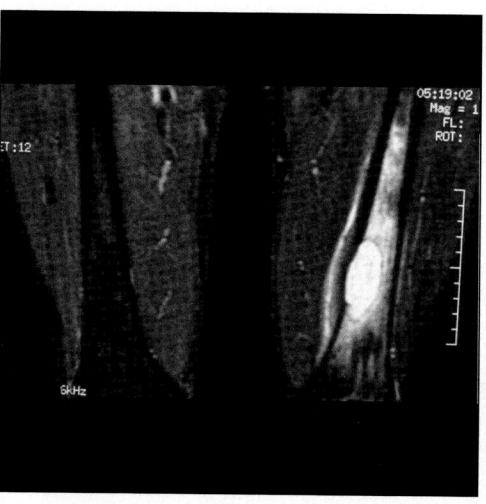

(Left) Coronal T1WI MR shows oval diaphyseal lesion of low signal involving the left femur. Surrounding bone marrow edema is hypointense. *(Right)* Coronal FS T2 FSE MR shows oval hyperintense lesion in the femoral diaphysis. Surrounding hyperintense bone marrow and soft tissue edema is noted.

EWING SARCOMA

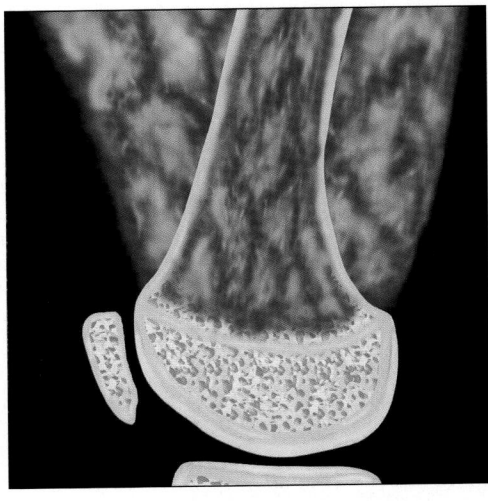

Sagittal graphic shows tumor involvement of the medullary cavity in the femoral metadiaphysis. Large extraosseous soft tissue component is shown in brown.

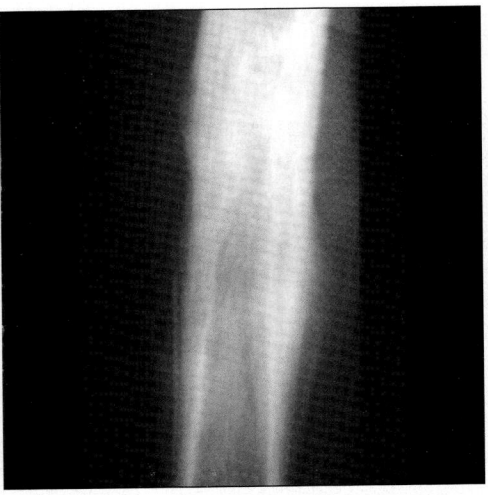

Anteroposterior radiography shows poorly defined diaphyseal lesion with permeative bone destruction and aggressive periosteal reaction.

TERMINOLOGY

Abbreviations and Synonyms
- Ewing's sarcoma, Ewing tumor

Definitions
- Round cell sarcoma of bone involving predominately long bones of skeletally immature patients

IMAGING FINDINGS

General Features
- Best diagnostic clue: Ill-defined intramedullary lesion with permeative bone destruction
- Location
  - Every bone can be affected
  - Diaphysis of long bones: 70%
  - Flat bones (sacrum, scapula): 25%
  - Ribs: 6%
  - Vertebral body: 5%
- Size: 3-20 cm long
- Morphology: Ill-defined lesion in diaphysis of long bones

Radiographic Findings
- Radiography
  - Ill-defined, lytic intramedullary lesion with permeative/moth eaten bone destruction
  - Prominent periosteal reaction of "onion skin" or "sunburst" type, Codman triangle
  - Cortical erosion, sclerosis, thickening
  - Saucerization of cortex due to periosteal destruction and extrinsic pressure from soft tissue mass
  - Penetration into soft tissue with extraosseous, noncalcified, soft tissue mass (50%)
  - No tumor matrix
  - Can be sclerotic in flat bones

CT Findings
- NECT
  - Intramedullary mass
  - Aggressive periosteal reaction
  - Associated soft tissue mass
  - Extraosseous (soft tissue) Ewing sarcoma: Rare
    - Nonspecific soft tissue mass
- CECT: Heterogeneous enhancement

MR Findings
- T1WI
  - Intermediate to low signal intensity
  - Hypointense compared to surrounding bone marrow
- T2WI
  - High signal intensity
  - Hyperintense compared to muscle
- STIR
  - High signal intensity
  - Helpful to show tumor extent and peritumor edema

DDx: Ewing Sarcoma

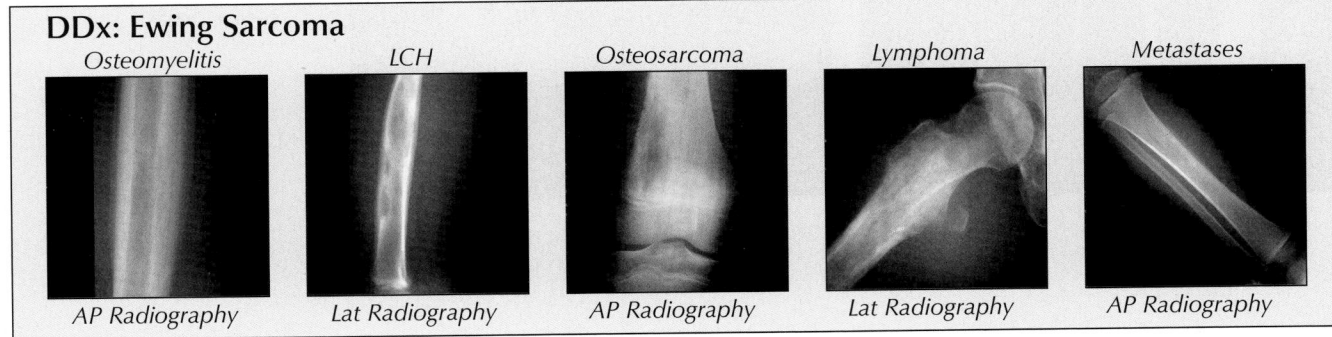

Osteomyelitis	LCH	Osteosarcoma	Lymphoma	Metastases
AP Radiography	Lat Radiography	AP Radiography	Lat Radiography	AP Radiography

EWING SARCOMA

Key Facts

Imaging Findings
- Best diagnostic clue: Ill-defined intramedullary lesion with permeative bone destruction

Top Differential Diagnoses
- Osteomyelitis
- Langerhans Cell Histiocytosis (LCH)
- Osteosarcoma
- Lymphoma
- Metastatic Neuroblastoma
- Primitive Neuroectodermal Tumor (PNET)

Pathology
- 6-8% of all primary malignant bone tumors
- 6th most common malignant bone tumor

Clinical Issues
- Localized pain
- Soft tissue mass
- Fever, leukocytosis, elevated ESR in disseminated disease (simulating osteomyelitis)
- Highly malignant neoplasm, 3rd leading cause of death in children between 10-14 years
- Metastases to lung, regional lymph nodes, and other bones in 30% at presentation
- Poor prognostic signs include increased age, large tumor, increased ESR and leucocytosis at presentation
- Adjuvant and neoadjuvant chemotherapy
- Surgical resection with wide margins in case of good response to chemotherapy
- Radiation therapy for surgically inaccessible lesions, stage III disease, poor response to chemotherapy

---

- T1 C+
  - To differentiate tumor from peritumoral edema
  - Enhancement of cellular areas
- To assess intra- and extraosseous extent

Angiographic Findings
- Hypervascular mass

Nuclear Medicine Findings
- Bone Scan
  - Intense radiotracer uptake
  - For evaluation of skeletal metastases
- PET
  - Increased FDG uptake of tumor and metastases
  - Helpful in assessing response to therapy
  - To differentiate tumor recurrence from post therapeutic changes

Imaging Recommendations
- Best imaging tool: MRI
- Protocol advice
  - Radiographs to detect aggressive periosteal reaction
  - MRI to determine extent of tumor
  - T1, FS T2W MR, STIR, T1 C+

DIFFERENTIAL DIAGNOSIS

Osteomyelitis
- May look identical
- Duration of symptoms usually shorter (< 2 weeks)

Langerhans Cell Histiocytosis (LCH)
- Solid periosteal reaction
- Less aggressive appearance

Osteosarcoma
- Usually involves metaphyses
- Bone formation within destructive lesion and soft tissue

Lymphoma
- Older age group
- Late cortical destruction

Metastatic Neuroblastoma
- Patients younger than 5 years
- Multifocal

Primitive Neuroectodermal Tumor (PNET)
- Clinically, radiologically, and histologically very similar to Ewing sarcoma
- Can not be differentiated from Ewing sarcoma by imaging

PATHOLOGY

General Features
- General path comments: Prototype of non-hematologic small round cell tumor
- Genetics
  - Reciprocal translocation of chromosomes 11 and 22 involving bands q24 and q12 in 90% of cases
  - Expression of new chimeric EWS/FLI-1 protein
- Etiology
  - Derived from undifferentiated mesenchymal cells of bone marrow or primitive neuroectodermal cells (small round cell tumor)
  - Associated with PNET
- Epidemiology
  - 6-8% of all primary malignant bone tumors
  - 6th most common malignant bone tumor

Gross Pathologic & Surgical Features
- Intraosseous component: Firm, gray-white, moist intramedullary mass
- Can involve large portion of medullary cavity without cortical disruption
- Cortex permeated by small nests of tumor, which penetrate cortex and grow subperiosteally
- Extraosseous component: Softer and more friable, may be considerably larger than intraosseous tumor

Microscopic Features
- Proliferation of undifferentiated mesenchymal cells
- Densely packed, small, uniform cells with round nuclei replacing medullary cavity

EWING SARCOMA

- Clear cytoplasm and nuclei with prominent cytoplasmic glycogen
- Two cell types
  - Principal type (light, open intact chromatin)
  - Secondary type (dark, condensed chromatin)
- Necrosis common
- Paucity of stromal elements
- No microscopic evidence of matrix production

Staging, Grading or Classification Criteria
- Surgical staging system for malignant musculoskeletal tumors
  - Stage IA: Low grade, intracompartmental
  - Stage IB: Low grade, extracompartmental
  - Stage IIA: High grade, intracompartmental
  - Stage IIB: High grade, extracompartmental
  - Stage IIIA: Low or high grade, intracompartmental, metastases
  - Stage IIIB: Low or high grade, extracompartmental, metastases

CLINICAL ISSUES

Presentation
- Most common signs/symptoms
  - Localized pain
  - Soft tissue mass
- Clinical profile
  - Most patients present with stage IIB lesion
  - Fever, leukocytosis, elevated ESR in disseminated disease (simulating osteomyelitis)
  - Pathologic fracture in 5-15%

Demographics
- Age
  - 5-25 years; peak: 15 years
  - 90% of patients present before 20 years
- Gender: M:F = 2:1
- Ethnicity: Caucasians: 96%

Natural History & Prognosis
- Highly malignant neoplasm, 3rd leading cause of death in children between 10-14 years
- Metastases to lung, regional lymph nodes, and other bones in 30% at presentation
- Presence of metastases best prognostic factor
  - Localized resectable disease treated with resection and chemotherapy: 5-year survival 70%
  - Disseminated disease: 5-year survival 30%
- Post-therapy necrosis important prognostic factor
  - 90-100% of necrosis strong predictor of long-term survival
- Poor prognostic signs include increased age, large tumor, increased ESR and leucocytosis at presentation

Treatment
- Adjuvant and neoadjuvant chemotherapy
  - Chemotherapy at time of diagnosis
  - If response is satisfactory (decrease of tumor size, pain relief, resolution of systemic symptoms) resection or radiation therapy
- Surgical resection with wide margins in case of good response to chemotherapy

- If solitary lesion involves expendable bone (long bones of upper and lower extremity, clavicle)
- In case of pathologic fracture
- In case of recurrence after chemo- and radiation therapy
- Radiation therapy for surgically inaccessible lesions, stage III disease, poor response to chemotherapy
  - Try to avoid radiating actively growing physis (risk of growth disturbance)
- Combination of chemotherapy, surgical resection, and radiation therapy in high-risk patients

DIAGNOSTIC CHECKLIST

Consider
- FDG PET useful to assess response to therapy potentially obviating repeated biopsies

Image Interpretation Pearls
- Can look and present clinically identical to osteomyelitis

SELECTED REFERENCES

1. Rodriguez-Galindo C et al: Treatment of Ewing sarcoma family of tumors: Current status and outlook for the future. Med Pediatr Oncol 40:276-87, 2003
2. Hawkins DS et al: Evaluation of chemotherapy response in pediatric bone sarcomas by -fluorodeoxy-D-glucose positron emission tomography. Cancer 94:3277-84, 2002
3. Devoe K et al: Immunohistochemistry of small round-cell tumors. Semin Diagn Pathol 17:216-24, 2000
4. Dorfman HD et al: Bone tumors. 1st ed. St. Louis MO, Mosby, 607-631, 1998
5. Llombart-Bosch A et al: Histology, immunohistochemistry, and electron microscopy of small round cell tumors of bone. Semin Diagn Pathol 13:153-70, 1996
6. Downing JR et al: Detection of the (11;22)(q24;q12) translocation of Ewing's sarcoma and peripheral neuroectodermal tumor by reverse transcription polymerase chain reaction. Am J Pathol 143:1294-300, 1993
7. Eggli KD et al: Ewing's sarcoma. Radiol Clin North Am 31:325-37, 1993
8. Oestreich AE: Imaging of the skeleton and soft tissues in children. Curr Opin Radiol 4:55-61, 1992
9. Bacci G et al: Long-term results in 144 localized Ewing's sarcoma patients treated with combined therapy. Cancer 36:1477-86, 1989
10. Boyko OB et al: MR imaging of osteogenic and Ewing's sarcoma. Am J Roentgenol 148:317-22, 1987

EWING SARCOMA

IMAGE GALLERY

Typical

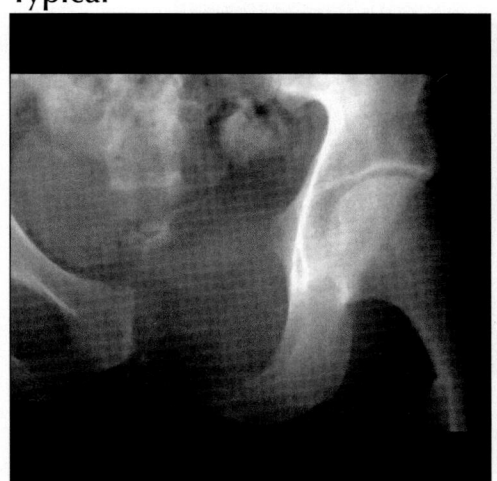
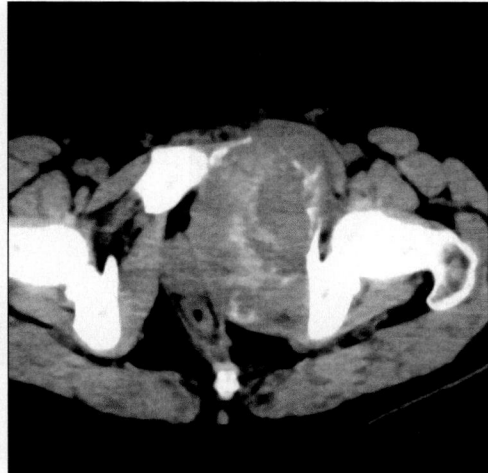

(**Left**) Anteroposterior radiography shows destruction of the left pubic rami with large associated soft tissue mass. Involvement of the flat pelvic bones is common in Ewing sarcoma and uncommon in other primary bone tumors in children. (**Right**) Axial NECT shows destruction of the pubic rami with large associated soft tissue component causing mass effect on the pelvic organs. Areas of calcification within the mass represent residual bone.

Typical

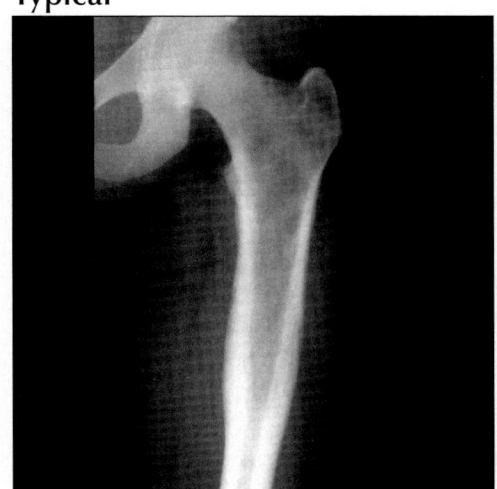
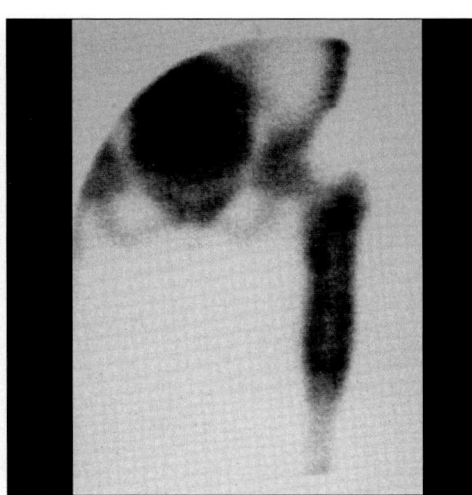

(**Left**) Anteroposterior radiography shows permeative bone destruction and aggressive lamellated periosteal reaction in the proximal femoral diaphysis. (**Right**) Anteroposterior bone scan shows increased uptake of radiotracer in the proximal femoral diaphysis. There is expansion of the involved bone.

Typical

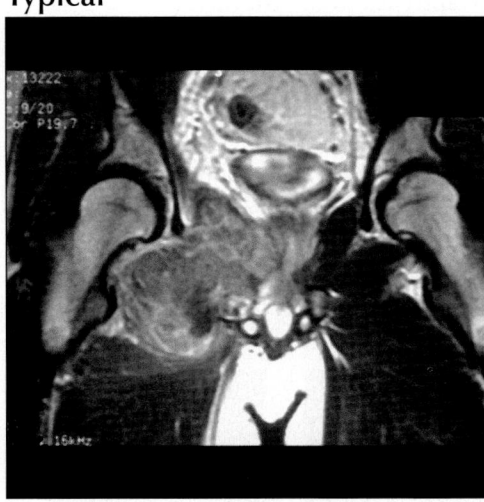
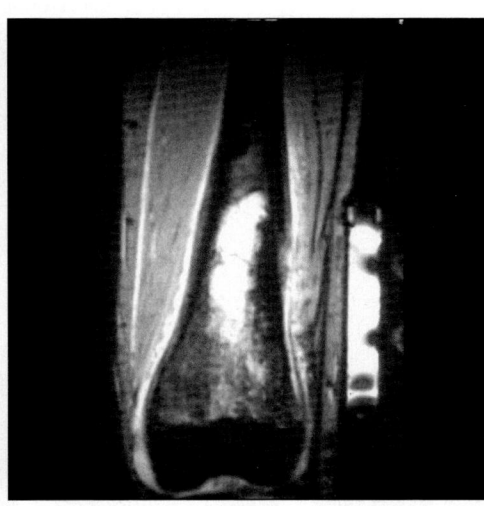

(**Left**) Coronal T1 C+ MR shows large soft tissue mass with heterogeneous enhancement in the right hemipelvis. Destruction of the pubic rami was seen on additional images. (**Right**) Coronal FS T2 FSE MR shows abnormal high signal in the distal femoral diaphysis, consistent with tumor involvement. Note associated soft tissue mass and cortical destruction.

LEUKEMIA

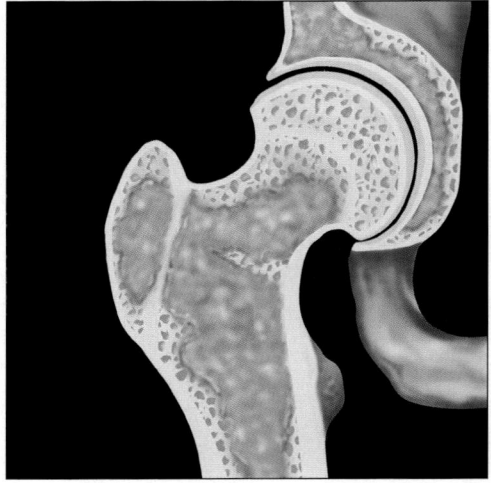

Coronal graphic shows leukemic infiltration of red marrow.

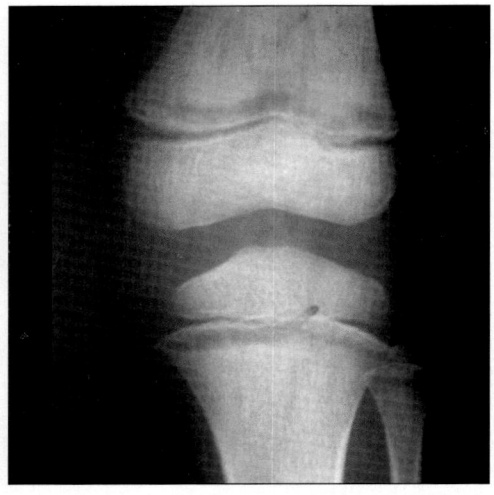

Anteroposterior radiography shows transverse radiolucent lines in the distal femoral and proximal tibial and fibular metaphyses (leukemic lines).

TERMINOLOGY

Abbreviations and Synonyms
- Acute lymphocytic leukemia (ALL), chronic lymphocytic leukemia (CLL), acute myelogenous leukemia (AML), chronic myelogenous leukemia (CML)
- Granulocytic sarcoma, chloroma

Definitions
- Neoplastic disorder of white blood cells that can be myeloid or lymphoid in origin and acute or chronic
- Granulocytic sarcoma (chloroma) represents extramedullary tumor of immature granulocytic cells in association with leukemia

IMAGING FINDINGS

General Features
- Best diagnostic clue: Moth eaten bone destruction +/- radiolucent transverse metaphyseal bands (leukemic lines)
- Location
  - Children
    - Femur: 24%
    - Humerus: 11%
    - Ilium: 17%
    - Spine: 14%
    - Tibia: 9%
    - Scapula: 4%
  - Adults: Axial skeleton
- Size: 3-10 cm
- Morphology: Moth eaten bone destruction

Radiographic Findings
- Radiography
  - Radiographically detectable bone lesions most common in children with acute leukemia
  - Diffuse osteopenia of spine and long bones
    - Radiographs can look normal
    - Coarse trabeculation of spongiosa
    - Collapsed vertebral bodies (vertebra plana)
  - "Leukemic lines": 40-53% in ALL
    - Transverse, radiolucent metaphyseal bands (most common in region of knee and humerus)
    - Horizontal bands in vertebral bodies
    - Dense metaphyseal lines post therapy
    - In patients < 2 years radiolucent lines are usually due to malnutrition, severe systemic disease
  - Focal destruction of flat/tubular bones
    - Multiple small well-defined osteolytic lesions
    - Moth eaten appearance
    - Lytic lesions distal to knee or elbow in children suggestive of leukemia
    - Blastic or mixed blastic-lytic lesions (rare)

DDx: Leukemia

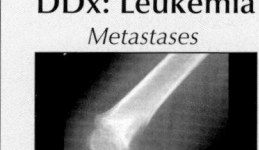 Metastases	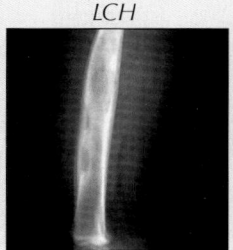 LCH	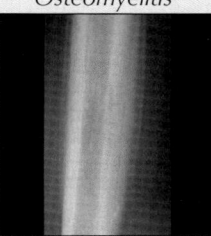 Osteomyelitis	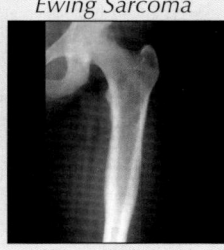 Ewing Sarcoma	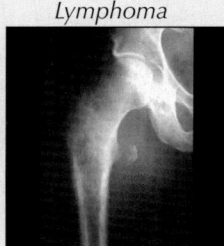 Lymphoma
Lat Radiography	*Lat Radiography*	*AP Radiography*	*AP Radiography*	*AP Radiography*

LEUKEMIA

Key Facts

Imaging Findings
- Best diagnostic clue: Moth eaten bone destruction +/- radiolucent transverse metaphyseal bands (leukemic lines)

Top Differential Diagnoses
- Metastases
- Langerhans Cell Histiocytosis (LCH)
- Osteomyelitis
- Ewing Sarcoma
- Lymphoma

Pathology
- Most common malignancy of childhood
- 20th most common cause of cancer death in all age groups

Clinical Issues
- Localized or diffuse bone pain
- Sharp, localized, recurrent paraarticular arthralgias (75%)
- Fever, elevated ESR
- May be confused with acute rheumatic fever, rheumatoid arthritis, osteomyelitis
- 5-year survival of all leukemias combined: 25-30%
- Children with ALL: Complete remission in 90%
- Adults with ALL: Remission in 60-80%
- Chemotherapy
- Intrathecal chemotherapy in case of CNS involvement
- Combined chemo- and radiation therapy
- Bone marrow transplant

- Sutural widening, prominent convolutional markings of skull
  - Periostitis of long bones: 12-25%
    - Smooth, lamellated, sunburst pattern of periosteal reaction
  - Pathologic fractures
    - Occur through abnormal metaphyses
    - Can result in slipped capital femoral epiphysis
  - Granulocytic sarcoma: Destructive lytic lesion

CT Findings
- NECT
  - Permeative bone destruction
  - Helpful in demonstrating localized mass in case of granulocytic sarcoma

MR Findings
- T1WI: Leukemic infiltrate of low signal, replacing high signal marrow fat
- T2WI: Increased signal intensity of leukemic marrow
- STIR: Increased signal intensity of leukemic marrow
- Most sensitive imaging modality, often positive when radiographs show no abnormalities

Nuclear Medicine Findings
- Bone Scan
  - Increased radiotracer uptake of involved areas
  - Often underestimates extent of disease

Imaging Recommendations
- Best imaging tool: MRI
- Protocol advice: T1, FS T2, whole body STIR MR

DIFFERENTIAL DIAGNOSIS

Metastases
- Metastatic neuroblastoma, rhabdomyosarcoma
- Bone involvement similar to leukemia
  - Metaphyseal bands, moth eaten bone destruction
- Multifocal

Langerhans Cell Histiocytosis (LCH)
- Lytic lesion

- Periosteal reaction
- Endosteal scalloping
- Soft tissue mass

Osteomyelitis
- Can have systemic symptoms similar to leukemia
- Periosteal reaction, soft tissue extension

Ewing Sarcoma
- No metaphyseal lucent lines
- Marked periosteal reaction
- Associated soft tissue mass

Lymphoma
- Older patients
- Large associated soft tissue mass

PATHOLOGY

General Features
- General path comments
  - Arises from primitive stem cell either de novo or from preexisting preleukemic state
  - Clone of malignant cells can arise at any stage of maturation
- Genetics
  - Patients with trisomy 21 and chromosomal translocations are at high risk of developing ALL
  - Trisomy 12 in patients with CLL
  - 90% of patients with CML have acquired chromosomal abnormality
    - Philadelphia chromosome, translocation between chromosomes 9 and 22
- Etiology
  - External factors: Alkylating drugs, ionizing radiation, chemicals (benzene)
  - Internal factors: Chromosomal abnormalities
  - Predisposing hematological disorders: Aplastic anemia, chronic myeloproliferative disorders
- Epidemiology
  - Most common malignancy of childhood
    - ALL: 75%, AML: 15-20%, CML: 5%

LEUKEMIA

○ 20th most common cause of cancer death in all age groups

Gross Pathologic & Surgical Features
- Hyperemic/hemorrhagic bone marrow with destruction of bony trabeculae
- Areas of bone infarction

Microscopic Features
- Diffuse infiltration of bone marrow by poorly-differentiated blast cells
- ALL: Infiltrates of small blue cells
- AML: Auer rods diagnostic
  ○ Condensed lysosomal cytoplasmatic rod shaped structures
- CLL: Mature lymphocytes, < 55% atypical cells
- CML: Leukocytosis with increase in basophils, eosinophils, neutrophiles
  ○ Philadelphia chromosome t(9;22)

CLINICAL ISSUES

Presentation
- Most common signs/symptoms
  ○ Localized or diffuse bone pain
  ○ Sharp, localized, recurrent paraarticular arthralgias (75%)
- Clinical profile
  ○ Fever, elevated ESR
  ○ May be confused with acute rheumatic fever, rheumatoid arthritis, osteomyelitis
  ○ Hepatosplenomegaly, lymphadenopathy
  ○ Joint effusion
  ○ Petechial hemorrhage, retinal hemorrhage
  ○ Anemia
  ○ Frequent infections
  ○ Proptosis, diplopia in orbital involvement
  ○ Patients with chronic leukemias can be asymptomatic

Demographics
- Age
  ○ ALL: Most common leukemia of childhood, peak: 2-10 years
  ○ AML: 15-20% of childhood leukemias, peak > 65 years
  ○ CML: Rare in childhood (< 5%), peak > 40 years
  ○ CLL: 50-70 years
- Gender: M:F = 2:1
- Ethnicity: More common in Caucasians

Natural History & Prognosis
- 5-year survival of all leukemias combined: 25-30%
- Children with ALL: Complete remission in 90%
  ○ 80% disease free 5 years after treatment
- Adults with ALL: Remission in 60-80%
  ○ 20-30% disease free 5 years after treatment
- AML: 5-year survival 45%
- CLL: Median survival 6 years
- CML: Median survival 5 years

Treatment
- Chemotherapy

○ Induction phase, consolidation phase, maintenance therapy phase
○ Intrathecal chemotherapy in case of CNS involvement
- Combined chemo- and radiation therapy
- Bone marrow transplant

DIAGNOSTIC CHECKLIST

Image Interpretation Pearls
- If leukemia is suspected MRI should be performed in case of negative radiographs or inconclusive laboratory findings

SELECTED REFERENCES

1. Beckers R et al: Acute lymphoblastic leukaemia presenting with low back pain. Eur J Paediatr Neurol 6:285-7, 2002
2. Barr RD et al: Impact of age and cranial irradiation on radiographic skeletal pathology in children with acute lymphoblastic leukemia. Med Pediatr Oncol 30:347-50, 1998
3. Greaves MF: Aetiology of acute leukaemia. Lancet 349:344-9, 1997
4. Gallagher DJ et al: Orthopedic manifestations of acute pediatric leukemia. Orthop Clin North Am 27:635-44, 1996
5. Heinrich SD et al: The prognostic significance of the skeletal manifestations of acute lymphoblastic leukemia of childhood. J Pediatr Orthop 14:105-11, 1994
6. Rivera GK et al: Treatment of acute lymphoblastic leukemia. 30 years' experience at St. Jude Children's Research Hospital. N Engl J Med 329:1289-95, 1993
7. Oestreich AE: Imaging of the skeleton and soft tissues in children. Curr Opin Radiol 4:55-61, 1992
8. McKinstry CS et al: Bone marrow in leukemic and aplastic anemia: MR imaging before, during, and after treatment. Radiology 162:701-7, 1987
9. Neiman RS et al: Granulocytic sarcoma: A clinicopathologic study of 61 biopsied cases. Cancer 48:1426-37, 1981

LEUKEMIA

IMAGE GALLERY

Typical

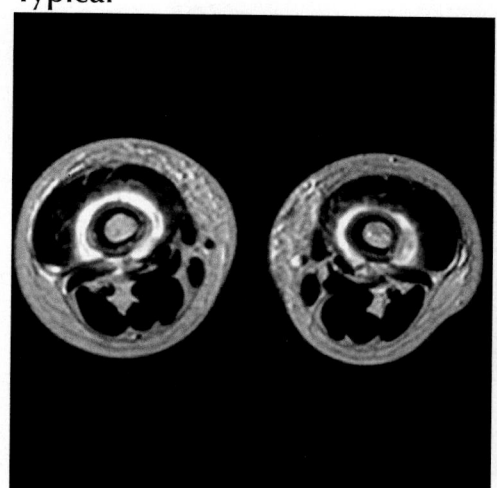

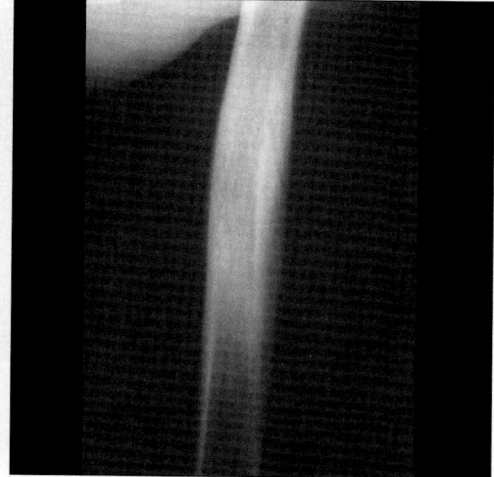

(Left) Axial T2WI MR shows abnormal hyperintense bone marrow and cortex of the femoral metaphyses. Note the surrounding hyperintense edema. *(Right)* Anteroposterior radiography shows permeative bone destruction and lamellated periosteal reaction.

Typical

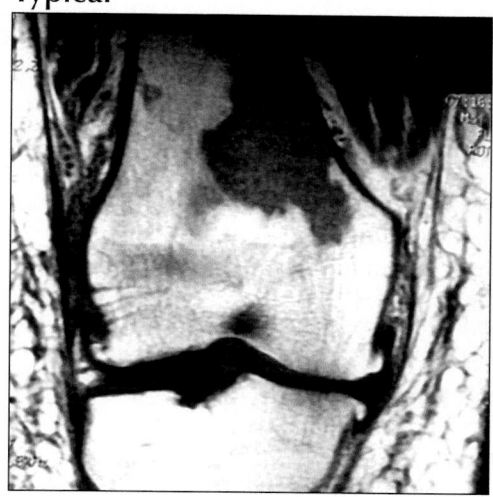

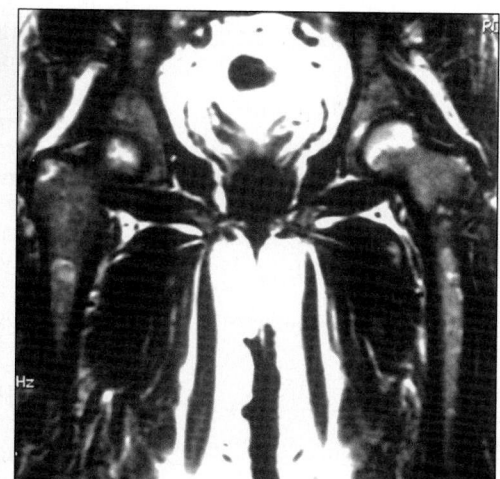

(Left) Coronal T1WI MR shows hypointense bone marrow infiltration of the distal femur in a patient with AML. *(Right)* Coronal T1WI MR shows diffuse hypointense bone marrow infiltration of the femoral metadiaphyses and iliac bones. Note the relative sparing of the epiphyses which contain predominately yellow marrow.

Other

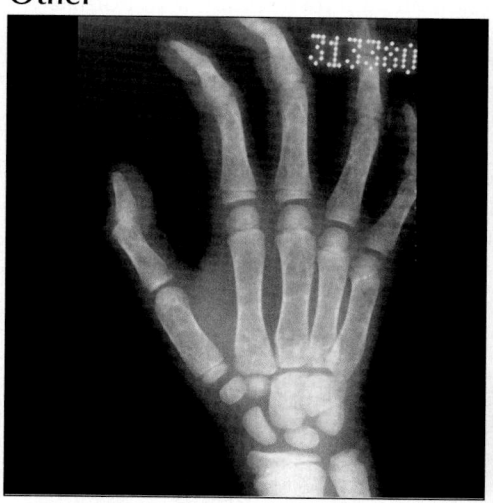

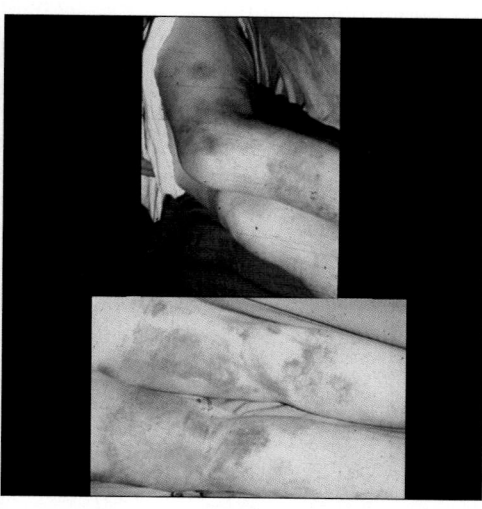

(Left) Anteroposterior radiography shows multiple small well-defined osteolytic lesions in the metacarpal and phalangeal bones in a child with ALL. *(Right)* Clinical photography shows red-violet nodules and plaques involving the lower extremities of a patient with AML. These findings represent leukemic infiltration of the skin and are usually a sign of disseminated disease.

LYMPHOMA

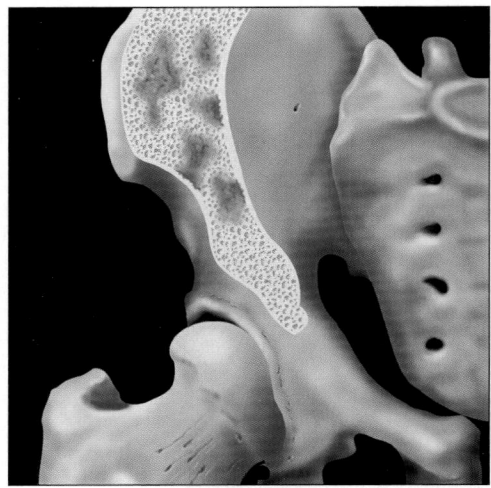

Coronal graphic shows lymphomatous bone marrow infiltration of the iliac crest.

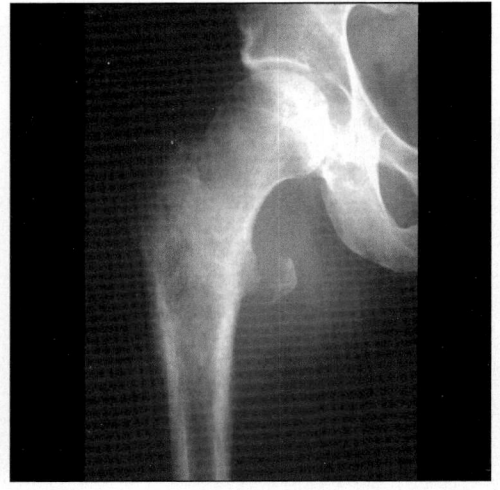

Anteroposterior radiography shows permeative bone destruction with periosteal reaction and large associated soft tissue mass. Note the pathologic fracture of the lesser trochanter.

TERMINOLOGY

Abbreviations and Synonyms
- Primary lymphoma of bone, reticulum cell sarcoma, lymphosarcoma

Definitions
- Lymphoma within medullary cavity of single bone without concurrent lymph node or visceral involvement for at least six months following diagnosis
- Must be distinguished from skeletal involvement in systemic lymphoma

IMAGING FINDINGS

General Features
- Best diagnostic clue
  - Mottled permeative pattern of bone destruction often with disproportionally large soft tissue component
  - Intact cortex despite soft tissue extension
- Location
  - Long tubular bones: 48%
    - Femur: 24%
    - Tibia: 10%
    - Humerus: 10%

- Pelvis: 20%
- Spine: 14%
- Skull: 7%
- Scapula: 5%
- Metadiaphysis
- Can involve entire bone with extension to subchondral bone
- Multifocal: 10-40%
  - Several foci in one bone, simultaneous involvement of multiple bones
- Size: 3-25 cm, mean: 5-10 cm
- Morphology: Permeative bone marrow infiltration with associated soft tissue mass

Radiographic Findings
- Radiography
  - Often normal
  - Cancellous bone erosion (earliest sign)
  - Mottled permeative pattern of bone destruction
  - Edges of lesion blend imperceptibly with normal bone
    - Radiographs often underestimate tumor extent
  - Mixed lytic-sclerotic lesions in 30%
  - Bone sequestrum: 11%
  - Late cortical destruction
  - Soft tissue component often disproportionally large
  - Sclerosis ("ivory bone") in vertebrae or flat bones (in secondary involvement from Hodgkin disease)

DDx: Lymphoma

Ewing Sarcoma	Osteomyelitis	Leukemia	Metastases	Multiple Myeloma
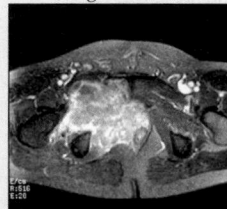	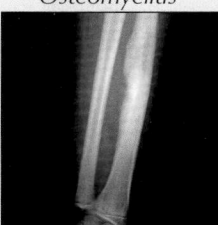	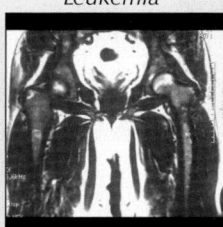	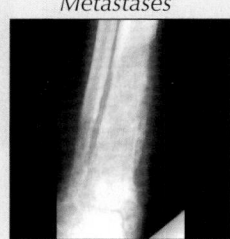	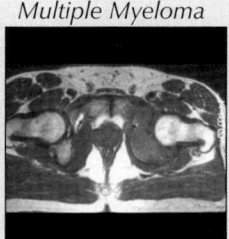
Ax T1 C+ MR	*AP Radiography*	*Cor T1WI MR*	*AP Radiography*	*Ax T1WI MR*

LYMPHOMA

Key Facts

Imaging Findings
- Mottled permeative pattern of bone destruction often with disproportionally large soft tissue component
- Intact cortex despite soft tissue extension

Top Differential Diagnoses
- Ewing Sarcoma
- Osteomyelitis
- Osteosarcoma
- Leukemia
- Metastases
- Multiple Myeloma
- Fibrosarcoma

Pathology
- 3-4% of all malignant primary bone tumors

Clinical Issues
- Localized dull/aching bone pain
- Few clinical symptoms despite extensive disease
- Primary osseous lymphoma without soft tissue involvement has best prognosis of all osseous malignancies
- 5-year survival for combined chemo- and radiation therapy: 60-80%
- Combined chemo- and radiation therapy

Diagnostic Checklist
- Important to distinguish primary lymphoma of bone from secondary involvement, which has worse prognosis and is treated differently

CT Findings
- NECT
  - To determine bone destruction and soft tissue involvement
  - Can detect bony sequestrum

MR Findings
- T1WI: Diffuse infiltration of low signal intensity
- T2WI
  - Heterogeneous signal intensity
  - Can be hyper-, iso- or hypointense
  - Hypointense areas correspond to fibrosis
- STIR: High signal intensity
- T1 C+: Enhancement
- Helpful to evaluate extent and associated soft tissue component
- Cortex can be intact despite soft tissue extension

Nuclear Medicine Findings
- Bone Scan
  - Increased radiotracer uptake
  - Central cold areas correspond to necrosis

Imaging Recommendations
- Best imaging tool: MRI
- Protocol advice
  - T1, T2, STIR or FS T2 FSE, T1 C+ MR
  - CT of chest, abdomen, pelvis to evaluate extent and to exclude primary lymphoma

DIFFERENTIAL DIAGNOSIS

Ewing Sarcoma
- Systemic symptoms
- Younger patients
- Lamellated/onion skin periosteal reaction

Osteomyelitis
- Can have similar radiographic picture
- Systemic symptoms

Osteosarcoma
- Less medullary extension
- New bone formation
- Younger patients

Leukemia
- Diffuse osteopenia, coarse trabeculae
- Leukemic lines
- Vertebral compression fractures, vertebra plana

Metastases
- Multifocal disease
- Cortical destruction

Multiple Myeloma
- No surrounding sclerosis or periosteal reaction
- Endosteal scalloping
- Cold on bone scan

Fibrosarcoma
- Well-defined to destructive lytic lesion +/- soft tissue mass
- No calcified matrix, minimal periosteal reaction
- Osseous sequestrum

PATHOLOGY

General Features
- General path comments
  - Most primary lymphomas of bone are due to non-Hodgkin lymphoma, 6% are due to Hodgkin lymphoma
  - Lymphoblastic cells produce osteoclast-stimulating factors that cause bone destruction
- Genetics: Translocation of chromosomes 14 and 18 and chromosomes 8 and 14
- Etiology
  - Unknown, might be due to viral infection or immunosuppression
  - Can occur as posttransplant lymphoproliferative disease in immunocompromised patients, often occurs in AIDS patients
- Epidemiology
  - 3-4% of all malignant primary bone tumors
  - 1% of all non-Hodgkin lymphomas

LYMPHOMA

○ Secondary involvement of bone in 35-50% of non-Hodgkin lymphoma and 13% of Hodgkin lymphoma

Gross Pathologic & Surgical Features
- Gray-white, soft, fleshy, intraosseous component (centered in metaphyses)
  ○ Mixture of bone spicules and marrow fat and areas of necrosis
- Reactive sclerosis: Firm ivory-like areas
- Cortical disruption and extension into soft tissues common
- Extraosseous tissue with tan/white appearance, resembles lymphomatous lymph nodes

Microscopic Features
- Sheet-like aggregates of malignant, small, round, lymphocytic cells that fill marrow spaces
- Majority of B cell type
  ○ Mixed small-and-large cell type (35%), diffuse large cell type (32%), immunoblastic type (3%)
- Diffuse growth pattern
  ○ Bone marrow permeation by round tumor cells
- Hodgkin lymphoma: Reed-Sternberg cells

Staging, Grading or Classification Criteria
- Modified Ann Arbor staging system
  ○ Stage I: One bone lesion with or without soft tissue extension
  ○ Stage II: Two bone lesions on the same side of the diaphragm or one bone lesion with regional lymph node involvement
  ○ Stage III: Involvement on both sides of diaphragm
  ○ Stage IV: Involvement of central or peripheral nervous system or bone marrow

CLINICAL ISSUES

Presentation
- Most common signs/symptoms
  ○ Localized dull/aching bone pain
  ○ Diagnostic requirement for primary lymphoma of bone
    ■ Interval of 4-6 months between skeletal manifestation and development of extraskeletal disease
- Clinical profile
  ○ Few clinical symptoms despite extensive disease
  ○ 50% of patients have symptoms for over one year
  ○ Occasionally palpable mass
  ○ Fever uncommon, no lymphadenopathy, or hepatosplenomegaly
  ○ Pathologic fractures in 25%
  ○ Hypercalcemia in some pediatric patients (poor prognosis)

Demographics
- Age: 20-70 years, peak: 35-45 years
- Gender: M:F = 1.5-2:1

Natural History & Prognosis
- Primary osseous lymphoma without soft tissue involvement has best prognosis of all osseous malignancies

- 5-year survival for combined chemo- and radiation therapy: 60-80%
- 5-year survival in children after aggressive chemotherapy: > 90%
- Metastases (lung, liver, brain)
- Local recurrence rare
- Poor prognostic factors
  ○ Advanced stage at diagnosis (lymph node, soft tissue involvement),
  ○ Advanced age (> 60 years)
- 5-year survival for secondary lymphoma is worse

Treatment
- Radiation therapy
  ○ Risk of growth disturbance if used in children, radiation induced sarcoma
- Chemotherapy
- Combined chemo- and radiation therapy
- Allogenic bone marrow transplantation for refractory cases
- Internal fixation in case of pathologic fractures or to prevent pathologic fracture
- Surgical resection rarely indicated

DIAGNOSTIC CHECKLIST

Consider
- Important to distinguish primary lymphoma of bone from secondary involvement, which has worse prognosis and is treated differently

Image Interpretation Pearls
- Combination of normal radiographs and positive bone scan should suggest possibility of osseous lymphoma

SELECTED REFERENCES

1. Gianelli U et al: Lymphomas of the bone: A pathological and clinical study of 54 cases. Int J Surg Pathol 10:257-66, 2002
2. Heyning FH et al: Primary non-Hodgkin's lymphoma of bone: A clinicopathological investigation of 60 cases. Leukemia 13:2094-8, 1999
3. Greenspan A et al: Differential diagnosis of tumors and tumor-like lesions of bones and joints. 1st ed. Philadelphia PA, Lippincott-Raven, 267-75, 1998
4. Melamed JW et al: Imaging of primary multifocal osseous lymphoma. Skeletal Radiol 26:35-41, 1997
5. Hillemanns M et al: Malignant lymphoma. Skeletal Radiol 25:73-5, 1996
6. Hicks DG et al: Primary lymphoma of bone. Correlation of magnetic resonance imaging features with cytokine production by tumor cells. Cancer 75:973-80, 1995
7. Mulligan ME at al: Sequestra in primary lymphoma of bone: Prevalence and radiologic features. Am J Roentgenol 160:1245-8, 1993
8. Malloy PC et al: Lymphoma of bone, muscle, and skin: CT findings. Am J Roentgenol 159:805-9, 1992
9. Bragg DG: Radiology of the lymphomas. Curr Probl Diagn Radiol 16:177-206, 1987

LYMPHOMA

IMAGE GALLERY

Typical

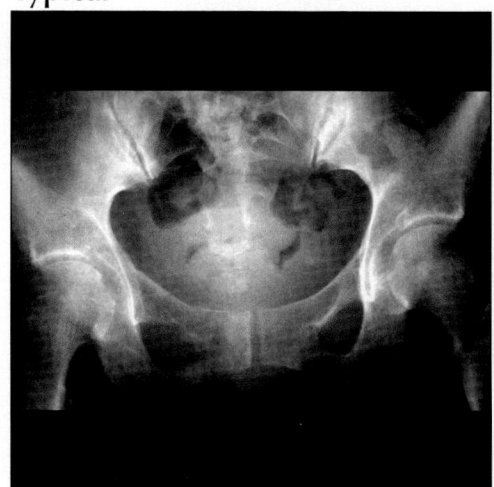
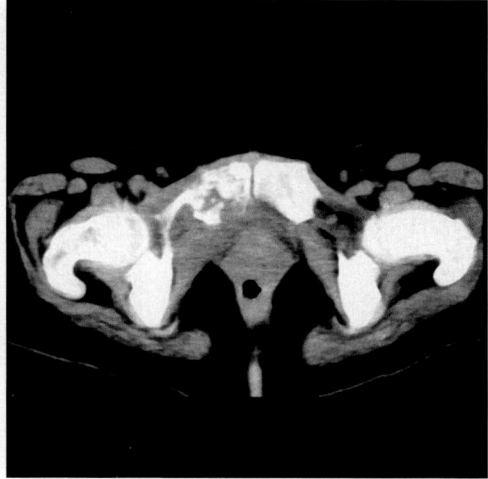

(Left) Anteroposterior radiography shows permeative bone destruction of the right superior pubic ramus. (Right) Axial NECT of the same patient shows destruction of the right inferior pubic ramus with associated soft tissue mass which was not visualized on the radiograph. Note the bony sequestrum at the medial aspect.

Typical

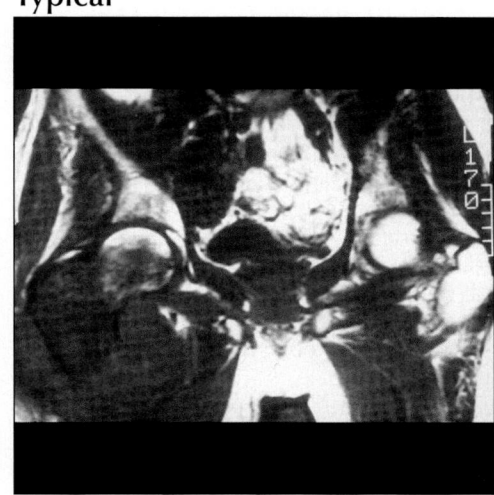
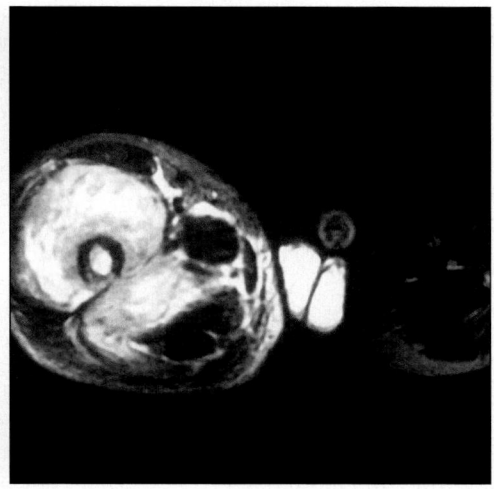

(Left) Coronal T1WI MR shows hypointense bone marrow infiltration of right proximal femur. Note the large surrounding hypointense soft tissue mass. (Right) Axial FS T2 FSE MR shows abnormal hyperintense bone marrow signal in the right femur with large surrounding hyperintense soft tissue mass. Note the relative lack of cortical destruction with abnormal signal at the posterior cortex.

Typical

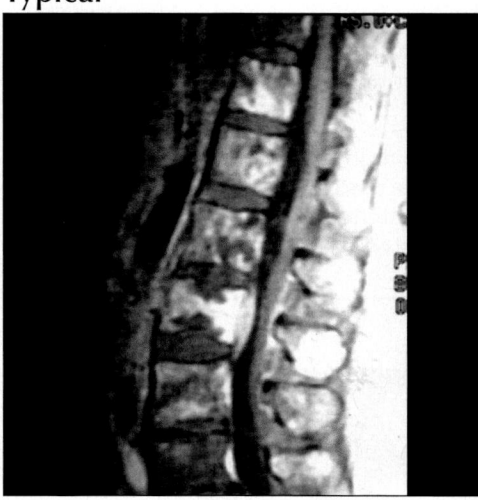
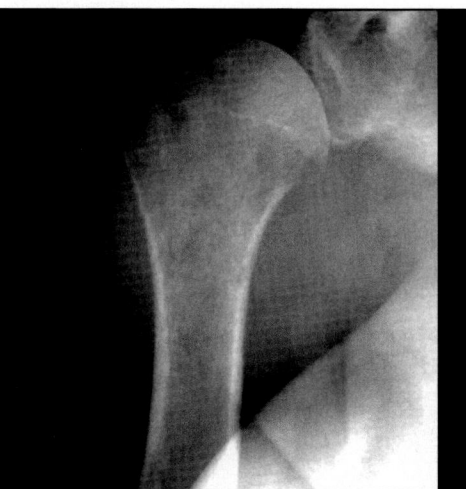

(Left) Sagittal T1WI MR shows diffuse, mottled hypointense bone marrow infiltration of the thoraco lumbar spine in a patient with disseminated non-Hodgkin lymphoma. (Right) Anteroposterior radiography shows mottled appearance of the proximal humerus with associated soft tissue mass. Subtle cortical destruction is seen medially.

MULTIPLE MYELOMA

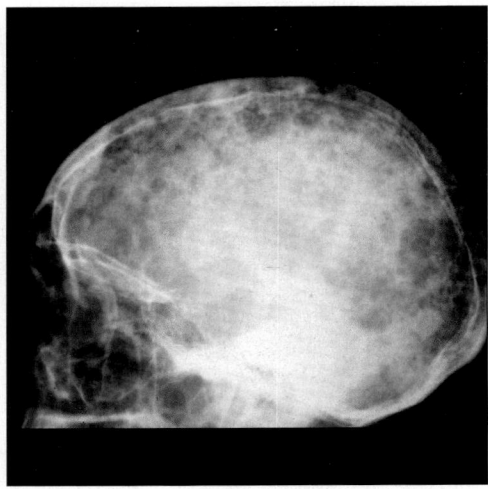

Sagittal graphic shows multiple small lytic "punched-out" lesions in the calvarium. Note scalloping of the inner cortical margin and lack of sclerotic borders.

Lateral radiography shows multiple lytic lesions without surrounding sclerosis involving the calvarium.

TERMINOLOGY

Abbreviations and Synonyms
- Myeloma, solitary myeloma, plasmacytoma, extraskeletal myeloma

Definitions
- Monoclonal, neoplastic proliferation of plasma cells involving bone marrow

IMAGING FINDINGS

General Features
- Best diagnostic clue: Multiple, well-defined, intramedullary lytic lesions
- Location
  - Any bone containing red marrow can be involved
  - Axial skeleton
    - Spine: 34%
    - Ribs: 20%
    - Femur: 18%
    - Pelvis: 15%
    - Humerus: 12%
  - Extraskeletal myeloma (rare)
    - Lungs, nasopharynx, oral cavity
- Size: Range from mms to several cms

- Morphology: Multifocal, sharply demarcated lytic intramedullary foci

Radiographic Findings
- Radiography
  - Multiple, well-defined, punched-out lesions
  - Plasmacytoma: Solitary, large, expansile lesion
    - Represents early stage of multiple myeloma
  - Endosteal scalloping
  - Cortical erosions
  - No periosteal new bone formation
  - Soft tissue mass adjacent to bone destruction
  - Diffuse osteoporosis or osteolysis, accentuated trabecular pattern
  - Expansile osteolytic lesion (ribs, pelvis, long bones)
  - Spine: Vertebral collapse
    - Sparing of posterior elements
    - Paraspinal soft tissue mass, extradural extension
  - Sclerosis after therapy

CT Findings
- NECT: Helpful in evaluating intra- and extraosseous extent, cortical destruction

MR Findings
- T1WI: Intermediate to low signal intensity compared to surrounding bone marrow
- T2WI: High signal intensity
- STIR: High signal intensity

DDx: Multiple Myeloma

Metastases	Osteoporosis	Hemangioma	Leukemia	Gaucher Disease
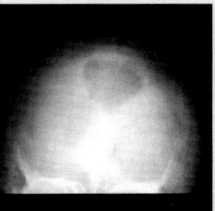	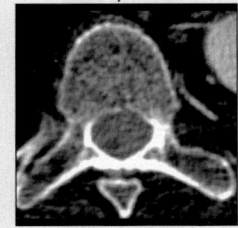	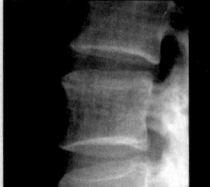	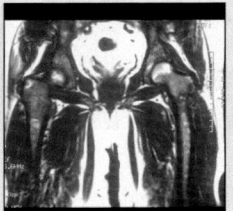	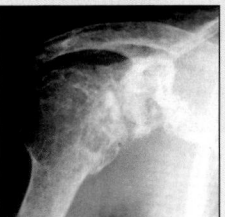
AP Radiography	Ax NECT	Lat Radiography	Cor T1WI MR	AP Radiography

MULTIPLE MYELOMA

Key Facts

Imaging Findings
- Best diagnostic clue: Multiple, well-defined, intramedullary lytic lesions

Top Differential Diagnoses
- Metastases
- Osteoporosis
- Hemangioma
- Lymphoma
- Leukemia
- Langerhans Cell Histiocytosis
- Gaucher Disease

Pathology
- Most common primary bone tumor
- 27-40% of all primary bone tumors

Clinical Issues
- Mild transient bone pain, worsened by activity (75%)
- Fatal disease, death usually 1-5 years after diagnosis
- Chemotherapy: Transient remission in 50-70%
- Radiation to control disease locally
- Osteoclast inhibiting agents: Bisphosphates
- Internal fixation for pathologic fractures or prevention of pathologic fractures

Diagnostic Checklist
- If patient presents with single lytic lesion (plasmacytoma) look carefully for additional lesions
- More than one lesion changes prognosis from stage I to stage III

- T1 C+: Enhancement
- Signal abnormalities can be focal or diffuse
- Associated soft tissue mass

Nuclear Medicine Findings
- Bone Scan
  - Normal scan in majority of cases
    - Due to bone destruction with minimal new bone formation
  - Increased radiotracer uptake in 10% of lesions
  - Can be hot due to hyperemia or cold due to replacement of marrow by myeloma cells
- PET: FDG-PET might be useful to assess extent of disease

Imaging Recommendations
- Best imaging tool: MRI
- Protocol advice: Skeletal survey and MRI of the spine to evaluate extent

DIFFERENTIAL DIAGNOSIS

Metastases
- Pedicles involved first (late involvement in myeloma)
- Increased activity on bone scan
- Ill-defined bone destruction

Osteoporosis
- No endosteal scalloping
- No cortical destruction or associated soft tissue mass

Hemangioma
- Vertical striations, honeycomb appearance
- Areas of high signal intensity on T1 and T2WI MR, corresponding to vascular components
- No soft tissue mass

Lymphoma
- "Ivory bone" in vertebrae or flat bones
- Cancellous bone erosion (earliest sign)
- Late cortical destruction

Leukemia
- Multiple small clearly-defined osteolytic lesions

- Coarse trabeculation of spongiosa
- Smooth, lamellated, sunburst pattern of periosteal reaction

Langerhans Cell Histiocytosis
- Younger patients
- Self limiting disease

Gaucher Disease
- Younger patients
- Generalized osteopenia or honeycombed appearance
- Erlenmeyer flask deformity
- No associated soft tissue mass

PATHOLOGY

General Features
- General path comments: Malignant hematological disorder characterized by bone marrow infiltration with neoplastic plasma cells
- Genetics: Translocation of chromosomes 11, 14
- Etiology
  - Uncontrolled proliferation of plasma cells (subset of B cells) within bone marrow
  - Secretion of nonfunctional monoclonal immunoglobulins that suppress benign polyclonal plasma cells
  - Myeloma cells produce osteoclast stimulating factor
  - Suppressed osteoblastic response resulting in demineralization and bone destruction
- Epidemiology
  - Most common primary bone tumor
  - 27-40% of all primary bone tumors
  - Second most common hematopoietic neoplasm
  - 1% of all malignant neoplasms
- Associated abnormalities
  - POEMS syndrome
    - Polyneuropathy, organomegaly, endocrine disorders, monoclonal gammopathy, skin changes
    - Enthesopathies
    - Sclerotic foci resembling bone islands or ivory vertebral bodies

MULTIPLE MYELOMA

○ Amyloidosis: 10-15%
  ▪ Amyloid deposited in bone marrow, kidneys, heart, GI tract, liver, spleen, muscle, skin, CNS

Gross Pathologic & Surgical Features
- Red-gray soft tumor replacing bone marrow
- Growth in discrete nodules, circumscribed or confluent (advanced stage)
- Extension into surrounding soft tissues

Microscopic Features
- Aggregates of neoplastic plasma cells
  ○ Infiltrate and completely replace normal hematopoietic and fatty marrow
- Myeloma cells: Eccentric, round, hyperchromatic nucleus with "cartwheel" distribution of chromatin
  ○ Expression of plasma cell associated antigen
- Drug resistant myeloma: Expression of p-170 (P glycoprotein)
  ○ Resistance to vincristine-doxorubicin, Adriamycin, dexamethasone (VAD) protocol

Staging, Grading or Classification Criteria
- Clinical staging system for multiple myeloma (Durie and Salmon)
  ○ Stage I: Up to one lytic bone lesion
    ▪ Hemoglobin: > 10 g/dL
    ▪ Serum calcium: < 12 mg/dL
    ▪ Low immunoglobin production: IgG < 5g/dL or IgA < 3 g/dL
  ○ Stage II: Patients in between stage I and stage III
  ○ Stage III: More than one lytic bone lesion
    ▪ Hemoglobin: < 8.5 g/dL
    ▪ Serum calcium: > 12 mg/dL
    ▪ High immunoglobulin production: IgG > 7g/dL, IgA > 5g/dL

CLINICAL ISSUES

Presentation
- Most common signs/symptoms
  ○ Mild transient bone pain, worsened by activity (75%)
    ▪ Predominately in weight bearing sites
    ▪ Duration of pain usually < 6 months
- Clinical profile
  ○ Palpable mass (extraosseous extension, associated hemorrhage)
  ○ Anemia, fever, weight loss
  ○ Bleeding diathesis
  ○ Hypercalcemia
  ○ Frequent infections
  ○ Bence Jones proteins in urine
  ○ Renal failure
  ○ Electrophoresis: Monoclonal gammopathy (IgA/IgG peak)
  ○ Pathologic fractures
  ○ Peripheral neuropathy in sclerotic form (POEMS syndrome)

Demographics
- Age: 40-80 years, peak: 64 years
- Gender: M:F = 3:2

Natural History & Prognosis
- Fatal disease, death usually 1-5 years after diagnosis
  ○ Stage I: Median survival 10 years
  ○ Stage II: Median survival 1-5 years
  ○ Stage III: Median survival < 2 years
- Solitary form (plasmacytoma) usually converts to multiple myeloma

Treatment
- Chemotherapy: Transient remission in 50-70%
  ○ Only used in patients with disseminated disease
- Radiation to control disease locally
  ○ Rapid decompression of vital structures (spinal canal)
  ○ For pain relief
- Osteoclast inhibiting agents: Bisphosphates
- Internal fixation for pathologic fractures or prevention of pathologic fractures
- Decompressive laminectomy for symptomatic spine involvement (compressive myelopathy)
- Vertebroplasty for vertebral compression fractures

DIAGNOSTIC CHECKLIST

Consider
- If patient presents with single lytic lesion (plasmacytoma) look carefully for additional lesions
- More than one lesion changes prognosis from stage I to stage III

Image Interpretation Pearls
- Punched out lytic lesions in ribs and skull of adults usually due to multiple myeloma

SELECTED REFERENCES

1. Schirrmeister H et al: Initial results in the assessment of multiple myeloma using 18F-FDG PET. Eur J Nucl Med Mol Imaging 29:361-6, 2002
2. Dimopoulos MA et al: Solitary plasmocytoma of bone and asymptomatic multiple myeloma. Blood 96:2037-44, 2000
3. Lecouvet FE et al: Skeletal survey in advanced multiple myeloma: Radiographic versus MR imaging survey. Br J Haematol 106:35-9, 1999
4. Ludwig H et al: Multiple myeloma: An update on biology and treatment. Ann Oncol 6:31-43, 1999
5. Dorfman HD et al: Bone tumors. 1st ed. St. Louis MO, Mosby, 664-79, 1998
6. Moulopoulos LA et al: Prognostic significance of magnetic resonance imaging in patients with asymptomatic multiple myeloma. J Clin Oncol 13:251-6, 1995
7. Libshitz HI et al: Multiple myeloma: Appearance at MR imaging. Radiology 182:833-7, 1992
8. Moulopoulos LA et al: Multiple myeloma: Spinal MR imaging in patients with untreated newly diagnosed disease. Radiology 185:833-40, 1992
9. Bataille R et al: Bone scintigraphy in plasma cell myeloma. A prospective study of 70 patients. Radiology 145:801-4, 1982

MULTIPLE MYELOMA

IMAGE GALLERY

Typical

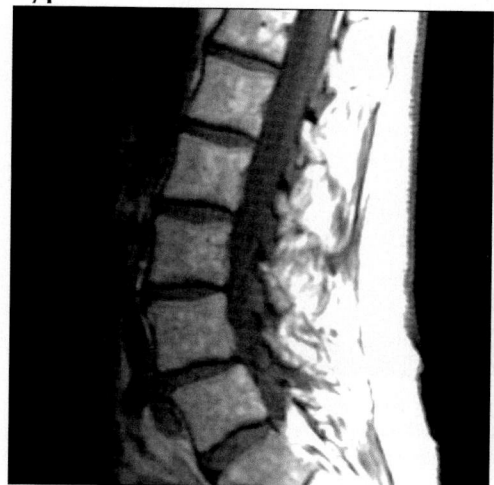 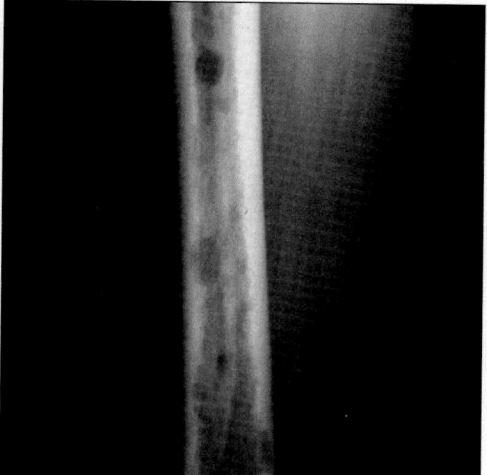

(Left) Sagittal T1WI MR shows heterogeneous bone marrow of the lumbar spine. Radiographs were normal in this patient with multiple myeloma. *(Right)* Lateral radiography of the femur shows multiple osteolytic lesions with endosteal scalloping of the cortex.

Typical

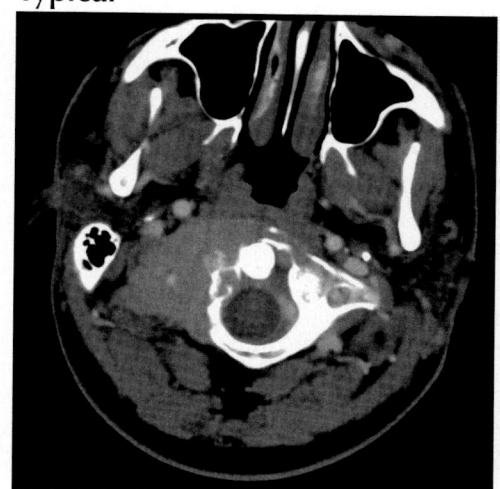 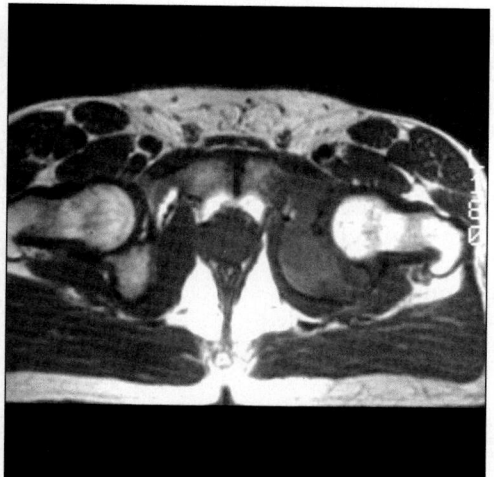

(Left) Axial CECT shows destruction of the C1 vertebral body with large associated soft tissue mass. *(Right)* Axial T1WI MR shows abnormal hypointense bone marrow signal involving the left pubis & ischium with associated expansion of bone.

Variant

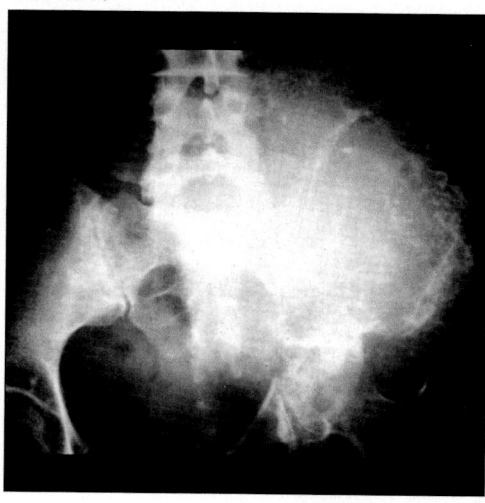 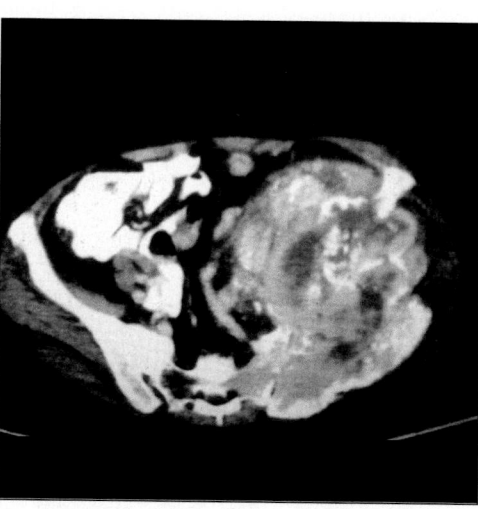

(Left) Anteroposterior radiography shows large lytic lesion with destruction of the left iliac bone in a patient with plasmacytoma. *(Right)* Axial CECT shows destruction of the left iliac bone and sacrum. There is heterogeneous replacement of bone marrow of the left hemipelvis with large associated soft tissue mass in a patient with plasmacytoma.

21

SICKLE CELL ANEMIA

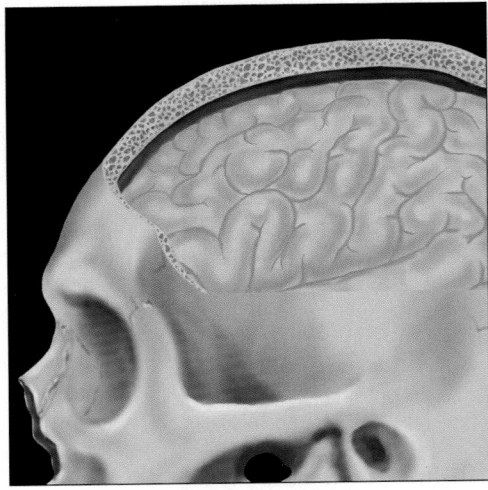

Sagittal graphic shows widening of the medullary cavity with thinning of the outer table.

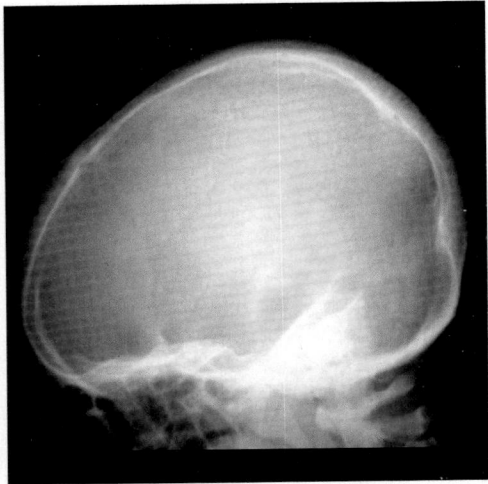

Lateral radiography shows widening of the medullary cavity and decreased width of the outer table. Vertical hair-on-end striations are also noted.

TERMINOLOGY

Abbreviations and Synonyms
- Sickle cell disease, hemoglobin HbSS disease, sickle cell trait, HbSA disease, HbSC disease

Definitions
- Systemic hereditary disease characterized by anemia due to replacement of fetal hemoglobin by abnormal S hemoglobin
- Homozygous: HbSS (sickle cell anemia)
- Heterozygous: HbSA (sickle cell trait), HbSC (less severe form)

IMAGING FINDINGS

General Features
- Best diagnostic clue
  - Hyperplasia of erythropoietic bone marrow
  - Multiple bone infarcts
- Location
  - Any bone can be involved
  - Long bones
    - Femur: 96%; humerus: 48%
  - Small tubular bones of hands and feet: 20-50%
  - Spine: 43-70%
  - Skull: 25%
  - Metaphysis, subchondral bone of long bones involved in adults
  - Diaphyses of small tubular bones of hands and feet involved in children
- Size: 3-10 cm
- Morphology
  - Expanded medullary cavity
  - Bone infarctions

Radiographic Findings
- Radiography
  - Marrow hyperplasia
    - Widened medullary space, thinning of cortex
    - Osteoporosis with thinning of trabeculae
    - Coarsened trabecular pattern
    - Skull: Widening of diploe, decreased width of outer table
    - Hair-on-end appearance of skull (vertical striations)
    - Biconcave "fish" vertebra (bone softening)
    - Pathologic fractures
  - Bone infarction/diminished blood supply
    - Avascular necrosis (AVN) in medullary spaces of long bones, hands, growing epiphyses
    - Osteolysis in acute infarct
    - Dystrophic medullary calcifications
    - Periosteal reaction: Bone-within-bone appearance
    - Juxtacortical sclerosis
    - H-shaped vertebrae

DDx: Sickle Cell Anemia

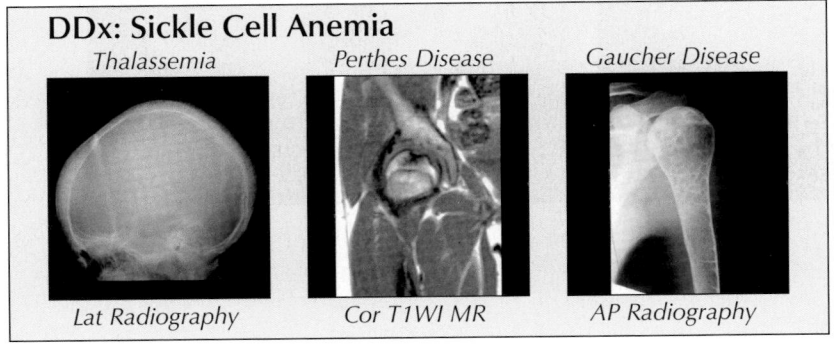

Thalassemia — Lat Radiography | Perthes Disease — Cor T1WI MR | Gaucher Disease — AP Radiography

7

22

SICKLE CELL ANEMIA

Key Facts

Imaging Findings
- Hyperplasia of erythropoietic bone marrow
- Multiple bone infarcts
- Hair-on-end appearance of skull (vertical striations)
- Biconcave "fish" vertebra (bone softening)
- Avascular necrosis (AVN) in medullary spaces of long bones, hands, growing epiphyses

Top Differential Diagnoses
- Thalassemia
- Legg-Calvé-Perthes
- Gaucher Disease

Pathology
- 1% of African Americans
- 8-13% of African Americans carry sickling factor (HbS)

Clinical Issues
- Sickle cell crisis: Sudden onset of severe bone, abdominal, chest pain
- Sickle cell crisis often as result of infection, temperature change, hypoxia (flight)
- Skeletal pain (bone infarction, osteomyelitis, cellulitis)
- Osteomyelitis (staphylococcus, salmonella)
- Repeated episodes lead to progressive bone infarction
- Death < 48 years in sickle cell disease
- Sickle cell crisis treatment: Oxygen, hydration, pain management
- No prophylactic measure to prevent bone infarcts

  - ▪ Collapse of femoral head
  - ▪ Premature epiphyseal closure resulting in growth defect
  - ▪ Epiphyseal deformity, cupped metaphyses
  - ▪ Dactylitis (hand-foot syndrome): Bone infarcts of hands and feet
  - ▪ Calcaneal erosions (represent microinfarction)
  - ○ Infections
    - ▪ Periostitis; septic arthritis

CT Findings
- NECT: Sclerotic bone infarction

MR Findings
- T1WI
  - ○ Low signal intensity of bone marrow (hematopoietic marrow replacing fatty marrow)
  - ○ Focal areas of low signal intensity (acute marrow infarction)
- T2WI
  - ○ Intermediate - low signal intensity of bone marrow (hematopoietic marrow replacing fatty marrow)
  - ○ Focal areas of increased signal intensity (acute marrow infarction)
- T1 C+
  - ○ Acute infarct: Thin, linear rim enhancement
    - ▪ Osteomyelitis: Geographic, irregular marrow enhancement
- To evaluate extent of disease
- Helpful in differentiating between infarcts and osteomyelitis

Nuclear Medicine Findings
- Bone Scan
  - ○ Marked expansion of hematopoietic marrow
  - ○ Increased radiotracer uptake in areas of infarction
  - ○ Bone marrow defects (old infarction)
  - ○ More sensitive than radiographs in detecting early AVN

Imaging Recommendations
- Best imaging tool: Radiographs diagnostic
- Protocol advice
  - ○ Radiographs

  - ○ T1, T2W MR to evaluate extent of disease
  - ○ T1 C+ to differentiate between osteomyelitis and bone marrow infract

DIFFERENTIAL DIAGNOSIS

Thalassemia
- Expanded bone marrow space
- AVN less common than in sickle cell anemia
- Paravertebral masses (extramedullary hematopoiesis)

Legg-Calvé-Perthes
- Idiopathic AVN of femoral head in children
- Rare in African Americans
- Femoral epiphysis of affected hip smaller than normal contralateral side
- Sclerosis, collapse of femoral epiphysis

Gaucher Disease
- AVN of hip and shoulder
- Erlenmeyer flask deformity
- Marrow expansion
- Cortical thinning, periostitis
- Lytic lesions

PATHOLOGY

General Features
- General path comments: Sickle cell disease HbSS associated with many bone findings, sickle cell trait HbAS occasionally associated with bone infarcts
- Genetics: Mutation resulting in substituting thymine for adenine in the 6th codon of beta-chain gene GAG to GTG
- Etiology
  - ○ Structural defect in hemoglobin HbS: Glutamic acid in position 6 substituted with valine
  - ○ Altered shape and plasticity of red blood cells under lowered oxygen tension leads to increase of blood viscosity, stasis
  - ○ Occlusion of small blood vessels leads to infarction, necrosis

SICKLE CELL ANEMIA

○ Children are protected for the first 6 months by elevated levels of fetal Hb (HbF)
○ HbS protects from malaria
• Epidemiology
  ○ 1% of African Americans
  ○ 8-13% of African Americans carry sickling factor (HbS)
  ○ 3% of African Americans are HbC carrier
  ○ 1:40 with sickle cell trait will manifest sickle cell anemia (HbSS)
  ○ 1:120 with sickle cell trait will manifest HbSC disease
• Associated abnormalities: Can coexist with thalassemia

Gross Pathologic & Surgical Features
• Areas of infarction: Dense, hard, sclerotic bone
• Yellow marrow replaced by hyperplastic red hematopoietic marrow
• Infarcted marrow spaces filled with clotted blood

Microscopic Features
• Areas of infarction: Thickened trabeculae, acellular necrotic bone
• Trabeculae have multiple concentric cement lines
• Proliferation of fibrovascular repair tissue
• No osteoclastic activity
• Marrow spaced filled with granular basophilic cell debris

CLINICAL ISSUES

Presentation
• Most common signs/symptoms
  ○ Sickle cell crisis: Sudden onset of severe bone, abdominal, chest pain
    ▪ Sickle cell crisis often as result of infection, temperature change, hypoxia (flight)
    ▪ +/- Fever, leukocytosis
    ▪ May last hours to days
• Clinical profile
  ○ Skeletal pain (bone infarction, osteomyelitis, cellulitis)
  ○ Osteomyelitis (staphylococcus, salmonella)
  ○ Chronic hemolytic anemia
  ○ Jaundice
  ○ Abdominal pain
  ○ Splenomegaly (in children), later splenic atrophy
  ○ Growth retardation
  ○ High incidence of infections
    ▪ Pneumococcal septicemia, meningitis are leading causes of death
  ○ Chest pain (acute pulmonary crisis, rib infarcts)
  ○ CNS involvement: Stroke
  ○ Dactylitis: 20-50% of children with with SS disease (between 6 months to 2 years)
    ▪ Swelling of hands and feet
    ▪ Decreased range of motion
    ▪ Self limiting after days to weeks

Demographics
• Age: Manifests in second half of first year of life; persists lifelong

• Gender: M:F = 1:1
• Ethnicity
  ○ Majority of cases found in African Americans
  ○ Less frequently in eastern Mediterranean and Middle Eastern populations

Natural History & Prognosis
• Sickle cell crisis begins at 2-3 years of life
• Repeated episodes lead to progressive bone infarction
• Premature arthritis due to AVN
• Poor prognostic factors: Dactylitis before 1 year, Hb levels < 7 g/dL, leukocytosis in absence of infection
• Death < 48 years in sickle cell disease
• Patients with sickle cell trait (HbSA) have normal life expectancy

Treatment
• Systemic treatment
• Sickle cell crisis treatment: Oxygen, hydration, pain management
• High-dose methylprednisolone can reduce duration of pain in children
• Hydroxyurea possibly helpful in increasing total Hb concentration, reducing vaso-occlusive complications
• No prophylactic measure to prevent bone infarcts
• AVN of femoral head: Varus osteotomy, total hip replacement
  ○ Transfusion of packed red blood cells to lower percentage of HbS < 45% (pre-operative)

DIAGNOSTIC CHECKLIST

Consider
• Patients should be educated about risk factors that precipitate sickle cell crisis

Image Interpretation Pearls
• Important to distinguish acute infarction from osteomyelitis

SELECTED REFERENCES
1. Steinberg MH: Hydroxyurea treatment for sickle cell disease. ScientificWorldJournal 25:1706-28, 2002
2. Lonergan GJ et al: Sickle cell anemia. Radiographics 21:971-94, 2001
3. States LJ: Imaging of metabolic bone disease and marrow disorders in children. Radiol Clin North Am 39:749-72, 2001
4. Jean-Baptiste G et al: Osteoarticular disorders of haematological origin. Baillieres Best Pract Res Clin Rheumatol 14:307-23, 2000
5. Umans H et al: The diagnostic role of gadolinium enhanced MRI in distinguishing between acute medullary bone infarct and osteomyelitis. Magn Reson Imaging 18:255-62, 2000
6. Hernigou P et al: Abnormalities of the adult shoulder due to sickle cell osteonecrosis during childhood. Rev Rhum Engl Ed 65:27-32, 1998
7. Rothschild BM et al: Microfoci of avascular necrosis in sickle cell anemia: Pathophysiology of the dot dash pattern. Clin Exp Rheumatol 15:663-6, 1997

SICKLE CELL ANEMIA

IMAGE GALLERY

Typical

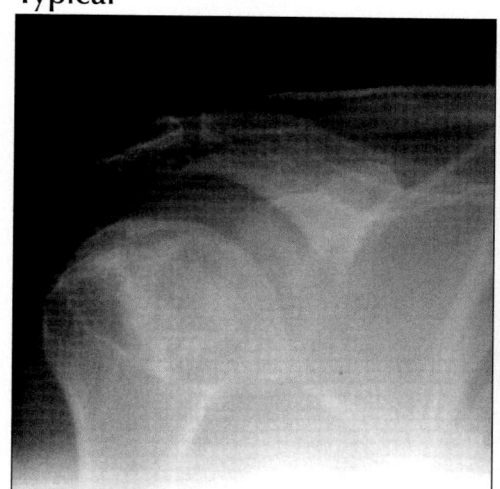

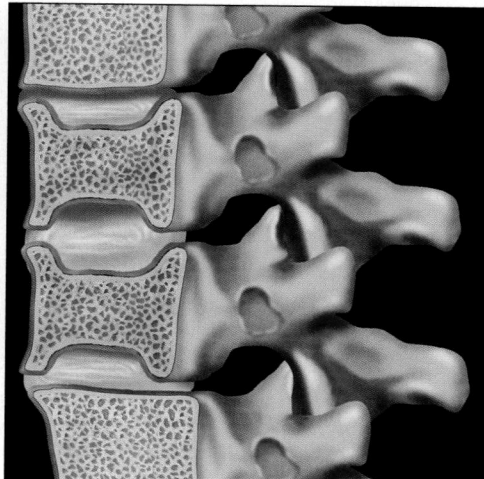

(Left) Anteroposterior radiography shows sclerosis of the humeral head, consistent with AVN. *(Right)* Sagittal graphic shows step-like endplate depression of the vertebral bodies (H-vertebra) as a result of infarction and bone softening.

Typical

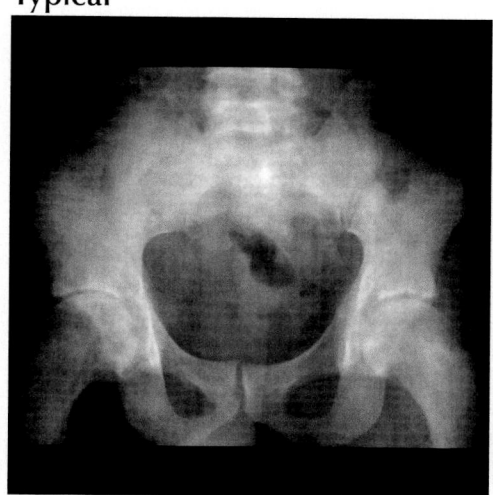

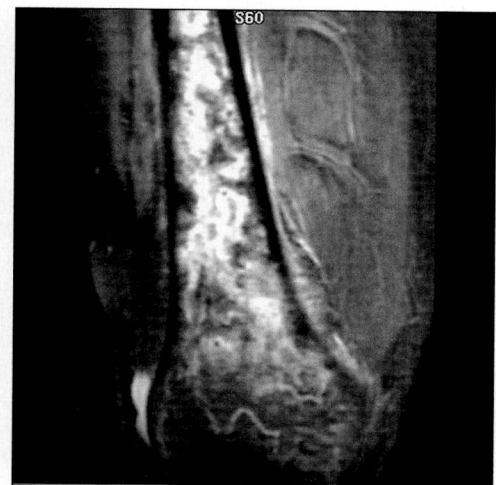

(Left) Anteroposterior radiography shows patchy sclerosis involving the entire pelvis and femoral heads, consistent with extensive bone marrow infarction. *(Right)* Coronal FS T2 FSE MR shows hyperintense bone marrow edema of the distal femur in a patient with acute infarction.

Variant

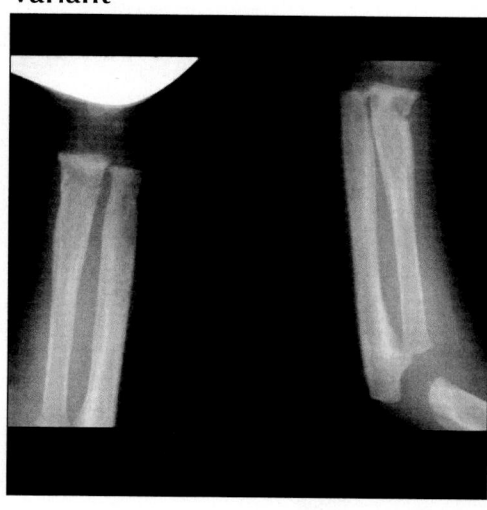

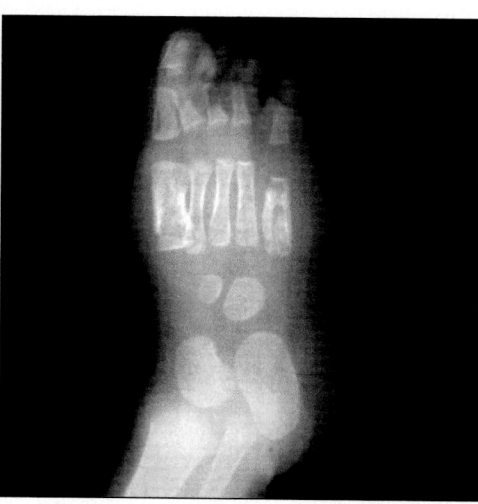

(Left) Anteroposterior radiography in a child with fever & leukocytosis shows lytic lesions with periosteal reaction and cortical destruction of the distal radius & ulna. This was found to represent osteomyelitis due to salmonella. *(Right)* Anteroposterior radiography shows patchy sclerosis of metatarsals & phalanges, consistent with bone infarcts in a child with hand-foot syndrome. Often impossible to distinguish osteomyelitis from bone infarction.

THALASSEMIA

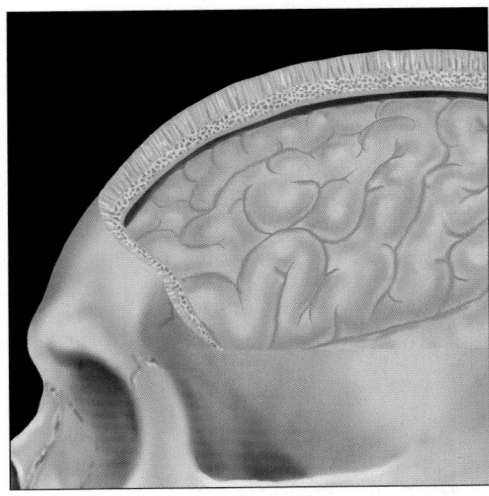

Sagittal graphic shows thickened calvarium. New bone formation in the diploic space is manifested by hair-on-end appearance.

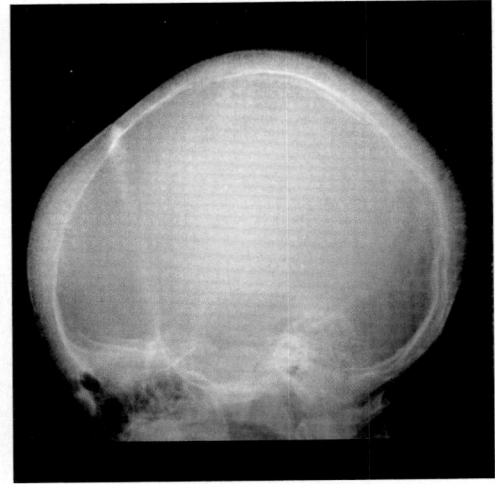

Lateral radiography shows widening of calvarium with hair-on-end appearance. Note the relative sparing of occipital bone due to lack of hematopoietic marrow.

TERMINOLOGY

Abbreviations and Synonyms
- Thalassemia major, thalassemia minor, Cooley anemia, thalassemia intermedia, Mediterranean anemia, hereditary leptocytosis, erythroblastic anemia

Definitions
- Hereditary group of disorders involving hemoglobin synthesis with decreased production of either alpha chains of hemoglobin resulting in varying degrees of anemia

IMAGING FINDINGS

General Features
- Best diagnostic clue
  - Expansion of medullary cavity, thinning of cortical bone, resorption of cancellous bone
  - Extramedullary hematopoiesis
- Location
  - Axial and proximal appendicular skeleton (hematopoietic marrow) in adults
  - Axial and appendicular skeleton in infants and children (equal distribution of hematopoietic marrow)
  - Femur

  - Humerus
  - Spine
  - Skull
  - Small bones of hands and feet
- Size: Involvement of entire bone
- Morphology: Expanded marrow cavity

Radiographic Findings
- Radiography
  - Skull
    - Widened diploic space, coarsened trabeculae, thinning of outer table
    - Hair-on-end appearance
    - Occipital bone usually spared (lacks hematopoietic marrow)
    - Impaired pneumatization of paranasal sinuses
    - Lateral displacement of orbits
    - Rodent facies: Ventral displacement of teeth due to marrow expansion of maxilla
  - Long bones
    - Widened medullary space, thinning of cortex, resorption of cancellous bone
    - Osteoporosis, coarsened trabeculae
    - Undertubulation of long bones (Erlenmeyer flask deformity)
    - Premature fusion of epiphysis (proximal humerus, distal femur, proximal tibia, proximal femur)
    - Cortical erosions due to subperiosteal proliferation of marrow

DDx: Thalassemia

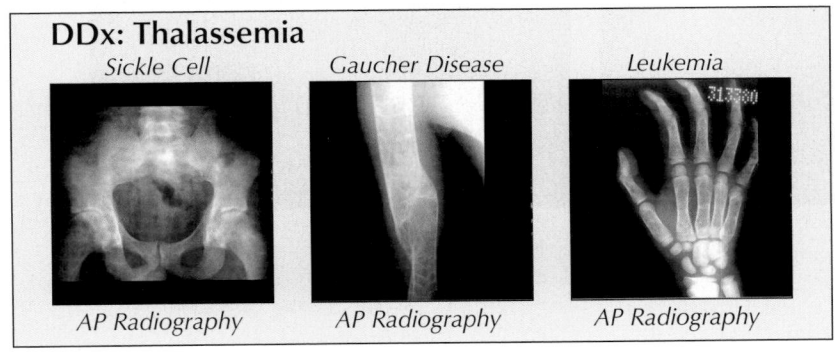

Sickle Cell	Gaucher Disease	Leukemia
AP Radiography	*AP Radiography*	*AP Radiography*

THALASSEMIA

Key Facts

Imaging Findings
- Expansion of medullary cavity, thinning of cortical bone, resorption of cancellous bone
- Extramedullary hematopoiesis

Top Differential Diagnoses
- Sickle Cell Anemia
- Gaucher Disease
- Leukemia

Pathology
- Thalassemia major (homozygote): 10% in high risk areas (Mediterranean islands)
- Thalassemia minor (heterozygote): 2.5% of Italian Americans, 7-10% of Greek Americans

Clinical Issues
- Most common signs/symptoms: Hypochromic microcytic anemia
- Hepatosplenomegaly due to extramedullary hematopoiesis
- Endocrine abnormalities due to iron overload of pituitary gland
- Cardiomegaly, congestive heart failure due to hemochromatosis
- Thalassemia major: Hemolysis and severe anemia
- Death within 1st decade of life if untreated
- Thalassemia minor: Normal life expectancy
- Transfusion of packed red blood cells to maintain physiologic Hb level
- Chelation therapy to prevent iron accumulation, promote iron excretion

---

- - Arthropathy (due to hemochromatosis, calcium pyrophosphate dihydrate deposition (CPPD))
  - Deferoxamine induced bone dysplasia
  - Spine
    - Thickened vertebral trabeculae, paucity of horizontal trabeculae (striated appearance)
    - Compression fractures
    - Paravertebral masses (extramedullary hematopoiesis)
  - Ribs
    - Expanded posterior aspect of ribs, thinned cortex
    - Rib-within-a-rib appearance: Linear density within medullary cavity of middle and anterior aspects of ribs

CT Findings
- NECT
  - Expanded medullary cavity
  - Extramedullary hematopoiesis: Soft tissue masses
- CECT: Enhancement of areas of extramedullary hematopoiesis
- To evaluate complex anatomic structures (craniofacial bones)
- To define extent of extramedullary hematopoiesis

MR Findings
- T1WI
  - Low-intermediate signal intensity of bone marrow
  - Extramedullary hematopoiesis: Active lesions intermediate signal
    - Inactive lesions: Low signal due to iron deposition, high signal due to fatty replacement
- T2WI: Low-intermediate signal intensity of bone marrow
- T2* GRE: Helpful to diagnose hemochromatosis
- T1 C+: Marked enhancement of areas of extramedullary hematopoiesis
- Deferoxamine-induced bone dysplasia: Blurred physeal-metaphyseal junction, physeal widening, metaphyseal signal changes
- To evaluate complications from extramedullary hematopoiesis (i.e. cord compression)

Nuclear Medicine Findings
- Bone Scan
  - Marked expansion of hematopoietic marrow
  - Increased overall skeletal radiotracer activity

Imaging Recommendations
- Best imaging tool: Radiographs diagnostic
- Protocol advice: MRI, CT for evaluation of disease and therapy induced complication (hemochromatosis, cord compression)

DIFFERENTIAL DIAGNOSIS

Sickle Cell Anemia
- Bone infarcts with avascular necrosis (AVN)
- Extramedullary hematopoiesis less common

Gaucher Disease
- Erlenmeyer flask deformity
- AVN of hip and shoulder
- Lytic lesions
- Cortical thinning, periostitis
- No extramedullary hematopoiesis

Leukemia
- Diffuse osteopenia of spine and long bones
- Leukemic lines
- Moth eaten pattern of bone destruction
- Collapsed vertebral bodies (vertebra plana)

PATHOLOGY

General Features
- General path comments
  - Physiologic hemoglobin in adulthood: HbA (98%, 2 alpha and 2 beta chains)
  - Physiologic hemoglobin in fetal life: HbF (2 alpha and 2 gamma chains)
  - Beta chain production starts at 8 weeks of gestation, switch to adult hemoglobin completed at 4 months of age

THALASSEMIA

- Genetics
  - Autosomal recessive inheritance
  - Beta globin chain gene: Chromosome 11p15.5
  - Type of mutation specific to ethnic group
- Etiology
  - Alpha thalassemia: Decreased synthesis of alpha chains leading to excess of beta and gamma chains
    - Disease begins in intrauterine life since no fetal hemoglobin (HbF) is produced
    - Homozygote form is lethal (no oxygen transport)
  - Beta thalassemia: Decreased synthesis of beta chains leading to excess of alpha and gamma chains (fetal hemoglobin)
    - Disease manifests in early infancy, after 4 months of life
    - Homozygote defect: Thalassemia major (Cooley anemia), early onset, thalassemia intermedia, later onset
    - Heterozygote defect: Thalassemia minor
  - Decrease of hemoglobin synthesis resulting in hypochromic anemia
  - Alpha chains precipitate as insoluble inclusion bodies
    - Increased erythrocyte hemolysis
- Epidemiology
  - Thalassemia major (homozygote): 10% in high risk areas (Mediterranean islands)
  - Thalassemia minor (heterozygote): 2.5% of Italian Americans, 7-10% of Greek Americans
  - Alpha thalassemia (heterozygote): 30% in Southeast Asia and Africa
- Associated abnormalities: Can coexist with sickle cell anemia

Gross Pathologic & Surgical Features
- Hyperplastic hematopoietic bone marrow
- Marrow spaces filled with clotted blood

Microscopic Features
- Microcytic anemia, normal low serum iron, decreased haptoglobin, hemopexin
- Normocellular hematopoiesis, erythroid predominance, megakaryocytosis

CLINICAL ISSUES

Presentation
- Most common signs/symptoms: Hypochromic microcytic anemia
- Clinical profile
  - Growth retardation
  - Hyperbilirubinemia (gallstones)
  - Hepatosplenomegaly due to extramedullary hematopoiesis
  - Skin hyperpigmentation
  - Endocrine abnormalities due to iron overload of pituitary gland
  - Cardiomegaly, congestive heart failure due to hemochromatosis
  - Liver failure, cirrhosis, pancreatic insufficiency, diabetes mellitus due to hemochromatosis
  - Increased infection rate
  - Bleeding diathesis
  - Thalassemia minor usually asymptomatic except for periods of stress (infection, pregnancy)

Demographics
- Age
  - Alpha thalassemia: Begins in utero
  - Beta thalassemia: Develops after newborn period, usually after 4-6 months
  - Persists lifelong
- Gender: M:F = 1:1
- Ethnicity
  - Alpha thalassemia: Southeast Asia and China
  - Beta thalassemia: People from Mediterranean origin, less frequently in Chinese and other Asians, African Americans

Natural History & Prognosis
- Thalassemia major: Hemolysis and severe anemia
  - Death within 1st decade of life if untreated
- Thalassemia intermedia: Milder clinical form with longer life expectancy
- Thalassemia minor: Normal life expectancy

Treatment
- No treatment necessary for heterozygote patients
- Treatment for homozygote patients
- Transfusion of packed red blood cells to maintain physiologic Hb level
  - Complications: Hepatitis B, hemosiderosis, hypersplenism
- Chelation therapy to prevent iron accumulation, promote iron excretion
  - Deferoxamine: Iron balance in growing children, negative iron balance in older patients
  - Complications: Erythema, pruritus, visual impairment (cataracts, poor color vision), sensorineural hearing loss
- Bone marrow transplant
- Splenectomy in case of hypersplenism

DIAGNOSTIC CHECKLIST

Consider
- Genetic counseling if both parents have disease or are carriers

Image Interpretation Pearls
- Imaging is important to detect serious complications from extramedullary hematopoiesis (cord compression) or frequent transfusions (hemochromatosis)

SELECTED REFERENCES

1. Ball LM et al: Paediatric allogeneic bone marrow transplantation for homozygous beta-thalassaemia, the Dutch experience. Bone marrow transplant 31:1081-7, 2003
2. Chaston TB et al: Iron chelators for the treatment of iron overload disease: Relationship between structure, redox activity, and toxicity. Am J Hematol 73:200-10, 2003
3. Orofino MG et al: Fetal HLA typing in beta thalassaemia: Implications for haemopoietic stem-cell transplantation. Lancet 362:41-2, 2003

THALASSEMIA

IMAGE GALLERY

Typical

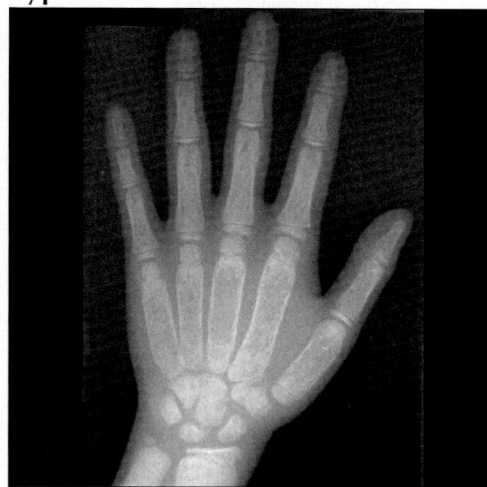

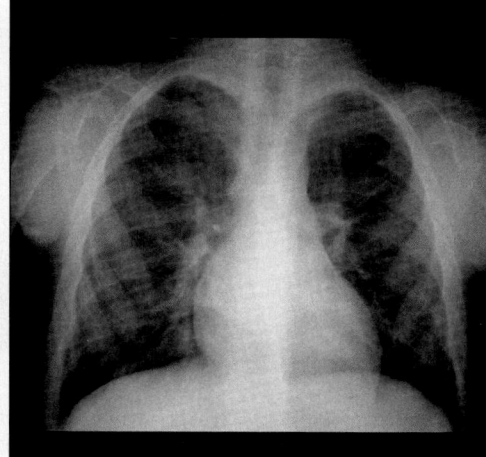

(Left) Anteroposterior radiography shows generalized osteopenia, coarsened trabeculae, and cortical thinning of the phalanges. Widening of the medullary cavity resulting in squaring of the metacarpals. *(Right)* Anteroposterior radiography shows widening of the ribs and clavicles. Linear densities overlapping the anterior ribs result in "rib-within-a-rib" appearance.

Typical

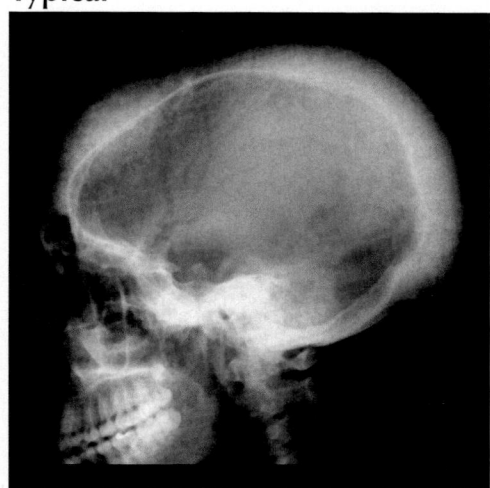

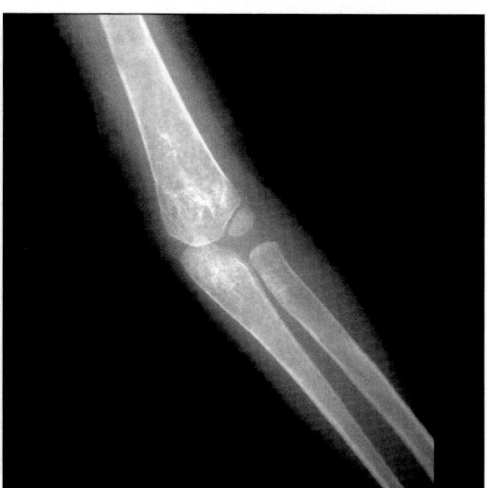

(Left) Lateral radiography shows marked expansion of the calvarium and hair-on-end appearance. Note the enlarged impressions of the calvarial vessels. *(Right)* Anteroposterior radiography shows expansion of the medullary cavity with coarsened trabeculae and cortical thinning.

Typical

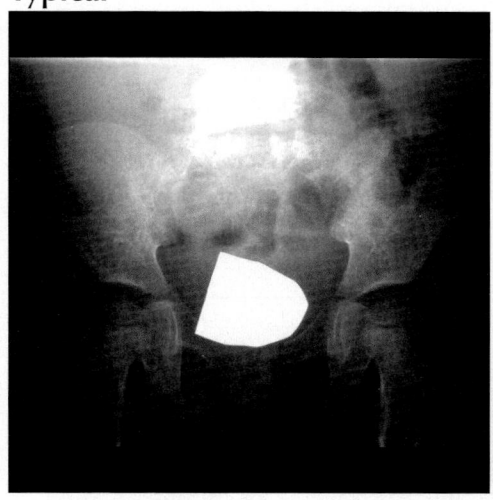

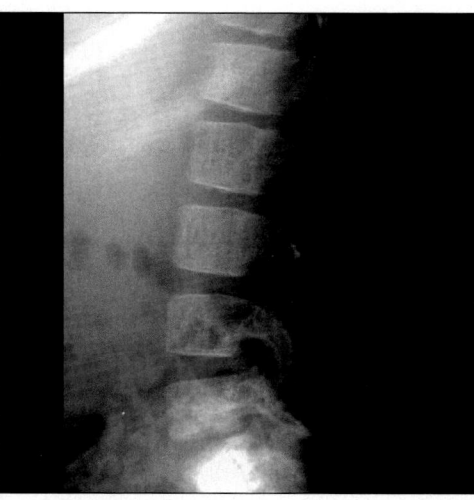

(Left) Anteroposterior radiography shows coarsening and osteopenia of the pelvis with expansion of the medullary cavity. *(Right)* Lateral radiography shows thickened vertical trabeculae with paucity of horizontal trabeculae resulting in a striated appearance. Note expansion of the medullary cavity.

GAUCHER'S DISEASE

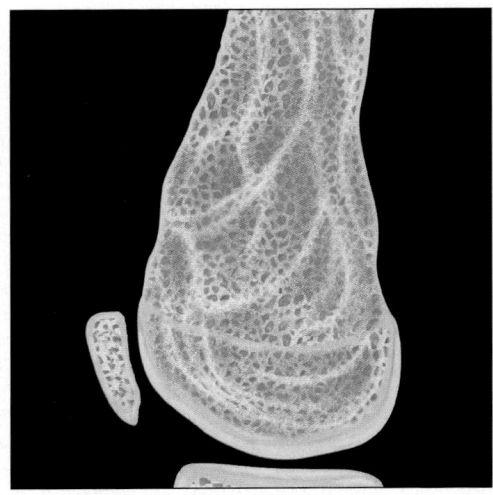

Sagittal graphic shows expansion of the medullary cavity with coarsened trabeculae and cortical thinning. Note undertubulation of the distal femur resulting in Erlenmeyer flask deformity.

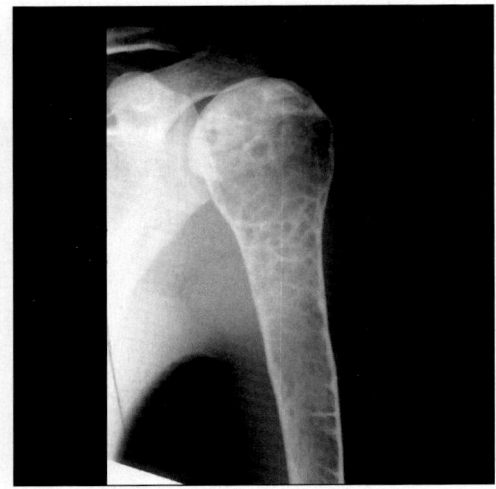

Anteroposterior radiography shows widening of the proximal humerus with osteopenia, coarse trabeculae, and cortical thinning.

TERMINOLOGY

Abbreviations and Synonyms
- Gaucher disease, acid beta-glucocerebrosidase deficiency

Definitions
- Hereditary disease characterized by deposition of glucocerebroside in cells of the reticuloendothelial system (RES) due to deficiency of beta-glucocerebrosidase

IMAGING FINDINGS

General Features
- Best diagnostic clue
  - Expansion of medullary cavity with generalized osteopenia
  - Erlenmeyer flask deformity
- Location
  - Axial skeleton
  - Long bones
  - Pelvis
  - Relative sparing of epiphyses
- Size: Involvement of entire bone
- Morphology: Widened medullary cavity with generalized osteopenia

Radiographic Findings
- Radiography
  - Generalized osteopenia
  - Coarsened trabeculae (honeycombing)
  - Erosion of inner cortex and widened medullary cavity
  - Endosteal scalloping
  - Multiple circumscribed lytic lesions
  - Expansion of metadiaphysis of long bones: Erlenmeyer flask deformity
  - Weakened subchondral bone, degenerative arthritis
  - Spinal compression fractures: H-shaped vertebrae (10%)
  - Avascular necrosis of femoral head (20%), humeral head (10%), ankle, wrist
  - Medullary bone infarcts
  - Dual-energy X-ray absorptiometry (DEXA) useful in evaluation of osteopenia

MR Findings
- T1WI: Bone marrow infiltration of low signal intensity
- T2WI
  - Bone marrow infiltration of low signal intensity
  - Areas of high signal represent acute disease
- STIR: Increased signal intensity
- MR helpful to evaluate for complication
  - Avascular necrosis (AVN), cord compression

DDx: Gaucher's Disease

Multiple Myeloma	Hurler's	Morquio	Thalassemia	Legg-Perthes
AP Radiography	AP Radiography	Lat Radiography	AP Radiography	Cor T1WI MR

GAUCHER'S DISEASE

Key Facts

Imaging Findings
- Expansion of medullary cavity with generalized osteopenia
- Erlenmeyer flask deformity

Top Differential Diagnoses
- Multiple Myeloma
- Hurler Syndrome
- Morquio Syndrome
- Thalassemia
- Legg-Calvé-Perthes
- Nieman Pick Disease

Pathology
- 60% of Ashkenazi Jewish population are homozygote for mild mutation

Clinical Issues
- Most common signs/symptoms: Splenomegaly, bleeding diathesis
- Pancytopenia (hypersplenism)
- Bone involvement in 75%
- Type 1: Longest time of survival
- Type 2: Death during first 2 years of life
- Type 3: Death in childhood, early adulthood
- Enzyme replacement therapy for type 1 disease

Diagnostic Checklist
- Bone crises with severe swelling and pain are frequently mistaken for synovitis or osteomyelitis

---

- Dixon chemical shift imaging helpful in quantifying bone marrow involvement

Nuclear Medicine Findings
- Bone Scan: Increased radiotracer uptake in region of proximal humeri, distal femora, proximal tibiae
- Positive bone scan in 60% of patients

Imaging Recommendations
- Best imaging tool: Radiographs diagnostic
- Protocol advice: T1, T2WI MR to evaluate disease extent and complications (AVN, cord compression)

DIFFERENTIAL DIAGNOSIS

Multiple Myeloma
- Older age group
- Soft tissue mass adjacent to bone destruction

Hurler Syndrome
- Shortened extremity bones
- Normal/increased vertebral body height
- Vertebral inferior beak
- Hypoplastic pelvis

Morquio Syndrome
- Platyspondyly (vertebra plana)
- Ovoid vertebral bodies with central anterior beak
- "Wine glass pelvis"

Thalassemia
- Extramedullary hematopoiesis
- "Hair-on-end" appearance of skull
- AVN less common

Legg-Calvé-Perthes
- Idiopathic AVN of femoral head in children
- Femoral epiphysis of affected hip smaller than normal contralateral side
- Sclerosis, collapse of femoral epiphysis

Nieman Pick Disease
- Erlenmeyer flask deformity
- Severe mental retardation

PATHOLOGY

General Features
- General path comments: Glucosylceramide (accumulated glycolipid) derived from phagocytosis and degeneration of leukocytes and erythrocyte membranes
- Genetics
  - Most common genetic lysosomal storage disorder
  - Autosomal recessive inheritance
  - Gene for glucocerebrosidase located on chromosome 1q21
- Etiology
  - Deficiency of beta-glucocerebrosidase leads to accumulation of glucosylceramide within cells of RES
  - Glucosylceramide storage in bone marrow, liver, spleen, lungs lead to pancytopenia, hepatosplenomegaly, diffuse pulmonary disease
  - Type 2 and 3: Neural cell loss due to accumulation of glucosphingosine from severe deficiency of acid beta-glucocerebrosidase
- Epidemiology
  - Carrier frequency 1 in 15, disease frequency 1 in 855 in Jewish people from Eastern European descent (type 1)
  - 60% of Ashkenazi Jewish population are homozygote for mild mutation

Gross Pathologic & Surgical Features
- Infiltration of cancellous bone with pale yellow tissue distinguishable from fatty marrow
- Secondary infarction: Dense sclerotic bone

Microscopic Features
- Infiltration of bone marrow with Gaucher cells (kerasin-laden histiocytes)
- Gaucher cell: Large, pale, polyhedral cell, eccentric nucleus, weakly eosinophilic cytoplasm containing striations ("wrinkled tissue paper" appearance)

GAUCHER'S DISEASE

Staging, Grading or Classification Criteria
- Type 1: Most common, no central nervous system involvement
- Type 2: Rare, involves central nervous system
- Type 3: Rare, involves central nervous system

CLINICAL ISSUES

Presentation
- Most common signs/symptoms: Splenomegaly, bleeding diathesis
- Clinical profile
  - Neurologic symptoms (type 2, 3): Seizures, mental retardation, spasticity
  - Hepatosplenomegaly due to accumulation of glucosylceramides
  - Pancytopenia (hypersplenism)
  - Fatigue, weight loss
  - Bone involvement in 75%
    - Bone crises: Bone pain from infarction
    - Pathologic fractures, vertebral compression fractures, cord compression
    - AVN of femoral and humeral head, wrist, ankle
    - Osteomyelitis
    - Osteoarthritis
    - Growth retardation
    - Repeated pulmonary infections

Demographics
- Age
  - Adult form (type 1): May present in childhood or adulthood
  - Infantile form (type 2): 1-12 months
  - Juvenile form (type 3): 2-6 years
- Gender: M:F = 1:1
- Ethnicity
  - Type 1: Most common genetic disorder among Ashkenazi Jewish population
  - Type 3 frequently found in Sweden

Natural History & Prognosis
- Type 1: Longest time of survival
  - Patients of non Ashkenazi Jewish descent have worse prognosis
- Type 2: Death during first 2 years of life
- Type 3: Death in childhood, early adulthood

Treatment
- Enzyme replacement therapy for type 1 disease
  - Recombinant enzyme imiglucerase (Cerezyme)
  - Can reverse visceral and hematologic manifestations
    - Skeletal disease responds slowly
- Beta-glucosidase mannose substitution
  - Substitution of mannose to the enzyme glucosidase causes destruction of the accumulated glucosylceramide
- AVN: Bed rest, analgesics, total hip replacement in advanced cases
- Splenectomy in case of severe splenomegaly

DIAGNOSTIC CHECKLIST

Consider
- Bone crises with severe swelling and pain are frequently mistaken for synovitis or osteomyelitis

SELECTED REFERENCES

1. Zhao H et al: Gaucher's disease: Identification of novel mutant alleles and genotype-phenotype relationships. Clin Genet 64:57-64, 2003
2. Cabrera-Salazar MA et al: Gene therapy for the lysosomal storage disorders. Curr Opin Mol Ther 4:349-58, 2002
3. Maas M et al: Quantification of skeletal involvement in adults with type I Gaucher's disease: Fat fraction measured by Dixon quantitative chemical shift imaging as a valid parameter. Am J Roentgenol 179:961-5, 2002
4. Weinreb NJ et al: Effectiveness of enzyme replacement therapy in 1028 patients with type 1 Gaucher disease after 2 to 5 years of treatment: A report from the Gaucher Registry. Am J Med 113:112-9, 2002
5. Poll LW et al: Magnetic resonance imaging of bone marrow changes in Gaucher disease during enzyme replacement therapy: First German long-term results. Skeletal Radiol 30:496-503, 2001
6. Kelman CG et al: Metaphyseal undertubulation in Gaucher disease: Resolution at MRI in a patient undergoing enzyme replacement therapy. J Comput Assist Tomogr 24:173-5, 2000
7. Hermann G et al: Gaucher disease: Assessment of skeletal involvement and therapeutic responses to enzyme replacement. Skeletal Radiol 26:687-96, 1997
8. Terk MR et al: MR imaging of patients with type 1 Gaucher's disease: Relationship between bone and visceral changes. Am J Roentgenol 165:599-604, 1995
9. Oestreich AE: Imaging of the skeleton and soft tissues in children. Curr Opin Radiol 4:55-61, 1992

GAUCHER'S DISEASE

IMAGE GALLERY

Typical

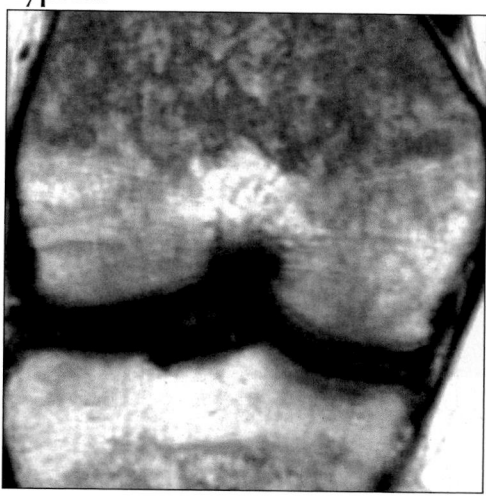
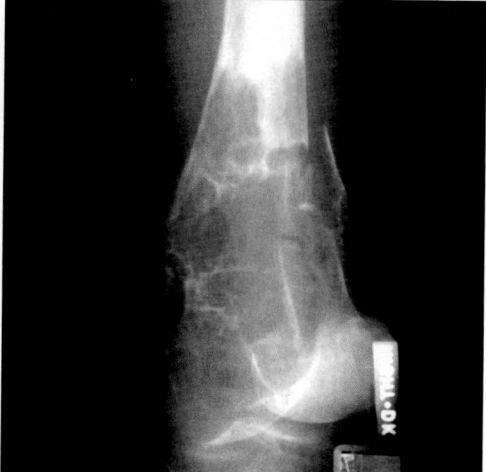

(Left) Coronal T1WI MR shows diffuse hypointense bone marrow infiltration of the distal femur. Hypointense signal represents lipid in reticuloendothelial cells. *(Right)* Anteroposterior radiography shows multiple lytic lesions involving the distal femur with associated pathologic fracture. This lytic appearance may be mistaken for metastatic disease.

Typical

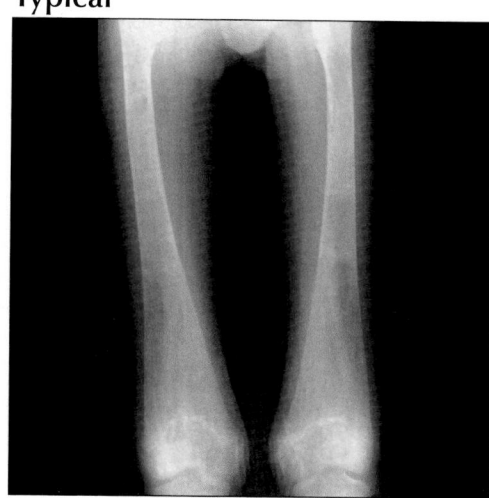
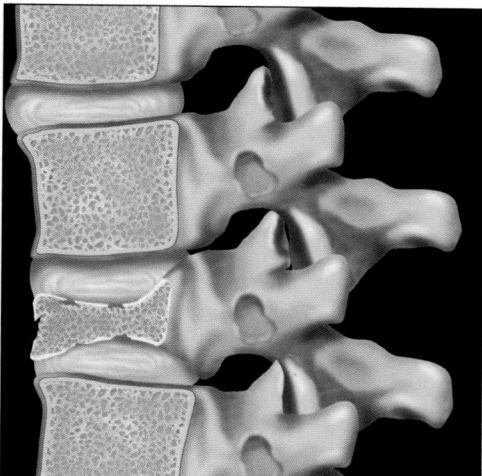

(Left) Anteroposterior radiography shows classic undertubulation (widening) of the distal femoral metadiaphyses (Erlenmeyer flask deformity). Diffuse osteopenia is noted. *(Right)* Sagittal graphic shows vertebral compression fracture.

Typical

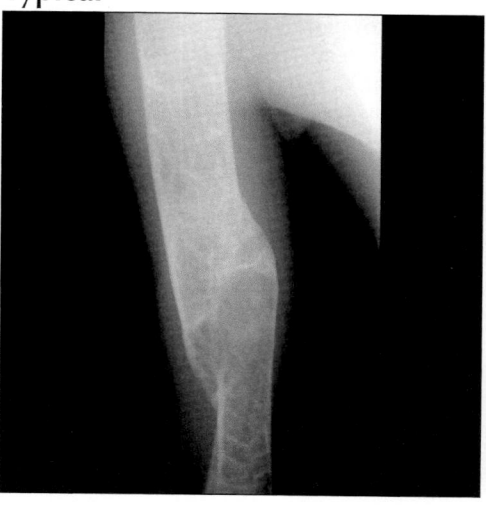
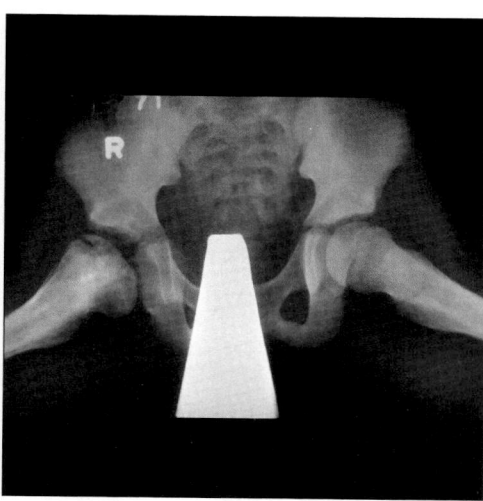

(Left) Anteroposterior radiography shows expansion of the humeral medullary cavity with osteopenia and coarsened trabeculae (honeycombing). *(Right)* Anteroposterior radiography shows avascular necrosis with significant associated osseous deformity involving the right femoral head.

METASTASES, BONE MARROW

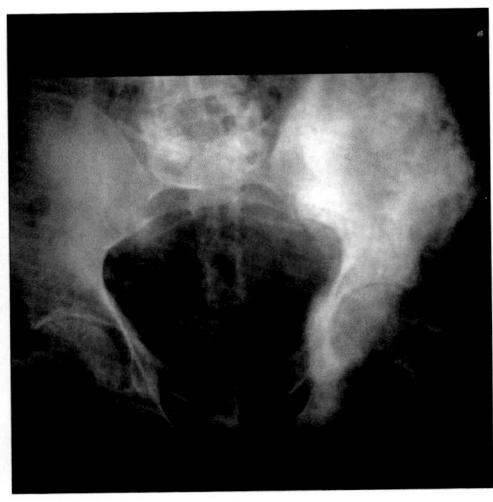

Sagittal graphic shows metastatic bone marrow infiltration of a thoracic vertebral body. Note cortical destruction and associated anterior soft tissue mass.

Anteroposterior radiography shows osteoblastic metastases from prostate cancer involving the pelvis.

TERMINOLOGY

Abbreviations and Synonyms
- Skeletal metastases, bone metastases

Definitions
- Spread of cancer from one part of the body to another

IMAGING FINDINGS

General Features
- Best diagnostic clue: Permeative pattern of bone destruction, osteolytic and/or osteoblastic lesions
- Location
  - Axial and proximal appendicular skeleton most frequently involved
    - Persistence of red marrow
    - Spine, ribs, pelvis, skull
    - Femur, humerus
  - Widespread disease in children (more red marrow)
    - Neuroblastoma, leukemia most common
  - Distal bones rarely affected: Lung, breast, renal cancer
    - Small tubular bones of hands and feet: Can be affected in lung cancer
- Size: < 5 cm in length

- Morphology: Single/multiple osteolytic or blastic lesions of variable size

Radiographic Findings
- Radiography
  - Insensitive for detecting early metastatic disease
    - At lease 30-50% of normal bone must be lost before metastases are visible
  - Multiple areas of bone destruction
    - Moth eaten, permeative, geographic pattern
  - Osteolytic lesions: 70%
    - Primary: Kidney, breast, thyroid, GI tract
  - Osteoblastic lesions: 15%
    - Primary: Prostate, breast, cervix, ovary, urinary bladder, carcinoid, osteosarcoma
  - Mixed osteoblastic and osteolytic lesions: 10%
    - Any primary, most common in breast, lung
  - +/- Cortical destruction, periosteal new bone formation
  - +/- Extension into soft tissue
  - Spine: Destruction of pedicles, endplate deformity
    - Joint spaces and intervertebral spaces preserved (cartilage resistant to invasion)
  - Increased sclerosis and decrease in size with healing

CT Findings
- NECT
  - Lytic or blastic bone marrow infiltration
  - Cortical destruction

DDx: Metastases, Bone Marrow

Multiple Myeloma	Lymphoma	Paget Disease	Hemangioma	MFH
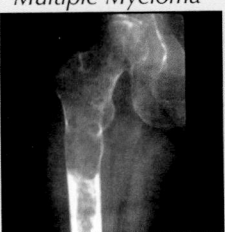	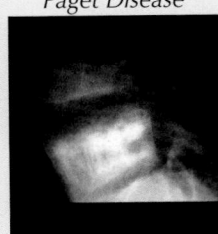	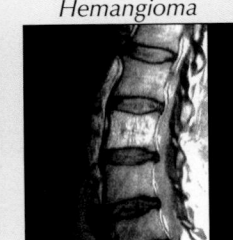		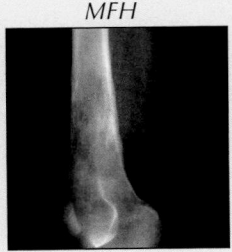
AP Radiography	Sag T1WI MR	Lat Radiography	Sag T1WI MR	Lat Radiography

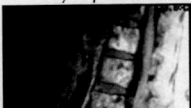

METASTASES, BONE MARROW

Key Facts

Imaging Findings
- Best diagnostic clue: Permeative pattern of bone destruction, osteolytic and/or osteoblastic lesions

Top Differential Diagnoses
- Multiple Myeloma
- Lymphoma
- Paget Disease
- Hemangioma
- Malignant Fibrous Histiocytoma (MFH)

Pathology
- Bone marrow: Third most common site of metastatic disease
- Skeletal metastases in 30-70% of patients with malignancy at autopsy

- Metastases to bone 25 times more common than primary skeletal neoplasms

Clinical Issues
- Most common signs/symptoms: Pain (70%), weight loss, anemia
- Pathologic fractures
- Osteoclast inhibiting agents: Bisphosphates (alendronate, etidronate, pamidronate, clodronate)
- Radiation therapy
- Internal fixation in case of pathologic fracture or to prevent pathologic fracture

Diagnostic Checklist
- Multiple bone lesions in patients over 50 years are usually due to metastases

---

- Useful in evaluating radiographically negative areas when metastases are suspected

MR Findings
- T1WI
  - Lytic metastases
    - Low signal intensity
  - Osteoblastic metastases
    - Low signal intensity
  - Mixed metastases
    - Heterogeneous signal intensity
- T2WI
  - Lytic metastases
    - High signal intensity
  - Osteoblastic metastases
    - Low signal intensity
  - Mixed metastases
    - Heterogeneous intermediate-high signal intensity
- STIR
  - Lytic metastases: High signal intensity
  - Osteoblastic metastases: Low signal intensity
  - Mixed metastases: Heterogeneous intermediate-high signal intensity
  - Whole body STIR to evaluate entire skeleton for metastases
- DWI: Helpful in differentiating benign osteoporotic from malignant compression fractures
- T1 C+: Variable enhancement
- Helpful in evaluating associated soft tissue components, complications (cord compression)

Angiographic Findings
- Hypervascular
- Preoperative embolization of hypervascular metastases

Nuclear Medicine Findings
- Bone Scan
  - High sensitivity for many metastatic tumors (breast, lung, prostate)
    - Increased radiotracer uptake in > 90%
    - Normal bone scan: 5%
    - Decreased activity in metastases with low metabolic activity or destruction but no new bone formation

- Multiple asymmetric areas of increased radiotracer uptake
- Superscan: Widespread bone marrow metastases produce diffusely increased uptake
  - Absence of normal activity in kidneys and urinary bladder
- "Healing flare" phenomenon: Transient increased activity under therapy during healing
- False positives: 10%

Imaging Recommendations
- Best imaging tool: Bone scan, MRI
- Protocol advice
  - Bone scan to detect extent of metastatic disease
  - MRI to evaluate complications

7

35

DIFFERENTIAL DIAGNOSIS

Multiple Myeloma
- Late involvement of pedicles (pedicles involved first in metastases)
- Cold on bone scan
- Sclerosis extremely rare
- Endosteal scalloping

Lymphoma
- Permeative bone destruction
- Cortical destruction occurs late in disease
- Lamellated, sunburst periosteal reaction

Paget Disease
- Thickened cortex and trabeculae
- Marrow replacement not mass like
- No cortical destruction

Hemangioma
- Multiloculated lytic foci
- Vertical striations, honeycomb appearance

Malignant Fibrous Histiocytoma (MFH)
- Permeative bone destruction
- Solitary lesion

METASTASES, BONE MARROW

PATHOLOGY

General Features
- General path comments
  - Metastases: Late event in process of cancer development
  - Every malignancy can metastasize to bone
    - Cancers metastasize more common than sarcomas
    - Cancers most likely to metastasize to bone: Breast, lung, prostate, thyroid, kidney
    - Children: Neuroblastoma
- Etiology
  - Hematogenous spread through arterial circulation to vascular red marrow
  - Hematogenous spread through retrograde venous flow (prostate)
  - Direct extension (uncommon)
- Epidemiology
  - Bone marrow: Third most common site of metastatic disease
  - Skeletal metastases in 30-70% of patients with malignancy at autopsy
  - Metastases to bone 25 times more common than primary skeletal neoplasms

Gross Pathologic & Surgical Features
- Firm, white tumor with or without necrotic, hemorrhagic areas
- Cortical disruption
- Invasion into adjacent soft tissues

Microscopic Features
- Replacement of bone marrow by carcinoma cells depending on origin of primary tumor
- Excretion of osteoclast-stimulating factors and necrotic factors with direct lytic activity by metastatic cells
- Tumor cells with increased levels of laminin and fibronectin surface receptors have high metastatic potential
- Increased type IV collagenase of tumor cells correlates with increased metastatic potential
  - Type IV collagenase degrades major component of basement membrane (type IV collagen)

CLINICAL ISSUES

Presentation
- Most common signs/symptoms: Pain (70%), weight loss, anemia
- Clinical profile
  - Swelling in region of affected bone
  - Pathologic fractures
  - Hypercalcemia (10%), elevated alkaline phosphatase
  - Neurologic impairment with spinal metastases

Demographics
- Age: > 40 years, unless known primary
- Gender: Dependent on primary cancer

Natural History & Prognosis
- Initial metastasis usually occurs within two years after diagnosis of primary malignancy
- Patients with lung cancers and bone metastases have median survival of < 6 months

Treatment
- Osteoclast inhibiting agents: Bisphosphates (alendronate, etidronate, pamidronate, clodronate)
- Radiation therapy
- Strontium-89 for bone pain (palliative)
- Vertebroplasty for spinal compression fractures
- Internal fixation in case of pathologic fracture or to prevent pathologic fracture
- Important to determine etiology of malignant lesion prior to fixation
  - If lesion represents primary mesenchymal sarcoma, increased risk of tumor seeding during internal fixation (may convert limb salvage procedure into amputation)
  - If lesion is due to metastatic carcinoma, low risk of tumor seeding during internal fixation

DIAGNOSTIC CHECKLIST

Image Interpretation Pearls
- Multiple bone lesions in patients over 50 years are usually due to metastases

SELECTED REFERENCES

1. Vanel D et al: MRI of bone marrow disorders. Eur Radiol 10:224-9, 2000
2. Traill ZC et al: Magnetic resonance imaging versus radionuclide scintigraphy in screening for bone metastases. Clin Radiol 54:448-51, 1999
3. Vanel D et al: MRI of bone metastases. Eur Radiol 8:1345-51, 1998
4. Yamaguchi T et al: Intertrabecular pattern of tumors metastatic to bone. Cancer 78:1388-94, 1996
5. Papac RJ: Bone marrow metastases. A review. Cancer 74:2403-13, 1994
6. Scher HI et al: Bone metastases: Improving the therapeutic index. Sem Oncol 21:630-56, 1994
7. Stetler-Stevenson WG et al: Tumor cell interactions with the extracellular matrix during invasion and metastasis. Annu Rev Cell Biol 9:541-73, 1993
8. Asdourian PL et al: The pattern of vertebral involvement in metastatic vertebral breast cancer. Clin Orthop 250:164-70, 1990
9. Gold RI et al: An integrated approach to the evaluation of metastatic bone disease. Radiol Clin North Am 28:472-83, 1990

IMAGE GALLERY

Typical

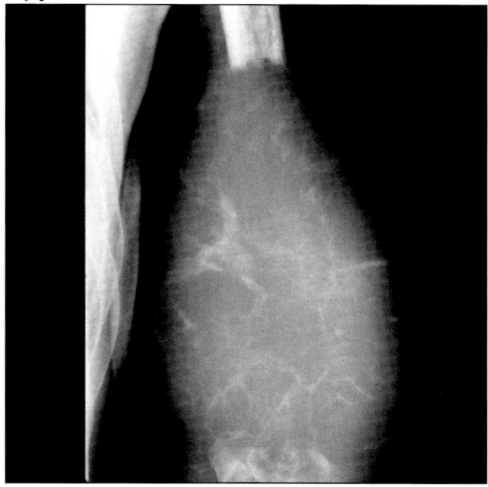
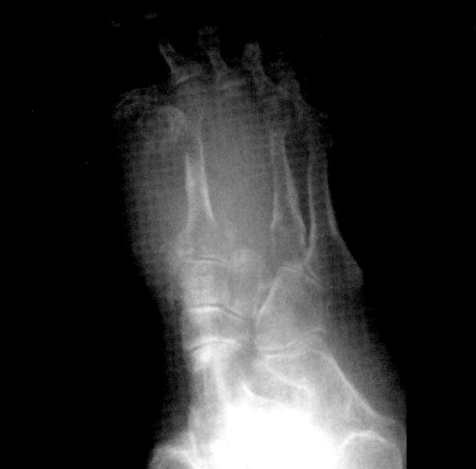

*(**Left**) Anteroposterior radiography shows large lytic expansile lesion involving the humerus in a patient with renal cell cancer. Metastases from renal cell cancer are hypervascular and can lead to severe hemorrhage during surgery. (**Right**) Anteroposterior radiography shows destruction of multiple tarsal and metatarsal bones in a patient with lung cancer. Metastases to the feet are uncommon but can be seen with lung cancer.*

Typical

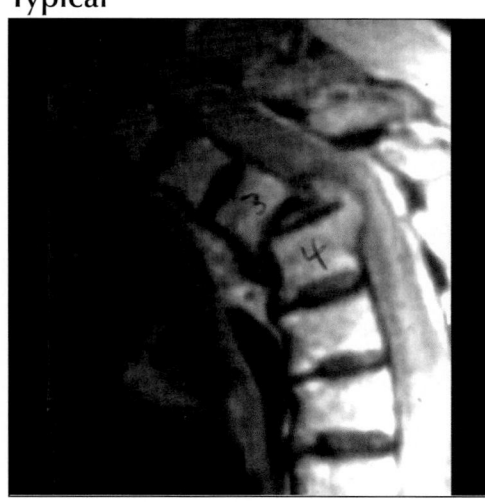
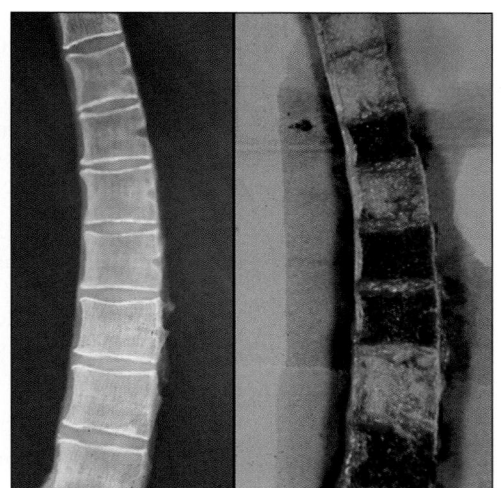

*(**Left**) Sagittal T1WI MR shows vertebral collapse with associated soft tissue mass and marked kyphotic angulation causing cord compression in a patient with colon cancer. (**Right**) Coronal radiography (resected specimen) shows normal thoracic vertebral bodies. Corresponding gross specimen shows multiple bone marrow metastases in a patient with breast cancer. This shows the low sensitivity of radiographs in metastases.*

Typical

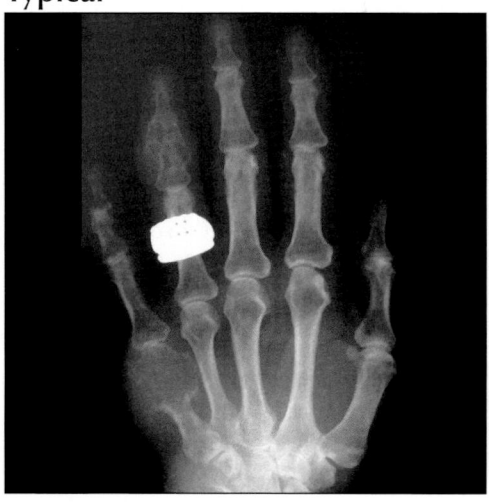
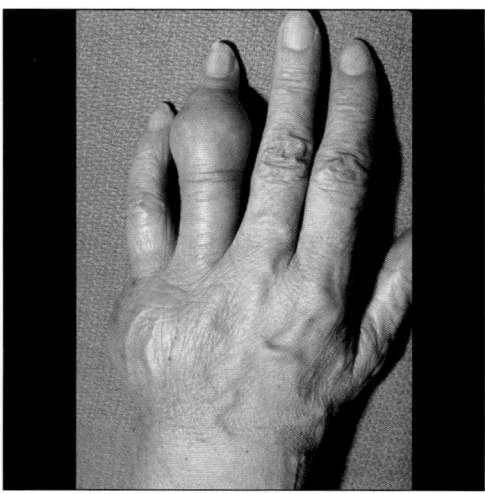

*(**Left**) Anteroposterior radiography shows expansile lytic lesions in the metacarpal bones and phalanges in a patient with thyroid cancer. (**Right**) Clinical photograph shows expansile masses in the metacarpals and phalanges corresponding to lytic metastases from thyroid cancer.*

PAGET DISEASE

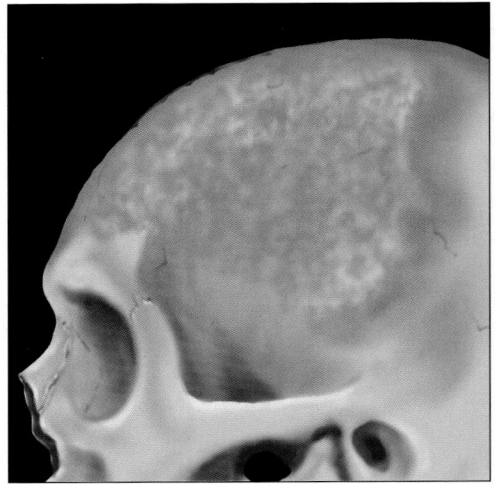

Sagittal graphic shows osteolytic phase of Paget disease (osteoporosis circumscripta) involving the frontal bone.

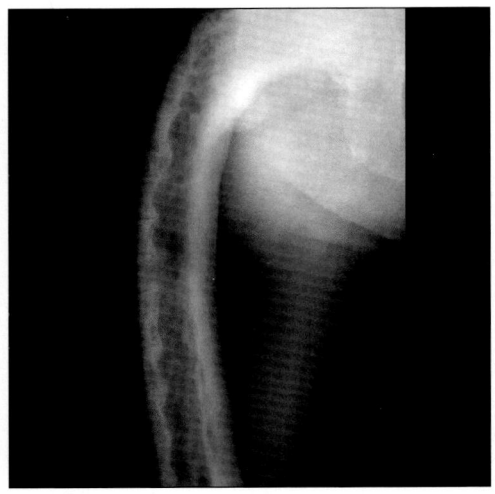

Lateral radiography shows cortical and trabecular thickening, expansion of the femur with multiple transverse stress fractures in the lateral cortex. The lesions extend to the end of bone.

TERMINOLOGY

Abbreviations and Synonyms
- Osteitis deformans, Paget's disease

Definitions
- Chronic skeletal disease characterized by abnormal osteoblastic and osteoclastic activity resulting in abnormal bone remodeling

IMAGING FINDINGS

General Features
- Best diagnostic clue
  - Enlarged bone with thickened and coarse trabeculae
  - Starts at one end of bone and progresses along shaft
- Location
  - Pelvis: 73%
  - Spine: 58%
  - Skull: 42%
  - Proximal long bones: 25-30%
  - Scapula: 24%
  - Clavicle: 11%
  - Long bones: Lesion starts at one end of bone, extends along shaft
    - Usually unilateral involvement, contralateral bone normal or minimally affected
  - Polyostotic: 70%
  - Monostotic: 10-35%
- Size
  - 2-3 cm in early stage
  - Involvement of entire bone in late phase
- Morphology: Expanded bone with thickened trabeculae

Radiographic Findings
- Radiography
  - Pelvis
    - Thickening of iliopectineal line
    - Thickened trabeculae, coarse cortex
    - Acetabular protrusion
  - Skull
    - Diploic widening: Inner and outer table involved
    - Osteoporosis circumscripta: Well-defined lytic lesions (destructive active stage)
    - Usually frontal bone involvement
    - Cotton-wool appearance: Mixed lytic and blastic pattern of thickened calvarium (late stage)
    - Basilar invagination with narrowing of foramen magnum
  - Long bones
    - "Candle flame" lysis: V-shaped lytic defect originating subarticular and advancing to diaphysis of long bone
    - Banana fractures: Small, horizontal stress fractures in weight bearing bones (on convex surface)

DDx: Paget Disease

Metastases	Lymphoma	Fibrous Dysplasia	Multiple Myeloma	Hemangioma
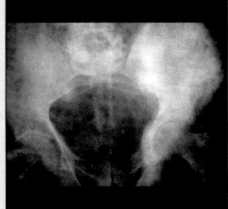	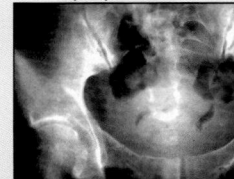	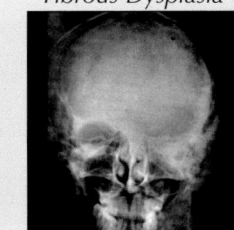	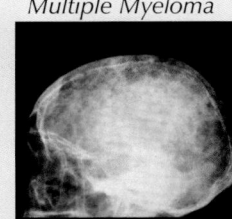	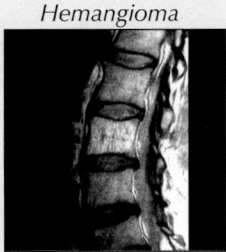
AP Radiography	AP Radiography	AP Radiography	Lat Radiography	Sag T1WI MR

PAGET DISEASE

Key Facts

Imaging Findings

- Enlarged bone with thickened and coarse trabeculae
- Starts at one end of bone and progresses along shaft
- Osteoporosis circumscripta: Well-defined lytic lesions (destructive active stage)
- Cotton-wool appearance: Mixed lytic and blastic pattern of thickened calvarium (late stage)

Top Differential Diagnoses

- Osteoblastic Metastases
- Lymphoma
- Fibrous Dysplasia
- Multiple Myeloma
- Hemangioma
- Myelofibrosis

Pathology

- Affects 3% of individuals > 40 years
- Affects 10% of individuals > 80 years

Clinical Issues

- Insidious onset, asymptomatic for many years
- Bowed and enlarged femur and tibia
- Compression fractures (soft bone despite increased density)
- Peripheral nerve compression, neurological disorders from compression of brainstem
- Elevated serum alkaline phosphatase and urine hydroxyproline
- Sarcomatous transformation (< 1%)
- Bisphosphates: Alendronate, etidronate
- Calcitonin

- Lateral bowing of femur, anterior bowing of tibia
- Acetabular protrusio
- Spine
    - Picture-frame vertebral body: Enlarged, square, vertebral body with thickened, peripheral trabeculae and radiolucent inner portion
    - Ivory vertebra: Increased density
    - Ossification of spinal ligaments
- Progression from active osteolytic phase to sclerotic phase
    - Reversion form sclerotic phase to lytic phase possible
    - However, lytic lesion in previously sclerotic pagetoid bone is suspicious for malignant degeneration
- Rarely associated with multiple giant cell tumors

CT Findings

- NECT: Enlarged sclerotic bone with thickened coarse trabeculae
- CECT: Dense enhancement in lytic phase
- Helpful in complex anatomic areas (skull, spine)

MR Findings

- T1WI
    - Low signal intensity
        - Yellow marrow/fat
        - Marrow replacement not mass like
- T2WI
    - Active phase: High signal intensity
    - Low signal intensity (sclerosis)
        - Marrow replacement: Parallels signal intensity of fat
- T1 C+: Enhancement in lytic phase
- Coarsened appearance of bone marrow
- Helpful in evaluating spine (cord, nerve root compression)
- For evaluation of sarcomatous degeneration

Angiographic Findings

- Involved bone is hypervascular

Nuclear Medicine Findings

- Bone Scan

- Increased radiotracer uptake in lytic phase
- Normal scan in sclerotic, burned-out lesions
- Abnormal before radiographs
- Helpful to assess distribution

Imaging Recommendations

- Best imaging tool: Radiographs diagnostic
- Protocol advice
    - Radiographs diagnostic, MRI and CT to evaluate for complications
    - Bone scan useful in determining extent of disease

DIFFERENTIAL DIAGNOSIS

Osteoblastic Metastases

- May be indistinguishable
- Often diffuse, bilateral (Paget usually unilateral)

Lymphoma

- Cancellous bone erosion
- Cortical destruction with soft tissue mass
- High signal on T2W MR of involved areas

Fibrous Dysplasia

- Ground glass appearance
- Cranial lesions may be indistinguishable

Multiple Myeloma

- Multiple well-defined lytic lesions
- Sclerosis extremely rare
- Endosteal scalloping
- Soft tissue mass adjacent to bone destruction

Hemangioma

- Vertical striations, honeycomb appearance
- Multiloculated lytic foci
- No trabecular thickening

Myelofibrosis

- Sclerosis without bone enlargement
- Bilateral involvement

PAGET DISEASE

PATHOLOGY

General Features
- General path comments
  - Increased osteoclastic activity resulting in progressive multifocal bone resorption followed by bone formation
  - High rate of bone turnover with rapid bone growth can lead to mutations and genomic deletions leading to malignant transformation
- Genetics: Mutations in gene encoding sequestosome 1 (SQSTM1) in familial and sporadic Paget disease
- Etiology
  - Chronic disease of osteoblasts and osteoclasts
  - Possible viral etiology (parvomyxovirus)
  - Regional difference in disease prevalence supports environment influence
- Epidemiology
  - Affects 3% of individuals > 40 years
  - Affects 10% of individuals > 80 years

Gross Pathologic & Surgical Features
- Newly formed bone abnormally soft and deformed
- Increased vascularity
- Disorganized trabecular pattern
- Thickened trabeculae with small marrow cavities

Microscopic Features
- Active phase (osteolytic phase)
  - Aggressive bone resorption with lytic lesions
  - Replacement of hematopoietic bone marrow by fibrous connective tissue
  - Increased vascular channels
  - Osteoblastic rimming
- Inactive phase (quiescent phase)
  - Decreased bone turnover with skeletal sclerosis and coarse trabeculae
  - Loss of excessive vascularity
  - Irregular cement lines
- Mixed pattern
  - Mixture of lytic and sclerotic phase
  - Intracytoplasmatic inclusions

CLINICAL ISSUES

Presentation
- Most common signs/symptoms
  - Insidious onset, asymptomatic for many years
  - Full clinical picture with characteristic bone deformities after 20-30 years
- Clinical profile
  - Fatigue
  - Bowed and enlarged femur and tibia
  - Skin over affected bones warm, erythematous
  - Secondary arthritis
  - Compression fractures (soft bone despite increased density)
  - Peripheral nerve compression, neurological disorders from compression of brainstem
    - Hearing loss, blindness, facial palsies
  - Enlarged hat size
  - Elevated serum alkaline phosphatase and urine hydroxyproline

- High output congestive heart failure (rare)

Demographics
- Age: 55-85 years, unusual < 40 years
- Gender: M:F = 2:1
- Ethnicity
  - Highest incidence in the United Kingdom, New Zealand, Australia
  - Uncommon in Asia, Africa (excluding South Africa)

Natural History & Prognosis
- Sarcomatous transformation (< 1%)
  - Osteosarcoma (22-90%)
  - Fibrosarcoma/malignant fibrous histiocytoma (MFH) (29-51%)
  - Chondrosarcoma (1-15%)
  - Poor prognosis, 5-year survival for osteosarcoma: 8%

Treatment
- Bisphosphates: Alendronate, etidronate
- Calcitonin
- Mithramycin
- Joint replacement in case of arthritis
- Fixation of pathologic fractures
- Radical resection of sarcomatous transformed bone, amputation often necessary

DIAGNOSTIC CHECKLIST

Consider
- Delayed diagnosis of sarcomatous degeneration may affect prognosis for prolonged survival

Image Interpretation Pearls
- In a patient with malignancy, metastases will preferentially involve pagetic bone

SELECTED REFERENCES

1. Hocking LJ et al: Domain-specific mutations in sequestosome 1 (SQSTM1) cause familial and sporadic Paget's disease. Hum Mol Genet 11:2735-9, 2002
2. Whitehouse RW: Paget's disease of bone. Semin Musculoskelet Radiol 6:313-22, 2002
3. Boutin RD et al: Complications in Paget disease at MR imaging. Radiology 209:641-51, 1998
4. Mirra JM et al: Paget's disease of bone: Review with emphasis on radiologic features. Part 1. Skeletal Radiol 24:163-71, 1995
5. Gallacher SJ: Paget's disease of bone. Curr Opin Rheumatol 5:351-6, 1993
6. Roberts MC et al: Paget disease: MR imaging findings. Radiology 173:341-5, 1989
7. Meunier PJ et al: Skeletal distribution and biochemical parameters of Paget's disease. Clin Orthop 217:37-44, 1987
8. Frame B et al: Paget disease: A review of current knowledge. Radiology 141:21-4, 1981

PAGET DISEASE

IMAGE GALLERY

Typical

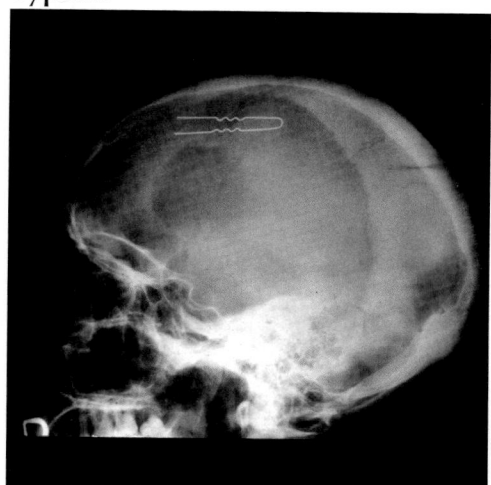
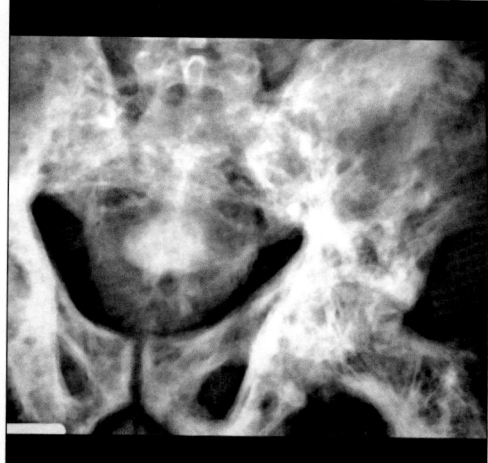

(Left) Lateral radiography shows osteolytic lesion involving the anterior calvarium, consistent with osteoporosis circumscripta (lytic phase). *(Right)* Anteroposterior radiography shows marked cortical thickening and coarse trabecular pattern of the pelvis in the cold phase of the disease.

Typical

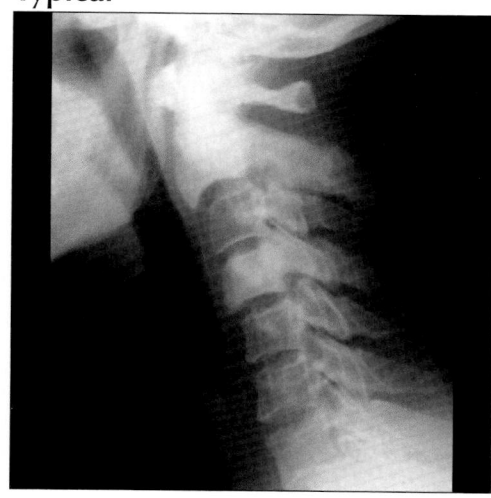
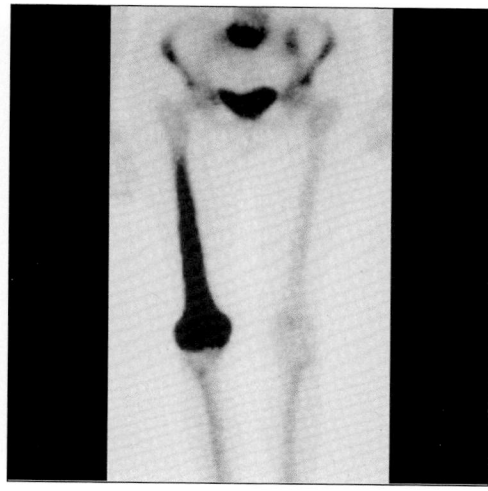

(Left) Lateral radiography shows increased density of the C2 and C4 vertebral bodies (ivory vertebral body). *(Right)* Anteroposterior bone scan shows markedly increased radiotracer uptake extending from the distal femoral epiphysis to the proximal diaphysis. Expansion of the femur is noted.

Other

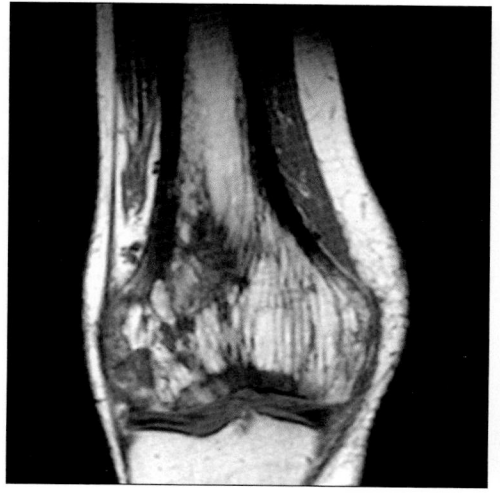
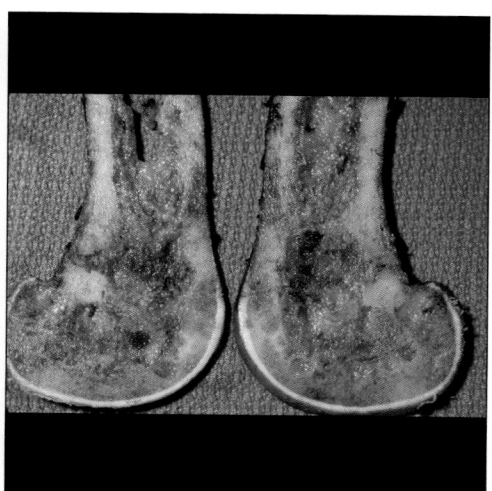

(Left) Coronal T1WI MR shows enlargement of the distal femur with cortical thickening and coarse cancellous trabeculae of low signal. *(Right)* Coronal gross pathology, section shows involvement of the distal femur with cortical thickening and coarse trabeculae.

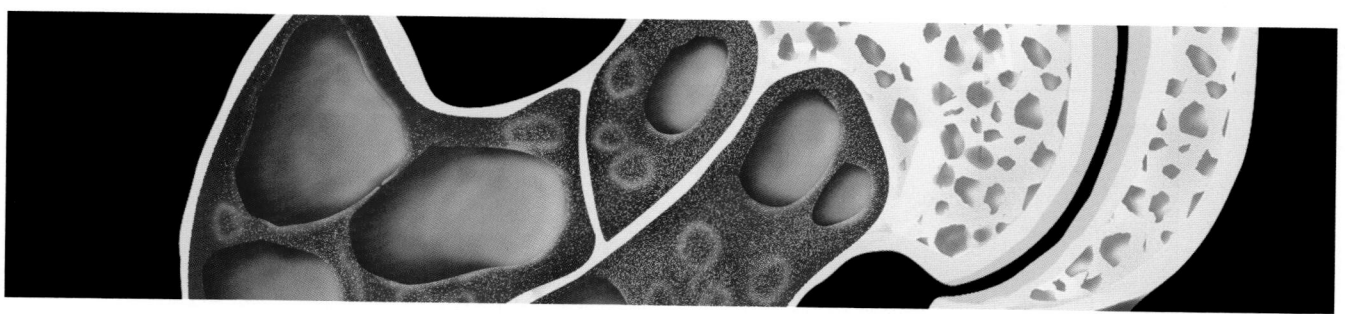

SECTION 8: Bone Tumors

OSTEOMA

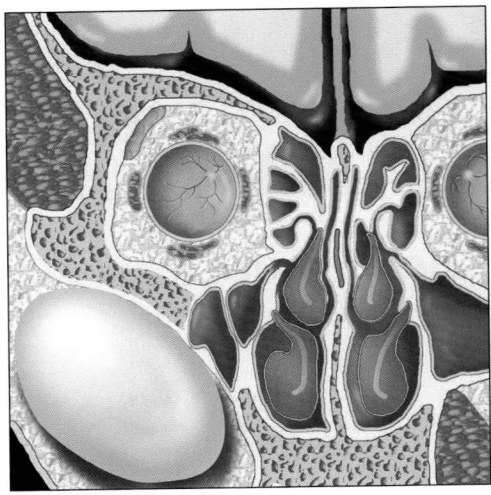

Coronal graphic show sclerotic ivory-like osteoma arising from the right mandible. The tumor abuts the orbital floor and maxillary sinus. There is no invasion or cortical destruction.

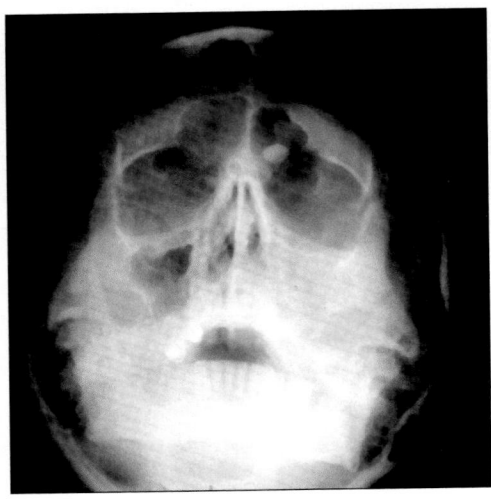

Anteroposterior radiography of the skull shows a round well-defined sclerotic lesion located in the left frontal sinus.

TERMINOLOGY

Abbreviations and Synonyms
- Ivory exostosis

Definitions
- Benign, slow growing hamartomatous lesion consisting of well-differentiated mature bone

IMAGING FINDINGS

General Features
- Best diagnostic clue: Well-defined round dense sclerotic lesion attached to underlying bone
- Location
  ○ Frontal and ethmoid sinuses: 75%
  ○ Sphenoid sinus: 1-4%
  ○ Inner/outer table of calvarium
  ○ Mandible
  ○ Rare in long and flat bones
  ○ Parosteal (not intramedullary)
  ○ May be multiple
- Size: 1-5 cm, usually < 2 cm
- Morphology: Dense sclerotic well-defined mass

Radiographic Findings
- Radiography
  ○ Dense, ivory-like sclerotic mass

○ Lesion attached to bone
○ Bone mass is arising from surface of bone
○ Well-defined margins
○ No associated osseous destruction
○ No satellite lesions
○ Mild periosteal reaction can be seen
○ Cranial osteomas
  ■ Intraparenchymal: No connection to dura or bone
  ■ Dural: No bony attachment, arise from falx
  ■ Skull base: Occur in paranasal sinuses, maxilla, mandible, temporal bone
  ■ Skull vault: Arise from outer table of skull (exostotic) or inner table (enostotic)

CT Findings
- NECT
  ○ Homogeneous calcific hemispheric mass
  ○ Lesion is arising from external surface of the cortex
  ○ Periosteal reaction can be seen
  ○ Helpful in demonstrating lack of cortical invasion and lack of medullary continuity with host bone
- CECT: No enhancement

MR Findings
- T1WI
  ○ Low signal intensity
  ○ Attached to underlying bone
- T2WI
  ○ Low signal intensity

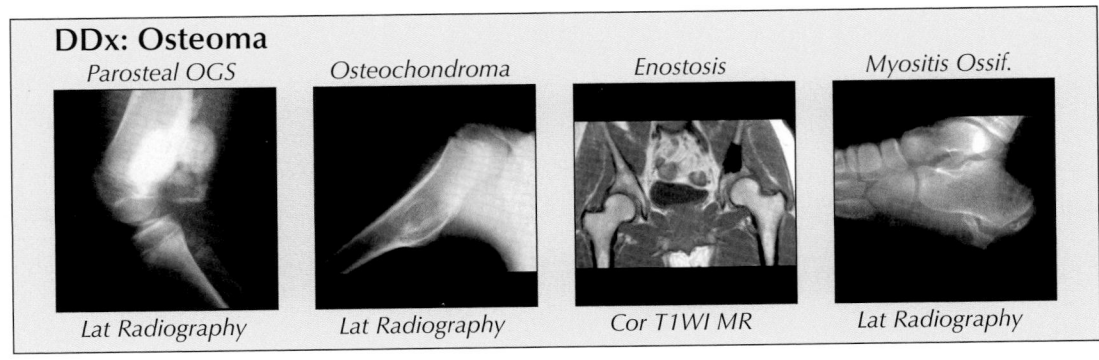

DDx: Osteoma

Parosteal OGS	Osteochondroma	Enostosis	Myositis Ossif.
Lat Radiography	Lat Radiography	Cor T1WI MR	Lat Radiography

OSTEOMA

Key Facts

Imaging Findings
- Best diagnostic clue: Well-defined round dense sclerotic lesion attached to underlying bone

Top Differential Diagnoses
- Parosteal Osteosarcoma
- Sessile Osteochondroma
- Enostosis (Bone Island)
- Juxtacortical Myositis Ossificans

Pathology
- Extracranial osteoma: 0.03% of biopsied primary bone lesions
- Gardner's Syndrome: Autosomal dominant
- Multiple osteomas, intestinal polyposis, soft tissue desmoid tumors

Clinical Issues
- Small lesions are usually asymptomatic
- Large paranasal sinus tumors may obstruct nasal ducts
- Tumors near orbit can cause exophthalmus, double vision, vision loss
- Benign lesion
- Asymptomatic lesions require no treatment

Diagnostic Checklist
- Multiple osteomas or osteomas outside craniofacial bones, think of Gardner's Syndrome
- Heterogeneous lesion, cortical destruction, consider parosteal osteosarcoma

---

- ○ Attached to underlying bone
- ○ FS T2 FSE
  - ▪ Low signal intensity
- STIR: Low signal intensity
- T1 C+: No enhancement

Nuclear Medicine Findings
- Bone Scan
  - ○ Increased radiotracer uptake of active lesions
  - ○ No increased uptake of latent lesions

Imaging Recommendations
- Best imaging tool: Radiographs, CT
- Protocol advice: CT to evaluate anatomic complex areas (craniofacial bones)

DIFFERENTIAL DIAGNOSIS

Parosteal Osteosarcoma
- Zone of decreased density at periphery
- Less dense and homogeneous than osteoma
- Incomplete cleft between lesion and adjacent cortex

Sessile Osteochondroma
- Cortex of lesion merges without interruption with cortex of host bone
- Cancellous portion continuous with host medullary cavity

Enostosis (Bone Island)
- Intramedullary location
- Blends with surrounding trabecular bone
- Irregular spiculated margins
- Small: < 1 cm

Juxtacortical Myositis Ossificans
- Zonal phenomenon
- Lucent center, dense ossified periphery

PATHOLOGY

General Features
- General path comments: Dysplastic developmental anomaly
- Genetics: Gardner's Syndrome (mutations involving adenomatous polyposis coli gene mapped to chromosome 5q21)
- Etiology
  - ○ Defect in bone resorption or formation during skeletal maturation
  - ○ Arises beneath endosteum from inner surface of cortex
  - ○ Elevation of periosteum form underlying bone causes surrounding reactive bone formation
    - ▪ Lesion grows inwards from the periphery
- Epidemiology
  - ○ Extracranial osteoma: 0.03% of biopsied primary bone lesions
  - ○ Paranasal sinus osteomas: Incidence 0.4%
- Associated abnormalities
  - ○ Gardner's Syndrome: Autosomal dominant
    - ▪ Multiple osteomas, intestinal polyposis, soft tissue desmoid tumors
    - ▪ Bone lesions may precede intestinal polyposis
    - ▪ Multiple osteomas, solitary osteoma of mandible, or osteomas in appendicular skeleton raise suspicion of Gardner's Syndrome

Gross Pathologic & Surgical Features
- Circumscribed, juxtacortical bone mass
- Periosteum easily removed from underlying lesion (serves as capsule)
- Similar to normal cortical bone
- Peripheral reactive bone formation

Microscopic Features
- Cancellous type: Cancellous, trabecular architecture
  - ○ Active bone formation with transformation to lamellar bone
- Lamellar bone: Composed of layers of mature matrix with densely packed collagen fibers

- Woven bone: Consists of mature matrix with collagen fibers
- Compact type: Dense, compact, mature lamellar bone
- Overlying periosteum: Layer of mature, fibrous, connective tissue and proliferating osteoblasts

Staging, Grading or Classification Criteria

- Surgical staging system for benign musculoskeletal tumors
  - Stage 1: Latent
  - Stage 2: Active
  - Stage 3: Aggressive

CLINICAL ISSUES

Presentation

- Most common signs/symptoms
  - Small lesions are usually asymptomatic
  - Palpable enlarging osseous mass
- Clinical profile
  - Large paranasal sinus tumors may obstruct nasal ducts
    - Can erode wall of cranial fossa and dura
    - Can cause mucoceles, sinusitis, nasal discharge, headache, pain
  - Tumors near orbit can cause exophthalmus, double vision, vision loss
  - Tumors in craniofacial bones can cause enlargement of cheeks ("cherubism")

Demographics

- Age: 10-79 years, peak: 4th-5th decade
- Gender: M:F = 1:1
- Ethnicity: No racial predilection

Natural History & Prognosis

- Benign lesion
- No malignant degeneration
- Lesion undergoes involution from active stage 2 lesion to latent stage 1 lesion

Treatment

- Asymptomatic lesions require no treatment
- Symptomatic lesions: En bloc resection with marginal margins
- Sinonasal endoscopy

DIAGNOSTIC CHECKLIST

Consider

- Multiple osteomas or osteomas outside craniofacial bones, think of Gardner's Syndrome

Image Interpretation Pearls

- Heterogeneous lesion, cortical destruction, consider parosteal osteosarcoma

SELECTED REFERENCES

1. Eppley BL et al: Large osteomas of the cranial vault. J Craniofac Surg 14:97-100, 2003
2. Haddad FS et al: Cranial osteomas: Their classification and management. Report on a giant osteoma and review of the literature. Surg Neurol 48:143-7, 1997
3. Peyser AB et al: Osteoma of the long bones and the spine: A study of eleven patients and a review of the literature. J Bone Joint Surg 78A:1172-80, 1996
4. Sundaram M et al: Surface osteomas of the appendicular skeleton. Am J Roentgenol 167:1529-33, 1996
5. Bertoni F et al: Parosteal osteoma of bones other than of the skull and face. Cancer 75:2466-73, 1995
6. Davies DR et al: Severe Gardner syndrome in families with mutations restricted to a specific region of the APC gene. Am J Hum Genet 57:1151-8, 1995
7. Greenspan A: Benign bone-forming lesions: Osteoma, osteoid osteoma, and osteoblastoma. Skeletal Radiol 22:485-500, 1993
8. O'Connell JX et al: Solitary osteoma of a long bone. J Bone Joint Surg 75A:1830-4, 1993
9. Greenspan A: Sclerosing bone dysplasias - a target-site approach. Skeletal Radiol 20:561-83, 1991
10. Cervilla V et al: Case report 596. Parosteal osteoma of the acetabulum. Skeletal Radiol 19:135-7, 1990
11. Sadry F et al: The potential aggressiveness of sinus osteomas. A report of two cases. Skeletal Radiol 17:427-30, 1988
12. Jacobson HG: Dense bone - too much bone: Radiological considerations and differential diagnosis. Part I. Skeletal Radiol 13:1-20, 1985
13. Jacobson HG: Dense bone - too much bone: Radiological considerations and differential diagnosis. Part II. Skeletal Radiol 13:97-113, 1985
14. Stern PJ et al: Giant metacarpal osteoma. A case report. J Bone Joint Surg 67A:487-9, 1985
15. Dolan K et al: Gardner's syndrome. A model for correlative radiology. Radium Ther Nucl Med 119:359-64, 1973

OSTEOMA

IMAGE GALLERY

Typical

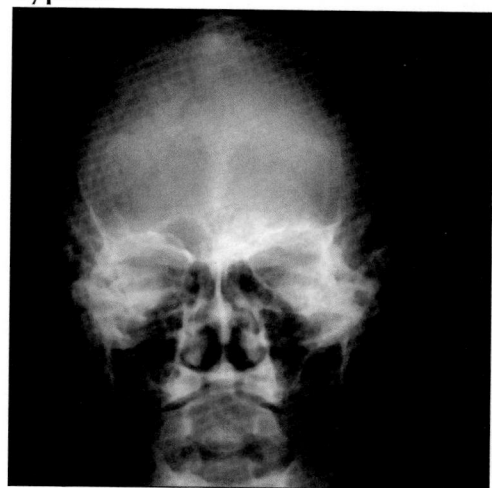

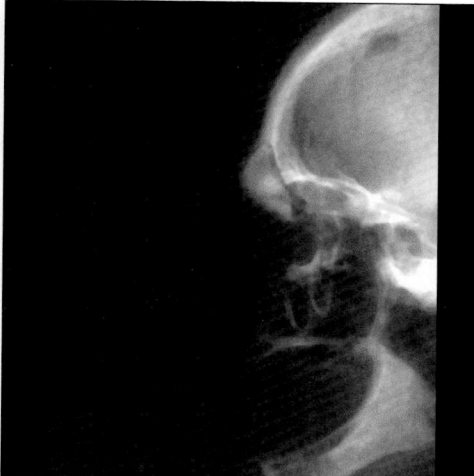

(Left) Anteroposterior radiography shows round sclerotic lesion in the left frontal sinus. *(Right)* Lateral radiography shows well-defined sclerotic mass in the frontal sinus.

Variant

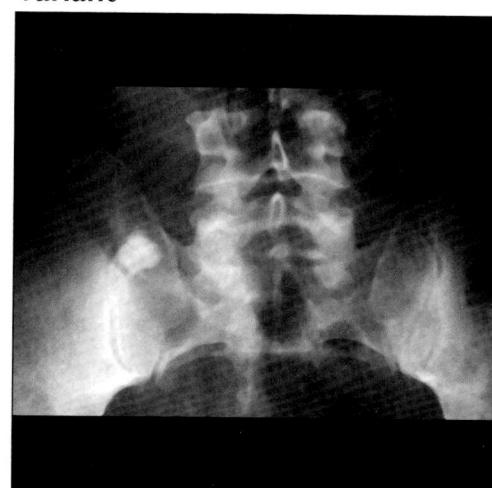

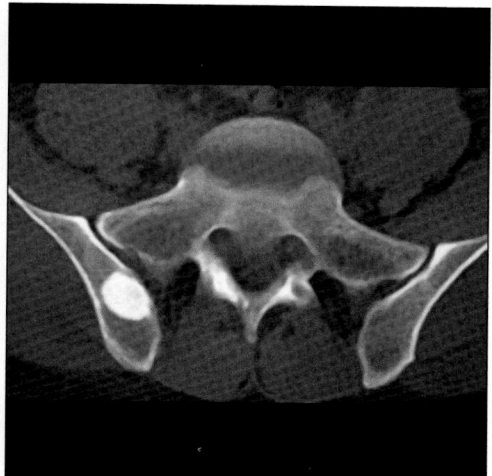

(Left) Anteroposterior radiography of the pelvis shows round, circumscribed, sclerotic lesion in the right iliac bone. *(Right)* Axial NECT shows round, well-defined sclerotic lesion in the right iliac bone, adjacent to the right SI joint. There is no osseous destruction or periosteal reaction.

Typical

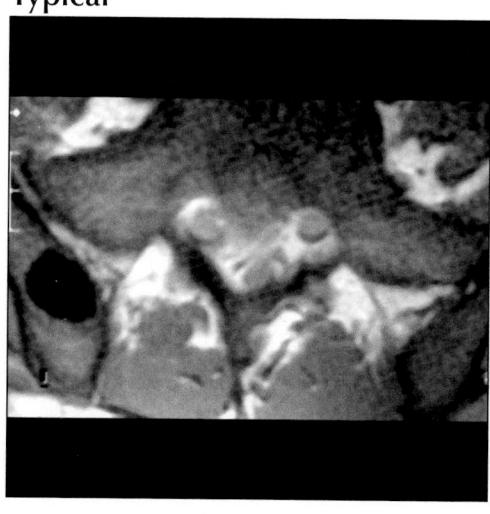

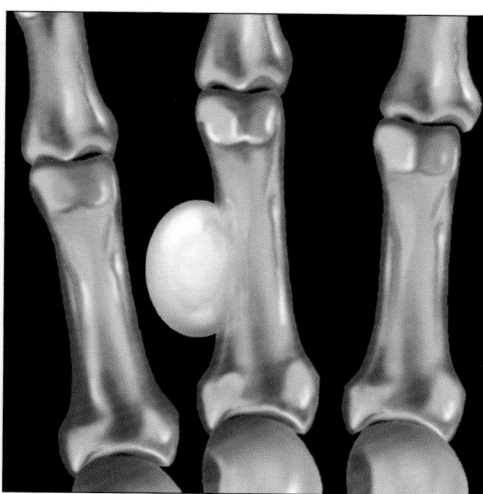

(Left) Axial T2WI MR shows a round area of signal void in the right iliac bone, consistent with sclerosis. Note absence of bone marrow edema or cortical disruption. *(Right)* Coronal graphic shows round ivory mass attached to the cortex of the proximal phalanx.

OSTEOID OSTEOMA

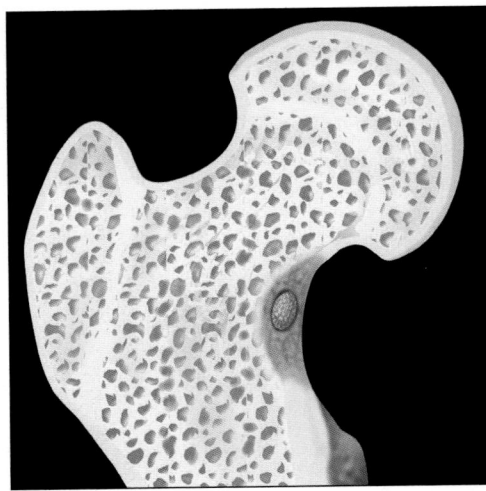

Coronal graphic shows intracortical osteoid osteoma in the femoral neck. Nidus (in red) and surrounding sclerosis are shown.

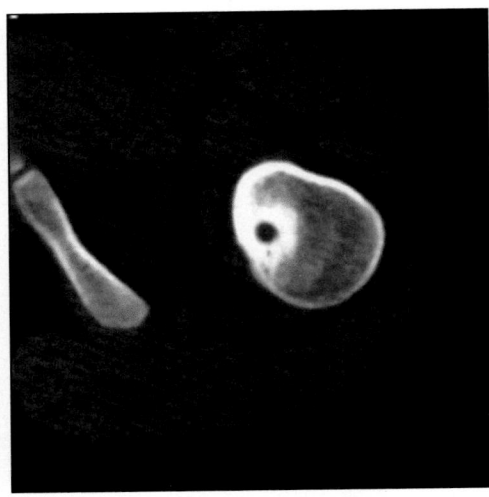

Axial NECT shows well-defined radiolucent nidus with surrounding sclerosis involving the subtrochanteric femur.

TERMINOLOGY

Abbreviations and Synonyms
- Osteoid Osteoma (OO)

Definitions
- Benign lesion characterized by less than 2 cm nidus of osteoid/woven bone in vascular tissue

IMAGING FINDINGS

General Features
- Best diagnostic clue: Well-defined lytic to sclerotic lesion with surrounding sclerosis
- Location
  - Metaphysis/diaphysis of long bones: 65-80%
    - Femur, tibia: 53-60%
  - Phalanges of hands and feet: 21%
  - Spine: 9%
    - Posterior elements: 90%
    - Vertebral body: 10%
  - Extremely rare in skull and facial bones
  - Cortical: 70-80%
    - Long bone diaphysis
  - Cancellous: 25%
    - Femoral neck, hands and feet
    - Often intraarticular
  - Subperiosteal: Rare
- Size: Nidus: < 1.5-2 cm
- Morphology: Lucent nidus with marked surrounding periosteal reaction

Radiographic Findings
- Radiography
  - Cortical lesion
    - Radiolucent central nidus < 1.5 cm with surrounding dense sclerosis
    - Periosteal reaction may be present
  - Cancellous/intraarticular lesion
    - Mild reactive sclerosis
    - Associated periostitis away from lesion
    - Joint effusion, synovitis
  - Subperiosteal lesion
    - Round soft tissue mass adjacent to cortex
    - Surrounding reactive changes usually absent
  - Limb overgrowth in children if located near growth plate

CT Findings
- NECT
  - Small, well-defined, round/oval nidus surrounded by sclerosis
  - Use thin sections (1-2 mm)

MR Findings
- T1WI: Nidus isointense to muscle

DDx: Osteoid Osteoma

Osteomyelitis	Enostosis	Stress Fracture	Osteoblastoma	Osteoma
AP Radiography	Cor T1WI MR	Ax NECT	Ax NECT	Ax NECT

OSTEOID OSTEOMA

Key Facts

Imaging Findings
- Best diagnostic clue: Well-defined lytic to sclerotic lesion with surrounding sclerosis

Top Differential Diagnoses
- Osteomyelitis (Brodie's Abscess)
- Enostosis (Bone Island)
- Stress Fracture
- Osteoblastoma
- Osteoma

Pathology
- Nidus has limited growth potential
- 4% of primary bone tumors
- 12% of benign bone tumors

Clinical Issues
- Most common signs/symptoms: Local pain worse at night, decreased by salicylates in less than 30 minutes (75%)
- Local swelling and point tenderness
- Spinal involvement: Painful scoliosis with concavity of curvature toward side of lesion
- No malignant potential
- No growth progression
- Can regress spontaneously
- Surgical en-block resection of nidus curative if nidus completely removed
- Percutaneous removal (CT guided)
- Percutaneous radio-frequency ablation (CT guided)
- Medical management: Nonsteroidal antiinflammatory drugs

- T2WI: Radiolucent areas of nidus: Intermediate to high signal intensity
- T1 C+
  - Dynamic imaging: Peak enhancement during arterial phase, early partial washout
    - Slower, progressive enhancement of adjacent bone marrow
- Low signal on all pulse sequences if nidus is completely mineralized
- May have extensive bone marrow edema which can obscure nidus
- Can show synovitis and joint effusion with intraarticular lesion

Ultrasonographic Findings
- Color Doppler
  - Increased vascularity of nidus
  - Can be used to localize lesion for biopsy

Angiographic Findings
- Intense blush of nidus during early arterial phase that persists during venous phase

Nuclear Medicine Findings
- Bone Scan
  - Increased uptake
  - Double density sign: Small focus of increased activity (nidus) surrounded by larger area of less intense activity (reactive sclerosis)
- PET: Can be used to detect osteoid osteoma in anatomic complex areas (posterior elements of spine)

Imaging Recommendations
- Best imaging tool: CT study of choice for identifying nidus
- Protocol advice: MRI in difficult cases to evaluate for joint effusion, synovitis

DIFFERENTIAL DIAGNOSIS

Osteomyelitis (Brodie's Abscess)
- Linear, serpentine tract, extends away from abscess cavity

- Cortical destruction

Enostosis (Bone Island)
- No increased activity on bone scan
- Thorny radiations
- Low signal on T2WI MR

Stress Fracture
- Radiolucency more linear and perpendicular to cortex (rather than parallel)

Osteoblastoma
- Larger (> 2-2.5 cm)
- Progresses, no regression

Osteoma
- Cold on bone scan
- No periosteal reaction
- No nidus

PATHOLOGY

General Features
- General path comments
  - Benign tumor consisting of osteoblastic mass (nidus) surrounded by zone of reactive sclerosis
    - Zone of sclerosis not integral part of tumor, represents secondary reversible change
    - Nidus has limited growth potential
  - Prostaglandin E2 elevated 100-1000 times within nidus (likely cause of pain and vasodilatation)
  - Tumor can regress spontaneously, possibly secondary to infarction
- Etiology
  - Unknown: May be inflammatory, traumatic, vascular, viral
  - Benign, highly vascular osteoblastic proliferation
- Epidemiology
  - 4% of primary bone tumors
  - 12% of benign bone tumors

Gross Pathologic & Surgical Features
- Nidus: Red/tan mass of gritty osseous tissue

- Easily separated from surrounding reactive bone
- Less than 1 cm in greatest dimension

Microscopic Features

- Nidus composed of osteoid tissue or mineralized, immature, woven bone
- Osteoid matrix and bone form trabeculae
  - Surrounded by highly vascular, fibrous stroma with osteoblastic and osteoclastic activity
- Sclerosis surrounding lesion composed of dense bone
- Adjacent synovium may be thickened and infiltrated with inflammatory cells and lymphoid follicles
  - Lymphofollicular synovitis; can simulate rheumatoid arthritis

Staging, Grading or Classification Criteria

- Surgical staging system for benign musculoskeletal tumors
  - Stage 1: Latent
  - Stage 2: Active
  - Stage 3: Aggressive

CLINICAL ISSUES

Presentation

- Most common signs/symptoms: Local pain worse at night, decreased by salicylates in less than 30 minutes (75%)
- Clinical profile
  - Local swelling and point tenderness
  - Pain exacerbated by alcohol
  - Average duration of symptoms: 3 years
  - Spinal involvement: Painful scoliosis with concavity of curvature toward side of lesion
    - Idiopathic scoliosis: Never painful
    - Scoliosis improves/resolves if nidus is resected within 15 months after diagnosis
    - Neurologic abnormalities in 6% of patients with spine involvement
  - Intraarticular lesion: Symptoms of arthritis
  - Elevated urinary excretion of major prostacyclin metabolite (2,3-dinor-6-keto-PGF 1 α)
    - Returns to normal after removal of nidus

Demographics

- Age: 10-35 years
- Gender: M:F = 2-3:1
- Ethnicity: Rare in African Americans

Natural History & Prognosis

- No malignant potential
- No growth progression
- Can regress spontaneously
- Regression of active stage 2 lesion to latent stage 1 lesion: 3 years (average)

Treatment

- Surgical en-block resection of nidus curative if nidus completely removed
  - Recurrence due to incomplete resection of nidus
  - Tetracycline and radionuclide labeling for lesion location at surgery
- Percutaneous removal (CT guided)
- Percutaneous radio-frequency ablation (CT guided)
  - Under general or spinal anesthesia
- Percutaneous thermocoagulation (CT guided)
- Medical management: Nonsteroidal antiinflammatory drugs
  - Can induce permanent relief of symptoms and regression of nidus

DIAGNOSTIC CHECKLIST

Consider

- Consider medical management as initial treatment since lesions can regress spontaneously
- Image guided therapy often more successful than surgical resection

SELECTED REFERENCES

1. Liu PT et al: Imaging of osteoid osteoma with dynamic gadolinium-enhanced MR imaging. Radiology 227:691-700, 2003
2. DeFriend DE et al: Percutaneous laser photocoagulation of osteoid osteoma under CT guidance. Clin Radiol 58:222-6, 2003
3. Dorfman HD et al: Bone tumors. 1st ed. St. Louis MO, Mosby, 85-103, 1998
4. Greenspan A et al: Differential diagnosis of tumors and tumor-like lesions of bones and joints. 1st ed. Philadelphia PA, Lippencott-Raven, 36-46, 1998
5. Assoun J et al: Osteoid osteoma: MR imaging versus CT. Radiology 191:217-23, 1994
6. Bilchik T et al: Osteoid osteoma: The role of radionuclide bone imaging, conventional radiography and computed tomography in its management. J Nucl Med 33:269-71, 1992
7. Cassar-Pullicino VN et al: Intra-articular osteoid osteoma. Clin Radiol 45:153-60, 1992
8. Greco F et al: Prostaglandins in osteoid osteoma. Int Orthop 15:35-7, 1991
9. Azouz EM et al: Osteoid osteoma and osteoblastoma of the spine in children. Report of 22 cases with brief literature review. Pediatr Radiol 16:25-31, 1986
10. Cohen MD et al: Osteoid osteoma: 95 cases and a review of the literature. Semin Arthritis Rheum 12:265-81, 1983

OSTEOID OSTEOMA

IMAGE GALLERY

Typical

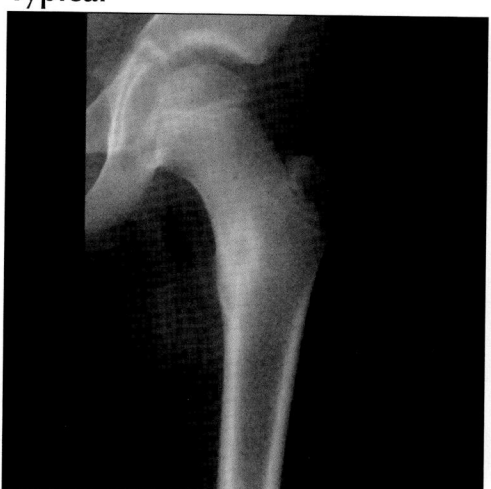
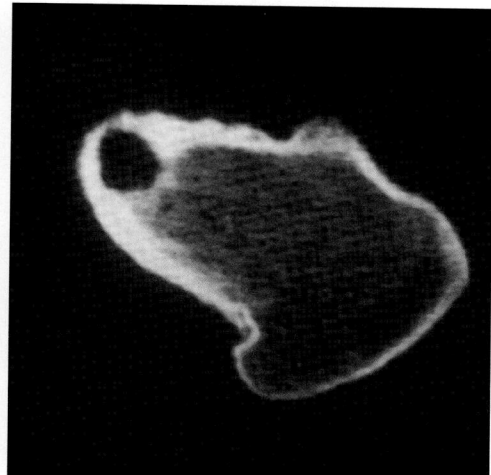

(Left) Anteroposterior radiography shows radiolucent nidus with surrounding sclerosis in the right femoral intertrochanteric region. *(Right)* Axial NECT shows lucent intracortical nidus with surrounding sclerosis in the proximal femur.

Typical

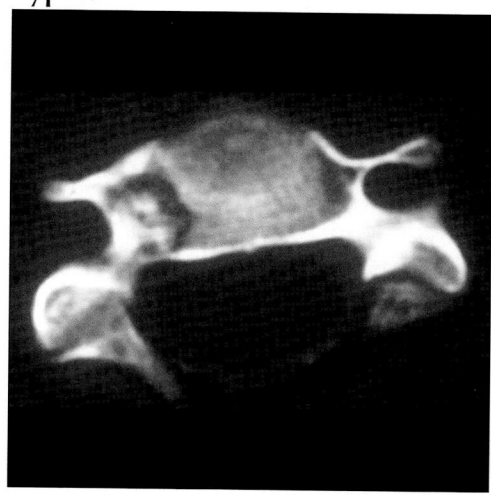
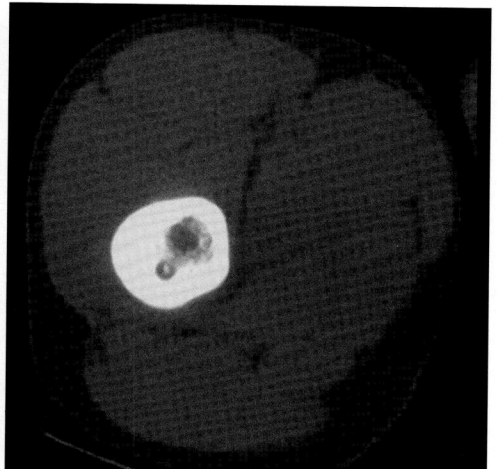

(Left) Axial NECT shows low attenuation nidus with central calcifications in the right pedicle of C4 extending into the lamina. *(Right)* Axial NECT shows radiolucent nidus with central sclerosis and surrounding periosteal reaction in the femoral cortex.

Other

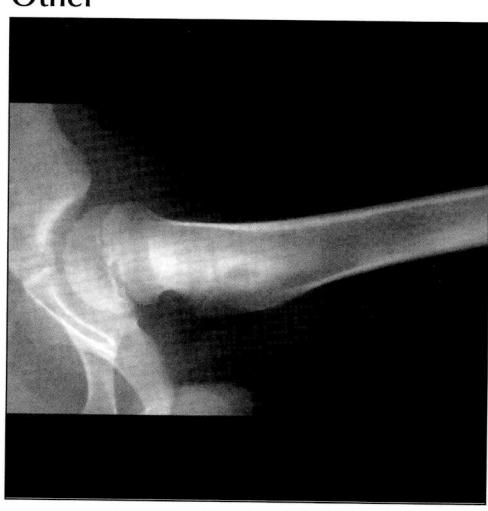
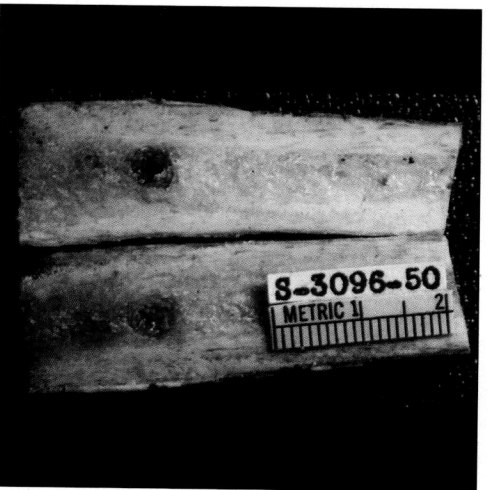

(Left) Lateral radiography shows radiolucent nidus with surrounding periosteal reaction in the proximal femoral metaphysis. *(Right)* Coronal gross pathology shows round, sharply demarcated, reddish nidus, surrounded by sclerotic bone.

OSTEOBLASTOMA

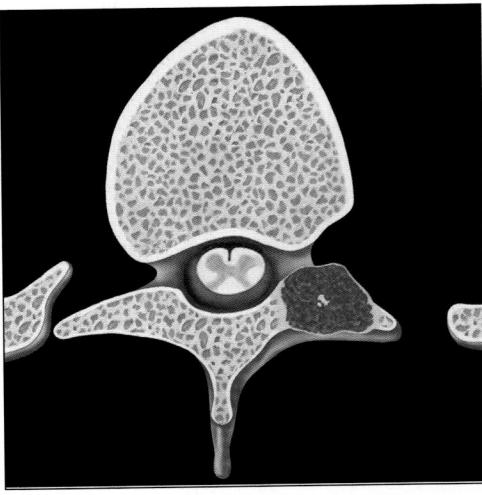

Axial graphic shows osteoblastoma (in red) involving the posterior elements. Central calcifications are shown in white.

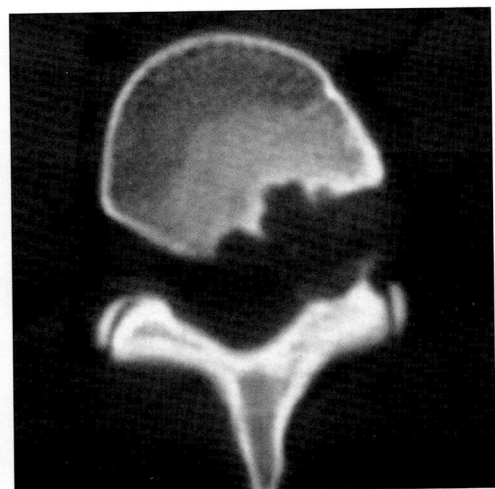

Axial NECT shows an expansile circumscribed lytic lesion with scalloped margins involving the vertebral body and posterior elements.

TERMINOLOGY

Abbreviations and Synonyms
- Giant osteoid osteoma, osteogenic fibroma

Definitions
- Benign osseous tumor, characterized by production of osteoid and woven bone

IMAGING FINDINGS

General Features
- Best diagnostic clue: Expansile, circumscribed lytic lesion involving extremities and posterior elements of spine
- Location
  - Spine: 40%
    - Posterior elements: > 60%
    - Posterior elements with extension into vertebral body: 25%
    - Vertebral body: 15%
  - Long bones: 30%
  - Hands and feet: 15%
  - Skull and face (jaw): 15%
  - Pelvis: 5%
  - Diaphysis: 58%
  - Metaphysis: 42%
  - Eccentric: 46%
  - Intracortical: 42%
  - Periosteal: Extremely rare
- Size: Greater than 1.5 - 2 cm
- Morphology: Expansile lytic lesion

Radiographic Findings
- Radiography
  - Expansile, circumscribed, lytic lesion
  - Reactive sclerosis: 60%
  - Variable central calcification and matrix
  - Can rapidly increase in size
  - Cortical expansion: 75-94%
  - Cortical destruction: 20-22%
  - Radiolucent nidus > 1.5 - 2 cm
  - Surrounding sclerosis, periostitis: 50%
  - Secondary aneurysmal bone cyst (ABC) component: 16%
  - Can have adjacent soft tissue mass

CT Findings
- NECT
  - Expansile lytic lesion with or without matrix mineralization
  - Adjacent periosteal reaction, sclerosis, cortical erosions
  - To evaluate mineralized matrix and nidus
  - Can show soft tissue mass

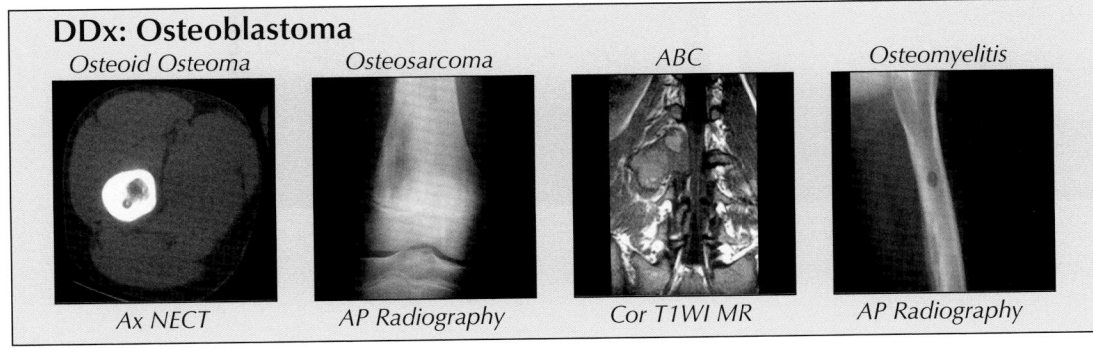

DDx: Osteoblastoma

Osteoid Osteoma	Osteosarcoma	ABC	Osteomyelitis
Ax NECT	AP Radiography	Cor T1WI MR	AP Radiography

OSTEOBLASTOMA

Key Facts

Imaging Findings
- Best diagnostic clue: Expansile, circumscribed lytic lesion involving extremities and posterior elements of spine

Top Differential Diagnoses
- Osteoid Osteoma
- Osteosarcoma
- Aneurysmal Bone Cyst (ABC)
- Osteomyelitis (Bone abscess)
- Chondromyxoid Fibroma

Pathology
- < 1% of all primary bone tumors
- 3% of all benign bone tumors
- Aggressive osteoblastoma: Epithelioid osteoblasts

Clinical Issues
- Dull, localized pain of insidious onset
- Localized swelling, tenderness, decreased range of motion
- Painful scoliosis with vertebral involvement
- Benign neoplasm, no malignant transformation
- Recurrence after resection: 10-25%
- Aggressive osteoblastoma: Recurrence in 50%
- Marginal en bloc excision of symptomatic lesions
- Radiation and chemotherapy in cases of aggressive and surgically unresectable lesions

Diagnostic Checklist
- Look for calcified matrix in spinal osteoblastomas to differentiate from ABC

- o Aggressive osteoblastoma disrupts cortex and has soft-tissue component

MR Findings
- T1WI
  - o Low-intermediate signal intensity
  - o Foci of signal void
    - Corresponding to calcifications
- T2WI
  - o Intermediate-high signal intensity
  - o Foci of signal void
    - Corresponding to calcifications
- T1 C+: Enhancement of tumor and surrounding inflammatory reaction
- To evaluate bone and soft tissue extent, adjacent edema
- May simulate malignant process due to extensive inflammatory response

Angiographic Findings
- Hypervascularity

Nuclear Medicine Findings
- Bone Scan: Intense uptake of radiotracer

Imaging Recommendations
- Best imaging tool: Radiographs, CT
- Protocol advice: CT imaging modality of choice to demonstrate exact size and areas of ossification within lesion

DIFFERENTIAL DIAGNOSIS

Osteoid Osteoma
- Smaller (< 2 cm)
- Predilection for axial skeleton
- Can regress spontaneously
  - o Osteoblastoma tends to progress

Osteosarcoma
- Cortical destruction
- Mineralized matrix
- Soft tissue component

Aneurysmal Bone Cyst (ABC)
- Fluid-fluid levels
- No matrix calcification
- Osteoblastoma often has secondary ABC component

Osteomyelitis (Bone abscess)
- Periosteal reaction
- Serpentine tract
- Sequestrum

Chondromyxoid Fibroma
- Expansile lytic lesion with sclerotic margin
- Matrix calcification rare
- Rare in spine
- No periosteal reaction

PATHOLOGY

General Features
- General path comments
  - o Lesion size > 1.5 cm
  - o Smaller lesions classified as osteoid osteoma
- Etiology
  - o Unknown
  - o Histologically similar to osteoid osteomas, producing osteoid and primitive woven bone
- Epidemiology
  - o < 1% of all primary bone tumors
  - o 3% of all benign bone tumors

Gross Pathologic & Surgical Features
- Circumscribed mass, often surrounded by shell of cortical bone or periosteum
- Sharp interface between the lesion and cancellous bone
  - o Often marked by a thin rim of reactive bone
- Nidus: 2-10 cm, friable, deep red (high vascularity)
  - o Well-demarcated at periphery
- Prominent cystic spaces may indicate secondary ABC formation

OSTEOBLASTOMA

Microscopic Features
- Similar to osteoid osteoma, greater osteoid production and vascularity
- Numerous, multinucleated giant cells (osteoclasts)
- Very vascular connective tissue stroma with interconnecting trabecular bone
- No cartilage
- Aggressive osteoblastoma: Epithelioid osteoblasts

Staging, Grading or Classification Criteria
- Surgical staging system for benign musculoskeletal tumors
  - Stage 1: Latent
  - Stage 2: Active
  - Stage 3: Aggressive

CLINICAL ISSUES

Presentation
- Most common signs/symptoms
  - Dull, localized pain of insidious onset
  - Pain rarely interferes with sleep
- Clinical profile
  - Localized swelling, tenderness, decreased range of motion
  - Response to salicylates in 7%
  - Painful scoliosis with vertebral involvement
  - Pathologic fractures rare
  - Can cause tumor associated osteomalacia
  - Toxic osteoblastoma: Extremely rare (two cases reported)
    - Severe systemic manifestations: Fever, weight loss, anemia, clubbing, hyperdynamic circulation, systemic periostitis

Demographics
- Age: 5-45 years, peak: 2nd decade
- Gender: M:F = 2-3:1
- Ethnicity: No racial predilection

Natural History & Prognosis
- Benign neoplasm, no malignant transformation
- Cases of malignant degeneration reported
  - These lesions likely represented undiagnosed osteosarcoma
- Presents as active, slow growing stage 2 lesion
- Can have foci of aggressive stage 3 lesion (prone to ABC formation, pathologic fracture)
- Recurrence after resection: 10-25%
  - Aggressive osteoblastoma can recur after excision of conventional osteoblastoma
- Aggressive osteoblastoma: Recurrence in 50%

Treatment
- Marginal en bloc excision of symptomatic lesions
  - Recurrence of stage 3 lesions: 30-50%
- Curettage with bone graft
- Radiation and chemotherapy in cases of aggressive and surgically unresectable lesions

DIAGNOSTIC CHECKLIST

Consider
- Consult orthopedic surgeon before biopsy of presumed osteoblastoma
- If histology reveals osteosarcoma, biopsy-induced contaminated needle tract can mandate different surgical approach

Image Interpretation Pearls
- Look for calcified matrix in spinal osteoblastomas to differentiate from ABC

SELECTED REFERENCES

1. Ozaki T et al: Osteoid osteoma and osteoblastoma of the spine: Experience with 22 patients. Clin Orthop 397:394-402, 2002
2. Dale S et al: Severe toxic osteoblastoma of the humerus associated with diffuse periostitis of multiple bones. Skeletal Radiol 30:464-8, 2001
3. Sulzbacher I et al: Periosteal osteoblastoma: A case report and a review of the literature. Pathol Int 50:667-71, 2000
4. Papagelopoulos PJ etal: Clinicopathologic features, diagnosis, and treatment of osteoblastoma. Orthopedics 22:244-7, 1999
5. Shaikh MI et al: Spinal osteoblastoma: CT and MR imaging with pathological correlation. Skeletal Radiol 28:33-40, 1999
6. Dorfman HD et al: Bone tumors. 1st edition. St. Louis MO, Mosby, 103-17, 1998
7. Greenspan A: Differential diagnosis of tumors and tumor-like lesions of bones and joints. 1st ed. Philadelphia PA, Lippincott-Raven, 46-59, 1998
8. Della Rocca C et al: Osteoblastoma: Varied histological presentations with a benign clinical course. An analysis of 55 cases. Am J Surg Pathol. 20:841-50, 1996
9. Crim JR et al: Widespread inflammatory response to osteoblastoma: The flare phenomenon. Radiology 177:835-6, 1990
10. Kroon HM et al: Osteoblastoma: Clinical and radiologic findings in 98 new cases. Radiology. 175:783-90, 1990
11. Gitelis S et al: Osteoid osteoma and osteoblastoma. Orthop Clin North Am 20:313-25, 1989
12. Azouz EM et al: Osteoid osteoma and osteoblastoma of the spine in children. Report of 22 cases with brief literature review. Pediatr Radiol 16:25-31, 1986
13. Kenan S et al: Aggressive osteoblastoma. A case report and review of the literature. Clin Orthop 195:294-8, 1985
14. DeSouza DL et al: Osteoid osteoma - osteoblastoma. Cancer 33:1075-81, 1974

OSTEOBLASTOMA

IMAGE GALLERY

Typical

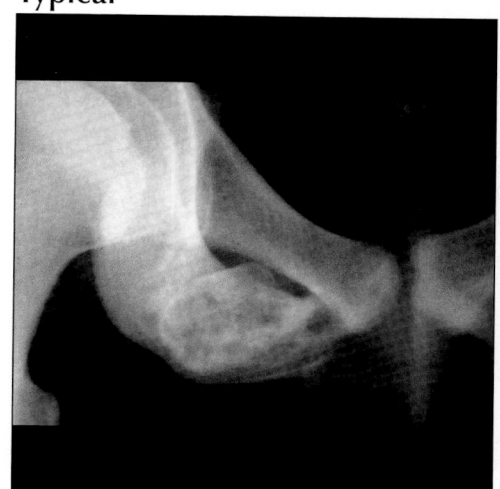
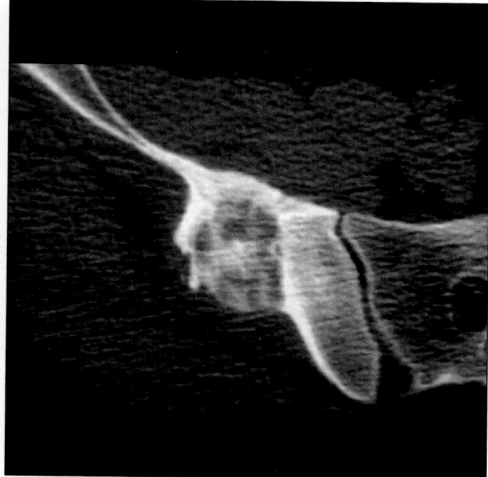

(Left) Anteroposterior radiography shows a circumscribed lesion with central ossifications involving the inferior pubic ramus. *(Right)* Axial NECT shows a lytic expansile lesion with central ossification of the right iliac bone. Note cortical thinning at the posterior aspect of the lesion.

Typical

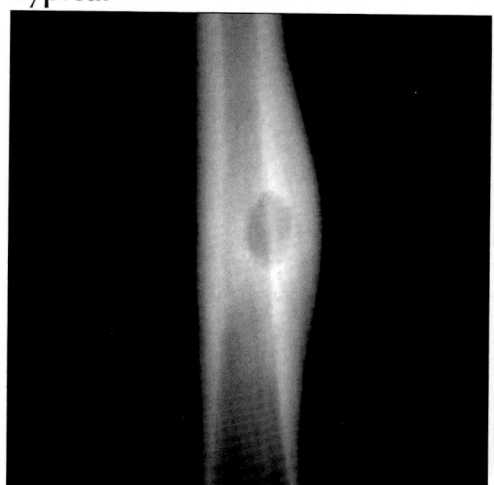
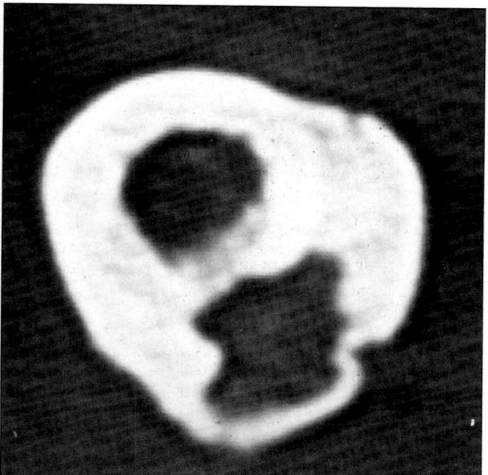

(Left) Anteroposterior radiography shows radiolucent lesion of the femoral diaphysis surrounded by sclerotic bone. *(Right)* Axial NECT *(same patient)* shows a well defined lytic lesion with surrounding sclerosis involving the femoral diaphysis.

Typical

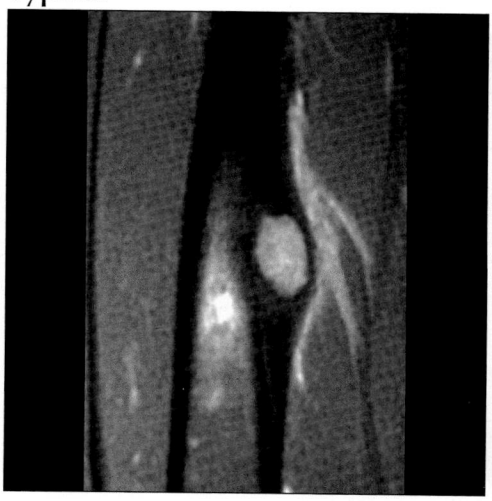
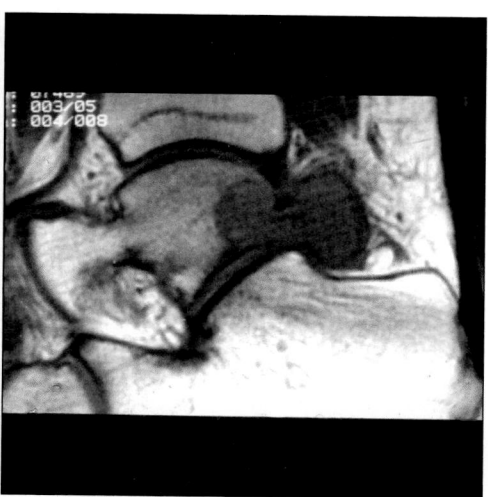

(Left) Sagittal FS T2 FSE MR shows a lesion of high signal in the femoral diaphysis. Note surrounding bone marrow edema. *(Right)* Sagittal T1WI MR shows eccentric lesion of low signal arising from the posterior calcaneus. There is cortical destruction and extension of the tumor into the adjacent soft tissues.

OSTEOSARCOMA

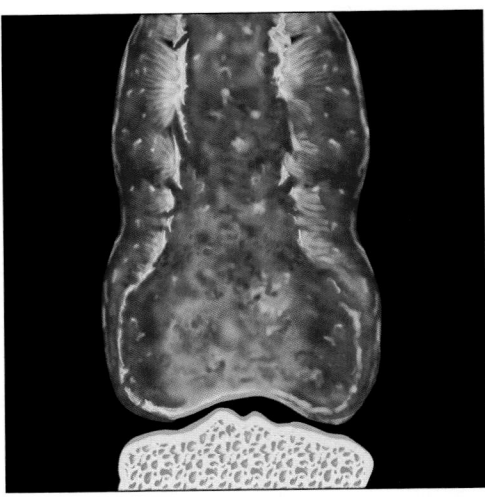

Coronal graphic shows osteosarcoma in the distal femur.

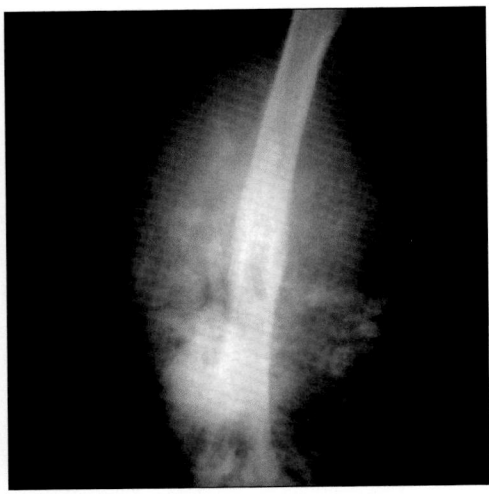

Lateral radiography of the femur shows medullary and cortical bone destruction with associated periosteal reaction of sunburst type. Soft tissue extension with new bone formation is present.

TERMINOLOGY

Abbreviations and Synonyms
- Osteogenic sarcoma (OGS)

Definitions
- Malignant tumor with ability to produce osteoid directly from neoplastic cells

IMAGING FINDINGS

General Features
- Best diagnostic clue: Bone destruction with associated tumor bone formation and aggressive periosteal reaction
- Location
  - Around knee: 55%
  - Metaphyses of long tubular bones: 80%
  - Extension into epiphysis: 75%
  - Flat bones, vertebral bodies: 20%
  - In older patients (> 50 years), axial skeleton and flat bones: 40%
- Size: 5-10 cm
- Morphology: Destructive lesion with osteoid formation

Radiographic Findings
- Radiography

- Conventional osteosarcoma: 85%
  - Poorly-defined, intramedullary mass, extends through cortex
  - Moth-eaten bone destruction
  - Aggressive periosteal reaction: Codman triangle, sunburst pattern
  - Indistinct borders with wide zone of transition
  - Soft tissue mass +/- tumor calcification
- Telangiectatic osteosarcoma: < 5%
  - Was thought to have worst prognosis, but prognosis is likely similar to conventional OGS
  - Purely lytic lesion
  - Cystic cavities filled with blood/necrosis
  - Fluid levels (may mimic aneurysmal bone cyst - ABC)
- Multicentric osteosarcoma: 1%
  - Synchronous osteoblastic osteosarcoma at multiple sites (usually symmetric)
  - Exclusively in children (5-10 years)
  - Extremely poor prognosis
- Parosteal osteosarcoma: 3%
  - Low grade osteosarcoma in older age group (20 - 50 years)
  - Posterior distal femur
  - Attached to underlying cortex at origin
- Periosteal osteosarcoma: 1%
  - Intermediate-grade osteosarcoma
  - Most common diaphyseal

DDx: Osteosarcoma

Ewing Sarcoma	Chondrosarcoma	Osteomyelitis	ABC	Myositis Ossif.
AP Radiography	AP Radiography	AP Radiography	Ax T2WI MR	Lat Radiography

OSTEOSARCOMA

Key Facts

Imaging Findings
- Best diagnostic clue: Bone destruction with associated tumor bone formation and aggressive periosteal reaction

Top Differential Diagnoses
- Ewing Sarcoma
- Osteomyelitis
- Chondrosarcoma
- Lymphoma
- Aneurysmal Bone Cyst (ABC)
- Myositis Ossificans

Pathology
- Most common malignant primary bone tumor in young adults and children
- 20% of all primary bone malignancies

Clinical Issues
- Progressive pain
- Soft tissue mass, swelling
- Pathologic fracture
- Pulmonary metastases common, can cause pneumothorax (calcifying)
- 5-year survival: 41%
- 5-year survival in patients with resectable tumor and without metastases: 60-70%
- Surgical resection with wide margins
- Adjuvant and neoadjuvant chemotherapy

Diagnostic Checklist
- Always image adjacent joints and use bone scan to detect skip lesions, metastases, multifocal OGS

- No medullary involvement
- Cortical thickening
  - Gnathic osteosarcoma: 5-9%
    - Involvement of mandible, maxilla
    - Sclerotic, lytic, mixed
    - Periosteal reaction
    - Soft tissue extension
  - Secondary osteosarcoma: 5%
    - Arises in association with preexisting lesion of bone such as Paget disease, prior radiation, bone infarct

CT Findings
- NECT
  - Helpful in imaging surface OGS
  - Can show complex anatomy in gnathic OGS
- CECT
  - Enhancement of solid components
    - Helpful in differentiating telangiectatic OGS from ABC
    - Telangiectatic OGS: Nodular peripheral enhancement

MR Findings
- T1WI
  - Low signal intensity: Mineralized tumor
  - Low-intermediate signal intensity: Solid, nonmineralized tumor
- T2WI
  - Low signal intensity: Mineralized tumor
  - High signal intensity: Nonmineralized tumor, soft tissue mass
- STIR: Helpful in imaging entire bone to detect skip lesions, multicentric OGS

Nuclear Medicine Findings
- Bone Scan
  - Increased uptake
  - For staging, detection of skip lesions, metastases
- PET
  - Useful in evaluating tumor recurrence
  - Helpful in imaging patients with protheses

Imaging Recommendations
- Best imaging tool: Radiographs first imaging modality to detect bone destruction and periosteal reaction
- Protocol advice
  - Radiographs to detect bone destruction and periosteal reaction
  - MR to determine
    - Extent of tumor within bone marrow and soft tissue
    - Relationship to vessels and nerves
  - Bone scan to detect skip lesions
  - MRI should be performed prior to biopsy

DIFFERENTIAL DIAGNOSIS

Ewing Sarcoma
- Diaphysis of long bone
- Large soft tissue mass

Osteomyelitis
- No bone formation
- Sequestrum

Chondrosarcoma
- Ring and arc calcifications
- Thickened cortex, endosteal scalloping

Lymphoma
- Moth-eaten lytic bone destruction
- No periosteal new bone formation

Aneurysmal Bone Cyst (ABC)
- Can look similar to telangiectatic OGS
- Purely lytic
- No periosteal reaction

Myositis Ossificans
- Bone formation in periphery, zonal phenomenon
  - Surface OGS: Central bone formation
- Cleft between osseous mass and cortex

OSTEOSARCOMA

PATHOLOGY

General Features
- General path comments
  - Malignant tumor with ability to produce osteoid directly from neoplastic cells
  - Frequency of tumor occurrence corresponds to greatest growth rate during adolescence
- Genetics
  - Overexpression of P-glycogen in OGS cells with propensity for metastases and treatment failure
  - Alterations of Rb genes in OGS that develops in association with retinoblastoma
- Etiology
  - Majority of OGS of unknown etiology = primary OGS
  - Secondary to predisposing factors (Paget disease, bone infarct, radiation) = secondary OGS
- Epidemiology
  - Most common malignant primary bone tumor in young adults and children
  - 20% of all primary bone malignancies

Gross Pathologic & Surgical Features
- Heterogeneous mass with ossified and non-ossified components
- Ossified areas: Yellow-white, firm, may be as hard as cortical bone
- Less ossified areas: Soft, tan, with foci of hemorrhage and necrosis
- Penetration of cortex with often large extraosseous tumor mass
- Periosteal reaction: Lamellae of new bone at periphery of lesion

Microscopic Features
- Highly pleomorphic, spindle-shaped tumor cells producing different forms of osteoid
- Three histologic subtypes depending on sarcomatous component
  - Osteoblastic, chondroblastic, fibroblastic OGS

Staging, Grading or Classification Criteria
- Surgical staging for malignant musculoskeletal tumors
  - Stage Ia: Low grade, intracompartmental
  - Stage Ib: Low grade, extracompartmental
  - Stage IIa: High grade, intracompartmental
  - Stage IIb: High grade, extracompartmental
  - Stage IIIa: Low or high grade, intracompartmental, metastases
  - Stage IIIb: Low or high grade, extracompartmental, metastases

CLINICAL ISSUES

Presentation
- Most common signs/symptoms
  - Progressive pain
  - Soft tissue mass, swelling
- Clinical profile
  - Pathologic fracture
  - Pulmonary metastases common, can cause pneumothorax (calcifying)
  - Increased serum alkaline phosphatase
  - Patients with OGS often taller than their peers
    - Increased levels of somatomedin

Demographics
- Age
  - Bimodal age distribution
    - First peak: 2nd-3rd decade, corresponds to peak of skeletal growth
    - Second peak: > 6th decade
- Gender: M:F = 1.3-1.6:1
- Ethnicity: Slightly more common in African Americans

Natural History & Prognosis
- Very aggressive tumor
- Prognosis depends on OGS type, size, location, resectability, presence of metastases
  - Central OGS worse prognosis than juxtacortical type
- 5-year survival: 41%
- 5-year survival in patients with resectable tumor and without metastases: 60-70%

Treatment
- Surgical resection with wide margins
- Adjuvant and neoadjuvant chemotherapy
- Amputations may be necessary
- Biopsies must be planned with future tumor excision in mind

DIAGNOSTIC CHECKLIST

Consider
- Always consult orthopedic surgeon before biopsy of possible OGS

Image Interpretation Pearls
- Always image adjacent joints and use bone scan to detect skip lesions, metastases, multifocal OGS

SELECTED REFERENCES

1. Goorin AM et al: Presurgical chemotherapy compared with immediate surgery and adjuvant chemotherapy for nonmetastatic osteosarcoma: Pediatric Oncology Group Study POG-8651. J Clin Oncol 21:1574-80, 2003
2. Bredella MA et al: Value of FDG PET in conjunction with MR imaging for evaluating therapy response in patients with musculoskeletal sarcomas. Am J Roentgenol 179:1145-50, 2002
3. Dorfman HD et al: Bone tumors. 1st ed. St. Louis MO, Mosby, 128-252, 1998
4. Onikul E et al: Accuracy of MR imaging for estimating intraosseous extent of osteosarcomas. Am J Roentgenol 167:1211-5, 1996
5. Baldini N et al: Expression of P-glycoprotein in high grade osteosarcoma in relation to clinical outcome. N Engl J Med 333:1380-5, 1995
6. Dorfman HD et al: Bone cancers. Cancer 75:203-10, 1995
7. Rosenberg ZS et al: Osteosarcoma: Subtle, rare, and misleading plain film features. Am J Roentgenol 165:1209-14, 1995
8. Bloem JL et al: Osseous lesions. Radiol Clin North Am 31:261-78, 1993

OSTEOSARCOMA

IMAGE GALLERY

Typical

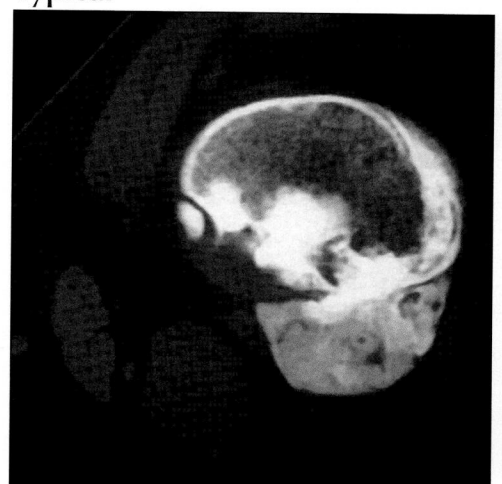
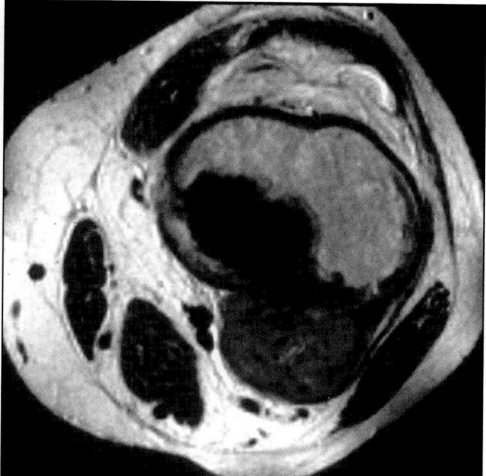

(Left) Axial NECT shows densely mineralized tumor in the medullary canal with cortical destruction and mineralized soft tissue component. *(Right)* Axial T1WI MR shows low signal intensity in the medullary cavity, corresponding to mineralized portions of osteosarcoma. Cortical disruption and extension into the posterior soft tissues is noted.

Variant

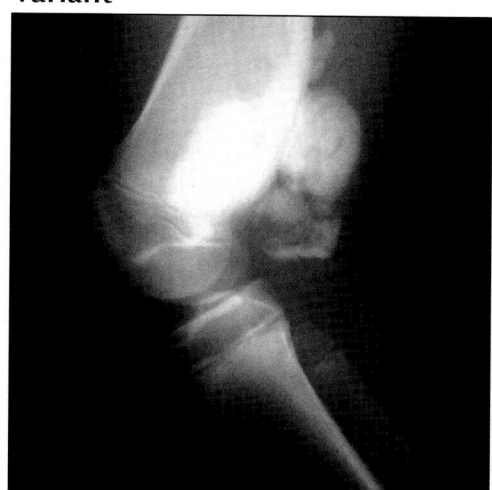
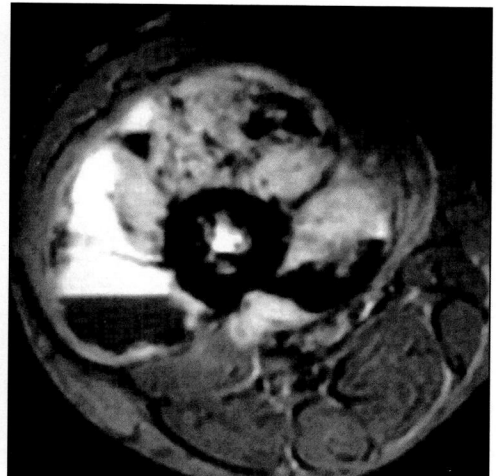

(Left) Lateral radiography shows lobulated sclerotic mass arising from the metaphyseal surface of the posterior distal femur, consistent with parosteal osteosarcoma. *(Right)* Axial FS T2 FSE MR shows abnormal bone marrow SI and large extraosseous soft tissue component with fluid-fluid levels, consistent with telangiectatic osteosarcoma.

Other

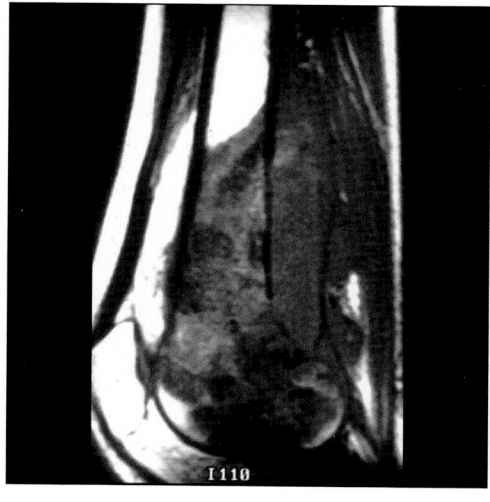
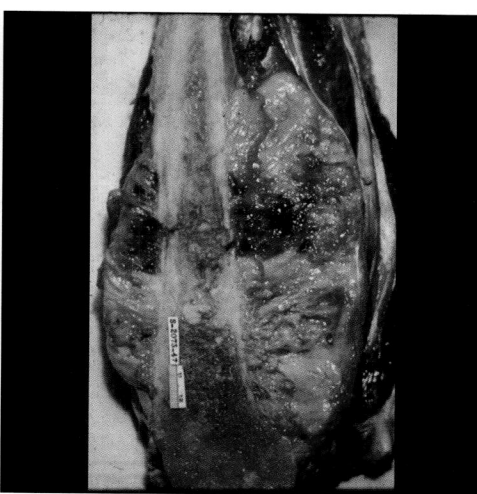

(Left) Sagittal T1WI MR shows heterogeneous tumor involving the distal femoral meta-diaphysis. Areas of low signal correspond to mineralized tumor, nonmineralized areas are of intermediate signal. *(Right)* Coronal gross pathology, section shows yellow-brown tumor with hemorrhagic areas in the femoral meta-diaphysis with cortical destruction and extraosseous extension.

ENCHONDROMA

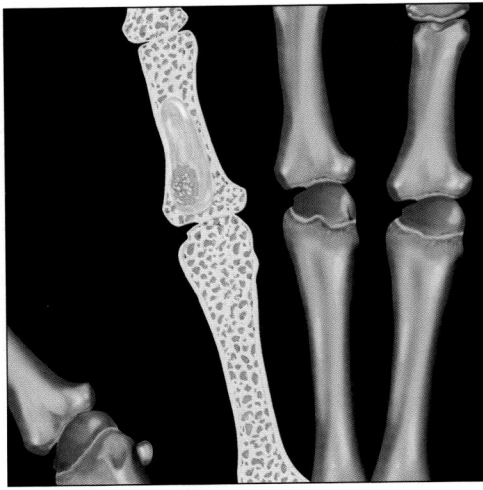

Coronal graphic shows enchondroma (in blue) involving the proximal 2nd phalanx.

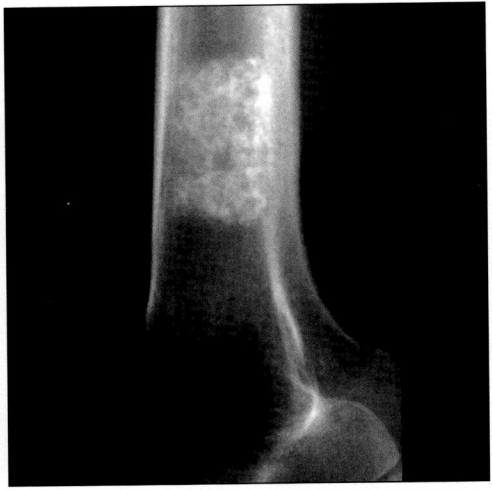

Lateral radiography shows radiolucent lesion in the distal femoral metaphysis containing chondroid matrix (rings and arcs calcifications).

TERMINOLOGY

Abbreviations and Synonyms
- Chondroma

Definitions
- Common benign intramedullary neoplasm composed of mature cartilage

IMAGING FINDINGS

General Features
- Best diagnostic clue: Well-defined lytic lesion with chondroid matrix (rings and arcs calcifications)
- Location
  - Any bone formed by enchondral ossification can be involved
  - Short, tubular bones of hands and feet: 60%
    - Most common tumor of phalanges of the hand
  - Long tubular bones: 25-45%
    - Metaphysis, proximal/distal end of diaphysis
    - Femur: 17%
    - Humerus: 7%
  - Pelvis: < 3%
  - Spine, scapula, ribs: rare
- Size: < 3 cm

- Morphology: Localized, radiolucent lesion with punctate or stippled calcification

Radiographic Findings
- Radiography
  - Short, tubular bones: Radiolucent lesion
  - Long bones: Chondroid calcification ("rings and arcs," "popcorn" type)
  - Scalloped inner cortical margins
  - Expansion of cortex without cortical break
  - No periosteal reaction or soft tissue mass
    - Cortical break, soft tissue mass suggest malignant transformation
  - Progressive calcification
    - Focal loss of calcification suggests malignant transformation
  - Rapid growth suggestive of malignant transformation

CT Findings
- NECT
  - Helpful in detecting chondroid matrix
  - Intact cortex

MR Findings
- T1WI
  - Low to intermediate signal intensity
  - Calcification: Signal void
- T2WI

DDx: Enchondroma

Bone Infarct	Chondrosarcoma	Epidermoid	Chondroma

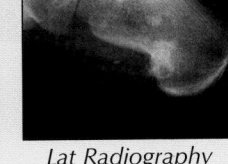 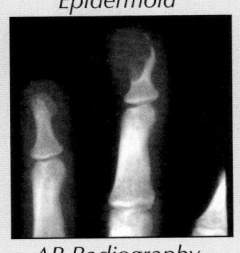 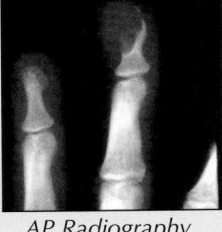 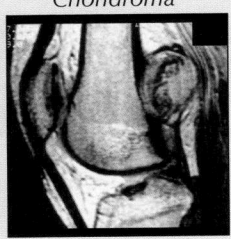

Cor T1WI MR	Lat Radiography	AP Radiography	Sag T2WI MR

ENCHONDROMA

Key Facts

Imaging Findings
- Best diagnostic clue: Well-defined lytic lesion with chondroid matrix (rings and arcs calcifications)
- Best imaging tool: Radiographs usually diagnostic
- Protocol advice: CT best imaging modality to detect chondroid matrix

Top Differential Diagnoses
- Bone Infarct
- Chondrosarcoma
- Epidermoid Inclusion Cyst
- Juxtacortical Chondroma

Pathology
- Second most common benign bone tumor
- 2-10% of all bone tumors

Clinical Issues
- Usually asymptomatic
- Painless swelling
- Pain, unexplained by injury or fracture, should raise suspicion of malignancy
- Heal after curettage and bone grafting
- Recurrence of incompletely curetted lesions in short bones of hands
- Recurrence of long bone lesions suggests malignancy
- Asymptomatic lesions require no treatment
- Painful or worrisome lesions require curettage and careful microscopic evaluation

Diagnostic Checklist
- In absence of a fracture, painful enchondroma is considered malignant until proven otherwise

---

- ○ High signal intensity
- ○ Calcification: Signal void
- T1 C+: No significant enhancement
- Helpful in evaluating exact size and extent of lesion

Nuclear Medicine Findings
- Bone Scan: No increased uptake unless fractured

Imaging Recommendations
- Best imaging tool: Radiographs usually diagnostic
- Protocol advice: CT best imaging modality to detect chondroid matrix

DIFFERENTIAL DIAGNOSIS

Bone Infarct
- Well-defined, densely sclerotic, serpiginous borders
- No endosteal scalloping

Chondrosarcoma
- Clinical findings (primarily pain) better indicator of chondrosarcoma than radiographic findings
- Periosteal reaction, soft-tissue mass
- Size: > 4 cm suggests malignancy

Epidermoid Inclusion Cyst
- Phalangeal tuft
- History of trauma

Juxtacortical Chondroma
- Involves surface of bone
- Can erode underlying cortex
- Periosteal new bone formation

PATHOLOGY

General Features
- General path comments: Occurs in bones that form by enchondral ossification (not skull)
- Genetics: Mutant parathyroid hormone related protein (PTH/PTHrP) type I receptor in enchondromatosis
- Etiology

- ○ Develop from abnormal zone of dysplastic chondrocytes in growth plate
  - Fail to undergo normal enchondral ossification
- Epidemiology
  - ○ Second most common benign bone tumor
  - ○ 12-24% of benign bone tumors
  - ○ 2-10% of all bone tumors
- Associated abnormalities
  - ○ Ollier disease: Non-hereditary rare developmental bone dysplasia
    - Multiple enchondromas
    - Predilection for appendicular skeleton; involvement of trunk bones in severe cases
    - Mostly unilateral monomelic distribution
    - Growth disparity with leg/arm shortening: Affected bones grow more slowly
    - Sarcomatous transformation: 25-30%
    - Osteosarcoma (young adults), chondrosarcoma/fibrosarcoma (older patients)
  - ○ Maffucci syndrome: Non-hereditary rare disorder characterized by enchondromatosis and soft tissue hemangiomas
    - Multiple enchondromas and multiple soft tissue cavernous hemangiomas
    - Unilateral involvement of hands and feet
    - Very large enchondromas, projecting into soft tissue
    - Phleboliths within hemangiomas
    - Malignant transformation of enchondroma into chondrosarcoma: 15-25%
    - Transformation of soft tissue hemangioma into vascular sarcoma: 3-5%
    - Associated ovarian and pancreatic malignancies
  - ○ Metachondromatosis: Autosomal-dominant
    - Multiple enchondromas and osteochondromas
    - Transformation into chondrosarcomas: 50%

Gross Pathologic & Surgical Features
- Most enchondromas treated by curettage; resected specimens rare
- Composed of confluent lobules of mature hyaline cartilage

ENCHONDROMA

- Tumor fragments consist of blue-white, glistering hyaline cartilage, mixed with yellow, calcified foci

Microscopic Features
- Lobules of mature hyaline cartilage with translucent intercellular matrix (little collagen)
- Tumor cells located in lacunae
- Lobules separated by normal bone marrow spaces
- Calcification common (correspond to matrix calcifications/enchondral ossification)
- Small bones of hands and feet can contain foci of myxoid tissue
  - Prominent myxoid changes suspicious of malignancy
- Immunohistochemistry: Positive for S-100 protein and vimentin

CLINICAL ISSUES

Presentation
- Most common signs/symptoms
  - Usually asymptomatic
  - Painless swelling
- Clinical profile
  - May present as pathologic fracture
  - Patient should be instructed to report symptoms:
    - Pain, unexplained by injury or fracture, should raise suspicion of malignancy

Demographics
- Age: 15-40 years; peak: 10-30 years
- Gender: M:F = 1:1
- Ethnicity: No racial predilection

Natural History & Prognosis
- Heal after curettage and bone grafting
- Recurrence of incompletely curetted lesions in short bones of hands
- Recurrence of long bone lesions suggests malignancy
- Malignant transformation of long bone enchondroma into chondrosarcoma rare
- Malignant transformation in Ollier disease, Mafucci syndrome, metachondromatosis: 15-50%

Treatment
- Asymptomatic lesions require no treatment
- Painful or worrisome lesions require curettage and careful microscopic evaluation
  - Important to evaluate entire lesion
  - Limited sampling may miss malignant foci
- Suspicious lesions of trunk and flat bones require wide local excision
  - Reduces tissue contamination and recurrence if lesion turns out to be malignant
- Curettage and bone grafting of large lesions

DIAGNOSTIC CHECKLIST

Consider
- Presence/absence of pain
- In absence of a fracture, painful enchondroma is considered malignant until proven otherwise

Image Interpretation Pearls
- Focal lucency in densely calcified enchondromas requires biopsy to exclude malignant transformation

SELECTED REFERENCES

1. Hopyan S et al: A mutant PTH/PTHrP type I receptor in enchondromatosis. Nat Genet 30:306-10, 2002
2. Unni KK: Cartilaginous lesions of bone. J Orthop Sci 6:457-72, 2001
3. Dorfman HD et al: Bone tumors. 1st ed. St. Louis MO, Mosby, 253-96, 1998
4. Greenspan A et al: Differential diagnosis of tumors and tumor-like lesions of bones and joints. 1st ed. Philadelphia PA, Lippincott-Raven, 125-46, 1998
5. Murphey MD et al: Enchondroma versus chondrosarcoma in the appendicular skeleton: Differentiating features. Radiographics 18:1213-37, 1998
6. Geirnaerdt MJ et al: Usefulness of radiography in differentiating enchondroma from grade 1 chondrosarcoma. Am J Roentgenol 169:1097-104, 1997
7. Geirnaerdt MJ et al: Cartilaginous tumors: Correlation of gadolinium-enhanced MR imaging and histopathologic findings. Radiology 186:813-7, 1993
8. Aoki J et al: MR of enchondroma and chondrosarcoma: Rings and arcs of Gd-DTPA enhancement. J Comput Assist Tomogr 15:1011-6, 1991
9. Greenspan A: Tumors of cartilage origin. Orthop Clin North Am 20:347-66, 1989
10. Resnik CS et al: Case report 522. Concurrent adjacent osteochondroma and enchondroma. Skeletal Radiol 18:66-9, 1989
11. Unger EC et al: MR imaging of Maffucci syndrome. Am J Roentgenol 150:351-3, 1988
12. Liu J e al: Bone sarcomas associated with Ollier's disease. Cancer 59:1376-85, 1987
13. Goodman SB et al: Ollier's disease with multiple sarcomatous transformations. Hum Pathol 15:91-3, 1984
14. Nakamura Y et al: S-100 protein in tumors of cartilage and bone: An immunohistochemical study. Cancer 52:1820-4, 1983

ENCHONDROMA

IMAGE GALLERY

Typical

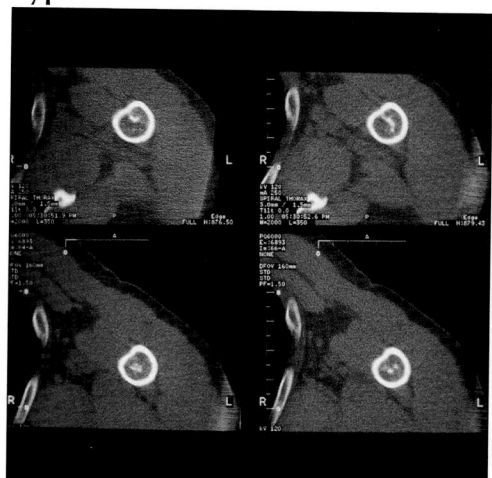
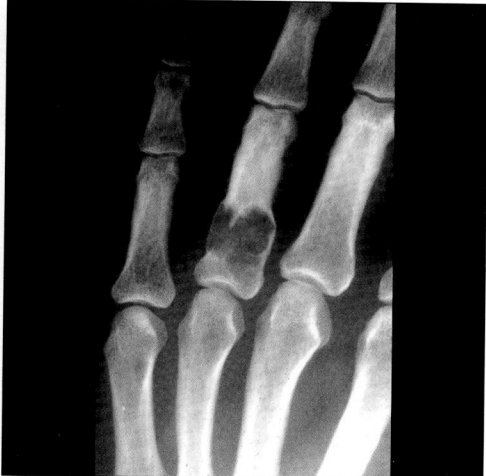

(Left) Axial NECT shows calcified lesion with chondroid matrix involving the proximal humerus. *(Right)* Anteroposterior radiography show expansile purely lytic lesion at the base of the proximal phalanx of the 4th digit. The radiolucent appearance is typical for enchondromas of the hands.

Typical

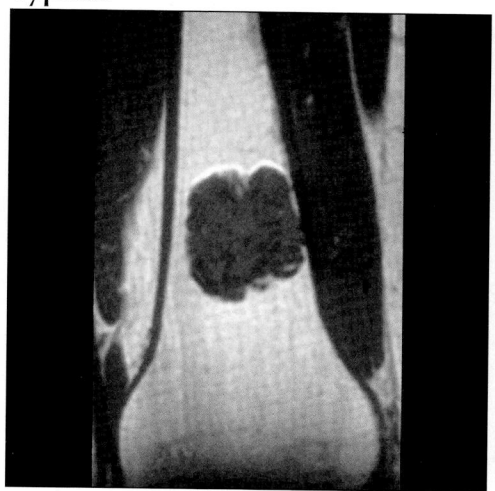
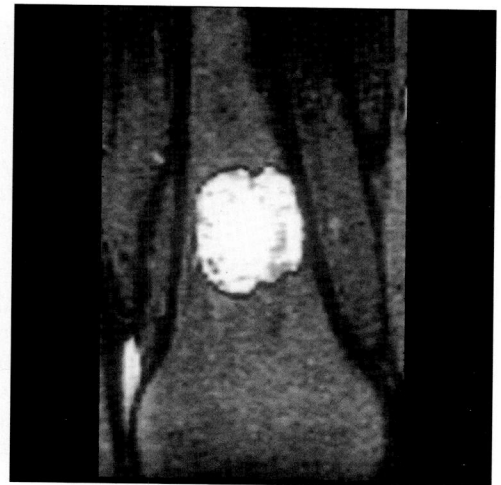

(Left) Coronal T1WI MR shows circumscribed, lobulated lesion of intermediate SI in the distal femoral metaphysis. *(Right)* Coronal FS T2 FSE MR shows circumscribed, lobulated femoral lesion of high signal. Areas of high signal represent cartilaginous matrix.

Variant

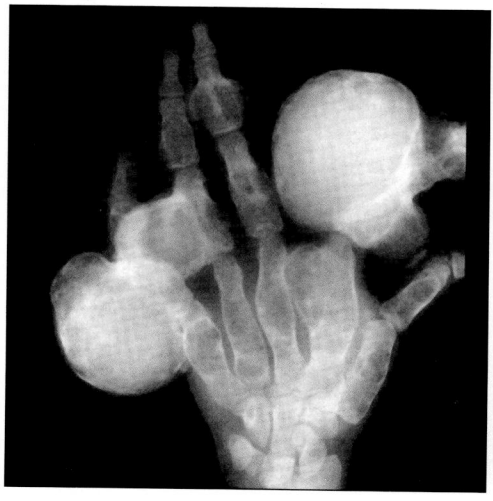
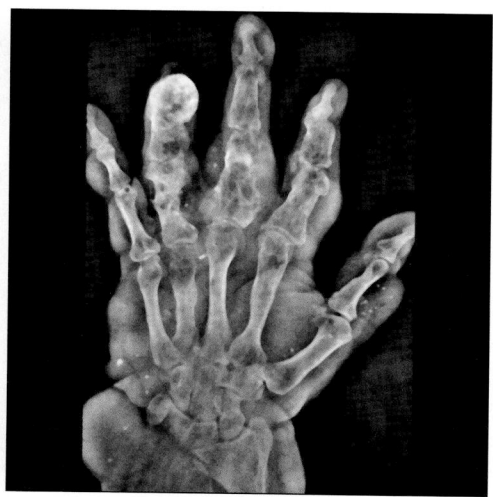

(Left) Anteroposterior radiography shows multiple large lobulated cartilaginous masses with associated bone deformity in a patient with Ollier disease. *(Right)* Anteroposterior radiography in a patient with Maffucci syndrome shows multiple enchondromas and associated phleboliths in soft tissue hemangiomas.

OSTEOCHONDROMA

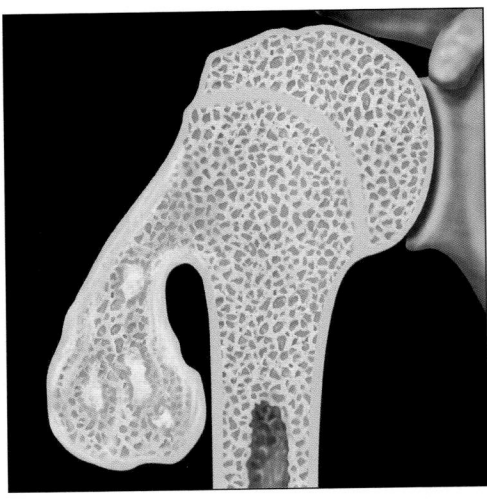

Coronal graphic shows pedunculated osteochondroma arising from the humeral metaphysis. Continuity with host bone is shown.

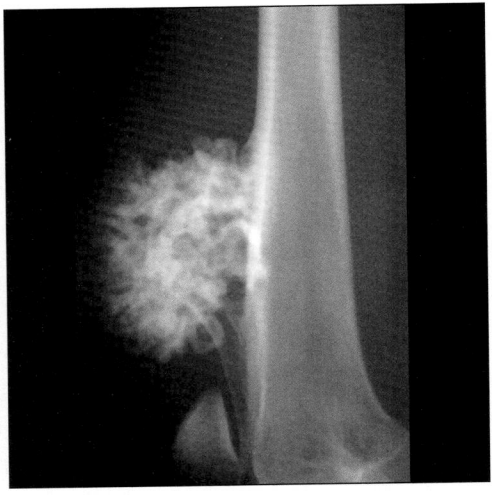

Lateral radiography shows heavily mineralized pedunculated osteochondroma arising from the distal femoral metaphysis.

TERMINOLOGY

Abbreviations and Synonyms
- Exostosis, osteocartilaginous exostosis

Definitions
- Developmental osseous anomaly resulting in exophytic outgrowth on surface of bone

IMAGING FINDINGS

General Features
- Best diagnostic clue: Exostosis with continuity of bone cortex and medullary marrow space to host bone
- Location
  - Any bone with enchondral ossification can be involved
  - Metaphysis of long bones: 70%
    - Femur: 30%
    - Tibia: 20%
    - Humerus: 20%
  - Hands and feet: 10%
  - Pelvis: 5%
  - Scapula: 4%
- Size: 1-15 cm, mean: 3-7 cm
- Morphology: Pedunculated or sessile

Radiographic Findings
- Radiography
  - Cartilage covered bony projection (exostosis) on external surface of bone
    - Calcification of hyaline cartilage cap
  - Pedunculated type: Slender pedicle directed away from joint
    - Lesion grows at right angles to long axis of host bone
  - Sessile type: Broad-based attachment to cortex
  - Undertubulation of long bones (Erlenmeyer flask deformity)
  - Malignant degeneration
    - Development of thick, bulky, cartilaginous cap (thickness > 1 cm by CT, > 2 cm by MRI)
    - Dispersed calcifications within cartilaginous cap
    - Development of soft tissue mass

CT Findings
- NECT
  - To demonstrate continuity of cortical and medullary portions of lesion with host bone
  - To demonstrate thickness of cartilaginous cap
  - Helpful in showing bursa formation

MR Findings
- T1WI: Intermediate signal intensity
- T2WI

DDx: Osteochondroma

Chondrosarcoma	Parosteal OGS	Myositis Ossific.	Chondroma	Subung. Exostosis
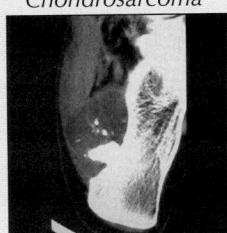	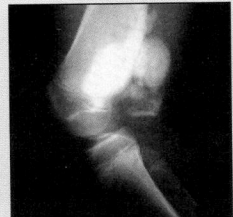	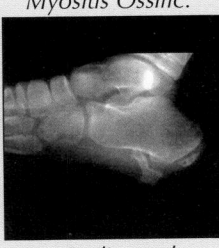	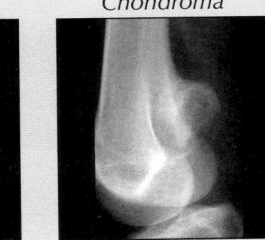	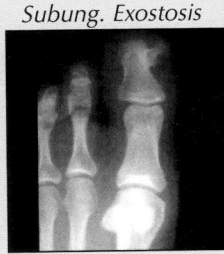
Ax NECT	Lat Radiography	Lat Radiography	Lat Radiography	AP Radiography

OSTEOCHONDROMA

Key Facts

Imaging Findings
- Best diagnostic clue: Exostosis with continuity of bone cortex and medullary marrow space to host bone

Top Differential Diagnoses
- Parosteal Osteosarcoma
- Periosteal Chondroma
- Chondrosarcoma
- Juxtacortical Myositis Ossificans
- Subungual Exostosis

Pathology
- Most common benign bone tumor
- 12% of all bone tumors
- Multiple hereditary osteochondromas (MHE): Autosomal dominant hereditary disorder

- Multiple osteochondromas associated with bone deformities of affected sites

Clinical Issues
- Most common signs/symptoms: Usually painless mass, present for many years
- Painful with impingement on nerves/blood vessels
- Bursa can form over cap
- Pain in absence of fracture, nerve compression, or bursitis considered malignant until proven otherwise
- Benign lesion with self-limited growth
- Malignant transformation: 1-2% of solitary lesions
- Malignant transformation of MHE: 3-5%
- Surgical resection of symptomatic lesions
- If entire cartilage cap removed recurrence unlikely (< 5%)

- o Cartilaginous cap: High signal intensity
- o Band of low signal surrounding cap (represents perichondrium)
- To evaluate thickness of cartilaginous cap and overlying bursa formation

Imaging Recommendations
- Best imaging tool: Radiographs diagnostic
- Protocol advice
  - o Radiographs for initial diagnosis
  - o CT or MRI to evaluate thickness of cartilaginous cap

DIFFERENTIAL DIAGNOSIS

Parosteal Osteosarcoma
- Osseous destruction

Periosteal Chondroma
- Can simulate sessile osteochondroma
- Intact cortex

Chondrosarcoma
- Cortical destruction
- Thick, bulky, cartilaginous cap
  - o > 1 cm by CT, > 2 cm by MRI

Juxtacortical Myositis Ossificans
- Intact cortex
- No continuity between abnormal ossification and host bone

Subungual Exostosis
- Intact cortex
- No flaring of cortical bone into lesion

PATHOLOGY

General Features
- General path comments
  - o Lesions have own growth plate and stop growing with skeletal maturity

- o Bursa formation as response to friction in moving body parts
- Genetics
  - o Genetic alterations in patients with multiple hereditary exostoses
    - Point mutation of EXT1 gene leading to premature translation stop
    - Alteration of EXT2 gene in families with chromosome 11p11-13 defect
- Etiology
  - o Arises from aberrant epiphyseal development with displacement of physeal cartilage through perichondral fibrous ring
    - Displaced peripheral chondroblasts act as ectopic growth plate
  - o Can be induced by implanting epiphyseal tissue into cortex
  - o Can arise after external radiation for non-osseous neoplasm
- Epidemiology
  - o Most common benign bone tumor
  - o 45% of all benign bone tumors
  - o 12% of all bone tumors
- Associated abnormalities
  - o Multiple hereditary osteochondromas (MHE): Autosomal dominant hereditary disorder
    - Multiple osteochondromas associated with bone deformities of affected sites
    - Involves knee, hip, ankle, shoulder (usually symmetric involvement)
    - Knees almost always affected: Knee radiographs for initial screening
    - Involvement of multiple sites in severe cases
    - Growth disturbance and bowing deformities of affected bones
    - Can result in pseudo-Madelung deformity of forearm (ulnar shortening, bowing of radius)
    - Sessile form more common
    - Increased risk of malignant transformation into chondrosarcoma

OSTEOCHONDROMA

Gross Pathologic & Surgical Features

- Normal cortical bone with cartilaginous cap covered by thin, fibrous membrane (perichondrium)
  - Perichondrium continuous with periosteum covering stalk
  - Thickness of cap 1-3 mm, rarely up to 1 cm
  - Greater thickness may imply malignant transformation
- Continuity of lesion with marrow and cortex of host bone (hallmark)
- Zone of provisional calcification of epiphyseal plate at junction of cap and underlying spongiosa

Microscopic Features

- Cartilage cap containing a basal surface with enchondral ossification
  - Represents epiphyseal growth plate
- Bursa at periphery of some osteochondromas attached to perichondrium of cap
  - Bursa wall lined by synovium
  - Can be associated with cartilaginous loose bodies in bursa

CLINICAL ISSUES

Presentation

- Most common signs/symptoms: Usually painless mass, present for many years
- Clinical profile
  - Painful with impingement on nerves/blood vessels
  - Pathologic fracture, usually at base of stalk, rarely presenting symptom
  - Bursa can form over cap
    - Can become inflamed, accumulate synovial fluid or loose bodies
  - Pain in absence of fracture, nerve compression, or bursitis considered malignant until proven otherwise

Demographics

- Age: 10-35 years
- Gender: M:F = 1.8-2:1

Natural History & Prognosis

- Benign lesion with self-limited growth
  - Growth ceases after skeletal maturation
- Recurrence: < 5%
- Malignant transformation: 1-2% of solitary lesions
  - Suspect if
    - Growth of lesion after skeletal maturation
    - Pain in absence of fracture, bursitis, nerve compression
- Malignant transformation of MHE: 3-5%

Treatment

- Surgical resection of symptomatic lesions
- Marginal excision including cartilaginous cap and overlying perichondrium
- Cartilaginous cap should not be traumatized during resection
- Osseous base has minimal activity and may be removed piecemeal
- If entire cartilage cap removed recurrence unlikely (< 5%)

DIAGNOSTIC CHECKLIST

Consider

- Pain in absence of fracture, nerve compression, bursitis suspicious of malignancy

Image Interpretation Pearls

- Cartilage thickness: Best measured on CT, MRI

SELECTED REFERENCES

1. Ahmed AR et al: Secondary chondrosarcoma in osteochondroma: Report of 107 patients. Clin Orthop 411:193-206, 2003
2. Trebicz-Geffen M et al: The short-lived exostosis induced surgically versus the lasting genetic hereditary multiple exostoses. Exp Mol Pathol 74:40-8, 2003
3. Murphey MD et al: Imaging of osteochondroma: Variants and complications with radiologic-pathologic correlation. Radiographics 20:1407-34, 2000
4. Dorfman HD et al: Bone tumors. 1st ed. St. Louis MO, Mosby, 331-52, 1998
5. Greenspan A et al: Differential diagnosis of tumors and tumor-like lesions of bones and joints. 1st ed. Philadelphia PA, Lippincott-Raven, 146-59, 1998
6. Mehta M et al: MR imaging of symptomatic osteochondromas with pathologic correlation. Skeletal Radiol 27:427-33, 1998
7. Karasick D et al: Symptomatic osteochondromas: Imaging features. AJR 168: 507-12, 1997
8. Le Merrer M et al: A gene for hereditary multiple exostoses maps to chromosome 19p. Human Molecular Genetics 3:717-22, 1994
9. Griffiths HJ et al: Bursitis in association with solitary osteochondromas presenting as mass lesion. Skeletal Radiol 20:513-6, 1991
10. Hudson TM et al: Benign exostoses and exostotic chondrosarcomas: Evaluation of cartilage thickness by CT. Radiology 152:595-9, 1984
11. Milgram JW: The origin of osteochondromas and enchondromas. Clin Orthop 174:264-84, 1983

OSTEOCHONDROMA

IMAGE GALLERY

Typical

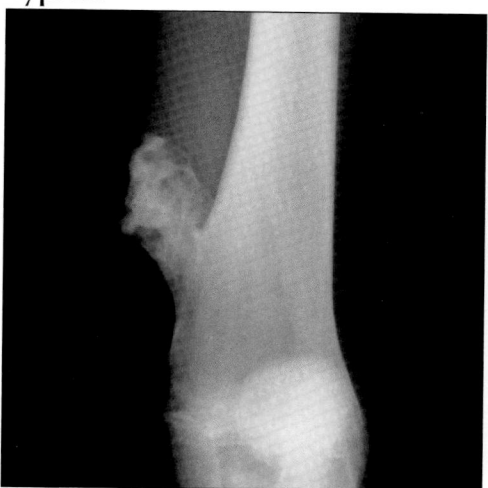
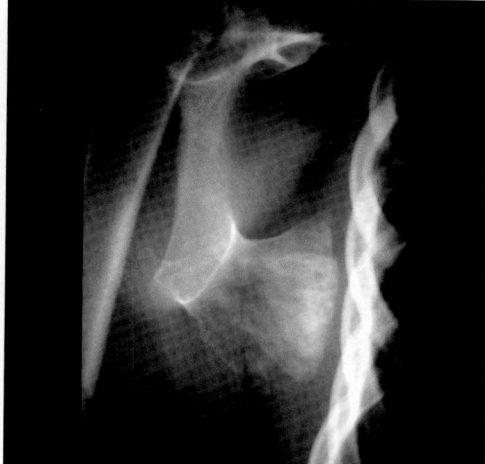

(Left) Anteroposterior radiography shows pedunculated osteochondroma arising from the distal femoral metaphysis. Note the continuity of cortical and cancellous bone. Pedunculated osteochondromas usually point away from closest joint. *(Right)* Anteroposterior radiography shows a large calcified broad based osteochondroma arising from the scapula.

Typical

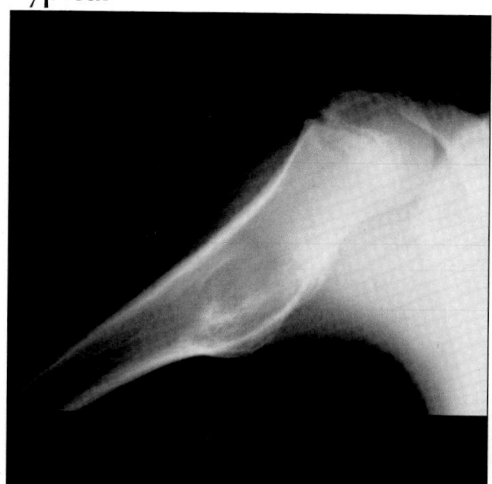
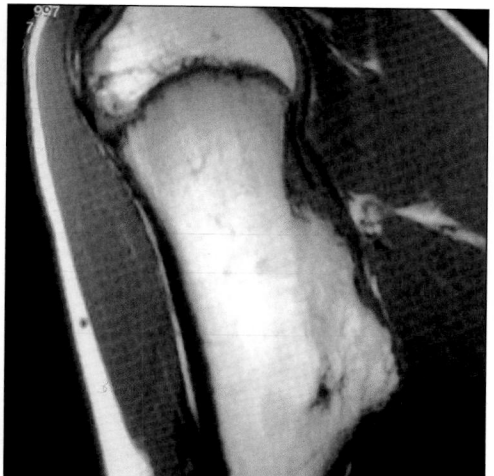

(Left) Anteroposterior radiography show sessile osteochondroma arising from the medial cortex of the proximal humeral diaphysis. Note the continuity of the lesion with the underlying cortex. *(Right)* Sagittal T1WI MR shows sessile osteochondroma arising from the proximal humeral meta-diaphysis. Note similar SI of medullary cavity of lesion and host bone. Thin hypointense rim surrounding the lesion represents perichondrium.

Variant

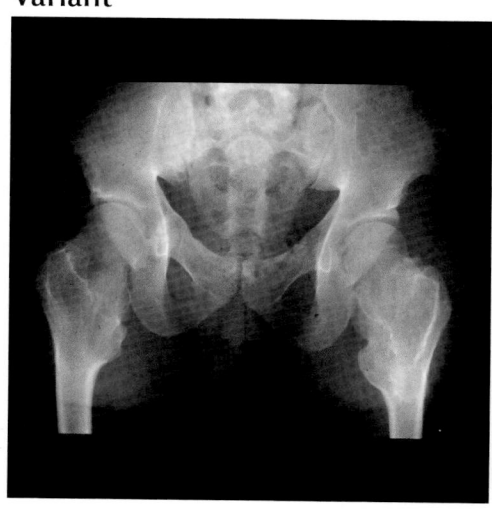
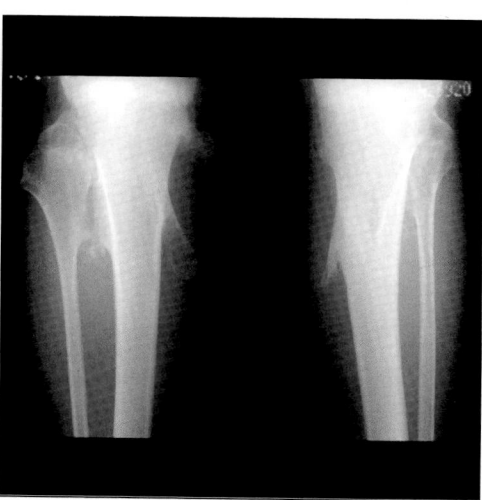

(Left) Anteroposterior radiography in a patient with MHE shows irregular dense undulations of the proximal femoral metaphyses. *(Right)* Anteroposterior radiography shows multiple osteochondromas arising from the proximal tibia and fibula in a patient with MHE.

CHONDROBLASTOMA

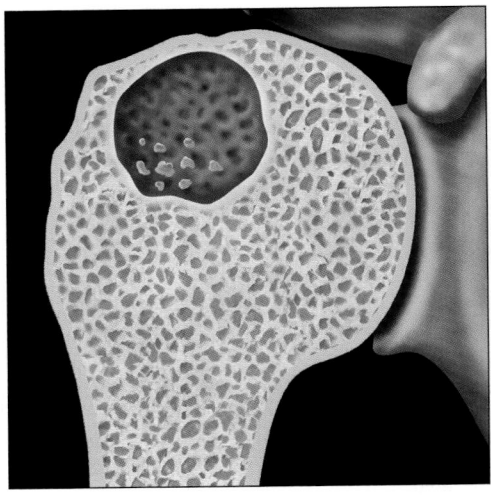

Coronal graphic shows lytic epiphyseal lesion with chondroid matrix (in white) involving the humeral head. Well-defined sclerotic margin is shown.

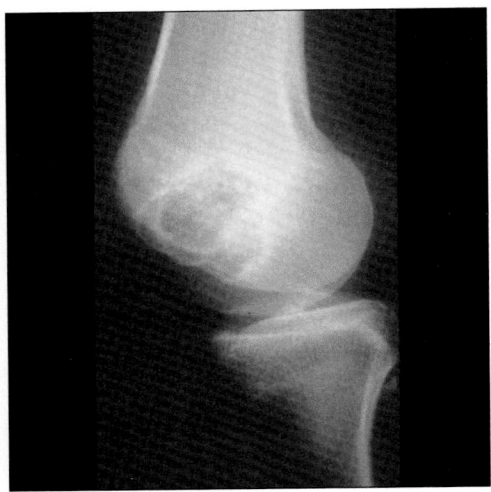

Lateral radiography shows a well-defined lytic lesion in the femoral epiphysis.

TERMINOLOGY

Abbreviations and Synonyms
- Codman tumor

Definitions
- Benign cartilage neoplasm, characterized by immature cartilage cells and extracellular matrix component

IMAGING FINDINGS

General Features
- Best diagnostic clue: Well-defined lytic lesion centered in epiphyses of skeletally immature patients
- Location
  - Long bones: 80%
    - Proximal femur and greater trochanter: 23%
    - Distal femur: 20%
    - Proximal tibia: 17%
    - Proximal humerus: 18%
  - Hands and feet: 10%
    - Tubular bones
    - Ankle (talus, calcaneus)
  - Craniofacial bones (base of skull and temporal fossa): 16%
  - Spine, clavicle, sternum: Rare
  - Epiphyses/apophyses: 40%
    - Apophyses: Greater trochanter, greater tuberosity, patella (most common tumor affecting patella)
    - Epiphyseal-equivalent site of flat bones: Acetabulum, iliac crest
  - Epiphyses and metaphyses: 55%
  - Metaphyses: 5%
- Size: 2-6 cm
- Morphology: Well-defined round/oval lytic defect with thin sclerotic rim

Radiographic Findings
- Radiography
  - Well-defined, eccentrically or centrally located lytic lesion
  - Rarely expansile
  - Thin sclerotic margin
    - Margins: Smooth (63%), scalloped (27%), lobulated (10%)
  - Geographic pattern of bone destruction
  - Stippled calcifications in 40-50%
  - Periosteal reaction away from lesion outside joint capsule: 50%
  - Bone expansion with secondary aneurysmal bone cyst formation: 15-20%
  - Stage 3 lesion may extend through growth plate into metaphysis or through cartilage into joint
  - Usually seen in immature skeleton

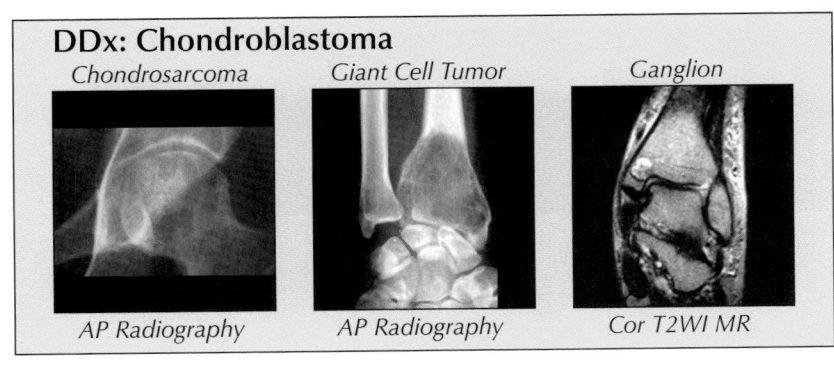

DDx: Chondroblastoma

Chondrosarcoma	Giant Cell Tumor	Ganglion
AP Radiography	AP Radiography	Cor T2WI MR

CHONDROBLASTOMA

Key Facts

Imaging Findings
- Best diagnostic clue: Well-defined lytic lesion centered in epiphyses of skeletally immature patients
- Radiographs diagnostic
- MRI might suggest aggressive/malignant lesion due to extensive surrounding edema

Top Differential Diagnoses
- Clear-Cell Chondrosarcoma
- Giant Cell Tumor
- Langerhans Cell Histiocytosis (LCH)
- Intraosseous Ganglion
- Aneurysmal Bone Cyst (ABC)
- Avascular Necrosis of the Femoral or Humeral Head
- Osteomyelitis (Abscess)
- Pseudotumor of the Greater Humeral Tuberosity

Pathology
- Less than 1% of all primary bone tumors
- 9% of benign bone tumors

Clinical Issues
- Mild joint pain, tenderness, swelling
- Benign tumor
- May become locally aggressive
- Curettage and packing with bone graft, polymethylmethacrylate

Diagnostic Checklist
- Location (epiphyses/apophyses), age (immature skeleton)

CT Findings
- NECT
  - Helpful in evaluating calcified chondroid matrix
  - Fluid-fluid levels

MR Findings
- T1WI
  - Low to intermediate signal intensity
  - Bone marrow edema: Low signal intensity
- T2WI
  - Intermediate to low signal intensity (solid components)
  - Bone marrow edema: High signal intensity
- T1 C+: Enhancement of edematous areas
- Prominent soft tissue and bone marrow edema
  - Overestimates extent and aggressiveness of lesion
- Joint effusions: 30-50%
- Fluid-fluid levels

Imaging Recommendations
- Best imaging tool: Radiographs
- Protocol advice
  - Radiographs diagnostic
  - MRI might suggest aggressive/malignant lesion due to extensive surrounding edema

DIFFERENTIAL DIAGNOSIS

Clear-Cell Chondrosarcoma
- May be indistinguishable
- Exhibits same benign pattern
- More heavily calcified
- Both may be seen in immature skeleton

Giant Cell Tumor
- Usually larger and less well-demarcated
- No calcified matrix
- Older age group with closed growth plate
- May expand epiphysis and diaphysis

Langerhans Cell Histiocytosis (LCH)
- No calcified matrix
- Variable margins, less well-defined
- Multiple lesion

Intraosseous Ganglion
- Eccentric location
- Radiolucent
- No calcified matrix

Aneurysmal Bone Cyst (ABC)
- No calcified matrix
- Thinned cortex

Avascular Necrosis of the Femoral or Humeral Head
- More irregular
- Crescent sign

Osteomyelitis (Abscess)
- Less well-defined
- Serpentine tract
- No calcified matrix

Pseudotumor of the Greater Humeral Tuberosity
- Lucency due to increase amount of cancellous bone
- Pseudotumor, no sclerotic margin or internal matrix

PATHOLOGY

General Features
- General path comments: Benign cartilage neoplasm, characterized by proliferation of immature cartilage cells
- Etiology: Originates from chondroblasts in epiphyseal cartilage plate
- Epidemiology
  - Less than 1% of all primary bone tumors
  - 9% of benign bone tumors

Gross Pathologic & Surgical Features
- Well-demarcated, gray-tan mass
- Blue-gray foci represent chondroid matrix
- Foci of calcification and hemorrhage

CHONDROBLASTOMA

- Large, blood-filled, multiloculated cyst-like areas: Secondary ABC formation
- Larger tumors may break into metaphysis or through cortex

Microscopic Features
- Nodules of mature cartilage matrix surrounded by undifferentiated tissue of chondroblast-like cells
- Contains multinucleated giant cells of osteoclast type
- "Chicken wire" calcification (pericellular deposition of calcification) pathognomonic
- ABC component: 5-15%
- Immunohistochemistry: Positive for S-100 protein and vimentin
- Receptor activator of NF-κB ligand (RANKL) involved in osteolytic bone destruction

Staging, Grading or Classification Criteria
- Surgical staging for benign musculoskeletal tumors
  - Stage 1: Latent
  - Stage 2: Active
  - Stage 3: Aggressive

CLINICAL ISSUES

Presentation
- Most common signs/symptoms
  - Mild joint pain, tenderness, swelling
    - Due to involvement of articular cartilage and synovium (epiphyseal lesion)
    - Symptoms can range from months to several years (> 10 years)
- Clinical profile
  - Joint effusion: 30%
  - Pathologic fractures rare
  - Elevated ESR

Demographics
- Age
  - 5-59 years; peak: 5-25 years
  - Occurs before cessation of enchondral bone growth
- Gender: M:F = 2:1

Natural History & Prognosis
- Benign tumor
  - May become locally aggressive
- Pulmonary "metastases" (pulmonary implants): Rare
  - No histologic evidence of malignancy
  - May be due to hematogenous spread of tumor cells during operative manipulation
  - Should be resected due to growth potential

Treatment
- Curettage and packing with bone graft, polymethylmethacrylate
  - Tumor may seed to adjacent joints or lungs if spilled
  - Recurrence: 5-10%
- Stage 3 lesions usually not amenable to curettage (50% recurrence rate)
  - En-bloc excision
- Excision of pulmonary nodules

DIAGNOSTIC CHECKLIST

Consider
- Location (epiphyses/apophyses), age (immature skeleton)

Image Interpretation Pearls
- MRI can be misleading (suggests aggressive lesion)

SELECTED REFERENCES

1. Huang L et al: Receptor activator of NF-κB ligand (RANKL) is expressed in chondroblastoma: Possible involvement in osteoclastic giant cell recruitment. Mol Pathol 56:116-20, 2003
2. Masui F et al: Chondroblastoma: A study of 11 cases. Eur J Surg Oncol 28:869-74, 2002
3. Greenspan A et al: Differential diagnosis of tumors and tumor-like lesions of bones and joints. 1st ed. Philadelphia PA, Lippincott-Raven, 158-63, 1998
4. Weatherall PT et al: Chondroblastoma: Classic and confusing appearance at MR imaging. Radiology 190:467-74, 1994
5. Turcotte RE et al: Chondroblastoma. Hum Pathol 24:944-9, 1993
6. Edel G et al: Chondroblastoma of bone: A clinical, radiological, light and immunohistochemical study. Virchows Arch 421:355-66, 1992
7. Brower AC et al: The frequency and diagnostic significance of periostitis in chondroblastoma. Am J Roentgenol 154:309-14, 1990
8. Bloem JL: Chondroblastoma: A clinical and radiological study of 104 cases. Skeletal Radiol 14:1-9, 1985
9. Huvos AG et al: Aggressive chondroblastoma: Review of the literature on aggressive behavior and metastases with report of one new case. Clin Orthop 126:266-72, 1977
10. Dahlin DC et al: Benign chondroblastoma: A study of 125 cases. Cancer 30:401-13, 1972

IMAGE GALLERY

Typical

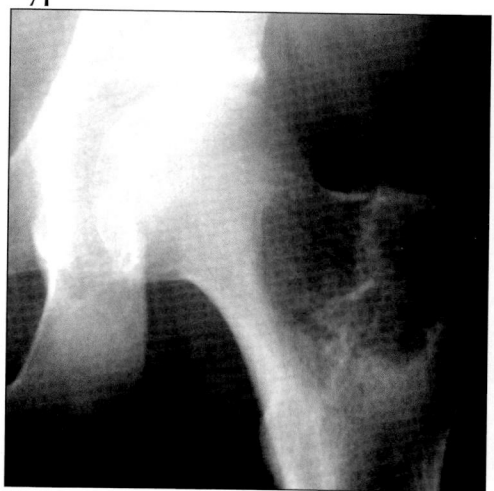
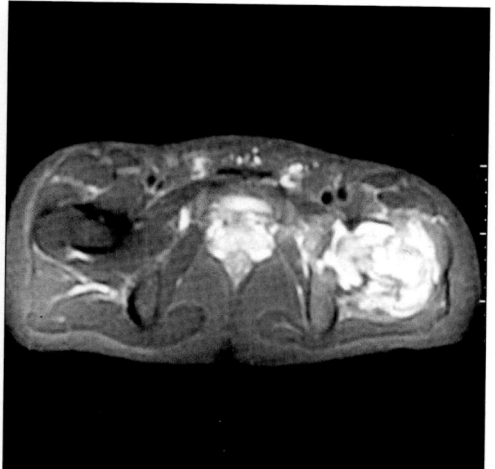

(Left) Anteroposterior radiography of the left proximal femur shows a well-defined lytic lesion involving the greater trochanter (epiphysis equivalent). *(Right)* Axial FS T2 FSE MR shows marked edema surrounding the chondroblastoma in the left greater trochanter.

Typical

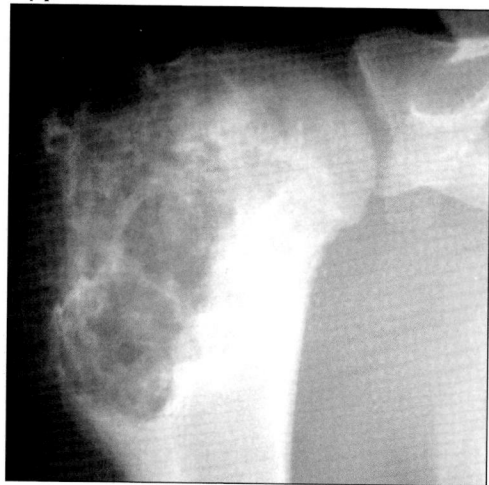
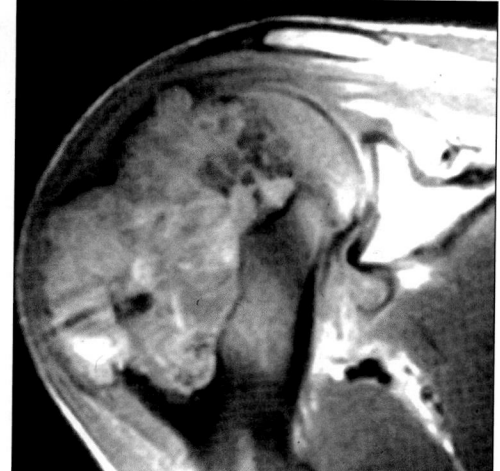

(Left) Anteroposterior radiography shows a multilobulated lytic expansile lesion with chondroid matrix in the humeral epiphysis. *(Right)* Coronal FS T2 FSE MR shows heterogeneous signal in the expansile lesion centered in the humeral epiphysis.

Typical

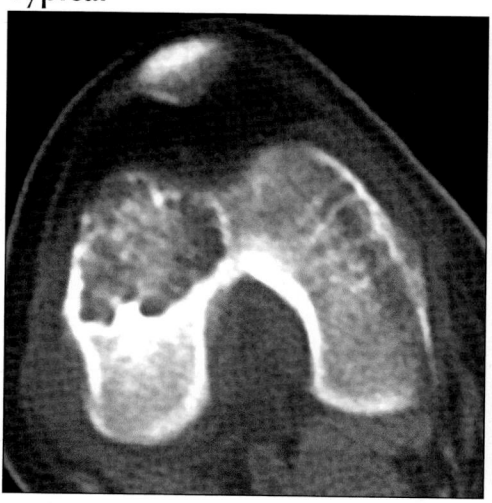
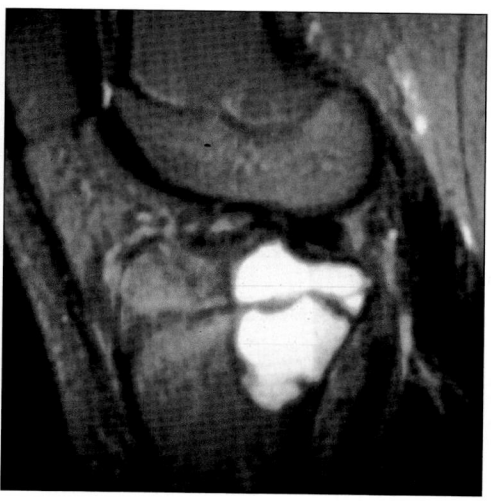

(Left) Axial NECT shows a lytic lesion with chondroid matrix in the distal femoral epiphysis. *(Right)* Sagittal FS T2 FSE MR shows a high signal lesion in the tibial epiphyseal which is crossing the growth plate. Findings are consistent with secondary ABC formation.

CHONDROMYXOID FIBROMA

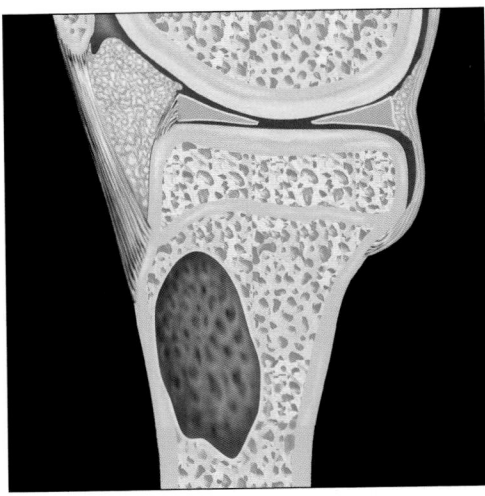

Sagittal graphic shows lytic, slightly lobulated lesion with thin sclerotic margin involving the tibial metaphysis.

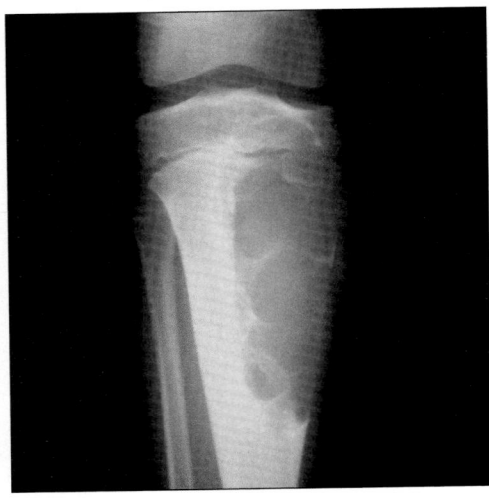

Anteroposterior radiography shows a radiolucent, lobulated lesion in tibial metadiaphysis, exhibiting geographic type of bone destruction, sclerotic scalloped borders, and internal septa.

TERMINOLOGY

Abbreviations and Synonyms
- CMF, fibromyxoid chondroma, myxofibrous chondroma

Definitions
- Benign tumor composed of immature myxoid mesenchymal tissue with features of primitive cartilaginous differentiation

IMAGING FINDINGS

General Features
- Best diagnostic clue
  - Well-defined expansile lytic metaphyseal lesion with geographic pattern of bone destruction and sclerotic margin
  - Predilection for proximal tibia
- Location
  - Long bones: 60%
    - About knee: 55%
    - Proximal tibia: 30%
  - Short tubular bones of hands and feet: 25%
    - Involvement of feet more common
  - Pelvis: 8%
  - Metaphyses: 95%
  - Diaphyses: 5%
  - Apophyses can be involved
- Size: 1-10 cm, mean: 3-4 cm
- Morphology
  - Expansile lytic lesion with well-defined sclerotic margin
  - Matrix calcification rare

Radiographic Findings
- Radiography
  - Round-ovoid eccentric lytic lesion
    - Long axis of lesion parallel to long axis of host bone
  - Geographic pattern of bone destruction
  - Septa within lesion occasionally seen
  - Scalloped, sclerotic margins
  - Small tumors: Thin sclerotic margins
    - No calcification or trabeculation
  - Cortical thickening can extend short distance beyond lesion
  - Partial cortical erosions
  - No visible periosteal reaction (unless fractured)
  - Matrix calcification rare
  - Can break through cortex and infiltrate into surrounding soft tissues (rare)

CT Findings
- NECT
  - Well-defined lytic lesion +/- matrix calcification

DDx: Chondromyxoid Fibroma

Fibroxanthoma	Fibrous Dysplasia	ABC	Chondroblastoma	Chondrosarcoma
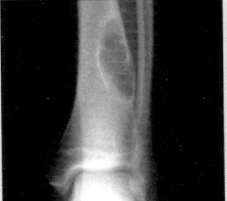	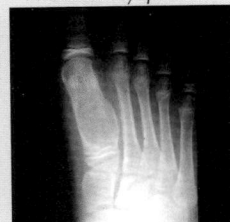	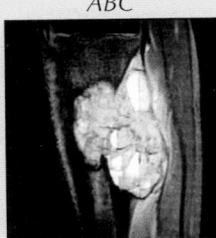	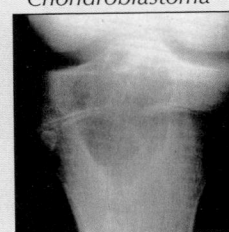	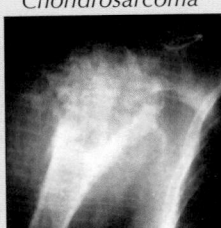
AP Radiography	*AP Radiography*	*Sag T2WI MR*	*AP Radiography*	*AP Radiography*

CHONDROMYXOID FIBROMA

Key Facts

Imaging Findings
- Well-defined expansile lytic metaphyseal lesion with geographic pattern of bone destruction and sclerotic margin
- Cortical expansion and soft tissue extension covered by thin layer of periosteal new bone

Top Differential Diagnoses
- Fibroxanthoma
- Fibrous Dysplasia
- Aneurysmal Bone Cyst (ABC)
- Chondroblastoma
- Chondrosarcoma
- Adamantinoma

Pathology
- 0.5% of all primary bone tumors

- 2% of all benign bone tumors

Clinical Issues
- Most common signs/symptoms: Local swelling and pain
- Can be asymptomatic, incidental finding in 10%
- Pathologic fracture: 2-5%
- Benign tumor
- Can cause damage by continued growth and extension into soft tissues
- Malignant degeneration rare
- Curettage and bone grafting for stage 2 lesions
- Recurrence (25%) likely due to incomplete curettage
- En bloc resection with marginal margin for stage 3 lesions

- o Cortical expansion and soft tissue extension covered by thin layer of periosteal new bone
- o To visualize chondroid matrix calcification
- o CT most sensitive modality to evaluate chondroid matrix calcifications
- CECT: Enhancement

MR Findings
- T1WI: Intermediate to low signal intensity
- T2WI
  - o High signal intensity
  - o Heterogeneous intermediate to high signal intensity
  - o Hypointense rim
- STIR: High signal intensity
- T1 C+: Heterogeneous enhancement
- Heterogeneous signal due to chondroid, myxoid, fibrous components +/- hemorrhage
- To demonstrate soft tissue extension

Angiographic Findings
- Minimal neovascularity

Nuclear Medicine Findings
- Bone Scan: Increased uptake of radiotracer

Imaging Recommendations
- Best imaging tool: Radiographs diagnostic
- Protocol advice
  - o CT to demonstrate thin overlying periosteal bone formation, matrix calcification
  - o MRI to demonstrate soft tissue extent

DIFFERENTIAL DIAGNOSIS

Fibroxanthoma
- No cortical ballooning or cortical destruction
- Periosteal reaction only in cases of fracture

Fibrous Dysplasia
- Central location
- Internal septations rare
- No periosteal reaction

- Osteofibrous dysplasia: Limited to anterior cortex of tibia
  - o More sclerotic
  - o Peak age: 1st decade of life

Aneurysmal Bone Cyst (ABC)
- Fluid-fluid levels
- Periosteal new bone formation
- No matrix mineralization

Chondroblastoma
- Epiphyseal lesion
- Calcified matrix in 50%

Chondrosarcoma
- Chondroid matrix
- Cortical destruction
- Soft tissue extension

Adamantinoma
- Predilection for tibia
- Cortical destruction
- Aggressive periosteal reaction
- Older patients

PATHOLOGY

General Features
- General path comments
  - o Benign tumor composed of mixture of chondroid, myxoid, and fibrous tissues
  - o Cases reported as osseous myxomas/myxofibromas probably represent CMF
- Genetics: Pericentric inversions of chromosome 6
- Etiology: Originates from cartilage-forming connective tissue
- Epidemiology
  - o 0.5% of all primary bone tumors
  - o 2% of all benign bone tumors

Gross Pathologic & Surgical Features
- Rubbery, bluish-gray, translucent tumor, resembles hyaline cartilage

CHONDROMYXOID FIBROMA

- Lobulated and well-marginated
- Surrounding bone shows sclerotic changes
- Hemorrhagic and cystic foci can be seen

Microscopic Features
- Large lobulated areas of spindle-shaped cells within myxoid or chondroid intercellular material
- Separated by septum-like zones of more cellular tissue that may contain giant cells
- Matrix: Dense chondroid; matrix stains basophilic
  - Loose myxoid matrix; stains eosinophilic
- Large pleomorphic and hyperchromatic cells occasionally seen
  - Can lead to confusion with diagnosis of chondrosarcoma
- Immunohistochemistry: Expression of type II collagen, S100B

Staging, Grading or Classification Criteria
- Surgical staging for benign musculoskeletal tumors
  - Stage 1: Latent
  - Stage 2: Active
  - Stage 3: Aggressive

CLINICAL ISSUES

Presentation
- Most common signs/symptoms: Local swelling and pain
- Clinical profile
  - Most cases present as stage 2 lesions
  - Can be asymptomatic, incidental finding in 10%
  - Pathologic fracture: 2-5%
  - Case report of oncogenic osteomalacia (hypophosphatemia, phosphaturia, low 1,25-dihydroxyvitamin D3)

Demographics
- Age
  - 5-79 years, peak: 2nd-3rd decade
  - 75% younger than 30 years
- Gender: M:F = 1.5 - 2:1
- Ethnicity: No racial predilection

Natural History & Prognosis
- Benign tumor
- Can cause damage by continued growth and extension into soft tissues
- Malignant degeneration rare
  - After radiation
- Recurrence in 25% after curettage
  - Recurrence more frequent in young patients (< 20 years)
- Rare cases of recurrence as chondrosarcoma reported

Treatment
- Curettage and bone grafting for stage 2 lesions
  - Recurrence (25%) likely due to incomplete curettage
- En bloc resection with marginal margin for stage 3 lesions
- Radiation therapy contraindicated due to risk of malignant transformation

DIAGNOSTIC CHECKLIST

Consider
- Location: Metaphysis of lower extremity, proximal tibia
- Morphology: Expansile, matrix calcification rare

SELECTED REFERENCES

1. Park HR et al: Expression of collagen type II, S100B, S100A2 and osteocalcin in chondroblastoma and chondromyxoid fibroma. Oncol Rep 9:1087-91, 2002
2. Park JM et al: Oncogenic osteomalacia associated with soft tissue chondromyxoid fibroma. Europ J Radiol 39:69-72, 2001
3. Durr HR et al: Chondromyxoid fibroma of bone. Arch Orthop Trauma Surg 120:42-7, 2000
4. Safar A et al: Recurrent anomalies of 6q25 in chondromyxoid fibroma. Hum Pathol 31:306-11, 2000
5. Greenspan A et al: Differential diagnosis of tumors and tumor-like lesions of bones and joints. 1st ed. Philadelphia PA, Lippincott-Raven, 164-69, 1998
6. Wu CT et al: Chondromyxoid fibroma of bone: A clinicopathologic review of 278 cases. Hum Pathol 29:438-46, 1998
7. Yamaguchi T et al: Radiographic and histologic patterns of calcification in chondromyxoid fibroma. Skeletal Radiol 27:559-64, 1998
8. O'Connor PJ et al: Chondromyxoid fibroma of the foot. Skeletal Radiol 25:143-8, 1996
9. White PG et al: Chondromyxoid fibroma. Skeletal Radiol 25:79-81, 1996
10. Wilson AJ et al: Chondromyxoid fibroma: Radiographic appearance in 38 cases and a review of the literature. Radiology 179:513-8, 1991
11. Zillmer DA et al: Chondromyxoid fibroma of bone: Thirty-six cases with clinicopathologic correlation. Hum Pathol 20:952-64, 1989
12. Schajowicz F: Chondromyxoid fibroma: Report of three cases with predominant cortical involvement. Radiology 164:783-6, 1987
13. Beggs IG et al: Chondromyxoid fibroma of bone. Clin Radiol 33:671-9, 1982
14. Rahimi A et al: Chondromyxoid fibroma: A clinicopathologic study of 76 cases. Cancer 30:726-36, 1972
15. Feldman F et al: Chondromyxoid fibroma of bone. Radiology 94:249-60, 1970

CHONDROMYXOID FIBROMA

Typical

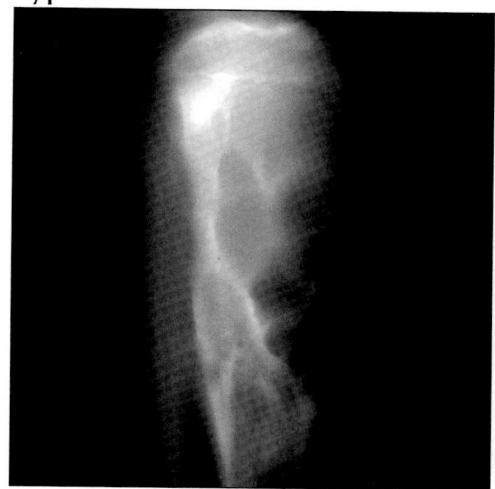
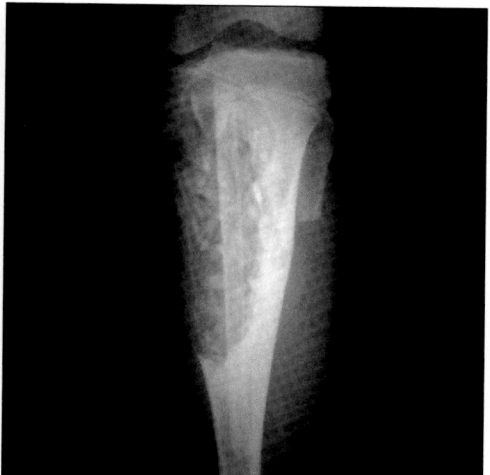

(Left) Lateral radiography (tomogram) shows a radiolucent, lobular lesion with internal septations in the proximal tibial metaphysis. *(Right)* Lateral radiography shows bone graft in tibial chondromyxoid fibroma.

Variant

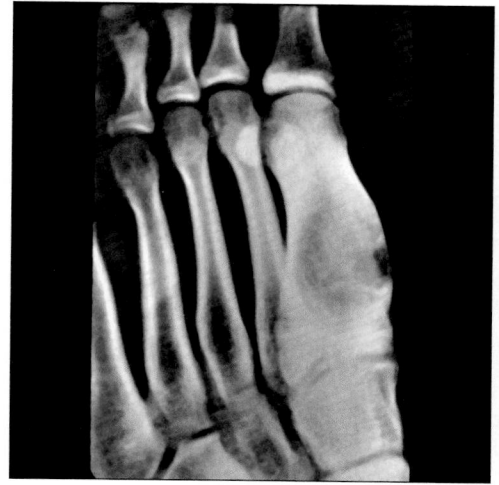
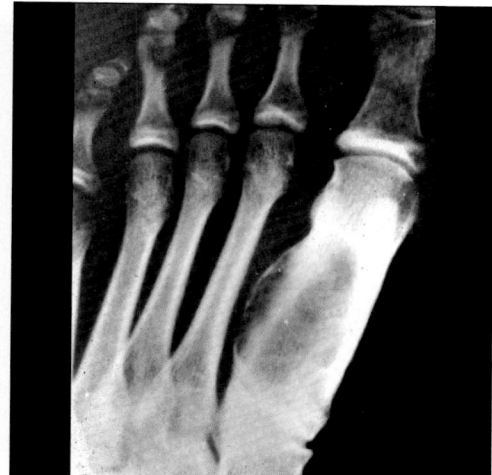

(Left) Anteroposterior radiography show a radiolucent, slightly lobulated lesion with thin sclerotic margin in the first metatarsal bone. Note cortical disruption which led to pain and local swelling. *(Right)* Anteroposterior radiography shows expansive lytic lesion in the metadiaphysis of the first metatarsal bone. Note thinned but intact cortex. This was thought to represent an enchondroma, however, biopsy revealed a CMF.

Other

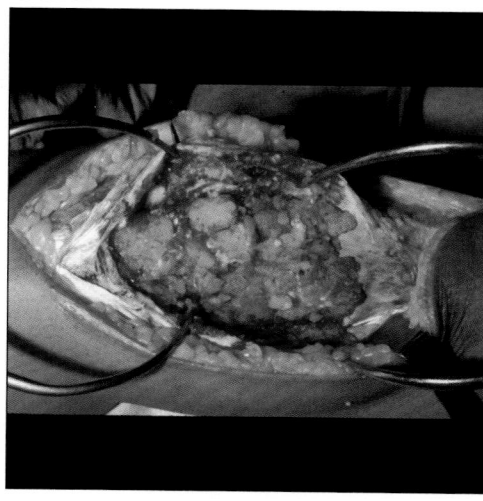
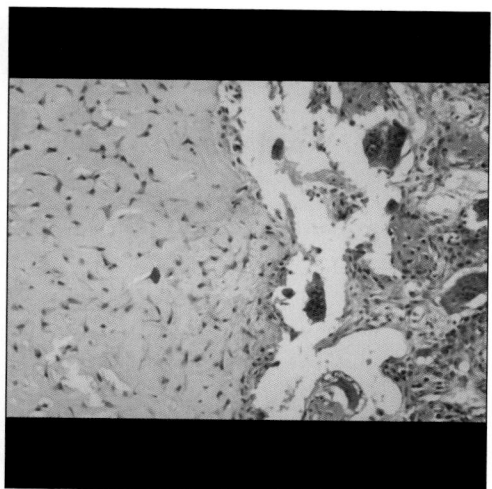

(Left) Coronal intra-operative photograph shows cartilaginous, lobulated, well marginated mass. *(Right)* Micropathology, low power, H&E stain shows lobules of chondromyxoid tissue (left) and cellular fibrous tissue (right).

CHONDROSARCOMA

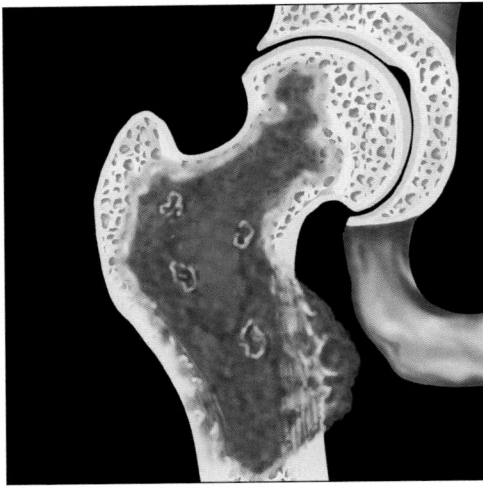

Coronal graphic shows chondrosarcoma in the proximal femur. Ring like calcifications are shown in white. There is cortical destruction and tumor extension through the cortex medially.

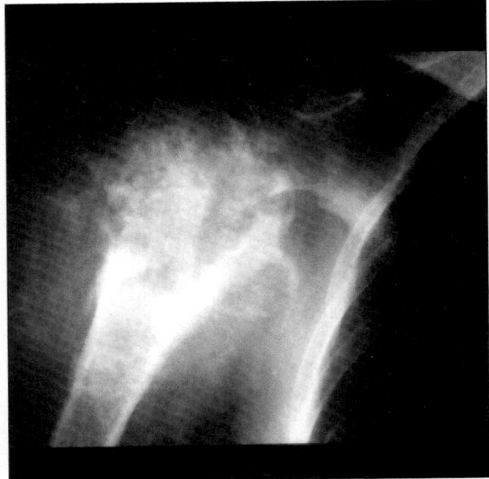

Anteroposterior radiography shows a destructive lesion in the proximal humerus with areas of ring and arc like calcifications, cortical destruction, and associated soft tissue extension.

TERMINOLOGY

Abbreviations and Synonyms
- Conventional chondrosarcoma, dedifferentiated chondrosarcoma, mesenchymal chondrosarcoma

Definitions
- Malignant tumor of connective tissue, characterized by formation of cartilage matrix by tumor cells

IMAGING FINDINGS

General Features
- Best diagnostic clue: Lytic mass with or without chondroid matrix, cortical disruption and extension into soft tissues
- Location
  - Flat bones
    - Pelvis: 25%
    - Ilium: 15%
    - Pubis and ischium: 9%
    - Scapula: 5%
  - Ribs and sternum: 12%
  - Metaphysis/diaphysis of long bones, may extend into epiphysis
    - Femur: 15%
    - Tibia: 5%
    - Humerus: 10%
  - Craniofacial bones: 2%, can arise from laryngeal cartilage
  - Spine and sacrum: 5%
  - Soft tissues (extraskeletal chondrosarcoma)
- Size: 1-40 cm, mean: 10 cm
- Morphology: Ill-defined lytic lesion with or without chondroid matrix

Radiographic Findings
- Radiography
  - Lytic mass with or without chondroid matrix
  - Medullary (central) chondrosarcoma: 85%
    - Expansion of medullary cavity
    - Thickening of cortex with endosteal scalloping
    - Popcorn-like ring and arc calcification
    - Cortical disruption with extension into soft tissue in advanced stages
  - Exostotic (peripheral) chondrosarcoma
    - Thickening of cortex and soft tissue mass at site of attachment to bone
    - Chondroid matrix
    - Late destruction of bone
  - Dedifferentiated chondrosarcoma: 10%
    - Ill-defined, lytic lesion in continuity with cartilaginous tumor
    - Abrupt transition between cartilaginous tumor and dedifferentiated lytic component
  - Mesenchymal chondrosarcoma: < 1%

DDx: Chondrosarcoma

Enchondroma	Chondroblastoma	Osteosarcoma	MFH
AP Radiography	AP Radiography	Lat Radiography	Ax NECT

8

34

CHONDROSARCOMA

Key Facts

Imaging Findings
- Best diagnostic clue: Lytic mass with or without chondroid matrix, cortical disruption and extension into soft tissues
- Chondroid matrix mineralization of "rings and arcs" (characteristic)

Top Differential Diagnoses
- Enchondroma
- Chondroblastoma
- Osteosarcoma (OGS)
- Malignant Fibrous Histiocytoma (MFH)

Pathology
- Can occur as primary chondrosarcoma or as malignant degeneration of osteochondroma or enchondroma

- Third most common primary malignant bone tumor
- 10-25% of all primary bone sarcomas
- Extraskeletal chondrosarcoma: 2% of all soft tissue sarcomas

Clinical Issues
- Dull aching pain at rest, may be severe at night
- Soft tissue swelling, mass
- Prognosis depends on location, size, and histologic grade
- Overall 5-year survival: 48-60%
- 5-year survival 90% for grade 1, 81% for grade 2, 29% for grade 3 tumors
- Wide surgical excision
- Biopsies must be planned with future tumor excision in mind

---

- Aggressive lytic bone destruction
- Predilection for mandible, femur, ribs
- Clear cell chondrosarcoma: 5%
  - Round, sharply-marginated, lytic lesion
  - Involves epiphysis of long bones
  - May contain calcifications
  - Surrounding sclerosis
  - Indistinguishable from chondroblastoma (slow growth over years)
- Extraskeletal chondrosarcoma
  - Lobulated soft tissue mass with and without calcification
  - Extremities (thigh) most common

CT Findings
- NECT
  - Chondroid matrix mineralization of "rings and arcs" (characteristic)
  - Nonmineralized portions of tumor hypodense to muscle
    - High water content of hyaline cartilage

MR Findings
- T1WI: Low to intermediate signal intensity
- T2WI: High signal (hyaline cartilage), areas of low signal intensity (mineralization)
- T1 C+
  - Enhancement of septa with ring and arc pattern
  - Nonenhancing areas represent hyaline cartilage, cystic mucoid tissue, necrosis
- To determine intramedullary extent and soft tissue invasion

Nuclear Medicine Findings
- Bone Scan
  - Increased uptake of radiotracer
  - Overestimates extent of lesion due to surrounding hyperemia and edema

Imaging Recommendations
- Best imaging tool: Radiographs diagnostic, show calcification, periosteal reaction, endosteal scalloping
- Protocol advice

- CT to evaluate for chondroid matrix, cortical destruction, intra- and extraosseous extension
- MRI to evaluate intramedullary extent and relationship to neurovascular bundle

DIFFERENTIAL DIAGNOSIS

Enchondroma
- No periosteal reaction or cortical destruction
- No soft tissue mass
- Development of pain and swelling in previously asymptomatic enchondroma suspicious for malignant degeneration

Chondroblastoma
- May be indistinguishable from clear cell chondrosarcoma
- Both occur in epiphyses and can occur before skeletal maturity

Osteosarcoma (OGS)
- Osteoid matrix
- No chondroid matrix
- Usually younger patients

Malignant Fibrous Histiocytoma (MFH)
- Often purely lytic
- Can have areas of sclerosis, no chondroid matrix
- No significant periosteal reaction

PATHOLOGY

General Features
- General path comments: Malignant tumor in which neoplastic cells form cartilage
- Genetics
  - Grade 1 chondrosarcomas: Diploid
  - Grade 2 and 3 chondrosarcomas: Aneuploid, correlate with aggressive behavior
  - High grade lesions: Complex chromosomal aberration with nonreciprocal translocations and deletions

CHONDROSARCOMA

- Accumulation of p53 protein, may be indicator of poor prognosis
- Etiology
  - Can occur as primary chondrosarcoma or as malignant degeneration of osteochondroma or enchondroma
  - Exostotic (peripheral) chondrosarcoma
    - Malignant degeneration of hereditary multiple exostoses, Ollier disease
    - Can arise in cartilage cap of a previously benign osteochondroma
- Epidemiology
  - Third most common primary malignant bone tumor
  - 10-25% of all primary bone sarcomas
  - Extraskeletal chondrosarcoma: 2% of all soft tissue sarcomas

Gross Pathologic & Surgical Features

- Lobulated tumor composed of translucent hyaline nodules (resemble normal cartilage)
  - Mineralization at periphery of nodules
- Focal ivory-like areas represent extensive enchondral ossification
- Hemorrhagic necrosis, especially in high-grade tumors
- Central lesions erode and destroy cortex with extension into surrounding soft tissue
  - Cortical disruption earlier in flat bones due to narrow medullary cavity
- Extraosseous component grows on outer bone surface
  - Encircles affected bone

Microscopic Features

- Irregular-shaped lobules of cartilage
- May be separated by narrow, fibrous bands
- Chondrocytes arranged in clusters, can be mononuclear or multinucleated
- Matrix: Mature hyaline cartilage or myxoid stroma
- Immunohistochemistry: Positive for S-100 protein and vimentin
- Dedifferentiated chondrosarcoma: Two components that coexist in one tumor
  - High grade sarcoma +/- heterologous elements (MFH, OGS)
  - Low-grade cartilaginous lesion

Staging, Grading or Classification Criteria

- Grade 1 chondrosarcoma: Slowly growing, locally aggressive, indolent course
  - Recurrent growth potential, no metastatic spread
  - Diagnosis requires supportive evidence from clinical and radiographic data
- Grade 2 chondrosarcoma: Locally aggressive tumor with great potential for local recurrence
  - Metastases in 10-15%
- Grade 3 chondrosarcoma: Highly aggressive, rapidly growing
  - Metastases in over 50%

CLINICAL ISSUES

Presentation

- Most common signs/symptoms
  - Dull aching pain at rest, may be severe at night

- Duration of symptoms - several months to years
- Clinical profile
  - Soft tissue swelling, mass
  - If lesion is close to joint, restricted range of motion

Demographics

- Age: 20-90 years, peak: 40-60 years
- Gender: M:F = 2:1

Natural History & Prognosis

- Prognosis depends on location, size, and histologic grade
  - Overall 5-year survival: 48-60%
  - 5-year survival 90% for grade 1, 81% for grade 2, 29% for grade 3 tumors
- Recurrence 5-10 years after surgery
  - Recurrence can be associated with increased histologic grade and more aggressive behavior
- Metastases (lung, lymph nodes, liver, kidneys, brain): 66% (grade 3 chondrosarcomas)
- Degeneration into fibrosarcoma, malignant fibrous histiocytoma, osteosarcoma in 10%
- Pelvic chondrosarcoma may invade bladder or colon
- Pathologic fractures rare

Treatment

- Wide surgical excision
- Limited role for chemotherapy or radiation therapy
  - For high grade chondrosarcomas
- Biopsies must be planned with future tumor excision in mind

DIAGNOSTIC CHECKLIST

Consider

- Enlarging or painful enchondroma or osteochondroma suspicious for sarcomatous transformation
- Clear cell chondrosarcoma may be indistinguishable from benign chondroid lesions (chondroblastoma, enchondroma)
- Always consult orthopedic surgeon before biopsy of possible chondrosarcoma

SELECTED REFERENCES

1. Bjornsson J et al: Primary chondrosarcoma of long bones and limb girdles. Cancer 83:2105-19, 1998
2. Dorfman HD et al: Bone tumors. 1st ed. St. Louis MO, Mosby, 353-440, 1998
3. Greenspan A et al: Differential diagnosis of tumors and tumor-like lesions of bones and joints. 1st ed. Philadelphia PA, Lippincott-Raven, 169-98, 1998
4. Swarts SJ et al: Chromosomal abnormalities in low grade chondrosarcoma and a review of the literature. Cancer Genet Cytogenet 98:126-30, 1997
5. Mercuri M et al: Dedifferentiated chondrosarcoma. Skeletal Radiol. 24:409-16, 1995
6. Aoki J et al: MR of enchondroma and chondrosarcoma: Rings and arcs of Gd-DTPA enhancement. J Comput Assist Tomogr 15:1011-6, 1991

CHONDROSARCOMA

IMAGE GALLERY

Typical

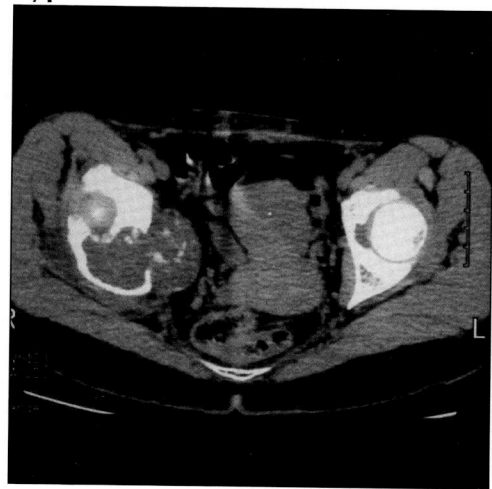
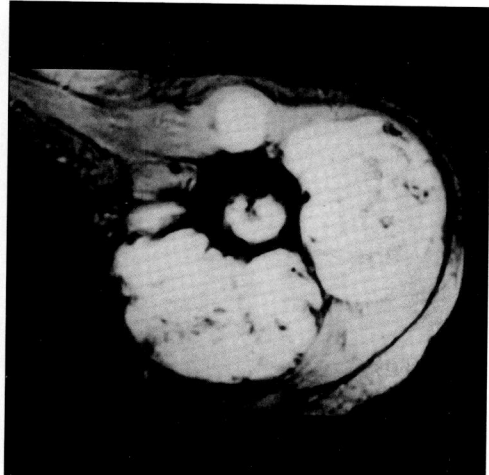

(Left) Axial NECT shows a destructive lesion in the right acetabulum with cortical destruction and associated soft tissue mass. Note the calcified matrix. *(Right)* Axial FS T2 FSE MR shows intramedullary tumor with large associated soft tissue mass displaying high signal corresponding to chondroid matrix. Areas of low signal are consistent with calcifications.

Variant

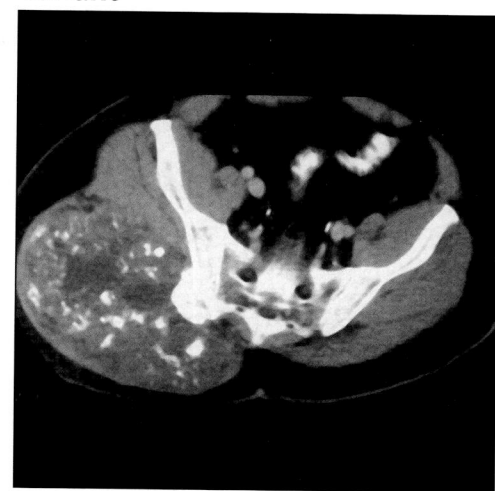
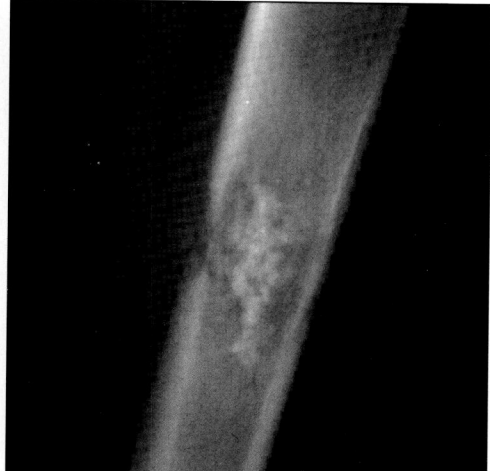

(Left) Axial NECT shows a large, partially calcified mass adjacent to the right sacrum, consistent with a soft tissue chondrosarcoma. *(Right)* Lateral radiography shows cortical destruction adjacent to an enchondroma, consistent with sarcomatous transformation.

Other

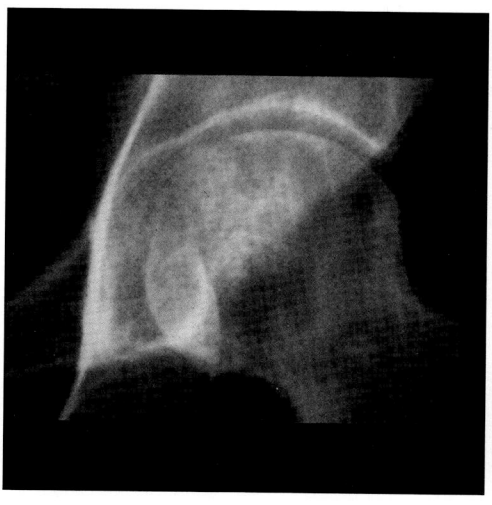
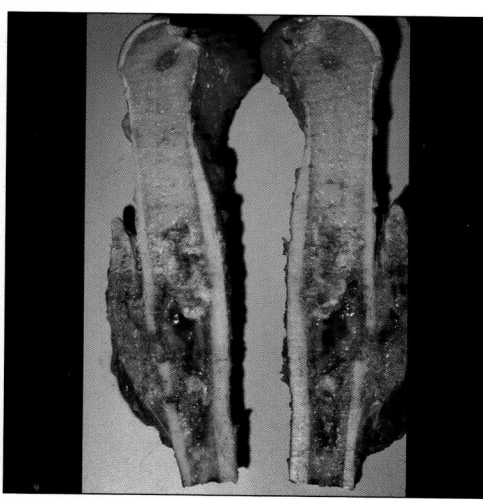

(Left) Anteroposterior radiography shows a lytic lesion with calcification of the femoral epiphysis. Biopsy revealed clear cell chondrosarcoma. *(Right)* Coronal gross pathology shows lobulated, cartilaginous tumor with ill defined margins, and soft tissue extension.

FIBROUS DYSPLASIA

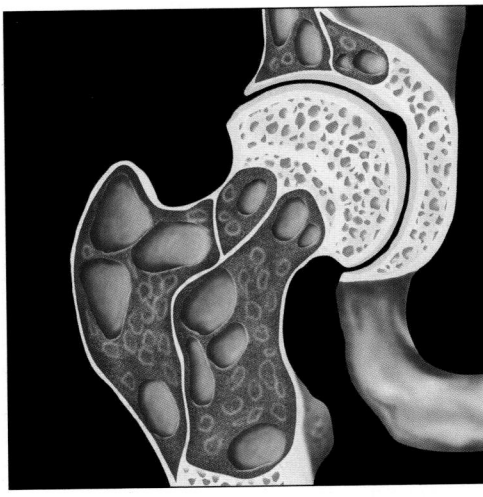

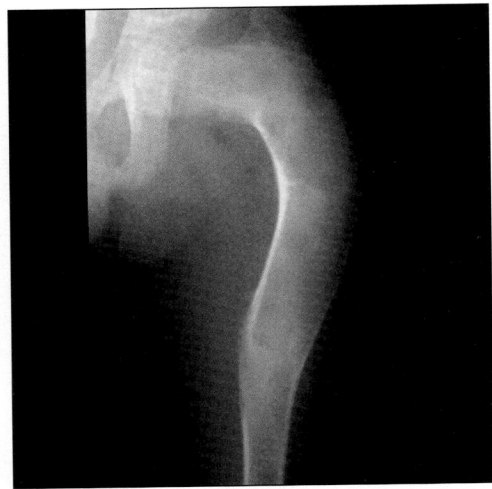

Coronal graphic shows polyostotic fibrous dysplasia involving the proximal femur and acetabular roof. Cystic changes are shown in red, ground glass appearance in brown.

Anteroposterior radiography shows bowing deformity of the proximal femur (shepherd's crook deformity). Note expansion of bone with ground glass appearance.

TERMINOLOGY

Abbreviations and Synonyms
- Osteitis fibrosa

Definitions
- Developmental anomaly of bone formation

IMAGING FINDINGS

General Features
- Best diagnostic clue: Expansile marrow lesion with "ground glass" appearance
- Location
  - Meta-diaphysis of long bones, sparing of epiphysis
  - Monostotic form: 85%
    - Femur: 35-40%
    - Tibia: 20%
    - Skull and facial bones: 10-25%
    - Ribs: 10%
    - Hands, feet, spine: Rare
  - Polyostotic form: 15%
    - Skull and facial bones: > 50%
    - Pelvis, long bones, ribs
    - Unilateral or monomelic
  - Osteofibrous dysplasia
    - Tibia: > 90%

- Fibula: 15%
- Size: 1-30 cm
- Morphology: Expansile lytic medullary lesion

Radiographic Findings
- Radiography
  - Radiolucent, expansile, medullary lesion
  - Ground glass appearance
    - Due to woven bone in bone marrow cavity
  - Well-defined sclerotic margins, endosteal scalloping
  - No periostitis
  - Bowing deformities of long bones (shepherd's crook deformity)
  - Growth disturbance (polyostotic form)
  - Craniofacial involvement: Mixed lytic and sclerotic lesions
    - Sclerosis in lesion involving skull base
    - Expanded calvarium with greater involvement of outer table
    - Frontal bossing, facial asymmetry
  - Osteofibrous dysplasia: Lytic lesion in anterior cortex of tibial diaphysis
    - May involve medullary cavity
    - Bowing, pathologic fracture, pseudoarthrosis

CT Findings
- NECT
  - No mineralized matrix
  - 70-400 HU, due to microscopic ossification

DDx: Fibrous Dysplasia

Paget Disease	UBC	ABC	CMF	Adamantinoma
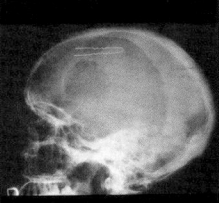	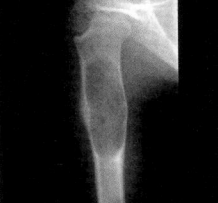	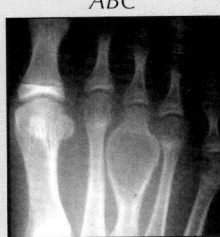	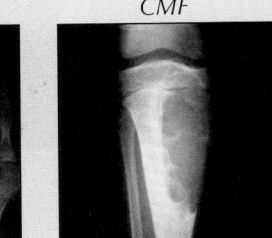	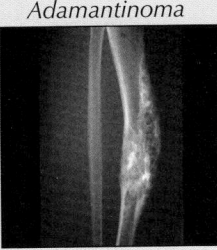
Lat Radiography	AP Radiography	AP Radiography	Lat Radiography	Lat Radiography

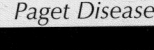

8

38

FIBROUS DYSPLASIA

Key Facts

Imaging Findings
- Best diagnostic clue: Expansile marrow lesion with "ground glass" appearance

Top Differential Diagnoses
- Neurofibromatosis
- Paget Disease
- Unicameral Bone Cyst (UBC)
- Chondromyxoid Fibroma (CMF)
- Aneurysmal Bone Cyst (ABC)
- Adamantinoma

Pathology
- 1% of biopsied primary bone tumors
- Most common benign lesion of the rib
- McCune Albright syndrome
- Mazabraud syndrome

Clinical Issues
- Monostotic form: Usually asymptomatic
- Polyostotic form: 2/3 symptomatic by age 10
- Leg pain, limp, pathologic fracture
- Endocrine disorders: Hyperthyroidism, hyperparathyroidism, diabetes mellitus, acromegaly
- No progression of monostotic to polyostotic form
- Malignant transformation: 0.5% into osteosarcoma (most common), chondrosarcoma, fibrosarcoma
- No treatment for asymptomatic lesions
- Curettage and bone grafting of large lesions at risk for pathologic fracture

Diagnostic Checklist
- Evaluate patient for endocrine abnormalities in polyostotic form

---

- o No soft tissue mass
- o Helpful in evaluating skull lesions
- CECT: Enhancement of active lesions

MR Findings
- T1WI: Homogeneous low signal, thin rim of low signal
- T2WI: High signal in 60%, mixed signal, thin rim of low signal
- T1 C+: Enhancement of active lesions

Nuclear Medicine Findings
- Bone Scan
  - o To determine activity and extent of involvement
  - o Increased uptake in majority of lesions
  - o Decrease in radiotracer activity implies that lesion has become inactive

Imaging Recommendations
- Best imaging tool: Radiographs diagnostic
- Protocol advice: Bone scan to determine if disease is monostotic or polyostotic

DIFFERENTIAL DIAGNOSIS

Neurofibromatosis
- Long bone deformities without intramedullary changes
- Pseudoarthrosis poor prognosis
  - o Pseudoarthrosis has good therapeutic response in fibrous dysplasia

Paget Disease
- Calvarium: Expansion of inner and outer table
  - o Greater involvement of outer table in fibrous dysplasia

Unicameral Bone Cyst (UBC)
- Centrally located
- "Fallen fragment" sign in case of fracture

Chondromyxoid Fibroma (CMF)
- Geographic pattern of bone destruction
- Periosteal new bone formation

Aneurysmal Bone Cyst (ABC)
- Marked expansion of affected bone
- Fluid-fluid levels

Adamantinoma
- Older patients
- Eccentrically located (osteofibrous dysplasia involves anterior tibial cortex)
- Destructive features

PATHOLOGY

General Features
- General path comments
  - o Inability of bone-forming tissue to produce mature lamellar bone
    - ▪ Even if osteoid is produced it cannot mature to lamellar bone
- Genetics
  - o Predisposition to somatic mutations of skeleton-forming mesenchymal tissue
    - ▪ Clonal structural alterations involving chromosomes 3, 8, 10, 12, 15
    - ▪ Heterozygous deactivating GNAS1 mutations
    - ▪ Increased levels of c-fos oncoprotein in lesions of fibrous dysplasia
- Etiology
  - o Benign developmental abnormality in which medullary cavity is replaced with fibrous tissue
    - ▪ Fibrous tissue contains immature woven bone
- Epidemiology
  - o 1% of biopsied primary bone tumors
  - o Most common benign lesion of the rib
- Associated abnormalities
  - o McCune Albright syndrome
    - ▪ Polyostotic unilateral fibrous dysplasia
    - ▪ Endocrine abnormalities (precocious puberty, hyperthyroidism)
    - ▪ Cafe-au-lait spots ("coast of Maine")
    - ▪ Female predominance
  - o Mazabraud syndrome

FIBROUS DYSPLASIA

- Multiple fibrous and myxomatous soft tissue tumors in association with polyostotic fibrous dysplasia

Gross Pathologic & Surgical Features
- Centrally located lesion of firm, fibrous, white or red tissue
- Variable gritty consistency, depending on the amount of mineralized bone
- Expanded thinned cortex
- Secondary blood-filled cyst formation common

Microscopic Features
- Medullary cavity replaced by spindle cells in storiform arrangement and irregular trabeculae of immature woven bone
- Various levels of bone trabeculae maturation
- Curved, branching trabeculae without surface osteoblasts: Resemble chinese characters
- Foci of cartilage in 10%

CLINICAL ISSUES

Presentation
- Most common signs/symptoms
  - Monostotic form: Usually asymptomatic
    - Can present with pathologic fracture
    - Painful stress fractures common in femoral neck
    - Dysplastic callus formation after fracture
  - Polyostotic form: 2/3 symptomatic by age 10
    - Leg pain, limp, pathologic fracture
    - Abnormal vaginal bleeding (25%)
    - Endocrine disorders: Hyperthyroidism, hyperparathyroidism, diabetes mellitus, acromegaly
    - Hypophosphatemic rickets
    - McCune Albright syndrome (precocious puberty)
- Clinical profile
  - Hyperpigmentation of skin (cafe-au-lait spots)
    - Often corresponds to sites of skeletal involvement
  - Soft tissue myxomas
  - Cherubism: Autosomal dominant
    - Symmetric involvement of mandible and maxilla
  - Leontiasis ossea (craniofacial fibrous dysplasia)
    - Involvement of facial and frontal bones
    - Leonine facies (resembling a lion)
    - Cranial nerve palsies

Demographics
- Age: 5-50 years; peak: 10-20 years
- Gender: M:F = 1:1

Natural History & Prognosis
- No progression of monostotic to polyostotic form
- Monostotic form: Growth of lesion usually stabilizes during puberty
- Enlargement of lesions during pregnancy
- Polyostotic form: Lesions remain active after puberty
- Malignant transformation: 0.5% into osteosarcoma (most common), chondrosarcoma, fibrosarcoma

Treatment
- No treatment for asymptomatic lesions
- Curettage and bone grafting of large lesions at risk for pathologic fracture
- Surgery with curettage associated with high rate of local recurrence: 20-100%
- Straightening of angular deformities and grafting with cortical bone
- Treatment of underlying endocrine abnormalities
- Bisphosphonates to decrease pain and prevent pathologic fractures
  - Can lead to partial resolution of lesions

DIAGNOSTIC CHECKLIST

Consider
- Evaluate patient for endocrine abnormalities in polyostotic form

SELECTED REFERENCES

1. Ippolito E et al: Natural history and treatment of fibrous dysplasia of bone: A multicenter clinicopathologic study promoted by the European Pediatric Orthopaedic Society. J Pediatr Orthop B 12:155-77, 2003
2. Rickard SJ et al: Analysis of GNAS1 and overlapping transcripts identifies the parental origin of mutations in patients with sporadic Albright hereditary osteodystrophy and reveals a model system in which to observe the effects of splicing mutations on translated and untranslated messenger RNA. Am J Hum Genet 72:961-74, 2003
3. Lane JM et al: Bisphosphonate therapy in fibrous dysplasia. Clin Orthop 382:6-12, 2001
4. Dorfman HD et al: Bone tumors. 1st ed. St. Louis MO, Mosby, 441-91, 1998
5. Greenspan A et al: Differential diagnosis of tumors and tumor-like lesions of bones and joints. 1st ed. Philadelphia PA, Lippincott-Raven, 215-30, 1998
6. Choi KH et al: Fibrous dysplasia: MR imaging characteristics with radiopathologic correlation. Am J Roentgenol 167:1523-7, 1996
7. Ruggieri P et al: Malignancies in fibrous dysplasia. Cancer 73:1411-24, 1994
8. Inamo Y et al: Findings on magnetic resonance imaging of the spine and femur in a case of McCune-Albright syndrome. Pediatr Radiol 23:15-8, 1993
9. Utz JA et al: MR appearance of fibrous dysplasia. J Comput Assist Tomogr 13:845-51, 1989
10. Campanacci M et al: Osteofibrous dysplasia of the tibia and fibula. J Bone Joint Surg 63(3):367-75, 1981

FIBROUS DYSPLASIA

IMAGE GALLERY

Typical

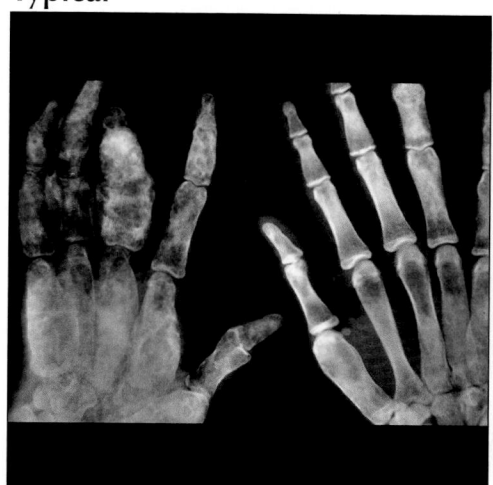
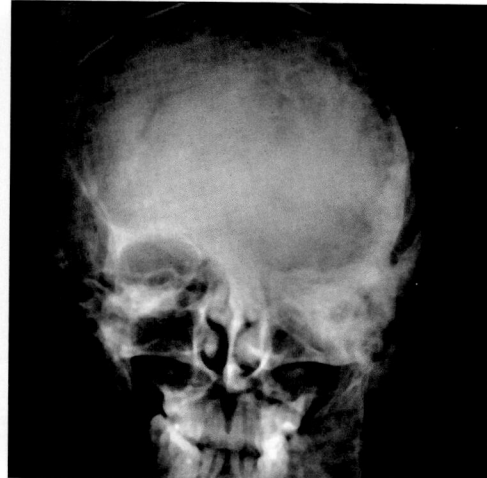

(Left) Anteroposterior radiography shows multiple circumscribed expansile lytic lesions involving the right hand in a patient with polyostotic fibrous dysplasia. Normal left hand for comparison. *(Right)* Anteroposterior radiography shows marked craniofacial involvement in a patient with McCune Albright syndrome. Note obliteration of the left orbit.

Typical

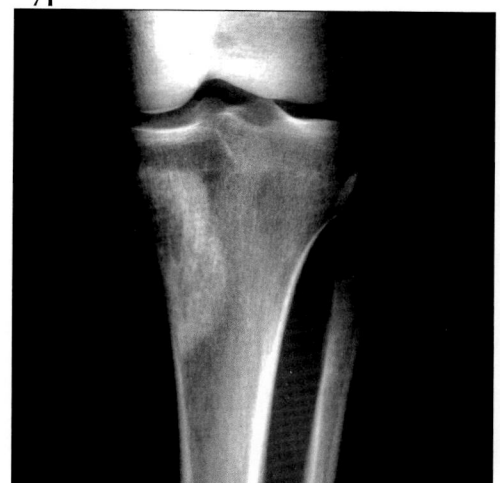
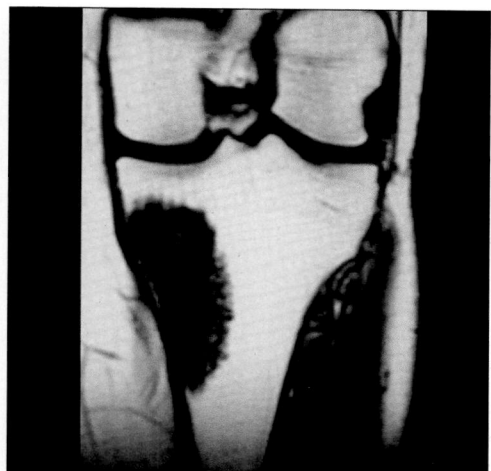

(Left) Anteroposterior radiography shows circumscribed mixed, predominately sclerotic and lytic lesion in the proximal tibial metaphysis. *(Right)* Coronal T1WI MR shows low signal lesion of the proximal femoral metaphysis with peripheral spiculation corresponding to areas of sclerosis.

Other

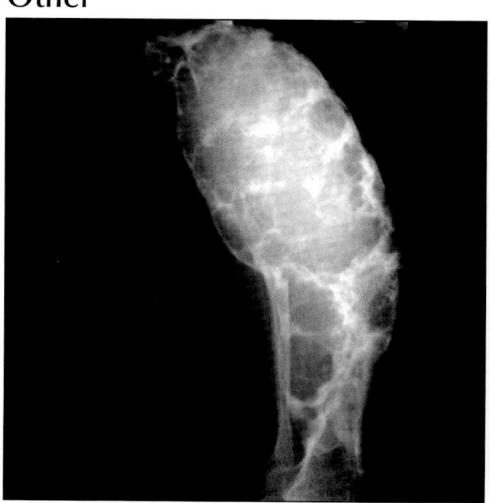
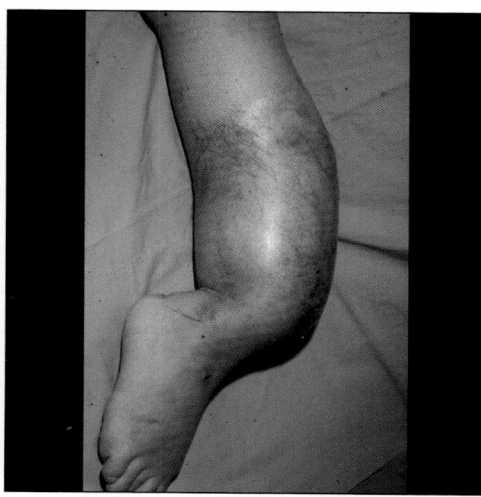

(Left) Anteroposterior radiography in a patient with polyostotic fibrous dysplasia shows marked deformity of the tibia and fibula with multiple expansile lytic lesions. *(Right)* Clinical photograph shows marked deformity of the lower extremity in a patient with polyostotic fibrous dysplasia.

FIBROXANTHOMA

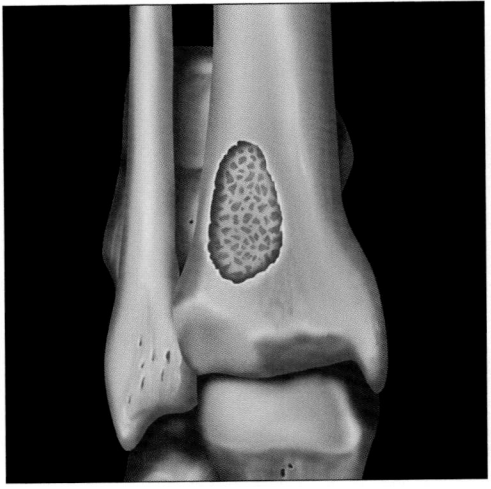

Coronal graphic shows eccentric lytic lesion with scalloped sclerotic margins in the tibial metaphysis.

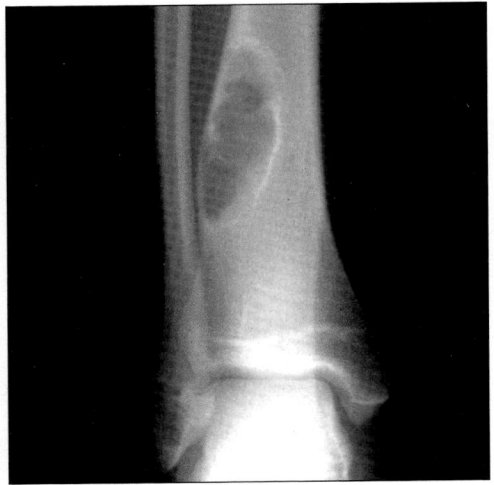

Anteroposterior radiography shows an eccentric well-defined lytic lesion with sclerotic scalloped borders in the distal tibial metaphysis.

TERMINOLOGY

Abbreviations and Synonyms
- Metaphyseal fibrous defect, benign fibrous histiocytoma, nonossifying fibroma, fibrous cortical defect

Definitions
- Benign asymptomatic hamartomatous lesion of children
- Fibroxanthoma comprises
  - Nonossifying fibroma (NOF)
  - Fibrous cortical defect (FCD)

IMAGING FINDINGS

General Features
- Best diagnostic clue: Well-defined expansile eccentric lytic lesion with scalloped sclerotic margins in metaphyses of long bones
- Location
  - Metaphysis of long bones (postero-medial): 90%
    - Close to growth plate
    - Distance from growth plate increases with age
  - Tibia: 43%
  - Femur: 38%
  - Fibula: 8%
  - Less common in upper extremity: 8%
    - Humerus: 5%
  - Multifocal: 50%
- Size: 0.5-7 cm
- Morphology: Eccentric cortical based lytic lesion

Radiographic Findings
- Radiography
  - Eccentric, cortical lytic lesion with thin or scalloped sclerotic margins
  - FCD: < 2 cm, within the cortex
  - NOF: > 2 cm, encroach medullary cavity
  - Can extend or primarily involve medullary cavity
  - Expansion of overlying cortex
  - Cortex may be thinned but intact
  - No matrix mineralization
  - Trabeculation in periphery of lesion
  - Increased mineralization in healing stages
    - Begins at diaphyseal end and progresses to growth plate
  - Long axis of lesion is parallel to long axis of bone

CT Findings
- NECT
  - Well defined lytic lesion with surrounding sclerosis
  - Helpful in showing medullary involvement and pathologic fractures
  - If lesion involves > 50% of transverse diameter of bone, increased risk of fracture

DDx: Fibroxanthoma

Cortical Desmoid	ABC	UBC	Fibrous Dysplasia	CMF
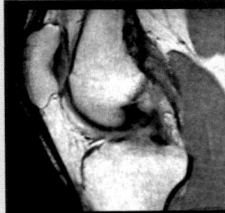	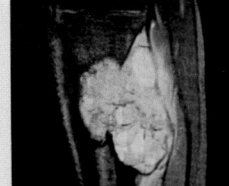	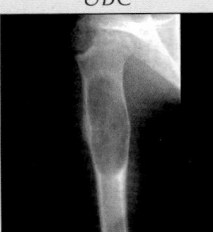	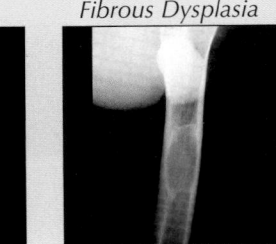	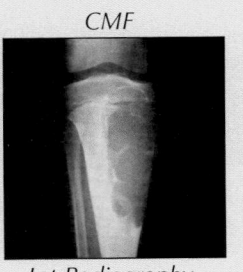
Sag T1WI MR	Sag FS T2 MRI	AP Radiography	AP Radiography	Lat Radiography

FIBROXANTHOMA

Key Facts

Imaging Findings
- Best diagnostic clue: Well-defined expansile eccentric lytic lesion with scalloped sclerotic margins in metaphyses of long bones
- FCD: < 2 cm, within the cortex
- NOF: > 2 cm, encroach medullary cavity
- Best imaging tool: Radiographs diagnostic

Top Differential Diagnoses
- Cortical Desmoid
- Aneurysmal Bone Cyst (ABC)
- Unicameral Bone Cyst (UBC)
- Fibrous Dysplasia
- Chondromyxoid Fibroma (CMF)

Pathology
- Most common fibrous lesion of bone

- Occurs in 20-30% of normal population during 1st and 2nd decades of life
- Jaffe-Campanacci syndrome
- Neurofibromatosis type 1

Clinical Issues
- Most common signs/symptoms: Usually asymptomatic
- May cause pain, pathologic fracture
- Benign lesion, no malignant transformation
- Spontaneous regression
- Usually does not require treatment
- Curettage with bone grafting of larger lesions at risk for fracture

Diagnostic Checklist
- Don't touch lesion

- HU slightly higher than normal bone marrow
- CECT: Enhancement

MR Findings
- T1WI
  - Low signal intensity
  - Peripheral hypointense rim (reactive sclerosis)
- T2WI
  - Low to intermediate signal intensity
  - Septations
  - Peripheral hypointense rim (reactive sclerosis)
- T1 C+: Enhancement

Nuclear Medicine Findings
- Bone Scan
  - Increased radiotracer uptake of active lesions
  - Decreased uptake corresponds to involution

Imaging Recommendations
- Best imaging tool: Radiographs diagnostic
- Protocol advice
  - Radiographs
  - CT for preoperative planning
  - Larger lesions require radiographic follow-up to assess progression and fracture risk
    - Radiographs every 4-6 months

DIFFERENTIAL DIAGNOSIS

Cortical Desmoid
- At tendinous insertion
- Typically posterior distal femur

Aneurysmal Bone Cyst (ABC)
- Marked expansion of affected bone
- Fluid-fluid levels
- Periosteal new bone formation

Unicameral Bone Cyst (UBC)
- Centrally located
- "Fallen fragment" sign in case of fracture

Fibrous Dysplasia
- Expansile medullary lesion

- Ground glass appearance

Chondromyxoid Fibroma (CMF)
- Geographic pattern of bone destruction
- Periosteal new bone formation

PATHOLOGY

General Features
- General path comments
  - Non-neoplastic process that occurs in the juxtaepiphyseal region of long bones
  - NOF results from proliferation of FCD that has expanded medullary cavity
- Etiology
  - Developmental defect arising in trabeculae of tubular bones
    - Migrates toward diaphysis as bone grows in length
  - May be result of periosteal injury
- Epidemiology
  - Most common fibrous lesion of bone
  - Occurs in 20-30% of normal population during 1st and 2nd decades of life
  - FCD: 30-40% of children develop one or more lesions
  - NOF: 2% of biopsied primary bone tumors
- Associated abnormalities
  - Jaffe-Campanacci syndrome
    - Multifocal fibroxanthoma with extraskeletal manifestations in children
    - Cafe-au-lait spots
    - Mental retardation
    - Hypogonadism, cryptorchidism
    - Congenital cardiovascular defects
  - Neurofibromatosis type 1
    - Multifocal fibroxanthoma of long bones
    - May be bilateral and symmetric

Gross Pathologic & Surgical Features
- Eccentric, cortically based lesion with demarcated and scalloped inner boundary
- Fibrous, fleshy tissue with shades of grey and yellow

FIBROXANTHOMA

○ Color dependent on relative proportions of fibrous tissue and foamy histiocytes
- Cystic changes, hemorrhage, necrosis in larger lesion with pathologic fracture
- Involuted lesions: Replacement of fibrous component by cholesterol

Microscopic Features
- NOF and FCD are histologically identical
- Bundles of spindle-shaped fibroblasts, scattered multinucleated giant cells, and foamy histiocytes
- Foam cells more common in older lesions
- Hemosiderin pigment in stromal cells
- Arranged in storiform pattern

Staging, Grading or Classification Criteria
- Surgical staging for benign musculoskeletal tumors
  ○ Stage 1: Latent
  ○ Stage 2: Active
  ○ Stage 3: Aggressive

CLINICAL ISSUES

Presentation
- Most common signs/symptoms: Usually asymptomatic
- Clinical profile
  ○ During adolescence fibroxanthoma represents active stage 2 lesion
  ○ May cause pain, pathologic fracture
    ■ Increased risk of pathologic fracture if lesion is larger than 3.3 cm or involves > 50% of weight bearing bone
  ○ Hypophosphatemic vitamin D resistant rickets, osteomalacia
    ■ Tumor may secrete substance that increases renal tubular resorption of phosphorus

Demographics
- Age: 2-20 years, peak: 10-15 years
- Gender: M:F = 2:1

Natural History & Prognosis
- Benign lesion, no malignant transformation
- Presents during childhood, disappears in adolescence
- Spontaneous regression
  ○ Involution over 2-4 years
- Heal by membranous ossification
- Bone island in adult may be residue of incompletely involuted fibroxanthoma

Treatment
- Usually does not require treatment
- Curettage with bone grafting of larger lesions at risk for fracture
  ○ Risk of growth disturbance from injury to growth plate
- Casting after pathologic fracture to avoid injury to physis during surgery
  ○ Lesion may heal after fracture

DIAGNOSTIC CHECKLIST

Consider
- If detected on radiographs no further work up required (no biopsy)
- Don't touch lesion

SELECTED REFERENCES

1. Yanagawa T et al: The natural history of disappearing bone tumors and tumour like conditions. Clin Radiol 56:877-86, 2001
2. Smith SE et al: Primary musculoskeletal neoplasms of fibrous origin. Semin Musculoskel Radiol 4:73-88, 2000
3. Dorfman HD et al: Bone tumors. 1st ed. St. Louis MO, Mosby, 205-15, 1998
4. Greenspan A et al: Differential diagnosis of tumors and tumor-like lesions of bones and joints. 1st ed. Philadelphia PA, Lippincott-Raven, 492-514, 1998
5. Friedland JA et al: Quantitative analysis of the plain radiographic appearance of nonossifying fibroma. Invest Radiol 30:474-9, 1995
6. Araki Y et al: MRI of fibrous cortical defect of the femur. Radiat Med 12:93-8, 1994
7. Sethi A et al: Allograft in the treatment of benign cystic lesions of bone. Arch Orthop Trauma Surg 112:167-70, 1993
8. Hudson TM et al: Fibrous lesions of bone. Radiol Clin North Am 31:279-97, 1993
9. Unni KK et al: Fibrous and fibrohistiocytic lesions of bone. Semin Orthop 6:177-86, 1991
10. Kransdorf MJ et al: MR appearance of fibroxanthoma. J Comput Assist Tomogr 12:612-5, 1988
11. Mirra JM et al: Disseminated nonossifying fibromas in association with cafe-au-lait spots (Jaffe-Campanacci syndrome). Clin Orthop 168:192-205, 1982

FIBROXANTHOMA

IMAGE GALLERY

Typical

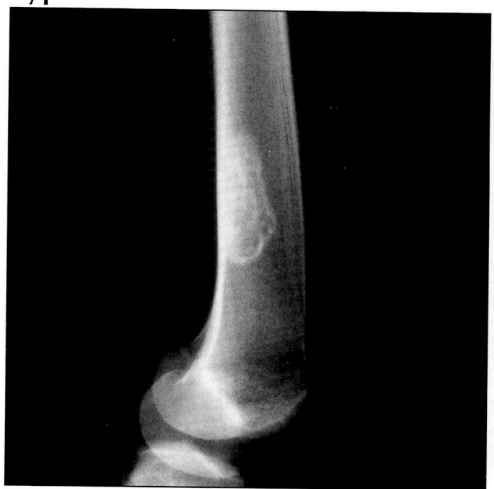

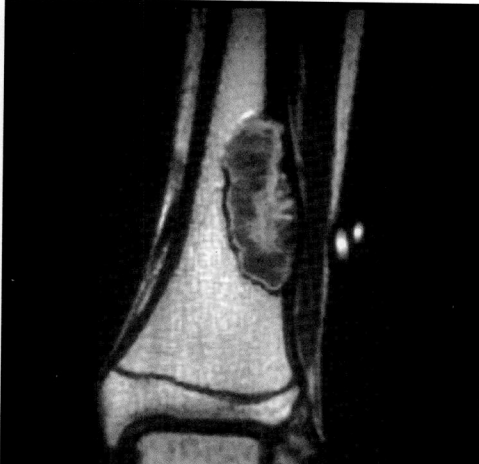

(Left) Lateral radiography shows predominantly sclerotic lesion in the posterior femur with scalloped sclerotic borders. *(Right)* Coronal T1WI MR shows well-defined, lobulated, eccentric lesion of low-intermediate SI in the distal tibial diaphysis.

Typical

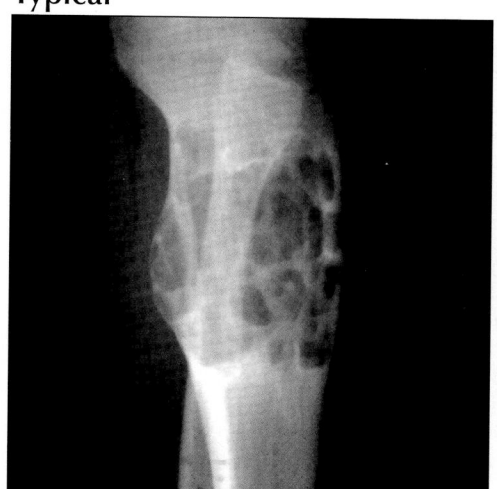

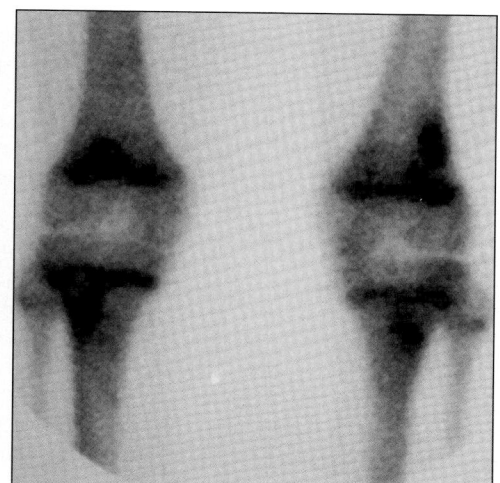

(Left) Lateral radiography shows well-demarcated expansile lytic lesion with trabeculation of the proximal tibia. *(Right)* Anteroposterior bone scan shows eccentric area of increased uptake in the left femoral metadiaphysis. Normal right side for comparison.

Variant

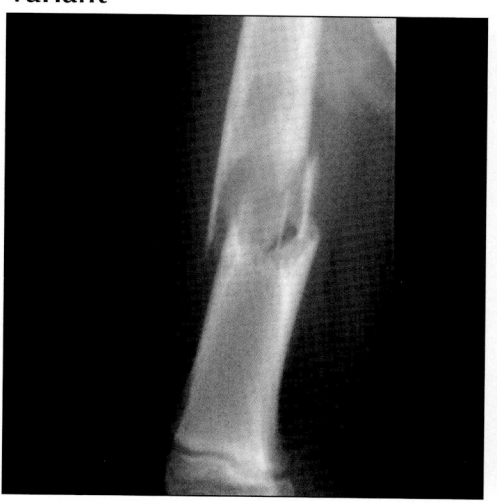

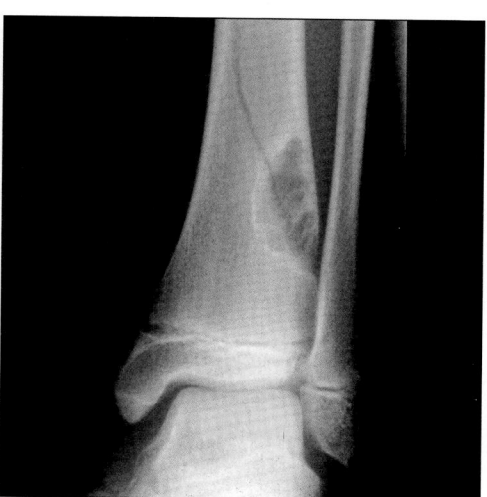

(Left) Anteroposterior radiography of the femur shows fibroxanthoma with pathologic fracture. *(Right)* Anteroposterior radiography shows fibroxanthoma of the distal tibial metaphysis with pathologic fracture.

MALIGNANT FIBROUS HISTIOCYTOMA, BONE

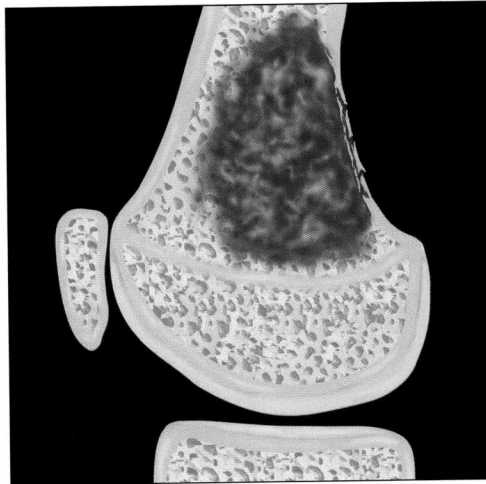

Sagittal graphic shows permeative tumor involving the distal femoral metaphysis. Cortical destruction is shown posteriorly.

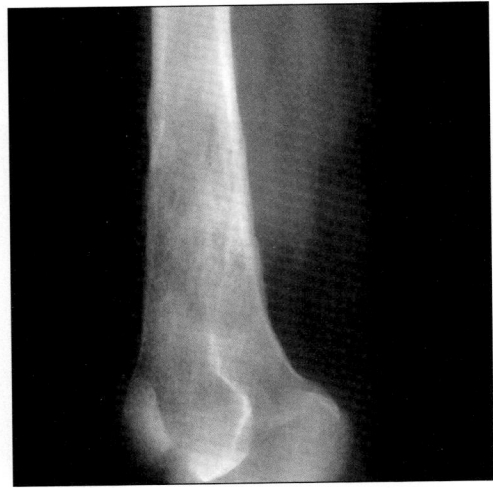

Lateral radiography shows destructive osteolytic lesion with moth-eaten pattern of bone destruction involving the distal femoral meta-diaphysis.

TERMINOLOGY

Abbreviations and Synonyms
- MFH, malignant fibrous xanthoma, malignant histiocytoma

Definitions
- Malignant neoplasm of bone characterized by mixture of spindle and pleomorphic cells

IMAGING FINDINGS

General Features
- Best diagnostic clue
  - Lytic ill-defined metaphyseal lesion with permeative bone destruction and cortical disruption
  - Frequently occurs as secondary sarcoma in area of abnormal bone
- Location
  - Long tubular bones
    - About knee: 50%
    - Femur: 45%
    - Tibia: 20%
    - Humerus: 10%
  - Pelvis
    - Ilium: 10%
    - Sacrum: 6%
  - Craniofacial bones: 9-14%
  - Spine: 5%
  - Rare in small bones of hands and feet
  - Metaphyses, central: 90%
  - Diaphyses, eccentric: 10%
- Size: 2-10 cm
- Morphology: Lytic ill-defined osseous lesion

Radiographic Findings
- Radiography
  - Lytic, ill-defined intramedullary lesion
  - Geographic, permeative, moth-eaten patterns of bone destruction
  - Cortical disruption
  - Extension into soft tissue
  - Little periosteal new bone formation
  - Lamellated periosteal reaction in presence of pathologic fracture
  - Secondary MFH: Occurs in areas of abnormal bone
    - Paget disease, bone infarct, chronic osteomyelitis
  - Presence of calcification suggests secondary MFH

CT Findings
- NECT
  - Density similar to muscle
  - Hypodense areas represent necrosis
- CECT: Variable enhancement

DDx: Malignant Fibrous Histiocytoma, Bone

Fibrosarcoma	Osteosarcoma	GCT	Lymphoma	Metastasis
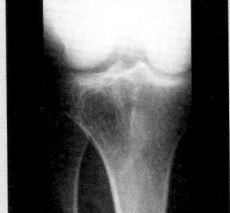	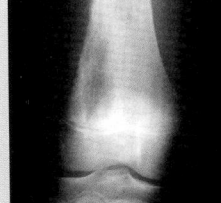	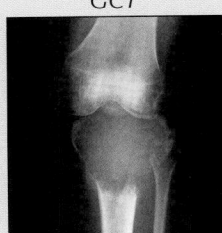	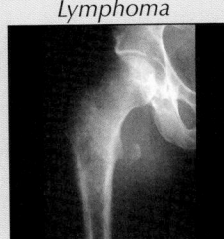	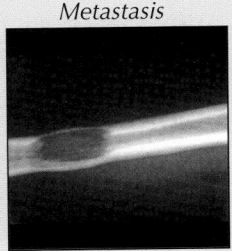
AP Radiography	AP Radiography	AP Radiography	AP Radiography	AP Radiography

MALIGNANT FIBROUS HISTIOCYTOMA, BONE

Key Facts

Imaging Findings

- Lytic ill-defined metaphyseal lesion with permeative bone destruction and cortical disruption
- Frequently occurs as secondary sarcoma in area of abnormal bone

Top Differential Diagnoses

- Fibrosarcoma
- Osteosarcoma
- Metastases
- Giant Cell Tumor (GCT)
- Lymphoma
- Multiple Myeloma

Pathology

- Epidemiology: 2-10% of primary malignant bone tumors

Clinical Issues

- Most common signs/symptoms: Pain with or without swelling
- Pathologic fracture: 23%
- Aggressive neoplasms with tendency to recur and metastasize
- Local recurrence: 31-44%
- Metastases: 42%
- 5 year survival: 52%
- Surgical resection with wide margins
- Neoadjuvant and adjuvant chemotherapy

Diagnostic Checklist

- 20% of all osseous MFH occur in areas of abnormal bone

MR Findings

- T1WI: Intermediate-low signal intensity
- T2WI
  - Heterogeneous signal
  - High signal intensity
- STIR: High signal intensity
- T1 C+: Variable enhancement
- To show intra- and extraosseous extent

Nuclear Medicine Findings

- Bone Scan: Increased radiotracer uptake, predominately in periphery of tumor

Imaging Recommendations

- Best imaging tool: Radiographs, MRI
- Protocol advice
  - Radiographs to diagnose osseous destruction
  - MRI to evaluate intra- and extraosseous extent

DIFFERENTIAL DIAGNOSIS

Fibrosarcoma

- Often indistinguishable
- Osseous sequestrum

Osteosarcoma

- Osseous matrix
- Aggressive periosteal reaction
- Can occur secondary to Paget disease

Metastases

- Multifocal
- Associated soft tissue mass
- Can be lytic, sclerotic, mixed

Giant Cell Tumor (GCT)

- Epiphyseal lesion
- No soft tissue mass
- Well-defined lytic lesion

Lymphoma

- Can be sclerotic ("ivory vertebra")
- Late cortical destruction

Multiple Myeloma

- Multifocal
- Cold on bone scan

PATHOLOGY

General Features

- General path comments: Resembles high-grade fibrosarcoma
- Genetics: Loss of chromosome 13
- Etiology
  - Derived from monocyte-macrophage precursors
  - Controversial if tumor represents specific entity or microscopic pattern common to heterogeneous group of sarcomas
  - Can occur secondary to preexisting lesion:
    - Paget disease, bone infarct, chronic osteomyelitis
  - Can arise after radiation therapy for unrelated tumor
- Epidemiology: 2-10% of primary malignant bone tumors

Gross Pathologic & Surgical Features

- Gray with fleshy yellow areas
- Soft-fibrous mass
- Irregular, ill-defined borders
- Cortical disruption, infiltration into adjacent soft tissues
- Areas of necrosis and hemorrhage

Microscopic Features

- Fibroblast like spindle cells and giant cells resembling histiocytes in pleomorphic-storiform pattern
- Necrotic foci common
- Storiform/pleomorphic type: 50-60%
- Myxoid type: 25%
- Giant cell type: 5-10%
- Inflammatory type: 5-10%

Staging, Grading or Classification Criteria

- Surgical staging system for musculoskeletal tumors
  - Stage IA: Low grade, intracompartmental
  - Stage IB: Low grade, extracompartmental

MALIGNANT FIBROUS HISTIOCYTOMA, BONE

- ○ Stage IIA: High grade, intracompartmental
- ○ Stage IIB: High grade, extracompartmental
- ○ Stage IIIA: Low or high grade, intracompartmental, metastases
- ○ Stage IIIB: Low or high grade, extracompartmental, metastases

CLINICAL ISSUES

Presentation
- Most common signs/symptoms: Pain with or without swelling
- Clinical profile
  - ○ Symptoms usually present for several months
  - ○ Most patients present with aggressive stage IIB lesion
  - ○ Pathologic fracture: 23%

Demographics
- Age
  - ○ 10-90 years, peak: 50 years
  - ○ 10% < 20 years
- Gender: M:F = 1-1.5:1
- Ethnicity: More frequent in Caucasians

Natural History & Prognosis
- Aggressive neoplasms with tendency to recur and metastasize
- Prognosis depends on tumor size, histologic subtype
- Secondary MFH (arising in preexisting condition) more aggressive than primary MFH
- Local recurrence: 31-44%
- Metastases: 42%
  - ○ Lung: 90%, lymph nodes: 4-12%, bone: 8%, liver: 1%
- 5 year survival: 52%
- 10 year survival: 41%

Treatment
- Surgical resection with wide margins
- Neoadjuvant and adjuvant chemotherapy
- Radiation and chemotherapy
- Radiation therapy for inoperable tumors
  - ○ Risk of radiation-induced sarcoma

DIAGNOSTIC CHECKLIST

Consider
- 20% of all osseous MFH occur in areas of abnormal bone

SELECTED REFERENCES

1. Bielack SS et al: Malignant fibrous histiocytoma of bone: A retrospective EMSOS study of 125 cases. European Musculo-Skeletal Oncology Society. Acta Orthop Scand 70:353-60, 1999
2. Mairal A et al: Loss of chromosome 13 is the most frequent genomic imbalance in malignant fibrous histiocytomas. A comparative genomic hybridization analysis of a series of 30 cases. Cancer Genet Cytogenet 111:134-8, 1999
3. Dorfman HD et al: Bone tumors. 1st ed. St. Louis MO, Mosby, 531-52, 1998
4. Greenspan A: Differential diagnosis of tumors and tumor-like lesions of bones and joints. 1st ed. Philadelphia PA, Lippincott-Raven, 1998
5. Nishida J et al: Malignant fibrous histiocytoma of bone. A clinicopathologic study of 81 patients. Cancer 79:482-93, 1997
6. Lin WY et al: The role of Tc-99m MDP and Ga-67 imaging in the clinical evaluation of malignant fibrous histiocytoma. Clin Nucl Med 19:996-1000, 1994
7. Murphey MD et al: From the archives of the AFIP. Musculoskeletal malignant fibrous histiocytoma: Radiologic-pathologic correlation. Radiographics 14:807-26, 1994
8. Yokoyama R et al: Prognostic factors of malignant fibrous histiocytoma of bone: A clinical and histopathologic analysis of 34 cases. Cancer 72:1902-9, 1993
9. Pezzi CM et al: Prognostic factors in 227 patients with malignant fibrous histiocytoma. Cancer 69:2098-103, 1992
10. Boland PJ et al: Malignant fibrous histiocytoma of bone. Clin Orthop 204:130-4, 1986
11. Huvos AG et al: The pathology of malignant fibrous histiocytoma of bone. A study of 130 patients. Am J Surg Pathol 9:853-71, 1985
12. Ros PR et al: Malignant fibrous histiocytoma: Mesenchymal tumor of ubiquitous origin. Am J Roentgenal 142:753-9, 1984
13. Weiss SW et al: Malignant fibrous histiocytoma: An analysis of 200 cases. Cancer 41:2250-60, 1978
14. Feldman F et al: Primary malignant fibrous histiocytoma (fibrous xanthoma) of bone. Skeletal Radiol 1:145-60, 1977
15. Spanier SS et al: Primary malignant fibrous histiocytoma of bone. Cancer 36:2084-98, 1975

IMAGE GALLERY

Typical

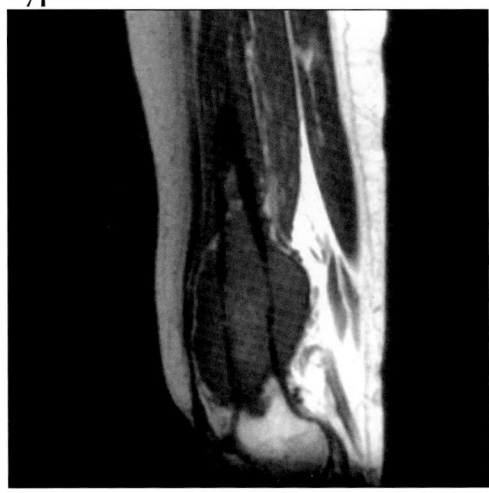
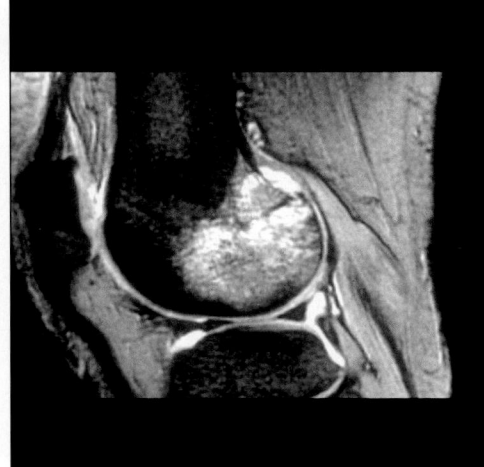

(Left) Sagittal T1WI MR shows heterogeneous intermediate signal with soft tissue extension involving the distal femoral meta-diaphysis. *(Right)* Sagittal FS T2 FSE MR shows high signal tumor in the distal femoral epiphysis. Note posterior cortical disruption.

Typical

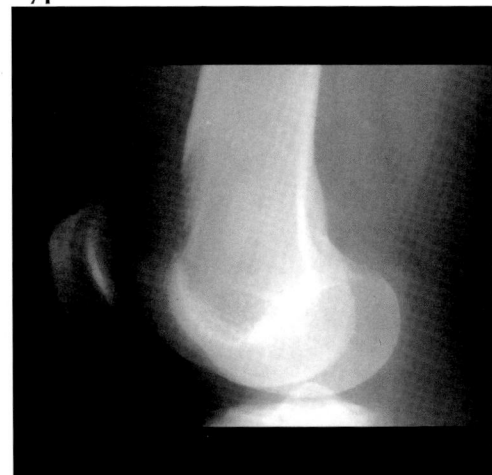
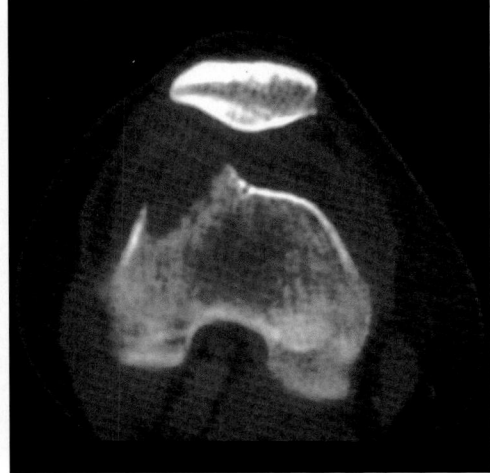

(Left) Lateral radiography shows ill-defined lytic lesion with anterior cortical destruction involving the distal femoral metaphysis. *(Right)* Axial NECT shows permeative osteolytic lesion with anterior cortical disruption and soft tissue extension.

Other

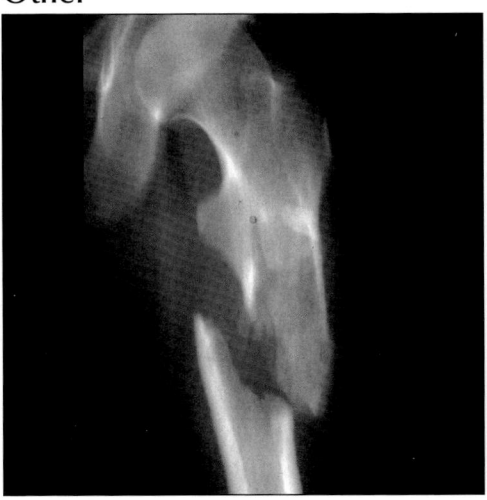
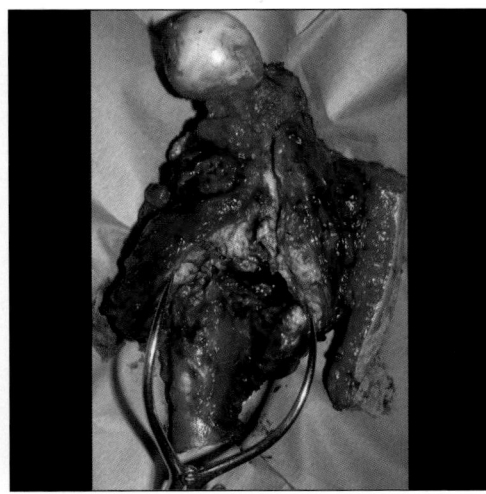

(Left) Anteroposterior radiography of the left proximal femur demonstrates pathologic fracture through ill-defined destructive lesion. *(Right)* Coronal surgical pathology shows hemorrhagic tumor with associated soft tissue mass involving the proximal femur.

FIBROSARCOMA

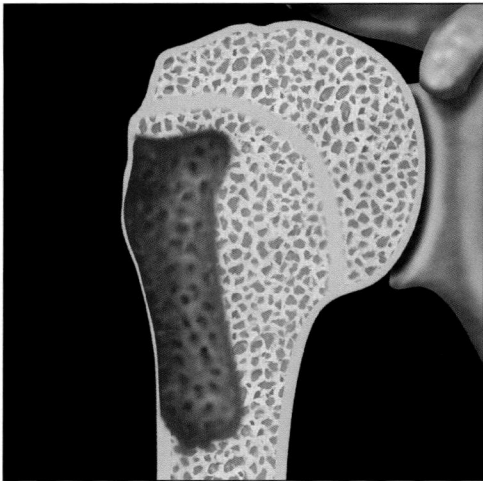

Coronal graphic shows eccentric destructive osteolytic lesion in the proximal femur. Note the lack of periosteal reaction.

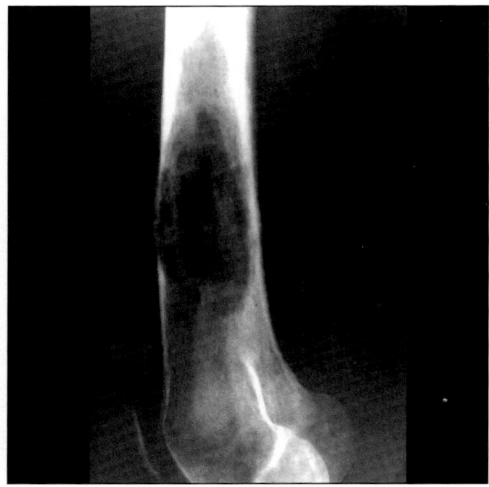

Lateral radiography shows ill-defined lytic lesion involving the distal femoral meta-diaphysis. Note the permeative pattern of bone destruction and wide zone of transition.

TERMINOLOGY

Abbreviations and Synonyms
- Fibroblastic malignancy, mesenchymal sarcoma

Definitions
- Spindle-cell sarcoma characterized by myofibroblastic differentiation and absence of osteoid production

IMAGING FINDINGS

General Features
- Best diagnostic clue
  - Low grade lesion: Circumscribed lytic lesion with irregular lobulated cortex, osseous sequestrum
  - High-grade lesion: Lytic ill-defined lesion with permeative bone destruction, cortical disruption, soft tissue mass
- Location
  - Long tubular bones
    - Femur: 40%
    - Tibia: 15%
    - About knee: 30-50%
    - Humerus: 9%
  - Pelvis: 15%
  - Craniofacial bones: 9%
  - Spine: 5%
  - Rare in small bones of hands and feet
  - Eccentric in metaphysis: 85%
  - Extension into diaphysis, epiphysis
  - Multifocal lesions: Rare
- Size: 2-10 cm
- Morphology: Well-defined to destructive lytic lesion +/- soft tissue mass

Radiographic Findings
- Radiography
  - Intramedullary (central) fibrosarcoma
    - Lytic lesion with permeative, moth-eaten, geographic pattern of bone destruction
    - Low-grade tumors: Circumscribed lytic lesion with sclerotic rim
    - Loculated "soap bubble" appearance
    - High-grade tumors: Large lytic lesion with cortical destruction, soft tissue extension
    - Associated soft tissue mass: 85%
    - Osseous sequestrum
    - Minimal periosteal reaction
    - No calcified matrix
    - Presence of calcification suggests secondary fibrosarcoma
  - Periosteal fibrosarcoma (rare)
    - Irregular cortex
    - Periosteal reaction
  - Secondary fibrosarcoma: Occurs in areas of abnormal bone

DDx: Fibrosarcoma

MFH	Osteosarcoma	GCT	Lymphoma	Multiple Myeloma

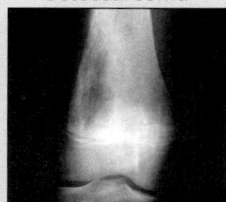 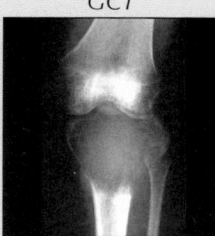 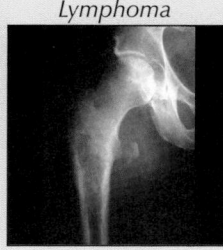 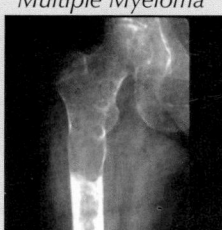

Lat Radiography	AP Radiography	AP Radiography	AP Radiography	AP Radiography

FIBROSARCOMA

Key Facts

Imaging Findings
- Low grade lesion: Circumscribed lytic lesion with irregular lobulated cortex, osseous sequestrum
- High-grade lesion: Lytic ill-defined lesion with permeative bone destruction, cortical disruption, soft tissue mass

Top Differential Diagnoses
- Malignant Fibrous Histiocytoma (MFH)
- Giant Cell Tumor (GCT)
- Lymphoma
- Metastases
- Multiple Myeloma
- Aneurysmal Bone Cyst (ABC)
- Osteosarcoma

Pathology
- Epidemiology: 4% of all primary bone tumors

Clinical Issues
- Mass with or without swelling
- Pathologic fractures: 15-23%
- Low-grade type: 10-year survival 80%
- High-grade type: 5-year survival 35-40%
- Stage Ia lesion: Limb salvage resection with wide surgical margins
- Stage IIb lesion: Radical resection with wide margins
- Adjuvant and neoadjuvant chemotherapy

Diagnostic Checklist
- 30% of all fibrosarcomas occur in areas of abnormal bone

  - Paget disease, bone infarct, chronic osteomyelitis, giant cell tumor
  - After radiation of giant cell tumor, lymphoma, malignancy unrelated to bone
  - Dedifferentiation of chondrosarcoma
- Infantile fibrosarcoma: Rare
  - Excellent prognosis

CT Findings
- NECT
  - Osseous mass of muscle density
  - Low density areas correspond to necrosis
- CECT: Variable enhancement

MR Findings
- T1WI: Intermediate-low signal intensity
- T2WI
  - Heterogeneous signal
  - High signal intensity
- STIR: High signal intensity
- T1 C+: Variable enhancement

Nuclear Medicine Findings
- Bone Scan: Increased radiotracer uptake

Imaging Recommendations
- Best imaging tool: Radiographs, MRI
- Protocol advice
  - Radiographs/CT to show bone destruction
  - MRI to evaluate intra- and extraosseous extent

DIFFERENTIAL DIAGNOSIS

Malignant Fibrous Histiocytoma (MFH)
- Radiographically indistinguishable from high-grade fibrosarcoma

Giant Cell Tumor (GCT)
- Epiphyseal lesion
- Well-defined borders
- Trabeculation within tumor matrix
- No marginal sclerosis

Lymphoma
- Can be sclerotic
- Late cortical destruction

Metastases
- Multifocal
- Associated soft tissue mass common

Multiple Myeloma
- Multifocal
- Cold on bone scan

Aneurysmal Bone Cyst (ABC)
- Can resemble low-grade fibrosarcoma
- Fluid-fluid levels
- No cortical destruction

Osteosarcoma
- Calcified matrix
- Aggressive periosteal reaction
- Associated soft tissue component

PATHOLOGY

General Features
- General path comments: Clinically and radiographically resembles MFH
- Etiology
  - Comprises low-grade end of spectrum that includes MFH at high-grade end
  - Can occur secondary to preexisting lesion
    - Paget disease, bone infarct, chronic osteomyelitis
  - Can be radiation induced
  - Patients with neurofibromatosis have 10% risk of developing fibrosarcoma
- Epidemiology: 4% of all primary bone tumors

Gross Pathologic & Surgical Features
- Fleshy-fibrous tumor
- Foci of tan-gray soft tissue
- Myxoid, hemorrhagic areas
- High grade tumors: Hemorrhagic, friable, necrotic
- Cortical break

FIBROSARCOMA

Microscopic Features

- Interlacing spindle cells arranged in "herringbone" pattern
- Permeative invasion of bony trabeculae
- No bone or cartilage matrix
- Low-grade tumors: Abundant collagen, hypocellular
- High-grade tumors: More cellular, less collagen production

Staging, Grading or Classification Criteria

- Surgical staging system for malignant musculoskeletal tumors
  - Stage Ia: Low grade, intracompartmental
  - Stage Ib: Low grade, extracompartmental
  - Stage IIa: High grade, intracompartmental
  - Stage IIb: High grade, extracompartmental
  - Stage IIIa: Low or high grade, intracompartmental, metastases
  - Stage IIIb: Low or high grade, extracompartmental, metastases

CLINICAL ISSUES

Presentation

- Most common signs/symptoms
  - Mass with or without swelling
  - Dull pain
- Clinical profile
  - Pathologic fractures: 15-23%
  - Metastases: 42%

Demographics

- Age: 10-90 years, peak: 3rd-5th decade
- Gender: M:F = 1.2:1
- Ethnicity: No racial predilection

Natural History & Prognosis

- Prognosis depends on tumor size, histologic subtype
- Low-grade type: 10-year survival 80%
- High-grade type: 5-year survival 35-40%
- Local recurrence: 60%

Treatment

- Stage Ia lesion: Limb salvage resection with wide surgical margins
- Stage IIb lesion: Radical resection with wide margins
  - Amputation may be required
  - Adjuvant and neoadjuvant chemotherapy
- Radiation therapy for surgically inaccessible lesion
  - Risk of radiation-induced sarcoma
- Resection of pulmonary metastases

DIAGNOSTIC CHECKLIST

Consider

- 30% of all fibrosarcomas occur in areas of abnormal bone

SELECTED REFERENCES

1. Saito T et al: Low-grade fibrosarcoma of the proximal humerus. Pathol Int 53:115-20, 2003
2. Papagelopoulos PJ et al: Clinicopathologic features, diagnosis, and treatment of fibrosarcoma of bone. Am J Orthop 31:253-7, 2002
3. Smith SE et al: Primary musculoskeletal tumors of fibrous origin. Semin Musculoskelet Radiol 4:73-88. 2000
4. Dorfman HD et al: Bone tumors. 1st ed. St. Louis MO, Mosby, 552-5, 1998
5. Nashida J et al: Malignant fibrous histiocytoma of bone. A clinicopathologic study of 81 patients. Cancer 79:482-93, 1997
6. Hudson TM et al: Fibrous lesions of bone. Radiol Clin North Am 31:279-97, 1993
7. Suh CH et al: Fibrosarcoma: Observations on the ultrastructure. Ultrastructural Pathol 17:221-9, 1993
8. Wiklund TA et al: Postirradiation sarcoma: Analysis of a nationwide cancer registry material. Cancer 68:524-31, 1991
9. Wetzel LH et al: A comparison of MR imaging and CT in the evaluation of musculoskeletal masses. Radiographics 7:851-74, 1987
10. Aisen AM et al: MRI and CT evaluation of primary bone and soft-tissue tumors. Am J Roentgenol 146:749-756, 1986
11. Bertoni F et al: Primary central (medullary) fibrosarcoma of bone. Semin Diagn Pathol 1:185-98, 1984
12. Taconis WK et al: Fibrosarcoma and malignant fibrous histiocytoma of long bones: Radiographic features and grading. Skeletal Radiol 11:237-45, 1984
13. Larsson SE et al: Fibrosarcoma of bone: A demographic, clinical and histopathological study of all cases recorded in the Swedish cancer registry from 1958 to 1968. J Bone Joint Surg 588-B:412-17, 1976
14. Huvos AG et al: Primary fibrosarcoma of bone: A clinicopathologic study of 130 patients. Cancer 35:837-47, 1975
15. Eyre-Brook AL et al: Fibrosarcoma of bone: Review of fifty consecutive cases from the Bristol Bone Tumour Registry. J Bone Joint Surg 51-B:20-37, 1969

FIBROSARCOMA

IMAGE GALLERY

Typical

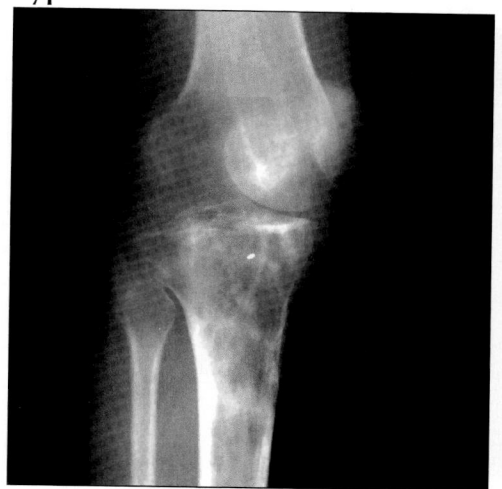

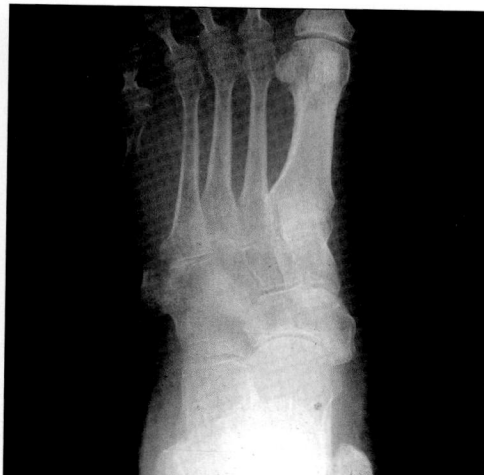

(Left) Lateral radiography shows destructive lytic lesion involving the proximal tibia. *(Right)* Anteroposterior radiography shows large lytic lesion involving the 5th metatarsal bone. Cortical destruction with no periosteal new bone formation is noted.

Variant

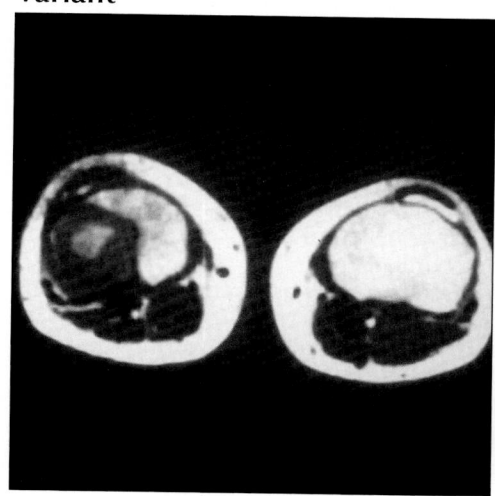

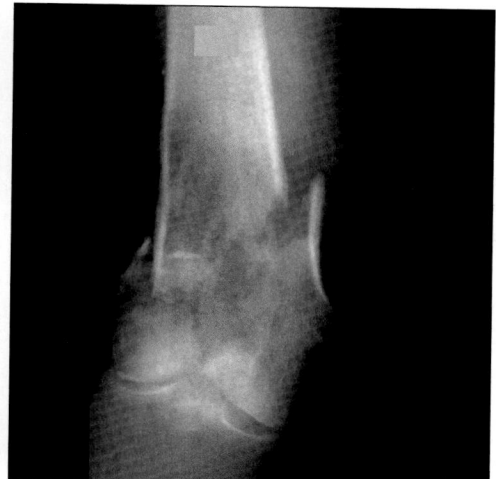

(Left) Axial T1WI MR shows eccentric tumor of low signal in the distal right femur. *(Right)* Anteroposterior radiography shows pathologic fracture through lytic destructive femoral lesion.

Other

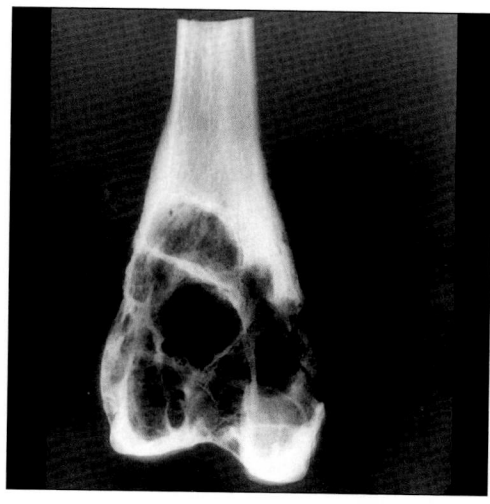

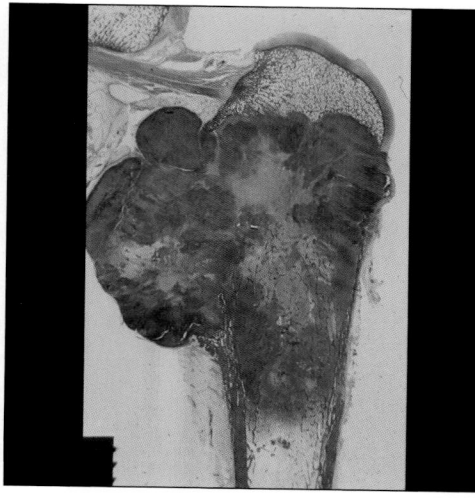

(Left) Anteroposterior radiography of resected specimen shows lytic lobulated tumor with cortical destruction. This was found to represent a low-grade fibrosarcoma. *(Right)* Coronal micropathology, low power shows infiltrating fibrosarcoma with cortical disruption involving the proximal femur.

GIANT CELL TUMOR

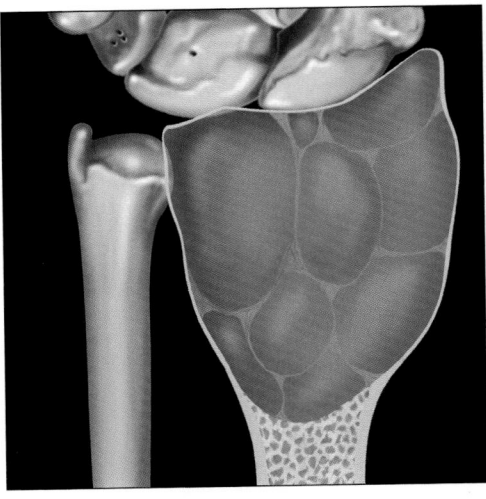

Coronal graphic shows expansile lytic lesion with trabeculations extending to subchondral bone. Thinned but intact cortex is shown.

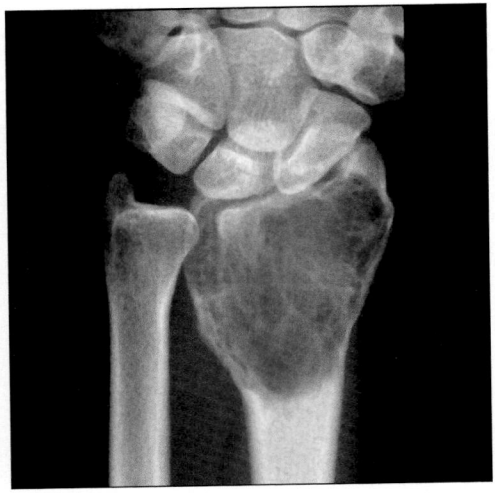

Anteroposterior radiography shows a large lytic expansile lesion with trabeculation involving the distal radius with extension to subchondral bone.

TERMINOLOGY

Abbreviations and Synonyms
- Giant cell tumor (GCT)

Definitions
- Locally aggressive neoplasm composed of osteoclast like giant cells involving the epiphyses in skeletally mature patients

IMAGING FINDINGS

General Features
- Best diagnostic clue
  - Lytic epiphyseal lesion extending to subchondral bone without surrounding sclerosis
  - Occurs typically in skeletally mature patients
- Location
  - Originates in metaphyseal side of growth plate
    - Centered in meta-epiphysis
    - Subsequent growth to subchondral bone
  - Long bones: 75-90%
    - About knee: 50-65%
    - Radius: 10%
    - Humerus: 6%
  - Spine: 7%
  - Hands and feet: 5%
  - Pelvis: 4%
  - Multifocal: 0.5-1% with Paget disease
- Size: 2-20 cm, mean: 5-7 cm
- Morphology: Eccentric lytic lesion without matrix extending to subchondral bone

Radiographic Findings
- Radiography
  - Eccentric, lytic bone lesion
  - Well-defined borders
  - Expansile remodeling with apparent cortical permeation: 20-50%
  - Conspicuous peripheral trabeculae without tumor matrix ("soap bubble" appearance)
  - Septations
  - No marginal sclerosis
  - Periosteal reaction: 10-30%

CT Findings
- NECT
  - Soft tissue attenuation, foci of low attenuation (hemorrhage/necrosis)
  - May break through cortex with cortical thinning, soft tissue invasion

MR Findings
- T1WI
  - Low-intermediate signal intensity
  - Best to see intramedullary portion of tumor

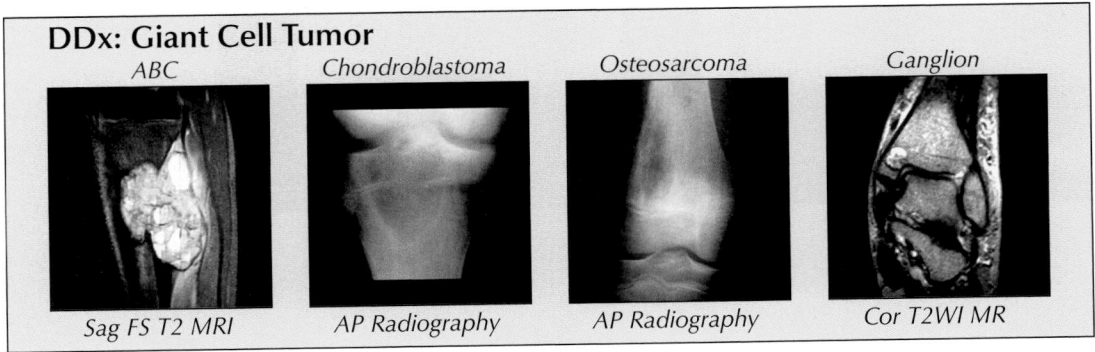

DDx: Giant Cell Tumor

ABC	Chondroblastoma	Osteosarcoma	Ganglion
Sag FS T2 MRI	AP Radiography	AP Radiography	Cor T2WI MR

GIANT CELL TUMOR

Key Facts

Imaging Findings
- Lytic epiphyseal lesion extending to subchondral bone without surrounding sclerosis
- Occurs typically in skeletally mature patients

Top Differential Diagnoses
- Aneurysmal Bone Cyst (ABC)
- Intraosseous Ganglion
- Chondroblastoma
- Osteosarcoma
- Giant Cell Reparative Granuloma

Pathology
- 5% of all primary bone tumors
- 6th most common primary bone tumor

Clinical Issues
- Pain and swelling at affected area, relieved by decreased activity
- Pathologic fracture in 30%
- Locally aggressive: 12-50% recurrence rate
- Can undergo sarcomatous transformation, spontaneously or in response to radiation therapy
- Curettage with cryotherapy, phenol, liquid nitrogen to reduce recurrence rate
- Surgical resection with filling of resection cavity with bone graft or methylmethacrylate
- Radiation only for cases of unresectable tumor (risk of sarcomatous degeneration)
- Resection of pulmonary implants

- T2WI
  - Low-intermediate signal intensity
  - Fluid-fluid levels
  - To evaluate extraosseous component of tumor

Angiographic Findings
- Neovascularity: 80%
- Intense, heterogeneous capillary blush

Nuclear Medicine Findings
- Bone Scan
  - Doughnut sign: Intense uptake around periphery with little activity in central portion
  - May help in detection of multicentric giant cell tumor

Imaging Recommendations
- Best imaging tool: Radiographs diagnostic
- Protocol advice: MRI to evaluate extraosseous component

DIFFERENTIAL DIAGNOSIS

Aneurysmal Bone Cyst (ABC)
- Rarely affects articular end of bone
- Younger age group
- May coexist with giant cell tumor

Intraosseous Ganglion
- Sclerotic borders
- Eccentric location

Chondroblastoma
- Calcified
- Younger age group

Osteosarcoma
- Aggressive periosteal reaction
- Osseous matrix

Giant Cell Reparative Granuloma
- Benign reparative lesions in small bones of hands and feet

PATHOLOGY

General Features
- General path comments: Solitary lesion characterized by osteoclast like giant cells and stroma cells originating at metaphyseal site of growth plate
- Genetics
  - Chromosomal aberrations with telomeric fusion may correlate with aggressive features
    - High recurrence rate
    - Metastatic potential
- Etiology
  - Unknown
  - Mononuclear cells from mesenchymal origin fuse to form giant cells
- Epidemiology
  - 5% of all primary bone tumors
  - 6th most common primary bone tumor
- Associated abnormalities
  - Goltz syndrome (focal dermal hypoplasia)
    - Rare condition characterized by multiple anomalies of skin, teeth, and bone

Gross Pathologic & Surgical Features
- Soft, friable, fleshy, red-brown tumor with yellow areas
- Tumor tissue well-demarcated, can extend to articular cartilage
- Can be hemorrhagic, ABC-like formation: 10-15%
- Surrounding bone is expanded with thinning of the cortex
- Delineated in periphery by thin layer of fibrous and reactive bone tissue

Microscopic Features
- Multinucleated osteoclastic giant cells intermixed throughout spindle cell stroma
- Osteoclastic giant cells not apposed to bone surfaces
  - Do not participate in bone resorption
- No bone or cartilage matrix production in multiloculated giant cells

Staging, Grading or Classification Criteria
- Surgical staging of benign musculoskeletal tumors

GIANT CELL TUMOR

- o Stage 1: Latent
- o Stage 2: Active
- o Stage 3: Aggressive

CLINICAL ISSUES

Presentation
- Most common signs/symptoms
  - o Pain and swelling at affected area, relieved by decreased activity
    - ■ Can mimic internal derangement of the knee
- Clinical profile
  - o Pathologic fracture in 30%
  - o Limited range of motion of joint adjacent to affected area
  - o Pulmonary metastases (benign pulmonary implants) in 1-2%
    - ■ Histologically identical to primary tumor

Demographics
- Age
  - o 20-55 years, occurs after skeletal maturity
  - o Rare in children: 1%
- Gender: F:M = 2:1
- Ethnicity: More common in Chinese population

Natural History & Prognosis
- Clinical behavior cannot be predicted on basis of radiological and histologic features
- Locally aggressive: 12-50% recurrence rate
- Can undergo sarcomatous transformation, spontaneously or in response to radiation therapy
- Pulmonary metastases (pulmonary implants): 1-2%
  - o Occurs in patients with stage 3 disease
  - o Within 3 years after removal of primary GCT, can be seen without prior surgery
  - o Self limited growth potential, histologically benign
  - o May regress spontaneously
  - o Cases of death reported due to progressive growth of non-resected lung lesions (rare)
- Tumor involving distal radius often more aggressive than in other locations
- Primary malignant GCT extremely rare

Treatment
- Curettage with cryotherapy, phenol, liquid nitrogen to reduce recurrence rate
  - o Stage 1 and 2 lesions
- Surgical resection with filling of resection cavity with bone graft or methylmethacrylate
  - o Stage 3 lesions
- Curettage alone associated with high rate of recurrence
- Wide excision in case of recurrence
- Radiation only for cases of unresectable tumor (risk of sarcomatous degeneration)
- Arterial embolization of GCT involving the sacrum
- Resection of pulmonary implants

DIAGNOSTIC CHECKLIST

Consider
- Location: Extends to subchondral bone
- Age: Fused growth plate

SELECTED REFERENCES

1. Boons HW et al: Oncologic and functional results after treatment of giant cell tumors of bone. Arch Orthop Trauma Surg 122:17-23, 2002
2. Lackman RD et al: The treatment of sacral giant-cell tumours by serial arterial embolization. J Bone Joint Surg 84(B):873-7, 2002
3. Dorfman HD et al: Bone tumors. 1st ed. St. Louis MO, Mosby, 559-606, 1998
4. Meis JM et al: Primary malignant giant cell tumor of bone: "Dedifferentiated" giant cell tumor. Mod Pathol 2:541-6, 1995
5. Manaster BJ et al: Giant cell tumor of bone. Radiol Clin North Am 31:299-323, 1993
6. Schutte HE et al: Giant cell tumor in children and adolescents. Skeletal Radiol 22:173-6, 1993
7. Tubbs WS et al: Benign giant-cell tumor of bone with pulmonary metastases: Clinical findings and radiologic appearance of metastases in 13 cases. Am J Roentgenol 158:331-4, 1992
8. Aoki J et al: Giant cell tumors of bone containing large amounts of hemosiderin: MR-pathologic correlation. J Comput Assist Tomogr. 15:1024-7, 1991
9. Bridge JA et al: Cytogenetic findings and biologic behavior of giant cell tumors of bone. Cancer 65:2697-703, 1990
10. Tanaka H et al: The Goltz syndrome associated with giant cell tumor of bone: A case report. Int Orthop 14:179-81, 1990
11. Carrasco CH et al: Giant cell tumors. Orthop Clin North Am 20:395-405, 1989

GIANT CELL TUMOR

IMAGE GALLERY

Typical

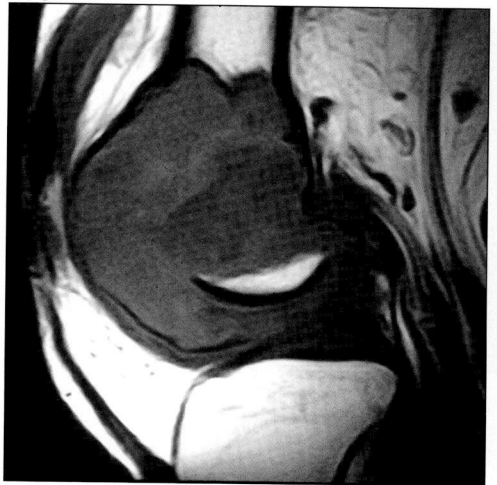
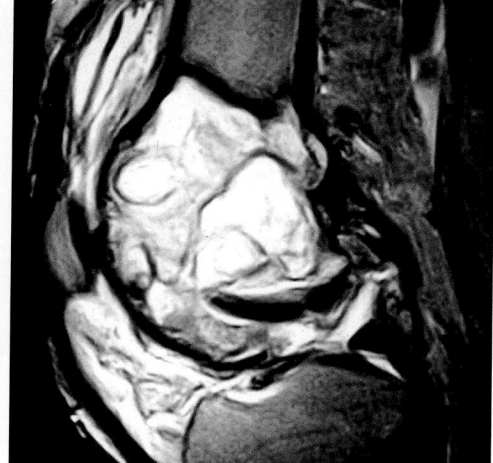

(Left) Sagittal T1WI MR shows tumor of low-intermediate SI involving the distal femoral meta-epiphysis. The tumor has penetrated the cortex. *(Right)* Sagittal T2WI MR shows high SI tumor with surrounding edema and cortical penetration.

Typical

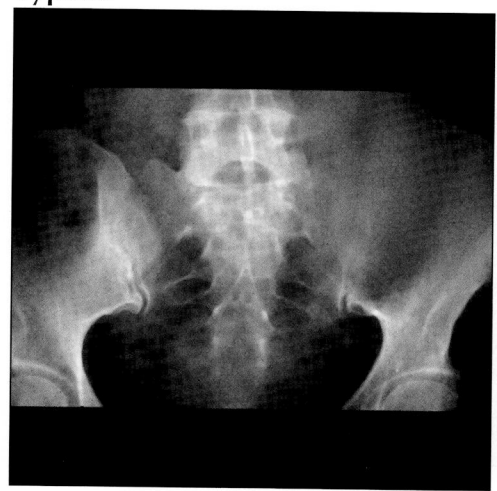
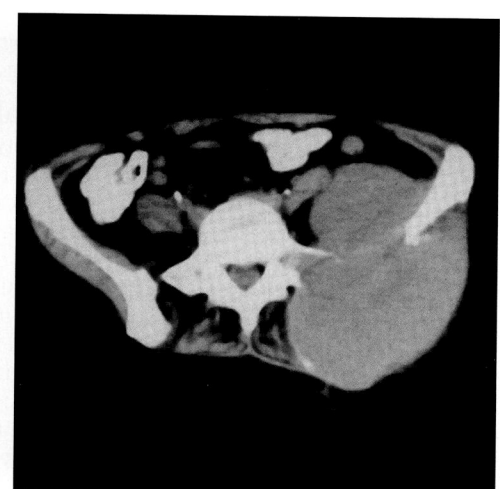

(Left) Anteroposterior radiography shows a large lytic lesion with cortical destruction involving the left hemipelvis. *(Right)* Axial NECT shows extensive destruction of the sacrum and ilium with large associated soft tissue mass.

Other

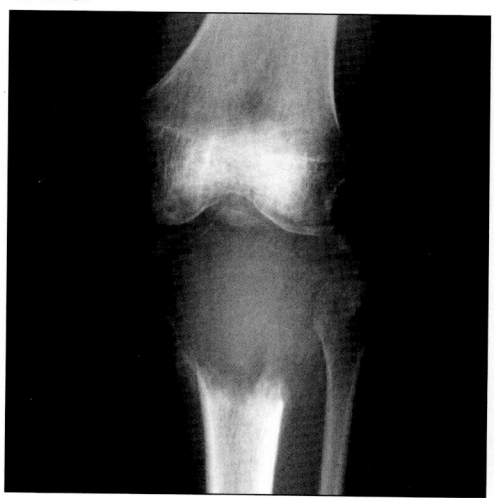
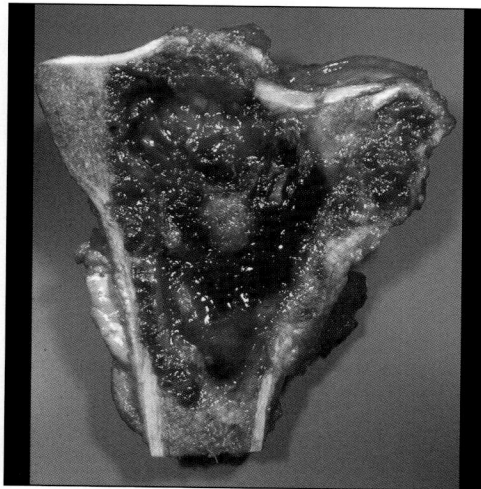

(Left) Sagittal T1WI MR shows a purely lytic lesion with non sclerotic margin and cortical destruction involving the proximal tibia. The lesion extends to subchondral bone. *(Right)* Coronal gross pathology shows brown-reddish tumor involving the proximal tibia with extension to subchondral bone and through the cortex. Areas of hemorrhage and cyst formation are noted.

INTRAOSSEOUS HEMANGIOMA

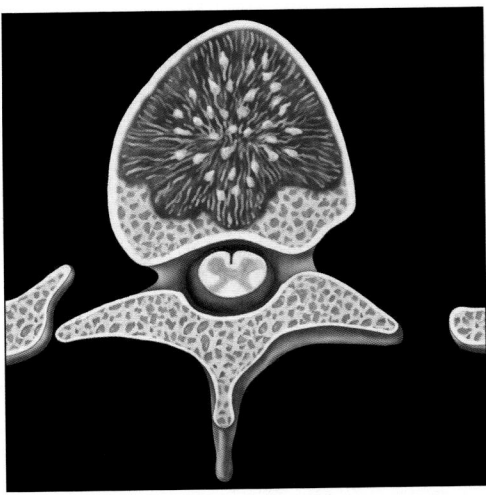

Axial graphic of the vertebral body shows radiating spicules and coarse trabeculations in a polka-dot pattern.

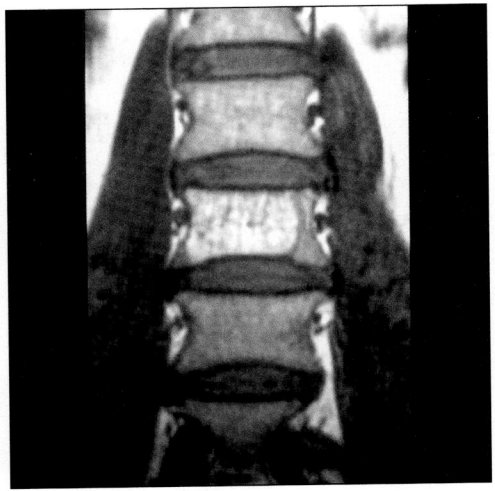

Coronal T1WI MR shows area of high signal involving the L2 vertebral body. Note the prominent trabeculations.

TERMINOLOGY

Abbreviations and Synonyms
- Hemangioma of bone

Definitions
- Benign lesion composed of newly formed blood vessels

IMAGING FINDINGS

General Features
- Best diagnostic clue
  - MRI: Areas of high signal on T1 and T2WI MR
  - Radiographs and CT: Vertical/radial striations, spoke wheel/polka-dot appearance
- Location
  - Spine: 28%
    - Vertebral body, may extend into lamina, spinous process (rare)
  - Calvarium: 20%
    - Occurs in diploic space
  - Flat bones: Rib, clavicle, mandible
  - Long bones
  - Intraosseous, intracortical, periosteal
  - Intraarticular (synovial)
  - Can be multifocal

- Size: 1-7 cm
- Morphology: Lytic lesion with radiating trabecular thickening

Radiographic Findings
- Radiography
  - Coarse striations
  - Multifocal lytic areas
  - Periosteal and intracortical type
    - Lytic, cortical erosions, periosteal reaction
  - Vertebral body: Vertical striations, honeycomb appearance
    - Multiloculated lytic foci
    - May have associate soft tissue mass or pathologic fracture
  - Calvarium: Small, round, circumscribed lytic lesion
    - Diploe: Greater expansion of outer than inner table
    - Radiating thickened trabeculae, spoke wheel pattern
    - Multicentric: 15%
  - Long bones: Expansile lesion, thinning of cortex
    - Honeycomb, "hole-within-hole" appearance
    - Radial trabecular thickening
    - Spiculated periosteal reaction
  - Flat bones: Radiating thickened trabeculae, spoke wheel pattern
    - Lesions usually larger

DDx: Intraosseous Hemangioma

Osteoporosis	Paget Disease	Multiple Myeloma	Metastases	LCH

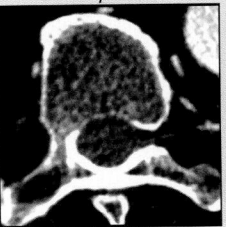
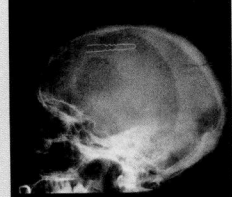
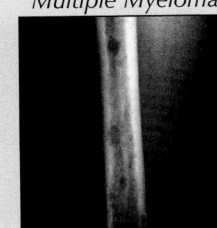
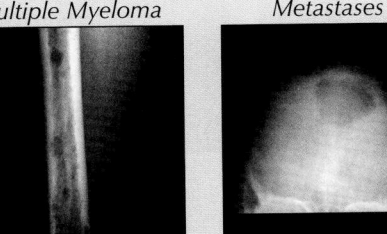
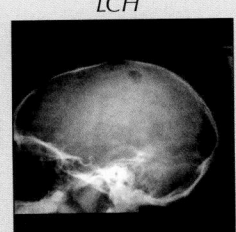

Ax NECT	Lat Radiography	Lat Radiography	AP Radiography	Lat Radiography

INTRAOSSEOUS HEMANGIOMA

Key Facts

Imaging Findings
- MRI: Areas of high signal on T1 and T2WI MR
- Radiographs and CT: Vertical/radial striations, spoke wheel/polka-dot appearance

Top Differential Diagnoses
- Osteopenia
- Fibrous Dysplasia
- Paget Disease
- Multiple Myeloma
- Metastases
- Langerhans Cell Histiocytosis (LCH)

Pathology
- Lesion with high degree of fat will less likely be symptomatic
- Incidence: 10%

- 1% of biopsied primary bone tumors

Clinical Issues
- Mostly asymptomatic
- Local pain and swelling with involvement of skull and ribs
- Vertebral hemangiomas can extend to spinal canal and cause cord compression
- Usually stabilizes in growth
- May undergo spontaneous regression
- Small asymptomatic lesions require no treatment
- Curettage and bone grafting for symptomatic lesions

Diagnostic Checklist
- Can look aggressive on radiographs, look for high signal on T1WI MRI

CT Findings
- NECT: Vertebral body: Multiple sclerotic dots ("polka dot" appearance)
- CECT: Enhancement

MR Findings
- T1WI
  - Areas of high signal intensity, corresponding to vascular components
    - Areas of low signal intensity, corresponding to trabecular thickening
- T2WI
  - Areas of high signal intensity, corresponding to vascular components
    - Areas of low signal intensity, corresponding to trabecular thickening
- T1 C+: Enhancement
- Helpful in demonstrating possible extension into spinal canal

Nuclear Medicine Findings
- Bone Scan
  - Moderate uptake
  - Photopenia

Imaging Recommendations
- Best imaging tool: MRI, CT
- Protocol advice: MRI to evaluate potential complications (e.g., cord compression)

DIFFERENTIAL DIAGNOSIS

Osteopenia
- Can be indistinguishable on CT
- No focal high signal on T1
- Diffuse, no focal mass

Fibrous Dysplasia
- Lytic lesion
- Ground glass appearance
- Expansile

Paget Disease
- Enlarged vertebral body
- Sclerotic endplates
- Diploic widening
- Osteoporosis circumscripta

Multiple Myeloma
- Destructive lesion
- Associated soft tissue mass
- Multiple lesions

Metastases
- Cortical destruction
- Often associated soft tissue mass
- Multifocal

Langerhans Cell Histiocytosis (LCH)
- Calvarium: Well-defined lytic lesion
  - Outer table of skull more destroyed than inner table
  - Button sequestrum
- Usually multifocal

PATHOLOGY

General Features
- General path comments
  - Vascular proliferation that may be congenital, developmental, or acquired
  - Lesion with high degree of fat will less likely be symptomatic
- Etiology
  - Vascular malformation
  - Likely hamartomatous condition rather than true neoplasm
- Epidemiology
  - Incidence: 10%
  - 1% of biopsied primary bone tumors
- Associated abnormalities
  - Hemangiomatosis
    - Multiple hemangiomas involving two or more non contiguous sites
  - Gorham disease

INTRAOSSEOUS HEMANGIOMA

- Progressive bone resorption in association with multiple hemangiomas or lymphangiomas

Gross Pathologic & Surgical Features
- Well-demarcated soft, friable, brown-red intramedullary lesion
- Can be intracortical or subperiosteal
- Bony trabeculae coursing through lesion
- Variable degree of sclerosis
- Some lesions composed exclusively of vascular tissue, contain no bone

Microscopic Features
- Hemangiomatous tissue spreads between bone trabeculae without causing bone distortion
- Capillary type: Small vessels, consist of flat epithelium, surrounded by only basilar membrane
  - Most common in vertebral body
- Cavernous type: Composed of dilated, blood-filled spaces lined by flat endothelium and basilar membrane
  - Most common in calvarium
- Venous type: Composed of thick-walled spaces with muscle layer, frequently contain phleboliths
- Arteriovenous type: Abnormal communication between arteries and veins
  - Rare in bones, common in soft tissues

CLINICAL ISSUES

Presentation
- Most common signs/symptoms
  - Mostly asymptomatic
  - Pathologic fracture rare
- Clinical profile
  - Local pain and swelling with involvement of skull and ribs
  - Vertebral hemangiomas can extend to spinal canal and cause cord compression

Demographics
- Age
  - 1-80 years
  - 75% diagnosed between 20-60 years
- Gender: F:M = 1.5-2:1
- Ethnicity: No racial predilection

Natural History & Prognosis
- Benign, no malignant degeneration
- Usually stabilizes in growth
- Can progress, causing tissue destruction
- May undergo spontaneous regression

Treatment
- Small asymptomatic lesions require no treatment
- Curettage and bone grafting for symptomatic lesions
  - Can cause severe hemorrhage during surgery
  - Preoperative arteriography and embolization
- Symptomatic spinal lesions: Decompression laminectomy
- CT guided intralesional injection of ethanol
- Hemangiomas of calvarium and facial bones: En bloc excision
- Surgically inaccessible lesions: Radiation therapy
  - Risk of radiation induced sarcoma

DIAGNOSTIC CHECKLIST

Consider
- Can look aggressive on radiographs, look for high signal on T1WI MRI
  - Malignant lesions are usually low signal on T1WI MRI

SELECTED REFERENCES

1. Doppman JL et al: Symptomatic vertebral hemangiomas: Treatment by means of direct intralesional injection of ethanol. Radiology 21:341-8, 2000
2. Wenger DE et al: Benign vascular lesions of bone: Radiologic and pathologic features. Skeletal Radiol 29:63-74, 2000
3. Greenspan A et al: Differential diagnosis of tumors and tumor-like lesions of bones and joints. 1st ed. Philadelphia PA, Lippincott-Raven, 289-96, 1998
4. Friedman DP: Symptomatic vertebral hemangiomas: MR findings. Am J Roentgenol 167:359-64, 1996
5. Lomasney LM et al: Multifocal vascular lesions of bone: Imaging characteristics. Skeletal Radiol 25:255-61, 1996
6. Murphey MD et al: From the archives of the AFIP. Musculoskeletal angiomatous lesions: Radiologic-pathologic correlation. Radiographics 15:893-917, 1995
7. Assoun J et al: CT and MRI of massive osteolysis of Gorham. J Comput Assist Tomogr 18:981-4, 1994
8. Suh JS et al: Soft tissue hemangiomas: MR manifestations in 23 patients. Skeletal Radiol 23:621-5, 1994
9. Conway WF et al: Miscellaneous lesions of bone. Radiol Clin North Am 31:339-58, 1993
10. Hawnaur JM et al: Musculoskeletal hemangiomas: Comparison of MRI with CT. Skeletal Radiol 19:251-8, 1990
11. Laredo JD et al: Vertebral hemangiomas: Fat content as a sign of aggressiveness. Radiology 177:467-72, 1990
12. Makhija M et al: Hemangioma: A rare cause of photopenic lesion on skeletal imaging. Clin Nucl Med 13:661-2, 1988
13. Moreno AJ et al: Hemangioma of bone. Clin Nucl Med 13:668-9, 1988
14. Cohen JW et al: Arteriovenous malformations of the extremities: MR imaging. Radiology 158:475-9, 1986
15. Laredo JD et al: Vertebral hemangiomas: Radiologic evaluation. Radiology 161:183-9, 1986
16. Faria SL et al: Radiotherapy in the treatment of vertebral hemangiomas. Int J Radiat Oncol Biol Phys 11:387-90, 1985

Typical

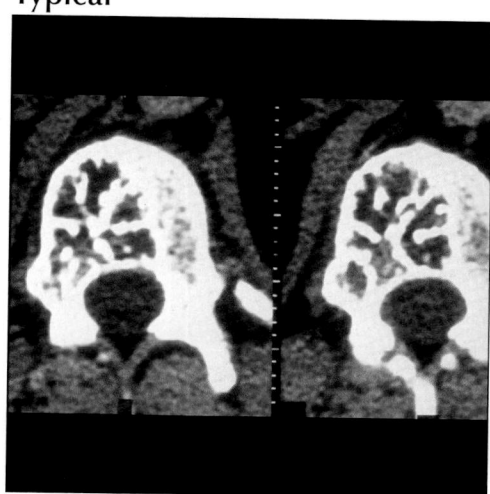 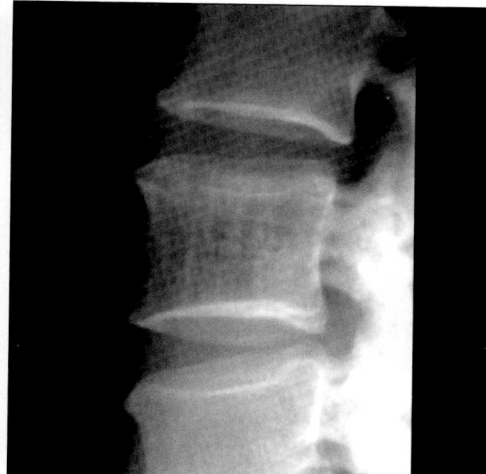

(Left) Axial NECT shows coarse dots that indicate reinforced trabeculae of cancellous bone ("polka-dots"). *(Right)* Lateral radiography shows increased vertical striations of the L2 vertebral body.

Typical

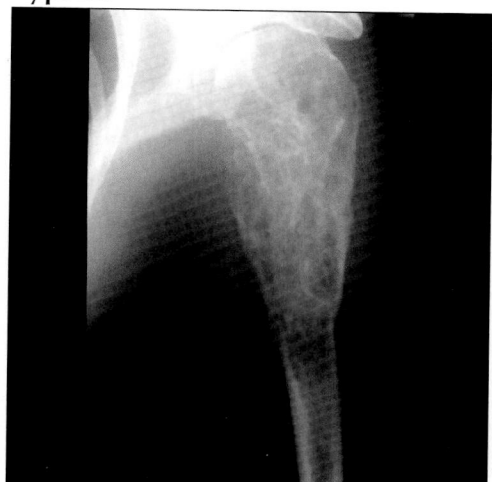 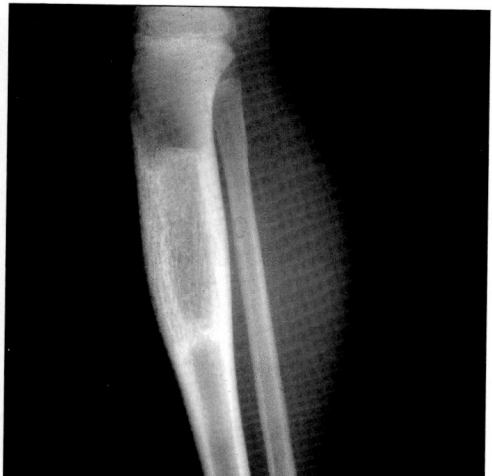

(Left) Anteroposterior radiography shows a large expansile trabeculated lytic lesion (honeycomb pattern) involving the proximal humerus. *(Right)* Lateral radiography shows slight anterior bowing, increased striations, and multiple small lucencies involving the tibial diaphysis.

Typical

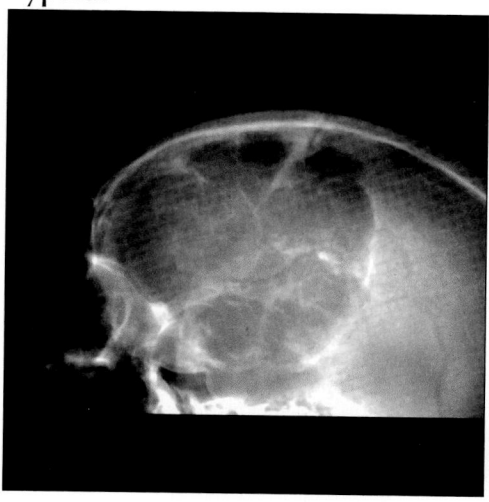 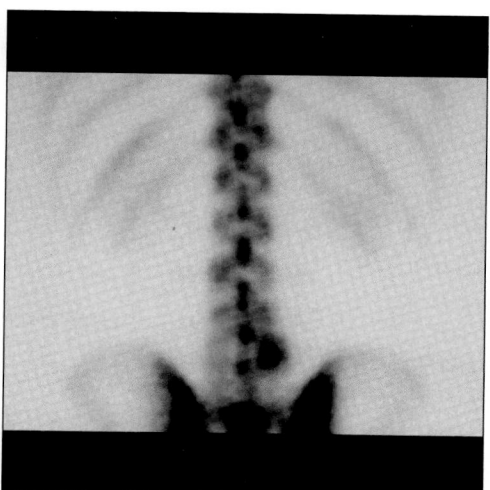

(Left) Lateral radiography shows a large lytic lesion with vertical trabeculation involving the calvarium. *(Right)* Anteroposterior bone scan shows increased radiotracer uptake in the L4 vertebral body.

UNICAMERAL BONE CYST

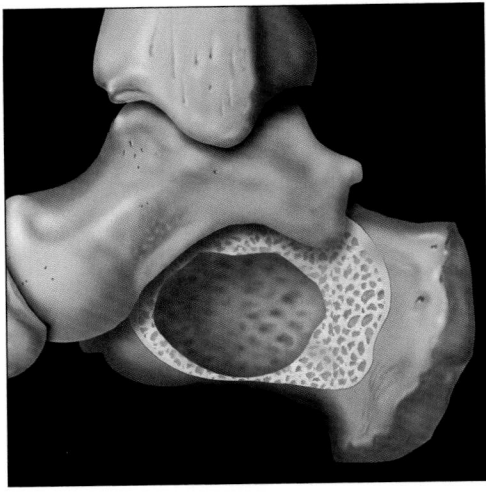

Sagittal graphic shows a unicameral bone cyst in the calcaneus. Note the lack of periosteal reaction and cortical destruction.

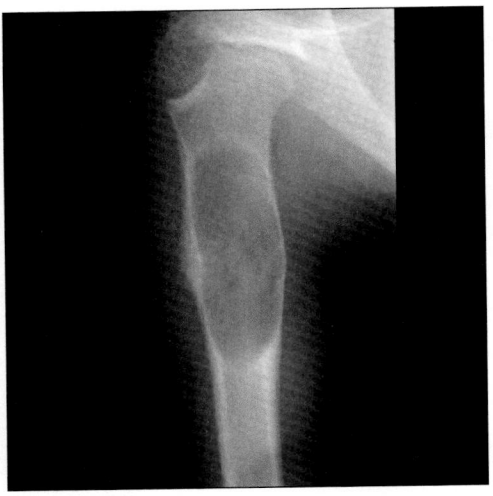

Anteroposterior radiography shows a well-defined lytic lesion in the central humeral metaphysis. Note the cortical thinning and lack of periosteal reaction.

TERMINOLOGY

Abbreviations and Synonyms
- Solitary or simple bone cyst

Definitions
- Tumor-like lesion of unknown etiology, attributed to local disturbance of bone growth

IMAGING FINDINGS

General Features
- Best diagnostic clue: Well-defined central lytic lesion
- Location
  - Humerus and femur: 60-80%
  - Calcaneus, talus, ilium: 50% (in older patients)
  - Spine, sacrum, craniofacial bones: Rare
  - Proximal metaphysis, adjacent to epiphyseal cartilage (during active phase)
  - Migration into diaphysis with growth (during latent phase)
  - Does not cross growth plate
- Size: 2-15 cm, mean: 6-8 cm
- Morphology
  - Well-defined lytic lesion
  - Migrates into diaphysis with bone growth

Radiographic Findings
- Radiography
  - Centrally located, well-defined, expansile, lucent lesion
  - Long axis parallel to long axis of host bone
  - Sclerotic margin
  - Scalloping of underlying cortex
  - Cortex never completely disrupted
  - Fluid-filled cavity (fluid/fluid levels)
  - No periosteal reaction unless fractured
  - No extension into soft tissues
  - Fallen fragment sign secondary to pathologic fracture (pathognomonic)
    - Fragment migrates to dependent portions of cyst
  - Increased density/sclerosis after steroid injection

CT Findings
- NECT
  - Fluid-filled cavity
    - HU: 15-20
    - Can have fluid-fluid levels
  - Helpful in evaluating anatomic complex areas (pelvis, spine)
  - To determine extent
- CECT
  - No enhancement
  - Helpful in differentiating cyst from solid lesion

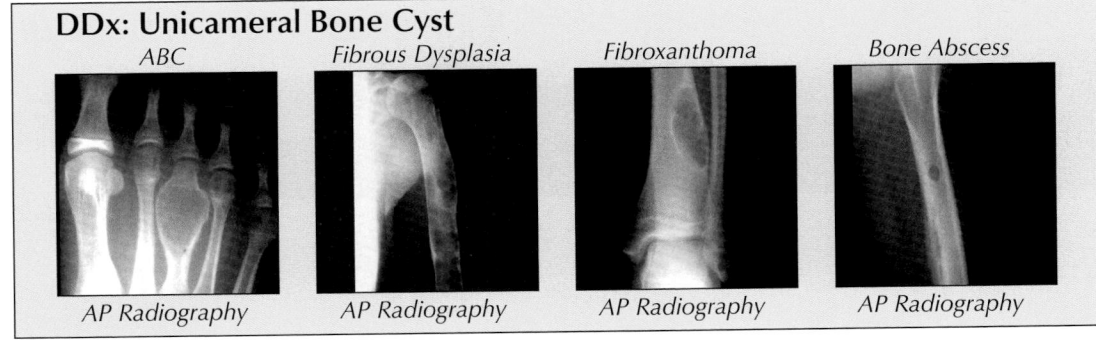

DDx: Unicameral Bone Cyst

ABC	Fibrous Dysplasia	Fibroxanthoma	Bone Abscess
AP Radiography	AP Radiography	AP Radiography	AP Radiography

UNICAMERAL BONE CYST

Key Facts

Imaging Findings
- Best diagnostic clue: Well-defined central lytic lesion
- Fallen fragment sign secondary to pathologic fracture (pathognomonic)

Top Differential Diagnoses
- Aneurysmal Bone Cyst (ABC)
- Fibrous Dysplasia
- Fibroxanthoma
- Bone Abscess
- Enchondroma
- Langerhans Cell Histiocytosis
- Brown Tumors

Pathology
- Epidemiology: 3% of primary bone lesions

Clinical Issues
- Most lesions asymptomatic
- Pain, swelling, stiffness at closest joint
- 66% of cysts present with pathologic fractures
- Spontaneous regression in majority of cases
- Recurrence rate after injection, curettage: 20-45%
- Dual needle aspiration and percutaneous injection of corticosteroids (80-200 mg methylprednisolone)
- Open curettage with bone graft in weight bearing bones

Diagnostic Checklist
- Starts at one end of bone, migrates towards diaphysis with bone growth

MR Findings
- T1WI: Low to intermediate signal intensity
- T2WI
  - High signal intensity
  - Heterogeneous signal in case of fracture (blood products)
- T1 C+
  - No enhancement
  - To differentiate cyst from solid lesions
- Fluid-fluid levels
- Septations

Nuclear Medicine Findings
- Bone Scan
  - Increased peripheral radiotracer uptake
  - Decreased central radiotracer uptake
  - May be normal

Imaging Recommendations
- Best imaging tool: Radiographs diagnostic
- Protocol advice: CT for anatomic complex areas (spine, pelvis)

DIFFERENTIAL DIAGNOSIS

Aneurysmal Bone Cyst (ABC)
- Eccentric, expansile lesion
- Periosteal reaction
- Geographic type of bone destruction
- Surrounding edema
- Prominent fluid-fluid levels

Fibrous Dysplasia
- No trabeculation
- Ground glass, smoky appearance
- No "fallen-fragment sign" in case of fracture

Fibroxanthoma
- Eccentric lesion
- Thin or scalloped sclerotic margins

Bone Abscess
- Periosteal reaction
- Cortical destruction
- Sinus tract

Enchondroma
- Calcified matrix
- Lytic in hands

Langerhans Cell Histiocytosis
- Destructive lesion
- Surrounding bone marrow edema

Brown Tumors
- Hyperparathyroidism (HPT)
- Associated with other features of HPT
  - Subperiosteal resorption, osteopenia

PATHOLOGY

General Features
- General path comments
  - Fluid containing lesion lined by mesenchymal cells
  - Only primary true cyst of bone that conforms to pathologic definition of cyst
- Genetics: Case report of translocation (16;20) (p11.2;q13)
- Etiology
  - Unknown
  - Appears to be reactive or developmental rather than neoplastic
  - Possibly due to lymphatic or venous obstruction or synovial rests that produce joint fluid
  - Venous obstruction in area of rapidly growing and remodeling bone
- Epidemiology: 3% of primary bone lesions

Gross Pathologic & Surgical Features
- Intact specimens rarely seen
- Intramedullary cavity filled with clear or yellow fluid with low viscosity
- Fluid under pressure
- Septation with multiple cavities occasionally seen
- Spongy component composed of multiple smaller cysts can be present

UNICAMERAL BONE CYST

- Wall composed of paper thin (1 mm), tan-yellow fibrous tissue with bony ridges
- Intact periosteum

Microscopic Features
- Wall of lesion has no epithelial lining
  - Fibrous and granulation tissue, hemosiderin deposits and small lymphocytes within cyst wall
  - Giant cells of osteoclastic type in cyst wall
  - Fibrinous debris may undergo calcification simulating cementum
- Fluid usually shows elevated alkaline phosphatase
- Fluid contains prostaglandins and interleukins (can cause bone resorption)
- Blood products in cyst fluid in case of prior fracture

CLINICAL ISSUES

Presentation
- Most common signs/symptoms
  - Most lesions asymptomatic
  - Pain, swelling, stiffness at closest joint
- Clinical profile
  - 66% of cysts present with pathologic fractures
    - Sudden onset of pain, often during exercise (playing tennis, soccer)
  - Growth arrest in 10% of patients
    - Due to pathologic fracture (+/- surgical curettage), extension to physeal plate
  - Older patients with involvement of atypical sites (calcaneus, talus, ilium) usually asymptomatic

Demographics
- Age: 10-20 years, 3-14 years: 80%
- Gender: M:F = 2-3:1

Natural History & Prognosis
- Benign lesion, no malignant transformation
- Enlarge during skeletal growth
- Inactive, latent after skeletal maturity
- Spontaneous regression in majority of cases
- Recurrence rate after injection, curettage: 20-45%

Treatment
- Trephination: Drilling multiple holes into lesion +/- irrigation
  - Performed in the operating room under general anesthesia
- Dual needle aspiration and percutaneous injection of corticosteroids (80-200 mg methylprednisolone)
  - 1-3 injection at 2 months interval
- Percutaneous injection of demineralized bone matrix and autogenous bone marrow
- Open curettage with bone graft in weight bearing bones
  - Recurrence 40-45%
  - Damage to growth plate may result in growth arrest
- Subtotal resection, allografting, packing with synthetic materials

DIAGNOSTIC CHECKLIST

Consider
- Starts at one end of bone, migrates towards diaphysis with bone growth

Image Interpretation Pearls
- Fallen fragment sign is pathognomonic, indicates that lesion is fluid-filled

SELECTED REFERENCES

1. Richkind KE et al: Translocation (16;20) (p11.2;q13): Sole cytogenetic abnormality in a unicameral bone cyst. Cancer Genet Cytogenet 137:153-5, 2002
2. Rougraff BT et al: Treatment of active unicameral bone cyst with percutaneous injection of demineralized bone matrix and autogenous bone marrow. J Bone Joint Surg 84-A:921-9, 2002
3. Wilkins RM: Unicameral bone cysts. J Am Acad Orthop Surg 8:217-24, 2000
4. Greenspan A et al: Differential diagnosis of tumors and tumor-like lesions of bones and joints. 1st ed. Philadelphia PA, Lippincott-Raven, 322-9, 1998
5. Lokiec F et al: Simple bone cyst: Etiology, classification, pathology, and treatment modalities. J Pediatr Orthop B 7:262-73, 1998
6. Capanna R et al: Unicameral and aneurysmal bone cysts. Orthop Clin North Am 27:605-14, 1996
7. Kransdorf MJ et al: Aneurysmal bone cyst: Concept, controversy, clinical presentation, and imaging. Am J Roentgenol 164:573-80, 1995
8. Conway WF et al: Miscellaneous lesions of bone. Radiol Clin North Am 31:339-58, 1993
9. Mylle J et al: Simple bone cysts: A review of 59 cases with special reference to their treatment. Arch Orthop Trauma Surg 111:297-300, 1992
10. Rud B et al: Simple bone cysts in children treated with methylprednisolone acetate. Orthopedics 14:185-7, 1991
11. Struhl S et al: Solitary (unicameral) bone cyst. The fallen fragment sign revisited. Skeletal Radiol 18:261-5, 1989
12. Blumberg ML: CT of iliac unicameral bone cysts. Am J Roentgenol 136:1231-2, 1981
13. McGlynn FJ et al: The fallen fragment sign in unicameral bone cyst. Clin Orthop 156:157-9, 1981
14. Weisel A et al: Development of a unicameral bone cyst. J Bone Joint Surg 62A:664-6, 1980
15. Norman A et al: Simple bone cyst: Factors of age dependency. Radiology 124:779-82,1977

UNICAMERAL BONE CYST

Typical

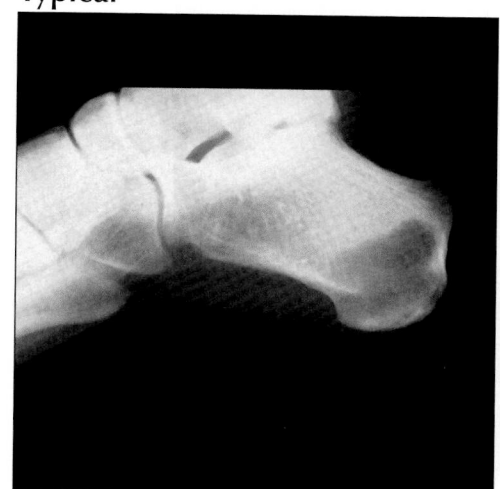

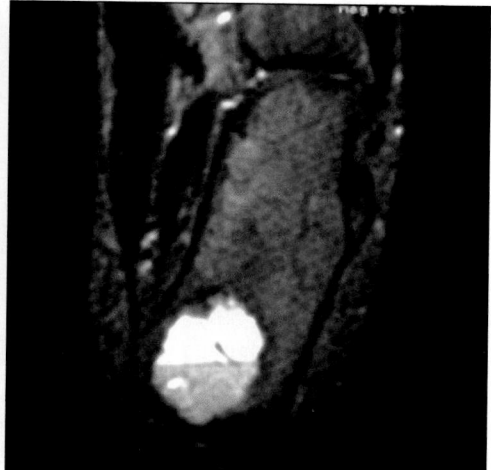

(Left) Lateral radiography shows a well-defined lytic lesion in the calcaneus. *(Right)* Axial FS T2 FSE MR shows a hyperintense lesion in the calcaneus with fluid-fluid levels.

Typical

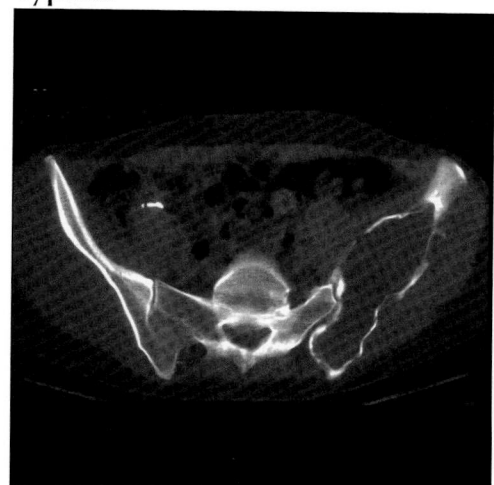

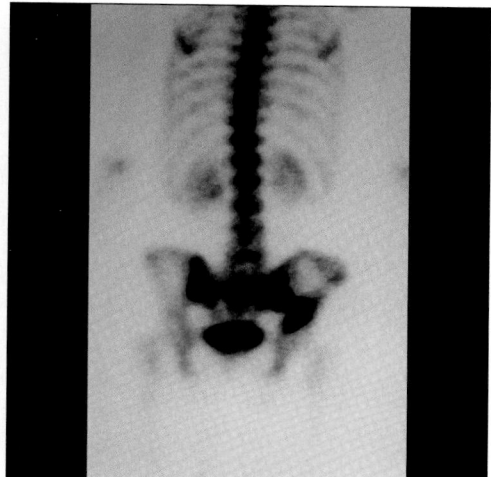

(Left) Axial NECT shows a lytic expansile lesion in the central iliac bone. Cortical thinning without periosteal reaction is noted. *(Right)* Anteroposterior bone scan shows expansion of the left iliac wing with decreased radiotracer uptake.

Variant

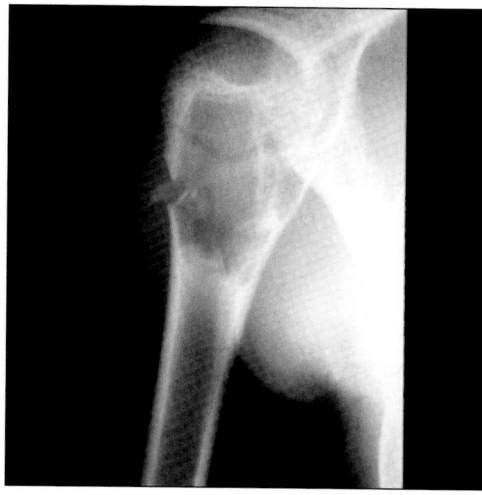

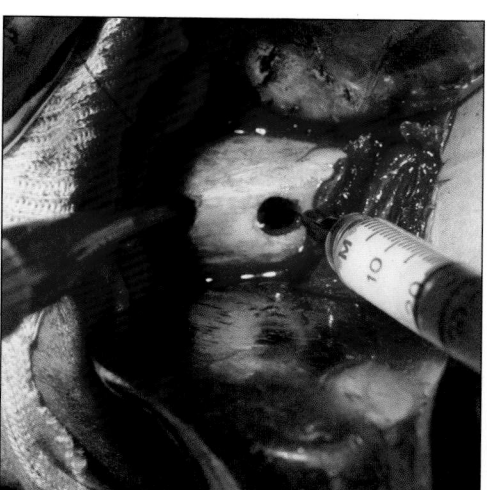

(Left) Anteroposterior radiography shows a lytic lesion in the proximal humerus with pathologic fracture. Note the osseous fragment in the dependent portion of the cyst (fallen fragment sign). *(Right)* Intra-operative photograph shows injection of corticosteroids into an UBC.

ANEURYSMAL BONE CYST

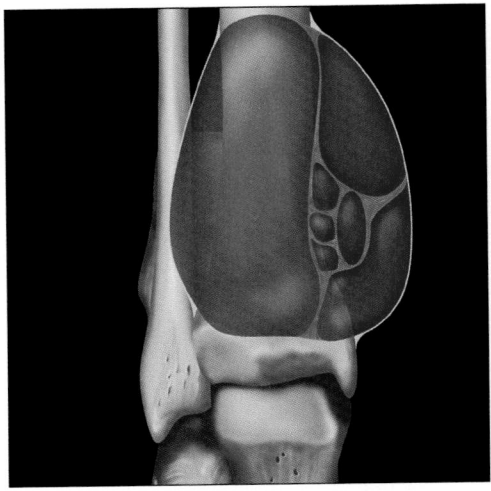

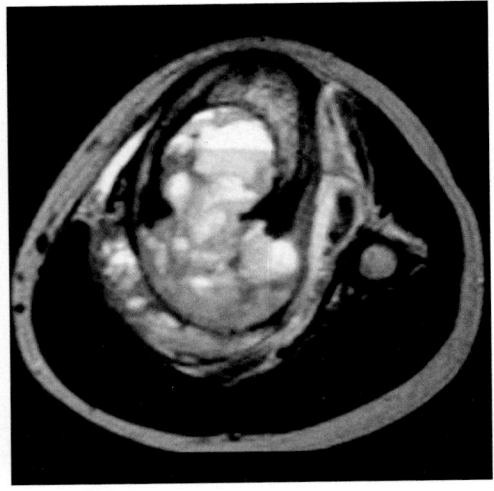

Coronal graphic shows an expansile, septated lesion in the distal tibia. Thinned but intact cortex is shown.

Axial T2WI MR shows an expansile lesion with fluid-fluid levels involving the proximal tibia. Note the surrounding edema.

TERMINOLOGY

Abbreviations and Synonyms
- Aneurysmal bone cyst (ABC)

Definitions
- Expansile lesion of bone containing thin-walled blood filled cystic cavities

IMAGING FINDINGS

General Features
- Best diagnostic clue
  - Radiographs: Expansile lytic lesion with septations
  - MRI: Fluid-fluid levels
- Location
  - Long tubular bones: 70-80%
  - Pelvis: 5-10%
  - Spine (posterior elements): 15%
    - May cross intervertebral disk to involve more than one vertebra
  - Hands: 10-15%
  - Metaphysis: 80-90%
  - Diaphysis: 10-20%
  - Intramedullary (most common)
  - Intracortical, intraperiosteal (rare)
- Size: 2-20 cm; mean: 5-8 cm

- Morphology: Eccentric geographic lytic lesion

Radiographic Findings
- Radiography
  - Multicystic, eccentric expansion of bone with thin periosteal reaction
  - Geographic type of bone destruction with narrow zone of transition
  - Sclerotic margin
  - Trabeculation within lesion
  - Internal calcification rare
  - Phase of rapid growth with marked bone destruction can be mistaken for malignant neoplasm

CT Findings
- NECT
  - Helpful in delineating extent, soft tissue involvement
  - Can show trabeculations
  - Intact, thin cortex
  - HU: 20-78
  - Fluid-fluid levels
- CECT: No enhancement of cystic components

MR Findings
- T1WI: Cyst of different signal intensity (different stages of blood products)
- T2WI

8

66

DDx: Aneurysmal Bone Cyst

Giant Cell Tumor	CMF	Osteosarcoma	UBC	Metastases
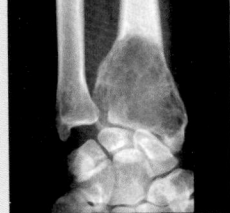	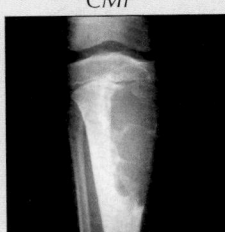	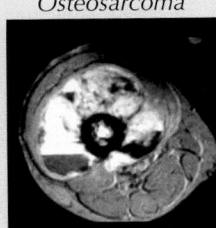	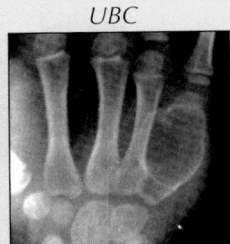	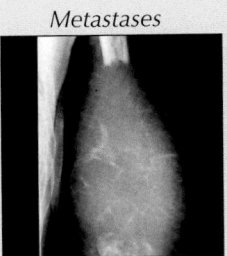
AP Radiography	Lat Radiography	Ax FS T2WI MR	AP Radiography	AP Radiography

ANEURYSMAL BONE CYST

Key Facts

Imaging Findings
- Radiographs: Expansile lytic lesion with septations
- MRI: Fluid-fluid levels

Top Differential Diagnoses
- Unicameral Bone Cyst (UBC)
- Chondromyxoid Fibroma (CMF)
- Telangiectatic Osteosarcoma
- Giant Cell Tumor (GCT)
- Metastases
- Osteoblastoma

Pathology
- Primary ABC
- Arises de-novo in bone without recognizable pre-existing lesion
- Secondary ABC

- Arises in preexisting lesion (benign or malignant neoplasm)
- Epidemiology: 6% of primary bone lesions

Clinical Issues
- Most common signs/symptoms: Progressive pain and swelling
- Locally destructive
- Recurrence in 10-20%
- No malignant transformation
- Curettage, cryosurgery, bone grafting

Diagnostic Checklist
- In case of recurrence, thorough examination of original radiographs and pathology specimens should be performed to exclude underlying neoplasm

---

  - Cysts of different signal intensity (different stages of blood products)
  - Surrounding edema: High signal
- T1 C+
  - No enhancement of cystic components
  - Septal components can enhance ("honeycomb" appearance)
- Well-defined lesion, lobulated contour
- Cystic cavities with fluid-fluid levels
- Internal septations
- Rim of low signal intensity surrounding lesion, represents intact thickened periosteal membrane

Angiographic Findings
- Hypervascular periphery of lesions

Nuclear Medicine Findings
- Bone Scan
  - Doughnut sign
    - Increased peripheral uptake, photopenic center

Imaging Recommendations
- Best imaging tool: Radiographs diagnostic, MRI to detect fluid-fluid levels

DIFFERENTIAL DIAGNOSIS

Unicameral Bone Cyst (UBC)
- Central location
- Little or no expansion
- Fallen fragment sign in case of fracture

Chondromyxoid Fibroma (CMF)
- May be indistinguishable
- Eccentric, expansile
- Metaphyseal
- MR: Solid lesion, no fluid-fluid levels

Telangiectatic Osteosarcoma
- Can be purely lytic
- Soft tissue extension

Giant Cell Tumor (GCT)
- Extends to subchondral bone

- No surrounding sclerosis/periosteal reaction

Metastases
- Usually multifocal
- Destructive

Osteoblastoma
- Can look identical in the spine
- Calcified matrix

PATHOLOGY

General Features
- General path comments
  - Benign lesion characterized by cyst-like walls of fibrous tissue filled with blood
  - Can be easily mistaken for malignant neoplasm (pathologically and radiographically)
- Genetics: (6:17) (p21;p13) gene translocation reported
- Etiology
  - Represents neither cyst nor neoplasm
  - Represents reparative process triggered by tumor or trauma induced vascular process
    - Osseous arterio-venous malformation, venous obstruction
  - Primary ABC
    - Arises de-novo in bone without recognizable pre-existing lesion
    - Can be caused by trauma
  - Secondary ABC
    - Arises in preexisting lesion (benign or malignant neoplasm)
    - Benign tumors: Giant cell tumor, osteoblastoma, chondroblastomas, fibrous dysplasia
    - Malignant tumors: Osteosarcoma, chondrosarcoma, malignant fibrous histiocytoma (MFH)
- Epidemiology: 6% of primary bone lesions

Gross Pathologic & Surgical Features
- Cavernous blood-filled spaces lined by fibrous walls
- "Blood-filled sponge"

ANEURYSMAL BONE CYST

- Fluid-fluid levels represent sedimentation of red blood cells and serum within cystic cavities

Microscopic Features

- Blood-filled spaces alternating with more solid areas
- Lined by single layer of flat undifferentiated cells
  - Endothelial lining rarely seen
- Fibrous lining contains giant cells
- Solid tissue composed of fibrous, highly vascular, connective tissue

CLINICAL ISSUES

Presentation

- Most common signs/symptoms: Progressive pain and swelling
- Clinical profile
  - Rapid increase of pain over 6-12 weeks
  - Spinal lesions may cause cord compression (radiculopathy, quadriplegia), nerve root impingement
    - Scoliosis: 10%
  - Pathologic fracture: 20%
  - Limited range of motion if close to joint
  - History of trauma

Demographics

- Age
  - 10-30 years old
  - < 20 years in 76%
- Gender: M:F = 1:1.2

Natural History & Prognosis

- Benign
- Locally destructive
- Recurrence in 10-20%
- Recurrence increased in young patients with open growth plate
- No malignant transformation
- Never metastasizes

Treatment

- Options, risks, complications
  - Important to identify underlying lesion which will change treatment
  - Curettage, cryosurgery, bone grafting
  - Resection
    - Risk of bleeding during surgery
    - Preoperative embolization
  - Embolotherapy
    - Complications: Aseptic necrosis
  - Percutaneous Ethibloc injection
  - Radiation therapy
    - Risk of sarcomatous degeneration

DIAGNOSTIC CHECKLIST

Consider

- In case of recurrence, thorough examination of original radiographs and pathology specimens should be performed to exclude underlying neoplasm

Image Interpretation Pearls

- Only osseous neoplasm named for its radiologic appearance

SELECTED REFERENCES

1. Mahnken AH et al: Aneurysmal bone cyst: Value of MR imaging and conventional radiography. Eur Radiol 13:1118-24, 2003
2. Falappa P et al: Aneurysmal bone cysts: Treatment with direct percutaneous Ethibloc injection: Long term results. Cardiovasc Intervent Radiol 25:282-90, 2002
3. Woertler K et al: Imaging features of subperiosteal aneurysmal bone cyst. Acta Radiol 43:336-9, 2002
4. Greenspan A et al: Differential diagnosis of tumors and tumor-like lesions of bones and joints. 1st ed. Philadelphia PA, Lippincott-Raven, 329-39, 1998
5. Kransdorf MJ et al: Aneurysmal bone cyst: Concept, controversy, clinical presentation, and imaging. Am J Roentgenol 164:573-80, 1995
6. Freiberg AA et al: Aneurysmal bone cyst in young children. J Pediatr Orthop 14:86-91, 1994
7. Wojno KJ et al: Fibro-osseous lesions of the face and skull with aneurysmal bone cyst formation. Skeletal Radiol 23:15-8, 1994
8. Gipple JR et al: Solid aneurysmal bone cyst. Orthopedics 15:1433-6, 1992
9. Murphy WA et al: Transcatheter embolization therapy of an ischial aneurysmal bone cyst. J Bone Joint Surg 64B:166-8, 1992
10. Vergel de Dios AM et al: Aneurysmal bone cyst. A clinicopathologic study of 238 cases. Cancer 69:2921-31, 1992
11. Martinez V et al: Aneurysmal bone cyst: A review of 123 cases including primary lesions and those secondary to other bone pathology. Cancer 61:2291-304, 1988

ANEURYSMAL BONE CYST

Typical

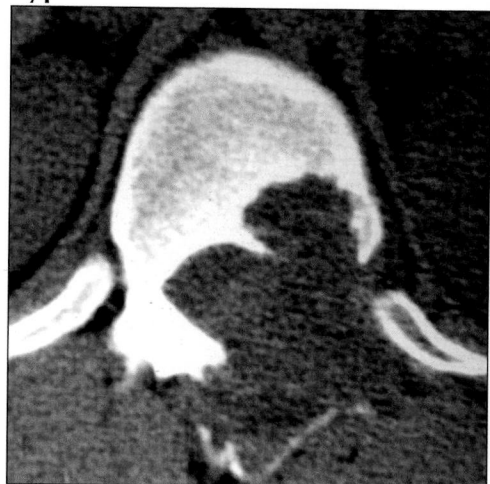
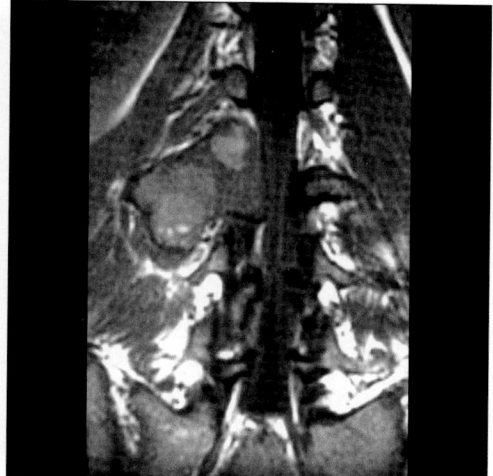

(Left) Axial NECT shows a lytic expansile lesion involving the posterior elements of a thoracic vertebra. There is no mineralized matrix. The lesion is surrounded by a thin shell of bone. *(Right)* Coronal T1WI MR shows expansile lesion with fluid-fluid levels involving the right posterior elements of L3.

Variant

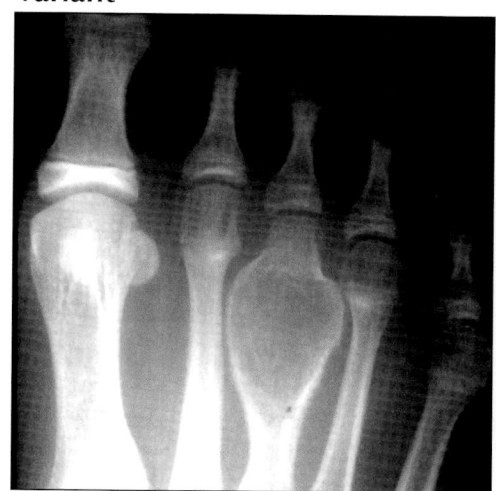
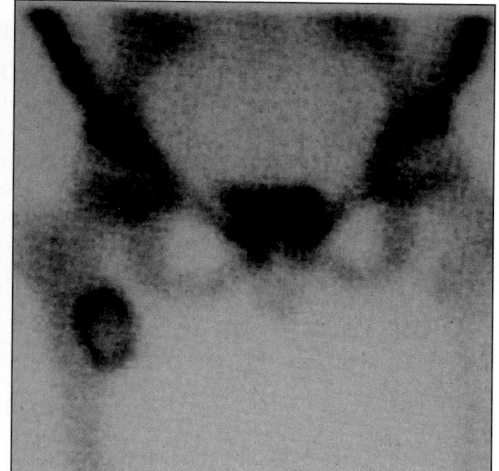

(Left) Anteroposterior radiography shows a lytic expansile lesion involving the third metatarsal bone. There is a thin shell of periosteal bone surrounding the lesion. *(Right)* Anteroposterior bone scan shows increased radiotracer uptake in the periphery of the femoral metaphysis and decreased uptake in the central portion (doughnut sign).

Other

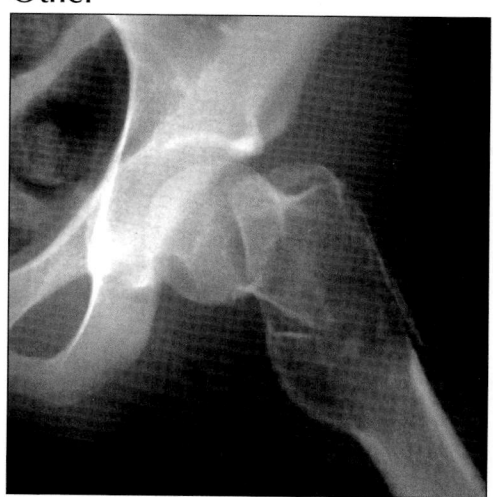
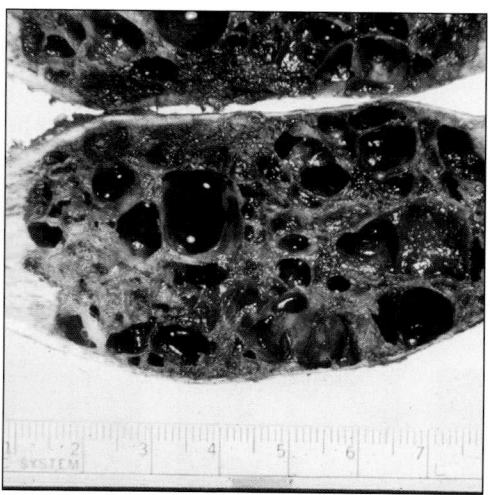

(Left) Anteroposterior radiography shows a lytic expansile lesion in the proximal femoral metaphysis with pathologic fracture. *(Right)* Gross pathology shows hemorrhagic and cystic lesion with multiple septations ("blood-filled sponge").

INTRAOSSEOUS LIPOMA

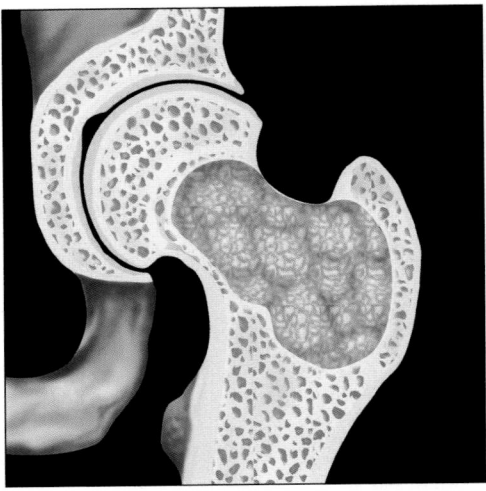

Coronal graphic shows lipomatous tumor (in yellow) involving the proximal femoral metaphysis. There is no cortical destruction or extraosseous extension.

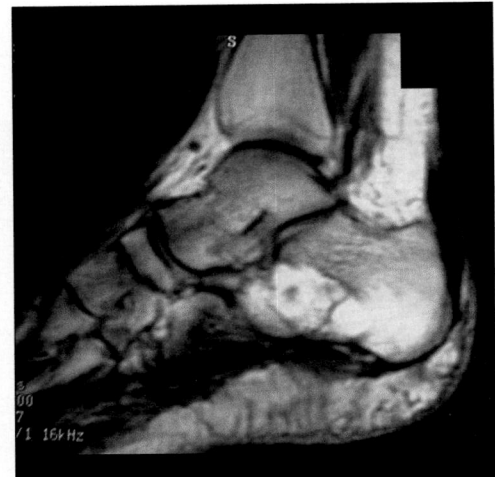

Sagittal T1WI MR shows calcaneal lesion almost entirely composed of fat. Central area of low SI is consistent with calcification. This corresponds to a Stage 1 lesion.

TERMINOLOGY

Abbreviations and Synonyms
- Lipoma of bone

Definitions
- Bone tumor comprised of mature adipose tissue

IMAGING FINDINGS

General Features
- Best diagnostic clue
  - MRI: Follows signal intensity of subcutaneous fat on all pulse sequences
  - CT: -40 to -100 HU (fat)
- Location
  - Metaphysis of long bones: 60%
    - Femur (inter-subtrochanteric area), tibia, fibula, humerus
  - Calcaneus: 10%
  - Ribs: 10%
  - Craniofacial bones: 10%
  - Pelvis: 6%
  - Spine: 4%
  - Solitary lesion
  - Intramedullary
  - Parosteal

- Size: 2-15 cm, mean: 3-6 cm
- Morphology: Expansile lesion containing fat

Radiographic Findings
- Radiography
  - Lytic lesion with trabeculation
  - Bone expansion with thinned, intact cortex
  - No periosteal reaction
  - Central calcifications (dystrophic calcification from fat necrosis)
  - Sclerotic, osseous pedicle in parosteal lipoma
    - Grows from bone surface into adipose tissue

CT Findings
- NECT
  - -40 to -100 HU
  - Central cyst formation: 0-20 HU
  - Peripheral calcification
- CECT: No enhancement

MR Findings
- T1WI
  - Tumor: High signal intensity
  - Cysts: Intermediate signal intensity
  - Peripheral rim of low signal intensity (calcification)
- T2WI
  - Tumor: Intermediate signal intensity
  - Cyst: High signal intensity
  - FS T2 FSE

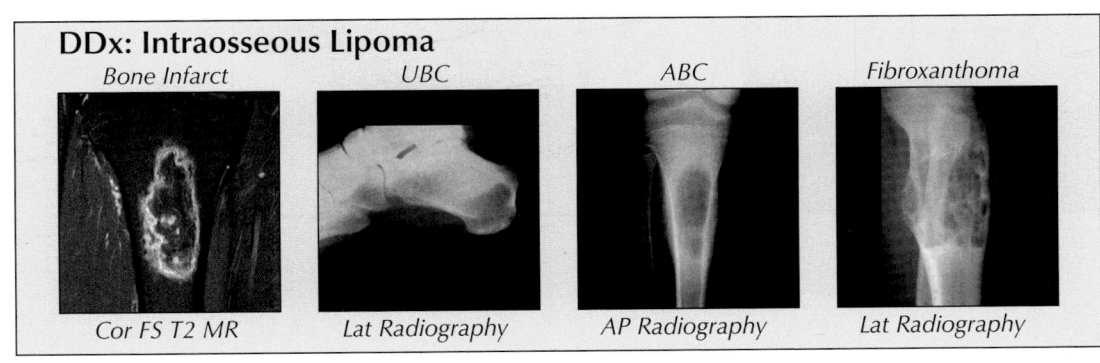

DDx: Intraosseous Lipoma

Bone Infarct	UBC	ABC	Fibroxanthoma
Cor FS T2 MR	Lat Radiography	AP Radiography	Lat Radiography

INTRAOSSEOUS LIPOMA

Key Facts

Imaging Findings
- MRI: Follows signal intensity of subcutaneous fat on all pulse sequences
- CT: -40 to -100 HU (fat)

Top Differential Diagnoses
- Medullary Bone Infarct
- Unicameral Bone Cyst (UBC)
- Aneurysmal Bone Cyst (ABC)
- Fibroxanthoma
- Pseudotumor

Pathology
- Controversial if lesion represents true benign tumor of fat or is end result of involution of other bone lesions
- Reported incidence: 0.1% of all primary bone tumor

- Likely more frequent with the advent of CT and MRI

Clinical Issues
- Most common signs/symptoms: Usually asymptomatic
- Pain, swelling
- Slow growing benign tumor
- Malignant transformation extremely rare
- Asymptomatic lesions require no treatment
- Curettage and packing with bone graft in large lesions with risk of fracture

Diagnostic Checklist
- Areas of osteoporosis and prominent trabeculae may mimic intraosseous lipoma
- Follows signal intensity of fat on all pulse sequences

- Tumor: Dark (fat suppression)
- Cyst: High signal intensity
  - T2 FSE
    - Tumor: High signal intensity
    - Cysts: High signal intensity
- STIR
  - Tumor: Dark
  - Cyst: Bright
- T2* GRE: Areas of low signal intensity (calcifications)
- T1 C+: No enhancement
- Follows signal intensity of subcutaneous fat on all pulse sequences
- Homogeneous in majority of cases
  - Heterogeneous in cases of hemorrhage, myxomatous degeneration
- Helpful in demonstrating intraosseous extension

Nuclear Medicine Findings
- Bone Scan
  - Variable
  - Can be normal
  - Peripheral increased uptake

Imaging Recommendations
- Best imaging tool: MRI
- Protocol advice: MRI with and without fat suppression

DIFFERENTIAL DIAGNOSIS

Medullary Bone Infarct
- Dense serpiginous peripheral calcifications
  - Lipoma: Central calcifications
- No osseous expansion
- Can be multifocal

Unicameral Bone Cyst (UBC)
- Well-defined, central, lucent lesion
- Scalloping of underlying cortex
- Fluid-filled
- Fallen fragment sign in case of fracture (excludes solid lesion)
- No fat on CT/MRI

Aneurysmal Bone Cyst (ABC)
- Eccentric, expansile lesion
- Fluid-fluid levels
- No fat on CT/MRI

Fibroxanthoma
- Eccentric location
- Thin scalloped sclerotic margins
- No central calcifications
- No fat on CT/MRI

Pseudotumor
- Normal zone of porosity in anterior calcaneus, subtrochanteric femur
- No discrete mass
- No margins

PATHOLOGY

General Features
- General path comments
  - Tumor composed of mature fat cells
    - Variable small quantities of fat necrosis, cysts formation, and dystrophic calcifications
- Etiology
  - Controversial if lesion represents true benign tumor of fat or is end result of involution of other bone lesions
    - May be the result of involuting bone infarcts, infection, other inflammatory processes
- Epidemiology
  - Reported incidence: 0.1% of all primary bone tumor
  - Likely more frequent with the advent of CT and MRI
- Associated abnormalities
  - Multiple lipomatosis:
    - Fat deposition due to associated endocrine abnormalities (Type IV hyperlipoproteinemia)

Gross Pathologic & Surgical Features
- Circumscribed lobular mass, composed of yellow, soft adipose tissue
- Tumor may be encapsulated

INTRAOSSEOUS LIPOMA

- Central areas of necrosis and dystrophic calcifications may be present

Microscopic Features
- Consists of lobules of mature lipocytes
  - Lipocytes slightly larger than non-neoplastic fat cells
- Fat necrosis with dystrophic calcifications can be present
  - Bone cysts may form in calcified regions

Staging, Grading or Classification Criteria
- Milgram staging system
  - Stage I: Viable mature lipocytes interspersed with fine bony trabeculae
    - Fat identical to subcutaneous fat, no cellular atypia
    - Areas of remodeling, intact cortex
  - Stage II: Expansion of lipocytes within trabeculae
    - Areas of infarction, necrotic adipose tissue, calcifications
  - Stage III: Extension of infarction to involve entire lesion
    - Necrotic fat, calcifications, cyst formation, reactive new bone formation
    - Resembles bone infarct

CLINICAL ISSUES

Presentation
- Most common signs/symptoms: Usually asymptomatic
- Clinical profile
  - Pain, swelling
  - Micro-trabecular fractures in area of weakened bone

Demographics
- Age: 5-75 years, mean: 38 years
- Gender: M:F = 1:1
- Ethnicity: No racial predilection

Natural History & Prognosis
- Slow growing benign tumor
- Malignant transformation extremely rare

Treatment
- Asymptomatic lesions require no treatment
- Curettage and packing with bone graft in large lesions with risk of fracture

DIAGNOSTIC CHECKLIST

Consider
- Areas of osteoporosis and prominent trabeculae may mimic intraosseous lipoma

Image Interpretation Pearls
- Follows signal intensity of fat on all pulse sequences

SELECTED REFERENCES

1. Campbell RS et al: Intraosseous lipoma: Report of 35 new cases and a review of the literature. Skeletal Radiol 32:209-22, 2003
2. Goto T et al: Intraosseous lipoma: A clinical study of 12 patients. J Orthop Sci 7:274-80, 2002
3. Jebson PJ et al: Intraosseous lipoma of the proximal radius with extraosseous extension and a secondary posterior interosseous nerve palsy. Am J Orthop 31:413-6, 2002
4. Propeck T et al: Radiologic-pathologic correlation of intraosseous lipomas. Am J Roentgenol 175:673-8, 2000
5. Greenspan A et al: Differential diagnosis of tumors and tumor-like lesions of bones and joints. 1st ed. Philadelphia PA, Lippincott-Raven, 339-42, 1998
6. Greenspan A et al: Intraosseous lipoma of the calcaneus. Foot Ankle Int 18:53-6, 1997
7. Levin MF et al: Intraosseous lipoma of the distal femur: MRI appearance. Skeletal Radiol 25:82-4, 1996
8. Blacksin MF et al: Magnetic resonance imaging of intraosseous lipomas: A radiologic-pathologic correlation. Skeletal Radiol 24:37-41, 1995
9. Rhodes RD et al: Intraosseous lipoma of the os calcis. J Am Podiatr Med Assoc 83:288-92, 1993
10. Williams CE et al: Intraosseous lipomas. Clin Radiol 47:348-50, 1993
11. Milgram JW: Intraosseous lipoma: Radiologic and pathologic manifestations. Radiology 167:155-60, 1988
12. Dooms GC et al: Lipomatous tumors and tumors with fatty component: MR imaging potential and comparison of MR and CT results. Radiology 157:479-83, 1985
13. Ramos A et al: Intraosseous lipoma: CT appearance. Radiology 157:615-9,1985
14. Milgram JW: Intraosseous lipomas with reactive ossification in the proximal femur. Report of eight cases. Skeletal Radiol 7:1-13, 1981
15. Freiberg RA et al: Multiple intraosseous lipomas with type-IV hyperlipoproteinemia. A case report. J Bone Joint Surg 56-A:1729-32, 1974
16. Zorn DT et al: Intraosseous lipoma of bone involving the sacrum. J Bone Joint Surg 53-A:1201-4, 1971

INTRAOSSEOUS LIPOMA

IMAGE GALLERY

Typical

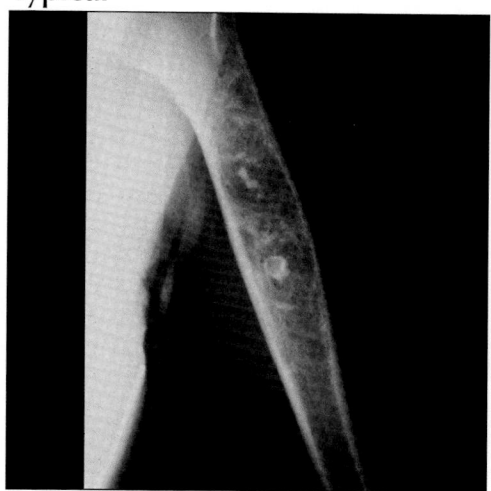

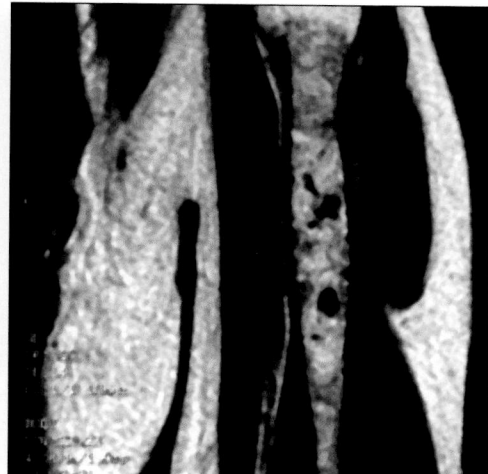

(Left) Anteroposterior radiography shows a lytic lesion with central calcifications in the humeral diaphysis. *(Right)* Coronal T1WI MR shows the humeral diaphyseal lesion to be of heterogeneous SI with areas following SI of fat and calcifications.

Typical

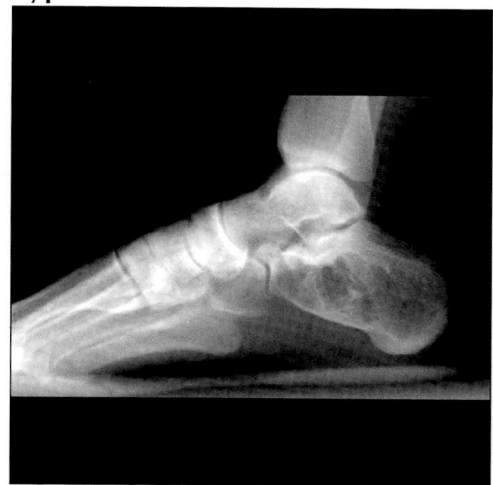

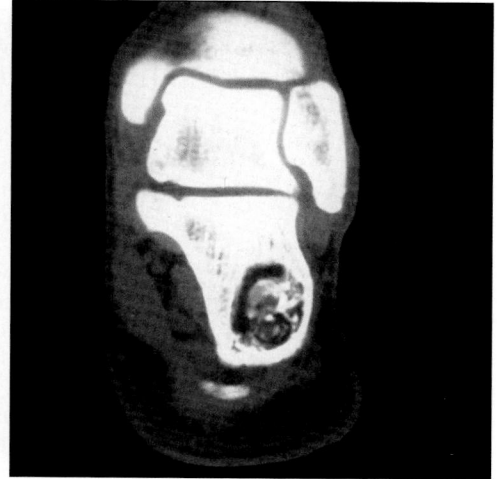

(Left) Lateral radiography shows lytic lesion in the calcaneus of fat density with central calcification. *(Right)* Axial NECT shows a calcaneal lesion of fat density with central calcifications and cyst formation.

Typical

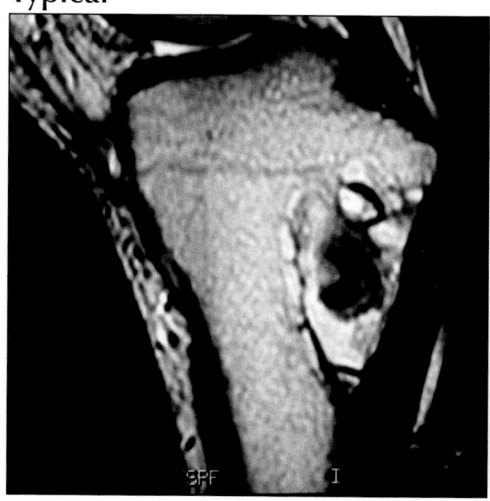

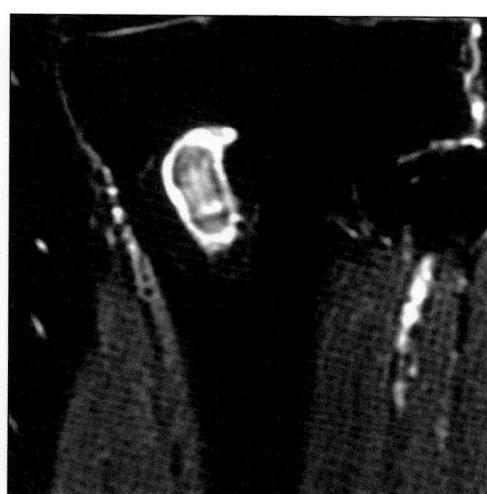

(Left) Sagittal T1WI MR shows a lesion in the tibial metaphysis with SI of fat and central areas of low SI, consistent with calcification. *(Right)* Sagittal FS T2 FSE MR shows saturation of previously noted areas of high SI, corresponding to fat. Central area of intermediate SI with surrounding rim of high SI corresponds to calcifications and fluid.

ADAMANTINOMA

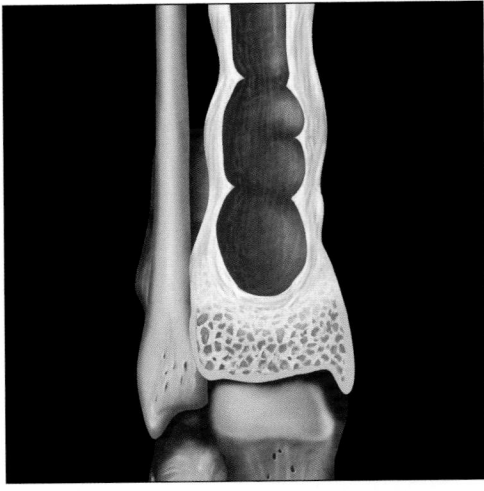

Coronal graphic shows lobulated expansile tumor in the tibial metadiaphysis.

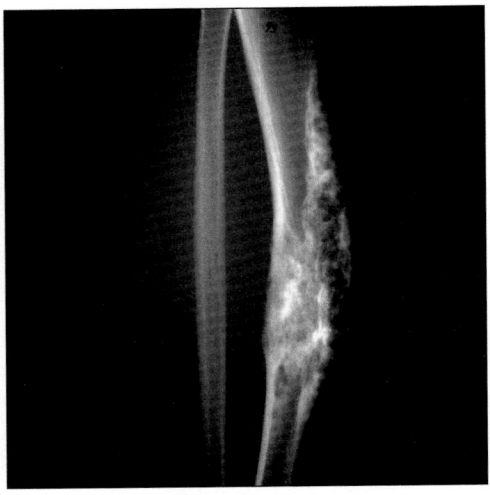

Lateral radiography shows multiple, confluent lytic lesions with areas of sclerosis involving the tibial diaphysis.

TERMINOLOGY

Abbreviations and Synonyms
- Angioblastoma, malignant angioblastoma, differentiated adamantinoma

Definitions
- Low-grade malignant tumor with preferential involvement of the tibia

IMAGING FINDINGS

General Features
- Best diagnostic clue: Large, lobulated, expansile lytic lesion in tibial meta-diaphysis
- Location
  - Tibia: 80%
  - Tibia and fibula: 5%
  - Femur: 5%
  - Humerus: 4%
  - Ulna: 3%
  - Fibula: 1%
  - Anterior metadiaphysis
- Size: 3-16 cm, mean: 11 cm
- Morphology
  - Eccentric, expansile, lytic lesion
  - Can break through cortex, soft tissue extension

Radiographic Findings
- Radiography
  - Well-defined, eccentric lesion in anterior tibial metadiaphysis
    - Can extend to ends of bone
  - Multiple lytic lesions with sclerotic intervening bone
  - Additional foci in continuity with dominant lesion
  - Sclerotic, ground glass appearance in long standing lesions
  - Can have soap bubble appearance
  - Expansion and destruction of cortex
    - Saw-toothed pattern of cortical destruction
    - Soft tissue mass
  - Bowing deformity of tibia
  - Intracortical or intramedullary involvement
  - Classic adamantinoma: Destructive growth
    - Older patients (> 20 years)
  - Differentiated adamantinoma: Intracortical, multicentric
    - Osteofibrous dysplasia-like pattern
    - Younger patients (< 20 years)

CT Findings
- NECT
  - Expansile lytic intramedullary lesion
    - Low attenuation lesion
  - Helpful in demonstrating cortical disruption and associated soft tissue mass

DDx: Adamantinoma

Fibrous Dysplasia	CMF	Metastases	Fibroxanthoma	Osteomyelitis
Lat Radiography	Lat Radiography	AP Radiography	AP Radiography	Lat Radiography

ADAMANTINOMA

Key Facts

Imaging Findings
- Best diagnostic clue: Large, lobulated, expansile lytic lesion in tibial meta-diaphysis

Top Differential Diagnoses
- Osteofibrous Dysplasia
- Fibroxanthoma
- Chondromyxoid Fibroma (CMF)
- Osteomyelitis
- Metastases

Pathology
- Possibly related to osteofibrous dysplasia
- Epidemiology: 0.1% of all primary bone tumors

Clinical Issues
- Dull aching pain

- Swelling near shin
- History of trauma in 60%
- Low grade malignancy
- Locally aggressive
- Local recurrence: 31%
- Metastases: 15-20%
- 10 year survival: 10-65%
- En bloc excision with wide surgical margins, bone graft

Diagnostic Checklist
- Location: Anterior tibia
- Age: Fused growth plate
- Important to differentiate adamantinoma from osteofibrous dysplasia (different management, prognosis)

MR Findings
- T1WI: Low signal intensity
- T2WI: High signal intensity
- T1 C+: Intense enhancement of some foci
- To determine extent of osseous and extraosseous involvement

Nuclear Medicine Findings
- Bone Scan: Increased uptake of radiotracer

Imaging Recommendations
- Best imaging tool: Radiographs diagnostic
- Protocol advice: MRI to evaluate intraosseous extent and soft tissue involvement

DIFFERENTIAL DIAGNOSIS

Osteofibrous Dysplasia
- Younger age
- Involves anterior tibial cortex
  - Adamantinoma more eccentric
- Well-defined
- Less aggressive
- No cortical destruction

Fibroxanthoma
- Lobulated, well-defined lesion with sclerotic borders
- No cortical invasion
- Periosteal reaction only in case of fracture

Chondromyxoid Fibroma (CMF)
- Expansile lytic lesion with sclerotic margins
- Geographic pattern of bone destruction
- No cortical invasion
- Matrix calcification rare

Osteomyelitis
- Periosteal reaction
- Sequestrum

Metastases
- Often multifocal
  - Use bone scan to look for additional lesions

- Isolated metastasis to tibia extremely rare

PATHOLOGY

General Features
- General path comments
  - Low grade malignant tumor characterized by formation of epithelial cells surrounded by spindle cell fibrous tissue
  - Stromal component with fibrous dysplasia-like features present in many cases
  - Resembles ameloblastoma (adamantinoma) of jaw
- Genetics: Translocation in region 13q14
- Etiology
  - Epithelial origin
  - Possibly related to osteofibrous dysplasia
- Epidemiology: 0.1% of all primary bone tumors

Gross Pathologic & Surgical Features
- Gray-white tumor of firm to soft consistency
- Smooth or lobulated
- Circumscribed at periphery
- Cystic degeneration, areas of hemorrhage
- May contain spicules of bone, cystic cavities, or straw colored fluid
- Involvement of cortex and periosteum common
- Can extent into soft tissues

Microscopic Features
- Epithelial component admixed with fibrous component
- Epithelial component: Islands of polyhedral cells
  - Peripheral nuclear palisading
  - Palisading and columnar arrangement of peripheral cells with stellate central cells
    - Resembles ameloblastoma of the jaw
  - Prominent keratin staining
- Hypocellular fibrous connective tissue in spaces between epithelioid islands
- Epithelial spaces and stroma may be highly vascular
  - Lesion may resemble vascular neoplasm
- May have foci of Ewing-like areas (worse prognosis)

ADAMANTINOMA

- May have osteofibrous dysplasia-like areas

Staging, Grading or Classification Criteria
- Surgical staging system for malignant musculoskeletal tumors
  - Stage IA: Low grade, intracompartmental
  - Stage IB: Low grade, extracompartmental
  - Stage IIA: High grade, intracompartmental
  - Stage IIB: High grade, extracompartmental
  - Stage IIIA: Low or high grade, intracompartmental, metastases
  - Stage IIIB: Low or high grade, extracompartmental, metastases

CLINICAL ISSUES

Presentation
- Most common signs/symptoms
  - Dull aching pain
  - Swelling near shin
- Clinical profile
  - Duration of symptoms: Months to years
  - Firm tender mass
  - History of trauma in 60%
  - Two case reports of paraneoplastic hypercalcemia

Demographics
- Age: 11-70 years, mean: 35 years
- Gender: M:F = 1.7:1
- Ethnicity: No racial predilection

Natural History & Prognosis
- Low grade malignancy
- Locally aggressive
- Local recurrence: 31%
  - Tumor can recur up to 7 years following diagnosis
- Metastases: 15-20%
  - Metastasizes to lungs, other bones, lymph nodes, liver
  - Metastases occur late, 2-5 years after diagnosis
- 10 year survival: 10-65%
- Highest mortality rate in young women

Treatment
- En bloc excision with wide surgical margins, bone graft
- Simple excision with marginal margins has high recurrence rate
- Amputation might be necessary in case of recurrence
- Radiation therapy and chemotherapy not useful

DIAGNOSTIC CHECKLIST

Consider
- Location: Anterior tibia
- Age: Fused growth plate

Image Interpretation Pearls
- Important to differentiate adamantinoma from osteofibrous dysplasia (different management, prognosis)

SELECTED REFERENCES

1. Kahn LB: Adamantinoma, osteofibrous dysplasia and differentiated adamantinoma. Skeletal Radiol 32:245-58, 2003
2. Torriani M et al: Magnetic resonance imaging of tibial classic adamantinoma at 2 tesla. J Comput Assist Tomogr 26:855-9, 2002
3. Dorfman HD et al: Bone tumors. 1st ed. St. Louis MO, Mosby, 949-73, 1998
4. Greenspan A et al: Differential diagnosis of tumors and tumor-like lesions of bones and joints. 1st ed. Philadelphia PA, Lippincott-Raven, 347-50, 1998
5. Zehr RJ et al: Adamantinoma. Skeletal Radiol 24:553-5, 1995
6. Benassi MS et al: Cytokeratin expression and distribution in adamantinoma of the long bones and osteofibrous dysplasia of tibia and fibula. An immunohistochemical study correlated to histogenesis. Histopathology 25:71-6, 1994
7. Hazelbag HM et al: Adamantinoma of the long bones. A clinicopathological study in thirty-two patients with emphasis on histological subtype, precursor lesion, and biological behavior. J Bone Joint Surg 76A:1482-99, 1994
8. Sweet DE et al: Cortical osteofibrous dysplasia of long bone and its relationship to adamantinoma. A clinicopathologic study of 30 cases. Am J Surg Pathol 16:282-90, 1992
9. Adler CP: Case report 587: Adamantinoma of the tibia mimicking osteofibrous dysplasia. Skeletal Radiol 19:55-8, 1990
10. Sozzi G et al: Involvement of the region 13q14 in a patient with adamantinoma of the long bones. Hum Genet 85:513-5, 1990
11. Keeney GL et al: Adamantinoma of long bones. A clinicopathologic study of 85 cases. Cancer 64:730-37, 1989
12. Moon NF et al: Adamantinoma of the appendicular skeleton-updated. Clin Orthop 204:215-37, 1986
13. Alguacil-Garcia A et al: Osteofibrous dysplasia (ossifying fibroma) of the tibia and fibula and adamantinoma. A case report. Am J Clin Pathol 82:470-4, 1984
14. Weiss SW et al: Adamantinoma of long bone. An analysis of nine new cases with emphasis on metastasizing lesions and fibrous dysplasia-like changes. Hum Pathol 8:141-53, 1977

ADAMANTINOMA

IMAGE GALLERY

Typical

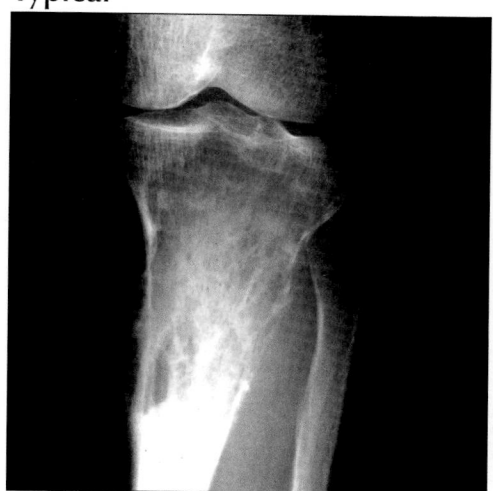

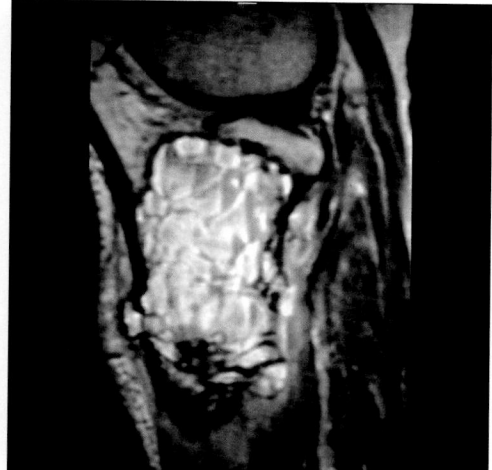

(Left) Anteroposterior radiography shows a lytic expansile lesion involving the proximal tibia. *(Right)* Sagittal T2WI MR shows expansile lesion with increased T2 signal involving the proximal tibia.

Typical

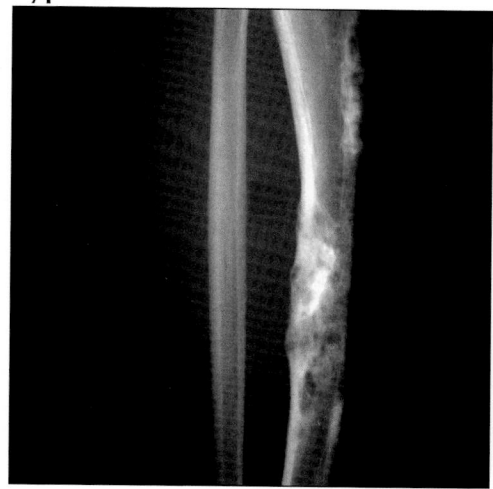

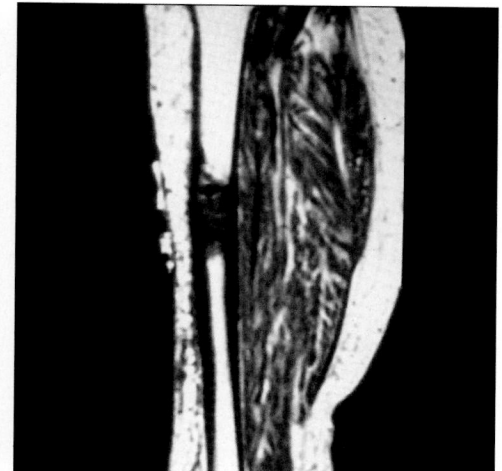

(Left) Lateral radiography shows a mixed sclerotic and lytic lesion with surrounding sclerosis in the mid-tibial diaphysis. *(Right)* Sagittal T1WI MR shows low signal of the mid-tibial diaphyseal lesion. Intraosseous extent is well seen on MRI.

Other

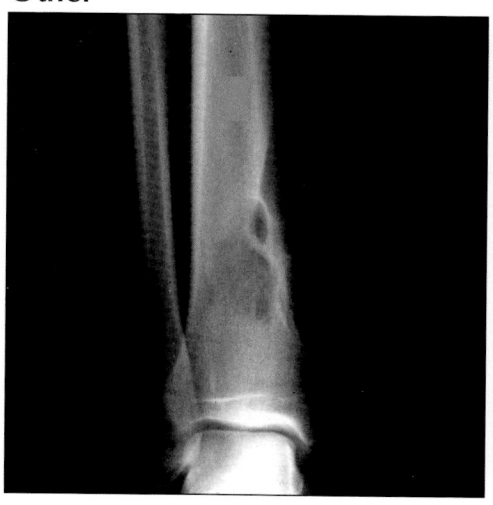

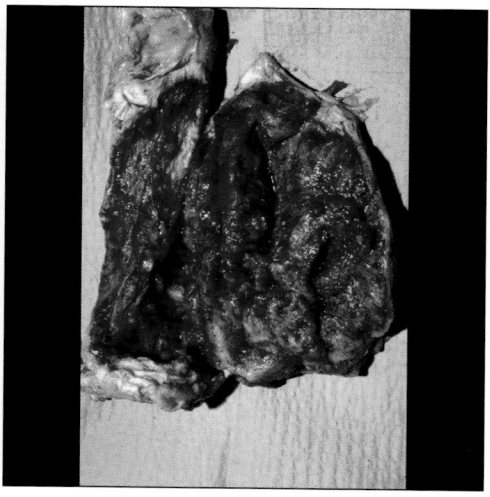

(Left) Anteroposterior radiography shows multiple lytic lesions involving the distal tibial diaphysis. *(Right)* Coronal gross pathology shows lobulated hemorrhagic lesion involving the distal tibia.

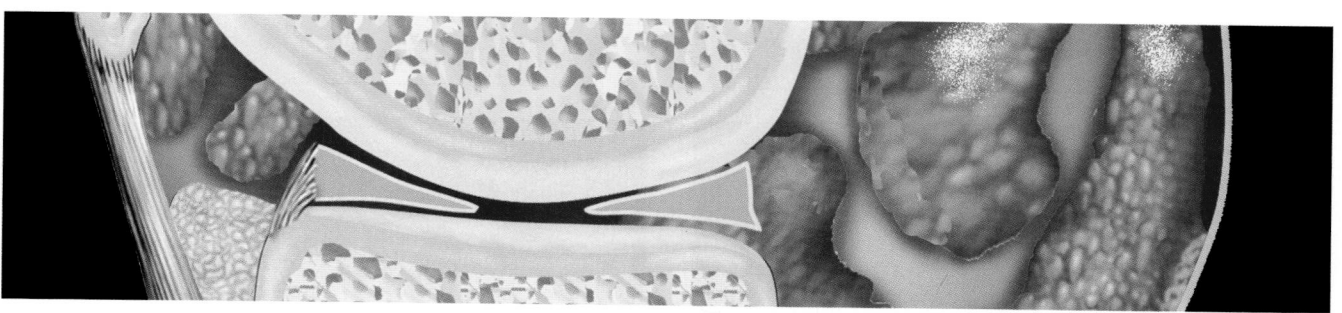

SECTION 9: Soft Tissue Tumors

FIBROSARCOMA, SOFT TISSUE

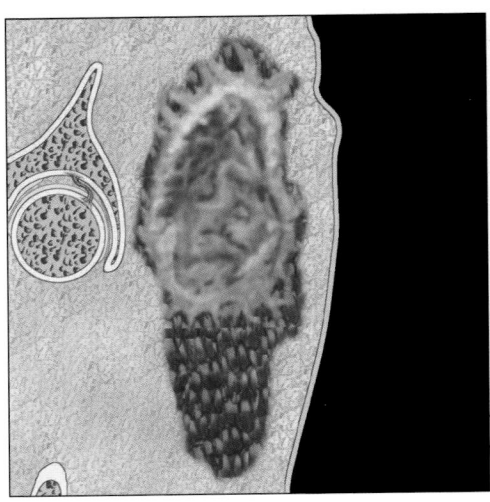

Sagittal graphic shows intramuscular fibrosarcoma in the posterior aspect of the hip. Surrounding pseudocapsule is shown in white.

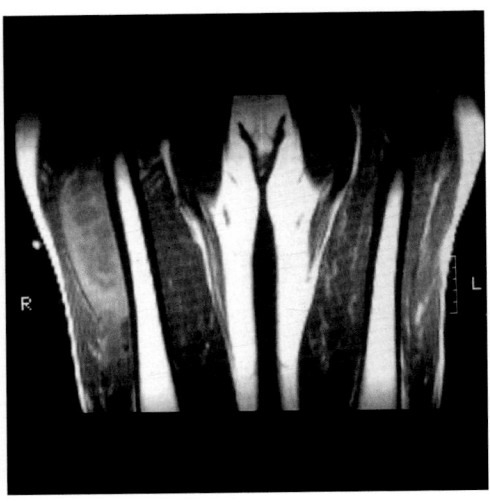

Coronal T1 C+ MR shows a heterogeneous, enhancing, deep soft tissue mass in the lateral right thigh.

TERMINOLOGY

Abbreviations and Synonyms
- Fibroblastic malignancy, mesenchymal sarcoma

Definitions
- Malignant mesenchymal tumor composed of fibroblasts

IMAGING FINDINGS

General Features
- Best diagnostic clue: Heterogeneous hemorrhagic deep soft tissue mass
- Location
  o Deep in large muscle groups of extremities: 75%
    ▪ Lower extremity: 45%
    ▪ Upper extremity: 28%
  o Trunk: 17%
  o Head and neck: 10%
  o Originates from intra- and intermuscular fibrous tissue, aponeuroses, tendons
- Size: 3-10 cm
- Morphology: Heterogeneous, deep soft tissue mass

Radiographic Findings
- Radiography
  o Soft tissue mass

o Poorly defined curvilinear/punctate peripheral calcifications in 5-20%
o Cortical erosions of adjacent bone

CT Findings
- NECT
  o Lobulated soft tissue mass with attenuation similar to muscle
  o Central hypodense areas
    ▪ Correspond to necrosis
  o High attenuation areas
    ▪ Correspond to hemorrhage
- CECT
  o Hypo- or hypervascular
  o Enhancement of solid components

MR Findings
- T1WI
  o Intermediate signal intensity
  o Areas of low signal
    ▪ Correspond to calcifications
- T2WI
  o High signal intensity
  o Areas of low signal
    ▪ Correspond to calcifications
- STIR: High signal intensity
- T1 C+
  o Enhancement of solid components

DDx: Fibrosarcoma, Soft Tissue

MFH	Fibromatosis	Synovial Sarcoma	Liposarcoma	MPNST

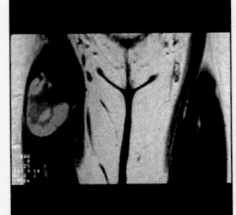
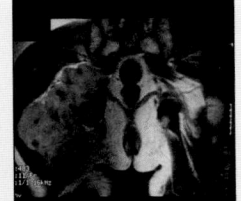
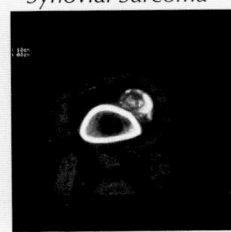
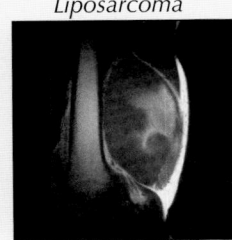
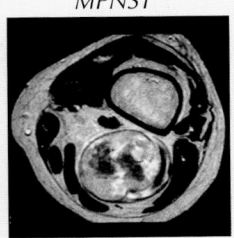

Cor T1WI MR	Cor T1 C+ MR	Ax NECT	Sag T1WI MR	Ax T2WI MR

FIBROSARCOMA, SOFT TISSUE

Key Facts

Imaging Findings

- Best diagnostic clue: Heterogeneous hemorrhagic deep soft tissue mass

Top Differential Diagnoses

- Malignant Fibrous Histiocytoma (MFH)
- Fibromatosis
- Synovial Sarcoma
- Liposarcoma
- Malignant Peripheral Nerve Sheath Tumor (MPNST)
- Hematoma

Pathology

- Clinically and radiographically similar to malignant fibrous histiocytoma
- Epidemiology: 5% of soft tissue sarcomas

Clinical Issues

- Most common signs/symptoms: Enlarging soft tissue mass
- Pain in 30-50%
- 5 year survival: 39-79%
- Local recurrence: 12-42%
- Metastases (lung, spine, skull, lymph nodes): 34-63%
- Surgical resection with wide margins
- Adjuvant radiation therapy
- Adjuvant chemotherapy for high grade fibrosarcomas

Diagnostic Checklist

- Always consult orthopedic surgeon before biopsy
- Biopsies must be planned with future tumor excision in mind

---

- ○ Helpful in differentiating fibrosarcoma from hematoma
- Heterogeneous often well defined soft tissue mass
  - ○ Pseudocapsule
- Areas of hemorrhage can obscure underlying tumor

Ultrasonographic Findings

- Well-defined hypoechoic solid mass

Angiographic Findings

- Hypervascular soft tissue mass

Nuclear Medicine Findings

- Bone Scan: Early blood pool images can show mildly increased radiotracer uptake

Imaging Recommendations

- Best imaging tool: MRI
- Protocol advice: T1, T2WI MR, T1 C+ MR

DIFFERENTIAL DIAGNOSIS

Malignant Fibrous Histiocytoma (MFH)

- Radiographically similar to fibrosarcoma
- Areas of extensive hemorrhage common

Fibromatosis

- Predominately low signal on T1 and T2WI MR
- No metastases

Synovial Sarcoma

- In proximity to joint
- Calcifications
- Cortical erosions
- Younger patients

Liposarcoma

- Presence of fat in > 40%
- Calcifications rare

Malignant Peripheral Nerve Sheath Tumor (MPNST)

- Related to neurovascular bundle

Hematoma

- No enhancing solid components
- Surrounding edema

PATHOLOGY

General Features

- General path comments
  - ○ Clinically and radiographically similar to malignant fibrous histiocytoma
  - ○ Comprises low-grade end of spectrum that includes malignant fibrous histiocytoma at high-grade end
- Genetics: Rearrangements of RET oncogene in radiation induced fibrosarcomas
- Etiology
  - ○ Possibly related to prior trauma
    - Can arise in scar tissue or at site of prior injury
  - ○ Can be radiation induced
  - ○ Can form dedifferentiated portion of dedifferentiated chondrosarcoma
- Epidemiology: 5% of soft tissue sarcomas
- Associated abnormalities: Patients with neurofibromatosis have 10% risk of developing fibrosarcoma

Gross Pathologic & Surgical Features

- Soft-firm, gray-white, yellow, fleshy lobulated mass
- Pseudocapsule
- Large tumors infiltrate surrounding tissues

Microscopic Features

- Anaplastic spindle cells with varying degrees of differentiation
- Cells arranged in herringbone pattern
- Well-differentiated type: Marked fibrogenesis, rich in mature collagen, herringbone pattern
  - ○ Osseous, cartilaginous metaplasia
- Poorly differentiated fibrosarcoma: Herringbone pattern less distinct
  - ○ Areas of necrosis, hemorrhage
- Sclerosing epithelioid type: Rare variant
  - ○ Hypocellular, densely hyalinized stroma

9

3

- ○ Epithelioid tumor cells arranged in nests, strands
- ○ Sarcomatous spindle cells

Staging, Grading or Classification Criteria
- Surgical staging system for malignant musculoskeletal tumors
  - ○ Stage Ia: Low grade, intracompartmental
  - ○ Stage Ib: Low grade, extracompartmental
  - ○ Stage IIa: High grade, intracompartmental
  - ○ Stage IIb: High grade, extracompartmental
  - ○ Stage IIIa: Low or high grade, intracompartmental, metastases
  - ○ Stage IIIb: Low or high grade, extracompartmental, metastases

CLINICAL ISSUES

Presentation
- Most common signs/symptoms: Enlarging soft tissue mass
- Clinical profile
  - ○ Pain in 30-50%
  - ○ Superficial lesions can cause skin ulcerations
  - ○ Hypoglycemia due to excretion of insulin-like substances
  - ○ Infantile fibrosarcoma: Rapidly growing soft tissue mass

Demographics
- Age
  - ○ 30-70 years, peak: 35-55 years
  - ○ Infantile fibrosarcoma: < 10 years
- Gender: M:F = 1.5:1
- Ethnicity: More frequent in Caucasians

Natural History & Prognosis
- Prognosis depends on tumor size, histologic subtype, location, metastases
- 5 year survival: 39-79%
- Local recurrence: 12-42%
- Reduced recurrence rate in case of postoperative radiation therapy
- Metastases (lung, spine, skull, lymph nodes): 34-63%
- Secondary fibrosarcomas have worse prognosis
- Infantile fibrosarcoma: Excellent prognosis, 5-year survival: 80%

Treatment
- Options, risks, complications
  - ○ Surgical resection with wide margins
  - ○ Adjuvant radiation therapy
    - ■ Recurrence: 12-30%
  - ○ Adjuvant chemotherapy for high grade fibrosarcomas
  - ○ Amputation may be necessary

DIAGNOSTIC CHECKLIST

Consider
- Always consult orthopedic surgeon before biopsy
- Biopsies must be planned with future tumor excision in mind

Image Interpretation Pearls
- Radiologically often indistinguishable from malignant fibrous histiocytoma

SELECTED REFERENCES

1. Fletcher CD et al: Clinicopathologic re-evaluation of 100 malignant fibrous histiocytomas: Prognostic relevance of subclassification. J Clin Oncol 19:3045-50, 2001
2. Weiss SW et al: Enzinger and Weiss's soft tissue tumors, 4th ed. St.Louis MO, CV Mosby, 409-39, 2001
3. Patel SC et al: Sarcomas of the head and neck. Top Magn Reson Imaging 10:362-75, 1999
4. Borman H et al: Fibrosarcoma following radiotherapy for breast carcinoma: A case report and review of the literature. Ann Plast Surg 41:201-4, 1998
5. Delpla PA et al: Soft tissue tumors following traumatic injury: Two observations of interest for the medicolegal causality. Am J Forensic Med Pathol 19:152-6, 1998
6. Ito T et al: In vitro irradiation is able to cause RET oncogene rearrangement. Cancer Res 53:2940-3, 1993
7. Wiklund TA et al: Postirradiation sarcoma: Analysis of a nationwide cancer registry material. Cancer 68:524-31, 1991
8. Scott SM et al: Soft tissue fibrosarcoma. A clinicopathologic study of 132 cases. Cancer 64:925-31, 1989
9. Wetzel LH et al: A comparison of MR imaging and CT in the evaluation of musculoskeletal masses. Radiographics 7:851-874, 1987
10. Ninane J et al: Congenital fibrosarcoma. Cancer 58:1400-6, 1986
11. Petasnick JP et al: Soft tissue masses of the locomotor system: Comparison of MR imaging with CT. Radiology 160:125-33, 1986
12. Lindberg RD et al: Conservative surgery and postoperative radiotherapy in 300 adults with soft tissue sarcomas. Cancer 47:2391-7, 1981
13. Chung EB et al: Infantile fibrosarcoma. Cancer 38:729-39, 1976
14. Pritchard DJ et al: Fibrosarcoma - a clinicopathologic and statistical study of 199 tumors of the soft tissues of the extremities and trunk. Cancer 33:888-97, 1974
15. Exelby PR et al: Soft-tissue fibrosarcoma in children. J Pediatr Surg 8:415-20, 1973

IMAGE GALLERY

Typical

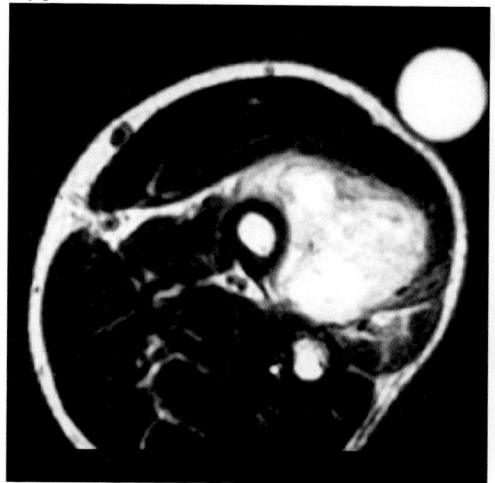
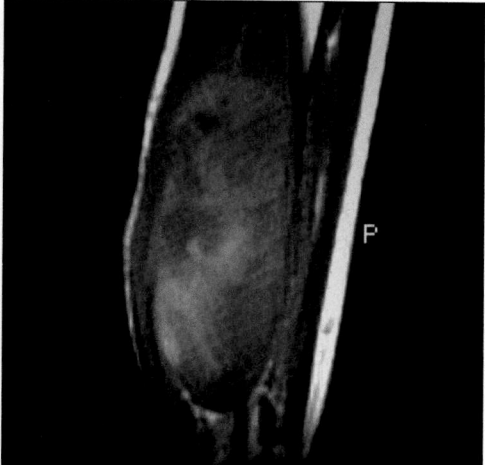

(Left) Axial T1 C+ MR show marked enhancement of the deep soft tissue mass involving the forearm. *(Right)* Sagittal T1WI MR shows large heterogeneous soft tissue mass in the forearm. Areas of high signal correspond to hemorrhage.

Typical

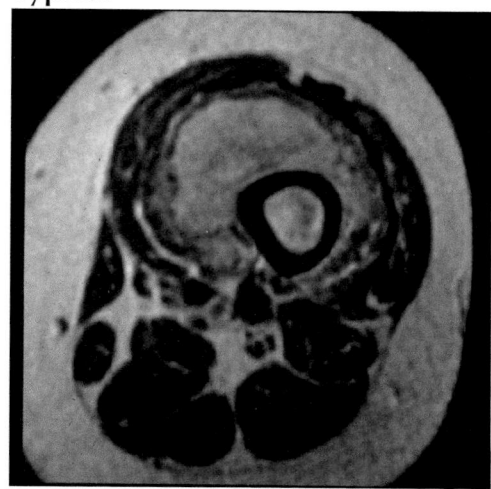
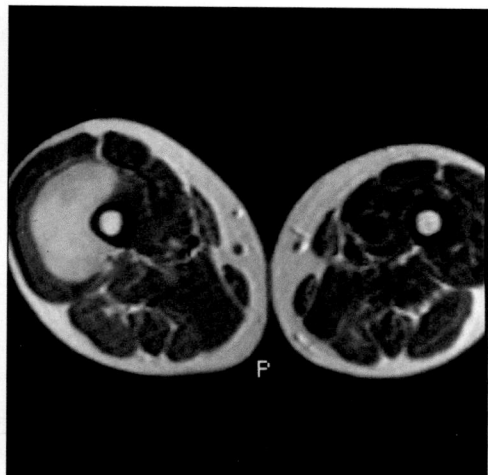

(Left) Axial PD FSE MR shows tumor of intermediate to high SI involving the thigh. *(Right)* Axial T1 C+ MR shows homogeneous, enhancing soft tissue mass in the right thigh.

Other

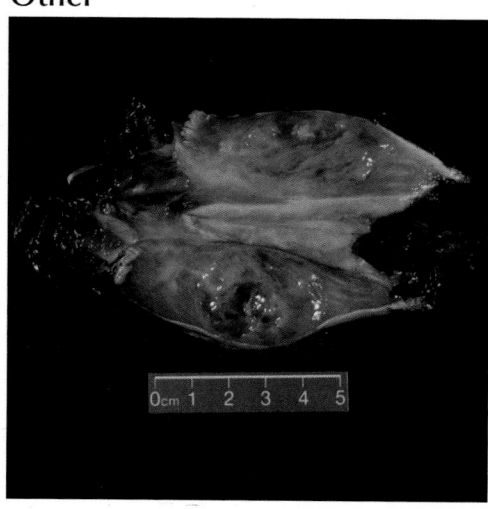
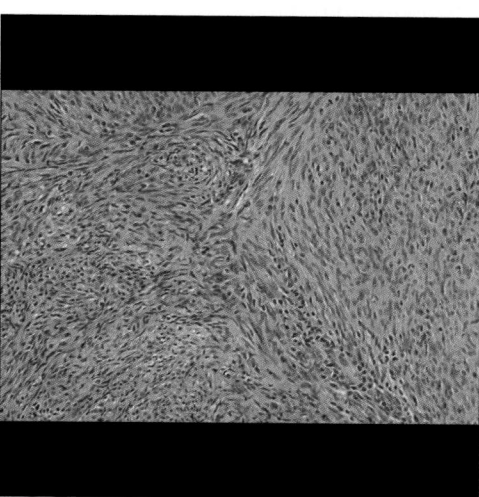

(Left) Coronal gross pathology shows brown fleshy soft tissue mass with small areas of hemorrhage. *(Right)* micropathology shows fibroblasts arranged in distinct intersecting fascicles ("herringbone" pattern).

FIBROMATOSIS

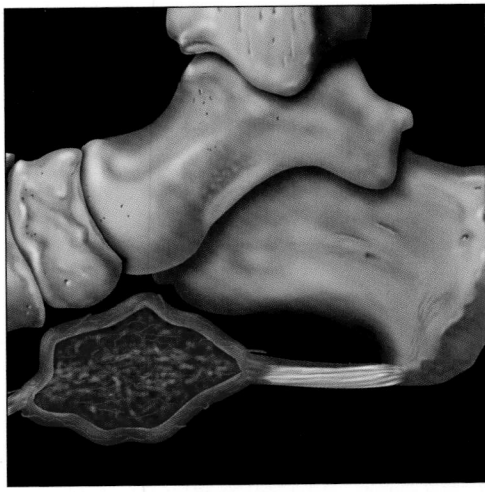

Sagittal graphic shows fibromatosis (in red) arising from the medial plantar aponeurosis.

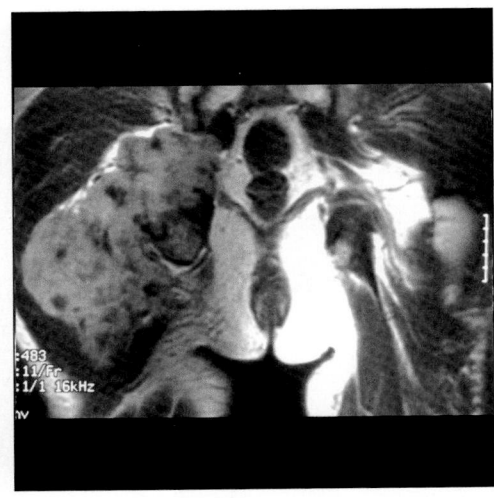

Coronal T1 C+ MR shows large enhancing soft tissue mass centered in the medial thigh with areas of low signal.

TERMINOLOGY

Abbreviations and Synonyms
- Non-metastasizing fibrosarcoma, aggressive fibromatosis, desmoid tumor

Definitions
- Group of benign disorders characterized by fibrous growth, tendency to infiltrate adjacent tissues and to recur

IMAGING FINDINGS

General Features
- Best diagnostic clue
  - Soft tissue mass invading soft tissue planes
  - Predominately low signal on T1 and T2WI MR
- Location
  - Superficial fibromatosis: Slowly growing, small, often multiple lesions
    - Palmar fibromatosis (Dupuytren contracture)
    - Plantar fibromatosis (Ledderhose disease)
    - Penile fibromatosis (Peyronie disease)
    - Arises from superficial fasciae, aponeuroses
  - Deep fibromatosis: Rapidly growing, large
    - Extraabdominal fibromatosis (extraabdominal desmoid)
    - Extremities: 60%
    - Abdominal fibromatosis (abdominal desmoid)
    - Mesenteric/intraabdominal fibromatosis in Gardner syndrome
    - Arises from deep structures (muscles of trunk and extremities)
  - Infantile fibromatosis
    - Solitary lesion most common
    - Multicentric lesions: 5-15%
- Size
  - Superficial type: 1-5 cm
  - Deep type: 5-10 cm, rarely > 20 cm
- Morphology: Soft tissue mass with invasion of adjacent tissues

Radiographic Findings
- Radiography
  - Soft tissue mass
  - Osseous involvement: 6-37%
    - "Frondlike" periosteal reaction, erosions, scalloping

CT Findings
- NECT
  - Iso-, hypo-, hyperdense to muscle
  - If close to bone: Erosion, periosteal reaction
- CECT: Enhancement during active phase

DDx: Fibromatosis

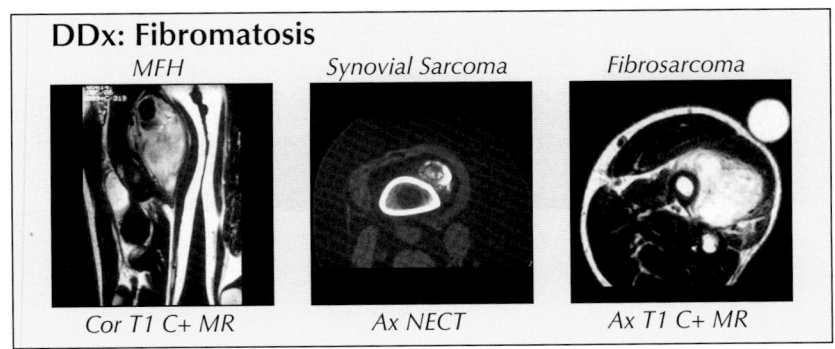

MFH	Synovial Sarcoma	Fibrosarcoma
Cor T1 C+ MR	Ax NECT	Ax T1 C+ MR

FIBROMATOSIS

Key Facts

Imaging Findings
- Soft tissue mass invading soft tissue planes
- Predominately low signal on T1 and T2WI MR

Top Differential Diagnoses
- Malignant Fibrous Histiocytoma (MFH)
- Synovial Sarcoma
- Fibrosarcoma

Pathology
- Dupuytren contracture: Incidence 1-2% in general population, 20% in patients > 65 years
- Concomitant palmar and plantar fibromatosis: 10-65%
- Intra-abdominal fibromatosis associated with Gardner syndrome: 15%

- Palmar and plantar fibromatosis: Associated with diabetes, epilepsy, alcohol induced liver disease

Clinical Issues
- Most common signs/symptoms: Soft tissue mass
- Biologic behavior intermediate between benign fibrous lesions and fibrosarcoma
- Local recurrence: 20-77%
- Self limited disease, no metastases
- Fatalities from direct invasion of chest wall or neck, and infiltration of vital organs
- Surgical excision with wide margins
- Radiation therapy in aggressive recurrent lesions

Diagnostic Checklist
- Can look very aggressive and may be mistaken for sarcoma

MR Findings
- T1WI
  - Iso- hypointense to muscle
  - Dupuytren contracture: Low signal intensity
    - If intermediate signal on T1, higher rate of recurrence
    - Contracture of 4th and 5th metacarpophalangeal joints
- T2WI
  - Intermediate - low signal intensity (fibrous components)
  - Areas of high signal
  - Dupuytren contracture: Low signal intensity
    - If intermediate signal on T2 higher rate of recurrence
- STIR: Hyper - isointense compared to surrounding muscle
- T1 C+
  - Intense enhancement during active phase
    - Enhancement of cellular areas
  - No significant enhancement during latent phase
- Poorly defined
- Invasion of fat/muscle
- Thickening of plantar aponeurosis

Ultrasonographic Findings
- Soft tissue mass of variable echogenicity
- Smooth well-defined margins

Imaging Recommendations
- Best imaging tool: MRI
- Protocol advice: T1, T2WI MR, T1 C+ MR

DIFFERENTIAL DIAGNOSIS

Malignant Fibrous Histiocytoma (MFH)
- Arises in deep soft tissues
- Calcifications
- Metastases

Synovial Sarcoma
- In proximity to joint

- Amorphous calcifications

Fibrosarcoma
- High signal on T2WI MR
- Areas of hemorrhage, necrosis
- Metastases

PATHOLOGY

General Features
- General path comments: Soft tissue lesion characterized by proliferation of fibrous tissue, surrounded by abundant collagen
- Genetics
  - Superficial fibromatoses: Trisomies of chromosome 7, 8, 14
  - Fibromatosis associated with Gardner syndrome: Abnormality of adenomatous polyposis coli (APC) gene
- Etiology
  - Superficial fibromatoses: Possibly caused by repetitive microtrauma or microvascular injury
  - Deep fibromatoses: Posttraumatic, postradiation
    - Abdominal fibromatosis: Endocrine abnormalities (tumor occurs after pregnancy)
- Epidemiology
  - Dupuytren contracture: Incidence 1-2% in general population, 20% in patients > 65 years
  - Concomitant palmar and plantar fibromatosis: 10-65%
- Associated abnormalities
  - Intra-abdominal fibromatosis associated with Gardner syndrome: 15%
  - Palmar and plantar fibromatosis: Associated with diabetes, epilepsy, alcohol induced liver disease

Gross Pathologic & Surgical Features
- Firm, gray-white mass
- Streaky, scar like cross section
- No capsule or pseudocapsule
- May appear circumscribed, microscopically ill-defined borders

FIBROMATOSIS

- Interdigitating, infiltrative growth into surrounding muscle or soft tissue

Microscopic Features
- Proliferation of uniform fibroblastic cells
- Early proliferative phase: Immature fibroblasts
- Late mature phase: Fibrocytes with abundant dense collagenous stroma
- No cellular atypia
- Myxoid changes, areas of hemorrhage, and focal inflammation
- Resembling hypertrophic scar tissue

Staging, Grading or Classification Criteria
- Surgical staging system for benign musculoskeletal tumors
  - Stage 1: Latent
  - Stage 2: Active
  - Stage 3: Aggressive

CLINICAL ISSUES

Presentation
- Most common signs/symptoms: Soft tissue mass
- Clinical profile
  - Subcutaneous nodules
  - Flexion contracture
  - Pain in case of nerve compression
  - Deep lesions usually non tender
  - Penile fibromatosis: Plaque-like scar tissue on penile shaft
  - Abdominal fibromatosis: Occurs after pregnancy, regression with menopause

Demographics
- Age
  - 20-40 years, peak: 23 years
  - Infantile fibromatosis: 0-2 years
- Gender
  - M:F = 1:1
  - Palmar fibromatosis: M:F = 4-7:1
  - Plantar fibromatosis: M:F = 1:1
  - Deep fibromatosis: M < F
- Ethnicity: More common in Caucasians

Natural History & Prognosis
- Biologic behavior intermediate between benign fibrous lesions and fibrosarcoma
  - No malignant transformation into fibrosarcoma
- Local recurrence: 20-77%
  - Younger patients have higher recurrence rate
- Self limited disease, no metastases
- Fatalities from direct invasion of chest wall or neck, and infiltration of vital organs

Treatment
- Early surgery should be avoided due to increased risk of recurrence
- Surgical excision with wide margins
  - Predisposition for local regrowth if excision is incomplete
  - Recurrence: 40-70%
- Release of flexion contracture
- Radiation therapy in aggressive recurrent lesions
- Amputation occasionally necessary
- Surgical excision with adjuvant radiation therapy
  - Recurrence: 20-30%
- Plantar fibromatosis: Well molded and padded shoes
  - Transference of weight away from nodules

DIAGNOSTIC CHECKLIST

Image Interpretation Pearls
- Can look very aggressive and may be mistaken for sarcoma

SELECTED REFERENCES

1. Breiner JA et al: Trisomy 8 and trisomy 14 in plantar fibromatosis. Cancer Genet Cytogenet 108:176-7, 1999
2. Arkkila PE et al: Dupuytren's disease: Association with chronic diabetic complications. J Rhematol 24:153-9, 1997
3. Kransdorf MJ et al: Imaging of soft tissue tumors. 1st ed. Philadelphia PA, W.B. Saunders, 160-75, 1997
4. Romero JA et al: Different biologic features of desmoid tumors in adults and juvenile patients: MR demonstration. J Comput Assist Tomogr 19:782-7, 1995
5. Yacoe ME et al: Dupuytren's contracture: MR imaging findings and correlation with MR signal intensity and cellularity of lesions. Am J Roentgenol 160:813-7, 1993
6. Liu P et al: MRI of fibromatosis: With pathologic correlation. Pediatr Radiol 22:587-9, 1992
7. Quinn SF et al: MR imaging in fibromatosis: Results in 26 patients with pathologic correlation. Am J Roentgenol 156:539-42, 1991
8. O'Keefe F et al: Magnetic resonance imaging in aggressive fibromatosis. Clin Radiol 42:170-3, 1990
9. Enneking WF: A system of staging musculoskeletal neoplasms. Clin Orthop 204:9-24, 1986
10. Hudson TM et al: Aggressive fibromatosis: Evaluation by computed tomography and angiography. Radiology 150:495-501, 1984

FIBROMATOSIS

IMAGE GALLERY

Typical

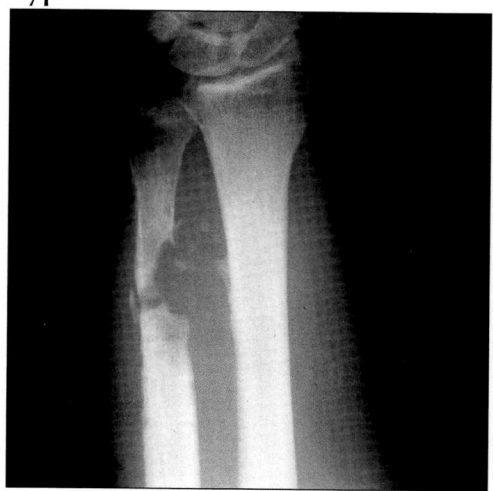
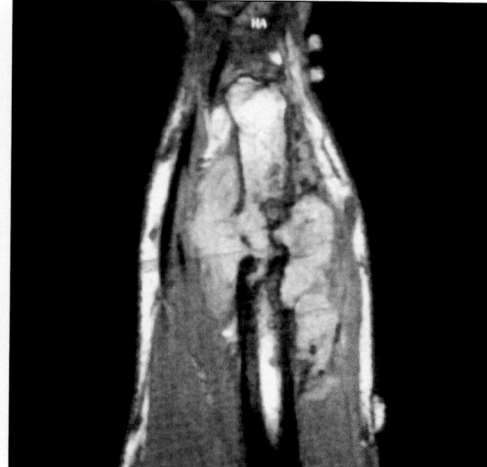

(Left) Anteroposterior radiography shows soft tissue mass and osseous destruction of the ulna in a patient with recurrent fibromatosis. *(Right)* Sagittal T1 C+ MR shows infiltrating enhancing soft tissue mass with associated osseous destruction.

Typical

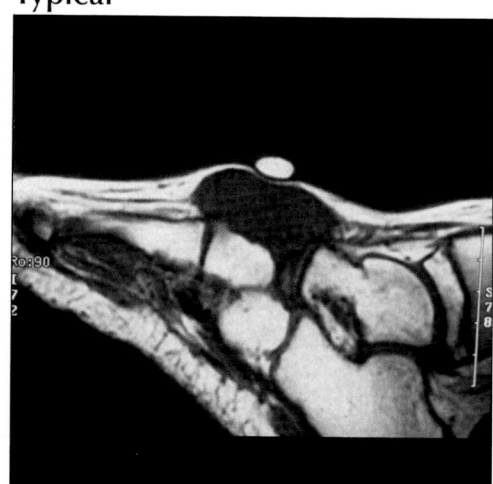
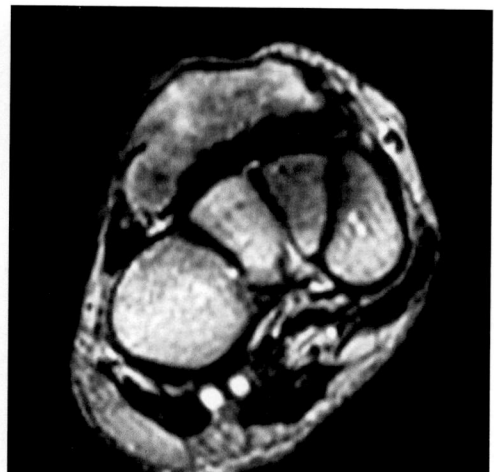

(Left) Sagittal T1WI MR shows well-defined soft tissue mass of low SI involving the dorsal aspect of the foot. *(Right)* Axial T2WI MR of the foot shows heterogeneous soft tissue mass with areas of intermediate - low signal and foci of high signal.

Typical

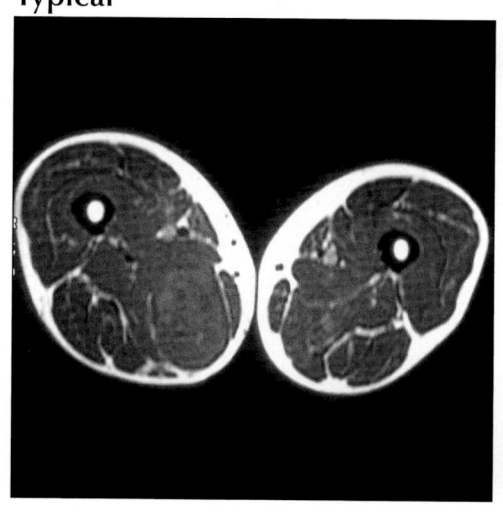
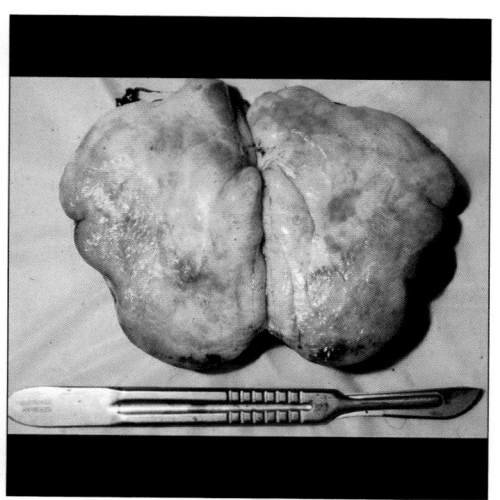

(Left) Axial T1WI MR shows well-defined soft tissue mass isointense to muscle in the posterior right thigh. *(Right)* Gross pathology shows circumscribed white tumor with coarsely trabeculated surface.

MALIGNANT FIBROUS HISTIOCYTOMA

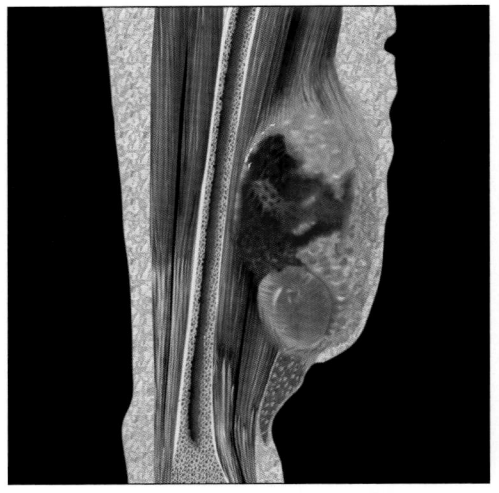

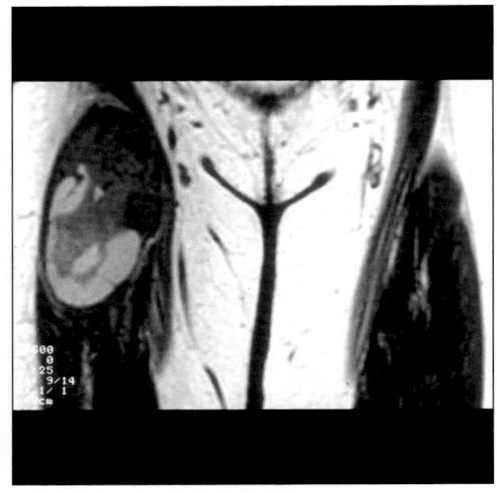

Sagittal graphic shows MFH arising in the deep soft tissues of the posterior thigh. Areas of calcifications are shown in white. Hemorrhage is shown in red.

Coronal T1WI MR shows hemorrhagic deep seated mass in the medial right thigh.

TERMINOLOGY

Abbreviations and Synonyms
- MFH, malignant fibrous xanthoma, xanthosarcoma, malignant histiocytoma

Definitions
- Sarcoma composed of spindle and pleomorphic cells demonstrating myofibroblastic differentiation

IMAGING FINDINGS

General Features
- Best diagnostic clue
  - Heterogeneous hemorrhagic deep soft tissue mass
  - Any patient with spontaneous musculoskeletal hemorrhage should be evaluated for underlying MFH
- Location
  - Extremities: 75%, involves deep large muscle groups
    - Lower extremity: 50%
    - Upper extremity: 25%
  - Retroperitoneum: 15%
  - Head and neck: 5%
  - Chest wall
  - Arises deep to the deep fascia
- Size: 5-15 cm

- Morphology: Heterogeneous, hemorrhagic, deep soft tissue mass

Radiographic Findings
- Radiography
  - Deep soft tissue mass
  - Curvilinear/punctate peripheral calcifications: 5-20%
  - Cortical erosions of adjacent bone

CT Findings
- NECT
  - Large lobulated soft tissue mass
  - Isodense to muscle
  - Central hypodense areas, corresponding to myxoid regions or necrosis
  - High attenuation areas, corresponding to hemorrhage
  - Punctate/curvilinear calcifications
  - Cortical erosions
  - Retroperitoneal tumor: Heterogeneous mass, invasion of abdominal wall
- CECT
  - Hypo- or hypervascular
  - Enhancement of solid components

MR Findings
- T1WI: Low to intermediate signal intensity
- T2WI: High signal intensity, especially myxoid type

DDx: Malignant Fibrous Histiocytoma

Fibrosarcoma	Fibromatosis	Hematoma	Liposarcoma	MPNST
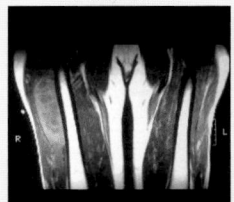	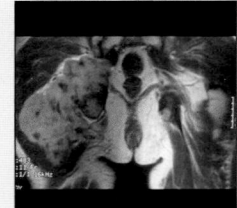	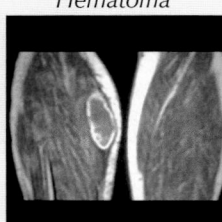	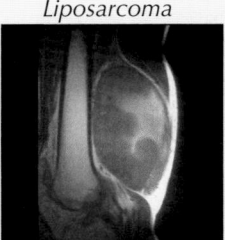	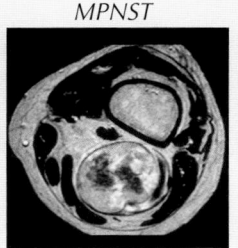
Cor T1 C+ MR	Cor T1 C+ MR	Cor T1WI MR	Sag T1WI MR	Ax T2WI MR

MALIGNANT FIBROUS HISTIOCYTOMA

Key Facts

Imaging Findings

- Heterogeneous hemorrhagic deep soft tissue mass
- Any patient with spontaneous musculoskeletal hemorrhage should be evaluated for underlying MFH
- Extensive areas of hemorrhage can obscure underlying neoplasm

Top Differential Diagnoses

- Fibrosarcoma
- Synovial Sarcoma
- Fibromatosis
- Hematoma
- Liposarcoma
- Malignant Peripheral Nerve Sheath Tumor (MPNST)

Pathology

- Most common primary malignant soft-tissue tumor of late adult life
- 20-30% of all soft tissue sarcomas

Clinical Issues

- Most common signs/symptoms: Painless soft tissue mass with progressive enlargement over several months
- Aggressive neoplasms with tendency to recur and metastasize
- 5-year survival: 65-70%, retroperitoneal tumors: 15-20%
- Stage I: Surgical resection with wide margins
- Stage II: Surgical resection with adjuvant radiation or chemotherapy

---

- T1 C+: Nodular enhancement
- Heterogeneous often well defined soft tissue mass
  - Pseudocapsule
- Areas of calcification, hemorrhage, necrosis
- Extensive areas of hemorrhage can obscure underlying neoplasm
  - Fluid-fluid levels in areas of hemorrhage

Ultrasonographic Findings

- Well-defined heterogeneous solid mass
- Hypoechoic areas correspond to necrosis

Angiographic Findings

- Hypervascular soft tissue mass

Nuclear Medicine Findings

- Bone Scan: Increased radiotracer uptake on blood pool images

Imaging Recommendations

- Best imaging tool: MRI
- Protocol advice: T1, T2WI, T1 C+ MR

DIFFERENTIAL DIAGNOSIS

Fibrosarcoma

- Radiographically often indistinguishable

Synovial Sarcoma

- In proximity to joints
- Cortical erosions
- Younger patients

Fibromatosis

- Predominately low signal on T1 and T2WI MR
- No metastases

Hematoma

- Nonenhancing solid components
- Surrounding soft tissue edema

Liposarcoma

- Presence of fat in > 40%
- Calcifications rare

Malignant Peripheral Nerve Sheath Tumor (MPNST)

- Related to neurovascular bundle

PATHOLOGY

General Features

- General path comments: Clinically and radiographically similar to fibrosarcoma
- Genetics: Imbalances in DNA sequence copy number
- Etiology
  - Derived from primitive mesenchyme with fibro- or myofibroblastic differentiation
  - Controversial if tumor represents specific entity with uniform pathogenesis or heterogeneous group of undifferentiated sarcomas
  - Can be radiation induced
- Epidemiology
  - Most common primary malignant soft-tissue tumor of late adult life
  - 20-30% of all soft tissue sarcomas
  - Most common radiation induced sarcoma
- Associated abnormalities: Hematological diseases: Lymphoma, multiple myeloma

Gross Pathologic & Surgical Features

- Multilobulated, gray-brown fleshy mass, attached to adjacent structures
- Focal areas of hemorrhage and necrosis
- Size at diagnosis usually over 5 cm

Microscopic Features

- Storiform/pleomorphic type: 50-60%
  - Fibroblast like spindle cells and giant cells resembling histiocytes, arranged in pleomorphic-storiform pattern
  - Most common in extremities
- Myxoid type: 25%
  - More than 50% of tumor must have myxoid stroma
  - Myxoid tissue: Large amount of mucoid material

MALIGNANT FIBROUS HISTIOCYTOMA

- ■ Extracellular mucopolysaccharide and hyaluronic acid
- ○ Most common in extremities and retroperitoneum
- Giant cell type: 5-10%
  - ○ Osteoclast-like giant cells
  - ○ Necrotic and hemorrhagic foci common
  - ○ Osteoid in 50%
  - ○ Most common in extremities
- Inflammatory type: 5-10%
  - ○ Inflammatory and foam cells
  - ○ Can present with fever and leukocytosis
  - ○ Most common in retroperitoneum

Staging, Grading or Classification Criteria
- Surgical staging system for malignant musculoskeletal tumors
  - ○ Stage Ia: Low grade, intracompartmental
  - ○ Stage Ib: Low grade, extracompartmental
  - ○ Stage IIa: High grade, intracompartmental
  - ○ Stage IIb: High grade, extracompartmental
  - ○ Stage IIIa: Low or high grade, intracompartmental, metastases
  - ○ Stage IIIb: Low or high grade, extracompartmental, metastases

CLINICAL ISSUES

Presentation
- Most common signs/symptoms: Painless soft tissue mass with progressive enlargement over several months
- Clinical profile
  - ○ Any deep-seated invasive intramuscular mass in a patient > 50 years is most likely MFH
  - ○ Any patient with spontaneous musculoskeletal hemorrhage should be evaluated for underlying MFH
  - ○ Patients with retroperitoneal MFH: Fever, malaise, weight loss, increased abdominal pressure

Demographics
- Age: 10-90 years, peak: 50 years
- Gender: M:F = 2:1
- Ethnicity: More common in Caucasians

Natural History & Prognosis
- Aggressive neoplasms with tendency to recur and metastasize
- Prognosis depends on tumor size, depth, location, histologic subtype
- Local recurrence: 19-31%
- Metastases: 35-41%
  - ○ Lung: 90%, lymph nodes: 4-12%, bone: 8%, liver: 1%
- 5-year survival: 65-70%, retroperitoneal tumors: 15-20%
- Tumor < 5 cm: 80% 5-year survival
- Tumor 5-10 cm: 65% 5-year survival
- Tumor > 10 cm: 40-50% 5-year survival

Treatment
- Stage I: Surgical resection with wide margins
- Stage II: Surgical resection with adjuvant radiation or chemotherapy
- Neoadjuvant and adjuvant chemotherapy
- Intra-arterial chemotherapy
- Radiation therapy

DIAGNOSTIC CHECKLIST

Consider
- Always consult orthopedic surgeon before biopsy
- Biopsies must be planned with future tumor excision in mind

Image Interpretation Pearls
- Spontaneous intramuscular hemorrhage in adult patient suspect underlying MFH

SELECTED REFERENCES

1. Mairal A et al: Loss of chromosome 13 is the most frequent genomic imbalance in malignant fibrous histiocytomas. A comparative genomic hybridization analysis of a series of 30 cases. Cancer Genet Cytogenet 111:134-8, 1999
2. Salo JC et al: Malignant fibrous histiocytoma of the extremity. Cancer 85:1765-72, 1999
3. Larramendy ML et al: Comparative genomic hybridization of malignant fibrous histiocytoma reveals a novel prognostic marker. Am J Pathol 151:1153-61, 1997
4. Miller TT et al: MRI of malignant fibrous histiocytoma of soft tissue: Analysis of 13 cases with pathologic correlation. Skeletal Radiol 23:271-5, 1994
5. Murphey MD et al: From the archives of the AFIP. Musculoskeletal malignant fibrous histiocytoma: Radiologic-pathologic correlation. Radiographics 14:807-26, 1994
6. Fletcher CD: Pleomorphic malignant fibrous histiocytoma: Fact or fiction? A critical reappraisal based on 159 tumors diagnosed as pleomorphic sarcoma. Am J Surg Pathol 16:213-28, 1992
7. Iwasaki H et al: Malignant fibrous histiocytoma: A tumor of facultative histiocytes showing mesenchymal differentiation in cultured cell lines. Cancer 69;437-47, 1992
8. Pezzi CM et al: Prognostic factors in 227 patients with malignant fibrous histiocytoma. Cancer 69:2098-103, 1992
9. Panicek DM et al: Hemorrhage simulating tumor growth in malignant fibrous histiocytoma at MR imaging. Radiology 181:398-400, 1991
10. Sanchez RB et al: Musculoskeletal neoplasms after intraarterial chemotherapy: Correlation with MR images with pathologic specimens. Radiology 174:237-40, 1990

IMAGE GALLERY

Typical

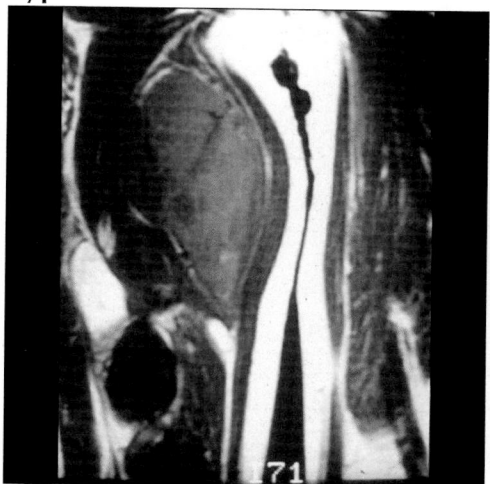 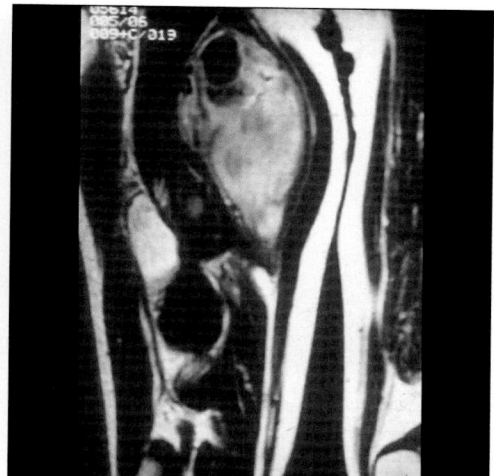

(Left) Coronal T1WI MR shows encapsulated (pseudocapsule) large soft tissue mass in the medial right thigh. Areas of high and low signal correspond to hemorrhage and necrosis, respectively. *(Right)* Coronal T1 C+ MR shows marked enhancement of the soft tissue mass. Nonenhancing areas correspond to necrosis.

Typical

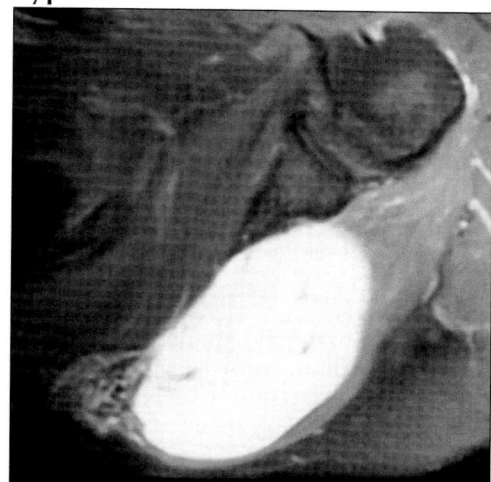 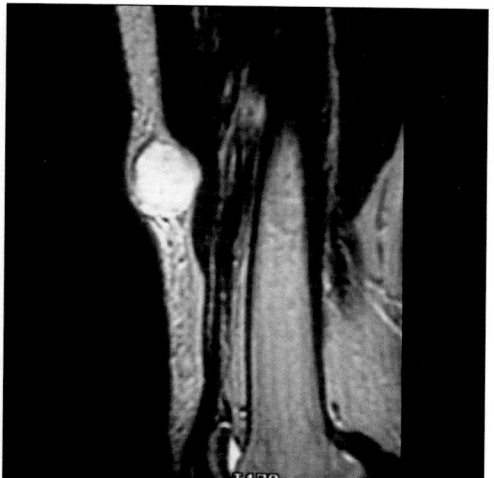

(Left) Axial T1 C+ MR shows homogeneously enhancing intramuscular mass in the left shoulder. *(Right)* Sagittal T2WI MR shows well defined round hyperintense lesion in the superficial soft tissues of the thigh.

Other

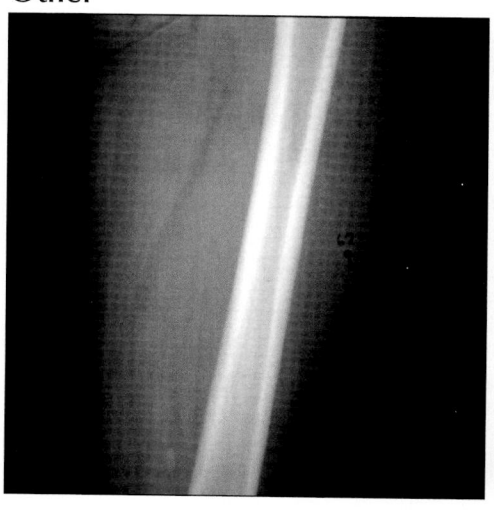 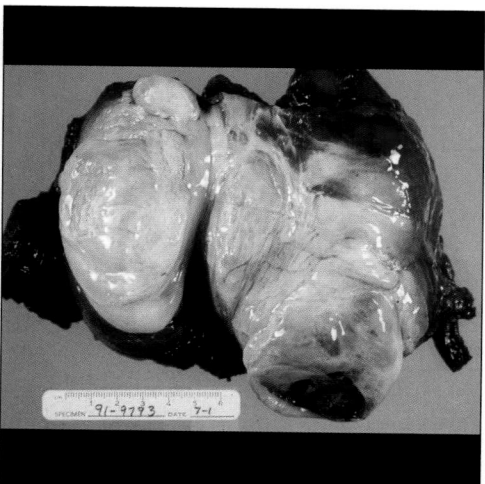

(Left) Anteroposterior radiography shows large soft tissue mass involving the thigh. Note areas of calcification at the inferior aspect of the mass. *(Right)* Gross pathology shows circumscribed, yellow-white, multilobulated, fleshy mass.

9

13

PIGMENTED VILLONODULAR SYNOVITIS

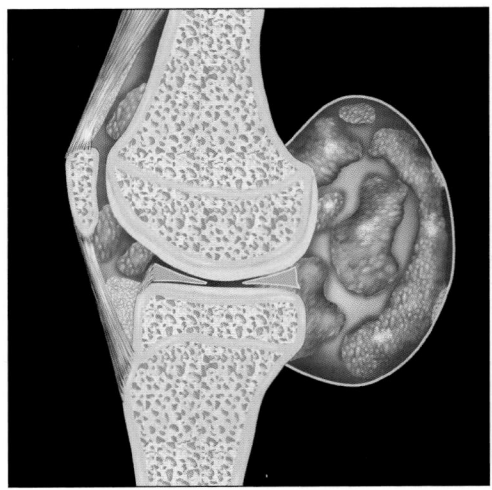

Sagittal graphic shows intraarticular mass with hypertrophied synovium (in brown).

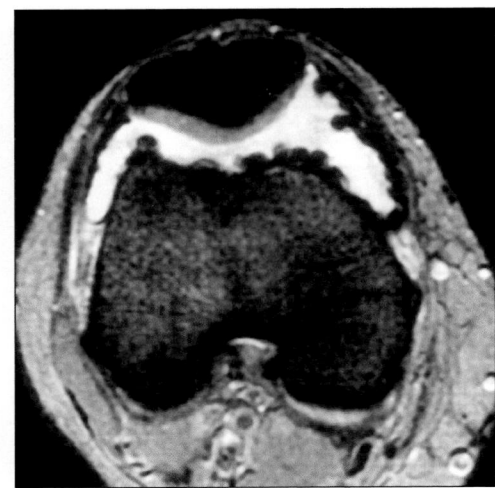

Axial T2* GRE MR shows frond-like projections of low SI.

TERMINOLOGY

Abbreviations and Synonyms
- PVNS, giant cell tumor of the tendon sheath (GCTTS), benign synovioma

Definitions
- Family of benign proliferative lesions originating in synovium of the joint, bursa, and tendon sheath
- GCTTS (nodular tenosynovitis): Localized form, extraarticular
- PVNS: Diffuse form, intraarticular

IMAGING FINDINGS

General Features
- Best diagnostic clue
  - MRI: Low signal on all pulse sequences
  - Radiographs/CT: Dense intra-articular soft tissue mass without calcifications
    - Subchondral erosions with preserved joint space
- Location
  - GCTTS
    - Hand and wrist (65-89%): Volar aspect of digits
    - Foot and ankle (5-15%): First and second toe
    - Usually solitary lesion
  - PVNS: Involves large joints
    - Knee: 80%
    - Hip, ankle, shoulder, elbow
    - Usually monoarticular
- Size
  - GCTTS: 2-4 cm
  - PVNS: Larger, irregular
- Morphology: Villonodular frond-like proliferation of synovial membrane

Radiographic Findings
- Radiography
  - GCTTS: Soft tissue mass
    - Pressure erosions of underlying bone: 15%
    - Calcifications may mimic synovial chondromatosis, calcific tendinitis
  - PVNS: Noncalcified, dense, soft tissue mass (hemosiderin deposits)
    - Joint effusion
    - Bony erosion: 50%
    - Erosions in joints with tight capsule: Hip (93%), shoulder (75%), knee (26%)
    - Erosions, subchondral cysts on both sides of joint
    - Joint space preserved
    - Secondary degenerative changes with concentric joint space narrowing, osteophytes in chronic disease
    - Normal mineralization
    - Calcifications rare

DDx: Pigmented Villonodular Synovitis

Synovial Sarcoma	Chondromatosis	Hemophilia	RA	Lipoma Arboresc.
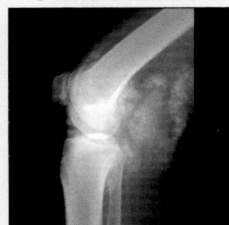	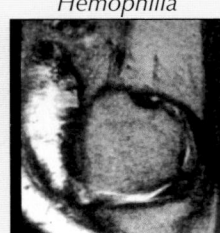	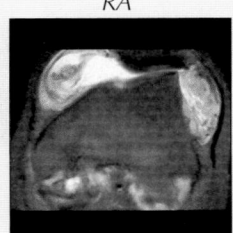	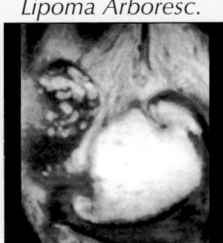	
Ax FS PD FSE MR	Lat Radiography	Sag T2WI MR	Ax FS PD MR	Sag T1WI MR

PIGMENTED VILLONODULAR SYNOVITIS

Key Facts

Imaging Findings
- MRI: Low signal on all pulse sequences
- Radiographs/CT: Dense intra-articular soft tissue mass without calcifications
- Subchondral erosions with preserved joint space

Top Differential Diagnoses
- Synovial Sarcoma
- Synovial Chondromatosis
- Hemophilia
- Rheumatoid Arthritis (RA)
- Posttraumatic Synovitis
- Lipoma Arborescence

Pathology
- 5% of all primary soft tissue tumors

Clinical Issues
- Most common signs/symptoms: Limited joint mobility
- Sudden increase in pain due to torsion of synovial nodules
- Rapid accumulation of joint fluid after aspiration
- Benign, locally aggressive lesion
- Progressive destruction of articular cartilage and subchondral bone results in severe osteoarthritis
- PVNS: Recurrence 20-50%
- Complete synovectomy (open): Recurrence 20%
- Arthroscopic synovectomy (often piecemeal, incomplete): Recurrence 50%
- Total joint replacement

CT Findings
- NECT
  - Soft tissue mass
  - Sharply defined erosions with sclerotic margins
  - Increased attenuation, relative to muscle due to hemosiderin
  - Joint effusion
- CECT: Enhancement of synovium

MR Findings
- T1WI
  - GCTTS: Low signal intensity
  - PVNS: Nodular mass iso/hypointense to muscle
    - Foci of high signal represent lipid laden macrophages
- T2WI
  - GCTTS: Heterogeneous
  - Signal intensity equal to or lower than fat
  - PVNS: Iso/hypointense to muscle, scattered areas of hyperintensity
- PD/Intermediate: Low signal intensity
- T1 C+: Intense enhancement
- GCTTS: Well-defined soft tissue mass adjacent to tendon
- PVNS: Heterogeneous well-defined synovium-based mass
  - Margins may be obscured and difficult to separate from adjacent muscle
  - Extends away from joint space
  - Septations
  - Subchondral erosions
  - Low signal on all pulse sequences characteristic (due to presence of hemosiderin)

Angiographic Findings
- Hypervascular soft tissue mass

Nuclear Medicine Findings
- Bone Scan: Increased uptake on blood pool images can be seen

Imaging Recommendations
- Best imaging tool: MRI
- Protocol advice: T1, T2WI MR, T1 C+ MR

DIFFERENTIAL DIAGNOSIS

Synovial Sarcoma
- Arises outside joint
- Areas of calcifications
- MRI: Shorter T1 and longer T2 than PVNS

Synovial Chondromatosis
- Multiple intraarticular bodies
- Can be calcified or noncalcified

Hemophilia
- Usually affects multiple joints
- Can cause growth disturbance

Rheumatoid Arthritis (RA)
- No hemosiderin deposits
- Periarticular osteoporosis
- Joint space narrowing

Posttraumatic Synovitis
- High signal on T2WI MR

Lipoma Arborescence
- Composed of hypertrophic villi distended with fat
- Follows signal intensity of fat on all pulse sequences

PATHOLOGY

General Features
- General path comments: Locally destructive fibrohistiocytic proliferation and villonodular protrusions of synovial membranes, affecting joints, bursae, tendon sheaths
- Genetics
  - Clonal chromosomal aberrations, aneuploidy
    - Trisomies 5 and 7
- Etiology
  - Controversial: Reactive inflammatory process
  - Low-grade, locally aggressive neoplasm

PIGMENTED VILLONODULAR SYNOVITIS

- Epidemiology
  - 5% of all primary soft tissue tumors
  - GCTTS: Second most common soft tissue mass of hand

Gross Pathologic & Surgical Features

- GCTTS: Small rubbery, encapsulated multinodular mass
  - Yellow-brown color, due to excessive deposits of lipid and hemosiderin
- PVNS: Joint filled with unclotted dark blood
  - Villonodular frond like proliferation of synovial membrane
  - Cut surface: Yellow-brown due to iron pigment (hemosiderin)

Microscopic Features

- GCTTS: Synovial proliferation
  - Multinucleated giant cells, macrophages, fibroblasts, xanthoma cells
  - Hemosiderin
- PVNS: Synovial hyperplasia
  - Multinucleated giant cells, hemosiderin-laden macrophages
    - Intra- and extracellular hemosiderin
  - Lipid laden histiocytes

CLINICAL ISSUES

Presentation

- Most common signs/symptoms: Limited joint mobility
- Clinical profile
  - GCTTS
    - Slowly enlarging, mobile, soft tissue mass
    - Pain increased with activity
  - PVNS
    - Joint swelling, pain of insidious onset
    - Increased skin temperature
    - Pain increased with motion, improved by rest
    - Sudden increase in pain due to torsion of synovial nodules
    - Decreased range of motion, joint locking
    - Joint effusion: Serosanguineous/xanthochromic fluid
    - Recurrent sanguinous effusions without history of trauma
    - Rapid accumulation of joint fluid after aspiration
    - Pathologic fracture secondary to subchondral bone invasion can be seen

Demographics

- Age
  - GCTTS: 30-50 years, mean: 32 years
  - PVNS: 30-40 years, childhood appearance reported
- Gender
  - GCTTS: M:F = 1:1
  - PVNS: F:M = 2:1

Natural History & Prognosis

- Benign, locally aggressive lesion
- Progressive destruction of articular cartilage and subchondral bone results in severe osteoarthritis
- PVNS: Recurrence 20-50%

Treatment

- Complete synovectomy (open): Recurrence 20%
  - Knee: Anterior and posterior synovectomy to reduce recurrence rate
- Arthroscopic synovectomy (often piecemeal, incomplete): Recurrence 50%
- Intraarticular yttrium-90 radiation synovectomy (experimental)
- Synovectomy combined with low dose radiation
- Total joint replacement
- Joint fusion in patients with advanced disease

DIAGNOSTIC CHECKLIST

Image Interpretation Pearls

- Can look like hemophilia but is monoarticular

SELECTED REFERENCES

1. Blanco CE et al: Combined partial arthroscopic synovectomy and radiation therapy for diffuse pigmented villonodular synovitis of the knee. Arthroscopy 17:527-31, 2001
2. De Beuckeleer L et al: Magnetic resonance imaging of localized giant cell tumour of the tendon sheath (MRI of localized GCTTS). Eur Radiol 7:198-201, 1997
3. Cotten A et al: Pigmented villonodular synovitis of the hip: Review of radiographic features in 58 patients. Skeletal Radiol 24:1-6, 1995
4. Hughes TH et al: Pigmented villonodular synovitis: MRI characteristics. Skeletal Radiol 24:7-12, 1995
5. Abdul-Karim EW et al: Diffuse and localized tenosynovial giant cell tumor and pigmented villonodular synovitis: A clinicopathologic and flow cytometric DNA analysis. Hum Pathol 23:729-35, 1992
6. Besette PR et al: Gadolinium-enhanced MRI of pigmented villonodular synovitis of the knee. J Comput Assist Tomogr 16:992-4, 1992
7. Fletcher JA et al: Trisomy 5 and trisomy 7 are non random aberrations in pigmented villonodular synovitis: Confirmation of trisomy 7 in uncultured cells. Genes Chromosomes Cancer 4:264-6, 1992
8. Karasick D et al: Giant cell tumor of tendon sheath: Spectrum of radiologic findings. Skeletal Radiol 21:219-24, 1992
9. Ogilvie-Harris DJ et al: Pigmented villonodular synovitis of the knee. The results of total arthroscopic synovectomy, partial, arthroscopic synovectomy, and arthroscopic local excision. J Bone Joint Surg Am 74(1):119-23, 1992
10. Butt WP et al: Pigmented villonodular synovitis of the knee: Computed tomographic appearances. Skeletal Radiol 19:191-6, 1990

PIGMENTED VILLONODULAR SYNOVITIS

IMAGE GALLERY

Typical

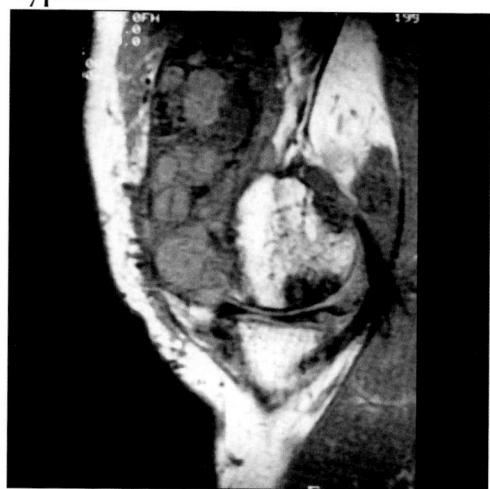
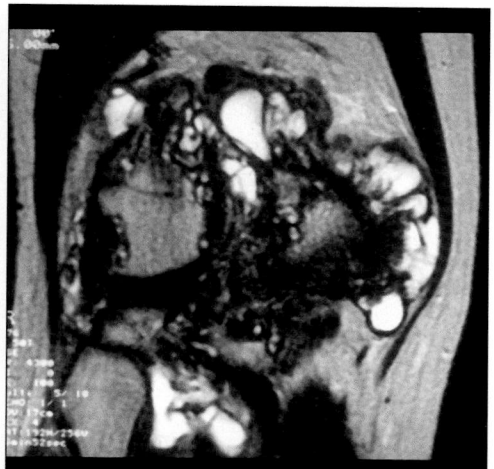

(Left) Sagittal T1WI MR of the knee shows lobulated masses of low signal intensity. *(Right)* Coronal T2WI MR shows heterogeneous lobulated mass with areas of high and low signal. Osseous erosions are noted.

Typical

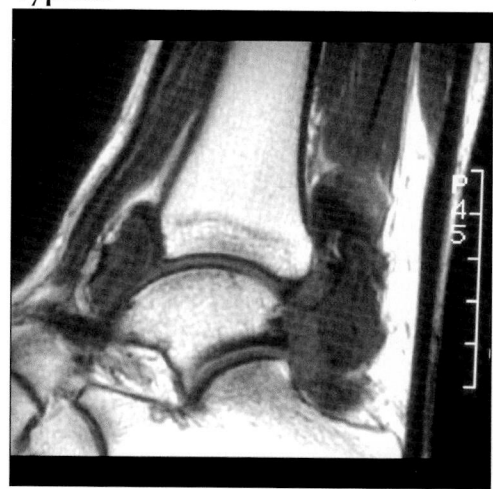
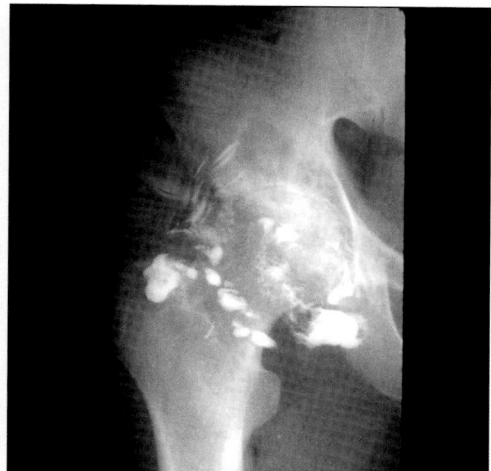

(Left) Sagittal T1WI MR shows lobulated mass of low signal involving the anterior and posterior aspect of the ankle. *(Right)* Anteroposterior radiography shows lytic lesions on both sides of the joint. There is joint space narrowing. Residual contrast from prior arthrogram is noted.

Other

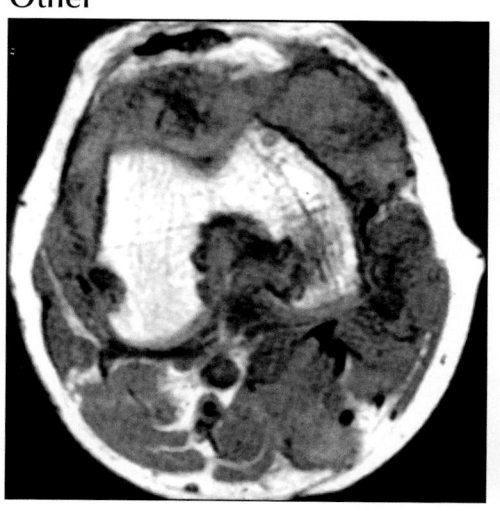
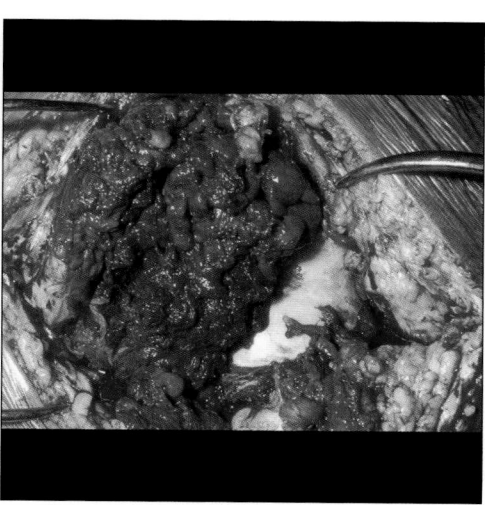

(Left) Axial T1WI MR shows large lobulated mass of low signal causing cortical erosions. *(Right)* Intra-operative photograph shows red-brown villonodular fronds.

SYNOVIAL SARCOMA

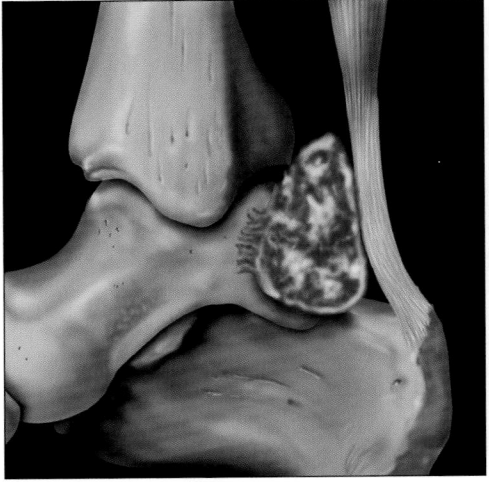

Sagittal graphic shows heterogeneous synovial sarcoma posterior to the talus. Cortical invasion is shown in the anterior aspect of the lesion.

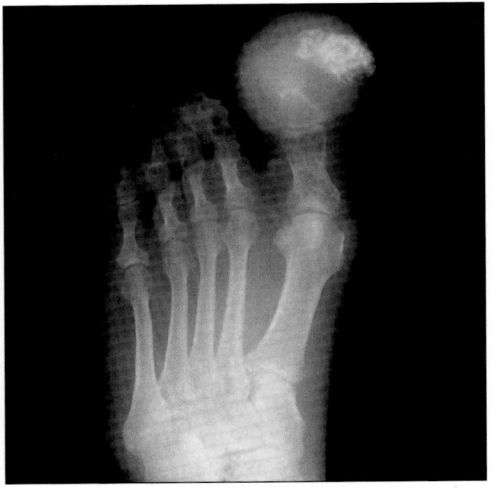

Anteroposterior radiography shows large soft tissue mass with coarse calcifications eroding the great toe.

TERMINOLOGY

Abbreviations and Synonyms
- Synovioma, tendosynovial sarcoma

Definitions
- Sarcoma of mesenchymal origin occurring in para-articular regions of extremities

IMAGING FINDINGS

General Features
- Best diagnostic clue
  - Radiographs, CT: Soft tissue mass with calcifications in proximity to joints
  - T2WI MR: Heterogeneous mass with triple signal intensity
- Location
  - Extremities: 80-95%
    - Lower extremity: 60%, knee and foot
    - Upper extremity: 15%
  - Head and neck: 10%
  - Trunk: 5-10%
  - Juxta-articular soft tissues, tendon sheaths
    - Within 5 cm of joint
  - Intraarticular: 5-10%
    - Extension from extraarticular site into joint
  - Deep soft tissues
- Size: 3-8 cm
- Morphology: Well-defined round or lobulated soft tissue mass

Radiographic Findings
- Radiography
  - Soft tissue mass close to joint
  - Amorphous calcifications: 25-30%
  - Bone invasion: 10-20%
    - Periosteal reaction, invasion of cortex, massive bone destruction rare
  - Juxta-articular osteoporosis

CT Findings
- NECT
  - Soft tissue mass isodense to muscle
  - Areas of hemorrhage, necrosis, cysts, calcifications
  - Useful to identify soft tissue calcification and osseous involvement
  - To evaluate pulmonary metastases, can be calcified
- CECT
  - Marked enhancement
  - IV contrast helpful to differentiate from adjacent muscle, neurovascular bundle

MR Findings
- T1WI
  - Heterogeneous septated mass

9

18

DDx: Synovial Sarcoma

Myositis Ossific.	PVNS	Fibromatosis	Osteosarcoma	Chondroma

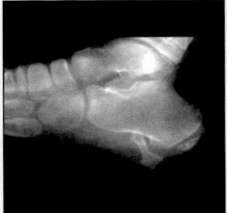
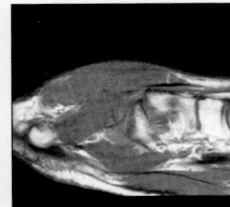
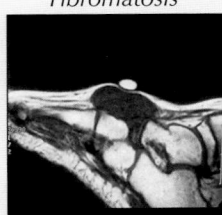
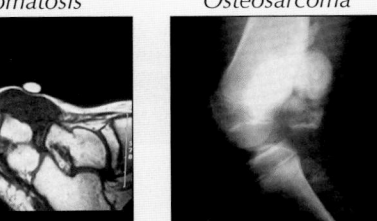
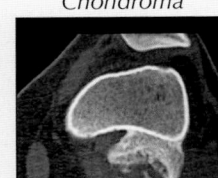

Lat Radiography	Sag T1WI MR	Sag T1WI MR	Lat Radiography	Ax NECT

SYNOVIAL SARCOMA

Key Facts

Imaging Findings
- Radiographs, CT: Soft tissue mass with calcifications in proximity to joints

Top Differential Diagnoses
- Soft Tissue Chondrosarcoma
- Myositis Ossificans
- Pigmented Villonodular Synovitis (PVNS)
- Parosteal Osteosarcoma
- Malignant Fibrous Histiocytoma (MFH)
- Juxtacortical Chondroma
- Fibromatosis

Pathology
- 8-10% of all soft tissue sarcomas
- Most common soft tissue sarcoma of hands and feet

Clinical Issues
- Slow growing palpable soft tissue mass
- Progressive pain
- Metastases in 80%
- Size less than 5 cm, young age (15 years or younger) have favorable prognosis
- 5 year survival rate: 27-76%, up to 82% in heavily calcified tumors
- 10 year survival rate: 20-63% (reflects relative high incidence of late metastases)
- Surgical resection with wide margins
- Local recurrence in 20-25%
- Surgical resection with preoperative radiation therapy
- Local recurrence: < 10%

  - Low - intermediate signal
  - Small lesions have homogeneous intermediate signal, isointense to muscle
- T2WI
  - Heterogeneous mass with hyperintense, isointense, and hypointense areas
  - Triple signal intensity: 30%
    - Mixture of cystic and solid elements with hemorrhage and fibrous tissue
  - Cystic components with fluid-fluid levels: 18%
- T1 C+: Marked enhancement
- Infiltrative margins
- Bone erosion and destruction
- To differentiate from surrounding muscles and neurovascular bundle

Ultrasonographic Findings
- Well-defined soft tissue mass
- Heterogeneous echogenicity +/- cystic components

Angiographic Findings
- Hypervascular soft tissue mass

Nuclear Medicine Findings
- Bone Scan: Increased radiotracer uptake around areas of calcification
- PET: Helpful in differentiating recurrent tumor from post-therapeutic changes

Imaging Recommendations
- Best imaging tool: MRI
- Protocol advice
  - MRI to evaluate extent
  - CT/radiographs to evaluate for calcification

DIFFERENTIAL DIAGNOSIS

Soft Tissue Chondrosarcoma
- Arises in proximal part of extremities and buttocks
- Aggressive appearance with invasion of adjacent skeletal structures

Myositis Ossificans
- Distinctive zoning phenomenon
- Lucent center, dense ossified periphery

Pigmented Villonodular Synovitis (PVNS)
- Rarely calcifies
- Low signal on T1 and T2WI MR

Parosteal Osteosarcoma
- Periosteal reaction
- Incomplete cleft between lesion and adjacent cortex

Malignant Fibrous Histiocytoma (MFH)
- Rarely calcified
- Older patients

Juxtacortical Chondroma
- Involves surface of bone
- Can erode subchondral bone
- Periosteal new bone formation

Fibromatosis
- Predominately low signal on T1 and T2WI MR

PATHOLOGY

General Features
- General path comments: Tumor of high malignancy but slow growth
- Genetics: Chromosome translocation t(X;18)(p11.2;q11.2)
- Etiology
  - Does NOT arise from synovial tissue
  - Likely originates from undifferentiated mesenchymal tissue (pluripotent mesenchyme of the limb bud)
- Epidemiology
  - 8-10% of all soft tissue sarcomas
  - 4th most common soft tissue sarcoma
  - Most common soft tissue sarcoma of hands and feet

SYNOVIAL SARCOMA

Gross Pathologic & Surgical Features
- Solid, sharply circumscribed, yellow, grey-white fleshy mass
- Smooth pseudocapsule
- Attached to surrounding tendons, tendon sheaths, joint capsule
- Areas of necrosis or hemorrhage
- Occasional spotty areas of calcification

Microscopic Features
- Biphasic type (most common): Spindle cell and epithelial component
  - Spindle and epithelial cells arranged in glandular or nest-like structure
- Monophasic type: Interdigitating fascicles formed by spindle cells
  - Only small number of epithelial cells
- Poorly differentiated type: Can be superimposed on other subtype
  - More aggressive, metastasizes earlier
  - Rich vascular pattern with thin walled vascular spaces, resembles hemangiopericytoma
- Foci of calcification usually in areas of hyalinization, periphery of tumor
- Chondroid and osseous metaplasia possible

Staging, Grading or Classification Criteria
- Surgical staging system for malignant musculoskeletal tumors
  - Stage Ia: Low grade, intracompartmental
  - Stage Ib: Low grade, extracompartmental
  - Stage IIa: High grade, intracompartmental
  - Stage IIb: High grade, extracompartmental
  - Stage IIIa: Low or high grade, intracompartmental, metastases
  - Stage IIIb: Low or high grade, extracompartmental, metastases

CLINICAL ISSUES

Presentation
- Most common signs/symptoms
  - Slow growing palpable soft tissue mass
  - Mass is firm and fixed to deeper structures
- Clinical profile
  - Progressive pain
  - Sensory/motor dysfunction distal to lesion
  - Long duration of symptoms: Average 2-4 years
    - Can be misdiagnosed as arthritis or synovitis
  - Metastases present at initial diagnosis in 25%

Demographics
- Age: 10-50, mean: 32 years
- Gender: M:F = 1.2:1

Natural History & Prognosis
- Slow growing malignant tumor with invasion of adjacent soft tissues and bone
- Lesions in hands and feet grow slower than lesions in more proximal extremities or trunk
- Metastases in 80%
  - Lungs: 60-90%
  - Lymph nodes: 5-20%
- Bones: 8-11%
- Lesions with calcification have better prognosis
- Size less than 5 cm, young age (15 years or younger) have favorable prognosis
- 5 year survival rate: 27-76%, up to 82% in heavily calcified tumors
- 10 year survival rate: 20-63% (reflects relative high incidence of late metastases)

Treatment
- Surgical resection with wide margins
  - Local recurrence in 20-25%
  - Occurs in excision scar/amputation stump
- Surgical resection with preoperative radiation therapy
  - Local recurrence: < 10%
- High grade lesions: Radical resection and radiation therapy
- Chemotherapy in metastatic cases
- Neoadjuvant chemotherapy successful in some cases

DIAGNOSTIC CHECKLIST

Image Interpretation Pearls
- Does NOT arise from joint
- Often misdiagnosed as benign lesion (e.g., ganglion)

SELECTED REFERENCES

1. Weiss SW et al: Enzinger and Weiss's soft tissue tumors. 4th ed. St. Louis MO, CV Mosby, 1483-509, 2001
2. Bergh P et al: Synovial sarcoma: Identification of low and high risk groups. Cancer 85:2596-607, 1999
3. Hirsch RJ et al: Synovial sarcomas of the head and neck: MR findings. Am J Roentgenol 169:1185-8, 1997
4. De Leeuw B et al: Identification of a yeast artificial chromosome (YAC) spanning the synovial sarcoma specific t(x;18)(p11.2;q11.2) breakpoint. Genes Chromosomes Cancer 6:182-9, 1993
5. Jones BC et al: Synovial sarcoma: MR imaging findings in 34 patients. Am J Roentgenol 161:827-30, 1993
6. Kampe CE et al: Synovial sarcoma: A study of intensive chemotherapy in 14 patients with localized disease. Cancer 72:2161-9, 1993
7. McKinney CD et al: Intraarticular synovial sarcoma. Am J Surg Pathol 16:1017-20, 1992
8. Menendez LR et al: Synovial Sarcoma: A clinicopathologic study. Orthop Rev 21:465-71, 1992
9. Morton MJ et al: MR imaging of synovial sarcoma. Am J Roentgenol 156: 337-40, 1991
10. Ryan JR et al: The natural history of metastatic synovial sarcoma. The experience of the southwest oncology group. Clin Orthop 164:257-, 1982
11. Varela-Duran J et al: Calcifying synovial sarcoma. Cancer 50:345-52, 1982

SYNOVIAL SARCOMA

Typical

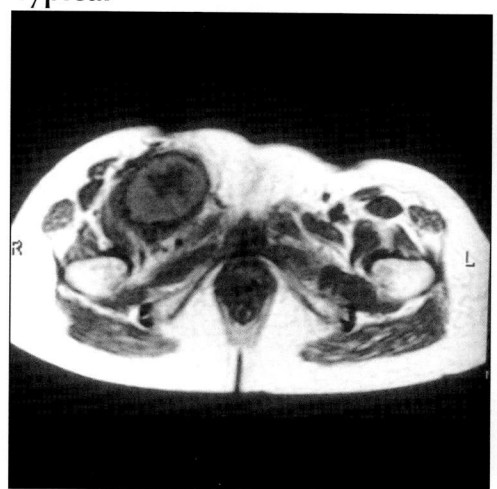
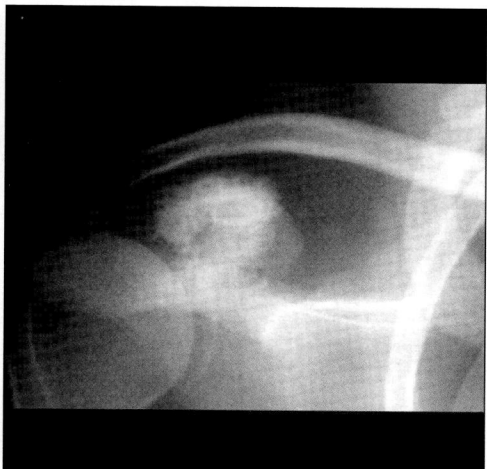

(Left) Axial T1WI MR shows round well-defined soft tissue mass of intermediate and central low signal in the anterior right thigh. *(Right)* Anteroposterior radiography shows calcified soft tissue mass in the right shoulder region.

Typical

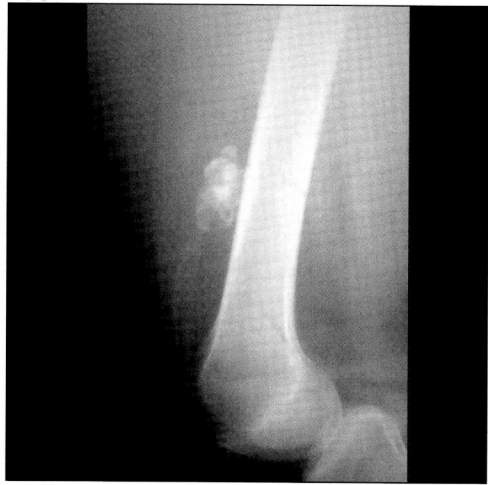
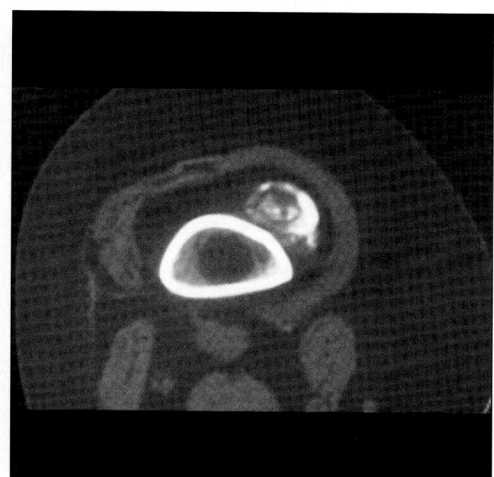

(Left) Lateral radiography shows soft tissue mass in the thigh with coarse calcifications. *(Right)* Axial NECT shows calcified soft tissue mass in the anterior thigh.

Typical

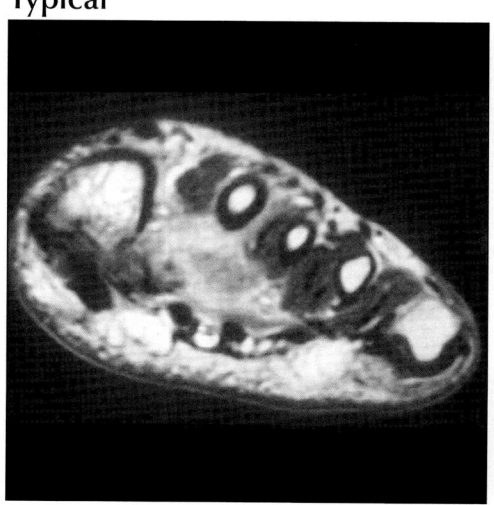
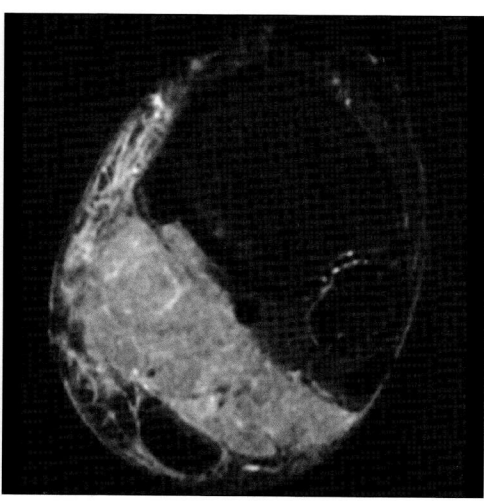

(Left) Axial T1 C+ MR shows heterogeneous enhancing mass at the plantar surface of the foot. *(Right)* Axial FS T2 FSE MR shows heterogeneous soft tissue mass of intermediate signal in the posterior ankle. Note areas of low and high signal.

LIPOMA, SOFT TISSUE

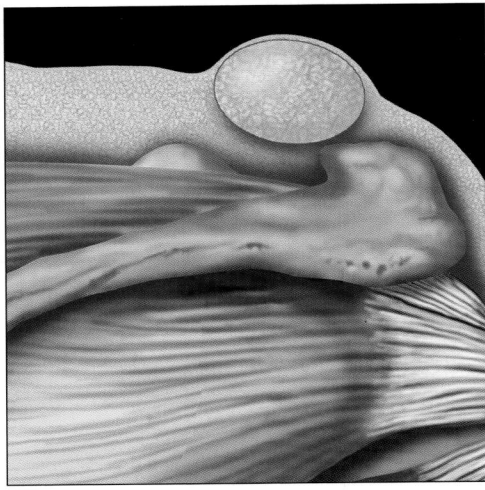

Coronal graphic shows well defined subcutaneous lipoma.

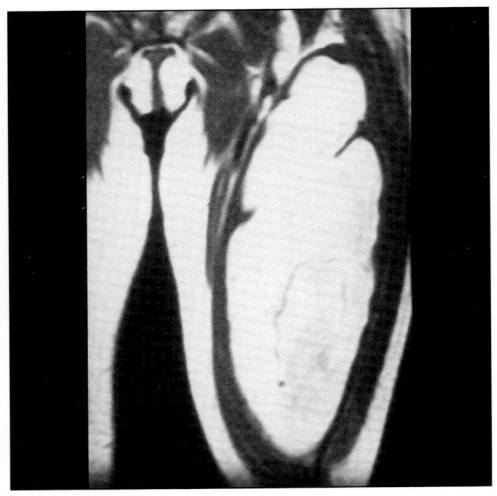

Coronal T1WI MR shows large homogeneous mass of fat SI involving the left thigh. Thin septations within the mass are noted.

TERMINOLOGY

Abbreviations and Synonyms
- Soft tissue lipoma

Definitions
- Benign soft tissue tumor composed of mature adipose tissue

IMAGING FINDINGS

General Features
- Best diagnostic clue: Parallels signal intensity of subcutaneous fat on all pulse sequences
- Location
  - Can occur anywhere in the body
  - Superficial/subcutaneous (most common): Posterior trunk, neck, proximal extremities
  - Deep: Retroperitoneum, chest wall, deep soft tissues of hands and feet
  - Multifocal: 5-8%
- Size
  - < 5 cm: 80%
  - > 10 cm rare
- Morphology: Well-defined homogeneous fatty soft tissue mass

Radiographic Findings
- Radiography
  - Hypodense soft tissue mass
  - Calcifications occasionally seen

CT Findings
- NECT
  - Well-defined, homogeneous soft tissue mass: Low attenuation (-65 to 120 HU)
    - Comparison with attenuation of surrounding fat helpful (fat attenuation can vary between different locations)
  - Occasional ossification within tumor
  - May cause cortical thickening when close to bone
  - Bone erosions rare
- CECT: No significant enhancement

MR Findings
- T1WI: High signal intensity
- T2WI: Intermediate signal intensity
- STIR: Low signal intensity
- T1 C+: No significant enhancement
- Parallels signal intensity of subcutaneous fat on all pulse sequences
- Differentiation from other lesions by fat suppression
- Well-defined and homogeneous, often with septations
- Intramuscular lipoma may be poorly marginated and infiltrate muscle planes

DDx: Lipoma, Soft Tissue

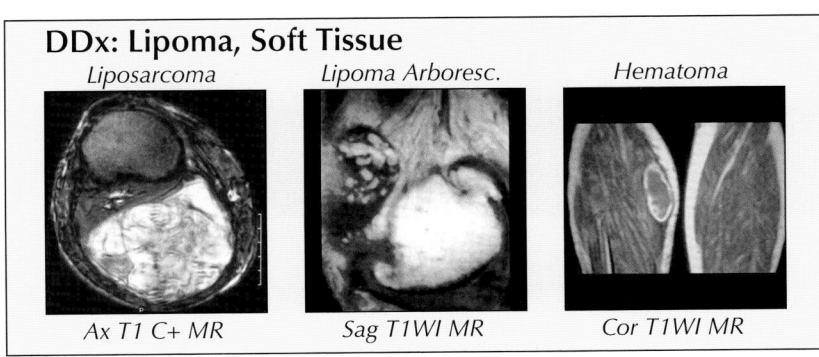

Liposarcoma	Lipoma Arboresc.	Hematoma
Ax T1 C+ MR	Sag T1WI MR	Cor T1WI MR

LIPOMA, SOFT TISSUE

Key Facts

Imaging Findings
- Best diagnostic clue: Parallels signal intensity of subcutaneous fat on all pulse sequences
- Well-defined, homogeneous soft tissue mass: Low attenuation (-65 to 120 HU)
- Use fat suppression sequences to differentiate from other lesions

Top Differential Diagnoses
- Liposarcoma
- Lipoma Arborescence
- Hematoma

Pathology
- Fat unavailable for systemic metabolism, does not change in size during starvation
- Most common soft tissue tumor

- 50% of all soft tissue tumors
- Familial multiple lipomas

Clinical Issues
- Most common signs/symptoms: Usually asymptomatic
- Slowly growing mobile soft mass
- Can produce pain by compression of nerves
- Benign tumor
- Marginal en bloc excision of large or symptomatic lesions
- Recurrence: 5%

Diagnostic Checklist
- If palpable tumor not easily identified on MRI the diagnosis is often subcutaneous lipoma

---

- Fibrolipoma: Contains fibrous tissue
  - Septations of low signal
- Lipoblastoma: Cellular, immature lipoma, occurs in childhood, rare
  - Mixed lipomatous and nonspecific non-lipomatous components
  - Resembles liposarcoma
- Angiolipoma: Composed of fatty and vascular tissue
  - Can have flow voids, phleboliths
- Spindle cell lipoma: Contains large amounts of collagen forming spindle cells
  - Spindle cell elements: Low signal intensity
- Infiltrating lipoma: Extends between muscle fibers
  - Associated with muscle atrophy
- Neural fibrolipoma: Enlargement of nerve by fibrofatty tissue
  - Longitudinal serpiginous signal voids separated by areas of fat signal

Angiographic Findings
- Hypovascular soft tissue mass

Imaging Recommendations
- Best imaging tool: MRI, CT
- Protocol advice
  - Use fat suppression sequences to differentiate from other lesions
  - Place marker over subcutaneous lesion
  - Comparison with contralateral side/extremity to identify subtle asymmetry

DIFFERENTIAL DIAGNOSIS

Liposarcoma
- Heterogeneous mass with fat and soft-tissue components
- Enhancement after IV contrast administration

Lipoma Arborescence
- Composed of hypertrophic villi distended with fat
- Likely reactive process to chronic synovitis
- Monoarticular
- Villous frondlike mass on MRI

- Signal intensity of fat on all pulse sequences

Hematoma
- Heterogeneous
- Surrounding edema

PATHOLOGY

General Features
- General path comments
  - Tumor tissue similar to ordinary body fat
  - Fat unavailable for systemic metabolism, does not change in size during starvation
- Genetics
  - Translocation between 12q13-15
  - HMGI-C gene part of high morbility group protein gene family, mapped to 12q15
- Etiology
  - Mesenchymal neoplasm
  - More common in obese patients and diabetics, often increases during weight gain
  - Blunt trauma or radiation can lead to overgrowth of fat indistinguishable from lipoma
  - Multiple lipomas reported in diabetic patients at the site of insulin injection
- Epidemiology
  - Most common soft tissue tumor
  - 50% of all soft tissue tumors
  - Occurs in 1% of population
- Associated abnormalities
  - Familial multiple lipomas
    - Autosomal dominant inheritance
    - Multiple subcutaneous lipomas
    - Hypercholesterolemia in some cases
  - Cowden syndrome: Autosomal dominant
    - Multiple hamartoma syndrome
    - Multiple lipomas, hemangiomas, papillomatous lesions of skin and mucosa
    - Multinodular goiter
    - Gastrointestinal polyps
  - Proteus syndrome
    - Rare hamartomatous disorder

LIPOMA, SOFT TISSUE

- Multiple lipomas, venous, lymphatic malformations, nevi
- Partial gigantism with limb overgrowth

Gross Pathologic & Surgical Features
- Soft, well-encapsulated, yellow lobulated mass
- Thin surrounding capsule
- Consists of yellow, grossly normal-appearing fat
- Greasy, myxoid cut surface

Microscopic Features
- Mature, uniform fat cells (adipocytes), slightly larger than non-neoplastic fat cells
- Fibrous connective tissue, associated with capsule or septations
- Well vascularized, vessels compressed by distended adipocytes

Staging, Grading or Classification Criteria
- Surgical staging system for benign musculoskeletal tumors
  - Stage 1: Latent
  - Stage 2: Active
  - Stage 3: Aggressive

CLINICAL ISSUES

Presentation
- Most common signs/symptoms: Usually asymptomatic
- Clinical profile
  - Slowly growing mobile soft mass
  - Deep intramuscular tumors can have firm consistency
  - Mass can harden after application of ice
  - Deep seated tumors can reach large size before diagnosis
  - Superficial lesions can be differentiated from cystic lesions by inability to transmit light
  - Can produce pain by compression of nerves

Demographics
- Age: 5-75 years; peak: 40-60 years
- Gender: M:F = 1:1

Natural History & Prognosis
- Benign tumor
- Commonly presents as active stage 2 lesion, becomes latent over time
- Deep lesions can become remarkably large
- Displaces adjacent tissues, no invasion of fascial planes
- Malignant transformation reported in few cases
  - Subtle features of malignancy in these cases probably missed at initial presentation

Treatment
- Marginal en bloc excision of large or symptomatic lesions
  - Recurrence: 5%
- Liposuction

DIAGNOSTIC CHECKLIST

Consider
- Lipoma variants can resemble liposarcoma and may require biopsy for diagnosis

Image Interpretation Pearls
- If palpable tumor not easily identified on MRI the diagnosis is often subcutaneous lipoma

SELECTED REFERENCES

1. Weiss SW et al: Enzinger and Weiss's soft tissue tumors. 4th ed. St.Louis MO, CV Mosby, 571-639, 2001
2. Willen H et al: Comparison of chromosomal patterns with clinical features in 165 lipomas: A report of CHAMP study group. Cancer Genet Cytogenet 102:46-9 , 1998
3. Kransdorf MJ et al: Imaging of soft tissue tumors. 1st ed. Philadelphia PA, W.B. Saunders, 57-79, 1997
4. Munk PL et al: Lipoma and liposarcoma: Evaluation using CT and MR imaging. Am J Roentgenol 169:589-94 , 1997
5. Stoll C et al: Multiple familial lipomatosis with polyneuropathy, an inherited dominant condition. Ann Genet 39:193-6, 1996
6. Schoenmakers EF et al: Recurrent rearrangements in the high mobility group protein gene, HMGI-C, in benign mesenchymal tumors. Nat Genet 10:436-44, 1995
7. Kransdorf MJ: Benign soft tissue tumors in a large referral population: Distribution of diagnoses by, age, sex, and location. Am J Roentgenol 164:395-402, 1995
8. Gelineck J et al: Evaluation of lipomatous soft tissue tumors by MR imaging. Acta Radiol 35:367-70, 1994
9. Mrozek K et al: Chromosome 12 breakpoints are cytogenetically different in benign and malignant lipogenetic tumors: Localization of breakpoints in lipoma to 12q15 and in myxoid liposarcoma to 12q13.3. Cancer Res 53:1670-5, 1993
10. Kransdorf MJ et al: Fat containing soft tissue masses of the extremities. Radiographics 11:81-106, 1991
11. Solvonuk PF et al: Correlation of morphologic and biochemical observations in human lipomas. Lab Invest 51:469-74, 1984

LIPOMA, SOFT TISSUE

IMAGE GALLERY

Typical

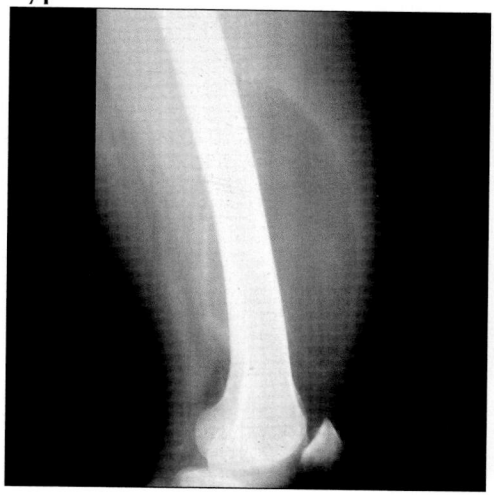
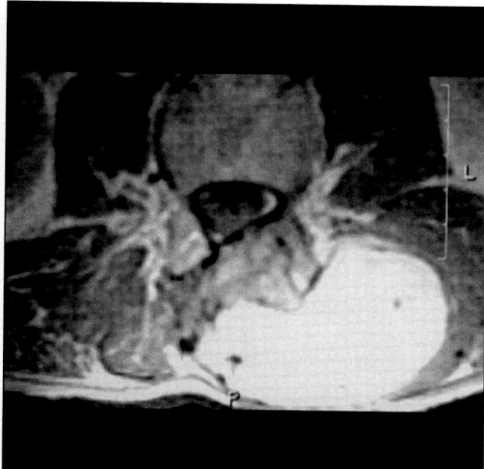

(Left) Lateral radiography shows large mass of fat density in the anterior thigh. *(Right)* Axial T1WI MR shows hyperintense mass of fat signal in the posterior paraspinous soft tissues.

Variant

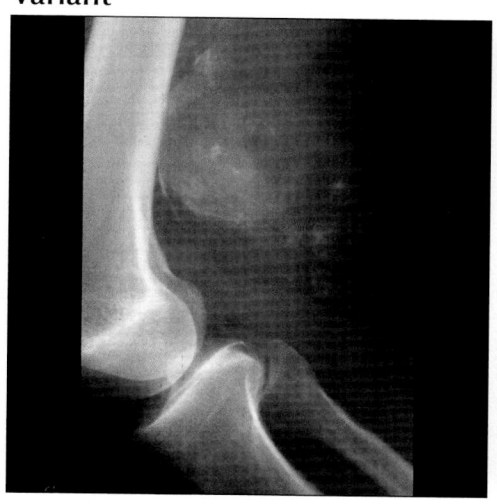
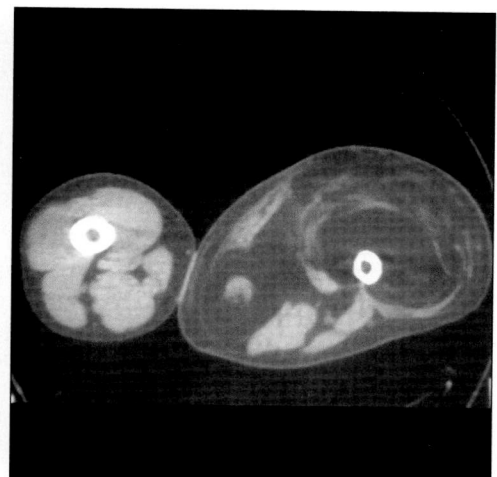

(Left) Lateral radiography shows soft tissue mass of fat density with areas of calcifications in the posterior thigh. *(Right)* Axial NECT in a patient with lipomatosis shows multiple lipomas replacing almost entire musculature of the left thigh.

Other

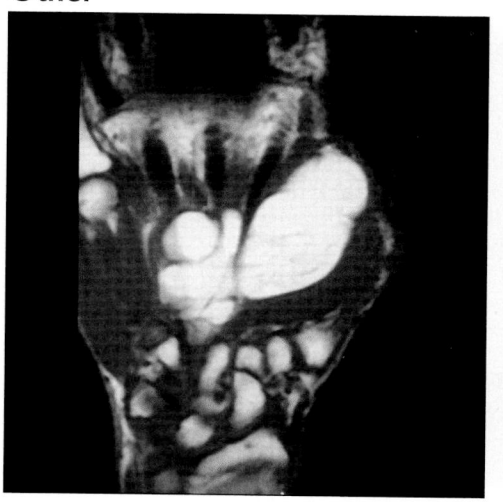
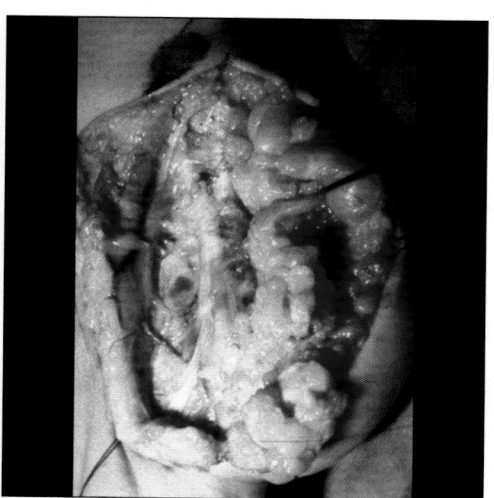

(Left) Coronal T1WI MR shows multiple lipomas of the hand in a patient with lipomatosis. *(Right)* Intra-operative photograph shows multiple lobulated yellow masses involving the hand.

LIPOSARCOMA, SOFT TISSUE

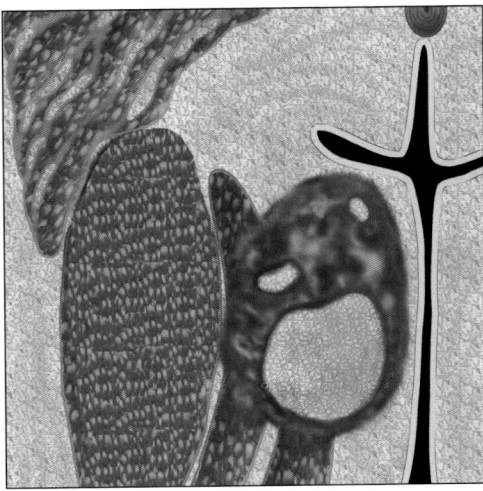

Coronal graphic shows infiltrating soft tissue mass in the medial thigh. Areas of mature fat are shown in yellow.

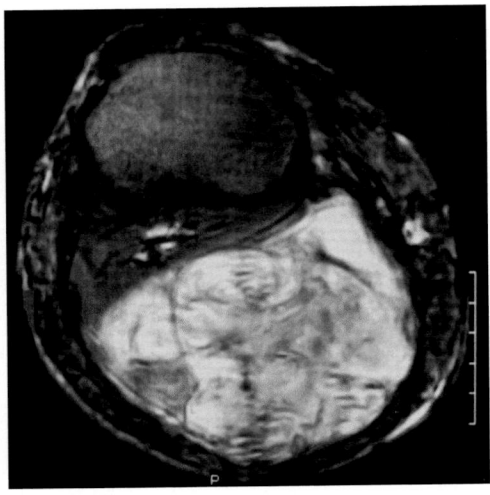

Axial T1 C+ MR show heterogeneous, enhancing soft tissue mass with septations posterior to the proximal tibia. Surgery revealed a high grade liposarcoma.

TERMINOLOGY

Abbreviations and Synonyms
- Soft tissue liposarcoma

Definitions
- Malignant mesenchymal tumor with microscopic appearance of adipose tissue

IMAGING FINDINGS

General Features
- Best diagnostic clue: Large, enhancing, septated mass with fatty and soft tissue components
- Location
  - Trunk/retroperitoneum: 42%
  - Lower extremity: 41%
    - Buttocks
    - Medial thigh
    - Popliteal fossa
    - Adductor canal
  - Upper extremity: 11%
    - Shoulder
    - Upper arms
  - Head and neck: 6%
  - Arises along neurovascular bundle, between muscles
- Size
  - 2-30 cm, may be > 30 cm
  - Retroperitoneal tumors can weigh several pounds
- Morphology: Heterogeneous soft tissue mass with or without fat

Radiographic Findings
- Radiography
  - Nonspecific soft tissue mass
  - Ossification within tumor: 10%

CT Findings
- NECT
  - Heterogeneous soft tissue mass
  - Fatty and soft tissue components
  - Fat frequently radiologically not detectable
  - Calcifications
- CECT: Enhancement

MR Findings
- T1WI
  - Hypo- hyperintense
  - Septations: Hypointense
- T2WI
  - Hyperintense, near water density (myxoid cells)
  - Septations: Hyperintense
- T1 C+: Enhancing components
- Fat may or may not be present
- The more differentiated, the more the signal intensity of tumor approaches fat

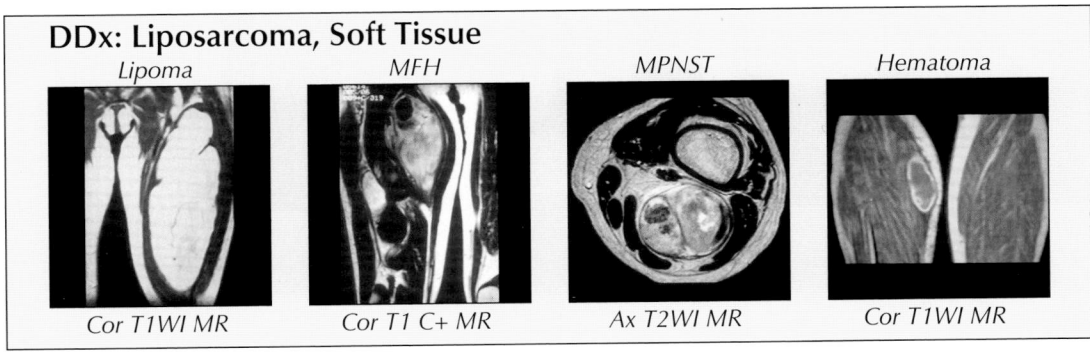

DDx: Liposarcoma, Soft Tissue

Lipoma	MFH	MPNST	Hematoma
Cor T1WI MR	Cor T1 C+ MR	Ax T2WI MR	Cor T1WI MR

LIPOSARCOMA, SOFT TISSUE

Key Facts

Imaging Findings

- Best diagnostic clue: Large, enhancing, septated mass with fatty and soft tissue components
- The more differentiated, the more the signal intensity of tumor approaches fat

Top Differential Diagnoses

- Lipoma
- Malignant Fibrous Histiocytoma (MFH)
- Peripheral Nerve Sheath Tumors: Malignant (MPNST), Benign (BPNST)
- Hematoma
- Intraabdominal Desmoid

Pathology

- 2nd most common soft tissue sarcoma in adults
- 16-20% of all malignant soft tissue tumors

Clinical Issues

- Most common signs/symptoms: Usually painless mass
- Can cause symptoms from compression of neurovascular bundle, abdominal organs
- Weight loss despite large soft tissue mass
- Biologic behavior and prognosis determined by histologic type and size
- Metastases in 50%
- Overall 5-year survival: 60%
- Stage I lesions: Surgical resection with wide margins
- Stage II lesions: Surgical resection with wide margins and radiation therapy

---

- Irregular thickened septa

Ultrasonographic Findings

- Hyperechoic heterogeneous soft tissue mass

Angiographic Findings

- Hypervascular soft tissue mass

Nuclear Medicine Findings

- PET: Increased FDG uptake

Imaging Recommendations

- Best imaging tool: MRI
- Protocol advice: T1, T2WI MR, T1 C+ MR

DIFFERENTIAL DIAGNOSIS

Lipoma

- Homogeneous soft tissue mass
- Occurs more commonly in subcutaneous tissues (liposarcoma: Deep soft tissues)
- No enhancement after IV contrast administration

Malignant Fibrous Histiocytoma (MFH)

- No fat components
- Often hemorrhagic

Peripheral Nerve Sheath Tumors: Malignant (MPNST), Benign (BPNST)

- Related to neurovascular bundle
- HU less than muscle
- May mimic fatty tissue (lipid rich Schwann cells)
- Entrapment of adjacent adipose tissue by plexiform neurofibromas

Hematoma

- Signal on T1 and T2WI MR longer than fat
- T1WI MR: Darker than fat
- T2WI MR: Brighter than fat
- Surrounding edema

Intraabdominal Desmoid

- No fat components

PATHOLOGY

General Features

- General path comments
  - Mesenchymal sarcoma with different subtypes that shows wide range of behavior and prognosis
    - Non metastasizing neoplasm to high grade sarcoma with metastatic potential
- Genetics
  - Myxoid and round cell type: Reciprocal translocation between chromosome 12 and 16
  - Breakpoint 12q13.3
- Etiology
  - Malignant tumor of mesenchymal origin with fat-forming cells (lipoblasts)
  - Relationship to trauma has been reported
- Epidemiology
  - 2nd most common soft tissue sarcoma in adults
  - 16-20% of all malignant soft tissue tumors

Gross Pathologic & Surgical Features

- Circumscribed, lobular tumor with smooth surface
- Color and consistency varies with histologic composition
  - Soft, bright yellow, fleshy, firm
  - Can have large areas of necrosis and hemorrhage

Microscopic Features

- Well-differentiated type: 15%, best prognosis
  - Large, mature lipocytes with varying degrees of nuclear atypia
- Myxoid type: 40-50%
  - Proliferating fibroblasts, plexiform capillary pattern, myxoid matrix, fat amount < 10%
  - Metastasizes to serosal and pleural surfaces, subcutis, spine
- Pleomorphic type: 20%, highly anaplastic tumor, pleomorphic cells growing in disorderly fashion
  - Voluminous cytoplasm filled with lipid vacuoles, displace and distort nuclei ("scalloped" effect)
- Round cell type: < 10%, poorly differentiated, highly cellular tumor

LIPOSARCOMA, SOFT TISSUE

- o Primitive, small, round cells with sporadic lipoblastic differentiation
- o Areas of hemorrhage and necrosis common
- Immunohistochemistry: S-100 positive

Staging, Grading or Classification Criteria
- WHO classification: Well differentiated, dedifferentiated, myxoid, pleomorphic, round cell type
- Surgical staging system for malignant musculoskeletal tumors
  - o Stage Ia: Low grade, intracompartmental
  - o Stage Ib: Low grade, extracompartmental
  - o Stage IIa: High grade, intracompartmental
  - o Stage IIb: High grade, extracompartmental
  - o Stage IIIa: Low or high grade, intracompartmental, metastases
  - o Stage IIIb: Low or high grade, extracompartmental, metastases

CLINICAL ISSUES

Presentation
- Most common signs/symptoms: Usually painless mass
- Clinical profile
  - o Painful in 10-15%
  - o Can cause symptoms from compression of neurovascular bundle, abdominal organs
  - o Patients with involvement of extremities present 5-10 years earlier than patients with retroperitoneal tumors
  - o Weight loss despite large soft tissue mass
  - o Metastases to lung (50%), visceral organs

Demographics
- Age
  - o 50-60 years
  - o Patients with liposarcomas involving extremities 10-15 years younger than patients with retroperitoneal liposarcomas
- Gender: M:F = 1:1, M > F

Natural History & Prognosis
- Biologic behavior and prognosis determined by histologic type and size
- Well differentiated type: Best prognosis, can recur locally, does not metastasize
  - o 5-year survival: 80-100%
- Pleomorphic and round cell type: Poor prognosis, recur, metastasize
  - o 5-year survival: 50%
- Size > 15 cm poor prognosis
- Metastases in 50%
- Overall 5-year survival: 60%

Treatment
- Stage I lesions: Surgical resection with wide margins
  - o Resection with marginal margins, neoadjuvant radiation therapy
  - o Recurrence in 60%
- Stage II lesions: Surgical resection with wide margins and radiation therapy
  - o Radical resection, possible amputation
- Surgical resection with radiation and chemotherapy for high grade stage III lesions

DIAGNOSTIC CHECKLIST

Image Interpretation Pearls
- Liposarcoma often does not contain visible fat

SELECTED REFERENCES

1. Weiss SW et al: Enzinger and Weiss's soft tissue tumors. 4th ed. St. Louis MO, CV Mosby, 641-43, 2001
2. Arkun R et al: Liposarcoma of soft tissue: MRI findings with pathologic correlation. Skeletal Radiol 26:167-72, 1997
3. Kransdorf MJ et al: Imaging of soft tissue tumors. 1st ed. Philadelphia PA, W.B. Saunders, 79-101, 1997
4. Fletcher CD et al: Correlation between clinicopathological features and karyotype in lipomatous tumors: A report of 178 cases from the chromosomes and morphologic (CHAMP) collaborative study group. Am J Pathol 148:623-630, 1996
5. Kilpatrick SE et al: The clinicopathologic spectrum of myxoid and round cell liposarcoma: A study of 95 cases. Cancer 77:1450-8, 1996
6. Kransdorf MJ: Malignant soft tissue tumors in a large referral population: Distribution of diagnoses by age, sex and location. Am J Roentgenol 164:129-34, 1995
7. Jelinek JS et al: Liposarcoma of the extremities: MR and CT findings in the histologic subtypes. Radiology 186:455-9, 1993
8. Mrozek K et al: Chromosome 12 breakpoints are cytogenetically different in benign and malignant lipogenetic tumors: Localization of breakpoints in lipoma to 12q15 and in myxoid liposarcoma to 12q13.3. Cancer Res 53:1670-5, 1993
9. Crim JR et al: Diagnosis of soft-tissue masses with MR imaging: Can benign masses be differentiated from malignant ones? Radiology 185:581-6, 1992.
10. Sundaram M et al: Myxoid liposarcoma: Magnetic resonance imaging appearances with clinical and histological correlation. Skeletal Radiol 19:359-62, 1990.
11. Bolen JW et al: Liposarcomas: A histogenetic approach to the classification of adipose tissue neoplasms. Am J Surg Pathol 8:3-17, 1984

LIPOSARCOMA, SOFT TISSUE

Typical

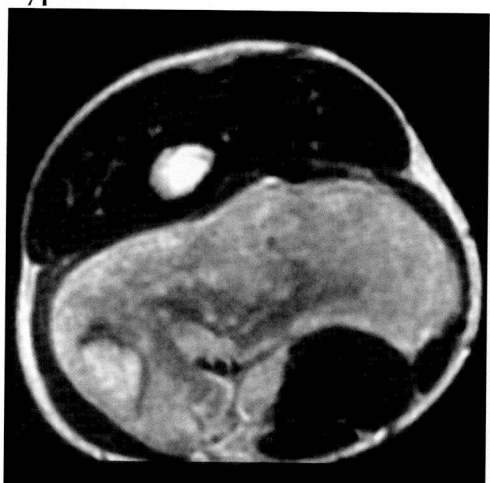
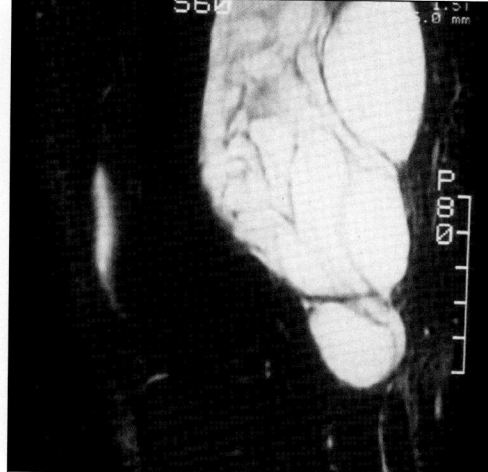

(Left) Axial T1 C+ MR shows heterogeneous, enhancing soft tissue mass in the posterior upper arm, which was found to be a liposarcoma of round-cell type. *(Right)* Sagittal FS T2 FSE MR shows hyperintense, septated soft tissue mass in the posterior thigh. Surgery revealed a myxoid liposarcoma.

Typical

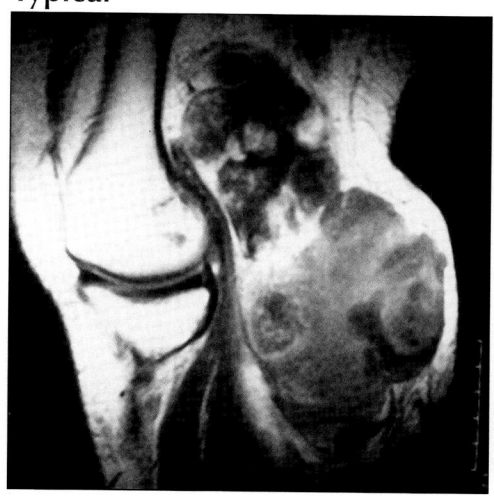
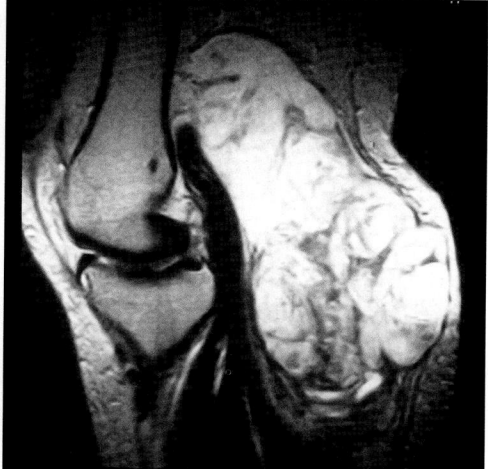

(Left) Sagittal T1WI MR shows heterogeneous mass with lipomatous components in the posterior thigh. Surgery revealed a high-grade liposarcoma. *(Right)* Sagittal T2WI MR of the high-grade liposarcoma shows marked hyperintensity of the tumor. Septations are better visualized on this T2 WI MR.

Other

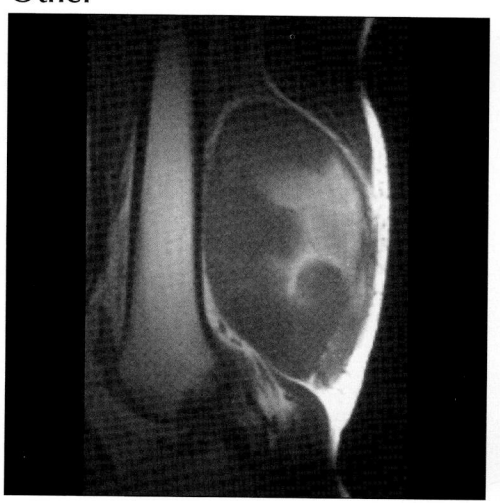
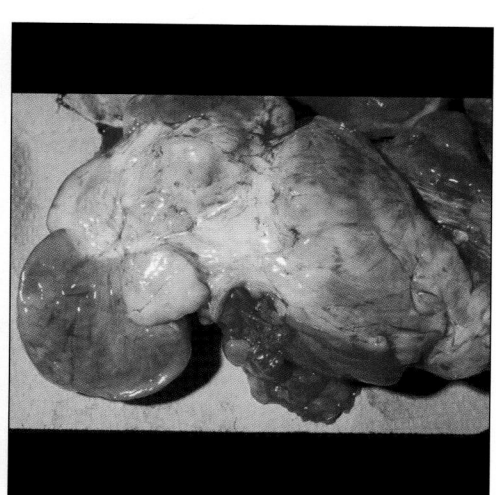

(Left) Sagittal T1WI MR shows well-defined mass in the posterior thigh with lipomatous components (hyperintense). Surgery revealed a well-differentiated liposarcoma. *(Right)* Gross pathology shows lobular tumor with yellow and fleshy areas.

BENIGN PERIPHERAL NERVE SHEATH TUMOR

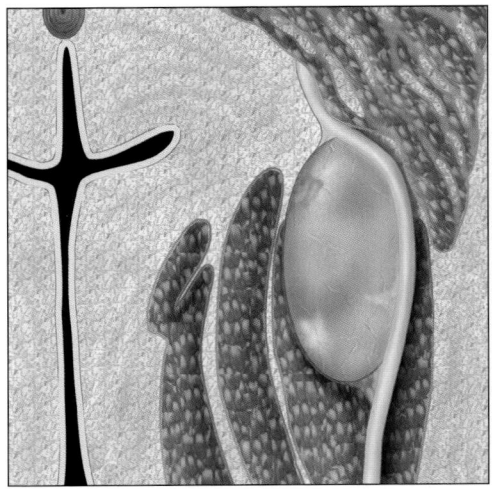

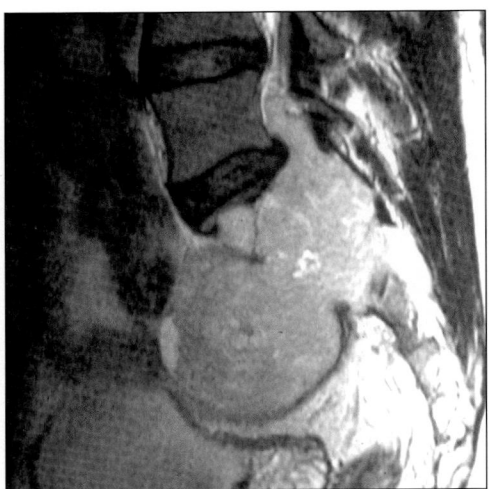

Coronal graphic shows BPNST in the medial thigh. The lesion is eccentric to the nerve consistent with Schwannoma. Surrounding epineurium is shown in yellow.

Sagittal PD FSE MR shows sacral dumbbell-shaped nerve sheath tumor of intermediate signal .

TERMINOLOGY

Abbreviations and Synonyms
- Benign peripheral nerve sheath tumors (BPNST) divided into
  - Schwannoma (neurilemmoma)
  - Neurofibroma

Definitions
- Benign lesion of neural origin that may occur in peripheral nerves, soft tissue, skin, or bone

IMAGING FINDINGS

General Features
- Best diagnostic clue
  - Circumscribed fusiform mass entering and exiting nerve
  - Best seen on long-axis MRI
- Location
  - Schwannoma
    - Cutaneous nerves of head and neck
    - Flexor surfaces of extremities (peroneal and ulnar nerves commonly involved)
    - Posterior mediastinum
    - Retroperitoneum
  - Neurofibroma
    - Neural plexus, peripheral, or spinal nerve
    - Cutaneous nerves most commonly involved
  - Neurofibroma
    - Solitary in 90%
  - Schwannoma
    - Mostly solitary
    - Multiple in 5%
- Size
  - < 5 cm
  - Deep lesions associated with large nerves: Up to 15 cm
- Morphology: Soft tissue mass related to neurovascular bundle

Radiographic Findings
- Radiography
  - Deep or superficial soft tissue mass
  - Mineralization within tumor uncommon
  - Erosion of adjacent bone

CT Findings
- NECT
  - Hypodense (20-30 HU) soft tissue mass, between muscle bundles associated with neurovascular bundle
  - Isodense to skeletal muscle
- CECT: Large lesions show marked enhancement

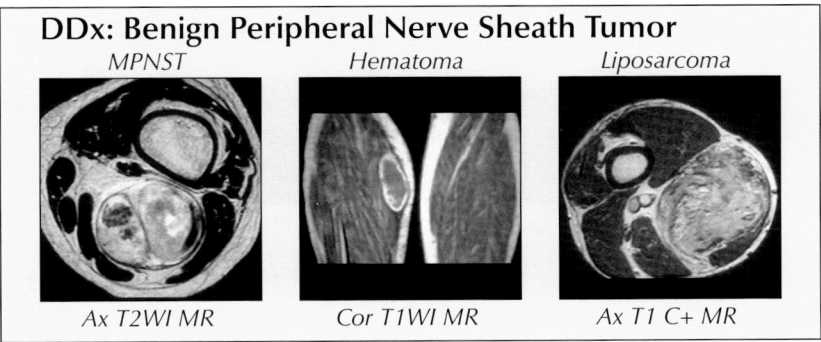

DDx: Benign Peripheral Nerve Sheath Tumor

MPNST	Hematoma	Liposarcoma
Ax T2WI MR	*Cor T1WI MR*	*Ax T1 C+ MR*

BENIGN PERIPHERAL NERVE SHEATH TUMOR

Key Facts

Imaging Findings
- Circumscribed fusiform mass entering and exiting nerve
- Best seen on long-axis MRI
- Best imaging tool: MRI

Top Differential Diagnoses
- Malignant Peripheral Nerve Sheath Tumor (MPNST)
- Hematoma
- Liposarcoma

Pathology
- Schwannoma: 5% of all benign soft tissue tumors
- Neurofibroma: Slightly more than 5% of all benign soft tissue tumors

Clinical Issues
- Most common signs/symptoms: Slowly growing painless mass
- Involvement of large nerves often produces neurologic symptoms
- Associated with NF-1: Neurofibromas, Lisch nodules, café-au-lait spots
- Only 10% of patients with neurofibromas have NF-1
- Schwannoma: Recurrence unusual
- Potential for malignant transformation: 4% in NF-1, rare in solitary tumors
- Surgical excision of symptomatic lesions

MR Findings
- T1WI: Soft tissue mass isointense to muscle
- T2WI
  - Soft tissue mass hyperintense compared to surrounding fat
  - "Target sign": Center of low signal (due to collagen and condensed Schwann cells)
- T1 C+
  - Variable enhancement
  - Often peripheral enhancement
- Well-defined fusiform mass
- Spinal involvement
  - Intradural extramedullary mass
  - Well-defined dumbbell shaped mass (extradural component extends through neural foramen)
  - Widening of intervertebral foramina
    - Erosion of pedicles
    - Scalloping of vertebral bodies
- Peripheral nerve involvement
  - Related to neurovascular bundle, nerve entering and exiting mass
  - Peripheral rim of fat ("split-fat" sign)
  - Can cause displacement of associated neurovascular bundle
  - Large masses can cause venous obstruction and hypertrophy of feeding vessels
  - Muscle atrophy can be seen
- Schwannoma
  - Nerve is eccentric to mass
  - Fibrous pseudocapsule
- Neurofibroma
  - Indistinct margins

Ultrasonographic Findings
- Hypoechoic well-defined mass

Imaging Recommendations
- Best imaging tool: MRI
- Protocol advice: T1, T2WI, T1C+ MR

DIFFERENTIAL DIAGNOSIS

Malignant Peripheral Nerve Sheath Tumor (MPNST)
- Involves major nerve trunks
- Sudden enlargement of pre-existing neurofibroma in NF-1
- Usually > 5 cm

Hematoma
- Surrounding edema
- No enhancement of solid components

Liposarcoma
- Not related to neurovascular bundle
- BPNST may mimic fatty tissue: Lipid rich Schwann cells
  - Entrapment of adjacent adipose tissue by plexiform neurofibromas

PATHOLOGY

General Features
- General path comments: Most important benign soft tissue tumors in which malignant transformation is acknowledged phenomenon
- Genetics
  - Neurofibromatosis Type 1 (NF-1), Von Recklinghausen's disease
    - Autosomal dominant, one of most common genetic diseases
    - High rate of penetrance
    - 50% of cases from new mutations
    - Genetic abnormality on chromosome 17
    - Tumor suppressor gene producing protein neurofibromin
- Etiology
  - Arises from tissue of neuroectodermal or neural crest origin
  - Schwannoma and neurofibroma contain cells that are closely related to normal Schwann cells
  - Might arise from Schwann cells

BENIGN PERIPHERAL NERVE SHEATH TUMOR

- Epidemiology
  - Schwannoma: 5% of all benign soft tissue tumors
  - Neurofibroma: Slightly more than 5% of all benign soft tissue tumors
- Associated abnormalities
  - NF-1: Multiple neurofibromas
    - Skeletal abnormalities
    - Kyphoscoliosis
    - Lambdoid suture defects
    - Pseudarthrosis (tibia)
    - Rib deformities
    - Meningoceles
    - Optic nerve gliomas, astrocytoma

Gross Pathologic & Surgical Features
- Schwannoma
  - True capsule composed of epineurium
  - Involvement of large nerves: Tumor eccentric to nerve, nerve displaced to periphery of mass
  - Involvement of small nerves: Nerve often obliterated by mass
  - Degenerative changes with cyst formation, calcification, hemorrhage
- Neurofibroma
  - Firm, gray-white mass often without capsule
  - Lesion cannot be separated from involved nerve
  - Nerve may be seen entering and exiting fusiform tumor mass
  - Extension of tumor outside epineurium of small nerves
  - Solitary neurofibroma: Well-delineated, firm, white shiny
  - Plexiform neurofibroma: Multifocal myxoid lesions, "bag of worms", diagnostic of NF-1

Microscopic Features
- Schwannoma
  - Intermixed Antoni A cells: Cellular, arranged in short bundles or interlacing fascicles
  - Antoni B cells: Less cellular and organized, more myxoid component
- Neurofibroma
  - Does not contain Antoni A or B cells
  - Composed of interlacing bundles of Schwann cells, fibroblasts, with involvement of nerve fibers
  - Immunohistochemistry: Variable S-100 expression

Staging, Grading or Classification Criteria
- Surgical staging system for benign musculoskeletal tumors
  - Stage 1: Latent
  - Stage 2: Active
  - Stage 3: Aggressive

CLINICAL ISSUES

Presentation
- Most common signs/symptoms: Slowly growing painless mass
- Clinical profile
  - Schwannoma
    - Painless mass
    - No neurologic symptoms
  - Neurofibroma
    - Superficial painless mass
    - Involvement of large nerves often produces neurologic symptoms
    - Associated with NF-1: Neurofibromas, Lisch nodules, café-au-lait spots
    - Only 10% of patients with neurofibromas have NF-1

Demographics
- Age: 20-30 years
- Gender: M:F = 1:1

Natural History & Prognosis
- Schwannoma: Recurrence unusual
  - Malignant degeneration extremely rare
- Neurofibroma
  - Potential for malignant transformation: 4% in NF-1, rare in solitary tumors

Treatment
- Surgical excision of symptomatic lesions
- Schwannoma
  - Resection with sparing of associated nerve
- Neurofibroma
  - Excision of involved nerve necessary
  - Incomplete excision of neurologically important nerves to decrease neurological impairment

DIAGNOSTIC CHECKLIST

Consider
- Malignant transformation in patients with NF-1 with enlarging neurofibroma

SELECTED REFERENCES

1. Weiss SW et al: Enzinger and Weiss's soft tissue tumors. 4th ed. St. Louis MO, CV Mosby, 1111-207, 2001
2. Beggs I: Pictorial review: Imaging of peripheral nerve tumors. Clin Radiol 52:8-17, 1997
3. Gutmann DH et al: The diagnostic evaluation and multidisciplinary management of neurofibromatosis 1 and neurofibromatosis 2. JAMA 278:51-7, 1997
4. Kransdorf MJ et al: Imaging of soft tissue tumors, 1st ed. Philadelphia PA, W.B. Saunders, 238-54, 1997
5. Pollack IF et al: Neurofibromatosis 1 and 2. Brain Pathol 7:823-36, 1997
6. Bass JC et al: Retroperitoneal plexiform neurofibromas: CT findings. Am J Roentgenol 163:617-20, 1994
7. Suh JS et al: Peripheral (extracranial) nerve tumors: Correlation of MR imaging and histologic findings. Radiology 183:341-6, 1992
8. Stull M et al: Magnetic resonance appearance of peripheral nerve sheath tumors. Skeletal Radiol 20:9-14,1991
9. Sundaram M et al: Magnetic resonance imaging of soft tissue masses: An evaluation of fifty-three histologically proven tumors. Magn Reson Imaging 6:237-48, 1988

BENIGN PERIPHERAL NERVE SHEATH TUMOR

IMAGE GALLERY

Typical

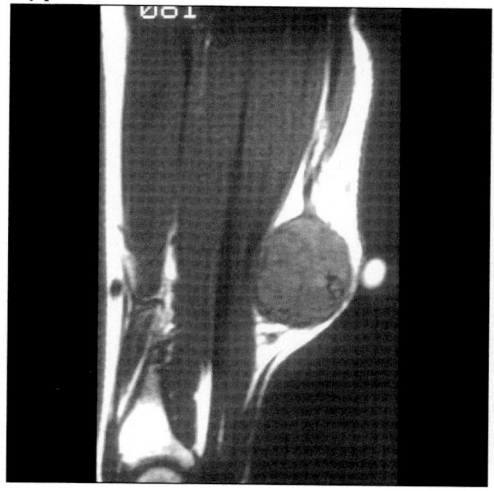
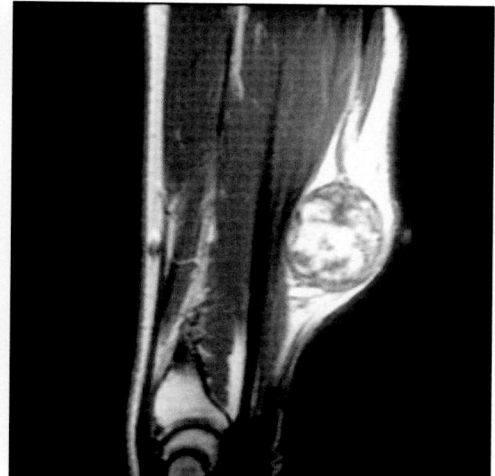

(Left) Sagittal T1WI MR shows well-defined round BPNST of intermediate signal involving the ulnar nerve. *(Right)* Sagittal T1 C+ MR show heterogeneous enhancement of the ulnar nerve sheath tumor.

Variant

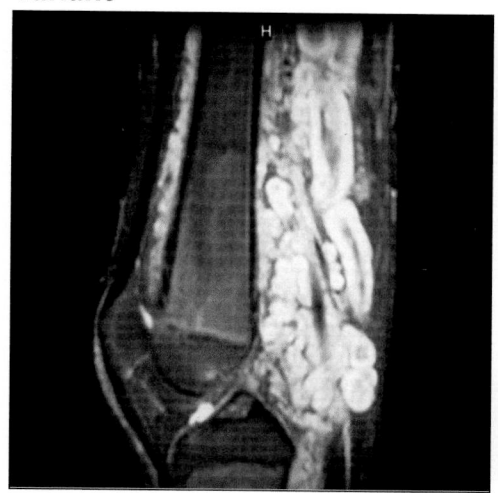
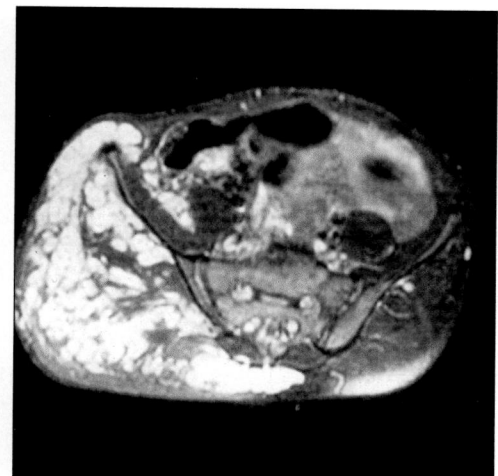

(Left) Sagittal FS T2 FSE MR shows hyperintense plexiform neurofibroma in a patient with NF1. *(Right)* Axial FS T2 FSE MR shows hyperintense plexiform neurofibroma in a patient with NF1.

Other

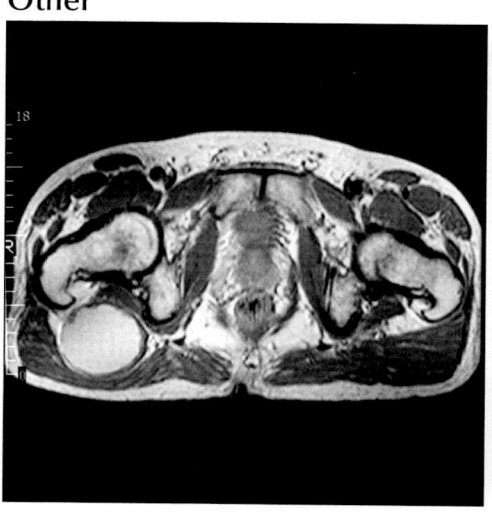
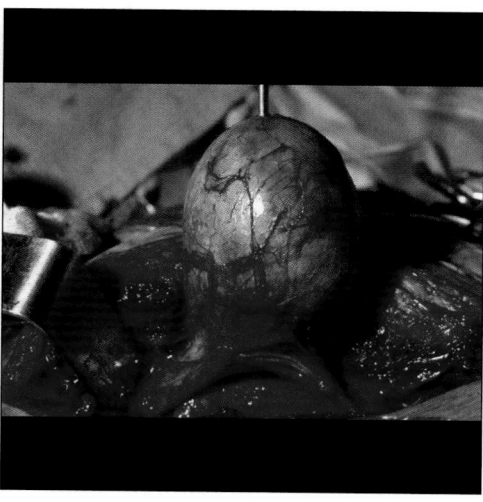

(Left) Axial T2WI MR shows hyperintense BPNST of the sciatic nerve. *(Right)* Intra-operative photograph show round well-defined BPNST of the sciatic nerve.

MALIGNANT PERIPHERAL NERVE SHEATH TUMOR

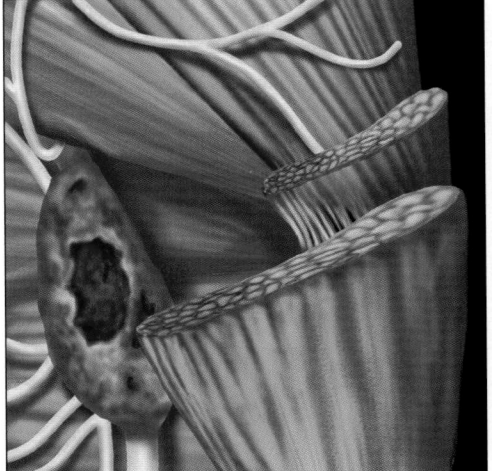

Coronal graphic shows a fusiform mass arising from the sciatic nerve. Areas of hemorrhage and necrosis are shown in the center of the lesion.

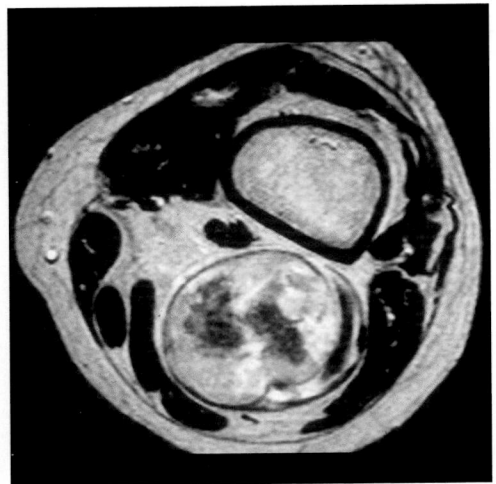

Axial T2WI MR shows heterogeneous MPNST in the posterior thigh.

TERMINOLOGY

Abbreviations and Synonyms
- Malignant peripheral nerve sheath tumors (MPNST) divided into
  - Malignant schwannoma
  - Neurofibrosarcoma

Definitions
- Malignant lesion of neural origin that may occur in peripheral nerves, soft tissue, skin, or bone

IMAGING FINDINGS

General Features
- Best diagnostic clue
  - Large infiltrative often hemorrhagic soft tissue mass related to neurovascular bundle
  - Best seen on long-axis MRI
- Location
  - Neural plexus, peripheral, spinal nerves
  - Posterior mediastinum
  - Retroperitoneum
  - Proximal portion of extremities
- Size: > 5 cm
- Morphology: Infiltrative soft tissue mass related to neurovascular bundle

Radiographic Findings
- Radiography
  - Deep or superficial soft tissue mass
  - Calcifications common

CT Findings
- NECT
  - Soft tissue mass hypodense to muscle
  - Heterogeneous areas corresponding to hemorrhage and necrosis
  - Calcifications
- CECT: Marked enhancement

MR Findings
- T1WI: Soft tissue mass isointense to muscle
- T2WI
  - Hyperintense compared to surrounding fat
  - T2 FSE: Hyperintense
- STIR: Hyperintense
- T1 C+: Marked enhancement
- Heterogeneous soft tissue mass with indistinct margins
- Areas of hemorrhage (fluid-fluid levels)
- Involves major nerve trunks, related to neurovascular bundle
- Can cause displacement of associated neurovascular bundle
- Nerve entering and exiting through mass

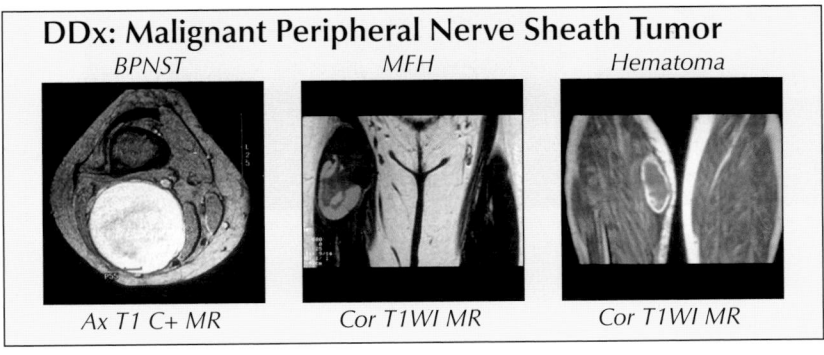

DDx: Malignant Peripheral Nerve Sheath Tumor

BPNST — Ax T1 C+ MR

MFH — Cor T1WI MR

Hematoma — Cor T1WI MR

MALIGNANT PERIPHERAL NERVE SHEATH TUMOR

Key Facts

Imaging Findings
- Large infiltrative often hemorrhagic soft tissue mass related to neurovascular bundle
- Best seen on long-axis MRI

Top Differential Diagnoses
- Benign Peripheral Nerve Sheath Tumor (BPNST)
- Malignant Fibrous Histiocytoma (MFH)
- Hematoma

Pathology
- 5-10% of all malignant soft tissue tumors
- 25-75% occur in association with NF-1
- NF-1: 3-5% of patients develop MPNST

Clinical Issues
- Most common signs/symptoms: Enlarging soft tissue mass
- Involves major nerve trunks, e.g., sciatic nerve, brachial or sacral plexus
- Pain and neurologic symptoms (motor weakness and sensory paresthesia)
- Sudden enlargement of preexisting neurofibroma in NF-1
- High grade sarcoma
- Local recurrence: 40%
- Metastases: 65% (lung, bone, pleura)
- Surgical resection
- Usually presents as stage IIb lesion: Requires radical resection
- Amputation often necessary

- Nutrient vessels connected to proximal and distal poles of the nerve
- Infiltration of surrounding soft tissues
- Muscle atrophy can be seen
- Spinal involvement: Intradural extramedullary mass, dumbbell configuration
  - Widening of intervertebral foramina
    - Erosion of pedicles
    - Scalloping of vertebral bodies

Angiographic Findings
- Hypervascular soft tissue mass

Nuclear Medicine Findings
- Bone Scan: Increased radiotracer uptake on blood pool and delayed images
- PET
  - Increased FDG uptake
  - To detect malignant changes in plexiform neurofibroma

Imaging Recommendations
- Best imaging tool: MRI
- Protocol advice: T1, T2WI MR, T1 C+ MR

DIFFERENTIAL DIAGNOSIS

Benign Peripheral Nerve Sheath Tumor (BPNST)
- No invasion of surrounding structures
- Variable enhancement
- Sudden enlargement of pre-existing neurofibroma in NF1 suspicious for MPNST

Malignant Fibrous Histiocytoma (MFH)
- Not related to neurovascular bundle
- Often hemorrhagic

Hematoma
- No enhancing solid components
- Surrounding edema

PATHOLOGY

General Features
- General path comments: Tumor of nerve sheath, composed of Schwann cells and fibroblasts
- Genetics
  - Neurofibromatosis Type 1 (NF-1), Von Recklinghausen's disease
    - Autosomal dominant, one of the most common genetic diseases
    - High rate of penetrance
    - 50% of cases from new mutations
    - Genetic abnormality on chromosome 17
    - Increased Ras activity due to loss of NF-1 gene product, neurofibromin
  - Increased expression of CD44 family transaminase glycoproteins
    - Might be responsible for tumor cell invasion and metastatic potential
- Etiology
  - Arise from tissue of neuroectodermal or neural crest origin
  - Occurs in 25-70% in association with NF-1
  - Radiation induced in 11% (latency period: 10-20 years)
- Epidemiology
  - 5-10% of all malignant soft tissue tumors
  - 25-75% occur in association with NF-1
- Associated abnormalities
  - NF-1: 3-5% of patients develop MPNST
    - Skeletal abnormalities
    - Kyphoscoliosis
    - Lambdoid suture defects
    - Pseudoarthrosis (tibia)
    - Rib deformities
    - Meningoceles
    - Optic nerve gliomas, astrocytoma

Gross Pathologic & Surgical Features
- Large fusiform mass associated with major nerve
- Often contains areas of hemorrhage and necrosis
- Infiltrate surrounding soft tissues
- Spreads along perineurium and epineurium

MALIGNANT PERIPHERAL NERVE SHEATH TUMOR

Microscopic Features

- Heterotopic epithelioid or mesenchymal elements (mature foci of bone and cartilage): 10-15%
- Components of rhabdomyosarcoma may be present (malignant Triton tumor, often seen in NF-1)
- Resembles fibrosarcoma

Staging, Grading or Classification Criteria

- Surgical staging system for malignant musculoskeletal tumors
  - Stage Ia: Low grade, intracompartmental
  - Stage Ib: Low grade, extracompartmental
  - Stage IIa: High grade, intracompartmental
  - Stage IIb: High grade, extracompartmental
  - Stage IIIa: Low or high grade, intracompartmental, metastases
  - Stage IIIb: Low or high grade, extracompartmental, metastases

CLINICAL ISSUES

Presentation

- Most common signs/symptoms: Enlarging soft tissue mass
- Clinical profile
  - Involves major nerve trunks, e.g., sciatic nerve, brachial or sacral plexus
    - Pain and neurologic symptoms (motor weakness and sensory paresthesia)
  - Sudden enlargement of preexisting neurofibroma in NF-1
  - Associated with NF-1: Neurofibromas, optic nerve gliomas, Lisch nodules, café-au-lait spots

Demographics

- Age
  - 20-50 years
  - If associated with NF-1: 10-50 years
- Gender
  - M:F = 1:1
  - In NF-1: M > F

Natural History & Prognosis

- High grade sarcoma
- Local recurrence: 40%
- Metastases: 65% (lung, bone, pleura)
- 5-year survival: 50%
- Patient with NF-1 might have worse prognosis

Treatment

- Surgical resection
  - Local recurrence: 40%
- Usually presents as stage IIb lesion: Requires radical resection
  - Amputation often necessary
- Preoperative radiation therapy, resection with wide margins

DIAGNOSTIC CHECKLIST

Consider

- Malignant transformation when preexisting neurofibroma enlarges

SELECTED REFERENCES

1. Lang-Lazdunski L et al: Malignant "Triton" tumor of the posterior mediastinum: Prolonged survival after staged resection. Ann Thorac Surg 75:1645-8, 2003
2. Su W et al: Malignant peripheral nerve sheath tumor cell invasion is facilitated by Src and aberrant CD44 expression. Glia 42:350-8, 2003
3. Weiss SW et al: Enzinger and Weiss's soft tissue tumors. 4th ed. St.Louis MO, CV Mosby, 1209-63, 2001
4. Ferner RE et al: Evaluation of (18) fluorodeoxyglucose positron emission tomography ((18) FDG PET) in the detection of malignant peripheral nerve sheath tumours arising from within plexiform neurofibromas in neurofibromatosis 1. J Neurol Neurosurg Psychiatry 68:353-7, 2000
5. Beggs I: Pictorial review: Imaging of peripheral nerve tumours. Clin Radiol 52:8-17, 1997
6. Kransdorf MJ et al: Imaging of soft tissue tumors, 1st ed. Philadelphia PA, W.B. Saunders, 240-54, 1997
7. Bass JC et al: Retroperitoneal plexiform neurofibromas: CT findings. Am J Roentgenol 163:617-20, 1994
8. Suh JS et al: Peripheral (extracranial) nerve tumors: Correlation of MR imaging and histologic findings. Radiology 183:341-6, 1992
9. Stull M et al: Magnetic resonance appearance of peripheral nerve sheath tumors. Skeletal Radiol 20:9-14,1991
10. Riccardi VM et al: Neurofibrosarcoma as a complication of von Recklinghausen neurofibromatosis. Neurofibromatosis 2:152-65, 1989
11. Sundaram M et al: Magnetic resonance imaging of soft tissue masses: An evaluation of fifty-three histologically proven tumors. Magn Reson Imaging 6:237-48, 1988

Typical

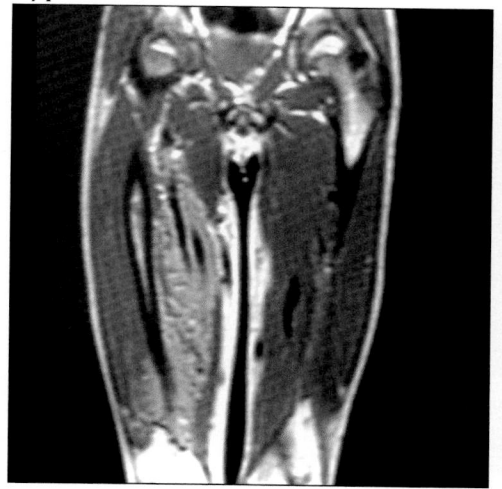 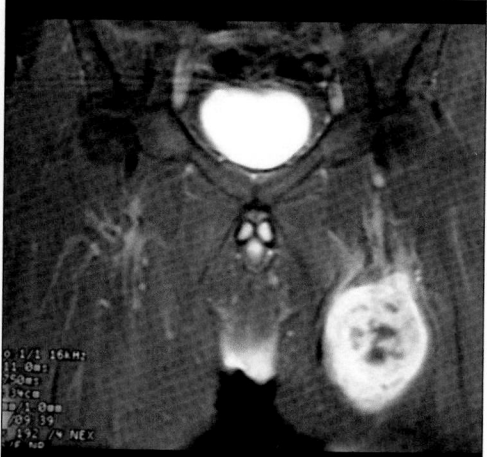

(Left) Coronal PD/Intermediate MR shows large soft tissue mass, hyperintense to muscle, in the region of the femoral nerve in a patient with NF-1. The mass was rapidly increasing in size and was found to represent a MPNST at surgery. *(Right)* Coronal T1 C+ MR shows enhancing mass in the right medial thigh. Central nonenhancing areas are consistent with necrosis.

Typical

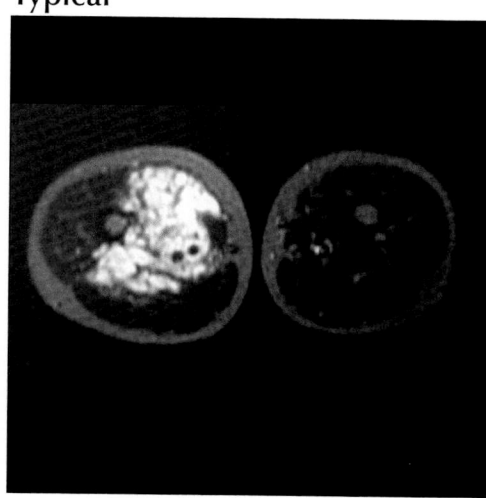 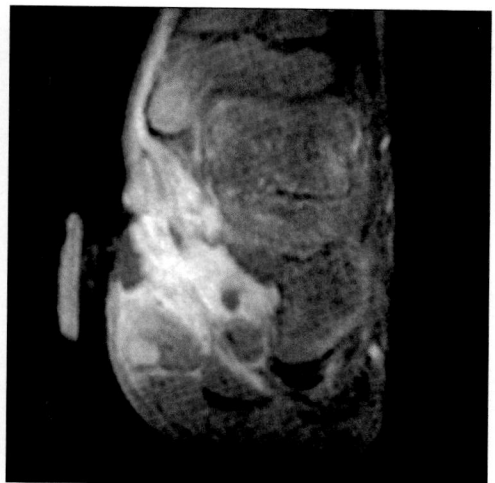

(Left) Axial FS T2 FSE MR in a patient with NF-1 shows hyperintense mass associated with the femoral nerve. Note irregular projection into surrounding soft tissues, encasement and displacement of the femoral artery and vein. *(Right)* Coronal T1 C+ MR shows infiltrative enhancing mass in the region of the medial malleolus with involvement of the medial side of the plantar arch, medial flexor tendons, and neurovascular bundle. Nonenhancing necrotic foci are present.

Other

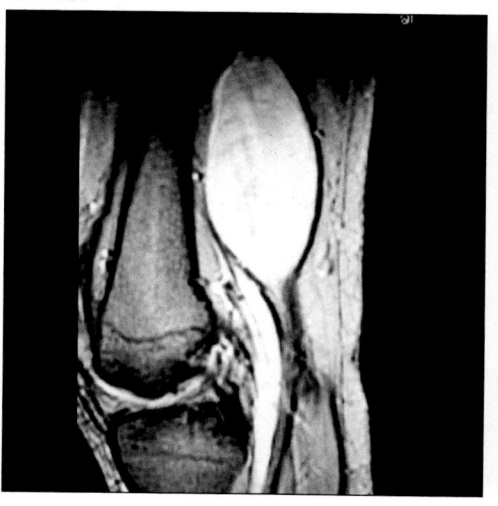 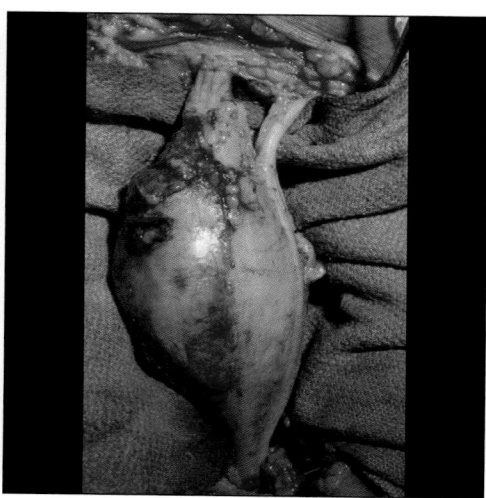

(Left) Sagittal FS T2 FSE MR show fusiform hyperintense tumor arising from the femoral nerve. This was found to represent a malignant schwannoma at surgery. *(Right)* Intra-operative photograph shows large fusiform mass arising from the femoral nerve. Note the enlarged nerve entering and exiting the tumor.

9

37

RHABDOMYOSARCOMA, SOFT TISSUE

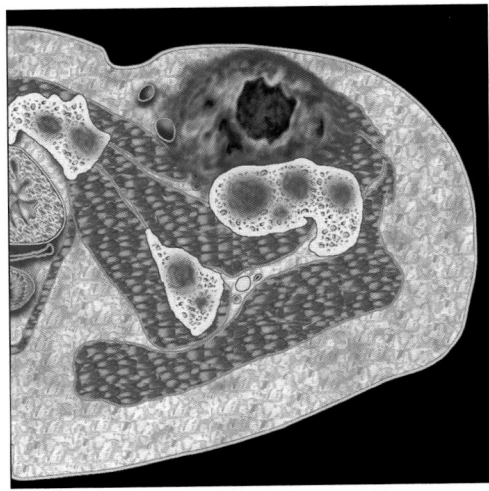

Axial graphic shows heterogeneous soft tissue mass anterior to the femoral neck. Areas of hemorrhage are shown in red. Note the osseous metastases (in brown).

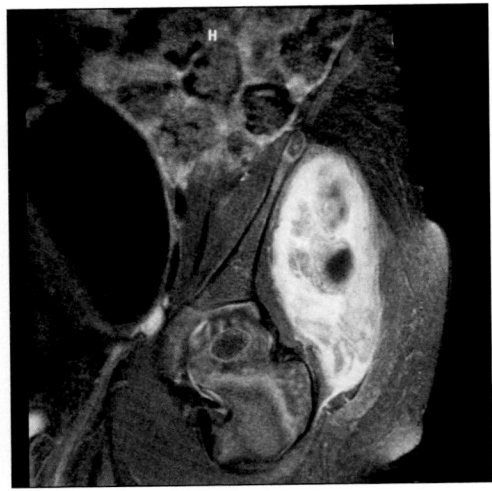

Sagittal T1 C+ MR shows heterogeneous, enhancing mass in the gluteus musculature.

TERMINOLOGY

Abbreviations and Synonyms
- RMS, sarcoma botryoides

Definitions
- Mesenchymal sarcoma occurring in children characterized by rhabdomyoblastic differentiation

IMAGING FINDINGS

General Features
- Best diagnostic clue: Soft tissue mass isointense to muscle
- Location
  ○ Head and neck: 44%
    - Orbit, sinuses, nasopharynx
  ○ Genitourinary system: 20-25%
    - Deep pelvic structures in region of pelvic floor, bladder, vulva, vagina, testicle
  ○ Extremities: 15%
  ○ Retroperitoneum and trunk: 15%
- Size
  ○ 3-4 cm
  ○ Pleomorphic type: > 10 cm
- Morphology: Soft tissue mass resembling muscle

Radiographic Findings
- Radiography
  ○ Nonspecific soft tissue mass
  ○ Local bone invasion: 24%
  ○ Permeative pattern of bone destruction
  ○ Bone metastases: Ill-defined lytic lesions in metaphyses of long bones

CT Findings
- NECT
  ○ Isodense to muscle
  ○ Orbit: Large soft tissue mass with ill-defined margins
    - Destruction of orbital wall
    - Extension into preseptal space, sinuses, intracranial cavity
    - Associated sclerosis and periosteal reaction
- CECT: Heterogeneous enhancement

MR Findings
- T1WI: Isointense to muscle
- T2WI: Hyperintense, can also be iso-hypointense to muscle
- STIR: High signal intensity
- T1 C+: Heterogeneous enhancement
- Prominent vascularity with serpentine vessels
- Areas of hemorrhage

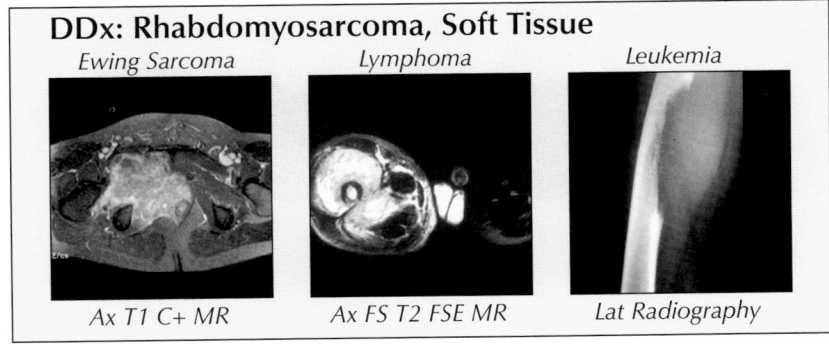

DDx: Rhabdomyosarcoma, Soft Tissue

Ewing Sarcoma	Lymphoma	Leukemia
Ax T1 C+ MR	Ax FS T2 FSE MR	Lat Radiography

RHABDOMYOSARCOMA, SOFT TISSUE

Key Facts

Imaging Findings
- Best diagnostic clue: Soft tissue mass isointense to muscle

Top Differential Diagnoses
- Neuroblastoma
- Ewing Sarcoma
- Lymphoma
- Leukemia

Pathology
- Most common soft tissue malignancy in children
- 19% of all childhood soft tissue sarcomas

Clinical Issues
- Most common signs/symptoms: Soft tissue mass

- Rapidly progressive exophthalmos, proptosis with orbital involvement
- Abdominal pain, distension (from bladder outlet obstruction)
- Metastases in 20% at presentation
- High grade malignancy with rapid growth, local recurrence and metastases
- 5-year survival for patients < 21 years: 30-80%
- 2-year survival for adults: 20-50%
- Survival following relapse: 32% at 1 year, 17% at 2 years
- Tumor of orbit and GU tract: Best prognosis
- Retroperitoneal tumors: Worst prognosis
- Resection with wide margins
- Adjuvant and neoadjuvant chemotherapy

Ultrasonographic Findings
- Isoechoic to muscle
- High diastolic flow

Angiographic Findings
- Hypervascular soft tissue mass

Nuclear Medicine Findings
- Bone Scan: Increased radiotracer uptake on blood pool images
- PET
  - Increased FDG uptake
  - Helpful in differentiating tumor recurrence from post therapeutic changes

Imaging Recommendations
- Best imaging tool: MRI
- Protocol advice
  - T1, T2WI MR, T1 C+ MR
  - Whole body STIR for staging

DIFFERENTIAL DIAGNOSIS

Neuroblastoma
- Coarse calcifications within tumor (40-70%)
- Located along sympathetic neural chain
- Catecholamine production

Ewing Sarcoma
- Originates in bone marrow
- Extension into soft tissues common

Lymphoma
- Lymphadenopathy
- Orbital lymphoma often presents without systemic disease
- Well-defined high density mass
- Osseous lymphoma can have associated soft tissue component

Leukemia
- Can infiltrate lacrimal glands, extraocular muscles

- Leukemic involvement of bones can look similar to metastases from rhabdomyosarcoma
- Can have associated soft tissue component

PATHOLOGY

General Features
- General path comments
  - Mesenchymal sarcoma that can arise anywhere in the body
    - Predominantly involving head and neck, genitourinary tract, retroperitoneum, and extremities
- Genetics
  - Abnormalities of short arm of chromosome 11
  - Translocation of (2;13) or (1;13)
- Etiology
  - Primary mesenchymal tumor with rhabdomyoblastic differentiation
    - Originally thought to arise from striated muscle
  - Increased incidence in patients with neurofibromatosis
- Epidemiology
  - Most common soft tissue malignancy in children
  - 19% of all childhood soft tissue sarcomas

Gross Pathologic & Surgical Features
- Firm rubbery gray-white to pink soft tissue mass
- Infiltration into surrounding tissues
- Areas of necrosis, cystic degeneration

Microscopic Features
- Embryonal type: Most common: 49-70%, best prognosis
  - Small cells with spindle-shaped hyperchromatic nuclei, eosinophilic cytoplasm (rhabdomyoblasts)
- Alveolar type: 18-45%, worst prognosis, high rate of early regional and distant metastases
  - Small round cells forming nests separated by fibrous connective tissue
- Pleomorphic type: Rare
  - Large tumor cells with eosinophilic cytoplasm

RHABDOMYOSARCOMA, SOFT TISSUE

○ Resembles malignant fibrous histiocytoma
○ Myo-D1 antibodies

Staging, Grading or Classification Criteria
• National cancer institute classification
  ○ Embryonal rhabdomyosarcoma (favorable): Conventional, pleomorphic, leiomyomatous
  ○ Alveolar rhabdomyosarcoma (unfavorable): Conventional, solid alveolar
  ○ Pleomorphic rhabdomyosarcoma
  ○ Rhabdomyosarcoma, "other"
• Surgical staging system for malignant musculoskeletal tumors
  ○ Stage Ia: Low grade, intracompartmental
  ○ Stage Ib: Low grade, extracompartmental
  ○ Stage IIa: High grade, intracompartmental
  ○ Stage IIb: High grade, extracompartmental
  ○ Stage IIIa: Low or high grade, intracompartmental, metastases
  ○ Stage IIIb: Low or high grade, extracompartmental, metastases

CLINICAL ISSUES

Presentation
• Most common signs/symptoms: Soft tissue mass
• Clinical profile
  ○ Symptoms depend on tumor location
  ○ Most patients present with stage IIb lesion
  ○ Rapidly progressive exophthalmos, proptosis with orbital involvement
  ○ Abdominal pain, distension (from bladder outlet obstruction)
  ○ Metastases in 20% at presentation
  ○ Bone/joint pain from osseous metastases
  ○ Anemia, thrombocytopenia, neutropenia

Demographics
• Age
  ○ Embryonal type
    ▪ Birth to 15 years, peak: 8 years
  ○ Alveolar type: Adolescents and young adults
    ▪ 10-25 years, peak: 16 years
  ○ Pleomorphic type: Adults
    ▪ > 45 years
• Gender
  ○ M:F = 1.4-1.7:1
  ○ GU tract: M:F = 2-3:1
  ○ Extremities: M:F = 1:1.2
  ○ Orbit: M:F = 1:1.2
• Ethnicity: More common in Caucasians

Natural History & Prognosis
• High grade malignancy with rapid growth, local recurrence and metastases
• 5-year survival for patients < 21 years: 30-80%
• 2-year survival for adults: 20-50%
• Survival following relapse: 32% at 1 year, 17% at 2 years
• Tumor of orbit and GU tract: Best prognosis
• Retroperitoneal tumors: Worst prognosis
• Hematogenous metastases
  ○ Lungs, pleura (most common)

○ Bone (long bones, spine, ribs, skull), bone marrow
○ Liver
○ Lymph nodes

Treatment
• Resection with wide margins
• Adjuvant and neoadjuvant chemotherapy
• Adjuvant radiation therapy
  ○ Risk of radiation induced sarcomas
• Amputation may be necessary

DIAGNOSTIC CHECKLIST

Consider
• Rhabdomyosarcoma in young adults with soft tissue mass

SELECTED REFERENCES

1. Bredella MA et al: Value of FDG PET in conjunction with MR imaging for evaluating therapy response in patients with musculoskeletal sarcomas. Am J Roentgenol 179:1145-50, 2002
2. Mazumdar A et al: Whole body fast inversion recovery MR imaging of small cell neoplasms in pediatric patients: A pilot study. Am J Roentgenol 179:1261-6, 2002
3. Weiss SW et al: Enzinger and Weiss's soft tissue tumors, 4th ed. St.Louis MO, CV Mosby, 785-835, 2001
4. Kransdorf MJ et al: Imaging of soft tissue tumors, 1st ed. Philadelphia PA, W.B. Saunders, 226-33, 1997
5. Yang WT et al: Imaging of pediatric head and neck rhabdomyosarcoma with emphasis on magnetic resonance imaging and a review of the literature. Pediatr Hematol Oncol 14:243-57, 1997
6. Wesche WA et al: Immunhistochemistry of Myo-D1 in adult pleomorphic soft tissue sarcomas. Am J Surg Pathol 19:261-9, 1995
7. Hays DM: Rhabdomyosarcoma. Clin Orthop 289:36-49, 1993
8. Shapeero LG et al: Bone metastases as the presenting manifestation of rhabdomyosarcoma in childhood. Skeletal Radiol 22:433-8, 1993
9. Tsokos M et al: Rhabdomyosarcoma: A new classification scheme related to prognosis. Arch Pathol Lab Med 116:847-55, 1992
10. Dillon E et al: The role of diagnostic radiology in the diagnosis and management of rhabdomyosarcoma in young persons. Clin Radiol 29:53-9, 1978

RHABDOMYOSARCOMA, SOFT TISSUE

IMAGE GALLERY

Typical

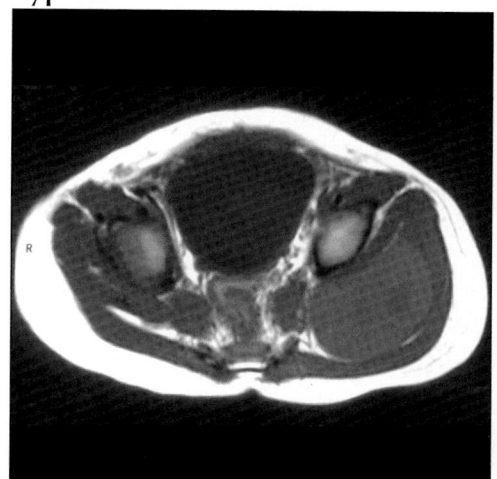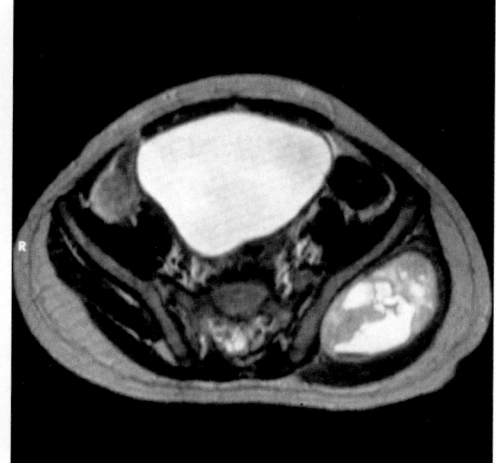

(Left) Axial T1WI MR shows soft tissue mass, isointense to muscle, anterior to left gluteus maximus. *(Right)* Axial T2WI MR shows well defined soft tissue mass with areas of hyperintense and intermediate signal.

Typical

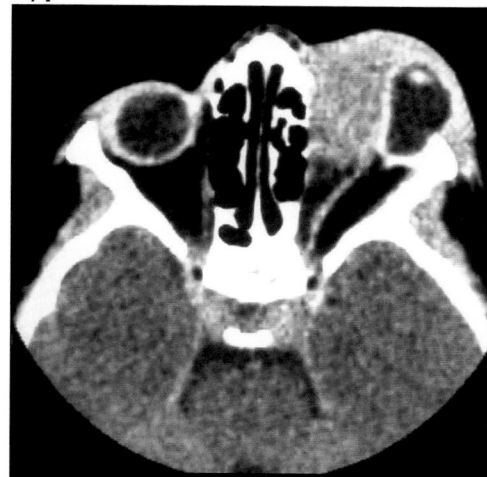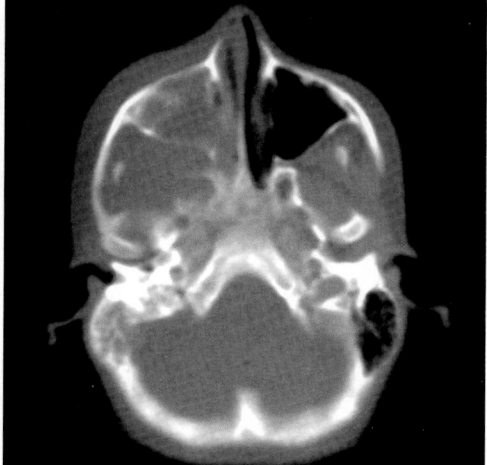

(Left) Axial NECT shows rhabdomyosarcoma involving the left orbit and causing deformity of the left globe and left sided exophthalmus. *(Right)* Axial NECT shows rhabdomyosarcoma arising in the right pterygopalatine fossa.

Variant

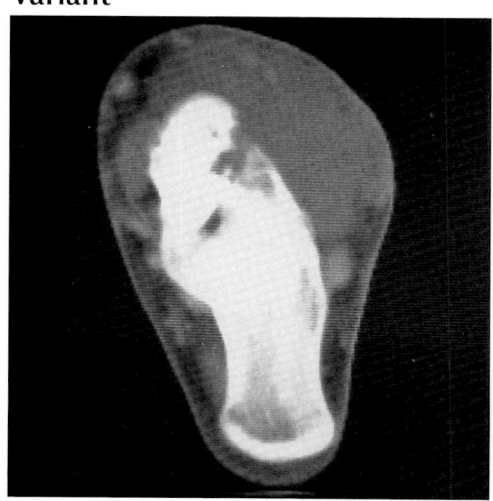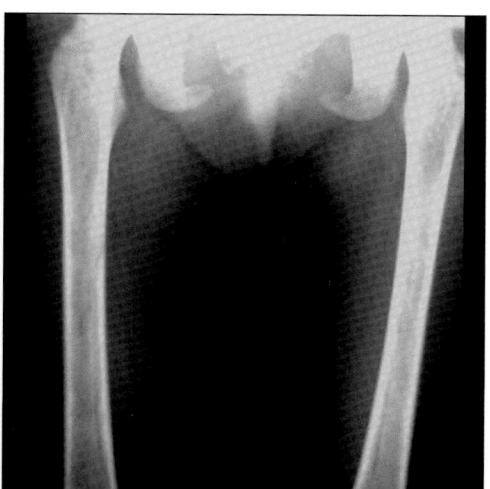

(Left) Axial NECT shows soft tissue mass involving the ankle. Note the underlying osseous destruction. *(Right)* Anteroposterior radiography shows mottled appearance of both femurs representing metastases in a patient with alveolar rhabdomyosarcoma of the upper extremity.

HEMANGIOMA, SOFT TISSUE

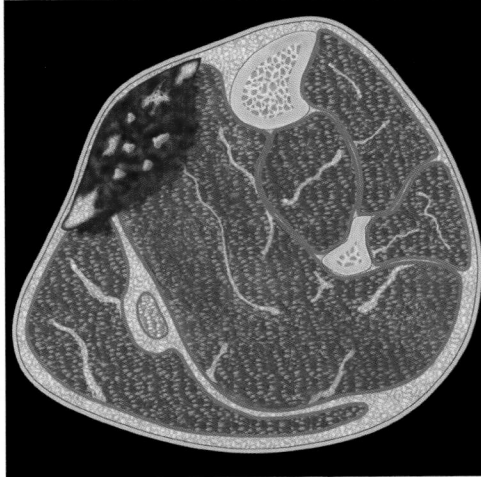

Axial graphic shows intramuscular mass with phleboliths (white) and vascular elements (red). Peripheral fat overgrowth is shown in yellow.

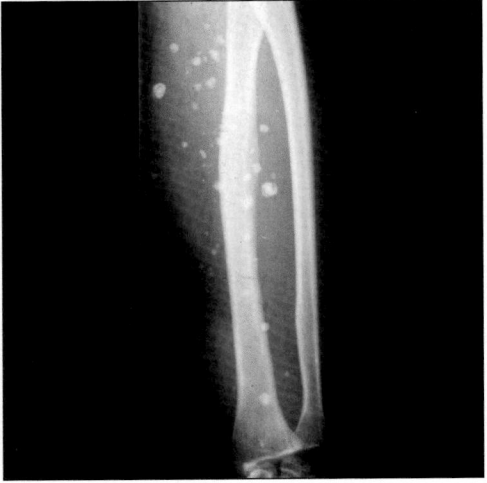

Anteroposterior radiography shows soft tissue mass in the forearm with multiple phleboliths, consistent with cavernous hemangioma.

TERMINOLOGY

Abbreviations and Synonyms
- Capillary, cavernous hemangioma, soft tissue hemangioma

Definitions
- Benign lesion that resembles normal blood vessels

IMAGING FINDINGS

General Features
- Best diagnostic clue
  - Soft tissue mass of muscle-fat density on radiographs or CT, phleboliths (diagnostic)
  - Areas of high signal on T1 and T2WI MR with flow voids
- Location
  - Superficial: Skin, subcutaneous tissue
    - Predilection for head and neck
  - Deep: Intramuscular
  - Synovial (rare)
  - Localized or multifocal
- Size: 1-15 cm
- Morphology: Soft tissue mass containing blood vessels

Radiographic Findings
- Radiography
  - Nonspecific soft tissue mass
  - Phleboliths: Most common in cavernous hemangiomas (30-50%)
  - Curvilinear, amorphous calcifications
  - May extend into bone
  - Bone overgrowth

CT Findings
- NECT
  - Poorly defined soft tissue mass, attenuation similar to muscle
  - Areas of fat attenuation
  - Phleboliths
  - Periosteal reaction in lesions adjacent to bone
- CECT: Serpentine enhancement

MR Findings
- T1WI
  - Poorly marginated heterogeneous mass
  - Isointense to muscle
  - Areas of high signal intensity (fat, slow flowing blood)
- T2WI
  - Well-marginated heterogeneous mass
  - Areas of intermediate and very high signal intensity
  - FS PD/T2 FSE: High signal intensity
- T2* GRE: Helpful to detect high (arterial) flow
- T1 C+
  - Marked enhancement

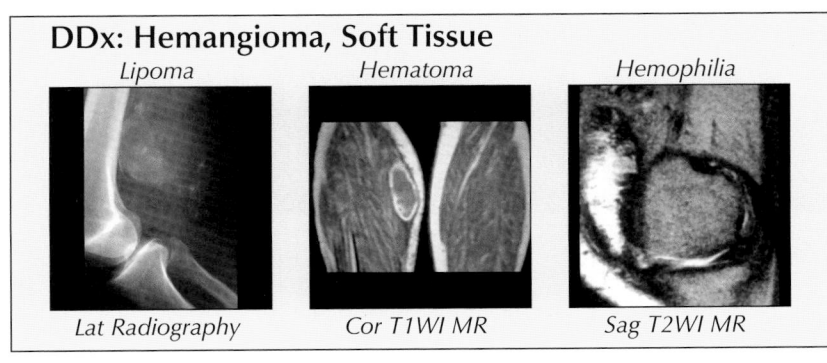

DDx: Hemangioma, Soft Tissue

Lipoma	Hematoma	Hemophilia
Lat Radiography	Cor T1WI MR	Sag T2WI MR

HEMANGIOMA, SOFT TISSUE

Key Facts

Imaging Findings
- Soft tissue mass of muscle-fat density on radiographs or CT, phleboliths (diagnostic)
- Areas of high signal on T1 and T2WI MR with flow voids

Top Differential Diagnoses
- Lipoma
- Hematoma
- Hemophilia

Pathology
- 7% of all benign tumors
- Most common tumor of infancy and childhood

Clinical Issues
- Most hemangiomas are asymptomatic

- Superficial lesions: Purple discoloration of overlying skin
- Intramuscular lesions: Pain after exercise
- Synovial lesion: Recurrent episodes of joint pain, swelling, effusion
- Benign lesion, no malignant transformation
- 90% of juvenile capillary hemangiomas involute by age 7
- Cavernous hemangiomas do not involute, can cause local destruction by increased pressure
- Capillary hemangiomas: Followed clinically
- Cavernous hemangiomas: Often require surgical resection with wide margins

---

  - Prominent draining veins
- Infiltration of adjacent tissue
- Joint effusion and hemorrhage in synovial hemangioma

Ultrasonographic Findings
- Complex mass
- Acoustic shadowing may be caused by phleboliths
- High flow on color Doppler

Angiographic Findings
- Vascular soft tissue mass, may be high or low flow
- Blood vessels oriented parallel to each other
- Important for pre-treatment planning if embolization is considered

Nuclear Medicine Findings
- Bone Scan: Little or no increased uptake of radiotracer

Imaging Recommendations
- Best imaging tool: MRI
- Protocol advice
  - T1, T2WI MR, FS PD/T2, T2* GRE, T1 C+
  - Use radiographs or CT to evaluate for phleboliths

DIFFERENTIAL DIAGNOSIS

Lipoma
- Homogeneous soft tissue mass
- Fat containing
- No enhancement

Hematoma
- Surrounding edema
- No enhancement

Hemophilia
- Repetitive bleeding of synovial hemangioma into joint can mimic hemophilia
- Polyarticular

PATHOLOGY

General Features
- General path comments
  - Benign lesion with increased number of normal or abnormal appearing vessels
  - Can increase in size during pregnancy: Endothelial cells responsive to circulating hormones
- Genetics
  - Capillary hemangioma can be familial (rare)
  - Mutation of chromosome 5
- Etiology
  - Vascular malformation that may be congenital, developmental, or acquired
  - Likely hamartomatous condition rather than true neoplasm
- Epidemiology
  - 7% of all benign tumors
  - Most common tumor of infancy and childhood
- Associated abnormalities
  - Kasabach-Merritt syndrome: Rapidly enlarging cavernous hemangiomas, hemangioendotheliomas, angiosarcomas
    - Usually located in extremity
    - Intravascular coagulation and sequestration of platelets
    - Petechiae and ecchymoses involving skin and internal organs
    - Death from hemorrhage: 30%
  - Maffucci syndrome: Mesodermal dysplasia with multiple hemangiomas and enchondromas
    - Cavernous hemangiomas
  - Osler-Weber-Rendu syndrome: Hereditary hemorrhagic telangiectasia
    - Autosomal dominant
    - Systemic vascular dysplasia, resulting in aneurysms, telangiectasia, arteriovenous malformations
    - Involves skin, lung, visceral organs
    - Repeated episodes of hemorrhage
  - Klippel-Trenaunay-Weber syndrome: Non-hereditary
    - Anomalies of deep venous system

- Bone and soft tissue hypertrophy, varicose veins, cutaneous hemangiomas
- Unilateral

Gross Pathologic & Surgical Features

- Blue-red soft tissue mass composed of large vessels
- Nonvascular elements: Fat, smooth muscle, fibrous tissue, bone
- Fat overgrowth may lead to misdiagnosis of lipoma

Microscopic Features

- Resembles normal blood vessels
- Nonvascular elements: Fat, smooth muscle, fibrous tissue, bone, hemosiderin
  - Capillary type: Small vessels lined by flattened endothelium
    - Occur in skin and subcutaneous tissues
  - Cavernous type: Dilated spaces filled with blood, lined by flattened epithelium
    - Involve deep structures
  - Arterio-venous type: Abnormal communication of arteries and veins, persistence of capillary bed
  - Venous type: Vessels with thick muscular walls

CLINICAL ISSUES

Presentation

- Most common signs/symptoms: Painful mass, intermittent change in size
- Clinical profile
  - Most hemangiomas are asymptomatic
  - Superficial lesions: Purple discoloration of overlying skin
  - Intramuscular lesions: Pain after exercise
    - Relative hypoxia of surrounding muscle
  - Synovial lesion: Recurrent episodes of joint pain, swelling, effusion
  - Arterio-venous type: Enlarged extremity
    - Reflex bradycardia after compression (Branham sign)
  - Can increase in size during pregnancy

Demographics

- Age: 1 month - 36 years; most hemangiomas involute by age 10
- Gender: F:M = 1.5-2:1

Natural History & Prognosis

- Benign lesion, no malignant transformation
- 90% of juvenile capillary hemangiomas involute by age 7
- Cavernous hemangiomas do not involute, can cause local destruction by increased pressure
- Limited growth potential
- Local recurrence: 15-50%

Treatment

- Capillary hemangiomas: Followed clinically
  - Symptomatic lesions with compression of critical structures (airways)
    - Systemic glucosteroid, interferon α
- Cavernous hemangiomas: Often require surgical resection with wide margins
  - Preoperative arteriography and embolization
  - Recurrence < 10%
  - Marginal excision: Recurrence > 25%
- Chemotherapy in hemangiomatosis has been tried with variable success

DIAGNOSTIC CHECKLIST

Image Interpretation Pearls

- Obtain radiographs if MRI is non-diagnostic, phleboliths might be missed with MRI

SELECTED REFERENCES

1. Walter JW et al: Genetic mapping of a novel familial form of infantile hemangioma. Am J Genet 82:77-83, 1999
2. Greenspan A et al: Synovial hemangioma: Imaging features in eight histologically proven cases, review of the literature, and differential diagnosis. Skeletal Radiol 24:583-590, 1995
3. Murphey MD et al: Musculoskeletal angiomatous lesions: Radiologic-pathologic correlation. Radiographics 15:893-917, 1995
4. Ezekowitz RA et al: Interferon alpha-2a therapy for life-threatening hemangiomas of infancy. N Engl J Med 326:1456-63, 1992
5. Greenspan A et al: Imaging strategies in the evaluation of soft tissue hemangiomas of the extremities: Correlation of the findings of plain radiography, CT, MRI, and ultrasonography in 12 histologically proven cases. Skeletal Radiol 21:11-8, 1992
6. Rak KM et al: MR imaging of symptomatic peripheral vascular malformations. Am J Roentgenol 159:107-112, 1992
7. Buetow PC et al: Radiologic appearance of intramuscular hemangioma with emphasis on MR imaging. Am J Roentgenol 154:563-7, 1990
8. Nelson MC et al: Magnetic resonance imaging of peripheral soft-tissue hemangiomas. Skeletal Radiol 19:447-82, 1990
9. Cohen EK et al: MR imaging of soft-tissue hemangiomas: Correlation with pathologic findings. Am J Roentgenol 150:1079-81, 1988

IMAGE GALLERY

Typical

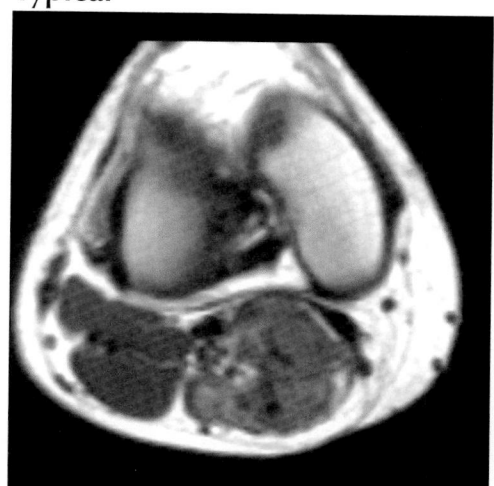
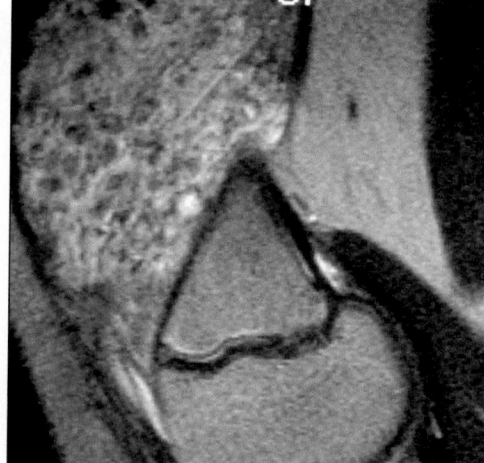

(Left) Axial T1WI MR shows soft tissue mass of intermediate signal in the gastrocnemius. Foci of high and low signal are seen within the mass. *(Right)* Sagittal T2WI MR shows heterogeneous mass in the vastus medialis. Areas of high signal correspond to slow flowing blood, intermediate signal corresponds to fat overgrowth.

Typical

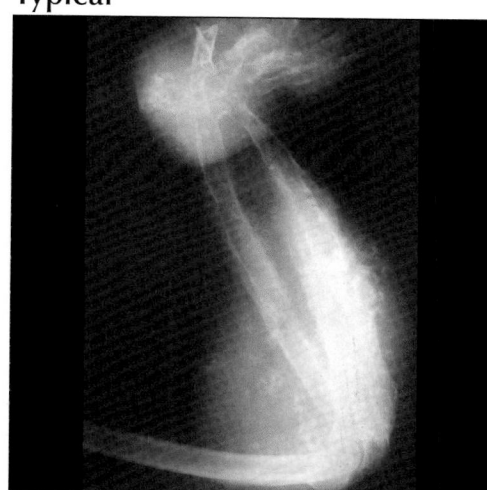
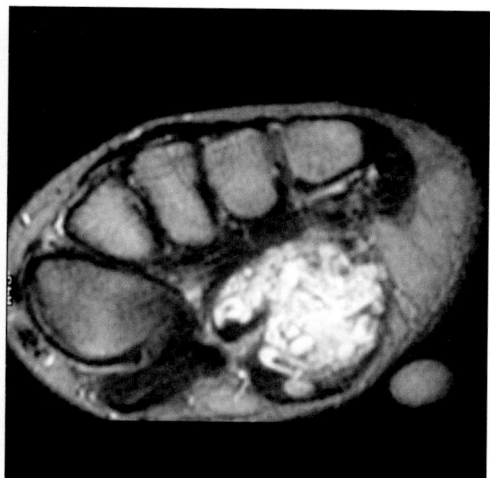

(Left) Anteroposterior radiography shows multiple osseous and soft tissue hemangiomas in a patient with hemangiomatosis. *(Right)* Axial T2WI MR shows hyperintense soft tissue mass at the plantar aspect of the foot. Serpentine areas of high signal correspond to slow flowing blood in vascular channels.

Typical

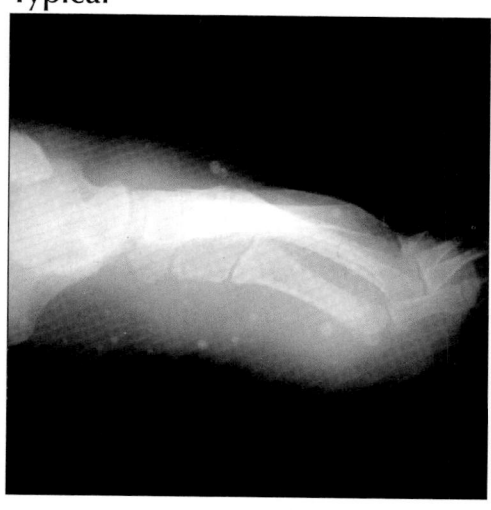
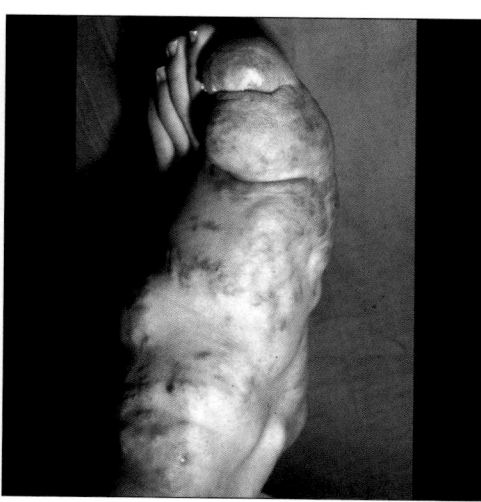

(Left) Lateral radiography of the foot reveals soft tissue mass and multiple phleboliths. Deformity of the first phalanx secondary to the soft tissue mass is noted. *(Right)* Clinical photograph shows marked enlargement and purple-bluish discoloration of the first phalanx (same patient).

9

45

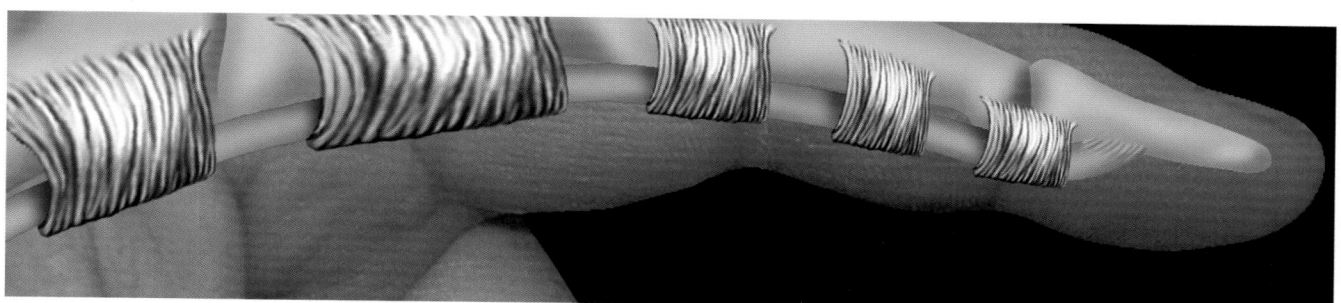

INDEX

A

INDEX

ii

INDEX

i

v

INDEX

INDEX

INDEX

INDEX

INDEX

INDEX

INDEX

INDEX

INDEX

INDEX

INDEX

INDEX

INDEX

INDEX

INDEX

INDEX